Schmidek & Sweet

Operative Neurosurgical Techniques

VOLUME
2

Schmidek & Sweet

Operative Neurosurgical Techniques

INDICATIONS, METHODS, AND RESULTS

Henry H. Schmidek, MD, FACS

David W. Roberts, MD

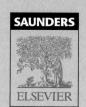

SAUNDERS

ELSEVIER

FIFTH EDITION

SAUNDERS
ELSEVIER

1600 John F. Kennedy Blvd.
Suite 1800
Philadelphia, PA 19103-2899

SCHMIDEK & SWEET OPERATIVE
NEUROSURGICAL TECHNIQUES:
INDICATIONS, METHODS, AND RESULTS
Copyright © 2006, Elsevier Inc. All rights reserved.

Part number 9997627121 (vol.1)
Part number 999762713x (vol.2)
ISBN-13: 978-0-7216-0340-7
ISBN-10: 0-7216-0340-8

Previous editions copyrighted 2000, 1995, 1988, 1982 by W. B. Saunders.

Library of Congress Cataloging-in-Publication Data

Schmidek & Sweet operative neurosurgical techniques : indications, methods, and results /
[edited by] Henry H. Schmidek, David W. Roberts.—5th ed.
p. ; cm.
Includes bibliographical references and index.
ISBN-13: 978-0-7216-0340-7 (set)   ISBN-10: 0-7216-0340-8 (set)
1. Nervous system—Surgery. I. Title: Schmidek and Sweet operative neurosurgical techniques.
II. Title: Operative neurosurgical techniques. III. Schmidek, Henry H. IV. Roberts, David W.
[DNLM: 1. Neurosurgical Procedures—methods. 2. Craniocerebral Trauma—surgery. 3. Nervous System
Diseases—surgery. WL 368 S348 2006]
RD593.O63 2006
617.4'8—dc22

2005043215

Acquisitions Editor: Rebecca Schmidt Gaertner
Developmental Editor: Agnes Hunt Byrne
Editorial Assistant: Suzanne Flint

Set ISBN-13: 978-0-7216-0340-7 (set)
Set ISBN-10: 0-7216-0340-8 (set)

Printed in the United States of America.

Last digit is the print number: 9 8 7 6 5 4 3 2

To William Herbert Sweet, MD, DSc, FACS

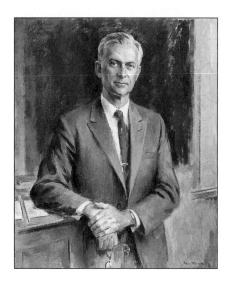

Dr. William Sweet died in his home in Brookline, Massachusetts, on January 22, 2001, after a long siege with Parkinson's disease complicated by dementia. It was as if a meteor that had traveled a lifetime of luminous miles was suddenly gone.

Dr. Sweet was passionate about astronomy, radio-astronomy, particle physics, classical music, history, and medicine, but especially those disciplines with the prefix "neuro." Life was a continual intellectual feast. It took an enormous amount of energy to feed this voracious intellect. He subscribed to, and read, each issue of over 60 journals. His private library contained at least 5000 books reflecting his interests in the basic neurosciences, neurosurgery, neurology, psychiatry, neuropathology, and surgery.

In his funeral oration, Pericles intoned, "the whole world is a sepulchre of the illustrious man." Sweet did indeed travel the world seeking knowledge at its premier clinical and research facilities. From a multitude of disciplines he translated observations into solutions of problems encountered in the nervous system.

Dr. Sweet was an intensely private person: he could be warm and charming when relaxed but he would never be confused with the touchy, feely, sensitive man now in vogue. He was a man of his own times and traditions. Like the majority of academic neurosurgeons of his generation, he grew up in rural America, was the son of a doctor, excelled scholastically, went to the local land grant university, and then migrated to one of the major east coast research universities to further his career. As a youth in Washington state his precocious intelligence and curiosity were already apparent. In high school he could easily have been made the principal and run the institution but his teachers preferred to graduate him at the age of 14. At age 18 he graduated from the University of Washington first in a class of 1000. He loved the classical piano: it was mathematical, ordered, controlled, yet creative. He also loved aviation: it was full of risks, challenge, and exhilaration. He debated being a concert pianist and considered being a naval aviator. He decided against the piano because he felt he would never attain world-class stature in this area.

In the late 1920s the major powers were all at peace so being a military officer and fighter pilot did not seem a fruitful endeavor. So when the time came for him to choose a career, he decided to follow in his father's footsteps: he became a doctor and then a surgeon. In 1930 he enrolled in the Harvard Medical School.

Dr. Cushing was at the time the senior professor of surgery at Harvard and was at the height of his fame. Between 1930 and 1932 Sweet had the opportunity to take Cushing's measure. Here was the personification of the focused, single-minded individual trying to understand and deal with pathology within the most complex system known to man—the human brain. To Sweet this was a challenge worth emulating. After his sophomore year in medical school, and with a Rhodes scholarship to Magdalen College, Oxford, he spent the next two years in Sherrington's laboratory, as had Cushing and as had Penfield.

Although he was the world's leading neurophysiologist, Sherrington stopped working and was never to return to his laboratory following the sudden and unexpected death of Lady Sherrington. As a result, Sweet found himself in England with an empty closet-sized laboratory, without guidance, and without a project. Fortunately, John Fulton and John Eccles were also in the laboratory at that time, and with their help Sweet obtained a bachelor's degree in neurophysiology rather than the doctorate he had planned to work toward. Still not sure of his path, he returned to the Harvard Medical School and at night and on weekends worked at the Boston Psychopathic Hospital so that he could gain some insight into psychiatry. After a year and a half at this endeavor he said he found this field "far too nebulous" and—with typical Sweetian syntax—"a complete morass of ignorance." Still in medical school, he did an elective rotation in neurosurgery at the Massachusetts General Hospital with Drs. Jason Mixter and J. C. White. Because one of the residents, Henry Heyl (subsequently Chief of Neurosurgery at Dartmouth and editor of the *Journal of Neurosurgery*), had left the service and the lab was short-staffed, Sweet was given a great deal of responsibility, and he thrived in this environment. This experience crystallized his decision to make neurosurgery his life's work. After graduating from medical school, six years after enrolling, he went to the University of Chicago to train with Percival Bailey, Earl Walker, and Paul Bucy. Bailey was to become his intellectual role model. Bailey was Cushing-trained in neurosurgery, he was trained in psychiatry, he was trained in neurology, and he had a doctorate in neurophysiology. Sweet was to immerse himself in these same disciplines.

After the University of Chicago Sweet returned to England to train in neurology just as England was going to war. Sweet described how within a 24-hour period after World War II was declared the National Hospital at Queen's Square removed its patients to outlying hospitals and made ready to receive the wounded. With the British neurosurgeons going into the military, Sweet volunteered to take over as *the* consultant neurosurgeon to the Queen Elizabeth Hospital in Birmingham—serving a community of 4.5 million inhabitants in the British midlands. For the next four years he enjoyed a surgical bonanza, and when needing advice with a difficult case, turned to another neurosurgeon who was to have a brilliant career, Sir Geoffrey Jefferson, the neurosurgeon in Manchester. Sweet and Jefferson shared many of the same attributes, and they were to remain lifelong friends.

As medicine had fed his mind, England nurtured his soul. He had great respect for the stoicism of the English people, and he loved England, with its beautiful Gothic architecture and its verdant and manicured gardens. He loved the controlled, understated, ever-articulate British with their droll humor. He remained a committed Anglophile and over the subsequent years made innumerable trips back to England.

In 1945 Dr. Sweet, 35 years old, returned home to the Massachusetts General Hospital ready to continue his academic career. He was to be tremendously productive and prolific. In 1961 he was named Chief of the Neurosurgical Service at the MGH and Professor of Surgery at the Harvard Medical School. I am reminded here of Winston Churchill's characterization of T. E. Lawrence: "Here was a man in whom existed an immense capacity for service. He reigned over those with whom he came in contact, and they felt themselves in the presence of an extraordinary being. They felt that the latent reserves of force and willpower were beyond measurement. When he roused himself to action, who could say what crisis he could not surmount or quell" (or, in Dr. Sweet's case, sometimes precipitate). As a chief, every day there were crises to surmount, committees to cajol, residents to be reined in, aneurysms to be clipped, research to be directed, funds to be procured, journals to be devoured, and more planes to be boarded. It just kept going and going. To this maelstrom of 110–120 hour work weeks, Sweet brought a penetrating unemotional intellect. He was also supremely confident of his surgical abilities. He raised more money for research than any other MGH surgical service. He established laboratories staffed with full-time

scientists working within neurosurgery in electron microscopy, neurophysiology, immunology, neurochemistry, experimental neuropathology, and biophysics. He transformed the MGH Neurosurgical Service from what Dr. Churchill, then Chief of Surgery, characterized as an "intellectual backwater" to a service of international renown. This did not always endear him to those around him, especially if one did not reach his standards or if someone was competing with him for resources and influence within the hospital—for he was a tough and tenacious competitor.

Sweet's qualities enabled him to attract an extraordinary group of men to train. During his 16 years as chief he trained 13 residents who became full professors and chiefs of neurosurgical services in the United States alone. He also was instrumental in the training of dozens of others who went on to distinguished careers both in neurosurgery and in the basic sciences. He provided advice to study sections of the NIH, to NASA, to the Neurosciences Research Program at MIT, and to the Brookhaven National Laboratory. He was routinely asked for advice on the careers of neurosurgeons worldwide. It was largely because of the discussions between Sweet and his friend Hugo Krayenbuhl, then Chief of Neurosurgery in Zurich, that Gazi Yasargil found himself in Burlington, Vermont, working with Pete Donaghy, and there laying the foundation of microvascular neurosurgery.

Dr. Sweet's interests are reflected in his 538 publications and 15 books. A major effort was devoted to investigating the uses of various forms of radiation to study (for example) CSF production, brain tumor localization, and treatment of glioblastomas, and to produce focal intracranial lesions. He published widely on stereotactic and functional neurosurgery in epilepsy, and in movement and behavioral disorders. He and J. C. White produced two classic monographs on the neurosurgical management of pain. To him is owed the concept of the production of focal lesions in the nervous system with the radiofrequency current. He made a major advance in the treatment of trigeminal neuralgia with the technique of differential thermal rhizotomy. He also made contributions in vascular neurosurgery: it was under his direction that the service performed the first operations on the brain at body temperatures of 24°C to 27°C. In 1954 he carried out one of the first carotid endarterectomies ever performed. He was the first to report the routine use of intracarotid pressure measurements with carotid occlusion for treatment of aneurysms. He published a remarkable series on the radical removal of craniopharyngiomas in adults. In addition, he was on the committee that defined the Harvard Brain Death criteria and devoted considerable effort to helping a large number of neurosurgeons with their medicolegal problems.

Anecdotes about Dr. Sweet abound, and everyone who spent time with him had a war story. I will share with you two of my stories. Presented with an annoying situation, Dr. Sweet could be surprisingly creative in how he dealt with it or avoided dealing with it. Consider this example, when he was called to participate in a gripe-session in which the pediatricians were to vent their dissatisfaction about the management of a case. This meeting was scheduled for a Monday morning at 8 AM in the Vincent Burnham Building of the MGH. As Dr. Sweet's resident, I arrived at 7:50 AM to meet with him in his office in the

White Building. I reminded him of the meeting—he invited me to have a cup of coffee. At 8:15 AM I again reminded him of the meeting—he suggested some more coffee. It was dawning on me that something was afoot. At about 8:20 AM we made our way down one elevator and up another and ten minutes later entered a room full of disgruntled pediatricians.

Dr. Sweet strode to the front of the room and began a monologue that had something of the following flavor: "I have just returned from the desert in New Mexico, where at an altitude of 2124 meters, a latitude of 30.4 degrees north, longitude of 107.37 degrees west, sits the world's premier radioastronomical observatory. This observatory consists of an array of 27 antennas, each antenna is 81 feet in diameter and sits on railroad tracks so the position can be changed. When dispersed this array is spread over 36 kilometers and when these antennae are combined electronically at a frequency of 43 gigaherz they give a resolution of 0.04 seconds—sufficient to see a golf ball 100 miles away." He continued this tutorial on radioastronomy. Promptly at 9:00 AM he glanced at his wristwatch, thanked the dumbstruck and silent audience for their attention, said that he had to be in the Operating Room forthwith and that he was delighted to have had an opportunity to join them at their conference. He walked out of the room. At the elevator he smiled and one could almost hear him say "check-mate."

Another anecdote involved a famous vascular surgeon who came to the MGH to present his successes with carotid endarterectomy at Surgical Grand Rounds. Sweet was in the audience along with the other MGH surgical "greats." The visitor held forth. During the discussion following the presentation this high-pitched voice emanated from the front row and it began: "Sir, could I please see slide ___ again." After the mandatory fumbling at the projector, a lateral projection of a carotid angiogram with a high grade extracranial internal carotid stenosis was shown. "Well, how did this patient do?" "Oh, very well, Dr. Sweet." "Really!" There was a pause, "Tell me, do you find it a useful tactic to revascularize glioblastomas?" On the angiogram one could see a part of the head and there was the tumor blush—unnoticed by anyone else in the room.

Churchill also said of T. E. Lawrence that he was "one of those men whose pace of life was faster and more intense than what is normal, such as an airplane only flies by its speed and pressure against the air, so he flew best and easiest in the hurricane." Through this hurricane of activity, this intense pressure of life, Elizabeth assisted with the focus, structured the chaos, and found humor in the pathos. She ran the service on a day-to-day basis during his chiefship, and when Dr. Sweet left the chiefship in 1977, she traveled the rest of the miles with him. He never retired but slowed as the infirmities accumulated. His last papers were published in 1997. In describing his parents' relationship in the last years of Sweet's life, I paraphrase their son David: As his giant mind and indomitable world broke apart and ebbed away into eternity, all those around him who knew him found this terribly painful to watch. One person, Elizabeth, had the love and the strength to take care of him—at home—for every one of those difficult days. She did this so well, she knew him so well, she guarded and shielded him so well that he never fully recognized the degree of his impairment, for she could always fill in the blanks for him.

Sweet was proud of the honorary fellowships, memberships, prizes, and decorations from the world's medical, scientific, and general learned societies, and also from national governments. As he looked back over his life, he felt he had accomplished his goal: as Cushing was the dominant neurosurgeon of his era and Penfield was of his, Sweet was the leading intellect of the third generation of neurosurgeons; he was once again first in his class.

He was an extraordinary person, and it was a privilege to have known him as teacher, mentor, colleague, and friend.

Henry H. Schmidek, MD, FACS
Dartmouth Medical School
Lebanon, New Hampshire

CONTRIBUTORS

KHALID M. ABBED, MD
Chief Resident, Neurosurgery, Academic Fellow,
Department of Neurosurgery, Harvard Medical School,
Massachusetts General Hospital, Boston, Massachusetts
  Surgical Management of Cerebellar Astrocytomas in Adults

DIANA L. ABSON KRAEMER, MD
Clinical Associate Professor, University of Washington,
Swedish Medical Center, Seattle, Washington
  *Diagnostic Techniques in Surgical Management of Epilepsy:
  Strip Electrodes, Grids, and Depth Electrodes*

CHRIS B. T. ADAMS, MChir, FRCS
Radcliffe Infirmary, Department of Neurological Surgery,
Oxford, England
  Transcranial Surgery for Pituitary Macroadenomas

JOHN R. ADLER, JR., MD
Professor, Department of Neurosurgery; Director,
Radiosurgery and Stereotactic Surgery, Stanford University
School of Medicine, Stanford, California
  CyberKnife Radiosurgery for Spinal Lesions

MANISH AGHI, MD, PhD
Resident in Neurosurgery, Harvard Medical School,
Massachusetts General Hospital, Boston, Massachusetts
  Surgical Management of Intracerebral Hemorrhage

ARUN P. AMAR, MD
Assistant Professor and Director of Endovascular
Neurosurgery, Yale University School of Medicine,
New Haven, Connecticut
  *Surgical Management of Growth Hormone–Secreting and
  Prolactin-Secreting Pituitary Adenomas*

SEPIDEH AMIN-HANJANI, MD
Assistant Professor, Department of Neurosurgery,
University of Illinois at Chicago, Chicago, Illinois
  *Surgical Management of Cavernous Malformations of the
  Nervous System*

JOSHUA M. AMMERMAN, MD
Resident, Department of Neurosurgery, The George
Washington University Medical Center, Washington, DC
  Video-Assisted Thoracoscopic Discectomy

JULIO ANTICO, MD
Professor, University of Buenos Aires; Chairman,
Department of Radiosurgery, University Hospital,
Buenos Aires, Argentina
  Sphenoid Ridge Meningiomas

TOOMAS ANTON, MD
Resident, Department of Neurosurgery, Henry Ford
Hospital, Detroit, Michigan
  Posterior Fossa Meningiomas

RONALD I. APFELBAUM, MD
Professor, Department of Neurosurgery, University of Utah
Health Sciences Center, Salt Lake City, Utah
  *Neurovascular Decompression in Surgical Disorders of
  Cranial Nerves V, VII, IX, and X*

JEFFREY E. ARLE, MD, PhD
Assistant Professor, Department of Neurosurgery,
Tufts University School of Medicine, Boston,
Massachusetts; Director, Functional Neurosurgery,
Lahey Clinic, Burlington, Massachusetts
  Current Management of Cervical Dystonia

TAKAO ASANO, MD, DMSc
Professor, Department of Neurosurgery, Saitama Medical
School, Saitama, Japan
  *Surgical Management of Ossification of the Posterior
  Longitudinal Ligament*

ERIK-OLOF BACKLUND, MD, PhD
Professor Emeritus, Department of Neurosurgery,
Linköping University Hopsital, Linköping,
Sweden
  *Stereotactic Radiosurgery for Pituitary Adenomas and
  Craniopharyngiomas*

JOACHIM BAEHRING, MD
Assistant Professor of Neurology and Neurosurgery,
Yale University School of Medicine; Attending
Neurologist, Yale New Haven Hospital, New Haven,
Connecticut
  Approaches to Lateral and Third Ventricular Tumors

PERRY A. BALL, MD
Associate Professor, Departments of Surgery and
Anesthesiology, Dartmouth Medical School; Staff
Neurosurgeon, Dartmouth-Hitchcock Medical Center,
Lebanon, New Hampshire
  *Spinal Cord Stimulation and Intraspinal
  Infusions for Pain*

JONATHAN J. BASKIN, MD
Atlantic NeuroSurgical Specialists, Morristown,
New Jersey
  *Surgical Techniques for Stabilization of the Subaxial
  Cervical Spine (C3–C7)*

ARMANDO BASSO, MD, PhD
Professor Emeritus, University of Buenos Aires School of
Medicine; Director, Neurosciences Institute, University
Hospital, Buenos Aires, Argentina
*Transcranial Approach to Lesions of the Orbit; Sphenoid
Ridge Meningiomas*

ULRICH BATZDORF, MD
Professor of Neurosurgery, Division of Neurosurgery,
UCLA Medical Center, Los Angeles, California
*Microsurgery of Syringomyelia and Syringomyelia Cord
Syndrome*

DONALD P. BECKER, MD
Professor of Surgery, Division of Neurosurgery, David
Geffen School of Medicine at UCLA; Director of UCLA
Neurosurgery Brain Tumor Program, UCLA Medical
Center, Los Angeles, California
Surgical Management of Severe Closed Head Injury in Adults

JOSHUA BEDERSON, MD
Professor, Department of Neurosurgery, Mount Sinai
School of Medicine, New York, New York
*Surgical Management of Spinal Cord Tumors and
Arteriovenous Malformations*

RUDOLF BEISSE, MD
Adjunct Professor, Department of Neurosurgery,
University of Utah, Salt Lake City, Utah; Head Trauma
Surgeon and Vice Chairman, Berufsgenossenchaftliche
Unfallklinik Muranau, Muranau, Germany
*Endoscopically Assisted Surgical Management of Thoracic
and Lumbar Fractures*

ALIM LOUIS BENABID, MD, PhD
Professor of Biophysics; Director, Laboratory of Neuro-
biophysics; Director, INSERM Preclinical Neurobiology,
Joseph Fourier University Medical School, Grenoble, France
Multilobar Resections in Epilepsy Surgery

LUDWIG BENES, MD
Neurosurgeon, Department of Neurosurgery, Philipps
University Marburg, Marburg, Germany
*Surgical Management of Aneurysms of the Vertebral and
Posterior Inferior Cerebellar Artery Complex*

VALLO BENJAMIN, MD
Professor, Department of Neurosurgery, New York
University School of Medicine; Attending Physician,
New York University Tisch Hospital, Bellevue Hospital,
New York, New York
*Surgical Management of Tuberculum Sellae and Medial
Sphenoid Ridge Meningiomas*

EDWARD C. BENZEL, MD
Chairman, Cleveland Clinic Spine Institute, Cleveland, Ohio
Surgical Management of Cervical Spondylotic Myelopathy

HELMUT BERTALANFFY, MD
Neurosurgeon, Professor, and Chairman, Department of
Neurosurgery, Philipps University Marburg, Marburg,
Germany
*Surgical Management of Aneurysms of the Vertebral and
Posterior Inferior Cerebellar Artery Complex*

SANAT N. BHAGWATI, MBBS, MS
Professor, Department of Neurosurgery, University of
Bombay; Senior Consultant Neurosurgeon,
Bombay Hospital and Medical Research Centre,
Mumbai, India
*Surgical Management of Fungal Infections of the Central
Nervous System*

RAVI BHATIA, MS, MCh
Professor of Neurosurgery, Department of Neurosurgery,
Indraprastha Apollo Hospital, New Delhi, India
*Surgical Management of Tuberculous Infections of the
Nervous System*

MARK H. BILSKY, MD
Attending Neurosurgeon, Memorial Sloan-Kettering
Cancer Center, New York, New York
Superior Sulcus Tumors

KEITH L. BLACK, MD
Director, Division of Neurosurgery; Director, Maxine
Dunitz Neurosurgical Institute, Ruth and Lawrence
Harvey Chair in Neurosciences, Cedars-Sinai Medical
Center, Los Angeles, California
Current Surgical Management of High-Grade Gliomas

LEWIS S. BLEVINS, JR., MD
Associate Professor of Medicine and Neurological
Surgery, Department of Neurological Surgery,
Vanderbilt University School of Medicine,
Nashville, Tennessee
*Endocrinologic Approach to the Evaluation and
Management of the Patient Undergoing Surgery for a
Pituitary Tumor*

NIKOLAS BLEVINS, MD
Assistant Professor, Department of Otolaryngology–Head
and Neck Surgery, Stanford University;
Attending Surgeon, Stanford Hospital and Clinics,
Lucile Packard Children's Hospital, Stanford,
California
Surgical Management of Glomus Jugulare Tumors

GEORGE T. BLIKE, MD
Associate Professor, Department of Anesthesia, Dartmouth
Medical School, Dartmouth-Hitchcock Medical Center,
Lebanon, New Hampshire
*Ensuring Patient Safety in Surgery—
"First Do No Harm"*

GÖRAN C. BLOMSTEDT, MD, PhD
Associate Professor, Docent of Neurosurgery, Helsinki
University; Vice Chairman, Helsinki University Hospital,
Helsinki, Finland
Considerations of Infections after Craniotomy

MAXWELL BOAKYE, MD
Assistant Professor, Department of Neurosurgery,
Stanford University Medical Center, Stanford,
California
Treatment of Odontoid Fractures

JAMES M. BORTHWICK, BSc, MB, ChB, FRCA
Honorary Clinical Senior Lecturer, University of Glasgow;
Consultant Anaesthetist, Department of
Neuroanaesthesia, Institute of Neurological Sciences,
Southern General Hospital, Glasgow, Scotland
  Surgical Management of the Rheumatoid Cervical Spine

ANNE BOULIN, MD
Department of Neuroradiology, Hôpital Foch,
Suresnes, France
  Transbasal Approach to Tumors Invading the Skull Base;
  Surgical Management of Endocrinologically Silent Pituitary
  Tumors

CHRISTOPHER M. BOXELL, MD
Clinical Assistant Professor, The University of Oklahoma
College of Medicine; Attending Physician, St. John
Medical Center, Tulsa Spine and Specialty Hospital, Tulsa,
Oklahoma
  Cervical Laminoplasty

ALBINO BRICOLO, MD
Professor and Chairman, Department of Neurosurgery,
University of Verona Medical School, University Hospital
of Verona, Verona, Italy
  Petroclival Meningiomas

RONALD BRISMAN, MD
Associate Professor of Clinical Neurosurgery, Columbia
University; Neurosurgeon, New York Presbyterian
Hospital, New York, New York
  Gamma Knife Radiosurgery for Trigeminal Neuralgia

GAVIN W. BRITZ, MD, MPH
Assistant Professor, Department of Neurological Surgery,
University of Washington School of Medicine;
Harborview Medical Center, Seattle, Washington
  Craniofacial Resection for Anterior Skull Base
  Tumors; Surgical Management of Moyamoya Disease
  in Adults

JASON A. BRODKEY, MD
Neurosurgeon, Michigan Brain and Spine Institute,
Ypsilanti, Michigan
  Transtemporal Approaches to the Posterior
  Cranial Fossa

JACQUES BROTCHI, MD, PhD
Professor of Neurosurgery, Faculty of Medicine, Université
Libre de Bruxelles; Chairman and Head, Department of
Neurosurgery, Erasme Hopsital, Brussels, Belgium
  Surgical Management of Intramedullary Spinal Cord
  Tumors in Adults

JEFFREY N. BRUCE, MD
Professor of Neurological Surgery, Columbia University
College of Physicians and Surgeons; Attending Physician
in Neurological Surgery, New York Presbyterian Hospital,
New York, New York
  Surgical Management of Intraorbital Tumors;
  Pineal Region Masses: Clinical Features and
  Management; Supracerebellar Approach for Pineal
  Region Neoplasms

FRANZ XAVER BRUNNER, MD
Professor, Zentralklinikum Augsburg, Augsburg,
Germany
  Surgical Management of Trauma Involving the Skull Base
  and Paranasal Sinuses

JOHN C. M. BRUST, MD
Professor, Department of Neurology, Columbia University
School of Medicine; Director, Harlem Hospital Neurology
Service, Harlem Hospital Center, New York, New York
  Surgical Management of Intracranial Aneurysms Caused by
  Infection

KIM J. BURCHIEL, MD, FACS
Professor and Chair, Department of Neurological Surgery;
Professor, Department of Anesthesiology and Perioperative
Medicine, Oregon Health and Science University School
of Medicine, Portland, Oregon
  Deep Brain Stimulation in the Management of Parkinson's
  Disease and Disabling Tremor

JAMES A. BURNS, MD
Assistant Professor, Division of Laryngology,
Department of Otolaryngology-Head and Neck
Surgery, University of Virginia, Charlottesville,
Virginia
  Transnasal Endoscopic Repair of Cranionasal Fistulas

RICHARD W. BYRNE, MD
Associate Professor, Rush University Medical School;
Associate Attending Physician, Rush University Medical
Center, Chicago, Illinois
  Multiple Subpial Transection for Epilepsy

PAOLO CAPPABIANCA, MD
Professor and Chairman of Neurological Surgery,
Department of Neurological Sciences, Federico II
University School of Medicine, Naples, Italy
  Repair of the Sella Turcica after Transsphenoidal
  Surgery

ANTHONY J. CAPUTY, MD, FACS
Professor and Chairman, Department of Neurosurgery,
The George Washington University, Washington, DC
  Video-Assisted Thoracoscopic Discectomy

FRANCESCO CARDINALE, MD
"Claudio Munari" Epilepsy Surgery Center, Niguarda
Hospital, Milan, Italy
  Multilobar Resections in Epilepsy Surgery

THOMAS P. CARLSTEDT, MD
Professor of Neurosurgery, University College London,
Consultant Orthopaedic Surgeon, The Royal National
Orthopaedic Hospital, Stanmore, England
  Surgical Management of Spinal Nerve Root Injuries

ANTONIO G. CARRIZO, MD, PhD
Professor, University of Buenos Aires School of Medicine;
Chairman, Department of Neurosurgery, University
Hospital, Buenos Aires, Argentina
  Transcranial Approach to Lesions of the Orbit; Sphenoid
  Ridge Meningiomas

BOB S. CARTER, MD, PhD
Assistant Professor of Surgery, Department of
Cerebrovascular Surgery, Harvard Medical School;
Attending Neurosurgeon, Massachusetts General Hospital,
Boston, Massachusetts
*Decompressive Craniectomy: Physiologic Rationale,
Clinical Indications, and Surgical Considerations;
Management of Dissections of the Carotid and Vertebral
Arteries; Surgical Management of Intracerebral
Hemorrhage*

ADRIAN CASEY, MD
Consultant Neurosurgeon, National Hospital for
Neurology and Neurosurgery, London, England
Innovations in Anterior Cervical Spine Surgery

LAURA CASTANA, MD
"Claudio Munari" Epilepsy Surgery Center, Niguarda
Hospital, Milan, Italy
Multilobar Resections in Epilepsy Surgery

STEVEN D. CHANG, MD
Assistant Professor, Department of Neurosurgery;
Director, CyberKnife Radiosurgery, Stanford University
School of Medicine, Stanford, California
CyberKnife Radiosurgery for Spinal Lesions

E. THOMAS CHAPPELL, MD
Associate Clinical Professor, University of California,
Irvine, University of California, Irvine Medical Center,
Orange, California
*Neurosurgical Management of HIV-Related Focal Brain
Lesions*

CLARK CHEN, MD, PhD
Post-Doctoral Fellow, Radiation Oncology, Dana-Farber
Cancer Institute, Harvard Medical School; Resident,
Department of Neurosurgery, Massachusetts General
Hospital, Boston, Massachusetts
*Decompressive Craniectomy: Physiologic Rationale,
Clinical Indications, and Surgical Considerations*

P. ROC CHEN, MD
Fellow in Endovascular Neurosurgery and Interventional
Neuroradiology, Department of Neurosurgery, Brigham and
Women's Hospital, Harvard Medical School, Boston,
Massachusetts
Management of Unruptured Cerebral Aneurysms

SAMUEL H. CHESHIER, MD, PhD
Resident, Department of Neurosurgery, Stanford
University School of Medicine, Stanford, California
CyberKnife Radiosurgery for Spinal Lesions

E. ANTONIO CHIOCCA, MD, PhD
Dardinger Family Endowed Chair in Oncological
Neurosurgery, Professor and Chairman, Department of
Neurosurgery, The Ohio State University Medical
Center/James Cancer Hospital, Columbus, Ohio
*Surgical Management of Cerebellar Astrocytomas
in Adults*

RAY M. CHU, MD
Attending Neurosurgeon, Maxine Dunitz Neurosurgical
Institute, Cedars-Sinai Medical Center, Los Angeles,
California
Current Surgical Management of High-Grade Gliomas

IVAN S. CIRIC, MD
Professor, Department of Neurological Surgery,
Northwestern University Feinberg School of Medicine,
Chicago, Illinois; Division of Neurosurgery, Evanston
Hospital, Evanston, Illinois
Complications of Transsphenoidal Microsurgery

ALAN R. COHEN, MD
Professor, Departments of Neurological Surgery and
Pediatrics, Reinberger Chair in Pediatric Neurological
Surgery, Case Western Reserve University School of
Medicine; Surgeon-in-Chief and Chief of Pediatric
Neurosurgery, Rainbow Babies and Children's Hospital,
University Hospitals of Cleveland, Cleveland, Ohio
Surgical Management of Tumors of the Fourth Ventricle

G. REES COSGROVE, MD, FRCS(C)
Professor, Department of Neurosurgery, Tufts University
School of Medicine, Boston, Massachusetts; Chairman,
Department of Neurosurgery, Lahey Clinic, Burlington,
Massachusetts
Cingulotomy for Intractable Psychiatric Illness

MASSIMO COSSU, MD
"Claudio Munari" Epilepsy Surgery Center, Niguarda
Hospital, Milan, Italy
Multilobar Resections in Epilepsy Surgery

PAUL R. COSYNS, MD
Professor and Chairman, Department of Psychiatry,
University of Antwerp, Wilrijk, Belgium, University
Hospital Antwerp, Edegem, Belgium
Neurosurgery for Psychiatric Disorders

WILLIAM T. COULDWELL, MD, PhD
Professor and Chairman, Department of Neurosurgery,
University of Utah Medical Center, Salt Lake City, Utah
*Surgical Management of Growth Hormone–Secreting and
Prolactin-Secreting Pituitary Adenomas*

SEAN P. CULLEN, MD
Instructor, Department of Radiology, Brigham and
Women's Hospital, Boston, Massachusetts
*Surgical and Endovascular Management of Aneurysms and
Fistulas Involving the Cavernous Sinus*

T. FORCHT DAGI, MD, MPH, MTS, FACS, FCCM
Department of Health Sciences and Technology,
Harvard-MIT Health Science and Technology Program,
Boston, Massachusetts
Management of Cerebrospinal Fluid Leaks

RONAN M. DARDIS, MD
Consultant Neurosurgeon, University Hospital Coventry
and Warwickshire, Warwickshire, England
Innovations in Anterior Cervical Spine Surgery

ARTHUR L. DAY, MD
Professor of Surgery, Department of Neurosurgery, Harvard
Medical School; Program Director and Vice Chairman,
Department of Neurosurgery, Brigham and Women's
Hospital, Boston, Massachusetts
*Perioperative Management of Severe Traumatic Brain
Injury in Adults; Surgical and Endovascular Management
of Aneurysms and Fistulas Involving the Cavernous Sinus;
Management of Unruptured Cerebral Aneurysms*

J. DIAZ DAY, MD
Clinical Assistant Professor, Department of Neurological
Surgery, University of Southern California; Director,
Neurological Surgery, Hoase Ear Clinic, Los Angeles,
California
*Surgical Management of Tumors Involving the Cavernous
Sinus*

ENRICO DE DIVITIIS, MD
Professor and Chairman of Neurological Surgery;
Chief, Department of Neurological Sciences, Frederico II
University School of Medicine, Naples, Italy
Repair of the Sella Turcica after Transsphenoidal Surgery

JACQUEZ CHARL DE VILLIERS, MD
Emeritus Professor, Department of Neurosurgery,
University of Cape Town, Cape Town, South Africa
*Surgical Management of Arteriovenous Malformations of
the Scalp*

VEDRAN DELETIS, MD, PhD
Associate Professor, Albert Einstein College of Medicine
of Yeshiva University, Bronx, New York; Director of
Intraoperative Neurophysiology, St. Luke's Roosevelt
Medical Center, New York, New York
*Intraoperative Neurophysiology: A Tool to Prevent and/or
Document Intraoperative Injury to the Nervous System*

ROBERT DERUTY, MD
Professor, Department of Neurosurgery, Laennec
University, Neurological Hospital, Lyon, France
*Surgical Management of Cerebral Arteriovenous
Malformations*

HAREL DEUTSCH, MD
Assistant Professor, Department of Neurosurgery, Rush
University, Chicago, Illinois
Endoscopic and Minimally Invasive Surgery of the Spine

JESSICA KOCH DEVIN, MD
Clinical Fellow in Endocrinology, Vanderbilt University
School of Medicine, Vanderbilt University Medical
Center, Nashville, Tennessee
*Endocrinologic Approach to the Evaluation and Management
of the Patient Undergoing Surgery for a Pituitary Tumor*

HARGOVIND DEWAL, MD
Fellow, Spine Surgery, Cleveland Clinic Foundation,
Cleveland, Ohio
*Surgical Management of Degenerative Lumbar Stenosis and
Spondylolisthesis*

P. C. TAYLOR DICKINSON, MD
Good Samaritan Hospital, New York, New York
*Surgical Management of Intracranial Aneurysms
Caused by Infection*

CURTIS A. DICKMAN, MD
Associate Chief, Spine Section; Director, Spinal Research,
Division of Neurological Surgery, Barrow Neurological
Institute, Phoenix, Arizona
*Surgical Techniques for Stabilization of the Subaxial
Cervical Spine (C3–C7)*

**ZAYNE DOMINGO, MBChB(Natal), FCS(SA), MMed(UCT),
DPhil(OXON)**
Specialist Neurosurgeon, Constantiaberg Mediclinic,
Wynberg, South Africa
*Surgical Management of Arteriovenous Malformations of
the Scalp*

CHARLES G. DRAKE, MD, FACD, FRCS†
*Surgical Techniques of Terminal Basilar and Posterior
Cerebral Artery Aneurysms*

JAMES M. DRAKE, BSE, MBBCh, MSc, FRCSC, FACS
Professor of Surgery, University of Toronto;
Neurosurgeon-in-Chief, Hospital for Sick Children,
Toronto, Ontario, Canada
*Cerebrospinal Fluid Shunting and Management of Pediatric
Hydrocephalus*

THOMAS B. DUCKER, MD
Professor of Neurosurgery, Johns Hopkins University
School of Medicine and Hospital, Baltimore, Maryland
Circumferential Spinal Fusion (Cervical)

ANNE-CHRISTINE DUHAIME, MD
Professor of Neurosurgery, Dartmouth Medical School;
Director, Pediatric Neurosurgery, Children's Hospital At
Dartmouth (CHAD), Dartmouth-Hitchcock Medical
Center, Lebanon, New Hampshire
Craniopharyngiomas: A Summary of Data—Commentary

IAN F. DUNN, MD
Resident in Neurosurgery, Department of Neurosurgery,
Harvard Medical School, Bringham and Women's
Hospital and Children's Hospital, Boston,
Massachusetts
*Perioperative Management of Severe Traumatic Brain
Injury in Adults; Surgical and Endovascular
Management of Aneurysms and Fistulas Involving the
Cavernous Sinus*

SUSAN R. DURHAM, MD
Assistant Professor, Department of Neurosurgery,
Dartmouth Medical School, Dartmouth-Hitchcock
Medical Center, Lebanon, New Hampshire
Surgical Management of Sciatic Nerve Lesions

---

†Deceased.

JOSHUA R. DUSICK, MD
Resident and Research Fellow, Division of Neurosurgery,
David Geffen School of Medicine, University of
California, Los Angeles, Los Angeles, California;
Department of Physical Therapy, Mount St. Mary's
College, Newburgh, New York
*Surgical Management of Severe Closed Head Injury in
Adults*

KURT M. EICHHOLZ, MD
Resident, University of Iowa College of Medicine,
Iowa City, Iowa
Management Options in Thoracolumbar Fractures

ALAA EL-NAGGAR, MD
Lecturer, Neurosurgery Department, Faculty of Medicine,
University of Alexandria, Egypt
*Orbitozygomatic Infratemporal Approach to Parasellar
Meningiomas*

DILANTHA B. ELLEGALA, MD
Clinical Fellow in Surgery, Department of Neurosurgery,
Brigham and Women's Hospital, Boston, Massachusetts,
Department of Neurological Surgery, Oregon Health and
Sciences University, Portland, Oregon
*Surgical and Endovascular Management of Aneurysms and
Fistulas Involving the Cavernous Sinus*

PAMELA ELY, MD, PhD
Associate Professor of Medicine, Director, Lymphoma
Clinical Oncology Group, Dartmouth-Hitchcock Medical
Center, Lebanon, New Hampshire
*Management of Primary Central Nervous System
Lymphomas*

JOSEPH A. EPSTEIN, MD
Clinical Professor Emeritus of Neurological Surgery,
The Albert Einstein College of Medicine, Bronx,
New York; The North Shore-Long Island Jewish Health
System, Manhasset and New Hyde Park; Long Island
Neurological Associates, P.C., New Hyde Park,
New York
*Far Lateral Lumbar Disc Herniations: Diagnosis and
Surgical Management*

NANCY E. EPSTEIN, MD, FACS
Clinical Professor of Neurosurgery, The Albert Einstein
College of Medicine, Bronx, New York; Chief, Division of
Spinal Neurosurgery, Winthrop University Hospital,
Mineola, New York
*Far Lateral Lumbar Disc Herniations: Diagnosis and
Surgical Management*

THOMAS J. ERRICO, MD
Associate Professor, Departments of Orthopaedic Surgery
and Neurosurgery, New York University School of
Medicine; Chief, Spine Service; Director, Spine
Fellowship Program; Attending Physician, NYU Hospital
for Joint Diseases; Attending Physician, Tisch Hospital,
New York, New York
*Surgical Management of Degenerative Lumbar Stenosis and
Spondylolisthesis*

R. FRANCISCO ESCOBEDO, MD†
Neurosurgical Aspects of Neurocysticercosis

CLIFFORD J. ESKEY, MD, PhD
Asssistant Professor, Department of Radiology, Dartmouth
Medical School; Director, Interventional Neuroradiology,
Dartmouth-Hitchcock Medical Center, Lebanon,
New Hampshire
Vertebroplasty and Kyphoplasty

CAMILO E. FADUL, MD
Associate Professor of Medicine, Dartmouth Medical
School, Dartmouth-Hitchcock Medical Center, Lebanon,
New Hampshire
*Management of Primary Central Nervous System
Lymphomas*

RUDOLF FAHLBUSCH, MD
Chairman and Professor, Department of Neurosurgery,
University of Erlangen-Nuremberg, Erlangen,
Germany
*Surgical Management of Convexity, Parasagittal,
and Falx Meningiomas*

GILBERT J. FANCIULLO, MD, MS
Associate Professor, Dartmouth Medical School;
Director, Section of Pain Medicine, Dartmouth-
Hitchcock Medical Center, Lebanon, New
Hampshire
*Spinal Cord Stimulation and Intraspinal Infusions
for Pain*

RICHARD G. FESSLER, MD, PhD
Professor and Chief, Section of Neurosurgery,
The University of Chicago, Chicago, Illinois
*Primary Reconstruction for Spinal Infections;
Surgical Approaches to the Cervicothoracic Junction*

GEORGES FISCHER, MD, PhD
Professor of Neurosurgery, Faculty of Medicine R. T. H.
Leannec; National Expert in Neurosurgery,
Domaine Scientifique de la Doua, Université Claude
Bernard Lyon 1, Lyon, France
*Surgical Management of Intramedullary Spinal Cord
Tumors in Adults*

NORMAN D. FISHER-JEFFES, MD
Department of Orthopedic Surgery, University of Natal,
Durban, South Africa
*Surgical Management of Arteriovenous Malformations of
the Scalp*

IAN G. FLEETWOOD, MD, FRCS(C)
Assistant Professor of Neurosurgery, Dalhousie
University; Director of Cerebrovascular Surgery,
Co-Director of Stereotactic Radiosurgery,
Queen Elizabeth II Health Sciences Centre, Halifax,
Nova Scotia, Canada
*Surgical Management of Midbasilar and Lower Basilar
Aneurysms*

†Deceased.

JOHN C. FLICKINGER, MD, FACR
Professor, Department of Radiation Oncology,
University of Pittsburgh School of Medicine; Radiation
Oncologist, UPMC-Presbyterian Hospital, Pittsburgh,
Pennsylvania
Radiosurgery of Vestibular Schwannomas

KEVIN T. FOLEY, MD
Professor, Department of Neurosurgery, University of
Tennessee School of Medicine, Semmes-Murphey Clinic,
Memphis, Tennessee
Image-Guided Spine Surgery

DARYL R. FOURNEY, MD, FRCSC
Assistant Professor, Division of Neurosurgery,
University of Saskatchewan, Royal University Hospital,
Saskatoon, Saskatchewan, Canada
Sacral Resection and Stabilization

STEFANO FRANCIONE, MD
"Claudio Munari" Epilepsy Surgery Center, Niguarda
Hospital, Milan, Italy
Multilobar Resections in Epilepsy Surgery

STEPHEN R. FREIDBERG, MD
Chair Emeritus, Division of Surgery; Chairman Emeritus,
Department of Neurosurgery, Lahey Clinic, Burlington,
Massachusetts
*Surgical Management of Cerebrospinal Fluid Leakage after
Spinal Surgery*

KAI FRERICHS, MD, PhD
Assistant Professor of Surgery, Department of
Neurosurgery, Harvard Medical School; Endovascular
Neurosurgery, Brigham and Women's Hospital, Boston,
Massachusetts
*Perioperative Management of Severe Traumatic Brain Injury
in Adults; Management of Unruptured Cerebral Aneurysms*

JONATHAN A. FRIEDMAN, MD
Assistant Professor, Dartmouth Medical School; Staff
Neurosurgeon, Dartmouth-Hitchcock Medical Center,
Lebanon, New Hampshire
*Surgical Management of Posterior Communicating,
Anterior Choroidal, and Carotid Bifurcation Aneurysms*

GERHARD M. FRIEHS, MD
Associate Professor of Neurosurgery, Department of Clinical
Neurosciences Program in Neurosurgery, Brown Medical
School; Director, Trauma and Functional Neurosurgery,
Rhode Island Hospital, Providence, Rhode Island
*Surgical Management of Injuries of the Cervical Spine and
Spinal Cord; Surgical Management of Segmental Spinal
Instability*

DAVID M. FRIM, MD, PhD
Associate Professor of Surgery and Pediatrics,
Biological Sciences Division, The University of Chicago;
Chief, Pediatric Neurosurgery, The University of Chicago
Children's Hospital, Chicago, Illinois
*Surgical Management of Adult Hydrocephalus; Surgical
Treatment of Neurofibromatosis*

AARON M. FROM, MD
Resident, Department of Internal Medicine, Mayo Clinic,
Rochester, Minnesota
*Ankylosing Spondylitis and Management of Spinal
Complications; Management Options in Thoracolumbar
Fractures*

TAKANORI FUKUSHIMA, MD, DMSc
Professor of Neurosurgery, Duke University Medical
Center, Durham, North Carolina; West Virginia
University Medical Center, Morgantown, West Virginia
*Surgical Management of Tumors Involving the
Cavernous Sinus*

MICHAEL R. GAAB, MD, PhD
Professor of Neurosurgery, Hannover Medical School;
Head, Department of Neurosurgery, Hannover Nordstadt
Hospital, Hannover, Germany
Neuroendoscopic Approach to Intraventricular Tumors

STEPHAN GAILLARD, MD
Department of Neurosurgery, Hôpital Foch, Suresnes, France
*Transbasal Approach to Tumors Invading the Skull Base;
Surgical Management of Endocrinologically Silent Pituitary
Tumors*

GALE GARDNER, MD
Clinical Professor, Department of Otolaryngology,
University of Tennessee College of Medicine, Memphis,
Tennessee
*Transtemporal Approaches to the Posterior Cranial Fossa;
Surgical Management of Glomus Jugulare Tumors*

BERNARD GEORGE, MD
Professor, Department of Neurosurgery, University of Paris;
Head, Department of Neurosurgery, Lariboisiere Hospital,
Paris, France
Meningiomas of the Foramen Magnum

VENELIN GERGANOV, MD
Department of Neurosurgery, Sofia Medical University,
Sofia, Bulgaria
Surgical Management of Craniopharyngiomas

CARL A. GEYER, MD
Assistant Professor of Radiology, Tufts University Medical
School; Clinical Lecturer, Harvard Medical School,
Boston; Neuroradiologist, Lahey Clinic, Burlington,
Massachusetts
Intraspinal Cerebrospinal Fluid Cysts

RENATO GIUFFRÈ, MD[†]
Surgical Management of Low-Grade Gliomas

ZIYA L. GOKASLAN, MD, FACS
Professor of Neurosurgery, Oncology, and Orthopedic
Surgery; Vice Chairman, Department of Neurosurgery;
Director, Neruosurgical Spine Program, Johns Hopkins
University, Baltimore, Maryland
Sacral Resection and Stabilization

[†]Deceased.

ALFREDO GOMEZ-AVINA, MD
Instituto Nacional de Neurología y Neurocirugía,
Mexico City, Mexico
Neurosurgical Aspects of Neurocysticercosis

SERGEY K. GORELYSHEV, MD
Professor and Chief, Department of Pediatric
Neurosurgery, Burdenko Neurosurgical Institute, Moscow,
Russia
*Surgical Management of Brain Stem, Thalamic,
and Hypothalamic Tumors*

TAKEO GOTO, MD
Lecturer, Department of Neurosurgery, Osaka City
University Graduate School of Medicine, Osaka, Japan
*Orbitozygomatic Infratemporal Approach to Parasellar
Meningiomas*

CHARLES W. GROSS, MD
Professor Emeritus, Rhinology, Departments of
Otolaryngology-Head and Neck Surgery and Pediatrics,
University of Virginia, Charlottesville, Virginia
Transnasal Endoscopic Repair of Cranionasal Fistulas

ROBERT G. GROSSMAN, MD
Chairman, Department of Neurosurgery; Director,
The Neurological Institute, The Methodist Hospital,
Houston, Texas
Temporal Lobe Operations for Drug-Resistant Epilepsy

DANIEL J. GUILLAUME, MD
Chief Resident, Neurosurgery, Roy J. and
Lucille A. Carver College of Medicine, University of
Iowa Hospitals and Clinics, Iowa City, Iowa
*Diagnosis and Management of Traumatic Intracranial
Aneurysms*

RICHARD W. GULLAN, MD
Senior Neurosurgeon, King's College Hospital, London,
England
Innovations in Anterior Cervical Spine Surgery

NIHAL T. GURUSINGHE, MBBS, FRCSE
Clinical Lecturer, Department of Neurosurgery, University
of Lancashire, Preston, Lancashire; Senior Consultant
Neurosurgeon, Preston Acute Hospitals, Preston, England
*Surgical Management of Fungal Infections of the Central
Nervous System*

BARTON L. GUTHRIE, MD
Associate Professor, University of Alabama, Birmingham
Medical Center, Birmingham, Alabama
*Neurosurgical Management of HIV-Related Focal Brain
Lesions*

JAN M. GYBELS, MD, PhD
Professor Emeritus of Neurology and Neurosurgery,
Laboratory of Experimental Neurosurgery and
Neuroanatomy, Katholieke Universiteit Leuven; Member,
Royal Academy of Medicine of Belgium, Leuven,
Belgium
Neurosurgery for Psychiatric Disorders

FUAD S. HADDAD, MD
Professor of Neurosurgery, American University of Beirut,
Beirut, Lebanon
*Diagnosis and Management of Traumatic Intracranial
Aneurysms*

GEORGES F. HADDAD, MD
Clinical Associate Professor of Neurosurgery, American
University of Beirut, Beirut, Lebanon
*Diagnosis and Management of Traumatic Intracranial
Aneurysms*

REGIS W. HAID, JR., MD
Atlanta Brain and Spine Care, Atlanta, Georgia
Treatment of Odontoid Fractures

STEPHEN J. HAINES, MD
Professor, Department of Neurosurgery, University of
Minnesota, Twin Cities, Minneapolis, Minnesota
Assessing Surgical Innovation

STEN HÅKANSON, MD, PhD
Former Head, Pediatric Neurosurgery, Karolinska
University Hospital, Stockholm, Sweden
Retrogasserian Glycerol Rhizolysis in Trigeminal Neuralgia

AKIRA HAKUBA, MD†
*Orbitozygomatic Infratemporal Approach to Parasellar
Meningiomas*

MARK G. HAMILTON, MD, FRCS(C)
Associate Professor of Neurosurgery, Departments of
Neurosciences, Pediatrics, and Surgery, University of
Calgary; Director, Division of Pediatric Neurosurgery and
Pediatric Neurosciences, Alberta Children's Hospital;
Co-Director, Surgical Neuro-oncology Program, Foothills
Hospital, Calgary, Alberta, Canada
*Surgical Management of Midbasilar and Lower Basilar
Aneurysms*

WINIFRED J. HAMILTON, PhD, SM
Assistant Professor, Departments of Medicine and
Neurosurgery, Baylor College of Medicine, Houston, Texas
Temporal Lobe Operations for Drug-Resistant Epilepsy

JOSEPH K. HAN, MD
Director of Rhinology and Sinus Surgery, Associate
Professor, Division of Rhinology and Endoscopic Sinonasal
Surgery, Department of Otorhinolaryngology–Head and
Neck Surgery, University of Virginia, Charlottesville, Virginia
Transnasal Endoscopic Repair of Cranionasal Fistulas

J. FREDERICK HARRINGTON, JR., MD
Assistant Professor of Neurosurgery, Department of
Clinical Neurosciences Program in Neurosurgery,
Brown Medical School; Surgeon-in-Charge, Spinal
Neurosurgery, Rhode Island Hospital, Providence,
Rhode Island
Surgical Management of Segmental Spinal Instability

---

†Deceased.

BRENT T. HARRIS, MD, PhD
Neuropathologist, Dartmouth-Hitchcock Medical Center,
Lebanon, New Hampshire
Frame-Based Stereotactic Brain Biopsy

GRIFFITH R. HARSH IV, MD
Professor of Neurological Surgery, Stanford Medical
School, Stanford, California
Surgical Management of Recurrent Gliomas

ROGER HARTL, MD
Assistant Professor, Department of Neurological Surgery,
Weill Cornell Medical College, New York, New York
*Surgical Techniques for Stabilization of the Subaxial
Cervical Spine (C3–C7)*

ADAM O. HEBB, MD
Resident, Department of Neurosurgery, University of
Minnesota, Twin Cities, Minneapolis, Minnesota
Assessing Surgical Innovation

CARL B. HEILMAN, MD
Associate Professor, Department of Neurosurgery, Tufts-
New England Medical Center, Boston, Massachusetts
Surgical Management of Glomus Jugulare Tumors

STEFAN HEINZE, MD
Neurosurgeon, Department of Neurosurgery, Philipps
University Marburg, Marburg, Germany
*Surgical Management of Aneurysms of the Vertebral and
Posterior Inferior Cerebellar Artery Complex*

DIETER HELLWIG, MD, PhD
Neurosurgeon, Department of Neurosurgery, Philipps
University Marburg, Marburg, Germany
*Surgical Management of Arachnoid, Suprasellar, and
Rathke's Cleft Cysts; Neuronavigation in Neuroendoscopic
Surgery*

STEPHEN J. HENTSCHEL, MD
Fellow, Department of Neurosurgery, The University of
Texas MD Anderson Cancer Center, Houston,
Texas
Surgical Management of Cerebral Metastases

JUHA HERNESNIEMI, MD, PhD
Professor and Chairman, Department of Neurosurgery,
University Hospital of Helsinki, Helsinki, Finland
*Surgical Management of Aneurysms of the Middle Cerebral
Artery; Surgical Techniques of Terminal Basilar and
Posterior Cerebral Artery Aneurysms*

SHIGERU HIRABAYASHI, MD, DMSc
Associate Professor, Saitama Medical School, Saitama, Japan
*Surgical Management of Ossification of the Posterior
Longitudinal Ligament*

PATRICK W. HITCHON, MD
Professor of Neurosurgery and Biomedical Engineering,
University of Iowa College of Medicine; Chief,
Neurosurgery Service, Veterans Administration Medical
Center, Iowa City, Iowa

*Diagnosis and Management of Traumatic Intracranial
Aneurysms; Ankylosing Spondylitis and Management of
Spinal Complications; Management Options in
Thoracolumbar Fractures*

BERND M. HOFMANN, MD
Neurosurgeon, Department of Neurosurgery, University of
Erlangen-Nuremberg, Erlangen, Germany
*Surgical Management of Convexity, Parasagittal, and
Falx Meningiomas*

BRIAN L. HOH, MD
Clinical Instructor of Surgery, Harvard Medical School;
Attending Neurosurgeon, Massachusetts General Hospital,
Boston, Massachusetts
*Management of Dissections of the Carotid and Vertebral
Arteries*

LANGSTON T. HOLLY, MD
Ruth and Raymond Stotter Chair in Neurosurgery,
Assistant Professor of Neurosurgery, UCLA School of
Medicine, Los Angeles, California
Image-Guided Spine Surgery

ROBERT N. N. HOLTZMAN, MD, PC
Associate Clinical Professor, Department of Neurological
Surgery, Columbia University School of Medicine,
New York, New York
*Surgical Management of Intracranial Aneurysms Caused by
Infection*

JOHN H. HONEYCUTT, JR., MD
Assistant Professor, Department of Neurosurgery,
University of Oklahoma, Oklahoma City, Oklahoma
*Surgical Management of Extracranial Carotid
Artery Disease*

EDGAR M. HOUSEPIAN, MD
Professor Emeritus, Clinical Neurological Surgery,
Columbia University College of Physicians and Surgeons;
Special Lecturer, Columbia Presbyterian Medical Center,
New York, New York
Surgical Management of Intraorbital Tumors

JASON H. HUANG, MD
University of Pennsylvania School of Medicine,
The Hospital of the University of Pennsylvania,
Philadelphia, Pennsylvania
Surgical Management of Sciatic Nerve Lesions

ALAN R. HUDSON, MD
President and CEO, Cancer Care Ontario, Toronto,
Ontario, Canada
Surgical Management of Peripheral Nerve Tumors

JAMES E. O. HUGHES, MD
Assistant Clinical Professor, Department of Neurological
Surgery, Columbia University School of Medicine,
Harlem Hospital Center, New York, New York
*Surgical Management of Intracranial Aneurysms
Caused by Infection*

MARK R. IANTOSCA, MD
Assistant Clinical Professor, University of Connecticut, Farmington; Director, Connecticut Children's Medical Center, Hartford, Connecticut
Cerebrospinal Fluid Shunting and Management of Pediatric Hydrocephalus

KEISUKE ISHII, MD, PhD
Associate Professor, Faculty of Medicine, University of Oita; Chief, Emergency Department, University Hospital of Oita, Oita, Japan
Surgical Management of Aneurysms of the Middle Cerebral Artery; Surgical Techniques of Terminal Basilar and Posterior Cerebral Artery Aneurysms

IVO P. JANECKA, MD, MBA
Senior Lecturer, Harvard Medical School, Brigham and Women's Hospital, Boston, Massachusetts
Anterior Midline Approaches to the Skull Base

MOHSEN JAVADPOUR, MB, BCh, FRCS(SN)
Consultant Neurosurgeon, Walton Centre for Neurology and Neurosurgery, Liverpool, England
Surgical Management of Cranial Dural Arteriovenous Fistulas

LOUIS G. JENIS, MD
Assistant Clinical Professor, Department of Orthopaedic Surgery, Tufts University School of Medicine; The Boston Spine Group, New England Baptist Hospital, Boston, Massachusetts
Surgical Management of Segmental Spinal Instability

DAVID H. JHO, BA
University of Illinois at Chicago College of Medicine, Chicago, Illinois
Endoscopic Transsphenoidal Surgery

HAE-DONG JHO, MD, PhD
Professor of Neurosurgery, Drexel University College of Medicine, Philadelphia; Director, Jho Institute for Minimally Invasive Neurosurgery, Allegheny General Hospital, Pittsburgh, Pennsylvania
Endoscopic Transsphenoidal Surgery

PATRICK JOHNSON, MD
Director, Institute for Spinal Disorders, Cedars-Sinai Medical Center, Los Angeles, California
Thoracoscopic Sympathectomy for Hyperhidrosis

FRANCIS G. JOHNSTON, MB, ChB
Consultant, St. George's Healthcare NHS Trust, London, England
Craniofacial Resection for Anterior Skull Base Tumors

ROBIN A. JOHNSTON, MD, FRCS
Honorary Senior Lecturer, University of Glasgow; Consultant Neurosurgeon, Institute of Neurological Sciences, Southern General Hospital, Glasgow, Scotland
Surgical Management of the Rheumatoid Cervical Spine

PETER JUN, MD
Department of Neurological Surgery, University of California, San Francisco, School of Medicine, San Francisco, California
Microsurgical Management of Anterior Communicating Artery Aneurysms

SILLOO B. KAPADIA, MD
Professor of Pathology and Surgery, Penn State College of Medicine, State College; Director of Surgical Pathology, Department of Anatomic Pathology, Milton S. Hershey Medical Center, Hershey, Pennsylvania
Anterior Midline Approaches to the Skull Base

AYSE KARATAS, MD
Department of Neurosurgery, University Hospital of Helsinki, Helsinki, Finland
Surgical Techniques of Terminal Basilar and Posterior Cerebral Artery Aneurysms

ANTHONY M. KAUFMANN, MD, BSc (Med), MSc, FRCS(C)
Associate Professor, Division of Neurological Surgery, University of Manitoba, Winnipeg, Manitoba, Canada
Microvascular Decompression Surgery for Hemifacial Spasm

MICHAEL KAZIM, MD
Associate Clinical Professor of Ophthalmology and Surgery, Columbia University College of Physicians and Surgeons; Associate Attending Physician in Opthalmology and Surgery, New York Presbyterian Hospital, New York, New York
Surgical Management of Intraorbital Tumors

DANIEL F. KELLY, MD
Professor of Neurosurgery, David Geffen School of Medicine, University of California; Director, UCLA Pituitary Tumor and Neuroendocrine Program; Co-Director of Clinical Brain Injury Program, UCLA Medical Center, Los Angles, Harbor-UCLA Medical Center, Torrance, California
Surgical Management of Severe Closed Head Injury in Adults

PATRICK J. KELLY, MD
Joseph Ransohoff Professor of Neurosurgery; Chairman, Department of Neurosurgery, New York University, New York, New York
CT/MRI-Based Computer-Assisted Volumetric Stereotactic Resection of Intracranial Lesions

SANFORD KEMPIN, MD
Director of Clinical Research, Department of Medical Oncology, St. Vincent's Comprehensive Cancer Center, New York, New York
Disorders of the Spine Related to Plasma Cell Dyscrasias

SAAD KHAIRI, MD
Fellow, Institute for Spinal Disorders, Cedars-Sinai Medical Center, Los Angeles, California
Thoracoscopic Sympathectomy for Hyperhidrosis

ELENA A. KHUHLAEVA, MD, PhD
Chief Neurologist, Department of Pediatric Neurosurgery, Burdenko Neurosurgical Institute, Moscow, Russia
Surgical Management of Brain Stem, Thalamic, and Hypothalamic Tumors

DANIEL H. KIM, MD
Associate Professor, Director, Spinal Neurosurgery and Reconstructive Peripheral Nerve Surgery, Stanford University Medical Center, Stanford, California
Surgical Approaches to the Cervicothoracic Junction; Surgical Management of Peripheral Nerve Tumors

DONG H. KIM, MD
Associate Professor, Department of Neurosurgery, Dana-Farber Cancer Institute, Harvard Medical School; Cerebrovascular and Skull Base Surgery, Brigham and Women's Hospital, Boston, Massachusetts
Perioperative Management of Severe Traumatic Brain Injury in Adults; Surgical and Endovascular Management of Aneurysms and Fistulas Involving the Cavernous Sinus; Management of Unruptured Cerebral Aneurysms

HIROYUKI KINOUCHI, MD, PhD
Associate Professor, Department of Neurosurgery, Akita University School of Medicine, Akita, Japan
Intraoperative Endovascular Techniques in the Management of Intracranial Aneurysms

RIKU KIVISAARI, MD
Radiologist, Resident in Neurosurgery, Department of Neurosurgery, University Hospital of Helsinki, Helsinki, Finland
Surgical Management of Aneurysms of the Middle Cerebral Artery

DAVID G. KLINE, MD
Boyd Professor and Chair, Department of Neurosurgery, Louisiana State University Health Science Center, New Orleans, Louisiana
Surgical Management of Peripheral Nerve Tumors

SHIGEAKI KOBAYASHI, MD, PhD
Professor Emeritus, Department of Neurosurgery, Shinshu University School of Medicine, Matsumoto, Japan; Director, Komoro Kosei General Hospital, Komoro, Japan
Surgical Management of Paraclinoid Aneurysms

DOUGLAS KONDZIOLKA, MD, FACS, FRCS(C)
Professor, Departments of Neurological Surgery and Radiation Oncology, University of Pittsburgh School of Medicine; Director, Specialized Neurosurgical Center, UPMC-Presbyterian Hospital, Pittsburgh, Pennsylvania
Radiosurgery of Vestibular Schwannomas

ALEXANDER N. KONOVALOV, MD
Professor and Director, Burdenko Neurosurgical Institute, Moscow, Russia
Surgical Management of Brain Stem, Thalamic, and Hypothalamic Tumors

MARK D. KRIEGER, MD
Assistant Professor, Keck School of Medicine at the University of Southern California, Childrens Hospital of Los Angeles, Los Angeles, California
Surgical Management of Growth Hormone–Secreting and Prolactin-Secreting Pituitary Adenomas

AJIT A. KRISHNANEY, MD
Resident, Departments of Neurosurgery and Orthopedic Surgery, The Cleveland Clinic Foundation, Cleveland, Ohio
Surgical Management of Cervical Spondylotic Myelopathy

JAMES T. KRYZANSKI, MD
Assistant Professor, Tufts University School of Medicine, Neurosurgeon, Tufts-New England Medical Center, Boston, Massachusetts
Distal Anterior Cerebral Artery Aneurysms

KAZUHIKO KYOSHIMA, MD, PhD
Department of Neurosurgery, Shinshu University School of Medicine, Matsumoto; Medical Advisor, Neurosurgery, Nadogaya Hospital, Kashiwa, Japan
Surgical Management of Paraclinoid Aneurysms

MAUREEN LACY, PhD
Assistant Professor of Psychiatry, The University of Chicago, Chicago, Illinois
Surgical Management of Adult Hydrocephalus

SANTOSH D. LAD, MBBS, MS
Clinical Tutor, Department of Neurosurgery, Sultan Qaboos University; Senior Consultant Neurosurgeon, Head of Department of Neurosurgery, National Neurosurgical Centre, Muscat, Sultanate of Oman
Surgical Management of Fungal Infections of the Central Nervous System

JESUS LAFUENTE, MD, PhD
Senior Registrar, National Hospital for Neurology and Neurosurgery, London, England
Innovations in Anterior Cervical Spine Surgery

FREDERICK F. LANG, MD, FACS
Associate Professor and Director of Clinical Research, Department of Neurosurgery, The University of Texas MD Anderson Cancer Center, Houston, Texas
Surgical Management of Cerebral Metastases

FRANÇOISE LAPIERRE, MD
Professor, Department of Neurosurgery, Poitiers University Medical School; Chief Neurosurgeon, University Hospital, Poitiers, France
Management of Cauda Equina Tumors

MICHAEL T. LAWTON, MD
Associate Professor, Department of Neurological Surgery, University of California, San Francisco, San Francisco, California
Microsurgical Management of Anterior Communicating Artery Aneurysms

HOANG N. LE, MD
Fellow, Department of Neurosurgery, Stanford University
Medical Center, Stanford, California
  Surgical Approaches to the Cervicothoracic Junction

KENDALL H. LEE, MD, PhD
Neurosurgery Resident, Dartmouth-Hitchcock Medical
Center, Lebanon, New Hampshire
  Frame-Based Stereotactic Brain Biopsy

MAX C. LEE, MD
Fellow in Spine Surgery, Department of Neurosurgery,
Stanford University Medical Center, Stanford, California
  Primary Reconstruction for Spinal Infections

ADAM I. LEWIS, MD
Jackson Neurosurgery Clinic, Jackson, Mississippi
  *Surgical Management of Brain Stem Vascular
  Malformations*

ROGER LICHTENBAUM, MD
Resident, Department of Neurosurgery, New York
University, New York, New York
  *CT/MRI-Based Computer-Assisted Volumetric Stereotactic
  Resection of Intracranial Lesions*

BENGT LINDEROTH, MD, PhD
Professor, Section of Functional Neurosurgery, Karolinska
Institute; Head, Section of Functional Neurosurgery,
Karolinska University Hospital, Stockholm, Sweden
  *Retrogasserian Glycerol Rhizolysis in Trigeminal Neuralgia;
  Spinal Cord Stimulation for Chronic Pain*

CHRISTER LINDQUIST, MD, PhD
Consultant Neurosurgeon, Director, Gamma Knife Center,
Cromwell Hospital, London, England
  *Gamma Knife Surgery for Cerebral Vascular
  Malformations, Tumors, and Functional Disorders*

MICHAEL J. LINK, MD
Department of Neurosurgery, Mayo Clinic, Rochester,
Minnesota
  Surgical Management of Brain Stem Vascular Malformations

KENNETH LITTLE, MD
Chief Resident, Division of Neurosurgery, Duke University
Medical Center, Durham, North Carolina
  *Spinal Infections: Vertebral Osteomyelitis and Spinal
  Epidural Abscess*

ALI LIU, MD
Professor, Capital University of Medical Sciences; Chief
Doctor, The Gamma Knife Center, Beijing Neurosurgical
Institute, Beijing, China
  *Surgical Management of Nonglomus Tumors of the Jugular
  Foramen*

JAMES K. LIU, MD
Department of Neurosurgery, University of Utah School of
Medicine, Salt Lake City, Utah
  *Surgical Management of Growth Hormone–Secreting and
  Prolactin-Secreting Pituitary Adenomas*

GIORGIO LO RUSSO, MD
Chief, "Claudio Munari" Epilepsy Surgery Center,
Niguarda Hospital, Milan, Italy
  Multilobar Resections in Epilepsy Surgery

CHRISTOPHER M. LOFTUS, MD
Professor and Chair, Department of Neurosurgery,
Temple University Hospital, Philadelphia,
Pennsylvania
  *Surgical Management of Extracranial
  Carotid Artery Disease*

S. SCOTT LOLLIS, MD
Division of Neurosurgery, Dartmouth Medical School,
Dartmouth-Hitchcock Medical Center, Lebanon,
New Hampshire
  Entrapment Neuropathies of the Lower Extremities

DONLIN M. LONG, MD, PhD
Distinguished Service Professor, Department of
Neurosurgery, Johns Hopkins University, Johns Hopkins
Hospital, Baltimore, Maryland
  *Management of Persistent Symptoms after Lumbar
  Disc Surgery*

RUSSELL R. LONSER, MD
Staff Neurosurgeon, Surgical Neurology Branch,
National Institute of Neurological Disorders
and Stroke, National Institutes of Health, Bethesda,
Maryland
  *Neurovascular Decompression in Surgical Disorders of
  Cranial Nerves V, VII, IX, and X*

WOLF LÜDEMANN, MD
Consultant, International Neuroscience Institute (INI),
Hannover, Germany
  Surgical Management of Craniopharyngiomas

L. DADE LUNSFORD, MD, FACS
Professor and Chair, Department of Neurological Surgery,
University of Pittsburgh School of Medicine; Chair,
Department of Neurological Surgery, UPMC-Presbyterian
Hospital, Pittsburgh, Pennsylvania
  Radiosurgery of Vestibular Schwannomas

JOSEPH R. MADSEN, MD
Associate Professor of Surgery, Harvard School of
Medicine, Children's Hospital, Bringham and Women's
Hospital, Boston, Massachusetts
  *Treatment of Intractable Epilepsy by Electrical Stimulation
  of the Vagus Nerve*

SUBU N. MAGGE, MD
Assistant Professor, Tufts University School of
Medicine, Boston; Lahey Clinic, Burlington, Massachusetts
  Microsurgery of Ruptured Lumbar Intervertebral Disc

ASHOK K. MAHAPATRA, MBBS, MS, MCh
Professor, Department of Neurosurgery, All India Institute
of Medical Sciences, New Delhi, India
  *Surgical Management of Fungal Infections of the Central
  Nervous System*

KHALID MAHLA, MD
Assistant, Faculty of Medicine R. T. H. Laennec, Université Claude Bernard Lyon 1; Assistant, Neurochirurgie "B", Hôpital Neurologique et Neurochirurgical Pierre Wertheimer, Lyon, France
Surgical Management of Intramedullary Spinal Cord Tumors in Adults

ROBERTO MAI, MD
"Claudio Munari" Epilepsy Surgery Center, Niguarda Hospital, Milan, Italy
Multilobar Resections in Epilepsy Surgery

GIULIO MAIRA, MD
Professor and Department Head, Department of Neurosurgery, Catholic University School of Medicine, Rome, Italy
Surgical Management of Lesions of the Clivus

DAVID G. MALONE, MD
Neurosurgeon, Oklahoma Spine and Brain Institute, Tulsa, Oklahoma
Cervical Laminoplasty

MITCHELL D. MARTINEAU, MS
Oklahoma Spine and Brain Institute, Tulsa, Oklahoma
Cervical Laminoplasty

ROBERT L. MARTUZA, MD
Professor of Surgery, Harvard Medical School; Chief, Neurosurgical Service, Massachusetts General Hospital, Boston, Massachusetts
Surgical Management of Olfactory Groove Meningiomas; Suboccipital Transmeatal Approach to Vestibular Schwannoma

JOHN E. McGILLICUDDY, MD
Professor of Neurosurgery and Orthopedics, University of Michigan, University of Michigan Hospitals, Ann Arbor, Michigan
Thoracic Outlet Syndrome

ARNOLD H. MENEZES, MD, FACS, FAAP
Professor and Vice Chairman, Department of Neurosurgery, Roy J. and Lucille A. Carter College of Medicine; Professor of Neurosurgery, University of Iowa Hospitals and Clinics, Iowa City, Iowa
Craniovertebral Abnormalities and Their Neurosurgical Management; Ankylosing Spondylitis and Management of Spinal Complications

ALI H. MESIWALA, MD
Maxine Dunitz Neurosugical Institute, Cedars-Sinai Medical Center, Los Angeles, California
Surgical Management of Moyamoya Disease in Adults

FREDRIC B. MEYER, MD
Professor and Chair, Department of Neurologic Surgery, Mayo Clinic College of Medicine, Rochester, Minnesota
Surgical Management of Lesions in Eloquent Areas of Brain

JONATHAN P. MILLER, MD
Resident, University Hospitals of Cleveland, Cleveland, Ohio
Surgical Management of Tumors of the Fourth Ventricle

JOHN MISLOW, MD
Resident, Department of Neurological Surgery, Harvard Medical School, Brigham and Women's Hospital, Boston, Massachusetts
Primary Reconstruction for Spinal Infections

KAZUO MIZOI, MD
Professor and Chairman, Department of Neurosurgery, Akita University School of Medicine, Akita, Japan
Intraoperative Endovascular Techniques in the Management of Intracranial Aneurysms

A. ALEX MOHIT, MD, PhD
Resident, Department of Neurological Surgery, University of Washington School of Medicine, Seattle, Washington
Craniofacial Resection for Anterior Skull Base Tumors

CHAD J. MORGAN, MD
Chief Resident, Department of Neurosurgery, University of Cincinnati College of Medicine, Cincinnati, Ohio
Percutaneous Stereotactic Rhizotomy in the Treatment of Intractable Facial Pain

PRAVEEN V. MUMMANENI, MD
Assistant Professor, Neurosurgery, Emory University, Atlanta, Georgia
Treatment of Odontoid Fractures

CLAUDIO MUNARI, MD[†]
Multilobar Resections in Epilepsy Surgery

AURANGZEB NAGY, MD
Department of Neurosurgery, University Medical Center, Las Vegas, Nevada
Surgical Management of Peripheral Nerve Tumors

DAVID W. NEWELL, MD
Executive Director, Swedish Neurological Institute, Seattle, Washington
Surgical Management of Moyamoya Disease in Adults

MIKA NIEMELÄ, MD
Professor and Chairman, Department of Neurosurgery, University Hospital of Helsinki, Helsinki, Finland
Surgical Techniques of Terminal Basilar and Posterior Cerebral Artery Aneurysms

DIMITRIOS C. NIKAS, MD
Division of Neurosurgery, Dartmouth Medical School, Dartmouth-Hitchcock Medical Center, Lebanon, New Hampshire
Entrapment Neuropathies of the Lower Extremities

LINO NOBILI, MD
"Claudio Munari" Epilepsy Surgery Center, Niguarda Hospital, Milan, Italy
Multilobar Resections in Epilepsy Surgery

[†]Deceased.

RICHARD B. NORTH, MD
Professor, Departments of Neurosurgery, Anesthesiology, and Critical Care Medicine; Director, Functional Spinal Neurosurgery, Department of Neurosurgery, Johns Hopkins University School of Medicine, Baltimore, Maryland
Spinal Cord Stimulation for Chronic Pain

W. JERRY OAKES, MD
Professor of Neurosurgery and Pediatrics, University of Alabama at Birmingham, Children's Hospital, Birmingham, Alabama
Tethered Cord Syndrome in the Adult

JOACHIM M. K. OERTEL, MD, PhD
Associate Professor of Neurosurgery, Hannover Medical School; Attending Neurosurgeon, Department of Neurosurgery, Hannover Norstadt Hospital, Hannover, Germany
Neuroendoscopic Approach to Intraventricular Tumors

CHRISTOPHER S. OGILVY, MD
Professor of Neurosurgery, Harvard Medical School; Attending Neurosurgeon, Director of Cerebrovascular Surgery, Massachusetts General Hospital, Boston, Massachusetts
Decompressive Craniectomy: Physiologic Rationale, Clinical Indications, and Surgical Considerations; Management of Dissections of the Carotid and Vertebral Arteries; Surgical Management of Intracerebral Hemorrhage; Surgical Management of Cavernous Malformations of the Nervous System

KENJI OHATA, MD
Associate Professor, Department of Neurosurgery, Osaka City University Graduate School of Medicine, Osaka, Japan
Orbitozygomatic Infratemporal Approach to Parasellar Meningiomas

ROBERT G. OJEMANN, MD
Professor, Department of Neurosurgery, Harvard Medical School; Visiting Neurosurgeon, Massachusetts General Hospital, Boston, Massachusetts
Surgical Management of Olfactory Groove Meningiomas; Suboccipital Transmeatal Approach to Vestibular Schwannoma; Surgical Management of Cavernous Malformations of the Nervous System

EDWARD H. OLDFIELD, MD
Chief, Surgical Neurology Branch, National Institute of Neurological Disorders and Stroke, National Institutes of Health, Bethesda, Maryland
Management of Cushing's Disease

S. BULENT OMAY, MD
Resident, Department of Neurosurgery, Yale University School of Medicine, New Haven, Connecticut
Approaches to Lateral and Third Ventricular Tumors

RICHARD K. OSENBACH, MD
Assistant Professor, Division of Neurological Surgery, Duke University Medical Center, Durham, North Carolina
Spinal Infections: Vertebral Osteomyelitis and Spinal Epidural Abscess

ROBERTO PALLINI, MD
Assistant Professor, Department of Neurosurgery, Catholic University School of Medicine, Rome, Italy
Surgical Management of Lesions of the Clivus

JON PARK, MD
Assistant Professor, Stanford University, Stanford, California
Surgical Approaches to the Cervicothoracic Junction

MICHAEL C. PARK, MD, PhD
Neurosurgery Resident, Department of Clinical Neurosciences Program in Neurosurgery, Brown Medical School, Rhode Island Hospital, Providence, Rhode Island
Surgical Management of Segmental Spinal Instability

FRANCESCO S. PASTORE, MD
Assistant Professor, Institute of Neurosurgery, Department of Neuroscience, University of Rome "Tor Vergata," Rome, Italy
Surgical Management of Low-Grade Gliomas

RANA PATIR, MS, MCh (Neurosurg)
Senior Consultant, Sir Ganga Ram Hospital, New Delhi, India
Surgical Management of Tuberculous Infections of the Nervous System

SANJAY J. PAWAR, MBBS, MS, MCh
Visiting Consultant Neurosurgeon, Wanless Hospital, Meeraj Medical College; Consultant Neurosurgeon, Poona Hospital, Ruby-Hall Hospital, Jahangir Hospital, Maharastra, India
Surgical Management of Fungal Infections of the Central Nervous System

SYDNEY J. PEERLESS, MD
Retired, Punta Gorda, Florida
Surgical Techniques of Terminal Basilar and Posterior Cerebral Artery Aneurysms

ISABELLE PELISSOU-GUYOTAT, MD, PhD
Head, Department of Emergency Neurosurgery, Neurological Hospital, Lyon, France
Surgical Management of Cerebral Arteriovenous Malformations

PAUL M. PELOSO, MD
Associate Professor, Department of Internal Medicine, University of Iowa Hospitals and Clinics, Iowa City, Iowa
Ankylosing Spondylitis and Management of Spinal Complications

PHILIPPE PENCALET, MD
Department of Neurosurgery, Hôpital Foch, Suresnes, France
Transbasal Approach to Tumors Invading the Skull Base; Surgical Management of Endocrinologically Silent Pituitary Tumors

RICHARD PENN, MD
Professor of Neurosurgery, The University of Chicago, Chicago, Illinois
Surgical Management of Adult Hydrocephalus

NOEL PERIN, MD
Director, Spine and Minimally Invasive Surgery, Department of Neurosurgery, St. Luke's-Roosevelt Hospital Center, New York, New York
Surgical Management of Spinal Cord Tumors and Arteriovenous Malformations

MARK A. PICHELMANN, MD
Chief Resident Associate, Department of Neurologic Surgery, Mayo School of Graduate Medical Education; Chief Resident of Neurologic Surgery, Mayo Clinic College of Medicine, Rochester, Minnesota
Surgical Management of Lesions in Eloquent Areas of Brain

JOSEPH PIEPMEIER, MD
Professor, Yale University School of Medicine, New Haven, Connecticut
Approaches to Lateral and Third Ventricular Tumors

JOHN M. D. PILE-SPELLMAN, MD
Professor, Departments of Radiology, Neurological Surgery, and Neurology; Director, Academic Interventional Neuroradiology; Vice-Chair of Research, Department of Radiology, Colombia University School of Medicine, New York, New York
Surgical Management of Intracranial Aneurysms Caused by Infection

RICK J. PLACIDE, MD, PT
Spinal and Orthopaedic Surgeon, West End Orthopaedic Clinic, Richmond, Virginia
Surgical Management of Cervical Spondylotic Myelopathy

CHARLES E. POLETTI, MD
Hartford Hospital, Hartford, Connecticut
Open Cordotomy and Medullary Tractotomy

KALMON D. POST, MD
Department of Neurosurgery, Mount Sinai School of Medicine, New York, New York
Surgical Management of Spinal Cord Tumors and Arteriovenous Malformations

LARS POULSGAARD, MD
Associate Professor, University Clinic of Neurosurgery, The Neuroscience Center, University of Copenhagen, Copenhagen, Denmark
Translabyrinthine Approach to Vestibular Schwannomas

PATRICIA B. QUEBADA, MD
Resident, Section of Neurosurgery, Dartmouth-Hitchcock Medical Center, Lebanon, New Hampshire
Surgical Management of Chronic Subdural Hematoma in Adults

ALFREDO QUIÑONES-HINOJOSA, MD
Resident, Department of Neurological Surgery, University of California School of Medicine, San Francisco, California
Microsurgical Management of Anterior Communicating Artery Aneurysms

ANTONINO RACO, MD
Associate Professor of Neurosurgery, Department of Neurolocal Sciences, "La Sapienza" Univeristy of Rome; Policlinico Umberto I, Rome, Italy
Surgical Management of Cerebellar Hemorrhage and Cerebellar Infarction

JOHN RATLIFF, MD
Assistant Professor, Department of Neurosurgery, Rush University, Chicago, Illinois
Endoscopic and Minimally Invasive Surgery of the Spine

AFSHIN E. RAZI, MD
Assistant Professor, Department of Orthopaedic Surgery, New York University School of Medicine; Attending Physician, NYU Medical Center, Hospital for Joint Diseases, New York, New York
Surgical Management of Degenerative Lumbar Stenosis and Spondylolisthesis

JAAKKO RINNE, MD, PhD
Associate Professor of Neurosurgery, Faculty of Medicine, University of Kuopio; Head of Division, Director, Neurovascular Surgery Group, Department of Neurosurgery, Kuopio University Hospital, Kuopio, Finland
Surgical Management of Aneurysms of the Middle Cerebral Artery

DAVID W. ROBERTS, MD
Professor of Surgery (Neurosurgery), Alma Hass Milham Distinguished Chair in Clinical Medicine, Dartmouth Medical School, Hanover; Chief, Section of Neurosurgery, Dartmouth-Hitchcock Medical Center, Lebanon, New Hampshire
Frame-Based Stereotactic Brain Biopsy; Section of the Corpus Callosum for Epilepsy

JON H. ROBERTSON, MD
Professor and Chairman, Department of Neurosurgery, University of Tennessee College of Medicine; Member, Semmes-Murphey Neurologic and Spine Institute, Memphis, Tennessee
Transtemporal Approaches to the Posterior Cranial Fossa; Surgical Management of Glomus Jugulare Tumors

JACK P. ROCK, MD
Senior Neurosurgical Staff, Henry Ford Hospital, Detroit, Michigan
Posterior Fossa Meningiomas

GERALD E. RODTS, JR., MD
Professor, Neurosurgery, Emory University, Atlanta, Georgia
Treatment of Odontoid Fractures

AXEL ROMINGER, MD
Treatment of Intractable Epilepsy by Electrical Stimulation of the Vagus Nerve

SETH I. ROSENBERG, MD
Clinical Assistant Professor, University of Pennsylvania, Philadelphia, Pennsylvania; Clinical Assistant Professor, University of South Florida; Sarasota Memorial Hospital, Lakewood Ranch Hospital, Venice Hospital, Sarasota, Florida
Vestibular Nerve Section in the Management of Intractable Vertigo

GUY ROSENTHAL, MD
Clinical Instructor, Department of Neurosurgery, Hebrew University Medical School, Hadassah University Hospital, Jerusalem, Israel
Penetrating Brain Injuries

SALVADOR RUIZ-GONZALEZ
Mexico City, Mexico
Neurosurgical Aspects of Neurocysticercosis

STEPHEN M. RUSSELL, MD
Assistant Professor, Department of Neurosurgery, New York University School of Medicine, New York, New York
Surgical Management of Tuberculum Sellae and Medial Sphenoid Ridge Meningiomas

SAMUEL RYU, MD
Senior Staff, Director, Center for Radiosurgery, Departments of Radiation Oncology and Neurosurgery, Henry Ford Hospital, Detroit, Michigan
Posterior Fossa Meningiomas

STEPHEN I. RYU, MD
Resident, Department of Neurosurgery, Stanford University School of Medicine, Stanford, California
CyberKnife Radiosurgery for Spinal Lesions

FRANCESCO SALA, MD
Attending Physician, Neurosurgeon, Department of Neurological Sciences and Vision, Verona University Hospital, Verona, Italy
Intraoperative Neurophysiology: A Tool to Prevent and/or Document Intraoperative Injury to the Nervous System

AMIR SAMII, MD, PhD
Associate Professor, Department of Neurosurgery, Medical School of Hannover; Vice Director, Department of Neurosurgery, International Neuroscience Institute (INI), Hannover, Germany
Surgical Management of Craniopharyngiomas

MADJID SAMII, MD, PhD
President, International Neuroscience Institute (INI), Hannover, Germany
Surgical Management of Craniopharyngiomas

PRAKASH SAMPATH, MD
Assistant Professor, Brown University, Rhode Island Hospital, Providence, Rhode Island
Surgical Management of Injuries of the Cervical Spine and Spinal Cord

RENE O. SANCHEZ-MEJIA, MD
Resident, University of California at San Francisco, San Francisco, California
Microsurgical Management of Anterior Communicating Artery Aneurysms

KEIJI SANO, MD
Emeritus Professor, Department of Neurosurgery, University of Tokyo; Director, Fuji Brain Institute Hospital, Fujinomiya City, Japan
Alternate Surgical Approaches to Pineal Region Neoplasms

IVANA SARTORI, MD
"Claudio Munari" Epilepsy Surgery Center, Niguarda Hospital, Milan, Italy
Multilobar Resections in Epilepsy Surgery

PAUL D. SAWIN, MD
Florida Neurosurgical Consultants, PA, Orlando, Florida
Surgical Techniques for Stabilization of the Subaxial Cervical Spine (C3–C7)

ALEXANDRA K. SCHMIDEK, MD
Division of Plastic Surgery, Department of Surgery, Harvard Medical School, Massachusetts General Hospital, Boston, Massachusetts
Surgical Management of Median Nerve Compression at the Wrist by Open Technique

HENRY H. SCHMIDEK, MD, FACS
Senior Neurosurgeon, Dartmouth-Hitchcock Medical Center, Dartmouth Medical School, Lebanon, New Hampshire
Surgical Management of Chronic Subdural Hematoma in Adults; Suppurative Intracranial Infections

HENRY W. S. SCHROEDER, MD, PhD
Professor of Neurosurgery; Director, Department of Neurosurgery, Ernst-Moritz-Arndt-Universität, Greifswald, Germany
Neuroendoscopic Approach to Intraventricular Tumors

DIRK MICHAEL SCHULTE, MD
Resident and Instructor, Department of Neurosurgery, Philipps University Marburg, Marburg, Germany
Surgical Management of Arachnoid, Suprasellar, and Rathke's Cleft Cysts; Neuronavigation in Neuroendoscopic Surgery

VOLKER SEIFERT, MD, PhD
Director, Klinik und Poliklinik für Neurochirurgie, Johann Wolfgang Goethe-Universität, Frankfurt, Germany
Anterior Approaches in Multisegmental Cervical Spondylosis

RICARDO SEGAL, MD
Senior Neurosurgeon, Department of Neurosurgery,
Hadassah University Hospital, Jerusalem, Israel
Penetrating Brain Injuries

DILIP K. SENGUPTA, MD, PhD
Department of Orthopaedics, Spine Center,
Dartmouth-Hitchcock Medical Center, Lebanon,
New Hampshire
Ankylosing Spondylitis and Management of Spinal Complications

REWATI RAMAN SHARMA, MBBS, MS, DNB
Clinical Tutor, Department of Neurosurgery,
Sultan Qaboos University; Chairman, Staff Development;
Senior Consultant Neurosurgeon, National Neurosurgical
Centre, Khoula Hospital, Muscat, Sultanate of Oman
Surgical Management of Fungal Infections of the Central Nervous System

JASON SHEEHAN, MD, PhD
Assistant Professor of Neurological Surgery and
Neuroscience, University of Virginia, Charlottesville,
Virginia
Gamma Knife Surgery for Cerebral Vascular Malformations, Tumors, and Functional Disorders

BASSEM SHEIKH, MD, FRCS, FKFU(NS)
Associate Professor, Department of Neurosurgery,
King Faisal University, Dammam, Saudi Arabia;
Consultant Neurosurgeon and Acting Chairman,
Department of Neurosurgery, King Fahd Teaching
Hospital, Al-Khobar, Saudi Arabia
Orbitozygomatic Infratemporal Approach to Parasellar Meningiomas

HU SHEN, MD
Senior Neurosurgeon, Department of Neurosurgery,
Nanshan Hospital, Shenzhen, Guangdong, China
Surgical Management of Aneurysms of the Middle Cerebral Artery

MASATO SHIBUYA, MD, PhD
Clinical Professor, Nagoya University School of Medicine,
Director, Chukyo Hospital, Nagoya, Japan
Surgical Management of Paraclinoid Aneurysms

PRISCILLA SHORT, MD
Clinical Associate in Neurosurgery, The University of
Chicago Pritzker School of Medicine, Chicago, Illinois
Surgical Treatment of Neurofibromatosis

WILLIAM A. SHUCART, MD
Professor and Chair, Department of Neurosurgery, Tufts
University School of Medicine, Chief of Neurosurgery,
Tufts-New England Medical Center, Boston,
Massachusetts
Distal Anterior Cerebral Artery Aneurysms

ADRIAN M. SIEGEL, MD
Department of Neurology, University Hospital of Zurich,
Zurich, Switzerland
Section of the Corpus Callosum for Epilepsy

HERBERT SILVERSTEIN, MD
Clinical Professor of Otorhinolaryngology, University of
Pennsylvania School of Medicine, Philadelphia,
Pennsylvania; University of South Florida, Sarasota
Memorial Hospital, Sarasota, Florida
Vestibular Nerve Section in the Management of Intractable Vertigo

NATHAN E. SIMMONS, MD
Assistant Professor, Section of Neurosurgery, Dartmouth-
Hitchcock Medical Center, Lebanon, New Hampshire
Surgical Techniques in the Management of Thoracic Disc Herniations

MARC P. SINDOU, MD, DSc
Professor, Department of Neurosurgery, University of Lyon
Medical School: Chairman, Department of Neurosurgery,
Hospital Neurologique Pierre Wertheimer, Lyon, France
Microsurgical DREZotomy

ROBERT J. SINGER, MD
Neurosurgeon, Neurological Surgeons, PC, Nashville,
Tennessee
Management of Dissections of the Carotid and Vertebral Arteries

EDWARD R. SMITH, MD
Instructor, Department of Neurosurgery, Harvard Medical
School; Assistant Professor, Neurosurgery, Children's
Hospital, Boston, Massachusetts
Decompressive Craniectomy: Physiologic Rationale, Clinical Indications, and Surgical Considerations

BRIAN E. SNELL, MD
Clinical Instructor, Department of Neurosurgery, Medical
College of Wisconsin; Spinal Surgery Fellow, Froedtert
Memorial Lutheran Hospital, Milwaukee, Wisconsin
Surgical Management of Extracranial Carotid Artery Disease

VOLKER K. H. SONNTAG, MD
Clinical Professor, Department of Neurosurgery, University
of Arizona, Tucson; Vice Chairman, Division of
Neurological Surgery, Barrow Neurological Institute;
Director, Residency Program, Chairman, BNI Spine
Section, Barrow Neurological Institute, Phoenix, Arizona
Surgical Techniques for Stabilization of the Subaxial Cervical Spine (C3–C7)

RENATO SPAZIANTE, MD
Professor of Neurosurgery and Chairman, University of
Genoa Medical School; Chairman, Department of
Neurosurgery, San Martino University Hospital,
Genoa, Italy
Repair of the Sella Turcica after Transsphenoidal Surgery

ROBERT F. SPETZLER, MD, FACS
Division of Neurosurgery, University of Arizona College of
Medicine, Tucson; Director, Barrow Neurological Institute,
St. Joseph's Hospital, Phoenix, Arizona
Surgical Management of Midbasilar and Lower Basilar Aneurysms

BENNETT M. STEIN, MD
Bernardsville, New Jersey
Surgical Management of Spinal Cord Tumors and Arteriovenous Malformations

LADISLAU STEINER, MD, PhD
Professor of Neurological Surgery, University of Virginia, Charlottesville, Virginia
Gamma Knife Surgery for Cerebral Vascular Malformations, Tumors, and Functional Disorders

MELITA STEINER, MD
Research Professor of Neurosurgery, University of Virginia, Charlottesville, Virginia
Gamma Knife Surgery for Cerebral Vascular Malformations, Tumors, and Functional Disorders

MICHAEL P. STEINMETZ, MD
Resident, Departments of Neurosurgery and Orthopedic Surgery, The Cleveland Clinic Foundation, Cleveland, Ohio
Surgical Management of Cervical Spondylotic Myelopathy

BERTIL STENER, MD, PhD[†]
Technique of Complete Spondylectomy in the Thoracic and Lumbar Spine

MATEI STROILA, PhD
Assistant Professor, Department of Neursurgery, Lars Leksell Center for Gamma Surgery, University of Virginia Health System, Charlottesville, Virginia
Gamma Knife Surgery for Cerebral Vascular Malformations, Tumors, and Functional Disorders

NARAYAN SUNDARESAN, MD
Central Park Neurosurgery, New York, New York
Disorders of the Spine Related to Plasma Cell Dyscrasias

ULRICH SURE, MD
Neurosurgeon and Associate Professor, Department of Neurosurgery, Philipps University Marburg, Marburg, Germany
Surgical Management of Aneurysms of the Vertebral and Posterior Inferior Cerebellar Artery Complex

BROOKE SWEARINGEN, MD
Assistant Professor of Surgery, Harvard Medical School, Associate Visiting Neurosurgeon, Massachusetts General Hospital, Boston, Massachusetts
Transsphenoidal Approach to Pituitary Tumors

WILLIAM H. SWEET, MD, DSc, FACS[†]
Craniopharyngiomas: A Summary of Data; Cervicothoracic Ankylosing Spondylitis

TOSHIHIRO TAKAMI, MD
Lecturer, Department of Neurosurgery, Osaka City University Graduate School of Medicine, Osaka, Japan
Orbitozygomatic Infratemporal Approach to Parasellar Meningiomas

PRAKASH NARAIN TANDON, MD, MS, FRCS
Emeritus Professor, All India Institute of Medical Sciences, New Delhi, India
Surgical Management of Tuberculous Infections of the Nervous System

EDWARD C. TARLOV, MD
Associate Professor, Department of Neurosurgery, Tufts University School of Medicine, Boston; Neurosurgeon, Lahey Clinic, Burlington, Massachusetts
Intraspinal Cerebrospinal Fluid Cysts; Microsurgery of Ruptured Lumbar Intervertebral Disc

RONALD R. TASKER, MD, FRCS(C)
Professor Emeritus, Department of Surgery, University of Toronto; Honorary Neurosurgeon, University Health Network, Toronto Western Hospital, Toronto, Ontario, Canada
Surgical Treatment of the Dyskinesias

LAURA TASSI, MD
"Claudio Munari" Epilepsy Surgery Center, Niguarda Hospital, Milan, Italy
Multilobar Resections in Epilepsy Surgery

JULIA K. TERZIS, MD, PhD
Professor of Surgery, Department of Surgery, Division of Plastic and Reconstructive Surgery, Eastern Virginia Medical School; Senior Surgeon, Sentara Norfolk General Hospital, Norfolk, Virginia
Surgical Management of Brachial Plexus Injuries in Adults

JOHN M. TEW, JR., MD
Professor, Department of Neurosurgery, University of Cincinnati College of Medicine; Medical Director, The Neuroscience Institute, Mayfield Clinic, Cincinnati, Ohio
Surgical Management of Brain Stem Vascular Malformations; Percutaneous Stereotactic Rhizotomy in the Treatment of Intractable Facial Pain

ISSADA THONGTRANGAN, MD
Fellow, Stanford University, Stanford, California
Surgical Approaches to the Cervicothoracic Junction

WUTTIPONG TIRAKOTAI, MD, MSc
Neurosurgeon, Siriraj Hospital, Mahidol University, Bangkok, Thailand, Clincal Fellow, Department of Neurosurgery, Philipps University Marburg, Marburg, Germany
Surgical Management of Arachnoid, Suprasellar, and Rathke's Cleft Cysts; Neuronavigation in Neuroendoscopic Surgery; Surgical Management of Aneurysms of the Vertebral and Posterior Inferior Cerebellar Artery Complex

GIUSTINO TOMEI, MD
Professor of Neurosurgery, Department of Surgical Sciences, University of Insubria-Varese, Varese, Italy
Transcallosal Approach to Tumors of the Third Ventricle

JAMES H. TONSGARD, MD
Associate Professor of Pediatrics and Neurology,
The University of Chicago Pritzker School of Medicine,
Chicago, Illinois
Surgical Treatment of Neurofibromatosis

JAMES C. TORNER, PhD
Professor, University of Iowa College of Public Health,
Iowa City, Iowa
Management Options in Thoracolumbar Fractures

NGUYEN VAN TUAN, MD
Associate Professor, University Formation Center;
Neurosurgeon, Bênh Viên Nhân Dân 115, Ho Chi Minh
City, Vietnam
Management of Cauda Equina Tumors

R. SHANE TUBBS, PA-C, PhD
Assistant Professor of Cell Biology and Neurosurgery,
University of Alabama at Birmingham, Children's
Hospital, Birmingham, Alabama
Tethered Cord Syndrome in the Adult

SERGIO TURAZZI, MD
Chief, Division of Neurosurgery, University Hospital of
Verona, Verona, Italy
Petroclival Meningiomas

FRANCIS TURJMAN, MD, PhD
Professor, Department of Neuroradiology, Laennec
University, Head, Interventional Radiology, Department
of Radiology, Neurological Hospital, Lyon, France
*Surgical Management of Cerebral Arteriovenous
Malformations*

PETER F. ULLRICH, JR., MD
Medical Director, NeuroSpine Center of Wisconsin,
Appleton, Wisconisn
*Anterior Lumbar Interbody Fusion: Mini-Open
Laparotomy Approach*

FELIX UMANSKY, MD
Professor of Neurosurgery, Hebrew University Medical
School; Professor and Chairman, Department of
Neurosurgery, Hadassah University Hospital, Jerusalem,
Israel
Penetrating Brain Injuries

JOHN C. VAN GILDER, MD
Professor, Department of Neurosurgery, Roy J. and
Lucille A. Carver College of Medicine, University of
Iowa Hospitals and Clinics, Iowa City, Iowa
*Craniovertebral Abnormalities and Their Neurosurgical
Management*

MARIOS D. VEKRIS
Lecturer in Orthopaedics, Ioannina University Medical
School, Attending in Orthopaedic Department,
University Hospital of Ioannina, Ioannina, Greece; Senior
Fellow in Microsurgery, Microsurgical Research Center,
Eastern Virginia Medical School, Norfolk, Virginia
Surgical Management of Brachial Plexus Injuries in Adults

PAUL VESPA, MD
Associate Professor , Director, Neurocritical Care Program,
Department of Neurology, Division of Neurosurgery,
David Geffen School of Medicine at UCLA, University of
California at Los Angeles, Los Angeles, California
Surgical Management of Severe Closed Head Injury in Adults

ROBERTO M. VILLANI, MD
Professor of Neurosurgery, Department of Neurological
Sciences, University of Milan, Milan, Italy
Transcallosal Approach to Tumors of the Third Ventricle

ANDRÉ VISOT, MD, AIHP, ACCA
Chief of Department of Neurosurgery, Hôpital Foch,
Suresnes, France
*Transbasal Approach to Tumors Invading the Skull Base;
Surgical Management of Endocrinologically Silent Pituitary
Tumors*

FRANK D. VRIONIS, MD, PhD
Associate Professor of Neurosurgery, ENT, and Oncology,
University of South Florida College of Medicine; Director,
Skull Base Oncology, H. Lee Moffitt Cancer Center and
Research Institute, Tampa, Florida
*Transtemporal Approaches to the Posterior
Cranial Fossa*

MICHEL P. WAGER, MD
Neurosurgeon, Poitiers University Medical School,
University Hospital, Poitiers, France
Management of Cauda Equina Tumors

M. CHRISTOPHER WALLACE, MD, MSc, FRCSC, FACS
Professor and Program Director, Division of Neurosurgery,
Faculty of Medicine, University of Toronto; Toronto
Western Hospital, Toronto, Ontario, Canada
*Surgical Management of Cranial Dural Arteriovenous
Fistulas*

CHUNG-CHENG WANG, MD, PhD
Professor, Capital University of Medical Sciences,
Director, Beijing Neurosurgical Institute, Beijing, China
*Surgical Management of Nonglomus Tumors of the Jugular
Foramen*

THOMAS N. WARD, MD
Associate Professor, Department of Neurology, Dartmouth
Medical School; Staff Neurologist, Dartmouth-Hitchcock
Medical Center, Lebanon, New Hampshire
Current Management of Cervical Dystonia

JOSEPH C. WATSON, MD
Assistant Professor, Albert Einstein College of Medicine;
Chief of Neurosurgery, Jacobi Medical Center and North
Central Bronx Hospital, Bronx, New York
Management of Cushing's Disease

HOWARD L. WEINER, MD
Associate Professor of Neurosurgery, New York University,
New York, New York
*CT/MRI-Based Computer-Assisted Volumetric Stereotactic
Resection of Intracranial Lesions*

MARTIN H. WEISS, MD
Professor of Neurology and Neurosurgery,
Department of Neurological Surgery, Keck School of
Medicine of University of Southern California, Los
Angeles, California
*Surgical Management of Growth Hormone–Secreting and
Prolactin-Secreting Pituitary Adenomas*

WILLIAM C. WELCH, MD, FACS, FICS
Professor, Departments of Neurological Surgery,
Orthopaedic Surgery, and Rehabilitation Science and
Technology, University of Pittsburgh; Chief, Neurological
Surgery, UPMC Health System, Pittsburgh, Pennsylvania
Thoracoscopic Sympathectomy for Hyperhidrosis

WALTER W. WHISLER, MD, PhD
Professor and Chairman Emeritus, Rush University
Medical School, Senior Attending Physician Emeritus,
Rush University Medical Center, Chicago, Illinois
Multiple Subpial Transection for Epilepsy

LOUIS A. WHITWORTH, MD
Assistant Professor, Department of Neurosurgical Surgery,
The University of Texas Southwestern, The University of
Texas Southwestern Medical Center at Dallas, Dallas, Texas
*Deep Brain Stimulation in the Management of Parkinson's
Disease and Disabling Tremor*

MARSHALL F. WILKINSON, MSc, PhD
Neurophysiologist, Inoperative Monitoring Program,
Health Sciences Centre, Winnipeg, Manitoba, Canada
Microvascular Decompression Surgery for Hemifacial Spasm

JONATHAN M. WINOGRAD, MD
Instructor in Surgery, Department of Surgery, Harvard
Medical School, Division of Plastic and Reconstructive
Surgery, Massachusetts General Hospital, Boston,
Massachusetts
*Surgical Management of Median Nerve Compression at the
Wrist by Open Technique*

MICHAEL L. WOLAK, MD, PhD
Department of Neurosurgery, Dartmouth-Hitchcock
Medical Center, Lebanon, New Hampshire
Cervicothoracic Ankylosing Spondylitis—Commentary

MICHAEL WOYDT, MD
Associate Professor, Neurosurgical Department,
University of Basel, Basel, Switzerland
Ultrasound in Neurosurgery

BAKHTIAR YAMINI, MD
Assistant Professor of Neurosurgery, The University
of Chicago Pritzker School of Medicine, Chicago,
Illinois
Surgical Treatment of Neurofibromatosis

MICHAEL J. YAREMCHUK, MD
Professor of Surgery, Harvard Medical School,
Chief of Craniofacial Surgery, Massachusetts General
Hospital, Boston, Massachusetts
Surgical Repair of Major Defects of the Scalp and Skull

DANIEL YOSHOR, MD
Assistant Professor, Department of Neurosurgery, Baylor
College of Medicine, Houston, Texas
Temporal Lobe Operations for Drug-Resistant Epilepsy

CHUN-JIANG YU, MD, PhD
Professor, Capital University of Medical Sciences;
Doctor, Department of Neurosurgery, Beijing Tiantan
Hospital, Beijing, China
*Surgical Management of Nonglomus Tumors of the Jugular
Foramen*

SETH M. ZEIDMAN, MD
Assistant Professor of Neurological Surgery and Neurology,
University of Rochester Medical Center, Rochester,
New York; Uniformed Services University of the Health
Sciences, Bethesda, Maryland
Circumferential Spinal Fusion (Cervical)

VASILIOS A. ZERRIS, MD, MPH, MMSc
Clinical Instructor, Brown University, Rhode Island
Hospital, Providence, Rhode Island
*Surgical Management of Injuries of the Cervical Spine and
Spinal Cord*

MICHAEL ZIMMERMANN, MD, PhD
Associate Professor, Department of Neurosurgery,
Johann Wolfgang Goethe University, Frankfurt,
Germany
*Anterior Approaches in Multisegmental Cervical
Spondylosis*

GIANLUIGI ZONA, MD, PhD
Attending Neurosurgeon, Department of Neurosurgery,
San Martino University Hospital, Genoa, Italy
Repair of the Sella Turcica after Transsphenoidal Surgery

PREFACE

In 1977 Dr. Sweet and I coedited a single volume entitled *Current Techniques in Operative Neurosurgery*, which reflected our own interests in a spectrum of neurosurgical procedures, with emphasis on those at the forefront of contemporary neurosurgical practice. Conceptually, we attempted in this and the subsequent three editions to provide the working neurosurgeon with information which would be useful when taking an adult patient with a particular brain, spine, or peripheral nerve problem to the operating room. The chapters provided an overview of the topic, a discussion of available options and results. In many cases, alternative surgical and nonsurgical options were included for dealing with a particular clinical situation. It was our goal to provide a single source that would allow a neurosurgeon to develop a surgical plan for the patient. The chapter references would be up-to-date and allow further immersion in the topic as needed. The success of these volumes, along with the recent translation of the fourth edition into Chinese, places *Operative Neurosurgical Techniques: Indications, Methods, and Results* among the most widely used neurosurgical texts worldwide. David W. Roberts has been added to the roster as a coeditor, and the current edition is dedicated to the memory of Dr. Sweet.

The fifth edition continues to reflect the same underlying vision for the book and attempts to keep up to date with the rapidly evolving changes in neurosurgery. The fifth edition consists of 168 chapters authored by 380 contributors representing neurosurgical services from 22 different countries. As scientific advances are being made worldwide, the book has attempted to reflect these contributions and their origins and to perpetuate the idea of an international text in neurosurgery. Approximately 40% of the chapters deal with material not previously addressed in this text, and, where appropriate, chapters published in earlier editions have been extensively rewritten. All the chapters have been reviewed to ensure that they reflect the current state of the art.

This edition could not have been accomplished without the enthusiastic participation of the contributors who, to the delight of the editors, completed their chapters in record time. To each of these individuals I extend my sincerest thanks. Every effort has been made to produce a product worthy of the contributions. This could only have been accomplished with the professionalism of Rebecca Schmidt Gaertner, Agnes Hunt Byrne, and Joan Sinclair at Elsevier, and of the staff at P. M. Gordon Associates. All deserve the sincerest thanks for a job well done, which I extend to them on behalf of the contributors and the editors.

Henry H. Schmidek, MD, FACS
Lebanon, New Hampshire

Color Plate

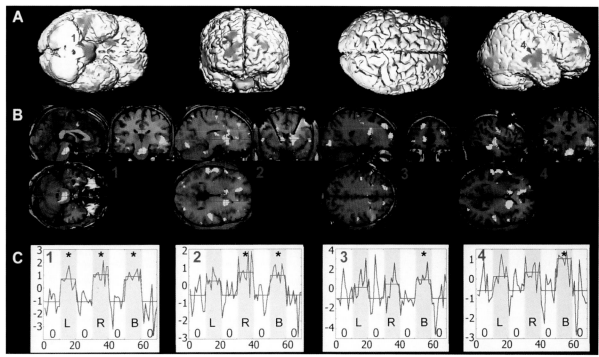

FIGURE 102-4   fMRI studies showing cortical and subcortical activation in patient 4 when brain activity is subtracted during the stimulation-off condition from brain activity shown during the stimulation-on condition, superimposed onto surface reconstructions (*A*) and sections of the patient's brain (*B*). Regions are labeled as follows: the midline focus in the pons (1), the striatum (2), the focus in the right frontal cortex (3), and the left superior temporal gyrus (4). In the brain sections, the left hemisphere is shown on the right or at the bottom. *C,* Percentage fMRI signal change (*blue line*) and statistically modeled signal change (*red line*) during left (*L*), right (*R*), simultaneous (*B*), and no stimulation (*0*) in the four labeled regions. Conditions for which stimulation versus no stimulation was significant ($p < 0.05$ corrected for multiple comparisons) are indicated by asterisks. (From Nuttin BJ, Gabriels LA, Cosyns PR, et al: Long-term electrical capsular stimulation in patients with obsessive-compulsive disorder. Neurosurgery 52:1263–1274, 2003.)

FIGURE 102-5   Digital subtraction analysis was performed with [^{18}F]2-fluoro-2-desoxy-D-glucose positron computed tomographic (PET) images before electrode implantation and after 3 months in the stimulation-on condition for patients 1 (*upper*), 2 (*middle*), and 3 (*lower*). The magnetic resonance imaging (MRI) scan and the preoperative and postoperative PET images were coregistered by using an automated algorithm[47] and were subtracted after normalization for global counts. Only the voxels (color) in the postoperative PET scan with decreased glucose metabolism of more than 2 standard deviations are combined with the coregistered MRI scan (patients 1 and 3) or with the preoperative PET scan (patient 2). The coregistered MRI scan and the preoperative PET scan are displayed in gray scale. Red represents the strongest reduction in glucose metabolism. The left hemisphere is shown in the images in the right column. (From Nuttin BJ, Gabriels LA, Cosyns PR, et al: Long-term electrical capsular stimulation in patients with obsessive-compulsive disorder. Neurosurgery 52:1263–1274, 2003.)

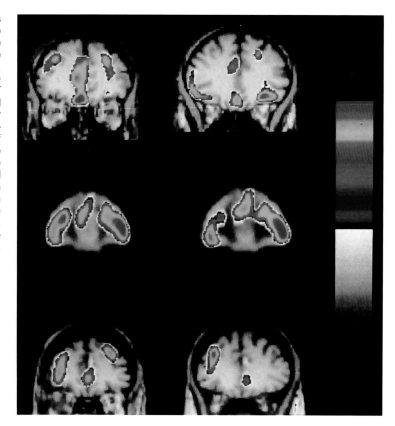

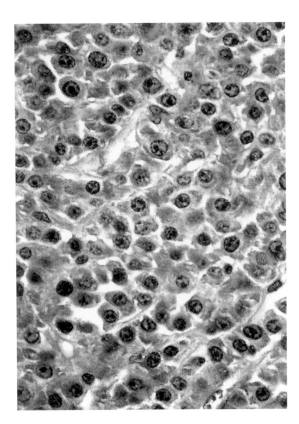

FIGURE 129-2 Plasmacytoma by light microscopy.

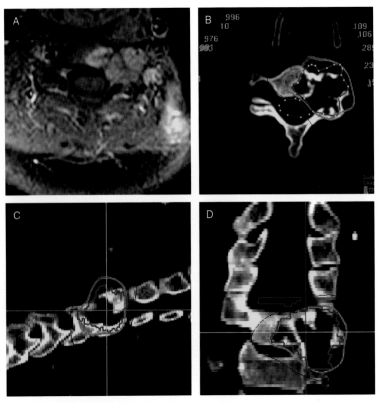

FIGURE 138-4 Treatment plan example in a patient with large malignant neuroendocrine tumor at C5–6 treated with 20 Gy to the 76% isodose line in two stages. (*A*), Pretreatment axial T1 postcontrast magnetic resonance imaging. Axial (*B*), sagittal (*C*), and coronal (*D*) postcontrast computed tomography images used in treatment planning are demonstrated. Red lines (with or without solid squares) demarcate the outline of the lesion, solid green lines demarcate the 76% isodose curve, and the purple lines demarcate the 50% isodose cure. The green line with squares demarcates the critical structure, the spinal cord.

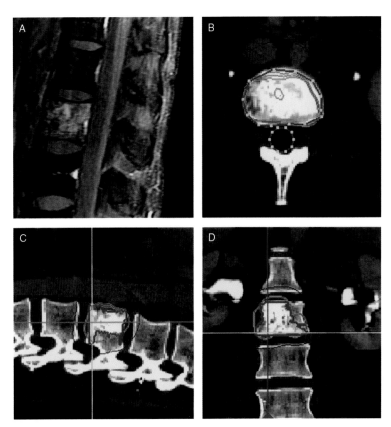

FIGURE 138-5 Treatment plan example in a patient with metastatic breast cancer to the L2 vertebral body treated with 20 Gy to the 83% isodose line in two stages. (*A*), Pretreatment sagittal T1-weighted postcontrast magnetic resonance imaging. Axial (*B*), sagittal (*C*), and coronal (*D*) postcontrast computed tomography images used in treatment planning are demonstrated. Red lines (with or without solid squares) demarcate the outline of the lesion, the solid green lines demarcate the 83% isodose curve, and the purple lines demarcate the 50% isodose cure. The green line with squares demarcates the critical structure, the spinal cord.

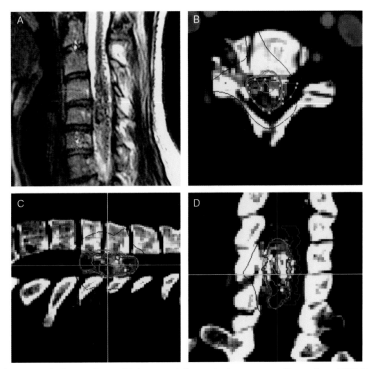

FIGURE 138-6 Treatment plan example in a patient with intramedullary arteriovenous malformation at C5–6 treated with 20 Gy to the 85% isodose line in two stages. (*A*), Pretreatment sagittal T2-weighted magnetic resonance imaging. Axial (*B*), sagittal (*C*), and coronal (*D*) postcontrast computed tomography images used in treatment planning are demonstrated. Red lines (with or without solid squares) demarcate the outline of the lesion, the solid green lines demarcate the 85% isodose curve, and the purple lines demarcate the 50% isodose cure. The green line with squares demarcates the critical structure, the spinal cord.

CONTENTS

Management of Intracranial Malformations

88 Surgical Management of Cerebral Arteriovenous Malformations

ROBERT DERUTY, FRANCIS TURJMAN, and ISABELLE PELISSOU-GUYOTAT

Since the late 1970s, the treatment of cerebral arteriovenous malformations (AVMs) has undergone considerable modification.[1] Until the 1980s, the only available treatment for cerebral AVM was surgical resection. Therefore, the debate over the proper management of these lesions concerned whether to pursue surgical or conservative treatment. A new treatment option arrived with the technique of cerebral blood vessel embolization. Begun in the 1960s, embolization became more prevalent in the late 1970s and early 1980s. This technique was initially used during surgery but later was done preoperatively. Today, cerebral embolization by the retrograde femoral route is widely used, and discussion about the management of AVMs has focused on whether to use either surgery or embolization, or to use both in a "combined treatment" modality. The most recent technique applied to the treatment of cerebral AVMs is stereotactic radiosurgery (RS). From its beginnings in the mid-1970s, RS developed during the 1980s and the 1990s to become the main competitor to surgery in the management of small AVMs. The management options available to the clinician who has diagnosed a cerebral AVM include surgical excision, endovascular embolization, stereotactic RS (used alone in a single-modality treatment), a combination of two or more of the previous techniques (multimodality treatment), or, in some difficult cases, conservative treatment. This chapter discusses these management options.

SURGICAL RESECTION OF BRAIN ARTERIOVENOUS MALFORMATIONS

History

Several authors have dealt thoroughly with the history of the surgical treatment of brain AVMs,[2,3] and several principles have been stressed. Partial excision is unsatisfactory because it does not reduce the danger of recurrent bleeding. AVMs should be totally removed when they are "significantly symptomatic," that is, when there are progressive neurologic deficits, incapacitating seizures, recurrent hemorrhage, intractable headache, or mental deterioration.[2]

The indication for surgery may be restricted for deep-seated AVMs and for those in eloquent areas of the brain. With increased experience, however, and by using modern techniques, the indications for surgery in these cases should increase. In a previous report,[4] the authors reviewed

the surgical management of AVMs between 1970 and 1990. During this period, the indications for surgical resection changed dramatically. During the 1970s, standard practice was to advise surgery for every AVM regardless of its location or the patient's symptoms. Gradually, some contraindications were recognized, particularly when the patient's age and the anatomic features of the AVM were taken into account. Eventually, in the 1980s, more realistic schemes for surgical intervention were proposed. Excluded were those patients presenting with epilepsy well controlled by anticonvulsants, those with large AVMs, those no older than their 50s or 60s, and all cases in which the risk of surgery exceeded that of the natural history of the disease.

Surgical Technique

The basic principles and techniques for the surgery of AVMs[5,6] are described in the following sections.

Approach

The approach is tailored to the site of the AVM. In all cases, the bone flap should encompass the entire cortical aspect of the malformation and should allow for the complete identification of normal structures surrounding the AVM. The dural opening should be performed very carefully because there are often thickened arachnoid strands that attach the external aspect of the AVM to the internal aspect of the dura. Great care should be taken gently to retract the dural flap, identify the arachnoid adhesions, and coagulate and cut them before opening the dura further. In addition, the surgeon should be aware that large draining veins may be adherent to the dura or even incorporated in it before draining into the dural sinuses.[5]

Dissection of the Nidus

Bipolar coagulation, the operating microscope, and gentle suction are the main tools used for dissection of the nidus.

Discrimination between arterial feeders and draining veins is not always easy. The draining veins usually run on the surface of the brain. A good way to approach the nidus is to recognize a draining vein and dissect it backward from the cortex.[6] The vein will lead the dissection close to the nidus itself.

Dissection of the nidus should be performed in a circumferential pattern, layer by layer. It is dangerous to go too deep on one side of the nidus before completing the dissection all around the malformation. This top-to-bottom dissection has been called spiral-like dissection.[5]

All feeding vessels should be sacrificed as soon as possible, but not all draining veins should be eliminated. At least one major draining vein should be preserved intact from the beginning to the end of the dissection, thus allowing for sufficient venous drainage and avoiding swelling and rupture of the nidus. At the end of the dissection, when all feeders have been interrupted, this remaining vein becomes bluish, which proves that all feeders have been eliminated. The nidus is then attached only to this vein, which can be safely sacrificed.

Almost all feeder arteries and draining veins can be coagulated with the bipolar forceps and cut without using hemoclips.[5,6] Only large feeding vessels should be clipped to avoid future bleeding. There may be some difficulty in distinguishing a feeding vessel from a normal artery. In such a case, interruption of the vessel should be delayed until its nature has been verified.

The difficulty of dissection increases from the cortical aspect to the depths of the white matter. There may be small vessels (either feeding or draining vessels) that are very thin and that have fragile walls. During dissection and coagulation, these may stick to the bipolar forceps and rupture, after which they usually retract into the white matter. Their hemostasis is difficult and requires patience. Sometimes, a coating with hemostatic material is required. Many supratentorial AVMs have a conical shape with the base at the surface and the apex next to, or in, the ventricle.[5] The deep feeding vessels coming toward the tip of the cone are particularly difficult to treat and require special attention.

In addition to the main nidus there may be smaller, residual, "daughter" niduses completely hidden in the white matter. These are connected to the main nidus by their feeding and draining vessels. If these daughter niduses are not removed, they may prove dangerous and become the source of catastrophic postoperative bleeding. Particularly dangerous are those daughter niduses that are first supplied distally and then drain toward the main nidus.[6] After complete resection of the main nidus, therefore, careful reexamination of the AVM bed should be undertaken. Continued bleeding from an unidentified source is highly suggestive of a residual daughter nidus.[5] The surgeon should look for it and remove it, even if this resection necessitates entry into a functional brain area.[6]

During dissection of the nidus, it is often necessary to retract the brain. In most cases, this retraction should be kept to a minimum. The surgeon should dissect as closely as possible to the external aspect of the nidus to avoid unnecessary resection of surrounding brain. In some cases, however, the external walls of the nidus are irregular, which creates the danger of entering the nidus itself. This mistake is responsible for considerable hemorrhage, which may be difficult to stop. Therefore, when there is any doubt about the exact limits of the nidus, it is recommended that the site of dissection be changed (i.e., dissect deeper on the other sides of the nidus and come back later to the area causing difficulty).

After complete resection of the nidus and after ensuring that no residual daughter nidus is hidden in the deep white matter, the surgeon should carefully reexamine the bed of the nidus. Additional coagulation may be necessary. The walls of the bed should be coated extensively with hemostatic material. Retraction on the surrounding brain is progressively and gently released before coating the cavity. In large cavities, tissue glue may be added to fix the hemostatic material and to ensure perfect hemostasis.

Technical Improvements

Over the years, several additional techniques were proposed to improve the resection of difficult brain AVMs. Intraoperative angiography[7,8] was found useful not only to localize small AVMs but mainly to disclose an unexpected residual nidus (in 8% to 19% of cases). Thus this technique may allow intraoperative assessment of outcome of surgery but does not replace postoperative angiography because of false negative findings, which may occur in 18% of cases.[8] Endoscope-assisted microsurgery[9] was proposed to enhance magnification, illumination, and technical precision during the dissection. This technique could help while the neurosurgeon is dissecting the AVM core vessels and while operating on AVMs extending into the ventricle. Computer-assisted surgery[10] or frameless-stereotaxy,[11] so-called neuronavigation techniques, may help the neurosurgeon in various ways (e.g., to plan the optimal trajectory, to minimize the skin and bone approach, to confirm the AVM margins, and to identify deep vascular structures during dissection).

The technique of dissection itself is under discussion.[12] Surgical resection of cerebral AVMs is often complicated by persistent bleeding from the nidus. This difficult hemostasis has been ascribed to the fragile and pathologic nature of the vessels. But it could be[12] that coagulation of the surface of the nidus may cause obstruction of intranidal drainage, and that this may cause increased intranidal pressure. Avoiding such coagulation of the nidus could diminish hemorrhagic problems. Hypotension and hypothermia were proposed in difficult cases.[13] One key to successful surgical resection of cerebral AVMs is control of bleeding and cerebral swelling. Induced hypotension was proposed as one of the most valuable means of achieving this control. This induced hypotension with mild hypothermia was obtained by using a percutaneous cardiopulmonary support system during the resection of a high-flow AVM. This resection could be total, with no hemostatic difficulties.

Postoperative Care

All patients should be cared for in the intensive care unit after surgery. When surgery has not been very difficult (e.g., in cases with small or medium-sized AVMs with minimal bleeding), there is no need to sedate or ventilate the patient. The patient should be extubated as soon after surgery as possible. By contrast, in more dangerous situations (e.g., with large and deep AVMs, or when surgery was difficult and coating necessary), sedation and ventilation should be maintained for 24 hours or longer, if necessary. Postoperative computed tomography (CT) scans help in deciding when to reduce sedation and allow the patient to breathe spontaneously.

Complications of Surgery

Complications occurring during and after surgical resection may or may not be based on cerebral hemodynamics.[14] Among the complications not related to hemodynamics are resection of eloquent brain, postretraction edema and hemorrhage, rupture of occult retained niduses, new onset of seizures, and retrograde thrombosis of the feeding arteries. Complications based on hemodynamics are unique to this lesion and are related to the circulatory disturbances created by the malformation itself. These complications consist of brain edema or hemorrhage, both intraoperative and postoperative, and do not have a precise anatomic basis. Two theories have been postulated to explain these complications:

1. The normal perfusion pressure breakthrough (NPPB) theory.[15] According to this theory, the circulatory disturbances created by the AVM induce a loss of autoregulation and a state of vasomotor paralysis in the surrounding brain. After resection of the malformation, the ischemic hemisphere returns to a normal perfusion pressure. The paralyzed vessels are unable to adjust to this new pressure. The result is capillary disruption and breakthrough, resulting in edema and hemorrhage in the adjacent brain.

2. Disturbances of the AVM's drainage. Inadvertent occlusion of major draining veins, or of the veins that drain the surrounding brain, could be responsible for most of the complications occurring after resection. These venous disturbances have been called venous overload[16] or occlusive hyperemia.[17] These disturbances are apt to produce hyperemia and engorgement of the cerebral circulation with subsequent edema and hemorrhage.

Outcome of Surgery

There are several ways to evaluate the outcome after surgical resection of AVMs. The main goal of surgery is to eliminate the future risk of hemorrhage, especially when surgery is performed after an initial bleed. It is generally agreed that partial resection of the AVM does not protect against the risk of fresh hemorrhage, and that only complete excision can eliminate such a risk. A rare case of regrowth of a malformation and subsequent bleeding was reported in an adult patient after an angiographically confirmed complete excision.[18]

The outcome of surgery for AVM in patients with epilepsy is more controversial.[4] In a review spanning two decades, the authors found that epilepsy is reported to be cured in only 2% to 4% of cases, and is reportedly unchanged in 11% to 33% of cases (average, 25%). The consensus was that surgery is indicated only in cases with intractable epilepsy, provided the AVM is readily accessible and hence without excessive surgical risk. More recent studies are more optimistic. One of these[19] reports a low incidence of new seizure disorder after surgery (6% of operated cases) and a good chance of resolution or control of a preexisting seizure disorder (83% seizure-free after 2 years of follow-up). Another study[20] demonstrates that complete cure of epilepsy may be achieved in 70% of cases provided surgery is directed not only at resection of the AVM but at removal of epileptic foci remote from the AVM area.

Regarding other signs and symptoms, opinions vary concerning the outcome of surgery. An ischemic deficit does not seem to be greatly influenced by resection; in effect, surgery makes little difference or even increases the deficit in cases of large malformations. Some, however, are more optimistic[19] and find on follow-up a good capacity for recovery of previous or new deficits.

The overall outcome of surgical resection should be assessed by comparing the patient's preoperative and postoperative clinical status. In particular, this is the only way to assess outcome in those patients in whom the AVM was diagnosed after minor symptoms (headache) or in patients who were asymptomatic and had their AVM discovered fortuitously. Several outcome scales can be found in the literature. The scale "good, fair, poor outcome, death" does not take into account preoperative clinical status. Similarly, the Glasgow Outcome Scale should be linked with preoperative status. One way to assess the benefit of surgery is to evaluate the clinical outcome in terms of deterioration caused by treatment after a follow-up of at least 6 months[21] as follows: no complication, minor complication, and severe complication. Severe complications include permanent neurologic deficit, vegetative survival, and death.

In the authors' study covering two decades (1972 to 1992), considerable variations in outcome were found in the published series. Roughly, the results were good outcome (or no deterioration), 52% to 82%; fair outcome (or minor deterioration), 4% to 29%; poor outcome (major deterioration), 2% to 8%; and death, 1% to 14%.

More recently, there has been a tendency to evaluate surgical outcome separately in two different groups of AVMs: (1) small and medium-sized AVMs, even those deeply situated or adjacent to cortical areas, as well as large malformations located in silent areas; and (2) large malformations with deep extension, located in or adjacent to critical areas. In the first group,[22] the combined mortality and morbidity rate with surgery was approximately 10%. However, in a series consisting only of microsurgical resection of small malformations (less than 3 cm in diameter), the morbidity and mortality rates dropped as low as 1.5% and 0%, respectively.[23] In the second group, the rate of serious morbidity/mortality was as high as 50%.[22]

INTERVENTIONAL RADIOLOGIC TREATMENT

Historical Background

In 1960, Luessenhop and Spence[24] first described embolization for the treatment of cerebral AVMs; development has been continuous since then. Embolic agents have changed from dura mater to silicone beads, and to the tissue adhesive N-butyl cyanoacrylate (NBCA). Improved delivery systems have led to a change from balloons with calibrated leak, to flow-guided microcatheters injected by means of a propelling chamber, to flow-guided microcatheters (Magic, Balt, Montmorency, France), "over-the-wire" microcatheters, and to the last generation of mixed microcatheters (Ultraflow, MTI, Irvine, CA).

Pretherapeutic Evaluation

Functional

Intranidal catheter placement for brain AVM embolization is supposed to avoid untoward occlusion of the pedicles feeding the normal brain and the resulting neurologic complications. Such ideal placement is not guaranteed.

Theoretically, knowledge of normal cerebrovascular functional anatomy should allow the interventionist to predict brain damage and neurologic deficit subsequent to the occlusion of a given pedicle. Cerebral AVMs may distort the normal functional anatomy of the brain and alter the results of vessel occlusion. The gold standard of functional evaluation of the brain has been implanted electrodes, but this is an invasive technique. Progress has been made in understanding the brain harboring an AVM, and pretherapeutic functional imaging can noninvasively assess the location of functional centers and help answer the question of whether the occlusion of a given pedicle will cause a new focal neurologic deficit. Various functional imaging techniques have been proposed for preoperative evaluation of cerebral AVMs.

Noninvasive Techniques

Functional Magnetic Resonance Imaging

Functional magnetic resonance imaging (fMRI) takes advantage of the local increase in oxyhemoglobin concentration that occurs as a result of the increase in the flow rate and blood volume in the eloquent cortex undergoing specific stimulation. The technique is noninvasive, and preliminary reports support cortical reorganization associated with cerebral AVMs because they are congenital lesions.[25,26] These results need further validation with accepted techniques for functional cortical mapping before fMRI can be used for routine evaluation. Some authors[26] suggest that fMRI may help predict the development of a post-therapy deficit. In addition, a study with normal subjects using fMRI demonstrated extensive left prefrontal activation with language tasks; the investigators noted that fMRI techniques do not distinguish between critical areas and those that participate in a task.[25–27] A recent study suggests that preoperative fMRI is highly sensitive in the identification of cortical areas essential for language.[28]

Whereas some data suggest that flow abnormalities may interfere with language lateralization assessment with functional MR imaging,[29] data from functional MRI with diffusion-weighted, perfusion-weighted and neuronal activation highlight abnormal brain areas near the AVM nidus. They demonstrate hemodynamic and neuronal adaptive phenomena involved in brain plasticity, and reflect the instantaneous hemodynamic brain conditions.

Positron Emission Tomography

Experimental studies using positron emission tomography (PET) have led to the development of stimulation paradigms used for fMRI. PET suffers from a lack of availability, from high cost, and from a lack of good spatial resolution. Short series of patients with AVMs successfully treated after functional evaluation with PET have been reported.[30,31]

Magnetoencephalography

Magnetoencephalography (MEG) provides temporal resolution in milliseconds because it is based on the flux of a magnetic field, but it also has limited availability and high expense. Localization techniques combining MEG and MRI are quite good.[32] Sensory and motor mapping were performed successfully in patients with brain AVMs by Hund and colleagues.[33] MEG data were superimposed on an MRI scan. The correlation between noninvasive MEG localization and intraoperative electrocorticographic findings is good.

MEG data were used in combination with 3-dimensional cerebral angiography to provide a simultaneous 3-dimensional perspective of the angioarchitecture of an AVM and its relationship to the sensorimotor cortex.[34]

Invasive Technique: Superselective

Amobarbital Test

The application of Wada's test to the selective study of a vessel before embolization of AVM feeding vessels has seen considerable development. The amobarbital sodium test was positive in 23 of 109 injections,[35] and in 11 tests of 66 vessels evaluated.[36] In all patients, the arteries undergoing superselective testing were those feeding the AVM. Superselective amobarbital sodium tests also have been performed in vessels remote from the lesions.[37] The results strongly suggest a posterior-to-anterior extension of some language skills in patients with left-sided AVMs.

This technique is helpful when intranidal microcatheter placement is not obtained.

Angioarchitecture

Careful analysis of cerebral AVM angioarchitecture helps in the selection of the best therapeutic management of brain AVMs by permitting a more accurate assessment of potentially hemorrhagic components of the lesion.[38] Once an endovascular approach is decided on, identifying weak points helps in planning the endovascular procedure itself.

Aneurysms associated with AVMs are a common angiographic finding. Depending on site, these aneurysms are classified as either proximal to the AVM or intranidal. Such aneurysms have been reported with a high frequency.[39]

Irregularly shaped, aneurysm-like vascular cavities with stagnation of contrast medium, in previously ruptured AVMs, are called pseudoaneurysms or false aneurysms. False aneurysms may have an endothelium but not a normally structured vessel wall. Pseudoaneurysms usually form after rupture at the point where an artery and vein make contact because the site is weak.[40]

Intranidal aneurysms are thin-walled structures exposed to the same pressures as arterial components of the AVM. Pressure monitoring during and after embolization has shown an increase in pressure in the vessel supplying the AVM during occlusion. When a choice of vascular pedicles exists for embolization, those pedicles supplying intranidal aneurysms should be embolized first to reduce the risk of hemorrhage.[41]

Sometimes, AVM-associated arteriovenous fistulas are discovered in the nidus that may require specific embolic material (detachable polymerizing balloons or fast histoacrylic glue [NBCA]) to decrease the chances of untoward embolization of the AVM's venous drainage or of the pulmonary circulation.

Technique

Standard Procedure

Cerebral AVMs are most commonly embolized using NBCA under general anesthesia and anticoagulation.

Before endovascular treatment, the patient must be prepared. During the patient's pretherapeutic visit, the objectives and risks of embolization are explained. The goal is to achieve a permanent and as complete an occlusion as possible. Endovascular therapy may be as effective as neurosurgery, and as hazardous as well. The patients must be prepared psychologically. Anxiolytic therapy may also help. Some authors suggest prescription of nimodipine weeks before the treatment.

The surgeon begins the procedure by inserting a No. 6 French gauge sheath into the femoral artery. The procedure is performed under general anesthesia to ensure the patient remains motionless. A No. 6 French gauge guiding catheter is then advanced into the internal carotid or vertebral artery. Anticoagulation is accomplished by injection of a bolus of heparin (60 IU/kg) controlled by intraprocedural testing of coagulation (twice the normal), and possibly followed by a second heparin injection of one third of the bolus 2 hours later.

Intravascular Navigation

Intravascular navigation is accomplished using a No. 1.5 French gauge flow-guided microcatheter, unless the diameter of the feeders is obviously too small for it. Injection through the microcatheter requires a 3-mL syringe; the high pressures obtained with a 1-mL syringe may damage the microcatheter. To ease its progression through the vascular curvature, the microcatheter is steam shaped. Various techniques (e.g., manual compression of the contralateral carotid artery to reach the anterior cerebral artery, use of a 0.010-inch microguide wire, or increasing the systemic blood pressure) may also help. On rare occasions, direct puncture of the internal carotid artery may be useful. Reaching the intranidal target may require the use of a microcatheter with a smaller distal outer diameter (e.g., No. 1.2 French gauge). These catheters are fragile and must be handled carefully. Enlargement of the microcatheter tip may help in cases of high-flow AVMs with tortuous feeders. Careful analysis of the circle of Willis may demonstrate the advantage of indirect catheterization toward the AVM. For example, a lenticulostriate feeder may be reached easily through the vertebral artery, a posterior cerebral artery through the posterior communicating artery, and an anterior cerebral artery through the anterior communicating artery.

Identification of the Embolization Point

Glue injection may be performed in three different situations: (1) when the tip of the microcatheter is inside the nidus; (2) when the tip of the microcatheter is inside a feeder to the nidus, without demonstration of a pedicle to the normal brain, and the nidus itself seems reachable through the remaining pedicle; and (3) when the tip of the microcatheter is inside a feeder to the nidus that seems reachable with embolization, but a pedicle to the normal brain is opacified and pretherapeutic functional evaluation or an intraoperative, hyperselective Wada's test demonstrates lack of functional significance of this vessel. Even without any change in the location of the microcatheter tip or the rate of injection, the surgeon must be aware that, because of the glue's viscosity, discrepancies may appear between the opacification demonstrated by hyperselective angiography and the progression of the embolic mixture.

Injection of the Embolic Material

Intranidal AVM occlusion is performed with NBCA (Histoacryl bleu, Braun, Melsungen, Germany). This has been demonstrated to be an effective and permanent cure for intracerebral AVMs. Before glue injection, the microcatheter is flushed with a nonionic solution to prevent early polymerization. Resistance during glue injection indicates obstruction of the catheter and cannot be overcome. Various parameters influence penetration of the glue inside the nidus.

Histoacryl Dilution

Histoacryl is mixed with Lipiodol (Guerbet, Aulnay, France) to adjust the polymerization time and ensure the mixture's opacity. This dilution is extremely important: pure Histoacryl polymerizes almost instantaneously, whereas a mixture of 20% Histoacryl/80% Lipiodol hardens in more than 2 minutes. Various parameters such as temperature and homogeneity of the mixture influence its polymerization time. The mixture is protected from ionic solution. Glue dilution is determined according to the distance between the tip of the microcatheter and the nidus and other parameters such as the flow inside the AVM. Intranidal injection usually requires a 17% to 40% dilution of the glue. Homogeneity of the liquid is ensured by careful mixing of its two constituents.

Injection Speed

Ideal casting of the nidus is achieved by slow injection of the polymer. Each tiny drop of glue exits the catheter and migrates into the vessels of the nidus; diluted glue permits prolonged injection times of up to several minutes without gluing the tip of the microcatheter to the vessel wall.

Geometry of the Vessels

Tortuosity of the vessels may slow the progression of the embolization mixture. En-passage vessels or side vessels usually are not filled with the mixture.

Flow inside the Nidus

Flow is of paramount importance in the progression of the glue. For example, true direct fistulas inside the AVM are easily reached by the liquid. During its progression inside the vessels, the tip of the microcatheter may eventually be large enough to prevent blood from filling the distal vessels. Such a situation is called flow control and may be used to advantage in embolization of the nidus. Thus when the mixture is injected, almost no blood comes in contact with the embolic material, and this technique allows for prolonged distal progression of the glue.

Stopping the Injection

The polymer injection is stopped either when the polymer has progressed through the nidus to the vein or if there is backflow of the polymer toward the microcatheter. Untoward embolization also leads to immediate cessation of the injection. Once the surgeon decides to stop the embolization, the microcatheter is vigorously and quickly removed.

Concomitant removal of the guiding catheter may help to ease the friction caused by quick removal of the microcatheter.

Procedural Variants

Anesthesia

There are advantages of neuroleptic analgesia, such as reduced aggressiveness and availability of intraoperative neurologic evaluation

However, many teams perform AVM occlusion under general anesthesia (GA); they do not rely on a superselective amobarbital test. Obviously, GA ensures a motionless patient even in prolonged procedures (up to 3 hours). Embolization under GA is assessed on control angiograms. Only minor complications without immediate therapeutic consequences may remain hidden; major complications are immediately identified on the angiograms. Management of an endovascular complication is much easier in a patient under GA.

Other Embolic Agents

Histoacryl remains the most popular embolic agent because of its ability to penetrate deeply into the AVM nidus and to occlude it permanently. The safe manipulation of NBCA requires intensive training because incorrect handling of this material produces disastrous complications. Recently, the Food and Drug Administration has approved NBCA for the treatment of cerebral AVMs.[42] Late recanalization of a nidus embolized with glue has been reported.[43,44] The current opinion is that complete nidus embolization is permanent, but that opacification of the glue may disappear with time. A new chemical presentation of NBCA with radical polymerization (versus anionic in histoacryl) is being used more often in the endovascular occlusion of AVMs.[45]

Various other embolic agents have been used in the occlusion of cerebral AVMs, such as polyvinyl alcohol (PVA), Ethibloc, silk, ethylene vinyl alcohol (EVAL), and microcoils, often in combination. These products are easier to handle than NBCA, but usually provide only temporary occlusion of the AVM and unsatisfactory casting of the nidus. PVA particles have been available for several years, and their embolic properties are well known. PVA usually produces temporary occlusion of the vessels for up to 1 month, and is used in the preoperative occlusion of AVMs. After occlusion of the nidus with small-diameter particles, it is advisable to occlude the pedicle with microcoils[46] or larger particles. PVA is useful in the occlusion of perforators or terminal branches; it does not penetrate the smallest and most distal branches,[47] and thus results in fewer neurologic complications. Ethibloc, a mixture widely used in the endovascular or percutaneous treatment of ear, nose, and throat lesions, has been used in the treatment of cerebral AVMs.[48] Ethibloc permanently occludes the vessels. Some precautions in its use (e.g., using several small doses of Ethibloc for each injection and avoiding withdrawal of the microcatheter within 10 minutes after the end of the embolization) are mandatory. Ethibloc can be difficult to inject through microcatheters because of its viscosity. Other agents (e.g., silk, EVAL, and microcoils) have also been used in the occlusion of these lesions. Silk suture is a very thrombogenic agent but is not visible under fluoroscopy and does not produce a good casting of the nidus.[49–51]

The most innovative and promising embolic material for AVM is ONYX (Micro interventional Therapeutics, Irvine, CA).[52] The Onyx liquid embolic system is a nonadhesive material. It is supplied in ready-to-use vials containing ethylene-vinyl alcohol copolymer (EVOH), dimethyl sulfoxide (DMSO), and tantalum. Onyx 6-0% contains 6% copolymer and 94% DMSO and is manufactured as Onyx 18. The microcatheter used for Onyx embolization must be DMSO compatible. Onyx can be used only after intranidal placement of the microcatheter tip.

The advantage of using Onyx is that it is a liquid embolic material that is opaque, is easily injected through a microcatheter, and is nonadhesive. Injections are slower and more controlled than with NBCA, resulting in easier control of the delivery of the embolic agent.

Prolonged injections up to 40 minutes are common, allowing multiple compartments of the AVM to be reached through the one initially catheterized. The initial drawbacks of Onyx (e.g., toxicity of DMSO and lack of radiopacity) have been overcome by refinements of the technique.

Gluing of the microcatheter is not possible, but entrapment of the microcatheter tip is; this must be prevented by carefully monitoring the reflux around the microcatheter. In a recent study,[53] complete endovascular occlusion of the AVM with Onyx alone was obtained in 25%, and complete occlusion of AVM with Onyx and surgery or radiotherapy was performed in 49 out of 52 cases.

Outcome

Results of AVM embolization are difficult to assess from the literature. Each cerebral AVM is unique, depending on its size, location, clinical presentation, and angioarchitecture. Furthermore, in the evaluation of any therapeutic technique in which better results entail higher risks, it useful to quote relative efficacy, which is a ratio of cure rate divided by combined morbidity/mortality. Efficacy of embolization must be considered the initial aim of endovascular treatment.

There are four objectives for embolic therapy: (1) complete and permanent embolization and cure, (2) partial embolization for preoperative devascularization, (3) diminution of nidus size to allow for RS, or (4) palliation in a symptomatic patient with a nonresectable AVM.

Complete and Permanent Cure

Complete and permanent cure of a cerebral AVM has been achieved in between 0% to 32% of patients as reported in the literature. A 5% overall total cure rate was reported in a 1995 review of the literature since 1990[54]; another study reported a 7% rate of occlusion,[55] which improved to 32% for the period 1994 to 1996.[56] This rate of complete occlusion may be increased by the use of intranidal embolization.

Partial Embolization for Preoperative Devascularization

The ultimate goal of embolization is to reduce the overall morbidity and mortality of treatment rather than to make excisional surgery easier.

Does embolization reduce the rate of complications after AVM resection? The fact that embolization may favor the development of smaller, deep-feeding vessels, which could increase the difficulty of surgery, seems well accepted. In the authors' experience, no hemodynamic complications were observed after surgery with or without embolization. Various opinions are expressed in the recent literature. Some authors report that in their experience, no normal perfusion pressure breakthrough or intraoperative hemorrhage has occurred since the introduction of selective embolization.[57,58] In another study,[59] one case of hyperperfusion on single photon emission CT (SPECT) was observed 2 weeks after embolization, together with a normal perfusion pressure breakthrough phenomenon occurring at the end of the operation, which was performed 3 weeks after embolization. The conclusion was that the hyperemic state caused by embolization probably continues for 2 to 3 weeks after embolization. In a series of patients with AVM treated by staged embolization followed by surgical excision,[60] the authors concluded that this mode of treatment did not completely eliminate postoperative intracranial hypertension, which was observed in 28% of cases, and more commonly in AVMs greater than 6 cm in maximum diameter, but with no mortality.

Preoperative embolization has been used to make inoperable AVMs operable or to make surgically treacherous lesions more manageable. It was demonstrated that preoperative embolization with NBCA enabled the surgeon safely to resect AVMs of higher Spetzler grade, thus achieving the same results as with lower-grade, nonembolized lesions.[61] Several studies suggest that preoperative embolization with NBCA reduced operative time and blood loss.[62,63] Others, however, noted no difference after embolization.[64,65] In the past, IBCA-embolized malformations were considered to be solid masses difficult to manipulate and cut. In contrast, NBCA-treated AVMs are easy to handle, and NBCA is currently the choice for AVM occlusion.

Partial Embolization for Diminution of Nidus Size before Radiosurgery

Embolization may play a role in small malformations that are suitable for treatment with RS in two ways: (1) reducing the weakness of the angioarchitecture and, it is hoped, affording protection during the RS latency period; and (2) further reducing the volume of the lesion (the smaller the volume, the more effective the RS).

Partial Embolization for Palliation in Nonresectable Arteriovenous Malformations

Palliation may be obtained in various ways.

DECREASING THE STEAL PHENOMENON

The angiographically demonstrated suppression of intracranial steal caused by an AVM is a common finding even after partial eradication, although this phenomenon may be transient. A case was reported demonstrating correction of the steal phenomenon and restoration to normal of a visual field defect after partial embolization.[66] A study using SPECT to investigate the effects of embolization on cerebral hemodynamics in AVMs confirmed that there is an acute flow redistribution immediately after incomplete embolization of AVMs.[59] This improvement in cerebral perfusion was particularly marked in patients with no history of hemorrhage, when the embolization had caused no new infarction in the surrounding normal brain, or when the nidus itself was occluded (particularly with liquid embolization agents such as NBCA).

TARGETED APPROACH

Partial embolization may be used in a targeted approach to correct angioarchitectural weak spots in the malformation (e.g., intranidal aneurysms) or to reduce the pressure in veins that have an outflow restriction.

A diminution in the hemorrhagic risk after targeted embolization has been demonstrated.[67]

SYMPTOMATIC APPROACH

Partial embolization of AVMs has been proposed to reduce severe headaches in patients with an external carotid supply to the AVM.

Complications

Technical complications of embolization may result in severe, temporary, or permanent neurologic deficit, or death. They include the following: (1) intracranial hemorrhage caused by rupture of an arterial feeder, (2) brain ischemia or infarct because of the accidental embolization of a normal artery, (3) gluing of a microcatheter inside a feeding artery, and (5) specific hemodynamic complications caused by the embolization procedure itself. Immediate and delayed complications of embolization have been reported, very similar to those described in the authors' experience.[21] The rupture of several AVMs several days to weeks after transfemoral embolization that converted a large AVM into a smaller one has been described.[65] This complication was explained by the AVM feeding artery pressure: after embolization of a large AVM, the resistance to flow increases and the feeding artery pressure in the remaining lesion is elevated. Finally, a common mechanism causing bleeding is occlusion of the venous drainage.

In a review of the literature since 1990,[54] the overall mortality rate was 1% (0% to 7%), and the permanent morbidity rate after embolization was 8%. These complications occurred mainly in high-grade AVMs. In a recent study, the rate of permanent complications and death after treatment of cerebral AVMs independently assessed in 233 patients was respectively 2% and 1%.[68]

Spontaneous hemorrhage after NBCA embolization has recently been reported with a 3% rate.[69]

The risk involved in the treatment of high-grade AVMs has shifted from surgical resection toward endovascular embolization, which is now the procedure of first choice for difficult cases in the authors' multidisciplinary approach.[21] Long-term toxicity associated with embolization has not been demonstrated.

STEREOTACTIC RADIOSURGERY

Historical Background

The principles of RS were first developed by Leksell in 1951.[70] The first clinical application was reported by Leksell using a cyclotron-generated proton beam. Technical advances led to the development of the gamma knife in 1968. Most recently, to increase the availability of RS, the linear accelerator was developed.[71] A single dose of radiation is delivered under stereotactic conditions to the target, thus avoiding irradiation of the normal surrounding tissue. The aim of RS in the treatment of cerebral AVMs is to produce progressive thrombosis of the nidus. Progressive occlusion corresponds with the histopathologic findings of intimal hyperplasia.[72,73]

Technique

Three different techniques have been developed using radiosurgical principles:

1. The gamma knife, using 201 gamma ray–emitting sources of ^{60}Co. The beams are directed toward a common target point using collimator helmets with beam channels of various diameters.
2. Heavy particles (proton, helium ion, neutron) have the physical property of a Bragg peak effect: most of the energy is deposited at a predictable depth in the tissue. The availability of this method is restricted by the cost of the cyclotron that produces the particle beams.
3. The modified linear accelerator uses x-rays that are virtually equivalent in energy to the photons produced in the gamma unit. Multiple, noncoplanar arcs of radiation are focused on the target, so a minimal dose is delivered to the normal brain and a maximum dose is delivered to the target.

Initial controversies arose concerning the efficacy, accuracy, and precision of these techniques. Published results on obliteration of AVMs and complications after treatment were similar whatever the technique used.[74–77] Moreover, a recent analysis of the results of an AVM series using different treatment modalities showed that the results were not related to the type of machine used.[78]

Two main problems must be resolved in the radiosurgical treatment of AVMs: (1) the definition of the target, and (2) the optimal dose to be delivered to the target.

Definition of the target remains a problem, with many authors reporting on the difficulties involving the spatial configuration of AVMs.[79,80] All reports emphasize the importance of complete nidus irradiation when treating AVMs.[81,82]

Different techniques are used in order to attempt the highest accuracy in target definition: stereotactic biplanar angiography with MRI or CT data,[83] nonstereotactic 3-dimensional rotational angiography with stereotactic CT with image fusion,[84] and stereotactic MR angiography.[85] This is particularly important when treating medium-sized AVMs.

It is more difficult to evaluate the nidus when a hematoma is associated with AVM rupture, and in cases of partially embolized AVMs.[86]

In cases of hemorrhage, stereotactic definition of the target is performed after resorption of the hematoma to avoid incomplete visualization of the nidus. In partially embolized AVMs, recognition of the nidus is difficult because of the presence of embolic material, and angiographic subtraction is necessary. In addition, embolization may produce fragmentation of the nidus, leading to an AVM with a more irregular shape or with multiple niduses.[80]

Stereotactic angiographic studies must be complete, including superselective and external carotid artery injections, to visualize all of the nidus compartments.[81] Greater conformality with more isocenters seems to lead to more target misses and lower radiologic obliterations rates (but also to lower complication rates).[87]

The adequate dose for treatment of AVMs is still unknown. Ten to 35 Gy is delivered, with an average dose of 20 to 25 Gy depending on the teams, the volume irradiated, and the location of the AVMs. Moreover, there is no unanimity of opinion in the literature regarding the isodose chosen when reporting the doses delivered to the AVMs. For some authors, the dose is expressed by the 70% isodose line; for others, it is expressed by the 50% isodose line; and, for still others, it is expressed by the "margins" of the nidus.

Repeat RS may be performed for incompletely obliterated AVM with good results.[88]

Complications

Hemorrhage

Hemorrhage after radiosurgical treatment may occur before complete obliteration (8% to 10%).[87,88]

Controversy exists regarding the risk of hemorrhage after RS in nonobliterated AVMs. A decreased risk was reported after a period of 2 years[89] and after 5 years.[90,91] However, most of the authors asserted that there was no difference between the hemorrhage rates in patients with nonobliterated irradiated AVMs and the expected natural history rates for untreated AVMs.[92–96]

Because postradiosurgical obliteration of an AVM requires 2 to 3 years or more,[82,97,98] predictive risk factors of hemorrhage are interesting. Studies have shown these factors to include single venous drainage, inversion of the venous drainage, reflux in deep veins, intranidal aneurysm or venous aneurysm, and the ratio of afferent:efferent drainage.[95,99–101] Given that prior hemorrhage led to an increased risk of bleeding during the first year after the hemorrhage,[94] and combining this with the poor rate of early AVM obliteration after RS, some have come to reject RS treatment for such an AVM if it is amenable to other treatment.[21]

Radiation-Induced Complications

The risk of delayed radiation-induced brain injury has been widely reported. Caution is necessary when comparing these reports, however, because treatment methods varied widely in terms of dosage, treatment modalities, and categories of patients.

First, it is important to separate transient complications from permanent deficits.

Postradiosurgical MRI changes were seen commonly, in up to 30% of cases,[102] but were transient in most cases and resolved within 3 years. These changes were symptomatic in only 10% of cases.[96] The occurrence of MRI changes may depend on the irradiated volume, and the risk of symptomatic MRI changes is related both to the volume and the location.[87,102,103] Concerning the risk of postradiosurgical complications, a lower risk of complication was reported in cases that had a previous hemorrhage.[104] This may be because the peripheral tissue had been damaged by the hemorrhage, and thus the peripheral radiation-induced damage remained asymptomatic.

A 1% to 10% rate of permanent complications is reported in the literature.[87,105,106] A definite correlation between lesion size, radiation dose to the lesion, and complications was reported. A 3% risk line (i.e., a mathematically derived line relating the delivered dose to the lesion diameter) was described.[107] Following this isorisk line, larger lesions are treated with lower doses. Symptoms are location dependent and develop within 18 months after treatment.[88] In the authors' personal series, no complication developed after 12 months.[21]

Other than the aforementioned delayed complications, headaches were commonly reported by patients after RS.[108] The mechanism of this headache syndrome remains unknown. Concerning epilepsy, some authors have reported exacerbation of seizure activity immediately after RS. Few reports, however, deal with the role of RS in AVMs diagnosed because of seizures.[90,109,110] Recent reports corroborate the possible curative effect of RS on AVM-related epilepsy.[110,111]

Second tumors after RS have been recently reported, with a 0.07% estimated risk of a radiation-induced neoplasm after RS.[88,112] Although the estimated risk is quite low, continual surveillance of treated patient should be considered.

Results

The goal of RS is complete obliteration of the AVM to eliminate the risk of future bleeding.

It is generally accepted that a bleeding risk persists as long as the nidus is not obliterated.[80,81] The outcome of RS for cerebral AVMs has classically been assessed after 2 years of follow-up, although more and more authors recognize the possibility of later obliteration at 3 years or more.[81,96–98]

Methods for assessment of obliteration are also controversial. Although some authors have based their eradication rates on complete obliteration as demonstrated by MRI[95] and MR angiography, most of the radiosurgical teams believe that evaluation must be done with angiography using the Lindquist and Steiner criteria.[75,89] In the recommendation for management of AVM published by the American Stroke Association, angiography is still the standard to confirm complete obliteration.[96] Obliteration rates in the literature varied between 15% and 100% if all types of AVMs were considered. Most series reported obliteration rates of 60% to 85%, even at long-term evaluation.[88]

Many studies were devoted to the factors that affect the obliteration rates of irradiated AVMs. Despite the fact that some authors[113] reported that the rate of obliteration at 2 years was independent of the AVM volume, most authors considered small malformations (less than 3 cm) and large ones separately[82,89,92,93] because the AVM's size seemed to be the main factor affecting the obliteration rate.

For small AVMs (less than 3 cm), the obliteration rate was reported to be between 70% and 100% with a dose of 20 to 25 Gy: 80% at 2 years in a series of 273 patients treated with a minimum dose of at least 25 Gy[114]; 75% at 2 years, strongly correlated with the size of the AVM[82]; 81.3% in AVMs less than 3 cm in diameter[106]; and a 71.6% obliteration rate in a series of 120 patients treated by the French SALT group between January 1990 and July 1992.[81]

For larger AVMs (greater than 3 cm), the obliteration rate with a dose of 15 to 20 Gy ranges from 15% to 60%, even when using Bragg peak proton beam treatment.[115] Higher obliteration rates could be obtained with a higher radiation dose, but this carries a higher complication rate.[76] The obliteration rate may increase with dose and decrease with increased AVM volume.[104]

Dosage is correlated with obliteration rate.[74,86,98] Furthermore, a higher dose shortened the latency between treatment and obliteration.[114] However, others[102] found no correlation with the AVM volume or maximum dose, although the minimum target dose was related to the obliteration rate. One study[80] reported four factors associated with successful AVM RS: (1) a smaller volume, (2) a single draining vein, (3) a hemispheric AVM location, and (3) a younger patient. Younger age had been reported previously, together with a faster obliteration rate in children.[116] Recently a new RS-based grading system for AVM was proposed to predict outcome after RS. The score is based on AVM volume, patient age, and AVM location.[117]

With regard to AVM location, it was found that no AVM in a cisternal or ventricular location was obliterated at 2 years, and that peripheral AVMs were obliterated less often at 2 years than were deep-seated, hemispheric AVMs.[79] There was no precise explanation for this. AVM angioarchitecture seemed to be another predictive factor: high-flow AVMs seemed less sensitive to RS.[79] For these authors, this was an argument for initial embolic obliteration of the AVM zones, where the flow was highest.

GENERAL MANAGEMENT OF BRAIN ARTERIOVENOUS MALFORMATIONS

There are three techniques available to treat brain AVMs: (1) conservative treatment, (2) single-modality treatment, and (3) multimodality treatment.[96,118]

AVMS Grading Scale

To assess the outcome of the management of cerebral AVMs, and to compare the various series, a pretreatment grading scale is necessary. A grading scale should include reliable prognostic factors, encompass every possible type of AVM, and be widely accepted. Over the years several grading systems have been proposed.[96,119] Eventually, the most widely accepted and regularly used in the papers is the Spetzler-Martin grading scale,[120] which considers the AVM size (under 3 cm, from 3 to 6 cm, and over 6 cm), the venous drainage as superficial or deep, and the function of the brain area as eloquent or noneloquent. The sum of the assigned points gives five grades, from grade I to grade V (grade I, II, III are low-grade AVMs, grades IV and V are high-grade AVMs).

Despite the wide acceptance of this grading scale, there were some criticisms concerning the so-called grade III AVMs. Some authors[121] named grade III A those malformations with a large size but located in a noneloquent area, and grade III B those with a small size but located in an eloquent area. Other authors[122] found that these grade III malformations are highly variable in terms of surgical risk; therefore, they introduced a modification of the grading scale. Grade III AVMs may be split in four groups according to the combination of size (S), venous drainage (V), and eloquence of the area (E). Grade III AVMs (S1 V1 E1) have a surgical risk similar to that of low-grade AVMs and can be treated safely with microsurgical resection. Grade III AVMs (S2 V1 E0) have intermediate surgical risk and require judicious selection for surgery. Grade III+ AVMs (S2 V0 E1) have a surgical risk similar to that of high grade AVMs, and are best managed conservatively. Last of all, Grade III* AVMs (S3 V0 E0) are either exceedingly rare, with a surgical risk that is unclear, or theoretical lesions with no clinical relevance.

Conservative Treatment

There are two goals in the treatment of brain AVMs: (1) complete removal of the malformation, and (2) preservation of neurologic function.[23,123] Regarding the latter, aphasia carries a very special onus and may sometimes be intolerable socially and professionally,[22,97] so that special attention should be paid to this particular risk.

Given the requirement of maximum preservation of neurologic function, the first and most difficult question is whether an intact patient should undergo aggressive treatment at all.[22,97] The risk of the treatment should not be greater than that of the disease's natural history, namely an annual rate of hemorrhage from 2% to 4%, rising to 6% during the year after an initial bleed (mean interval of 7 to 8 years between two episodes of hemorrhage); and an annual rate of morbidity of 3% and mortality, 1% for each hemorrhagic episode.[22,23,95,124,125] These figures should be kept in mind when considering aggressive treatment for difficult malformations.

Single-Modality Treatment

Small or medium-sized malformations (3 cm or less in diameter), regardless of location or functionality, superficial or deep, are treatable by any of the three available techniques. These malformations may be operated on, embolized, or irradiated. The choice of technique depends on several factors: (1) who sees the patient first (e.g., neurologist, neurosurgeon, interventional radiologist, or surgical radiotherapist); (2) the experience of the physician, whatever his or her specialty; (3) the way the physician works, singly or in a multidisciplinary team; and (4) the wishes of the patient, who has become increasingly more aware of the various techniques of treatment and of their risks. The controversy is particularly acute between microsurgery and RS.[23,126–131] Defenders of surgery point out that immediate protection against rebleeding and the avoidance of delayed radiation-related brain injury offer distinct advantages over RS. In a series of patients operated on for AVM smaller than 3 cm,[131] an angiographic obliteration was obtained in 99% of cases, with a worsening rate of 4.3% when AVM was located in an eloquent area, and of 1.6% in noneloquent area. The neurologic deficit tended to be transient in the majority of cases. In the authors opinion, direct microsurgery is recommended for small and readily accessible malformations. RS should be considered for small malformations that are deeply situated in a functional area, thus necessitating a dangerous surgical approach. For small brain stem AVMs, however, RS is not recommended because of the catastrophic consequences of possible radionecrosis.

In a attempt to make more precise this discussion between surgery and RS, a decision analysis model was developed.[132] The result is sensitive to only two variables: surgical morbidity and surgical mortality. Surgery confers a large clinical benefit over RS because surgery protects the patient from hemorrhage earlier and with greater success. However, the preferred treatment strategy changes to favor RS when the rate of permanent neurologic morbidity resulting from surgery exceeds 12% or when the surgical mortality rate exceeds 4%.

In the same prospect, and to support the decision-making process for low Spetzler-Martin grade AVMs,[133] a mathematic model was designed to describe patient survival rates after treatment with either surgery or radiosurgery. Conventional surgery and radiosurgery definitely produced better survival than observation. For unruptured AVMs, RS was equivalent to surgery, with a combined morbidity and mortality rate of 3% to 7% for a 20-year-old patient (mortality rate, 1% to 2%). For ruptured AVMs, those rates became slightly higher with mortality at 2% to 3% and combined morbidity/mortality at 5% to 9%.

Embolization should be considered only when there is a reasonably high likelihood of complete obliteration of the AVM. This occurs in only a few cases. For small or medium-sized AVMs in which reductive therapy is not absolutely necessary, untoward effects of embolization certainly increase the risk of this treatment.

Multimodality Treatment

For large malformations (greater than 3 cm in diameter), especially those located in eloquent or deep areas, multimodality treatment is increasingly the treatment of choice. Most authors, including us, recommend endovascular embolization first to devascularize and diminish the size of the nidus, after which treatment is continued with either surgical resection or RS. The benefit of embolization before surgical resection or RS has been described by many authors. The actual benefit rate, however, is not known precisely. Endovascular embolization is assumed to improve the surgical and radiosurgical cure rates of cerebral AVMs by 25%.[97] In cases of surgical resection, this benefit is ascribed to reducing the size and volume of the malformation, reducing the intraoperative blood loss, and possibly allowing for normalization of hemodynamics in adjacent cortex.[134] This would allow for a more precise plane of dissection closer to the nidus, and thus reduce undue parenchymal resection.[22] The authors are in complete agreement with those opinions. The main benefit of embolization before RS is that of reducing the size and volume of the lesion. Decreasing the total radiation dose needed to obtain complete obliteration, and possibly shortening the period of latency before obliteration, have also been cited as advantages.[135]

In a study about the comprehensive management of AVMs (involving 344 patients over 10 years),[121] it was found that the treatment of AVMs can achieve better results (compared with the natural history) if managed by a well-trained group of specialists led by an experienced neurosurgeon. The strategy was surgery for grade I and II AVMs, embolization for grade III A (large size, silent area), radiosurgery for grade III B (small size, eloquent area), and conservative for grades IV and V. The following surgical results were obtained: good (85.8%), fair (12.5%), bad (0.6%), and died (1.2%). In an attempt to quantify the need for different modalities of treatment, a population-based analysis of AVM treatment was conducted[136] on a population of 1 million people. Figures for surgeries performed ranged from 6 to 10 operations per year. Embolization as well as gamma knife surgery procedures ranged from 2 to 7 per year, depending of the strategy at hand. When using nonsurgical approaches for grades I to III lesions, the number of patients requiring treatment with more than one method for obliteration increases drastically as does the potential risk for procedure-related complications.

Some authors do not like to embolize a malformation before RS,[137] preferring to treat with RS only those lesions that can be completely covered in the radiosurgical field. The efficacy of the association between embolization and RS, however, has been well demonstrated.[100] A study was designed to determine the safety and efficacy of embolization of brain AVMs prior to RS, and to evaluate the total obliteration rate achieved.[138] The endovascular treatment of brain AVMs prior to RS proved safe and effective, and must be considered in either high-grade or incidental AVMs. The obtained size reductions ranged from 10% to 95% (mean, 63%). However, in this study, AVM obliteration after embolization and RS is less commonly achieved than after stereotactic irradiation of primarily small AVMs.

Another scheme of combined management[139] is to use RS first, or combined embolization and RS, to treat those portions of large AVMs located in the deep and eloquent areas of the brain; then, to wait for obliteration to be complete and plan for microsurgical resection of the more superficial components of the nidus several years later. An example is given in a case of giant AVM,[140] in which three staged radiosurgical treatments of different portions of the AVM were performed, spaced 6 months apart, followed by delayed microsurgical removal of the much-reduced residual AVM 3 years later. This is proposed as a treatment strategy for the management of a grade V malformation that might be untreatable by any single method used alone. The combination of embolization first, followed with radiosurgery and then with surgical resection, was also recently reported.[140]

Arteriovenous malformations located in the basal ganglia and thalamus can be treated successfully with multimodality treatment.[141] In treating deep AVMs, it has been recommended to treat aggressively only those patients presenting with severe or repeat hemorrhage, and to treat conservatively those patients presenting with seizures, symptoms of vascular steal, or headache.[123]

As to the result on seizures, it was reported that a multimodality treatment approach for brain AVMs can achieve excellent seizure control.[110] Factors associated with Engel class I outcomes (seizure-free patient), included surgical resection and complete AVM obliteration. When only completely obliterated AVMs were considered, there was no statistically significant differences between surgery, radiosurgery, and embolization.

Very Large and Diffuse Malformations

Despite the modern technical improvements discussed previously,[13,140] many controversies continue to swirl about the treatment of very large and complex malformations, those with deep extension, or those located in eloquent brain areas.

Despite some optimistic reports,[141–143] there is a tendency, which the authors share, to evaluate the indications carefully and to refrain from aggressive treatment when the symptomatology is not life threatening. Sometimes, in large AVMs, embolization results only in breaking the nidus into several peripherally located parts without reducing the overall diameter, and thus does not allow for subsequent irradiation. Recently a series of giant intracranial AMVs managed by means of multimodality treatment was reported.[144] In this series, the cure rate was found lower, and the morbidity rate

higher, than those reported in series of smaller AVMs; but the authors believe that certain patients with symptomatic AVMs, especially young patients, should be treated aggressively.

However, in very large and complex malformations, controversy remains over whether to undertake any treatment at all.[97] For grades IV and V malformations, an intention to treat analysis was reported.[145] In this prospective series, the authors recommend no treatment for 75% of patients, partial treatment in 10%, and complete surgical removal in only 5%. They found an overall retrospective hemorrhage rate of 1.5% per year. This annual risk of hemorrhage rose to 10.4% among patients who had received incomplete treatment. Thus the authors recommend that no treatment be given for most grade IV and V malformations, and that no evidence indicates that partial treatment reduces a patient's risk of hemorrhage. In fact, partial treatment may worsen the natural history of an AVM. The authors do not support palliative treatment except in case of arterial or intranidal aneurysms, or with progressive neurologic deficits related to vascular steal.

Other authors[146] agree with these conclusions and confirm that these grade IV and V AVMs are treated when the patient already has the deficit likely to be produced by surgery, or has a progressive deficit that could be attributed to steal. Additional indications for treatment include associated aneurysms, intractable headaches attributed to dilated dural feeders, and multiple hemorrhages associated with accumulating neurologic deficits.

Personal Experience

Patients and Techniques

From 1989 to 2001, 129 patients with cerebral AVM were treated in the authors' department of neurosurgery (13 years, average 10 patients per year). Ages ranged from 11 to 69 years. The patient groups were 64% male and 36% female. The malformations were classified according to the Spetzler-Martin scale in five grades. Overall, 73% were low-grade and 27% were high-grade malformations (grade I, 7%; grade II, 29%; grade III, 36%; grade IV, 22.5%; and grade V, 5%).

The first choice of treatment was surgical resection in 32 patients (25%), endovascular embolization in 81 patients (63%), and radiosurgery in 16 patients (12%). In several cases, however, surgical resection and endovascular embolization required adjunctive treatment to achieve complete cure. Thus surgical resection had to be completed in some cases with radiosurgery, and endovascular embolization had to be completed in many cases either with surgical resection or with radiosurgery. Overall, 69 AVMs were managed with single modality treatment (53.5%), and 60 were managed with multimodality treatment (46.5%). Precisely, the distribution of the various types of management was: surgery alone, 22%; embolization alone, 19%; radiosurgery alone, 12%; embolization plus surgery, 27%; embolization plus radiosurgery, 16%; and surgery plus radiosurgery, 3%.

Cure Rate

The cure rate was based on angiography. For irradiated patients, results were assessed on the 2-year post-treatment angiogram. Some 108 patients (84%) underwent post-treatment angiography; the other 16% include those irradiated patients who have not yet reached this 2-year delay for angiography, or who did not came back for angiography, and some operated patients who had no postoperative angiogram. The cure rates are calculated on these 108 patients with adequate follow-up.

Overall, a 77% rate of complete angiographic eradication was obtained. However, the rate of eradication is strongly related to the grade of the malformation. For low-grade AVMs, the eradication rate rises as high as 88%; for high-grade AVMs, it is only 45.5%. The respective rate of eradication for each technique of treatment is as follows: after surgery in the first place, 86%; after embolization in the first place, 5%; after radiosurgery in the first place, 100%; after embolization plus surgical resection, 97%; after embolization plus radiosurgery, 80%; and after surgical resection plus radiosurgery, 100%.

Clinical Outcome

The clinical outcome was evaluated in terms of deterioration attributable to treatment, with a follow-up of at least 6 months. Three groups of results may be described: no complication (72%), minor complication (16%), and severe complication (11.5%). Severe complications include permanent neurologic deficit (7%), vegetative survival (2.3%), and death (2.3%). The figures are actually different for low-grade (no complication, 78%; minor complications, 15%; and severe complication, 7%) and high-grade malformations (no complication, 57%; minor complication, 20% and severe complication, 23%).

Overall, the authors observed severe complications in 11.5% of all cases (7% in low-grade and 23% in high-grade AVMs). These severe complications are diversely related to the technique of treatment. Complications caused by surgical resection were motor deficits (3% of surgical cases). Complications caused by radiosurgery were either motor deficit (5%) or vegetative survival (2.5%) in an overall 7.5% of all irradiated patients. Complications caused by endovascular embolization were deficit (6%), vegetative survival (2.5%), or death (4%) in an overall 12.5% of all embolized patients. These postembolization complications were caused by hemorrhage (7.5%) or ischemia (5%). All death cases (3 patients) were caused by postembolization hemorrhage.

CONCLUSIONS

Despite the recent progresses, the treatment of cerebral AVMs remains a challenge for any specialist dealing with this pathology. Several things are known:

- Direct excision of large AVMs remains a formidable procedure, full of dangers intra- and postoperatively. At present, the authors do not agree with this attitude of direct surgical treatment for such large malformations.
- Direct surgical excision of small and medium-sized AVMs remains possible and with an acceptable risk, even in eloquent areas, provided their access is simple.
- Radiosurgery of small AVMs gives excellent outcome. Radiosurgery of large AVMs cannot make them disappear. Complications of radiosurgery are more and more often reported, and this technique cannot be presented as completely safe.

- Endovascular embolization alone gives a very low rate of complete occlusion for AVMs. Such a complete occlusion may happen for small AVMs but certainly does not happen for large ones. Embolization is very useful for both surgical excision and radiosurgery in the treatment of medium-sized and large malformations. Endovascular embolization is, and should be, widely used as a first stage in this treatment, despite the rate of complications related to this technique. The severe post-treatment complications that once occurred during and after surgical excision are now the consequence of endovascular embolization: the risk of the treatment has almost quite naturally shifted from surgery toward endovascular embolization. Despite this rate of complications, the authors recommend that this endovascular embolization be widely used, to prepare for either surgery or radiosurgery in a second stage.
- The problem of very large malformations is not solved. These AVMs, with a large volume, many arterial feeders, and many draining veins, are not cured with repeat embolization procedures.
The number of large feeders may be reduced, or the volume of the nidus may be reduced. However, these malformations are still not fit for either surgical excision or for radiosurgery. The treatment remains partial, and such a partial treatment does not protect the patient against further bleeding. This partial treatment may reduce the intracranial steal, and so temporarily protect the patient against ischemic neurologic deficit. But we know that this protection does not last very long, and during the next months or years there may be a repermeation phenomenon through new feeders coming from both internal and external arteries.

Acknowledgment

The authors thank Edward Katz, MD (Twin Falls, Idaho), for his help with this chapter.

REFERENCES

1. Deruty R, Pelissou-Guyotat I, Mottolese C, et al: The combined management of cerebral arteriovenous malformations. Acta Neurochir (Wien) 123:101–112, 1993.
2. French LA: Surgical treatment of arteriovenous malformations: A history. Clin Neurosurg 24:22–33, 1976.
3. Yasargil MG: Microneurosurgery, vol III A: AVM of the Brain. Stuttgart: Georg Thieme Verlag, 1987, pp 3–21.
4. Deruty R, Pelissou-Guyotat I, Amat D, et al: Multidisciplinary treatment of cerebral arteriovenous malformations. Neurol Res 17:169–177, 1995.
5. Yasargil MG: Microneurosurgery, vol III B: AVM of the Brain. Stuttgart: Georg Thieme Verlag, 1988, pp 25–53.
6. Sugita K: Microneurosurgical Atlas. Berlin: Springer-Verlag, 1985, pp 136–177.
7. Pietila TA, Stendes R, Jansons J, et al: The value of intra-operative angiography for surgical treatment of cerebral AVMs in eloquent brain areas. Acta Neurochir (Wien) 140:1161–1165, 1998.
8. Munshi I, Macdonald RL, Weir BKA: Intra-operative angiography of brain AVMs. Neurosurgery 45:491–499, 1999.
9. Yamada S, Iacono RP, Mandybur GT, et al: Endoscopic procedures for resection of arterio-venous malformations. Surg Neurol 51:641–649, 1999.
10. Muacevic A, Steiger HJ: Computer-assisted resection of cerebral AVMs. Neurosurgery 45:1164–1171, 1999.

11. Russel SM, Woo HH, Joseffer SS, et al: Role of frameless stereotaxy in the surgical treatment of cerebral AVMs: Technique and outcome in a controlled study of 44 consecutive patients. Neurosurgery 51:1101–1331, 2002.

12. Hashimoto N: Microsurgery for cerebral AVMs: Dissection technique and its theoretical implications. Neurosurgery 48:1278–1281, 2001.

13. Iwama T, Hashimoto N, Todaka T, et al: Resection of a large high-flow AVM during hypotension and hypothermia induced by a percutaneous cardiopulmonary support system. J Neurosurg 87:440–444, 1997.

14. Morgan MK, Johnston IH, Hallinan JM, et al: Complications of surgery of AVMs of the brain. J Neurosurg 78:176–182, 1993.

15. Spetzler RF, Wilson CB, Weinstein PH, et al: Normal perfusion pressure breakthrough theory. Clin Neurosurg 25:651–672, 1977.

16. Wilson CB, Hieshima G: Occlusive hyperemia: A new way to think about an old problem. J Neurosurg 78:165–166, 1993.

17. Al Rhodan NRF, Sundt TM Jr, Piepgras DG, et al: Occlusive hyperemia: A theory for the hemodynamic complications following resection of intracerebral AVMs. J Neurosurg 78:167–175, 1993.

18. Gabriel EM, Samson JH, Wilkins RH: Recurrence of a cerebral AVM after surgical excision. J Neurosurg 84:879–882, 1996.

19. Piepgras DG, Sundt TM Jr, Ragoowansi AT, et al: Seizure outcome in patients with surgically treated arteriovenous malformations. J Neurosurg 78:5–11, 1993.

20. Yeh HS, Kashiwai S, Tew JM Jr, et al: Surgical management of epilepsy associated with cerebral AVMs. J Neurosurg 72:216–223, 1990.

21. Deruty R, Pelissou-Guyotat I, Amat D, et al: Complications after multidisciplinary treatment of cerebral arteriovenous malformations. Acta Neurochir (Wien) 138:119–131, 1996.

22. Nusbaum ES, Heros RC, Camarata PJ: Surgical treatment of intracranial arteriovenous malformations, with an analysis of cost-effectiveness. Clin Neurosurg 42:348–369, 1995.

23. Sisti MB, Kader A, Stein BM: Microsurgery for 67 intracranial AVMs less than 3 cm in diameter. J Neurosurg 79:653–661, 1993.

24. Luessenhop AJ, Spence WT: Artificial embolization of cerebral arteries: Report of use in a case of arteriovenous malformation. JAMA 172:1153–1155, 1960.

25. Latchaw RE, Hu X, Ugurbil K, et al: Functional magnetic resonance imaging as a management tool for cerebral arteriovenous malformations. Neurosurgery 37:619–626, 1995.

26. Maldjian J, Atlas SW, Howard RS II, et al: Functional magnetic resonance imaging of regional brain activity in patients with intracerebral arteriovenous malformations before surgical or endovascular therapy. J Neurosurg 84:477–483, 1996.

27. Binder JR, Frost JA, Hammerke TA, et al: Human brain language areas identified by functional magnetic resonance imaging. J Neurosci 17:353–362, 1997.

28. Pouratian N, Bookheimer SY, Rex DE, et al: Utility of preoperative functional magnetic resonance imaging for identifying language cortices in patients with vascular malformations. J Neurosurg 97:21–32, 2002.

29. Lehericy S, Biondi A, Sorour N, et al: Arteriovenous brain malformations: Is functional MR imaging reliable for studying language reorganization in patients? Initial observations. Radiology 223:672–682, 2002.

30. Hojo M, Miyamoto S, Nakahara I, et al: A case of arteriovenous malformation successfully treated with functional mapping of the language area by PET activation study. Neurol Surg 23:537–541, 1995.

31. Leblanc R, Meyer E, Bub D, et al: Language localization with activation positron emission tomography scanning. Neurosurgery 31:369–373, 1992.

32. Sobel DF, Gallen CC, Scharwtz BJ, et al: Locating the central sulcus: Comparison of MR anatomic and magnetoencephalographic functional methods. AJNR Am J Neuroradiol 14:915–925, 1993.

33. Hund M, Rezai AR, Kronberg E, et al: Magnetoencephalographic mapping: Basis of a new functional risk profile in the selection of patients with cortical brain lesions. Neurosurgery 40:936–943, 1997.

34. Kamirya T, Cappell J, Kronberg E, et al: Interactive use of cerebral and magnetoencephalography in arteriovenous malformations: Technical note. Neurosurgery 4:903–910, 2002.

35. Rauch RA, Vinuela F, Dion J, et al: Preembolization functional evaluation in brain arteriovenous malformations: The superselective amytal test. AJNR Am J Neuroradiol 13:303–308, 1992.

36. Han MH, Chang KH, Han DH, et al: Preembolization functional evaluation in supratentorial cerebral arteriovenous malformations with superselective intra-arterial injection of thiopental sodium solution. Acta Radiol 35:212–216, 1993.

37. Lazar RM, Marshall RS, Pile-Spellman J, et al: Anterior translocation of language in patients with left cerebral arteriovenous malformation. Neurology 49:802–808, 1997.

38. Muller-Forell W, Valavanis A: How angioarchitecture of cerebral arteriovenous malformations should influence the therapeutic considerations. Minim Invasive Neurosurg 38:32–40, 1995.

39. Turjman F, Massoud TF, Vinuela F, et al: Aneurysms related to cerebral arteriovenous malformations: Superselective angiographic assessment in 58 patients. AJNR Am J Neuroradiol 15:1601–1605, 1994.

40. Khayata MH, Zabramski JM, Johnson PC, et al: False aneurysm associated with rupture of an arteriovenous malformation: Implications for treatment: Case report. Neurosurgery 33:753–756, 1993.

41. Marks MP, Lane B, Steinberg GK, et al: Intranidal aneurysms in cerebral arteriovenous malformations: Evaluation and endovascular treatment. Radiology 183:355–360, 1992.

42. Kerber CW, Wong W: Liquid acrylic adhesive agents in interventional neuroradiology. Neurosurg Clin N Am 11:85–99, 2000.

43. Rao VRK, Mandalam KR, Gupta AK, et al: Dissolution of isobutyl 2-cyanoacrylate on long-term follow-up. AJNR Am J Neuroradiol 10:135–141, 1989.

44. Gruber A, Mazal PR, Bavinzski G, et al: Repermeation of partially embolized cerebral arteriovenous malformations: A clinical, radiologic and histologic study. AJNR Am J Neuroradiol 17:1323–1331, 1996.

45. Levrier O, Mekkaoui C, Rolland PH, et al: Efficacy and low vascular toxicity of embolization with radical versus anionic polymerisation of N-butyl-2-cyanoacrylate (NBCA): An experimental study in the swine. J Neuroradiol 2:95–102, 2003.

46. Purdy PD, Samson D, Hunt Batjer H, et al: Preoperative embolization of cerebral arteriovenous malformations with polyvinyl alcohol particles: Experience in 51 adults. AJNR Am J Neuroradiol 11:501–510, 1990.

47. Dowd CF, Halbach VV, Barnwell SL, et al: Particulate embolization of the anterior choroidal artery in the treatment of cerebral arteriovenous malformations. AJNR Am J Neuroradiol 12:1055–1061, 1991.

48. Grzyska U, Westphal M, Zanella F, et al: A joint protocol for the neurosurgical and neuroradiologic treatment of cerebral arteriovenous malformations: Indications, technique, and results in 76 cases. Surg Neurol 40:476–484, 1993.

49. Schmutz F, McAuliffe W, Anderson DM, et al: Embolization of cerebral arteriovenous malformations with silk: Histopathologic changes and hemorrhagic complications. AJNR Am J Neuroradiol 18:1233–1237, 1997.

50. Terada T, Nakamura Y, Nakai K, et al: Embolization of arteriovenous malformations with peripheral aneurysms using ethylene vinyl alcohol copolymer. J Neurosurg 75:655–660, 1991.

51. Hara Y, Nakamura M, Ehara K, et al: Transarterial embolization of cerebrospinal lesions with liquid coils. Intervent Neuroradiol 3(Suppl 2):201–204, 1997.

52. Jahan R, Murayama Y, Gobin YP, et al: Embolization of arteriovenous malformations with Onyx: Clinicopathological experience in 23 patients. Neurosurgery 5:984–997, 2001.

53. Hammani N, Mounayer C, Spelle L, et al: Traitement des malformations artérioveineuses par ONYX à propos d'une série de 68 cas. Oral presentation: SFNR Paris, Mars 2004.

54. Frizzel RT, Fisher WS III, Heros RC, et al: Cure, morbidity, and mortality associated with embolization of brain arteriovenous malformations: A review of 1246 patients in 32 series over a 35-year period. Neurosurgery 37:1031–1040, 1995.

55. Vinuela F: Functional evaluation and embolization of intracranial arteriovenous malformations. In Vinuela F, Van Halbach VV, Dion JE (eds): Interventional Neuroradiology of the Central Nervous System. New York: Raven Press, 1992, pp 77–87.

56. Wikholm G, Lundqvist C, Svendsen P: Transarterial embolization of cerebral arteriovenous malformations: How few can you do? Intervent Neuroradiol 3:119–123, 1997.

57. Morgan MK, Johnston IH, Hallinan JM, et al: Complications of surgery of AVMs of the brain. J Neurosurg 78:176–182, 1993.

58. Young WL, Pile-Spellman J, Prohovnik I, et al: Evidence for adaptive autoregulatory displacement in hypotensive cortical territories adjacent to arteriovenous malformations. Neurosurgery 34:601–611, 1994.

59. Takeuchi S, Abe H, Nishimaki K, et al: Cerebral haemodynamic changes after endovascular treatment of arteriovenous malformations: Evaluation by single-photon emission CT. Acta Neurochir (Wien) 127:142–150, 1994.

60. Awad JA, Magdinec M, Schubert A: Intracranial hypertension after resection of cerebral arteriovenous malformations: Predisposing factors and management strategy. Stroke 25:611–620, 1994.

61. Jafar JJ, Davis AJ, Berenstein A, et al: The effect of embolization with N-butyl cyanoacrylate prior to surgical resection of cerebral arteriovenous malformations. J Neurosurg 78:60–69, 1993.

62. Cromwell LD, Harris AB: Treatment of cerebral arteriovenous malformations: A combined neurosurgical and neuroradiological approach. J Neurosurg 52:705–708, 1980.

63. Debrun G, Vinuela F, Fox A, et al: Embolization of cerebral arteriovenous malformations with bucrylate: Experience in 46 cases. J Neurosurg 56:615–627, 1982.

64. Peerless SJ, Friedman WA, Sypert GW, et al: Successful treatment of the normal perfusion pressure breakthrough syndrome. Neurosurgery 11:625–630, 1982.

65. Spetzler RF, Martin NA, Carter LP, et al: Surgical management of large AVMs by staged embolization and operative excision. J Neurosurg 67:17–28, 1987.

66. Sugita M, Takahashi A, Ogawa A, et al: Improvement of cerebral blood flow and clinical symptoms associated with embolization of a large arteriovenous malformation: Case report. Neurosurgery 33:748–752, 1993.

67. Meisel HJ, Mansmann U, Alvarez H, et al: Effect of partial targeted N-butyl-cyano-acrylate embolization in brain AVM. Acta Neurochir (Wien) 9:879–887, 2002.

68. Hartman A, Pile-Spellman J, Stapf C, et al: Risks of endovascular treatment of brain arteriovenous malformations. Stroke 7:1816–1820, 2002.

69. Picard L, Da Costa E, Anxionnat R, et al: Acute spontaneous hemorrhage after embolization of brain arteriovenous malformation with N-butyl cyanoacrylate. J Neuroradiol 3:147–165, 2001.

70. Leksell L: The stereotaxic method and RS of the brain. Acta Chir Scand 102:316–319, 1951.

71. Betti OO, Derechinsky VE: Irradiations stereotaxiques multifaisceaux. Neurochirurgie 28:53–56, 1982.

72. De Salles AAF, Solberg TD, Mischel P, et al: Arteriovenous malformation animal model for radiosurgery: The rete mirabile. AJNR Am J Neuroradiol 17:1451–1458, 1996.

73. Szeifert GT, Kemeny AA, Timberley WR, et al: The potential role of myofibroblasts in the obliteration of AVMs after radiosurgery. Neurosurgery 40:61–66, 1997.

74. Betti OO, Munari C, Roster R: Stereotactic radiosurgery with the linear accelerator: Treatment of arteriovenous malformations. Neurosurgery 24:311–321, 1989.

75. Lindquist C, Steiner L: Stereotactic radiosurgical treatment of malformations of the brain. In Lunsford LD (ed): Modern Stereotactic Neurosurgery. Boston: Martinus Nijhoff, 1988, pp 491–506.

76. Steinberg GK, Famkant JL, Marks MP, et al: Stereotactic heavy-charged particle Bragg peak radiation for intracranial arteriovenous malformations. N Engl J Med 323:96–101, 1990.

77. Becker G, Kortmann R, Kaulich TW, et al: Gamma knife versus stereotaktische linarbeschleunigerbestrauhlung: Durchfuhrung, klinisher ergebnisse und Kosten-Nutzen-relation. Radiologe 30:345–353, 1996.

78. Schwarte M, Sixel K, Young C, et al: Prediction of obliteration of arteriovenous malformations after radiosurgery: The obliteration prediction index. Can J Neurol Sci 24:106–109, 1997.

79. Meder JF, Oppenheim C, Trystram D, et al: Radiotherapic stereotaxique des malformations arterioveineuses cerebrales: Place de la neuroradiologie. J Neuroradiol 24:126–133, 1997.

80. Pollock BE, Flickinger JC, Lunsford LD, et al: Factors associated with successful arteriovenous malformation radiosurgery. Neurosurgery 42:1239–1247, 1998.

81. Gallina P, Merienne L, Meder JF, et al: Failure in radiosurgery treatment of cerebral AVMs. Neurosurgery 42:996–1004, 1998.

82. Colombo F, Pozza F, Chiereg G, et al: Linear accelerator radiosurgery of cerebral AVMs: An update. Neurosurgery 34:14–21, 1994.

83. Tercier PA, Coucke P, Fandhauser H, et al: Transfer of information between angiographic films and CT images: H techniques to control the drawing of target volumes. Radiother Oncol 45:263–269, 1997.

84. Colombo F, Cavedon C, Francescon P, et al: Three-dimensional angiography for radiosurgical treatment planning for arteriovenous malformations. J Neurosurg 98:536–543, 2003.

85. Kondziolka D, Lunsford LD, Kanal E, et al: Stereotactic magnetic resonance angiography for targeting in arteriovenous malformations radiosurgery. Neurosurgery 35:585–591, 1994.

86. Flickinger JC: Kondziolka D, Maitz AH, et al: An analysis of the dose response for arteriovenous malformation radiosurgery and other factors affecting obliteration. Radiother Oncol 63:347–354, 2002.

87. Friedman WA, Bova FJ, Bollampally S, et al: Analysis of factors predictive of success or complication in arteriovenous malformative radiosurgery. Neurosurgery 52:296–307, 2003.

88. Pollock BE, Gorman DA, Coffey RJ: Patient outcomes after arteriovenous malformation radiosurgical management: Results based on a 5- to 14-year follow-up study. Neurosurgery 52:1291–1296, 2003.

89. Kjellberg RN: Proton beam therapy for arteriovenous malformations of the brain. In Schmidek HH, Sweet WH (eds): Operative Neurosurgical Techniques. New York: Grune & Stratton, 1988, pp 911–915.

90. Steiner L, Lindquist C, Adler JR, et al: Clinical outcome of radiosurgery for cerebral AVMs. J Neurosurg 77:1–8, 1992.

91. Karlsson B, Lindquist C, Steiner L: Effects of the gamma knife surgery on the risk of rupture prior to AVM obliteration. Minim Invasive Neurosurg 39:21–27, 1996.

92. Kondziolka D, Lunsford LD, Kanale, et al: Gamma knife stereotactic radiosurgery for cerebral vascular malformations. In Alexander E III, Loeffler JS, Lunsford LD (eds): Stereotactic Radiosurgery. New York: McGraw-Hill, 1993, pp 136–146.

93. Steinberg GK, Levy RP, Marks MP, et al: Charged particle radiosurgery. In Alexander E III, Loeffler JS, Lunsford LD (eds): Stereotactic Radiosurgery. New York: McGraw-Hill, 1993, pp 122–135.

94. Friedman WA, Blatt DL, Bova FJ, et al: The risk of hemorrhage after radiosurgery for AVMs. J Neurosurg 84:912–919, 1996.

95. Pollock BE, Flickinger JC, Lunsford LD, et al: Factors that predict the bleeding risk of cerebral arteriovenous malformations. Stroke 27:1–6, 1996.

96. Ogilvy CL, Stieg PE, Awad I, et al: Recommendations for the management of intracranial arteriovenous malformations: A statement for health care professionals from a special writing group of stroke council, American Stroke Association. Stroke 32:1458–1471, 2001.

97. Fischer WS III: Therapy of AVMs: A decision analysis. Clin Neurosurg 42:294–312, 1995.

98. Yamamoto Y, Coffey RJ, Nichols DA: Interim report on the radiosurgical treatment of cerebral AVMs: The influence of size, dose, time, and technical factors on obliteration rate. J Neurosurg 83:832–837, 1995.

99. Nataff J, Meder JF, Roux FX, et al: Angioarchitecture associated with hemorrhage in cerebral arteriovenous malformations: A prognostic statistical model. Neuroradiology 39:52–58, 1997.

100. Gobin P, Laurent A, Merienne L, et al: Treatment of brain arteriovenous malformations by embolization and radiosurgery. J Neurosurg 85:19–28, 1996.

101. Inoue HK, Ohye C: Hemorrhage risks and obliteration rates of arteriovenous malformations after gamma knife radiosurgery. J Neurosurg 97:474–476, 2002.

102. Flickinger JC, Kondziolka D, Pollock BE, et al: Complications from arteriovenous malformation radiosurgery: Multivariate analysis and risk modeling. Int J Radiat Oncol Biol Phys 38:485–490, 1997.

103. Flickinger JC, Kondziolka D, Maitz AH, et al: Analysis of neurological sequelae from radiosurgery of arteriovenous malformations: How location affects outcome. Int radiat Oncol Biol Phys 40:273–278, 1998.

104. Karlson B, Lax I, Soderman M: Factors influencing the risk for complications following gamma knife radiosurgery for cerebral AVMs. Radiother Oncol 43:275–280, 1997.

105. Steiner L: Radiosurgery in cerebral arteriovenous malformations. In Fem JM, Flamm ES (eds): Cerebrovascular Surgery, vol 4. Berlin: Springer-Verlag, 1984, pp 116–215.

106. Pica A, Ayzac L, Sentenac J, et al: Stereotactic radiosurgery for AVM of the brain using a standard LINAC: The Lyon experience. Radiother Oncol 40:51–54, 1996.

107. Flickinger JC, Schell MC, Larson DA: Estimation of complications for linear accelerator: Radiosurgery with the integrated logistic formula. Int J Radiat Oncol Biol Phys 19:143–148, 1990.

108. Rozen TD, Swanson JW: Post gamma knife headache: A new headache syndrome. Headache 37:180–183, 1997.

109. Gerszten PC, Adelson PD, Kondziol KAD, et al: Seizure outcome in children treated for AVMs using gamma knife radiosurgery. Pediatr Neurosurg 24:139–144, 1996.

110. Hoh BL, Chapman PH, Loeffler JS, et al: Results of multimodality treatment for 141 patients with brain arteriovenous malformations

and seizures: Factors associated with seizures incidence and seizures outcomes. Neurosurgery 51:303–309, 2002.

111. Falkson CB, Chakrabarti KB, Doughty D, et al: Stereotactic multiple arc radiotherapy. III: Influence of treatment of arteriovenous malformations on associated epilepsy. Br J Neurosurg 11:12–15, 1997.

112. Loeffler JS, Niemierko A, Chapman PH: Second tumors after radiosurgery. Neurosurgery 52:1436–1443, 2003.

113. Friedman WA, Bova FJ: Linear accelerator radiosurgery for arteriovenous malformations. J Neurosurg 77:832–841, 1992.

114. Karlzzon B, Lindquist C, Steiner L, et al: Prediction of obliteration after gamma knife surgery for cerebral AVMs. Neurosurgery 40:425–431, 1997.

115. Seifert V, Stolke D, Medhorn M, et al: Clinical and radiological evaluation of long-term results of stereotactic proton beam radiosurgery in patients with cerebral AVMs. J Neurosurg 81:683–689, 1994.

116. Tanaka T, Kobayashi T, Kida Y, et al: The comparison between adult and pediatric AVMs treated by gamma knife radiosurgery. Neurol Surg 23:773–777, 1995.

117. Pollock BE, Flickinger JC: A proposed radiosurgery-based grading system for arteriovenous malformations. J Neurosurg 97:474–476, 2002.

118. Deruty R, Pelissou-Guyotat I, Morel C, et al: Reflection on the management of cerebral arteriovenous malformations. Surg Neurol 50:245–256, 1998.

119. Deruty R, Pelissou-Guyotat I, Mottolese C, et al: Prognostic value of the Spetzler's grading system in a series of cerebral AVMs treated by a combined management. Acta Neurochir (Wien) 131:169–175, 1994.

120. Spetzler RF, Martin NA: A proposed grading system for AVMs. J Neurosurg 65:476–483, 1986.

121. De Oliveira E, Tedeschi H, Raso J: Comprehensive management of AVMs. Neurological Research 20:673–683, 1998.

122. Lawton MT: Spetzler-Martin grade III AVMs: Surgical results and a modification of the grading scale. Neurosurgery 52:740–749, 2003.

123. Lawton MT, Hamilton MG, Spetzler RF: Multimodality treatment of deep AVMs: Thalamus, basal ganglia, and brain stem. Neurosurgery 37:29–36, 1995.

124. Friedman WA: Radiosurgery for arteriovenous malformations. Clin Neurol Surg 42:328–347, 1995.

125. Kondziolka D, McLaughlin MR, Kestle JRW: Simple risk prediction for arteriovenous malformation hemorrhage. Neurosurgery 37:851–855, 1995.

126. Pollock BE, Lundsford LD, Kondziolka D, et al: Patient outcomes after stereotactic radiosurgery for "operable" AVMs. J Neurosurg 35:1–8, 1994.

127. Robinson JR, Brown AP, Spetzler RF: Patient outcome after stereotactic radiosurgery for "operable" AVMs. Neurosurgery 36:433–434, 1995.

128. Steiner L, Linquist C, Cail W, et al: Microsurgery and radiosurgery in brain AVMs. J Neurosurg 79:647–652, 1993.

129. Pikus HJ, Beach ML, Harbaugh RF: Microsurgical treatment of arteriovenous malformations: Analysis and comparison with stereotactic radiosurgery. J Neurosurg 88:641–646, 1998.

130. Schaller C, Schramm J: Microsurgical results for small AVMs acessible for radiosurgical or embolization treatment. Neurosurgery 40:664–674, 1997.

131. Pik JHT, Morgan MK: Microsurgery for small AVMs of the brain: Results in 110 consecutive patients. Neurosurgery 47:571–577, 2000.

132. Porter PJ, Shin AY, Detsky AS, et al: Surgery versus stereotactic radiosurgery for small, operable cerebral AVMs: A clinical and cost comparison. Neurosurgery 41:757–766, 1997.

133. Chang HS, Nihei H: Theoretical comparison of surgery and radiosurgery in cerebral AVMs J Neurosurg 90:709–719, 1999.

134. Standard SC, Hopkins LN: Comments on: Embolization of cerebral AVMs. II: Aspects of complications and late outcome (Lundquist C, Wikholm G, Svensen P). Neurosurgery 39:467–468, 1996.

135. Yoshimoto T, Takahashi A, Kinouchi H, et al: Role of embolization in the management of arteriovenous malformations. Clin Neurosurg 42:313–327, 1995.

136. Hillman J: Population-based analysis of arteriovenous malformation treatment. J Neurosurg 95:633–637, 2001.

137. Heros C: Comments on: Cure, morbidity and mortality associated with embolization of brain AVMs (Frizzel RT, Fisher WS III). Neurosurgery 37:1039, 1995.

138. Henkes H, Nahser HC, Berg-Damer E, et al: Endovascular therapy of brain AVMs prior to Radiosurgery. Neurol Res 20:479–492, 1998.

139. Steinbeck GK, Chang SD, Levy RP, et al: Surgical resection of large incompletely treated intracranial AVMs following stereotactic radiosurgery. J Neurosurg 84:920–928, 1996.

140. Firlik AD, Levy EI, Kondziolka D, et al: Staged volume radiosurgery followed by microsurgical resection: A novel treatment for giant cerebral AVMs. Neurosurgery 43:1223–1228, 1998.

141. Sasaki T, Kurita H, Saito I: Arteriovenous malformations in the basal ganglia and thalamus: Management and results in 101 cases. J Neurosurg 88:285–292, 1998.

142. Sadasivan B, Hwang PYK: Large cerebral AVMs: Experience with 27 cases. Surg Neurol 45:245–249, 1996.

143. Tew JM, Lewis AJ, Reichert KW: Management strategies and techniques for deep-seated supratentorial AVMs. Neurosurgery 36:1065–1072, 1995.

144. Chang SD, Marcellus ML, Marks MP, et al: Multimodality treatment of giant intracranial AVMs. Neurosurgery 53:1–13, 2003.

145. Han JP, Ponce FA, Spetzler RF: Intention to treat analysis of Spetzler-Marin grade IV and V AVMs: Natural history and treatment paradigm. J Neurosurg 98:3–7, 2003.

146. Heros RC: Spetzler-Martin grade IV and BV arteriovenous malformations. J Neursurg 98:1–2, 2003.

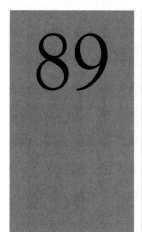

89 | Surgical Management of Arteriovenous Malformations of the Scalp

ZAYNE DOMINGO, NORMAN D. FISHER-JEFFES,
and JACQUEZ CHARL DE VILLIERS

INTRODUCTION

Arteriovenous fistulas of the scalp are remarkable lesions that have never failed to excite interest; they occur mostly on the scalp, and therefore attract the attention of both the patient and those around him or her. It has even been suggested that some ancient examples may have given rise to the legend of the serpent hair of the gorgon Medusa.[1] It is an uncommon disorder with many clinical manifestations, from an innocuous looking subcutaneous scalp lump to a large, grotesque, pulsatile mass with skin necrosis and a propensity to massive hemorrhage.

Arteriovenous fistulas were first described by William Hunter in 1757.[1] The term cirsoid aneurysm (from the Greek kirsos, "varix-like") was first used in 1833 by Brescht and describes a fistulous connection between the arterial feeding vessels of the scalp and the corresponding draining veins, without an intervening capillary bed.[1] The essential components of the lesion are a nidus, with dilated feeding arteries; and draining veins (Fig. 89-1). These draining veins are often grossly dilated and create the cosmetic deformity, which probably accounts for the great interest in these lesions. The nomenclature used to describe these lesions has been complex and inconsistent, with various names applied to the malformation including aneurysma cirsoide, aneurysma serpentinum, aneurysma racemosum, plexiform angioma, arteriovenous fistula, arteriovenous aneurysm, and arteriovenous malformation.[1-3]

Although uncommon, this type of lesion was the subject of a fairly constant stream of communications in the late 19th and early 20th centuries. More recently, with the development of endovascular techniques for obliteration of the malformation, there has been renewed interest in these lesions.[4-9] The obvious appearance and apparently obvious cause of these malformations have tended to make their treatment by obliteration of the nidus, either by surgical excision or endovascular occlusion, seem simple. Lack of understanding of the exact nature of the pathologic process or development, the high shunt flow, complicated vascular anatomy, and cosmetic considerations have continued to challenge the surgeon, and there is still no standard form of therapy.

This chapter focuses on the surgical approach to these challenging lesions and reviews the authors' treatment strategy and policy for scalp arteriovenous malformations.

These approaches and results were originally reported in Neurosurgery in 1995, with experience based on 24 patients seen over a 25-year period.[10]

CLINICAL SERIES

Patients

Twenty-four patients, 14 male and 10 female, with a mean age of 35 years (range, 4 to 70 years), were treated over a 25-year period. Trauma to the head occurring 2 to 15 years (mean, 8 years) before the development of the mass was reported in 9 patients (38%). In one patient, the trauma was a surgical excision of an avascular scalp lesion. The remainder were the result of blunt, nonpenetrating trauma to the head.

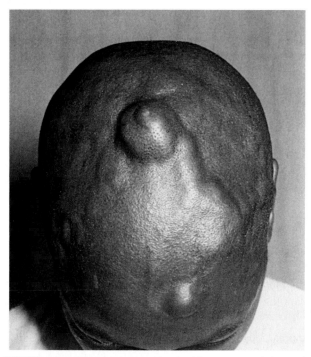

FIGURE 89-1 This post-traumatic cirsoid aneurysm of the scalp shows the nidus and large draining veins.

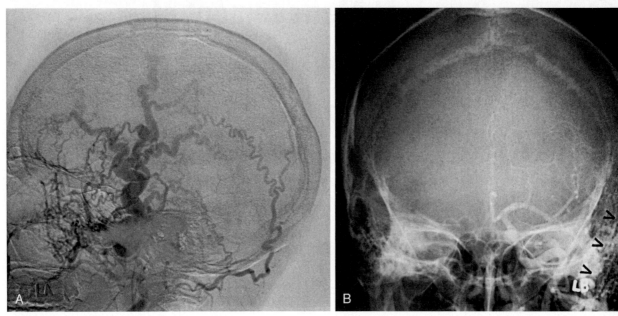

FIGURE 89-2 *A,* Selective external carotid angiography showing the arteriovenous fistula, draining veins, and dilated varix. *B,* Carotid angiography showing the filling of abnormal vessels within the substance of the temporalis muscle. These vessels are filled via the deep temporal arteries, and care must be taken to ensure that they are removed at the time of surgery.

Clinical Presentation

All 24 patients were symptomatic, complaining of a pulsatile mass on the head. Eleven patients had disturbing tinnitus, 3 had focal headaches, and 2 presented after a bleed. In all patients, there was an obvious, pulsatile swelling of the scalp, with dilated vessels leading into the lesion and an audible bruit on auscultation. Compression of the ipsilateral carotid or of the main feeding vessel caused the lesion to shrink and diminished the bruit. Three patients had precordial flow murmurs owing to an increase in cardiac output, but none demonstrated features of high-output cardiac failure. Three patients presented with recurrent cirsoid aneurysms after treatment at other institutions, 2 having had ligation of the superficial temporal artery alone, and 1 having had embolization with multiple coils.

The vascular malformation was temporal in 11 patients, frontal in 5, occipital in 4, supraorbital in 3, and over the vertex in 1. The lesions were equally distributed on either side of the head.

Radiologic Investigations

Plain Skull Radiographs

These showed enlargement of the diploic channels in 2 patients. In the remaining 22 patients, skull radiographs revealed no abnormality.

Computed Tomographic Scan

Aside from an increase in the soft tissue on the side of the arteriovenous malformation, computed tomography (CT) scanning revealed nothing abnormal, and no associated intracranial pathologic process was noted.

Angiography

Selective internal and external carotid angiography was performed in all patients to isolate the feeding vessels, define

the extent of the lesion, and reveal any intracranial component of the malformation (Fig. 89-2). The surgical scalp flap is also planned based on angiographic results.

In 17 patients, the malformation had only one feeding vessel (the superficial temporal artery in 13 and the occipital artery in 4). In addition to the occipital and superficial temporal artery, the remaining 7 malformations had a contribution from the ophthalmic artery in 3, the deep temporal artery in 2, and the facial and maxillary arteries in 2.

The pericranial component of the anomaly, which the authors believe to be an important factor in treatment and recurrence, is fed by the dural arteries and can be very difficult to demonstrate. The technique used in this series was to place a tourniquet around the head just above the level of the ears. With a common carotid injection, the anomaly does not fill as a result of occlusion of the superficial scalp-feeding vessels, but the maxillary and meningeal vessels do fill. A tangential radiograph of the scalp at the site of the cirsoid aneurysm then demonstrates the pericranial component as well as any filling of the malformation by the middle meningeal vessels (Fig. 89-3). This is important for deciding the extent of surgical excision.

Treatment

Three patients refused surgical treatment and were lost to follow-up. Twenty-one patients had the lesion surgically excised. Three patients required a second operation, and 1 required a third operation to complete the excision of the lesion. Preoperative embolization was not performed in this series because this was thought to increase the risk of scalp necrosis.

Surgical Technique

The technique is standard for all patients. An inverted U-shaped or "question-mark" flap is carefully marked out with its base across the main feeding vessels. After infiltration with

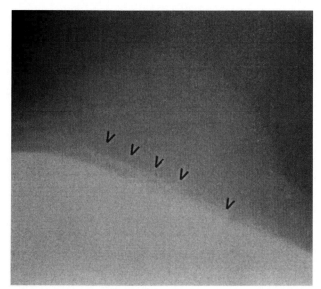

FIGURE 89-3 Tangential radiograph of the scalp showing a branch of the middle meningeal artery passing through the bone into the pericranial component of the malformation (*arrowheads*). Filling of the superficial temporal artery has been obliterated with the use of a tourniquet.

ornithine vasopressin, a vasoconstrictor, the incision is made in short segments with careful hemostasis obtained by ligation or coagulation of the feeding vessels or by draining veins as they are encountered. Greater than average bleeding occurs, and this must be adequately controlled to prevent

troublesome or unnoticed blood loss during the remainder of the procedure. The scalp flap is then carefully raised, with coagulation of vessels running from the pericranial component through the galea and into the malformation lying in the subcutaneous tissue.

Once the scalp flap is raised, the pericranial component of the malformation becomes obvious. It is circumscribed with a cutting diathermy, and the pericranium containing the malformation is removed. The brisk bleeding encountered from the bone is controlled with bone wax and cautery. In this series, a pericranial component was seen in 15 patients (71%), and removal of this is an essential part of the operation (Fig. 89-4). Histologic examination of the excised pericranium revealed an increase in the size and number of vessels.

An incision is then made into the galea at the base of the flap. The feeding vessels of the malformation are isolated and divided between ligatures. At this stage, the malformation is completely devascularized and can be excised from the subcutaneous tissue. Care must be taken not to breach the skin, which may be extremely thin in areas. In those patients in whom the malformation overlies the temporalis muscle, large, tortuous vessels are seen entering the bulk of the muscle, so that the muscle has a spongy consistency. It is important that these vessels be completely removed because they form an important collateral supply from the deep temporal arteries to the malformation. If they are inadequately dealt with or are not totally removed, they become an important collateral supply for revascularization of the malformation after surgery. Six of the 21 patients treated surgically (29%) had involvement of the temporalis muscle,

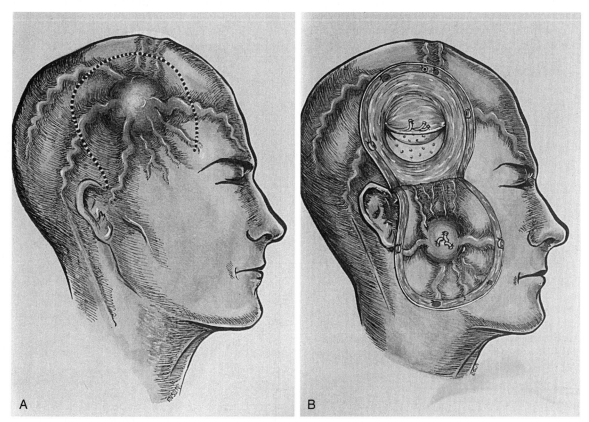

FIGURE 89-4 *A,* Schematic representation of the malformation and planned flap. *B,* The elevated flap contains the malformation within the subcutaneous tissue as well as the pericranial component, which is partially removed.

with feeding vessels coming through the muscle into the scalp component of the malformation.

Complications

Six patients (29%) had postoperative complications. In 4, there was sufficient devascularization to result in partial necrosis of the scalp. This healed on conservative treatment in 3, with only 1 patient requiring skin grafts and rotation flaps to cover the defect. One patient bled into the scalp, and 1 had wound sepsis.

Recurrence

Four patients had recurrence of the malformation after surgical excision. In 2 patients, this was caused by incomplete devascularization of the lesion owing to the contribution from the ophthalmic artery. In the other 2 patients, recurrence was the result of the temporalis muscle component, which was inadequately removed. Repeat angiography in this group of patients showed that the arterial supply was from the ophthalmic artery, deep temporal artery, and the opposite superficial temporal artery, and could be effectively treated at reoperation.

DISCUSSION

Etiology

Although controversy still exists regarding the etiology of these arteriovenous malformations, it is generally accepted that they may be either of congenital or traumatic origin. The congenital cause is held to be the more common etiology, yet if the case history of affected patients is examined, it is uncommon to find the history of a preexisting anomaly. In addition, familial scalp fistulas are extremely rare and have been reported only in two siblings of one family.[2,3] Various theories are postulated for their congenital occurrence, including persistence of primitive arteriovenous fistulas, as a sequel to vascular hamartomas, and formation at a site of arteriovenous crossing.[11-14]

Trauma, usually nonpenetrating, is a less common cause, and in the authors' series 38% of lesions could be directly related to trauma (blunt, nonpenetrating trauma in most). If the frequency with which trauma to the head occurs is compared with the rarity of cirsoid aneurysms, the disparity is remarkable. Penetrating trauma as a cause is well described,[15,16] including iatrogenic fistulas after hair transplantation,[17-22] arthroscopy of the temporomandibular joint,[23] and craniotomy for intracranial procedures.[24] The period from trauma to the development of the malformation may vary from immediate to 13 years.

The components of the malformation vary from patient to patient, and this may reflect the underlying etiology. Traumatic fistulas tend to be less complex than the congenital varieties. It is therefore important to establish the components of the anomaly before surgery.

Pathology

A cirsoid aneurysm of the scalp is an abnormal arteriovenous communication lying within the subcutaneous fatty layer of the scalp, with its feeding arteries derived from vessels normally supplying the scalp. The malformation is drained by the corresponding scalp veins in the anatomic plane where these vessels normally occur. All these vessels are enlarged and tortuous. The draining veins may in part show variceal dilatation. There is no capillary bed between the feeding arteries and the draining veins. These malformations must be distinguished from other vascular lesions of the scalp (e.g., sinus pericranii, vascular hamartomas, and hemangiomas) (Fig. 89-5).

An important aspect of these anomalies is their potential to evolve, with the recruitment of feeding vessels and draining veins. With the large, plexiform anomalies related to trauma, it is likely that functionally nonpatent fistulas and hemangiomatous capillaries existed before the trauma but were not clinically apparent. The trauma, in some unknown way, activates or opens the fistula. Once the shunt is established, because of the rich vascular supply to the scalp, feeding vessels are recruited and the malformation enlarges.

Although the lesion lies predominantly in the subcutaneous layer of the scalp, the smaller pericranial component is of vital importance at surgery.[1,25-29] This component has been variously described by most authors, but its surgical importance is often underplayed. Clairmont[30] (1908) describes these vessels as emissary vessels distributed over a small area underlying the anomaly. Vessels running between the scalp abnormality and the skull were mentioned by Searby[31] (1931), and Clunie[32] (1936) mentions vessels passing into the bone, which showed erosion by the mass. Rundle[29] (1937) found a few emissary vessels in a nontraumatic case and described the skull as slightly depressed over this area. The communication is difficult to demonstrate angiographically, but the authors have managed to do so on a few occasions by applying a tourniquet around the skull, parallel to the base,

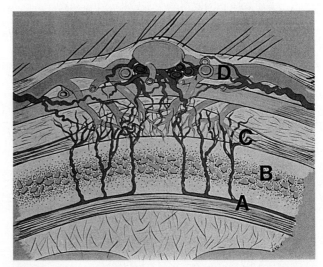

FIGURE 89-5   An artist's impression of a cross section through a cirsoid aneurysm, demonstrating the important pathologic points. One can easily see (A) the perforating vessels, branches of the meningeal arteries passing through the skull (B) to enter the pericranial component of the malformation (C). Dilated arteries and veins pass through the subgaleal space to enter the nidus (D) of the malformation within the subcutaneous tissue.

while injecting the external carotid artery. The filling of the pericranial component by the middle meningeal vessels can then be demonstrated. The authors have also histologically proven the presence of arteriovenous malformation in the pericranium. Small vessels perforate the bone over an area of 2 to 3 cm in diameter and superficially drain into the scalp veins.

Clinical Presentation

Almost all patients present with a small subcutaneous scalp swelling, sometimes from birth or after trivial injury. Although the malformation may be situated anywhere on the scalp, it most commonly occurs just in front of or behind the ear. The swelling increases in size slowly, producing a disfiguring, pulsatile mass. More rapid increases in size have been reported to occur at puberty[33,34] or at the time of menstruation.[27] A more commonly described aggravating circumstance is pregnancy.[28,32,35–37]

Hemorrhage has been described in the past but tends to occur only with neglected, very large lesions or after trauma.[13,38] Associated symptoms and signs include pain, throbbing headaches, and bruits.[39–41] Pain, either at the site of the nidus or more diffusely situated, is rarely severe and is more often of an unpleasant, pulsating sensation. Severe, incapacitating pain, however, can occur. Large lesions have also been associated with scalp necrosis.[3] High-output cardiac failure as a result of large fistulas has been reported but is rare.[42]

Investigation

The diagnosis is clinical and obvious in most patients. Further investigation is undertaken accurately to delineate the lesion and plan the therapeutic approach.

Plain radiographs of the skull usually show no abnormality apart from soft-tissue swelling at the sites of maximal development of the anomaly. If there is an intracranial component fed by dural vessels, the middle meningeal grooves may be enlarged on plain radiography. This was probably first described by Clairmont[30] in a congenital cirsoid aneurysm. In the surgical note for this particular patient, it is stated that some of the vessels that crossed the subgaleal space were as thick as a man's finger. This raises the possibility of an associated primary dural abnormality. In the authors' experience, the pericranial component has been small yet is significant in the latter condition.

Computed tomographic scans do not add much to the diagnosis. The soft-tissue scalp swelling is delineated and an associated intracranial pathologic process excluded. Contrast-enhanced CT scans have been described as useful in differentiating vascular anomalies from other congenital tumors (e.g., encephalocele, dermoid, neurofibroma, hemangioma, lymphangioma, and lipoma).[43]

Angiography is undertaken to delineate the lesion and to exclude an intracranial component.[44–46] This takes the form of an enlarged middle meningeal artery with fine feeding vessels running through the bone and feeding the malformation.[2,47] Involvement of the cerebral blood vessels has rarely been described; it represents an anomalous communication because the cerebral vessels have a different embryonic source.[2]

Treatment Options

Indications for treatment are cosmetic relief of the pulsatile disfiguring mass (the main concern of the patient), headache, and tinnitus, and the prevention of hemorrhage. It is also important that the anomalous arteriovenous communication be completely eliminated because recurrence or enlargement is inevitable after incomplete treatment. Incomplete treatment can also cause scalp necrosis and bleeding. Treatment options include surgical excision,[11,47–52] ligation of the feeding vessels,[39,53,54] transarterial and transvenous embolization,[4–6,8,9,20,51,55] injection of sclerosant into the nidus,[7,26,56,57] and electrothrombosis.[58] Radical surgical excision with total removal of the fistulas is necessary to obtain complete cure: this has been the most common method of dealing with the lesion and, in the authors' experience, is the treatment of choice.[1,2,11,25,27,47,48,50] The other, nonsurgical techniques do not reliably provide complete cure.

Surgical Excision

The evolution of a surgical method of treatment could hardly be followed more clearly than in the history of the treatment of cirsoid aneurysms of the scalp. These lesions inspired dread in the surgeon who had to deal with them before 1940. Before 1900, almost any method had to be tried before surgery was resorted to, and it was only the introduction of the method of excision by means of the scalp flap by Krause in 1898 that changed the attitude of surgeons to this condition. Radical excision, although regarded as the best form of treatment, was a lengthy procedure to undertake at a time when any form of anesthesia was a grave risk. Add to this the fact that there was no blood replacement, and one can understand why only the very skillful and very brave attempted surgery. As late as the 1930s, patients still died of blood loss.[34]

Despite the use of a scalp flap, the surgeon still has to contend with torrential hemorrhage, and various techniques have been used to reduce this danger. Siegmund (1904) suggested that a head tourniquet be used to reduce the blood flow. This, however, resulted in local scalp necrosis caused by prolonged compression of the scalp, as well as torrential hemorrhage from the edges of the flap from vessels not seen at the time of the operation. Keppler[27] (1912) used a double layer of interlocking sutures with the incision placed between them. Searby[31,59] (1931) used a tourniquet in the initial phases and then put an intestinal clamp over the base of the flap for a few days, removing the malformation as a second-stage procedure a few days later. All these techniques, however, have a fairly high risk of scalp necrosis.

The authors' surgical technique can be described as follows. First, the scalp flap must be carefully planned so that its base lies across the feeding vessels, and care must be taken to allow sufficient blood supply to maintain the viability of the flap after removal of the malformation. The scalp flap must be of sufficient size to encompass the entire lesion.

Infiltration of the flap with ornithine vasopressin is followed by a stepwise incision with careful pressure control by the surgeon and assistant, with ligation of vessels crossing the line of incision in the subcutaneous tissues of the scalp. The authors believe this is the best method of controlling blood loss while ensuring flap viability. The edges of the flap are held back in the standard neurosurgical manner with clips applied to the galea. The scalp flap containing the malformation is slowly lifted. Once the surgeon gets to the area of the main scalp anomaly, it is possible to palpate the spongy thickening of the underlying pericranium. From this region, vessels of considerable size may cross the subgaleal space. These vessels are of arterial and venous nature and, depending on their size, are dealt with by diathermy or double ligation and division. If this is done carefully, there is no undue loss of blood. If there is an accidental tear of a vessel, the subgaleal part is controlled by pressure while the scalp component is dealt with first. With the scalp flap turned downward on its base, it can for the moment be ignored and the pericranial anomaly dealt with.

The pericranial component is circumscribed with cutting diathermy and removed. The pericranial anomaly is then elevated from the underlying skull, which usually shows a slight depression. Histologic study of this tissue confirms the increase in size and number of vessels in the pericranium, which feed the malformation from the meningeal vessels (Fig. 89-6). This is an important part of the surgery. Brisk bone bleeding is controlled with the use of bone wax. Failure to adequately remove the pericranial component results in the recurrence of the lesion with opening of the middle meningeal feeders, making subsequent surgery more difficult.

Next, the feeding vessels of the malformation are exposed by an incision into the galea at the base of the flap. This is again done in a slow, stepwise manner. The vessels are divided between ligatures, completely devascularizing the lesion. The surgeon can then incise the galea over the anomaly and excise the devascularized malformation from the subcutaneous tissue.

If present, abnormal, large, tortuous vessels in the temporalis muscle, fed from the deep temporal arteries, must be completely removed. Once hemostasis has been secured, the flap is turned back into position and held with a double layer of sutures through galea and skin in the standard fashion.

Careful attention to each stage of the excision ensures complete removal while minimizing the risk of torrential hemorrhage, scalp necrosis, and recurrence. Ligation, embolization, and the sclerosis of feeding vessels have not been effective in the treatment of cirsoid aneurysms.[7,13,26,39,53,54,57] Not only is the nidus inadequately treated, but these methods allow collateral feeding vessels to develop, making the lesion far more complex and difficult to treat. In addition, access to the feeding vessels is denied if endovascular treatment is considered.

Endovascular Obliteration

With improvements in catheter technology and the development of newer embolic material, endovascular obliteration of the malformation has become an important treatment modality.[4–9,26,60–62] Results of treatment vary, but in most series the follow-up period is not long enough to adequately assess the results of treatment. Despite improved endovascular techniques and materials, large series still report surgery as

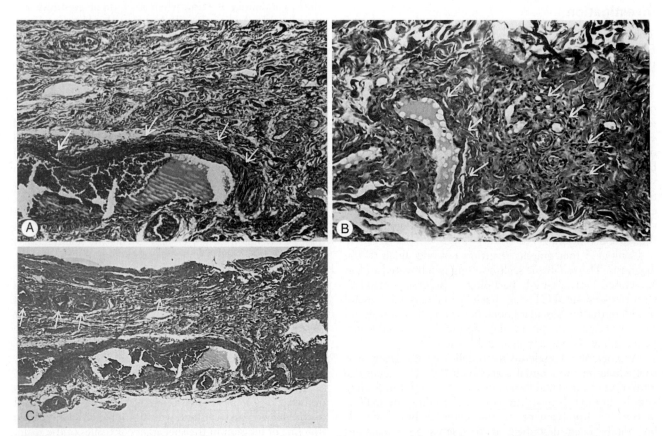

FIGURE 89-6   Elastic tissue stains (von Gieson) of the excised pericranial component of the arteriovenous malformation. There is an increase in the number and size of the vessels in the pericranium (*arrows*) of patients with the arteriovenous malformation fed via the meningeal vessels.

the cornerstone of treatment.[2,10,63] In the authors' experience, this form of therapy does not deal with the pericranial component, and therefore the risk of recurrence must be high. In addition, surgery is neither difficult nor dangerous and has excellent results.[2,10,63] However, endovascular intervention does have a role, and the patient selection, based on angiography, is important. In patients where a single feeding artery with either a proximal fistulous communication (Yokouchi and colleagues Type A)[64] or distal fistulous communication (Yokouchi and colleagues Type B)[64] is demonstrated, then a transarterial technique may be sufficient. However, in those patients with a plexiform malformation with multiple fistulas (Yokouchi and colleagues Type C),[64] direct puncture and embolization may have a role in reducing the vascularity of very large lesions before surgery.[62,63] There are few reports of complete obliteration of the fistula with embolization techniques alone. Embolic materials vary and include liquid (n-butyl cyanoacrylate), pledgets of gelatin sponge, polyvinyl alcohol particles, detachable balloons, and metal coils. Access to the malformation may be through a transarterial route, or venous occlusion through a direct percutaneous puncture or a femoral transvenous approach.

Definitive embolization therapy requires permanent and complete occlusion of the fistula site. Occluding the feeding vessels alone is insufficient and results in recurrence because of vascular recruitment. Mechanical compression of the draining veins may be required during embolization to prevent the escape of embolic material into the venous circulation and to trap the embolic material within the malformation, thereby improving the degree of penetration of the abnormal vascular channels within the lesion and improving the efficacy of closure of the shunt.[61,62] The authors' experience suggests that these patients return at a later date with a far more complex recurrence, making cure less likely. We therefore strongly advocate a surgical approach to the treatment of these complex lesions.

REFERENCES

1. Elkin DC: Cirsoid aneurysm of the scalp with the report of an advanced case. Ann Surg 80:332–340, 1924.
2. Khodadad G: Arteriovenous malformations of the scalp. Ann Surg 177:79–85, 1973.
3. Khodadad G: Familial cirsoid aneurysms of the scalp. J Neurol Neurosurg Psychiatry 34:664–667, 1971.
4. Barnwell SL, Halbach VV, Dowd CF, et al: Endovascular treatment of scalp arteriovenous fistulas associated with a large varix. Radiology 173:533–539, 1989.
5. Djindjian R, Cophignon J, Theron J, et al: Embolization by superselective angiography from the femoral route in neuroradiology: Review of 60 cases. Neuroradiology 6:20–26, 1973.
6. Kasdon DL, Altemus LR, Stein BM: Embolization of a traumatic arteriovenous fistula of the scalp with radiopaque Gelfoam pledgets. J Neurosurg 44:753–756, 1976.
7. Mourao GS, Hodes JE, Gobin YP, et al: Curative treatment of scalp arteriovenous fistula by direct puncture and embolization with absolute alcohol. J Neurosurg 75:634–637, 1991.
8. Olcott C, Newton TH, Stoney RJ, et al: Intra-arterial embolization in the management of arteriovenous malformations. Surgery 79:3–12, 1976.
9. Stillman RM, Powers JC, Fitzgerald JF: Cosmetic excision of an isolated extracranial arteriovenous malformation using Gelfoam embolization. Br J Surg 64:784–785, 1977.
10. Fisher-Jeffes ND, Domingo Z, Madden M, et al: Arteriovenous malformations of the skull. Neurosurgery 36:656–660, 1995.
11. Davies-Colley R: Cirsoid aneurysm. Guys Hosp Rep 90:134–148, 1940–1941.
12. Komatsu Y, Narushima K, Kobayashi E, et al: Congenital arteriovenous malformation of the scalp: Case report. Neurol Med Chir (Tokyo) 29:230–234, 1989.
13. Malan E, Azzolini A: Congenital arteriovenous malformations of the face and scalp. J Cardiovasc Surg (Torino) 9:109–137, 1968.
14. Maroun FB, Jacob JC, Markesteyn TH, et al: Congenital venous malformations of the scalp associated with plexiform neurofibroma and skull defects. J Neurosurg 31:465–467, 1969.
15. Badejo L, Rockwood P: Traumatic arteriovenous fistula of the scalp. J Neurosurg 66:773–774, 1987.
16. Danziger J, Bloch S, Podlas H: Trauma to the arterial supply to the brain visualised by angiography. S Afr Med J 50:11–14, 1976.
17. Barros D'sa AAJ, Heard GE: Arteriovenous fistula after hair transplantation. BMJ 1:340–341, 1978.
18. Davis AJ, Nelson PK: Arteriovenous fistula of the scalp secondary to punch autograft hair transplantation: Angioarchitecture, histopathology, and endovascular and surgical therapy. Plast Reconstr Surg 100:242–249, 1997.
19. Lanzieri CF, Sacher M, Som PM, et al: Arteriovenous fistula after hair transplantation. AJNR Am J Neuroradiol 6:111–112, 1985.
20. Mathis JM, DeNardo AJ, Jensen ME, et al: Arteriovenous fistula of the scalp after hair transplantation treated by endovascular embolisation. Ann Plast Surg 33:633–637, 1994.
21. Semashko DC, Schwartz ME, Kaynan A, et al: Arteriovenous fistula following punch-graft hair transplantation. J Dermatol Surg Oncol 15:754–755, 1989.
22. Williams LR, Robinson JK, Yao JS: Hair transplantation producing arteriovenous fistulization. Ann Vasc Surg 1:241–243, 1986.
23. Preisler SA, Koorbusch GF, Olson RAJ: An acquired arteriovenous fistula secondary to temporomandibular joint arthroscopy. J Oral Maxillofac Surg 49:187–190, 1991.
24. Morioka T, Nishio S, Hikita T: Traumatic arteriovenous fistulae of the scalp at the area of previous craniotomy. Surg Neurol 30:404–407, 1988.
25. Berger H: Die Estirpation des Angioma arteriale racemosum aus Kopfes. Beitr Klin Chir 22:129, 1898.
26. Fite P: Cirsoid aneurysm of the scalp. South Med J 26:816–821, 1933.
27. Keppler M: Zur Behandlung des Aneurysma arteriole racemosum. Beitr Klin Chir 78:521–536, 1912.
28. Kummel H: Zur Behandlung des Angioma arteriole racemosum. Arch Klin Chir 28:184–213, 1883.
29. Rundle F: A case of cirsoid aneurysm of the scalp. Br J Surg 25:872–878, 1937.
30. Clairmont P: Zur Behandlug des Angioma racemosum. Arch Klin Chir 85:549, 1908.
31. Searby H: Cirsoid aneurysm of the scalp. Aust N Z J Surg 1:209, 1931.
32. Clunie T: Cirsoid aneurysm of the scalp. BMJ 2:1183, 1936.
33. Muller H: Ein Fall von arteriellem Rankenangiom des Kopfes. Beitr Klin Chir 8:79, 1892.
34. Schlorchetzki H: Ein Beitrag zur Pathologie und Klinik des Randenangiome der Kopschroote. Beitr Klin Chir 35:157, 1933.
35. Coley WB: Cirsoid aneurysms successfully treated by excision after ligation of the external carotid. Ann Surg 34:414, 1901.
36. Cosman B: Traumatic arterial malformations of the scalp: A review of the literature and two case reports. Ann Surg 150:1032–1040, 1959.
37. Dandy WE: Arteriovenous aneurysms of the brain. Arch Surg 17:190, 1928.
38. Gauger GE, Herrmann PW: Cranial arteriovenous malformation: Suicide by exsanguination. J Forensic Sci 33:283–286, 1988.
39. Brodie BC: An account of a case of aneurysm by anastomosis of the forehead treated by the application of ligatures. Med Chir Trans 15:177–185, 1829.
40. Dandy W: Arteriovenous aneurysms of the scalp and face. Arch Surg 52:1–32, 1946.
41. Fukuta K, Smith RJ, Jackson IT: Arteriovenous fistula formation after punch graft hair transplantation in the frontal region. Plast Reconstr Surg 93:587–589, 1994.
42. Sugrue M, McCollum P, O'Driscoll K, et al: Congenital arteriovenous malformation of the scalp with high output cardiac failure: A case report. Ann Vasc Surg 3:387–388, 1989.
43. Silbergleit R, Gabrielsen TO: Arteriovenous malformation simulating encephalocele: CT findings. J Comput Assist Tomogr 11:522–524, 1987.
44. Verbiest H: Extracranial and cervical arteriovenous aneurysms of the carotid and vertebral arteries. Johns Hopkins Med J 122:350–357, 1968.

45. Verbiest H: Results of arterial slow flow angiography with arteriovenous aneurysms in the supply area of the external or internal carotid arteries. AJR Am J Roentgenol 116:1–15, 1972.
46. Wilson CB: Aneurysms of the superficial temporal artery. AJR Am J Roentgenol 105:331–333, 1969.
47. Irving AD, Thakur A, Walker WF: Cirsoid aneurysm of the scalp. J R Coll Surg Edinb 27:115, 1982.
48. Forbes WS: Successful treatment of a large cirsoid aneurism of the scalp. Med News Phila 66:663–664, 1895.
49. Korte W: Beitrag sur Lehre vom Angioma arteriale racemosum. Dtsch Z Chir 13:24–42, 1880.
50. Meyer W: Excision of cirsoid aneurysm of the temporal region. NY Med J 56:214–215, 1892.
51. Nagasaka S, Fukushima T, Goto K, et al: Treatment of scalp arteriovenous malformation. Neurosurgery 38:671–677, 1996.
52. Shepard RH: Cirsoid arteriovenous malformations of the scalp. J Neurol Neurosurg Psychiatry 38:827–828, 1975.
53. Mussey RD: Aneurismal tumours upon the ear, successfully treated by ligation of both carotids. Am J Med Sci 26:333–335, 1853.
54. Mynter H: Extensive cirsoid aneurism of the scalp obliterated by multiple ligatures. Ann Surg 11:83–95, 1890.
55. Komiyama M, Nishikawa M, Kitano S, et al: Non-traumatic arteriovenous fistulas of the scalp treated by a combination of embolisation and surgical removal. Neurol Med Chir (Tokyo) 36:162–165, 1996.
56. Hendrix LE, Meyer GA, Erickson SJ: Cirsoid aneurysm treated by percutaneous injection of sodium tetradecyl sulfate. Surg Neurol 46:557–560, 1996.
57. Mullan S, Beckman F, Vailati G: Simplified thrombosis of a large hypertrophic hemangioma of the scalp. J Neurosurg 21:68–72, 1964.
58. Gardner AMN, Stewart IA: Treatment of arteriovenous malformation by endarterial electrocoagulation. Br J Surg 59:146–148, 1972.
59. Oldfield MC, Addison NV: Cirsoid aneurysms of the scalp. BMJ 2:23–24, 1962.
60. Marotta TR, Berenstein A, Zide B: The combined role of embolisation and tissue expanders in the management of arteriovenous malformations of the scalp. AJNR Am J Neuroradiol 15:1240–1246, 1994.
61. Duncan IC, Fourie PA: Circumferential flow reduction during percutaneous embolotherapy of extracranial vascular malformations: The "cookie-cutter" technique. Am J Neuroradiol 24:1453–1455, 2003.
62. Moon Hee Han, Su Ok Seong, Hong Dae Kim, et al: Craniofacial arteriovenous malformation: Pre-operative embolization with direct puncture and injection of n-butyl cyanoacrylate. Radiology 211:661–666, 1999.
63. Muthukamar N, Rajagopal V, Manoharan AV, et al: Surgical management of cirsoid aneurysms. Acta Neurochir (Wien) 144:349–356, 2002.
64. Yokouchi T, Iwabuchi S, Tomiyama A, et al: Embolization of scalp AVF. Interventional Neuroradiology 5(Suppl)1:115–120, 1999.

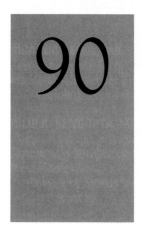

90

Surgical Management of Cranial Dural Arteriovenous Fistulas

MOHSEN JAVADPOUR and M. CHRISTOPHER WALLACE

Dural arteriovenous fistulas (DAVFs) are abnormal arteriovenous shunts within the dural leaflets. They are usually located within or near the wall of a dural venous sinus, which is often narrowed or obstructed. The nidus of arteriovenous shunting is contained solely within the dural leaflets, and this characteristic distinguishes DAVFs from pial arteriovenous malformations. The arterial supply is usually derived from dural arteries and less frequently from osseous branches. Venous drainage occurs via a dural venous sinus, retrogradely through leptomeningeal (cortical) veins, or both. Shunting of arterial blood from the meningeal arteries into venous sinuses and/or cortical veins results in venous hypertension, which is the main cause of clinical symptoms related to DAVFs. Drainage into cortical veins is referred to as cortical venous reflux (CVR).

DAVFs account for approximately 5% to 20% of all intracranial vascular malformations.[1,2] They can occur at any age, but the mean age at presentation in most studies lies between the sixth and seventh decades of life.[2,3] The term dural arteriovenous malformation has been applied by some authors to all types of DAVFs, both pediatric and adult. However, malformation implies a congenital origin. We prefer to use the term DAVF because, at least in adults, there is good evidence that these lesions are acquired rather than congenital.[4-6] The rare exception is in the pediatric age group in whom congenital malformations of dural venous sinuses are associated with high-flow arteriovenous fistulas.[7]

PATHOGENESIS

The etiologic factors and mechanisms involved in the pathogenesis of DAVFs are poorly understood. DAVFs are associated with several conditions including head injury, previous craniotomy, and dural venous sinus thrombosis, suggesting that they are acquired rather than congenital lesions.[4,7] According to the most popular theory, DAVFs are formed as a consequence of thrombosis and subsequent recanalization of dural venous sinuses.[8,9] Venous hypertension is thought to play an important role in this process. Indeed animal studies have shown that venous hypertension, even in the absence of sinus thrombosis, can elicit the formation of DAVFs.[6] Whether sinus thrombosis is in fact the initial event in the genesis of DAVFs is controversial.[8] Only a small number of patients with sinus thrombosis go on to

develop DAVFs, and not all DAVFs are associated with sinus thrombosis.[4,10]

What follows sinus thrombosis and venous hypertension is also controversial. Two hypotheses have been proposed. The first suggests that DAVFs arise from opening up of preexisting microscopic vascular channels within the dura mater. These preexisting channels are thought to open up or enlarge as a result of venous hypertension secondary to sinus thrombosis.[7] The second hypothesis suggests that DAVFs result from the formation of new vascular channels in the dura, a process stimulated and regulated by angiogenic factors. To support this, surgical DAVF specimens have been shown to contain basic fibroblastic growth factor and vascular endothelial growth factor, which were absent in control specimens.[11,12] Angiogenic factors may originate either directly as part of the inflammatory process that occurs during organization and recanalization of a thrombosed sinus or indirectly as a result of cerebral ischemia secondary to venous hypertension.[13] If the angiogenic theory is true, antiangiogenic agents may provide an adjuvant therapy for patients with untreatable DAVFs.[8]

Many cranial DAVFs ultimately undergo spontaneous resolution. The exact mechanism for this is unknown, but it is thought to result from progressive thrombosis of the involved dural sinus. This is paradoxical in that the cause of the abnormality is also thought to be the curing process. In some cases, however, spontaneous resolution has occurred despite sinus patency.[14]

CLASSIFICATION

Ideally, a classification system should predict the clinical behavior of a lesion and aid in therapeutic decision making. Several classification schemes have been devised for DAVFs.[15-19] The most commonly used are those of Borden and colleagues[16] (Borden classification) and Cognard and colleagues[17] (Cognard classification) (Table 90-1 and Fig. 90-1). Both are based on the pattern of venous drainage of the lesion, the factor that best predicts the clinical presentation and natural history of DAVFs. The Cognard classification, which is a modification of the classification of Djindjian and colleagues,[18] divides cranial DAVFs into five types, based on the presence or absence of CVR, sinusal drainage, and direction of flow in the involved dural sinus.[17]

TABLE 90-1 ▪ **Venous Drainage Pattern of Dural Arteriovenous Fistulas According to Borden and Cognard Classification Schemes**

Borden Classification	Cognard Classification
Type I: Drainage into dural venous sinus or meningeal vein only	Type I: Drainage into dural venous sinus only, with normal antegrade flow Type IIa: Drainage into dural venous sinus only, with retrograde flow
Type II: Drainage into dural venous sinus or meningeal vein + CVR	Type IIb: Drainage into dural venous sinus (antegrade flow) + CVR Type IIa + b: Drainage into dural venous sinus (retrograde flow) + CVR
Type III: CVR only	Type III: CVR only without venous ectasia Type IV: CVR only with venous ectasia Type V: Drainage into spinal perimedullary veins

CVR, cortical venous reflux (this has also been referred to as cortical venous drainage,[3] retrograde leptomeningeal venous drainage,[20] and drainage into subarachnoid veins[16]).

Data from Borden JA, Wu JK, Shucart WA: A proposed classification for spinal and cranial dural arteriovenous fistulous malformations and implications for treatment. J Neurosurg 82:166–179, 1995; Cognard C, Gobin YP, Pierot L, et al: Cerebral dural arteriovenous fistulas: Clinical and angiographic correlation with a revised classification of venous drainage. Radiology 194:671–680, 1995.

The Borden classification[16] is a more simplified scheme with three types based on the presence or absence of CVR and sinusal drainage, without taking into account the direction of flow in the venous sinus. In a study by the University of Toronto Brain Vascular Malformation Study Group, Davies and colleagues[19] validated the classification systems of Borden and of Cognard with respect to clinical presentation. Aggressive presentation (i.e., intracranial hemorrhage [ICH], focal neurologic deficit, or death) occurred in 2% of the Borden classification type I, 39% of type II, and 79% of type III cranial DAVFs. Similar correlation was found between the Cognard classification and clinical presentation (Table 90-2).[19] Subsequent studies by our group have demonstrated that the pattern of venous drainage and in particular the presence or absence of CVR also correlate with the natural history of DAVFs after the initial presentation.[3,20]

DAVFs were previously classified according to their anatomic location.[21] Anterior cranial fossa and tentorial lesions were associated with a higher risk of aggressive clinical behavior than lesions in other locations.[1,19] However, it was later shown that the poor prognosis of lesions in these "dangerous" locations was purely a function of their pattern of venous drainage.[19,22] It is the presence of CVR, not the anatomic location per se, that leads to aggressive clinical behavior.[1,19] Hemodynamically, DAVFs may be classified into high-flow or low-flow fistulas. The classification of Barrow and colleagues[23] is described later in the section on carotid cavernous fistulas. The classification of pediatric DAVFs is not discussed in this chapter.

CLINICAL PRESENTATION

Other than pulsatile tinnitus, the symptoms of DAVFs are related to venous hypertension.[7,24] This may lead to venous congestion, cerebral edema, cerebral infarction, and ICH. The clinical features of cranial DAVFs are shown in Table 90-3. ICH, nonhemorrhagic neurologic deficit (NHND), and death are considered aggressive.[1,19] The most significant risk factor for aggressive clinical presentation is the presence of CVR.[1,17,19] Therefore, type II and III lesions of the Borden classification are frequently associated with aggressive clinical behavior, whereas type I lesions are rarely so (see Table 90-2). ICH associated with DAVFs typically results from rupture of an arterialized cortical vein and is usually intraparenchymal but may also occur into the subarachnoid, subdural, and intraventricular spaces (Fig. 90-2). NHND is caused by cerebral ischemia secondary to venous congestion. This category does not include ophthalmoplegia secondary to cranial nerve dysfunction. The neurologic deficit may be focal or global.

Benign symptoms include pulsatile tinnitus and orbital symptoms. Pulsatile tinnitus is produced by turbulent flow in the diseased dural sinus.[4] Objective bruit is heard in 40% of patients with tinnitus. Ophthalmologic symptoms and signs are most commonly seen with cavernous sinus DAVFs, but they can also occur with lesions in other locations, if the venous drainage involves the cavernous sinus and ophthalmic veins.[25] The symptoms are caused by venous congestion.[4,26] The ophthalmologic symptoms may be progressive and disabling and may even lead to blindness and therefore may not be considered benign by the patient. In infants, heart failure and craniomegaly may occur.

RADIOGRAPHIC EVALUATION

Computed Tomography and Magnetic Resonance

In cases of DAVF without CVR, computed tomography and magnetic resonance imaging (MRI) of the brain parenchyma are typically normal. However, MRI and magnetic resonance angiography may show the stenosis or occlusion of the dural sinuses.[7] Hydrocephalus may be seen in any DAVF that causes venous hypertension in the superior sagittal sinus. In cases of DAVF with CVR, computed tomography and MRI of the brain may show ICH, engorged pial vessels, and diffuse white matter edema secondary to venous congestion. The ICH is usually intraparenchymal but may also have subdural, subarachnoid, or intraventricular components (see Fig. 90-2). The pattern of hemorrhage is not specific to DAVFs, and a high index of suspicion is required. Dilated pial vessels and white matter edema are more likely to be seen on MRI than on computed tomography.[7] On T2-weighted MRI, dilated pial vessels are seen as flow voids on the surface of the brain, and diffuse white matter edema is seen as hyperintensity in the cerebral or cerebellar hemispheres, brain stem, or spinal cord (Fig. 90-3). Recent reports have demonstrated improvements in the

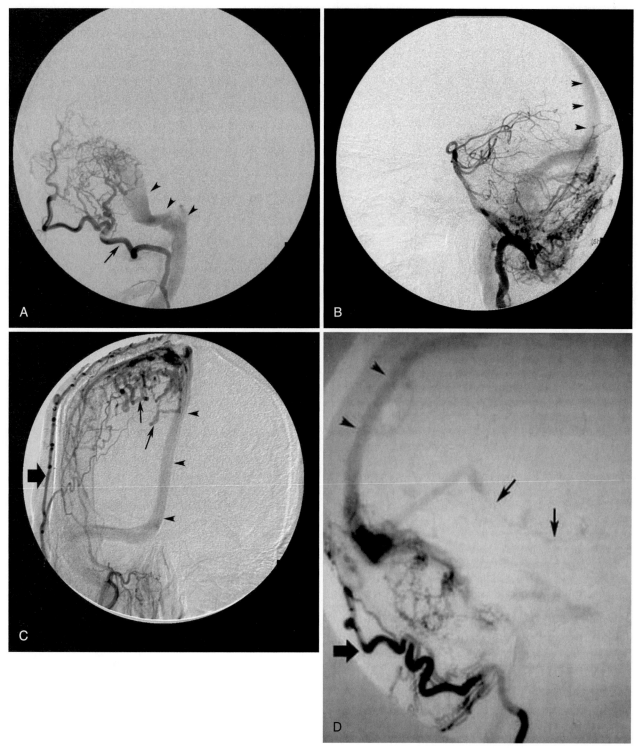

FIGURE 90-1 Cerebral angiograms showing the different types of DAVFs categorized according to the Borden and Cognard classifications. *A,* Borden type I/Cognard type I. Selective right occipital artery (*arrow*) angiogram, lateral projection, shows a right transverse/sigmoid sinus dural arteriovenous fistula (DAVF) with antegrade drainage into the transverse/sigmoid sinuses (*arrowheads*). *B,* Borden type I/Cognard type IIa. Left vertebral artery angiogram, lateral projection, shows a transverse/sigmoid sinus DAVF, with retrograde drainage into the transverse and superior sagittal sinuses (*arrowheads*). The direction of flow in the sinuses is retrograde. *C,* Borden type II/Cognard type IIb. Left external carotid artery (ECA) angiogram, anteroposterior projection, shows a superior sagittal sinus DAVF, fed by branches of the superficial temporal artery (*thick arrow*), with antegrade drainage into the superior sagittal sinus (*arrowheads*), and cortical venous reflux (*small arrows*). *D,* Borden type II/Cognard type IIa + b. Left ECA angiogram, lateral projection, shows a transverse sinus DAVF, fed by the posterior branch of the occipital artery (*thick arrow*), with retrograde drainage in the transverse sinus (*arrowheads*) and cortical venous reflux (*arrows*). The direction of flow in the sinuses is retrograde.

(Continued)

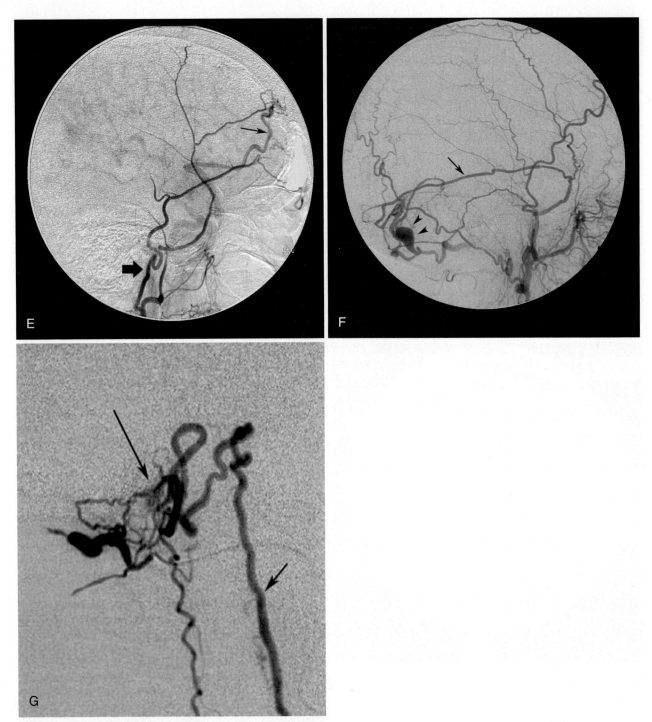

FIGURE 90-1 Cont'd *E*, Borden type III/Cognard type III. Right ECA angiogram, lateral projection, shows a convexity DAVF fed by branches of the superficial temporal artery (*thick arrow*) and draining solely into a cortical vein (*small arrow*). *F*, Borden type III/Cognard type IV. Right ECA angiogram, lateral projection, shows a torcular DAVF, fed by the posterior branch of the middle meningeal artery (*small arrow*), and refluxing into an ectatic cortical vein (*arrowheads*). *G*, Borden type III/Cognard type V. Foramen magnum DAVF (*long arrow*) with cortical venous drainage via spinal cord (*arrow*).

TABLE 90-2 ▪ **Relationship between Aggressive Clinical Presentation and Classification of 102 Cranial Dural Arteriovenous Fistulas (DAVFs)**

Classification and Type	% of DAVFs with Aggressive Clinical Presentation (i.e., ICH or NHND)
Borden type I (n = 55)	2
Cognard type I (n = 40)	0
Cognard type IIa (n = 15)	7
Borden type II (n = 18)	39
Cognard type IIb (n = 8)	38
Cognard type IIa + b (n = 10)	40
Borden type III (n = 29)	79
Cognard type III (n = 13)	69
Cognard type IV (n = 12)	83
Cognard type V (n = 4)	100

ICH, intracranial hemorrhage; NHND, nonhemorrhagic neurologic deficit.

From Davies MA, TerBrugge K, Willinsky R, et al: The validity of classification for the clinical presentation of intracranial dural arteriovenous fistulas. J Neurosurg 85:830–837, 1996.

ability of magnetic resonance angiography to diagnose DAVFs and to detect CVR.[27] However, these results have been reported in small selected series and require further study. At present, the diagnosis of DAVFs cannot be excluded with negative computed tomography, MRI, or magnetic resonance angiography. If clinically suspected, catheter angiography is required to confirm or exclude the presence of a DAVF.

Intra-arterial Catheter Angiography

This is the gold standard method for diagnosis and evaluation of DAVFs. The characteristic angiographic feature of DAVFs is premature visualization of intracranial veins or venous sinuses during the arterial phase (see Fig. 90-3C; Fig. 90-4A).[28] This is caused by shunting of arterial blood into the venous system through the fistula. To obtain the necessary information regarding the arterial supply and venous drainage of the DAVF and the venous drainage of the brain,

TABLE 90-3 ▪ **Clinical Manifestations of Dural Arteriovenous Fistulas**

Intracranial hemorrhage
Focal neurologic deficit (e.g., motor weakness, aphasia, cerebellar signs, progressive myelopathy)
Global neurologic deficit (e.g., dementia)
Pulsatile tinnitus, objective bruit
Proptosis, conjunctival injection, chemosis
Ophthalmoplegia (secondary to extraoccular muscle swelling, or compression of cranial nerves III, IV, VI)
Visual loss (secondary to orbital congestion and increased intraocular pressure, retinal hemorrhages, or optic neuropathy)
Glaucoma
Papilledema (secondary to hydrocephalus or pseudotumour cerebri caused by impaired venous drainage)
Facial pain (secondary to compression of the first and second divisions of the trigeminal nerve in the lateral wall of the cavernous sinus)

imaging must start in the ultraearly arterial phase and be carried well into the late venous phase. Selective angiography with magnification and subtraction techniques is essential. The study should include injections of both internal carotid arteries (ICAs), both external carotid arteries (ECAs), and both vertebral arteries. This is because a single DAVF may have multiple feeding arteries (see Figs. 90-3 and 90-4) and also because 8% of patients have multiple DAVFs.[29] Detailed knowledge of dural arterial anatomy is essential in angiographic evaluation of DAVFs. Meningeal arteries that are invisible or difficult to see on normal angiograms may be dilated and clearly visible when supplying a DAVF. For example, the tentorial branch of the meningohypophyseal trunk of the ICA (the artery of Bernasconi and Cassinari) or the meningeal branch of the posterior cerebral artery (the artery of Davidoff and Schecter) may be dilated and easily seen on the angiograms (see Fig. 90-3C).

The nidus of a DAVF is the site of arteriovenous shunting and refers to that part of the dura where there is convergence of all feeding arteries and the origin of venous draining channels. The best views of the nidus are often obtained during the ultraearly arterial phase of the angiogram and by injections of distant arterial feeders.[28] Images obtained when injecting the main arterial feeders, particularly in the later arterial phase or in the venous phase, are often obscured by engorged feeding arteries and draining veins.

Assessment of the venous drainage pattern of DAVFs is extremely important as this factor determines the natural history of the lesion and aids in selecting the most appropriate management strategy. The presence or absence of CVR, venous sinus occlusion, direction of flow in the venous sinuses, and the venous drainage pattern of the brain must be determined. The exact site of CVR must be determined to allow treatment planning.[7] At angiography, a delayed circulation time is compatible with venous congestion.[30] Focal areas of delayed venous drainage in the brain correspond to the site of CVR.[7] In some cases, tortuous, dilated pial veins may be seen that develop as a result of venous hypertension (see Fig. 90-3F). Willinsky and colleagues[30] have described this finding as the pseudophlebitic pattern, which is a sign of venous congestion of the brain and may be associated with an aggressive natural history.[7]

NATURAL HISTORY

The natural history of a disease refers to the disease course after presentation if left untreated. Knowledge of the natural history is essential in patient management. The results and complications of available treatment strategies must be compared with the outcome of the natural history of the disease. Recently, our group reported the results of the largest prospective natural history studies of patients with cranial DAVFs.[3,20] The results, summarized in the following, showed that the presence of CVR is the most significant predictive factor for an aggressive natural history.[3,20]

Dural Arteriovenous Fistulas with Cortical Venous Reflux

Of 236 cranial DAVFs, 119 had CVR (Borden classification type II or III and Cognard classification type IIb, IIa + b,

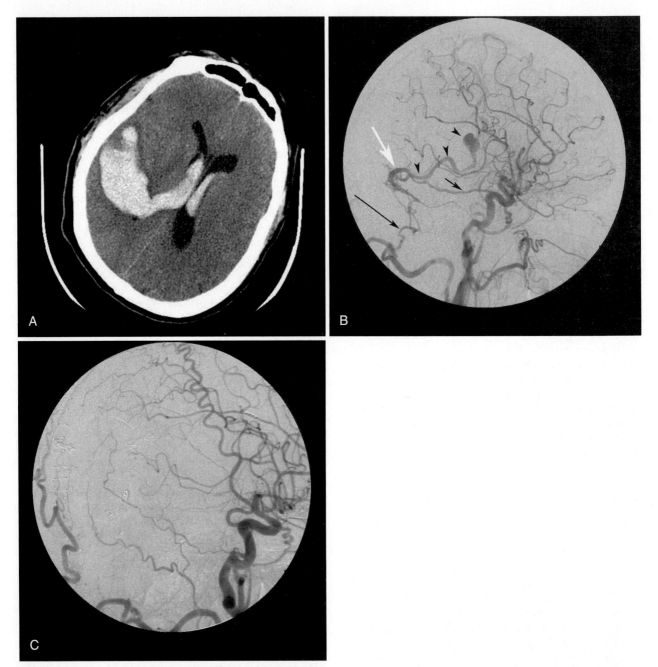

FIGURE 90-2   *A,* Axial computed tomography scan of a 56-year-old man who presented with sudden headache followed by loss of consciousness shows intracerebral and intraventricular hemorrhage. *B,* Right common carotid artery angiogram, lateral projection, shows a transverse sinus dural arteriovenous fistula (DAVF), fed by branches of the right middle meningeal artery (*arrow*) and the right occipital artery (*large arrow*). Venous drainage was by reflux into a cortical vein (*white arrow*) leading to an ectasia (*arrowheads*). There was no sinusal drainage, making this a Borden type III/Cognard type IV DAVF. In this patient, selective angiography was not possible because of severe atherosclerosis and tortuosity of the carotid arteries. *C,* Postoperative angiogram after right occipital craniotomy exposing the transverse sinus. The dura was opened and reflected inferiorly based on its attachment to the transverse sinus. The DAVF was treated by coagulation and division of this vein close to the transverse sinus, at the site shown by the *white arrow* in Figure 90-3*B.*

III, or IV). Of these, 96 patients successfully underwent curative treatment, and three patients were lost to follow-up. Van Dijk and colleagues[20] followed the remaining 20 patients with persistent CVR (14 patients who refused treatment and 6 who had partial treatment only) for a mean follow-up period of 4.3 years (86.9 patient-years). In these 20 patients,

the annual risks of ICH and NHND (disregarding aggressive events at presentation) were found to be 8.1% and 6.9%, respectively, adding up to an annual event rate (i.e., ICH and NHND) of 15%. The annual mortality rate was 10.4%. These results demonstrate that DAVFs with CVR have an aggressive natural history.

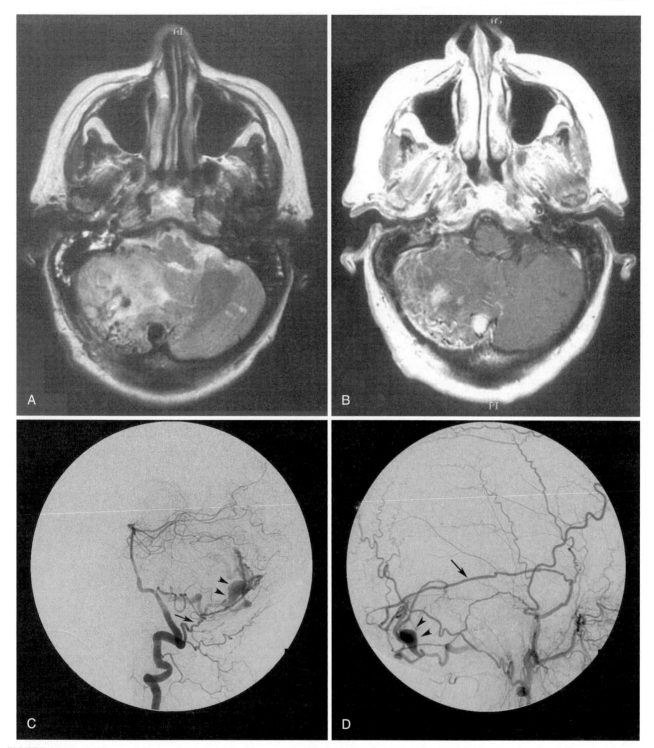

FIGURE 90-3 A 67-year-old woman presented with severe headache and subsequent deterioration in conscious level. Computed tomography scan showed a right cerebellar hematoma that was evacuated. *A,* Axial T2-weighted magnetic resonance imaging (MRI) shows a central area of hyperintensity in the right cerebellar hemisphere. Tortuous dilated vessels appearing as flow voids in the right cerebellar hemisphere indicate the presence of cortical venous reflux. *B,* Axial gadolinium-enhanced T1-weighted MRI shows peripheral enhancement surrounding the hyperintense region seen on the T2-weighted image. *C,* Left vertebral artery angiogram, lateral projection DAVF with ectasia (*arrowheads*) fed by dural branch of vertebral artery (*arrow*). *D,* Right external carotid artery (ECA) angiogram, lateral projection, same ectasia (*arrowheads*) fed by posterior branch of middle meningeal artery (*arrow*).

(Continued)

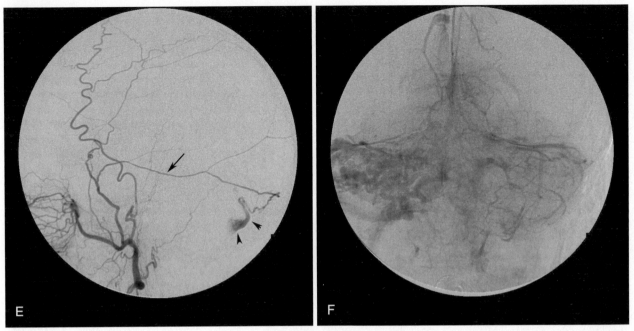

FIGURE 90-3 Cont'd (*E*), show a torcular dural arteriovenous fistula (DAVF), fed by branches of the left vertebral artery (*arrow*), and right and left middle meningeal arteries (*arrowheads*). The fistula drains into a cortical vein (*curved arrows*), with a varix (*open curved arrow*), making this a Borden type III/Cognard type IV DAVF. *F,* The venous phase of the angiogram demonstrates tortuous, dilated pial veins, referred to as a pseudophlebitic pattern. This fistula was successfully cured by transarterial embolization.

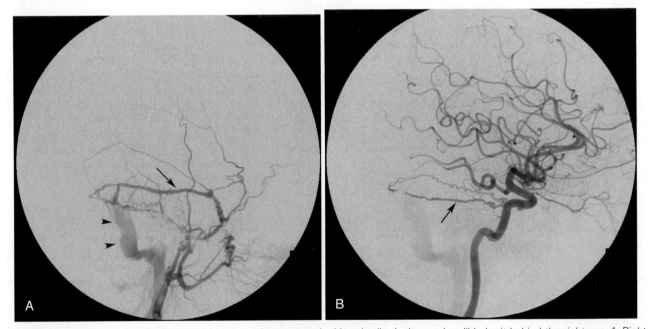

FIGURE 90-4 Angiograms of a 52-year-old woman who presented with pulsatile tinnitus and audible bruit behind the right ear. *A,* Right external carotid artery angiogram, lateral projection shows premature appearance of the sigmoid sinus (*arrowheads*) in the ultraearly arterial phase of the angiogram. A transverse sinus dural arteriovenous fistula (DAVF) is shown, fed by the posterior branch of the right middle meningeal artery (*arrow*) and draining antegradely into the transverse/sigmoid sinus (*arrowheads*) without any cortical venous reflux (CVR) (Borden type I, Cognard type I). The same DAVF is shown in Figure 90-1*A* being fed also by the right occipital artery. *B,* Right internal carotid artery angiogram, lateral projection, revealed a hypertrophied artery of Bernasconi and Cassinari, also supplying the DAVF (*arrow*). As there was no CVR, the patient was managed with observation alone.

Dural Arteriovenous Fistulas without Cortical Venous Reflux

Of the 236 cranial DAVFs, 117 had no CVR (Borden type I, Cognard type I or IIa). Five patients were lost to follow-up. The remaining 112 patients were followed up clinically for a median of 27.9 months (range, 1 month to 17.5 years), amounting to 348 patient-years. Of these, 68 underwent observation alone, and 44 underwent palliative treatment for symptomatic control (43 endovascular, 1 surgery). Palliative treatment, never aimed at cure, was performed if the patient had intolerable symptoms or if there was persistent high intraocular pressure or decreasing visual acuity. Using this conservative management strategy, 98% of patients had a benign and well-tolerated clinical course, without any ICH or NHND.[3] Long-term angiographic follow-up in 50 patients showed that DAVFs without CVR have a 2% to 3% risk of developing CVR.[3]

INDICATIONS FOR TREATMENT

Decisions regarding treatment of DAVFs should be guided by their natural history. Therefore, DAVFs with CVR should be treated to eliminate the risk of hemorrhage and neurologic deficit. The aim of treatment in these cases is elimination of CVR or complete cure if possible. Lesions without CVR do not require treatment unless they are associated with intolerable symptoms such as intolerable tinnitus and ophthalmologic symptoms including visual deterioration and pain. For these lesions, the aim of treatment is not cure, but palliative symptom control.

MANAGEMENT OPTIONS

Several options are available for the management of cranial DAVFs. In many cases, a combination of methods may be required.

Observation

DAVFs without CVR usually behave in a benign manner and are rarely associated with hemorrhage or neurologic deficit. Therefore, observation is the most appropriate management option for these patients if they are asymptomatic or are tolerating their symptoms.[4,7] As they have a 2% to 3% chance of developing CVR, all patients should be followed up clinically and radiographically. Any change in symptoms (worsening or improvement) may be a warning signal for development of CVR and should prompt repeat cerebral angiography.[3,7] In patients with a stable clinical condition, serial MRI and magnetic resonance angiography and a conventional angiogram after 3 years is advised.[7] Observation is not a valid treatment option for DAVFs with CVR.

Compression Therapy

Intermittent manual carotid compression by the patient has been used by Halbach and colleagues,[8,31] to treat DAVFs of the cavernous sinus in patients with no evidence of carotid atherosclerosis. The patient is instructed to compress the carotid-jugular area ipsilateral to the DAVF, with the contralateral hand for as long as 30 minutes per session.

The compression should be terminated if any weakness develops.[8] Halbach and colleagues[8,31] reported a cure rate of 27% with this technique after 4 to 6 weeks. However, this treatment has been the subject of debate because the 27% cure rate in the short term may reflect the natural history of the disease.[7]

Transarterial Embolization

Superselective embolization of the dural feeding vessels to a DAVF can be an effective treatment in some cases.[8] The ideal goal is to cure the DAVF by occluding the fistula itself. To achieve this from the arterial side, a microcatheter must be navigated into the distal part of a feeding artery and wedged, so that cyanoacrylate glue can be pushed through the nidus and into the most proximal venous outlet. This is essentially a venous treatment performed through the arterial side. Liquid adhesive agents (e.g., n-butyl cyanoacrylate), the rate of polymerization of which can be controlled, are the best agents to permanently occlude a fistula.[7] Successful occlusion of the fistula using this technique has been reported in a small number of patients.[7,32]

In most cases, transarterial embolization involves occlusion of the feeding arteries without occlusion of the fistula. This may decrease flow through the fistula but is rarely curative because most DAVFs have multiple small feeding arteries that are not amenable to transarterial embolization. Furthermore, in most cases, the lesion will continue to recruit feeding arteries from other sources, leading to recurrence.[8,32] Transarterial embolization is commonly used as an adjunct before surgical treatment or transvenous embolization of DAVFs. It is also used as palliative treatment for benign DAVFs with intolerable symptoms. Preoperative embolization of large feeding arteries, particularly in the external carotid territory, carries a relatively low risk and helps to reduce intraoperative blood loss. Particles (e.g., polyvinyl alcohol) may be used for this purpose.[7]

Endovascular therapy is not without risk. Knowledge of the important anastomoses between the external carotid, internal carotid, and vertebrobasilar systems is crucial for safe embolization.[33] Embolic agents can inadvertently travel through these anastomoses and lead to occlusion of important branches. Embolization of feeding arteries that arise directly from the ICA or vertebral artery may lead to reflux of embolic material into the parent artery and result in stroke. In the case of benign DAVFs, it is important to ensure that the embolic material does not flow past the fistula site and obstruct venous outflow. If this occurs, venous drainage may be diverted to cortical veins, thereby converting a benign fistula to an aggressive one.

Transvenous Embolization

Transvenous embolization is increasingly used in the management of cranial DAVFs.[34,35] This involves a retrograde approach through the veins with deposition of materials such as coils into the venous compartment at the fistula site. Usually the transfemoral route is employed. In the majority of cases, transvenous embolization involves sacrificing the involved dural venous sinus. This can only be performed if detailed study of the venous phase of the cerebral angiogram has shown that the involved dural sinus is not being used by the brain and that alternate pathways for venous drainage of the brain have developed.[7] In some cases it may be possible to use a retrograde transvenous approach to disconnect CVR without sacrificing the dural sinus. However, in most cases this is not possible because of the difficulty in access to the refluxing cortical veins and the tortuosity of these veins.

In some cases of transverse/sigmoid sinus DAVFs, the lesion may be draining into a venous pouch, parallel to and separate from the transverse sinus. The University of California–San Francisco interventional neuroradiology group have reported 10 such cases and named this entity the parallel venous channel. In their series, transvenous embolization was used to occlude the parallel venous channel and cure the fistula in all 10 cases while preserving the transverse/sigmoid sinus.[36] Identification of this separate venous channel is important as it may allow curative treatment of the fistula without sacrificing the transverse sinus. However, this type of channel has been identified in a small number of cases only.

The mainstay of transvenous embolization is occlusion of the affected venous sinus. Neurologic complications after embolization occur if outflow to normally draining veins is obstructed, resulting in venous hypertension and venous infarction. After embolization of cavernous sinus DAVFs, paradoxical worsening of ophthalmologic symptoms may develop secondary to excessive thrombosis and venous hypertension involving the ophthalmic veins. Other complications include guidewire injury to the wall of dural sinuses resulting in subarachnoid hemorrhage and injury to cranial nerves.[34]

Surgery

Although endovascular therapy is increasingly used to treat intracranial DAVFs, surgery still plays an important role in the management of these lesions. We recommend surgery for DAVFs with CVR when endovascular therapy fails or is technically not feasible. Three different surgical strategies exist for treatment of intracranial DAVFs. The first is to obtain venous access for direct packing of the involved dural venous sinus. The second is complete excision of the DAVF. The third is to disconnect the arterialized leptomeningeal veins (CVR) only, without attempting to excise the entire lesion. These strategies are discussed in the following sections.

Surgery to Obtain Venous Access

In some cases, the usual venous access routes may not be available for transfemoral transvenous embolization. This can occur due to thrombosis or steno-occlusive disease of the dural venous sinuses. In these cases, access may be gained to the fistula by direct surgical exposure and catheterization of the involved sinus. Direct packing of the sinus can then be performed using coils or other thrombogenic materials such as Gelfoam and silk sutures.[37]

Surgical Excision

Traditionally, the goal of surgery for aggressive DAVFs has been complete excision of the lesion. This involves interruption of the arterial feeders, extensive coagulation, and excision of the pathologic dural leaflet, and disconnection

of arterialized leptomeningeal veins (i.e., CVR). In some cases, the involved dural venous sinus is also excised if it is not participating in the venous drainage of normal brain. We use preoperative transarterial embolization of the arterial feeders whenever possible to reduce intraoperative blood loss. Prophylactic intravenous antibiotics are given at induction. Intraoperative mannitol and cerebrospinal fluid drainage using a lumbar spinal drain may be used when necessary to reduce the need for brain retraction. Under general endotracheal anesthesia, the scalp incision and craniotomy are fashioned in the appropriate location. Frameless or frame-based stereotaxy may be helpful in localizing the lesion, particularly if enlarged cortical veins or a venous varix can be visualized on computed tomography or MRI. Once the pathologic region of dura has been exposed, the involved dura and feeding arteries are extensively coagulated. If the involved venous sinus can be sacrificed, the dura is incised on both sides of, and parallel to, the sinus. Feeding arteries are coagulated or occluded using hemostatic clips as they are encountered. The involved segment of the venous sinus can then be ligated proximally and distally and excised together with the pathologic dura. All arterialized leptomeningeal veins are coagulated or clipped at their entrance into the sinus and divided. Intraoperative angiography is used to ensure complete obliteration of the fistula.

If the sinus is being used for normal venous drainage of the brain, it should be skeletonized and left in situ.[38] Skeletonization of the sinus involves interruption of the dural arterial supply to the fistula, and excision of dural segments on both sides of the sinus, while preserving the venous sinus and the nonarterialized cortical veins. In cases of transverse/sigmoid or superior sagittal sinus DAVFs, the tentorium or the falx adjacent to the sinus should also be coagulated and cut to ensure complete interruption of arterial supply to the fistula.

The extensive procedures used for total excision of DAVFs may be associated with significant complications. Access may be difficult when the lesion is in a deep location (e.g., tentorial and posterior fossa lesions) and may require extensive skull base procedures. Significant hemorrhage may occur at any stage of the procedure. Torrential hemorrhage may occur from engorged vessels when incising the scalp and from engorged osseous and dural vessels when performing the craniotomy.[39] Bleeding from bone should be controlled using bone wax. Bleeding from the enlarged dural arteries feeding the fistula should be controlled using extensive coagulation or hemostatic clips. Preoperative transarterial embolization of the feeding vessels is extremely helpful in reducing intraoperative hemorrhage.

Disconnection of Cortical Venous Reflux Alone

The goal of treatment for aggressive DAVFs is to eliminate the risk of ICH and neurologic deficit. Because CVR is the predisposing factor for aggressive natural history, it has been suggested that a procedure limited to disconnection of arterialized leptomeningeal veins (CVR) is sufficient in the treatment of aggressive lesions and that complete excision of the involved dural leaflet and the venous sinus is not necessary.[7,40–42] Disconnection of CVR is a simpler procedure with less morbidity and changes the natural history of the lesion from aggressive to benign. There are now several reports showing that this technique is effective, and we now use it in preference to complete excision in most cases.[43]

The surgical procedure involves exposure of the pathologic dural leaflet as explained previously. Any dural feeding arteries are coagulated or occluded with hemostatic clips. The dura is then opened, and with careful dissection, the arterialized leptomeningeal veins are exposed. These veins are then coagulated or clipped and divided at their entrance into the dural venous sinus or as close to the fistula site as possible. It is important to ensure that the vein is adequately coagulated before division. The adjacent dural areas should be examined to ensure that all arterialized leptomeningeal veins have been disconnected. "Blue" nonarterialized cortical veins should be preserved. The dura is then closed, the bone flap replaced, and the wound closed in the usual manner.

Stereotactic Radiosurgery

There is a limited number of reports on the radiosurgical treatment of intracranial DAVFs.[44-49] Pan and colleagues[47] reported complete angiographic resolution of the nidus in 47% of 19 transverse/sigmoid sinus DAVFs, after a median follow-up of 19 months. Pollock and colleagues[45,46] have used a combination of stereotactic radiosurgery and transarterial embolization. Although radiosurgery is effective in obliterating some DAVFs, its main disadvantage is the long interval between treatment and the expected therapeutic effects. In patients with CVR, this delay is not acceptable because of the high risk of ICH and neurologic deficit (15% per year) while waiting for obliteration of the lesion.[7,20,42] In patients without CVR, curative treatment is not required because of the benign natural history of these lesions. Most of these patients can be managed by observation alone or by palliative transarterial embolization. The risk of radiosurgery

in these patients may not be acceptable, especially in view of the limited data available on the efficacy of this treatment.[3,7] Therefore, the role of radiosurgery in the management of intracranial DAVFs is currently unclear.

COMPREHENSIVE MANAGEMENT STRATEGY

This section outlines a comprehensive management strategy for the treatment of intracranial DAVFs. The specific features of individual DAVFs in different locations are dealt with later in the chapter. As a general principle, the management strategy is based on the pattern of venous drainage of the lesion because this determines the natural history of DAVFs.

Dural Arteriovenous Fistulas without Cortical Venous Reflux (Benign Fistulas: Borden Type I, Cognard Types I and IIa)

For patients with DAVFs without CVR who are asymptomatic or have tolerable symptoms, observation is the most appropriate treatment option.[4,7] If the patient has intolerable symptoms, such as tinnitus or ophthalmologic symptoms, treatment may be indicated. In these cases, curative treatment is not necessary as the patient is not at risk of ICH or neurologic deficit. Palliative treatment in the form of transarterial embolization of the feeding arteries is usually effective in symptom control and is associated with fewer complications compared with curative transvenous embolization or surgery. All patients should be followed up clinically and radiographically, and any change in symptoms (deterioration or improvement) should prompt repeat conventional angiography to look for development of CVR (Fig. 90-5).

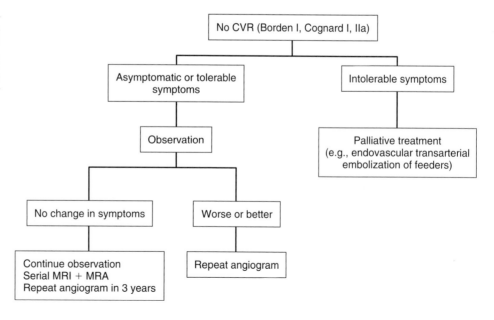

FIGURE 90-5 Management strategy for dural arteriovenous fistulas without cortical venous reflux (CVR) (benign dural arteriovenous fistulas, Borden type I and Cognard types I and IIa). MRA, magnetic resonance angiography; MRI, magnetic resonance imaging.

Dural Arteriovenous Fistulas with Cortical Venous Reflux (Aggressive Fistulas: Borden Types II and III, Cognard Types IIb through V)

These lesions must be treated aggressively because they are associated with a 15% annual risk of hemorrhage and neurologic deficit.[20] Treatment should be performed soon after the diagnosis has been made.[4] There is evidence that rebleeding may occur early after an initial hemorrhagic presentation. In one series, 35% of patients had a rebleed within 2 weeks after the first hemorrhage.[50] Complete obliteration of the fistula is ideal but not critical because there is increasing evidence that disconnection of CVR alone results in long-term protection against hemorrhage and neurologic deficit.[4,40–43,51]

Treatment of cranial DAVFs with CVR requires a multidisciplinary approach. A combination of transarterial embolization, transvenous embolization, and surgery may be required in some cases. The primary goal of treatment, whether endovascular or surgical, is to eliminate CVR. Endovascular embolization is usually the primary treatment modality and often begins with transarterial embolization. This is rarely curative and is usually followed by transvenous embolization. If endovascular therapy is not feasible or fails, then surgery is indicated.

For lesions with CVR only without any sinusal drainage (Borden type III and Cognard types III, IV, and V), CVR disconnection alone is all that is required. Transvenous embolization is rarely successful in these cases because the adjacent venous sinus cannot be used for access to the refluxing cortical vein. Most of these cases therefore require surgical disconnection of CVR. Before disconnection, it must be decided whether it is safe to interrupt the veins involved in CVR. This is particularly important when the vein to be disconnected is a major cortical draining vein,

such as the vein of Labbé. The venous phase of the cerebral angiograms must be studied in detail to ensure that normal brain is not draining into the concerned veins and that other venous routes are being used by the brain (Fig. 90-6).

The management of DAVFs that have both CVR and sinusal drainage (Borden type II and Cognard types IIb and IIa + b) is more complex. The management strategy for these lesions requires a detailed knowledge of the venous drainage of the brain as well as that of the fistula. If the involved dural sinus is being used only by the DAVF and is not being used for venous drainage of the brain, then it may be sacrificed. This can be achieved by transvenous embolization or by surgical packing or excision of the sinus. The decision regarding the safety of sinus sacrifice is based on preoperative clinical and angiographic assessment of the patient. If the patient is neurologically intact, and the venous phase of the cerebral angiogram shows that the involved venous sinus is not used for drainage of the brain and that other pathways have developed for venous drainage of the brain, the sinus may be sacrificed. However, if angiography shows that the sinus is used for venous drainage of the brain, treatment must be limited to CVR disconnection alone without obliteration or excision of the sinus. This converts Borden type II (Cognard types IIb and IIa + b) lesions to Borden type I (Cognard types I and IIa) lesions, which have a benign natural history.

The most difficult situation arises in patients with preoperative neurologic deficit. In these patients, an assumption that the sinus can be sacrificed, based solely on angiographic findings may be incorrect. In other words, the patient's neurologic deficit may be a consequence of the retrograde flow in the sinus and the resulting venous hypertension, which may improve if normal flow in the sinus can be reestablished. Occlusion of the sinus or the refluxing cortical veins in these cases would eliminate the chance of recovery of neurologic function and may lead to venous infarction.

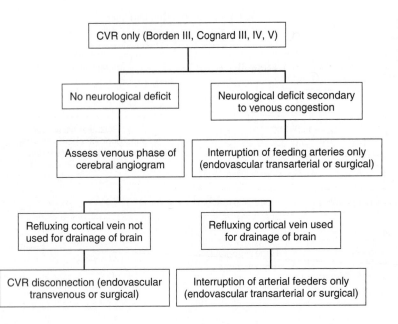

FIGURE 90-6 Management strategy for dural arteriovenous fistulas with cortical venous reflux (CVR) only (aggressive dural arteriovenous fistulas, Borden type III and Cognard types III, IV and V).

FIGURE 90-7 Management strategy for dural arteriovenous fistulas with cortical venous reflux (CVR) and sinusal drainage (aggressive dural arteriovenous fistulas, Borden type II and Cognard types IIb and IIa + b).

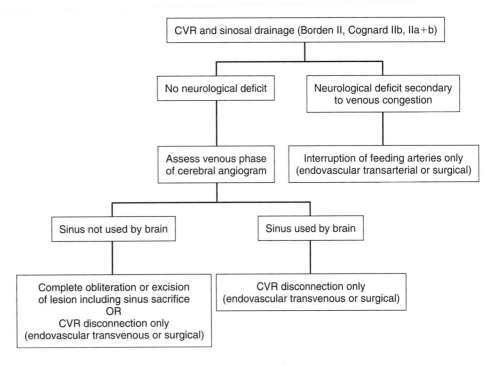

In these patients, the safest option may be to limit the procedure to the arterial side of the lesion. This can be achieved by extensive transarterial embolization of the feeding arteries or by surgical skeletonization of the sinus. All cortical veins and the venous sinuses should be left intact. Fortunately, this situation arises rarely (Fig. 90-7).

In all patients with DAVFs and CVR, treatment should continue until all CVR has been eliminated. Simply reducing the size of the nidus without eliminating CVR does not eradicate the risk of future hemorrhage or neurologic deficit. All patients, particularly those in whom complete obliteration of the fistula has not been achieved, require lifelong follow-up, with a routine delayed angiogram at 3 years to check for recurrence of CVR. Patients would also require an angiogram if there is any change (deterioration or improvement) in their symptoms.

ANATOMIC CONSIDERATIONS FOR DURAL ARTERIOVENOUS FISTULAS IN SPECIFIC LOCATIONS

In itself, anatomic location of a DAVF has no direct correlation with aggressive clinical events, although this has been suggested in the past.[3,19] DAVFs in any location can develop CVR (Table 90-4).[1,19] However, DAVFs in particular locations such as the anterior cranial fossa and the tentorium are more often associated with CVR and are therefore more likely to behave aggressively than are lesions in other locations. This reflects the pattern of regional venous anatomy in these locations. For example, anterior cranial fossa DAVFs cannot drain into any venous sinuses and can only drain into cortical veins and are therefore always associated with CVR.[19] Table 90-4 shows the anatomic location of intracranial DAVFs. They are named according to the dural sinus with which they are associated.[52] This section deals

with the anatomy and surgical management of DAVFs in specific locations.

Transverse/Sigmoid Sinus Dural Arteriovenous Fistulas

Transverse/sigmoid sinus DAVFs are the most common intracranial DAVFs, accounting for 4% to 60% of cases (see Table 90-4).[28,36,43] Their arterial supply is derived mainly from branches of the ECA, namely, the transmastoid branches of the occipital artery, the posterior auricular artery, the posterior branch of the middle meningeal artery, and the neuromeningeal division of the ascending pharyngeal artery. They may also receive arterial supply from the posterior meningeal branch of the vertebral artery, the tentorial branch of the meningohypophyseal trunk of the ICA, and the petrous bone.[8,28] Venous drainage may be through the ipsilateral transverse/sigmoid sinuses or through the contralateral side if the ipsilateral sinus is occluded. Occasionally, these lesions drain into the diploic veins, which may lead to significant hemorrhage during craniotomy. CVR may occur through temporal, occipital, and cerebellar veins.[4,7]

If endovascular therapy fails, surgery should be performed in cases with CVR. Preoperative transarterial embolization is very helpful in reducing intraoperative bleeding and should be used whenever possible. The patient is placed in the park-bench position with the side of the lesion up. It is important to have access to the region between the inion and the mastoid. A lazy "S"-shaped incision is made two fingerbreadths behind the ear. The occipital and posterior auricular arteries, which are usually enlarged, should be doubly ligated and divided. In some cases, this interrupts the main arterial supply to the DAVF. The nuchal muscles are incised using monopolar cautery, leaving a small cuff of fascia at the superior nuchal line. The muscles are then scraped off

TABLE 90-4 ▪ Anatomic Location of 236 Dural Arteriovenous Fistulas Managed by the University of Toronto Brain Vascular Malformation Study Group

Anatomic Location	No. (% of all DAVFs)	No. with CVR (% of DAVFs in This Location)
Transverse sigmoid	100 (42.4)	38 (38)
Cavernous sinus	79 (33.5)	29 (36.7)
Deep venous/tentorial incisural	20 (8.5)	20 (100)
Superior sagittal sinus and convexity	12 (5.1)	12 (100)
Foramen magnum	11 (4.6)	9 (81.8)
Anterior cranial fossa	9 (3.8)	9 (100)
Temporal fossa	4 (1.7)	1 (25)
Superior petrosal sinus	1 (0.4)	1 (100)

CVR, cortical venous reflux; DAVFs, dural arteriovenous fistulas.

the bone using subperiosteal dissection. A craniotomy is performed to expose the transverse sinus and the dura superior and inferior to it. Great care must be taken to prevent a dural laceration while performing the craniotomy as this may lead to torrential hemorrhage from enlarged dural feeding arteries. The cutting bit of a high-speed drill may be used for performing the craniotomy. The bone is gradually removed along the margin of the bone plate until the dura can be seen through a thin layer of bone. The dura is gently separated from the bone flap, and the bone flap is elevated using a periosteal elevator.[39] Significant hemorrhage from the dura when elevating the bone flap may be controlled by placing a large piece of Gelfoam or Surgicel over the dura and applying pressure with a wet sponge for a few minutes. Dural feeders can be coagulated using bipolar cautery or occluded using hemostatic clips.

The remainder of the procedure depends on the goal of treatment, which should have been decided preoperatively. If the goal of treatment is CVR disconnection only, then the dura is incised above or below the transverse sinus depending on the location of CVR (i.e., temporal/occipital or cerebellar). The dural flap is reflected on a base along the transverse sinus. The arterialized leptomeningeal vein or veins should then be identified, coagulated or clipped, and divided as close to the fistula as possible. It is important to ensure that all arterialized leptomeningeal veins are disconnected. The dura is then closed in the usual manner. If the mastoid air cells have been entered, they should be obliterated using bone wax. The bone flap is then replaced, and muscle, fascia, and scalp are closed as usual.

If the goal of treatment is complete excision of the fistula and the sinus can be sacrificed, then after performing the craniotomy as described previously, the mastoid and posterolateral portion of the petrous bone are removed using a diamond burr on a high-speed drill to expose the dura lateral and anterior to the sigmoid sinus.[38,39] Knowledge of the anatomy of this region or assistance from an otolaryngologist is important to avoid damage to hearing or to the facial nerve during this stage of the procedure.[38] At this point, bleeding is mainly from arterial feeders contained within the petrous bone, which should be controlled using bone wax. The dura is incised above and below the transverse sinus and parallel to its long axis. Feeding arteries are coagulated or clipped as they are encountered. The transverse sinus is then occluded medially using two curved hemostats placed approximately 2 cm apart. The sinus is cut between the two hemostats, the ends are closed using 3-0 silk

transfixion sutures, and the hemostats are removed. The dural incisions above and below the sinus are then continued laterally. Gentle retraction on the occipital lobe and the cerebellum exposes the tentorium, which should also be cut in a medial to lateral direction to interrupt any tentorial feeding arteries. All arterialized leptomeningeal veins are also coagulated and divided. The dural and tentorial incisions are extended laterally, distal to the junction of the transverse and sigmoid sinuses, which is usually the site of the fistula. The skeletonized sinus is resected distal to this site. The sigmoid sinus is then evaluated for patency. If there is a significant vein of Labbé, the sigmoid sinus should be left patent to drain it. However, if the vein of Labbé is arterialized and is not used for venous drainage of the brain, it can be clipped and divided, and the sigmoid sinus is then packed with Surgicel or Gelfoam and ligated. Duraplasty using fascia lata, pericranium, or synthetic dura is then performed to close the dural defect. The mastoid air cells are completely obliterated using bone wax, and the bone flap is replaced. The nuchal muscles and fascia are closed in multiple layers to prevent cerebrospinal fluid leak. The scalp is closed in the usual manner. Intraoperative angiography is used to ensure complete excision of the nidus.

Cavernous Sinus Dural Arteriovenous Fistulas

These are the second most common intracranial DAVFs, accounting for a third of all lesions in our series (see Table 90-4).[8,28,43] They are supplied by branches from the ICAs, ECAs, or both. Venous drainage is via the cavernous sinus, with subsequent anterior drainage into the superior and inferior ophthalmic veins, posterior drainage into the superior and inferior petrosal sinuses (IPSs), or cortical venous drainage into the sphenoparietal sinus, sylvian, uncal, and anterior pontomesencephalic veins.[7,28] Barrow and colleagues[23] classified carotid cavernous fistulas into four categories based on the type of feeding arteries detected on angiography. Type A fistulas are direct fistulas between the ICA and the cavernous sinus. Types B, C, and D are DAVFs involving the cavernous sinus. Type B are fed by meningeal branches of the ICA, type C by meningeal branches of ECA, and type D by meningeal branches of both ICA and ECA. Type A fistulas are high-flow fistulas and usually result from a traumatic tear in the cavernous ICA or spontaneously from a rupture of an intracavernous ICA aneurysm. These high-flow fistulas rarely resolve spontaneously and require treatment to prevent progressive visual loss, intolerable bruit, or pain.[19] They are almost always treated by endovascular embolization and are not dealt with in this chapter. Most spontaneous carotid cavernous fistulas are of the low-flow types B, C, or D and are referred to as cavernous sinus DAVFs. They are usually idiopathic and occur most commonly in middle-aged women. They may present with proptosis, chemosis, diplopia, visual loss, pulsatile bruit, retro-orbital pain, and facial pain.[35] Cavernous sinus DAVFs may present with ophthalmologic symptoms on the contralateral side. Unlike type A fistulas, a significant proportion of these low-flow fistulas undergo spontaneous resolution.

Cavernous sinus DAVFs can also be classified according to the pattern of venous drainage based on the Borden or Cognard classification. As with other DAVFs, it is the presence or absence of CVR that determines the natural history of these lesions. CVR occurs in 19% to 37% of patients with cavernous sinus DAVFs (see Table 90-4).[35,53] CVR is more common in patients with bilateral orbital signs but can also occur in those with unilateral signs. In a study of 118 patients with cavernous sinus DAVFs, 43% of patients with bilateral orbital signs and 9% of those with unilateral orbital signs had CVR.[53] Cavernous sinus DAVFs without CVR usually have a benign clinical course. Many of these lesions undergo spontaneous involution, with symptom resolution over weeks or months.[28] The majority of patients can be managed conservatively but must be followed up closely by a neuro-ophthalmologist. Although these lesions have been referred to as benign, in some cases, spontaneous venous thrombosis and venous hypertension may result in increased intraocular pressure and progressive visual loss.[7] Medical therapy including topical agents, oral corticosteroids, and systemic anticoagulation may be used to prevent blindness. However, if medical therapy fails to control intraocular pressure and deteriorating vision, prompt endovascular treatment is indicated.[7] Transarterial embolization using particles may be tried first to slow down the flow through the fistula. If this fails, transvenous embolization is required.

If CVR exists, these DAVFs must be treated with the same aggressiveness as DAVFs in other locations. This is usually done using transvenous embolization. Before this, transarterial embolization may be performed, particularly if there is significant supply through ECA branches. For transvenous embolization, access to the cavernous sinus is usually obtained by the femoral route through the internal jugular vein and the IPS. This venous approach may be difficult or impossible in cases in which the IPS is partially or completely thrombosed. However, with improved materials and experience, some surgeons have successfully navigated an angiographic catheter, even through a thrombosed IPS.[54] If access through the IPS is not possible or has failed, other routes may be employed. These may involve endovascular and/or surgical techniques. The approach depends on the direction of venous drainage of the fistula and may use the superior ophthalmic vein (SOV), the facial and angular veins, the pterygoid plexus, the superior petrosal sinus, the refluxing cortical veins, or direct surgical puncture of the cavernous sinus.[34] The goal of transvenous embolization is to occlude the venous side of the lesion. This is usually achieved by placing coils into the cavernous sinus.

Obliteration of the venous side of the lesion can result in the total disappearance of the fistula.[28] However, in some cases of successful treatment, thrombosis may extend into the orbital veins, and this may lead to venous hypertension and paradoxical visual deterioration.[7] This may require treatment with oral corticosteroids, antiplatelet therapy, or anticoagulation.

If endovascular therapy fails, surgery is indicated in cases with persistent CVR or when vision is at risk. The role of surgery in the treatment of cavernous sinus DAVFs is mainly in providing venous access to the cavernous sinus in cases in which access through the femoral route is not possible. Several options are available, including cannulation of the SOV, cannulation of refluxing intracranial veins such as the sylvian veins, or direct exposure of the cavernous sinus.[34]

The SOV approach is often performed by a team consisting of an ophthalmologist, a neurosurgeon, and a neuroradiologist.[55] The procedure is performed under general anesthesia and under fluoroscopic guidance. A sheath is placed in a common femoral artery to allow intraoperative angiography. The skin incision is made in the nasal part of the superior sulcus of the upper eyelid, under magnification provided by an operating microscope.[55] The incision is carried down through the orbicularis oculi muscle. The orbital septum is then opened, exposing the retroseptal orbital fat. The SOV is then identified and cleaned of the surrounding orbital fat to expose a segment of vein 5 to 20 mm in length. Two ligatures (2-0 silk suture) are placed around the vein approximately 1 cm apart. A sheath is then inserted into the vein between the ligatures, and thrombogenic material (such as platinum coils) is injected into the cavernous sinus under fluoroscopy. At the end of the procedure, an intraoperative angiogram is performed through the femoral sheath to ensure complete closure of the fistula. The SOV sheath is then removed, the vein is suture ligated, and the lid incision is closed. Alternatives to surgical exposure of the SOV have been reported and include direct percutaneous puncture of the SOV under angiographic guidance, direct percutaneous puncture of the facial vein under sonographic guidance, and transvenous transfemoral access to the facial vein.[34,35] In cases in which the facial vein is catheterized, the catheter is advanced into the angular vein, then into the SOV, and finally into the cavernous sinus.

In rare instances, a cavernous sinus DAVF may only drain by retrograde flow into cortical veins, and there may be no access through the IPSs, the ophthalmic veins, or the pterygoid plexus. In such cases, access to the cavernous sinus may be achieved via the refluxing cortical vein (e.g., a refluxing sylvian vein). This has been described using the percutaneous transfemoral technique and also by surgical exposure of the cortical vein.[34]

Direct microsurgery of cavernous sinus DAVFs has also been described,[9,56–58] but with advances in endovascular embolization, these techniques are rarely required. These procedures require surgical experience and detailed knowledge of the anatomy of the cavernous sinus. The cavernous sinus is approached through triangles that are formed by convergence and divergence of the cranial nerves in the region of the cavernous sinus and the middle fossa.[25] The selection of approach is determined by the pattern of venous drainage of the fistula, and the degree of familiarity of the surgeon. The two main approaches used are described below.

The anteroinferior extradural approach to the cavernous sinus is suitable for anteriorly draining fistulas and is performed through a standard pterional craniotomy. After administration of intravenous mannitol, the dura is reflected away from the anterior and anteromedial walls of the middle fossa to expose the lateral wall of the cavernous sinus. The posterior aspect of the orbital roof is then drilled all the way to the lateral aspect of the anterior clinoid process. The superior orbital fissure region is exposed, the periorbita is opened, and the cranial nerves are identified. The superior or inferior orbital vein is then identified. An intraoperative Doppler probe may be used to localize the high arterial flow in these veins.[58] An atraumatic intravenous cannula is then inserted into the vein, and a guidewire is directed posteriorly into the cavernous sinus. A catheter is then introduced over the guidewire into the cavernous sinus and used to introduce thrombogenic material such as coils to obliterate the fistula. An intraoperative angiogram is performed to confirm adequate obliteration of the sinus. It must be noted that it may be difficult to identify the ophthalmic veins in a low-flow fistula.[9]

The posterosuperior approach is appropriate for posteriorly draining fistulas. It is performed through a pterional craniotomy. After opening the dura, the sylvian fissure is split widely to allow gentle retraction of the frontal and temporal lobes. The oculomotor nerve is then identified as a landmark. Underneath the oculomotor nerve, the superior petrosal sinus is identified and followed proximally to its origin from the cavernous sinus. Thrombogenic material is injected through the superior petrosal sinus into the cavernous sinus.[9] If the superior petrosal sinus cannot be identified, the cavernous sinus can be packed through Parkinson's triangle, bounded by the lower margin of the trochlear nerve, the upper margin of the ophthalmic division of trigeminal nerve, and a line connecting the point of entry of trochlear nerve into the dura to the point of entry of trigeminal nerve into Meckel's cave.[25] An intraoperative angiogram is performed to confirm complete occlusion of the fistula. The dura is closed as usual, the bone flap is repositioned, and the temporalis muscle, galea, and skin are closed in layers. Combined and more extensive approaches to the cavernous sinus, with opening and packing of all triangles, have been described but are rarely necessary.[56]

Anterior Cranial Fossa Dural Arteriovenous Fistulas

The arterial supply to the anterior cranial fossa dura is derived mainly from the ICA through the ophthalmic artery, which gives off the anterior and posterior ethmoidal arteries within the orbit. The ethmoidal arteries leave the orbit to enter the ethmoidal air cells. The smaller of the two, the posterior ethmoidal artery, supplies the dura in the region of planum sphenoidale. The anterior ethmoidal artery gives origin to the falcine artery and supplies the dura of the medial and inferior portions of the anterior cranial fossa. As well as supply from the ethmoidal arteries, DAVFs in this region may also recruit dural arterial supply via the anterior division of the middle meningeal arteries from both dural convexities and transcranial arterial supply via engorged scalp arteries.[28] The venous drainage of anterior cranial fossa DAVFs is always via cortical venous drainage through the frontal and olfactory veins.[4,7] The cortical veins may often be variceal. This constant presence of CVR explains the high incidence of aggressive clinical behavior for lesions in this location. They must therefore be treated aggressively to eliminate CVR. Anterior fossa DAVFs are rarely cured by endovascular means. Transarterial embolization is usually limited to ECA branches. Embolization of ophthalmic artery branches is usually avoided as it carries the risk of central retinal artery occlusion and visual compromise.[59] Transvenous embolization has been described in case reports[60] but is not possible for most lesions in this location due to lack of venous access. Surgery is associated with high cure rates and low complication rates and is the treatment of choice for most anterior fossa DAVFs.[59] This is performed through a low unilateral frontal craniotomy in the supine position with minimal retraction of the frontal lobes. A unilateral craniotomy allows disconnection of leptomeningeal veins on both sides via the transfalcine route. Alternatively, a bifrontal craniotomy may be performed. The next step is to disconnect the arterialized leptomeningeal veins, which should be coagulated and divided. Excision of the dura involved with the fistula is not necessary.[59]

Superior Sagittal Sinus (Convexity) Dural Arteriovenous Fistulas

The arterial supply to these lesions is from the middle meningeal arteries. The venous drainage may be into the superior sagittal sinus, into cortical veins, or both. If CVR exists, the lesion must be treated to prevent future hemorrhage or neurologic deficit. Few cases of successful curative endovascular treatment have been reported.[8,61] Surgical treatment is therefore required in most cases and involves disconnection of CVR. The lesion is usually approached through a unilateral craniotomy on the side of the fistula. Preoperative transarterial embolization is used to reduce the amount of hemorrhage from scalp and dura.

In some cases without CVR, there may be a high-flow fistula that shunts into a patent superior sagittal sinus. These lesions may be associated with papilledema.[28] These cases may be managed with extensive transarterial embolization or surgical skeletonization of the superior sagittal sinus to reduce the flow through the fistula. Other options include the use of lumboperitoneal shunting or optic nerve sheath decompression for treatment of papilledema.[28]

Deep-Seated and Posterior Fossa Dural Arteriovenous Fistulas

This group consists of lesions associated with the deep veins (tentorial incisura), superior petrosal sinus, IPS, or the marginal sinus (foramen magnum). As with DAVFs in other locations, deep-seated and posterior fossa lesions without CVR can be observed or treated palliatively by transarterial embolization of the arterial feeders. Lesions with CVR should be treated aggressively until all CVR is disconnected. This may be achieved by endovascular or surgical means.[42,43,52] Extensive resection of the nidus, which was performed in the past, often requires complex skull base approaches, carries significant risk of morbidity, and is unnecessary. If endovascular treatment fails to eliminate

CVR, surgical disconnection can be performed with relatively little risk to the patient.[42,43]

Deep Venous (Tentorial Incisura) Dural Arteriovenous Fistulas

These lesions are located at the tentorial incisura and involve the deep venous system. They may extend along the straight sinus to involve the falx. Their arterial supply may be bilateral and is derived from the tentorial dural branches of the ECA, ICA, and vertebral and posterior cerebral arteries. Angiography may reveal hypertrophy of embryonic dural arteries, including the artery of Bernasconi and Cassinari (tentorial branch of the meningohypophyseal trunk of the ICA) and the artery of Davidoff and Schecter (dural branch of the posterior cerebral artery).[28] Venous drainage is almost always leptomeningeal and involves the basal vein of Rosenthal, the lateral mesencephalic veins, and the vein of Galen.[7,8] Fistulas at this location may have infra- or supratentorial cortical venous drainage or drainage into spinal medullary veins.[42] The presence of CVR explains the high incidence of ICH and neurologic deficit with these lesions. Drainage into the spinal medullary veins may be associated with progressive quadriparesis.[62] Surgical exposure of these lesions may be performed using a posterior parasagittal craniotomy and interhemispheric approach with the trajectory posterior to the splenium of the corpus callosum.[63] Surgical treatment consists of CVR disconnection.

Superior Petrosal Sinus Dural Arteriovenous Fistulas

These lesions are often included in the same group as the deep venous DAVFs and together are referred to as tentorial DAVFs. Other authors have grouped them separately because they are located at the petrous ridge and involve the superior petrosal sinus.[8,52] The arterial supply is from dural branches of the ECA, ICA, and the vertebrobasilar system. Most cases are associated with thrombosis of the superior petrosal sinus on either side of the fistula site, with venous drainage diverted into cortical veins.[8,52] ICH is the most common mode of presentation. In a series of 18 patients reported by Ng and colleagues,[52] 17 (94%) had CVR and 9 (50%) presented with ICH. Ocular symptoms may occur if there is venous reflux into the cavernous sinus and the SOV. Trigeminal neuralgia may occur secondary to irritation of the trigeminal ganglion in Meckel's cave by dilated tortuous feeding arteries or compression of the trigeminal nerve at the root entry zone by a dilated petrosal vein. Surgical excision of this type of DAVF may require an extensive skull base approach consisting of subtemporal craniotomy, posterior petrosectomy, and suboccipital craniotomy.[63] These extensive procedures are usually unnecessary, and treatment should focus on disconnection of CVR only.

Inferior Petrosal Sinus Dural Arteriovenous Fistulas

The main arterial supply to these lesions is usually from the dural and muscular branches of the vertebral arteries and dural branches from the ascending pharyngeal, middle meningeal, and occipital branches of the ECA.

Venous drainage may be retrograde up the IPS and into the cavernous sinus. This may result in presentation with ocular symptoms similar to those of cavernous sinus DAVFs. Alternatively, venous drainage may flow into the ipsilateral jugular bulb, resulting in pulsatile tinnitus.[8] Retrograde flow up the ipsilateral sigmoid and transverse sinuses and into the contralateral transverse/sigmoid sinuses or into the straight and superior sagittal sinuses may also occur.[63] Surgical exposure may be performed using the far lateral suboccipital approach.[63] Treatment consists of CVR disconnection.

Marginal Sinus (Foramen Magnum Region) Dural Arteriovenous Fistulas

These lesions are rare. The marginal sinus encircles the foramen magnum and communicates with the basal venous plexus of the clivus anteriorly and with the occipital sinus posteriorly. It normally drains to the sigmoid sinus or jugular bulb through a series of small sinuses.[64] Fistulas in this area have often been grouped together with posterior fossa DAVFs or referred to as foramen magnum region DAVFs. Their arterial supply is usually from the muscular branches of the vertebral artery, the transmastoid perforators of the occipital artery, the neuromeningeal division of the ascending pharyngeal artery, and the posterior clival dural branches of the meningohypophyseal trunk of the ICA.[64] Venous drainage may be into the sigmoid sinus/jugular vein, in which case the patient may complain of pulsatile tinnitus, or into the IPS, which may lead to venous engorgement in the ipsilateral cavernous sinus and ocular symptoms.[28,64] CVR may lead to ICH, and reflux into the spinal medullary veins may result in progressive myelopathy and quadriparesis.[65] These lesions are surgically approached through a posterior paramedian craniocervical exposure, with the patient in the semiprone position. The venous plexus surrounding the vertebral artery may be arterialized and require meticulous hemostasis during exposure. Suboccipital craniotomy and laminectomy at the appropriate levels are then performed. The dura is extensively coagulated and opened. Refluxing leptomeningeal veins communicate with arterialized tortuous posterior and/or anterior medullary veins. The refluxing leptomeningeal veins are coagulated or clipped and divided, whereas the anterior and posterior medullary veins should be left intact.

OUTCOME AND COMPLICATIONS OF TREATMENT

Between 1984 and 2001, 236 cranial DAVFs have been managed by the University of Toronto Brain Vascular Malformation Study Group. Of these, 117 did not have CVR (Borden type I and Cognard types I and IIa) and were managed by observation alone or by palliative treatment. Of these patients, 98% had a benign clinical course.[3] The other 119 patients had DAVFs with CVR (Borden types II and III, and Cognard type IIb, IIa + b, III, or IV). Three patients were lost to follow-up after initial assessment, and 14 patients declined treatment. The remaining 102 patients were treated.[43] Forty-seven patients (46.1%) were treated by disconnection of CVR, 49 (48%) had complete obliteration of the fistula, and 6 (5.9%) were partially treated. The six partially treated patients had persistent CVR but

TABLE 90-5 ▪ Complications of Treatment in 102 Patients with Cranial Dural Arteriovenous Fistulas with Cortical Venous Reflux

Complication	Surgery (74 Procedures)	Endovascular Embolization (120 Procedures)
Significant blood loss	8	0
Memory dysfunction	1	1
Seizures	1	0
Cranial nerve deficit	1	0
Hemorrhage	1	0
Meningitis	1	0
Embolic transient ischemic attack	0	1
Groin hematoma	0	1

From Van Dijk JM, Ter Brugge KG, Willinsky RA, Wallace MC: Selective disconnection of cortical venous reflux as treatment for cranial dural arteriovenous fistulas. J Neurosurg 101:31–35, 2004.

refused or were physically unable to undergo further treatment. Therefore, complete obliteration of the fistula or CVR disconnection was achieved in 94.1% of patients. This was achieved by endovascular treatment alone in 26 patients (25.5%), by surgery alone in 25 patients (24.5%), and by a combination of endovascular and surgical treatments in 45 patients (44%). Multiple treatment sessions were required in some patients, resulting in 120 endovascular and 74 surgical procedures. The complications of treatment were all transient and are outlined in Table 90-5. No deaths or permanent neurologic deficits occurred in this series. The mean follow-up period was 3.7 years (741 patient-years). Control angiography was performed in 93 patients (91.2%). CVR disconnection was equally effective in lowering the risk of aggressive events as total obliteration of the fistula.[43]

SUMMARY

The clinical presentation and natural history of DAVFs are determined by their pattern of venous drainage. Lesions without CVR behave in a benign fashion and do not require curative treatment. Lesions with CVR have a 15% annual adverse event rate (ICH and NHND) and a 10% annual mortality rate and should be managed aggressively with the aim of eliminating all refluxing cortical veins. Treatment of DAVFs should be performed in a multidisciplinary setting and may consist of transarterial embolization, transvenous embolization, surgery, or a combination of these. Endovascular treatment should be tried first. If surgery is indicated, CVR disconnection is effective in eliminating the risk of future aggressive clinical events and carries less morbidity compared with complete excision of the lesion. All patients should be followed up for life, and any change in symptoms (deterioration or improvement) should be investigated with repeat cerebral angiography to look for development of CVR.

REFERENCES

1. Awad IA, Little JR, Akarawi WP, et al: Intracranial dural arteriovenous malformations: Factors predisposing to an aggressive neurological course. J Neurosurg 72:839–850, 1990.
2. Al-Shahi R, Bhattacharya JJ, Currie DG, et al: Prospective, population-based detection of intracranial vascular malformations in adults: The Scottish Intracranial Vascular Malformation Study (SIVMS). Stroke 34:1163–1169, 2003.
3. Satomi J, van Dijk JM, Terbrugge KG, et al: Benign cranial dural arteriovenous fistulas: Outcome of conservative management based on the natural history of the lesion. J Neurosurg 97:767–770, 2002.
4. Sarma D, ter Brugge K: Management of intracranial dural arteriovenous shunts in adults. Eur J Radiol 46:206–220, 2003.
5. Herman JM, Spetzler RF, Bederson JB, et al: Genesis of a dural arteriovenous malformation in a rat model. J Neurosurg 83:539–545, 1995.
6. Terada T, Higashida RT, Halbach VV, et al: Development of acquired arteriovenous fistulas in rats due to venous hypertension. J Neurosurg 80:884–889, 1994.
7. van Dijk JM, Willinsky RA: Venous congestive encephalopathy related to cranial dural arteriovenous fistulas. Neuroimaging Clin N Am 13:55–72, 2003.
8. Malek AM, Halbach VV, Higashida RT, et al: Treatment of dural arteriovenous malformations and fistulas. Neurosurg Clin N Am 11:147–166, 2000.
9. Mullan S: Treatment of carotid-cavernous fistulas by cavernous sinus occlusion. J Neurosurg 50:131–144, 1979.
10. Hamada Y, Goto K, Inoue T, et al: Histopathological aspects of dural arteriovenous fistulas in the transverse-sigmoid sinus region in nine patients. Neurosurgery 40:452–458, 1997.
11. Terada T, Tsuura M, Komai N, et al: The role of angiogenic factor bFGF in the development of dural AVFs. Acta Neurochir (Wien) 138:877–883, 1996.
12. Uranishi R, Nakase H, Sakaki T: Expression of angiogenic growth factors in dural arteriovenous fistula. J Neurosurg 91:781–786, 1999.
13. Lawton MT, Jacobowitz R, Spetzler RF: Redefined role of angiogenesis in the pathogenesis of dural arteriovenous malformations. J Neurosurg 87:267–274, 1997.
14. Luciani A, Houdart E, Mounayer C, et al: Spontaneous closure of dural arteriovenous fistulas: Report of three cases and review of the literature. AJNR Am J Neuroradiol 22:992–996, 2001.
15. Lalwani AK, Dowd CF, Halbach VV: Grading venous restrictive disease in patients with dural arteriovenous fistulas of the transverse/sigmoid sinus. J Neurosurg 79:11–15, 1993.
16. Borden JA, Wu JK, Shucart WA: A proposed classification for spinal and cranial dural arteriovenous fistulous malformations and implications for treatment. J Neurosurg 82:166–179, 1995.
17. Cognard C, Gobin YP, Pierot L, et al: Cerebral dural arteriovenous fistulas: Clinical and angiographic correlation with a revised classification of venous drainage. Radiology 194:671–680, 1995.
18. Djindjian R, Merland JJ, Theron J: Superselective Arteriography of the External carotid Artery. New York: Springer-Verlag, 1977.
19. Davies MA, TerBrugge K, Willinsky R, et al: The validity of classification for the clinical presentation of intracranial dural arteriovenous fistulas. J Neurosurg 85:830–837, 1996.
20. van Dijk JM, terBrugge KG, Willinsky RA, et al: Clinical course of cranial dural arteriovenous fistulas with long-term persistent cortical venous reflux. Stroke 33:1233–1236, 2002.
21. Aminoff MJ: Vascular anomalies in the intracranial dura mater. Brain 96:601–612, 1973.
22. Malik GM, Pearce JE, Ausman JI, et al: Dural arteriovenous malformations and intracranial hemorrhage. Neurosurgery 15:332–339, 1984.
23. Barrow DL, Spector RH, Braun IF, et al: Classification and treatment of spontaneous carotid-cavernous sinus fistulas. J Neurosurg 62:248–256, 1985.
24. Lasjaunias P, Chiu M, ter Brugge K, et al: Neurological manifestations of intracranial dural arteriovenous malformations. J Neurosurg 64:724–730, 1986.
25. Rhoton AL, Jr: The cavernous sinus, the cavernous venous plexus, and the carotid collar. Neurosurgery 51:S375–S410, 2002.
26. Stiebel-Kalish H, Setton A, Nimii Y, et al: Cavernous sinus dural arteriovenous malformations: Patterns of venous drainage are related to clinical signs and symptoms. Ophthalmology 109:1685–1691, 2002.
27. Noguchi K, Melhem ER, Kanazawa T, et al: Intracranial dural arteriovenous fistulas: Evaluation with combined 3D time-of-flight MR angiography and MR digital subtraction angiography. AJR Am J Roentgenol 182:183–190, 2004.
28. Awad IA: Dural arteriovenous malformations. In Carter LP, Spetzler RF, Hamilton MG (eds): Neurovascular Surgery. New York: McGraw-Hill, 1995, pp 905–932.

29. van Dijk JM, TerBrugge KG, Willinsky RA, et al: Multiplicity of dural arteriovenous fistulas. J Neurosurg 96:76–78, 2002.
30. Willinsky R, Goyal M, terBrugge K, et al: Tortuous, engorged pial veins in intracranial dural arteriovenous fistulas: Correlations with presentation, location, and MR findings in 122 patients. AJNR Am J Neuroradiol 20:1031–1036, 1999.
31. Halbach VV, Higashida RT, Hieshima GB, et al: Dural fistulas involving the cavernous sinus: Results of treatment in 30 patients. Radiology 163:437–442, 1987.
32. Nelson PK, Russell SM, Woo HH, et al: Use of a wedged microcatheter for curative transarterial embolization of complex intracranial dural arteriovenous fistulas: Indications, endovascular technique, and outcome in 21 patients. J Neurosurg 98:498–506, 2003.
33. Lasjaunias P, Berenstein A, ter Brugge K: Surgical Neuroangiography: Clinical Vascular Anatomy and Variations, vol 1, 2nd ed. Berlin: Springer-Verlag, 2001.
34. Klisch J, Huppertz HJ, Spetzger U, et al: Transvenous treatment of carotid cavernous and dural arteriovenous fistulae: Results for 31 patients and review of the literature. Neurosurgery 53:836–857, 2003.
35. Meyers PM, Halbach VV, Dowd CF, et al: Dural carotid cavernous fistula: Definitive endovascular management and long-term follow-up. Am J Ophthalmol 134:85–92, 2002.
36. Caragine LP, Halbach VV, Dowd CF, et al: Parallel venous channel as the recipient pouch in transverse/sigmoid sinus dural fistulae. Neurosurgery 53:1261–1267, 2003.
37. Houdart E, Saint-Maurice JP, Chapot R, et al: Transcranial approach for venous embolization of dural arteriovenous fistulas. J Neurosurg 97:280–286, 2002.
38. Ojemann RG, Heros RC, Crowell RM: Dural arteriovenous malformations. In Surgical Management of Cerebrovascular Disease, 2nd ed. Baltimore: Williams & Wilkins, 1988, pp 415–425.
39. Sundt TM, Jr, Piepgras DG: The surgical approach to arteriovenous malformations of the lateral and sigmoid dural sinuses. J Neurosurg 59:32–39, 1983.
40. Collice M, D'Aliberti G, Arena O, et al: Surgical treatment of intracranial dural arteriovenous fistulae: Role of venous drainage. Neurosurgery 47:56–67, 2000.
41. Thompson BG, Doppman JL, Oldfield EH: Treatment of cranial dural arteriovenous fistulae by interruption of leptomeningeal venous drainage. J Neurosurg 80:617–623, 1994.
42. Tomak PR, Cloft HJ, Kaga A, et al: Evolution of the management of tentorial dural arteriovenous malformations. Neurosurgery 52:750–762, 2003.
43. Van Dijk JM, Ter Brugge KG, Willinsky RA, Wallace MC: Selective disconnection of cortical venous reflux as treatment for cranial dural arteriovenous fistulas. J Neurosurg, 101:31–35, 2004.
44. Shin M, Kurita H, Tago M, et al: Stereotactic radiosurgery for tentorial dural arteriovenous fistulae draining into the vein of Galen: Report of two cases. Neurosurgery 46:730–734, 2000.
45. Friedman JA, Pollock BE, Nichols DA, et al: Results of combined stereotactic radiosurgery and transarterial embolization for dural arteriovenous fistulas of the transverse and sigmoid sinuses. J Neurosurg 94:886–891, 2001.
46. Pollock BE, Nichols DA, Garrity JA, et al: Stereotactic radiosurgery and particulate embolization for cavernous sinus dural arteriovenous fistulae. Neurosurgery 45:459–467, 1999.
47. Pan DH, Chung WY, Guo WY, et al: Stereotactic radiosurgery for the treatment of dural arteriovenous fistulas involving the transverse-sigmoid sinus. J Neurosurg 96:823–829, 2002.
48. O'Leary S, Hodgson TJ, Coley SC, et al: Intracranial dural arteriovenous malformations: Results of stereotactic radiosurgery in 17 patients. Clin Oncol (R Coll Radiol) 14:97–102, 2002.
49. Guo WY, Pan DH, Wu HM, et al: Radiosurgery as a treatment alternative for dural arteriovenous fistulas of the cavernous sinus. AJNR Am J Neuroradiol 19:1081–1087, 1998.
50. Duffau H, Lopes M, Janosevic V, et al: Early rebleeding from intracranial dural arteriovenous fistulas: Report of 20 cases and review of the literature. J Neurosurg 90:78–84, 1999.
51. Collice M, D'Aliberti G, Talamonti G, et al: Surgical interruption of leptomeningeal drainage as treatment for intracranial dural arteriovenous fistulas without dural sinus drainage. J Neurosurg 84:810–817, 1996.
52. Ng PP, Halbach VV, Quinn R, et al: Endovascular treatment for dural arteriovenous fistulae of the superior petrosal sinus. Neurosurgery 53:25–33, 2003.
53. Stiebel-Kalish H, Setton A, Berenstein A, et al: Bilateral orbital signs predict cortical venous drainage in cavernous sinus dural AVMs. Neurology 58:1521–1524, 2002.
54. Benndorf G, Bender A, Lehmann R, et al: Transvenous occlusion of dural cavernous sinus fistulas through the thrombosed inferior petrosal sinus: Report of four cases and review of the literature. Surg Neurol 54:42–54, 2000.
55. Miller NR, Monsein LH, Debrun GM, et al: Treatment of carotid-cavernous sinus fistulas using a superior ophthalmic vein approach. J Neurosurg 83:838–842, 1995.
56. Day JD, Fukushima T: Direct microsurgery of dural arteriovenous malformation type carotid-cavernous sinus fistulas: Indications, technique, and results. Neurosurgery 41:1119–1126, 1997.
57. Tu YK, Liu HM, Hu SC: Direct surgery of carotid cavernous fistulae and dural arteriovenous malformations of the cavernous sinus. Neurosurgery 41:798–806, 1997.
58. Krisht AF, Burson T: Combined pretemporal and endovascular approach to the cavernous sinus for the treatment of carotid-cavernous dural fistulae: Technical case report. Neurosurgery 44:415–418, 1999.
59. Lawton MT, Chun J, Wilson CB, Halbach VV: Ethmoidal dural arteriovenous fistulae: An assessment of surgical and endovascular management. Neurosurgery 45:805–811, 1999.
60. Defreyne L, Vanlangenhove P, Vandekerckhove T, et al: Transvenous embolization of a dural arteriovenous fistula of the anterior cranial fossa: preliminary results. AJNR Am J Neuroradiol 21:761–765, 2000.
61. Fukai J, Terada T, Kuwata T, et al: Transarterial intravenous coil embolization of dural arteriovenous fistula involving the superior sagittal sinus. Surg Neurol 55:353–358, 2001.
62. Ricolfi F, Manelfe C, Meder JF, et al: Intracranial dural arteriovenous fistulae with perimedullary venous drainage. Anatomical, clinical and therapeutic considerations. Neuroradiology 41:803–812, 1999.
63. Lewis AI, Rosenblatt SS, Tew JM, Jr: Surgical management of deep-seated dural arteriovenous malformations. J Neurosurg 87:198–206, 1997.
64. McDougall CG, Halbach VV, Dowd CF, et al: Dural arteriovenous fistulas of the marginal sinus. AJNR Am J Neuroradiol 18:1565–1572, 1997.
65. Pierot L, Chiras J, Meder JF, et al: Dural arteriovenous fistulas of the posterior fossa draining into subarachnoid veins. AJNR Am J Neuroradiol 13:315–323, 1992.

91 Surgical Management of Cavernous Malformations of the Nervous System

SEPIDEH AMIN-HANJANI, ROBERT G. OJEMANN, and CHRISTOPHER S. OGILVY

INTRODUCTION

Cavernous malformations (CMs) have long been recognized as one of the major clinicopathologic categories of vascular malformations of the nervous system.[1-3] Because no abnormal vascularity is seen on angiography, CMs have been included in the descriptions of cryptic or occult vascular malformations, a term that has been used to describe any vascular malformation that cannot be seen on angiography.[4-9] The term cavernous angioma was used by Russell and Rubinstein[3] in their excellent description of the pathology of these lesions. CMs have also been called cavernous hemangiomas or cavernomas, but more recently the term cavernous malformation has become more widely accepted, explicitly distinguishing these lesions from true vascular neoplasms as suggested by the term angioma.

Before computed tomography (CT), the diagnosis of CMs was rarely made before operation or autopsy. CT suggested the diagnosis in some patients; however, when high-field magnetic resonance imaging (MRI) became available, a picture characteristic of CMs was defined, allowing the diagnosis to be established in many cases. Furthermore, the advances in imaging have not only improved diagnosis of symptomatic lesions but have also resulted in increasing reports of incidental CMs.

The management of patients with CMs usually includes a consideration of surgical treatment or of observation. Rarely, radiosurgery is considered, but high complication rates and poor definition of end points for therapy have discouraged the use of this technique. With emerging knowledge of the natural history of CMs, the indications and guidelines for management decisions continue to evolve. This chapter reviews the surgical management of 121 cases of CMs seen by the authors at the Massachusetts General Hospital (MGH). From this information and from a review of the literature, recommendations are made for treating patients with this disorder.

PATHOLOGIC FEATURES

CMs can occur throughout the brain or spinal cord parenchyma, as well as on cranial and spinal nerves.[10,11] The lesions, which may be multiple, can range in size from a few millimeters to several centimeters. Often an associated venous malformation of the brain may be present; rarely, similar lesions may be found in other parts of the body.[3,12]

How a CM develops is unknown. In some patients, the lesions are clearly acquired, appearing in areas of brain that were normal on prior MRI studies.[9] These include patients with familial lesions and those in whom the CM has developed in an area of previously irradiated brain tissue or even developed sporadically.[13-17] Wilson[9] has proposed a possible pathogenesis for the development of acquired lesions.

The lesion is well defined and usually has a lobulated appearance. There is often a characteristic gross appearance that has been likened to a mulberry, characterized by a dark red or purple color. Inside the lesion is a honeycomb of thin-walled vascular spaces.[2] Small hemorrhages adjacent to or within the lesion may occur, but large hemorrhages are rare. A variable number of small blood vessels enter the lesion. Gliotic tissue surrounds the mass, and it is usually stained yellow. In some patients, the lesion may gradually enlarge as a result of small hemorrhages, progressive hyalinization, thickening of the vascular walls, or gradual thrombosis.[11,18]

Irregular sinusoidal spaces are visible on microscopic examination and many contain areas of thrombosis and organization with thin walls devoid of elastic tissue and muscle. These walls consist of a single layer of endothelium with varying amounts of extraluminal connective tissue. No intervening or neural tissue is present except that at the periphery, which is a layer of gliotic tissue that contains hemosiderin-packed macrophages adjacent to the lesion. There also may be seen hematomas of varying ages; extensive calcification; and, on the surface, collections of capillaries.

RADIOLOGIC FEATURES

High-quality CT scans suggest the diagnosis of CM in some patients. The characteristic findings are a roughly circular or irregularly shaped lesion located in the brain parenchyma; this lesion shows high density on the noncontrast scan and slight or no contrast enhancement. In some patients, extensive calcification is noted. Other types of occult vascular malformations, and some tumors associated with hemorrhage, also have the same CT appearance.

MRI accurately establishes the diagnosis in most cases and often is the only study needed. The criteria for MRI diagnosis is a well-circumscribed lesion with a combination of a reticulated or mottled core of mixed signal intensity and a prominent surrounding rim of decreased signal intensity (Fig. 91-1).[19] Hemorrhages of different ages may be seen within or around the lesion, and an associated venous

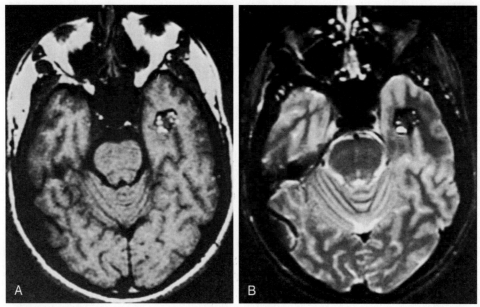

FIGURE 91-1   Temporal cavernous malformation in a 34-year-old man presenting with a seizure. Removal of the lesion was followed by a normal recovery. Magnetic resonance imaging axial T1- and T2-weighted images (*A* and *B*, respectively) show a well-circumscribed lesion in the left temporal lobe with a mottled core of mixed signal intensity and a surrounding rim of decreased signal intensity.

anomaly may be seen. On T2-weighted images, an increased signal may be present in the adjacent brain as a result of edema. Usually little or no enhancement follows the administration of gadolinium. Although appearance on MRI has a high correlation with the diagnosis of CM, occasionally an occult arteriovenous malformation or a tumor can have a similar appearance.[9,20,21] Significant enhancement suggests the possibility of a tumor.

The angiographic results are almost always normal because the lesion has small blood vessels with low flow and no hypertrophied feeding arteries or early draining veins. Rarely an avascular mass or capillary blush can be identified.[19,22] Since the development of MRI, angiography is rarely indicated. Occasionally, angiography is needed to obtain information regarding the vascular anatomy to help plan a surgical approach. If the MRI scan suggests an association with another vascular malformation, or if the diagnosis is in doubt, angiography should be done.

FAMILIAL OCCURRENCE AND GENETICS

CMs are known to be present in both sporadic and familial forms.[17,23,24] The familial form of the disease affects up to 30% to 50% of patients harboring a CM[19,23] and seems most common among Hispanic Americans.[17] Studies have shown that familial CMs are more prevalent than previously believed, and there is a greater incidence of multiple lesions (Fig. 91-2).[17] Rigamonti and colleagues[24] estimated a 73% familial incidence of multiple CMs of the brain, compared with a 10% to 15% incidence in the sporadic form. Further reports have indicated that familial CMs can be found in diverse ethnic groups including the Japanese and French.[25,26] Familial and sporadic forms of the disease appear to be similar clinically[27]; however, as many as 75% of patients who present with multiple CMs likely harbor the hereditary form of the disease.[25]

An autosomal dominant pattern of inheritance with variable penetrance was first described in a 122-member Hispanic pedigree of whom 5 harbored symptomatic lesions.[23] This autosomal pattern of inheritance was confirmed by a subsequent description of six unrelated Hispanic families.[17] Subsequent study of other families utilizing MR to detect silent lesions revealed a more complete expression than previously suspected.[25] The location of the responsible gene was mapped to the long arm of chromosome 7, to a locus named CCM1.[28,29] CCM1 locus homogeneity was identified in an analysis of 14 Hispanic families with CMs[30] but did not extend to kindreds of different ethnicity. Investigation of 20 non-Hispanic Caucasian families revealed linkage to two additional loci: CCM2 at chromosome 7p, and CCM3 at chromosome 3q.[31] The clinical, radiographic, and pathologic characteristics of the disease in kindreds mapping to these other loci does not appear to differ from those seen in kindreds mapping to the CCM1 locus. Linkage to one of these three loci (i.e., 7q, 7p, or 3q) accounted for inheritance in all 20 Caucasian kindreds studied. In fact, CCM1 was felt to be the locus involved in only 40% of non-Hispanic kindreds, with the remaining pedigrees linked to CCM2 (20%) or to CCM3 (40%).[31] Subsequent analysis of further kindreds seems to confirm that about 40% of familial CMs are attributable to CCM1 mutations.[32] The discovery of genetic heterogeneity in familial CMs has important implications both for the ability to provide reliable genetic testing in presymptomatic diagnosis and for understanding the pathogenesis of the disease. It has been suggested that there may be locus-specific differences in the penetrance of the disease, although such differences may also be attributable to the particular mutation involved.[31]

The responsible gene associated with CCM1, at the chromosome 7q locus, has been identified as human KRIT 1 (Krev interaction trapped 1). Mutations in KRIT 1 were first identified in a study of 57 French kindreds

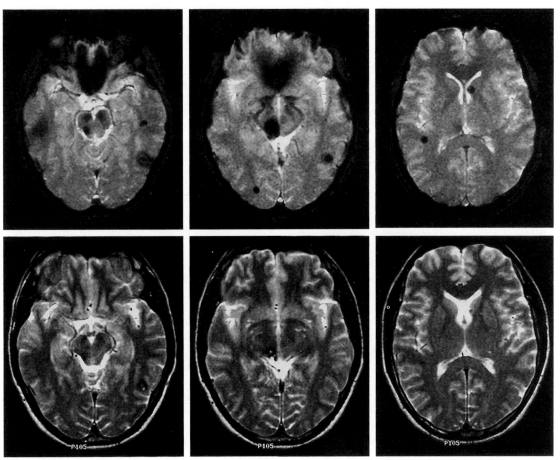

FIGURE 91-2   Magnetic resonance imaging (MRI) in a middle-aged male with a family history of CMs, who presented with seizures. T2-weighted images (*bottom panel*) reveal well-circumscribed lesions with a reticulated or mottled core of mixed signal intensity, typical for CMs. Susceptibility MR images (*top panel*) demonstrate further lesions showing the multiplicity of CMs. (From Amin-Hanjani S: The genetics of cerebrovascular malformations. Seminars in Cerebrovascular Diseases and Stroke 2(1):73–81, 2002.)

with CMs; 12 different mutations were discovered.[33] Further KRIT 1 mutations have been described in families of different ethnicities.[34,35] Although the exact function of KRIT 1 remains unknown, its interaction with Krev/rap1a (a ras family GTPase) and integrin cytoplasmic domain associated protein-1 alpha, and evidence that KRIT1 is a microtubule-associated protein, suggest a role in endothelial cell matrix interactions that could play a role in abnormal vascular development.[36] Gene products associated with CCM2 have been recently reported as a protein with potential involvement in integrin signaling encoded by a gene MGC4607[37]; a gene product associated with CCM3 has not been identified to date. However, because the resulting disease is phenotypically identical to CCM1, mutations at all three loci may result in changes that converge at the molecular level to result in abnormal endothelial cell proliferation. Presumably, different gene mutations result in the same abnormality via a common pathophysiologic pathway.

Based on the identified genetic abnormalities, it could be proposed that familial CMs result from inherited mutations and that sporadic CMs result from either a germline mutation in an individual or from a somatic mutation in a single cell. There are reports both for de novo germline mutations[38] and for somatic cell mutations in KRIT1 leading to sporadic CMs.[39] Support for the notion of somatic mutations

may be found in the development of CMs following radiation therapy, where cerebral lesions have been described within the irradiated field and were not present prior to treatment.[14] The possibility of radiation-induced mutagenesis resulting in CM formation is one explanation for this observation.

CLINICAL PRESENTATION

In 1976, Voigt and Yasargil[40] analyzed 163 cases reported up to 1974. They found that these lesions occurred in every age group and that the gender incidence was equal. In 1988, Simard and colleagues[41] reviewed 126 cases published since 1960 and added 12 of their own. The male-to-female ratio was 0.9:1, and the ages ranged from neonate to 75 years. In 1991, two publications were based on the analysis of consecutive MRI scans performed over several years.[42,43] In the report by Robinson and co-workers[42] of 66 patients, the male-to-female ratio was 1.2:1, and the age ranged from 4 months to 84 years (mean, 34.6 years). In the report of 32 patients by Curling and associates,[43] the male-to-female ratio was 1.1:1, the age ranged from 16 to 72 years (mean, 37.6 years), and multiple lesions were present in 6 patients (19%). Scott and colleagues[44] reported a series of 19 children ranging in age from 7 months to 17 years. In the MGH series of 116 patients, age ranged from 4 to 69 years (mean, 35.5 years), with a male-to-female ratio of 1:1.2. Multiple lesions were present in 12 patients (10.3%), and associated venous malformations were present in 9 patients (7.8%).

Most CMs that come to attention are supratentorial in location[40]; the distribution of CMs within the central nervous system seems to reflect the volume of tissue, without specific predilection for any particular location. The locations of the 121 operated CMs in the authors' series of 116 patients is shown in Table 91-1.

The four general categories of clinical presentation are seizures, headache, neurologic deficit, and asymptomatic presentation.[40–43] Seizure is the most common presenting symptom, affecting 35% to 55% of patients.[24,41–43,45,46] In many patients, more than one symptom is present. Within each of the symptomatic categories, some patients have had a hemorrhage into the adjacent brain parenchyma. The hemorrhages are usually small but on rare occasion can be large, with the patient having rapid deterioration. In some patients, the CM gradually enlarges, and the lesion can act as a mass that causes a progressive neurologic deficit. The clinical symptoms arising from the 121 CMs in the MGH surgical series are presented in Table 91-2; among the intracranial lesions, seizures were the presenting symptom in 45%, followed by neurologic deficits (38%) and headaches (17%).

NATURAL HISTORY

In 1985, Wilkins[8] reviewed the natural history of vascular malformations. He concluded that not enough information was present in the literature to describe the natural history of cavernous angiomas. In 1991, two reports of CMs diagnosed in large consecutive series of MRI scans gave some information about the short-term natural history,[42,43] and data from familial cases have also contributed to knowledge.[17]

Most hemorrhages are noncatastrophic, but there are occasional exceptions. Zimmerman and co-workers[47] reported one patient who died from rehemorrhage of a tectal CM. There are consequences, however, even of repeated small hemorrhages.

TABLE 91-1 ▪ Location of Cavernous Malformation

Location	No.	Percent
Cerebrum	84	69.4
Frontal	36	
Parietal	16	
Temporal	28	
Occipital	4	
Brain stem	17	14.0
Mesencephalon	2	
Pontomesencephalon	4	
Pons	8	
Pontomedullary	2	
Medulla	1	
Cerebellum	8	6.6
Cranial nerves	4	3.3
Spinal cord	8	6.6
Cervicomedullary	2	
Cervical	3	
Thoracic	2	
Lumbar	1	
Total	121	

TABLE 91-2 ▪ Presenting Symptoms of Cavernous Malformation

Location	No.	Presenting Symptoms, No.		No. of Overt Hemorrhage (%)*
Cerebrum	84	Seizure	51	28 (54.9)
		Neurologic deficit	15	13 (86.6)
		Headache	18	16 (88.9)
Brain stem	17	Neurologic deficit	17	12 (70.6)
Cerebellum	8	Neurologic deficit	7	7 (100)
		Headache	1	0 (0)
Cranial nerves	4	Neurologic deficit	4	1 (25)
Spinal cord	8	Neurologic deficit	8	6 (75)

*Percentage of patients with a particular clinical presentation who experienced overt hemorrhage.

Progressive deterioration with successive hemorrhages has been described,[6] and Robinson and associates[48] found a strong association between hemorrhage and neurologic disability in patients with CMs. Knowledge regarding the long-term risk of hemorrhage is of importance in management decisions, especially for CMs presenting incidentally or with minimal symptoms.

Overall, available estimates of the risks of initial hemorrhage from CMs have indicated low hemorrhage rates. In a retrospective study, Curling and colleagues[43] reported a 0.25% per person-year and 0.1% per lesion-year hemorrhage rate among 32 patients with 76 lesions. Robinson and colleagues[42] followed 57 symptomatic patients with 66 lesions for a mean of 26 months and observed only 1 hemorrhage in 143 lesion-years, resulting in a 0.7% per lesion-year hemorrhage rate. Porter and associates[46] reported a 1.6% per person-year hemorrhage rate among 110 patients followed for a mean of 46 months. In 68 prospectively followed patients, Moriarty and colleagues reported an overall 3.1% per person-year hemorrhage rate.[49] The risk of bleeding may be higher in deep or brain stem CMs.[46] In their cohort of 110 prospectively followed patients, Porter and colleagues found a 10-fold higher hemorrhage rate amongst infratentorial lesions at 3.8% per year compared with supratentorial lesions at 0.4% per year. This may reflect the eloquence of the surrounding tissue, with even small brain stem hemorrhages being more likely to be clinically manifest than lesions in the cerebral hemispheres.

The risk of hemorrhage in familial CMs appears to be similar to that in nonfamilial CMs, when considering the increased frequency of lesion multiplicity. In their follow-up of six families with familial CMs, Zabramski and colleagues[17] found a 1.1% per lesion-year (6.5% per person-year) rate of bleeding over a follow-up period of 26 months. In 40 patients with familial CMs, Labauge and colleagues reported a 2.5% per lesion-year hemorrhage risk.[50]

Several reports suggest a higher risk of bleeding after a first hemorrhage. Kondziolka and colleagues[51] followed 122 patients for 34 months and noted a low 0.6% per person-year hemorrhage rate among those without history of prior hemorrhage but a higher 4.5% per person-year rate among those with a previous hemorrhage. Kim and colleagues also reported a slightly higher recurrent hemorrhage rate of 3.8% per person-year compared with 2.3% per person-year for first hemorrhage.[52] For brain stem lesions, Kupersmith and colleagues reported bleeding rate of 2.5% per person-year, with a rebleeding rate of 5.1% per person-year.[53] Tung and co-workers[6] reported recurrent hemorrhage occurring in seven patients whose diagnosis of CM was confirmed at surgery. The median interval from the initial hemorrhage to the recurrent hemorrhage was 12 months, and only 2 months until a second rebleed. Aiba and associates[54] also found a much higher incidence of hemorrhage in those with prior bleeds at 22.9% per lesion-year versus 0.4% per lesion-year in those without prior bleeds. There is also evidence for temporal clustering of hemorrhages, with rates of rehemorrhage initially as high as 2% per month in a selected population but decreasing to less than 1% per month after 2 to 3 years.[55]

Information regarding the long-term risk of seizure development is scarce. Kondziolka and colleagues[51] reported that 4 of 94 patients without seizures developed seizures over the mean 34-month follow-up. Curling and associates[43] estimated the risk of seizure development to be 1.5% per person-year based on 32 patients. In Zabramski and colleagues'[17] group of patients with familial CMs followed over a mean period of 2.2 years, one of six asymptomatic individuals developed seizures. The rate of new seizures in the 68 patients reported by Moriarity and colleagues was 2.4% per person-year.[49]

The natural history of familial CMs has been addressed in several reports. Zabramski and associates[17] reported 6 families with familial CMs; 31 patients among these families harbored CMs, 21 of whom were followed clinically and with serial imaging. A total of 128 CMs were identified radiographically in these patients. During the mean follow-up of 2.2 years, 5 lesions were found to change in size, 13 lesions showed changes in signal characteristics, and 17 new lesions were identified in 6 patients. Given the dynamic nature of the CMs, the authors recommended serial MRI at 12-month intervals for symptomatic individuals, in addition to screening of family members. This approach can clarify the risk of morbidity in these patients and the need for close radiographic and clinical follow-up while providing data regarding the natural history. Labauge and colleagues noted 23 new lesions in 11 patients (27.5%) during follow-up of 40 patients with familial CM harboring 232 CMs over a mean follow-up of 3.2 years.[50] Nine lesions (3.9%) changed in size, and signal change was observed in 14 lesions (6%) over the same follow-up period.

De novo lesions have been described in nonfamilial cases of CMs also. The primary risk factor which has been identified has been radiation therapy, with reports of de novo development of CMs in the spinal cord[56] and the brain[14,15] years following irradiation. However, cases without an identifiable risk factor have also been documented.[57,58]

Little information is available about asymptomatic patients and their risks for developing symptoms. In the report by Robinson and co-workers,[42] four of nine asymptomatic patients developed symptoms related to the cavernous malformation over a relatively short follow-up period of 6 months to 2 years (mean, 18 months).

MANAGEMENT CONSIDERATIONS

Treatment for patients with CMs is based on careful comparison of the benefits and risks associated with the treatment options, usually either surgery or observation.

Occasionally, radiosurgery has been used. The age and medical condition of the patient are considered in this decision. Because knowledge and experience are still in the cumulative stage, only guidelines can be offered.

Surgery

The current, well-established indications for surgical resection of CMs are recurrent hemorrhage, progressive neurologic deterioration, and intractable epilepsy, unless the location is associated with an unacceptably high surgical risk.[42,43,59] When the surgical risk is high, observation or radiosurgery should be considered. Because the risk of surgery is low for lesions in many locations, there are groups of patients (e.g., those with CMs of the cerebrum or cerebellum with a single overt hemorrhage, those with the onset of a seizure disorder, and those who are worried about the presence of the lesion) in whom surgery should be considered.[60] In children, Scott and co-workers[44] have a "policy to recommend surgery for patients with cavernous angiomas if the lesion is safely accessible, is currently symptomatic either by mass effect and/or hemorrhage or seizure, or shows evidence of having bled in the past."

In a special category is the young woman who wants to become pregnant (Fig. 91-3). Robinson and colleagues[42] noted that two of their six patients with acute hemorrhage were in the first trimester of pregnancy. They suggested that in women contemplating pregnancy, one of the indications for surgical excision was an accessible lesion. Other authors have also commented on the possible role of hormonal influences as a contributing factor.[16,54] Aiba and associates[54] reported that women predominated in the group of patients presenting with hemorrhage, and that young women had a higher rate of subsequent hemorrhage.

When surgical excision of a CM is indicated, the lesion can usually be totally removed with low morbidity. This procedure is facilitated by microsurgical dissection in the gliotic tissue that surrounds the lesion, allowing a distinct plane of cleavage to be developed through microsurgical techniques, bipolar coagulation, and the use of fine-regulated suction. When the lesion is exposed, internally decompressing the mass and retracting the capsule into the area of the decompression may help avoid pressure on the surrounding normal parenchyma. When the lesion is densely calcified, an ultrasonic surgical aspirator may be used for debulking. Bleeding is usually not a significant problem.

In some patients, splitting a cortical fissure may be possible rather than performing a full corticectomy to approach the lesion. For lesions in critical areas, cortical mapping and stimulation may be used. When removal of a CM in the deep portions of the cerebral hemispheres is indicated, the lesion is localized with stereotactic techniques and intraoperative ultrasound.[6,44,61] For brain stem lesions, special monitoring with evoked potential responses may be helpful, and arrangements for temporary cardiac pacing may be prudent.

Radiosurgery

Stereotactic radiosurgery has been used to treat patients with CMs thought to be inoperable and associated with progressive worsening of neurologic symptoms because of mass effect or recurrent hemorrhage. There is difficulty, however,

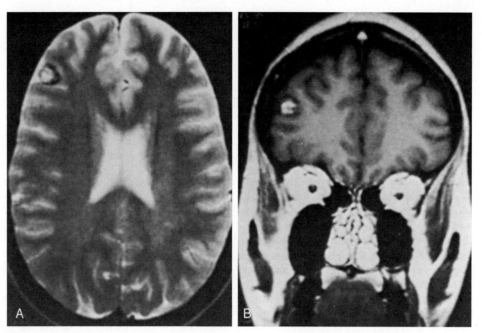

FIGURE 91-3 Frontal cavernous malformation in a 34-year-old physician presenting with seizures. The seizures were controlled with medication, but she wanted to become pregnant and requested surgical excision. Removal of the lesion was followed by normal recovery. Magnetic resonance imaging axial T2- and coronal T1-weighted images (*A* and *B*, respectively) show a superficial right frontal lesion with no parenchymal hemorrhage.

in establishing valid end points for therapeutic success because the natural history is poorly understood, because complications can be related to either minor rebleeding or to delayed radiation-induced injury, and because MRI results may not change significantly during the follow-up period.

Kondziolka and associates[62] reported on the gamma knife use in the treatment of 47 patients with surgically inaccessible lesions with at least 1 prior hemorrhage. Over the mean follow-up of 3.6 years, they found a significant decline in hemorrhage rates from 32% per lesion-year pretreatment to 1.1% per lesion-year at 2 years after treatment. There was a high incidence of radiation-induced complications after the treatment with mean center doses of 32 Gy (range, 20 to 40 Gy): 12 of the 42 patients (27%) were affected, although only 2 patients (4%) were reported to suffer permanent deficits. In a subsequent report from the same institution, 82 patients were analyzed. Again, a reduction in hemorrhage risk was reported from 33.9%, down to 12.3% during the first 2 years post-treatment, and 0.76% per patient-year thereafter.[63] Overall incidence of radiosurgical morbidity was 13.4%. Karlsson and colleagues[64] also reported experience with gamma knife, treating 22 patients with symptomatic CMs using maximum doses of 11 to 60 Gy (mean and median, 33 Gy) and minimum doses of 9 to 35 Gy (mean and median, 18 Gy). Over the mean follow-up of 6.5 years, they noted a decreasing trend in hemorrhages 4 years after treatment. However, they also found a high rate of morbidity, with six patients (27%) suffering radiation-related complications, and in five of them (23%) these led to permanent deficits. Pollock and co-authors also noted a high incidence of radiation-related complications, occurring in 41% of their 17 patients with deep lesions, although hemorrhage rates did decline from 40.1% pretreatment to 2.9% more than 2 years after treatment.[65] Another series of gamma knife radiosurgery noted a reduced frequency of seizures following

treatment, with 18 of 28 patients (64%) who had a chief complaint of seizure experiencing this benefit.[66]

Stereotactic charged-particle radiosurgery, both helium-ion radiosurgery and proton beam therapy, has also been used to treat cavernous angiomas. Fabrikant and associates[67] noted that the clinical results after helium-ion radiosurgery for cavernous angiomas were not as good as those for arteriovenous malformations. Radiosurgery using a linear accelerator has also been reported but with small numbers of patients treated and lack of long-term data.[68] Chang and colleagues[69] summarized the results of 57 patients treated using helium ion (47 patients) or linear accelerator (10 patients). All patients harbored CMs that had bled previously and were treated with mean doses of 18 GyE. Hemorrhage rates decreased 3 years after treatment to 1.6% per patient-year. Five patients (9%) suffered radiation-related edema or necrosis, resulting in permanent deficits in two patients (4%). Analysis of Kjellberg's experience at the Harvard cyclotron using proton beam therapy revealed a decline in hemorrhage rates from 17.3% per lesion-year before treatment to 4.5% per lesion-year after a latency period of 2 years.[70] Among the 98 lesions treated with a median center dose of 18 Gy, 26 (26.5%) were associated with radiation-related complications, 16 of which were permanent and 3 of which resulted in mortality.

Because the long-term natural history of CMs is not well defined, current evidence favors expectant management, given the high rates of complications with radiosurgery. The risk of radiation-related complications appears to be significantly higher than that found for AVMs of similar size and location[65]; although the basis for this is unknown, a role for the potential radiosensitizing properties of the hemosiderin ring around CMs has been proposed.[71] The decline in hemorrhage rates observed in most studies cannot definitively be ascribed to the treatment because it may reflect the poorly characterized natural history of bleeding in these lesions.

Temporal clustering of hemorrhages, with a spontaneous 2.4-fold decline in hemorrhage rates after 2 years, has been observed and may affect the interpretation of hemorrhage risk reduction in radiosurgical series.[55] This modality is presently considered only rarely for deep, inaccessible lesions associated with repeated hemorrhage and progressive neurologic deficit.

Observation

Some patients with CMs should be followed conservatively. Almost all asymptomatic lesions are observed because they can remain asymptomatic indefinitely, and if a hemorrhage occurs, it is usually small without major neurologic deficit. Another group that may be observed is those with symptomatic lesions in a deep or critical area when the risks of surgery are judged to be significant and neither recurrent hemorrhage nor an increasing neurologic deficit is present. Some patients with seizures or headache, in whom no hemorrhage has occurred, have been observed, but subsets of these patients are also candidates for surgery, as discussed in the following. The decision of which treatment is appropriate depends on a detailed evaluation of the clinical problem and on discussion with the patient.

No clear guidelines exist on how often the MRI scan should be repeated. The authors generally perform MRI on the patient at 6-month intervals for 2 years; then, if the lesion is stable, the scan is repeated once a year.

CAVERNOUS MALFORMATIONS OF THE CEREBRUM

Management

Patients Presenting with Seizures

The treatment of patients with CMs presenting with seizures continues to evolve. With the good results of surgical removal, the indications for operation have expanded beyond conditions in which medical control of seizures is difficult and in which the diagnosis is in question (more common before the advent of MRI). Surgery is recommended in most patients who have had a parenchymal hemorrhage and in many patients who have not had a hemorrhage when the surgical risk is low. These patients are usually in their 20s to 40s but are sometimes younger, and they are often concerned about the presence of the lesion. Although the seizures can often be controlled with medication, the removal of the CM and the adjacent gliotic yellow-stained tissue may reduce the long-term frequency and severity of seizures and allow the patients to discontinue their medications.[2,42,43] Robinson and colleagues[42] reported that all 18 patients who did not have surgery continued to require medical control of their seizures. In the surgically treated group, 50% had no more seizures, and the others had a reduction in seizure frequency.

Rengachary and Kalyan-Raman[2] described a possible basis for recommending surgery. They suggest that slow lysis of red cells sequestrated in the cavernous spaces allows red cell pigment to diffuse out of the lesion into the adjacent tissue. This pigment seems to induce gliosis, which may contribute to the development of a seizure focus. The authors quote experimental studies that suggest that chemical compounds containing iron play important roles in inducing a seizure focus.

In the MGH series, a seizure was the primary presenting symptom in 51 of 84 (61%) patients with lesions of the cerebrum (see Table 91-2). Some of these patients also had other symptoms (usually headache), and slightly more than half had an associated parenchymal hematoma. Patients with CMs presenting with seizure are shown in Figure 91-1 (temporal), Figure 91-3, Figure 91-4 (frontal), Figure 91-5 (parietal), and Figure 91-6 (motor-sensory cortex).

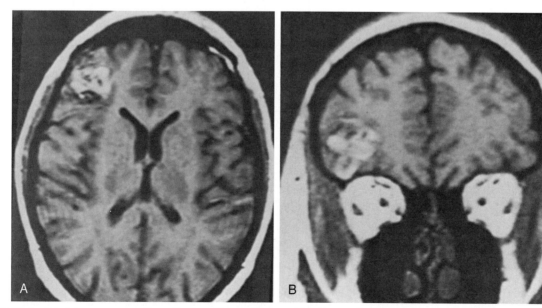

FIGURE 91-4 Frontal cavernous malformation in a 45-year-old man with a history of mild frontal headache for several weeks who then presented with a seizure. After the malformation was removed, the patient had a normal recovery. T1-weighted axial and coronal images (*A* and *B*, respectively) show findings consistent with a cavernous angioma but no hematoma in the adjacent parenchyma. These findings were confirmed at operation, but there was yellow staining in the adjacent cerebral tissue.

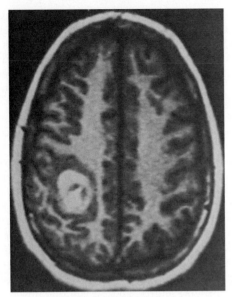

FIGURE 91-5 A parietal cavernous malformation in a 19-year-old man who presented with a seizure. Removal of the lesion was followed by full recovery of the patient. A magnetic resonance imaging axial T1-weighted image showed the circumscribed mottled core with adjacent hematoma and edema.

Patients Presenting with Headache

If the headache is a new symptom or is recurrent, it can often be related to the CM. In these patients, MRI often shows a recent hemorrhage. In the authors' series, 16 of 18 patients with headache (89%) had a parenchymal hemorrhage (see Table 91-2). Surgery is indicated in most of these patients to avoid future neurologic disability from recurrent hemorrhage (except in patients with unacceptably high surgical risk because of a critical anatomic location). An example is illustrated in Figure 91-7.

Patients Presenting with Neurologic Deficit

In most patients with a progressive or acute neurologic deficit, there is an associated hematoma, and surgical removal of the lesion is indicated to prevent further neurologic damage and to help restore neurologic function. Some of these patients also have had headaches. In the patient whose deficit is improving, observation can be the initial strategy used. If the surgical risks are judged to be relatively low, however, the lesion should be electively removed to prevent the effects of rehemorrhage. These patients are generally younger than 60 years old and are at risk for repeated hemorrhages and neurologic deficits.[6] Involvement of the speech or motor-sensory cortex should not preclude the consideration of surgery, but a final decision should include an assessment of the surgical accessibility of the lesion.

In the authors' series, most patients (13 of the 15, or 87%) presenting with a neurologic deficit had an associated acute hemorrhage. The indications for surgery were progressive neurologic deficit, sudden severe neurologic deficit, recurrent episodes of neurologic deficits lasting days to weeks, and history of a hemorrhage followed by recovery. An example is illustrated in Figure 91-8.

Results

Several reports documented good results in the surgical treatment of CMs of the cerebral hemispheres.[9,40,44,45,60,72–77]

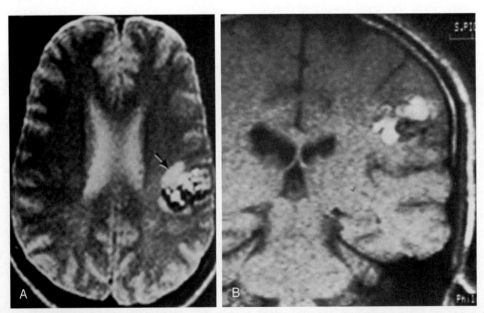

FIGURE 91-6 Frontoparietal cavernous malformation in a 36-year-old neurosurgeon who had a focal seizure involving the right hand and right side of the face. After another seizure occurred 4 months later, magnetic resonance imaging axial T2-weighted and coronal T1-weighted images (*A* and *B*, respectively) show the cavernous angioma in the left inferior motor-sensory cortex and an area of new hemorrhage (*arrow*) that was not seen on the scan after the first seizure. The patient carefully considered the treatment options and concluded (as had the authors) that further hemorrhage entailed a risk of ending his career with damage to his dominant hand. Also, he wanted to reduce the probability of a seizure and to stop taking medications. Surgical removal was followed by the patient's complete recovery with no focal neurologic deficit and with resumption of neurosurgical practice.

FIGURE 91-7 Temporal cavernous malformation in a 26-year-old man who had the onset of headache with weight lifting. The headaches started to increase. A magnetic resonance imaging (MRI) scan showed a left temporal cavernous angioma with hemorrhage. Angiography showed no abnormal vascularity or stain. The patient was followed up, and his headaches persisted. The patient's neurologic examination remained normal, but repeat MRI axial T1- and T2-weighted images (A and B, respectively) showed an increase in the size of the hematoma. Surgical removal of the left temporal cavernous malformation and hematoma was followed by the patient's complete recovery with no speech difficulty.

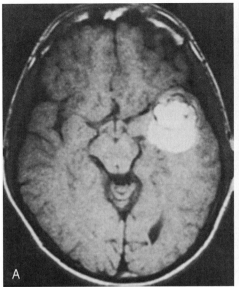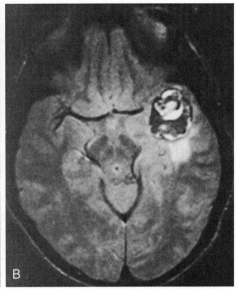

With accessible lesions, surgical morbidity is minimal, and mortality is almost zero. Acciarri and co-workers[72] found a 90% incidence of good outcomes in 55 patients with hemispheric lesions, with 0% mortality. Smaller series have found similarly favorable results, with good results in 100% of patients.[45,75,76] Chadduck and co-workers[78] reviewed patients with intraventricular CMs. Although they found good outcomes, particularly in patients with lateral ventricular lesions, 2 of 15 (13%) surgically treated patients died, and 1 patient was rendered comatose. Acciarri and co-workers[72] reported 2 deaths among 4 patients with intraventricular lesions.

The treatment of CMs of the basal ganglia and thalamus has been controversial, and these lesions (along with brain stem lesions) may be considered dangerous to excise. Some practitioners suggest that surgery be considered when there are recurrent episodes of hemorrhage or progressive worsening neurologic deficit.[44,79] Lorenzana and associates[80] reported a patient with a CM that involved the anterior third of the lentiform nucleus and a large part of white matter anterior to the nucleus. The patient was cured by use of CT-assisted stereotactic craniotomy with an approach through the second frontal sulcus. In other case reports, the results of treatment of CMs in the thalamus were discouraging.[76,81] Bertalanffy and associates[82] found permanent neurologic complications in 6 of 12 patients (50%) after resection of deep-seated lesions within the basal ganglia, thalamus, and insula. Steinberg and colleagues reported worsening in 16 (29%) of a group of 56 patients with deep or brain stem lesions, of which 15 were located in the basal ganglia or thalamus; long-term outcome, however, was improved condition in 52%, unchanged in 43%, and worse in 5%.[83]

FIGURE 91-8 Parietal cavernous malformation in a 42-year-old man who had a brief episode of weakness in his left lower extremity 2 weeks before being examined. Nine days before admission to the hospital, he developed a limp because of weakness in his left lower extremity. The next day, his foot became weaker and then he noted weakness in his left upper extremity. The progression of the weakness stopped when he was given steroids. MRI axial T2-weighted and coronal images (A and B, respectively) show a hemorrhage associated with a cavernous angioma deep in the right parietal region. Stereotactic localization was performed, and the lesion was removed. The patient completely recovered except for a slight residual weakness in his foot.

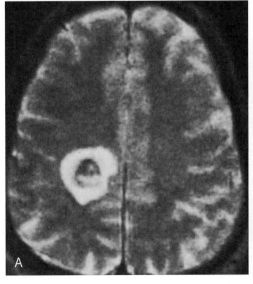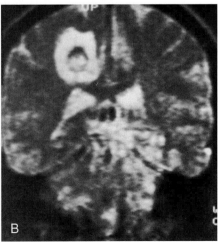

The effects of resection on seizure control are pertinent given the frequency of seizures among supratentorial CMs. Lesionectomy alone has resulted in favorable results.[72,84,85] Despite the implication of iron products as potential seizure foci, surgical removal of the surrounding hemosiderin ring has not shown a correlation with improved outcomes in small studies.[86,87] Length of seizure history and total number of seizures, however, do seem to affect surgical outcome negatively.[85,87,88] Retrospective studies reveal that 75% to 100% of patients with fewer than five seizures or shorter than a 12-month history of seizures are seizure-free after lesionectomy, as compared with 50% to 62.5% of patients with more than five seizures or a seizure history longer than 1 year.[85,88]

In the MGH series of 84 patients with CMs of the cerebrum outside the basal ganglia and thalamus, operative mortality was zero and all patients had complete removal of the lesion. Postoperatively, 81 of the 84 patients (96%) had an excellent or good outcome neurologically (i.e., were able to return to their previous level of activity) and, in most cases, had normal results on neurologic examination. Three patients (4%) were classified as fair because of residual disability. Neurologic outcome and comparison of presurgical and postsurgical neurologic status are shown in Table 91-3. Of the 52 patients presenting with seizures, 29 underwent surgery primarily for seizure control; the remainder underwent surgery to eliminate risk of further hemorrhage rather than primary treatment of the seizure disorder. Of the 52 patients, 50 (96%) were seizure-free on or off anticonvulsants after surgery. Of the 29 patients treated primarily for epilepsy, 26 (90%) experienced improvement in seizure control after surgery.

CAVERNOUS MALFORMATIONS OF THE BRAIN STEM

Management

Based on their experiences with 8 patients (4 of whom had surgery), Falbusch and colleagues[89] recommended that CMs of the brain stem that are associated with recurrent episodes of hemorrhage, MRI-confirmed diagnosis, negative angiographic results, and a progressive neurologic disability should be removed. Patients with recovery or stabilization of their neurologic deficit, or those who are asymptomatic, should be observed. The report by Zimmerman and associates[47] summarized 24 patients (16 of whom had surgery). They recommended that neurologically intact patients with CMs

that did not touch the pial surface should be observed. When the lesion was associated with repeated hemorrhages or with progressive neurologic deficit and was close to the pial surface, surgery was performed. They also suggested that any symptomatic lesion of the brain stem located superficially be considered for surgery if eloquent tissue could be spared. Based on the poor overall natural history of symptomatic CMs in brain stem location, resection is advocated for lesions abutting a pial surface or surrounded by only a thin rim of tissue.[90–94] The optimal timing of surgery following hemorrhage is less well defined. Operation in the subacute phase following hemorrhage (several days to a few weeks) may be preferable.[94–96] This allows time to stabilize the patient's condition while conferring the benefit of earlier reduction of mass effect by evacuation of hematoma. Furthermore, the presence of a subacute hematoma may create a better surgical plane than would be present after delayed surgery following complete clot resorption, or with acute surgery with a firm clot.[83] Mathiesen and colleagues found better outcomes among their patients with brain stem cavernomas if surgery was performed within 1 month of the hemorrhagic ictus.[95] On the other hand, Samii and colleagues reported that there was no difference in long-term outcomes based on the timing of surgery in 36 patients.[93]

In the past, some CMs of the brain stem were treated with radiosurgery when recurrent hemorrhages and increased neurologic deficit were present. The patient whose MRI scan is illustrated in Figure 91-9 was treated for this reason several years ago. The lesion did not become smaller, and recurrent hemorrhage with worsening symptoms occurred. The patient declined surgical management.

The indications for operation in the authors' patients were progressive or recurrent neurologic symptoms. The risk of surgery is probably lower when the lesion comes to the surface, obviating pial incision. The risk of surgery is probably higher when the lesion is large without associated hemorrhage, or when it is densely calcified, making removal more difficult.

Careful study of the MRI scan aids in planning of the precise corridor of exposure and resection. Neuronavigation can be of considerable help, especially for lesions that are covered by a thin rim of tissue and that are not directly visible on the surface.[96] Electrophysiologic monitoring (e.g., somatosensory evoked potentials, brain stem auditory evoked potentials, and fifth, seventh, and twelfth nerve function monitoring) can be utilized in an effort to minimize complications.[83,96] Pontomedullary CMs can be approached through a midline suboccipital craniotomy and exposure of the fourth ventricle. Lesions in the pontomesencephalic

Location	No.	Excellent (%)*	Good (%)*	Fair (%)*	Poor (%)*	Improved (%)	Stable (%)	Worse (%)
Cerebrum	84	68 (80.9)	13 (15.5)	3 (3.6)	0 (0)	4 (4.8)	76 (90.4)	4 (4.8)
Brain stem	17	1 (5.9)	10 (58.8)	4 (23.5)	2 (11.7)	5 (29.4)	9 (52.9)	3 (17.6)
Cerebellum	8	2 (25)	5 (62.5)	1 (12.5)	0 (0)	2 (25)	6 (75)	0 (0)
Cranial nerves	4	0 (0)	4 (100)	0 (0)	0 (0)	0 (0)	4 (100)	0 (0)
Spinal cord	8	0 (0)	6 (75)	2 (25)	0 (0)	5 (62.5)	3 (37.5)	0 (0)
Total	121	71 (58.7)	38 (31.4)	10 (8.3)	2 (1.6)	16 (13.2)	98 (81)	7 (5.8)

TABLE 91-3 ▪ **Neurologic Outcome after Surgical Resection**

*Excellent = no neurologic deficit. Good = free of major neurologic deficit and able to return to previous activity. Fair = independent but some neurologic disability. Poor = dependent with significant neurologic disability.

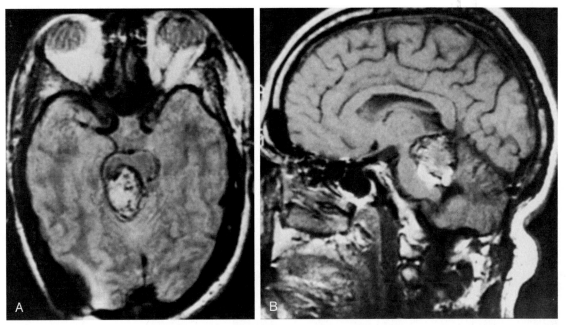

FIGURE 91-9 Brain stem cavernous angioma in a 27-year-old man treated with radiosurgery 4 years earlier presenting with increased dysarthria and ataxia. Magnetic resonance imaging T1-weighted axial (A) and sagittal (B) images show the lesion with new hemorrhage around the inferior margin. The patient declined to undergo surgery.

region are more difficult to manage but may be treated by a subtemporal or combined subtemporal-suboccipital approach. Falbusch and colleagues[89] used a supracerebellar infratentorial approach for midline pontomesencephalic lesions.

In the authors' patients, upper brain stem CMs were removed by a subtemporal approach (Fig. 91-10); in one patient, a laterally placed brain stem lesion was approached through the cerebellopontine angle between the fifth and seventh cranial nerves. In patients with lesions in the pons or medulla, a midline exposure through the floor of the fourth ventricle was used (Fig. 91-11).

Results

Zimmerman and co-workers[47] reported that among 16 patients who underwent surgery, some had transient postoperative worsening, but the outcome in all except one was the same or improved. Isamat and Louesa[97] had six patients with CMs in the pons or medulla that were in contact with the floor of the fourth ventricle and were removed through the floor of the ventricle. All patients returned to their previous activities and had improvement in their neurologic deficits. Three other patients are being followed because the lesion was completely surrounded by normal brain stem tissue.

Fritschi and colleagues[98] reviewed 93 cases of brain stem CMs treated operatively from their own experience and from the literature up to 1992. They found good outcomes in 84% of cases. The authors compared the surgical results with 30 patients treated conservatively without surgery. Although most nonoperative patients recovered completely or with minimal deficits (67%), 20% died, and 7% suffered poor outcomes. Porter and colleagues reported improved outcomes in 87% of 84 patients who underwent operation for brain stem CMs; 10% were worsened postoperatively, and 4% died.[90] A 12% incidence of severe or permanent

morbidity was reported. Despite successful resection of brain stem lesions, CMs within this location clearly carry a higher risk of operative morbidity and mortality. Rates of transient complications within the literature range from 25% to 70%,[47,82,91,95,99] rates of permanent complications are up to 25%,[82,90,91,99,100] and mortality rates are up to 6%.[47,82,90,98,101]

In the MGH series of 17 patients, 5 improved, but some residual neurologic deficits that had been present before surgery were usually persistent (see Table 91-3). Eight patients (47%) experienced transient postoperative neurologic deficits, all of which resolved to baseline within 1 month. Three patients (17.6%) experienced permanent postoperative deficits. One of these patients harbored a mesencephalic CM and initially presented with hemorrhage, in coma; clot evacuation and partial lesion resection was undertaken. He made a gradual recovery but had a small rehemorrhage 2 years later. He underwent reoperation, which resulted in poor outcome. Another patient presented with a progressive quadriparesis (see Fig. 91-11) and at operation, the large lesion was calcified and difficult to remove. Complete resection was achieved, but the patient had further neurologic deficits postoperatively, leaving her bedridden. The third patient had a pontomedullary CM and presented with progressive diplopia and ataxia. Postoperatively, the patient's condition was worse, with difficulty swallowing and hoarseness that improved but with residual effect.

CAVERNOUS MALFORMATIONS OF THE CEREBELLUM

Management

The general management guidelines for most cerebellar CMs are similar to those outlined for the cerebral hemisphere. Surgery is indicated because the patient has presented with

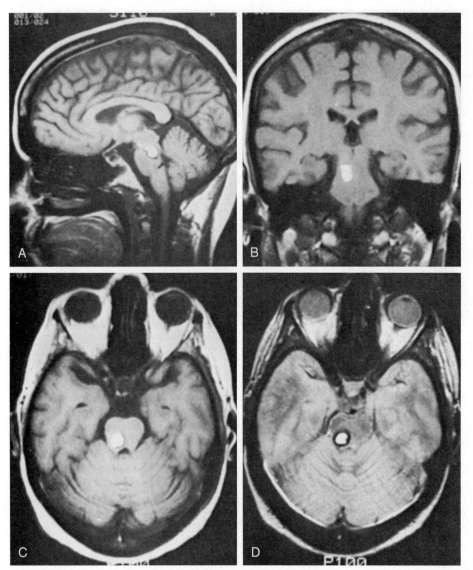

FIGURE 91-10 An upper brain stem cavernous malformation in a 37-year-old woman. Because of recurrent symptoms (second hemorrhage and inability to walk), the lesion was removed using a right subtemporal approach. Magnetic resonance imaging T1-weighted sagittal (*A*), coronal (*B*), axial (*C*), and T2-weighted axial (*D*) images. Note that the lesion almost comes to the surface and is localized to one side.

a neurologic deficit, there is an associated hemorrhage, the morbidity of removal is low, and the risk of significant neurologic disability with repeat hemorrhage is high.

Results

There were eight patients with CMs of the cerebellum in the MGH series: all made a good recovery and could be classified as having excellent or good outcomes (see Table 91-3) except one patient classified as a fair outcome secondary to persistence of a preoperative deficit. One patient had an associated venous anomaly (Fig. 91-12). At operation, a typical CM was resected, and the large venous angioma was carefully preserved. The patient made an uneventful recovery. Another patient with a cerebellar CM and associated venous anomaly developed a venous infarction 1 month postoperatively, despite efforts to leave the venous anomaly intact. This complication required reoperation for cerebellar decompression, but the patient ultimately regained her preoperative neurologic status.

CAVERNOUS MALFORMATIONS OF THE CRANIAL NERVES

Management

CMs have been reported to involve cranial nerves in the following locations: optic nerves and chiasm, third nerve, seventh nerve in the temporal bone, and seventh and eighth nerves in the internal auditory canal.[102–106] The presenting symptoms relate to the nerve involved with the lesion. The MRI scan usually suggests the diagnosis, but in some patients, the pathology may not be evident until surgery. Surgery does not usually restore function in the involved nerve, although some improvement in deficit can be observed.[106] Surgery is indicated to prevent hemorrhage into adjacent neural structures or, as in a patient with a facial nerve lesion, to remove the malformation and place a sural nerve graft, which may restore some function. Gross total resection of the lesion is required to prevent progression of the cranial nerve dysfunction.

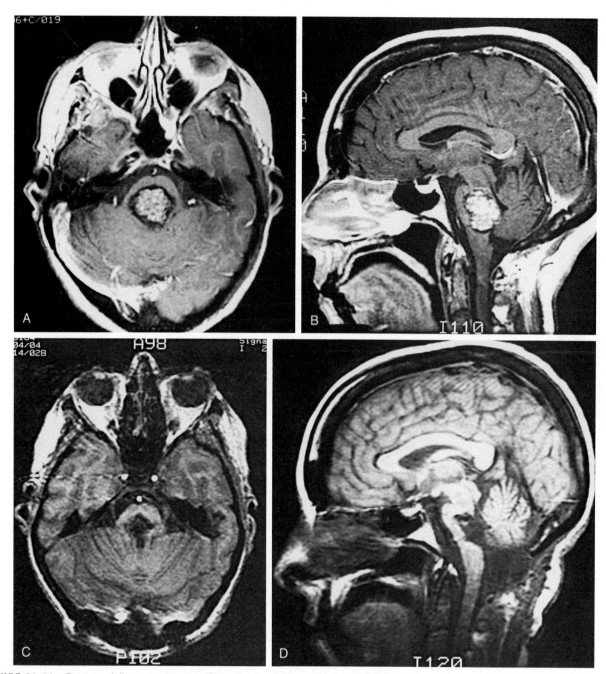

FIGURE 91-11 Pontomedullary cavernous malformation in a 53-year-old woman who presented with progressive neurologic deficits; she was quadriparetic and wheelchair-bound preoperatively. Axial and sagittal T1-weighted magnetic resonance images reveal the large brain stem lesion preoperatively (*A* and *B*), and after complete resection (*C* and *D*). Postoperatively, the patient deteriorated neurologically and was bedridden. (From Amin-Hanjani S, Ogilvy CS, Ojemann RG, et al: Risks of surgical management for cavernous malformations of the nervous system. Neurosurgery 42:1224, 1998.)

Results

Improvement in function has been documented with removal of cranial nerve CMs.[107] Others, however, report a low potential for restoration of function[103,104] and note that complete resection is difficult without incurring permanent nerve injury.[104,105]

In the MGH series of four patients (Table 91-4), one patient had a CM in the optic chiasm. A field deficit developed during pregnancy as a result of hemorrhage, then improved, only to worsen after a second hemorrhage a few months after delivery. The field deficit improved somewhat after removal of the lesion. Malik and colleagues[103] reported the partial removal of a CM from the underside of the optic nerve and chiasm in one patient. Vision did not improve, but no further symptoms occurred. Shibuya and colleagues[107] reported visual improvement after resection of a chiasmal CM. Deshmukh and colleagues reported visual improvement in all four of their patients with chiasmal CMs.[106]

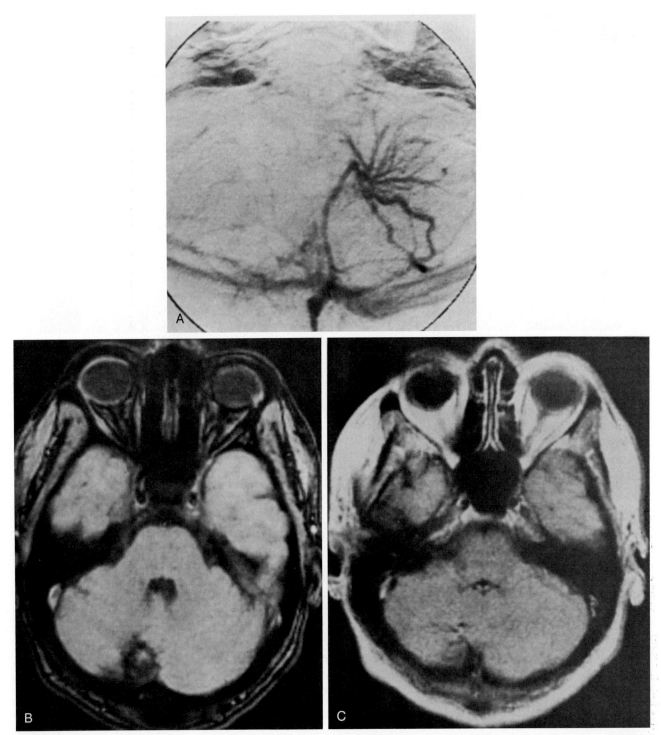

FIGURE 91-12   Cerebellar cavernous malformation in a 32-year-old woman who had a sudden severe headache with nausea and vomiting and severe ataxia. At another hospital, a computed tomography scan showed a right cerebellar hemorrhage; angiography (*A*) showed no early-filling veins but a large venous angioma. The patient recovered, and her neurologic examination was normal. Three months later, magnetic resonance axial T1-weighted images (*B* and *C*) showed evidence of the adjacent venous anomaly and the old hemorrhage with a mottled appearance within this area, supporting the diagnosis of cavernous malformation. Surgery was recommended because of the serious disability that resulted from the first hemorrhage. The venous angioma was not treated, and the patient had a good recovery.

One patient in this series had a lesion involving the seventh and eighth nerves in the internal auditory canal. Involvement in the internal auditory canal has been reported in four patients, including the one in the authors' series.[104,108] The eighth nerve could not be saved in any patient, but reasonable facial nerve function remained in three. When the facial nerve cannot be saved, a nerve graft is placed at operation. One patient in the MGH series had a malformation involving the seventh nerve in the temporal bone. The malformation and nerve were removed, and a sural nerve

TABLE 91-4 ▪ Cavernous Malformations of the Cranial Nerves

Age/Sex	Location	Clinical Course	Outcome
33/F	Optic chiasm	Developed visual field deficit during pregnancy, second hemorrhage after delivery	Good: residual visual field deficit
25/M	Third nerve	Progressive third nerve palsy	Good: third nerve palsy
53/M	Seventh nerve	Progressive facial weakness	Good: facial nerve graft placed with some recovery
27/F	Seventh and eighth nerves in internal auditory canal and posterior fossa	Fullness in ear, facial twitch	Good: loss of hearing, facial nerve graft placed with some recovery

graft was placed. The last patient in the series had a lesion of the third cranial nerve[105] that was extensively involved and was resected to remove the malformation. The case reported by Scott[109] was treated in the same way.

CAVERNOUS MALFORMATIONS OF THE SPINAL CORD

Clinical Presentation

Reviewing spinal cord CMs reported within the literature through 1991, Ogilvy and colleagues[11] described 36 patients with 37 spinal lesions, including 6 patients from the MGH series. The series included 25 (69%) women and 11 (31%) men. The locations of the lesions along the spinal axis were cervical medullary junction in 3 (8%), cervical in 12 (32%), thoracic in 20 (54%), lumbar spinal cord in 1 (3%), and conus medullaris in 1 (3%). Two patients had a history of familial CM, four had a CM at some other site in the central nervous system, and one had a second spinal lesion. The ages ranged from 12 to 62 years, and the most common age for the appearance of initial symptoms was in the 30s. Four clinical categories of symptoms were identified:

1. Thirteen patients presented with episodes of neurologic deterioration with variable degrees of neurologic recovery between episodes. The episodes lasted hours to days. The interval between events was often months to years.
2. Twelve patients had a clinical course characterized by slowly progressive neurologic deterioration. The duration of the progression was usually several years. Two patients had discrete episodes of gradual worsening separated by many years.
3. Eight patients had an acute onset of symptoms followed by neurologic worsening over several days.
4. Three patients had the acute onset of mild symptoms followed by weeks or months of deterioration of neurologic function.

Review of the brain imaging studies of 17 patients in a recent series of spinal CMs demonstrated a higher incidence of mutiple neuroaxis CMs, with 8 (47%) such patients harboring multiple CMs[110]; patients with spinal CMs may warrant complete neuroaxis imaging to evaluate for additional lesions.

Management

The diagnosis of a CM of the spinal cord is established by the characteristic MRI appearance (Fig. 91-13). There are no reports of long-term follow-up of untreated patients with CMs of the spinal cord. From the history obtained from symptomatic patients, it is evident that in some patients there can be intervals of several years between episodes of recurrent neurologic problems that presumably result from hemorrhage. In these intervals, a neurologic deficit is stable, or the patient is symptom-free. Also, in recurrent hemorrhages, the neurologic deficit often increases and does not always fully recover. Rehemorrhage rates as high as 66% per year have been reported, favoring resection of symptomatic lesions.[111]

In most patients, lesions present on the dorsal or dorsolateral aspect of the spinal cord. The authors usually recommend surgery. The findings at operation are similar to those found at operation in CMs of the brain. A well-defined gliotic plane exists around the lesion, which aids in the microsurgical removal. The use of fine sutures in the pia to retract the spinal cord when the lesion is deep, a fine-regulated suction, and microbipolar forceps facilitate the dissection. Gross total removal of the malformation should be the goal of surgical treatment.

Results

Several small case series have shown favorable results with complete resection of intramedullary CMs.[112,113] Transient neurologic complications in the early postoperative period can be prominent, however.[113,114] Spetzger and colleagues[113] noted such complications in five of nine (55%) patients but found that over long-term follow-up, eight of nine (88%) were normal or improved compared with preoperative status. Operative intervention for spinal cord CMs generally results in long-term improvement or stabilization of function.[11,111–116] Cantore and associates[117] found a correlation between surgical outcome and the severity and length of preoperative symptoms in six patients, and Canavero and co-workers[118] found that preoperative status was the most important factor affecting outcome from surgery.

In the MGH series of CMs involving the spinal cord, there were eight patients ranging in age from 31 to 61 years. The lesion was completely removed in all eight patients. On follow-up, all patients were ambulatory, and their conditions were as good as or better than before the operation. One patient had a previous subtotal removal at another institution and had a further small hemorrhage with a neurologic deficit that did not fully recover. In three patients, the CM protruded from the dorsal aspect of the spinal cord. In the others, a myelotomy was required, and in three of these patients, the lesion projected more to one side, and a myelotomy was placed in the dorsal root entry zone.

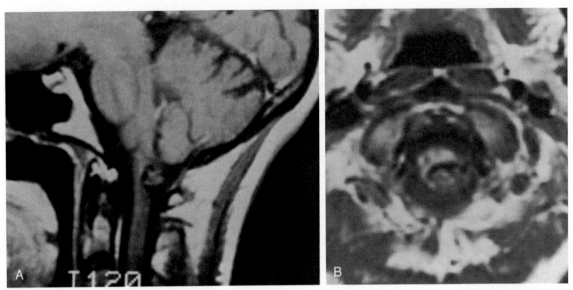

FIGURE 91-13 Cervical medullary junction cavernous malformation in a 36-year-old woman who had the onset of generalized headache 4 months before surgery. Twenty-four hours later, she noted numbness in the left lateral leg that progressed over the next week to involve the entire left lower extremity; this condition improved. A computed tomography scan of the head was normal. Two weeks later, the patient noted difficulty jogging because of discoordination in the left lower extremity. Magnetic resonance T1-weighted sagittal (*A*) and axial (*B*) images show a posteriorly placed lesion involving the midline and left side of the cervical medullary junction that is consistent with a cavernous angioma; the patient was followed. Ten days before she was admitted to the hospital, she had nausea and vomiting and increased numbness and weakness on the left side of her body. Complete excision of the lesion was followed by improvement in the left lower extremity function, temporary worsening of position sense in the left hand, and numbness in the left upper extremity. Subsequently, she had a good recovery; she was able to jog, and she returned to work.

CONCLUSIONS

The management of patients with CMs continues to evolve. Current recommendations for management are as follows:

1. Patients who are asymptomatic are observed.
2. Patients with acute severe or progressive neurologic deficits undergo surgical resection.
3. Patients presenting with medically uncontrolled seizures undergo surgical resection; patients with new-onset seizures may undergo resection, but some are observed, depending on the factors discussed in this chapter.
4. Patients with a single hemorrhage in the cerebrum, cerebellum, or spinal cord usually undergo surgical resection. When the hemorrhage is in the brain stem, thalamus, or basal ganglia, the patients are observed.
5. Patients with a recurrent hemorrhage usually undergo resection, but there are exceptions when the lesion is in a deep area with high surgical risk.

REFERENCES

1. McCormick WF: The pathology of vascular ("arteriovenous") malformations. J Neurosurg 24:807–816, 1966.
2. Rengachary SS, Kalyan-Raman UP: Other cranial intradural angiomas. In Wilkins RH, Rengachary SS (eds): Neurosurgery, vol 2. New York: McGraw-Hill, 1985, pp 1465–1472.
3. Russell DS, Rubinstein LJ: Pathology of Tumors of the Nervous System. London: Edward Arnold, 1959, pp 79–83.
4. Ogilvy CS, Heros RC, Ojemann RG, et al: Angiographically occult arteriovenous malformations. J Neurosurg 69:350–355, 1988.
5. Ojemann RG, Heros RG, Crowell RM: Surgical Management of Cerebrovascular Disease. Baltimore: Williams & Wilkins, 1988, pp 401–403.
6. Tung H, Giannotoa SL, Chandrasoma PT, et al: Recurrent intraparenchymal hemorrhage from angiographically occult vascular malformations. J Neurosurg 73:174–180, 1990.
7. Wakai S, Ueda Y, Inoh S, et al: Angiographically occult angiomas: A report of 13 cases with analysis of the cases documented in the literature. Neurosurgery 17:549–556, 1985.
8. Wilkins RH: Natural history of intracranial vascular malformations: A review. Neurosurgery 16:421–430, 1985.
9. Wilson CB: Cryptic vascular malformations. Clin Neurosurg 38:49–84, 1992.
10. Maraire JN, Awad IA: Intracranial cavernous malformations: Lesion behavior and management strategies. Neurosurgery 37:591–605, 1995.
11. Ogilvy CS, Louis DN, Ojemann RG: Intramedullary cavernous angiomas of the spinal cord: Clinical presentation, pathologic features and surgical management. Neurosurgery 31:219–230, 1992.
12. Rigamonti D, Spetzler RF: The association of venous and cavernous malformations: Report of four cases and discussion of the pathophysiological, diagnostic, and therapeutic implications. Acta Neurochir (Wien) 92:100–105, 1988.
13. Detwiler PW, Porter RW, Zabramski JM, et al: De novo formation of a central nervous system cavernous malformation: Implications for predicting risk of hemorrhage: Case report and review of the literature. J Neurosurg 87:629–632, 1997.
14. Larson JJ, Ball WS, Bove KE, et al: Formation of intracerebral cavernous malformations after radiation treatment for central nervous system neoplasia in children. J Neurosurg 88:51–56, 1998.
15. Pozzati E, Giangaspero F, Marliani F, et al: Occult cerebrovascular malformations after irradiation. Neurosurgery 39:677–682, 1996.
16. Pozzati E, Acciarri N, Tognetti F, et al: Growth, subsequent bleeding, and de novo appearance of cerebral cavernous angiomas. Neurosurgery 38:662–669, 1996.
17. Zabramski JM, Wascher TM, Spetzler RF, et al: The natural history of familial cavernous malformations: Results of an ongoing study. J Neurosurg 80:442–432, 1994.
18. Pozzati E, Giuliani G, Nuzzo G, et al: The growth of cerebral cavernous angiomas. Neurosurgery 25:91–97, 1989.
19. Rigamonti D, Drayer BP, Johnson PC, et al: The MRI appearance of cavernous malformations (angiomas). J Neurosurg 67:518–524, 1987.
20. Muras I, Confronti R, Scuotto A, et al: Cerebral cavernous angioma: Diagnostic considerations. J Neuroradiol 20:34–41, 1993.

21. Roda JM, Carceller F, Perez-Higueras A, et al: Encapsulated intracerebral hematoma: A defined entity. J Neurosurg 78:829–833, 1993.
22. Servo A, Porras M, Raininko R: Diagnosis of cavernous haemangiomas by computed tomography and angiography. Acta Neurochir (Wien) 71:273–282, 1984.
23. Hayman LA, Evans RA, Ferrell RE, et al: Familial cavernous angiomas: Natural history and genetic study over a 5-year period. Am J Med Genet 11:147–160, 1982.
24. Rigamonti D, Hadley MN, Drayer BP, et al: Cerebral cavernous malformations: Incidence and familial occurrence. N Engl J Med 19:343–347, 1988.
25. Labauge P, Laberge S, Brunereau L, et al: Hereditary cerebral cavernous angiomas: Clinical and genetic features in 57 French families. Societe Francaise de Neurochirurgie. Lancet 352:1891–1897, 1998.
26. Sunada I, Nakabayashi H, Tsuchida K, et al: A case of familial cerebral cavernous angioma and review of Japanese cases. No Shinkei Geka 29:359–365, 2001.
27. Siegel AM: Familial cavernous angioma: an unknown, known disease. Acta Neurol Scand 98:369–371, 1998.
28. Gil-Nagel A, Dubovsky J, Wilcox KJ, et al: Familial cerebral cavernous angioma: A gene localized to a 15–cm interval on chromosome 7q. Ann Neurol 39:807–810, 1996.
29. Gunel M, Awad IA, Anson J, et al: Mapping of a gene causing cerebral cavernous malformations to 7q11.2–q21. Proc Natl Acad Sci U S A 92:6620–6624, 1995.
30. Gunel M, Awad IA, Finberg K, et al: A founder mutation as a cause of cerebral cavernous malformation in Hispanic Americans. N Engl J Med 334:946–951, 1996.
31. Craig HD, Gunel M, Cepeda O, et al: Multilocus linkage identifies two new loci for a mendelian form of stroke, cerebral cavernous malformation, at 7p15–13 and 3q25.2–27. Hum Mol Genet 7:1851–1858, 1998.
32. Davenport WJ, Siegel AM, Dichgans J, et al: CCM1 gene mutations in families segregating cerebral cavernous malformations. Neurology 56:540–543, 2001.
33. Laberge-le Couteulx S, Jung HH, Labauge P, et al: Truncating mutations in CCM1, encoding KRIT1, cause hereditary cavernous angiomas. Nat Genet 23:189–193, 1999.
34. Zhang J, Clatterbuck RE, Rigamonti D, et al: Mutations in KRIT1 in familial cerebral cavernous malformations. Neurosurgery 46:1272–1277, 2000.
35. Marini V, Ferrera L, Dorcaratto A, et al: Identification of a novel KRIT1 mutation in an Italian family with cerebral cavernous malformations by the protein truncation test. J Neurol Sci 212:75–78, 2003.
36. Gunel M, Laurans MSH, Shin D, et al: KRIT1, a gene mutated in cerebral cavernous malformations, encodes a microtubule-associated protein. PNAS 99:10677–10682, 2002.
37. Liquori CL, Berg MJ, Siegel AM, et al: Mutations in a gene encoding a novel protein containing a phosphotyrosine-binding domain cause type 2 cerebral cavernous malformations. Am J Hum Genet 73:1459–1464, 2003.
38. Lucas M, Costa AF, Montori M, et al: Germline mutations in the CCM1gene, encoding KRIT1, cause cerebral cavernous malformations. Ann Neurol 49:529–532, 2001.
39. Kehrer-Sawatzki H, Wilda M, Braun VM, et al: Mutation and expression analysis of the KRIT1 gene associated with cerebral cavernous malformations (CCM1). Acta Neuropathol 104:231–240, 2002.
40. Voigt K, Yasargil MG: Cerebral cavernous haemangiomas or cavernomas: Incidence, pathology, localization, diagnosis, clinical features and treatment: Review of the literature and report of an unusual case. Neurochirurgia (Stuttg) 19:59–68, 1976.
41. Simard JM, Garcia-Bengochea F, Ballinger WE Jr, et al: Cavernous angioma: A review of 126 collected and 12 new clinical cases. Neurosurgery 18:162–172, 1986.
42. Robinson JR Jr, Awad IA, Little JR: Natural history of the cavernous angioma. J Neurosurg 75:709–719, 1991.
43. Curling OD Jr, Kelly DL, Elster AD, et al: An analysis of the natural history of cavernous angiomas. J Neurosurg 75:702–708, 1991.
44. Scott RM, Barnes P, Kupsky W, et al: Cavernous angiomas of the central nervous system in children. J Neurosurg 76:38–46, 1992.
45. Giombini S, Morello G: Cavernous angiomas of the brain: Account of 14 personal cases and review of the literature. Acta Neurochir (Wien) 40:61–82, 1978.
46. Porter PJ, Willinsky RA, Harper W, et al: Cerebral cavernous malformations: Natural history and prognosis after clinical deterioration with and without hemorrhage. J Neurosurg 87:190–197, 1997.
47. Zimmerman RS, Spetzler RF, Lee KS, et al: Cavernous malformations of the brain stem. J Neurosurg 75:32–39, 1991.
48. Robinson JR Sr, Awad IA, Magdinee M, et al: Factors predisposing to clinical disability in patients with cavernous malformations of the brain. Neurosurgery 32:730–736, 1993.
49. Moriarity JL, Wetzel M, Clatterbuck RE, et al: The natural history of cavernous malformations: A prospective study of 68 patients. Neurosurgery 44:1166–1171, 1999.
50. Labauge P, Brunereau L, Levy C, et al: The natural history of familial cerebral cavernomas: A retrospective MRI study of 40 patients. Neuroradiology 42:327–332, 2000.
51. Kondziolka D, Lunsford LD, Kestle JRW: The natural history of cerebral cavernous malformations. J Neurosurg 83:820–824, 1995.
52. Kim DS, Park YG, Choi JU, et al: An analysis of the natural history of cavernous malformations. Surg Neurol 48:9–17, 1997.
53. Kupersmith MJ, Kalish H, Epstein F, et al: Natural history of brain stem cavernous malformations. Neurosurgery 48:47–54, 2001.
54. Aiba T, Tanaka R, Koike T, et al: Natural history of intracranial cavernous malformations. J Neurosurg 83:56–59, 1995.
55. Barker FG, Amin-Hanjani S, Butler WE, et al: Temporal clustering of hemorrhages from untreated cavernous malformations of the central nervous system. Neurosurgery 49:15–25, 2001.
56. Narayan P, Barrow DL: Intramedullary spinal cavernous malformation following spinal irradiation: Case report and review of the literature. J Neurosurg 98(Suppl 1):68–72, 2003.
57. Massa-Micon B, Luparello V, Bergui M, et al: De novo cavernoma case report and review of the literature. Surg Neurol 53:484–487, 2000.
58. Ludemann W, Ellerkamp V, Stan AC, et al: De novo development of a cavernous malformation of the brain: Significance of factors with paracrine and endocrine activity: Case report. Neurosurgery 50:646–649, 2002.
59. Golfinos JG, Wascher TM, Zabramskik JM, et al: The management of unruptured intracranial vascular malformation. Barrow Neurol Inst Q 8:2–11, 1992.
60. Amin-Hanjani S, Ogilvy CS, Ojemann RG, et al: Risks of surgical management for cavernous malformations of the nervous system. Neurosurgery 42:1220–1227, 1998.
61. Esposito V, Oppido PA, Delfini R, et al: A simple method for stereotactic microsurgical excision of small deep-seated cavernous angiomas. Neurosurgery 34:515–519, 1994.
62. Kondziolka D, Lunsford LD, Flickinger JC, et al: Reduction of hemorrhage risk after stereotactic radiosourgery for cavernous malformations. J Neurosurg 83:825–831, 1995.
63. Hasegawa T, McInerney, Kondziolka D, et al: Long-term results after stereotactic radiosurgery for patients with cavernous malformations. Neurosurgery 50:1190–1197, 2002.
64. Karlsson B, Kihlstrom L, Lindquist C, et al: Radisourgery for cavernous malformations. J Neurosurg 88:293–297, 1998.
65. Pollock BE, Garces YI, Stafford SL, et al: Stereotactic radiosurgery for cavernous malformations. J Neurosurg 93:987–991, 2000.
66. Zhang N, Pan L, Wang BJ, et al: Gamma knife radiosurgery for cavernous hemangiomas. J Neurosurg 93(Suppl 3):74–77, 2000.
67. Fabrikant JI, Levy RP, Steinberg GK, et al: Charged-particle radiosurgery for intracranial vascular malformations. Neurosurg Clin N Am 3:99–139, 1992.
68. Alexander E III, Loeffler SS: Radiosurgery using a modified linear accelerator. Neurosurg Clin N Am 3:167–190, 1992.
69. Chang SD, Levy RP, Adler JR, et al: Stereotactic radiosurgery of angiographically occult vascular malformations: 14-year experience. Neurosurgery 43:213–220, 1998.
70. Amin-Hanjani S, Ogilvy CS, Candia GJ, et al: Stereotactic radiosurgery for cavernous malformations: Kjellberg's experience with proton beam therapy in 98 cases at the Harvard Cyclotron. Neurosurgery 42:1229–1238, 1998.
71. St George EJ, Perks J, Plowman PN: Stereotactic radiosurgery XIV: The role of the haemosiderin "ring" in the development of adverse reactions following radiosurgery for intracranial cavernous malformations: A sustainable hypothesis. Br J Neurosurg 16:385–391, 2002.
72. Acciarri N, Padovani R, Giulioni M, et al: Intracranial and orbital cavernous angiomas: A review of 74 surgical cases. Br J Neurosurg 7:529–539, 1993.
73. Little JR, Awad IA, Jones SC, et al: Vascular pressures and cortical blood flow in cavernous angioma of the brain. J Neurosurg 73:555–559, 1990.
74. Schneider RC, Liss L: Cavernous hemangiomas of the cerebral hemispheres. J Neurosurg 15:391–399, 1958.

75. Tagle P, Huete I, Mendez J, et al: Intracranial cavernous angioma: Presentation and management. J Neurosurg 64:720–723, 1986.

76. Vaquero J, Leunda G, Martinez R, et al: Cavernomas of the brain. Neurosurgery 12:208–210, 1983.

77. Yamasaki T, Hande H, Yamashita J, et al: Intracranial and orbital cavernous angiomas. J Neurosurg 64:197–208, 1986.

78. Chadduck WM, Binet EF, Farrell FW Jr, et al: Intraventricular cavernous hemangioma: Report of three cases and review of the literature. Neurosurgery 16:189–197, 1985.

79. Pozzati E: Thalamic cavernous malformations. Surg Neurol 53:30–39, 2000.

80. Lorenzana L, Cabezudo JM, Porras LF, et al: Focal dystonia secondary to cavernous angioma of the basal ganglia: Case report and review of the literature. Neurosurgery 31:1108–1112, 1992.

81. Roda JM, Alvarez F, Isla A, et al: Thalamic cavernous malformations. J Neurosurg 72:642–649, 1990.

82. Bertalanffy H, Gilsbach JM, Eggert HR, et al: Microsurgery of deep-seated cavernous angiomas: Report of 26 cases. Acta Neurochir (Wien) 108:91–99, 1991.

83. Steinberg GK, Chang SD, Gewirtz RJ, et al: Microsurgical resection of brain stem, thalamic and basal ganglia angiographically occult vascular malformation. Neurosurgery 46:260–271, 2000.

84. Bertalanffy H, Kuhn G, Scheremet R, et al: Indications for surgery and prognosis in patients with cerebral cavernous angiomas. Neurol Med Chir (Tokyo) 32:659–666, 1992.

85. Cohen DS, Zubay GP, Goodman RR: Seizure outcome after lesionectomy for cavernous malformations. J Neurosurg 83:237–242, 1995.

86. Casazza M, Broggi G, Franzini A, et al: Supratentorial cavernous angiomas and epileptic seizures: Preoperative course and postoperative outcome. Neurosurgery 39:26–34, 1996.

87. Zevgaridis D, van Velthoven V, Ebeling U, et al: Seizure control following surgery in supratentorial cavernous malformations: A retrospective study in 77 patients. Acta Neurochir (Wien) 138:672–677, 1996.

88. Cappabianca P, Alfieri A, Maiuri F, et al: Supratentorial cavernous malformations and epilepsy: Seizure outcome after lesionectomy on a series of 35 patients. Clin Neurol Neurosurg Psychiatry 99:179–183, 1997.

89. Falbusch R, Strauss C, Huk W, et al: Surgical removal of pontomesencephalic cavernous hemangioma. Neurosurgery 26:449–457, 1990.

90. Porter RW, Detwiler PW, Spetzler RF, et al: Cavernous malformations of the brain stem: Experience with 100 patients. J Neurosurg 90:50–58, 1999.

91. Bertalanffy H, Benes L, Miyazawa T, et al: Cerebral cavernomas in the adult: Review of the literature and analysis of 72 surgically treated patients. Neurosurg Rev 25:1–53, 2002.

92. Ziyal IM, Sekhar LN, Salas E, et al: Surgical management of cavernous malformations of the brain stem. Br J Neurosurg 13:366–375, 1999.

93. Samii M, Eghbal R, Carvalho GA, et al: Surgical management of brain stem cavernomas. J Neurosurg 95:825–832, 2001.

94. Wang C, Liu A, Zhang J, et al: Surgical management of brain stem cavernous malformations: Report of 137 cases. Surg Neurol 59:444–454, 2003.

95. Mathiesen T, Edner G, Kihlstrom L: Deep and brain stem cavernomas: A consecutive 8-year series. J Neurosurg 99:31–37, 2003.

96. Sandalcioglu IE, Wiedemayer H, Secer S, et al: Surgical removal of brain stem cavernous malformations: Surgical indications, technical considerations, and results. J Neurol Neurosurg Psychiatry 72:351–355, 2002.

97. Isamat F, Louesa G: Cavernous angioma of the brain stem. Neurosurg Clin N Am 4:507–518, 1993.

98. Fritschi JA, Reulen HJ, Spetzler RF, et al: Cavernous malformations of the brain stem. Acta Neurochir (Wien) 130:35–46, 1994.

99. Weil SM, Tew JM: Surgical management of brain stem vascular malformations. Acta Neurochir (Wien) 105:14–23, 1990.

100. Scott RM: Brain stem cavernous angiomas in children. Pediatr Neurosurg 16:281–286, 1990.

101. LeDoux M, Aronin PA, Odrezin GT: Surgically treated cavernous angiomas of the brain stem: Report of two cases and review of the literature. Surg Neurol 35:395–399, 1991.

102. Corboy JR, Galetta SL: Familial cavernous angiomas manifesting with an acute chiasmal syndrome. Am J Ophthalmol 108:245–250, 1989.

103. Malik S, Cohen BH, Robinson J, et al: Progressive vision loss: A rare manifestation of familial cavernous angiomas. Arch Neurol 49: 170–173, 1992.

104. Matias-Guiu X, Alejo M, Sole T, et al: Cavernous angiomas of the cranial nerves. J Neurosurg 73:620–622, 1990.

105. Ogilvy CS, Pakzaban P, Lee JM: Oculomotor nerve cavernous angioma in a patient with Robert's syndrome. Surg Neurol 33:39–47, 1993.

106. Deshmukh VR, Albuquerque FC, Zabramski JM, et al: Surgical management of cavernous malformations involving the cranial nerves. Neurosurgery 53:352–357, 2003.

107. Shibuya M, Baskaya MK, Saito K, et al: Cavernous malformations of the optic chiasm. Acta Neurochir (Wien) 136:29–36, 1995.

108. Sundaresan N, Ellen T, Civic I: Hemangiomas of the internal auditory canal. Surg Neurol 6:119–121, 1976.

109. Scott RM: Third nerve palsy in a 14-year-old boy due to cavernous hemangioma of the third nerve. In Raimond AJ (ed): Concepts in Pediatric Neurosurgery. New York: Karger, 1983, pp 100–107.

110. Vishteh AG, Zabramski JM, Spetzler RF: Patients with spinal cord cavernous malformations are at an increased risk for multiple neuraxis cavernous malformations. Neurosurgery 45:30–32, 1999.

111. Sandalcioglu IE, Wiedemayer H, Gasser T, et al: Intramedullary spinal cord cavernous malformations: Clinical features and risk of hemorrhage. Neurosurg Rev 26:253–256, 2003.

112. Gordon CR, Crockard HA, Symon L: Surgical management of spinal cord cavernoma. Br J Neurosurg 9:459–464, 1995.

113. Spetzger U, Gilsbach JM, Bertalanffy H: Cavernous angiomas of the spinal cord clinical presentation, surgical strategy, and postoperative results. Acta Neurochir (Wien) 134:200–206, 1995.

114. Anson JA, Spetzler RF: Surgical resection of intramedullary spinal cord cavernous malformations. J Neurosurg 78:446–451, 1993.

115. Cosgrove GR, Bertrand G, Fontaine S, et al: Cavernous angiomas of the spinal cord. J Neurosurg 68:31–36, 1988.

116. McCormick PC, Michelson WJ, Post KD, et al: Cavernous malformations of the spinal cord. Neurosurgery 23:459–463, 1988.

117. Cantore G, Delfini R, Cervoni L, et al: Intramedullary cavernous angiomas of the spinal cord: Report of six cases. Surg Neurol 43:448–452, 1995.

118. Canavero S, Pagni CA, Duca S, et al: Spinal intramedullary cavernous angiomas: A literature meta-analysis. Surg Neurol 41:381–388, 1994.

92

Surgical Management of Brain Stem Vascular Malformations

JOHN M. TEW, JR., MICHAEL J. LINK, and ADAM I. LEWIS

Historically, brain stem vascular malformations were considered inoperable because of their deep location and intimate relationship to complex neurovascular structures.[1] Nevertheless, the natural history of this disorder suggests that more than 50% of patients with deep-seated arteriovenous malformations (AVMs) experience significant morbidity or death from hemorrhage.[2] With the advent of magnetic resonance imaging (MRI), more brain stem vascular malformations are being discovered. Advances in microsurgical technique and refinement in skull-base approaches have expanded the operative domains of the neurosurgeon to include vascular malformations of the brain stem. Furthermore, intraoperative monitoring of brain stem tracts and stimulation of brain stem nuclei have helped reduce morbidity by avoiding injury to vital brain stem structures. The authors and others have shown that surgical excision of brain stem vascular malformations is a safe and effective mode of treatment in selected patients.[3–6]

CLASSIFICATION

Intracranial vascular malformations are classified pathologically as AVMs, cavernous malformations, venous malformations, and capillary telangiectasias.[7] Clinically, brain stem vascular malformations may be divided into angiographically visible and occult vascular malformations.[8] AVMs and cavernous malformations are the only vascular malformations that are amenable to operative intervention. McCormick and colleagues[9] reviewed 164 posterior fossa AVMs and found 38 telangiectasias. None of these lesions showed signs of hemorrhage, and all affected individuals were asymptomatic. In our experience, venous malformations do not cause intracranial hemorrhage. A retrospective review of MRIs found that venous angiomas are benign lesions that should be managed conservatively.[10] One prospective study by McLaughlin and colleagues[11] confirms that venous malformations have a benign natural history.

Most surgeons refer to the AVM classification for operative difficulty of Spetzler and Martin.[12] In this system, five surgical grades are based on the size of the AVM, the relationship to eloquent neural structures, and venous drainage. Results demonstrated that with each successive grade, the percentage of patients sustaining a permanent neurologic deficit related to surgery increased. Vascular malformations of the brain stem defy the classification system of Spetzler and Martin because venous characteristics and size have little connection with expected outcome.

NATURAL HISTORY

AVMs of the brain stem are rare, representing only 1% of all AVMs. They usually present with hemorrhage and neurologic deficit; once symptomatic, they tend to hemorrhage repeatedly. The natural history of symptomatic AVMs demonstrates a rate of major rebleeding of 4% per year. Combined major morbidity and mortality is 2.7% per year.[2] Each hemorrhagic episode carries a 10% mortality rate and a 30% major morbidity rate. Because brain stem AVMs are located in a densely packed area of vital brain tissue and have little space for an expanding hematoma, the deficits resulting from hemorrhage here are often more devastating than those for AVMs in other locations.

CLINICAL FEATURES

The initial presentation of brain stem vascular malformations varies greatly, and the clinical course may resemble that of low-grade gliomas, multiple sclerosis, or inflammatory disorders. Unlike most supratentorial cavernous malformations that present with seizures,[13] those in the brain stem present with parenchymal hemorrhage.

Once symptomatic, brain stem AVMs tend to hemorrhage repeatedly.[14,15] Although cavernous malformations also have a propensity toward recurrent hemorrhage, they rarely rupture into the subarachnoid space or the ventricular system. Further, cavernous malformations are low-flow lesions that produce less destruction than parenchymal AVMs when they rupture[8,16]; consequently, cavernous malformations tend to displace rather than destroy neural tissues.[17] In most cases, patients with cavernous malformations recover significant neurologic function if brain stem tolerance for the mass effect of the hematoma is not exceeded. By comparison, ruptured brain stem AVMs produce larger hematomas, and patients are less likely to recover neurologic function.[16] Finally, brain stem AVMs often produce subarachnoid or intraventricular hemorrhage because they are superficial or subpial to the brain stem surface.

Clinical signs and symptoms are related to the location of the malformation. In our series of 128 patients, presenting symptoms in order of frequency were diplopia, facial numbness, incoordination, gait difficulties, numbness and paresthesias, arm or leg weakness, and difficulty speaking and swallowing. Clinical signs included abducens and oculomotor palsy, internuclear ophthalmoplegia, nuclear facial palsy, nystagmus, facial hypoesthesia, hemisensory deficit, hyperreflexia, hemiparesis, and cerebellar ataxia (Table 92-1).

TABLE 92-1 ▪ **Clinical Findings in 128 Patients with Brain Stem Arteriovenous Malformations**

	No.	Percent
Hemorrhage	110	86
Cranial nerve palsy	90	70
Cerebellar ataxia	68	53
Sensory loss	46	36
Hemiparesis	32	25
Dysarthria-dysphagia	17	13
Neurologically intact	21	16

PREOPERATIVE EVALUATION

Angiography is the current standard for AVM evaluation. A complete angiographic evaluation includes a four-vessel study and sequential evaluation of all phases, including arterial, capillary, and venous phases. This sequence gives a clear understanding of vascular dynamics of the malformation, such as rate of blood flow, differential in regional flow (arterial steal), and patterns of collateral flow. Additional information includes nidus size and configuration as well as the position, number, and size of feeding arteries and associated aneurysms. Rotational angiography provides a 3-dimensional understanding of the anatomy.

Because most cavernous malformations are not visible by angiography, MRI is the best study for preoperative evaluation. MRI of cavernous malformations shows a consistent morphologic appearance: a central focus of mixed signal intensity representing hemorrhage of various ages. The nidus is surrounded by a hypointense rim on T2 of hemosiderin from chronic microhemorrhages. Venous malformations are associated with cavernous malformations in 15% of cases. For both malformation types, MRI describes the 3-dimensional location relative to the regional brain and bony anatomy. MRI also provides information regarding the presence of hemorrhage, the relative chronology of multiple hemorrhages, and the status of regional parenchyma in terms of mass effect, edema, and injury.[18]

Patients with recurrent hemorrhage and progressive neurologic deficit are candidates for surgery. Ideally, the lesion should be superficial to the brain stem surface. When the malformation is not subpial and the patient continues to deteriorate, a corridor of noneloquent tissue can be defined by use of intraoperative monopolar stimulation of brain stem nuclei. There are no data to indicate that treatment of asymptomatic lesions is warranted. Surgical intervention, in our experience, is associated with a transient neurologic deficit in more than 60% of cases and may not be advisable in a neurologically intact patient. We do not advocate surgery for patients with recurrent hemorrhage who have minimal or no neurologic deficits and whose malformation lies deep to the brain stem surface.

Some argue that surgery should be soon, before the clot retracts and limits access. We agree with others that the best time to operate is when the condition is subacute.[19,20] Allowing time for the patient to recover from the ictus and the hematoma to organize are the main reasons for operating within 1 to 4 weeks. The hematoma is well differentiated from the surrounding gliotic capsule, and a plane for dissection is easily defined. Operations performed emergently are avoided because the hematoma is not consolidated; the edematous neural tissue is friable; and the gliotic plane between the malformation and the brain stem is poorly defined. However, if the operation is delayed more than 1 month, the malformation may adhere to the gliotic capsule; removal of the malformation often leaves a ragged gliotic plane, which increases the potential for residual malformation. Furthermore, posthemorrhagic fibrosis occurs within the malformation after the subacute period and may require vigorous exploration and manipulation to remove.

Regional Surgical Anatomy

Mesencephalic AVMs are rare lesions that are usually located on the surface of the brain stem. Those that lie on the tectum produce disturbances in ocular motility and consciousness when hemorrhage occurs. More laterally placed lesions may lie at the junction of the upper fourth ventricle and the superior cerebellar peduncle in the pia-arachnoid space (above the root entry zone of the trigeminal nerve). Arterial supply arises from the superior cerebellar and anteroinferior cerebellar arteries. Contribution from the posterior cerebral artery branches is variable. Venous drainage is to the superior petrosal, mesencephalic, and superior vermian veins and the basal vein of Rosenthal. The trochlear nerve is often entangled in the malformation.

Cerebellopontine angle AVMs are supplied primarily from anteroinferior cerebellar artery and posteroinferior cerebellar artery branches. Feeding arteries are often intertwined with cranial nerves V through XII. Usually, these AVMs maintain an extrapial or superficially subpial location and may extend into the fourth ventricle. During resection, the fourth ventricle should be inspected for residual AVM. Venous drainage is to the superior petrosal, ependymal, and pontomesencephalic veins.

Pontomedullary AVMs are often embedded in the brain stem and have a vascular supply derived from the penetrating branches of the basilar artery and branches of the anteroinferior and posteroinferior cerebellar arteries. These vessels are often indistinct from those supplying normal brain. Additionally, pontomedullary AVMs may derive their blood supply from anteroinferior cerebellar and superior cerebellar artery branches. The nidus tends to be smaller and less accessible than that of other brain stem AVMs. Venous drainage is via lateral mesencephalic and pontomesencephalic veins. In our experience, brain stem AVMs supplied by penetrating branches of the basilar artery cannot be safely removed surgically.

Surgical Approaches

Four surgical approaches to brain stem vascular malformations exist: superior vermian, inferior vermian, lateral cerebellar, and combined subtemporal-suboccipital transtentorial (Fig. 92-1). The surgical approach is dictated by the most superficial location of the vascular malformation to the surface of the brain stem (Fig. 92-2). For midline approaches, the patient is positioned with the lesion side down to allow the widest angle of approach to the lesion and to avoid retraction of the brain stem (Fig. 92-3).

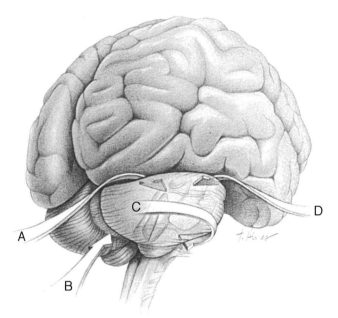

FIGURE 92-1 There are four approaches to brain stem vascular malformations illustrated in this drawing: superior vermian (*A*), inferior vermian (*B*), lateral cerebellar (*C*), and combined subtemporal-suboccipital transtentorial (*D*). The approach is dictated by the most superficial location of the malformation to the surface of the brain stem or fourth ventricle. (From Tew JM Jr, van Loveren HR: Atlas of Operative Microneurosurgery, vol 1. Philadelphia: WB Saunders, 1994.)

Anesthetic Considerations

Anesthesiologists serve an integral role for AVM resection. They reduce the patient's intracranial pressure, protect the brain from ischemia, and maintain hypotension during resection, which aids in hemostasis. Initially, the patient is hyperventilated to a P_{CO_2} of 25 to 30 mm Hg, and osmotic diuretics are administered to reduce intracranial pressure. Spinal drainage via a lumbar drain further relaxes the brain. A nitroprusside drip is titrated to mean arterial pressure of 60 mm Hg during the resection of the AVM. Induced hypotension is essential to control bleeding or intraoperative brain swelling during the resection of AVMs.

However, patients may be kept normotensive for resection of cavernous malformations. Cerebral protection with etomidate or barbiturates may be given during the operation to avoid ischemia to surrounding brain tissue.

Adjuncts to Surgery

Before surgery, baseline electrophysiologic monitoring, including brain stem auditory evoked responses and somatosensory evoked potentials are obtained. Stimulation of brain stem nuclei and motor cranial nerves with a monopolar electromyogram stimulator (Xomed Nerve Integrity Monitor-2, Xomed-Treace, Jacksonville, FL) defines a corridor of noneloquent tissue and prevents injury to vital brain stem tracts. Typically, the abducens, facial, vagal, and hypoglossal nuclei are monitored and stimulated bilaterally. Real-time intraoperative ultrasound precisely locates the malformation, avoids dissection of normal tissue, and ensures a complete surgical resection. Imaging is performed with an Ultramark 9 (High Density Imaging) real-time, color-flow ultrasound system (Advanced Technology Laboratories, Bothell, WA). The ultrasonic probe with an 8-mm diameter provides a 180-degree sweep with a frequency of 7 MHz. The high-density imaging boosts the effective frequency to 14 MHz. The combined potassium-titanium-phosphate (KTP) and neodymium:yttrium-aluminum-garnet (Nd:YAG) laser (Laserscope Surgical Systems, San Jose, CA) is particularly useful in defining a plane between the malformation and normal tissue. A focusing micromanipulator with coincident helium-neon laser for coaxial aiming is attached to the microscope (Opmilas YAG, Carl Zeiss). Bypassing the hand-held piece allows better visualization of deep regions in the brain stem.

Preoperative embolization of brain stem AVMs has been rarely successful. Advances in microcatheters and guidewires allow for improved navigation of the small intraluminal diameters and acute angles characteristic of feeding arteries. However, the lack of collateral vessels poses a high risk of producing brain stem infarction from inadvertent occlusion of normal arteries; therefore, a cure is never achieved.

Stereotactic radiosurgery is worthy of consideration for asymptomatic AVMs involving the tectum, for which surgical risk is high. There is no conclusive evidence that radiosurgery

FIGURE 92-2 This series of T1-weighted magnetic resonance imaging scans demonstrates three discrete hemorrhagic episodes from a pontine cavernous malformation. After the third hemorrhage, a complete surgical resection was performed with no new neurologic deficits. Surgical therapy is indicated if there is recurrent hemorrhage or progressive neurologic deficit or if the lesion is superficial to the brain stem surface.

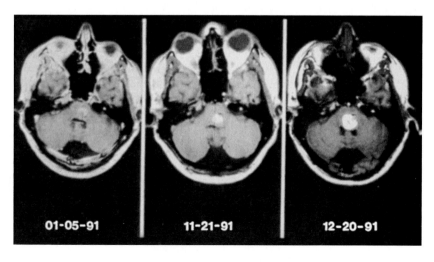

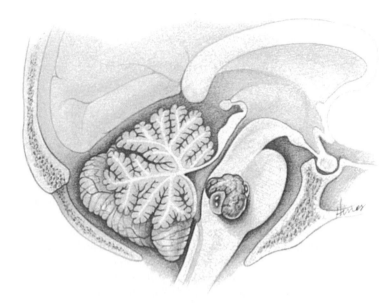

FIGURE 92-3 A sagittal view of the case presented in Figure 92-2 shows the relationship of the cavernous malformation to the fourth ventricle, pons, and cerebellum. The surgical approach to this lesion is midline with sectioning of the inferior vermis to expose the floor of the fourth ventricle. (From Tew JM Jr, van Loveren HR: Atlas of Operative Microneurosurgery, vol 1. Philadelphia: WB Saunders, 1994.)

is effective in preventing rebleeding of cavernous or venous malformations and may be associated with a significant risk of radionecrosis.

SURGICAL TECHNIQUE

The goal of surgery is complete excision of the malformation to eliminate the risk of hemorrhage. The patient undergoes general endotracheal anesthesia in the supine position. An armored endotracheal tube is placed to allow the neck to be flexed, facilitating exposure to the posterior fossa. The groin is prepared, and a femoral artery sheath is placed and maintained with heparin solution under pressure for intraoperative angiography. Intraoperative angiography is not planned for patients with cavernous malformations. A radial arterial line and urinary catheter are inserted, and pneumatic compression stockings are placed on the legs. Paired electrodes are placed in the lateral rectus, orbicularis oris, vocalis muscle, and hypoglossal muscles to monitor cranial nerve nuclei. The median and auditory nerves are also selected to evaluate somatosensory and brain stem auditory evoked responses, respectively. The patient is placed in the lateral oblique position with the thorax elevated 15 degrees to improve venous drainage. The head is held in slight lateral extension and cervical flexion with the radiolucent Mayfield three-point fixation device for intraoperative angiography (Ohio Medical Instrument Company, Cincinnati, OH). Appropriate padding is placed, including an axillary roll for protection of the brachial plexus. A lumbar drain is placed in the lumbar cistern for cerebrospinal fluid drainage, and hyperventilation to a PCO_2 of 25 to 30 mm Hg is maintained.

For tectal, pontine, and medullary vascular malformations, a midline suboccipital skin incision is made from the inion to the level of C2. A bilateral suboccipital craniotomy is performed with Midas Rex pneumatic instrumentation (Midas Rex Institute, Fort Worth, TX). The bony removal includes the foramen magnum and the posterior arch of C1. The dura is opened in a Y-shaped fashion with the incision based on the transverse sinus. The Budde Halo system of flexible arm, self-retracting blades is used to expose the vermis

in the midline (Ohio Medical Instrument Company, Cincinnati, OH). The cistern is opened, and the tonsils are retracted laterally with two 10-mm self-retaining retractors. For lesions of the pons or medulla, the lower one third of the vermis is split by use of bipolar electrocautery or focused carbon dioxide laser energy at 10 WC, which is delivered via a micromanipulator attached to the operating microscope (Fig. 92-4). For lesions of the mesencephalon, the upper vermis is sectioned. Microretractors are positioned to permit visualization from the median raphe to the lateral recesses of the fourth ventricle. In most cases, the vascular malformation is subependymal and distorts the floor of the fourth ventricle.

Monopolar stimulation of the floor of the fourth ventricle effectively maps the sixth, seventh, tenth, and twelfth cranial nerve nuclei (Fig. 92-5). In pontomedullary AVMs, the hematoma cavity is opened lateral to the seventh nerve nucleus with the carbon dioxide laser (Fig. 92-6). Suction is used to remove the liquefied portion of the cavity, and the KTP or Nd:YAG laser is used to remove the solid component. A plane of dissection is developed between the malformation and the gliotic capsule (Fig. 92-7). Feeding arteries are sacrificed while adequate venous drainage is preserved. Deep microscopic arteries that penetrate the bed of resection are obliterated with the impedance monitored bipolar forceps and laser (Fig. 92-8). Hypotension is continued throughout the dissection phase, at least until intraoperative angiography has proved that the AVM is completely excised.

Precise inspection of all bleeding points is mandatory because these vessels may have lost their autoregulation (i.e., ability to contract) and must be thoroughly obliterated by sealing of their collagen walls (Fig. 92-9). Application of a small pledget of absorbable gelatin sponge (Gelfoam) soaked with thrombin under a gently applied retractor can eliminate troublesome bleeding from capillaries and arterioles. Cavernous malformations may be subdivided by numerous trabeculae and pockets of malformation that can become embedded and hidden from view within the gliotic capsule. Intraoperative ultrasound is a useful first step to evaluate residual AVMs and is essential to detect residual cavernous malformations. Finally, a postoperative MRI (Fig. 92-10) or intraoperative angiography with digital subtraction in two

FIGURE 92-4 The dura is opened by cruciate incision. The cisterna magna is opened, and the tonsils are retracted laterally with two 10-mm self-retaining retractors. After the obex is exposed, the inferior vermis between distal branches of the posteroinferior cerebellar artery (PICA) is incised with focused laser energy. (From Tew JM Jr, van Loveren HR: Atlas of Operative Microneurosurgery, vol 1. Philadelphia: WB Saunders, 1994.)

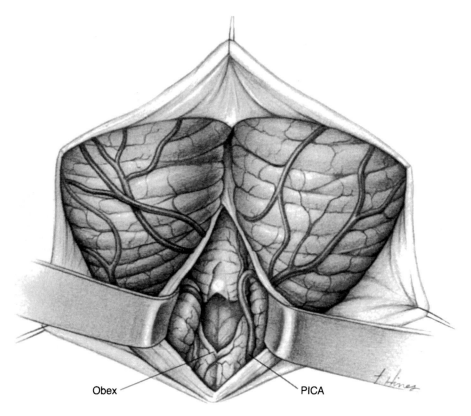

Obex   PICA

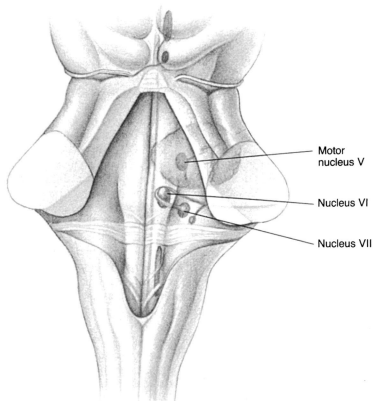

Motor nucleus V

Nucleus VI

Nucleus VII

FIGURE 92-5 Anatomy of the floor of the fourth ventricle is shown in relation to the distorted appearance of the operative view. The locations of the cranial nerve V, VI, and VII nuclei are mapped on the floor of the fourth ventricle by monopolar electrical stimulation in order to avoid injury during removal of the vascular malformation. In combination with somatosensory evoked potentials and brain stem auditory evoked responses, brain stem monitoring has helped to reduce postoperative morbidity. (From Tew JM Jr, van Loveren HR: Atlas of Operative Microneurosurgery, vol 1. Philadelphia: WB Saunders, 1994.)

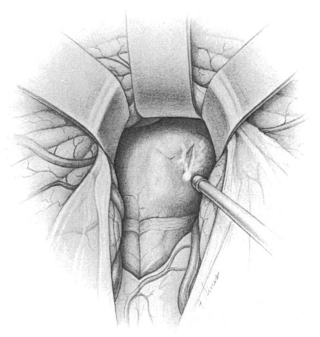

FIGURE 92-6 Retractors are positioned to permit visualization from the median raphe to the lateral recess of the right fourth ventricle. After mapping the floor of the fourth ventricle, an incision is made 1-cm superolateral to the site where stimulation elicited a facial response. (From Tew JM Jr, van Loveren HR: Atlas of Operative Microneurosurgery, vol 1. Philadelphia: WB Saunders, 1994.)

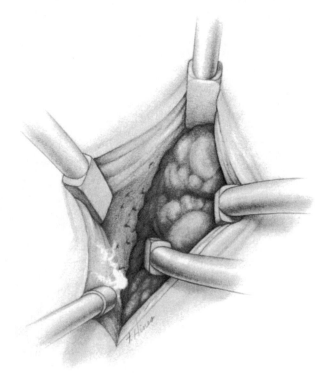

FIGURE 92-8 Initially, the liquefied portion of the hematoma is aspirated with atraumatic suction catheters. A plane is defined between the gliotic capsule and the malformation by coagulating arteriolar-like feeding arteries with bipolar forceps or laser energy. (From Tew JM Jr, van Loveren HR: Atlas of Operative Microneurosurgery, vol 1. Philadelphia: WB Saunders, 1994.)

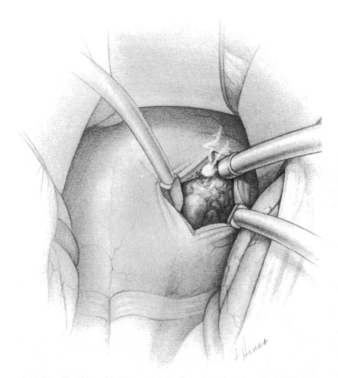

FIGURE 92-7 Opposing 2-mm retractors provide exposure of the thrombosed malformation. Later in the dissection, these retractors are very useful in allowing visualization of the entire cavity without undue manipulation of the brain stem tissues. (From Tew JM Jr, van Loveren HR: Atlas of Operative Microneurosurgery, vol 1. Philadelphia: WB Saunders, 1994.)

planes is essential to document complete removal of the AVMs. Physiologic preservation of the brain stem nuclei is confirmed by stimulation with the monopolar instrument.

Laterally placed vascular malformations in the cerebellopontine angle are resected through a lateral cerebellar approach. A straight incision over the mastoid notch that crosses the superior nuchal line and descends in the midline is performed. The superior and lateral myofascial cuff is retained, and the skin and muscle flaps are reflected inferiorly. A burr hole is made at the asterion, and a craniotomy is carried laterally to the edge of the sigmoid sinus and superiorly to the edge of the transverse sinus. The inferior margin extends to the foramen magnum to permit adequate decompression and removal of cerebrospinal fluid from the cisterna magna. A curvilinear incision is made in the dura after good cerebellar relaxation is achieved. The cerebellar hemisphere is retracted medially. The malformation and hematoma are dissected free from the gliotic cerebellum, and the pia-arachnoid membrane adjacent to the AVM is developed. Numerous branches of the superior cerebellar artery and anteroinferior cerebellar artery are coagulated and incised. Commonly, the AVM is entangled in the cranial nerves, but they can be preserved with precise dissection. The nidus of cerebellopontine angle AVMs usually remains superficial to the brain stem surface. Most of these upper prepontine AVMs are located in a pia-arachnoid plane and are readily excised. If they are embedded in the tissue of the brain stem, they may be unresectable.

A posterolateral approach to the brain stem is preferable for pontine cavernous malformations that do not present to

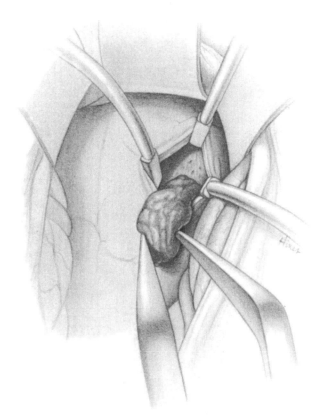

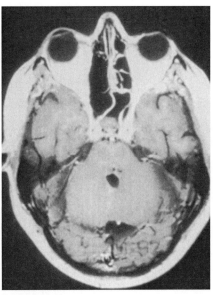

FIGURE 92-10 Postoperative T1-weighted magnetic resonance imaging scan of the patient depicted in Figure 92-2 shows no residual vascular malformation.

FIGURE 92-9 The shrunken malformation is removed from the cavity of the pons. The entire bed of the cavity is inspected for residual malformation. Real-time color-coded ultrasound is useful for identifying loculated areas of malformation that are embedded in the gliotic capsule. Electrophysiologic stimulation of the resection bed and floor of the fourth ventricle is repeated (after resection of the malformation) to confirm preservation of brain stem nuclei. (From Tew JM Jr, van Loveren HR: Atlas of Operative Microneurosurgery, vol 1. Philadelphia: WB Saunders, 1994.)

the ependymal surface of the floor of the fourth ventricle (Fig. 92-11). This approach has the advantage of allowing early interruption of the main feeding vessels to the lesion from the basilar artery. It also permits a longer myelotomy compared with opening the floor of the fourth ventricle, extending from the root entry zone of cranial nerve V to the root exit zone of nerve VII on the lateral pons.

A combined temporal-suboccipital craniotomy is performed, allowing access to both the posterior and middle cranial fossae. A mastoidectomy is then performed, and the dense cortical bone overlying the semicircular canals and the facial nerve is identified. This represents the limit of the anterior bone resection to expose the presigmoid dura (Fig. 92-12A). The presigmoid and middle fossa dura is opened, and the superior petrosal sinus is ligated and cut

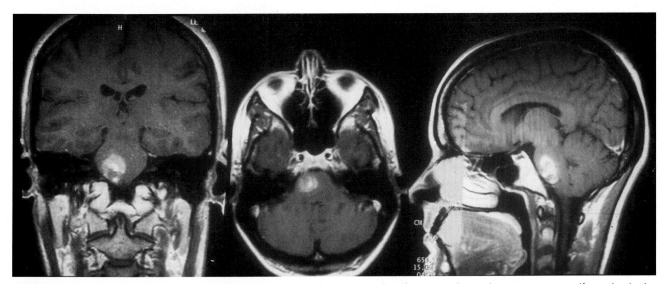

FIGURE 92-11 Coronal, axial, and sagittal T1-weighted magnetic resonance imaging scans show a large cavernous malformation in the right ventral pons. The patient presented with progressive left hemiparesis and sixth nerve palsy.

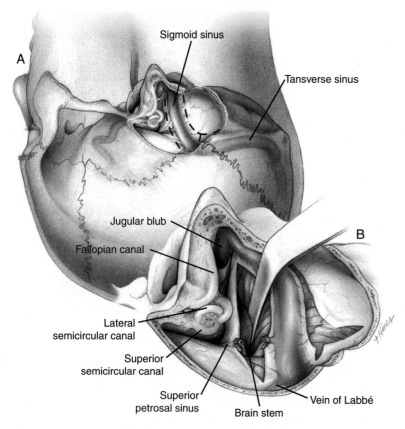

A

Sigmoid sinus

Tansverse sinus

Jugular blub

Fallopian canal

Lateral
semicircular canal

Superior
semicircular canal

Superior
petrosal sinus

Brain stem

Vein of Labbé

B

FIGURE 92-12   Posterior petrosectomy with preservation of the labyrinth and skeletonization of the fallopian canal (*A*). The mastoidectomy is expanded to expose the temporal lobe to facilitate sacrifice of the superior petrosal sinus, section of the tentorium cerebelli, and placement of relaxing incision above the transverse sinus, along with a small suboccipital (retrosigmoid) craniotomy. *Dashed lines* represent dural incisions. (From Tew JM Jr, van Loveren HR, Keller JT: Atlas of Operative Microneurosurgery, vol 2. Philadelphia: WB Saunders, in press.) The superior petrosal sinus is sacrificed between two titanium clips (*B*). Also shown is a possible opening of the retrosigmoid dura for possible exploration from a conventional suboccipital approach. (From Tew JM Jr, van Loveren HR, Keller JT: Atlas of Operative Microneurosurgery, vol 2. Philadelphia: WB Saunders, in press.)

(see Fig. 92-12*B*). The tentorium is incised ventrally toward the incisura in a course directed posterior to the trochlear nerve. By gently elevating the temporal lobe and retracting the cerebellum, an excellent avenue to the lateral brain stem is provided. A longitudinal incision is made in the brain stem between the fifth and seventh nerve root entry zones (Fig. 92-13). The cavernous malformation can then be removed by using the same principles as outlined in Figures 92-6 to 92-9. The mastoidectomy defect is obliterated with a fat graft taken from the abdomen and the incision closed in anatomic layers (Fig. 92-14). This approach is preferred over the midline suboccipital approach unless the lesion significantly breaches the floor of the fourth ventricle, thus effectively having made the myelotomy during hemorrhage. This approach is also useful for pial lesions laterally positioned on the upper pons (Fig. 92-15).

Alternative Treatments

Aspiration of brain stem cavernous malformations associated with major hematoma formation has been recommended by several authors.[21,22] Although aspiration of the hematoma relieves mass effect and may improve recovery, it has several disadvantages: (1) the risk that the probe may injure vital brain stem structures and incite new hemorrhage with puncture of the malformation[23,24]; (2) aspiration of the contents may be nondiagnostic, and recurrent hemorrhage may occur[25]; and (3) aspiration removes only the liquefied portion of the hematoma and not the solid portion of the malformation.[26]

Although stereotactic-guided approaches have greatly improved our ability to resect deep-seated vascular malformations, their role in surgery of brain stem vascular

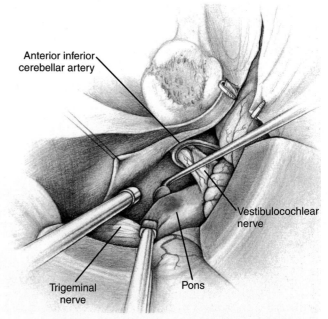

Anterior inferior
cerebellar artery

Vestibulocochlear
nerve

Trigeminal
nerve

Pons

FIGURE 92-13   The surgeon gently applies 10-mm self-retaining retractors to the posterior temporal lobe and lateral cerebellar hemisphere to expose the lateral pons, basilar artery, and cranial nerves V through VIII. A longitudinal incision is made in the brain stem between the V and VIII nerve root entry zones to expose the malformation. (Modified from Tew JM Jr, van Loveren HR: Atlas of Operative Microneurosurgery, vol 1. Philadelphia: WB Saunders, 1994.)

FIGURE 92-14 Postoperative sagittal and axial T1-weighted magnetic resonance imaging scans show complete resection of the pontine cavernous malformation. The fat placed in the right mastoidectomy defect creates a high signal on the axial view.

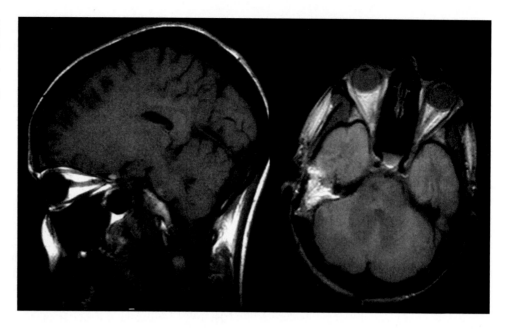

malformations is limited.[23,27] Stereotactic procedures do not account for pial planes in the posterior fossa. Coordinates plotted preoperatively may shift significantly with spinal fluid drainage, mannitol, and retraction; thereafter, these coordinates are no longer on target. We do find frameless stereotaxis helpful for intraparenchymal cavernous malformations in planning the myelotomy.

COMPLICATIONS

Intraoperative complications include hemorrhage, cerebral ischemia, and swelling of surrounding brain tissue.

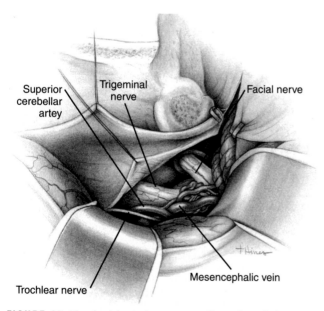

FIGURE 92-15 A pial arteriovenous malformation of the upper pons exposed through a posterior petrosectomy approach (Reprinted with permission from the Mayfield Clinic.)

Despite attempts to avoid manipulation of the brain stem, gentle tamponade and exploration of the gliotic capsule may be required to stop friable deep-feeding vessels that retract during rupture. Returning to the appropriate dissection plane and compressing the malformation medially maintains a drier resection bed.

When the cerebellum suddenly becomes tense and bulging, most commonly either cerebellar venous drainage has been disturbed or the patient is not being ventilated properly. The position and patency of the endotracheal tube should be assessed, and the patient's neck position should be examined. Alternatively, obstructive hydrocephalus or occult bleeding may cause brain swelling. Tissues surrounding AVMs may be asymptomatically ischemic from the hemodynamic effects of high-volume, low-pressure shunts, which steal blood flow from them. If the arterial feeders are occluded too rapidly, loss of normal autoregulation in the surrounding ischemic areas may lead to an oversupply of blood that results in swelling and hemorrhage. Staged resection of AVMs may permit autoregulation to return to these ischemic areas and prevent this catastrophe. Spetzler and colleagues[28] have described this phenomenon under the rubric "normal perfusion breakthrough theory." In our experience, breakthrough bleeding resulting from loss of cerebral autoregulation during removal of brain stem or deep-seated AVMs has not occurred and should be a diagnosis of exclusion. Most symptomatic ischemia results from inadvertent occlusion of normal arterial or venous vessels. Vasospasm with significant vessel stenosis is a rare cause of ischemia after surgical resection of AVMs.

Hemorrhage from poorly secured hemostasis, uncontrolled blood pressure, or residual tufts of malformation are the most devastating consequence of surgery on brain stem AVMs. A hematoma in the resection bed or cerebellum requires an urgent return to the operating room for its evacuation. Reperfusion phenomena from altered hemodynamics may cause ischemia and swelling to surrounding brain tissue. The tight confines of the brain stem tolerate very little edema formation, and transient obstructive hydrocephalus may develop. Obstructive hydrocephalus from brain stem swelling usually resolves and may be managed with a ventriculostomy.

Postoperative Management

All patients are treated in the neuroscience intensive care unit. Complications in the postoperative period can often be anticipated and are preventable. The primary cause of postoperative hemorrhage, residual malformation, has been mainly eliminated by use of intraoperative angiography and single-stage AVM removal. In the immediate postoperative period, regional cerebrovascular autoregulation may not protect the parenchyma surrounding large AVMs from reperfusion injury. We, therefore, maintain systemic hypotension for at least 72 hours postoperatively (mean arterial pressure, 60 to 70 mm Hg). Patients are susceptible to obstruction of the cerebral aqueduct from parenchymal swelling and may require steroids and a ventriculostomy. Recording of cranial nerves with injury action potentials during intraoperative monitoring alerts the surgeon to the possible need for a temporary tarsorrhaphy, tracheostomy, or gastrostomy postoperatively.

RESULTS

We have reviewed our experience (1984 to 1998) to evaluate the treatment and outcome of 128 patients with brain stem vascular malformations (Tables 92-2 and 92-3). Surgery was performed when the malformation was superficial to the brain stem surface or in cases of deteriorating neurologic status or repeat hemorrhage. The transvermian, lateral cerebellar, and posterior petrosal approaches were used in all cases. Resection of venous angiomas was avoided. Among 86 surgical patients, 48 (56%) had transient worsening of their neurologic status and 16 (19%) suffered permanent neurologic deficits. There were no operative deaths.

Most cases of neurologic worsening were caused by injury to the cranial nerve nuclei and cerebellar tracts. We sought to reduce these risks by using the lateral approach to the brain stem through a corridor between the root entry zones of the trigeminal and facial nerves. The surgical approach requires a posterior petrosectomy, sectioning of the tentorium cerebelli, and removal of pial AVMs and parenchymal cavernous malformations, which does not disturb the functional nuclei in the floor of the fourth ventricle (see Fig. 92-13).

TABLE 92-2 ▪ Types of Brain Stem Arteriovenous Malformations in 128 Patients

Type	No.	Percent
Cavernous malformation	61	48
Arteriovenous malformation	25	20
Venous malformation	21	16
Capillary telangiectasia	9	7
Mixed	12	9

TABLE 92-3 ▪ Location of Brain Stem Arteriovenous Malformations in 128 Patients

Location	No.	Percent
Medulla	13	10
Pons	83	65
Mesencephalon	18	14
Pia	14	11

SUMMARY

Symptomatic brain stem vascular malformations have a propensity toward repeated hemorrhage. Although patients often improve substantially, nevertheless, with each successive hemorrhage, they are less likely to recover function. The goal of therapy is to eliminate the risk of hemorrhage without causing significant neurologic injury. Surgical excision is currently the best treatment for brain stem vascular malformations that are subpial and present with progressive neurologic deficit from recurrent hemorrhage. With appreciation for transient deficit, these lesions can be excised with acceptable permanent morbidity and no mortality.

Acknowledgment

The authors thank Tonya Hines for illustrations and Don Thompson for editorial assistance.

REFERENCES

1. Logue V, Monckton G: Posterior fossa angiomas: A clinical presentation of 9 cases. Brain 77:252–273, 1954.
2. Ondra SL, Troupp H, George ED, et al: The natural history of symptomatic arteriovenous malformations of the brain: A 24-year follow-up assessment. J Neurosurg 73:387–391, 1990.
3. Drake CG, Friedman AH, Peerless SJ: Posterior fossa arteriovenous malformations. J Neurosurg 64:1–10, 1986.
4. Solomon RA, Stein BM: Management of arteriovenous malformations of the brain stem. J Neurosurg 64:857–864, 1986.
5. Weil SM, Tew JM Jr: Surgical management of brain stem vascular malformations. Acta Neurochir (Wien) 105:14–23, 1990.
6. Zimmerman RS, Spetzler RF, Lee KS, et al: Cavernous malformations of the brain stem. J Neurosurg 75:32–39, 1991.
7. Russell DS, Rubenstein LJ: Pathology of Tumors of the Nervous System, 5th ed. Baltimore: Williams & Wilkins, 1989, pp 727–765.
8. Abe M, Kjellberg RN, Adams RD: Clinical presentations of vascular malformations of the brain stem: Comparison of angiographically positive and negative types. J Neurol Neurosurg Psychiatry 52:167–175, 1989.
9. McCormick WF, Hardman JM, Boulter TR: Vascular malformations (angiomas) of the brain, with special reference to those occurring in the posterior fossa. J Neurosurg 28:241–251, 1968.
10. Garner TB, Curling OD Jr, Kelly DL, et al: The natural history of intracranial venous angiomas. J Neurosurg 75:715–722, 1991.
11. McLaughlin MR, Kondziolka D, Flickinger JC, et al: The prospective natural history of cerebral venous malformations. Neurosurgery 43:195–201, 1998.
12. Spetzler RF, Martin NA: A proposed grading system for arteriovenous malformations. J Neurosurg 65:476–483, 1986.
13. Robinson JR, Awad IA, Little JR: Natural history of cavernous angioma. J Neurosurg 75:709–714, 1991.
14. Humphries RP, Hendrick EB, Hoffman HJ: Arteriovenous malformations of the brain stem in childhood. Childs Brain 11:1–11, 1984.
15. Scott MR, Barnes P, Kupsky W, Adelman LS: Cavernous angiomas of the central nervous system in children. J Neurosurg 76:38–44, 1992.
16. Lobato RD, Rivas JJ, Gomez PA, et al: Comparison of the clinical presentation of symptomatic arteriovenous malformations (angiographically visualized) and occult vascular malformations. Neurosurgery 31:391–397, 1992.

17. La Torre E, Delitala A, Sorano V: Hematoma of the quadrigeminal plate. J Neurosurg 49:610–613, 1978.
18. Kashiwagi S, van Loveren HR, Tew JM Jr, et al: Diagnosis and treatment of vascular brain-stem malformations. J Neurosurg 72:27–34, 1990.
19. Bertalanffy H, Gilsbach JM, Eggert HR, Seeger W: Microsurgery of deep seated cavernous angiomas: Report of 26 cases. Acta Neurochir (Wien) 13:204–207, 1991.
20. Fahlbusch R, Strauss C, Huk W, et al: Surgical removal of pontomesencephalic cavernous hemangiomas. Neurosurgery 26:449–457, 1990.
21. Beatty RM, Zervas NT: Stereotactic aspiration of a brain stem hematoma. Neurosurgery 13:204–207, 1983.
22. Bosch DA, Beute GN: Successful stereotaxic evacuation of an acute pontomedullary hematoma: Case report. J Neurosurg 62:153–156, 1985.
23. Davis DH, Kelly PJ: Stereotactic resection of occult vascular malformations. J Neurosurg 72:698–702, 1990.
24. Ogilvy CS, Heros RC, Ojemann RG, et al: Angiographically occult arteriovenous malformations. J Neurosurg 69:350–355, 1988.
25. Batjer H, Samson D: Arteriovenous malformations of the posterior fossa. J Neurosurg 64:849–856, 1986.
26. Konovalov A, Spallone A, Makhmudov UB: Surgical management of hematomas of the brain stem. J Neurosurg 73:181–186, 1990.
27. Sisti MB, Solomon RA, Stein BM: Stereotactic craniotomy in the resection of small arteriovenous malformations. J Neurosurg 75:40–44, 1991.
28. Spetzler RF, Wilson CB, Weinstein P, et al: Normal perfusion pressure breakthrough theory. Clin Neurosurg 25:651–672, 1978.

93 Surgical Management of Spinal Cord Tumors and Arteriovenous Malformations

KALMON D. POST, JOSHUA BEDERSON,
NOEL PERIN, and BENNETT M. STEIN

INTRAMEDULLARY SPINAL CORD TUMORS

Although Von Eiselsberg totally excised a neurofibrosarcoma from the spinal cord in 1907 and Cushing operated on an 8-year-old child and completely removed an intramedullary ependymoma extending from C1 to T2 in 1924,[1] the first well-documented surgical effort to remove an intramedullary tumor was reported by Elsberg in 1925.[2] Of the 13 tumors that he reported on, three were totally removed and the remainder were partially removed. He stressed that because some of these tumors were infiltrating, they defied removal; nevertheless, he emphasized that the surgeon must search out those tumors with well-defined cleavage planes that permit total removal of the neoplasm. Considering his lack of magnification techniques and previous surgical experience with such tumors, these results were remarkable. When a definitive plane between the tumor and the spinal cord was not visible, Elsberg proposed a second operation when the tumor might present through the myelotomy, making total removal possible. Later, Matson[3] also advocated this technique. With the exception of these reports, little experience with two-stage removal has been published. After Elsberg's early reports, others[1,3–10] described successful removals of intramedullary tumors. Successful surgical removal of these tumors was mounted on a firm foundation when Greenwood[5] presented his experience with 10 intramedullary tumors, primarily ependymomas, which he removed totally with no fatalities. These results, with successful survivals, justified his enthusiasm for an aggressive surgical approach to these lesions. He also emphasized the use of magnification techniques and microsurgical instrumentation.

Guidetti[6] published his experience with a large group of intramedullary tumors and noted the difficulty in totally removing astrocytomas. In the presence of intramedullary ependymomas and other tumors, however, he thought that every effort should be made to achieve total removal, although only a line of cleavage between the normal spinal cord and the tumor would make this possible. Once a cleavage was established, gentle dissection separated the tumor from the normal spinal cord on each side; then the tumor could be lifted carefully by one end or the other and slowly dissected from its bed. Blood vessels were severed close to the tumor by bipolar cautery with irrigation.

Guidetti achieved an overall total removal of 24 of 71 tumors, representing a wide variety of histologic types, with a 10% operative mortality rate. In the famous case of Horrax and Henderson,[7] an intramedullary ependymoma extending the entire length of the spinal cord was totally enucleated during a series of operations, resulting in recovery and long-term survival.

Our initial series comprised 40 cases of intramedullary tumors.[4,10] A range of histology was represented, with astrocytoma and ependymoma being the most common tumors and teratomatous types found less frequently. No lipomas were included in this group. Some patients had undergone previous treatment, including decompressive laminectomy, tapping of cysts associated with the tumors, and radiotherapy. The effects of treatment other than total removal were difficult to evaluate. It was clear, however, that the degree of neurologic deficit caused by the disease process before surgery often determined the postoperative result.

We later reported a consecutive series[10a] of 23 patients who underwent removal of an intramedullary spinal cord ependymoma. Mild neurologic deficits were present in 22 patients initially. The location was predominantly cervical or cervicothoracic. Magnetic resonance imaging (MRI) had become the most valuable radiographic procedure. At operation, complete removal was achieved in all patients. No patient received postoperative radiation, and on follow-up for a mean period of 62 months, there were no recurrences. In this group, eight patients showed clinical improvement, 12 had no change, and only three had neurologic deterioration. These data supported the belief that long-term disease-free control of intramedullary spinal ependymomas with an acceptable morbidity rate could be achieved using microsurgical removal alone.[11]

Clinical Presentation

Although intramedullary tumors occur most commonly in adults,[2,4,6,10] a significant incidence has been reported in children.[3,12] The symptomatology in both age groups is similar. It is quite amazing at times to see an extensive tumor filling the majority of the intramedullary space yet causing few symptoms. Often, however, an end point is reached when compensatory ability fails, and marked neurologic deterioration develops rapidly. Persistent pain involving the dorsal root dermatomes in the area of tumor involvement is often the signature of an intramedullary neoplasm. Dysfunction of the posterior column may occur in a progressive fashion, with sensory dysesthesias in the arms, torso, and legs, depending on the site of the intraspinal neoplasm. Sacral sparing may be present and is not an invariable finding with intramedullary neoplasms. Lower motor neuron symptoms and signs usually occur at the level of the tumor. Well-defined central cord syndromes, as seen in syringomyelia, with disassociated sensory loss and the classic signs of anterior horn cell involvement may be lacking. Children often have a scoliosis. The symptomatology generally is progressive with few remissions or exacerbations. Symptoms are usually bilateral, but in rare instances neurologic abnormalities are confined to one extremity. The duration of symptoms generally is measured in years, although some neoplasms may have histories of 6 months or less.

Diagnostic Evaluation

The radiographic demonstration of these tumors had been dependent on myelography with either iohexal (a nonionic water-soluble agent) or iophendylate (Pantopaque),[13] although this is no longer routinely used for the diagnosis of intramedullary spinal cord tumors. A fusiform dilatation of the cord in the region of the tumor usually was seen, and a complete block was not generally present (Fig. 93-1). If a block was present, dye was also instilled from the opposite end of the spinal canal to define the complete extent of the tumor. Since the introduction of water-soluble contrast agents, radiographic definition has been improved significantly. Dilated venous channels at the caudal aspect of small intramedullary tumors had suggested the differential diagnosis of a vascular malformation. This differential is rarely a problem with high-definition MRI, and spinal angiography has not been of diagnostic value except for the identification of an intramedullary hemangioblastoma, or intramedullary arteriovenous malformation (AVM), which can mimic a vascular intramedullary tumor. Angiography has been carried out in the presence of dilated vessels and has been helpful in the diagnosis of hemangioblastoma and AVMs.[9]

Routine computed tomography of the spinal canal has not been of practical use in the diagnosis of these neoplasms. We have retrospectively scanned a number of patients with large tumors, failing to visualize these tumors. Computed tomography with water-soluble contrast agents aids in the diagnosis of a wide spinal canal. It also assists in the definitive diagnosis of syringomyelia. Computed tomography has shown metrizamide leaking into the fluid within a syrinx,[14,15] particularly with a 6-hour delayed scan.

MRI, without and with gadolinium, is the standard of care in the diagnostic evaluation of intramedullary tumors of the spinal cord. A fusiform dilatation of the cord in the region of the tumor with possible associated rostral and caudal cysts, especially in ependymomas and hemangioblastomas, was a typical finding on the T1-weighted images. The tumor typically enhanced with the administration of the gadolinium. An ependymoma was likely to be more centrally placed within the spinal cord as opposed to an astrocytoma and more often associated with rostral and caudal cysts. The ependymoma was more circumscribed and enhanced more uniformly with the contrast, but the astrocytoma was somewhat more diffuse and enhanced more irregularly. The hemangioblastoma presented on or close to the surface of the cord and enhanced brilliantly with contrast material and was always associated with a cyst. Intramedullary spinal cord tumors were more common in the cervical and cervicomedullary junction (Fig. 93-2).

Percutaneous cord puncture and myelocystography have been reported[16] and were performed once in our series. Our patent had a percutaneous puncture to distinguish a cord tumor from a syrinx rather than for relief of symptoms.

Surgical Pathology

Intramedullary spinal cord tumors account for one third of primary intraspinal neoplasms.[2,6,8,10,16] Astrocytomas and ependymomas constitute the largest group of intramedullary tumors and occur with approximately equal frequency, although astrocytomas are more common in childhood and ependymomas are more prevalent in the adult population. They are generally low grade and extend over many segments of the spinal cord. Astrocytomas most commonly appear in the cervical and thoracic regions of the spinal cord, whereas the ependymomas have a higher incidence in the caudal regions because of their prevalence in the conus medullaris and filum terminale.[17]

Tumors that occur less frequently include dermoids, epidermoids, teratomas, oligodendrogliomas, hemangioblastomas, and either primary or metastatic malignant tumors. Lipomas, common in children, have different growth patterns and therapeutic implications and are not discussed here.

Intramedullary ependymomas often have a distinct plane between the neoplasm and spinal cord tissue. These tumors generally are soft and solid, and have a pseudocapsule. They are not highly vascular and may have necrotic areas. Astrocytomas usually are infiltrative with an ill-defined margin between the neoplasm and the normal spinal cord tissue. Where a well-defined margin between the neoplasm and the normal spinal cord exists, a pseudocapsule is found. This variety is similar to the cerebellar astrocytoma, which has a uniformly soft consistency and minimal vascularity sometimes associated with cysts containing yellow fluid high in protein.

At times, astrocytomas may appear to have a plane between the tumor and the normal cord tissue, yet pathologically they demonstrate infiltration (Fig. 93-3).

The pathologic grade may also vary in different parts of the tumor, just as it does within brain tumors. Astrocytomas and ependymomas produce a fusiform enlargement of the spinal cord, often without any indication of their presence on the surface of the cord other than an occasional dilated vein at the caudal end of the tumor. In some cases the dorsal surface of the cord will be so thin that it will be transparent. Glioblastomas produce a discoloration of the cord and are associated with a plethora of enlarged arterialized veins and obvious feeding arteries. Ependymomas of the conus or filum terminale region often grow in an exophytic fashion from the intramedullary locus into the cauda equina, displacing and sometimes adhering to the nerve roots. Because of the expanding nature of these neoplasms, structural changes in the osseous spinal canal may be produced.

Teratomas and dermoid tumors have varying amounts of grumous material in their central portions, are frequently

FIGURE 93-1 *A,* Anteroposterior cervical myelogram shows widened spinal cord. *B,* Lateral cervical myelogram shows a widened spinal cord. *C,* Operative view of the exposed spinal cord at C2–T2. Note the widened full appearance. *D,* Operative view of the spinal cord after a cystic ependymoma was removed.

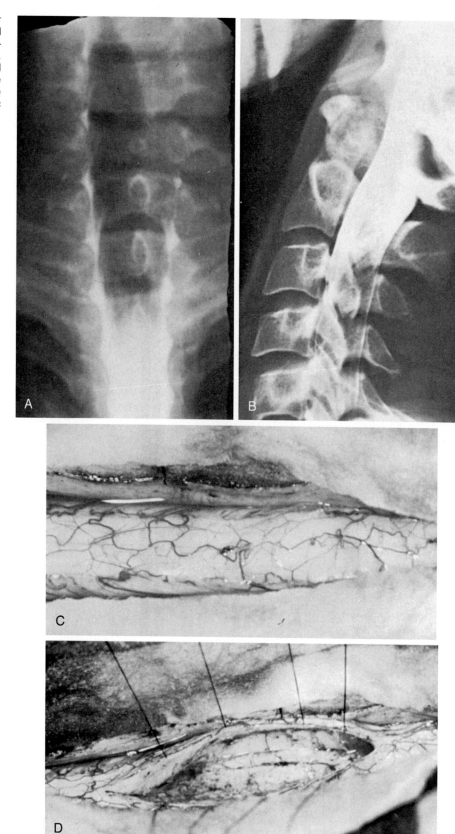

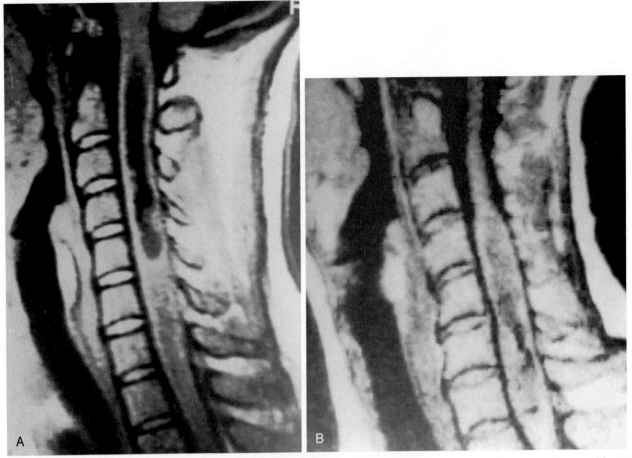

FIGURE 93-2 *A,* Sagittal magnetic resonance imaging (MRI) demonstrates a cyst within the cervical spinal cord and a mural hemangioblastoma at the C4–5 level. *B,* Sagittal MRI demonstrates a wide cervical spinal cord with an intramedullary tumor.

variegated, and have a capsule that is adherent to the surrounding spinal cord tissue; often there is a pedicle from a fibrous tract involving the dura and overlying bone and soft tissues. Radiographic defects may be present in the overlying bone if a fibrous tract is present.

Intramedullary tumors receive their blood supply from perforating branches of the anterior spinal artery that enter the ventral aspect of the tumor. These vessels are small and are not associated with a high degree of vascularity within the tumor. Small vessels also enter the tumor from the dorsal and lateral positions of the spinal cord. The tumors tend to be eccentric and located in the more dorsal portion of the spinal cord. Invariably there is a thin layer of compressed spinal cord tissue overlying the dorsal surface of these tumors, and they rarely present directly on the surface of the cord.

In our series, 80% of the tumors were divided almost equally between astrocytoma and ependymoma.[10,18] Fortunately, only three of the astrocytomas were glioblastomas. There were five cases of hemangioblastomas, a relatively rare intramedullary tumor. Four of these hemangioblastomas involved the cervical thoracic region while one involved the thoracolumbar region. Teratomas generally occurred in the lumbosacral region. A cavernous malformation occupied the lumbar region and gave rise to a 21-year history. A rare intramedullary pigmented neurofibroma

extending from the midcervical region to the obex of the medulla was successfully removed in an elderly patient.

Surgical Technique

Turnbull[1] stated: "A surgeon exploring a spinal cord for a suspected intramedullary tumor must be prepared to face a formidable problem and also have the courage of conviction to make every attempt to remove the tumor. Anything less than this, with a cursory inspection of the spinal cord or aspiration thereof, can only create problems of a more complex nature for the subsequent surgical effort to remove such tumors."

Surgery is the primary treatment for intramedullary tumors. Radiotherapy has little to offer, even for malignant tumors.[10,12,17–19] In timing surgery, the sooner the better in terms of tumor growth. There is nothing to be gained by allowing the tumor growth to devastate the patient while withholding surgery. The surgical results are generally predicated on the preoperative condition of the patient, no matter how large the tumor. If the patient preoperatively has minimal neurologic findings, then the postoperative course should be gratifying, especially if the tumor can be resected in toto. Those patients who arrive for surgery in a wheelchair or with severe paralysis or sensory loss may regain little of their lost function even after a successful operation.

The prone position is generally used for all intramedullary cord tumors, although early in our experience, the sitting position was used for some cervical cord tumors. The prone position is preferred now because it decreases the potential for vasomotor collapse, which can be significant when the autonomic pathways are compromised by the tumor or surgery; it also allows the assistant to take a more active role in the operation, providing traction, irrigation, or assistance with the dissection.

Some operations were carried out with evoked potential monitoring of dorsal column function. This had been of some use in guiding the surgery, although there were times when potentials were lost and surgery had to proceed. There did not appear to be enough correlation with the somatosensory evoked potentials and functional outcome. Therefore, we preferred not to use somatosensory evoked potentials but rather to rely on observations through the operation microscope as to the extent of dissection. We have begun to use with greater efficiency recordings from the corticospinal tract motor evoked potentials. It is too early in our experience to comment on their benefit. Although these recordings have been of some value in guiding the operation, clinical impression and judgment should dictate the decisions made during the tumor removal.

General anesthesia with endotracheal intubation is always used, and the endotracheal tube is frequently left in place for 24 to 48 hours after surgery on more extensive cervical intramedullary tumors.

The full extent of the tumor must be known before the surgery. This usually is well demonstrated on the preoperative MRI. Intraoperatively, once the dura is exposed, ultrasonography is used routinely to identify the extent of the solid tumor and associated cystic components. In the case of a suspected hemangioblastoma, the vasculature could be demonstrated by arteriography to aid in the surgical removal, but often the MRI is enough so that surgery will not be altered by an arteriogram. A wide laminectomy then is performed over the entire extent of the solid portion of the tumor, extending to a level above and below. The dura must be opened carefully because the pia arachnoid of the enlarged spinal cord often adheres to the underside of the dura. It is important to prevent any injury to the cord vasculature because hemorrhage during this phase of the operation will obscure all landmarks and significantly compromise the surgical effort. In the event of previous surgery, particularly if the dura has been left open, this early dissection is tedious, but care must be taken to reestablish all anatomic landmarks. In those cases, both with and without previous surgery, the initial appearance of the cords generally was similar; the cords appeared widened, often without evidence of tumor on the surface. The widening of the spinal cord and the presence of dilated veins at the caudal end of the tumor site were indications of the underlying pathologic process. When observing a widened spinal cord, the surgeon must not be misled in

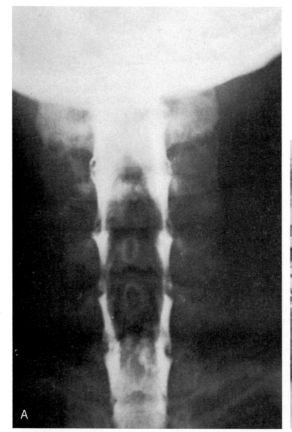
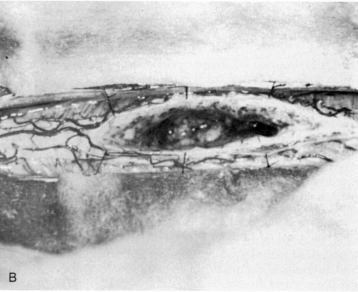

FIGURE 93-3 *A,* Cervical myelography (anteroposterior view) shows a widened spinal cord. *B,* Operative view of the exposed spinal cord during the first operation.

(Continued)

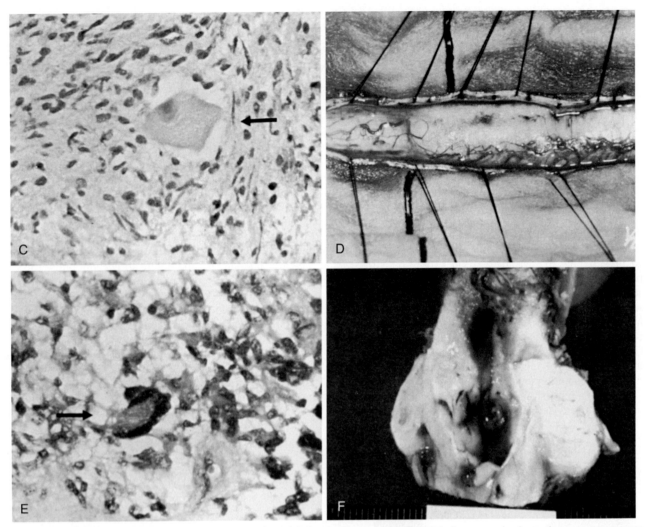

FIGURE 93-3 Cont'd   *C*, Microscopic picture of tissue removed during the first operation. The pathology was mixed ependymoma-astrocytoma grade II. Note the invasion with the tumor surrounding a neuron. *D*, Operative view of the exposed spinal cord during the second operation. Note the extreme fullness of the spinal cord. *E*, Microscopic picture of the tissue removed during the second operation. The pathology was a glioblastoma. Note the giant cell. *F*, Pathologic specimen, postmortem. Note the metastatic nodules along the floor of the fourth ventricle.

those rare instances of anterior extramedullary lesion in which the cord is splayed out over the lesion.[10,18]

The dorsal surface of the cord at the area of greatest enlargement then is inspected for the site of the myelotomy. Generally, myelotomies are performed in the midline with a preference for the thinnest and most avascular areas. When the spinal cord is rotated and the midline is difficult to identify, the dorsal root entry zones can be identified and thereby help to define the midline to perform the myelotomy. At times, however, it is more expeditious to use a paramedian approach (Fig. 93-4).

Some of the vasculature will be sacrificed during this myelotomy. An initial incision of approximately 1 to 2 cm is performed over the greatest enlargement of the spinal cord to evaluate the plane between the tumor and the spinal cord tissue. In some instances, the presence of a cyst associated with the tumor may be easily noted; if so, additional room may be gained by aspirating some of the cystic contents through a small-bore needle. To facilitate dissection,

however, these cysts should not be completely evacuated. Once it is determined that the neoplasm is cystic or has well-defined planes, the myelotomy is lengthened over the extent of the tumor. With teratomas, a stalk between the cord and the dura should be removed as an integral part of the lesion. With ependymomas extending from the conus, the extra-axial portion in the cauda equina may be removed first, providing adequate decompression and visualization of the residual tumor involving the intramedullary portion of the conus. The draining veins of intramedullary hemangioblastomas must be left until the latter part of the surgical resection.

Following the myelotomy, 6-0 or 7-0 traction sutures are placed through the pial margins on either side and sutured to the edges of the opened dura to expose the interior of the spinal cord (see Fig. 93-4). Generally, the tumor is visible a few millimeters under the dorsal surface of the spinal cord. There is often a soft gliotic interface between the tumor and the spinal cord proper. With the operating microscope and

FIGURE 93-4 *A,* A myelotomy over an intramedullary tumor. *B,* Removal of an intramedullary tumor. *C,* The open cord after removal of an intramedullary tumor.

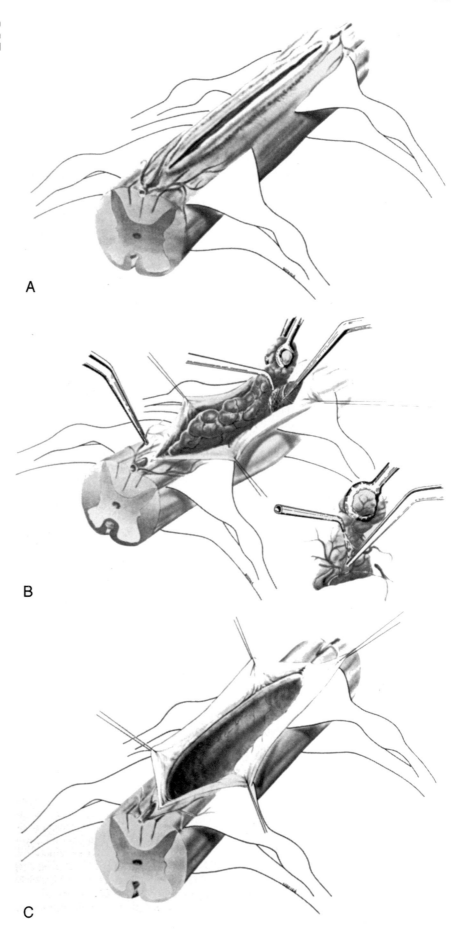

microsurgical techniques, using bipolar cautery, small suction tubes, and various dissectors, a plane is developed around the margin of the tumor, taking care to retract primarily on the tumor and not on the spinal cord. The surgeon works to one or the other end of the tumor. At the pole where the tumor is the narrowest, it may be possible to grasp the end and gently extract it from the interior of the cord. All the fine vascular adhesions to the spinal cord, especially on the ventral aspect of the tumor, should be cauterized with bipolar cautery and sharply divided. No blunt dissection should be carried out in areas where vascular channels connect the tumor to the spinal cord. Most tumors are amazingly avascular and present no threat of hemorrhage or the loss of control of large blood vessels. It is important to keep the operative field meticulously dry so that the plane between the tumor and the spinal cord may be readily identified (see Fig. 93-4).

If the tumor is too large to remove in toto or necessitates too much retraction on the spinal cord, its interior may be decompressed. We prefer to use an ultrasonic aspirator to debulk the tumor, facilitating dissection around its capsule and its removal. This has a minor disadvantage of spilling the contents of the tumor into the dissection plane or obscuring the dissection plane by bleeding. In most instances, however, the tumors are relatively avascular, and bleeding is not a major problem, even with the use of the ultrasonic aspirator. Gradually, the entire tumor may be removed. For those tumors (usually astrocytomas) that are infiltrating, a debulking procedure is valuable, especially in children. CO_2 and argon lasers have also been used for this.[20]

Cystic collections at the margins of the tumor, as in the case of ependymomas, facilitate the tumor resection. We make no attempt, however, to remove the wall of the cyst, which is thin and nonneoplastic. If there is any doubt about the totality of removal, small biopsies may be obtained from the margin of the resection and evaluated by frozen section during surgery. In most instances, the margins are well defined and there is no question about the removal of the tumor (see Figs. 93-4 and 93-6). Malignant tumors such as the glioblastoma respond poorly to surgery and do not appear to respond to radiation therapy. These cases are usually hopeless.

In children, the syndrome of holospinal cord widening is associated with extensive astrocytomas or localized astrocytomas and extensive cysts.[12] Here we must localize the tumor either through clinical or radiographic evaluation and remove it while only draining the cyst. A subtotal radical removal with the Cavitron or laser appears to pay dividends in these children with long-term remission of the disease process. Although these astrocytomas are histologically identical to those in adults, they may have different growth behavior related more to the child's development than to the histologic appearance.

Special attention is given to the removal of hemangioblastomas. These are highly vascular tumors and if they are decompressed or cut into, the bleeding will not only obscure the anatomic planes but may result in catastrophic problems. Therefore, even in large hemangioblastomas, we work around the margin of the tumor, interrupting the feeding arteries and finally the primary draining vein as the tumor is rolled out on the last venous pedicle. Often these tumors are associated with a cyst, facilitating their removal. They are identified by their characteristic orange-red appearance and in all instances extrude from the pial surface. Their presence is also identified by large dilated arterialized veins that often surround them. This will mimic an AVM on the myelogram and occasionally on spinal angiography. In some instances, hemangioblastomas may be multiple, and additional tumors may be removed if they are accessible. In rare instances, they will be associated with cranial tumors or the von Hippel-Lindau syndrome.

In cases in which the tumor has been treated with radiation previously, we have noted intense intramedullary gliosis by biopsy, distinctly separate from the margin of the tumor, usually at the caudal or rostral interface. It is assumed that this is an adverse effect of preoperative radiation. Previous surgery with aspiration of a cyst but without definitive removal of the intramedullary tumor has provided transient benefits and reaccumulation of the cyst fluid.

In teratomas, the border of the tumor, although well defined, may be densely adherent to the surrounding spinal cord. Every attempt should be made to remove this capsule, which is a potential source of regrowth. There may be extensive involvement of central areas of the spinal cord and the tumors may extend from the posterior to the anterior surface. Teratomatous tumors also may have a dumbbell configuration within the substance of the spinal cord, and the surgeon must be wary not to miss satellite portions of the primary tumor.

When the margins of the cord are allowed to fall back into position, the remarkable decompressive effect of tumor removal is quite apparent. The dorsal columns are often thin to the point of being transparent. If there has been minimal retraction on the cord, these fiber tracts function in a satisfactory way and will show progressive functional recovery. Rarely has the function of the spinal cord been made permanently worse by this dissection. Gentleness of dissection may be gauged by the vascular pattern on the dorsal surface of the cord at the completion of tumor resection. Distended veins that were present before removal, usually at the caudal end of the tumor on the surface of the spinal cord, will not be less prominent. No attempt has been made to sew the pial surfaces of the spinal cord together. The dura is closed in a watertight fashion; it is rarely necessary to use a fascial graft other than in those cases in which the dura was left open after previous surgery. If total removal of an intramedullary tumor is not feasible, the dura should be reconstructed, preferably with a fascial graft, so that subsequent surgical endeavors may be facilitated.

The most important factor determining the ease of the operation is the presence and nature of previous operations. In patients who have had previous surgery and in whom the dura mater was left open, the initial exposure of the tumor and the dissection of adjacent tissues from the spinal cord has prolonged the operation and made exposure more difficult. In those cases in which radiation was administered previously, gliotic areas in the dorsocentral portion of the spinal cord have been verified by biopsy. There have been no histologic changes in the tumor that were attributed to radiation. Similarly, none of the tumors that were previously irradiated showed malignant changes. Problems with wound healing also were encountered frequently in those cases in which radiotherapy was used previously.

A number of aspects concerning the surgical removal and management of intramedullary spinal cord tumors must be emphasized. The surgeon should assume that the majority of all intramedullary cord tumors are benign and resectable. Intraoperative judgment should be based on the gross rather than the histologic tumor characteristics because many low-grade astrocytomas are well circumscribed and resectable. An inadequate myelotomy may fail to reveal a clear plane, and frozen section specimens made from a small piece of tumor taken through a limited myelotomy may lead to an erroneous tissue diagnosis and be misleading. This problem often occurs with tanocytic ependymomas. On the other hand, if the histologic diagnosis is ependymoma, then every attempt must be made to remove the tumor in toto. This is particularly true for large tumors that initially seem infiltrative or that severely compress the surrounding spinal cord such that it is almost unrecognizable. It is sometimes amazing that this thin ribbon of cord tissue can function reasonably well and recover some of the lost function. Therefore, even very large and extensive ependymomas should not deter the surgeon from complete removal. Finally, it should be stressed as noted previously that reoperation for recurrent tumor or surgery after radiation is extremely difficult when planes are obscured by the gliosis.

Postoperative Treatment

Steroids are routinely used pre- and postoperatively in high doses (dexamethasone 4 to 8 mg intravenously every 4 hours or the Solu-Medrol spinal cord injury protocol) with a slow taper, depending on the neurologic condition. Prophylactic antibiotics are used intraoperatively. If the surgery involved extensive areas of the cervical region, the endotracheal tube is left in place for at least 24 hours, regardless of the patient's condition at the termination of surgery.

Radiation therapy is considered postoperatively for children with astrocytomas, but we generally wait with adults and consider reoperation if recurrence should occur.

Careful orthopedic follow-up and possible bracing are necessary for the pediatric patients.

Results

Removal of large intramedullary tumors can be performed with a fair degree of safety (Table 93-1) and can offer significant neurologic improvement in many situations. Generally, those patients with only mild to moderate neurologic deficit before surgery did extremely well, regardless of the size of the tumor. The total removal of these tumors offers a much improved outlook for patients who have not responded to previous decompressive laminectomy and radiotherapy. Our follow-up period in the astrocytoma and ependymoma group has been too short to draw definite conclusions regarding a recurrence rate, although many patients have reached 5 years or more after surgery without showing evidence of recurrence. Experience would indicate that the recurrence rate should be low after total removal.[2,5,7,8,11,18,21,22]

CASE REPORT

A 35-year-old woman was asymptomatic until 6 months before admission when she developed sharp pains radiating around the right breast, as well as progressive numbness in a suspended pattern over the right side from the nipple line to the umbilicus level. Subsequently, she developed numbness in the right V2 distribution as well as around the shoulders. Minimal weakness was present in the upper arms.

TABLE 93-1 ▪ Intramedullary Spinal Cord Tumors

Case No.	Patient Age	Location of Tumor	Histology	Removal	Result	Follow-up
1	26	C	Ependymoma	T	I	3 mo
2	24	Conus	Ependymoma	T	I	1 yr
3	49	C	Ependymoma	T	I	5 yr
4	28	C-D	Ependymoma	T	S	4 yr
5	38	C	Ependymoma	T	S	4 yr
6	45	Conus	Ependymoma	T	S	2 yr
7	35	Conus	Ependymoma	T	S	2 yr
8	20	Conus	Ependymoma	T	S	2 yr
9	35	C	Ependymoma	T	I	1 yr
10	12	C	Astrocytoma	P	S	6 mo
11	60	C-D	Astrocytoma	90%	S	6 yr
12	13	D-L	Astrocytoma	T	S	4 yr
13	3	C-D	Astrocytoma	95%	I	4 yr
14	48	C	Astrocytoma	T	I	4 yr
15	38	C	Astrocytoma	T	I	5 yr
16	7	C	Astrocytoma	T	I	1 yr
17	5	C-D-L-S	Astrocytoma	50%	S	1 yr
18	14	C	Malignant glioma	P	W	1 yr (died)
19	20	C	Malignant glioma	P	W	6 mo (died)
20	13	D	Teratoma	T	I	4 yr
21	12	Conus	Dermoid	T	I	11 yr
22	4 mo	Conus	Epidermoid	T	I	11 yr
23	28	D-L	Mixed	P	W	2 yr
24	52	D	Metastatic	P	S	1 mo (died)
25	57	C	Hemangioblastoma	T	I	2 mo

C, cervical; D, dorsal; L, lumbar; P, partial; I, improved; S, same; T, total; W, worse.

Examination showed hypalgesia in the right V1 and V2 distribution. Strength was uniformly good except for minimal weakness of the left biceps muscles. Sensory examination showed a marked suspended sensory level loss from T1 to T8, with a lesser loss extending up to C2. Posterior column function was good. Reflexes were decreased in the left biceps and slightly increased in the lower extremities. Babinski signs were absent.

Myelography was performed, which demonstrated a widened cord extending from T2 to C2 (see Fig. 93-1). Subsequently, a laminectomy from C2 through T2 was performed with myelotomy and total removal of a cystic ependymoma (see Fig. 93-1). Follow-up examination 4 years after surgery showed the patient to be functioning extremely well at home. She noted some numbness under the right breast and tingling in her left fingers. Examination showed full muscle power with a decreased left biceps and triceps reflex. Joint position sense and vibratory sensation were decreased in the lower extremities but normal in the upper extremities.

Radicular pain in the distribution of the nerve roots associated with the tumor has been a distressing postoperative problem. This pain has a burning quality, which is severely disturbing to the patient and extremely difficult to control. Derangement of the physiologic pathways for pain at the dorsal route entry zone has been postulated as the cause. Unfortunately, we have not had satisfactory results in the treatment of these postoperative dysesthetic or pain syndromes.

Our experience[4,10,11,18] and that of others[5,6] indicate that a decompressive laminectomy, whether or not a tumor cyst has been evacuated, with or without radiotherapy, has had little beneficial effect on the course of most intramedullary spinal cord tumors. Some reviews[6,23] of the effects of radiation on these tumors are clouded by incomplete knowledge of the pathologic process, the natural course of these tumors, and the number of associated variables, including decompression and partial surgical removals.

One report by Schwade and colleagues[24] retrospectively reviewed 34 patients, 25 of whom had confirmed histologic evidence of tumor. They recommend conservative surgery to remove as much tumor as is safely possible. Postoperative radiation therapy was given to 4500 to 5000 rads in 5 to 6 weeks, through portals that cover the tumor generously. Twelve of 12 patients with ependymomas were alive without recurrence with a minimum follow-up of 3 years. Five of six patients with low-grade astrocytomas survived longer than 3 years. Although encouraging, longer follow-up may be needed to evaluate this fully. In most reports, there has been little objective follow-up of reduction in tumor size after radiation therapy. A significant number of reports indicate that surgical removal is the treatment of choice.[3-6,8-12,18]

Improvement in the patient's condition, or at least an arrest of the neurologic deterioration, may be anticipated in most cases after surgery. The postoperative result is determined by the degree of preoperative neurologic involvement. Many surgeons have reported difficulty in totally removing astrocytomas. In our series, we were able to totally remove approximately half the astrocytomas with no more significant problems than those encountered in the removal of ependymomas.

Through the use of microsurgical techniques and strict attention to postoperative pulmonary function, negligible mortality and morbidity rates can be expected, even with removal of extensive tumors in the cervical region.

We have not used postoperative radiation for intramedullary tumors that have been totally removed and do not advocate postoperative radiation for benign intramedullary tumors that have been incompletely removed, except occasionally in children. The patient's course should be monitored closely with regularly spaced MRI scanning. A second surgical attempt should be made to remove the tumor at the time of recurrence. After this, radiation may be considered.

SPINAL CORD ARTERIOVENOUS MALFORMATIONS

AVMs of the spinal cord are relatively rare, being only one tenth as common as cerebral AVMs and one tenth as common as primary spinal neoplasms. They appear more commonly in males (4:1) and generally occur in an older age group than those of the brain. Eighty percent occur in the thoracolumbar spinal cord, although they may involve the entire cord from cervical to sacral levels.[25,26]

Anatomy and Terminology

The spinal branch of each intercostal artery divides into dural and radicular arteries after penetrating the outer dural layers covering the nerve roots in the intervertebral foramina. The dural arteries supply blood to the spinal and nerve root dura, and the radicular arteries supply the anterior and posterior nerve roots. A unique feature of the vascular supply to the spinal nerve root dura is the presence of arteriovenous anastomoses within the dura.[27] At some levels, the segmental artery also gives rise to a medullary branch that penetrates the nerve sheath dura, travels along the nerve roots, and supplies the anterior spinal artery or one of the paired posterolateral spinal arteries.[28] The venous drainage of the spinal cord is carried by a rich network of radially oriented veins with anastomotic connections to the coronal plexus and longitudinal veins. These are drained segmentally by radicular veins of varying caliber, which penetrate the dura near the axilla.[29] In childhood, the spinal cord surface veins generally correspond to the arterial pattern, with predominant anterior and paired dorsolateral vessels, and an additional median longitudinal venous channel exists dorsally. In adulthood, progressive ectasia and tortuosity occur, adding complexity to interpretation of the venous anatomy. One of the prominent and puzzling features of the spinal venous system is the difficulty of retrograde venous injections from the epidural to the intrathecal compartments. This has made anatomic studies of the venous system difficult and has suggested that a functional valvelike structure exists limiting reflux from the epidural compartment.[29-31]

Spinal AVMs can arise from any of the vascular components described previously, and this has led to a number of different classification schemes. The term malformation is inaccurate in some cases because the abnormality can be a discrete arteriovenous fistula rather than a true malformation.

The lesion types have been differentiated by fistula location, as determined by selective spinal angiography.

In the classifications of DiChiro[10] and Doppman,[32,33] type I lesions are the most common, and represent dural malformations, in which the nidus is an arteriovenous fistula located within the dura matter of the nerve root sleeve. The venous drainage is medullary, with myelopathy caused by venous hypertension transmitted to the spinal cord parenchyma.

Type II lesions are true intraparenchymal AVMs of the spinal cord. The malformations are angiographically and surgically well visualized and well defined[33,34] (Figs. 93-5 and 93-6). They occur with equal frequency in males and females.

Type III lesions, the juvenile type seen most commonly in children, are more diffuse AVMs and may encircle the spinal cord in a cuirass configuration (see Fig. 93-5). These lesions often permeate the spinal cord and adjacent vertebral bodies at multiple levels, making their obliteration impossible (see Fig. 93-5). They have varying degrees of arterial contributions that may be visualized at arteriography. Flow is rapid and the blood supply of the AVM and the cord may be closely related.

Type IV lesions represent the intrathecal perimedullary arteriovenous fistulas, originally described by Djindjian and colleagues,[35] later emphasized by Heros and colleagues,[36] and recently reviewed by Mourier and colleagues.[37] Type IV lesions are now recognized with increasing frequency as angiographic techniques become more precise. One source of confusion in the nomenclature of spinal AVMs is the further classification of type IV lesions into three subtypes, described by Mourier and colleagues as follows: (1) a single arteriovenous fistula of the conus medullaris or filum terminale fed by the anterior spinal artery, (2) a small group of arteriovenous fistulas of the conus medullaris fed by both anterior and posterior spinal arteries, and (3) a single giant arteriovenous fistula of the cervical or thoracic cord fed by both anterior and posterior spinal arteries. Combining the classifications of DiChiro and Doppman with Mourier, we refer to the three categories of type IV lesions as A, B, and C.

Distinction between type I (dural) and type IV (intrathecal) fistulas can be difficult. In general, type I lesions are thoracic and dorsal, whereas type IV lesions are near the cauda equina. We have recently shown that some type I lesions, with all the clinical and angiographic characteristics of dural fistulas, are in fact located intrathecally. Precise differentiation between the different types of spinal arteriovenous lesions can only be established histologically.

Other vascular lesions of the spinal cord include cavernous angiomas, which are not true AVMs. AVMs of the posterior fossa can have prominent and symptomatic spinal venous drainage[38] but are not truly spinal arteriovenous lesions. Vertebral artery epidural arteriovenous fistulas are typically post-traumatic lesions and are not discussed further in this chapter.

Clinical Presentation and Natural History

Spinal AVMs tend to occur more frequently in males (in a male:female ratio of 2:1 to 4:1) in the 30- to 70-year age group, primarily at the thoracolumbar levels.[25] Frequently, the diagnosis of an AVM is not considered, and tumor or disc problems are suspected. The specific clinical syndrome depends on the type of AVM. Type II and III lesions are true AVMs and, like their intracranial counterparts, produce symptoms by causing hemorrhage or arterial steal. Accordingly, deficits can be catastrophic and sudden in onset in the case of hemorrhage, or insidious and progressive in the case of steal. These patients are typically younger than 30 years old. Type I and IV lesions typically have an insidious onset in middle age with progressive and relentless deterioration. Pain, fever, extremity weakness, and urinary complaints are the most frequent symptoms. In the landmark papers of Aminoff and Logue, the clinical features of spinal AVMs were probably weighted toward type I and IV malformations. They found that 91% of patients had gait disturbance within 3 years of symptom onset, and 50% were severely disabled within 3 months of the onset of functional disturbance. Within 3 years of the onset of the disorder, 50% of the patients were severely disabled. Only 20% of the cases had sudden deterioration owing to subarachnoid hemorrhage. Since Aminoff and Logue, more recent reviews have confirmed the progressive nature of deficits and the generally poor prognosis once symptoms have occurred.[25,39] A small percentage of patients, probably less than 10%, present with subarachnoid hemorrhage or sudden neurologic deterioration. When it does occur, subarachnoid hemorrhage usually presents in younger patients with type IV (intrathecal) fistulas. In such instances, the onset may be devastating, with all the manifestations that go with a ruptured intracranial aneurysm.

The cause of symptoms in type I lesions is venous hypertension, a result of arterialized draining veins and obstruction of venous outflow at the dural exit zone. These lesions appear to produce symptoms because of ischemic changes in the spinal cord secondary to a vascular steal and the mass effect of the lesion.[40–42] On occasion, the arterialized veins that compose these malformations are layered four to five deep on the surface of the spinal cord (Fig. 93-7). When the lesions are removed, grooves from the dilated vascular channels can be noted on the surface of the spinal cord. Many of the symptoms associated with spinal AVMs may relate to increased venous pressure, altering the dynamics of blood flow within the spinal cord and leading to venous congestion and infarction within the substances of the spinal cord.

Diagnosis

The location of the pain, however, is often not a reliable indication of the levels of involvement.[25] Progressive upper or lower motor neuron involvement is the rule, with spasticity or absent reflexes, depending on location. Involvement of the dorsal columns with paresthesias, loss of position, and other sensory modalities is also part of the progressive picture.

On physical examination, two signs are helpful if present. A bruit over the spine is virtually diagnostic[43] of a type II or III AVM, and the presence of a cutaneous angioma may help to localize the level of the lesions.[44] Plain x-ray films of the spine generally are noncontributory. Cerebrospinal fluid evaluation shows some abnormality in 75% of patients, with protein elevation and pleocytosis being most common.[25,45]

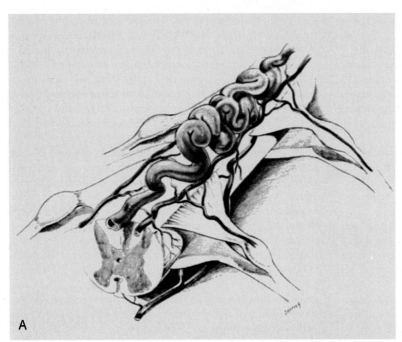

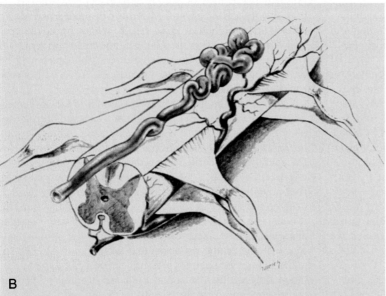

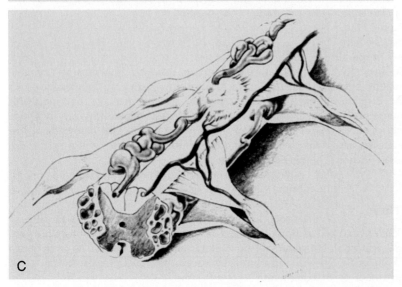

FIGURE 93-5 Arteriovenous malformations (AVMs) of the spinal cord. *A,* Abnormal arterialized tortuous veins cover the dorsal aspect of the cord (lighter and larger vessels). These veins are fed by numerous arterial branches at multiple levels (smaller and darker vessels). *B,* A nidus with a feeding artery (dark vessel) and a localized tangle of abnormal draining veins (lighter and larger vessels). *C,* This AVM lies both within and on the surface of the spinal cord. It consists of large cavernous channels and multiple arteriovenous shunts. (From Baker HL Jr, Love JG, Layton DD Jr: Angiographic and surgical aspects of spinal cord vascular anomalies. Radiology 88: 1078–1085, 1967.)

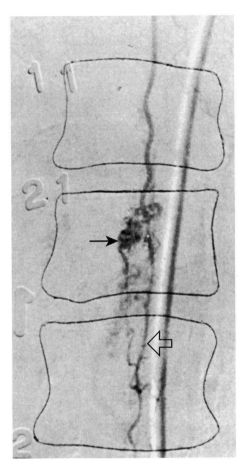

FIGURE 93-6 Anteroposterior spinal cord arteriograms with a subtraction technique. The nidus of the arteriovenous malformation is seen at the *small arrow*. The feeding artery is present at the *open arrow*. (From Kasdon DL, Wolpert SM, Stein BM: Surgical and angiographic localization of spinal arteriovenous malformations. Surg Neurol 5:279–283, 1976.)

In the past, spinal myelography with isophendylate (Pantopaque) was often diagnostic.[46-48] However, false-positive diagnoses were possible because of webbing or trabeculation of the dorsal arachnoid or occasionally tortuous nerve roots, spinal metastases, and dilated vessels associated with intramedullary tumors (Fig. 93-8). Myelography is now performed with water-soluble contrast agents and, together with computed tomography, facilitates diagnosis.[49]

Spinal angiography with selective injection of the relevant arteries and a serial study with subtraction technique are critical in determining the precise location of the malformation and are an invaluable part of preoperative planning. Spinal angiography must be comprehensive to be of use in evaluating a spinal AVM, and bilateral injections should be performed along the extent of the AVM. The critical features that should be angiographically defined are (1) precise definition of the level and location of all the arterial feeders, (2) determination of the predominant venous drainage pattern, (3) detection of venous and arterial aneurysms, and (4) delineation of the anterior and posterior spinal arteries in the region of the AVM. If there is no myelographic or MRI clue to the location of the AVM, the procedure can be painstaking.

Despite the great strides in spinal angiography, in some instances, arteriography may fail to define the precise arterial contribution to an extensive juvenile malformation of dilated arterialized veins extending over multiple segments of the spinal cord. In other instances, it may be difficult to tell from angiography whether the lesion is intra- or extramedullary in location.[50] We have shown that even superselective angiography may fail to distinguish between dural and intrathecal type IV spinal arteriovenous lesions.[51]

MRI has recently been added to the preoperative diagnostic armamentarium. Type I lesions are characterized by enlargement of the cauda equina, probably on an ischemic basis. However, vessels are poorly seen. Types II and III lesions can be difficult to define precisely with MRI, and it is unlikely that MRI will lead to as detailed an evaluation as angiography often accomplishes.

Evoked potentials have been most useful during surgery and radiographic procedures.[52] As a clinical tool before

FIGURE 93-7 Operative exposure of a large arteriovenous malformation of the spinal cord that consists principally of tortuous, distended, arterialized veins.

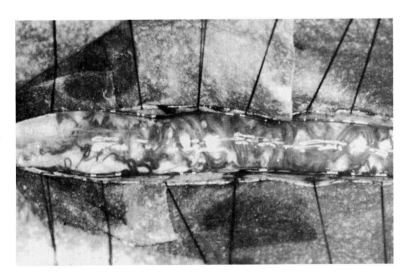

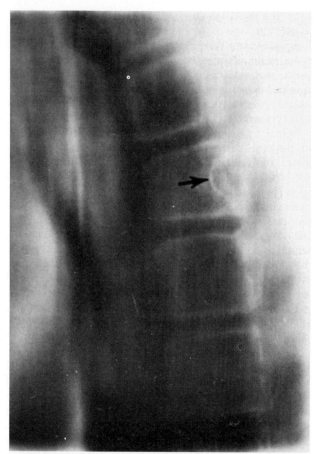

FIGURE 93-8 Lumbar thoracic myelogram demonstrates tortuous shadows suggestive of abnormal vascular channels but representing redundant nerve roots (*arrow*). (From Stein BM: Arteriovenous malformations of the brain and spinal cord. In Practice of Surgery. Hagerstown, MD: Harper & Row, 1979.)

operation, these studies have not shown great promise, especially in definitively locating and diagnosing the presence of a spinal AVM.

Treatment

Because the prognosis is poor for patients with spinal AVMs that are untreated or simply decompressed, we believe that definitive treatment should be attempted. The only completely satisfactory treatment for spinal AVMs is total obliteration or excision.

Embolization

Various techniques have been used, including a variety of materials that are placed via catheter into the feeding arteries.[53–55] The technical difficulties of embolization are due to the small size of the feeding arteries; the fact that these arteries, which are proximal to the lesion, may be significant contributors to the normal spinal cord circulation; and the frequently low-flow nature of the lesions, which precludes flow-directed embolization. The role of embolization varies with the type of AVM.

For type I lesions, embolization has been used both as primary treatment and as adjunctive treatment.[37] In a series of 70 patients treated at the Lariboisière Hospital in Paris,

30 (43%) were referred for surgery when embolization was considered dangerous or had been attempted unsuccessfully. In the remaining 40 patients, seven (10%) could be embolized successfully, and of those, 50% improved and 50% remained clinically stable. In the same series, surgical treatment resulted in a 100% obliteration rate, even in patients who had failed embolization.

Because of the high failure rates, the need for multiple procedures, the incidence of recanalization, and the high success rate of surgery, we believe that embolization is not generally the first procedure of choice in type I AVMs.

Type II intramedullary AVMs have been treated by embolization alone or in conjunction with surgery. The particulate embolization with PVA, silk, or other materials, results in a very high recanalization rate. In 31 patients subjected to 158 embolization procedures, none had complete angiography obliteration, 28 (80%) had recanalization on subsequent angiogram, and 20% experienced clinical deterioration as a result of embolization.[56] Recanalization has occurred after complete angiographic obliteration.[56,57]

Surgical Excision

The cornerstone of treatment for spinal AVMs is microsurgical obliteration.[40,50,58–63] The lesions lend themselves to surgery because the vast majority lie on the dorsal surface of the spinal cord and are thereby accessible (Figs. 93-9 and 93-10; see also Fig. 93-7). They also represent low-flow and low-pressure systems in which there is a limited arterial contribution with a significant venous component that is readily visualized on the surface of the spinal cord. Uncommonly, the lesion invades portions of the spinal cord. Even in such instances, the AVM occasionally may be removed microsurgically with satisfactory results.[33]

The axiom that the preoperative neurologic status is often related to the postoperative outcome is particularly pertinent in these lesions. Surgery should be accomplished early in the disease before major neurologic deficits. Function is unlikely to improve in the face of severe incapacitation.

The patient is prepared with dexamethasone before surgery. Malis[64] prefers to use the sitting position for those lesions located in the upper thoracic, cervical, and cervicomedullary region. This creates a certain degree of hypotension, which he considers potentially useful. It also minimizes the respiratory movement artifact. In those lesions located at the lower levels, he prefers an oblique position so as to limit respiratory excursions. Both of these positions preclude the effective use of an assistant during the operation, which we consider a major disadvantage. We prefer to operate on all these lesions in the prone position with the patient's abdomen and chest free for respiratory excursions. The surgeon and assistant work together across the operating table. The extent of the lesion as identified by myelography, and spinal angiography determines the exposure. The laminectomy should be moderately broad and the dura opened widely with preservation of the arachnoid until the extent of the lesion is determined by visualization through the arachnoid. The operating microscope is always used from the point of dural opening. The arachnoid is then opened widely with small scissors or arachnoidal knife. It may be necessary to rotate the cord, cutting the dentate ligament and grasping it to see the lateral supply to the malformation. In many cases of long dorsal AVMs, the malformation may

FIGURE 93-9 Surgical resection of an arteriovenous malformation shows meticulous cautery of the feeding arteries and gradual peeling away of the abnormal venous channels from the surface of the spinal cord. (From Stein BM: Arteriovenous malformations of the brain and spinal cord. In Practice of Surgery. Hagerstown, MD: Harper & Row, 1979.)

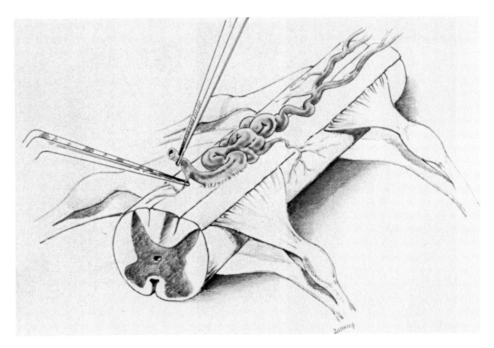

extend over different regions of the spinal cord, and a few cases have been described in which the lesion extends the entire length of the spinal cord. As reported recently,[63] it may not be necessary to remove the entire malformation. Interrupting the fistula between the major arterial supply and the arterialized venous system may suffice.[65]

However, there may be minor arterial contributions, and in such cases the malformation may remain turgid with the veins containing arterialized blood under pressure. It may be necessary to remove the entire arterialized venous system, interrupting even the smallest arterial contribution, in one or multiple stages.

Lesions of the juvenile variety or those that permeate the spinal cord will be easily identified by visualization of the dorsal, dorsolateral, and ventrolateral portion of the spinal cord. Lesions that are primarily intramedullary may be identified by a local bulge of the spinal cord with draining veins coming out over the dorsal surface of the spinal cord. Occasionally, discoloration due to old hemorrhage or thrombosis within the lesion is seen. These areas are treated by myelotomy and techniques similar to intramedullary tumor surgery.

Microbipolar cautery is used under constant moisture during the occlusion of the AVM vessels. Only the largest vessels are clipped, and from a practical point of view, this means none, one, or two arteries during the removal of the usual spinal AVM. It is extremely difficult to use the standard metallic clips in the removal of an intramedullary lesion, which must be accomplished by bipolar cautery. We prefer to approach the lesions from the arterial side first. The venous flow, even though arterialized, is often slow and can be managed easily should rupture occur on the venous side. We see no advantage in attacking the lesion primarily from the venous side if definitive arterial contributions are easily visualized. The lesion is generally peeled away from the spinal cord while additional arterial contributions are coagulated and divided (see Fig. 93-9). In general, malformations

located within the spinal cord are associated with large venous aneurysms, often partially thrombosed. These are rather dangerous "bombs," and we do not want to threaten the venous drainage or the aneurysm more than necessary to collapse it so that it may be removed safely from within the spinal cord. We have not been using hypotension during the removal, especially if the patient is in the sitting position. In the prone position, hypotension is not necessary because of the low flow in these systems. The dura is always closed, no matter what has been accomplished at the time of the operation.

Lesser surgical procedures such as decompressive laminectomy with or without opening the dura appear to have little or no merit in the treatment of these malformations. In fact, such operative "explorations" may be detrimental in that they make future definitive surgery more difficult. If the lesion is found to be inoperable and all that can be offered is decompression with opening of the dura, then the dura should be closed with a patch graft of fascia to prevent adhesions to the surface of the spinal cord. If there is a possibility that surgery will be performed in the future, it is mandatory to close the dura, because the adhesions that will otherwise form will preclude subsequent, definitive surgical ventures.

Special Considerations

Type I Malformations

The large coiled arterialized veins associated with these lesions are fed by one or two primary arteries, which are part of the dorsal radiculomedullary system. It has been previous practice to gradually sweep the entire "malformation" off the dorsal aspect of the cord, interrupting all arterial feeders to it until the venous system turns blue. This practice has been all but abandoned in favor of a more limited resection of the arteriovenous fistula in or near the dura,[59,65–67] based

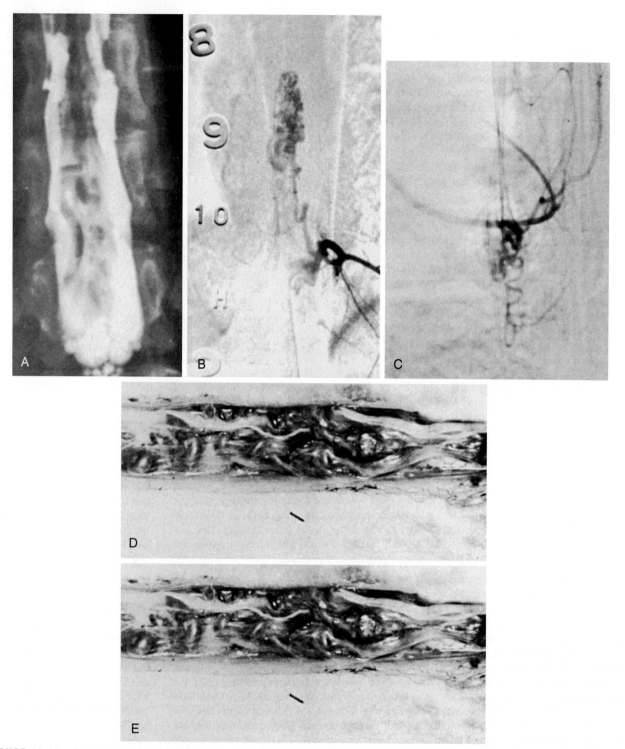

FIGURE 93-10   *A,* Low thoracic myelogram (anteroposterior [AP] projection) demonstrates a serpiginous filling defect suggestive of an arteriovenous malformation (AVM). *B,* Selective spinal arteriogram (AP view) demonstrates a spinal AVM opposite T8–10. *C,* Selective spinal arteriogram (lateral view) demonstrates a spinal AVM with components appearing dorsal, ventral, and possibly within the spinal cord. *D,* Operative exposure of the spinal cord from T7–11 with an extensive AVM. *E,* Operative view after the dorsal and lateral portions of the AVM were removed.

on the concept that the arteriovenous connection is in or near the dura. Clinically, this more limited procedure has led to dramatic improvement in many cases, and postoperative arteriographic studies have shown no visualization of the AVM in such cases.

At present, it is our recommendation that observations at surgery be considered in determining the extent of the surgery. In general, the major coils of veins do not need to be obliterated. There is some evidence that this stripping procedure may cause compromise of the normal cord blood supply and ischemic changes beyond the area of the malformation. After the stripping of large coiled veins from the dorsal surface of the cord, it appears significantly devascularized (see Fig. 93-10). When the major arterial fistula is interrupted the circulation has a more appealing appearance, and postoperative angiography demonstrates complete obliteration.[51]

Glomus Malformations

AVMs in the form of a nidus or glomus are the easiest to comprehend and treat. These lesions produce symptoms of mass hemorrhage or venous thrombosis. They can be circumscribed by interruption of their feeding arteries at the exact margin of the glomus. Interruption of the major venous drainage first may jeopardize the operation by creating intolerable intraluminal forces within the malformation, resulting in hemorrhage.

Malformations that are primarily intramedullary are usually glomus in configuration. A rare one will be associated with a long dorsal type of malformation in conjunction with the primary intramedullary lesion. They are managed in the fashion of removing a glomus from the dorsal or dorsolateral surface of the cord with the additional considerations akin to removal of an intramedullary tumor. The locus of the lesion is visualized as the cord is exposed. A myelotomy is made in a longitudinal direction from the polar aspects of the lesion, allowing visualization of the rostral and caudal margin of the lesion. Dissection is carried carefully around the appropriate margin depending on the anatomy of the venous drainage and arterial supply as determined by angiography and intraoperative observations. These lesions are preferably approached from the arterial side using bipolar cautery for interruption of the arterial feeders while the malformation is rolled toward the venous pedicle. Occasionally, the venous pedicle is in direct relationship to the major supply from the anterior spinal artery. It should be possible to approach the lesion from the arterial side, and once this is interrupted, the venous pedicle is easy to manage. Clips are rarely used. Sharp dissection is always preferred in the removal as opposed to blunt or a tearing type of dissection technique. These lesions are frequently associated with a large aneurysmal dilatation, often partially thrombosed, but still active and thin walled, predisposing to intraoperative hemorrhage secondary to excessive manipulation. Careful use of a broad bipolar tip under irrigation may be used to shrink venous aneurysms, but care must be taken that the wall is not violated. In many cases, the venous aneurysm may be gently teased out of the cord intact. The venous aneurysm is often on the edge of the shunt component of the malformation. The cavity left by removal of these lesions is similar in size and configuration to that left by the total removal of a large intramedullary tumor. It is remarkable how thin the surrounding cord structure can be and still result in a functional neurologic state.

Juvenile or Diffuse Malformations

These lesions are the most difficult to treat. They permeate the cord, and histologic examination indicates functional neural tissue interspersed with vascular channels of the malformation. It is obvious that they do not have well-defined margins permitting resection and that they comprehensively involve both the interior and exterior of the spinal cord over many segments. It is our opinion that confirmation of these lesions must be left to surgical exploration and that definitive knowledge as to their presence, which would preclude intraoperative interventions, cannot be obtained by the usual radiographic studies. Perhaps MRI will answer this question in the future. Although these lesions are nonresectable, in one instance under evoked potential monitoring, we were able to clip a major radicular artery and witness a rather remarkable clinical improvement in an individual who had been plagued by progressive deterioration of spinal cord function. In most cases, these lesions can be treated with little more than a decompressive procedure and perhaps, in exceptional cases, selective ligation of arteries under evoked potential monitoring. These maneuvers are of questionable benefit.

Results

In those patients in whom surgical obliteration or resection of the lesion has been accomplished, good results in terms of an improved neurologic status or arrested deterioration are seen in approximately 80% to 90% of the patients.[40,47,48,51,59,60,62,64]

Unfortunately, the results are often predicated on the preoperative condition of the patient, so that those with neurologic devastation or severe advanced disease are less apt to make gratifying recoveries after successful resection of the lesion. On the other hand, individuals who have mild or modest neurologic deficits before surgery will receive the most benefit and often return to normal or near normal status. Resection of these malformations precludes the possibility of devastating neurologic deficit from subsequent hemorrhage.

Luessenhop and Dela Cruz[58] reported, in a broad review of the literature, that decompressive procedures resulted in improvement in 19% and deterioration in 81%, and ligation of some feeders resulted in improvement in 34% and worsening in 66%. When these figures are compared with those of surgical resection, it is clear that the latter procedure, if feasible, is preferable. It is our view that decompression plays little role in the therapy of these lesions and may be deleterious, producing scar tissue that would make subsequent definitive operative procedures on these lesions difficult or impossible. A postoperative arteriogram should be obtained in all cases to define the completeness of resection.

In addition to the AVMs that directly involve the spinal cord, similar situations may exist in the meninges or parameningeal areas. These lesions are often represented by enormous arteriovenous communications involving the intercostal or cervical arteries and involving not only the dura and sometimes the spinal cord but also often extensively the muscles and surrounding soft tissues. These malformations are associated with bruits and may not manifest themselves with the spinal cord syndrome so familiar to true AVMs of the spinal cord. Unfortunately, these lesions, being extensive with large shunts between arteries and veins, are difficult to treat by embolization, surgery, or both. In many instances, emboli will traverse the fistula and enter into the systemic venous circulation. Because of the extensive nature of these lesions, it is often impossible to remove the entire lesion, even with thoracotomy and massive resection. They are similar to some of the soft tissue AVMs that involve the face and tissues at the base of the skull.

REFERENCES

1. Turnbull F: Intramedullary tumors of the spinal cord. Clin Neurosurg 8:237–247, 1962.
2. Elsberg CA: Tumors of the Spinal Cord. New York: Paul B. Hoeber, 1925, pp 206–239.
3. Matson DD: Neurosurgery of Infancy and Childhood. Springfield, IL: Charles C Thomas, 1969, pp 647–688.
4. Garrido E, Stein BM: Microsurgical removal of intramedullary spinal cord tumors. Surg Neurol 7:215–229, 1977.
5. Greenwood J Jr: Surgical removal of intramedullary tumors. J Neurosurg 26:276–282, 1967.
6. Guidetti BP: Intramedullary tumors of the spinal cord. Acta Neurochir 17, 1967.
7. Horrax G, Henderson D: Encapsulated intramedullary tumor involving whole spinal cord from medulla to conus: Complete enucleation with recovery. Surg Gynecol Obstet 68:814, 1939.
8. Malis LI: Intramedullary spinal cord tumors. Clin Neurosurg 25:512, 1978.
9. Yasargil MG, Antic J, Laciga R, et al: The microsurgical removal of intramedullary spinal hemangioblastomas: Report of twelve cases and a review of the literature. Surg Neurol 6:141, 1976.
10. Stein BM: Spinal Intradural Tumors. New York: McGraw-Hill, 1985, pp 1048–1061.
10a. McCormick PC, Toms R, Post KD, Stein BM: Intramedullary ependymoma of the spinal cord. J Neurosurg 72:523–532, 1990.
11. Rand RW, Rand CW: Intraspinal Tumors of Childhood. Springfield, IL: Charles C Thomas, 1960.
12. Epstein F, Epstein N: Surgical treatment of spinal cord astrocytomas of childhood: A series of 19 patients. J Neurosurg 57:685, 1982.
13. Tievsky AL, Davis DO: Radiology of spinal cord neoplasia. In Wilkins RH, Rengachary SS (eds): Neurosurgery. New York: McGraw-Hill, 1985, pp 1039–1048.
14. Vignaud J, Aubin MD, Jardin C: CT in 75 cases of syringomyelia. AJNR Am J Neuroradiol 2:199–204, 1981.
15. Kan S, Fox AJ, Vineula F, et al: Delayed CT metrizamide enhancement of syringomyelia secondary to tumor. AJNR Am J Neuroradiol 4, 1983.
16. Quencer RM, Tenner MS, Rothman LM: Percutaneous spinal cord puncture and myelocystography. Radiology 118, 1976.
17. Fischer G, Mansuy L: Total removal of intramedullary ependymomas: Follow-up study of 16 cases. Surg Neurol 14, 1980.
18. Stein BM: Surgery of intramedullary spinal cord tumors. Clin Neurosurg 26:529–542, 1979.
19. Guidetti B, Mercuri S, Vagnozzi R: Long-term results of the surgical treatment of 129 intramedullary spinal gliomas. J Neurosurg 54, 1981.
20. Powers SK, Edwards SB, Boggan JE, et al: Use of the argon surgical laser in neurosurgery. J Neurosurg 60:523, 1984.
21. Greenwood J Jr: Intramedullary tumors of the spinal cord: A follow-up study after total surgical removal. J Neurosurg 20, 1963.
22. Love JG, River MH: Thirty-one year cure following removal of intramedullary glioma of cervical portion of spinal cord: Report of case. J Neurosurg 19:906, 1962.
23. Wood EH, Berne AS, Taveras JM: The value of radiation therapy in the management of intrinsic tumors of the spinal cord. Radiology 63:11, 1954.
24. Schwade JG, Wara WM, Sheline GE, et al: Management of primary spinal cord tumors. Int J Radiat Oncol Biol Phys 4, 1978.
25. Tobin WD, Layton DD: The diagnosis and natural history of spinal cord arteriovenous malformations. Mayo Clin Proc 51, 1976.
26. Krayenbuhl H, Yasargil MG: Die varicosis spinalis und ihre Behandlung. Schweiz Arch Neurol Psychiatr 92:74, 1963.
27. Vuia O, Alexianu M: Arteriovenous shunt in the spinal cord circulation. Acta Neurol Scand 45:216–223, 1969.
28. Thron AK: Vascular Anatomy of the Spinal Cord. Neuroradiological Investigations and Clinical Syndromes. New York: Springer-Verlag, 1988.
29. Crock HV, Yoshizawa H: The Blood Supply of the Vertebral Column and Spinal Cord in Man. New York: Springer, 1977.
30. Tadie M, Hemet J, Aaron C, et al: Le dispositif protecteur anti-reflux des veines de la moelle. Neuro-Chir 25:28–30, 1979.
31. Domisse GF: The Arteries and Veins of the Human Spinal Cord from Birth. New York: Churchill Livingstone, 1975.
32. Doppman JL, DiChiro G, Ommaya AK: Selective Arteriography of the Spinal Cord. St. Louis: Warren Green, 1969.
33. Doppman JL: The nidus concept for spinal cord arteriovenous malformations. A surgical recommendation based on angiographic observations. Br J Radiol 44, 1971.
34. Cogen P, Stein BM: Spinal cord arteriovenous malformations with significant intramedullary components. J Neurosurg 59, 1983.
35. Djindjian M, Djindjian R, Hurth M, et al: Intradural extramedullary spinal arteriovenous malformations fed by the anterior spinal artery. Surg Neurol 8:85–93, 1977.
36. Heros R, Debrun G, Ojemann R, et al: Direct spinal arteriovenous fistula: A new type of spinal AVM. J Neurosurg 64:134–139, 1986.
37. Mourier KL, Gobin YP, George B, et al: Intradural perimedullary arteriovenous fistulae: Results of surgical and endovascular treatment in a series of 35 cases. Neurosurgery 32:885–891, 1993.
38. Mahagne MH, Rogopoulos A, Paquis P, et al: Intracranial dural arteriovenous fistula with spinal venous drainage. Rev Neurol (Paris) 148:789–792, 1992.
39. Herdt JR, DiChiro G, Doppman JL: Combined arterial and arteriovenous aneurysms of the spinal cord. Radiology 99, 1971.
40. Krayenbuhl H, Yasargil MG, McClintock HG: Treatment of spinal cord vascular malformations by surgical excision. J Neurosurg 30:427, 1969.
41. Kaufman HH, Ommaya AK, DiChiro G, et al: Compression vs. "steal." The pathogenesis of symptoms in arteriovenous malformations of the spinal cord. Arch Neurol 23, 1970.
42. Djindjian M, Djindjian R, Hurth M, et al: Steal phenomenon in spinal arteriovenous malformations. J Neuroradiol 5, 1978.
43. Matthews WB: The spinal bruit. Lancet 2, 1959.
44. Doppman JL, Wirth F Jr, DiChiro G, et al: Value of cutaneous angiomas in the arteriographic localization of the spinal cord arteriovenous malformations. N Engl J Med 281, 1969.
45. Yasargil MG: Diagnosis and treatment of spinal cord arteriovenous malformations. Prog Neurol Surg 4:355, 1971.
46. Wyburn MR: The Vascular Abnormalities and Tumors of the Spinal Cord and Its Membranes. London: Krimptom, 1943.
47. Aminoff MJ, Logue V: Clinical features of spinal vascular malformations. Brain 97, 1974.
48. Aminoff MJ, Logue V: The prognosis of patients with spinal vascular malformations. Brain 97, 1974.
49. DiChiro G, Doppman JL, Wener L: Computed tomography of spinal arteriovenous malformations. Radiology 123, 1977.
50. Kasdon DL, Wolpert SM, Stein BM: Surgical and angiographic localization of spinal arteriovenous malformations. Surg Neurol 5:279–283, 1976.
51. Bederson JB, Spetzler RF: Pathophysiology of type I spinal dural arteriovenous malformations. BNI Q 12:23–32, 1996.
52. Berenstein A, Young W, Ransohoff J, et al: Somatosensory evoked potentials during spinal angiography and therapeutic transvascular embolization. J Neurosurg 60, 1984.
53. Doppman JL, DiChiro G, Ommaya AK: Percutaneous embolization of spinal cord arteriovenous malformations. J Neurosurg 34, 1971.
54. Hilal SK, Sane P, Michelson WJ, et al: The embolization of vascular malformations of the spinal cord with low-viscosity silicone rubber. Neuroradiology 16, 1978.
55. Djindjian R: Embolization of angiomas of the spinal cord. Surg Neurol 4, 1975.
56. Biondi A, Merland JJ, Reizine D, et al: Embolization with particles in thoracic intramedullary arteriovenous malformations: Long-term angiographic and clinical results. Radiology 177:651–658, 1990.
57. Hall WA, Oldfield EH, Doppman JL: Recanalization of spinal arteriovenous malformations following embolization. J Neurosurg 70:714–720, 1989.
58. Luessenhop AJ, Dela Cruz T: Surgical excision of spinal intradural vascular malformations. J Neurosurg 30:552, 1969.
59. Ommaya AK, DiChiro G, Doppman JL: Ligation of arterial supply in the treatment of spinal cord arteriovenous malformations. J Neurosurg 30, 1969.
60. Houdart R, Djindjian R, Hurth M: Vascular malformations of the spinal cord; the anatomic and therapeutic significance of arteriography. J Neurosurg 24, 1966.
61. Kunc Z, Bret J: Diagnosis and treatment of vascular malformations of the spinal cord. J Neurosurg 30, 1969.

62. Yasargil RW, DeLong WB, Guarnaschelli JJ: Complete microsurgical excision of cervical extramedullary and intramedullary vascular malformations. Surg Neurol 4:211, 1975.
63. Latchaw TW, Harris RD, Chou S, et al: Combined embolization and operation in the treatment of cervical arteriovenous malformations. Neurosurgery 6, 1980.
64. Malis LI: Microsurgery for spinal cord arteriovenous malformations. Clin Neurosurg 26:543, 1979.
65. Oldfield EH, DiChiro G, Quindlen EA, et al: Successful treatment of a group of spinal cord arteriovenous malformations by interruption of dura fistula. J Neurosurg 59:1019–1030, 1983.
66. Bailey WL, Sperl MP: Angiomas of the cervical spinal cord. J Neurosurg 30:560–568, 1969.
67. Baker H Jr, Love JG, Layton D Jr: Angiographic and surgical aspects of spinal cord vascular anomalies. Radiology 88:1078–1085, 1967.

Section XV

Surgical Management of Epilepsy

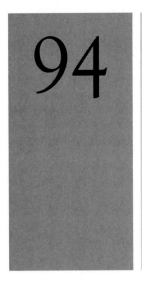

94 Diagnostic Techniques in Surgical Management of Epilepsy: Strip Electrodes, Grids, and Depth Electrodes

DIANA L. ABSON KRAEMER

SUMMARY

This chapter presents the techniques and indications for the placement of subdural strip and grid electrodes and intra-parenchymal depth electrodes. The traditional techniques for placement of these electrodes is discussed and then expanded with inclusion within each section of special considerations for electrode placement for unique circumstances. The use of both frame-based and frameless techniques for depth electrode placement are discussed. The chapter concludes with practical advise on techniques to minimize complications during surgery.

INDICATIONS

The presurgical evaluation for epilepsy has changed substantially in the past few decades, most notably since the advent of magnetic resonance imaging (MRI) and advanced neuroimaging techniques. The presurgical evaluation requires input from many members of an integrated team, which includes neurologists, electrophysiologists, neuropsychologists, social workers, radiologists, nurses, and the epilepsy neurosurgeon(s). Aspects of the presurgical evaluation include the patient's history and physical examination, family history and genetic background, social circumstances, seizure syndrome and severity, and diagnostic testing, including interictal electroencephalography (EEG), ictal scalp video EEG, MRI, positron emission tomography, single photon emission computed tomography, and subtraction ictal single photon emission computed tomography, magnetoencephalography, and neuropsychological data (Minnesota Multiphasic Personality Inventory, cognitive testing, and Wada evaluation) as indicated.[1-10] Usually, a surgical plan is developed using a team approach with all information being discussed in a conference format. This allows give and take between multiple experts so that a unique surgical approach is tailored to the individual's personal needs and epilepsy syndrome. When all presurgical information points to a unifying location and theory regarding focal seizure onset (also referred to as "concordant data"), then the patient may proceed directly to resective surgery. When data are inadequate to define a resective strategy, then diagnostic intracranial electrodes may be considered

to further define the syndrome or site of seizure onset before any resective surgery.

Invasive intracranial monitoring is indicated when

1. Seizures are lateralized but not localized (e.g., a left-sided, nonlesional frontotemporal onset)
2. Seizures are localized but not lateralized (e.g., bilateral temporal lobe epilepsy [TLE])
3. Seizures are neither localized nor lateralized (e.g., stereotypical complex partial seizures with diffuse late ictal changes or initial changes obscured by artifact)
4. Seizure localization is discordant with other data and electroencephalographic ictal scalp data are discordant with neuroimaging (e.g., MRI, positron emission tomography, single photon emission computed tomography) or neuropsychological data
5. The relationship of seizure onset to functional tissue must be determined (e.g., seizures with early involvement of language or motor function)
6. The relationship of seizure onset to a lesion(s) must be determined (e.g., dual pathology or multiple intracranial lesions)
7. Seizures are clinically suspected, but the presurgical evaluation is inadequate in defining seizures (e.g., pseudopseudoseizures[11])

The examples above do not represent the only indications for intracranial monitoring but are given as examples of when intracranial monitoring might be useful. The considerations for the treatment of epilepsy are unique to each patient and also to the center conducting the evaluation. The challenges of epilepsy surgery and the multiple options available to the treatment team are the appealing aspects of being involved in the surgical treatment of epilepsy.

Invasive intracranial monitoring and/or surgery will not lead to seizure freedom in every patient. Therefore, our understanding of epilepsy and techniques to treat it are limited at best. It is incumbent on the surgeon to question not only where electrodes should be placed based on the presurgical information available but also to consider what other alternative localization may also need to be included or excluded to obtain a positive outcome. The concept that epilepsy consists of a "focus" that can be removed has evolved into a more unifying theory in which the neural network, environment, genetic predisposition, and epileptogenic substrate must all be considered during the evaluation of the patient with epilepsy if surgery is to be effective.[12,13]

DEFINITIONS

Depth, strip, and grid electrodes are implantable intracranial devices used for recording bioelectrical central nervous system activity and for electrically stimulating cortex to determine function. Depth electrodes are multicontact, thin, tubular, rigid or semirigid electrodes that penetrate the brain substances for the purpose of recording from deep structures (Fig. 94-1A). Intracranial strip electrodes are a linear array of 2 to 16 multiple disc electrode contacts embedded in a strip of Silastic[14] (see Fig. 94-1B), or they can be tubular multicontact in structure, similar to depth electrodes.[15] Grid electrodes are parallel rows of similar numbers of electrode contacts that can be configured in standard or custom designs according to the preferences of the surgeon

and abilities of the manufacturer (see Fig. 94-1B and C). Grid and strip electrodes are designed to be in direct contact with the cortical surface. In most cases, electrodes are placed in the subdural space, although they may occasionally be used in the epidural space. All these electrode types are constructed from biologically inert materials (stainless steel, platinum, or platinum-iridium). Platinum electrodes are more easily seen on fluoroscopy than are stainless steel electrodes and are compatible with MRI so that postoperative diagnostic and localizing neuroimaging can be performed with electrodes in place.

OPERATIVE TECHNIQUES

Strip Electrodes

Strip electrodes are used most often to lateralize the side of seizure onset in frontal and temporal lobe epilepsy but may also be used to perform survey studies over all cortical surfaces of the brain. They are usually implanted with the

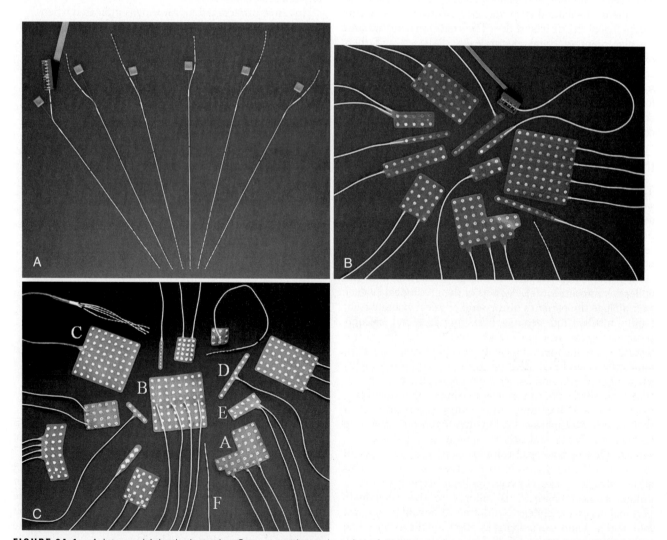

FIGURE 94-1 *A,* Intracranial depth electrodes. Contact spacing and number of contacts can be custom designed. *B,* Intracranial strip electrodes and standard Wyler subdural grid electrodes. *C,* Custom intracranial subdural strip and grid electrodes. A, Spencer grid for coverage of the lateral and inferior temporal neocortex; B, Doyle grid; C, custom grid with a single tail, used by some centers to reduce cerebrospinal fluid leak. Custom subdural strip (D) and grid (E) for placement in the interhemispheric fissure. F, a cylindrical subdural strip electrode. (Courtesy of Ad-Tech Corporation, Racine, WI.)

patient under general anesthesia. Skin incisions for strip electrodes should be made so that they can be incorporated into subsequent craniotomy incisions. A burr hole(s) is made at the desired location in the skull. Bleeding from the bone is controlled with monopolar cautery and then the dura is cauterized with bipolar cautery, after which the dura is opened with a cruciate incision. Foreign bodies, such as bone wax or absorbable gelatin sponge, are used temporarily and are left in place only if necessary because of the theoretical increased risk of infection. Electrodes are implanted according to the preoperative plan created by the epilepsy monitoring team. Electrodes can be directed over long distances within the cranium by "surfing" the electrodes over the brain surface using a fluid wave (see "Complication Avoidance"). Care must be taken when placing electrodes to sense for distal obstructions (dural adhesions or bridging veins); even minimal resistance to passage of the electrode should be respected and the electrode should be redirected. Electrodes can be safely directed over fairly long distances within the calvarium by using this technique (Fig. 94-2). Fluoroscopy is used to confirm placement before closure of the wound. The electrode wires are tunneled with a 13-gauge passing needle designed for that purpose (Ad-Tech Corporation, Racine, WI) to exit the skin several centimeters from the burr hole incision. Cerebrospinal fluid (CSF) is less likely to track along the electrodes when they are tunneled superior to the burr hole. It has not been the tradition at our center to place a cable-retaining suture in the scalp, as others have suggested,[16,17] because this increases the risk of breaking the electrode cable if pulled violently during a seizure. Instead, Ad-Tech quick-release connectors are used because these break apart easily if tugged.

The wound is closed in anatomic layers using absorbable braided suture material. No attempt is made to close the dura. The electrodes are tunneled so that they exit the wound deep to the temporalis muscle (if present) so that the muscle can be placed on tension to aid in hemostasis. The temporalis muscle, fascia, and galea are then closed in

anatomic layers with absorbable suture, and staples are placed in the skin. The wounds and electrode exit sites are dressed with antibiotic ointment and Telfa, and then a clean, dry towel is used as a loose head wrap to protect the electrodes while the patient is in the recovery room. The patient is then transferred to the monitoring unit for hookup, after which the EEG technicians create a formal head wrap. CSF may leak from around the electrode wires in the first 3 days after implantation. Because of this, the dressing is changed as often as needed.

Subdural strip electrodes are designed to be removed through the skin without requiring open surgical removal. Removal is performed in a dedicated anesthesia workroom using deep conscious sedation. The electrodes are removed using gentle but constant traction, with attention paid to ensure that none of the electrode pads fracture off and are left beneath the skin. Although this rarely occurs, open removal under general anesthesia is necessary; this is more likely to occur when the electrodes are being removed from the occipital fascia.

Although strip electrodes can be inserted epidurally[18,19] this practice is not advisable for routine cases because the exposure is limited to the lateral convexities of the brain. The epidural space in the temporal fossa does not allow the electrode to be advanced medially enough to record from the parahippocampal gyrus, and electrodes cannot be placed over mesial frontal lobe cortex. In most exploratory investigations, these locations should be sampled. However, epidural placement may be the most reasonable option when recording from a patient with a previous craniotomy because scarring may obliterate the subdural space.

Special Considerations for Strip Electrode Placement

TEMPORAL LOBE SURVEYS

Although TLE surgery can be highly successful in patients with hippocampal atrophy, approximately 30% will continue to have some seizures.[20] Patients with nonlesional TLE are no more likely to have a good surgical outcome than are patients with nonlesional TLE. Therefore, it is important when evaluating the patient with TLE to determine not only where seizures arise but to also target areas from which seizures might propagate. The surgeon should consider placing orbitofrontal and parietal electrodes in patients with nonlesional TLE because these regions readily propagate to the medial temporal lobe and can falsely localize.[21–25] An appropriate placement of the burr hole to reach all these sites can be made with an elliptical trough craniectomy (created by two burr holes placed side by side) in the low frontal region, approximately 7 cm above the zygoma. From this location, an eight-contact, 9.5-cm strip electrode can be directed in an anteroposterior direction so that the most medial electrodes overlie the entorhinal cortex of the parahippocampal gyrus.[26] Another eight-contact, 9.5-cm strip can be directed under the orbitofrontal cortex. Fluoroscopy is useful to confirm placement because these electrodes can deflect off of the pterion and be misdirected. Additional electrodes can be placed over the posterior temporal, frontal, parietal, and occipital lobes with ease. Coverage of the mesial frontal, parietal, and occipital lobes is difficult from this location and will usually require another burr hole if such coverage is desired.

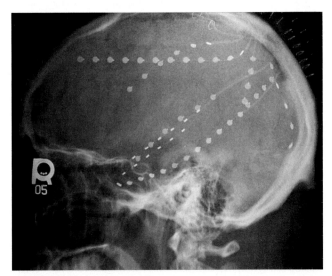

FIGURE 94-2 Radiograph of implanted intracranial electrodes placed for an occipitotemporal survey study. Electrodes were placed as far as 16 cm from the burr hole by "surfing" the electrodes into place (see text for details).

In our institution, patients with nonlesional temporal epilepsy receive bilateral strip electrodes over the anterior, middle, and posterior temporal cortices and orbitofrontal cortex in additional to intrahippocampal depth electrodes. Antiepileptic medications are withheld beginning the morning of surgery (except for benzodiazepines and barbiturates, which are reduced). Using this approach, 345 seizures were recorded in 44 patients (range, 1 to 70 seizures; average of 7.8 seizures per patient). Intracranial studies were performed for 3 to 16 days, with a median duration of electrode implantation of 6 days. In 29 patients with no or mild hippocampal atrophy, 5 had initial ictal discharges limited only to the neocortex.[27]

INTERHEMISPHERIC STRIP ELECTRODE PLACEMENT

A variety of interhemispheric strip electrodes and subdural grids have been devised to reach the interhemispheric fissure. Clinical seizures most commonly seen from the mediofrontal hemispheres are supplemental motor area seizures or, less commonly, focal motor seizures of the foot. Scalp electrographic changes may be delayed, diffused, or bilateral given the deep location of seizure onset. Interhemispheric electrode placement should be considered whenever a frontal lobe epilepsy syndrome is suspected that does not localize to the lateral convexity because supplemental motor area seizures do not always begin with classic fencing semiology.[28]

Interhemispheric subdural electrode strips can be directed into the interhemispheric fissure through either an anterior or a posterior burr hole. A high frontal parasagittal vertex burr hole can be used for placement; however, it can be difficult to direct strips from this position because of the presence of draining veins and arachnoidal villi, which obscure the subdural space. It can also be difficult to get an electrode to make the sharp bend between the frontal convexity and the interhemispheric space. Even if the strip electrode does negotiate this bend, the angle at which the electrode will deflect off the falx cerebri is unpredictable, and therefore it is difficult to reliably place electrodes over the supplemental motor area from this position unless one is willing to create a craniotomy flap.

Interhemispheric strip electrode placement from the occipital approach is performed as follows: The patient is placed in the semisitting position with the head flexed forward and held with either a radiolucent headholder or stereotactic head frame (used if depth electrodes are being placed simultaneously). Doppler sonography is placed to detect air embolism. The occipital region is prepared as described elsewhere in this chapter. A parasagittal burr hole is placed 2 to 3 cm from the midline, lateral enough to ensure that the initial burr hole does not tear the sagittal sinus during the initial opening. (This burr hole is higher and more medial than the location used for occipital depth electrode placement). The dura is opened and cauterized to avoid air embolism. A 1 × 12 contact, 13.5-cm subdural strip is directed medially and slightly superiorly. If the strip does not turn the "bend" between the occipital pole and interhemispheric fissure at the posterior falx, then the craniectomy must be extended superomedially with a Kerrison rongeur. The dura is opened upward and slightly medially toward the sagittal sinus in short, careful increments. An attempt is made to place the electrode after every few millimeters of dural opening until the electrode enters the

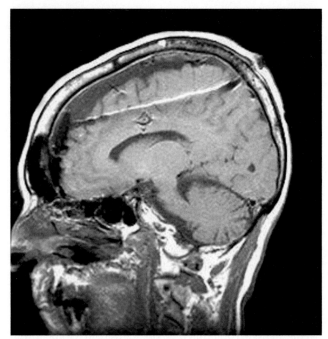

FIGURE 94-3 Placement of a 12-contact interhemispheric strip electrode through a high occipital burr hole. The patient had dual pathology, with a cavernous malformation in the cingulated gyrus and left hippocampal atrophy.

interhemispheric plane. The electrode can then usually be "surfed" easily along this plane until the distal contact rests on the anterior mesial frontal lobe. If resistance is met after the electrode has been inserted 5 to 6 cm, then it is likely that the electrode is abutting the posterior corpus callosum. The electrode should be withdrawn, and the craniectomy and dural incision should be enlarged more superiorly for another few millimeters, after which another pass is likely to be successful. Fluoroscopy can be used throughout this portion of the procedure to direct and confirm final electrode placement. Complete coverage of the length of mesial frontal and parietal lobes is provided with this approach (Fig. 94-3).

Intracranial grids have also been designed for interhemispheric use, including a grid with electrode contacts on both sides of the grid that can be implanted on one side of the brain (see Fig. 94-1C). These electrodes work well when one is already preparing a frontal craniotomy for grid implantation over the convexity. However, when a bilateral survey study is planned, bilateral interhemispheric 1 × 12 strip electrodes may be a better alternative.

STAGED PROCEDURES

A series of intracranial procedures may be necessary when presurgical scalp EEG is poorly lateralized. Some authors have noted an increase in complications with bilateral intracranial grids or with increasing numbers of electrodes.[29,30] Therefore, many centers will perform an intracranial survey study with bilateral strip electrodes to lateralize seizure onset to one hemisphere to avoid the placement of bilateral grids. The survey study may lateralize to one hemisphere and localize to a particular lobe (frontal, temporal, occipital) but may not provide sufficient information to allow focal cortical resection. In these cases, strips are removed and the patient is allowed to recover before returning for an intracranial grid implantation. These cases can be anticipated by the epilepsy team, and a series of intracranial surgeries may be planned and presented to the patient for discussion and education of the process involved.[31,32]

EPIDURAL PEG ELECTRODES

Some centers use epidural peg electrodes more often than others for invasive monitoring. Epidural peg electrodes can consist of titanium pegs or screws of different lengths that are inserted through trephine openings so that the electrode contact transverses the skull, improving the signal-to-noise ratio that complicates scalp electroencephalographic recording. Epidural peg or screw studies in general use fewer electrodes than intracranial studies and are limited in reaching mesial intracranial structures but may help to lateralize scalp recordings when the initial onset is obscured by artifact.

FORAMEN OVALE ELECTRODES

Foramen ovale electrodes are an invasive alternative to strip and depth electrodes when evaluating mesial TLE.[33–35] They are placed percutaneously into the foramen ovale where they enter the dura and lie adjacent to the mesial temporal lobe. The limitation of foramen ovale electrodes is that they sample only from the mesial temporal structures. The complication rate for foramen ovale electrodes is similar to that of subdural strips.

Subdural Grid Electrodes

Arrays of electrodes that are more than one column wide are considered to be intracranial grids. Practically speaking, electrode arrays that are two or three contacts wide will not pass easily for any substantial distance through a burr hole and will require a craniotomy. Once the decision to proceed with a craniotomy is made, grid arrays of five to eight rows of eight electrodes (40 to 64 contacts) are usually employed to maximize coverage over the craniotomy site. The craniotomy site will be determined by the presurgical evaluation; usually a large craniotomy will be performed to accommodate a grid as large as 8 × 8 cm. Prophylactic antibiotics and dexamethasone are used routinely. Mannitol is not used unless necessary because the putative space created by fluid shift could adversely contribute to hematoma formation after closure. The dura is opened, and the grid is inserted underneath the dural margins to cover as much of the cortex as possible. Sometimes the entire grid cannot be placed into position without buckling the array, deforming the brain, or impinging on adjacent vessels. If repositioning the grid does not resolve the problem, then its shape or contour can be altered by either cutting off columns or slicing the Silastic between electrode rows to allow some overlap of the grid on itself (Fig. 94-4). When making such cuts, the surgeon should avoid making sharp edges on the cut surfaces of the grid. Once the grid is placed, the grid is sutured to the dura to prevent motion (Fig. 94-5). The electrode tails are positioned so that the dura can be closed without placing torque on the leads, which might press the grid into the brain. Often, one or more strip electrodes are added to sample adjacent areas or lobes, such as the interhemispheric fissure or basal temporal lobe. The dura is closed with interrupted, braided, nonabsorbable sutures. Electrode tails are

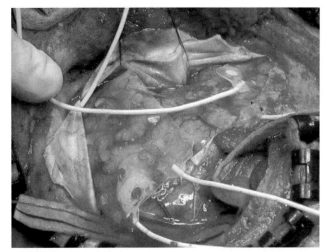

FIGURE 94-4 Placement of a Wyler subdural grid. A 64-contact grid has been cut into three pieces: one 4 × 8 grid covers the frontal pole, one 2 × 8 grid covers the orbitofrontal cortex, and one 2 × 8 grid covers the lateral temporal neocortex. The two dural tack-up sutures at the top of the photo are on either side of the pterion.

tunneled similarly to strip electrodes, and the bone flap is sutured into place. The scalp is closed in anatomic layers with absorbable sutures and skin staples. A clean, dry towel is used to cover the wound while the patient is in the recovery room before being transferred to the video EEG monitoring suite, where the patient is hooked up on the day of surgery. Acute nursing care is provided in the monitoring suite during the first 24 hours after craniotomy, similar to the level one would find in a neurologic step-down unit.

The grid is removed when sufficient data have been obtained to determine the site of ictal onset or, alternatively, determine that no more recording is likely to lead to satisfactory localization. If resective surgery is planned, then the grid's relationship to the underlying cortex must stay unchanged while the craniotomy is reopened. Details of the

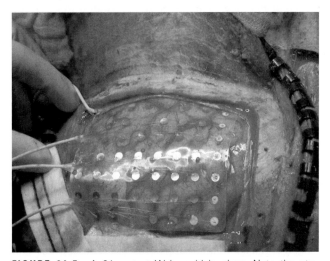

FIGURE 94-5 A 64-contact Wyler grid in place. Note the stay suture tied around the electrode tail in the upper left hand corner. This suture also goes through the plastic of the grid to immobilize the grid. The grid will slide under the dural margins of the craniotomy flap as the dural is closed, so bridging veins must be accommodated during planning to avoid venous compromise or hemorrhage.

initial stages of removing a grid are discussed under "Complication Avoidance, Infection." The dura is opened, leaving the grid-stabilizing sutures intact and keeping all relationships between electrode contacts and unique underlying cortical topography (such as blood vessels) undisturbed. Once these relationships have been documented and the surgeon has extrapolated the mapped data to the underlying cortex, the grid is removed and discarded. Resective surgery is performed as appropriate, with the epilepsy monitoring team present in the operating room (OR) as necessary. If resection is not performed at the time of grid removal (due to hemorrhage, edema, patient preference, or insufficient data), then pertinent landmarks may be documented for reoperation at a later date with digital photography or frameless stereotaxy, as appropriate.

Complication rates for intracranial grid electrodes have been associated with an increased number of electrode contacts, increased length of monitoring period, placement of burr holes in addition to the craniotomy, and multiple cable exit sites.[29,30] Grid implantation can be scheduled on a Monday for adults with removal/resection scheduled for the following Friday (postoperative day 4), although many institutions prefer a 7- or 8-day monitoring period. Most pediatric patients are scheduled for an implantation followed by explantation and resection 48 to 72 hours later. Two thirds of patients are ready for grid removal by the scheduled date. If the monitoring team is not entirely certain of the reliability of ictal onset data, then the grid removal is postponed until adequate data are obtained.

Special Considerations for Grid Implantation

CUSTOM GRIDS

Custom grids can be created to facilitate the investigation of specific clinical investigations (see Fig. 94-1C). For example, the Spencer grid is designed to conform to the temporal lobe, so that inferior and lateral temporal lobe coverage is obtained and extraoperative language mapping of the basal temporal lobe can be accomplished (Ad-Tech Corporation).[36] The grid is designed to avoid posterior temporal draining veins. A Kraemer modification of the Spencer grid extends more posteriorly and superiorly, so that the perisylvian cortex is also covered (not shown). Other modifications have also been made; the Doyle grid is a custom, 64-contact grid in which electrode tails arise from the center of the grid rather than from the side. This allows the grid to be placed through a relatively smaller craniotomy and dural opening and is particularly useful in pediatric cases. Its use should be limited to the lateral convexities to avoid injury to bridging veins during insertion. Although this author works routinely with Ad-Tech Corporation, other manufacturers may also create custom grids on request.

STAGED PROCEDURES

A second intracranial study may be considered for a number of reasons,[9,23,31,37-40] including the following:

1. Strip electrode survey study for lateralization and localization to a lobe, with a planned return at a later date for grid implantation for definition of the ictal onset zone and cortical mapping as necessary
2. Reimplantation of a second grid due to failed localization secondary to sampling error (seizures may

occur on the margin of the grid, be diffuse, or show variable propagation that makes seizure localization suspect)
3. Recurrent seizures after a previous intracranial study and resection

These procedures are typically performed months to years after the first intracranial study, either to give the wound time to heal or because seizures recur at some variable time after resective surgery. Often, an interim presurgical evaluation will be performed, including video electroencephalographic monitoring, ictal single photon emission computed tomography, MRI, and/or magnetoencephalography to re-explore the theory regarding a person's epilepsy and prepare a more effective intracranial study. Secondary grid implantations can be quite troublesome because dural adhesions are the rule rather than the exception. Therefore, when planning a second intracranial study, the surgeon should anticipate a difficult entry and use many of the strategies used for reoperation in other craniotomies, including enlarging the bone flap until pristine dura is encountered and opening the dura away from the previous operative site and away from functional cortex. An operating microscope should be reserved and used early in the dissection if adhesions are encountered: I routinely plan to spend 1 to 3 hours under the operating microscope when scheduling a reoperation for epilepsy. Even with tedious dissection, adhesions can limit the distal passage of electrodes and limit the effectiveness of a repeat intracranial study.

CONSECUTIVE GRID PLACEMENT

An alternative approach to delayed reoperation has been suggested by several authors.[41-43] These authors advocate immediate reimplantation during the same hospitalization if a first grid is nondiagnostic. Silverberg and Doyle[43] refer to this as a three-stage procedure, and Lee and colleagues[42] describe the same technique as a double grid. This technique has some advantages over delayed return for second grid implantation. First, adhesions will not obscure the subdural space, which can limit grid reimplantation. Second, cortical injury can be avoided because dissection of adhesions from functional tissue will not be necessary. Third, intracranial electroencephalographic changes can be compared with the previous study while the subtleties of the previous intracranial electrocorticogram are still fresh in the minds of the evaluating team. Doyle advocates performing a limited resection of the ictal onset zone seen with the first grid, as a partial resection of the epileptogenic region may help identify which additional areas are still contributing to seizure onset once the major site of ictal origin has been removed. Favorable seizure control was seen with no apparent increase in surgical morbidity in 42 three-stage procedures when compared with 369 traditional grid protocols[43] and in 18 double procedures compared with 165 routine intracranial procedures.[42]

Depth Electrodes

Depth electrodes are used most commonly for recording from the hippocampus. My preferred approach for hippocampal placement is the occipital, parasagittal route.[44,45] This trajectory allows for simultaneous implantation into the amygdala and anterior and posterior hippocampus using a single multicontact electrode. Placement is performed using either a frameless system, discussed later, or a stereotactic frame with adequate clearance at the back of the head. MRI is used with both frame-based and frameless stereotactic placement to allow direct visualization of the target and trajectory.[15,32,46–50]

Depth Electrode Placement Using Traditional Frame-Based Techniques

The stereotactic frame is secured using local anesthesia before MRI localization. Axial, sagittal, and coronal T1-weighted images are obtained perpendicular to the frame and then transferred to an adjacent workstation for offline calculations. Imaging is performed out of the plane of the encoding phase to minimize distortion artifact. The angle and trajectory of each hippocampus are visually inspected on parasagittal images: the hippocampus rises from anterior to posterior at an angle of 15 to 30 degrees, relative to the base of the frame, depending on the angle at which the frame is applied (Fig. 94-6). This angle is calculated and is useful for two purposes: First, it allows estimation of a tract for the entry point at the occiput. Second, injury to the thalamus will be avoided as long as the angle of approach is less than the angle of inclination of the hippocampus (Fig. 94-7). The target point is chosen in the inferior anterior amygdala on coronal images. This point should be slightly inferior to the plane of the hippocampus so that the electrode passes through the length of the hippocampus. This target should also be lateral enough to avoid the brain stem and posterior cerebral artery. Most MRI workstations provide software

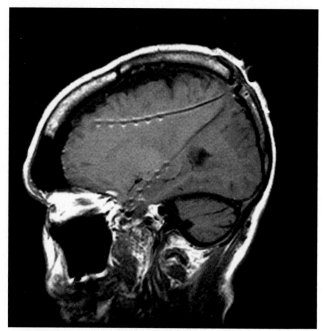

FIGURE 94-7 Misplacement of a depth electrode in a patient with dual pathology (cingulate lesion and hippocampal atrophy). This photograph illustrates several technical errors. The author attempted to use one burr hole for placement of a depth electrode and interhemispheric subdural strip (not seen). The angle of entry for the depth electrode is greater than the angle of rise of the hippocampus. The hippocampal depth electrode travels through the thalamus, misses the hippocampus, and enters the amygdala. The patient was asymptomatic. This patient has a second depth electrode placed into the parenchyma of the frontal lobe, just lateral to the cingulate lesion. In general, the author now avoids placing two depth electrodes through the same entry site to decrease risk of cortical hemorrhage.

that allows the surgeon to study the planned trajectory in relationship to these crucial landmarks (see additional comments under "Frameless Stereotaxy").

Electrodes are placed under general anesthesia with the patient in a semisitting position and the Leksell frame secured to a Mayfield holder. Doppler sonography and end-tidal CO_2 monitoring are used to observe for air embolus. The occiput is shaved from vertex to inion and scrubbed with alcohol and Betadine. A sterile, transparent ophthalmic drape is used to protect the operative field without obstructing frame access so that adjustments can be made as necessary. The entry point is determined and a 5-cm vertical incision is made (3 to 4 cm lateral to the midline is optimal). Because most electrode placements are bilateral, two vertical incisions are created. It is useful to place the occipital burr hole as superior as possible, accommodating for the inclination of the hippocampus to avoid interference from the frame. If the bone is particularly thick, the edges of the burr hole may obstruct the planned trajectory and should be considered when planning the entry point. A cruciate dural incision is opened, and the dura is cauterized to avoid air embolus. The underlying occipital lobe is inspected, and small adjustments in the entry point are made to avoid draining veins or sulci during electrode placement. The pia and arachnoid are cauterized before inserting the electrode. A flexible depth electrode with a semirigid, removable

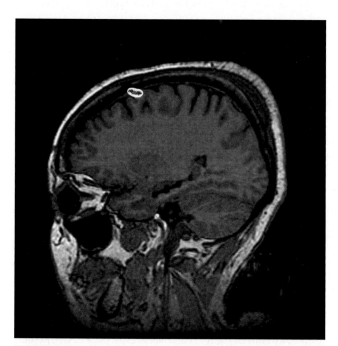

FIGURE 94-6 Placement of an intracerebral depth electrode along the long axis of the hippocampus. Not all electrode contacts can be seen because the electrode is not exactly parallel with the sagittal plane. The most anterior contacts of this electrode are implanted in the amygdala.

internal stylet is readied for placement. Even with this stylet, the electrode is pliable and can be easily deflected, particularly by the ependyma of the lateral ventricle at the atrium. To improve placement accuracy, a rigid guide cannula is inserted from the occipital cortex to a point just posterior to the hippocampal tail (CSF may drain from the cannula after placement). The depth electrode is then introduced through this guide tube. The surgeon often feels a subtle "pop" as the electrode breaches the ependyma. The electrode is then advanced gently to the target position. If resistance is encountered, the electrode should not be advanced further until all trajectory coordinates have been verified by an independent operator. When the electrode tip has been advanced to the target point, the stylet is removed and the guide cannula withdrawn from the brain without disturbing the electrode. The electrode has a tendency to back out during stylet and cannula removal, but this may be minimized with practice. Most electrode companies will add a black marker to the electrode near the cortical surface (13 cm from the tip) on request so that visual confirmation of electrode shift can be seen. Alternatively, a suture can be tied to the electrode at a convenient distance for the surgeon as a visual aid. Fluoroscopy is used to confirm satisfactory placement. After the supporting equipment is removed from the brain, the electrode is tunneled through a trocar to an exit site and then sutured to the skin with two separate nylon ligatures to prevent dislodgment. After implantation of the first electrode is completed, the stereotactic frame is adjusted to the coordinates for the second depth electrode.

It is increasingly common for depth electrodes to be placed using a combination of frame-based stereotaxy and frameless navigation.[51] An MRI suitable for frameless navigation is obtained with the frame in place. Most frameless stereotaxic units have software incorporated or available to seamlessly incorporate the frame into the guidance system. The surgeon then has the combined advantages of frame-based stability with the added enhancement of frameless navigation. Multimodality imaging of anatomic and angiographic studies can be merged to allow the surgeon to plan trajectories that avoid all pertinent deep vessels using both a trajectory-based and "probe's eye" view of the intended target and approach. It is likely that this additional neuronavigation adds to the safety of depth electrode placement.

Hippocampal depth electrodes can be placed orthogonally (temporal approach).[33,47,52] Care must be taken to place the frame as low as possible while still leaving room for the fiducial box. When targeting the temporal region, it is imperative that the anatomy of the middle cerebral arteries be kept in mind because the vessels of the middle cerebral artery can deviate quite inferiorly into the temporal lobe and are at risk of injury. Therefore, many orthogonal stereotactic techniques employ either stereotactic angiography or magnetic resonance angiography and venography. As previously mentioned, merging frame-based and frameless navigational techniques is likely to improve the margin of safety, particularly in avoiding the middle cerebral vessels. Electrodes are placed through twist drill or burr holes, secured to the bone or scalp, and tunneled through separate stab wound incisions.

Hippocampal depth electrodes can be placed from a coronal approach.[53,54] This technique is used less often as

the electrode traverses the internal capsule en route to the hippocampus. Occasionally, this approach might be useful when targeting another abnormality for depth electrode placement simultaneously (for example, deep cortical developmental malformation or hypothalamic hamartoma). The reader should be advised that false lateralization with depth electrodes to the temporal lobe in the presence of hypothalamic hamartoma has been described.[55]

Frameless Stereotaxy

Frameless stereotaxy is not required for placement of intracranial electrodes but can facilitate the operative time and accuracy of depth electrode placement. Frameless stereotaxy requires a frameless navigation system, an appropriate fixation arm for stabilizing the trajectory of the electrode, and a stylet/cannula system that will allow the depth electrode and its connecting wires to exit from the cannula without being retracted with the cannula system. The frameless system that one employs to place depth electrodes will be specific to the surgeon, the operative hardware available, and the trajectory of depth electrode placement. For example, some surgeons feel comfortable placing temporal depth electrodes into the hippocampus with a freehand technique using the orthogonal approach. Others have reported that they find the commercially available arms created for stereotactic biopsy to be adequate and have success using them to place electrodes in the hippocampus. Others use the IGN Frameless Trajectory Guide (Image-Guided Neurologics, Melbourne, FL). As discussed earlier, the vasculature of the Sylvian fissure and perimesencephalic cisterns must be kept in mind when planning an approach. Image fusion techniques allow the surgeon to visualize the trajectory to ensure that major arteries and veins are avoided. These systems will ultimately improve operative time and allow more facile placement of intracranial depths and grids.[17,48]

The current technology of navigational systems poses several limitations, particularly for the treatment of epilepsy. Most of the articulating arms of frameless systems have only two degrees of freedom; this may be sufficient for tumor biopsy but is less helpful for placing depth electrodes, particularly from the occipital approach, where small changes at the entry point can lead to large changes at the target point given the long trajectory of the electrode. Another limitation of frameless navigation is that it cannot image the path of a strip or depth electrode in real time once it enters the dura because the bony contour of the skull, brain parenchyma, or draining veins may deflect the electrode in unpredictable ways. Therefore, fluoroscopy is still preferable for determining accurate electrode placement in the OR: it is unclear whether stereotactic fluoroscopic systems under development will overcome these limitations. Several companies are working on magnetic guidance systems that will allow intracranial tracking of electrodes. Another limitation of intraoperative navigational systems that specifically relates to epilepsy is the use of fluid attenuated inversion recovery imaging (FLAIR). Many lesions in epilepsy surgery are seen only on FLAIR, which typically uses a 5-mm slice on a 1.5-T magnet. If the slice width is reduced to the maximal tolerance allowed for frameless navigation (2.5 to 3.0 mm), then the FLAIR abnormality may be lost due to signal-to-noise incompatibility.

Although such sequences can be "hand merged" onto the navigational systems, the resultant accuracy may not be useful, particularly around crucial structures such as motor pathways or optic radiations.

I have used a number of the frameless targeting systems that are commercially available. For the longer approach necessary for occipital placement of depth electrodes, a freehand trajectory is not possible. Of the rigid systems, both the IGN Navigus burr hole trajectory guide and the Navigus DBA Tower work well. The Navigus DBA Tower allows the surgeon to visualize the cortex and vessels of the brain slightly better than the burr hole attachment and allows more degrees of freedom of movement, which may justify the additional cost of the DBA Tower over the burr hole cap.

In our institution, we find the most accurate system to be a stereotactic head frame (Leksell) with image guidance provided with the Stealth Frame-Link System (Medtronic Sofamor-Danek, Minneapolis, MN). This allows for fine-tuning of the trajectory tract along the hippocampus, and the probe's eye view of the trajectory is useful to visualize occipital sulci on the initial entry and to avoid the posterior cerebral artery as one approaches the midbrain. Hippocampal depth electrodes, occipital strip electrodes, and interhemispheric strip electrodes can all be accomplished with the patient in the head frame without changing drapes. It is feasible but cumbersome to place frontotemporal strip electrodes through frontal burr holes while in the stereotactic frame. Therefore, once posterior electrode placement is completed, the stereotactic head frame is removed and the patient is repositioned and redraped for placement of additional strip or grid electrodes if indicated.

SPECIAL CONSIDERATIONS: COMPARISON OF STRIP AND DEPTH ELECTRODES

Intrahippocampal depth electrodes are more sensitive than subtemporal strip electrodes in lateralizing ictal onset in TLE, but subdural strip electrodes are often clinically sufficient to determine the lateralization of temporal lobe seizures, particularly when hippocampal atrophy is present.[45,56–58] However, intrahippocampal depth electrodes contradict subdural strip recordings in a small subset of patients, particularly when the subdural strips do not cover the parahippocampal gyrus.[4,59,60] Some authors have noted an increased failure rate in surgery when independent interictal spike or electrographic seizures occur bilaterally in depth electrodes.[3,25,61–63]

At our center, hippocampal depth electrodes are placed in all patients with nonlesional TLE to distinguish between mesial and lateral TLE and to determine interhemispheric propagation time.[24,63] Intracranial electrodes are not routinely placed in patients with hippocampal atrophy unless the presurgical evaluation suggests bitemporal seizures may be a concern. Indications for depth and strip electrode placement in patients with lesional TLE in our center have included dual pathology, failure of localization on scalp ictal EEG, apparent unilateral temporal scalp EEG onset with rapid spread contralaterally, seizures apparently arising independently over either temporal lobe on scalp EEG, contralateral temporal lobe scalp localization in the face of a structural lesion, and rapid bilateral temporal spread in patients with temporal lobe cortical dysplasia.

Rarely, intracranial studies began as strip surveys only, and depth electrodes were placed later in the hospital stay when it became apparent that the subdural strips survey might be inconclusive.

ELECTROENCEPHALOGRAPHIC MONITORING

Electroencephalographic monitoring in the chronic setting with intracranial electrodes is often referred to as chronic electrocorticography. Long-term electrocorticography allows the neurologist to evaluate interictal epileptiform activity, background activity, and ictal onset. Electroencephalographic data from all contacts should be recorded if possible; if not, then a strategy for a sampling from each electrode should be created to decrease the risk of sampling error. Electrocorticography can be analyzed by bipolar or referential montages; for the latter, a reference electrode is affixed to the scalp (parietal vertex, P_z) with collodion. Because of the significant electroencephalographic voltage difference between scalp and direct cortical recordings, the scalp reference is relatively inactive. The intracranial electrodes are then usually read referential to the P_z electrode. Most centers now have at least 64-channel recording capability per patient; however, more channels are frequently used for strip/grid combinations, particularly in nonlesional, extratemporal intracranial surveys.

There is some controversy over the relative accuracy of ictal versus interictal electrographic activity. When recording from a focal cortical dysplasia, distinctive interictal epileptiform patterns have been identified that may provide enough data to guide a resection based on interictal data only. However, interictal spikes are usually more diffuse than the ictal onset zone, and bilateral interictal spikes do not preclude a good surgical outcome. It is usually preferable to obtain ictal recordings to confirm the significance of interictal abnormalities. When monitoring a lesion with intracranial electrodes, seizure outcome is best when both the lesion and the ictal onset zone are completely resected; outcome is compromised when either the lesion or the ictal onset zone is incompletely resected.[21,64] In the case of nonlesional epilepsy, seizure freedom is more difficult to achieve, even in cases in which the ictal onset zone has been well studied with intracranial electrodes.

The number of seizures required to "complete" an intracranial study depends on the specific questions posed in treating a particular patient. In general, the arbitrary number of three of the patient's typical clinical seizures has been considered as a minimum that one should attempt to capture; however, exceptions to this rule abound.[31] For example, a patient with a posterior temporal or parietal lesion with scalp electroencephalographic localization to the anterior temporal lobe might be considered for an intracranial study to confirm the clinical suspicion that seizures are falsely localized to the anterior temporal lobe. In such a case, one or two seizure onsets with high-frequency beta activity directly over the lesion (with concomitant scalp electrodes showing a delayed scalp onset over the temporal lobe) might be sufficient to proceed to surgical resection, particularly if seizures occur infrequently and further monitoring could extend for days or weeks to capture additional seizures. Conversely, a patient with nonlesional epilepsy with bilateral ictal onset in both temporal lobes on preoperative scalp monitoring might require many more than three seizures to exclude bilateral temporal onset and/or establish a predominant side of onset. The number of seizures required may be influenced by the type of ictal onset recorded. Fewer seizures will need to be recorded in the patient with identical ictal onset patterns over the exact same electrode contacts in every seizure than in the patient with multifocal ictal onsets in different electrodes from seizure to seizure. Initial ictal changes at the beginning of a seizure are more important than are late changes and propagation patterns of the seizure. Seizures within seconds to minutes after a previous seizure may be disregarded as being potentially misleading.[31,65]

New computer-assisted prediction paradigms are being created that analyze not only the ictal onset, but changes in background electrical state, interictal spike frequency, confluence analysis, and chaos theory to predict seizure occurrence minutes to hours before ictal onset. It is likely that intracranial monitoring will need to adapt to accommodate these new technologies in the near future.[66–72]

DOCUMENTING THE INTRACRANIAL STUDY

Each intracranial study will be unique to the patient to for whom it is designed. Even "routine" intracranial cases will have subtle variations in electrode placement based on the patient's anatomy. Some sort of documentation of the intracranial study is advisable for a number of reasons, including confirmation of accuracy of placement, communication with the neurophysiology team, and correlation with gyral anatomy and/or intracranial lesions. This section discusses the possible options available for documentation, beginning with the simplest and proceeding to the more complicated.

When placing intracranial strip electrodes, the first, most vital piece of documentation regarding the study begins in the OR. As each electrode is inserted, the operating surgeon describes the identifying characteristics of that electrode (e.g., length, color coding, scalp exit site) and its intracranial position to an assistant, usually an OR nurse, who documents this information directly into the operative record or chart notes so that there is no room for confusion when electrodes are eventually hooked up. Most EEG technicians will appreciate a handwritten line diagram by the surgeon penned into the chart to assist them with the hookup and montage. This simple step can eliminate many potential sources of human error, particularly with extensive intracranial surveys, and facilitates communication between all members of the team. Another simple way to document the operative technique is for the monitoring team to use an anatomic brain diagram (Duvernoy[73] [pp 5 and 29] works well), and transparencies of the grid montage to create a mock-up of the surgery. The image created is compared with fluoroscopic images taken at surgery so that a relatively accurate rendition of the electrode placement is available within minutes on the day of the surgery. These images can be quite helpful in interpreting seizure onset and propagation during electroencephalographic monitoring. In more complicated cases, a member of the monitoring team is present in the OR to take digital photographs of the exposed cortex before and after grid placement. Digital photography identifies the relationship of a grid to the Sylvian fissure and is one of the best methods to document the fine anatomy of the brain, including sulcal and arteriolar anatomy that cannot be seen with advanced imaging techniques. These images are distributed to the hospital record, electrophysiology permanent files, and computer files so that there is redundancy within the system because it can be quite disappointing to return to a case at a later time and find that the data that one saved have been inadvertently erased. The above steps can be performed by all centers with a minimal amount of technology or cost.

More sophisticated imaging techniques exist and are being used with increasing frequency as advanced imaging software becomes more available. MRI can be safely performed in patients with intracranial grids and strip electrodes in place if a few safety considerations are kept in mind. Platinum electrodes are endorsed as being MRI compatible by most electrode manufacturers, although both platinum and stainless steel electrodes have been used without apparent patient injury. Since each center's procedures will differ, it is advisable to check the recommendations of the particular electrode manufacturer before performing MRI. In all cases, current loops can theoretically be created within a magnetic field if the electrode tails are allowed to contact one another. Therefore, all electrode tails should be isolated before MRI. This can be performed using plastic connectors if the patient is imaged before the electroencephalographic monitoring session, or, if performed at the end of monitoring, then ½-inch Steri-Strips work well.

Most MRI workstations or software packages allow for 3-dimensional reconstruction of images, which are often more useful than traditional MRI or computed tomographic images.[51,53,74] In addition, most frameless stereotaxic navigation systems allow for image reconstruction of a magnetic resonance image that can be merged with preoperative anatomic, functional, or angiographic imaging to create an accurate rendition of a grid in relation to the relevant operative anatomy.[17,74] If an operative frameless navigational system is used for image fusion, the epilepsy center should consider creating a system to archive these images independent of both the OR and radiology suite to protect these images for later reference.

CORTICAL MAPPING

Often, in addition to defining the location of the epileptogenic cortex, the surgeon must determine its relationship to functional cortex. This requires mapping the cortex underlying an implanted grid electrode.[36,75] The technique is similar to that performed acutely in the OR and requires a testing protocol appropriate to the cortical region investigated. Cortical stimulation is performed using commercially available constant-current generators so that studies of stimulation or afterdischarge threshold can be performed (afterdischarge potentials are repetitive spike discharges or electrical seizures directly provoked by electrical stimulation). Cortical mapping is performed by selecting two adjacent electrodes (1-cm intervals) rather than between an electrode and a common ground because bipolar stimulation provides more precise control of current flow. Bipolar pulses at 50 Hz are used for language, motor, and sensory mapping. Extraoperative cortical mapping has several advantages over acute intraoperative mapping. Functional mapping may be performed in multiple sessions if necessary, for example, if a seizure is generated during mapping that impairs function, the patient may be allowed to recover for several hours (or days) until proceeding with further mapping. Advanced paradigms may be performed over hours or days, which would not be possible in the acute intraoperative setting. If ictal onset occurs within a region of function, the patient, family, and surgeon will have time to discuss the potential risks/benefits of surgery and make decisions to accept or reject a functional loss that might be associated with surgery.

Stimulation occurs with a neuropsychologist and/or physician testing the patient and an electrophysiologist reviewing the electrocorticogram during stimulation to ensure that any disruption of neurologic function is directly correlated with the stimulation and not a result of focal afterdischarges (with or without spread to adjacent cortex). The amount of current needed to produce an effect varies between patients and between cortical regions. Enough current should be used to produce a reliable effect without causing afterdischarge. Occasionally, pain can result from current spread to the dura or a nearby cortical vessel. In such cases, a particular contact may not be suitable for mapping.

It is often useful for the surgeon to be present for extraoperative intracranial mapping, particularly early in his or her career. There are slight variations of mapping technique and interpretation that have subtle ramifications for the surgeon and that are different from those that a neurologist or neuropsychologist might appreciate. On some occasions, mapped cortical regions will vary from what one would expect from classic anatomic studies. On other occasions, mapping different pairs of electrodes in a specific region, such as motor or language areas, might allow the surgeon to appreciate the orientation of a crucial region relative to the orientation of the grid or adjacent contacts. On other occasions, subtle errors in naming or language may be present extraoperatively when the patient is off antiepileptic drugs that change when the patient resumes taking antiepileptic drugs.[76] Such subtleties of extraoperative mapping can be useful to the surgeon if observed personally before a resection.

Implanted grid arrays are excellent tools to identify the position of sensorimotor cortex through somatosensory evoked potentials. The rationale and technique have been reviewed by Allison and colleagues,[76–79] and clinical experience with subdural grids for this purpose has been discussed by others.[36,75,80–82] Briefly, somatosensory evoked potentials can be used during acute recording in the OR using subdural strip electrodes to identify primary motor cortex. The strip electrode must be positioned to traverse motor and sensory cortex and may need to be repositioned several times during intraoperative recording to optimize the signal. Therefore, when planning to perform somatosensory evoked potentials during extraoperative long-term monitoring, it is helpful to use a subdural grid to optimize the electrode arrays available for optimizing signal over the hand motor cortex. We have been relatively unsuccessful at achieving somatosensory evoked potential of the leg motor cortex using interhemispheric electrodes, despite multiple attempts using the array referred to in Figure 94-3.

Sometimes extraoperative mapping identifies that the ictal onset zone is close to or overlies critical motor or speech areas. On such occasions, it may be helpful to use the advantages of awake operative language mapping at the time of grid removal and resection of the epileptic focus. Although extraoperative mapping has many advantages, its spatial resolution is limited to an accuracy of 1 cm (i.e., the distance between two electrode pairs). Sometimes awake intraoperative mapping will help to confirm which electrode is the contact directly overlying cortical function. This can be particularly important when the two electrodes overlie or span a sulcus; in such cases, awake mapping may allow the surgeon to determine which gyrus is or is not involved in function.[80] In such cases, the epileptic zone may be resected up to the pial margin without disturbing function as long as the vascular structures within the pia are preserved.

COMPLICATIONS

Published series of infection rates from all types of intracranial electrodes range from 0 to 12%. The morbidity of surgery depends on the type of electrode implantation. Intracranial strip electrodes have the lowest morbidity and intracranial grid placement the highest.[14–16,29,30,32,36,45,57,83–90]

The most common cause of morbidity in subdural strip placement is infection. One randomized study by Wyler and colleagues[87,90] found a 0.85% rate of infection between groups treated with antibiotics before surgery compared with a 3% infection rate when no antibiotics were given. There was no difference in infection rate between those patients who received antibiotics for the entire time of strip electrode implantation compared with those who received only a single preoperative dose; therefore, a single dose of antibiotics may be given immediately before strip or grid implantation. Other complications of intracranial strip placement include cortical contusion, cerebral edema, brain abscess, subdural empyema and subdural hemorrhage, placement of electrodes into the brain parenchyma, accidental extraction of electrodes, and superficial wound infection. Many of these complications are minor and cause no long-term problems: permanent neurologic deficit is seen in less than 1% of patients implanted with intracranial strip electrodes.

Complications of grid implantation include infection, transient neurologic deficit, hematoma, cerebral edema with increased intracranial pressure, and infarction. Transient neurologic deficits can occur secondary to edema, hematoma, or mass effect from the grid. In most cases, the grid should be removed immediately in the face of neurologic compromise. Cerebral edema is more likely to occur with an increase in the length of the monitoring session or with a greater number of intracranial electrodes.[29,30] Some authors[91] have been concerned that pediatric patients are more likely to have increased intracranial pressure because there is theoretically less space to accommodate the mass of an intracranial grid, but others have not found this to be clinically evident.[29,50,64,92,93]

Complications from depth electrodes include intraparenchymal hemorrhage, subarachnoid hemorrhage, arterial spasm, and misplacement of the electrode. Permanent neurologic deficit from occipital depth electrodes has been reported at less than 1%.[58,94] The risk of hitting the brain stem or posterior cerebral artery with occipitally inserted depth electrodes may be decreased by (1) targeting tip placement in the lateral amygdala and lateral hippocampus, (2) making sure the occipital burr hole is not too medial, and (3) confirming the trajectory with an image guidance system before placing the electrode. Alternatively, one can attempt to place an occipital depth electrode in the lateral ventricle rather than in the hippocampus. To do so, a rigid guide cannula is placed in the ventricle (verified by identifying CSF flow from the cannula) and then the depth electrode is inserted in the ventricle; the electrode then lies in the temporal horn adjacent to the hippocampus with its tip entering the targeted amygdala. Ictal recording from the ventricle usually conducts signal well, with only occasional failure.[27] The signal obtained will amplify both hippocampal and parahippocampal ictal onsets and intraparenchymal amygdalar onset. The risk of subarachnoid hemorrhage may be minimized if the depth electrodes are placed under direct visualization through a burr hole rather than using a closed twist drill technique so that draining veins are avoided during placement.

COMPLICATION AVOIDANCE

Infection

Every surgeon has his or her own strategies to prevent infection, some based in the art and some based in the science of medicine. The science of wound infection was discussed previously, and this section deals with my preferences for attempting to control infection. On the night before surgery, patients are asked to wash their hair with Betadine several times before coming to the hospital in the morning. The entire head is *not* shaved. The surgical site(s) is shaved closely without using a sharp razor to avoid skin abrasion. A contiguous scalp area is prepared for electrodes to exit via separate stab would incisions; care is taken to place these exit sites superior to scalp incisions to decrease postoperative CSF leakage. The head is then scrubbed with Betadine by the surgeon, and the hair is directed away from the operative sites with Betadine solution and toothed nailbrushes. Then, while the surgeon is at the scrub sink, the circulating nurse performs another standard surgical scrub, so that they entire preoperative scrub time meets or exceeds 10 minutes. Preoperative antibiotics are infused by the time of the skin incision. The operative sites are then draped with iodoform-impregnated adhesive drapes, followed by standard sterile draping. Raney clips are placed on skin edges to decrease contact of the skin with the electrodes and to hold the iodoform-impregnated drapes in place. Electrodes are maintained in their sterile packaging until just before insertion and then placed in antibiotic-containing saline before placement in the head. Exit sites for electrode tails are created using a passing needle designed for that purpose (Ad-Tech Corporation). Care is taken to direct the needle so that it remains within muscle or scalp for as long a tract as possible to create a physical barrier to infection and CSF leakage and directed superiorly to decrease CSF leakage. A staple is placed just proximal to the exit site of the electrode tail (in such a way that the electrode is not impaled) to further decrease CSF leakage. If a purse-string suture is preferred at the exit site, then the

suture bites should be placed parallel to the electrode rather than underneath the buried electrode to avoid injury to the subcutaneous portion of the electrode.

Intracranial grids are treated in a similar manner for insertion. Care is taken to avoid tunneling electrodes across a suture line because this may help reduce exposure to infection. Instead, electrodes are passed through a trocar, as with subdural strips, creating as long a pass through muscle and scalp as possible and directing the electrodes superiorly whenever possible. Removal of the intracranial grid requires a secondary craniotomy later during the same hospital stay. No attempt is made to shampoo the hair on the night before reoperation. Instead, the patient is brought to the OR and local or general anesthesia is administered. Preoperative antibiotics are given so that infusion is completed by the time that the patient enters the OR. The head dressing is removed, usually revealing a suture line with blood encrusted between staples, with a short stubble of hair growing over the exposed scalp. The craniotomy site is scrubbed with nailbrushes and Betadine while the sutures are still in place to remove the majority of this debris, including collodion and stray hair as necessary. The electrode tails are scrubbed at their exit sites and saturated with Betadine. Once this initial cleaning is done, the staples are removed. The wound is then gently rescrubbed by the surgeon to clean the suture line itself; this usually results in a small amount of bleeding. The electrode tails are placed on gentle traction (without displacing the grid) while downward pressure is placed on the scalp with a pair of sterile scissors. Each electrode tail is then cut off at the scalp, and the intracranial portion then retracts several millimeters under the skin edge. The wound is rescrubbed by the circulating nurse so that the total scrub time is in excess of 10 minutes. The drapes must be stapled into place because the regrowth of hair means that adhesive drapes will not adhere to the scalp. An iodoform-impregnated drape is placed over the towels after which the usual craniotomy drapes are put into place. The wound is reopened with a separate table and instruments that are used until the grid is removed and are then retired from the field. As the wound is reopened, all intracranial sutures are removed and Raney clips are used to secure the crani-drape and iodoform drape to the skin edges, again to decrease exposure of the skin edges, which are likely colonized with bacteria. The most distal portions of the electrode tails are identified on the inner surface of the scalp and are cut off, and then these sections of electrode tail are immediately placed in wastebaskets to avoid contamination of the operating table. The wound is irrigated with antibiotic-laced saline. The bone flap is removed, scrubbed with a sterile toothbrush, placed into antibiotic-laced saline, then rescrubbed later in the case, and placed into a fresh solution of antibiotic saline. Any coagulated blood is removed from the epidural space, as is any Gelfoam and dural tack-up sutures. Any additional bone removal needed to optimize operative exposure is performed at this time, and these bone fragments are also scrubbed and soaked. The epidural space is irrigated, and then the dural sutures are removed in such a manner that the grid and its relationship to underlying brain can be visualized. Contacts overlying the ictal onset zone can be documented with digital photography, or, if the region is to be removed, a bipolar forceps can be slipped under the grid to cauterize pertinent landmarks. The grid and any final dural sutures are removed. All operative equipment used to this point is retired from the field, gloves are changed by all personnel, and the definitive procedure continues using the main operating worktable and equipment (the original drapes are not disturbed). This two-stage approach to grid removal may decrease infection and adds little extra time or equipment to the procedure. The intracranial procedure is performed according to the operative plan devised by the comprehensive epilepsy team. On closure, foreign materials are used as needed, including braided non-absorbable suture, duraplasty materials, Surgicel, Gelfoam, and titanium plating systems.

CSF leak while electrodes are in place may be a cause for concern, particular with prolonged intracranial monitoring periods. However, CSF leaks frequently occur without leading to infection, even when sutures are used. CSF leaks can be resistant to the surgeon's attempt to stop them, particularly outside the OR. Placing an additional staple or suture at the bedside to stop a leak will be painful for the patient, is unlikely to be sterile, and is often less than successful. It is more difficult to completely avoid CSF leaks in pediatric patients because the scalp is more fragile and creates less resistance to fluid flow. The best time to control potential CSF leaks is at the time of electrode placement in the OR. The surgeon should consider what degree of CSF leak is acceptable and adapt his or her operative technique to address this concern at the time of initial placement of strip or grid electrodes.

Intracranial Hematoma

Intracranial hematomas are potentially life-threatening risks to all intracranial procedures, including epilepsy surgery. Some techniques may be employed to reduce risk. When placing intracranial strips, focal contusion at the site of entry can lead to neurologic injury. This can occur with any electrode insertion but becomes more likely when multiple passes are made over one area of cortex. A Penfield No. 3 dissector can be used to depress the brain gently away from the burr hole to help initiate the insertion of a strip electrode into the subdural space. Enlargement of the burr hole to allow more working room or placement of two burr holes side by side to form an elliptical craniectomy to facilitate placement of multiple strips is particularly useful if more than three electrodes will be placed through one burr hole. The placement of intracranial electrodes entails most of the risks of a craniotomy, without the exposure to control complications. Bleeding from the middle meningeal artery may be encountered with larger craniectomies over the inferior frontal/superior temporal region. This can be dealt with using standard neurosurgical techniques, including enlarging the bony opening (and skin incision), cauterizing the artery (often not entirely successful in a confined space), placing Gelfoam between the dura and bone, and placing the dura on tension with a tack-up suture that can be draped off of a hemostat, Raney clip, or scalp retractor. Usually, by the end of the procedure, the suture can be removed. If bleeding persists, one may occasionally need to place a more formal dural tack-up suture by making a wire-pass hole in the bone adjacent to the burr hole (absorbable suture is adequate).

When passing any intracranial electrode, whether depth, strip or grid, it is critical that the electrode is never forced when resistance is met. This can be troublesome when attempting to pass electrodes over long distances. The surgeon can decrease the normal friction between the brain and dura using irrigation. To do this, the electrode is placed to a point where resistance is met, a nasal bulb irrigator is placed at the burr hole between the brain and the electrode, and a gentle stream of water is pulsed under the electrode. If this technique "surfs" the electrode further along its path, and then it is safe to continue advancement. However, if resistance is still met, then the electrode may be impinging on a vein and should be removed and redirected. Patient safety must always take precedence over completion of the preoperative plan. Usually, enlargement of the burr hole by 1 to 2 cm will lead to success; however, if an electrode is crucial to the study and cannot be placed via the initial approach, the surgeon can finish that portion of the procedure, close, and reprep and redrape the patient during the same anesthesia for another attempt at electrode placement. Despite one's best intentions, a bridging vein may be injured during strip placement, in which case, blood will begin to ooze from the subdural space. The best recourse is to remove the electrode, pause, and irrigate the brain until the bleeding ceases. No further electrode passes should be made along that trajectory.

Specific techniques can be performed during closure to decrease the risk of hemorrhage. When tunneling electrode tails of all types of electrodes, one should keep in mind that the electrode and the intracranial portion of the electrode can be repositioned (torqued, shifted, advanced, or removed) during manipulation of the tail. If an electrode does move, it may traumatize an adjacent vessel, leading to either hemorrhage or infarction. Therefore, the intracranial portion of the electrode requires attention during tunneling and externalization of the tails. Closure of the dura around an intracranial grid can lead to similar problems. An intracranial grid is a 2-dimensional structure being molded to a 3-dimensional space. The grid, although pliable, is still more rigid than the brain and vessels with which it interacts. The intracranial grid should be securely fastened to the dura with stay sutures to avoid shifting. In addition, the surgeon should anticipate that several millimeters of shift may occur during dural closure as tension is applied to the dura. Therefore, intracranial grids should not be placed close to draining veins or arterial trunks to avoid ischemia or hemorrhage.

With all types of intracranial electrode placement, the presence of the electrode tails will ensure that closure of the dura will not be complete. Any bleeding that occurs anywhere above the dura has real potential to track along the tails into the subdural space. Strict hemostasis of bone (using monopolar cautery to avoid bone wax), dura, temporalis muscle, and scalp, including puncture sites of electrode tail exit sites, should be performed with utmost care as even the "driest" closure will show some accumulation of hematoma at grid removal. Sodium valproate has been shown to cause platelet abnormalities that may interfere with hemostasis.[95] I prefer to wean patients off valproate, if possible, before intracranial strip, depth, or grid placement, particularly because the dura will not be intact after surgery.

Leaving the bone flap in during a grid placement is a judgment call (alternatives include freezing the bone flap or placing it in an abdominal pouch). Some surgeons believe that the added benefit of additional space to avoid increased intracranial pressure, particularly if a dural patch is used, warrants removal of the bone. However, the bone flap provides a solid structure to aid in hemostasis, which is a substantial benefit. I have performed grid implantations with both techniques, freezing the bone and leaving it in the cranium. My personal preference is to leave the bone flap in place, loosely tied to the adjacent calvarium because I find that the accumulation of hematoma is less when the bone flap is in place than when it is removed.

Standardization of postoperative routines can aid in the detection of postoperative hematomas. One comprehensive and thoughtful review on postoperative complications by Hamer and colleagues[29] from the Cleveland Clinic reports that new neurologic deficits referable to epidural hematoma (2.8%) and edema (8%) occurred from 1 to 9 days after grid implantation, with a median duration of 6 days. Therefore, anticipation of delayed neurologic deficits beyond the acute postoperative recovery phase is appropriate. Early normal MRI does not preclude late hemorrhage, as demonstrated in Figure 94-8. This patient was referred to our center for a second opinion regarding the cause of hematoma formation, which occurred after two secondarily generalized seizures. Although generalized seizures do not routinely cause intracranial hemorrhage, it may be that this occurred in this patient or that traction on the grid led to disruption of a draining vein. Nursing protocols that emphasize attention to late deterioration are appropriate. In addition, it is helpful to have in place protocols that prevent the inappropriate dosing of nonsteroidal medications such as ibuprofen or ketorolac by well-meaning novice practitioners and/or the insidious buildup of heparin dosing of which the surgeon is unaware. Antithrombotic sequential compression dressings are used routinely on all intracranial monitoring patients as prophylaxis against deep venous thrombosis.

Increased Intracranial Pressure/ Cerebral Edema

Symptoms of increased intracranial pressure may occur in as many as 12% patients with intracranial grids. Increased intracranial pressure may be a combination of mass effect from the grid itself,[96] accumulation of blood at the craniotomy site, and/or cerebral edema. Cerebral edema can occur in any intracranial electrode study but is more common with grid implantation than with strip electrodes. Symptoms of increased intracranial pressure can occur from 1 to 12 days after surgery and can lead to neurologic deterioration and potential herniation.

Several authors have described an increase in cerebral edema with prolonged monitoring periods. Hamer and colleagues[29] found that bilateral intracranial grid or more than 60 electrode contacts was associated with an increased risk of edema (but no increased risk in pediatric patients). Wiggins and colleagues[30] found an increase in cerebral edema when more than 100 contacts were used. Both studies recommend the use of short-term steroids to decrease the risk of cerebral edema, and this is widely practiced by many epilepsy centers. Many centers avoid placing bilateral intracranial grids, opting instead to perform a lateralizing study with bilateral strip electrodes as a staged procedure before placing an intracranial grid. Sometimes the side of predominant ictal onset is strongly suspected but cannot be confirmed; in such case, a unilateral intracranial grid on the side referable to clinical onset can be placed, whereas bilateral or multifocal seizures can be excluded with several contralateral strip electrodes.

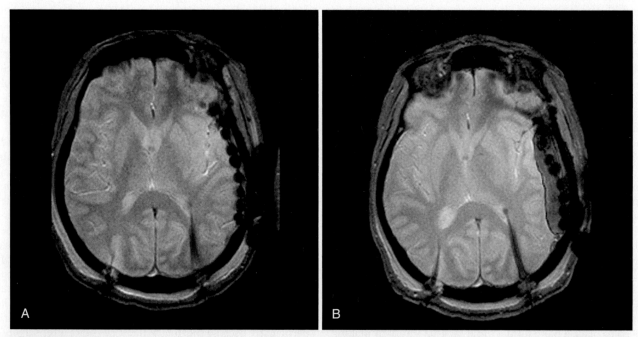

FIGURE 94-8 Delayed occurrence of a subdural hematoma. No hematoma was seen immediately after grid placement (A), but one was present on follow-up magnetic resonance imaging performed 6 days later (B). See text for details. (Courtesy of Brad Davis and Paul Gorsuch, Montana Epilepsy Program, Great Falls, MT.)

This type of approach will decrease the total number of intracranial contacts and may help prevent cerebral edema. In addition, compromise of a vessel by impingement of the grid could contribute to venous congestion or infarct and possibly worsen cerebral edema; therefore, grids should not be allowed to compress or place traction on a bridging vein. The grid can shift during closure of the dura; therefore, a relatively wide berth should be given to major draining veins within the surgical exposure.

The etiology of diffuse cerebral edema with intracranial grid electrodes is unknown but may be an idiosyncratic response to a foreign material. Cerebral edema occurs sporadically, is difficult to predict, and therefore must be anticipated as possible in all patients. It is useful to educate the nursing team to recognize this syndrome so that early intervention can be performed. With early intervention, cerebral edema from intracranial electrodes is completely reversible, unless complicated by infarction.

REFERENCES

1. Abosch A, Bernasconi N, Boling W, et al: Factors predictive of suboptimal seizure control following selective amygdalohippocampectomy. J Neurosurg 97:1142–1151, 2002.
2. Berg AT, Vickrey BG, Langfitt JT, et al: The multicenter study of epilepsy surgery: Recruitment and selection for surgery. Epilepsia 44:1425–1433, 2003.
3. Chung MY, Walczak TS, Lewis DV, et al: Temporal lobectomy and independent bitemporal interictal activity: What degree of lateralization is sufficient? Epilepsia 32:195–201, 1991.
4. Diehl B, Luders HO: Temporal lobe epilepsy: When are invasive recordings needed? Epilepsia 41(Suppl 3):S61–S74, 2000.
5. Dikmen SS, Hermann BP, Wilensky AJ, et al: Validity of the Minnesota Multiphasic Personality Inventory (MMPI) to psychopathology in patients with epilepsy. J Nerv Ment Dis 171:114–122, 1983.
6. Henry TR, Van Heertum RL: Positron emission tomography and single photon emission computed tomography in epilepsy care. Semin Nucl Med 33:88–104, 2003.
7. Lantz G, Grave de Peralta Menendez R, Gonzalez Andino S, et al: Noninvasive localization of electromagnetic epileptic activity. II. Demonstration of sublobar accuracy in patients with simultaneous surface and depth recordings. Brain Topogr 14:139–147, 2001.
8. Salanova V, Markand O, Worth R: Focal functional deficits in temporal lobe epilepsy on PET scans and the intracarotid amobarbital procedure: Comparison of patients with unitemporal epilepsy with those requiring intracranial recordings. Epilepsia 42:198–203, 2001.
9. Siegel AM, Jobst BC, Thadani VM, et al: Medically intractable, localization-related epilepsy with normal MRI: Presurgical evaluation and surgical outcome in 43 patients. Epilepsia 42:883–888, 2001.
10. So EL: Integration of EEG, MRI, and SPECT in localizing the seizure focus for epilepsy surgery. Epilepsia 41(Suppl 3):S48–S54, 2000.
11. Wilkus RJ, Thompson PM, Vossler DG: Bizarre ictal automatisms: Frontal lobe epileptic or psychogenic seizures? J Epilepsy 3:207–213, 1990.
12. Spencer SS: Neural networks in human epilepsy: Evidence of and implications for treatment. Epilepsia 43:219–227, 2002.
13. Spencer SS: Substrates of localization-related epilepsies: Biologic implications of localizing findings in humans. Epilepsia 39:114–123, 1998.
14. Wyler AR, Ojemann GA, Lettich E, et al: Subdural strip electrodes for localizing epileptogenic foci. J Neurosurg 60:1195–1200, 1984.
15. Dubeau F, McLachlan RS: Invasive electrographic recording techniques in temporal lobe epilepsy. Can J Neurol Sci 27(Suppl 1):S29–S34, 2000.
16. Rosenbaum TJ, Laxer KD, Vessely M, et al: Subdural electrodes for seizure focus localization. Neurosurgery 19:73–81, 1986.
17. Vives KP, Lee S, McCarthy K, et al: Intracranial monitoring. In Winn HR (ed): Youmans Neurological Surgery, 5th ed. Philadelphia: WB Saunders, 2004, pp 2551–2563.
18. Goldring S, Gergorie EM: Surgical management of epilepsy using epidural electrodes to localize the seizure focus: Review of 100 cases. J Neurosurg 60:457–466, 1984.
19. Kuzniecky RI, Faught E, Morawetz RB: Electroencephalographic correlations of extracranial and epidural electrodes in temporal lobe epilepsy. Epilepsia 32:335–340, 1991.
20. Wiebe S: A randomized, controlled trial of surgery for temporal-lobe epilepsy. N Engl J Med 345:311–318, 2001.
21. Awad IA, Rosenfeld J, Ahl J, et al: Intractable epilepsy and structural lesions of the brain: Mapping, resection strategies, and seizure outcome. Epilepsia 32:179–186, 1991.
22. Lieb JP, Dasheiff RM, Engel J: Role of the frontal lobes in the propagation of mesial temporal lobe seizures. Epilepsia 32:822–837, 1991.
23. Roberts DW, Jobst BC, Siegel AM, et al: Investigation of extra-temporal epilepsy. Stereotact Funct Neurosurg 77:216–218, 2001.
24. Weinand ME, Wyler AR, Richey ET, et al: Long-term ictal monitoring with subdural strip electrodes: Prognostic factors for selecting temporal lobectomy candidates. J Neurosurg 77:20–28, 1992.
25. Smith JR, Lee MR, Jenkins PD, et al: A 13-year experience with epilepsy surgery. Stereotact Funct Neurosurgery 73:98–103, 1999.
26. Cohen-Gadol AA, Spencer DD: Use of an anteromedial subdural strip electrode in the evaluation of medial temporal lobe epilepsy: Technical note. J Neurosurg 99:921–923, 2003.
27. Vossler DG, Kraemer DLA, Haltiner AM, et al: Intracranial EEG in temporal lobe epilepsy: Location of seizure onset relates to degree of hippocampal pathology. Epilepsia 45:497–503, 2004.
28. Chassagnon S, Minotti L, Kremer S, et al: Restricted frontomesial epileptogenic focus generating dyskinetic behavior and laughter. Epilepsia 44:859–863, 2003.
29. Hamer HM, Morris HH, Mascha MS, et al: Complications of invasive video-EEG monitoring with subdural grid electrodes. Neurology 58:97–103, 2002.
30. Wiggins GC, Elisevich K, Smith BJ: Morbidity and infection in combined subdural grid and strip electrode investigation for intractable epilepsy. Epilepsy Res 37:73–80, 1999.
31. Appendix II, Presurgical evaluation protocols: In Engel J Jr (ed): Surgical Treatment of the Epilepsies. New York: Raven Press, 1993, pp 707–754.
32. Ross DA, Brunberg JA, Drury I, et al: Intracerebral depth electrode monitoring in partial epilepsy: The morbidity and efficacy of placement using magnetic resonance image-guided stereotactic surgery. Neurosurgery 39:327–334, 1996.
33. Wieser HG, Bancaud J, Talairach J, et al: Comparative value of spontaneous and chemically and electrically induced seizures in establishing the lateralization of temporal lobe seizures. Epilepsia 20:47–59, 1979.
34. Alarcon G, Kissani N, Dad M, et al: Lateralizing and localizing values of ictal onset recorded on the scalp: Evidence from simultaneous recordings with intracranial foramen ovale electrodes. Epilepsia 42:1426–1437, 2001.
35. Kissani N, Alarcon G, Dad M, et al: Sensitivity of recordings at sphenoidal electrode site for detecting seizure onset: Evidence from scalp, superficial and deep foramen ovale recordings. Clin Neurophysiol 112:232–240, 2001.
36. Luders HO, Hahn JF, Lesser RP, et al: Basal temporal subdural electrodes in the evaluation of patients with intractable epilepsy. Epilepsia 30:131–143, 1989.
37. Kraemer DL: Reoperation for failed epilepsy surgery. In Wyler AR (ed): Techniques in Neurosurgery. New York: Raven Press, 1995, pp 58–62.
38. Salanova V, Wuesney LF, Rasmussen T, et al: Reevaluation of surgical failures and the role of reoperation in 39 patients with frontal lobe epilepsy. Epilepsia 35:70–80, 1994.
39. Schwartz TH, Spencer DD: Strategies for reoperation after comprehensive epilepsy surgery. J Neurosurg 95:615–623, 2001.
40. Siegel AM, Roberts DW, Thadani VM, et al: The role of intracranial electrode reevaluation in epilepsy patients after failed initial invasive monitoring. Epilepsia 41:571–580, 2000.
41. Devinsky O, Romanelli P, Orbach D, et al: Surgical treatment of multifocal epilepsy involving eloquent cortex. Epilepsia 44:718–723, 2003.
42. Lee SK, Kim KK, Nam H, et al: Adding or repositioning intracranial electrodes during presurgical assessment of neocortical epilepsy: Electrographic seizure pattern and surgical outcome. J Neurosurg 100:363–471, 2004.
43. Silverberg A, Doyle WK: Complications and outcomes in 1428 surgical procedures for epilepsy: A comprehensive review of contemporary epilepsy surgery from one epilepsy center. Epilepsia 44(Suppl 9):121(Abst.1.348), 2003.
44. McCarthy G, Spencer DD, Riker RJ: The stereotaxic placement of depth electrodes. In Luders H (ed): Epilepsy Surgery. New York: Raven Press, 1991, pp 385–393.
45. Spencer SS, Spencer DD, Williamson PD, et al: Combined depth and subdural electrode investigation in uncontrolled epilepsy. Neurology 40:74–79, 1990.

46. Blatt DR, Roper SN, Friedman WA: Invasive monitoring of limbic epilepsy using stereotactic depth and subdural strip electrodes: Surgical technique. Surg Neurol 48:74–79, 1997.

47. Levesque MF, Wilson CL, Behnke, EJ, et al: Accuracy of MR-guided stereotactic electrode implantation: 1. Preimplantation correlation with the Talairach system. Stereotact Funct Neurosurg 54/55:51–55, 1990.

48. Murphy MA, Morris KF, Cook MJ: Insertion of depth electrodes with or without subdural guidance using frameless stereotactic guidance system—technique and outcome. Br J Neurosurg 16:119–125, 2002.

49. Pillay PK, Barnett G, Awad I: MRI-guided stereotactic placement of depth electrodes in temporal lobe epilepsy. Br J Neurosurg 6:47–54, 1992.

50. Zaccariotti VA, Pannek HW, Holthausen H, et al: Evaluation with subdural plates in children and adolescents. Neurol Res 21:463–474, 1999.

51. Kamiryo T, Jackson T, Laws E Jr: A methodology designed to increase accuracy and safety in stereotactic brain surgery. Minim Invasive Neurosurg 43:1–3, 2000.

52. Levesque MF, Zhang JX, Wilson CL: Stereotactic investigation of limbic epilepsy using a multimodal image analysis system: Technical note. J Neurosurg 73:792–797, 1990.

53. Noordmans HJ, van Rijen PC, van Veelen CW, et al: Localization of implanted EEG electrodes in a virtual-reality environment. Comput Aided Surg 6:241–258, 2001.

54. Ray CD: A new multipurpose human brain depth probe. J Neurosurg 24:911–921, 1966.

55. Cascino GD, Andermann F, Berkovic SF, et al: Gelastic seizures and hypothalamic hamartomas: Evaluation of patients undergoing chronic intracranial EEG monitoring and outcome of surgical treatment. Neurology 43:747–750, 1993.

56. Sperling MR, O'Connor MJ: Comparison of depth and subdural electrodes in recording temporal lobe seizures. Neurology 39:1497–1504, 1989.

57. Barry E, Wolf AL, Huhn S, et al: Simultaneous subdural grid and depth electrodes in patients with refractory complex partial seizures. J Epilepsy 5:111–118, 1992.

58. Spencer SS: Depth versus subdural electrode studies for unlocalized epilepsy. J Epilepsy 2:123–127, 1989.

59. Alsaadi TM, Laxer KD, Barbaro NM, et al: False lateralization by subdural electrodes in two patients with temporal lobe epilepsy. Neurology 57:532–534, 2001.

60. Eisenschenk S, Gilmore RL, Cibula JE, et al: Lateralization of temporal lobe foci: Depth versus subdural electrodes. Clin Neurophysiol 112:836–844, 2001.

61. So NK, Olivier A, Andermann F, et al: Results of surgical treatment in patients with bitemporal epileptiform abnormalities. Ann Neurol 25:432–439, 1989.

62. So NK: Depth electrode studies in mesial temporal epilepsy. In Luders H (ed): Epilepsy Surgery. New York: Raven Press, 1991, pp 371–884.

63. Spencer SS, Williamson PD, Spencer DD, Mattson RH: Human hippocampal seizure spread studied by depth and subdural recording: The hippocampal commissure. Epilepsia 28:479–489, 1987.

64. Wyllie E, Luders HO, Morris HH, et al: Subdural electrodes in the evaluation for epilepsy surgery in children and adults. Neuropediatrics 19:80–86, 1988.

65. Schiller Y, Cascino GD, Busaker NE, et al: Characterization and comparison of local onset and remote propagated electrographic seizures recorded with intracranial electrodes. Epilepsia 39:380–388, 1998.

66. Asano E, Muzik O, Shah A, et al: Quantitative interictal subdural EEG analyses in children with neocortical epilepsy. Epilepsia 44:425–434, 2003.

67. Battiston JJ, Darcey TM, Siegel AM, et al: Statistical mapping of scalp-recorded ictal EEG records using wavelet analysis. Epilepsia 44:664–672, 2003.

68. D'Alessandro M, Esteller R, Vachtsevanos G, Schiff SJ: Epileptic seizure prediction using hybrid feature selection over intracranial EEG electrode contacts: A report of four patients. IEEE Trans Biomed Eng 50:603–615, 2003.

69. Iasemidis LD, Shiau D, Chaovalitwongse W, et al: Adaptive epileptic seizure prediction system. IEEE Trans Biomed Eng 50:616–627, 2003.

70. Litt B, Esteller R, Echauz J, et al: Epileptic seizures may begin hours in advance of clinical onset: A report of five patients. Neuron 30:51–64, 2001.

71. Richardson KA, Cluckman BJ, Weinstein SL, et al: In vivo modulation of hippocampal epileptiform activity with radial electric fields. Epilepsia 44:768–777, 2003.

72. Zaveri HP, Duckrow RB, de Lanerolle NC, et al: Distinguishing subtypes of temporal lobe epilepsy with background hippocampal activity. Epilepsia 42:725–730, 2001.

73. Duvernoy HM: The Human Brain. Wien: Springer-Verlag, 1991, pp 5, 29.

74. Murphy MA, O'Brien TJ, Morris K, et al: Multimodality image-guided surgery for the treatment of medically refractory epilepsy. J Neurosurg 100:452–462, 2004.

75. Lee BI, Luders HO, Lesser RP, et al: Cortical potentials related to voluntary and passive finger movements recorded from subdural electrodes in humans. Ann Neurol 20:32–37, 1986.

76. Laban O, Barr W, Doyle W, et al: False positive localization of language sites during electrical mapping near epileptic foci. Epilepsia 44(Suppl 9):146 (Abst.1.422), 2003.

77. Allison T, McCarthy G, Wood CC, et al: Human cortical potentials evoked by stimulation of the median nerve. I: Cytoarchitectonic areas generating short-latency activity. J Neurophysiol 62:694–710, 1989.

78. McCarthy G, Allison T, Spencer DD: Localization of the face area of human sensorimotor cortex by intracranial recording of somatosensory evoked potentials. J Neurosurg 79:874–884, 1993.

79. Wood CC, Spencer DD, Allison T, et al: Localization of human sensorimotor cortex during surgery by cortical surface recording of somatosensory evoked potentials. J Neurosurg 68:99–111, 1988.

80. Cohen-Gadol AA, Britton JW, Collignon FP, et al: Nonlesional central lobule seizures; use of awake cortical mapping and subdural grid monitoring for resection of seizure focus. J Neurosurg 98:1255–1262, 2003.

81. Lesser RP, Luders HO, Klem G, et al: Extraoperative cortical functional localization in patients with epilepsy. J Clin Neurophysiol 4:27–53, 1987.

82. Lim SH, Dinner DS, Pillay PK, et al: Functional anatomy of the human supplementary sensorimotor area: Results of extraoperative electrical stimulation. Electroencephalogr Clin Neurophysiol 91:179–193, 1994.

83. Rydenhag B, Silander HC: Complications of epilepsy surgery after 654 procedures in Sweden, September 1990–1995: A multicenter study based on the Swedish National Epilepsy Surgery Register. Neurosurgery 49:1–57, 2001.

84. Behrens E, Schramm J, Zentner J, et al: Surgical and neurological complications in a series of 708 epilepsy surgery procedures. Neurosurgery 41:1–10, 1997.

85. Espinosa J, Olivier A, Andermann F, et al: Morbidity of chronic recording with intracranial depth electrodes in 170 patients. Stereotact Funct Neurosurg 63:63–65, 1994.

86. Fernandez G, Hufnagel A, Van Roost D, et al: Safety of intrahippocampal depth electrodes for presurgical evaluation of patients with intractable epilepsy. Epilepsia 38:922–929, 1997.

87. Fullagar T, Wyler AR: Morbidity of long-term seizure monitoring using subdural strip electrodes: A follow-up. J Epilepsy 6:95–97, 1993.

88. Kramer U, Riviello JJ, Carmant L, et al: Morbidity of depth and subdural electrodes: Children and adolescents versus young adults. J Epilepsy 7:7–10, 1994.

89. Swartz BE, Rich JR, Dwan PS, et al: The safety and efficacy of chronically implanted subdural electrodes: A prospective study. Surg Neurol 46:87–93, 1996.

90. Wyler AR, Walker G, Somes GW: The morbidity of long-term seizure monitoring using subdural strip electrodes. J Neurosurg 74:734–737, 1991.

91. Wyler AR: Diagnostic techniques in surgical management of epilepsy: Strip electrodes, grids, and depth electrodes. In Schmidek HH (ed): Schmidek and Sweet Operative Neurosurgical Techniques. Philadelphia: Elsevier, 2000, pp 1429–1435.

92. Adelson PD, Black PM, Madsen JR, et al: Use of subdural grids and strip electrodes to identify a seizure focus in children. Pediatr Neurosurg 22:174–180, 1995.

93. Onal C, Otsubo H, Araki T, et al: Complications of invasive subdural grid monitoring in children with epilepsy. J Neurosurg 98:1017–1026, 2003.

94. Van Roost D, Solymosi L, Schramm J, et al: Depth electrode implantation in the length axis of the hippocampus for the presurgical evaluation of medial temporal lobe epilepsy: A computed tomography-based stereotactic insertion technique and its accuracy. Neurosurgery 43:819–827, 1998.

95. Zeller JA, Schlesinger S, Runge U, Kessler C: Influence of valproate monotherapy on platelet activation and hematologic values. Epilepsia 40:186–680, 1999.

96. Studholme C, Novotny E, Zubal IG, et al: Estimating tissue deformation between functional images induced by intracranial electrode implantation using anatomical MRI. Neuroimage 13:561–576, 2001.

95

Treatment of Intractable Epilepsy by Electrical Stimulation of the Vagus Nerve

JOSEPH R. MADSEN and AXEL ROMINGER

Epilepsy is estimated to affect approximately 50 million people worldwide,[1] with a higher incidence in children, estimated at 100 to 200 per 100,000 children per year, compared with 24 to 53 per 100,000 in adults.[2] While the overall prognosis of epilepsy is good, approximately 30% of patients do not respond adequately to antiepileptic drugs or ketogenic diet and suffer from medically intractable seizures.[2] More than half of these patients are not good candidates or are not controlled by resective surgery, subpial transection, or corpus callosotomy. The effect on health and quality of life, as well as impact on society, is enormous, so the establishment of a new surgical strategy for control of seizures is of significant interest to neurosurgeons. Vagus nerve stimulation (VNS) in the neck, approved since July 1997 by the Food and Drug Administration (FDA) and in much of the European community since 1994, has now been used to treat more than 20,000 patients in at least 26 countries.

Currently, the vagal nerve stimulator is indicated for treatment of partial seizures in patients aged 12 years and older. Many patients with generalized seizures and children younger than 12 years have also been treated "off label."

In the late 1930s, animal studies demonstrated that electrical stimulation of the vagus nerve altered electroencephalographic (EEG) activity. Over the next few decades, animal investigations verified the changes in the EEG and documented anticonvulsant activity. Human clinical trials were begun in the late 1980s, with the outcomes showing significant effects on seizure reduction and minimal side effects.

A brief history of VNS follows, with discussion of possible mechanisms of action, current uses, efficacy, and safety profile, as well as surgical technique.

BACKGROUND

The vagus nerve, the tenth cranial nerve, is composed of approximately 80% afferent visceral fibers[3] transmitting visceral sensory information from receptors in the heart, aorta, lungs, and gastrointestinal system to the central nervous system (CNS). Accordingly, it is not surprising that VNS can affect CNS activity. A small number of fibers pass directly to the spinal trigeminal nucleus and the reticular formation, but most vagal afferents originate from nodose ganglion neurons with projections primarily to the nucleus of the solitary tract, which has widespread projections to the cerebral cortex, basal forebrain, hypothalamus, dorsal raphe, and cerebellum,[4] and important areas for epileptogenesis such as amygdala, hippocampus, and thalamus.

There is also a direct pathway with viscerotopic representation to the insular cortex via the parabrachial nucleus in the pons.[5] This is probably the pathway that relays sensation from vagal stimulation to conscious perception.

Other axons from the parabrachial nucleus go to the thalamic intralaminar and midline nuclei, which have extensive and diffuse projections throughout the cerebral cortex. This pathway may represent the point at which vagal stimulation interacts with pathways traditionally believed to control cortical synchronization and desynchronization.

The parasympathetic nucleus lies beneath the floor of the fourth ventricle and receives afferent input from the hypothalamus and glossopharyngeal nerve (carotid sinus). The efferent output supplies involuntary muscles of the bronchi, esophagus, stomach, small intestine, part of the large intestine to the distal third of the transverse colon, and heart.

The motor nucleus of the vagus nerve is formed by the nucleus ambiguus in the reticular formation of the medulla and receives input from both cerebral hemispheres. This nucleus supplies the constrictor muscles of the pharynx and the intrinsic muscles of the larynx.

In addition to the anatomic studies of the vagus nerve showing the vast number of cortical projections, animal studies have demonstrated effects on the EEG with stimulation. Electrical stimulation of the vagus nerve in cats was first shown to cause EEG changes in 1938 by Bailey and Bremer.[6] Further studies have shown that, depending on the stimulation intensity and frequency, the cortical EEG can be synchronized or desynchronized.[7] Low frequency (1 to 16 Hz) and very high intensity synchronize (increase slow waves), and higher intensity and faster frequencies (greater than 70 Hz) desynchronize (arousal, rapid eye movement), as do high intensity and slower frequency (20 to 50 Hz).[8–10] This suggests that different afferent fibers are stimulated under different circumstances, affecting different pathways and connections, with ultimately differing effects on the cortical EEG.

ANIMAL STUDIES

Based on studies showing that the vagus nerve has a wide "connectivity" to the CNS,[11,12] various animal models have been used to investigate the effect of VNS on epilepsy.

Some of the early studies in cats, dogs, rats, and monkeys showed reduction or prevention of seizures using a variety of chemically induced seizures. Study of the stimulation parameters required showed maximal anticonvulsant effect with C-fiber stimulation.[13–16]

In addition, McLachlan[17] demonstrated reduction or abolition of interictal spike activity in an acute epilepsy model using rats. Secondarily generalized seizures were also reduced in duration, but only if VNS occurred within 3 seconds of the start of the seizure. After 3 seconds, VNS had no effect on duration. This was also borne out in studies by Woodbury and Woodbury,[14,15] who showed that the longer the delay in stimulating the vagal nerve, the longer the duration of a seizure. In the same study, it was also shown that the effect on interictal spiking was seen 1 to 2 seconds after the onset of VNS and could persist for 1 to 3 minutes beyond stimulation; therefore, the anticonvulsant effect appeared to outlast the stimulation. Koo[18] showed that during stimulation at the frequency of 20 to 30 Hz, there is synchronization of the epileptiform activity during the time when the stimulus is on, and suggested that there may be desynchronization of EEG results during the time when the stimulator is off. This may contribute to the mechanism of intermittent stimulation of the VNS as opposed to continuous stimulation.

Other parameters for optimal stimulation were assessed and shown in animal studies to be a stimulation of 10 to 20 Hz with a pulse width of 0.5 to 1 msec.[14,15,19] In practice, human stimulation is usually started with a pulse width of 0.25 msec (250 μsec).

HUMAN STUDIES AND EFFICACY

The first human implantation was in 1988, with FDA approval following five clinical studies, enrolling about 500 patients. These studies looked at efficacy, safety, stimulation frequency, and tolerability of VNS as an adjunctive treatment in refractory partial seizures in adults.

The data show that patients treated with high stimulation rates (5 minutes or less of "off time") had a mean decrease in seizure frequency of almost 30% versus a mean decrease of 15% in the low-stimulation-rate group (180 minutes off, used as an "active control"). Results also show that the responder rate of at least a 50% reduction in seizure numbers was 30% in the group with the high stimulation rate. The responder rate in the low-stimulation-rate group was 13%, which suggests that VNS works at both rates but the higher stimulation rates are optimal. The use of such "active control" strategies has been critical in minimizing potential placebo effects when interpreting the results of this modality.[20,21]

Long-term results from the first four studies reported a 95% continuation beyond the first year of implantation, with 82% and 69% beyond 2 and 3 years, respectively. Reduction in seizure frequency remained the same or improved over time, with pooled results showing a 40% reduction in seizures at 36 months. Thus it appears that the effects of VNS are cumulative without increased adverse effects.

There have been a few small studies suggesting that rapid-cycle (7 to 14 seconds on, 30 seconds off) stimulation may be effective in the patient who has not responded to slower cycling rates. This has shown some added efficacy in patients with Lennox-Gastaut syndrome and tuberous sclerosis.[22–24]

A few studies have included children also.[25,26] The numbers are small, but most children had a more than 50% reduction in seizure frequency and a significant number had more than 90% reduction.

A small number of patients with generalized seizures have been studied. These studies suggest that these patients may respond better, with a higher responder rate to VNS than patients with partial seizures. Of the 25 patients with generalized seizure, 11 had a more than 50% seizure reduction.

Since FDA approval of the stimulator device in 1997, over 250 children, adolescents, and young adults have received implants and have been studied at our institution. The age ranged from 3 to 33 years, and most had refractory mixed seizures and generalized seizures, with a few with partial-onset seizures. The children with generalized seizures have shown a greater than 50% reduction on seizure number in more than 50% of the group. The children with partial seizures have shown a 30% to 40% reduction in number in approximately one third of the group. In addition to reduction in seizure number, seizure severity and the postictal period are dramatically decreased in a large number of patients. Finally, the level of alertness and interaction improves significantly in many of these children according to parents' impressions.

MECHANISMS OF ACTION

Chronic VNS induces many physiologic changes in the brain. Naritoku and colleagues[27] have reported increases in neuronal *fos* expression with VNS. The increased activity was seen in areas of the medulla, hypothalamus, thalamus, amygdala, and cingulate with connectivity to the vagus nerve. The increased *fos* activity suggests increased neuronal activity.

Positron emission tomography scanning has also shown activation of CNS structures with VNS. Regional blood flow changes showing increases in the ipsilateral anterior thalamus and cingulate gyrus were reported by Garnett and co-workers,[28] and in another study, Ko and associates[29] found increased blood flow in the ipsilateral putamen and cerebellum with contralateral increases in the thalamus and temporal lobe.

In addition to reports of increased blood flow, concentrations of inhibitory neurotransmitters and amino acids have been shown to increase. Ben-Menachem and co-workers[30] reported increases in cerebrospinal fluid levels of total γ-aminobutyric acid and ethanolamine concentrations in chronic VNS.

PATIENT SELECTION

Selection criteria for VNS are broad and continue to evolve. Selected patients should have medically refractory epilepsy. VNS is not a first-line treatment for epilepsy and is thus reserved for patients who have already tried multiple treatments. In addition, a potentially curative surgical resection should be considered preferable to VNS, when possible. It is highly desirable that all patients undergoing consideration for vagal nerve surgery be evaluated by epileptologists and surgeons well versed in other surgical options. For many patients, stimulator implantation may be preferable to extratemporal surgery in an eloquent area, corpus callosotomy, or repeat craniotomy for those who have failed surgery before. The use of the stimulator in cases where a more risky surgical approach or a less effective procedure is the only option gives an alternative treatment option with low morbidity. The last inclusion criterion is that the patient's body size allow implantation of the device.

Seizure type is not an inclusion criterion. Studies have shown that the efficacy of VNS in generalized seizures and Lennox-Gastaut syndrome is comparable with that in partial seizures.[22,31] A clear definition of the best patients for use of this therapy is unknown. Initial studies focused primarily on patients with intractable partial epilepsy. Approximately 20% of the patients studied in this group had a 50% or greater reduction in the number of seizures, with another 50% of the patients having a significant decrease in seizure frequency of at least 20%. Many patients also reported a decrease in seizure intensity, which is more difficult to quantify.

Patients who have previously undergone left cervical or bilateral vagotomies are excluded. In addition, patients who have significant preexisting upper airway/pharyngeal, pulmonary, cardiac, or gastrointestinal problems, presence of a dysautonomia, history of vasovagal syncope, or concurrent brain stimulator should be approached with caution and may need more frequent follow-ups.

Once the patient has received the implant, the stimulator is activated at any time from surgery to 2 weeks postsurgery. There have been no adverse effects when activating the device on the day of surgery. At our institution, the device is routinely activated by the surgeon at the time of implantation with initial settings as follows: 0.25 mA output, 20 Hz, pulse width of 250 msec, on time of 30 seconds, and off time of 5 minutes. These minimal settings allow the patient to acclimate to the stimulation. Follow-up for reprogramming can then take place as frequently as once a week to once every few months.

The current stimulator device gives options for telemetrically changing the current intensity in milliamps, pulse width, length of time for stimulus train, and off time or time between stimulus trains. Reprogramming the stimulus output is usually the first parameter to adjust, and it can be increased in increments based on the patient's tolerance. Other parameters that are adjusted are stimulus on and off times, which can be shortened or lengthened. Changing the on time to as little as 7 seconds and the off time to as little as 30 seconds has been shown to improve seizure control in patients with Lennox-Gastaut syndrome who have shown no improvement with the usual settings.[22]

Follow-up examinations serve not only as an opportunity to reprogram and interrogate the device, but to begin adjustment of medications. Tapering of medications usually begins within a reasonable period after improved seizure control is observed. If improvement in seizure control is not seen, continued reprogramming and medication adjustment can be done.

ADVERSE EFFECTS

The most common adverse effects are intermittent voice alteration with the "on" period of stimulation. This has been described as a hoarseness or vibration of the voice, with the severity depending on the intensity of stimulation. Other, less common adverse effects that have been described by patients are pharyngeal paresthesias, coughing, increased drooling, and sensation of shortness of breath, all of which tend to improve or resolve shortly after activation

or increase in intensity during reprogramming. Very debilitated patients with little subcutaneous fat have a risk of skin breakdown over the device, and this should be considered a relative contraindication. The manufacturer supplies information suggesting that peptic ulcer disease and a history of certain cardiac problems should also be considered relative contraindications, although stimulation of the vagus nerve itself has not been reported to have an autonomic effect on heart rate or acid secretion in the stomach. This lack of side effects presumably relates to a lower threshold for stimulation of the afferent as opposed to the efferent neurons coursing through the vagus nerve.

SURGICAL TECHNIQUE

Implantation of the device is a fairly straightforward procedure and can be done in patients of all ages, including young children. The vagus nerve in the neck is located in the carotid sheath, usually between the carotid artery and the jugular vein. The nerve is usually invested in the tissue of the carotid sheath between the carotid and jugular vein, but it can be located anterior, lateral, or posterior to the carotid artery and is sometimes more intimately associated with the jugular vein than the artery. There are usually no macroscopic branches of the nerve in the lower cervical regions below the carotid bifurcation region where the exposure is made, which is important because placement of the coil electrodes around the nerve requires circumferential dissection of the nerve, and it is crucial not to devascularize or damage any branches of the vagus.

In animal experiments, the right vagus nerve tends to innervate the cardiac centers responsible for bradycardia to a significantly greater extent than the left. For this reason, the left vagus nerve is traditionally selected to be the side for stimulation, unless there is some significant anatomic contraindication such as a prior dissection in the region.

The patient is positioned supine with the neck in slight extension and with the head turned slightly to the right. If the neck is turned too severely, greater retraction is required on the sternocleidomastoid muscle to allow for the dissection, and a moderate degree of rotation gives the best exposure to a suitable length of the nerve.

For an anterior axillary incision, the arm is positioned with slight abduction to allow access to the anterior axillary fold, but without having the arm so far away from the body that it is difficult for the surgeon to stand near the patient. A rolled towel beneath the patient's scapulas allows the left arm to fall backward slightly, giving good access to the border of the pectoralis muscle. The surgeon stands on the left side of the patient with the assistant either across the table or just to the surgeon's right.

Two skin incisions are made (Fig. 95-1). The cervical incision is made in the direction of a skin crease centered over the anterior edge of the sternocleidomastoid muscle approximately two thirds of the way down from the angle of the jaw to the clavicle. It is helpful to keep the exposure low enough to be well below the carotid bifurcation to ensure the most straightforward dissection of the nerve. Adequate exposure of the nerve can be obtained through an incision 2.0 to 2.5 cm long in a thin patient, but in the presence of a thick neck or prior surgery a longer incision should be made. We prefer to divide the platysma in the direction of its fibers along the anterior border of the sternocleidomastoid

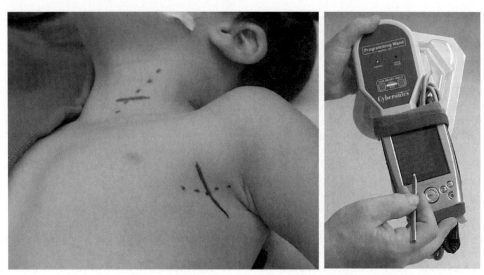

FIGURE 95-1 Positioning and incision location for vagal nerve stimulator placement. The neck is extended with the head turned slightly to the right for exposure of the left vagal nerve low in the neck. A short incision (2 to 3 cm long) is located at the anterior border of the sternocleidomastoid in the transverse direction of a skin crease. The left arm is abducted and extended so that the anterior axillary region can be well prepared. A 4-cm incision lateral and inferior to the pectoralis muscle allows the insertion of the pulse generator. Making this incision in the direction of natural skin creases also improves cosmesis. During induction of anesthesia and positioning, a hand-held programmer can be used to program the stimulator (*right*).

muscle, then follow this anterior border in the avascular plane down to the carotid sheath. A Cloward retractor, usually with the shortest blunt blades, gives excellent exposure of the carotid sheath, and the vagus nerve is identified within the sheath.

It is important to pay attention to the thickness and nature of the carotid sheath fascia while opening it on either side of the nerve, because this fascia is used for placing anchoring sutures to hold in the electrodes after they are placed on the vagus nerve. The nerve needs to be dissected clear of the sheath for a distance of approximately 3 cm, and this is facilitated by passing a plastic vessel loop around it and using it to elevate the nerve while using sharp dissection to open the sheath of either side of the nerve to free it up (Fig. 95-2). Blunt dissection is then used to open up space within the carotid sheath inferiorly for another 2 cm, because this will be used for a relaxing loop of cable to be fashioned later.

After the nerve is isolated, the subcutaneous pocket or subpectoral pocket is made (Fig. 95-3). Previously, an incision approximately 10 cm below and parallel to the clavicle was recommended, although the stimulator device can be easily implanted into the same pocket by making an incision just at the inferior and lateral border of the pectoralis muscle approximately 5 cm in length in the region of the anterior axillary line. We have further modified this technique to make the axillary incision more horizontal and slightly curved, to follow the natural skin creases. This results in improved cosmetic appearance of the scar. Dissection is carried down below all of the subcutaneous tissue and just above the fascia of the pectoralis muscle itself, if a subcutaneous pocket is desired, or deep to the

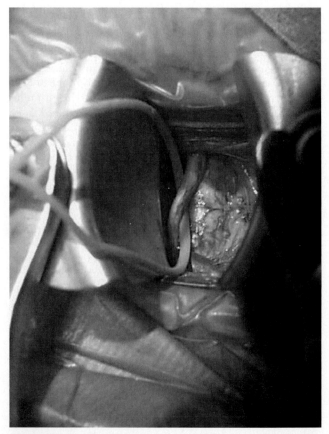

FIGURE 95-2 Exposure of the vagus nerve by division of the carotid sheath on either side. A Cloward retractor with short smooth blades affords adequate exposure to isolate 3 cm of the nerve.

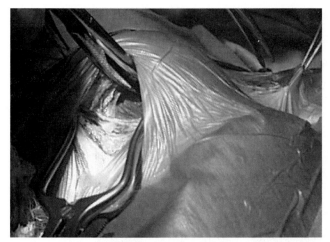

FIGURE 95-3 A pocket deep to the pectoralis major muscle is created by sharp and blunt dissection, or in some patients with significant breast tissue or subcutaneous fat, a pocket superficial to the muscle may be preferred.

pectoralis for subpectoral placement. The device is approximately 5 cm in diameter, and with practice the surgeon can readily determine when the pocket is large enough to admit the stimulator device in relation to the size of his or her hand. It is useful to have the pocket deep enough that the device is recessed 1 to 2 cm away from the skin incision.

After the pocket is fashioned, the tunneling device can be passed in either direction between the pocket and the surgical incision. We usually do this from the pocket to the cervical incision above (Fig. 95-4), with care taken to avoid injury to the exposed deep structures and with the ideal level of emergence of the tunneler just below the platysma.

At this point, the electrodes can be passed through the subcutaneous tunnel that has been created. It is important that the coil electrodes themselves not pass through the tunnel because they can be damaged with minor trauma. The electrode connectors can be passed into the plastic sheath of the tunneling device and then pulled from above to below without difficulty.

The next step involves putting the coil electrodes onto the vagus nerve (Fig. 95-5). Although this is conceptually simple, it can be frustrating if an attempt is made to put them on in the wrong orientation. We have found the simplest technique is to pull the cable inferiorly somewhat so there is no redundant cable below the coil devices. Starting with the lowest of the three coils (which is really just a retaining coil, and not an electrode), fine threads coming from the two ends of the Silastic coil are grasped and the superior of these is passed from lateral to medial, going deep to the vagus nerve. This is helped by having the assistant retract the nerve gently upward using the plastic loop. If the nerve is allowed to lay in a middle groove of the slightly opened coil, bringing the upper thread laterally and the

FIGURE 95-4 The electrode cable is tunneled the short distance from the pocket to a plane below the platysma but above the sternocleidomastoid. The one-pin contact of the Model 302 electrode fits snugly in the inner sheath of the tunneler.

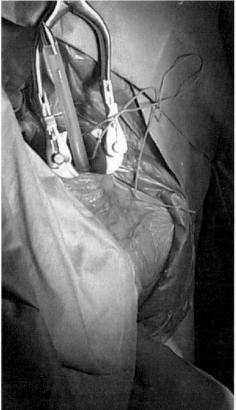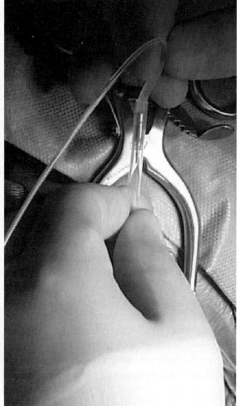

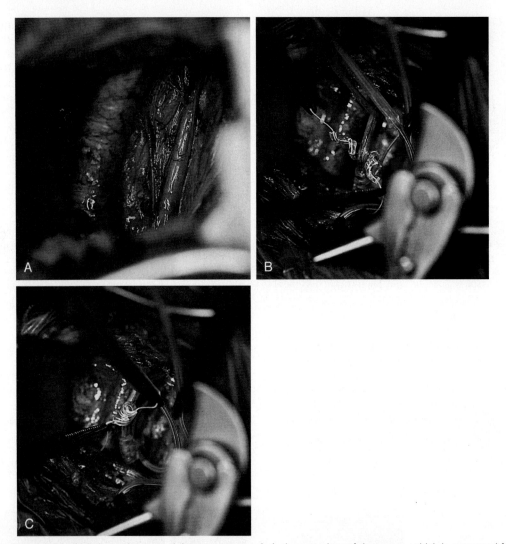

FIGURE 95-5   Coiling the helical electrodes around the vagus nerve. *A*, A close-up view of the vagus, which is separated from the carotid artery and sheath but without elevation by the vessel loop. *B*, With the lowest anchoring helix already in place, the superior part of the middle electrode is passed behind the nerve from lateral to medial and is grasped only by the supporting threads. *C*, Crossing the ends of the helix over the nerve concludes one and a half revolutions of the helix placement.

lower thread medially across that nerve completes one full revolution of the coil, and then releasing the coil causes it to snap back into a good position around the nerve. Usually one to one-and-a-half more revolutions of the helix need to be completed around the nerve, but this is relatively easily done. Each of the two other coils can then be placed around the nerve, and because the superior coils that contain electrodes are shorter and have fewer completed coils than the lower retaining coil, they often go in somewhat more easily. If the nerve is not dissected for an adequate length to begin with, the last coil may be more difficult because of the lack of adequate space.

Once the three cables are in place, the electrode wires leading away from the cables are secured in the neck. The wires leading away from the two electrodes are separate for a distance of several centimeters and then joined together at a bifurcation point. The separate cables can be slid down into the carotid sheath so that they are in line with the coil electrodes, which have already been placed.

The point of bifurcation then becomes a good place to secure the cables using a small plastic wing anchor. This can be sutured to the deep fascia of the neck using a 4-0 braided nylon or silk suture and a fine needle. Locating this deep fascia around the carotid sheath is important because suturing these anchors to any muscular fascia causes them to move when the patient has neck motion, and the aim is to keep them anchored with as little motion relative to the vagus nerve as possible. It is also important to keep the anchors away from the large vascular structures, including the carotid artery and jugular vein, to prevent erosion into these structures with late vascular complications. Two such tie-downs should be placed, one at the lower and one at the upper limit of the exposure of the deep cervical fascia. A third tie-down should then be placed after some additional free cable is passed upward above the exposure but deep to the platysma, so that it can be fastened onto the fascia of the sternocleidomastoid muscle deep to the platysma and at a level where it will not interfere with the incision, either above or below the skin incision. All of these anchoring sutures should be completed before any manipulation of the more distal part of the electrode cable to ensure that the electrodes on the nerve do not inadvertently come off of their siting.

At this point, the connector cable can be placed into the connection socket on the stimulator device. In the current design (Model 102), only one cable is used, but for replacements with the older, two-contact electrode cables it is important to note which cable is positive and which negative. The positive cable is marked with a white band and goes into the stimulator at the level of a port marked with a plus sign. When inserting the cables, a set screw may block the socket if the cable connector does not insert smoothly. Simply backing out the set screws solves this problem. Once these are in place and the set screws are tightened, the electrical integrity and correct impedance of the nerve electrodes can be tested with diagnostics supplied by the computer (Fig. 95-6). This is done by placing the wand of the computer (along with the hand-held programmer, if this is used instead of a laptop computer for programming) in a sterile plastic drape, such as a clear x-ray cassette cover, and passing it onto the field. The device can then be tested and even activated. We turn on the device at the time of

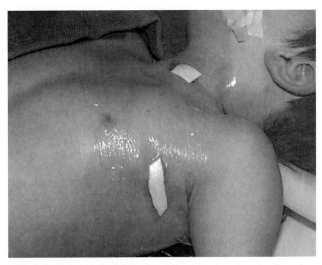

FIGURE 95-7 Completion of surgery with dressings in place. In a pediatric patient, the stimulator makes a noticeable bulge in the contour of the skin with a subcutaneous pocket, but less so when the device is subpectoral.

placement as noted above, but some clinicians prefer simply to leave it off for a few weeks to be certain that any postoperative symptoms the patient is having can be distinguished from symptoms related to stimulation.

The pulse generator is then inserted into the subcutaneous pocket and secured using a single 2-0 silk stitch to the pectoralis fascia, which keeps it anchored deeply into the pocket. It is useful to have the logo of the device facing toward the outside, which optimally orients the antenna for communication with the wand, especially in patients with thicker subcutaneous tissues. Once this is secured in place, both incisions can be closed with resorbable sutures to the deep fascia in the pocket and the platysma in the neck, followed by subcutaneous closure and subcuticular closure with paper strips to close the edges of the skin. Dry sterile dressings are placed, and we usually instruct patients to leave them on for 7 to 10 days to keep the incision completely dry (Fig. 95-7; Table 95-1).

CONCLUSION

Vagal nerve stimulation is a novel approach to treatment of refractory epilepsy in pediatric and adult patients. The spectrum of seizure type that has been shown to respond to chronic VNS includes both partial and generalized seizures and epilepsy syndromes such as Lennox-Gastaut syndrome.

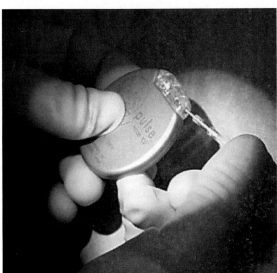

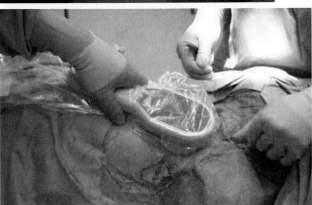

FIGURE 95-6 Lead test follows fixing the cable to the generator and placement of the generator in the pocket. Normal electrical impedance tested by diagnostic routine of the generator serves as a final test of cable integrity.

TABLE 95-1 ▪ Changes in Pulse Generator Size and Weight

Model Number	Face Size (diameter)	Thickness	Weight
100	55 mm	13.2 mm	65 g
101	54 mm	10 mm	38 g
102	52 mm	7 mm	25 g

REFERENCES

1. Brodie MJ, Shorvon SD, Canger R, et al: Commission on European Affairs: appropriate standards of epilepsy care across Europe: ILEA. Epilepsia 38:1245–1250, 1997.
2. Hauser WA: Incidence and prevalence. In Engel J, Pedley TA (eds): Epilepsy: a comprehensive textbook. Vol 1. Philadelphia: Lippincott-Raven, 1997, pp 47–48.
3. Agostoni E, Chinnock JE, Daly MD, Murray JG: Functional and histological studies of the vagus nerve and its branches to the heart, lungs and abdominal viscera in the cat. J Physiol 135:182–205, 1957.
4. Rutecki P: Anatomical, physiological, and theoretical basis for the antiepileptic effect of vagus nerve stimulation. Epilepsia 31(Suppl 2): 1–6, 1990.
5. Cechetto DF: Central representation of visceral function. Fed Proc 46:17–23, 1987.
6. Bailey P, Bremer F: A sensory cortical representation of the vagus nerve. J Neurophysiol 1:4405–4412, 1938.
7. Salinsky MC, Burchiel KJ: Vagus nerve stimulation has no effect on awake EEG rhythms in humans. Epilepsia 34:299–304, 1993.
8. Chase MH, Sterman MB, Clemente CD: Cortical and subcortical patterns of response to afferent vagal stimulation. Exp Neurol 16:36–49, 1966.
9. Chase MH, Nakamura Y, Clemente CD, et al: Afferent vagal stimulation: Neurographic correlates of induced EEG synchronization and desynchronization. Brain Res 5:236–249, 1967.
10. Magnes J, Moruzzi G, Pompeiano O: Synchronization of the EEG produced by very low frequency electrical stimulation of the region of the solitary tract. Arch Ital Biol 99:33–67, 1961.
11. Ricardo JA, Koh ET: Anatomical evidence of direct projections from the nucleus of the solitary tract to the hypothalamus, amygdala, and other forebrain structures in the rat. Brain Res 153:1–26, 1978.
12. Saper CB: Diffuse cortical projection systems: Anatomical organization and role in cortical function. In Plum F (ed): Handbook of Physiology: The Nervous System V. Bethesda, MD: American Physiological Society, 1987, pp 169–210.
13. Lockard JS, Congdon WC, DuCharme LL: Feasibility and safety of vagal stimulation in monkey model. Epilepsia 31(Suppl 2):20–26, 1990.
14. Woodbury DM, Woodbury JW: Effects of vagal stimulation on experimentally induced seizures in rats. Epilepsia 31(Suppl 2):7–19, 1991.
15. Woodbury JW, Woodbury DM: Vagal stimulation reduces the severity of maximal electroshock seizures in intact rats: Use of a cuff electrode for stimulating and recording. Pacing Clin Electrophysiol 1:94–107, 1991.
16. Zabara J: Inhibition of experimental seizures in canines by repetitive vagal stimulation. Epilepsia 33:1005–1012, 1992.
17. McLachlan RS: Suppression of interictal spikes and seizures by stimulation of the vagus nerve. Epilepsia 34:918–923, 1993.
18. Koo B: EEG changes with vagus nerve stimulation. J Clin Neurophysiol 18:434–441, 2001.
19. Takaya M, Terry WJ, Naritoku DK: Vagus nerve stimulation induces a sustained anticonvulsant effect. Epilepsia 37:1111–1116, 1996.
20. Amar AP, Heck CN, Levy ML, et al: An institutional experience with cervical vagus nerve trunk stimulation for medically refractory epilepsy: Rationale, technique, and outcome. Neurosurgery 43:1265–1280, 1998.
21. Handforth A, Degiorgio CM, Schachter SC, et al: Vagus nerve stimulation therapy for partial-onset seizures: A randomized active-control trial. Neurology 51:48–55, 1998.
22. Al-Jayyousi M, Helmers SL: Adjunctive treatment in Lennox-Gastaut syndrome using vagal nerve stimulation. Epilepsia 39(Suppl 6):169, 1998.
23. Ben-Menachem E, Hellstrom K, Runmarker B, Augustinsson L-E: A prospective single-center open-label trial of vagal nerve stimulation (VNS) in 59 patients for the treatment of refractory epilepsy. Epilepsia 38(Suppl 8):208, 1997.
24. Handforth A: Effect on seizure control of reducing current off period from 5 to 1.8 min in patients receiving cyclic vagus nerve stimulation. Epilepsia 38(Suppl 8):177, 1997.
25. Hornig GW, Murphy JV, Schallert G: Left vagus nerve stimulation in children with refractory epilepsy: An update. South Med J 90:484–488, 1997.
26. Murphy JV, Hornig G, Schallert G: Left vagal nerve stimulation in children with refractory epilepsy. Arch Neurol 52:886–889, 1995.
27. Naritoku DK, Terry WJ, Helfert RH: Regional induction of fos immunoreactivity in the brain by anticonvulsant stimulation of the vagus nerve. Epilepsy Res 22:53–62, 1995.
28. Garnett ES, Nahmias C, Scheffel A, et al: Regional cerebral blood flow in man manipulated by direct vagal stimulation. Pacing Clin Electrophysiol 15:1579–1580, 1992.
29. Ko D, Heck C, Grafton S, et al: Vagus nerve stimulation activates central nervous system structures in epileptic patients during PET H215O blood flow imaging. Neurosurgery 39:426–431, 1996.
30. Ben-Menachem E, Hamberger A, Hedner T, et al: Effects of vagus nerve stimulation on amino acids and other metabolites in the CSF of patients with partial seizures. Epilepsy Res 20:221–227, 1995.
31. Labar D, Nikolov B, Tarver B, Fraser R: Vagus nerve stimulation for symptomatic generalized epilepsy: A pilot study. Epilepsia 39:201–205, 1997.

96 Temporal Lobe Operations for Drug-Resistant Epilepsy

DANIEL YOSHOR, WINIFRED J. HAMILTON, and ROBERT G. GROSSMAN

Complex partial seizures (CPSs) of temporal lobe origin are the single most common type of seizure disorder, accounting for approximately 25% of all epilepsies and for approximately 70% of patients referred for surgical consideration.[1–3] Nearly one third of patients with temporal lobe epilepsy will have unsatisfactory control of their seizures with antiepileptic drug therapy,[4,5] and many patients exhibit signs of drug toxicity at the doses that they must take to reduce the frequency of seizures significantly. Frequent seizures and the side effects of medications may lead to secondary problems for patients with CPSs, including intellectual impairment and social and psychological disturbances.[6] For many patients with CPSs, resection of the anterior temporal lobe offers the possibility of a seizure-free, or nearly seizure-free, life and reduced dependency on antiepileptic drugs.[7,8]

The purpose of this chapter is to describe in detail an operative technique for anterior temporal lobectomy as well as to briefly discuss the issues involved in the selection of patients for surgery.

PATIENT SELECTION FOR TEMPORAL LOBECTOMY

It is beyond the scope of this chapter to fully discuss the variety of protocols that are used at different centers to select patients for anterior temporal lobectomy.[9–15] Briefly, there are two general criteria for patient selection: (1) the demonstration of intractability of the seizures to medical management and (2) the concordance of electrophysiologic, neurologic, neuropsychological, and imaging data that indicate the right or the left anterior temporal lobe as the site of origin of the patient's characteristic seizures. The necessary conditions in this concordance are the demonstration of the site of seizure origin during three or more of the patient's typical seizures and the localization of that site to structures that can be removed without producing unacceptable deficits. This demonstration requires correlation of the behavioral pattern of the seizure with electrical recordings from the temporal lobes, as well as recordings from the frontal, occipital, and parietal lobes.

The correlation of video recording of behavior and cerebral electrical activity is carried out initially by recording temporal lobe activity using standard scalp electrode locations. These scalp electrodes may be supplemented by percutaneously inserted sphenoidal electrodes, although the value of sphenoidal electrodes in improving seizure localization is unclear.[16–18] The findings of noninvasive recordings fall into one of four categories: (1) localization of the seizures to either the right or the left temporal lobe; (2) bilateral localization of the origin of the seizures; (3) posterior temporal or extratemporal, usually frontal, localization of the origin of the seizures; and (4) the inability to localize the site of onset of the seizures. In our experience, approximately 60% of patients who have undergone noninvasive electroencephalography have had recordings that fall into categories 1 to 3. Patients with recordings in category 1 are candidates for anterior temporal lobectomy. Patients with recordings in category 4 are candidates for direct recording from the medial temporal structures.[19–21] To accomplish this, we typically use subdural strip electrodes inserted through temporal burr holes[19,22] or depth electrodes that are stereotactically inserted in the hippocampus.[23,24] Each of these methods has its own benefits and risks.[25]

The next step in patient selection is to determine the concordance of the site of seizure origin with evidence of temporal lobe pathology on brain imaging studies. A high-quality magnetic resonance imaging (MRI) study of the brain is a requisite and should include a thin-section (minimum 3 mm, no gaps) coronal fluid-attenuated inversion recovery sequence. Recent technologic improvements in MRI allow demonstration of subtle brain abnormalities such as hippocampal sclerosis or focal cortical dysplasia.[26–30] If MRI findings are not clearly concordant with the electrophysiologic studies, positron-emission tomography and single photon emission computed tomography studies are often helpful in demonstrating the site of seizure origin.[31] Neuropsychological testing also offers valuable information about lateralized cognitive deficits, which often correlate well with the side of seizure origin.[32]

The final step is to determine the risk of the surgery producing speech or memory deficits, based on the data from neuropsychological testing and from the testing of memory during the suppression of temporal lobe function produced by intracarotid amobarbital (Amytal) injection (Wada test).[33]

RESECTION OF THE TEMPORAL LOBE FOR CONTROL OF COMPLEX PARTIAL SEIZURES

Extent of Tissue Resection

A discussion of the technique of anterior temporal lobectomy for the treatment of CPSs should consider (1) the anatomic structures within the temporal lobe that should be excised, (2) the preoperative planning for the surgery, and (3) the intraoperative techniques for performing the resection.

With respect to the structures to be excised, epileptic discharges can be recorded in patients with CPSs from the lateral temporal neocortex (the superior, middle, inferior, and fusiform temporal gyri), the parahippocampal gyrus, the hippocampal formation (Ammon's horn), the insula, the amygdala, and the uncus. All these structures are possible sites of resection for seizure control. Five questions about the resection of these structures to obtain control of CPSs should be considered: (1) Which of these anatomic structures must be excised to obtain seizure control? (2) Which specific areas and volumes of these structures must be removed? (3) Is intraoperative electrocorticography of value in defining the optimal extent of surgical resection? (4) What are the neurologic and neuropsychological deficits that can result from these resections? (5) What are the risks and benefits of the various techniques for performing the resections?

Definitive answers cannot be given to these questions at present. Although there are clear empirical data that demonstrate the utility of anterior temporal lobectomy in treating intractable CPSs,[7] the precise way in which this operation works to control seizures and, most importantly, the exact structures that must be resected for optimal seizure control, are unknown. The number of temporal resections for epilepsy that have been performed worldwide and reported in detail is still small, and the lack of uniform criteria for patient selection, the grading of outcome, postoperative verification with MRI of the structures removed, and the description of the pathology of the resected tissue has made it difficult to compare surgical series.[34,35] The organization of a common database for temporal lobe surgery would provide a basis for answering these questions.[14,36]

With this perspective in mind, we describe a surgical technique for the removal of a limited portion of the anterior lateral temporal neocortex, the anterior 3 cm of the parahippocampal gyrus, the anterior 3 cm of the hippocampal formation, and the amygdala. The resection can be modified based on electrocorticographic and neuroradiographic findings and represents an evolution in technique from the classic temporal lobectomy,[37,38] in which a much larger area of the lateral temporal lobe was resected. The operation can be considered to hold an intermediate position between a classic lobectomy and a selective amygdalohippocampectomy,[39–41] which limits the resection to mesial temporal structures and spares the lateral temporal neocortex.

The standard anterior temporal lobectomy technique described in this chapter was used in 149 consecutive anterior temporal lobectomies performed by one surgeon (R.G.G.), which have been followed for up to 20 years (Table 96-1). In this group, resection of these structures in the manner described here has provided excellent long-term control of seizures (defined as a reduction in the frequency of seizures of 95% or more) in 85% of patients with classic Ammon's horn sclerosis (AHS), with no mortality and minimal morbidity. The relationship of outcome to the pathology of the resected tissue suggests that the extent of temporal lobe resection necessary for the control of CPSs may vary with the underlying neuropathology that causes the seizures. AHS is the pathologic change that is found most frequently in temporal lobectomy specimens. AHS is found in 50% to 60% of specimens in most series, followed in frequency by low-grade tumors in 20% to 30% of cases, and neuronal loss and gliosis in a pattern not characteristic of AHS in approximately 10% of patients.[32,42,43] Vascular malformations, cortical dysplasias, infarcts, and various structural lesions of the temporal lobe comprise the remainder of the pathologic substrates of CPSs. It is possible that a more extensive resection of temporal tissue than described here may be needed to achieve control of seizures in some patients with diffuse pathologic changes in the lateral temporal neocortex. It is also possible that a more limited resection than described here, such as selective amygdalohippocampectomy or stereotactic radiosurgical ablation[44] of the anterior portion of Ammon's horn, might give equally good results in the control of CPSs in patients with AHS.

Recent improvements in MRI of the temporal lobe and hippocampus have dramatically enhanced the ability to preoperatively identify structural abnormalities in the mesial

TABLE 96-1 ■ **Outcome by Pathology after Anterior Temporal Lobectomy for Complex Partial Seizures (Follow-up Range, 6 Months to 20 Years, *n*=149)**

Pathology	Outcome Category			
	1	**2**	**3**	**4**
Classic AHS (*n*=79)	67 (85%)	8 (10%)	3 (4%)	1 (1%)
Low-grade tumor (*n* = 28)	16 (57%)	6 (22%)	3 (11%)	3 (11%)
GG (*n* = 24)				
DNET (*n* = 4)				
Atypical sclerosis (*n* = 21)	6 (29%)	6 (29%)	4 (19%)	5 (14%)
Other (*n* = 21)	11 (52%)	5 (24%)	3 (14%)	2 (10%)
Inconclusive (*n* = 9)				
Microdysgenesis (*n* = 4)				
AVM (*n* = 3)				
Classic AHS and GG (*n* = 2)				
Infarct (*n* = 2)				
Classic AHS and DNET (*n* = 1)				
Total (*n* = 149)	100 (67%)	25 (17%)	13 (9%)	11 (7%)

Outcome categories: 1 ≥ 95% reduction in seizures; 2 = 75% to 94% reduction in seizures; 3 = 50% to 74% reduction in seizures; and 4 = <50% reduction in seizures.

AHS = Ammon's horn sclerosis; AVM = arteriovenous malformation; DNET = dysembryoplastic neuroepithelial tumor; GG = ganglioglioma.

temporal lobe, the lateral temporal neocortex, or both (dual pathology).[26–28,45–48] For example, in many patients with CPSs, preoperative MRI reveals a shrunken hippocampus with increased T2 signal in fluid-attenuated inversion recovery images of the temporal lobe from where the seizures originate. The improvements in imaging have allowed us to modify our approach to the surgical treatment of temporal lobe epilepsy. In cases in which the preoperative MRI reveals hippocampal sclerosis, we now perform a smaller resection of the lateral temporal neocortex that is limited to the anterior-most portion (<3 cm) of the middle and inferior temporal gyri. This is followed by a relatively aggressive resection of the mesial temporal lobe that is tailored to intraoperative recordings. We and others[49,50] have found that even this limited lateral temporal neocortical resection provides generous exposure for the hippocampal resection. In cases involving the dominant temporal lobe, this approach also offers the benefit of sparing the anterior superior temporal gyrus, which exhibits eloquence for language in a small subset of patients studied with direct cortical stimulation mapping.[51]

This smaller lateral neocortical resection does not appear to affect outcome in patients in whom both the epileptiform activity and anatomic abnormality lie in the mesial temporal lobe, such as in the common situation of a patient with CPSs who is found to have AHS, although long-term outcome studies are needed to confirm this. However, for patients with CPSs in whom the preoperative imaging and other studies indicate that the seizure focus lies in the lateral temporal lobe, we now perform a tailored lateral temporal neocortical resection that is designed to maximally resect portions of the temporal lobe that exhibit epileptiform discharges during intraoperative electrocorticography. When seizure onset in the lateral neocortex of the dominant temporal lobe is suspected, this tailored temporal neocortical resection is done with the patient awake to permit language mapping. Alternatively, language mapping and electrocorticography for localization of a lateral neocortical seizure focus can be performed extraoperatively using surgically implanted subdural electrodes. Both of these techniques permit the surgeon to identify and resect epileptogenic areas (as defined by electrocorticography and imaging studies) of the lateral temporal neocortex (including the superior temporal gyrus) while sparing cortical sites essential for language. It is noteworthy that even in cases in which all evidence suggests that the seizure focus lies in the lateral temporal neocortex, we typically still record from the amygdalohippocampal complex and resect any regions that exhibit epileptiform activity, if the preoperative neuropsychological and Wada testing indicates that this can be done safely. For reasons that may relate to the complex circuitry of the mesial temporal lobe or to dual pathology, we and others have found that solely resecting the lesion in the lateral temporal neocortex while sparing the mesial structures is often ineffective in controlling seizures.[52,53]

Preoperative Preparation of the Patient

The patient's anticonvulsant drug regimen is continued until the time of surgery, with the possible exception of valproic acid or its derivatives (e.g., Depakote), which may interfere with platelet function, although temporal lobectomies have been performed without bleeding complications in patients taking valproate.[54] The patient may be typed and cross-matched for blood as a precautionary measure, but transfusion is rarely needed. Blood loss occurs almost exclusively during the opening of the craniotomy and at its closure, and the loss seldom exceeds 100 mL. A corticosteroid (dexamethasone) is given at the time of the induction of anesthesia and after surgery. The corticosteroids are tapered off postoperatively over approximately 10 days. A single dose of prophylactic antibiotic is given immediately before the start of surgery.

Anesthesia

The use of general anesthesia precludes testing for localization of speech and language function during the surgery. However, the risk of producing language dysfunction is small if only a limited portion of the lateral temporal neocortex is resected and if the arterial supply and the venous drainage of the cortex are respected, as discussed later. The benefits of general anesthesia include the certainty of lack of movement of the patient during microsurgery, which is performed adjacent to the posterior cerebral artery and to the brain stem, and absolute control of the patient's airway. We therefore reserve the use of awake craniotomy for those patients in whom lateral temporal neocortical seizure onset is suspected and a tailored resection of the lateral temporal neocortex of the dominant hemisphere is desired.

A description of the anesthesia techniques employed for awake craniotomy is beyond the scope of this chapter.[55] The general anesthesia protocol that we currently use includes propofol (Diprivan) for induction and desflurane (Suprane, 6.5% to 8.5% in oxygen), supplemented with small amounts of fentanyl, as the inhalational agent. Muscle paralysis is obtained with cisatracurium besylate (Nimbex). An arterial line is typically inserted for continuous monitoring of blood pressure.

Electrocorticography

A full discussion of the role of electrocorticography as a guide to surgical resection is beyond the scope of this chapter.[56] Electrocorticography has classically been used as a guide to tailoring the extent of the resection. Although some studies demonstrate that outcome after temporal lobectomy for intractable epilepsy is worse in patients in whom postresection epileptiform discharges were recorded intraoperatively,[57–59] other investigators found that the presence or absence of these discharges after resection has no prognostic significance.[60–62] In the surgical series summarized in Table 96-1,[32] electrocorticography was used primarily for correlation with outcome and only to a minor extent in tailoring the resection. We recently reviewed this surgical experience to study the prognostic significance of residual hippocampal spikes following resection electrocorticographic and found that in the subset of patients with AHS, the absence of postresection hippocampal spikes predicted a higher likelihood of a good outcome (94%) than if hippocampal spikes remained after resection (60%) ($p < 0.05$). We now use intraoperative electrocorticography to tailor temporal resections as described below.

Patients with neocortical epilepsy of the dominant temporal lobe are operated on using local anesthesia to allow language mapping, which facilitates a tailored neocortical resection. In these cases, electrocorticography is performed with the patient fully awake, and therefore anesthesia does not interfere with neurophysiologic recordings. If the surgery is performed using general anesthesia, the desflurane concentration is reduced to 2.5% to 3.0% before electrocorticography. The patient's blood pressure and the concentrations of the anesthetic gases are monitored. As the anesthesia lightens, the blood pressure increases but is not allowed to increase rapidly or to any significant degree, in the judgment of the anesthesiologist and the surgeon, before deepening the anesthesia again.

Electrocorticographic recordings from the lateral temporal neocortex are obtained using a coronet electrode array or a Silastic grid of electrodes spaced 1 cm apart. A strip electrode is also slipped over the lateral temporal lobe and under the inferior temporal gyrus to the parahippocampal gyrus to record from the mesial temporal lobe. In instances in which preoperative MRI and electroencephalographic studies suggest mesial temporal pathology, intraoperative electrocorticography is only used to a limited extent to guide the lateral neocortical resection. However, if the preoperative workup suggests that seizure onset is in the lateral temporal neocortex, electrocorticography plays a prominent role in tailoring this portion of the resection. After the neocortical recording is completed, the anesthesia is deepened and the lateral temporal resection, including opening the temporal horn of the lateral ventricle and exposing the hippocampus, is carried out. Hippocampal recording is done using a strip electrode with four or six contacts spaced 1 cm apart. This electrode strip is inserted in the temporal horn to lie on the ventricular surface of the hippocampus, extending posteriorly toward the occipital horn of the lateral ventricle. After this initial hippocampal recording is completed, a mesial resection is performed that is tailored to include structures that exhibit epileptiform activity. This tailored resection of mesial temporal structures generally includes the anterior 3 cm of the parahippocampal gyrus, the anterior 3 cm of the hippocampus, the inferior portion of the amygdala, and the uncus. A final recording is then obtained from the remaining posterior parahippocampal gyrus, lying at and posterior to the petrous ridge, and from the posterior hippocampus. After the initial mesial resection has been completed, patients may have residual spike discharges in the hippocampal stump adjacent to the resection. As noted previously, we are now relatively aggressive in resecting these spike-generating areas in an effort to enhance outcome.

Patient Positioning

The position used is similar to that used for a pterional craniotomy. The patient is positioned supine with a roll under the shoulder and the back of the table moderately elevated to bring the head above the heart. The head is slightly extended and is turned 45 degrees to bring the frontotemporal area uppermost. The head is held in place with three-point skull fixation. The table is rotated an additional 15 to 20 degrees to make the frontotemporal area more nearly horizontal.

OPERATIVE TECHNIQUE

The procedure can be divided into four stages: (1) craniotomy; (2) resection of the anterior lateral portion of the temporal lobe; (3) microsurgical resection of the amygdala, hippocampal formation, and parahippocampal gyrus; and (4) closure. Particular considerations are of primary importance in each of these stages.

Craniotomy

The major considerations in the design of the scalp and bone flaps are (1) providing adequate exposure of the temporal lobe and (2) obtaining a good cosmetic result. Because the objective of the operation is to return the patient, who is generally a young person, to as normal a life as possible, performing a craniotomy that is virtually undetectable by the patient and by others is of psychological benefit to the patient. A modified pterional craniotomy is used, as shown in Figure 96-1, using a smaller scalp flap than that described by Yasargil for the surgery of aneurysms of the circle of Willis.

The skin incision is started at the hairline at the anterior portion of the superior temporal line, is carried back parallel and just superior to the temporal line to a point above the ear, and is extended down along the anterior border of the ear to the root of the zygoma. The position of the superficial temporal artery is identified by palpation before making the incision. The artery is avoided by making the incision along the anterior border of the ear. The outer layer of the fascia of the temporalis muscle is incised sharply below its insertion on the superior temporal line to leave a small cuff of fascia for reattaching the temporalis muscle. The posterior limb of the fascial incision is carried down to the root of the zygoma using scissors. The temporalis muscle fibers are incised with cutting current to expose the root of the zygoma, which is the basal limit of the craniotomy (see Fig. 96-1, perforation 6). The anterior limb of the temporalis fascia incision is carried along the superior temporal line to expose the frontal process of the zygomatic bone. This exposure can usually be accomplished without extending the scalp incision onto the side of the forehead by cutting the galea with fine scissors beneath the skin. The temporalis muscle is elevated from the skull. The scalp and temporalis muscle, which are not separated from the galea, form a single flap, which is retracted with fishhook retractors attached to springs (Fig. 96-2A).

A free bone flap is made with a Gigli saw or a high-speed drill. To make the flap with the Gigli saw, multiple burr holes, approximately 3 cm apart, are made (see Fig. 96-1, perforations 1 to 6). Alternatively, the bone flap can be fashioned by making a single burr hole and then using a high-speed drill with a foot-plate adapter.

Once the bone flap is elevated, the middle meningeal artery is identified, cauterized, and cut. It is not necessary to drill down the lateral aspect of the sphenoid wing, as is done for exposure of the circle of Willis. Preserving the sphenoid wing maintains the normal temporal contour. Drill holes are made in the margins of the craniotomy, and the dura is tacked to the bone with 4-0 sutures. The dura is opened using a horseshoe-shaped flap, is retracted back over the temporalis muscle, and is protected with moist cottonoids

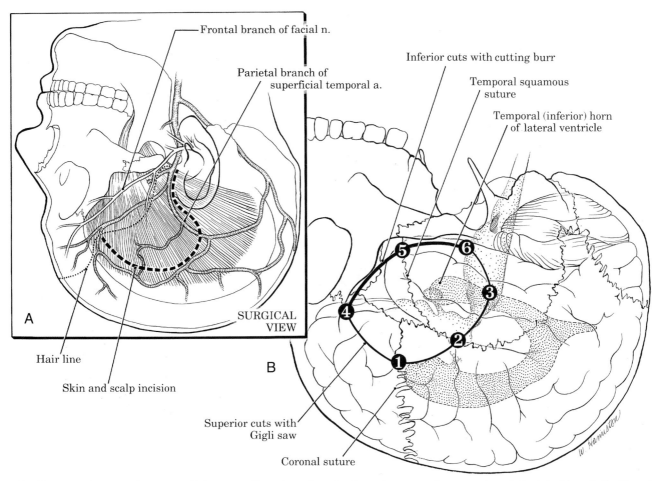

FIGURE 96-1 Right anterior temporal lobectomy. Operative orientation from the surgeon's perspective. *A,* Scalp incision. *B,* Position of the craniotomy in relationship to important anatomic structures and the order in which skull perforations are made.

to reduce shrinkage. The inferior frontal gyrus and 5 to 6 cm of the temporal lobe are exposed by the craniotomy. Electrocorticography may be carried out at this time as described earlier.

Resection of the Anterior Lateral Temporal Lobe

The major considerations in this portion of the operation are to avoid excision of too much of the lateral temporal lobe and to avoid interruption of the arteries and veins supplying the more posterior portions of the temporal lobe. Language deficits after temporal lobectomy can result from resection of the anterior superior temporal gyrus or from interruption of the branches of the middle cerebral artery, which leave the sylvian fissure and course over the superior and middle temporal gyri within the anterior 4 cm of the temporal lobe to ultimately supply the more posterior cortex.[63,64] The superior portion of the resection should be tailored to avoid damaging the superior temporal gyrus of the dominant hemisphere or interrupting these vessels. Labbé's vein, when present, lies 4 to 6 cm from the temporal tip. The vein should not be disturbed. The extent of the lateral temporal resection should be kept as small as possible, compatible with resection of epileptogenic lateral temporal neocortex and exposure of the hippocampus in the floor of

the temporal horn of the lateral ventricle. The size of the lateral resection should not be completely based on measurement of the length of the temporal lobe along its long axis, particularly in children. The entire configuration of the temporal fossa should be assessed, and the resection should be kept anterior to the petrous ridge. The area of the brain to be resected is demarcated by thin sheets of rubber or Telfa and covered with moist cottonoids.

The lateral cortical resection is usually more easily made under loupe magnification than under the operating microscope. The initial incision is made along the middle or superior temporal gyrus, using a fine microblade or microscissors to cut the pia-arachnoid (see Fig. 96-2, incisions 1a or 1b). Microbipolar cautery is used to coagulate vessels, and a fine suction tip is used to remove tissue. Suction tips with a rounded, closed tip and multiple side openings have been found to be very useful for atraumatic suction and dissection when working adjacent to delicate vessels and neural structures (Grossman Micro Suction system; Aesculap, South San Francisco, CA). The incision is started approximately 2 cm from the temporal tip and through the white matter of the temporal cortex. If a middle temporal gyrus incision is used (see Fig. 96-2, incision 1a), the incision is typically directed orthogonally to project toward the temporal horn. If a superior temporal gyrus incision is used (see Fig. 96-2, incision 1b), the incision is inclined slightly laterally (toward the

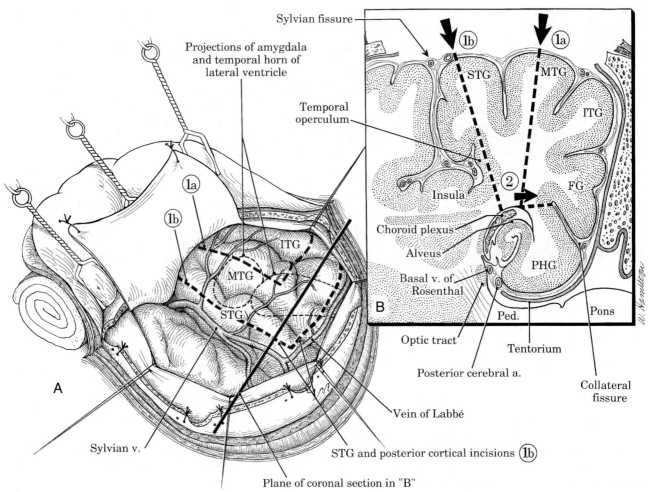

FIGURE 96-2   Lateral temporal resection. *A,* Exposure of the lateral temporal lobe. The positions of the amygdala and the temporal horn of the lateral ventricle are indicated, as are the cortical incisions. *B,* A coronal section through the right temporal lobe approximately 1 cm posterior to the tip of the hippocampal pes viewed from a posterior-to-anterior perspective. Cortical incision 1a through the middle temporal gyrus (MTG) is directed orthogonally through the subcortical white matter to enter the temporal horn of the lateral ventricle. Cortical incision 1b demarks the incision that we routinely used in the past. This incision was directed through the superior temporal gyrus (STG) and was angled slightly laterally (toward the floor of the middle fossa) through the gray matter of the temporal operculum to the temporal horn of the lateral ventricle. a., artery; FG, fusiform gyrus; ITG = inferior temporal gyrus; Ped., peduncle; PHG, parahippocampal gyrus; v., vein.

floor of the middle fossa), at a depth of 1 to 2 cm, the gray matter of the cortex adjacent to the sylvian fissure may be encountered, and a small amount of cerebrospinal fluid (CSF) is usually recognized, indicating that the line of resection is passing along the subarachnoid space of the sylvian fissure. The incision is then carried posteriorly, typically to a distance of 2 to 4 cm from the temporal tip.

The direction of the incision is then redirected at a right angle to cross the long axis of the temporal lobe, and the incision is carried across the middle and inferior temporal gyri. The incision is carried deep into the gyri, angling the incision slightly posteriorly until the temporal horn of the lateral ventricle is entered. A small cottonoid is placed in the horn. Semisharp dissection through the white matter with a Freer dissector is useful in finding the temporal horn. The depth of the temporal horn from the cortical surface should be determined from the MRI scan; it usually lies at a depth of 3 to 3.5 cm. Measurement of the depth of the incision with a ventricular cannula marked at 3.5 cm is useful as the incision is made. In some patients, the temporal horn

may be very thin and difficult to locate. If the temporal horn is not quickly found at the proper depth, it is best to bring in the operating microscope and to use self-retaining retractors to hold the incision apart. This allows one to dissect in the white matter with microsurgical instruments, observing for CSF flow when the wall of the ventricle is entered. It can also be helpful to follow the collateral fissure from its origin in the basal temporal lobe to the lateral ventricle. Ultrasound is not generally helpful in locating the temporal horn. Frameless stereotaxy, however, can be used for localization at this stage of the operation as there is little shift of structures at this point, although we do not use it unless there is a structural lesion such as a tumor that is to be resected.

The removal of tissue and CSF causes the anterior temporal lobe to retract away from the sphenoid wing, allowing better visualization of the tip of the temporal lobe. The incision along the superior or middle temporal gyrus is now extended anteriorly to the temporal tip. Veins draining from the sylvian fissure into the sphenoparietal sinus are preserved. The lateral temporal lobe is then removed by dissection parallel to the cortical surface in the white matter at the level of the temporal horn (see Fig. 96-2, incision 2). This incision will reach the collateral fissure and the fusiform gyrus on the floor of the middle fossa. Incision of the pia-arachnoid of the fusiform gyrus is started posteriorly and is carried anteriorly. The lateral temporal lobe is lifted upward, and the most anteromedial portion of the cortex is removed subpially. The pia-arachnoid of the anteromedial cortex is cut, and the specimen is removed. The insula and the hippocampus in the temporal horn are exposed. Recording is then carried out from the parahippocampal gyrus and the hippocampus.

Resection of the Amygdala, Hippocampus, and Parahippocampal Gyrus

This part of the operation is performed with the aid of the operating microscope. The major consideration is to avoid injury to the internal capsule lying medial to the temporal horn, the posterior cerebral artery, and the third and the fourth cranial nerves lying in the incisura. An understanding of the anatomy of the temporal lobe is essential.[65–67] There is an excellent illustration of the vascular anatomy in the paper by Yasargil and colleagues[68] on amygdalohippocampectomy. A second consideration is that a large amount of CSF is removed by suction during this stage of the surgery, which results in the cortex falling away from the dura and the stretching of draining cortical veins. This can result in avulsion of the posterior inferior temporal veins that drain into the petrosal sinus, causing profuse hemorrhage. Therefore, CSF should be replaced frequently by irrigation of the basal cisterns with saline or artificial CSF.

A third precaution is to avoid compressing the medial aspect of the temporal horn with a retractor blade, which can damage the internal capsule or the basal ganglia lying beneath the ventricle. The use of stable self-retaining retractors with tapered blades greatly facilitates this portion of the operation. In children, the temporal horn is generally smaller than in adults and resection of the hippocampus is correspondingly more difficult. The most anterior portion of the temporal horn is held open, with the retractor blades placed on the medial and lateral walls (Fig. 96-3B). The walls are protected with rubber strips (not shown in the figure). An incision is made, using the bipolar cautery and suction, from the tip of the choroid fissure to the anteromedial edge of the medial temporal lobe (see Fig. 96-3B, incision 3). The incision is carried through the amygdala, which is removed by aspiration, down to the pia-arachnoid of the anterior medial parahippocampal cortex. Through the pia-arachnoid, it is possible to see the tentorial edge and incisura and the oculomotor nerve and the posterior cerebral artery (see Fig. 96-3C). The pia-arachnoid is cut over the tentorium.

The retractors are then moved posteriorly to the level of the choroid plexus. A third retractor is placed posteriorly against the overlying temporal lobe to facilitate exposure. The medial retractor is placed on the choroid plexus, which is gently retracted medially, thereby exposing the pia-arachnoid of the choroid fissure. The fimbria and alveus are then removed from the body of the hippocampus with a No. 5 French closed suction cannula (see Fig. 96-3C).

The aspiration of these structures reveals the edge of the hippocampal fissure. A veil of arachnoid extends from the choroid fissure into the hippocampal fissure. The arachnoid surrounds a vein 2 to 3 mm in diameter. The vein is coagulated, and the vein and the arachnoid are cut with microscissors (see Fig. 96-3A and D, incision 5). This incision exposes the superior edge of the subiculum. Arterial branches also enter the hippocampal fissure posterior to the vein, and if the posterior hippocampus is resected, these vessels are also coagulated and cut.

The posterior cerebral artery and its branches that supply the undersurface of the temporal lobe have a variable relationship to the subiculum. The posterior cerebral artery can be strongly attached to the subiculum and can lie laterally. Great care should be taken to ascertain the course of the posterior cerebral artery as it travels posteriorly from the anterior incisura, where it can be easily seen. The hippocampus and subiculum could be removed en bloc at this point by detaching the subicular pia-arachnoid from the vasculature covering it. However, it is safer to remove these structures with a subpial subicular incision. This incision traverses the subiculum and reaches the pia-arachnoid of the parahippocampal gyrus (see Fig. 96-3A and E, incision 6). To make this incision, the hippocampus and parahippocampal gyrus are retracted slightly laterally so that they lie on the tentorium (see Fig. 96-3E). The subicular incision is started anteriorly at the rostral edge of the tentorium and is carried down to the tentorium (see Fig. 96-3E). The incision is continued posteriorly, keeping the incision on the tentorium. As branches of the posterior cerebral artery are encountered in the pia-arachnoid of the subiculum, they are coagulated and cut. The incision is carried posteriorly for 3 cm from the anterior tip of the pes in the temporal horn. The resection extends approximately 1 cm posterior to the vein entering the hippocampal fissure. This incision frees the medial edge of the specimen. The fourth nerve may be seen under an arachnoid veil at the edge of the tentorium. To completely detach the specimen, an incision is made at right angles to the long axis of the hippocampus, through the parahippocampal gyrus (starting laterally at the parahippocampus), and then going through the hippocampus (see Fig. 96-3E, incision 7, and F). In some cases, it is easier to reverse these last two steps and to perform the right-angle transection of the parahippocampal gyrus and hippocampus before making the subicular incision to detach the specimen along the edge of the tentorium.

The uncus can then be removed subpially with suction, taking care not to damage fine perforating vessels going to the brain stem from the posterior communicating, choroidal, and posterior cerebral arteries.

Recording from the hippocampal stump and the posterior parahippocampal cortex is carried out at this point. If epileptiform activity is recorded from a discrete region of the hippocampal stump, the resection is extended posteriorly using subpial suction. The bipolar electrocautery is carefully used for final hemostasis. The cut surfaces are then covered with a single layer of oxidized regenerated cellulose (Surgicel).

Closure

The subarachnoid space is filled with saline. The dura is closed in a watertight fashion with a running continuous

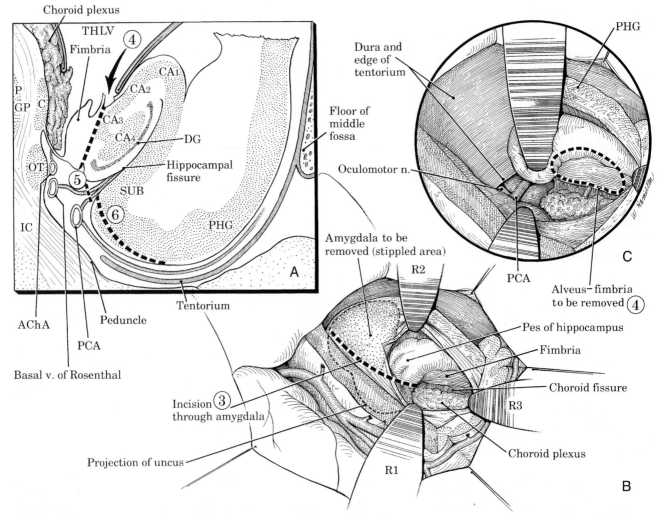

FIGURE 96-3 Microsurgical resection of the amygdala, hippocampus, and parahippocampal gyrus. *A,* Coronal section of the right mesial temporal lobe viewed from a posterior-to-anterior perspective shows orienting anatomy and incisions. *B,* Exposure of the amygdala and the hippocampus after removal of the anterior lateral temporal lobe. The temporal horn is opened, showing the pes of the hippocampus and the choroid plexus. Incision 3, from the choroid fissure through the amygdala, is indicated; the *stippled area* will be removed with suction. *C,* The amygdala and anterior medial parahippocampal gyrus have been removed, revealing the tentorium, posterior cerebral artery (PCA), and oculomotor nerve. The *dotted line* indicates where suction is used to remove the fimbria and alveus from the body of the hippocampus.

(Continued)

4-0 nonabsorbable suture. Occasionally, a small patch graft of lyophilized human dura or pericranium is required to obtain watertight closure. An epidural drain may be placed. The bone flap is secured in position with titanium miniplates. The temporalis muscle is closed with a 2-0 absorbable suture, and the muscle fascia closed with another layer of 2-0 suture. Generally, the entire craniotomy site is covered by the closure of the fascia. The galea is closed with 3-0 absorbable suture, and the skin is closed with staples.

OUTCOME

Complications

Serious complications after anterior temporal lobectomy are rare, but hemiplegia, oculomotor and trochlear palsies, and visual field deficits can occur.[69–71] Of the 149 consecutive anterior temporal lobectomies in our series detailed in Table 96-1, there were no deaths, infections, or hemiparesis after surgery. Three patients in this series, which preceded our current practice of avoiding resection of the dominant anterior superior temporal gyrus unless this is deemed to be safe by direct cortical stimulation mapping, exhibited aphasia that improved over time. Transient paresis of cranial nerves III or IV was seen in three patients. A recent neuro-ophthalmologic study indicates that subtle diplopia may be more common than generally recognized, but fortunately these deficits nearly always resolve spontaneously.[72] Two patients exhibited an acute psychotic reaction, a rare but well-recognized complication.[73,74] A state of anxiety, which generally responds to psychotropic medications, occurs in approximately 5% of patients in the weeks immediately after surgery.[75,76]

Contralateral superior quadrantanopsia has been reported to occur in approximately 50% of patients after temporal lobectomy.[77,78] This field defect is thought to result from

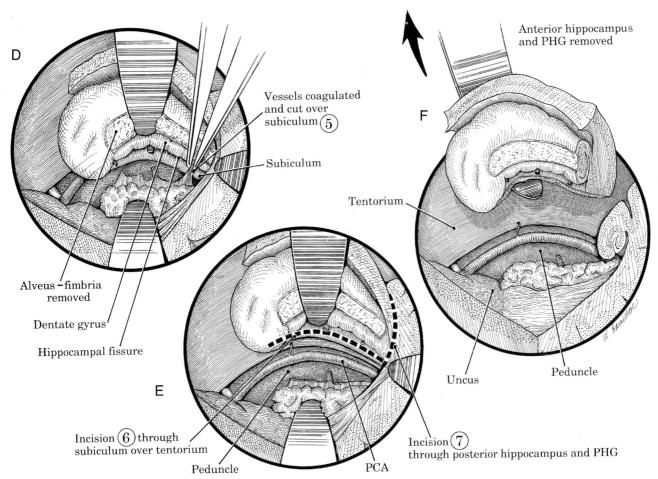

FIGURE 96-3 Cont'd *D,* The alveus-fimbria has been removed. The vein entering the hippocampal fissure is coagulated and cut, working over the subiculum (incision 5). *E,* The hippocampus is retracted very slightly laterally over the tentorium. The position of the PCA is kept in mind as the hippocampal specimen is detached medially (incision 6), and posteriorly (incision 7). *F,* The anterior hippocampus and parahippocampal gyrus are removed. AchA, anterior choroidal artery; C, tail of the caudate; CA1 to CA4, areas of Ammon's horn (cornu ammonis) of the hippocampus; DG, dentate gyrus; GP, globus pallidus; IC, intercommissural fibers; OT, optic tract; P, putamen; PHG, parahippocampal gyrus; R1 to R3, retractors 1 to 3; SUB, subiculum; THLV, temporal horn of the lateral ventricle.

interruption of the optic radiation fibers in Meyer's loop in the temporal lobe. The incidence of a field defect is lower when the amount of lateral temporal lobe resected is restricted to less than 4 cm.

Seizure Control

Accurate comparison of outcomes among various centers is difficult because different methodologies are used to select patients and to assess outcome.[79] Based on data from a worldwide survey, Engel[80] compiled seizure outcome data on 3579 patients from 100 epilepsy centers who underwent anterior temporal lobectomy for CPSs between 1986 and 1990. Of these patients, 2429 (68%) were seizure free after surgery and 860 (24%) were improved.

In our series of 149 patients who underwent standardized anterior temporal lobectomy for CPSs and who have been followed for periods ranging from 6 months to 19.7 years (mean, 8.3 years) (see Table 96-1),[32] 100 patients (67.1%) experienced a 95% or better reduction in their seizures after surgery. As a group, the patients with classic AHS

(hippocampal sclerosis in CA1, CA4, and the dentate gyrus) had the best outcome. Among the 79 patients with classic AHS, 67 (85%) experienced a 95% or better reduction in seizures after surgery. Of these 79 patients, 55 (70%) were entirely free of auras and seizures or had only rare seizures or auras with identifiable precipitating causes, generally as a result of stopping anticonvulsant medication. Of the 75 of 79 patients with AHS for whom we have medication follow-up data, 50 (67%) were taking significantly reduced levels (50% or more reduction) of antiepileptic medication at the time of their most recent follow-up, including 24 patients (32%) who were no longer taking antiepileptic medication.

As noted earlier, patients with pathologic findings other than AHS in general did less well. Of the patients with low-grade tumors (n = 28), who represent the second largest group of patients, 16 (57%) experienced a 95% or better reduction in the frequency of seizures. Patients whose specimen displayed atypical sclerotic changes (n = 21) had the poorest outcome, with six (29%) experiencing a reduction of 95% or better in the occurrence of seizures over the follow-up period.

Neuropsychological Outcome

A loss of material-specific memory is noted in most patients who undergo an anterior temporal lobectomy that includes the excision of mesial temporal structures. In our series of patients,[32] a comparison of preoperative and postoperative testing revealed that verbal memory was more affected than spatial memory and that, as expected, a decline in verbal memory was more likely to occur after a left temporal resection. Patients with a right-sided resection or with pathologic findings of AHS exhibited the least postoperative memory decline. This second finding concurs with several studies in which investigators found that patients with moderate or severe hippocampal sclerosis have significantly less change in their memory after anterior temporal lobectomy than do patients with no or mild hippocampal sclerosis.[81,82]

A significant increase in attention span and in perceptual organization was seen in nearly all patients with AHS and in most patients with a left-sided procedure after surgery. This is probably the reason that intelligence scores were modestly higher in most patients after surgery, although the change was not statistically significant. Other centers have reported similar findings.[83,84] In our series, patients with AHS showed greater improvement in intelligence scores after surgery than did patients with other types of pathology, although patients with AHS typically had slightly lower intelligence scores preoperatively.

Patients who were seizure free after surgery generally reported significantly decreased levels of anxiety and depression as well as a greater sense of self-confidence and independence. For many patients, obtaining a driver's license was particularly important and allowed them to expand their educational, employment, and social choices significantly. Patients with long-standing emotional and social problems often improved less than would be expected based on the postoperative control of their seizures, a finding that has been noted in other series.[76,85]

REFERENCES

1. Hauser WA, Annegers JF, Rocca WA: Descriptive epidemiology of epilepsy: Contributions of population-based studies from Rochester, Minnesota. Mayo Clin Proc 71:576–586, 1996.
2. Williamson PD, Engel J Jr: Complex partial seizures. In Engel J Jr, Pedley TA (eds): Epilepsy: A Comprehensive Textbook. Philadelphia/New York: Lippincott–Raven, 1998, pp 557–566.
3. Zimmerman RS, Sirven JI: An overview of surgery for chronic seizures. Mayo Clin Proc 78:109–117, 2003.
4. Kwong KL, Sung WY, Wong SN, et al: Early predictors of medical intractability in childhood epilepsy. Pediatr Neurol 29:46–52, 2003.
5. Singhvi JP, Sawhney IM, Lal V, et al: Profile of intractable epilepsy in a tertiary referral center. Neurol India 48:351–356, 2000.
6. Jacoby A, Baker GA, Steen N, et al: The clinical course of epilepsy and its psychosocial correlates: Findings from a U.K. community study. Epilepsia 37:148–161, 1996.
7. Wiebe S, Blume WT, Girvin JP, et al: A randomized, controlled trial of surgery for temporal-lobe epilepsy. N Engl J Med 345:311–318, 2001.
8. McIntosh AM, Wilson SJ, Berkovic SF: Seizure outcome after temporal lobectomy: Current research practice and findings. Epilepsia 42:1288–1307, 2001.
9. Doyle WK, Spencer DD: Anterior temporal resections. In Engel J Jr, Pedley TA (eds): Epilepsy: A Comprehensive Textbook, vol 2. Philadelphia/New York: Lippincott–Raven, 1998, pp 1819–1828.
10. Ojemann GA: Treatment of temporal lobe epilepsy. Annu Rev Med 48:317–328, 1997.
11. Anonymous: Presurgical evaluation protocols. In Engel J Jr (ed): Surgical Treatment of the Epilepsies, 2nd ed. New York: Raven Press, 1993, pp 707–750.
12. Salanova V, Markand O, Worth R, et al: Presurgical evaluation and surgical outcome of temporal lobe epilepsy. Pediatr Neurol 20:179–184, 1999.
13. Immonen A, Jutila L, Kalviainen R, et al: Preoperative clinical evaluation, outline of surgical technique and outcome in temporal lobe epilepsy. Adv Tech Stand Neurosurg 29:87–132, 2004.
14. Berg AT, Vickrey BG, Langfitt JT, et al: The multicenter study of epilepsy surgery: Recruitment and selection for surgery. Epilepsia 44:1425–1433, 2003.
15. Jones MW, Andermann F: Temporal lobe epilepsy surgery: definition of candidacy. Can J Neurol Sci 27(Suppl 1):S11–S21, 2000.
16. Sperling MR, Guina L: The necessity for sphenoidal electrodes in the presurgical evaluation of temporal lobe epilepsy: Pro position. J Clin Neurophysiol 20:299–304, 2003.
17. Kanner AM, Parra J, Gil-Nagel A, et al: The localizing yield of sphenoidal and anterior temporal electrodes in ictal recordings: A comparison study. Epilepsia 43:1189–1196, 2002.
18. Blume WT: The necessity for sphenoidal electrodes in the presurgical evaluation of temporal lobe epilepsy: Con position. J Clin Neurophysiol 20:305–310, 2003.
19. Spencer SS, Sperling MR, Shewmon DA: Intracranial electrodes. In Engel J Jr, Pedley TA (eds): Epilepsy: A Comprehensive Textbook, vol 2. Philadelphia/New York: Lippincott–Raven, 1998, pp 1719–1747.
20. Pacia SV, Ebersole JS: Intracranial EEG in temporal lobe epilepsy. J Clin Neurophysiol 16:399–407, 1999.
21. Dubeau F, McLachlan RS: Invasive electrographic recording techniques in temporal lobe epilepsy. Can J Neurol Sci 27(Suppl 1):S29–S52, 2000.
22. Weinand ME, Wyler AR, Richey ET, et al: Long-term ictal monitoring with subdural strip electrodes: Prognostic factors for selecting temporal lobectomy candidates. J Neurosurg 77:20–28, 1992.
23. Cascino GD, Trenerry MR, Sharbrough FW, et al: Depth electrode studies in temporal lobe epilepsy: Relation to quantitative magnetic resonance imaging and operative outcome. Epilepsia 36:230–235, 1995.
24. Schuh LA, Henry TR, Ross DA, et al: Ictal spiking patterns recorded from temporal depth electrodes predict good outcome after anterior temporal lobectomy. Epilepsia 41:316–319, 2000.
25. Eisenschenk S, Gilmore RL, Cibula JE, et al: Lateralization of temporal lobe foci: Depth versus subdural electrodes. Clin Neurophysiol 112:836–844, 2001.
26. Gilliam F, Faught E, Martin R, et al: Predictive value of MRI-identified mesial temporal sclerosis for surgical outcome in temporal lobe epilepsy: An intent-to-treat analysis. Epilepsia 41:963–966, 2000.
27. Kuzniecky RI, Burgard S, Bilir E, et al: Qualitative MRI segmentation in mesial temporal sclerosis: Clinical correlations. Epilepsia 37:433–439, 1996.
28. Lehericy S, Semah F, Hasboun D, et al: Temporal lobe epilepsy with varying severity: MRI study of 222 patients. Neuroradiology 39:788–796, 1997.
29. McBride MC, Bronstein KS, Bennett B, et al: Failure of standard magnetic resonance imaging in patients with refractory temporal lobe epilepsy. Arch Neurol 55:346–348, 1998
30. Ryvlin P, Coste S, Hermier M, et al: Temporal pole MRI abnormalities in temporal lobe epilepsy. Epileptic Disord 4(Suppl 1):S33–S39, 2002.
31. Henry TR, Van Heertum RL: Positron emission tomography and single photon emission computed tomography in epilepsy care. Semin Nucl Med 33:88–104, 2003.
32. York MK, Rettig GM, Grossman RG, et al: Seizure control and cognitive outcome after temporal lobectomy: A comparison of classic Ammon's horn sclerosis, atypical mesial temporal sclerosis, and tumoral pathologies. Epilepsia 44:387–398, 2003.
33. Spencer DC, Morrell MJ, Risinger MW: The role of the intracarotid amobarbital procedure in evaluation of patients for epilepsy surgery. Epilepsia 41:320–325, 2000.
34. So EL, Radhakrishnan K, Silbert PL, et al: Assessing changes over time in temporal lobectomy: Outcome by scoring seizure frequency. Epilepsy Res 27:119–125, 1997.
35. Vickrey BG, Hays RD, Engel J Jr, et al: Outcome assessment for epilepsy surgery: The impact of measuring health-related quality of life. Ann Neurol 37:158–166, 1995.
36. Engel J Jr, Van Ness PC, Rasmussen TB, et al: Outcome with respect to epileptic seizures. In Engel J Jr (ed): Surgical Treatment of the Epilepsies, 2nd ed. New York: Raven Press, 1993, pp 609–621.
37. Falconer MA, Taylor DC: Surgical treatment of drug-resistant epilepsy due to mesial temporal sclerosis: Etiology and significance. Arch Neurol 19:353–361, 1968.

38. Penfield W, Baldwin M: Temporal lobe seizures and the technic of subtotal temporal lobectomy. Ann Surg 136:625–634, 1952.
39. Park TS, Bourgeois BF, Silbergeld DL, et al: Subtemporal transparahippocampal amygdalohippocampectomy for surgical treatment of mesial temporal lobe epilepsy. J Neurosurg 85:1172–1176, 1996.
40. Wieser HG, Ortega M, Friedman A, et al: Long-term seizure outcomes following amygdalohippocampectomy. J Neurosurg 98:751–763, 2003.
41. Abosch A, Bernasconi N, Boling W, et al: Factors predictive of suboptimal seizure control following selective amygdalohippocampectomy. J Neurosurg 97:1142–1151, 2002.
42. Armstrong DD: The neuropathology of temporal lobe epilepsy. J Neuropathol Exp Neurol 52:433–443, 1993.
43. Armstrong DL, Bruton CJ: Postscript: What terminology is appropriate for tissue pathology? How does it predict outcome? In Engel J Jr (ed): Surgical Treatment of the Epilepsies. New York: Raven Press, 1987, pp 541–552.
44. Regis J, Bartolomei F, Rey M, et al: Gamma knife surgery for mesial temporal lobe epilepsy. J Neurosurg 93(Suppl 3):141–146, 2000.
45. Van Paesschen W, Sisodiya S, Connelly A, et al: Quantitative hippocampal MRI and intractable temporal lobe epilepsy. Neurology 45:2233–2240, 1995.
46. Trenerry MR, Westerveld M, Meador KJ: MRI hippocampal volume and neuropsychology in epilepsy surgery. Magn Reson Imaging 13:1125–1132, 1995.
47. Mitchell LA, Jackson GD, Kalnins RM, et al: Anterior temporal abnormality in temporal lobe epilepsy: A quantitative MRI and histopathologic study. Neurology 52:327–336, 1999.
48. Lee DH, Gao FQ, Rogers JM, et al: MR in temporal lobe epilepsy: Analysis with pathologic confirmation. Am J Neuroradiol 19:19–27, 1998.
49. Spencer DD, Spencer SS, Mattson RH, et al: Access to the posterior medial temporal lobe structures in the surgical treatment of temporal lobe epilepsy. Neurosurgery 15:667–671, 1984.
50. Fried I: Anatomic temporal lobe resections for temporal lobe epilepsy. Neurosurg Clin N Am 4:233–242, 1993.
51. Ojemann G, Ojemann J, Lettich E, et al: Cortical language localization in left, dominant hemisphere: An electrical stimulation mapping investigation in 117 patients. J Neurosurg 71:316–326, 1989.
52. Jooma R, Yeh HS, Privitera MD, et al: Lesionectomy versus electrophysiologically guided resection for temporal lobe tumors manifesting with complex partial seizures. J Neurosurg 83:231–236, 1995.
53. Cascino GD, Kelly PJ, Sharbrough FW, et al: Long-term follow-up of stereotactic lesionectomy in partial epilepsy: Predictive factors and electroencephalographic results. Epilepsia 33:639–644, 1992.
54. Ward MM, Barbaro NM, Laxer KD, et al: Preoperative valproate administration does not increase blood loss during temporal lobectomy. Epilepsia 37:98–101, 1996.
55. Costello TG, Cormack JR: Anaesthesia for awake craniotomy: A modern approach. J Clin Neurosci 11:16–19, 2004.
56. Kuruvilla A, Flink R: Intraoperative electrocorticography in epilepsy surgery: Useful or not? Seizure 12:577–584, 2003.
57. Fiol ME, Gates JR, Torres F, et al: The prognostic value of residual spikes in the postexcision electrocorticogram after temporal lobectomy. Neurology 41:512–516, 1991.
58. Jennum P, Dhuna A, Davies K, et al: Outcome of resective surgery for intractable partial epilepsy guided by subdural electrode arrays. Acta Neurol Scand 87:434–437, 1993.
59. McBride MC, Binnie CD, Janota I, et al: Predictive value of intraoperative electrocorticograms in resective epilepsy surgery. Ann Neurol 30:526–532, 1991.
60. Schwartz TH, Bazil CW, Walczak TS, et al: The predictive value of intraoperative electrocorticography in resections for limbic epilepsy associated with mesial temporal sclerosis. Neurosurgery 40:302–311, 1997.
61. Cascino GD, Trenerry MR, Jack CR Jr, et al: Electrocorticography and temporal lobe epilepsy: Relationship to quantitative MRI and operative outcome. Epilepsia 36:692–696, 1995.
62. Tran TA, Spencer SS, Marks D, et al: Significance of spikes recorded on electrocorticography in nonlesional medial temporal lobe epilepsy. Ann Neurol 38:763–770, 1995.
63. Schwartz TH, Devinsky O, Doyle W, et al: Preoperative predictors of anterior temporal language areas. J Neurosurg 89:962–970, 1998.
64. Ojemann GA: Cortical organization of language. J Neurosci 11:2281–2287, 1991.
65. Awad IA: Anatomic considerations in temporal lobe surgery. In Lüders H (ed): Epilepsy Surgery. New York: Raven Press, 1992, pp 547–558.
66. Renella RR: Microsurgery of the Temporo-medial Region. Wien/New York: Springer-Verlag, 1989.
67. Duvernoy HM: The Human Hippocampus: An Atlas of Applied Anatomy. Munich: J. F. Bergmann Verlag, 1988.
68. Yasargil MG, Teddy PJ, Roth P: Selective amygdalo-hippocampectomy: Operative anatomy and surgical technique. In Krayenbühl H (ed): Advances and Technical Standards in Neurosurgery, vol 12. New York: Springer-Verlag, 1985, pp 93–123.
69. Salanova V, Markand O, Worth R: Temporal lobe epilepsy surgery: Outcome, complications, and late mortality rate in 215 patients. Epilepsia 43:170–174, 2002.
70. Rydenhag B, Silander HC: Complications of epilepsy surgery after 654 procedures in Sweden, September 1990–1995: A multicenter study based on the Swedish National Epilepsy Surgery Register. Neurosurgery 49:51–57, 2001.
71. Behrens E, Schramm J, Zentner J, et al: Surgical and neurological complications in a series of 708 epilepsy surgery procedures. Neurosurgery 41:1–10, 1997.
72. Cohen-Gadol AA, Leavitt JA, Lynch JJ, et al: Prospective analysis of diplopia after anterior temporal lobectomy for mesial temporal lobe sclerosis. J Neurosurg 99:496–499, 2003.
73. Inoue Y, Mihara T: Psychiatric disorders before and after surgery for epilepsy. Epilepsia 42(Suppl 1):13–18, 2001.
74. Blumer D, Wakhlu S, Davies K, et al: Psychiatric outcome of temporal lobectomy for epilepsy: Incidence and treatment of psychiatric complications. Epilepsia 39:478–486, 1998.
75. Mayanagi Y, Watanabe E, Nagahori Y, et al: Psychiatric and neuropsychological problems in epilepsy surgery: Analysis of 100 cases that underwent surgery. Epilepsia 42(Suppl 6):19–23, 2001.
76. Bladin PF: Psychosocial difficulties and outcome after temporal lobectomy. Epilepsia 33:898–907, 1992.
77. Pathak-Ray V, Ray A, Walters R, et al: Detection of visual field defects in patients after anterior temporal lobectomy for mesial temporal sclerosis-establishing eligibility to drive. Eye 16:744–748, 2002.
78. Egan RA, Shults WT, So N, et al: Visual field deficits in conventional anterior temporal lobectomy versus amygdalohippocampectomy. Neurology 55:1818–1822, 2000.
79. Berg AT, Vickrey BG: Outcome Measures. In Engel J Jr, Pedley TA (eds): Epilepsy: A Comprehensive Textbook, vol 2. Philadelphia: Lippincott–Raven, 1998, pp 1891–1899.
80. Engel J Jr: Surgery for seizures. N Engl J Med 334:647–652, 1996.
81. Hermann BP, Seidenberg M, Dohan FC Jr, et al: Reports by patients and their families of memory change after left anterior temporal lobectomy: Relationship to degree of hippocampal sclerosis. Neurosurgery 36:39–45, 1995.
82. Davies KG, Bell BD, Bush AJ, et al: Naming decline after left anterior temporal lobectomy correlates with pathological status of resected hippocampus. Epilepsia 39:407–419, 1998.
83. Wachi M, Tomikawa M, Fukuda M, et al: Neuropsychological changes after surgical treatment for temporal lobe epilepsy. Epilepsia 42 (Suppl 6):4–8, 2001.
84. Westerveld M, Sass KJ, Chelune GJ, et al: Temporal lobectomy in children: Cognitive outcome. J Neurosurg 92:24–30, 2000.
85. Hermann BP, Wyler AR, Somes G: Preoperative psychological adjustment and surgical outcome are determinants of psychosocial status after anterior temporal lobectomy. J Neurol Neurosurg Psychiatry 55:491–496, 1992.

97 Multilobar Resections in Epilepsy Surgery

GIORGIO LO RUSSO, MASSIMO COSSU, LAURA TASSI,
FRANCESCO CARDINALE, STEFANO FRANCIONE,
LAURA CASTANA, ROBERTO MAI, IVANA SARTORI,
LINO NOBILI, ALIM LOUIS BENABID, and CLAUDIO MUNARI[†]

INTRODUCTION

Apparently, general agreement exists concerning the selection criteria of patients who are candidates for surgical treatment of severe, drug-resistant, focal epilepsies.[1] Several therapeutic surgical techniques are currently employed, varying from relatively limited resections,[2] such as the selective amygdalohippocampectomy,[3] to hemispherectomy.[4]

Multilobar resection was synonymous with total[5] or functional[6] hemispherectomy.[7] In the largest published series, this kind of intervention has been performed in percentages varying from 2.5% to 11% of the cases.[8] Such widely extended cortical resections were mainly performed in children with malformation-hamartomatous lesions, or encephalomalacia sequelae of anoxic-ischemic encephalopathy.[9] These resections, which have been progressively replaced by less aggressive procedures as hemispheric disconnections,[10] are generally not included among the surgical alternatives in patients with focal epilepsy that is either cryptogenic or symptomatic of a limited anatomic lesion.[11]

The rationale of curative resective procedures aiming at control of focal drug-resistant epilepsy is total excision of the epileptogenic zone (EZ), that is, the cortical region of onset and early spread of the ictal discharge.[12] In this regard, the main efforts must be performed in order to correctly localize the EZ. Considering the dynamic features of the ictal discharge, and therefore its spatial-temporal structure,[13] it is not surprising that in a number of patients the EZ may not be localized within the anatomic limits that mark the boundaries between the cerebral lobes.[14] Moreover, the extension of an anatomic lesion that may correlate with seizures does not necessarily correspond to that of the EZ. Indeed, lesions limited to a single lobe may be associated with a multilobar EZ, and anatomic abnormalities as wide as an entire hemisphere may be observed in patients with an EZ involving only a portion of a single lobe.

The presurgical diagnostic methodology that must be applied and, consequently, the type of cortical excision that can be performed are among the most controversial points in epilepsy surgery.[15–17] In patients with symptomatic focal epilepsy, the main problem consists in understanding the complex topographic and functional relationships between an anatomic (presumed to be epileptogenic) lesion and the EZ, and there is no general agreement concerning the strategy to adopt. In patients suffering from cryptogenic focal epilepsies, the identification and spatial definition of the EZ must be based on electrical and clinical findings.[18] Presurgical diagnostic approaches include noninvasive or invasive tools, or both. In several epilepsy surgery centers, intracranial electrodes are bilaterally, and often symmetrically, implanted in different standardized anatomic targets,[19–22] in accordance with Gloor's[23] 1991 statement that "intracranial recordings must be designed to avoid biasing the exploration strategy in favor of one's preferred localizing hypothesis."

As far as intracerebral electrodes are concerned, stereo-electroencephalography (SEEG)[24] should be distinguished from the so-called depth electrode recording, "since the purpose of the stereo-electroencephalography is to provide a 3-dimensional (3D) evaluation of the epileptogenic zone that requires placement of electrodes into deep, intermediate, and superficial planes of the brain."[7] The use of SEEG has been proposed as a method of verifying (either with or without evidence of an anatomic lesion) the previously elaborated hypothesis concerning the location and extent of the EZ. Such hypotheses need to be supported by the electroclinical study of spontaneous seizures and by a rigorous stereotactic and stereoscopic anatomic assessment.[25,26]

Careful pre-SEEG assessment of patients is probably at the origin of the following findings:

1. In most SEEG explorations, intracerebral electrodes are unilaterally implanted.[27] In our series of 250 SEEG investigations, more than 80% were unilateral, 18% were bilateral and asymmetrical, and only 2% were bilateral and symmetrical.
2. Intracerebral electrodes are generally implanted in several lobes, with the twofold aim of recording the initial ictal discharges and correlating their early spreading with the early sequence of ictal clinical symptoms.[28,29]

Among several important results obtained with this methodologic approach, we wish to emphasize the following:

1. The individual EZ may be observed extending beyond the classic landmarks of each cerebral lobe.
2. Multilobar partial cortical resections may then be proposed and performed in patients with focal

---

[†]Before his untimely death in 1999, Claudio Munari was the Chief of the Epilepsy Surgery Center of Ni Guardia Hospital and also the first author of this chapter in earlier editions of this book. We dedicate this chapter in this new edition to our master and friend, whose "unique blend of intellectual provocation and human warmth"[63] marked his life and affected all his pupils. His memory continuously inspires and strengthens our work.

epilepsies that are either cryptogenic or associated with limited anatomic lesions, and not only in focal epileptic patients with severe, extended, hemispheric anatomic lesions (i.e., as an alternative solution to hemispherectomy).

PREOPERATIVE EVALUATION

Noninvasive

Collection of historical and clinical information is mandatory in candidates for surgical treatment of drug-resistant focal epilepsy. Age at seizure onset must be assessed, as must seizure frequency and semeiology. Chronology of ictal symptoms must be accurately defined by carefully questioning the patients about subjective manifestations and witnesses about objective signs occurring during seizures. The possible occurrence of loss of contact must be assessed, as must the presence of postictal deficits. This initial step may provide crucial clues as to lateralization and/or gross localization of ictal onset.[30]

Interictal EEG is helpful in determining the side and site of epileptiform and of slow-wave activity. Long-term monitoring with scalp video-EEG recording, coupled with direct intensive surveillance of the patient allowing detailed ictal clinical examination, is mandatory when electroclinical correlates are needed.[31]

High-resolution magnetic resonance imaging (MRI) provides valuable anatomic information in these patients. The neuroradiologist must be aware of the electroclinical features of the patient to be evaluated, in order to tailor the study to the individual case. In patients suspected to have a temporal lobe involvement, transverse and coronal slices are oriented parallel and perpendicular to the major hippocampal axis, respectively. Images are oriented according to the bicommissural line when electroclinical data suggest an extratemporal epilepsy. Transverse double-echo, T2-weighted coronal turbo spin-echo (TSE), T2-weighted coronal TSE fluid-attenuation-inversion-recovery (FLAIR), and T1-weighted coronal inversion-recovery (IR) are acquired in all patients, with additional sequences and slices obtained when needed.[32] By these means, in more than 90% of the patients undergoing surgery in our center (regardless of the site of resection), an anatomic lesion has been demonstrated.

In multilobar epilepsies it is not infrequent to deal with highly functional areas and with cases presenting with altered anatomic patterns in eloquent regions (as often encountered in malformations of cortical development). In these cases, functional magnetic resonance imaging[33] (fMRI) is particularly helpful in defining the limits of activated areas by, for instance, motor[34] or speech tasks,[35] thus allowing the surgeon to minimize the risks for unacceptable new neurologic deficits.[36]

The correlation among anatomic, EEG, and clinical data, supported by a full neuropsychological evaluation and, when needed, by a Wada test for language lateralization, is then employed to formulate a coherent hypothesis as to the localization of the EZ. A high degree of correlation allows surgery to be offered to a large amount of patients (about 60% in our center) without the need for further invasive investigations.

Invasive

When noninvasive investigations alone fail to correctly define the EZ, and/or when the EZ (or the anatomic lesion) are suspected to involve highly functional regions, invasive recording with stereotactically implanted intracerebral electrodes is indicated. This further diagnostic step is required in approximately 40% of patients undergoing surgery in our center. For each patient, the strategy of intracerebral electrode placement is tailored according to previously acquired clinical, electrical, and anatomic data.

Planning of electrode trajectories is accomplished by using stereotactic and stereoscopic cerebral angiography, coregistered by landmark anatomic correlation with a 3D MRI (Spoiled Gradient Echo T1-weighted sequence, slice thickness 1 mm, no gap, matrix 512 × 512). The employment of these two imaging modalities enables the clinician both to identify the cerebral structures to be explored and to plan avascular trajectories, in order to minimize the risk for bleeding from injured vessels. Intracerebral multilead semiflexible platinum-iridium electrodes (diameter 0.8 mm; 5 to 18 contacts of 1.5 mm length, 2 mm apart) are implanted under general anesthesia, according to the Talairach methodology.[37] Titanium hollow screws are fixed to the bone following transcutaneous twist drill trephination, and the electrodes are then advanced to the desired targets under fluoroscopic control. Most of the trajectories are orthogonal to the sagittal plane of the Talairach's frame, but in many instances oblique trajectories are used, with the aid of either a manual or a robotized tool holder.[38] By these means, any superficial, intermediate, or deep/mesial structure, as well as anatomic lesions, may be sampled. Up to 20 electrodes per patient have been employed, with an average of 12 electrodes per patient. When bilateral (20% of explorations), intracerebral implants are rarely symmetrical, with a limited number of "sentinel" electrodes contralateral to the side of the suspected origin of the discharge when an early contralateral spread of the discharge is suggested by ictal surface EEG.

The temporal lobe and, respectively, the rolandic region (pre- and postcentral gyri with the corresponding portion of the operculum and paracentral lobule) have at least one implanted electrode in approximately 80% of procedures, the frontal and parietal lobes in 70%, and the occipital lobe in 40%. The insular cortex is sampled in less than 20% of implants, by electrodes inserted through the supra- or infrasylvian opercula or by a retroinsular trajectory with a frontopolar entry point (Fig. 97-1).

After implantation, a 3D MRI is obtained in order to verify the actual position of each electrode and to detect the possible occurrence of complications linked to the procedure. Some examples of exploration strategies are illustrated in Figures 97-2 and 97-3.

Once awake from anesthesia, the patient is moved to the EEG laboratory and video-stereo-EEG monitoring begins. Once the number of recorded habitual seizures is considered adequate for the single case under evaluation, low- and high-frequency electrical stimulations to contiguous leads are delivered, with the twofold aim of inducing seizures and performing a functional mapping of highly eloquent cortex and pathways.[39,40] At the end of monitoring (mean duration approximately 10 days), the electrodes are removed.

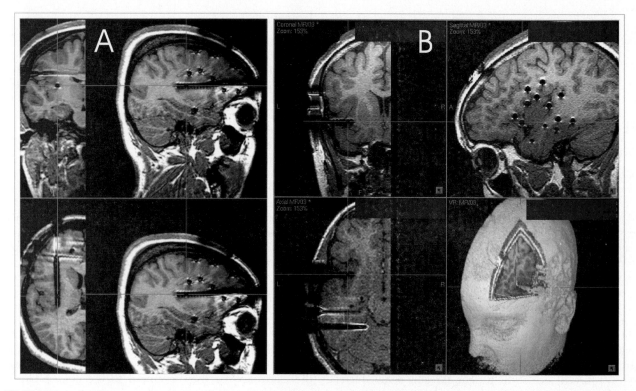

FIGURE 97-1 Insular cortex may be sampled by stereotactically implanted intracerebral electrodes employing either retroinsular trajectories with a frontopolar entry point (*A*) or transopercular-transcysternal trajectories (*B*).

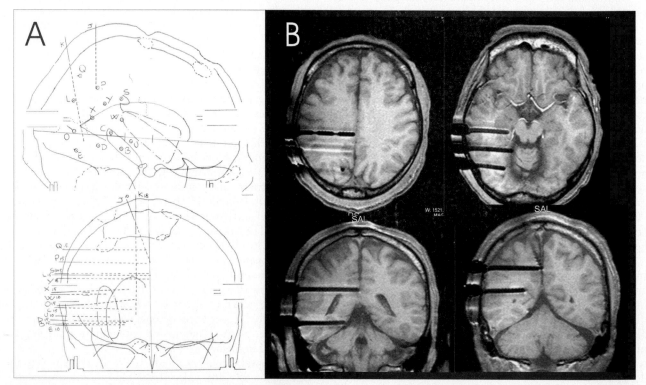

FIGURE 97-2 *A,* Stereotactic diagram (lateral and frontal views) obtained from stereotactic angiography of a stereoelectroencephalography exploration. In this 35-year-old man, who previously received callosotomy in another center with poor results on seizures, the noninvasive electroclinical findings suggested right parietotemporo-occipital origin of the ictal discharges, with magnetic resonance imaging (MRI) showing no definite abnormalities. The scheme outlines the main skull structures (including the margins of the previous frontal parasagittal craniotomy for callosotomy) and the vascular landmarks of the insula, sylvian fissure, central sulcus, and mesial aspect of the occipital lobe. The 15 intracerebral electrodes are indicated with upper-case letters, and they are represented either as circles or as dotted lines (each dot indicates single contacts of the electrode). The exploration was designed in order to sample the posterior portion of the temporal lobe and both occipital and parietal lobes. Each electrode records from lateral, intermediate, and mesial cortex. *B,* Postimplantation T1-weighted MRI sequences showing intracerebral electrodes. The explored structures are easily recognizable in these images.

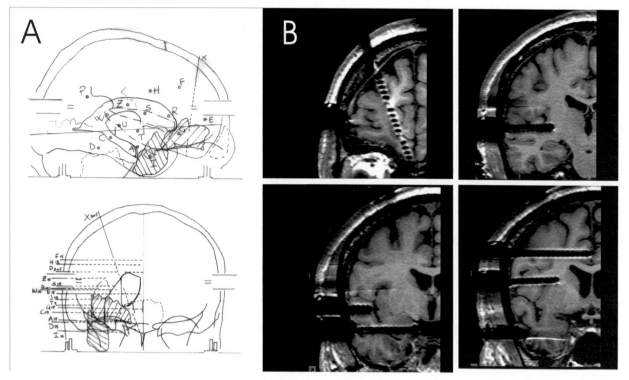

FIGURE 97-3 *A,* Stereotactic diagram showing a stereoelectroencephalography investigation with 16 intracerebral electrodes. This 36-year-old man suffered from posttraumatic epilepsy. Ictal electroencephalography showed early modifications on a wide frontocentraltemporal region of the right hemisphere. Magnetic resonance imaging (MRI) documented posttraumatic lesions in the frontobasal and temporopolar regions (*dashed areas*). For details see Figure 97-2. *B,* Postimplantation MRI showing intracerebral electrodes.

Review of the SEEG data is performed by at least two neurologists, and, based on the electrical features of the investigation, it leads to the definition of three distinct electrical entities: (1) the lesional zone, identified by depression of background activity and/or by the prevalence of slow wave activity; (2) the irritative zone, defined by the presence of epileptiform activity; and (3) the EZ, corresponding to the region of ictal onset and early spread of the discharge. The topographic relationships of the different zones with the possible anatomic lesion are also defined. On these grounds, a tailored surgical strategy is formulated and discussed with the patient, along with the chances of achieving control of seizures and the associated surgical risks.

This method can lead to the finding that in some cases initial ictal discharges do not respect the anatomic limits of a single cerebral lobe, therefore corresponding to the diagnosis of multilobar epilepsy. This has been the case in 37% of the patients undergoing surgery after SEEG recording in our center. On the other hand, only 7% of patients evaluated by noninvasive investigations underwent a multilobar resection.

SURGICAL MANAGEMENT

The larger the epileptogenic cortex to be removed, the harder the compromise to be reached between the desire to cure each patient and the fear of creating new neurologic or neuropsychological damage. The well-known concept of critical mass[41] does apply to epilepsy surgery, and the decision on the extent of the EZ in multilobar partial epilepsies raises several particular diagnostic and therapeutic problems. In surgical planning, several questions can be considered that have no standard solutions and could have different answers depending on the characteristic of each patient and the attitude, feelings, and experience of the different epilepsy surgery teams:

- What are the criteria for identifying the actual epileptogenic cortex?
- Should only the cortical areas that are affected by the ictal discharges at the onset of the seizures be removed?
- How long is the onset? One second? Five seconds? Or longer?
- If the initial clinical symptom occurs several seconds after the onset of the electrical discharge, is removal of the symptomatogenic cortex mandatory,[42] or will removal of only the initially affected cortical region be sufficient?
- What is the risk of removing all of the epileptogenic cortex?
- What kind of neurologic or neuropsychological deficits can be induced? Are all of them predictable?

ANESTHETIC CONSIDERATIONS

Resective surgery for treatment of focal epilepsy does not require anesthetic approaches substantially differing from those commonly employed in other intracranial procedures. In our center, resections are performed under general anesthesia, with the patient positioned according to the site of surgery. Prophylactic antibiotics (intravenous cephamezine 1 to 2 g) are given at anesthesia induction. Candidates for surgical treatment of severe partial epilepsy are commonly in very good physical conditions, and their interictal intracranial pressure (ICP) is not elevated.[43] Careful anesthesiologic management (mostly hyperventilation, diuretics, or barbiturates) can be helpful when the volume of the exposed brain suddenly increases. This transitory increase in ICP may suggest the occurrence of an epileptic seizure,[44] the clinical symptoms of which are masked by anesthesia. Except for this infrequent, transitory, and easily controlled incident, no other major intraoperative complications occur.

SURGICAL TECHNIQUE

As compared with classical approaches for unilobar resections, those adopted for multilobar excisions are tailored according to the site and extension of removal. The supine position is usually preferred even when surgery is performed on the posterior portions of the hemisphere, with the operating table being tilted and the head rotated in order to obtain a comfortable access to the surgical field. The prone position is used mainly when resection involves the mesial aspects of the parietal or occipital lobes. Both skin incision and bone flap are designed to fully expose the region to be removed as well as the surrounding cortical areas. In some instances, when a two-step procedure is likely, the surgeon must take into account the possible subsequent step when fashioning skin and bone flaps. In patients who have been previously evaluated by SEEG, the tracks of electrodes can be easily identified on the bone surface, and they are used as landmarks to plan the extent of the bone flap. While opening the dura mater, if an SEEG has been previously performed, care should be taken to separate the adhesions between the inner aspect of the dura and the cortical surface at the electrodes' entry points. Once the dura is opened, it is very useful to compare the vascular surgical anatomy with the stereoscopic angiograms obtained preoperatively, which provide an exquisite 3D view of the sulcal and gyral pattern

of the region.[45] Careful inspection of the exposed cortex enables the surgeon to identify the entry points of intracerebral electrodes, which are used to draw the borders of resection (Fig. 97-4).

Neuronavigation is helpful in optimizing precision and safety of the procedure, and it is routinely employed in our center. Skin markers are applied on the patient's head, and a 3D fast field echo (FFE) MRI sequence is obtained and imported in the neuronavigation workstation the day before surgery. Different anatomic and functional elements can then be included in the neuronavigational planning:

- The volume of either the lesion, the planned resection, any region of interest (e.g., the ventricular cavities), and highly functional areas as identified by intracerebral electrical stimulations
- The electrode trajectories of a previous SEEG, whose tracks are usually easily identified on the MRI
- The volume of cortical areas activated at fMRI (in the latter case, an additional data set is imported and coregistered to the data set employed for neuronavigation) (Fig. 97-5)

With the aid of the surgical microscope, resection is accomplished according to a few simple rules:

- Vessels crossing the region of resection but tributaries of, or draining from, regions outside its borders must be identified on the stereoscopic angiograms, isolated, and left intact.
- Subpial dissection should be preferred, especially in mesial regions and along the main fissures, in order to protect vascular and extra-axial nervous

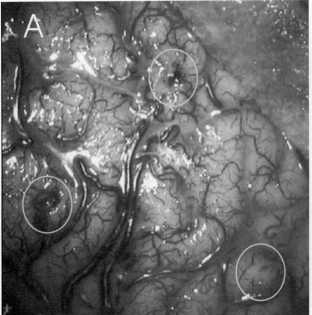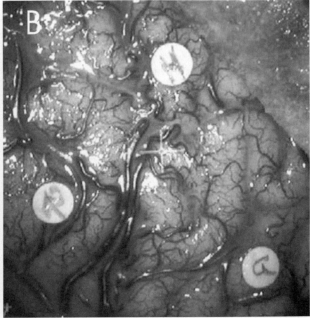

FIGURE 97-4   *A,* The tracks left by the multilead electrodes of a previous stereoelectroencephalography at the cortical entry point are still clearly visible at surgery several months after their removal. *B,* Before starting cortical excision, lettered paper tags are used to mark every electrode's entry point, in order to correctly draw the planned resection on the cortical surface.

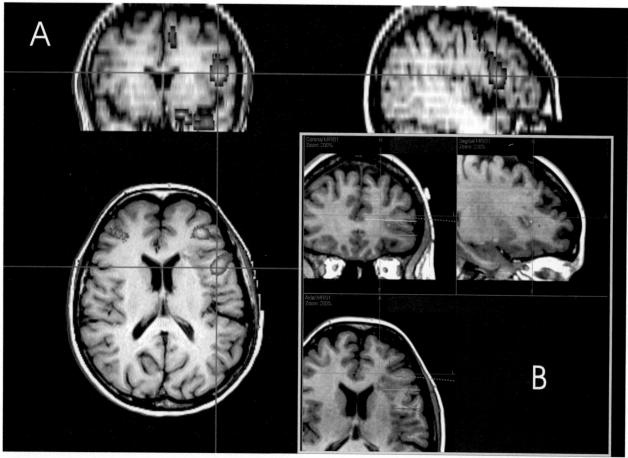

FIGURE 97-5 Functional magnetic resonance imaging data in neuronavigation planning. *A*, Multiplanar reconstruction of structural imaging (three-dimensional T1 FFE-weighted sequence) with functional overlay showing two areas of activation-obtained speech tasks. These two areas lie anteriorly and posteriorly to the lesion, a Taylor-type focal cortical dysplasia extending from the cortical convexity of the left inferior frontal gyrus to the lateral wall of the frontal horn. *B*, Multiplanar reconstruction of neuronavigation planning: the two activated areas are bordered with red dot lines, and the lesion with a green dot line. Fusion of the two sequences was obtained by point-to-point coregistration.

structures (e.g., those in the prepeduncular cistern during mesial temporal removal).

- Suction and bipolar coagulation should be avoided whenever possible, in order to obtain as many unaltered specimens as possible available for histopathologic evaluation.

At dural closure, intravenous phenytoin (10 to 15 mg/kg body weight) is administered over a 20-minute period. At the end of surgery the patient is moved to the intensive care unit, and anesthesia is progressively tapered. Habitual oral antiepileptic medicaments are given as soon as the patient can safely swallow.

The anatomofunctional basis of morbidity in multilobar resections does not differ substantially from that of unilobar resections, and it is strictly dependent on the site of surgery. So transient motor impairment, akinesia, and mutacism may occur after surgery in the posteromesial aspect of the frontal lobe as a consequence of removal of the supplementary motor area,[46] transient speech disturbances may be experienced following resections involving the neocortex of the dominant temporal lobe, and contralateral superior quadrantoanopia is usually a permanent and expected deficit in anterior temporal lobectomies. When temporo-occipital resections are performed, the risk for larger contralateral visual field defects is higher, as is also true in patients subjected to parietotemporal or parieto-occipital excisions. When removal is contiguous to the rolandic region, the risk for motor-sensory impairment is usually increased, and functional mapping by either intracerebral electrical stimulations at SEEG, as well as fMRI, are crucial tools employed to minimize the chances of unwanted postoperative deficits.

CLINICAL SERIES

From May 1996 to February 2004, 453 patients underwent resective surgery at our center for severe, drug-resistant focal epilepsy, and in 94 of them resection included cortical areas of two or more adjacent lobes (multilobar resections).

Three hundred eighty-two patients (including 80 with multilobar resections, 20.9%) with a postoperative follow-up of at least 12 months were available in order to evaluate surgical results on seizures. Their general characteristics are summarized in Table 97-1.

TABLE 97-1 ▪ General Features of the 382 Patients Who Received Resective Surgery and with a Follow-up of at Least 12 Months

	Sex (M/F)	Mean Age at Surgery (years)	Mean Age at Epilepsy Onset (years)	Mean Epilepsy Duration (years)	Median Seizure Frequency (no. per month)	Right/Left Epilepsies (no.)	Preoperative MRI (Positive/Negative)
Unilobar resections (302)	162/140	27.7 ± 11.8	8.8 ± 8.1	18.8 ± 11.2	10 (4–30)	168/134	91.1%–8.9%
Multilobar resections (80)	45/35	23.0 ± 13.7	5.8 ± 5.3	17.0 ± 11.5	35 (15–90)	49/31	85.0%–15.0%

SEEG investigation was performed in 82.5% of patients (66 of 80) with multilobar resections and in 34.4% of patients (104 of 302) with unilobar excisions (Table 97-2).

Sites of unilobar and, respectively, multilobar resections are summarized in Tables 97-3 and 97-4. Multilobar resections included the temporal lobe in 46 cases, and they were exclusively extratemporal in 34 patients (see Table 97-4).

Major surgical morbidity was detected in three patients. In two of these (one of whom presented with a platelet aggregation deficit) postoperative intracranial bleeding occurred, with full recovery after surgical evacuation of the clot. Following a wide cortical resection, another patient developed acute hydrocephalus, which was successfully treated with cerebrospinal fluid shunt. The only major unexpected neurologic complication was represented by permanent mild speech disturbances after a left-sided frontocentral resection.

The findings of histologic examination in both uni- and multilobar resections are indicated in Table 97-5. The most frequent diagnosis among malformative pathologies was focal cortical dysplasia (114 cases, 29.3%); among neoplastic lesions, gangliogliomas (39 cases, 10.2%) and dysembrioplastic neuroepithelial tumors (DNT) (34 cases, 8.9%) prevailed over other tumoral types.

In 21 patients (5.5%, 5 cases in multilobar and 16 cases in unilobar resections), no significant histologic abnormalities were found in the resected tissue. Mesial temporal sclerosis (MTS) was found in 129 patients (33.8%). In 38 of these (all unilobar resections), MTS was the only disclosed histologic abnormality. In other 21 patients, excessive fragmentation of the amygdalohippocampal specimens prevented an adequate histologic evaluation for MTS.

The postoperative results on seizures are reported in Tables 97-6 and 97-7, according to the Engel's classification.[47] Completely seizure-free patients (classes Ia and Ic) were 64.6% and 31.3% in unilobar and multilobar cases, respectively.

ILLUSTRATIVE CASE 1

This 15-year-old girl underwent repeated surgery (at 2.4 and 13 months of age, respectively) for a complex cardiac malformation, following several hypoxic-anoxic episodes occurring since birth.

At 4 years of age she started presenting with seizures, which became drug resistant despite different pharmacologic attempts.

When she was referred to our center at 15 years of age, seizures were clinically characterized by nonlateralized blurred vision, head and eye deviation toward the left side, loss of contact, and inconstant late oroalimentary automatisms. No peri-ictal speech disturbances were reported. Abrupt ictal falls with no prodromic symptoms were also described. Seizure frequency was three to four episodes daily.

Results of the neurologic examinations were normal, with a WISC-R (Wechler Intelligence Scale for Children–revised) score of 73 (verbal score 79; performance score 71).

Scalp video-EEG disclosed a slower background activity in the right hemisphere and interictal slow waves and spike and waves in the right temporo-occipital regions. Ictal EEG showed an early low-voltage fast activity in the right posterior leads, with late spread to the homologous contralateral regions. Brain MRI documented two separate lesions of a possible ischemic nature in the right hemisphere, involving, respectively, the basal occipital and the rolandic regions (Fig. 97-6A). An SEEG investigation was performed in order to evaluate the relationships between the occipital anatomic lesion and the EZ,

TABLE 97-2 ▪ Invasive Recording by Stereoelectroencepalography (SEEG) in Patients with Uni- and Multilobar Resections

	SEEG Performed	SEEG Not Performed
Unilobar resections	104 (34.4%)	198 (65.6%)
Multilobar resections	66 (82.5%)	14 (17.5%)

TABLE 97-3 ▪ Sites of Resection in 302 Patients with Unilobar Surgery

Lobe	No. (%)
Temporal	218 (72.2)
Frontal	66 (21.8)
Parietal	13 (4.3)
Occipital	3 (1.0)
Central	2 (0.7)

TABLE 97-4 ▪ **Sites of Resection in 80 Patients with Multilobar Surgery**

Lobes	No. (%)
Multilobar (T)	46 (57.5)
TO	16
TOP	15
TP	7
TF	4
TOPCF	2
TCF	2
Multilobar (extraT)	34 (42.5)
OP	16
CF	9
PCF	2
OPCF	2
OPC	2
PC	1
FI	1
CFI	1

T, multilobar resection including areas of the temporal lobe; extraT, multilobar extratemporal resections; TO, temporo-occipital; TOP, temporo-occipito-parietal; TP, temporo-parietal; TF, temporo-frontal; TOPCF, temporo-occipito-centro-frontal; OP, occipito-parietal; CF, centro-frontal; PCF, parieto-centro-frontal; OPCF, occipito-parieto-centro-frontal; OPC, occipito-parieto-central; PC, parieto-central; FI, fronto-insular; CFI, centro-fronto-insular.

which were suspected to also involve the parietal and temporal lobes on the basis of the electroclinical findings (see Fig. 97-6B). No electroclinical data indicated the need to sample the rolandic lesion by intracerebral electrodes. Electroclinical correlations obtained during SEEG recording localized the EZ in the inferior half of the occipital lobe (electrodes L and V), and in the posterior mesiobasal aspect of the temporal lobe (electrodes F and E) (see Fig. 97-6C). Surgical resection of the EZ was performed (see Fig. 97-6D), and histologic examination documented gliotic changes in the excised tissue corresponding to the MRI lesion. The patient was left with an expected and anticipated complete left-sided hemianopia, and she is seizure free since undergoing surgery after 3 years of follow-up.

ILLUSTRATIVE CASE 2

A maternal aunt of this 18-month-old young girl suffers from partial epilepsy. Partial placenta detachment at the

fourth month of pregnancy was reported. Since the age of 15 days, despite different pharmacologic treatments, multiple seizures started, occurring mostly at sleep onset. They were characterized by repeated bilateral arm raising, predominant to the right, then by bending on her left side, and finally by clonic jerks on the right side.

The neurologic examination at admittance in our Centre showed a right mild hemiparesis and failure to acquire deambulation.

Interictal scalp EEG showed asymmetric (better organized on the right side) background activity. The physiologic spindles and K complex were localized only in the right hemisphere, and continuous spiking and slow wave activity was observed in the left centroparietal region (Fig. 97-7A and B). Ictal EEG discharges, represented by a flattening followed by rhythmic slow spikes and waves, involved the left parietocentral region (see Fig. 97-7C).

The cerebral MRI (see Fig. 97-7D) demonstrated the presence of a cortical malformative lesion in the parasagittal parietocentral region of the left hemisphere.

On the basis of anatomoelectroclinical correlations, a lesionectomy was performed (see Fig. 97-7E). The histologic examination disclosed a Taylor-type focal cortical dysplasia. Postoperatively, she completely recovered from her preoperative right upper limb weakness. Since surgery (1 year follow-up) she is seizure free and she acquired autonomous deambulation, even of the lower limb paresis was substantially unchanged.

FINAL REMARKS

Presurgical investigations should provide a correct definition of the EZ (the cortical areas where the ictal discharges originate and whose removal results in abolition of seizures). As invasive EEG recording is potentially dangerous, time consuming, and expensive,[48,49] indications to surgery for epilepsy should be based, whenever possible, on non-invasive investigations. However, "general statements as to areas of possible agreement on whether noninvasive tests are sufficient should only be attempted after taking into consideration specific situations or goals."[50]

In most instances, an accurate presurgical evaluation of patients may allow the diagnosis of unilobar epilepsy with reasonable certainty. This is the case, for example, with central lobe seizures, which are easily recognized based only on the highly localizing value of ictal clinical signs, although surgery for these situations is hardly pursued for

TABLE 97-5 ▪ **Findings at Histologic Examination in the Resected Specimens, for both Uni- and Multilobar Surgery**

	Cryptogenetic	Malformation	Neoplastic	Degenerative/Flogistic
Unilobar resections	54 (17.9%) (MTS: 38)	155 (51.3%) (MTS: 66)	85 (28.2%) (MTS: 17)	8 (2.6%) (MTS: 1)
Multilobar resections	5 (6.3%) (MTS: 0)	44 (55.0%) (MTS: 3)	16 (20.0%) (MTS: 1)	15 (18.7%) (MTS: 3)

Association of histologically documented MTS is indicated in parentheses; MTS, mesial temporal sclerosis.

TABLE 97-6 ▪ Results on Seizures in 302 Unilobar Resections (According to Engel's Classification)

Class	No.	%
I	235	77.8
Ia+c	195	64.6
II	25	8.3
III	18	6.0
IV	24	7.9

Ia+c, completely seizure-free patients.

obvious functional reasons, unless a severe and stable neurologic deficit is already present. Similarly, patients in whom the origin of the discharge, with a limited local propagation, is suspected to involve the poles of the temporal, occipital, or frontal lobes, especially when associated with a clear and well-circumscribed anatomic lesion,[51] can benefit from a limited resection carried out in a single lobe with satisfactory results on seizures. In the same way, the more or less standardized surgical procedures advocated for temporal lobe epilepsy provide an excellent rate of complete benefit from seizures in a high percentage of patients.[1,52] Nevertheless, even in these apparently simple cases, a rate of noncured patients still exists,[53–56] raising the question as to the correct preoperative localization of the EZ. One of the possible answers to this question is that the ictal discharge originating in the resected areas of a single lobe actually may exceed its limits, involving the neighboring lobe(s). As a matter of fact, multilobar seizures may be suspected in cases with particularly complex clinical ictal patterns, suggestive of the participation of a widespread area of different regions, or when interictal and ictal EEG abnormalities involve an extended brain region, or when a large anatomic lesion is detected by MRI. It must be stressed that no one of these findings alone legitimates drawing definite conclusions as to the "multilobarity" of epilepsy in a given patient. In our opinion, anatomic, clinical, and electrical findings must be coherently correlated in order to formulate a hypothesis as to the localization of the EZ. In this view, a limited anatomic lesion may sustain a multilobar organization of the ictal discharge, and a limited extent of the EZ is demonstrated even in cases with a diffuse anatomic lesion. Incidentally, this latter statement raises the question as to whether all patients with diffuse, or even hemispheric, structural abnormalities should be considered for hemispheric resections or disconnections, or if some of them can benefit from more limited removals.

We have presented a series of patients with a preoperative diagnosis of multilobar epilepsy. Compared with a previous report on multilobar resections,[57] an increasing number of lesions have been demonstrated preoperatively, possibly because of the increasing ability of newer-generation high-resolution MRI to detect small-sized subtle abnormalities. Despite the increasing evidence of associated lesions in these patients, the definition of the EZ has relied heavily on electroclinical evidences. Actually, SEEG has been employed in 82.5% of patients who received multilobar resections, compared with 34.4% of cases with unilobar surgery, a figure that accounts for the complexity of these cases.

An increasing number of multilobar, "posterior" resections involving the temporal cortex is performed in our center. This can be explained with the increasing evidence that a number of patients exist in whom ictal symptoms of temporal lobe involvement actually are preceded by other subtle signs that, if adequately sought, may account for an initial involvement of the occipital or parietal lobes.[58] On the other hand, it is not uncommon that a discharge originating in the posterior aspect of the basal temporal cortex propagates to the basal occipital cortex. In this latter instance, it is not difficult to anticipate how a "standardized" temporal resection is doomed to failure.

It is not surprising that, as far as the histologic substrate of epilepsy is concerned, patients undergoing multilobar resection present with a higher rate of degenerative-flogistic abnormalities in the resected specimens, as compared with unilobar resections. Cerebral inflammatory pathologies are most often diffused, thus accounting for the involvement of large brain areas in the epileptogenic process.

Results on seizures of multilobar resections are by far less gratifying than those for unilobar, especially temporal lobe, resections (Table 97-8), with only 47.5% of patients in class I and 31.3% completely seizure free, and this rather disappointing figure is in good agreement with the data in the literature.[51,55,59–62] Slightly better results are observed in multilobar resections, including the temporal lobe. It must be stressed, however, that despite a complex epileptologic situation, which could hardly be improved by further drug regimens, patients can be cured or improved (classes I to III, approximately 75% in our series) with surgical treatment.

We feel that careful presurgical selection, carried out according to a rigorous evaluation of all the anatomic, clinical, and electrophysiological findings available, may provide remarkable improvement even to patients suffering from a challenging epileptic disorder such as multilobar epilepsy.

TABLE 97-7 ▪ Results on Seizures in 80 Multilobar Resections (According to Engel's Classification)

Class	All Multilobar Resections (80)		Multilobar (extraT) (34)		Multilobar (T) (46)	
	No.	%	No.	%	No.	%
I	38	47.5	15	44.1	23	50.0
Ia+c	25	31.3	10	29.4	15	32.6
II	14	17.5	3	8.8	11	23.9
III	7	8.8	4	11.8	3	6.5
IV	21	26.2	12	35.3	9	19.6

A separate evaluation of results in multilobar (T) and multilobar (extra T) cases is also reported (see text and Table 97-4).

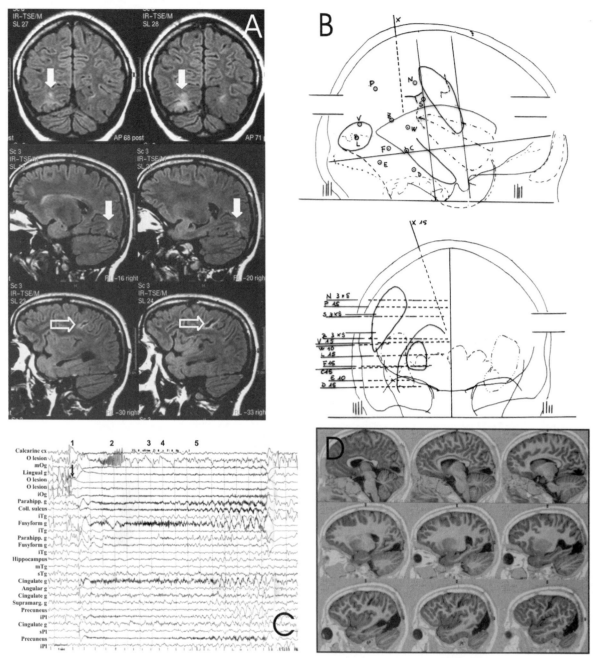

FIGURE 97-6 *A,* Brain magnetic resonance imaging (MRI) (coronal and sagittal sections, T2-weighted fluid-attenuation-inversion-recovery sequences) showing two separate mainly hyperintense lesions in the right rolandic region (*open arrows*) and in the basal aspect of the ipsilateral occipital lobe (*closed arrows*). Electroclinical noninvasive findings suggested a right occipito-parieto-temporal localization of the epileptogenic zone. *B,* Stereotactic scheme of the stereoelectroencephalography (SEEG) exploration, lateral and frontal views of the skull. Dashed areas indicate the sites of the lesions imported from the MRI coregistered with stereotactic angiography. The 16 stereotactically implanted intracerebral electrodes are indicated by letters. Explored structures were, from lateral to mesial, as follows: D, inferior temporal gyrus, fusiform gyrus, parahippocampal gyrus; E, inferior temporal gyrus, fusiform gyrus; C, middle temporal gyrus, posterior hippocampus, parahippocampal gyrus; F, inferior temporal gyrus, parahippocampal gyrus; W, posterior part of the superior temporal gyrus; L, inferior occipital gyrus, occipital lesion, lingual gyrus; V, middle occipital gyrus, lesion, calcarine cortex; Z, angular gyrus, posterior cingulated gyrus; S, supramarginal gyrus, postcentral cingulated gyrus; P, inferior parietal lobule, precuneus; N, supramarginal gyrus, precuneus; X, superior parietal lobule, precuneus, posterior cingulate gyrus. *C,* Ictal SEEG: the recorded spontaneous seizure showed a sequence of polyspikes well localized in the lingual gyrus and inferior calcarine cortex (on L1 and V1), followed by a low-voltage fast activity (*arrow*) on the same leads, and, with a delay of about 500 msec, the involvement of the fusiform and parahippocampal gyri (F1 and E1). The ictal discharge spreading to other structures appeared less prominent. The clinical symptomatology was characterized by an oculocephalic deviation toward the left, grimacing (1), then a further rotation of the head to the left (2), the patient calls her mother (3), raising a dystonic left arm (4), and finally a rotation of the trunk to the left appeared (5). No speech disturbance was observed in the postictal period. Cx, cortex; O, occipital; mOg, middle occipital gyrus; iOg, inferior occipital gyrus; Parahipp, parahippocampal; Coll, collateral; iTg, inferior temporal gyrus; mTg, middle temporal gyrus; sTg, superior temporal gyrus; Supramarg, supramarginal; iPl, inferior parietal lobule; sPl, superior parietal lobule. *D,* Postoperative brain MRI (sagittal T1-weighted inversion recovery sequences), showing resection of the mesiobasal and dorsolateral portions of the right occipital lobe as well as of the posterior mesiobasal cortex of the temporal lobe.

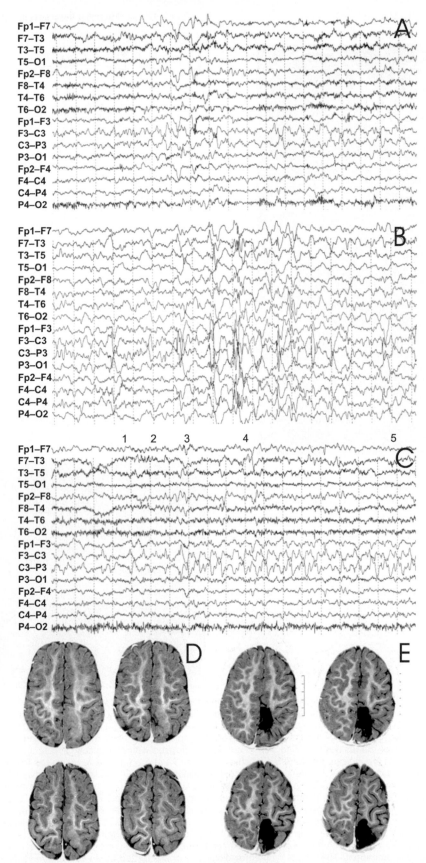

FIGURE 97-7 *A,* Scalp electroencephalogram (EEG) during wakefulness, showing a continuous pathologic activity localized on the left parietocentral region, characterized by delta slow waves intermingled by slow spikes. *B,* Scalp EEG: the same interictal activity on the left parietocentral region, emphasized by sleep. *C,* Scalp EEG: the spontaneous seizure was characterized by a flattening in the parietocentral region followed by rhythmic spikes and waves. The patient repetitively raises both upper limbs (1, 2, and 3), then she bends on the left side (4), and right clonic jerks appear in the late phases of the seizure (5). *D,* Axial T1-weighted inversion recovery magnetic resonance imaging (MRI) sequences, showing altered signal involving the left superior parietal lobule and the parasagittal portion of the two central convolutions, including the paracentral lobule. Signal abnormality was suggestive of a focal cortical dysplasia. *E,* Postoperative MRI, same sequence as in *B.* Resection was extended to the whole abnormal tissue. At histology a Taylor-type focal cortical dysplasia was diagnosed.

TABLE 97-8 ▪ Literature Evidence Reporting Seizure Outcome in Multilobar Resections (Publication Period 1998–2003)

Investigators	Described Population	Outcome: Seizure Free/Non–Seizure Free (Only Multilobar)
Francione et al, 2003[59]	10 pediatric patients with FCD	1/2 (50%)
Kral et al, 2003[51]	53 patients with FCD	0/1 (0%)
Bernasconi et al, 2001[60]	8 double cortex patients	1/2 (50%)
Edwards et al, 2000[61]	35 patients with MCD	6/11 (55%)
Paolicchi et al, 2000[55]	75 pediatric patients with DRFE	2/9 (22%)
Duchowny et al, 1998[62]	31 pediatric patients with DRFE	2/5 (40%)

FCD, focal cortical dysplasia; MCD, malformation of cortical development; DRFE, drug-resistant focal epilepsy.

REFERENCES

1. Engel J Jr, Shewmon DA: Overview: Who should be considered a surgical candidate? In Engel J Jr (ed): Surgical Treatment of the Epilepsies, 2nd ed. New York: Raven, 1993, pp 23–34.
2. Hardiman O, Burke T, Phillips J, et al: Microdysgenesis in resected temporal neocortex: Incidence and clinical significance in focal epilepsy. Neurology 38:1041–1047, 1988.
3. Yasargil MG, Teddy PJ, Roth P: Selective amygdalohippocampectomy: Operative anatomy and surgical technique. In Symon L, et al (eds): Advances and Technical Standards in Neurosurgery, vol 12. Vienna: Springer-Verlag, 1985, pp 93–123.
4. Villemure JG: Hemispherectomy techniques. In Lüders HO (ed): Epilepsy Surgery. New York: Raven, 1991, pp 569–578.
5. Krynauw RA: Infantile hemiplegia treated by removing one cerebral hemisphere. J Neurol Neurosurg Psychiatry 13:243–267, 1950.
6. Rasmussen T: Hemispherectomy for seizures revisited. Can J Neurol Sci 10:71–78, 1983.
7. Olivier A: Extratemporal cortical resections: Principles and methods. In Lüders HO (ed): Epilepsy Surgery. New York: Raven, 1991, pp 559–568.
8. Olivier A, Awad IA: Extratemporal resections. In Engel J Jr (ed): Surgical Treatment of the Epilepsies, 2nd ed. New York: Raven, 1993, pp 489–500.
9. Farrel MA, DeRosa MJ, Curran JG, et al: Neuropathologic findings in cortical resections (including hemispherectomies) performed for the treatment of intractable childhood epilepsy. Acta Neuropathol 83:246–259, 1992.
10. Villemure JG, Vernet O, Delalande O: Hemispheric disconnections: Callosotomy and hemispherotomy. Adv Tech Stand Neurosurg 26:25–78, 2000.
11. Commission on Classification and Terminology of the International League Against Epilepsy: Proposal for revisited classification of epilepsies and epileptic syndromes. Epilepsia 30:389–399, 1989.
12. Talairach J, Bancaud J, Szikla G, et al: Approche nouvelle de la neurochirurgie de l'épilepsie: Méthodologie stéréotaxique et résultats thérapeutiques. Neurochirurgie 20(Suppl 1):1–240, 1974.
13. Bancaud J, Talairach J, Bonis A, et al: Informations neurophysiopathologiques apportées par l'investigation fonctionnelle stéréotaxique (SEEG) dans les épilepsies. Rev Neurol 108:81–86, 1963.
14. Yasargil MG: Topographic anatomy for microsurgical approaches to intrinsic brain tumors. In Yasargil MG (ed): Microneurosurgery IV A. New York: Thieme, 1994, pp 1–114.
15. Ebner A: Preoperative evaluation in epilepsy surgery: Some principal considerations. In Lüders HO, Comair YG (eds): Epilepsy Surgery. Philadelphia: Lippincott Williams & Wilkins, 2001, pp 177–183.
16. Carreno M, Lüders HO: General principles of presurgical evaluation. In Lüders HO, Comair YG (eds): Epilepsy Surgery. Philadelphia: Lippincott Williams & Wilkins, 2001, pp 185–199.
17. Munari C, Lo Russo G, Minotti L, et al: Presurgical strategies and epilepsy surgery in children: Comparison of literature and personal experiences. Child's Nerv Syst 15:149–157, 1999.
18. Quesney LF, Gloor P: Localization of epileptic foci. Electroencephalogr Clin Neurophysiol 37(Suppl):165–200, 1985.
19. Engel J Jr, Crandall PH: Intensive neurodiagnostic monitoring with intracranial electrodes. In Gumnit R (ed): Intensive Neurodiagnostic Monitoring. New York: Raven, 1986, pp 85–106.
20. McCarthy G, Spencer DD, Riker RJ: The stereotactic placement of depth electrodes in epilepsy. In Lüders HO (ed): Epilepsy Surgery. New York: Raven, 1991, pp 385–393.
21. Olivier A, De LotbiniPre A: Stereotactic techniques in epilepsy. Neurosurgery State Art Rev 2:257–285, 1987.
22. Spencer SS: Depth electroencephalography in selection of refractory epilepsy for surgery. Ann Neurol 9:207–214, 1981.
23. Gloor P: Preoperative electroencephalographic investigation in temporal lobe epilepsy: Extracranial and intracranial recordings. Can J Neurol Sci 18:554–558, 1991.
24. Bancaud J, Talairach J, Bonis A, et al: La Stéréo-Électro-Encéphalographie dans L'épilepsie: Informations Neuro-Physio-Pathologiques Apportées par L'Investigation Fonctionnelle Stéréotaxique. Paris: Masson, 1965.
25. Szikla G, Bouvier G, Hori T, Petrov V: Angiography of the Human Brain Cortex: Atlas of Vascular Patterns and Stereotactic Cortical Localization. Berlin: Springer-Verlag, 1977.
26. Talairach J, Szikla G, Tournoux P, et al: Atlas D'Anatomie Stéréotaxique du Télencéphale: Etudes Anatomo-Radiologiques. Paris: Masson, 1967.
27. Munari C: Depth electrode implantation at hospital Sainte Anne, Paris. In Engel J Jr (ed): Surgical Treatment of the Epilepsies. New York: Raven, 1987, pp 583–588.
28. Munari C, Bancaud J: The role of stereo-electro-encephalography (SEEG) in the evaluation of partial epileptic patients. In Porter RJ, Morselli PL (eds): The Epilepsies. London: Butterworth, 1987, pp 267–306.
29. Wieser HG: Electroclinical Features of the Psychomotor Seizure. London: Butterworth, Gustave Fisher, 1983.
30. Wieser HG, Williamson PD: Ictal semeiology. In Engel J Jr (ed): Surgical Treatment of the Epilepsies, 2nd ed. New York: Raven Press, 1993, pp 161–171.
31. Munari C, Kahane P: Traitement neurochirurgical de l'épilepsie. Encycl Méd Chir. Neurologie, 17-700-D-10. Paris: Elsevier, 1998, p 14.
32. Colombo N, Tassi L, Galli C, et al: Focal cortical dysplasias: MR imaging, histopathologic, and clinical correlations in surgically treated patients with epilepsy. AJNR Am J Neuroradiol 24:724–733, 2003.
33. Moritz C, Houghton V: Functional MR imaging: Paradigms for clinical preoperative mapping. Magn Reson Imaging Clin North Am 11:529–542, 2003.
34. Alkadhi H, Crelier GR, Boendermaker SH, et al: Reproducibility of primary motor cortex somatotopy under controlled conditions. AJNR Am J Neuroradiol 23:1524–1532, 2002.
35. Springer JA, Binder JR, Hammeke TA, et al: Language dominance in neurologically normal and epilepsy subjects: A functional MRI study. Brain 122:2033–2045, 1999.
36. Heilbrun MP, Lee JN, Alvord L: Practical application of fMRI for surgical planning. Stereotact Funct Neurosurg 76:168–174, 2001.
37. Munari C, Giallonardo AT, Musolino A, et al: Specific neuroradiological examinations necessary for stereotactic procedures. In Wieser HG, Elger CE (eds): Presurgical Evaluation of Epileptics. Berlin: Springer-Verlag, 1987, pp 141–145.

38. Benabid AL, Cinquin P, Lavalle S, et al: Computer-driven robot for stereotactic surgery connected to CT scan and magnetic resonance imaging: Technological design and preliminary results. Appl Neurophysiol 50:153–154, 1987.

39. Kahane P, Tassi L, Francione S, et al: Manifestations électro-cliniques induites par la stimulation électrique intra-cérébrale par "chocs" dans les épilepsies temporales. Neurophysiol Clin 22:305–326, 1993.

40. Munari C, Kahane P, Tassi L, et al: Intracerebral low frequency electrical stimulation: A new tool for the definition of the "epileptogenic area"? Acta Neurochir Suppl (Wien) 58:181–185, 1993.

41. Rasmussen T: Cortical resection for medically refractory focal epilepsy: Results, lessons and questions. In Rasmussen T, Marino R (eds): Functional Neurosurgery. New York: Raven, 1979, pp 253–269.

42. Lüders HO, Engel J Jr, Munari C: General principles. In Engel J Jr (ed): Surgical Treatment of the Epilepsies, 2nd ed. New York: Raven, 1993, pp 137–153.

43. Munari C, Andreoli A, Frattarelli M, et al: Activation par l'Amitryptiline (remarques électrocliniques à propos de 120 patients épileptiques). Rev EEG Neurophysiol 7:194–197, 1977.

44. Penfield W, Jasper H: Epilepsy and the Functional Anatomy of the Human Brain. Boston: Little, Brown, 1954.

45. Yasargil MG: Introduction. In Yasargil MG (ed): Microneurosurgery IV B. New York: Thieme, 1996, pp xix–xxi.

46. Ainik A, Lehericy S, Duffau H, et al: Role of the supplementary motor area in motor deficit following medial frontal lobe surgery. Neurology 57:871–878, 2001.

47. Engel J Jr: Outcome with respect to epileptic seizures. In Engel J Jr (ed): Surgical Treatment of the Epilepsies. New York: Raven, 1987, pp 553–571.

48. Sperling MR, Mendius JR: Strategies for semi-invasive and invasive approaches. In Engel J Jr (ed): Surgical Treatment of the Epilepsies, 2nd ed. New York: Raven, 1993, pp 451–454.

49. Munari C, Hoffmann D, Francione S, et al: Stereo-electroencephalography methodology: Advantages and limits. Acta Neurol Scand (Suppl) 152:56–67, 1994.

50. Ajmone Marsan O: When are noninvasive tests enough? In Engel J Jr (ed): Surgical Treatment of the Epilepsies, 2nd ed. New York: Raven, 1993, pp 313–318.

51. Kral T, Clusmann H, Blumcke I, et al: Outcome of epilepsy surgery in focal cortical dysplasia. J Neurol Neurosurg Psychiatry 74:183–188, 2003.

52. Primrose DC, Ojemann G: Outcome of resective surgery for temporal lobe epilepsy. In Lüders HO (ed): Epilepsy Surgery. New York: Raven, 1991, pp 601–611.

53. Koszewsky W, Czarkwiani L, Bidzinski J: Multilobar resections in surgical treatment of medically intractable epilepsy. Neurol Neurochir Pol 32 (Suppl 2):81–94, 1998.

54. Leiphart JW, Peacock WJ, Mathern GW: Lobar and multilobar resections for medically intractable pediatric epilepsy. Pediatr Neurosurg 34:311–318, 2001.

55. Paolicchi JM, Jayakar P, Dean P, et al: Predictors of outcome in pediatric epilepsy surgery. Neurology 54:642–647, 2000.

56. Foldvary N, Nashold B, Mascha E, et al: Seizure outcome after temporal lobectomy for temporal lobe epilepsy: A Kaplan-Meier survival analysis. Neurology 54:630–637, 2000.

57. Munari C, Francione S, Kahane P, et al: Multilobar resections for the control of epilepsy. In Schmidek HH (ed): Operative Neurosurgical Techniques. Philadelphia: WB Saunders, 2000, pp 1473–1489.

58. Elisevich K, Smith BJ: Surgery for parieto-occipital epilepsy. In Lüders HO, Comair YG (eds): Epilepsy Surgery, 2nd ed. Philadelphia: Lippincott Williams & Wilkins, 2001, pp 705–718.

59. Francione S, Vigliano P, Tassi L, et al: Surgery for drug resistant partial epilepsy in children with focal cortical dysplasia: Anatomical-clinical correlations and neurophysiological data in 10 patients. J Neurol Neurosurg Psychiatry 74:1493–1501, 2003.

60. Bernasconi A, Martinez V, Rosa-Neto P, et al: Surgical resection for intractable epilepsy in "double cortex" syndrome yields inadequate results. Epilepsia 42:1124–1129, 2001.

61. Edwards JC, Wyllie E, Ruggeri PM, et al: Seizure outcome after surgery for epilepsy due to malformation of cortical development. Neurology 55:1110–1114, 2000.

62. Duchowny M, Jayakar P, Resnick T, et al: Epilepsy surgery in the first three years of life. Epilepsia 39:737–743, 1998.

63. Avanzini G. Obituary. Claudio Munari (1943–1999). Clin Neurophysiol 111:951–952, 2000.

98 Multiple Subpial Transection for Epilepsy

RICHARD W. BYRNE and WALTER W. WHISLER

Multiple subpial transection (MST) is a surgical technique designed to address the problem of seizure foci originating in eloquent cortex. In these areas, such as speech areas and sensorimotor cortex, surgical resection would result in unacceptable deficits. The technique is based on experimental evidence showing the following:

1. Human neocortex is functionally arranged in vertical columns.[1-4]
2. Epileptic discharges spread and synchronize horizontally along interconnecting cortical fibers.[5-8]
3. A minimal cortical area of 12.5 mm^2 is required to generate a synchronous paroxysmal seizure discharge.[9]
4. Vertical transection of eloquent cortex produces minimal, if any, permanent deficit.[10-13]

Based on the aforementioned concepts, Morrell and colleagues[10] conceived of the technique of MST. He found that focal seizures produced by a penicillin lesion in the motor cortex of the monkey could be stopped by subpial transection in the seizure focus at intervals of 5 mm perpendicular to the long axis of the gyrus. After the procedure, the monkey was clinically and electrographically seizure free for 1 year and did not suffer permanent loss of motor function after the transection. Later resection of this cortex caused paralysis.[14]

The clinical application and surgical technique of MST was then developed by Morrell and Whisler and used at the Rush Epilepsy Center in cases in which the seizure focus existed entirely in eloquent cortex or extended into eloquent cortex. The initial report of the series described promising results in a diverse population of patients, many of whom were previously considered inoperable.[10] Since the initial report, our experience with MST has grown to include more than 100 patients. This chapter reports our long-term experience and the experience of other centers.

PATIENT SELECTION

Patients considered for MST suffer medically intractable focal onset epilepsy in eloquent cortex. Patients undergo a thorough medical trial and evaluation, including video-electroencephalography, magnetic resonance imaging (MRI) with thin coronal sections, and neuropsychiatric evaluation. Positron emission tomography, ictal single photon emission computed tomography, functional MRI, Wada's test, methohexital suppression test, and intracranial epidural or subdural electrode recording and stimulation are done when appropriate. Further delineation of the epileptogenic zone and the eloquent cortex is performed at the time of surgery with electrocorticography, somatosensory evoked potential responses, and functional mapping. Patients who have mesial temporal or frontal onset of seizures without eloquent cortical involvement are treated by standard resective surgery. Patients with lesional epilepsy are first treated with removal of the lesion and the epileptogenic cortex, if it is greater than 1.5 cm from eloquent cortex. If electrocorticography shows further epileptogenic cortex in eloquent areas, MST is considered. Epileptogenic cortex is delineated either by ictal recording of seizure onset or by convergent interictal data and electrocorticography that show a clear seizure focus that displays an electrical field. This focus must be differentiated from mere spikes on electrocorticography, which are not appropriate for MST. This differentiation requires an experienced electrocorticographer.

Patients with Landau-Kleffner syndrome (LKS) (epileptic aphasia that develops in previously developmentally normal children) have also been treated by MST.[15-22] This acquired aphasia is thought to be secondary to continuous slow spike and wave epileptic discharge of focal onset in the parasylvian cortex affecting the speech areas.[23] MST of the epileptic trigger zone as delineated by electroencephalography, MRI, positron emission tomography, magnetoencephalography, and electrocorticography reduces or eliminates the slow spike and wave discharge on electrocorticography. Table 98-1 summarizes these and other indications for MST.

POSITIONING AND ANESTHESIA

Patients are given preoperative antibiotics and steroids. After intubation and the placement of a Foley catheter and leg compression boots, the patient is positioned laterally with Mayfield head fixation, and pressure points are padded. The head is kept true lateral in all cases, unless we anticipate opening the sylvian fissure or access to the midline is needed. Cases in which MST is being considered are usually extratemporal or posterior temporal and may require a large exposure. If surgery is being performed on an awake patient, all possible accommodations to patient comfort are made to help the patient endure a lengthy operation.

TABLE 98-1 ▪ Indications for Multiple Subpial Transection

Seizure focus arising in eloquent cortex
Persistent seizure activity in eloquent cortex after resection of noneloquent cortex
Landau-Kleffner syndrome
Epilepsia partialis continua—motor or sensory
Rasmussen's encephalitis in functional motor cortex (cases in which hemispherectomy is not yet appropriate)

Anesthesia is achieved with intravenous methohexital when general anesthesia is desired. Methohexital is known to induce seizure activity on electrocorticography but also may preferentially activate seizure foci.[24–26] Local anesthesia is used generously, particularly if surgery is performed on an awake patient. In cases of awake surgery, intravenous sedation is used to allow the patient to sleep through the opening and closing. The planned incision is infiltrated with a mixture of lidocaine 1% and 0.25% bupivacaine. A field block is also performed with particular attention to the origin of the scalp nerves. The operative area is then prepared and draped.

OPERATIVE PROCEDURE

An appropriately wide scalp flap is opened. A craniotomy and dural opening expose the involved cortex, as delineated by preoperative evaluation. Electrocorticography of the exposed cortex is performed before any surgical intervention. An electrocorticography grid and six contact cylindric electrodes placed subtemporally, subfrontally, or anywhere the preoperative evaluation deems necessary are used. Functional mapping is then performed, if not previously done with subdural grid placement.

In most cases in which MST is being considered, the epileptic focus, as delineated by preoperative testing and electrocorticography, overlaps eloquent and noneloquent cortex. In these cases the noneloquent cortex is first resected, then electrocorticography is repeated. If the resection of noneloquent cortex does not resolve the epileptic discharges from the adjacent eloquent cortex, MST is performed. In rare cases, the epileptic focus is entirely in eloquent cortex. In these cases, MST is the only choice and the only procedure done. In most cases of LKS, the seizure focus lies within the sylvian fissure, and the fissure is opened carefully before MST.

TRANSECTIONS

The area to be transected usually does not follow exact anatomic borders. The gyral and vascular anatomy are carefully inspected, and great care is taken to avoid vessels traversing the gyri or running deep in the sulci. The transections are performed starting in the more dependent regions. These areas are done first because subarachnoid blood gravitates to the dependent area and obscures these regions. To help drain this subarachnoid blood, a small hole is made in the pia arachnoid membrane.

Care is taken to ensure that the transections are perpendicular to the long axis of each gyrus. This transection pattern is not always possible in situations in which the gyri bend or in areas with a microgyral pattern.[27,28] Once a starting point is decided on, a 20-gauge needle is used to puncture a small hole in an avascular area of the pia at the edge of the gyrus. The subpial transection hook (Whisler-Morrell Subpial Transector, Redman Neurotechnologists, Lake Zurich, IL, U.S.A.), as seen in Figure 98-1, is held with the 4-mm point upward. The tip of the transector is introduced through the pial opening and advanced across the gray matter of the gyrus in a stepwise fashion (Fig. 98-2). The instrument has a malleable wire, which may be bent slightly to accommodate most angles. The hook of the wire is bent at 105 degrees to make snagging a vessel in a sulcus less likely. Once the contralateral sulcus is reached, the

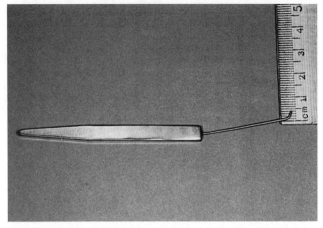

FIGURE 98-1 Whisler-Morrell Subpial Transector, Redman Neurotechnologists, Lake Zurich, Illinois.

instrument is retrieved along the same path with the tip visible beneath the pia. The pia is spared because much of the cortical blood supply runs in this layer. A small piece of gelatin sponge is placed over the pial opening, and a cottonoid is placed over the transection line. The next transection is made 5 mm away from the first transection and in a parallel direction. If bleeding from a previous transection obscures the area, transections are made on a separate gyrus while waiting for the first area to become clear again. If an area is covered by a confluence of veins or in the area of the vein of Labbé or sylvian fissure, it is not always possible to make transections safely at 5-mm intervals. In these instances, the anatomy of the region dictates the interval of transection. After the area is transected, further electrocorticography is done. The usual findings on electrocorticography after MST are a resolution or decrease in the epileptic activity and a depression of background rhythm. If further spiking occurs in the transected area, it usually occurs in an area that was incompletely transected. In some cases, it may be from deep within a sulcus. If this is the case, the sulci in the area can be transected. This situation requires caution not to disrupt the pial membranes of the sulcus and its blood vessels.

In cases in which transections are done in the sylvian fissure, deep sulci, or intrahemispheric area, it is useful to reverse the orientation of the transection hook so that the tip faces away from the pial surface.[29–31] This reversal makes it less likely that the tip will snag a vessel in these hard-to-visualize areas.

It is important that the hook of the instrument maintain a vertical orientation because only a small deviation from the vertical can cause extensive cortical undercutting. At the conclusion of the procedure, fine red parallel lines are seen on the cortical surface (Fig. 98-3). All intracortical and subpial bleeding resolves with Gelfoam sponge and gentle pressure. Several researchers have introduced modifications of this technique. Wyler proposed the introduction of the transection tip in an orientation with the tip pointing into the cortex instead of toward the pia.[32] In cases where initial transection did not resolve the epileptic discharge, Spencer and Schramm have both proposed additional transections in an orientation at right angles to the first set of transections.[33–35]

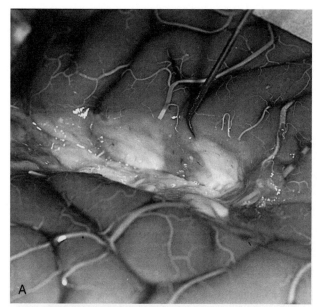

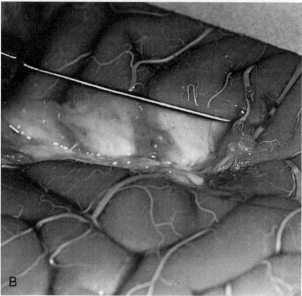

FIGURE 98-2 *A,* The subpial transector is introduced through the opened pia as seen in this cadaver specimen with a coronal section removed. *B,* The transector is carefully advanced through the gray matter with the tip pointed upward. This is done perpendicular to the long axis of the gyrus until the opposite sulcus is reached. The transector is then withdrawn along the same transection line with the tip visible beneath the pia.

RADIOLOGY

Early computed tomography and MRI findings in MST show fine lines of cortical blood and edema in the areas transected. MRI scans done at 6 months show these fine cortical lines with resolution of the edema. In some patients in whom substantial hemorrhage has occurred, these areas of hemorrhage have a cystic appearance by 6 months. They also show hemosiderin deposits and focal gyral atrophy (Fig. 98-4).

PATHOLOGY

Two studies have been done on the histologic changes that occur in cortex that has undergone subpial transection.

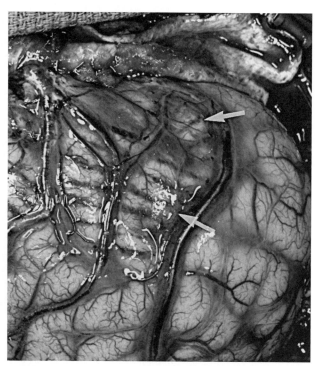

FIGURE 98-3 An operative photograph of subpial transection of the pre- and postcentral gyrus in a patient with a seizure focus localized to this area. *Arrows* point to the transection lines.

The first study showed acute and chronic changes secondary to MST.[27] Acutely, hemorrhage, edema, and some evidence of local cell injury were noted. Chronic changes showed gliosis, some microcystic changes, preservation of interval neuronal columns, and no regrowth of connections. The depth of transection corresponded well to the depth of the gray matter.

The second study showed that variability in cortical thickness, microgyral patterns, gyral angles, and variability in technique can lead to oblique transections, white matter transection, and more extensive cell loss.[28,29] As can be seen in Figure 98-4A, care must be taken to account for these variables, and the direction of the transections is adjusted accordingly.

RESULTS

Seizure Outcome

Outcome with respect to seizure control is best analyzed in the following categories to see the effect of MST:

1. Patients who underwent only MST for focal seizures
2. Patients who underwent only MST for LKS
3. Patients who underwent MST of eloquent cortex after resection of noneloquent areas

The first category gives the best indication of the effects of MST because resection is not a confounding variable (Table 98-2). In our series, 32 patients underwent only MST. Sixteen of these patients had focal seizures in the sensorimotor or speech areas. Six of these 16 patients became seizure free. Another six patients had rare seizures or greater than 90% reduction in seizures. In total, 75% of

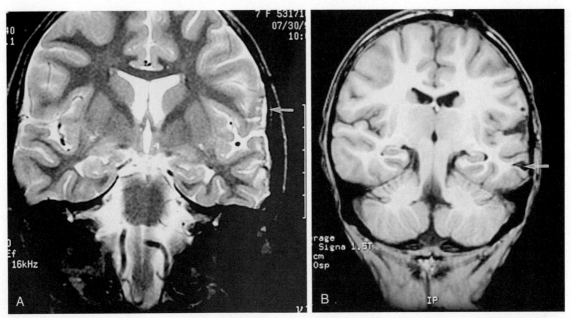

FIGURE 98-4 *A*, Postoperative coronal T2-weighted magnetic resonance image (MRI) showing the typical appearance of subpial transections in the left parasylvian cortex 6 months after surgery. *Arrows* point to the transection lines. *B*, Postoperative coronal T1-weighted MRI showing cystic changes in the temporal lobe after subpial transection in this region.

these patients who were considered medically intractable with seizures arising in unresectable eloquent cortex had a worthwhile 90% or greater improvement in seizure frequency (Engel class I through III). Because these patients were previously considered inoperable, these results should be compared with medical therapy in intractable epilepsy or with resection of eloquent cortex with its resultant deficits.

The second category for analysis is MST for LKS. As previously described, LKS is a seizure disorder manifested as an acquired epileptic aphasia of childhood in previously normal children. This stands in distinction from autistic children. Epileptic discharges in autistic children are likely an epiphenomenon of a more widespread brain disorder and are therefore not appropriate for surgical treatment. Although children with LKS do have seizures, it is thought that the aphasia results from the near-continuous bombardment and disruption of the speech areas by the slow spike-and-wave discharge characteristic of the syndrome. This discharge can be shown in most cases to be of focal onset in or near the sylvian fissure. Transection of this focus and the neighboring speech areas in our series resolved the continuous

discharge in 9 of 16 patients.[15] Thirteen of 16 patients were able to regain speech within 2 years. Of these children, seven regained age-appropriate speech. This is an improvement over the natural history of LKS, in which most patients have a permanent, severe, language deficit. Without intervention, the slow spike-and-wave discharge usually resolves by age 15, an average of 10 years after its onset.[15,16,23] By this age, if speech is not developed, it develops poorly at best.[15,16,23]

The final category for analysis is MST after resection of noneloquent cortex. In our series, this was the most common indication for MST because most seizure foci do not lie entirely in eloquent cortex. Because a resection is done adjacent to the transected area, it is difficult in these cases to determine if the resultant seizure control or morbidity is attributable to the resection or the transections. The data on MST alone, however, clearly show that MST does have an effect on seizure outcome. Overall, seizure control and morbidity attributed to transection and resection are shown in Table 98-2. These numbers include many extratemporal and posterior temporal neocortical cases, which were previously considered inoperable.

TABLE 98-2 ▪ Postsurgical Outcome in Patients with Partial Seizure Disorders Only

Surgical Procedure	n	Engel Classification				Neurologic Complication	
		Class I	Class II	Class III	Class IV	Transient	Permanent
MST only* (partial seizure disorder)	16	6 (37.5%)	4 (25%)	2 (12.5%)	4 (25%)	1 (6%)	3 (19%)
MST and resection of noneloquent cortex	68	33 (48.5%)	7 (10%)	16 (23.5%)	12 (18%)	7 (10%)	4 (6%)
Total	84	39 (46.5%)	11 (13%)	18 (21.5%)	16 (19%)	8 (9.8%)	7 (8.3%)

*The outcome of 16 children with Landau-Kleffner syndrome is presented in the text.
  MST, multiple subpial transection.
  From Morrell F, Kanner A, Whisler W: Multiple subpial transection. In Stefan H, Anderman F (eds): Plasticity in Epilepsy. Philadelphia: Lippincott-Raven, 1998.

TABLE 98-3 ▪ Epilepsy Center Multiple Subpial Transection Experience

Investigator	Year	Total No.	Pure	Plus Resection	Good Outcome (>75% Improvement)	Permanent Complications
Spencer Meta-analysis	2002	211	53	158	154/211	47
Schramm	2002	20	20	0	9/20	0
Mulligan	2001	12	4	8	5/12	0
Hufnagel	1997	22	6	16	15/22	5
Wyler	1995	6	4	2	5/6	0
Sawhney	1995	18	6	12	11/18	0

Many other centers have reported their outcomes from MST over the past 10 years.[34-44] Spencer and colleagues performed an international meta-analysis on the MST experience of six centers in 211 patients.[45] Their results showed an excellent outcome (>95% reduction in seizure frequency) in 68% of the 45 patients with simple partial seizures who underwent MST with resection. In patients who underwent MST alone for simple partial seizures, 63% had an excellent outcome. Similar outcomes were noted in patients who underwent MST for complex partial and generalized seizure disorders. Overall, 65% (35 of 54) of the patients who had MST as their only procedure had an excellent outcome in the meta-analysis.[45] At individual centers the published results show efficacy in seizure control, but complete seizure cessation is less common (Table 98-3). Wyler reported a series of six cases of uniform pathology where MST was the only procedure done.[33] Of the six patients, with at least 1 year follow-up, four had at least an Engel class III outcome (greater than 90% improved). Schramm and colleagues reported a series of 20 patients of nonuniform pathology who underwent MST as the only procedure.[35] Forty-five percent of patients achieved at least an Engel class III. A trend toward better outcome was noted in nonlesional cases and in cases of limited epileptogenic area. Mulligan and colleagues reported the Yale experience in 12 patients, 4 of whom had MST alone.[34] Patients in this series had nonuniform pathology, but most cases involved sensorimotor cortex. Five of the 12 patients had a greater than 75% reduction in their seizures. Two additional patients had a significant reduction in their seizure severity.

Morbidity

We have performed MST in more than 100 patients at the Rush Epilepsy Center. In the postoperative period, it is common to see subtle, transient dysfunction of the areas transected. These deficits almost always clear over the course of 2 to 4 weeks. If a computed tomography scan is done, it usually reveals only edema and small cortical or subcortical hemorrhage.

There has been no mortality associated with subpial transection in our series of more than 100 patients. In 20 cases, temporary (lasting more than 1 month) or permanent complications have occurred. Of these 20 complications, 14 were attributable to subpial transection. Of these 14, only 5 were permanent. These complications corresponded to the areas transected with the exception of one unrelated basal ganglia hemorrhage causing permanent hemiparesis.

These permanent complications include two patients with foot weakness after retraction and transection of parasagittal motor cortex, one patient with permanent worsening of a preoperative dysphasia, and one patient with a posterior temporal lobe hemorrhagic infarct. Transient complications in eight patients corresponded to the areas transected; these complications were hemiparesis,[3] monoparesis,[3] sensory loss,[1] and dyslexia.[1] One patient had an asymptomatic deep hemorrhage.

Other complications in our series corresponded to the resection of noneloquent brain or other surgical complications. Of these, only two (a visual field deficit and a mild sensory loss) were permanent. One case each of phlebitis, orchitis, meningitis, and sixth nerve palsy resolved. Our final complication rate in these MST cases, including all permanent deficits, was 7%. In Schramm's series of 20 cases of pure MST without resection, there was no significant permanent morbidity related to MST.[35] Transient morbidity related to the area transected was common. These deficits resolved over days to months. In the Yale series, all patients had a transient deficit that gradually resolved over 6 months.[34] In the meta-analysis, 10 of 53 patients who had MST as the only procedure had new deficits. Four had hemiparesis, one had a visual field deficit, and four had memory complaints.[45]

CONCLUSIONS

MST is a useful technique when applied to well-defined seizure foci residing in eloquent cortex. It can be performed with only a small risk of permanent morbidity in patients who were previously considered inoperable. Our initial success with the procedure has now been duplicated at many epilepsy centers throughout the world.[37-59] Further research into the effects of cortical transection and the physiology of seizure foci will likely make this technique even more safe and effective.

REFERENCES

1. Mountcastle VB: Modality and topographic properties of single neurons of cat's somatic sensory cortex. J Neurophysiol 20:408–434, 1957.
2. Mountcastle VB: The columnar organization of the neocortex. Brain 120:701–722, 1957.
3. Asanuma H: Recent developments in the study of the columnar arrangement of neurons within the motor cortex. Physiol Rev 55:143–156, 1975.
4. Hubel DH, Wiesel TN: Receptive fields, binocular interaction and functional architecture in the cat's visual cortex. J Physiol 160:106–154, 1962.

5. Morrell F: Microelectrode studies in chronic epileptic foci. Epilepsia 2:81–88, 1961.
6. Morrell F: Cellular pathophysiology of focal epilepsy. Epilepsia 10:495–505, 1969.
7. Morrell F: Secondary epileptogenic lesions. Epilepsia 1:538–560, 1959/1960.
8. Tharp BR: The penicillin focus: A study of field characteristics using cross-correlation analysis. Electroencephalogr Clin Neurophysiol 31:45–55, 1971.
9. Lueders H, Bustamente L, Zablow L, et al: The independence of closely spaced discrete experimental spike foci. Neurology 31:846–851, 1981.
10. Morrell F, Whisler WW, Bleck T: Multiple subpial transection: A new approach to the surgical treatment of focal epilepsy. J Neurosurg 70:231–239, 1989.
11. Sperry RW, Miner N: Pattern perception following insertion of mica plates into visual cortex. J Comp Physiol Psychol 48:463–469, 1955.
12. Sperry RW, Miner N, Myers RE: Visual pattern perception following subpial slicing and tantalum wire implantations in visual cortex. J Comp Physiol Psychol 48:50–58, 1955.
13. Sperry RW: Physiological plasticity and brain circuit theory. In Harlow HF, Woolsey CN (eds): Biological and Biochemical Bases of Behavior. Madison, WI: University of Wisconsin Press, 1958.
14. Morrell F, Whisler WW, Smith MC: Multiple subpial transection in Rasmussen's encephalitis. In Andermann F (ed): Chronical Encephalitis and Epilepsy: Rasmussen's Syndrome. Boston: Butterworth-Heinemann, 1981, pp 219–234.
15. Morrell F, Whisler WW, Smith MC, et al: Landau-Kleffner syndrome: Treatment with subpial intracortical transection. Brain 118:1529–1546, 1985.
16. Morrell F, Kanner AM, Hoeppner TJ, et al: Multiple subpial transection for selected cases of Landau-Kleffner syndrome. In Tuxhorn I, Holthausen H, Boenigk HE (eds): Pediatric Epilepsy Syndromes and Their Surgical Treatment. London: John Libbey (in press).
17. Rintahaka PJ, Chugani HT, Sankar R: Landau-Kleffner syndrome with continuous spikes and waves during slow-wave sleep. J Child Neurol 10:127–133, 1985.
18. Grote C, Van Slyke P, Hoeppner J-A: Language outcome following multiple subpial transection for Landau-Kleffner syndrome. Brain 122:561–566, 1989.
19. Irwin K, et al: Multiple subpial transection in Landau-Kleffner syndrome. Dev Med Child Neurol 43:248–252, 2001.
20. Otsubo H, et al: Malignant rolandic-sylvian epilepsy in children. Neurology 57:590–596, 2001.
21. Paetau R, et al: Magnetoencephalography in presurgical evaluation of children with Landau-Kleffner syndrome. Epilepsia 40:326–335, 1989.
22. Robinson R, et al: Landau-Kleffner syndrome: Course and correlates with outcome. Dev Med Child Neurol 43:243–247, 2001.
23. Landau W, Kleffner F: Syndrome of acquired aphasia with convulsive disorder in children. Neurology 7:523–530, 1957.
24. Wyler AR, Richey ET, Atkinson RA, et al: Methohexital activation of epileptogenic foci during acute electroencephalography. Epilepsia 28:490–494, 1987.
25. Hardiman O, Coughlan A, O'Moore B, et al: Interictal spike localization with methohexital: Pre-operative activation and surgical follow-up. Epilepsia 28:335–339, 1987.
26. Hufnagel A, Burr W, Elger CE, et al: Localization of the epileptical focus during methohexital-induced anesthesia. Epilepsia 33:271–284, 1982.
27. Pierre-Louis SJC, Smith MC, Morrell F, et al: Anatomical effects of multiple subpial transection. Epilepsia 34:104(Suppl), 1983.
28. Whisler WW: Letters to Editor. Epilepsia 38:258–260, 1987.
29. Kauffmann W, Kraus G, Uematsu S, et al: Treatment of epilepsy with multiple subpial transections: An acute histologic analysis in human subjects. Epilepsia 37:342–352, 1986.
30. Whisler WW: Multiple subpial transection. In Rengachary SS (ed): Neurosurgical Operative Atlas, vol 6. Park Ridge, IL: American Association of Neurological Surgeons, 1987, pp 125–129.

31. Whisler WW: Multiple subpial transection. In Kaye A, Black P (eds): Operative Neurosurgery. Edinburgh: Churchill Livingstone, 1987.
32. Morrell F, Kanner AM, Whisler WW: Multiple subpial transection. In Stefan H, Andermann F (eds): Plasticity in Epilepsy. Philadelphia: Lippincott-Raven, 1988.
33. Wyler A, Wilkins R, Rostad S, Vossler D: Multiple subpial transection for partial seizures on sensorimotor cortex. Neurosurgery 37:1122–1128, 1985.
34. Mulligan L, Spencer D, Spencer S: Multiple subpial transections: The Yale experience. Epilepsia 42:226–229, 2001.
35. Schramm J, Aliashkevich A, Grunwald T: Multiple subpial transactions: outcome and complications in 20 patients who did not undergo resection. J Neurosurg 97:39–47, 2002.
36. Schramm J, et al: Surgery to treat focal frontal lobe epilepsy in adults. J Neurosurg 51:644–655, 2002.
37. D'Giano C, et al: Treatment of refractory partial status epilepticus with multiple subpial transection: Case report. Seizure 10:382–385, 2001.
38. Hufnagel A, et al: Multiple subpial transection for control of epileptic seizures: Effectiveness and safety. Epilepsia 38:678–688, 1987.
39. Misra S, Sinch NN: Management of status epilepticus. J Ind Med Assoc 100:298–303, 2002.
40. Neville BG, et al: Surgical treatment of severe autistic regression in childhood epilepsy. Pediatr Neurol 16:137–140, 1987.
41. Polkey CE: Multiple subpial transection: A clinical assessment. Int Rev Neurobiol 45:547–569, 2001.
42. Rougier A, et al: Multiple subpial transection: Report of 7 cases. Epilepsy 24:57–63, 1986.
43. Smith M: Multiple subpial transection in patients with extratemporal epilepsy: An international met-analysis. Epilepsia 43:141–145, 2002.
44. Zimmerman R, Sirven J: An overview of surgery for chronic seizures. Mayo Clinic Proc 78:109–117, 2003.
45. Spencer S, et al: Multiple subpial transection for intractable partial epilepsy: An international met-analysis. Epilepsia 43:141–145, 2002.
46. Sugiyama S, Fugil M, Ito H: Electrophysiological effects of MST in the experimental model of epilepsy induced by cortical stimulation. Epilepsy Res 25:1–9, 1985.
47. Sawhney IMS, Robertson IJA, Polkey CE, et al: Multiple subpial transection: A review of 21 cases. J Neurol Neurosurg Psychiatry 58:344–349, 1985.
48. Hufnagel A, Zentner J, Fernandez G, et al: Multiple subpial transection for control of epileptic seizures: Effectiveness and safety. Epilepsia 38:678–688, 1987.
49. Devinsky O, Perrine K, Vazquez B, et al: Multiple subpial transections in the language cortex. Brain 117:255–265, 1984.
50. Pacia SV, Devinsky O, Perrine K, et al: Multiple subpial transection for intractable partial seizures: Seizure outcome. J Epilepsy 10:86–91, 1987.
51. Wyler AR, Wilkus RJ, Rotard SW, et al: Multiple subpial transection for partial seizures in sensorimotor cortex. Neurosurgery 37:1122–1128, 1985.
52. Rougier A, Sundstrom L, Claverie B, et al: Multiple subpial transection: Report of 7 cases. Epilepsy Res 24:57–63, 1986.
53. Patil A-A, Andrews RV, Torkelson R: Surgical treatment of intractable seizures with multilobar or bihemispherical seizure foci (MLBHSF). Surg Neurol 47:72–78, 1987.
54. Shimizu H, Suzuki I, Ishijima B, et al: Multiple subpial transection (MST) for the control of seizures that originated in unresectable cortical foci. Jpn J Psychiatr Neurol 45:354–356, 1981.
55. Honavar M, Janota I, Polkey CE: Rasmussen's encephalitis in surgery for epilepsy. Dev Med Child Neurol 34:1–4, 1982.
56. Neville BGR, Harkness WFJ, Cross JH: Surgical treatment of severe autistic regression in childhood epilepsy. Pediatr Neurol 16:137–140, 1987.
57. Zonghui L, Quanjun Z, Shiyue L, et al: Multiple subpial transection for treatment of intractable epilepsy. Chin Med J 108:539–541, 1985.
58. Tanaka T, Yonemasu Y: Basical and clinical approaches for surgical treatment of intractable epilepsies. Clin Neurol 34:1237–1239, 1984.
59. Patil A-A, Andrews R, Torkelson R: Minimally invasive surgical approach for intractable seizures. Stereotact Funct Neurosurg 65:86–89, 1985.

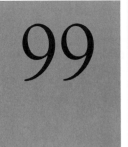

99 Section of the Corpus Callosum for Epilepsy

DAVID W. ROBERTS and ADRIAN M. SIEGEL

For most of the latter half of the 20th century, division of the corpus callosum for the treatment of intractable seizure disorders was an operation evolving from an uncommon but neuropsychologically fascinating surgery to a generally accepted management option for some patients with few therapeutic alternatives. With the introduction and widespread adoption of vagal nerve stimulation (VNS) as an option for refractory but nonresectable epilepsy, the number of corpus callosotomies being performed has decreased dramatically.[1] The less invasive and less morbid nature of VNS make this both understandable and for most patients only appropriate. Nevertheless, there remains a diminished but still recognized role for commissurotomy as an effective palliative procedure, particularly in patients whose seizure disorder has been insufficiently responsive to VNS and in particular other settings such as that of severe drop attacks or where, for a variety of economic, biologic, or other reasons, an implantable device is not a good option. This chapter reviews the larger corpus callosotomy experience, with an aim to better understand the operation's appropriate role today.

Since Horsley's[2] first craniotomy for the treatment of a seizure disorder in 1886, the most widely performed surgery for medically intractable epilepsy has shared the fundamental principle of removing a portion of resectable cerebral cortex presumed to represent the primary epileptogenic focus. In those patients in whom such a focus can be identified, the results of operative intervention are generally rewarding; successful outcome after anterior temporal lobectomy, for example, can be achieved in as many as 92% of patients selected for that procedure.[3] There is a large population of patients with poorly controlled seizures, however, in whom a resectable epileptic focus cannot be identified and who therefore are not candidates for resective surgery. For many of these patients, a palliative procedure, such as VNS, multiple subpial transection, deep brain stimulation, and corpus callosum section, may be of considerable benefit.

In the 1930s, Van Wagenen, having made the observation that patients with epilepsy who subsequently sustained a stroke involving the corpus callosum often had improvement in their seizure disorders, divided the corpus callosum in a small number of patients.[4] This was followed in the early 1960s by the report of Bogen and colleagues[5-7] of a small series of similarly operated patients with encouraging results, and the comparable success of Luessenhop and colleagues[8,9] in three of four children. In 1971, Wilson and colleagues[10-16] chose this procedure as an alternative to hemispherectomy in a 9-year-old boy with infantile hemiplegia and began a series of ultimately 20 patients that demonstrated an efficacy to the procedure, warranting its wider application.

The number of centers performing corpus callosotomy steadily increased over the following two decades, and today the majority of epilepsy centers offer this operation in their surgical armamentarium. Although some questions have remained regarding optimal selection criteria and long-term prognosis, most reported experiences confirm the outcomes of earlier series.[17-61]

Concurrent with the clinical application of commissurotomy, an extensive body of experimental data has developed. Although the effects of callosotomy in nonprimates had been investigated earlier, Erickson's[62] work remains a landmark for its demonstration of the major role played by the corpus callosum in the propagation of seizures in the monkey. The disruption of seizure generalization by division of the commissure has been demonstrated by numerous investigators,[63-69] and these data have often been cited in support of clinical application. Data suggesting no effect or worsening of seizures after commissurotomy also exist.[70,71] For further discussion of nonclinical investigations, the reader is referred to the excellent collection of papers presented at the 1982 Dartmouth Conference on the Corpus Callosum and Epilepsy (*Epilepsy and the Corpus Callosum*, edited by Reeves[72]) and to the review papers of Spencer and colleagues[53] and Blume.[73]

PATIENT SELECTION

In patients in whom a resectable epileptogenic focus can be defined, nearly all centers would agree that a resective procedure is the procedure of choice. The presence of such a definable focus represents perhaps the most important of exclusion criteria for a palliative procedure. Of those patients with refractory epilepsy and no resectable seizure focus, consideration for a palliative procedure, such as VNS, multiple subpial transection, or callosal section, may be appropriate. As noted earlier, VNS is the most common of these performed today, primarily because of its lesser degree of invasiveness and lower morbidity. The intuitive basis for proceeding with a disconnection procedure, conversely, has usually rested on the presumption that propagation of the spreading seizure discharge could be disrupted and the seizure thus confined to one hemisphere. Many early patients were selected for surgery because of secondarily generalized seizures in the setting of demonstrable nondiffuse pathology, such as infantile hemiplegia. Early clinical results suggested better outcome in these as well as in those with less severe but nonetheless confined disease.[10,12,14-16]

In addition to seizure disorders with secondary generalization, other generalized seizure types have been demonstrated to respond favorably to commissurotomy. Most notable among these are the atonic or akinetic seizures generally characterized by sudden drop attacks. Many series, including those of Dartmouth,[11,15] Minnesota,[26,27] and Yale[57] have found either elimination or attenuation of this seizure type in most patients with such spells, and intractability of this seizure type in the setting of no identifiable resective focus is the most favorable and common indication for commissurotomy. Patients incapacitated by this type of seizure should be seriously considered for callosotomy.

The distinction between truly primary generalized seizures and rapidly generalizing seizures may be exceedingly difficult clinically, and we have not excluded from surgery patients who failed to demonstrate evidence of focal onset. Tonic and tonic-clonic generalized seizures as well have been found to respond to commissurotomy and are common seizure disorders coming to such surgery. The majority of patients in callosotomy series have presented with multiple seizure types. Surgical results in terms of seizure type have been reported[11,45,53,57] and are reviewed here.

In an attempt to improve selection criteria, Williamson[74] reviewed surgical outcomes of various series in terms of clinical diagnoses. Classifying patients into groups of infantile hemiplegia, forme fruste infantile hemiplegia, Rasmussen's syndrome, Lennox-Gastaut syndrome, frontal lobe epilepsy, and focal/multifocal epilepsy, he found slightly better outcomes in the first two groups but sufficient improvement to justify surgical intervention in all categories.[74]

Electroencephalographic findings have also been correlated with surgical results.[29,53,54] Both Geoffroy and colleagues[29] and Spencer and colleagues[53] have reported better results in patients with lateralized electroencephalographic abnormalities. Bilaterally synchronous epileptiform activity has been present in the majority of patients and does not represent a necessarily bad prognostic sign.[75] The significance of bilaterally independent foci remains undetermined.

Our selection criteria include (1) medical intractability of at least 2 and usually 4 years' duration, with exhaustive anticonvulsant regimens and documented adequate serum anticonvulsant levels, (2) poor candidacy for VNS or inadequate response to previous VNS, (3) generalized seizures, usually but not necessarily major motor or akinetic in type, and (4) potential functional benefit if improvement in the seizure disorder is achieved. Although the likelihood of success may be less in some instances, we have not automatically excluded patients from surgery because of retardation, age, mixed hemisphere dominance, lack of demonstrable focal seizure onset, or bilaterally independent electroencephalographic abnormalities.

There is less consensus regarding the indications for proceeding to completion of the callosal section in those patients who have already undergone anterior section. The majority of clinical experiences with callosotomy demonstrate superior outcome with respect to seizure control in those patients who have had complete rather than partial section. The success rate of complete section in achieving a significant reduction in seizure frequency has been approximately twice that of partial section in several larger series.[59,76,77] The question of proceeding to completion of the callosal section is a slightly different one, however, and analysis of the incremental benefit derived by patients who go on to completion is required. Review of the experiences at both Dartmouth[76] and Yale[57] demonstrates a very clear benefit in proceeding to completion in those patients with persistent generalized seizures whose response to partial section has been disappointing (discussed further in "Results" section); there has been one report of a patient in whom completion of the section was not associated with such benefit.[24]

SURGICAL TECHNIQUE

Review of the early commissurotomy series shows comparable success rates regardless of whether division of the anterior commissure or one fornix was performed at the time of corpus callosotomy.[12–16] Although there may be individuals in whom these other structures play important roles in seizure propagation, we have restricted our procedure to division of the major commissure and underlying posterior hippocampal commissure only. Whether partial callosotomy is preferable to complete division as an initial procedure is less clear. We are currently advocating partial callosotomy in most patients, with division of two thirds to three fourths of the corpus callosum, unless there is evidence of a predominantly posterior focus. Many of these patients will subsequently require completion of the callosotomy (see later), but it appears preferable to spare those not requiring complete section the effects of greater disconnection.

The surgery is performed under general anesthesia, and intraoperative electroencephalographic recording, when performed, has been primarily for investigative purposes. At least one surgeon has tailored his length of resection based on intraoperative electroencephalographic information,[35] but given the frequency of insufficient electroencephalographic findings intraoperatively as well as the observation of subsequent seizure propagation across remaining adjacent callosal fibers, we have not adopted this practice. For most of our series, we have placed the patient supine on the operating table and secured the unturned head in a three-point pin fixation. For the anterior division, the neck has been left in a neutral position; for the posterior division, it has been flexed approximately 20 degrees. Spencer (personal communication) has described positioning the head laterally, allowing gravity to assist the hemisphere on the side of the approach to fall away and thereby minimize the amount of necessary retraction. We have increasingly used this strategy and can confirm its utility. Decadron (10 mg) and prophylactic antibiotic are administered before surgery.

We have used linear incisions and 2-inch trephinations (Figs. 99-1 and 99-2),[14,78,79] but the type of craniotomy is recognized as relatively unimportant. For the anterior procedure, a 9-cm transverse incision with one third of its length across the midline is placed 2 cm in front of the coronal suture. For the posterior procedure, a similar incision and trephination are employed at the level of the parietal eminence. The placement of the craniotomy across the sagittal sinus requires increased caution but facilitates later exposure down the interhemispheric fissure. The approach is generally on the side of the nondominant right hemisphere except for those instances in which significant pathology is well lateralized to the other.

Angiography for localization of parasagittal draining veins before transcallosal procedures has been advocated by some[80] but has not been a routine study in our series.

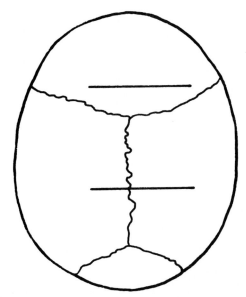

FIGURE 99-1 Anterior and posterior callosal sections are performed through respective 9-cm linear incisions and 2-inch trephinations. (From Roberts DW: Corpus callosotomy. In Reeves AG [ed]: Epilepsy and the Corpus Callosum. New York: Plenum Press, 1985, p 261.)

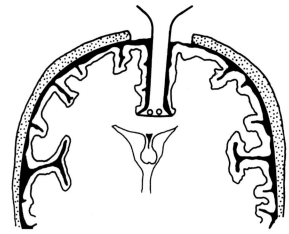

FIGURE 99-3 Minimal retraction is required on the nondominant hemisphere if at all. Retraction of the inferior aspect of the falx and the contralateral cingulate gyrus is occasionally useful. (From Roberts DW: Corpus callosotomy. In Reeves AG [ed]: Epilepsy and the Corpus Callosum. New York: Plenum Press, 1985, p 262.)

Using microsurgical technique, it has always been possible to work on either or both sides of such a vein without requiring its sacrifice. It is interesting and useful to note, nonetheless, the observation of Apuzzo and colleagues[80] that in 42 of 100 angiographic studies, significant veins were noted to enter the sagittal sinus within 2 cm of the coronal suture with 70% of these posterior to that suture. Angiographic information may be available in those patients who have previously undergone Amytal testing, and magnetic resonance angiography/magnetic resonance

venography (MRV) or computed tomography angiography can now delineate parasagittal venous structures.

The dura is opened in a curvilinear fashion and reflected on the sagittal sinus. Initial dissection down the interhemispheric fissure is performed under loupe magnification, and retraction is aided by the administration of mannitol (1 g/kg) during the opening. Pressed Gelfoam protects the exposed cortex, and the Greenberg's self-retaining retractor is placed before using the operating microscope. A single retractor blade gently retracts the ipsilateral hemisphere, and, when needed, an additional blade is used on the inferior aspect of the falx or contralateral cingulate gyrus (Fig. 99-3).

The glistening white appearance of the corpus callosum distinguishes it from the more superficial cingulate gyrus, and exposure along the length of callosum to be divided is obtained before entering the commissure. Adhesions between the hemispheres, especially common in the setting of previous infection or trauma, may make exposure difficult; approaching the callosum more posteriorly and using the deeper extension of the falx will prove helpful in this situation. The pericallosal arteries are easily identified overlying the callosum. The actual division of callosal fibers is carried out most often between these arteries, although division lateral to these vessels, when more convenient, can be performed (Fig. 99-4).

The magnification and illumination provided by the operating microscope are invaluable during the final exposure and actual sectioning. We currently use the Leica microscope–equipped Surgiscope system (Elekta AB, Stockholm, Sweden). Navigational assistance during surgery is not essential to this operation but, if available, facilitates the midline callosal division and helps confirm the length of section. The 300-mm objective lens provides a reasonable working distance to the field, and midlevel magnification is most commonly used. Small vessels supplying only the callosum itself may be coagulated using bipolar cautery. The actual division of callosal fibers is carried out using the microseptal or microsuction tip. As ultrasonic aspiration equipment becomes more refined and smaller, it may prove to be of greater utility in this step. Early descriptions of

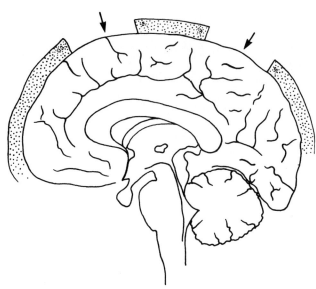

FIGURE 99-2 The anterior and posterior approaches provide direct and convenient access to the respective halves of the callosum. (From Roberts DW: Corpus callosotomy. In Reeves AG [ed]: Epilepsy and the Corpus Callosum. New York: Plenum Press, 1985, p 264.)

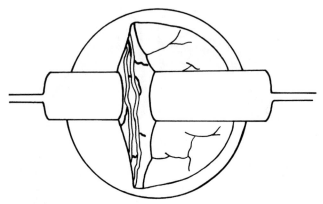

FIGURE 99-4   The pericallosal arteries are identified overlying the callosum, and the section is most often performed between them; section lateral to these arteries may sometimes prove more convenient during part of the section. (From Roberts DW: Corpus callosotomy. In Reeves AG [ed]: Epilepsy and the Corpus Callosum. New York: Plenum Press, 1985, p 262.)

callosal section describe the bluish appearance of the underlying ventricular ependymal surface and recommend this landmark as the ventral limit of division.[11,12] Over the course of our series, the advantages of identifying the midline during the division have become increasingly evident and include unequivocal assurance of completeness of fiber division, elimination of possible lateral deviation (especially in the frontal region), decreased likelihood of entering the lateral ventricle, and less operative time. A gentle sweeping from side to side of a blunt microinstrument as the callosum is nearly traversed will often expose the midline cleft between the lateral ventricles (Figs. 99-5 to 99-7). Once this cleft has been identified, the remainder of the section follows easily.

The direction of actual section is not critical, but identification of the midline during the anterior division is easiest at the posterior-most portion of the genu or the anterior

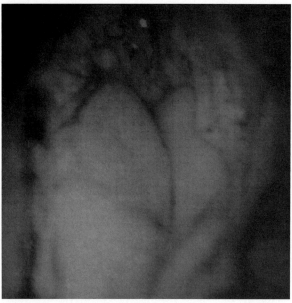

FIGURE 99-6   Intraoperative exposure of the divided genu. The ependymal surfaces of the frontal horns, the cut surfaces of the callosum, and the midline cleft are visualized (see Fig. 99-5).

portion of the body. Subsequent division around the genu and down the rostrum is performed extraventricularly as far as possible. At this point, the rostrum is nearly paper thin and any remaining fibers are insignificant. No attempt is made to divide the anterior commissure blindly.

Attention is now directed to the posterior extent of the division. If an attempt is being made to achieve success with a partial division, it is reasonable to carry the division through the anterior three fourths. When assurance of section and hemostasis is complete, a metal clip attached to a small piece of Gelfoam is placed at the posterior extent of the

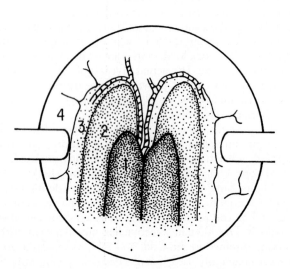

FIGURE 99-5   Division of the callosum at the level of the genu. 1 = Ependymal surfaces of the frontal horns of the lateral ventricles; 2 = cut surface of the genu; 3 = dorsal aspect of the genu; 4 = cingulate gyrus. The anterior cerebral arteries are visualized. (From Roberts DW: Corpus callosotomy. In Reeves AG [ed]: Epilepsy and the Corpus Callosum. New York: Plenum Press, 1985, p 263.)

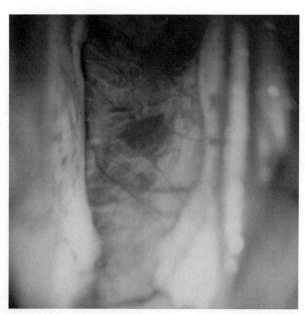

FIGURE 99-7   Intraoperative exposure of the divided splenium. The cut surfaces of the callosum and the underlying arachnoid are evident.

divided callosum. At subsequent surgery, gliosis may obscure the extent of previous resection and such a marker has often been greatly appreciated. It has not created undesirable magnetic resonance imaging artifact.

Division of the posterior corpus callosum is similarly performed. As previously mentioned, the more extensive falx cerebri often aids the more posterior exposure. The fibers of the splenium are divided with similar instrumentation, and under magnification, the completeness of the section is certain. The underlying arachnoid, beneath which lie the pineal and quadrigeminal cistern, is preserved. The posterior hippocampal commissure may be indistinguishable from the adjacent callosal fibers, but this is of no practical significance as it is divided as well. If an anterior section has been previously performed, the earlier placed clip is retrieved; if the posterior section is the initial commissurotomy procedure, a clip is left as a marker at the anterior-most extent of the section.

After confirmation of hemostasis, the dura is closed over Gelfilm using 4-0 Vicryl. The bone plug is secured through predrilled holes with 2-0 Ethilon, the galea aponeurosis is reapproximated using 2-0 Vicryl, and the skin is closed with either 4-0 Prolene or staples. The patient is observed in the neurosurgical observation unit overnight and usually transferred to the neurosurgical ward the following morning. Mobilization begins immediately, and the patient is typically discharged within 3 to 4 days. Anticonvulsant medication is generally left unaltered until at least subsequent follow-up. A decision regarding completion of the callosotomy is made a minimum of 2 months and more often 6 or more months after the first procedure.

RESULTS

Reporting on a total of 10 patients, Van Wagenen and Herren[4] reported significant improvement in 9. Wilson and colleagues[15,16] noted 16 of 20 patients to have greater than 50% reduction in overall seizure frequency, and Geoffroy and colleagues[29] similar success in six of nine patients. Rayport and colleagues[43] reported seven of nine patients significantly improved, Luessenhop and colleagues[8,9] three of four, Amacher[17] four of four, and Bouvier and colleagues[21] six of six. An outcome analysis in 183 patients from 14 centers[81] found 5.5% free of seizures, 73.5% improved, and 20.7% unimproved; the range of no improvement was 10% to 38%, and a follow-up survey in 1991 included 563 patients of whom 7.6% were reported to be seizure free and 60.9% improved.[3] Although these figures are not as good as those for temporal lobectomy or extratemporal cortical resection, the patient populations are distinct, with nearly all who underwent division of the corpus callosum having failed to fulfill the selection criteria for other surgery. More recent experiences, with similar outcomes, include those of Rutka[60] and van Veelen and colleagues.[61]

The great majority of patients undergoing callosal surgery for seizure control have had multiple seizure types, and it is useful to analyze outcome in terms of seizure classification. Tables 99-1 to 99-5 summarize outcome in the Dartmouth series of 83 evaluable patients with a mean follow-up of 10.4 years and range of 1 to 26.8 years.

Sixty-two of 83 patients preoperatively had major motor seizures, and of these, 21 have had elimination of

TABLE 99-1 ▪ Response of Major Motor Seizures to Commissurotomy in the 62 of 83 Patients Who Experienced Major Motor Seizures among Their Seizure Types Preoperatively

Seizure Response	No. of Patients (%)
No seizures	21 (34)
>80% reduction in frequency	10 (16)
50%–80% reduction in frequency	5 (8)
<50% reduction in frequency	2 (3)
No reduction in frequency	19 (31)
Worse	5 (8)

those seizures. An additional 10 patients have had greater than 80% reduction in their seizure frequency, and 5 a 50% to 80% reduction. Two have had less than 50% improvement; 19 have had no improvement in frequency, although in the majority seizures are less severe.

Forty-three of 83 patients had atonic seizures, generally characterized by sudden falls to the ground. In 22 patients, these have been eliminated and in another 6, reduction of greater than 80% has been achieved. Although frequency has been less successfully affected in the remaining 15, the actual seizure has been modified in 4 from a fall to head nod or other less injurious manifestation.

Absence spells were present in 37 of 83 patients, and although the procedure was not performed for this particular seizure type, 25 patients have had elimination or greater than 80% reduction in frequency of these spells.

The results in focal motor epilepsy, which might be presumed to remain unaffected by a procedure thought to be effective by disruption of propagation, are indeed less successful but nevertheless interesting in this subgroup of 24 patients. Five patients demonstrated no further focal seizure activity and an additional one had better than 80% reduction. One patient in this group had an increase in frequency for this seizure type, and 14 patients who had not experienced focal motor seizures developed them after surgery. A worsening of this seizure type after callosotomy has been described,[56] and the possibility of the procedure resulting in a loss of an inhibitory influence has been suggested.[53,56,73] Our data confirm the occurrence of increased or new-onset focal seizures, but they have nearly always occurred as the attenuated remnant of previously generalizing

TABLE 99-2 ▪ Response of Focal Motor Seizures to Commissurotomy in the 24 of 83 Patients Who Experienced Focal Motor Seizures among Their Seizure Types Preoperatively

Seizure Response	No. of Patients (%)
No seizures	5 (21)
>80% reduction in frequency	1 (4)
50%–80% reduction in frequency	3 (13)
<50% reduction in frequency	1 (4)
No reduction in frequency	13 (54)
Worse	1 (4)
New onset	14 (24)

TABLE 99-3 ▪ **Response of Atonic Seizures to Commissurotomy in the 43 of 83 Patients Who Experienced Atonic Seizures among Their Seizure Types Preoperatively**

Seizure Response	No. of Patients (%)
No seizures	22 (51)
>80% reduction in frequency	6 (14)
50%–80% reduction in frequency	3 (7)
<50% reduction in frequency	4 (9)
No reduction in frequency	7 (16)
Worse	1 (2)

TABLE 99-5 ▪ **Response of Complex Partial Seizures to Commissurotomy in the 31 of 83 Patients Who Experienced Complex Partial Seizures among Their Seizure Types Preoperatively**

Seizure Response	No. of Patients (%)
No seizures	13 (42)
>80% reduction in frequency	3 (10)
50%–80% reduction in frequency	3 (10)
<50% reduction in frequency	4 (13)
No reduction in frequency	8 (26)
Worse	0 (0)

seizure activity. In no instance has this represented a deterioration in overall functional outcome.

Corpus callosotomy has not been advocated as a substitute for temporal lobectomy in patients eligible for that procedure, but the results with regard to complex partial seizures in 31 of 83 patients are noteworthy.[82] Thirteen of 31 have had elimination of this seizure type and another 3 patients have had greater than 80% reduction in their frequency. In nine patients, the seizures have been significantly modified in severity. The role of this procedure in patients with only complex partial seizures but in whom investigations fail to define a resectable focus remains undefined.

In a report of their own experience, Spencer and colleagues[57] noted comparable success rates with atonic, tonic-clonic, and myoclonic seizures. In compiling reports on 330 patients from a number of institutions, they also note success rates (cure or marked improvement) for atonic seizures of 71% with anterior section and 74% with total section, for tonic-clonic seizures of 56% and 75%, respectively, for tonic seizures of 47% and 75%, respectively, and for absence of 33% and 64%, respectively.[57]

Incremental response to completion of the callosal section in those patients whose response to anterior section has been disappointing has been noted by both the Dartmouth[76] and Yale[57] groups. Of 27 patients who had undergone anterior callosal section at our institution but continued to experience generalized seizures at a greater than desired frequency and therefore underwent completion of their section, notable improvement was found for major motor, atonic, and complex partial seizures (Table 99-6). For all seizures together, the percentage of patients obtaining an 80% to 100% reduction in generalized seizures improved from 29% after anterior section to 62% after completion of callosal section.[76]

Surgical complications early in the Dartmouth series included hydrocephalus in three patients, but this subsequently has not been encountered; the present surgical technique of remaining extraventricular may be responsible. Wound or bone flap infections occurred in three patients. Sterile meningitis was noted in three patients, and septic meningitis was documented in one. One patient in whom surgery and the early postoperative course had been unremarkable died of a frontal lobe infarction 12 days after surgery. A second patient died of cardiopulmonary arrest after the development of status epilepticus, pneumonia, thrombophlebitis, and possible pulmonary embolus 3 months after surgery. The marked reduction in complication rate in the last 80 patients who have undergone callosal section illustrates the learning curve and improved technique familiar to all centers.

The behavioral and neuropsychological effects of commissurotomy have been studied extensively,[83–115] the most enlightening work in this area being that of Gazzaniga and colleagues.[91–98,105] The initial impression after the earliest series had been that callosotomy produced little alteration in cognitive function.[83,84] Subsequent and more sophisticated investigations have demonstrated numerous effects of disconnection,[91,97] but in general it has been unusual for these to represent significant handicaps. In almost all cases, the benefits in terms of seizure improvement have far exceeded any neuropsychological adverse effects.

TABLE 99-4 ▪ **Response of Absence Seizures to Commissurotomy in the 37 of 83 Patients Who Experienced Absence Seizures among Their Seizure Types Preoperatively**

Seizure Response	No. of Patients (%)
No seizures	17 (46)
>80% reduction in frequency	8 (22)
50%–80% reduction in frequency	0 (0)
<50% reduction in frequency	2 (5)
No reduction in frequency	8 (22)
Worse	2 (5)

TABLE 99-6 ▪ **Incremental Response to Completion of Corpus Callosum Section in 27 Patients with Suboptimal Response to Anterior Callosotomy**

Type of Seizure (No. of Patients with Seizure Type)	No. of Patients with at Least 80% Reduction in Seizure Frequency after Anterior Section	No. of Patients with at Least 80% Reduction in Seizure Frequency after Completion of Section
Major motor (21)	6	13
Atonic (16)	6	13
Focal motor (7)	1	1
Complex partial (8)	6	8

Data from reference 76.

With division of the anterior corpus callosum, decreased spontaneity of speech (ranging from subtle slowing to complete mutism) and decreased use of the nondominant hand and leg (sometimes described as a paresis or apraxia) may be seen and usually resolve over several days.[107] There remains discussion as to the relative contribution of surgical retraction versus acute disconnection in the etiology of these findings. The majority of patients exhibit no long-standing effects from anterior section, although exacerbation of previous lateralized deficits has been reported.[90]

Posterior callosal section, in contrast, produces a now well-recognized disconnection syndrome characterized by interhemispheric sensory dissociation. This can be demonstrated with somatosensory, auditory, and visual stimuli, with the language-dominant hemisphere not having direct access to information presented to the other hemisphere. With incomplete section, the language-dominant hemisphere may still gain access to contralateral hemisphere information, and the dissociation may not be demonstrable. With complete section, the sensory dissociation is complete and permanent.

The majority of patients in the Dartmouth series have improved or remained unchanged in their level of cognitive function. This has usually been the result of both diminished seizure activity and decreased anticonvulsant medication. Ferrell and colleagues[102] reported on formal neuropsychological testing in eight of the earliest patients and found improvement in six. The families of five patients have reported decreased cognitive ability, usually described as poorer memory or concentration, and this has been noted in other series as well.[88,103] Further investigation of this finding has suggested that it may be more of an attention disorder than actual memory dysfunction,[104] although more recent investigations have documented deficits in recall as well.[105] Speech and motor dysfunction has been frequently noted in the immediate postoperative period, but persistence of these deficits has been infrequent.[14,38,91] Antagonism between the right and left hemispheres, usually manifested as opposing actions of the right and left hands, has been similarly reported.[88] In only one patient in our series has this been a chronic difficulty.

CONCLUSIONS

Although the answers to important questions regarding indications and expectations for corpus callosotomy in the treatment of intractable epilepsy continue to evolve, the experience accumulated over more than 50 years allows a number of important points to be made. Perhaps most important is the recognition that for some patients who have failed medical management and who are not eligible for other seizure surgery, commissurotomy may successfully reduce seizure frequency and severity. Atonic seizures and secondarily generalized major motor seizures are most likely to be improved, but other seizure types may also respond.

Extraventricular division of the corpus callosum alone achieves the aforementioned success; complete callosotomy may not be required in all patients, and staging of the procedure remains a reasonable approach. As a microsurgical procedure, division of the corpus callosum can be safely and confidently performed.

Behavioral and neuropsychological sequelae of commissurotomy are well-recognized but uncommonly permanent disabilities. In the majority of patients, the benefits resulting from the procedure outweigh any such effects.

REFERENCES

1. Polkey CE: Alternative surgical procedures to help drug-resistant epilepsy—a review. Epileptic Disord 5:63–75, 2003.
2. Horsley V: Brain surgery. BMJ 2:670–675, 1886.
3. Engel J Jr, Van Ness PC, Rasmussen TB, et al: Outcome with respect to epileptic seizures. In Engel J Jr (ed): Surgical Treatment of the Epilepsies, 2nd ed. New York: Raven Press, 1993, pp 609–621.
4. Van Wagenen WP, Herren RY: Surgical division of the commissural pathways in the corpus callosum: Relation to spread of an epileptic attack. Arch Neurol Psych 44:740–759, 1940.
5. Bogen JE, Fisher ED, Vogel PJ: Cerebral commissurotomy: A second case report. JAMA 194:1328–1329, 1965.
6. Bogen JE, Sperry RW, Vogel PJ: Addendum: commissural section and propagation of seizures. In Jasper HH, Ward AA Jr, Pope A (eds): Basic Mechanisms of the Epilepsies. Boston: Little, Brown, 1969, p 439.
7. Bogen JE, Vogel PJ: Cerebral commissurotomy in man: Preliminary case report. Bull Los Angeles Neurol Soc 27:169–172, 1962.
8. Luessenhop AJ: Interhemispheric commissurotomy: (the split brain operation) as an alternative to hemispherectomy for control of intractable seizures. Am Surg 36:265–268, 1970.
9. Luessenhop AJ, dela Cruz TC, Fenichel GM: Surgical disconnection of the cerebral hemispheres for intractable seizures. JAMA 213:1630–1636, 1970.
10. Harbaugh RE, Wilson DH, Reeves AG, et al: Forebrain commissurotomy for epilepsy: Review of 20 consecutive cases. Acta Neurochir (Wien) 68:263–275, 1983.
11. Reeves AG, O'Leary PM: Total corpus callosotomy for control of medically intractable epilepsy. In Reeves AG (ed): Epilepsy and the Corpus Callosum. New York: Plenum Press, 1985, pp 269–280.
12. Wilson DH, Culver C, Waddington M, et al: Disconnection of the cerebral hemispheres: An alternative to hemispherectomy for the control of intractable seizures. Neurology 25:1149–1153, 1975.
13. Wilson DH, Reeves A, Gazzaniga M: Division of the corpus callosum for uncontrollable epilepsy. Neurology 28:649–653, 1978.
14. Wilson DH, Reeves A, Gazzaniga M: Corpus callosotomy for control of intractable seizures. In Wada JA, Penry JK (eds): Advances in Epileptology: The Xth Epilepsy International Symposium. New York: Raven Press, 1980, pp 205–213.
15. Wilson DH, Reeves AG, Gazzaniga MS: "Central" commissurotomy for intractable generalized epilepsy: Series two. Neurology 32:687–697, 1982.
16. Wilson DH, Reeves AG, Gazzaniga MS, et al: Cerebral commissurotomy for control of intractable seizures. Neurology 27:708–715, 1977.
17. Amacher AL: Midline commissurotomy for the treatment of some cases of intractable epilepsy. Childs Brain 2:54–58, 1970.
18. Andersen B, Rogvi-Hansen B, Kruse-Larsen C, et al: Corpus callosotomy: Seizure and psychosocial outcome: A 39-month follow-up of 20 patients. Epilepsy Res 23:77–85, 1996.
19. Avila JO, Radvany J, Huck FR, et al: Anterior callosotomy as a substitute for hemispherectomy. Acta Neurochir (Suppl) 30:137–143, 1980.
20. Behrens E, Schramm J, Zentner J, et al: Surgical and neurological complications in a series of 708 epilepsy surgery procedures. Neurosurgery 41:1–9, 1997.
21. Bouvier G, Mercier C, St. Hilaire JM, et al: Anterior callosotomy and chronic depth electrode recording in the surgical management of some intractable seizures. Appl Neurophysiol 46:52–56, 1983.
22. Cendes F, Ragazzo PC, da Costa V, et al: Corpus callosotomy in treatment of medically resistant epilepsy: Preliminary results in a pediatric population. Epilepsia 34:910–917, 1993.
23. Fiol ME, Gates JR, Mireles R, et al: Value of intraoperative EEG changes during corpus callosotomy in predicting surgical results. Epilepsia 34:74–78, 1993.
24. Fuiks KS, Wyler AR, Hermann BP, et al: Seizure outcome from anterior and complete corpus callosotomy. J Neurosurg 74:573–578, 1991.
25. Garcia-Flores E: Corpus callosum section for patients with intractable epilepsy. Appl Neurophysiol 50:390–397, 1987.
26. Gates JR, Leppik IE, Yap J, et al: Corpus callosotomy: Clinical and electroencephalographic effects. Epilepsia 25:308–316, 1984.

27. Gates JR, Maxwell R, Leppik IE, et al: Electroencephalographic and clinical effects of total corpus callosotomy. In Reeves AG (ed): Epilepsy and the Corpus Callosum. New York: Plenum Press, 1985, pp 315–328.
28. Gates JR, Rosenfeld WE, Maxwell RE, et al: Response of multiple seizure types to corpus callosum section. Epilepsia 28:28–34, 1987.
29. Geoffroy G, Lassonde M, Delisle F, et al: Corpus callosotomy for control of intractable epilepsy in children. Neurology 33:891–897, 1983.
30. Gilliam F, Wyllie E, Kotagal P, et al: Parental assessment of functional outcome after corpus callosotomy. Epilepsia 37:753–757, 1996.
31. Huck FR, Radvany J, Avila JO, et al: Anterior callosotomy in epileptics with multiform seizures and bilateral synchronous spike and wave EEG pattern. Acta Neurochir Suppl 30:127–135, 1980.
32. Lassonde M, Sauerwein C: Neuropsychological outcome of corpus callosotomy in children and adolescents. J Neurosurg Sci 41:67–73, 1997.
33. Maehara T, Shimizu H, Oda M, et al: Surgical treatment of children with medically intractable epilepsy—outcome of various surgical procedures. Neurol Medicochir 36:305–309, 1996.
34. Mamelak AN, Barbaro NM, Walker JA, et al: Corpus callosotomy: A quantitative study of the extent of resection, seizure control, and neuropsychological outcome. J Neurosurg 79:688–695, 1993.
35. Marino R Jr, Ragazzo PC: Selective criteria and results of selective partial callosotomy. In Reeves AG (ed): Epilepsy and the Corpus Callosum. New York: Plenum Press, 1985, pp 281–301.
36. Murro AM, Flanigin HF, Gallagher BB, et al: Corpus callosotomy for the treatment of intractable epilepsy. Epilepsy Rev 2:44–50, 1988.
37. Nordgren RE, Reeves AG, Viguera AC, et al: Corpus callosotomy for intractable seizures in the pediatric age group. Arch Neurol 48:364–372, 1991.
38. Oguni H, Olivier A, Andermann F, Comair J: Anterior callosotomy in the treatment of intractable epilepsies: A study of 43 patients with a mean follow-up of 39 months. Ann Neurol 30:357–364, 1991.
39. Phillips J, Sakas DE: Anterior callosotomy for intractable epilepsy: Outcome in a series of twenty patients. Br J Neurosurg 10:351–356, 1996.
40. Purves SJ, Wada JA, Woodhurst WB, et al: Results of anterior corpus callosum section in 24 patients with medically intractable seizures. Neurology 38:1194–1201, 1988.
41. Quattrini A, Papo I, Cesarano R, et al: EEG Patterns after callosotomy. J Neurosurg Sci 41:85–92, 1997.
42. Rappaport ZH, Lerman P: Corpus callosotomy in the treatment of secondary generalizing intractable epilepsy. Acta Neurochir 94:10–14, 1988.
43. Rayport M, Corrie WS, Ferguson SM: Corpus callosum section for control of clinically and electroencephalographically classified seizures. In Reeves AG (ed): Epilepsy and the Corpus Callosum. New York: Plenum Press, 1985, pp 329–337.
44. Rayport M, Ferguson SM, Corrie WS: Outcomes and indications of corpus callosum section for intractable seizure control. Appl Neurophysiol 46:47–51, 1983.
45. Reutens DC, Bye AM, Hopkins IJ, et al: Corpus callosotomy for intractable epilepsy: Seizure outcome and prognostic factors. Epilepsia 34:904–909, 1993.
46. Rossi G, Colicchio G, Marchese E, et al: Callosotomy for drug resistant generalized seizures. J Neurosurg Sci 41:37–40, 1997.
47. Rougier A, Claverie B, Pedespan JM, et al: Callosotomy for intractable epilepsy: Overall outcome. J Neurosurg Sci 41:51–57, 1997.
48. Sainte-Hilaire JM, Giard N, Bouvier G, et al: Anterior callosotomy in frontal lobe epilepsies. In Reeves AG (ed): Epilepsy and the Corpus Callosum. New York: Plenum Press, 1985, pp 303–314.
49. Sorenson JM, Wheless JW, Baumgartner JE, et al: Corpus callosotomy for medically intractable seizures. Pediatr Neurosurg 27:260–267, 1997.
50. Spencer DD, Spencer SS: Corpus callosotomy in the treatment of medically intractable secondarily generalized seizures of children. Cleve Clin J Med 56(Suppl 1):S69–S77, 1988.
51. Spencer SS: Corpus callosum section and other disconnection procedures for medically intractable epilepsy. Epilepsia 29(Suppl 2):S85–S99, 1988.
52. Spencer SS, Elquera ED, Williamson PD, et al: Evolution of seizure types after callosotomy. J Epilepsy 4:149–156, 1992.
53. Spencer SS, Gates JR, Reeves AG, et al: Corpus callosum section for uncontrolled epilepsy. In Engel J (ed): Surgical Treatment of Epilepsy. New York: Raven Press, 1987, pp 425–444.
54. Hanson RR, Risinger M, Maxwell R: The ictal EEG as a predictive factor for outcome following corpus callosum section in adults. Epilepsy Res 49:89–97, 2002.
55. Spencer SS, Katz A, Ebersole J, et al: Ictal EEG changes with corpus callosum section. Epilepsia 34:568–573, 1993.
56. Spencer SS, Spencer DD, Glaser GH, et al: More intense focal seizure types after callosal section: The role of inhibition. Ann Neurol 16:686–693, 1984.
57. Spencer SS, Spencer DD, Sass K, et al: Anterior, total, and two-stage corpus callosum section: Differential and incremental seizure responses. Epilepsia 34:561–567, 1993.
58. Spencer SS, Spencer DD, Williamson PD, et al: Effect of corpus callosum section on secondary bilaterally synchronous interictal EEG discharges. Neurology 35:1689–1694, 1985.
59. Spencer SS, Spencer DD, Williamson PD, et al: Corpus callosotomy for epilepsy. I: Seizure effects. Neurology 38:19–24, 1988.
60. Rutka J: Image-guided, frameless stereotactic sectioning of the corpus callosum in children with intractable epilepsy. Pediatr Neurosurg 34:286–294, 2001.
61. van Veelen CW, van Rijen PC, Debets RM, et al: [Dutch Collaborative Epilepsy Surgery Program: Reduction of seizures, operative complications and tapering of medication in 338 patients, 1973–1998]. Ned Tijdschr Geneeskd 17:2223–2228, 2001.
62. Erickson TE: Spread of the epileptic discharge: An experimental study of the after discharge induced by electrical stimulation of the cerebral cortex. Arch Neurol Psychiatry 43:429–452, 1940.
63. Marcus EM, Watson CW: Bilateral synchronous spike wave electrographic patterns in the cat. Arch Neurol 14:601–610, 1966.
64. Marcus EM, Watson CW: Symmetrical epileptogenic foci in monkey cerebral cortex: Mechanisms of interaction and regional variations in capacity for synchronous discharges. Arch Neurol 19:99–116, 1968.
65. Kopeloff N, Kennard MA, Pacella BL, et al: Section of the corpus callosum in experimental epilepsy in the monkey. Arch Neurol Psychiatry 63:719–727, 1950.
66. Crowell RM, Ajmone Marsan C: Topographical distribution and patterns of unit activity during electrically induced after-discharge. Electroenchaphalogr Clin Neurophysiol Suppl 31:59–73, 1972.
67. Mutani R, Bergamini L, Fariello R, et al: Bilateral synchrony of epileptic discharge associated with chronic asymmetrical cortical foci. Electroencephalogr Clin Neurophysiol 34:53–59, 1973.
68. Matsuo A, Ono T, Baba H, et al: Callosal role in generation of epileptiform discharges: Quantitative analysis of EEGs recorded in patients undergoing corpus callosotomy. Clin Neurophysiol 114:2165–2171, 2003.
69. Ono T, Fujimura K, Yoshida S, et al: Suppressive effect of callosotomy on epileptic seizures is due to the blockade of enhancement of cortical reactivity by transcallosal volleys. Epilepsy Res 51:117–121, 2002.
70. Stavraky GW: Supersensitivity Following Lesions of the Nervous System. Toronto: University of Toronto Press, 1961, pp 33–38.
71. Kusske JA, Rush JL: Corpus callosum and propagation of afterdischarge to contralateral cortex and thalamus. Neurology 28:905–912, 1978.
72. Reeves AG (ed): Epilepsy and the Corpus Callosum. New York: Plenum Press, 1985.
73. Blume WT: Corpus callosum section for seizure control: Rationale and review of experimental and clinical data. Cleve Clin Q 51:319–332, 1984.
74. Williamson PD: Corpus callosum section for intractable epilepsy: Criteria for patient selection. In Reeves AG (ed): Epilepsy and the Corpus Callosum. New York: Plenum Press, 1985, pp 243–257.
75. Oguni H, Andermann F, Gotman J, et al: Effect of anterior callosotomy on bilaterally synchronous spike and wave and other EEG discharges. Epilepsia 35:505–513, 1994.
76. Roberts DW, Reeves AG, Nordgren RE: The role of posterior callosotomy in patients with suboptimal response to anterior callosotomy. In Reeves AG, Roberts DW (eds): Epilepsy and the Corpus Callosum 2. New York: Plenum Press, 1995, pp 183–190.
77. Sakas DE, Phillips J: Anterior callosotomy in the management of intractable epileptic seizures: Significance of the extent of resection. Acta Neurochir (Wien) 138:700–707, 1996.
78. Roberts DW: Corpus callosotomy: Surgical technique. In Reeves AG (ed): Epilepsy and the Corpus Callosum. New York: Plenum Press, 1985, pp 259–267.
79. Roberts DW, Rayport M, Maxwell RE, et al: Corpus callosotomy. In Engel J Jr (ed): Surgical Treatment of the Epilepsies, 2nd ed. New York: Raven Press, 1993, pp 519–526.

80. Apuzzo MLJ, Chikovani OK, Gott PS: Transcallosal, interforniceal approaches for lesions affecting the third ventricle: Surgical considerations and consequences. Neurosurgery 10:547–554, 1982.
81. Engel J Jr: Outcome with respect to epileptic seizures. In Engel J Jr (ed): Surgical Treatment of the Epilepsies. New York: Raven Press, 1987, pp 553–571.
82. Roberts DW, Reeves AG: Effect of commissurotomy on complex partial epilepsy in patients without a resectable seizure focus. Appl Neurophysiol 50:398–400, 1987.
83. Akelaitis AJ: Studies on corpus callosum: Higher visual function in each hemisphere's field following complete section of the corpus callosum. Arch Neurol Psychiatry 45:786–796, 1941.
84. Akelaitis AJ: A study of gnosis, praxis and language following section of the corpus callosum and anterior commissure. J Neurosurg 1:94–102, 1944.
85. Gordon HW, Bogen JE, Sperry RW: Absence of deconnection syndrome in two patients with partial section of the neocommissures. Brain 94:327–336, 1971.
86. Campbell AL Jr, Bogen JE, Smith A: Disorganization and reorganization of cognitive and sensorimotor functions in cerebral commissurotomy: Compensatory roles of the forebrain commissures and cerebral hemispheres in man. Brain 104:493–511, 1981.
87. Oepen G, Schulz-Weiling R, Zimmermann P, et al: Long-term effects of partial callosal lesions: Preliminary report. Acta Neurochir (Wien) 77:22, 1985.
88. Ferguson SM, Rayport M, Corrie WS: Neuropsychiatric observations on behavioral consequences of corpus callosum section for seizure control. In Reeves AG (ed): Epilepsy and Corpus Callosum. New York: Plenum Press, 1985, pp 501–514.
89. Lassonde M, Sauerwein H, Geoffroy G, et al: Effects of early and late transection of the corpus callosum in children. Brain 109:953–967, 1986.
90. Sass KJ, Spencer DD, Spencer SS, et al: Corpus callosotomy for epilepsy. II: Neurologic and neuropsychological outcome. Neurology 38:24–28, 1988.
91. Gazzaniga MS: The Bisected Brain. New York: Appleton-Century-Crofts, 1970.
92. Gazzaniga MS, Risse GL, Springer SP, et al: Psychologic and neurologic consequences of partial and complete cerebral commissurotomy. Neurology 25:10, 1975.
93. Ledoux JE, Risse GL, Springer SP, et al: Cognition and commissurotomy. Brain 100:87–104, 1977.
94. Sidtis JJ, Volpe BT, Holtzman JD, et al: Cognitive interaction after staged callosal section: Evidence for transfer of semantic activation. Science 212:344–346, 1981.
95. Volpe BT, Sidtis JJ, Holzman JD: Cortical mechanisms involved in praxis: Observations following partial and complete section of the corpus callosum in man. Neurology 32:645–650, 1982.
96. Gazzaniga MS, Smylie CS: Dissociation of language and cognition: A psychological profile of two disconnected right hemispheres. Brain 107:145–153, 1984.
97. Gazzaniga MS: Some contributions of the split-brain studies to the study of human cognition. In Reeves AG (ed): Epilepsy and the Corpus Callosum. New York: Plenum Press, 1985, pp 341–348.
98. Gazzaniga MS: Perceptual and attentional processes following callosal section in humans. Neuropsychologia 25:119–133, 1987.
99. Clark CR, Geffen GM: Corpus callosum surgery and recent memory. Brain 112:165–175, 1989.
100. Sergent J: Furtive incursions into bicameral minds. Brain 113:537–568, 1990.
101. Sergent J: Processing of spatial relations within and between the disconnected cerebral hemispheres. Brain 114:1025–1043, 1991.
102. Ferrell RB, Culver CM, Tucker GJ: Psychosocial and cognitive function after commissurotomy for intractable seizures. J Neurosurg 58:374–380, 1984.
103. Zaidel E, Sperry RW: Memory impairment after commissurotomy in man. Brain 97:263–272, 1974.
104. Beniak TE, Gates JR, Risse GL: Comparison of selected neuropsychological test variables pre- and postoperatively on patients subjected to corpus callosotomy. Epilepsia 26:53, 1985.
105. Tramo MJ, Baynes K, Fendrich R, et al: Hemispheric specialization and interhemispheric integration: Insights from experiments with commissurotomy patients. In Reeves AG, Roberts DW (eds): Epilepsy and the Corpus Callosum 2. New York: Plenum Press, 1995, pp 263–295.
106. Quattrini A, Del Pesce M, Provinciali L, et al: Mutism in 36 patients who underwent callosotomy for drug-resistant epilepsy. J Neurosurg Sci 41:93–96, 1997.
107. Ross MK, Reeves AG, Roberts DW: Post-commissurotomy mutism. Ann Neurol 16:11, 1984.
108. Fabri M, Polonara G, Del Pesce M, et al: Posterior corpus callosum and interhemispheric transfer of somatosensory information: An fMRI and neuropsychological study of a partially callosotomized patient. J Cogn Neurosci 13:1071–1079, 2001.
109. Kennerley SW, Diedrichsen J, Hazeltine E, et al: Callosotomy patients exhibit temporal uncoupling during continuous bimanual movements. Nat Neurosci 5:376–81, 2002.
110. Lessard N, Lepore F, Villemagne J, et al: Sound localization in callosal agenesis and early callosotomy subjects: Brain reorganization and/or compensatory strategies. Brain 125:1039–1053, 2002.
111. O'Shea RP, Corballis PM: Binocular rivalry in split-brain observers. J Vision 3:610–615, 2003.
112. Corballis MC, Corballis PM, Fabri M: Redundancy gain in simple reaction time following partial and complete callosotomy. Neuropsychologia 42:71–81, 2004.
113. Devinsky O, Laff R: Callosal lesions and behavior: History and modern concepts. Epilepsy Behav 4:607–617, 2003.
114. Hausmann M, Corballis MC, Farbi M: Line bisection in the split brain. Neuropsychology 17:602–609, 2003.
115. Keenan JP, Wheeler M, Platek SM, et al: Self-face processing in a callostomy patient. Eur J Neurosci 18:2391–2395, 2003.

Surgical Management of Movement Disorders and Pain

100 Surgical Treatment of the Dyskinesias

RONALD R. TASKER

INTRODUCTION

This chapter reviews stereotactic surgery for involuntary movement disorders, but not open surgery, botulinum toxin therapy, microvascular decompression, or radiosurgery. The history of the development of these techniques has been so frequently reviewed that it does not require repetition here.[1] In most centers, Parkinson's disease remains the main indication, and the relevant operations have been steadily elaborated to their present state so as to maximize relief of the dyskinesia and minimize complications. There have, however, been no recent major conceptual advances. Often several options are available for each patient, the final choice being influenced by both the patient and the surgeon, keeping in mind that there is as yet no convincing evidence that any of the conventional stereotactic procedures described here alter the course of the disease; they are palliative. However, both thalamotomy[2] and subthalamic nucleus deep brain stimulation (DBS)[3] have been thought to slow the course of Parkinson's disease. Nevertheless, there is an active ongoing search for alternative procedures that might clearly influence the disease progress, particularly in the case of Parkinson's disease. Such a major conceptual advance probably still remains for the future.

SURGICAL TECHNIQUES AND INDICATIONS

There are six stereotactic procedures now in regular use for the treatment of Parkinson's disease: thalamotomy, thalamic DBS, pallidotomy, pallidal DBS, subthalamotomy, and subthalamic nucleus DBS (STN DBS). The thalamic procedures have been used in a variety of other involuntary movements as well, and the pallidal ones for dystonia. The stereotactic technique is essentially the same for all, with only the targets differing and either a DBS electrode is implanted at the target site or a radiofrequency (RF) lesion made.

To consider surgery in a movement disorder, the patient should not have a bleeding diathesis and should have significant life disability despite optimal nonsurgical therapy, and the disability should be caused by features of the movement disorder for which surgery offers reasonable chance of benefit. Significant cognitive disorders should not be present, and the patient should have sufficient physical resources to make use of the limited palliation provided by the surgery. In parkinsonian patients, surgery is probably not likely to help with symptoms that do not respond to treatment with L-dopa. Gait and speech deficits other than the speech deficits caused by tremor are less likely to be helped than others. Bilateral symmetrical lesions in any structure are more likely to cause complications than unilateral ones. In the thalamus and pallidum, bilateral lesions particularly result in speech disorders and in pallidum cognitive disorders. In general, the tremor of cerebellar disease responds less well than that of Parkinson's disease or essential tremor, whereas STN DBS[4] is the current preference for treating Parkinson's disease, although this is by no means universal. DBS is preferred to lesion making because it is reversible and its effects modifiable by parameter adjustment, although it incurs additional equipment management costs not seen after lesions are made and also is associated with the risks of equipment failure. In addition to the above advantages, it also avoids the risks of bilateral lesions if used contralaterally to a lesion or bilaterally.

Stereotactic Technique

A suitable stereotactic frame such as the Leksell G model is attached to the patient's head under local anesthetic as closely as possible to a nonrotated or tilted midsagittal position.[5–12] Although ventriculography or computed tomography scans are preferred by some surgeons for imaging, the author prefers magnetic resonance imaging or image fusion with computed tomography.[13] The 3-dimensional coordinates of anterior and posterior commissures are then read off using the magnetic resonance imaging software and used to construct a series of sagittal brain diagrams based on those in the Schaltenbrand and Wahren[14] brain atlas but redrawn to match the length of the patient's anteroposterior commissure line. They are then ruled in a 1-mm grid conforming to the Leksell frame coordinates. These diagrams are used for physiologic localization of the target. In some cases, the stereotactic target may be visible on the magnetic resonance imaging scan when its coordinates can be read off directly as they would be for stereotactic location of, say, a brain tumor. Some surgeons consider targets sufficiently consistently located that they can make localizations based on distance from visible anatomic structures when the target itself is not directly visible.

Physiologic Localization

A burr hole is now made under local anesthesia in the same sagittal plane as the intended target and the dura opened. Most stereotactic neurosurgeons prefer the added confidence provided for target localization by physiologic localization even if that target can be visualized on magnetic resonance imaging. Such physiologic localization may be restricted to the target alone or it may consist of a brain mapping procedure of the target territory from which the optimal target is selected. The three most common methods are macrostimulation, microstimulation, microelectrode recordings, or combinations thereof. This author prefers microelectrode recording of spontaneous and evoked neuronal activity and microstimulation for all targets, although truly scientific studies of the need for such physiologic localization or of the differences in results between the different techniques are not available.[7-10,15-18]

A microelectrode that is capable of recording single cell activity is directed through the dural opening toward the target and beyond it using a hydraulic microdrive with continual recording from approximately 10 to 15 mm above to approximately 10 mm below the target identifying spontaneous activity, effective stimuli, receptive fields, and parameters of stimulation.[5-12] Threshold microstimulation up to 100 μA is done every 1 mm and the reported response noted; this identifies the projected field. These data are mapped on a suitable chart such as in Figure 100-1, making use of what Woolsey termed figurine charts. Usually at least three trajectories are used, and there is at least one autopsy report showing that this technique does not damage the brain.[19] Excessive cerebrospinal fluid leakage around the microelectrode and any implanted DBS electrode that can cause brain shift is minimized by the use of fibrin glue.

Target Manipulation

Once the desired target is found, either a DBS electrode is inserted or an RF lesion made in such a position as to influence the movement disorder. The DBS electrode (Model 3387; Medtronic Corporation, Minneapolis, MN) is introduced with its stylet (to keep it stiff) and, once it has been confirmed to be in a suitable position, is anchored into the burr hole using a ring and cap device provided by Medtronic that prevents it from migrating proximally or distally. It is necessary to be certain that no such electrode movement takes place during the operation until the electrode is finally locked in place by applying "gunsights" symmetrically on each side of the frame and with the image intensifier adjusting their position on the frame until their images overlap one another and that of the active site on the DBS electrode. The proximal end of the electrode is now tunneled under the scalp away from the burr hole itself to minimize infection and brought out through a scalp stab wound to allow postoperative testing. It is later attached at a second operative procedure, with a subcutaneous lead, to a suitable stimulator pack placed in the infraclavicular area.

Lesion making is done with a 1.1-mm electrode insulated except for a 3-mm bare tip and activated with a suitable RF backup generator such as the OWL Universal RF system (Diros Technology, Toronto, Ontario, Canada). Lesioning starts at 50°C to 60°C for 60 seconds, gradually increased to 80°C to 90°C with serial testing of neurologic function and of the dyskinesia itself.

In general, the DBS and lesion targets are thought to be the same except that Kiss and colleagues[20] found the ideal thalamic DBS electrode stimulating site was located significantly anterior and dorsal to the ideal RF target.

THALAMIC SURGERY

Thalamotomy or thalamic DBS is currently done chiefly for the relief of essential tremor since STN DBS has largely

replaced other surgery for Parkinson's disease. This is because thalamotomy has no significant effect on parkinsonian bradykinesia but STN manipulation does. However, in a patient with slowly progressing Parkinson's disease with mainly tremor, thalamotomy or, better still, thalamic DBS may be very valuable. The ideal thalamic target site for either DBS or lesioning is among the kinesthetic or voluntary cells in the nucleus ventralis intermedius or oralis posterior that fire in time with tremor, with receptive fields and projected fields in the same body part as that of the disabling tremor. At the ideal target, the firing of the tremor cells is most tightly linked to the tremor electromyography and stimulation-induced tremor arrest is most striking[21] (see Fig. 100-1).

The mechanism of tremor control by stimulating or lesioning this area is unclear.[17,22] The fact that such surgery is effective in tremor of different origins (e.g., Parkinson's disease, essential tremor, cerebellar tremor) makes the pathophysiology difficult to understand. Tremor cells that fire synchronously with the tremor occur in all three of these diseases seem to be located at the same site in the thalamus in each, although rest tremor may be associated with a larger number of tremor cells in Parkinson's disease than occur in the other conditions.[23] In this author's opinion, thalamotomy and thalamic DBS are more likely to control parkinsonian tremor completely in the long term than the other tremor types.[5]

The mere passage of an electrode into the tremor target area is sufficient to arrest tremor in many patients, the microthalamotomy effect,[24,25] and the tremor relief may be very long lasting; the phenomenon is more common in Parkinson's disease than in essential or cerebellar tremor. The more profound the microthalamotomy effect is and the longer it lasts after the introduction of a DBS electrode, the more likely it is that DBS will be successful in the tremor control. This information suggests that at least one mechanism of tremor control in the thalamus may be blockage of the tremor cells' driving of the tremor.

The ideal tremor control area is 2 mm rostral to the rostral margin of the tactile cells and 2 to 3 mm above the anteroposterior commissure line.[22]

Outcome Data: Thalamic Deep Brain Stimulation

Long-term DBS does not appear to damage the brain.[26]

For tremor control, thalamic DBS is used at a higher frequency than would be used to control pain; 130 to 185 Hz with a pulse width of 60 to 120 μsec and 1 to 3 V. Typically, there is considerable discrepancy among reported outcomes in dyskinesia surgery, perhaps reflecting different lengths of follow-up as well as variations among patients, surgical techniques, and methods of assessment. Published series report 42% to 90% total or nearly total suppression of contralateral tremor; contralateral rigidity and dopa dyskinesia are less affected, and there is no ipsilateral effect.[15,24-41]

For essential tremor, results were not as good, there being significant tremor recurrence over time. Reduction of contralateral tremor was reported in 31% to 76% and total suppression in 14% to 31%.[22,31-33,35-37,42-45] In the author's experience, 14% of patients showed no tremor, 57% had minimal tremor at latest follow-up, and 57% were rendered

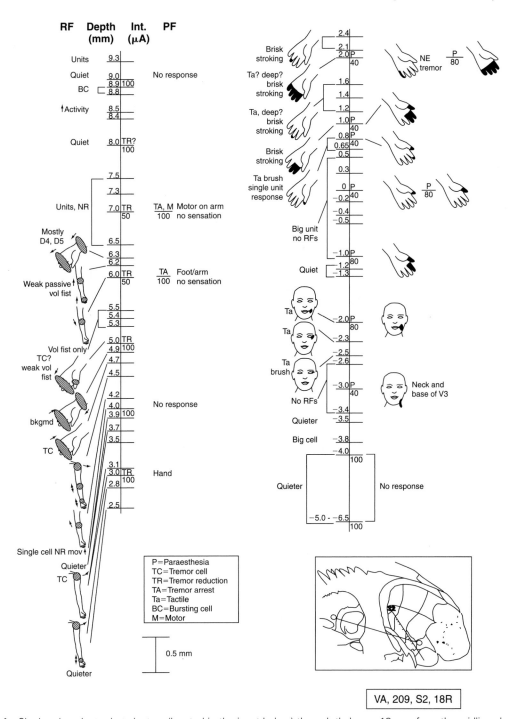

FIGURE 100-1 Single microelectrode trajectory (located in the inset below) through thalamus 18 mm from the midline showing receptive fields to the left and projected fields to the right of the trajectory. From 6.3 to 2.5 mm above the selected target point (depth 0), voluntary then kinesthetic cells are identified associated with various contralateral active (6.3 to 5 mm above) and passive (below 5) movements; some fire synchronously with tremor (TC). From 2.4 to 1 mm above the target, deep tactile cells are seen then tactile cells related to the contralateral hand and face. Projected fields with thresholds in microamperes are shown to the right, including tremor arrest and tremor reduction from 8 to 3 mm above the target.

able to drink. Midline tremor responded poorly, and there was no significant ipsilateral effect.

For cerebellar tremor,[35,36,43,46–49] 0 to 40% showed no tremor and 33% were able to drink postoperatively, but recurrence was more striking than with even essential tremor. Tremor reduction was often not necessarily accompanied by functional improvement.

Complications

These include 3% to 7% intracerebral hemorrhage, often without neurologic deficit, the incidence reported depending on whether a routine computed tomography scan was done postoperatively. Electrode migration affected 2% to 7%, epilepsy affected 2%, and various unwanted stimulation effects such as dysarthria, hand ataxia, gait disturbance affected up to 46.5%, often corrected readily by parameter change. Superficial infection occurred in up to 7%, persistent numbness up to 6%, equipment failure up to 6%, battery failure 9%, loose lead connection 6%, persistent dysarthria up to 12%, and dysequilibrium up to 3%. Complications were similar despite the diagnosis for which the surgery was done, although complications seemed to be more common in multiple sclerosis.[27,28,30,32,33,35,36,46]

THALAMOTOMY IN PARKINSON'S DISEASE

After thalamotomy, 79% of patients in published series enjoyed good contralateral tremor reduction, 60% transient, and 10% to 20% permanent complications in a review by Perry and Lenz.[50] In the literature review by Tasker and colleagues,[51] 45% to 92% of patients with Parkinson's disease enjoyed total abolition and 68% to 100% a significant reduction of contralateral tremor; 41% to 92% had total abolition and 50% to 100% significant reduction of contralateral rigidity. Manual dexterity was moderately improved, depending on whether the disability was caused by tremor. Speech, gait, stance, and bradykinesia were not significantly affected. Although thalamotomy reduces contralateral dopa dyskinesia, the effect is nowhere near as prominent as that from pallidal surgery. In the author's experience, 15% of thalamotomies had to be repeated because of recurrent tremor to achieve the above-mentioned result.[2,5,24,25,50–55]

Complications

Sixty percent of patients developed temporary and 10% to 20% permanent complications.[2,5,24,25,50–56] Intracranial hemorrhage affected 1.5% to 6%. Mortality ranged from 0 to 5%, and as many as 30% of procedures had to be repeated to achieve optimal tremor control. Cognitive problems affected up to 39% of patients, persistent in 0.8% to 11.2%; persistent hemiparesis occurred in 0 to 6.3%, persistent dysphagia in 0 to 3%, aggravation of dysarthria in 1% to 25%, hand ataxia in 1% to 3%, gait disturbance in 1.2% to 6%, persistent equinovarus and other ankle deformities in 3.5% to 5.3%, hyperkinesias in 0.3% to 9%, persistent numbness in 0.5% to 3.3%, epileptic seizures in 0.5% to 8%, infections in 0.5% to 2.7%, and pseudobulbar symptoms in 0.25% to 0.5%.

Is Thalamic Surgery Still Warranted in Parkinson's Disease?

Most parkinsonian patients have bradykinesia, and therefore most stereotactic surgeons favor surgery on the subthalamic nucleus, which improves most aspects of Parkinson's disease. However, parkinsonian cases do occur in which the disease is either arrested or is very slowly progressive, with tremor the main problem. This is particularly true in patients whose disease began before age 40 or who had postencephalitic Parkinson's disease. In these patients, thalamic surgery might well still be considered.[2]

Thalamotomy versus Thalamic Deep Brain Stimulation

The author is unaware of a properly documented comparison of the two procedures; in his own experience, the incidence of tremor relief is identical except that 15% of his thalamotomies had to be repeated because of recurrent tremor, but only 3% of thalamic DBS procedures had to be repeated to achieve this level of tremor control.[25,38]

Bilateral Thalamotomy for Parkinson's Disease

The complications of bilateral thalamotomy are essentially twice those of unilateral thalamotomy except for dysarthria, which occurred in 27.3% of the author's 55 patients. Published complications include mortality, 0 to 4.3%; persistent cognitive deficits, 1.8% to 34.8%; persistent dysphasia, 3.6%; persistent hemiparesis, 0.8% to 1.8%; dysphagia, 4.8% to 5.4%, persistent worsening of dysarthria, 18% to 60%; gait disturbance, 7.4%.[2,5] Osenbach and Burchiel[52] reported 39% cognitive deficit after unilateral thalamotomy and 60% after bilateral.

THALAMOTOMY FOR ESSENTIAL TREMOR

Essential tremor might be considered the ideal indication for thalamic surgery because the disability is almost entirely dependent on tremor. Unfortunately, there is a tendency for the tremor to recur postoperatively with time, termed "tolerance" by Benabid. Although immediately postoperatively, nearly 100% of patients have no tremor, only 62% will be that well at long-term follow-up, and although virtually 100% are able to drink with the operated hand immediately postoperatively, only 71% can do so later on.[5,57] Published results indicate 68% to 83% total or nearly total reduction of tremor, allowing most patients to return to work.[22] In the author's experience, 4.5% had an intracerebral hematoma that had to be evacuated, and 4.5% had persistent hemiparesis, dysarthria, or gait disturbance; 9.1% had persistent numbness, 9.1% had isolated epileptic seizures, 4.5% had superficial scalp infection, 4.5% had transient cognitive disturbance, 4.5% had transient dysarthria, and 13.6% had transient numbness.

THALAMOTOMY FOR CEREBELLAR TREMOR

Unlike Parkinson's disease, cerebellar tremor inflicts loss of manual dexterity, restoration of which is the aim of the surgery, not the cosmetic effects of persisting rest tremor, and although the immediate postoperative effects are very good as in Parkinson's disease and essential tremor, the tremor and loss of manual dexterity recur much more often and more rapidly and dramatically even than in essential tremor and much more so than in Parkinson's disease. Of the author's patients, 84.8% had no or only minor tremor immediately postoperatively, whereas this percentage dropped to 45% at the latest follow-up. Immediately postoperatively, 56.5% could drink with the operated hand, but at the latest follow-up, only 15.2% could do so and another

21% could drink with difficulty.[5,22,46,53,58] Published series report 11% to 50% of patients with multiple sclerosis were relieved of their tremor by thalamotomy and 44% to 90% enjoyed significant reduction of tremor. However, functional improvement is often not noted. Goldman and Kelly, on the other hand,[58] reported significant reduction of tremor in 65% of 131 patients with multiple sclerosis, 75% of 44 patients with post-traumatic tremor, and 100% of 29 patients with poststroke tremor; functional improvement occurred in 44%, 90%, and 33%, respectively, of these three groups; others have reported similarly encouraging data.

Although the complications are similar to those of thalamotomy for Parkinson's disease, in our hands, they seem more numerous: 0.2% intracerebral hemorrhage, 8.7% aggravation of multiple sclerosis, 4.3% persistent cognitive disturbance, 8.7% persistent mild hemiparesis, 4.3% persistent dysarthria, 4.3% persistent arm ataxia, 2.2% persistent gait disturbance, and 4.3% persistent numbness in the multiple sclerosis group.

PALLIDOTOMY AND PALLIDAL DEEP BRAIN STIMULATION

Introduction

After Laitinen drew attention to the efficacy of pallidotomy for bradykinesia in Parkinson's disease, interest in pallidotomy was rekindled.[59-64] The effect was explained by the DeLong model,[3,65,66] which attributed bradykinesia to increased output from striatum to the globus pallidus externa (GPe), reduced output from the GPe to the STN, globus pallidus interna (GPi), and substantia nigra pars reticulata (SNr) with disinhibitory activation of the STN, GPi, and SNr. This results in turn in excess inhibitory output of the GPi on thalamocortical circuitry causing bradykinesia. A pallidotomy would reduce the excess inhibition of the GPi on thalamocortical circuits relieving bradykinesia, a concept that was not widely thought of in the early days of pallidotomy when bradykinesia was looked on as a negative feature like paralysis that could not be improved by further lesioning. Suddenly, there was intent interest in pallidotomy for Parkinson's disease, surgery which had been abandoned in the 1960s in favor of thalamotomy. To be successful, pallidotomy had to involve the sensory motor portion of the GPi and spare the cognitive part, that is, lesioning Leksell's ventroposteromedial portion on which Laitinen focused attention.

Patient Selection

Patients with Parkinson's disease without cognitive impairment who were disabled by bradykinesia and who showed a response to L-dopa were the prime subjects considered for pallidotomy or pallidal DBS.[62,63] Tremor is less affected in this author's opinion than it is by thalamic or STN surgery, but because bradykinesia is so seldom absent in Parkinson's disease, it is the most important element to consider when planning surgery. There is still controversy as to the exact pallidal target; whether it should be in the pallidum itself and at which site or the ansa lenticularis; whether there are different sites for treating tremor, rigidity, bradykinesia,

and dopa dyskinesia; and whether somatotopographic organization within the GPi allows differential targeting for arm and leg function. Some authors advocated including the GPe in the lesion; others thought that the preferable target was the GPi. Some authors have found that the presence of cerebral atrophy or ischemic changes did not negate the benefits of pallidotomy. Merello and colleagues[67] found the results better if involuntary movements were seen as the lesion was being made. Taha and colleagues[68] found tremor control better if the lesion included the tremor synchronous cells.

Technique (Fig. 100-2)

The procedure is done as in other stereotactic surgery, most centers targeting the center of the medial portion of the GPi. Sierens and Bakay[59] suggested that before the era of L-dopa, the pallidotomy target was 15 to 17 mm from midline and 0 to 5 mm posterior to the anterior commissure, whereas the current target is 20 to 22 mm lateral and 2 to 6 mm ventral to the intercommissural plane and 0 to 4 mm anterior to the midpoint of the anterior and posterior commissures line. Although this target can be directly visualized, this author prefers to have the additional backup of physiologic localization, which usually requires two to three microelectrode trajectories to confirm the location of the optimal target.[8-12] The electrode passing from anterodorsally first passes through the GPe with high-voltage spontaneous activity consisting of either 10- to 20-Hz discharges interspersed with rapid bursts or 40 to 60 Hz with occasional pauses. As the electrode leaves the GPe and enters the GPi, "border cells" are encountered with regular slow or slowly fluctuating firing rates. In the GPi are found high-activity, rapidly firing (80 to 90 Hz) cells, sometimes with pauses, 25% of which respond with either an increase or a decrease in their firing rate to passive movements on chiefly the contralateral side but not usually to specific movements; they may fire synchronously with tremor. Leaving the GPi, typical cellular activity ceases, with the recording becoming quiet until, in the optic tract, one may record axonal discharges to contralateral light flashes or else contralateral phosphenes with microstimulation. In the internal capsule, recording silence is again seen and tetanizing responses occur with microstimulation. The general activity of GPi cells is thought to be greater in Parkinson's disease than it is normally, and it may be reduced in movement disorders such as dystonia. The ideal target must be located sufficiently far from optic nerve or internal capsule responses to avoid damage by the RF lesion or activation by the DBS electrode.

Outcome Data

Reported outcome data vary considerably.[32,59-63,68-98] Tremor is reduced in 33% to 90% of cases, rigidity in 25% to 92%, bradykinesia in 19% to 92%, and dopa dyskinesia in 61% to 82%; gait is improved in 7% to 30%, often only transiently, and activities of daily living in 23% to 33%. Although bilateral surgery is more effective than unilateral, it may incur speech and cognitive disorders. All observers note that dopa dyskinesia is the most dramatically reduced (82% to 92% reduction).

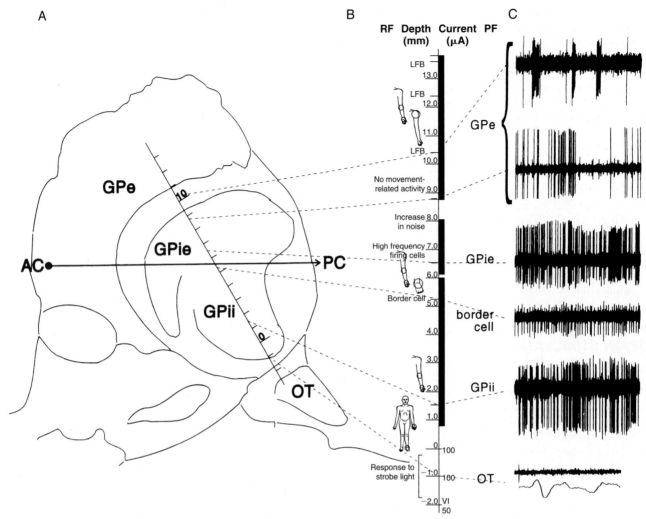

FIGURE 100-2 Physiologic data collected from one microelectrode trajectory through the globus pallidus mapped on a redrawn sagittal diagram from the Schaltenbrand and Wahren atlas. (RF, receptive field; PF, projected field.) Neuronal activity is shown at the right and receptive fields at the left of the trajectory. The axonal response to visual stimuli is shown in the bottom two traces. In the lower one of the two, appropriate filtering of the upper trace reveals the visual evoked potential unseen in the upper trace. (LFB, low-frequency bursting neuron; GPe, globus pallidus externa; GPie, globus pallidus interna external segment; GPii, globus pallidus interna internal segment; ACPC, anterior and posterior commissures). (From Germano IM [ed]: Neurosurgical Treatment of Movement Disorders. Park Ridge, IL: AANS, 1998, p 139.)

Complications

Permanent complications affected 1% to 37.5% of patients, being less in the larger series, especially affecting vision. Complications in the University Health Network series included 0% mortality or confusion, 5% facial weakness, 7.5% dysarthria, 5% dysphagia, 10% cognitive difficulties, 5% personality change, 0% paresis, 10% worsening of handwriting, 5% imbalance, 2.5% word finding difficulties, and 0% visual field defects. Obviously hemiparesis from encroachment on the capsule and visual field defects from encroachment on the optic tract are very real concerns during pallidotomy but can be avoided with careful imaging and physiologic monitoring.

Lang and colleagues[97] found subtle transient and persistent neuropsychological changes after unilateral pallidotomy such as word finding deficit in 69% of patients operated on the left side and 25% on the right. Various other impairments were seen, particularly verbal ones with left-sided lesions, 20% showed frontal or executive behavioral change, 28% had memory and concentration problems, and 27% of patient families noted neuropsychological behavioral changes that the patients did not notice but believed the benefits of the operation far outweighed the complications. Interestingly, 35% showed weight gain. Other observers found few neuropsychological abnormalities and, strangely, some observers found pallidotomy not useful in improving the Parkinson's score but only in controlling dopa dyskinesia. Alegret and colleagues[98] found that unilateral pallidotomy may produce transient changes in prefrontal and visual spatial function, but no permanent neuropsychological effects.

Pallidal Deep Brain Stimulation

DBS in the GPi gives essentially the same results as pallidotomy, whereas the complications are similar to those from stimulation at other sites.[99–102] Morello and colleagues[103] did a randomized study and found the results the same in unilateral GPi DBS and unilateral pallidotomy, whereas

Burchiel and colleagues[104] found no difference in reduction of akinetic rigid symptoms in Parkinson's disease or dyskinesias between STN- and GPi-stimulated patients. Volkmann and colleagues[105] found 54% ± 33.1% improvement in all motor function in the GPi DBS group, 67% ± 22.6% in the STN DBS group at 1-year follow-up, a significant difference. Moreover, the GPi patients continue to require the same medication doses postoperatively as they did before, whereas the STN patients have an average reduction of dopamimetic medication in the 65% range and equivalent improvement in off motor function. Carr and colleagues[73] noted that most patients who underwent unilateral left posteroventral pallidotomy for Parkinson's disease exhibited declines in learning, fluency, working memory, and speed at color naming, whereas Troster and colleagues[74] noted the most marked declines in lexical and semantic verbal fluency after left pallidotomy. The patients who underwent right pallidotomy did not exhibit significant cognitive decline, but fluency did decline in 71% of patients.

Pallidal DBS may be useful to avoid the cognitive difficulties of bilateral pallidotomy if performed contralateral to a previous destructive lesion.[106]

PALLIDAL SURGERY AND DYSTONIA

Introduction

This is not the place to review dystonia. Although most procedures available to treat dyskinesias have been applied to dystonia,[107,108] the dramatic effect of pallidal surgery on dopa dyskinesia, one particular form of drug-induced dystonia, has focused attention on pallidal surgery for dystonia in general. Dystonia associated with cerebral palsy[109–111] is common, but usually it is the cerebral palsy, and not the dystonia, that limits the patient's abilities and does not respond to surgery for dyskinesia. Similarly, in secondary dystonia, the operation will not benefit the primary lesion that causes the dystonia. As a result, attention here is focused on primary dystonia or dystonia musculorum deformans. The same issues apply as in Parkinson's disease with respect to contraindications to surgery, although there are some others. The normal brain of the patient with primary dystonia, in contrast to the parkinsonian patient with larger ventricles, may place the internal capsule at risk if one makes, say, a thalamic lesion 14 to 15 mm from the midline, which would be perfectly safe in Parkinson's disease,[112] and bilateral surgery can be just as dangerous in dystonia as in Parkinson's disease.

Thalamotomy

Thalamotomy has been used to treat dystonia for many years with good results in 22% to 62% and significant improvement in 14% to 54%.[113–123] Although sometimes the patient shows delayed improvement after the operation, usually the improvement occurs early and declines over time. Possibly patients do better who carry the DVT gene abnormality. It seemed to this author that limb dystonia, whether primary or secondary, improved better than axial dystonia. Andrew and colleagues[114] found segmental and focal dystonia did best. Secondary patients tended to be vulnerable to gait disturbance and shoulder dislocation after thalamotomy. In patients with dystonia, bilateral thalamotomy

resulted in dysarthria at greater than expected rates as well as a tendency to pseudobulbar disturbance. Patients whose disease was progressing rapidly did less well.

Pallidotomy for Dystonia

The procedure is done as it would be for Parkinson's disease. After pallidotomy, motor performance improved from 13% to 100% in different series after unilateral or bilateral pallidotomy,[123] but only small numbers of patients have been reported in these series. Axial symptoms require bilateral surgery. Sometimes the results can be spectacular.

Pallidal Deep Brain Stimulation

The procedure is done as in Parkinson's disease, and the target is the same as for pallidotomy in Parkinson's disease. Again, although the number of patients treated is small, this is clearly a beneficial method for treating this disabling condition with results similar to those of pallidotomy.[123–125]

Kupsch and colleagues[126] noted excellent results in pallidal DBS in patients with primary dystonia with the DYT1 gene abnormality. Other idiopathic generalized cases, myoclonus dystonia, tardive dystonia, and focal and secondary disease, fared less well. Yianni and colleagues[127] found that GPi DBS helped generalized dystonia and spasmodic torticollis. Krauss and colleagues[128] found GPi DBS a good treatment for generalized dystonia, including patients not harboring the DYT1 gene abnormality, but improvement in choreoathetosis was only modest.

SUBTHALAMIC NUCLEUS SURGERY

Introduction

The DeLong model calls for the STN, located in the indirect pathway, to also become hyperactive in Parkinson's disease just as the direct pathway does.[65] This being the case, STN surgery should have results similar to those of pallidal surgery in this condition. Fearing hemiballismus as produced by Carpenter and colleagues[129] in monkeys when STN lesions were made, Benabid and colleagues and others[130,131] started doing bilateral STN stimulation to control Parkinson's disease. Cautiously, Obeso and colleagues[132] and other groups[133–136] have also studied the effects of STN lesions, finding that hemiballismus is not an inevitable consequence and making the benefits of STN surgery available where DBS is not an economically practical activity. Perhaps the altered circuitry in Parkinson's disease makes hemiballismus less likely when the STN is lesioned. Whereas pallidotomy reduces the amount of dopa dyskinesia, STN surgery reduces the need for L-dopa, thus diminishing the incidence of dopa dyskinesia by reducing its intake.

Technique for Subthalamotomy and Subthalamic Deep Brain Stimulation

The procedure is performed as other stereotactic operations for dyskinesia are. The STN, which can often be seen directly on magnetic resonance imaging,[137] lies approximately 6 mm below the middle of the intercommissural line and 10 to 15 mm from midline The author prefers to confirm the location of the target with microelectrode recording. Typically, the electrode passes through structures dictated by the trajectory chosen, especially the rostral thalamus where cells fire at low frequency. Entry into the STN is marked by cells firing at 30 to 70 Hz with receptive fields for passive movement in contralateral limbs, some of which are tremor cells. Identification of proper position may be confirmed by microstimulation, which dramatically reduces contralateral rigidity (Fig. 100-3).

As a microelectrode is advanced, the ventral border of the STN is marked by reduction in electrical activity until the electrode enters the SNr anteriorly or the substantia nigra pars compacta (SNc) more posteriorly. SNr cells are small and fire in a regular high-frequency pattern of 60 to 80 Hz, and occasional cells respond to saccadic eye movements. SNr stimulation may cause eye deviation because of current spread into the oculomotor fascicles. Microstimulation is then done at 0.1 to 100 µA, 300 Hz, 100-µsec pulse width, proximity to the medial lemniscus being indicated by low-threshold paresthesia, whereas low-threshold muscle contractions indicate proximity to the internal capsule, which lies anterior and lateral to the STN. Usually, as at other sites, three or four microelectrode trajectories are necessary.

For STN DBS, the electrode and its pulse generator are inserted in the same way as for other DBS operations. Postoperative programming takes care and time, and the attempt to do so is usually delayed until the patient reaches preoperative baseline. Stimulation is then carried out with varying parameters until the best relief of symptoms without untoward effects is obtained. Monopolar, bipolar, or multipolar stimulation may be necessary, and the frequency of stimulation may range from 120 to 185 Hz, the pulse width from 60 to 90 µsec, and the amplitude from 2 to 3.5 V, although sometimes stimulation may have to be done well outside of this range.

Outcome

As in other dyskinesia procedures, reported outcomes vary,[138–144] with improvement in the Unified Parkinson's Disease Rating Scale motor score off medication ranging from 42% to 70%, reduction of L-dopa intake from 0% to 65% (usually at least 40%), tremor reduction of 74% to 97% (off), rigidity reduction of 33% to 68% (off), bradykinesia of 25% to 71% (off), and dopa dyskinesia, 0% to 67% (on). Improvement in axial symptoms of posture, gait, and speech varied widely, and time will tell the eventual story.

Complications

Complications were similar to those after other DBS procedures, with intracranial hemorrhage occurring in 0.6% to 3.5%, rarely resulting in death. Hardware problems with infection and erosion ranged from 2.5% to 23.4% and hardware malfunctions ranged from 5.8% to 17.7%. Lead migration affected 14.2% of patients in one series but was not mentioned in others.

Unwanted stimulation effects could generally be controlled by changing the stimulation parameters and included, in some series, depression, increased hypophonia and

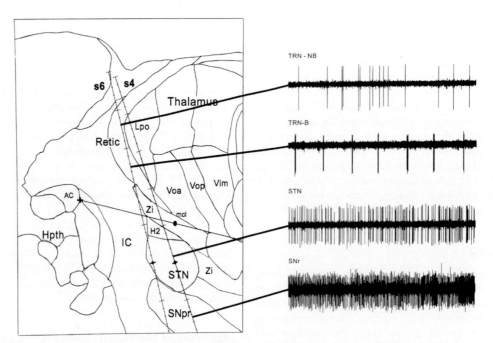

FIGURE 100-3 As in Figure 100-1, which shows a trajectory through the subthalamic nucleus to the left, recordings of spontaneous activity at four sites along the trajectory at the right. (S4, S6, fourth and sixth trajectory used; Lpo, lateropolar nucleus; Retic, reticular nucleus of the thalamus; Voa, Vop, anterior and posterior oral nuclei of the thalamus; Vim, ventral intermediate nucleus of the thalamus; AC, anterior commissure; Hpth, hypothalamus; IC, internal capsule; ZI, zona incerta; STN, subthalamic nucleus; H2, Forel's fields H2; SNpr, substantia nigra pars reticulata; mcl, intercommissural line.) The tracings at the right represent two types of spontaneous activity in the reticular nucleus of the thalamus (R type A, R type B) and one each from the subthalamic nucleus and the substantia nigra pars reticulata. (From Hutchison WD, Allan RJ, Opitz H, et al: Neurophysiological identification of the subthalamic nucleus in surgery for Parkinson's disease. Ann Neurol 44:622–628, 1998.)

dysarthria, and apraxia of eyelid opening. Confusion in the immediate postoperative phase occurred particularly in patients older than 60 years of age.

Subthalamotomy

STN lesions can be made at the same site at which DBS is done.

Outcome

There are now a number of published series of subthalamotomy.[132–136] Vilela Filho and Da Silva[134] noted, after unilateral subthalamotomy, a 68.2% reduction of bradykinesia, 83.9% of rigidity, 84.9% of tremor, 66.5% of postural disturbance, 44.2% of speech disturbance, and 74.2% of dyskinesia. L-Dopa intake was cut by 42.6%; 4.1% of their patients developed hemiballismus, abolished by lesions in posterior oral nucleus of the thalamus or the ventral intermediate nucleus of the thalamus at the same sitting, 38.1% had transient confusion, and 5% had interference with speech. Some procedures were done bilaterally. In other series of patients undergoing subthalamotomy, some bilaterally, as many as 25% developed postoperative dyskinesia or chorea, which usually subsided spontaneously. The Unified Parkinson's Disease Rating Scale motor off score improved as much as 58% in the off-medications state. Activities of daily living improved 25.1% and "on time," without significant dopa dyskinesia, doubled. Contralateral tremor, rigidity, and bradykinesia were reduced. The overall L-dopa dose required was reduced by 50%. Cognitive difficulties were not prominent.

Bilateral subthalamotomy was done either simultaneously or staged. The dramatic immediate motor improvements might deteriorate with time in these cases, possibly because the lesions were made smaller than in unilateral cases.

OTHER PROCEDURES

Unless bilateral STN DBS is proven to slow the progression of Parkinson's disease, as Benabid and colleagues[4] and others have recently suggested,[3] all the surgery discussed here is palliative. Various procedures have been studied but largely abandoned in attempts to find a technique to alter the course of the disease including adrenal cell and mesencephalic fetal cell implants, glial-derived nerve growth factor infusion into the cerebrospinal fluid, and motor cortex stimulation.

However, Gill and colleagues[145] infused glial-derived nerve growth factor directly into the putamen in five patients with Parkinson's disease (glial-derived nerve growth factor does not enter the brain from blood or cerebrospinal fluid) and found that after 1 year, there were no significant clinical complications but instead a 39% improvement in the off motor Unified Parkinson's Disease Rating Scale score, a 61% improvement in the activities of daily living, and 64% reduction in drug induced dyskinesia.

CONCLUSION

Palliative stereotactic dyskinesia surgery has been brought to a very high level of technical elaboration with, more recently, reasonably consistent results. In Parkinson's disease,

the chief interest is in bilateral STN DBS, but STN lesioning is also available and a detailed comparison with bilateral GPi DBS is awaited in a sufficient number of patients to indicate which is best. Thalamic DBS and thalamotomy are available and useful, particularly in essential tremor, but also in slowly progressing predominantly tremor cases of Parkinson's disease. These procedures are less successful in cerebellar tremor. In primary dystonia, pallidotomy and GPi DBS are the most effective treatments, although the numbers are still small in the reported series.

However, reliable procedures that reverse or slow the course of a dyskinesia are being eagerly sought and glial-derived nerve growth factor infusion into the putamen appears promising in Parkinson's disease.

REFERENCES

1. Benabid AL, Caparros-Lefebvre D, Pollak P: History of surgery for movement disorders. In Germano M (ed): Neurosurgical Treatment of Movement Disorders. Park Ridge, IL: AANS, 1998, pp 19–36.
2. Tasker RR, DeCarvalho GC, Li CS, et al: Does thalamotomy alter the course of Parkinson's disease? Adv Neurol 69:563–583, 1996.
3. Rodrigues MC, Obeso JA, Olanow CW: Subthalamic nucleus mediated excitotoxicity in Parkinson's disease: A target for neuroprotection. Ann Neurol 44:S175–S188, 1998.
4. Benabid AL, Pollak P, Gross C, et al: Acute and long-term effects of subthalamic nucleus stimulation in Parkinson's disease. Stereotact Funct Neurosurg 62:76–84, 1994.
5. Tasker RR: Thalamotomy for Parkinson's disease and other types of tremor. Part II: The outcome of thalamotomy for tremor. In Gildenberg PL, Tasker RR (eds): Textbook of Stereotactic and Functional Neurosurgery. New York: McGraw-Hill, 1998, pp 1179–1198.
6. Tasker RR, Dostrovsky JP: Invasive lesioning of the central nervous system for functional disorders. In Alexander EB, Maciunas RM (eds): Advanced Neurosurgical Navigation. New York: Thieme, 1999, pp 483–506.
7. Tasker RR, Davis KW, Hutchison WD, et al: Subcortical and thalamic mapping in functional neurosurgery. In Gildenberg PL, Tasker RR (eds): Textbook of Stereotactic and Functional Neurosurgery. New York: McGraw-Hill, 1998, pp 883–969.
8. Lozano A, Hutchison WD: Pallidotomy: Indications and technique. In Germano IM (ed): Neurosurgical Treatment of Movement Disorders. Park Ridge, IL: AANS, 1998, pp 131–141.
9. Lozano AM, Hutchison WD, Dostrovsky JO: Microelectrode monitoring of cortical and subcortical structures during stereotactic surgery. Acta Neurochir (Wien) 64(Suppl):30–34, 1995.
10. Lozano A, Hutchison W, Kiss Z, et al: Methods for microelectrode-guided posteroventral pallidotomy. J Neurosurg 84:194–202, 1996.
11. Hutchison WD, Lozano AM, Davis KD, et al: Differential neuronal activity in segments of globus pallidus in Parkinson's disease patients. Neuroreport 5:1533–1537, 1994.
12. Lozano AM, Lang AE, Hutchison WD, et al: Microelectrode recording-guided posteroventral pallidotomy in patients with Parkinson's disease. Adv Neurol 74:167–174, 1997.
13. Alterman RL, Kall BA, Cohen H, et al: Stereotactic ventrolateral thalamotomy: Is ventriculography necessary? Neurosurgery 37:717–722, 1995.
14. Schaltenbrand G, Wahren W: Atlas for Stereotaxy of the Human Brain. Stuttgart: Thieme, 1977.
15. Nordera GP, Mesiano T, Durisotti C, et al: Six years experience in deep brain stimulation in Parkinson's disease: Advantages and limitations of use of neurophysiological intraoperative microrecording. Neurol Sci 24:194, 2003.
16. Linhares MN, Tasker RR: Thalamotomy with microelectrode recordings. In Lozano AM (ed): Movement Disorder Surgery. Progress in Neurological Surgery, vol 15. Basel: Karger, 2000, pp 156–171.
17. Kaplitt MG, Hutchison WD, Lozano AM: Target localization in movement disorders surgery. In Tarsy D, Vitek JL, Lozano AM (eds): Surgical Treatment of Parkinson's Disease and Other Movement Disorders. Totowa, NJ: Humana, 2003, pp 89–98.

18. Priori A, Egidi M, Pesenti A, et al: Do intraoperative microrecordings improve subthalamic nucleus targeting in stereotactic neurosurgery for Parkinson's disease? J Neurosurg Sci 47:56–60, 2003.

19. Counclis GJ, Simuni T, Forman MS, et al: Bilateral subthalamic nucleus deep brain stimulation for advanced PD: Correlation of intraoperative MER and postoperative MRI with neuropathological findings. Mov Disord 18:1062–1065, 2003.

20. Kiss ZHT, Wilkinson M, Krcek J, et al: Is the target for thalamic DBS the same as for thalamotomy? Mov Disord 18:1169–1175, 2003.

21. Lenz FA, Normand SL, Kwan HC, et al: Statistical prediction of the optimal site for thalamotomy in parkinsonian tremor. Mov Disord 10:318–328, 1995.

22. Hua SE, Garonzik IM, Lee J-I, Lenz FA: Thalamotomy for tremor in surgical treatment of Parkinson's disease and other movement disorders. In Tarsy D, Vitek JL, Lozano AM (eds): Surgical Treatment of Parkinson's Disease and Other Movement Disorders. Totowa, NJ: Humana, 2003, pp 99–113.

23. Brodkey JA, Lozano AM, Tasker RR, et al: Tremor cells in the human thalamus: Differences among neurological disorders. J Neurosurg 101:43–47, 2004.

24. Tasker RR, Munz M, Junn FS, et al: Deep brain stimulation and thalamotomy for tremor compared. Acta Neurochir (Wien) 68(Suppl):49–53, 1997.

25. Tasker RR: Deep brain stimulation is preferable to thalamotomy for tremor suppression. Surg Neurol 49:145–154, 1998.

26. Caparros-Lefebvre D, Ruchoux MM, Blond S, et al: Long-term thalamic stimulation in Parkinson's disease: Postmortem anatomoclinical study. Neurology 44:1856–1860, 1994.

27. Hariz GM, Bergenheim AT, Hariz MI, et al: Assessment of ability/disability in patients treated with chronic thalamic stimulation for tremor. Mov Disord 13:78–83, 1998.

28. Benabid AL, Pollak P, Gao D, et al: Chronic electrical stimulation of the ventralis intermedius nucleus of the thalamus as a treatment of movement disorders. J Neurosurg 84:203–214, 1996.

29. Alterman RL, Kelly P: Magnetic resonance imaging guidance in surgery for Parkinson's disease. In Germano IM (ed): Neurosurgical Treatment of Movement Disorders. Park Ridge, IL: AANS, 1998, pp 195–205.

30. Alesch F, Pinter MM, Helscher RJ, et al: Stimulation of the ventral intermediate thalamic nucleus in tremor dominated Parkinson's disease and essential tremor. Acta Neurochir (Wien) 136:75–81, 1995.

31. Alesch F, Pinter MM, Koos WT: Chronic stimulation of the ventralis intermedius nucleus in patients with Parkinson's disease and essential tremor: The Vienna experience. Stereotact Funct Neurosurg 65:66, 1995.

32. Duff J, Sime E: Surgical interventions in the treatment of Parkinson's disease (PD) and essential tremor (ET): Medial pallidotomy in PD and chronic deep brain stimulation (DBS) in PD and ET. Axone 18:85–89, 1997.

33. Koller W, Pahwa R, Busenbark K, et al: High-frequency unilateral thalamic stimulation in the treatment of essential and parkinsonian tremor. Ann Neurol 42:292–299, 1997.

34. Defebvre L, Blatt JL, Blond S, et al: Effect of thalamic stimulation on gait in Parkinson's disease. Arch Neurol 53:898–890, 1996.

35. Tasker RR: Deep brain stimulation in thalamus. In Couldwell WT, Cosgrove GR (eds): Contemporary Surgical Management of Movement Disorders. St. Louis: Quality Medical Publishing (in press).

36. Broggi G: Chronic deep brain stimulation: Clinical results. In Germano IM (ed): Neurosurgical Treatment of Movement Disorders. Park Ridge, IL: AANS, 1994, pp 169–177.

37. Tarsy D, Norrogard T, Hubble J: Thalamic deep brain stimulation for Parkinson's disease and essential tremor. In Tarsy D, Vitek JL, Lozano AM (eds): Surgical Treatment of Parkinson's Disease and Other Movement Disorders. Totowa, NJ: Humana, 2003, pp 153–161.

38. Schuurman PR, Bosch DA, Bossuyi PM, et al: A comparison of continuous thalamic stimulation and thalamotomy for suppression of severe tremor. N Engl J Med 342:461–469, 2000.

39. Rehncrona S, Johnels B, Widner H, et al: Long-term efficacy of thalamic deep brain stimulation for tremor: Double-blind assessments. Mov Disord 18:163–170, 2003.

40. Tamma F, Rampini P, Egidi M, et al: Deep brain stimulation for Parkinson's disease: The experience of the Policlinico-San Paolo Group in Milan. Neurol Sci 24(Suppl 1):S41–S42, 2003.

41. Landi A, Parolin M, Piolti R, et al: Deep brain stimulation for the treatment of Parkinson's disease: The experience of the Neurosurgical Department in Monza. Neurol Sci 24(Suppl 1):S43–S44, 2003.

42. Hubble JP, Busenbark KL, Wilkinson S, et al: Deep brain stimulation for essential tremor. Neurology 46:1150–1153, 1996.

43. Hubble JP, Busenbark KL, Wilkinson S, et al: Effects of thalamic deep brain stimulation based on tremor type of diagnosis. Mov Disord 12:337–341, 1997.

44. Fields JA, Troster AI, Woods SP, et al: Neuropsychological and quality of life outcomes 12 months after unilateral thalamic stimulation for essential tremor. J Neurol Neurosurg Psychiatry 74:305–311, 2003.

45. Bryant JA, DeSalles A, Cabatan C, et al: The impact of thalamic stimulation on activities of daily living for essential tremor. Surg Neurol 59:479–484, 2003.

46. Geny C, Nguyen JP, Pollin B, et al: Improvement of severe postural cerebellar tremor in multiple sclerosis by chronic thalamic stimulation. Mov Disord 11:489–494, 1996.

47. Carpenter MA, Pahwa R, Miyawaki KL, et al: Reduction in voice tremor under thalamic stimulation. Neurology 50:796–798, 1998.

48. Whittle IR, Hooper J, Pentland B: Thalamic deep-brain stimulation for movement disorders due to multiple sclerosis. Lancet 351:109–110, 1998.

49. Katayama Y, Fukaya C, Yamamoto T: Control of post-stroke involuntary and voluntary movement disorders with deep brain or epidural cortical stimulation. Stereotact Funct Neurosurg 69:73–79, 1997.

50. Perry VL, Lenz FA: Ablative therapy for movement disorders: Thalamotomy for Parkinson's disease. Neurosurg Clin N Am 9:317–324, 1998.

51. Tasker RR, Siqueira J, Hawrylyshyn P, et al: What happened to VIM thalamotomy for Parkinson's disease? Appl Neurophysiol 46:68–83, 1983.

52. Osenbach RR, Burchiel RJ: Thalamotomy: Indications, techniques, and results. In Germano M (ed): Neurosurgical Treatment of Movement Disorders. Park Ridge, IL: AANS, 1998, pp 107–129.

53. Jankovic J, Cardoso F, Grossman RG, et al: Outcome after stereotactic thalamotomy for parkinsonian, essential, and other types of tremor. Neurosurgery 37:680–687, 1996.

54. Fox MW, Ahlskog JE, Kelly PJ: Stereotactic ventrolateral thalamotomy for medically refractory tremor in post-levodopa era Parkinson's disease patients. J Neurosurg 75:723–730, 1991.

55. Brophy BP, Kimber TJ, Thompson PD: Thalamotomy for parkinsonian tremor. Stereotact Funct Neurosurg 69:1–4, 1997.

56. Lund-Johansen M, Hugdahl K, Wester K: Cognitive function in patients with Parkinson's disease undergoing stereotaxic thalamotomy. J Neurol Neurosurg Psychiatry 60:564–571, 1996.

57. Shahzadi S, Tasker RR, Lozano A: Thalamotomy for essential and cerebellar tremor. Stereotact Funct Neurosurg 65:11–17, 1995.

58. Goldman MS, Kelly PJ: Symptomatic and functional outcome of stereotactic ventralis lateralis thalamotomy for intention tremor. J Neurosurg 77:223–229, 1992.

59. Sierens DK, Bakay RAE: Pallidotomy for Parkinson's disease. In Tarsy D, Vitak JL, Lozano AM (eds): Surgical Treatment of Parkinson's Disease and Other Movement Disorders. Totowa, NJ: Humana, 2003, pp 115–128.

60. Narabayashi H, Miyashita N, Hattori Y, et al: Posteroventral pallidotomy: Its effect on motor symptoms and scores of MMPI test in patients with Parkinson's disease. Parkinsonism Relat Disord 3:7–20, 1997.

61. Jacques DS, Eagle RS, Kopyov OV: Use of posteroventral pallidotomy for treatment of Parkinson's disease: Is pallidotomy still an experimental procedure? A review and commentary. Stereotact Funct Neurosurg 70:19–31, 1998.

62. Krauss JK, Jankovic J, Lai EC, et al: Posteroventral medial pallidotomy in levodopa-unresponsive parkinsonism. Arch Neurol 54:1026–1029, 1997.

63. Laitinen LV, Bergenheim AT, Hariz MI: Leksell's posteroventral pallidotomy in the treatment of Parkinson's disease. J Neurosurg 76:53–61, 1992.

64. Guiridi J, Lozano AM: A brief history of pallidotomy. Neurosurgery 41:1169–1183, 1997.

65. Wichmann T, DeLong MR: Models of basal ganglia function and pathophysiology of movement disorders. Neurosurg Clin N Am 9:223–236, 1998.

66. Lopez SS: Anatomy of movement disorders. In Gildenberg PL, Tasker RR (eds): Textbook of Stereotactic and Functional Neurosurgery. New York: McGraw-Hill, 1998, pp 1005–1014.

67. Merello M, Cammarota A, Betti O, et al: Involuntary movements during thermolesion predict a better outcome after microelectrode guided posteroventral pallidotomy. J Neurol Neurosurg Psychiatry 63:210–213, 1997.

68. Taha JM, Favre J, Baumann TK, et al: Tremor control after pallidotomy in patients with Parkinson's disease: Correlation with microrecording findings. J Neurosurg 86:642–647, 1997.

69. Starr PA, Vitek JL, Bakay RAE: Pallidotomy: Clinical results. In Germano M (ed): Neurosurgical Treatment of Movement Disorders. Park Ridge, IL: AANS, 1998, pp 143–156.

70. Alterman RL, Kelly PJ: Pallidotomy technique and results: The New York University experience. Neurosurg Clin N Am 9:337–343, 1998.

71. Shima F, Ishido K, Sun SJ, et al: Surgical control of akinesia in Parkinson's disease. Eur Neurol 36(Suppl 1):55–61, 1996.

72. Burzaco J: Stereotactic pallidotomy in extrapyramidal disorders. Appl Neurophysiol 48:283–287, 1985.

73. Carr JA, Honey CR, Sinden M, et al: A waitlist control-group study of cognitive mood and quality of life outcome after posteroventral pallidotomy in Parkinson's disease. J Neurosurg 99:78–88, 2003.

74. Troster AI, Woods SP, Fields JA: Verbal fluency declines after pallidotomy: An interaction between task and lesion laterality. Appl Neuropsychol 10:69–75, 2003.

75. Laitinen LV: Ventroposterolateral pallidotomy. Stereotact Funct Neurosurg 62:41–52, 1994.

76. Baron MS, Vitek JL, Bakay RA, et al: Treatment of advanced Parkinson's disease by posterior GPi pallidotomy: 1-year results of a pilot study. Ann Neurol 40:355–366, 1996.

77. Dogali M, Sterio D, Fazzini E, et al: Effects of posteroventral pallidotomy on Parkinson's disease. Adv Neurol 69:585–590, 1996.

78. Fazzini E, Dogali M, Sterio D, et al: Stereotactic pallidotomy for Parkinson's disease: A long-term follow-up of unilateral pallidotomy. Neurology 48:1273–1277, 1997.

79. Gross RE, Lozano AM, Lang AE, et al: The effects of pallidotomy on Parkinson's disease: Study design and assessment techniques. Acta Neurochir 68(Suppl):24–28, 1997.

80. Kishore A, Turnbull IM, Snow BJ, et al: Efficacy, stability and predictors of outcome of pallidotomy for Parkinson's disease: Six-month follow-up with additional 1-year observations. Brain 120:729–737, 1997.

81. Johansson F, Malm J, Nordh E, et al: Usefulness of pallidotomy in advanced Parkinson's disease. J Neurol Neurosurg Psychiatry 62:125–132, 1997.

82. Kopyov O, Jacques D, Duma C, et al: Microelectrode-guided posteroventral medial radiofrequency pallidotomy for Parkinson's disease. J Neurosurg 87:52–59, 1997.

83. Krauss JK, Grossman RG, Lai EC, et al: Medial posteroventral pallidotomy for the treatment of Parkinson's disease. Zentralbl Neurochir 58:153–162, 1997.

84. Lozano AM, Lang AE, Galvez-Jimenez N, et al: Effect of GPi pallidotomy on motor function in Parkinson's disease. Lancet 346:1383–1387, 1995.

85. Meyer CH: Unilateral pallidotomy for Parkinson's disease promptly improves a wide range of voluntary activities—especially gait and trunk movements. Acta Neurochir (Wien) 68(Suppl):37–41, 1997.

86. Ondo WG, Jankovic J, Lai EC, et al: Assessment of motor function after stereotactic pallidotomy. Neurology 50:266–270, 1998.

87. Samuel M, Caputo E, Brooks DJ, et al: A study of medial pallidotomy for Parkinson's disease: Clinical outcome, MRI location and complications. Brain 121:59–75, 1998.

88. Schuurman PR, de Bie RM, Speelman JD, et al: Posteroventral pallidotomy in movement disorders. Acta Neurochir (Wien) 68(Suppl):14–17, 1997.

89. Shannon KM, Penn RD, Kroin JS, et al: Stereotactic pallidotomy for the treatment of Parkinson's disease: Efficacy and adverse effects at 6 months in 26 patients. Neurology 50:434–438, 1998.

90. Uitti RJ, Wharen RE Jr, Turk MF, et al: Unilateral pallidotomy for Parkinson's disease: Comparison of outcome in younger versus elderly patients. Neurology 49:1072–1077, 1997.

91. Vitek JL, Bakay RA: The role of pallidotomy in Parkinson's disease and dystonia. Curr Opin Neurol 10:332–339, 1997.

92. Favre J, Taha JM, Nguyen TT, et al: Pallidotomy: A survey of current practice in North America. Neurosurgery 39:883–892, 1996.

93. Lang AE, Lozano AM, Montgomery E, et al: Posteroventral medial pallidotomy in advanced Parkinson's disease. N Engl J Med 337: 1036–1042, 1997.

94. Hariz MI, De Salles AA: The side-effects and complications of posteroventral pallidotomy. Acta Neurchir (Wien) 68(Suppl):42–48, 1997.

95. Alkhami A, Lozano AM: Pallidotomy for Parkinson's disease: A review of contemporary literature. J Neurosurg 94:43–49, 2001.

96. Fine J, Duff J, Chen R, et al: Long-term follow-up of unilateral pallidotomy in advanced Parkinson's disease. N Engl J Med 342: 1708–1714, 2000.

97. Lang AE, Lozano A, Tasker R, et al: Neuropsychological and behavioral changes and weight gain after medial pallidotomy. Ann Neurol 41:834–836, 1997.

98. Alegret M, Valldeoriola F, Tolosa E, et al: Cognitive effects of unilateral posteroventral pallidotomy: A 4-year follow-up study. Mov Disord 18:323–328, 2003.

99. Siegfried J: Deep brain stimulation for movement disorders. In Gildenberg PL, Tasker RR (eds): Textbook of Stereotactic and Functional Neurosurgery. New York: McGraw-Hill, 1998, pp 1081–1085.

100. Siegfried J, Lippitz B: Bilateral chronic electrostimulation of ventroposterolateral pallidum: A new therapeutic approach for alleviating all parkinsonian symptoms. Neurosurgery 35:1126–1130, 1994.

101. Siegfried J, Wellis G: Chronic electrostimulation of ventroposterolateral pallidum: Follow-up. Acta Neurochir (Wien) 68(Suppl):11–13, 1997.

102. Siegfried J, Lippitz B: Chronic electrical stimulation of the VL-VPL complex and of the pallidum in the treatment of movement disorders: Personal experience since 1982. Stereotact Funct Neurosurg 62:71–75, 1994.

103. Merello M, Nouzeilles MI, Kuzis G: Unilateral radiofrequency lesion versus electrostimulation of posteroventral pallidum: A prospective randomized comparison. Mov Disord 14:50–56, 1999.

104. Burchiel K, Anderson VC, Favre J: Comparison of pallidal and subthalamic nucleus deep brain stimulation for advanced Parkinson's disease: Results of a randomized, blinded pilot study. Neurosurgery 45:1375–1382, 1999.

105. Volkmann J, Allest N, Vogas J: Safety and efficacy of pallidal or subthalamic nucleus stimulation in advanced Parkinson's disease. Neurology 56:548–551, 2001.

106. Galvez-Jimenez N, Lozano A, Tasker R, et al: Pallidal stimulation in Parkinson's disease patients with a prior unilateral pallidotomy. Can J Neurol Sci 25:300–305, 1998.

107. Vitek JL: Surgery for dystonia. Neurosurg Clin N Am 9:345–366, 1998.

108. Bronte-Stewart H: Surgical therapy for dystonia. Curr Neurol Neurosci Rep 3:296–305, 2003.

109. Tasker RR: Surgical treatment of the dystonias. In Gildenberg PL, Tasker RR (eds): Textbook of Stereotactic and Functional Neurosurgery. New York: McGraw-Hill, 1998, pp 1015–1032.

110. Narabayashi H: Experiences of stereotaxic surgery on cerebral palsy patients. Acta Neurochir (Wien) 24(Suppl):3–10, 1977.

111. Narabayashi H: Stereotaxic surgery for athetosis or the spastic state of cerebral palsy. Confin Neurol 22:364–367, 1962.

112. Hawrylyshyn PA, Tasker RR, Organ LW: Third ventricular width and the thalamocapsular border. Appl Neurophysiol 39:34–42, 1976/1977.

113. Andrew J, Edwards JM, Rudolf N de M: The placement of stereotaxic lesion for involuntary movements other than in Parkinson's disease. Acta Neurochir (Wien) 21(Suppl):39–47, 1974.

114. Andrew J, Fowler GJ, Harrison MJG: Stereotaxic thalamotomy in 55 cases of dystonia. Brain 106:981–1000, 1983.

115. Cardoso F, Jankovic J, Grossman RG, et al: Outcome after stereotactic thalamotomy for dystonia and hemiballismus. Neurosurgery 36:501–507, 1995.

116. Kandel EI: Functional and Stereotactic Neurosurgery (Translated by Watts G, translation edited by Walker AE). New York: Plenum, 1989.

117. Cooper IS: 20-year followup study of neurosurgical treatment of dystonia musculorum deformans. Adv Neurol 14:423–452, 1976.

118. Cooper IS: Dystonia: Surgical approaches to treatment and physiologic implications. In Yahr MD (ed): The Basal Ganglia. New York: Raven, 1976, pp 369–383.

119. Cooper IS: Involuntary Movement Disorders. New York: Harper & Row, 1969, pp 160–292.

120. Gros C, Frerebeau PH, Perez-Dominguez E, et al: Long term results of stereotaxic surgery for infantile dystonia and dyskinesia. Neurochirugica 19:171–178, 1976.

121. Tasker RR, Doorly T, Yamashiro K: Thalamotomy in generalized dystonia. Adv Neurol 50:615–633, 1988.

122. Tasker RR: Thalamotomy for dystonia. In Tarsy D, Vitek VC, Lozano AM (eds): Surgical Treatment of Parkinson's Disease. Totowa, NJ: Humana, 2003, pp 259–264.

123. Abosch A, Vitek VL, Lozano AM: Pallidotomy and pallidal deep brain stimulation for dystonia. In Tarsy D, Vitek VC, Lozano AM (eds): Surgical Treatment of Parkinson's Disease and Other Movement Disorders. Totowa, NJ: Humana, 2003, pp 265–274.

124. Kupsch A, Klaffke S, Kuhn AA, et al: The effects of frequency in pallidal deep brain stimulation for primary dystonia. J Neurol 250:1201–1205, 2003.

125. Cif L, El Fertit H, Vayssiere N, et al: Treatment of dystonic syndromes by chronic electrical stimulation of the internal globus pallidus. J Neurosurg Sci 47:52–55, 2003.

126. Kupsch A, Kuehn A, Klaffke S, et al: Deep brain stimulation in dystonia. J Neurol 250(Suppl 1):147–152, 2003.

127. Yianni J, Bain PG, Gregory RP, et al: Post-operative progress of dystonia patients following globus pallidus internus deep brain stimulation. Eur J Neurol 10:239–247, 2003.

128. Krauss JK, Loher TJ, Weigel R, et al: Chronic stimulation of the globus pallidus internus for treatment of non-DYT1 generalized dystonia and choreoathetosis: 2-year follow up. J Neurosurg 98:785–792, 2003.

129. Carpenter MB, Whittier JR, Mettler FA: Analysis of choreoid hyper-kinesias in the rhesus monkey: Surgical and pharmacological analysis of hyperkinesias resulting from lesions in the STN. J Comp Neurol 92:293–331, 1950.

130. Pollak P, Benabid AL, Limousin P, et al: Subthalamic nucleus stimulation alleviates akinesia and rigidity in parkinsonian patients. Adv Neurol 69:591–594, 1966.

131. Guridi J, Obeso JA: The role of the subthalamic nucleus in the origin of hemiballism and parkinsonism: New surgical perspectives. Adv Neurol 74:235–247, 1997.

132. Obeso JA, Alvarez LM, Macias RJ, et al: Lesions of the subthalamic nucleus in Parkinson's disease. Neurology 48:A138, 1997.

133. Gill SS, Heywood P: Bilateral dorsolateral subthalamotomy for advanced Parkinson's disease. Lancet 350:1224, 1997.

134. Vilela Filho O, Da Silva DJ: Unilateral subthalamic nucleus lesioning: A safe and effective treatment for Parkinson's disease. Arg Neuropsiquiatr 60:935–948, 2002.

135. Gill SS, Patel NK, Heywood P: Subthalamotomy for Parkinson's disease. In Tarsy D, Vitek JL, Lozano AM (eds): Surgical Treatment of Parkinson's Disease and Other Movement Disorders. Totowa, NJ: Humana, 2003, pp 145–152.

136. Su PC, Tseng HM, Liu HM, et al: Treatment of advanced Parkinson's disease by subthalamotomy: One-year results. Move Disord 18:531–538, 2003.

137. Rampini PM, Locatelli M, Alimehmeti R, et al: Multiple sequential image-fusion and direct MRI localization of subthalamic lesions for deep brain stimulation. J Neurosurg Sci 47:33–39, 2003.

138. Landi A, Parolin M, Piolti R, et al: Deep brain stimulation for the treatment of Parkinson's disease: The experience of Neurosurgical Department in Monza. Neurol Sci 24(Suppl 1):S43–S44, 2003.

139. Limousin P, Krack P, Pollak P, et al: Electrical stimulation of the subthalamic nucleus in advanced Parkinson's disease. N Engl J Med 339:1105–1111, 1998.

140. Kleiner-Fisman G, Fisman DN, Sime E, et al: Long-term follow up of bilateral deep brain stimulation of the subthalamic nucleus in patients with advanced Parkinson's disease. J Neurosurg 99:489–495, 2003.

141. Limousin P, Pollak P, Benazzouz A, et al: Effect on Parkinsonian signs and symptoms of bilateral subthalamic nucleus stimulation. Lancet 345:91–95, 1995.

142. Krack P, Pollack P, Limousin P, et al: Stimulation of subthalamic nucleus alleviates tremor in Parkinson's disease. Lancet 350:1675, 1997.

143. Abosch A, Lang AE, Hutchison WD, Lozano AM: Subthalamic deep brain stimulation for Parkinson's disease. In Tarsy D, Vitek JL, Lozano AM (eds): Surgical Treatment of Parkinson's Disease and Other Movement Disorders. Totowa, NJ: Humana, 2003, pp 175–187.

144. Tamma F, Rampini P, Egidi M, et al: Deep brain stimulation for Parkinson's disease: The experience of the Policlinico-San Paolo Group in Milan. Neurol Sci 24(Suppl 1):S41–S42, 2003.

145. Gill SS, Patel NK, Hotton GR, et al: Direct brain infusion of glial cell line-derived neurotrophic factor in Parkinson's disease. Nat Med 9:589–595, 2003.

Deep Brain Stimulation in the Management of Parkinson's Disease and Disabling Tremor

LOUIS A. WHITWORTH and KIM J. BURCHIEL

HISTORY

The treatment of movement disorders has been a focus of neurosurgery since its inception. One of the first case reports, by Horsley[1] in 1909, described a resection of the precentral gyrus in a patient with hemiathetosis. The procedure completely relieved the patient of the athetosis but left him with a permanent hemiparesis and dyspraxia. A few decades passed before a renewed interest in this field led Bucy to perform a similar procedure for treatment of tremor. In 1937, Bucy and Case[2] resected the motor and premotor regions in a patient with an incapacitating post-traumatic tremor. The procedure completely abolished the tremor and led Bucy to apply the same technique to parkinsonian tremor. Although most effective in treating the tremor, the procedure left patients with impairment of dexterous movements and varying degrees of hemiparesis. Subsequently, locations were sought for interruption of the corticospinal tract that might be associated with less morbidity. Walker[3] described sectioning of the lateral two thirds of the cerebral peduncle to treat parkinsonian tremor. Again, this procedure was also associated with postoperative hemiparesis, although dexterity seems to have been less affected.

It was not until the 1940s that surgeons first performed surgery on the basal ganglia to treat movement disorders. Before then, most physicians shared Dandy's view that this region of the brain was the center of consciousness and that damage to the basal ganglia could lead to vegetative states. Meyers[4] performed the first direct operation on the basal ganglia in 1939 to treat a patient with postencephalitic tremor. In this procedure, via a transcortical, transventricular approach, he resected two thirds of the caudate nucleus, resulting in good control of the patient's contralateral tremor. Subsequent surgeries by Meyers for parkinsonism, hemiballism, and choreoathetosis included resections of the caudate along with portions of the putamen, globus pallidus, and/or the ansa lenticularis. By 1949, he had performed 58 such procedures.[5] Sixty-two percent of patients had significant improvement in their tremor and rigidity; however, there was a 12% rate of operative mortality. Meyers determined that the mortality rate was excessive for elective surgery and concluded that open surgery on the basal ganglia had a very limited role, although he showed that surgery in these regions did not lead to alterations in consciousness or coma.

A few years later, Cooper[6] discovered an alternate way of performing Meyers's procedure. While attempting to perform a pedunculotomy on a patient with Parkinson's disease (PD), he inadvertently transected the anterior choroidal artery and was forced to abandon the operation. However, when the patient awoke from surgery, he had no neurologic deficit and his tremor and rigidity were much improved. Cooper reasoned that sacrificing the artery led to a circumscribed infarct within the basal ganglia and the subsequent improvement of the patient's symptoms. He went on to perform anterior choroidal artery ligation in a series of 55 patients. Tremor and rigidity were improved in approximately 70% of patients; however, there was an 11% rate of postoperative hemiplegia and a 10% rate of operative mortality.[7] The high complication rate was attributed to the great variability in the vascular territory of the artery, and the procedure was soon abandoned.

Perhaps the most significant development in movement disorder surgery came in 1947 when Spiegel and Wycis[8] introduced their stereotactic apparatus. Their first cases involved pallidal lesions in patients with Huntington's chorea and choreoathetosis. This was followed by similar procedures for patients with Parkinson's disease and tremor. In their series of 50 patients, 78% had significant improvement in their tremor, whereas there was only a 4% rate of hemiplegia and 3% rate of operative mortality.[9] Spiegel and Wycis proved their stereotactic technique was at least as effective as open resections, with far less morbidity and mortality. They were soon followed by Hassler and Riechert[10] who performed the first stereotactic thalamotomy in 1952. The ventral lateral thalamus soon became the target of choice for the treatment of PD. Thalamotomy proved more effective than pallidotomy for treating tremor and was arguably as effective for rigidity.

The introduction of levodopa in the 1960s led to a sharp decline in surgery for PD. It was not until a few decades later, when the long-term complications of levodopa became apparent, that interest was rekindled in movement disorder surgery. Many technical advances have been made in the interim. The use of computed tomography and magnetic resonance imaging has supplanted ventriculography for target localization. The use of microelectrode recording (MER) has become more prevalent and provides an additional method for target confirmation. Even the targets for the lesions themselves have become better defined. The ventral intermediate nucleus (Vim), a portion of the ventral lateral nucleus, has become the preferred target for tremor control, and the posteroventral portion of the globus pallidus interna (GPi) the preferred target for bradykinesia and rigidity.

The use of subcortical or deep brain stimulation (DBS) is the most recent advance in the treatment of PD and other movement disorders. Since the introduction of stereotactic surgery, electrical stimulation has frequently been performed to improve target localization and predict potential adverse effects before creating a lesion. For example, it was recognized that high-frequency stimulation (>100 Hz) in the Vim could suppress tremor and represented an appropriate target for lesioning. Because of the risk of irreversible neurologic injury and the complications associated with bilateral thalamic lesions, Benabid and colleagues[11] carried out the first large-scale series of thalamic DBS for tremor. The safety and efficacy of this technique fueled interest in applying DBS to other targets such as GPi and the subthalamic nucleus (STN). The remainder of this chapter focuses on the use of DBS at these three sites to treat PD and disabling tremor.

PATHOPHYSIOLOGY OF PARKINSON'S DISEASE AND TREMOR

Parkinson's Disease

Although a comprehensive review of the extrapyramidal motor system is beyond the scope of this chapter, the reader should have a fundamental understanding of the basal ganglia and basal nuclei in regard to their physiologic function and the pathophysiology of movement disorders. The basal ganglia integrate and modulate cortical information along multiple parallel channels. Three main parallel systems can be delineated: sensorimotor, associative, and limbic.[12] The best understood functions of the basal ganglia are associated with the sensorimotor system. The role of the associative and limbic loops in causing the cognitive and behavioral disturbances associated with basal ganglia syndromes is less clear. These systems affect behavior indirectly by feedback to the cerebral cortex and directly by providing information to subcortical centers that influence movements. Their function is primarily through disinhibition of neural activity. Disruption of these channels by disease or injury results in disruption of movement and may be associated with significant deficits in cognition, perception, and mentation.

The basal ganglia can be divided into dorsal and ventral divisions. The dorsal basal ganglia include the caudate and putamen (neostriatum) and the globus pallidus (paleostriatum). Associated with the dorsal group are the substantia nigra (SN) and the STN. The ventral basal ganglia are located inferior to the anterior commissure and include the substantia innominata, nucleus basalis of Meynert, and the nucleus accumbens. The ventral region is intimately associated with the amygdala and the limbic system. The striatal complex (caudate and putamen) serves as the primary input into the motor circuit of the basal ganglia. The majority of afferent projections to the striatum are from the cerebral cortex, but there are also projections from the thalamus, SN pars compacta, and parabrachial pontine reticular formation. Afferents from the prefrontal area terminate preferentially in the caudate nucleus, whereas projections from the motor and sensory cortices terminate primarily in the putamen. The output nuclei of the basal ganglia consist of

the GPi and the SN pars reticulata (SNr). Output neurons from the GPi project primarily to the ventral anterior, ventral lateral, and centromedian nuclei of the thalamus. These fibers exit the GPi as two bundles: the ansa lenticularis and lenticular fasciculus. The ansa lenticularis originates from the lateral portion of the GPi and curves around the internal capsule to enter Forel's fields, whereas the lenticular fasciculus originates from the dorsomedial portion and traverses the internal capsule as small groups of axons. Within Forel's fields, these two fasciculi join to form the thalamic fasciculus, which courses dorsal to the zona incerta en route to the thalamus. The SNr has more diffuse projections, which provide afferent input to the thalamus, superior colliculus, and parabrachial pontine reticular formation.

Motor input to the striatum from the neocortex is via excitatory glutaminergic projections that terminate on spiny cells in the putamen; dopaminergic terminals from the SN pars compacta coterminate on these cells. Neurons within the putamen send inhibitory GABAergic axons to the globus pallidus externa, GPi, and SNr. Although a matter of some debate, it appears that dopamine increases striatal output to the GPi and SNr (the direct pathway) and decreases transmission to the globus pallidus externa (the indirect pathway) via D_1 and D_2 receptors, respectively[13] (Fig. 101-1A).

The direct pathway begins as an excitatory, glutaminergic projection from the cerebral cortex to the putamen. GABAergic projections from the putamen inhibit cells of the GPi and SNr. Cells of the GPi and SNr are also GABAergic and project to the ventral lateral thalamus. These fibers have a high rate of spontaneous activity and thus tonically inhibit thalamic neurons. Inhibition of these pallidal and nigral projections by afferents from the striatum decreases the inhibitory inputs to the thalamic neurons (thalamic disinhibition). Because the ventral lateral thalamic neurons have excitatory projections to the cerebral cortex, the net effect of the direct pathway is to increase the activity of the thalamus, excite the cortex, and facilitate movement. By contrast, the indirect pathway sends its GABAergic projections from the putamen to the globus pallidus externa, which in turn has projections to the STN. These pallidosubthalamic fibers are also GABAergic and tonically inhibit cells of the STN. Inhibition of these fibers by the striatum releases these subthalamic cells from their tonically inhibited state. The STN sends excitatory glutaminergic projections to the GPi, which increases the firing rates of pallidothalamic fibers. Because the fibers from the GPi to the thalamus are inhibitory, this leads to a decrease in thalamic output to the cortex (thalamic inhibition). The net effect of the indirect pathway is to decrease activity of the thalamus, and consequently, decrease activity of the cerebral cortex.

This represents a very simplified description of the basal ganglia motor loop and omits several pathways such as those from the cortex to the subthalamus or from the subthalamus to the external segment of the globus pallidus. It does, however, provide a basic framework for understanding the basal ganglia's role in the extrapyramidal system. A delicate balance exists between the direct and indirect pathways, with the former increasing thalamocortical activity (thalamic disinhibition) and the latter decreasing it (thalamic inhibition). It has been proposed that these two

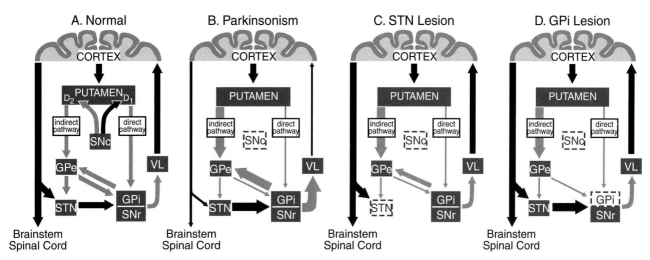

FIGURE 101-1 Functional anatomy of basal ganglia. *A*, Normal physiologic state with balance between the direct and indirect pathways. *B*, Parkinson's disease state. Loss of dopaminergic input from the substantia nigra pars compacta (SNc) leads to increased activity along indirect pathway and decreased activity along direct pathway, resulting in increased inhibitory input to the ventral lateral thalamic nucleus (VL). *C*, Effects of a subthalamic nucleus (STN) lesion in parkinsonism, decreasing inhibitory input to the VL. *D*, Effects of a globus pallidus interna (GPi) lesion in parkinsonism, decreasing inhibitory input to VL. *black arrows* indicate excitatory connections and *light gray arrows* indicate inhibitory connections. SNr, substantia nigra pars reticulata; GPe, globus pallidus externa; D$_1$, dopamine receptor subtype 1; D$_2$, dopamine receptor subtype 2.

pathways may be involved with scaling or termination of movements.[14] Striatal output would first inhibit GPi and SNr neurons via the direct pathway (facilitating movement) followed by disinhibition of the same neurons via the indirect pathway (terminating movement). Alternately, these pathways may be involved in the focusing of movements by simultaneously targeting separate populations of neurons in the GPi and SNr.[15] Activity along the direct pathway would lead to inhibition of select GPi and SNr neurons, facilitating an intended movement, whereas activity along the indirect pathway would target surrounding neurons in the GPi and SNr, inhibiting unintended movements.

PD, whose hallmarks include bradykinesia, akinesia, and rigidity, is the most common and best understood disorder of the basal ganglia. The disease correlates with a loss of dopaminergic neurons in the SN pars compacta that project to the striatum. According to the DeLong model,[16] this loss of dopaminergic input to the putamen leads to increased activity of the indirect pathway while decreasing activity along the direct pathway (see Fig. 101-1*B*). The net effect of this change results in overexcitation of GPi and SNr neurons, which in turn increases their tonic inhibition of thalamocortical cells. This deficit of dopamine in the basal ganglia circuitry leads to the development of the cardinal symptoms of PD. Positron emission tomography studies in parkinsonian patients have demonstrated decreased activity in the supplementary motor area, dorsal prefrontal cortex, and frontal association areas that receive subcortical input from the basal ganglia.[17]

According to the DeLong model, the increased basal ganglia output causing PD is primarily due to overactivity of the STN and GPi. As such, these nuclei have become the surgical targets for the correction of PD. Ablation of the GPi[18] and more recently the STN[19] has been shown to ameliorate many of the cardinal symptoms associated with the disease. The effects of such ablations in regard to the DeLong model can be seen in Figure 101-1*C* and *D*.

Recent surgical treatments have focused on the use of DBS in these nuclei to reduce their overactivity.

Tremor

The pathophysiologic basis of tremor is less well known. Animal models of PD, such as 1-methyl-4-phenyl-1,2,3,6-tetrahydropyridine (MPTP)-treated monkeys, rarely exhibit significant tremor, and no animal model exists for essential tremor (ET). In humans, tremor can manifest in a variety of conditions, with the most common being PD and ET. Tremor may also been seen in the setting of various injuries or insults to the central nervous system. These secondary tremor disorders, which often are associated with other neurologic deficits, include multiple sclerosis, cerebrovascular accident, and traumatic brain injury. The characteristics of the tremor vary by disease process. Parkinsonian tremor occurs at rest and has a frequency of 4 to 5 Hz. In contrast, ET is primarily a postural and/or action tremor with a slightly higher frequency. Secondary tremors (e.g., multiple sclerosis, traumatic brain injury) tend to be both postural and kinetic, have high amplitude with low frequency, and often affect the proximal limb as much as the distal. Interestingly, despite the varying etiologies and presentations, the same operations tend to benefit all types of tremor; the consensus is to target the Vim of the thalamus for ablation or high-frequency stimulation.

The Vim has been extensively mapped using MER during thalamic procedures. Two subsets of tremor cells have been identified: kinesthetic cells, which simply fire in response to somatotopographically organized contralateral movements, and autonomous tremor cells, which fire synchronously with the tremor.[20] Tremor cells can also be found in other brain structures, such as the GPi and STN, but their relationship to thalamic tremor cells is unclear. It is important to note that the Vim does not receive direct projections from the GPi and appears to receive principally cerebellar input. It has been proposed that Vim thalamotomy or thalamic stimulation may in fact be targeting pallidal outflow fibers en route to other thalamic regions.[21] Cells discharging at rates similar to the tremor have been identified in regions of the thalamus that receive input from the basal ganglia.[22] The increased inhibition on the thalamus from the GPi and SNr in parkinsonian patients may promote bursts in thalamocortical cells,[23] and periodic bursting of the reticular nucleus during periods of immobility may enhance this rhythmic oscillation.

Physiologic Effects of Stimulation

Despite its use for more than 20 years, little is known about the in vivo mechanism of action of DBS. Because high-frequency stimulation has demonstrated clinical effects comparable with lesioning, it has been postulated to exert its effect via a hyperpolarizing blockade of the cells within the target nucleus. However, work by Holsheimer and colleagues[24] and McIntyre and Grill[25] would suggest that, at the pulse widths and amplitudes used in DBS, stimulation is likely affecting myelinated axons as opposed to cell bodies. Fibers running parallel to the direction of the stimulating current would be preferentially activated as opposed to those running transversely. In addition, given the short refractory period of myelinated axons, frequencies in the 100- to 200-Hz range are unlikely to lead to inhibition of conduction. However, what is not known is the response of the postsynaptic neuron to this frequency of stimulus. There is evidence to suggest that postsynaptic potentials may start to fuse at frequencies of 100 to 200 Hz.[26] This synaptic depolarization can inactivate the spike-generating mechanism at the postsynaptic membrane, effectively inhibiting the postsynaptic cell. The relative contribution of this postsynaptic phenomenon remains unclear and does not take into account the potential effects of orthodromic stimulation on afferent fibers. Thus, although it appears that DBS preferentially stimulates axons, the ultimate effect that it produces is difficult to predict. The variable volume of the neuropil that is affected by stimulation further confounds this. Based on animal data, average stimulation currents used in DBS may excite neural elements for a distance of 2 to 5 mm from the active cathode.[27] As our clinical experience with DBS continues to grow, our fundamental understanding of its effects at the cellular level unfortunately lags far behind.

Patient Selection

Proper patient selection is one of the most important factors in ensuring successful outcomes after DBS. Although the ultimate decision to perform surgery is the responsibility of the neurosurgeon, input from the neurologist and the neuropsychologist is invaluable. Presurgical evaluation by a neurologist with experience in movement disorders ensures that the patient has undergone appropriate medical management before progressing to surgical intervention. In addition, they can screen for those patients with atypical parkinsonian syndromes such as progressive supranuclear palsy or multisystem atrophy. These "Parkinson plus" syndromes do not typically respond well to DBS. Neuropsychological evaluation can identify those patients with cognitive dysfunction, as this

may worsen postoperatively and compromise the likelihood of success.

Several criteria are generally accepted by movement disorder programs for their selection of surgical candidates, regardless of the proposed procedure.

1. Patients should have significant disability despite maximal medical therapy.
2. Patients should be in generally good health without significant cardiac, pulmonary, or renal risk factors. In addition, many centers use an age of 70 years as a cutoff, although this is becoming less stringent.
3. Patients should not be demented or have significant cognitive impairment, nor should they have uncontrolled psychiatric illness such as anxiety or mood disorders.
4. Patients should be able to comprehend the risks of the proposed procedure. In addition, they should have reasonable expectations concerning the outcome from surgery.
5. Patients should not have severe atrophy or extensive white matter disease on preoperative magnetic resonance imaging, as these findings may increase the risk of intracerebral hemorrhage or postoperative cognitive impairment.

Parkinson's Disease

The ideal candidate for STN or GPi stimulation is a patient with levodopa-responsive idiopathic PD. Patients should have disabling symptoms from their disease including bradykinesia, rigidity, and tremor and/or significant side effects from medication such as dyskinesias and *on/off* fluctuations. As mentioned previously, psychiatric disorders such as dementia, acute psychosis, and major depression are exclusion criteria. Patients who are no longer levodopa responsive or who have one of the Parkinson plus syndromes (e.g., progressive supranuclear palsy, multisystem atrophy) are generally poor candidates for surgery. With the exception of tremor, symptoms that do not respond to levodopa are not likely to improve significantly with stimulation.

Tremor

Disabling tremor occurs in a variety of neurologic disorders. It is seen most commonly in PD and ET. Extensive experience with thalamic DBS to treat PD and ET exists, and results are generally quite good. Patients who meet the above criteria and have undergone appropriate trials of medication are good candidates for stimulation. Tremor also occurs in the setting of various neurologic insults such as traumatic brain injury, stroke, and multiple sclerosis. These secondary tremor disorders are frequently associated with other significant neurologic deficits. Secondary tremor is often postural and/or kinetic and high amplitude with low frequency, often has a proximal component, and frequently affects the trunk and head. Although there is less experience in treating secondary tremor, the consensus is that it does not respond as well as PD or ET to surgery. Patients should have realistic expectations regarding outcome before undergoing DBS for one of these disorders. The best candidates for surgery have resting or action tremor that is most prominent in the distal upper extremity.

VENTRALIS INTERMEDIUS NUCLEUS STIMULATION

Introduction

Ablation of the Vim of the thalamus (thalamotomy) has been used as a treatment for both ET and parkinsonian tremor for more than 50 years. The procedure is highly effective, significantly reducing contralateral tremor in approximately 85% of patients.[28] However, thalamotomy is associated with a high rate of transient and, to a lesser degree, permanent neurologic deficits. Series have shown as many as 60% of patients experience transient deficits lasting as long as 3 months and permanent deficits in 23% of those treated.[29] These deficits include weakness, dysarthria, ataxia, and sensory deficits. The risks are even greater for bilateral thalamotomy, with more than 50% of patients experiencing bulbar and cognitive effects. Because of these complications, Andy[30] suggested that chronic stimulation of the thalamus might be preferable to lesioning. The use of intraoperative stimulation to identify lesioning targets was well established.[31] Stimulation of the Vim at low frequencies would exacerbate patients' tremor, whereas high-frequency stimulation (>100 Hz) in the same location would suppress the tremor. The efficacy of stimulation in suppressing tremor and the side effects associated

with bilateral thalamotomy led Benabid[11] to carry out the first large-scale trial of thalamic stimulation for parkinsonian and ET.

Targeting and Lead Placement

The authors' preferred target for Vim stimulation is at the level of the anterior commissure–posterior commissure line (AC-PC), 25% the length of the AC-PC line anterior to the PC, and 55% of the AC-PC length laterally (Fig. 101-2). Corrections are made based on imaging if the target is too close to the internal capsule or the patient has a particularly wide third ventricle. The lead is inserted under local anesthetic (see Surgical Technique section for further details) and macrostimulation is carried out to assess efficacy and side effects. Stimulation at frequencies of less than 5 Hz is used to look for motor effects that may indicate that the lead is too lateral or within the internal capsule. Next, stimulation is carried out at 50 Hz to assess the sensory threshold. Paraesthesias at less than 1 V indicate that the lead may be too posterior. Finally, stimulation is performed at 180 Hz to assess tremor suppression. Because of the consistency of anatomic targeting and simplicity of performing macrostimulation, we do not routinely perform microelectrode recordings

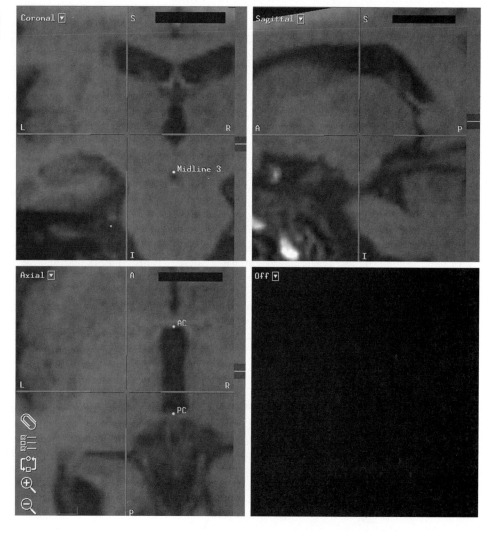

FIGURE 101-2 Axial, coronal, and sagittal views of the ventral intermediate nucleus target on magnetic resonance imaging.

TABLE 101-1 ▪ Thalamic Stimulation for Essential Tremor

Study	n	Good Result (%)	Tremor Free (%)
Benabid et al[32]	20	39	61
Koller et al[33]	29	69	31
Limousin et al[34]	37	89	NA

NA, not available.

TABLE 101-3 ▪ Thalamic Stimulation for Multiple Sclerosis Tremor

Study	n	Good Result (%)	Tremor Free (%)
Montgomery et al[35]	15	93	NA
Geny et al[36]	13	69	0
Schuurman et al[37]	5	60	40

NA, not available.

for Vim lead implants. The lead is then implanted so that the middle two contacts bracket the final target.

Outcomes

The original application of Vim stimulation as reported by Benabid[11] was for parkinsonian tremor in patients who had previously undergone contralateral thalamotomy. The technique, which proved to be as effective as thalamotomy, was subsequently used bilaterally in the treatment of both parkinsonian tremor and ET. Results for ET show good to excellent control of tremor in 89% to 100% of patients[32-34] (Table 101-1). One series reported 61% of patients to be tremor free at 6-month follow-up,[32] although there is some evidence that patients develop tolerance to stimulation over time. Equally impressive are the results for PD, which have good to excellent control in 85% to 100% of patients[32-34] (Table 101-2) with as many as 58% of patients being tremor free.[33] Tremor suppression appears to remain stable during 2-year follow-up. In general, resting tremor is better controlled than postural or action tremor, distal better than proximal or axial tremor, and upper better than lower extremity tremor. As expected, thalamic stimulation does little to improve rigidity or bradykinesia in patients with PD.[32] Vim DBS has also been used to treat secondary tremor from a variety of disorders including multiple sclerosis, cerebrovascular accidents, and traumatic brain injury. Secondary tremors are often severe, postural, and kinetic and have a major proximal component. Multiple sclerosis represents the majority of secondary tremor cases treated using DBS. Good results have been obtained in 60% to 93% of patients[35-37] (Table 101-3). However, the tremor is less consistently or effectively suppressed by thalamic DBS than ET or parkinsonian tremor.[32] Patients with multiple sclerosis also tend to develop tolerance to the effects of stimulation and require frequent reprogramming.[35] There are only sporadic reports of Vim DBS in the treatment of other secondary tremors. The consensus appears that it is less effective than stimulation for PD or ET. Nonetheless, given the severe disability of these patients and the lack of alternatives, DBS for secondary tremor may be gratifying.

SUBTHALAMIC NUCLEUS STIMULATION

Introduction

According to the DeLong model,[16] the motor symptoms seen in PD can be attributed to overactivity of the indirect pathway due to a deficiency of dopamine. This phenomenon occurs because the STN is released from its tonic inhibition and provides increased excitatory input to GPi and SNr. Appreciation of the STN's role in the pathophysiology of PD has led to interest in the STN as a target for the treatment of the disease. Bergman and colleagues[38] demonstrated that lesions of the STN in monkeys with MPTP-induced parkinsonism could improve their motor symptoms. Further animal studies demonstrated that high-frequency stimulation of the STN in MPTP monkeys reversed rigidity and akinesia.[39] Concerns of creating hemiballismus by lesioning the STN and the safety and efficacy of Vim stimulation for tremor prompted Benabid to attempt STN stimulation in parkinsonian patients.[40] Since this first publication, much interest has been generated in DBS of the STN, and it has become the procedure of choice for treating PD.

Targeting and Lead Placement

The authors' preferred target for STN stimulation is 4 mm below the level of the AC-PC line, 4 mm posterior to the midcommissural point, and 12 mm lateral to the AC-PC line (Fig. 101-3). Corrections are made to the final target if it appears too anterior within the cerebral peduncle or too medial with respect to the red nucleus. Physiologic mapping and lead placement are performed under local anesthetic (see Surgical Technique section for further details). MER is performed to identify the reticular nucleus of the thalamus, the zona incerta, STN, and the SNr. The reticular nucleus typically contains cells that exhibit brief bursts of spontaneous of activity. The subthalamic white matter is relatively electrically quiet except for the zona incerta, which shows some increased cellular activity. The STN is identified by high-frequency (30 to 70 Hz), irregularly firing cells that may respond to contralateral passive limb movements. Cells with an even high frequency and regular discharge pattern mark entrance into the SNr. Once the target nucleus has been identified, the permanent electrode is positioned so that the second (number 1) contact lies within the MER-defined center of the STN.

TABLE 101-2 ▪ Thalamic Stimulation for Parkinsonian Tremor

Study	n	Good Result (%)	Tremor Free (%)
Benabid et al[32]	80	50	39
Limousin et al[34]	73	85	NA
Koller et al[33]	24	42	58

NA, not available.

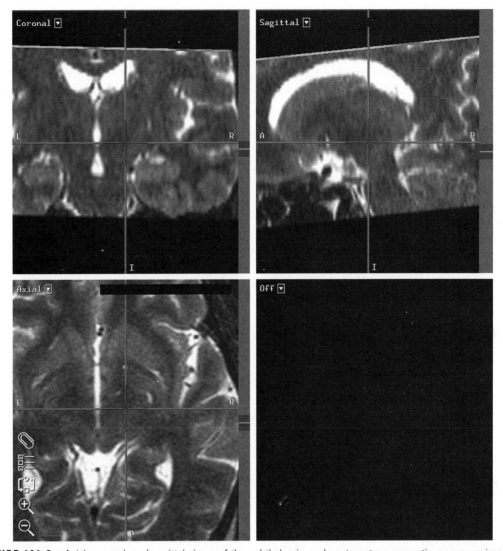

FIGURE 101-3 Axial, coronal, and sagittal views of the subthalamic nucleus target on magnetic resonance imaging.

Outcomes

STN stimulation has been reported to improve all the motor symptoms of PD including rigidity, bradykinesia, postural stability, and gait. Improvements in the scores in the motor section of the Unified Parkinson's Disease Rating Scale in the *off* medication state range from 50% to 74% in most series[41-44] (Table 101-4). However, the improvements in scores in the *on* medication state after STN DBS show little change (0% to 26%).[41,43,44] Given the fact that STN stimulation does little to improve *on* medication motor function, it is important to counsel patients that the effects of stimulation will likely be equal to their best *on* state. Much of the benefit derived from STN stimulation comes from reductions in *off* time and *on/off* fluctuations.[41] Time in the *off* state was reduced by more than 60% in one study.[41] In addition, STN DBS significantly increases *on* time without dyskinesias.[41,45] Overall, dyskinesia scores tend to decrease by 50% after stimulation. Much of the improvement in regards to dyskinesia may be related to significant reductions in levodopa requirements by patients after STN stimulation. Most series report a reduction in daily levodopa doses by approximately 40% to 60%.[41-44] Fewer studies have specifically measured the effects of STN stimulation on tremor; those that have typically show a 70% to 80% reduction of tremor in the *off* medication state.[41,45]

GLOBUS PALLIDUS INTERNA STIMULATION

Introduction

Pallidotomy has been used to treat the akinesia and rigidity associated with PD for more than five decades. However, with the introduction of levodopa in the 1960s, the procedure was largely abandoned. Despite advances in medical therapy, patients often developed severe medication-induced dyskinesias and motor fluctuations. In 1992, Laitinen and colleagues[46] reintroduced the procedure and found it to be effective in treating both the motor symptoms and the dyskinesias of PD. However, most patients with advanced PD have bilateral disease with prominent gait and balance disturbances. These symptoms are not adequately treated by unilateral surgery. Bilateral pallidotomy is only rarely performed due to the increased risk of cognitive impairment and speech disorders.[47] This prompted Siegfried and

TABLE 101-4 ▪ Subthalamic Nucleus Stimulation for Parkinson's Disease

Study	n	% Improvement mUPDRS *off* Medications	% Improvement mUPDRS *on* Medications	% Change in L-Dopa
Deep Brain Stimulation for Parkinson's Disease Study Group[41]	91	51%	26%	37% decrease
Houeto et al[42]	23	66%	55%	61% decrease
Limousin et al[43]	20	60%	10%	50% decrease
Rodriguez-Oroz et al[44]	15	74%	NS	55% decrease

mUPDRS, motor section of Unified Parkinson's Disease Rating Scale; NS, not significant; L-Dopa, levodopa.

Lippitz[48] to perform high-frequency bilateral GPi stimulation. Previous work by Benabid[11] had shown that thalamic stimulation had effects similar to those of thalamotomy and could safely be performed bilaterally. Pallidal DBS offered the ability to provide the therapeutic benefits of bilateral pallidotomy without the associated morbidity.

Targeting and Lead Placement

The authors' preferred target for GPi stimulation is 4 mm below the level of the AC-PC line, 2 mm anterior to the midcommissural point, and 21 mm lateral to the AC-PC line (Fig. 101-4). Corrections are made as necessary to ensure that final target does not abut the optic tract.

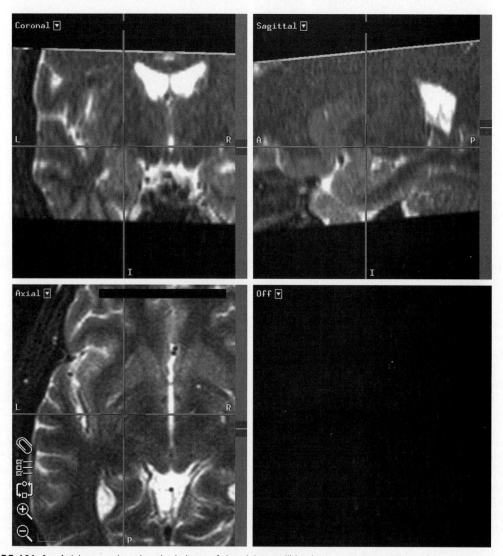

FIGURE 101-4 Axial, coronal, and sagittal views of the globus pallidus interna target on magnetic resonance imaging.

TABLE 101-5 ▪ Globus Pallidus Interna Stimulation for Parkinson's Disease

Study	n	% Improvement mUPDRS *off* Medications	% Improvement mUPDRS *on* Medications	% Change in L-Dopa
Deep Brain Stimulation for Parkinson's Disease Study Group[41]	36	33%	27%	3% increase
Volkmann et al[49]	11	51%	44%	27% decrease
Ghika et al[50]	6	50%	26%	35% increase
Durif et al[51]	6	36%	44%	6% increase

mUPDRS, motor section of Unified Parkinson's Disease Rating Scale; L-Dopa, levodopa.

Physiologic mapping and lead placement are performed under local anesthetic (see Surgical Technique section for further details). MER is performed to identify the external and internal segments of the globus pallidus as well as the subpallidal white matter. The globus pallidus externa typically displays large voltage spontaneous activity at low frequency interspersed with rapid bursts. The transition zone between the external and internal segments of the globus pallidus contains border cells demonstrating slow discharge rates. The GPi is marked by highly active, high-frequency (80 to 90 Hz) neurons. Once the target nucleus has been identified, the permanent electrode is implanted so that its distal most contact lies at the base of the GPi.

Outcomes

Much like STN stimulation, GPi DBS has been shown to be efficacious in treating the contralateral motor symptoms of PD. Improvements in *off* medication states show a 33% to 50% reduction in the motor section of the Unified Parkinson's Disease Rating Scale scores[41,49-51] (Table 101-5). These reductions were significant for tremor, rigidity, bradykinesia, gait, and postural stability. Improvements in the *on* medication state show a more modest reduction of 26% to 44%.[41,49-51] Unlike the case with STN stimulation, there is some evidence of a synergistic effect between pallidal stimulation and levodopa in the *on* state.[45] GPi stimulation also increases the length of the *on* period without dyskinesias.[41] In addition, patients' total *on* time increases along with a concomitant decrease in *on/off* fluctuations.[41] To date, there have been only two prospective, randomized studies comparing GPi with STN DBS.[45,52] The initial study with 10 patients and a following study with 20 patients showed no significant difference in benefit between the two therapies. The only outcome measure that was significantly different between the GPi and STN groups was medication use. The mean levodopa intake at 12 months was reduced by 50% in the STN group but remained unchanged in the GPi group. Similar effects on medication dosing have been noted by others[41,50,51] and suggest that the mechanism of interaction between levodopa and DBS may be very different at the two sites.

Surgical Technique

The Leksell Model G (Elekta, Stockholm, Sweden) stereotactic base ring and localizer are affixed to the patient's skull under local anesthesia. Magnetic resonance imaging is then performed using spoiled grass (Gradient Recalled Acquisition in the Steady State) and fast spin echo inversion recovery sequences. It is the authors' preference to use magnetic resonance imaging for targeting, but the use of positive-contrast ventriculography and computed tomography are well described. The images are then transferred to the Stealth Station (Medtronic Inc., Minneapolis, MN), and targeting is carried out with the aid of the system's Frame Link (Medtronic Inc.) software. The AC and PC are identified on axial images (Fig. 101-5), as are several midline structures. The target coordinates are then calculated based on fixed relationships to these structures (Table 101-6). The software superimposes the target onto corresponding axial, sagittal, and coronal magnetic resonance imaging slices. Modifications are then made if the target appears to be too close to critical structures (e.g., internal capsule, optic tract).

Patients are given a perioperative dose of antibiotics, and the first portion of the procedure is carried out using only a local anesthetic. The use of intravenous sedatives or analgesics may interfere with MER and may suppress symptoms such as tremor, making physiologic targeting more difficult. A single skin incision is made just anterior to the coronal suture, crossing the midline for bilateral procedures. A 14-mm burr hole is placed just anterior to the coronal suture and 1 to 3 cm lateral to the sagittal suture. The laterality is selected so that recording and implant trajectories will be parallel to the sagittal plane. Once the dura is opened, Gelfoam is placed in the burr hole to prevent loss of cerebrospinal fluid and subsequent shifting of the brain.

For STN and GPi implants, MER is performed using the MicroGuide (Alpha Omega, Nazareth, Israel) system. Recordings are begun using a single-channel electrode system, approximately 25 mm above the presumed target. Initial recordings are taken in 0.5-mm increments until the target nucleus is encountered and then are taken every 0.1 to 0.2 mm. Recordings continue until either the reticular portion of the SN (for the STN) or the subpallidal white matter (for the GPi) is identified. The authors do not routinely conduct MER for placement of electrodes within the Vim of the thalamus. The consistency of targeting based on anatomic structures and the ease of performing intraoperative macrostimulation to assess efficacy have, in our experience, made MER unnecessary in these cases. However, many physicians still advocate the use of MER for the placement of Vim electrodes.

Once the recordings and test stimulation are complete, the permanent lead is inserted so that the maximal number

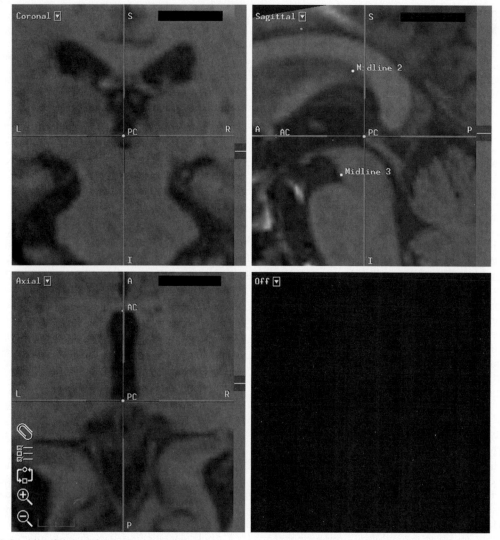

FIGURE 101-5 Identification of the anterior and posterior commissures on axial, coronal, and sagittal magnetic resonance imaging.

of contacts lies within the target nucleus. The lead is then secured to the skull using the Navigus (Image-Guided Neurologics, Melbourne, FL) cap system. Fluoroscopy is used to ensure that the electrode does not migrate during the anchoring process. The distal end of the lead is then coiled up within a subgaleal pocket and the incision is closed. The patient is then taken out of the stereotactic frame, and general endotracheal anesthesia is administered. The lead will then be connected, using an extension cable, to an implantable pulse generator, which is typically placed in an infraclavicular subcutaneous pocket.

Hardware

The lead currently used for implantation at our institution is the Medtronic model 3387 quadripolar DBS electrode with four platinum-iridium contacts, each 1.5 mm long and separated by 1.5 mm. Also available is the Medtronic model 3389 electrode with contacts spaced 0.5 mm apart. The lead comes with a central stylet to provide increased rigidity during insertion. Both electrodes allow for bipolar or monopolar stimulation. The lead is connected to the generator by extension cables of varying lengths. The Soletra (Medtronic Inc.) is a fully implantable pulse generator powered by a

TABLE 101-6 ▪ Deep Brain Stimulation Target Coordinates

Target	Lateral (x) to MCP	Anterior/Posterior (y) to MCP	Vertical (z) to MCP
Vim	0.55 (AC-PC length)	0.25 (AC-PC length) posterior	0
STN	12 mm	4 mm posterior	4 mm below
GPi	21 mm	2 mm anterior	4 mm below

AC, anterior commissure; GPi, globus pallidus interna; MCP, midcommissural point; PC, posterior commissure; STN, subthalamic nucleus; Vim, ventral intermediate nucleus.

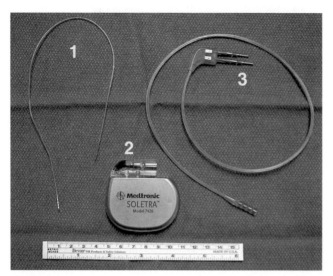

FIGURE 101-6 Deep brain stimulation hardware. 1, Electrode; 2, implantable pulse generator; 3, extension cable.

lithium battery. It is housed in a titanium casing with an epoxy heading where the extension cable inserts (Fig. 101-6).

The device allows for a wide range of stimulus parameters and is externally programmable. Frequencies can be set from 5 to 185 Hz, pulse widths from 30 to 450 μsec, and amplitudes up to 10 V. Typical stimulation parameters are a frequency of 185 Hz, pulse width of 60 to 90 μsec, and amplitude of 1 to 3 V. Given these settings, battery life averages approximately 3 to 5 years. The device comes with an external programmer to allow the patient to turn the device on or off as desired.

Programming

The process of deep brain stimulator programming can be time consuming and labor intensive in and of itself. In addition, patients frequently require concurrent adjustments in their medications. This can be particularly difficult soon after placement of the DBS electrodes, when microlesional effects are diminishing. For these reasons, at our institution, we have found that it is most efficient for the neurologists to conduct the majority of the programming. This allows for a single physician to manage both medical and stimulation therapies, which reduces the number of office visits for the patient and provides continuity of care.

Patients are typically admitted to the hospital and undergo implantation of both the electrode and generator during one operation. They are then observed in the hospital for 1 to 2 days postoperatively. During this period, the system is typically programmed in a "monopolar" configuration at very low amplitudes. Some patients exhibit a microlesional effect from the implantation of the electrode and may not receive any initial programming. These patients are then scheduled to follow-up with neurology 1 to 2 weeks postoperatively for the initial programming session. This allows the patient to recover from surgery and provides enough time for the transient lesional effects to resolve.

For their initial programming session, patients with PD have their medication held for at least 12 hours. Baseline motor assessments are then performed, evaluating the patient for rigidity, bradykinesia, gait, and postural stability.

The electrode contacts are then sequentially evaluated in a monopolar configuration. Frequency and pulse width are typically kept at constant settings of 180 Hz and 90 μsec, respectively. The amplitude is then steadily increased to the tolerance level of the patient or until side effects occur. Repeat motor evaluation is then performed to assess efficacy of stimulation. This process is carried out for each of the four electrode contacts. Ten to 15 minutes is allowed to pass between trials of separate contacts to allow for at least partial washout of any previous stimulation effects. If a satisfactory result cannot be achieved with monopolar stimulation, more complex arrays consisting of bipoles, tripoles, or multiple cathodes are tried. Once an effective program has been established, patients are given an appropriate dose of levodopa and are observed for dyskinesias. Further programming adjustments are then made as required to treat any perceived drug-induced dyskinesias.

The goals for successful programming of a deep brain stimulator are threefold. First, the stimulation parameters must provide therapeutic benefit for the patient. Second, the stimulation should produce minimal if any side effects. Third, attempts should be made to select a program that provides maximal benefits for the patient with minimal power drain on the battery. Although this may seem the least important of the three, the cost associated with repeated surgery for generator replacement cannot be overlooked. In addition, each time that the patient is subjected to an operation for replacement of the generator, there exists a risk of infecting the system.

Complications

The complications from DBS can be broken down into three main categories: (1) procedure related, (2) hardware related, and (3) stimulation related. The overall incidence of complications from DBS is approximately 30%,[41,53] but the majority is relatively minor or amenable to changes in stimulation parameters. Mortality rates are less than 1%, with intracerebral hemorrhage being the most common cause of death. The complication rates are essentially the same regardless of the target with the exception of some stimulation-related adverse events.

The most common surgical complications are intracerebral hemorrhage and infection. The incidence of intracerebral hemorrhage ranges between 1% and 5%.[41,53] Fortunately, most of these hemorrhages are small and cause minimal if any symptoms. As with any procedure involving the implantation of hardware, infection is a major concern. Reported infection rates range from 3% to 13%.[41,53] Superficial wound infections may be treated with intravenous antibiotics, but infections, which involve the device generally, require wound debridement and explantation of the stimulator. Care must also be taken to prevent a secondary infection of the stimulator; patients with DBS undergoing routine dental work and minor surgical procedures should be given prophylactic antibiotics.

Complications related to the hardware include lead fractures, lead migration, skin erosion, and hardware malfunctions. Reports of equipment failure range from approximately 5% to 13% in most series.[41,53] Fracture of the electrode is the most common cause of device failure. This is becoming less of a problem as newer electrodes are made entirely of platinum. In our early experience, lead fracture occurred most commonly just proximal to the connection with the extension cable. We found that ensuring this connection was placed over the skull, as opposed to the soft tissues of the neck, eliminated this problem. Another problem related to the hardware can be erosion of the skin overlying the device. Most often this occurs at the site of the electrode-extension cable connection but may also occur over the lead anchoring caps in individuals with thin scalps. The newer low profile extension cable will likely reduce the incidence of erosion at the connection site.

Stimulation-related complications are typically related to activation of adjacent nuclei or fiber tracts. Such adverse reactions generally respond to adjustments in stimulation parameters, although sometimes at the expense of therapeutic benefit. For thalamic stimulation, the most common reactions are paresthesia involving the face or limb, dysarthria, dysmetria, and ataxia.[32] Reported complications after STN stimulation include dysarthria, diplopia, apraxia of eyelid opening, and depression.[41,49] Stimulation of the globus pallidus has been reported to cause dyskinesia, dystonia, and ataxia.[41,49]

CONCLUSION

DBS represents a significant advance in the treatment of PD and other movement disorders. Numerous studies have shown these techniques to be both safe and efficacious. However, many questions remain to be answered. The optimal target (GPi vs. STN) to treat the cardinal symptoms of PD is yet to be determined. Is one clearly superior, or perhaps do differing clinical presentations favor one site over the other? What is the best method for localizing the target nuclei—anatomically based coordinates or direct radiographic imaging? Does the use of microelectrode recording for localization improve clinical outcomes? Questions like these can only be answered through large, prospective, randomized trials. Although our clinical experience with DBS has grown, our fundamental understanding of its effects on the cellular level remains somewhat of an enigma. A greater appreciation of the cellular response to stimulation may help us to better refine our stimulation parameters and even the targets themselves. This must be coupled with an improved understanding of the functional organization of the basal ganglia and its role in various disease states. The future of DBS will require the combined efforts of both clinicians and basic scientists to both design prospective outcome-based trials and further elucidate the cellular mechanisms underlying its effects.

REFERENCES

1. Horsley V: The function of the so-called motor area of the brain. BMJ 2:125–132, 1909.
2. Bucy PC, Case TJ: Tremor, physiologic mechanism and abolition by surgical means. Arch Neurol Psychiatry 41:721–746, 1939.
3. Walker AE: Cerebral pedunculotomy for the relief of involuntary movements: Parkinsonian tremor. J Nerv Ment Dis 116:766–775, 1952.
4. Meyers R: A surgical procedure for the alleviation of postencephalitic tremor, with notes on the physiology of the premotor fibers. Arch Neurol Psychiatry 44:455–459, 1940.
5. Meyers R: Historical background and personal experiences in the surgical relief of hyperkinesias and hypertonus. In Fields WS (ed): Pathogenesis and Treatment of Parkinsonism. Springfield, IL: Charles C Thomas, 1958, pp 229–270.
6. Cooper IS: Ligation of the anterior choroidal artery for involuntary movements of parkinsonism. Psychiatr Q 27:317–319, 1953.
7. Cooper IS: The Neurosurgical Alleviation of Parkinsonism. Springfield, IL: Charles C Thomas, 1956.
8. Spiegel EA, Wycis HT, Marks M, Lee AJ: Stereotactic apparatus for operations in the human brain. Science 106:349–350, 1947.
9. Wycis HT, Spiegel EA: Long range results of pallidoansotomy in paralysis agitans and parkinsonism. In Fields WS (ed): Pathogenesis and Treatment of Parkinsonism. Springfield, IL: Charles C Thomas, 294–298, 1958.
10. Hassler R, Riechert T: Indikationen an Lokalosations-methode der gezielten Hirnoperationen. Nervearzt 25:441–447, 1954.
11. Benabid AL, Pollak P, Loveau A, et al: Combined (thalamotomy and stimulation) stereotactic surgery of the VIM nucleus for bilateral Parkinson disease. Appl Neurophysiol 50:344–346, 1987.
12. Alexander GE, Crutcher MD: Functional architecture of basal ganglia circuits: Neural substrates for parallel processing. Trends Neurosci 13:266–271, 1990.
13. Gerfen CR: Dopamine receptor function in the basal ganglia. Clin Neuropharmacol 18:S162–S177, 1995.
14. Mink JW: The basal ganglia: Focused selection and inhibition of competing motor programs. Prog Neurobiol 50:381–425, 1996.
15. Wenger KK, Musch KL, Mink JW: Impaired reaching and grasping after focal inactivation of the globus pallidus pars interna in the monkey. J Neurophysiol 82:2049–2060, 1999.
16. DeLong MR: Primate models of movement disorders of basal ganglia origin. Trends Neurosci 13:281–285, 1990.
17. Brooks DJ: Functional imaging of Parkinson's disease: Is it possible to detect brain areas for specific symptoms? J Neural Transm 56:139–153, 1999.
18. Laitinen LV: Pallidotomy for Parkinson's disease. Neurosurg Clin N Am 6:105–112, 1995.
19. Su PC, Tseng HM, Liu HM, et al: Treatment of advanced Parkinson's disease by subthalamotomy: One-year results. Mov Disord 18:531–538, 2003.
20. Tasker RR, Davis KW, Hutchison WD, et al: Subcortical and thalamic mapping in functional neurosurgery. In Gildenberg PL, Tasker RR (eds): Textbook of Stereotactic and Functional Neurosurgery. New York: McGraw-Hill, 1998, pp 883–969.
21. DeLong MR, Wichmann T, Vitek JL: Pathophysiological basis of neurosurgical treatment of Parkinson's disease. In Gildenberg PL, Tasker RR (eds): Textbook of Stereotactic and Functional Neurosurgery. New York: McGraw-Hill, 1998, pp 1139–1146.
22. Pare D, Curro'Dossi R, Steriade M: Neuronal basis of the parkinsonian resting tremor: A hypothesis and its implications for treatment. Neuroscience 35:217–226, 1990.
23. Buzsaki G, Smith A, Berger S, et al: Petit mal epilepsy and parkinsonian tremor: Hypothesis of a common pacemaker. Neuroscience 36:1–14, 1990.
24. Holsheimer J, Demeulemeester H, Nuttin B, de Sutter P: Identification of the target neuronal elements in electrical deep brain stimulation. Eur J Neurosci 12:4573–4577, 2000.
25. McIntyre CC, Grill WM: Selective microstimulation of central nervous system neurons. Ann Biomed Eng 28:219–233, 2000.
26. Brock LG, Coombs JS, Eccles JC: The recording of potentials from motoneurons with an intracellular electrode. J Physiol 117:431–460, 1952.
27. Ranck JB: Which elements are excited in electrical stimulation of mammalian central nervous system: A review. Brain Res 98:417–440, 1975.
28. Jankovic J, Cardoso F, Grossman RG, Hamilton WJ: Outcome after stereotactic thalamotomy for parkinsonian, essential and other types of tremor. Neurosurgery 37:680–687, 1995.
29. Hallet M, Litvan I: A task force on surgery for Parkinson's disease. Evaluation of surgery for Parkinson's disease. Neurology 53:1910–1921, 1999.
30. Andy OJ: Thalamic stimulation for control of movement disorders. Appl Neurophysiol 46:107–111, 1983.
31. Cooper IS, Upton AR, Amin I: Reversibility of chronic neurologic deficits. Some effects of electrical stimulation of the thalamus and internal capsule in man. Appl Neurophysiol 43:244–258, 1980.
32. Benabid AL, Pollack P, Gao D, et al: Chronic electrical stimulation of the ventralis intermedius nucleus of the thalamus as a treatment of movement disorders. J Neurosurg 84:203–214, 1996.
33. Koller W, Pahwa R, Busenbark K, et al: High-frequency unilateral thalamic stimulation in the treatment of essential and parkinsonian tremor. Ann Neurol 42:292–299, 1997.

34. Limousin P, Speelman JD, Gielen F, et al: Multicentre European study of thalamic stimulation in parkinsonian and essential tremor. J Neurol Neurosurg Psychiatry 66:289–296, 1999.
35. Montgomery EB, Baker KB, Kinkel RP, Barnett G: Chronic thalamic stimulation for the tremor of multiple sclerosis. Neurology 53:625–628, 1999.
36. Geny C, Nguyen JP, Pollin B, et al: Improvement of severe postural cerebellar tremor in multiple sclerosis by chronic thalamic stimulation. Mov Disord 11:489–494, 1996.
37. Schuurman PR, Bosch DA, Bossuyt MM, et al: A comparison of continuous thalamic stimulation and thalamotomy for suppression of severe tremor. N Engl J Med 342:461–468, 2000.
38. Bergman H, Wichman T, DeLong MR: Reversal of experimental parkinsonism by lesions of the subthalamic nucleus. Science 249:1436–1438, 1990.
39. Benazzouz A, Gross C, Feger J, et al: Reversal of rigidity and improvement of motor performance by subthalamic high-frequency stimulation in MPTP-treated monkeys. Eur J Neurosci 5:382–389, 1993.
40. Limousin P, Pollak P, Benazzouz A, et al: Effect of parkinsonian signs and symptoms of bilateral subthalamic nucleus stimulation. Lancet 345:91–95, 1995.
41. Deep-Brain Stimulation for Parkinson's Disease Study Group: Deep-brain stimulation of the subthalamic nucleus or the pars interna of the globus pallidus in Parkinson's disease. N Engl J Med 345:956–963, 2001.
42. Houeto J, Damier P, Bejjani P, et al: Subthalamic stimulation in Parkinson's disease: A multidisciplinary approach. Arch Neurol 57:461–465, 2000.
43. Limousin P, Krack P, Polack P, et al: Electrical stimulation of the subthalamic nucleus in advanced Parkinson's disease. N Engl J Med 339:1105–1111, 1998.
44. Rodriguez-Oroz MC, Gorospe A, Guridi J, et al: Bilateral deep brain stimulation of the subthalamic nucleus in Parkinson's disease. Neurology 55:S45–S51, 2000.
45. Burchiel KJ, Anderson VC, Favre J, et al: Comparison of pallidal and subthalamic nucleus deep brain stimulation for advanced Parkinson's disease: Results of a randomized, blinded pilot study. Neurosurgery 45:1375–1382, 1999.
46. Laitinen LV, Bergenheim AT, Hariz MI: Leksell's posteroventral pallidotomy in the treatment of Parkinson's disease. J Neurosurg 76:53–61, 1992.
47. Favre J, Burchiel KJ, Taha JM, et al: Outcome of unilateral and bilateral pallidotomy for the treatment of Parkinson's disease: Patient assessment. Neurosurgery 46:344–353, 2000.
48. Siegfried J, Lippitz B: Bilateral chronic electrostimulation of ventroposterolateral pallidum: A new therapeutic approach for alleviating all parkinsonian symptoms. Neurosurgery 35:1126–1129, 1994.
49. Volkman J, Allert N, Voges J, et al: Safety and efficacy of pallidal or subthalamic nucleus stimulation in advanced PD. Neurology 56:548–551, 2001.
50. Ghika J, Villemure JG, Frankhauser H, et al: Efficiency and safety of bilateral contemporaneous pallidal stimulation (deep brain stimulation) in levodopa-responsive patients with Parkinson's disease with severe motor fluctuations: A 2-year follow-up review. J Neurosurg 89:713–718, 1998.
51. Durif F, Lemaire J, Debilly B, et al: Acute and chronic effects of anteromedial globus pallidus stimulation in Parkinson's disease. J Neurol Neurosurg Psychiatry 67:315–321, 1999.
52. Anderson VC, Burchiel KJ, Hogarth, et al: Pallidal vs subthalamic nucleus deep brain stimulation in Parkinson disease. Arch Neurol 62:554–560, 2005.
53. Levy R, Lamb S, Adams J: Treatment of chronic pain by deep brain stimulation: Long term follow-up and review of the literature. Neurosurg 21:885–893, 1987.

102 Neurosurgery for Psychiatric Disorders

JAN M. GYBELS and PAUL R. COSYNS

Operations in the brain for psychiatric disorders are the most controversial biologic treatments in psychiatry. Physicians familiar with these treatments are convinced, from their clinical experience, that highly selective stereotactic operations on the brain can benefit some carefully selected, chronically ill psychiatric patients with a low rate of unwanted side effects. These stereotactic interventions are aimed at different brain structures. Targets that are or have been used for the treatment of obsessive-compulsive disorders (OCDs) and depression include the medial frontal subcaudate white matter, the cingulum, and the anterior part of the capsula interna; for the treatment of aggressive conduct disorders, lesions are placed in the amygdala, the intralaminar nuclei of the thalamus, the posteromedial hypothalamus, and the fundus striae terminalis.

Moreover, a recent development, electrical stimulation of the capsula interna and possibly surrounding brain for the treatment of OCD, is discussed in some detail. This new surgical technique of deep brain stimulation (DBS) with implanted electrodes is reversible and allows, for the first time in this controversial domain, empirical research following the methodologic double-blind paradigm (stimulation on or off).

The present discussion emphasizes two sources of experience. The first one comes from a multidisciplinary review board on psychosurgery that was active from 1971 until the 1990s and supervised and coordinated functional stereotactic neurosurgery for mental disorders (NMD) in Belgium and the Netherlands. This experience is published in extensive detail elsewhere.[1] During this period we also noticed some timid resurgence of interest for psychosurgery (the term *psychosurgery* is inappropriate, the surgeon operates on the brain and not on the psyche of the patient) in the psychiatric literature, mainly for disorders like OCD, where abnormalities in metabolism have been reported in the orbitofrontal cortex that are influenced by psychosurgery.[2] The second source consists of a Belgian review board of NMD whose activity started in the 1990s.

This chapter is mainly concerned with subcaudate tractotomy and DBS in OCD.

PSYCHIATRIC DISORDERS SUITABLE FOR PSYCHOSURGERY

During the 1940s and 1950s, psychosurgery was performed on large and disparate categories of psychiatric patients. Then, with the tremendous development of psychopharmacotherapy and new forms of psychotherapy, there was a marked reduction in the patient stream treated by psychosurgery. Despite this progress in diagnostic and therapeutic modalities, however, psychiatrists remain confronted with a residual group of highly disturbed and suffering patients for whom the psychopharmacologic and psychotherapeutic treatments have proved to be of limited use. In countries where politics have not intruded too heavily on the decision-making process about psychosurgery, this form of treatment continues to be performed, albeit on a limited scale and on a small number of highly selected patients. In Europe, for instance, stereotactic neurosurgery for psychiatric disorders is still practiced by a small number of well-known neurosurgical teams, usually in university hospitals, working closely with appropriately experienced psychiatrists.

The scientific literature agrees on the following psychiatric disorders as indications, under certain circumstances, for psychosurgery: OCD, anxiety disorders, mood disorders (unipolar as well as bipolar), anorexia nervosa, and violent behavior in the mentally retarded. The caveat "under certain circumstances" is included because psychiatric diagnostic labels are necessary but not sufficient on their own for deciding to perform stereotactic surgery. In addition to the psychiatric diagnosis, the patient must fulfill several stringent criteria concerning the duration of the disorder, level of personal suffering, failure of previous usually adequate therapies for the disorder, and actual availability of postoperative long-term psychiatric management (see later section on Inclusion and Exclusion Criteria: Decision-Making Procedures for Neurosurgery for Mental Disorders).

Psychosurgery, as we conceive it, is not an end in itself or a substitute for careful psychiatric treatment, but it has a place in the treatment algorithm of some psychiatric disorders. In the preceding edition of this textbook (2000), we stated that psychosurgery is a treatment of last resort because of its irreversible nature and the impossibility to identify clear predicting factors of a good outcome. This statement must be revised, because neurostimulation is both reversible in nature, and proof-stimulation may be a predicting factor of good outcome, as has been clearly shown in Parkinson's disease and intractable pain.

Indications for Neurosurgery for Mental Disorders

Most studies published in the 1990s reported that over 40% of severe OCD patients obtain considerable benefit from psychosurgery.[3] Owing to the unusual severity of illness of this patient group, these results are clinically encouraging and significant. The most recent algorithms of OCD treatment published in psychiatric literature include neurosurgery as a last resort for refractory and debilitating OCD.[4,5]

For OCD, four targets and three surgical procedures are currently accepted as being effective. The explored targets are the substantia innominata (subcaudate tractotomy), the cingulum (anterior cingulotomy), the limbic leukotomy (a combination of subcaudate tractotomy and anterior cingulotomy),[6] and the anterior limb of the internal capsule (capsulotomy). The three surgical procedures are lesions in the mentioned target areas, DBS of the anterior limb of the internal capsule, or a radiosurgical lesion in the same area (gamma knife capsulotomy). The relative advantages and disadvantages of this noninvasive stereotactic radiosurgical approach remain undetermined.[7] Subcaudate tractotomy and DBS will be discussed in more detail later in this chapter.

Treatment resistant depression remains the most common indication for subcaudate tractotomy in the Geoffrey Knight Unit in London. Mood disorders have been found to improve gradually within 12 months in 34% to 68% of cases.[8] We notice that the proportion of patients with good outcome declined over the years, probably as a result of improvements in pharmacotherapy. These results suggest that the prefrontal cortex subserves an essential function in emotion and that disruption of its connections modifies mood and anxiety.

Patients with incapacitating anxiety disorders can also benefit from subcaudate tractotomy or capsulotomy. The Karolinska research group[9] published the long-term results of 26 patients suffering from generalized anxiety disorder, panic disorder, and social phobia. The reduction in anxiety ratings was significant both at 1 year and long-term follow-up (a positive response rate of 67%), but 7 of the 26 patients (27%) had adverse symptoms such as apathy and dysexecutive behavior.

The scientific evidence of positive results of NMD in anorexia nervosa is scarce but worth mentioning. Morgan and Crisp[10] published long-term positive results in three of five cases of intractable anorexia nervosa patients without long-term neuropsychiatric sequelae. They concluded that NMD is a justifiable recommendation of the last resort in some exceptionally severe and intractable cases. The mode of action remains puzzling because these patients present in the course of their chronic illness with anxiety, mood, and compulsive symptoms.

Indications Still in Dispute

Violent auto- or heteroaggressive behavior and aggressive conduct disorder in patients with profound mental retardation present delicate ethical problems. The patient is incompetent, and informed consent must be obtained from at least the legal guardian. These cases are always submitted by third parties, and a conflict of interest may exist between the safety requirements of this third party (or society) and the best interest of the incompetent patient. For this reason the French National Advisory Board of Health Ethics[11] does not recommend this indication, while the Belgian Review Board will review these cases, taking into account that the best interest of the patient must prevail.

The proposed targets for this indication are the posteromedial hypothalamus, the fundus striae terminalis, the amygdala, and the intralaminar and dorsomedial nuclei of the thalamus. Our research group has a limited experience of 13 patients with aggressive conduct disorder and mental retardation (IQ less than 50) treated by bilateral intralaminar

and dorsomedial thalamotomy or amygdalotomy. They all had protracted, severe, therapy-resistant autoaggressive or heteroaggressive behaviors. It concerns nine male and four female institutionalized patients with a mean age of 23 years (range, 10 to 37 years) and a mean follow-up period of 7 years (range, 4 to 11 years). At follow-up, the investigators reported an improvement of 50% for heteroaggressive violent behavior and of 53% for self-mutilation and autoaggressive behavior.

Kim and colleagues[12] operated on two patients with aggressive behavior with a combined lesion, bilateral amygdalotomy, and subcaudate tractotomy. They reported a significant decline of aggressive behavior with clinical improvement.

The limited scientific evidence allows further research in this area, but is not convincing enough to recommend it as an accepted standard procedure.

Not an Indication for Neurosurgery for Mental Disorders

Violent sexual aggression as an indication for stereotactic hypothalamotomy is a controversial issue.[13] For ethical reasons, we do not accept compulsorily admitted psychiatric patients or detained delinquents as candidates for psychosurgery. Constraints from civil or judicial authorities complicate the necessary respect we owe to the essentials of the informed consent doctrine and the decision-making capacity of the patient. There exist dissenting opinions on this matter, however, that argue that withholding effective treatment from a prisoner violates his or her right to treatment.[14]

Some authors accept stereotactic operations for violent behavior in patients with a normal IQ or in children (6 to 7 years of age) who are overactive, destructive, and self-mutilating even without a significant degree of mental retardation.[15,16] We have no experience of NMD in these situations, but stress the absolute necessity of an appropriate multidisciplinary review board to approve the indications for surgery.

Schizophrenia is a major psychosis for which no causal treatment is currently available. Since the early period of psychosurgery, a great number of schizophrenic patients have undergone surgery without showing convincing improvement. In the absence of any scientific evidence, we consider schizophrenic disorder a contraindication, but researchers such as Ballantine and Giriunas[17] have found it useful in "carefully selected cases . . . in whom depression, anxiety, or obsessions are very prominent accompanying symptoms." It is perhaps reasonable to initiate studies of neurostimulation in these conditions.

Personality disorders are not indications for psychosurgery. The neurosurgical treatment of addictive behavior must be considered experimental and not an accepted indication for stereotactic surgery in the current state of the art.

In Conclusion

The main indications for psychosurgery are therapy-resistant and disturbing anxiety-linked behaviors, such as obsessions or compulsions, and depressive mood disorders. Only some well-defined axis I disorders, as defined in the American Psychiatric Association's *Diagnostic and Statistical Manual of*

Mental Disorders, 4th revised edition (*DSM-IV*),[18] and never axis II disorders, can be taken into consideration.

An extensive overview of the field of surgery for psychiatric disorders in all its aspects can be found in *Neurosurgery Clinics of North America.* Eight groups of authors have contributed to this overview, which is edited by Rezai, Rasmussen, and Greenberg[19] and covers the lesioning techniques in different psychiatric disorders such as OCD, depression, neuropsychiatric thalamocortical dysrhythmia, electrical deep brain and cervical vagus nerve stimulation, neuroimaging and neurocircuitry models in psychiatric disorders, transcranial magnetic stimulation, and history's lessons for the ethical conduct and regulation of neuropsychiatric research.

INCLUSION AND EXCLUSION CRITERIA: DECISION-MAKING PROCEDURES FOR NEUROSURGERY FOR MENTAL DISORDERS

What is the frequency of NMD, what are the inclusion and exclusion criteria, and which decision-making procedures are recommended to fulfill ethical concerns associated with this therapy?

A multidisciplinary review board on psychosurgery is a necessary part of the decision-making process for this form of surgery. Given the low basic incidence of these psychiatric cases, most psychiatrists cannot develop sufficient experience during their professional career to establish accurate indications for psychosurgery. Neurosurgeons, on the other hand, should not operate on psychiatric patients without adequate psychiatric expert advice and proper psychiatric follow-up care. The Belgian Review Board of Neurosurgery for Mental Disorders consists of an independent group of individual experts: neurosurgeons, psychiatrists, lawyers, and ethicists from the medical schools of four different universities.

It functions as a third opinion for the patient and for his or her therapist, who submits the case for review. This review board assesses the indication for NMD for a selected patient, the competence of the surgeon, the appropriateness of the proposed surgical procedure, the adequacy of the patient's informed consent, and the quality of the planned psychiatric follow-up. The main ethical justification of the surgery rests in its aim to restore normal function and relieve patient's distress and suffering. NMD should only be performed to improve patients' lives and never for social, law enforcement, or political purposes.

The following requirements are considered by the review board in each case:

- Appropriate psychiatric diagnosis for NMD.
- Severity of patient's suffering, which results in marked impairment in social or occupational activities.
- Absence of contraindications:
  - No comorbidity with axis I diagnosis of *DSM-IV,*[18] such as delirium, dementia, amnestic and other cognitive disorders, substance-related disorders, or schizophrenia and other psychotic disorders.
  - No comorbidity with axis II diagnoses of DSM-IV,[18] mainly from clusters B and A, but not necessarily cluster C (when anxiety plays a major role and may be improved by the treatment).
  - No comorbidity with neurologic brain diseases.

- All adequate therapeutic measures have been applied and have proved to be ineffective.
- The proposed surgical procedure and target area in the brain are appropriate.
- The proposed neurosurgeon and surgical unit are competent to perform the planned surgical intervention.
- Adequate preoperative and postoperative psychiatric evaluation and treatment are available.
- The patient, the nearest relative, and the therapist consent to the surgical treatment after being duly informed.

Most of these criteria concerning indications and contradictions are in agreement with those of Bridges[20] and with Swedish[21] clinical research centers performing neurosurgical interventions for psychiatric disorders. They also fit the requirements of the OCD-DBS Collaborative Group concerning the ethics of DBS for psychiatric disorder.[22]

The patient's informed consent is an absolute condition for NMD. Some of our patients could not give it because of their psychopathology, some being too anxious to make such a decision, others too fixed in their doubts and indecision. Whenever a patient declines our advice for NMD or when the patient's consent is only questionable, we always accept and respect his or her choice, regardless of the motivation, healthy or pathologic. Prisoners and other involuntarily committed patients cannot be considered for surgery because they are not in a position to make free choices. For incompetent mentally retarded patients, the legally appointed guardian and therapist in charge must give their (informed) consent, and even in these cases, the patient's consent is requested. In our practice, NMD requires the consent of the patient, the nearest relative, and his or her therapist, as well as a positive recommendation from the review board of NMD.

Concerning the frequency of NMD, not many statistics are available, but where they are, the actual frequency of neurosurgery for psychiatric disorders is very low: for example, in Belgium and the Netherlands, 0.2 per million inhabitants (1982–1991); in the United Kingdom, 0.3 per million inhabitants (1985–1989); and in Australia and New Zealand, 0.2 per million inhabitants (1985–1989) (adapted from Hay and Sachdev[23]).

SUBCAUDATE TRACTOTOMY FOR OBSESSIVE-COMPULSIVE DISORDERS

Patient Selection

In addition to the previously discussed inclusion and exclusion criteria, the specific clinical criteria for patients with OCD are as follows:

- Persistent obsessions and/or compulsions of at least 4 years' duration with the symptoms constituting a source of severe personal distress and suffering for the patient and gross interference with normal daily routines. In fact, the duration of illness exceeds 10 to 15 years in most cases because surgery is a treatment of a last resort.
- Failure to achieve significant and lasting positive effects with existing and usual treatment procedures

over a sufficient period. Such treatments include intensive behavior therapy and psycho-pharmacotherapy, such as the use of clomipramine at high doses (250 to 300 mg) for at least 3 months, at least two specific serotonin reuptake inhibitors at high doses during a long time period and a trial of augmentation strategy. All of our patients undergoing surgery had been hospitalized during the course of their illness, mainly for intensive inpatient behavior therapy.

- Comorbidity with major depressive episodes or other mood disorders do not constitute a contraindication for NMD. The diagnosis of OCD implies that the core symptomatology should be present in the absence of any significant mood change.
- Comorbidity with schizophrenic or other psychotic disorders constitutes a contraindication for psychosurgery. Comorbidity with personality disorders of cluster B (*DSM-IV*), mainly the histrionic, borderline, and antisocial personality disorders, needs very close evaluation and generally means a contraindication for neurosurgery.
- The availability of intensive psychiatric treatment or rehabilitation programs following psychosurgery is also a prerequisite for a positive recommendation.

Target: The Substantia Innominata

In 1964, Knight[24] described the subcaudate tractotomy in which a lesion is placed in the medioposterobasal part of the frontal lobes. His rationale for this procedure was based on the favorable results, in some cases, of the orbital under-cutting operation described by Scoville.[25] The area destroyed has often been called the substantia innominata, the structure situated beneath the head of the caudate nucleus in the region overlying the agranular cortex of area 13 and part of 14; neuroanatomic research has shown that the lesion is in fact anterior to the substantia innominata.[26]

In an attempt to identify the fibers interrupted by this stereotactic intervention, Knight[24] cites the following anatomic data: "The relationship between the frontal cortex and the hypothalamus as described by Le Gros Clark and Meyer[27]; the presence of fibres from area 24 of the anterior cingulate cortex passing through the septal cortex en route to the posterior portion of area 14[28]; bilateral projections from the posterior orbital cortex of area 13 to the ventro-medial hypothalamic nuclei[29]; a projection from the amyg-daloid nucleus and the lobus pyriformis sweeping up and passing into the posterior substantia before turning back and running caudally towards the hypothalamus and the dorsal medial nucleus (MD) of the thalamus from where it is relayed to the frontal cortex." Because the lesion does not penetrate the substantia innominata, it is only the amygdaloid projection to the prefrontal cortex, and mainly area 13, that is interrupted in its terminal segment after it passes through the pars magnocellularis of the thalamic dorsomedial nucleus.

Technique

For subcaudate tractotomy, target localization can be performed using either bony landmarks, air encephalography,

ventriculography, and computed tomography (CT) or magnetic resonance imaging (MRI). Because most of our subcaudate tractotomies have been performed using bony landmarks, this method of target localization is described.

After fixation of the head in the stereotactic frame, bony landmarks are identified as reference structures for determining the coordinates. The target is localized 1 cm above the skull base plane (orbital roof and planum sphenoidale). It lies 5 mm anterior to the anterior border of the sella turcica (Fig. 102-1A). Initially, the target was situated at 3 mm anterior to the sella border, but since MRI showed the very near proximity of the anterior cerebral arteries, we have moved the target 2 mm forward (Fig. 102-1B). The technique originally described by Knight[24] involves the use of radio-active yttrium 90 rods. We make the lesion by producing a series of thermocoagulations at multiple points along three trajectories, creating a lesion between 10 and 20 mm from the midline and 2 cm rostrocaudally in front of the target. The lesion is always made in one session on both sides with the patient under local or general anesthesia. If necessary, a second operation to enlarge the lesion is performed at a later time; during this second intervention, two more trajectories, 10 and 22 mm lateral to the midline and 10 mm more anterior than the first target, are used. Figure 102-1C shows a sagittal MRI scan 6 months after the stereotactic procedure, and Figure 102-1D shows an axial MRI scan of the same lesion 1 day after the procedure.

Knight[30] stressed the importance of a low approach to prevent damage to the caudate nucleus. He described a case with a fatal outcome from a lesion that entered the striatum. Therefore, the bilateral frontal burr holes are made as low as possible in the supraorbital region 1.5 cm from the midline. For psychological reasons, we try to achieve an almost invisible scar by placing the incision in a skin crease. The burr hole can be filled by plastic buttons or by reinsertion of the bone dust, supported in and covered by Surgicel. Sometimes, the frontal sinuses can reach so far upward that in order to avoid infection, a subcaudate tractotomy is not indicated, and an anterior capsulotomy or cingulotomy is preferable. When local anesthesia is used (the usual procedure), stimulation (pulse width 1 msec, frequency range from 3 to 100 pulses per second, and amplitude 0.1 to 2 mA) in the different target points prior to coagulation in our experience does not elicit any psychic or emotional effect. Respiratory and cardiac accelerations have been observed on stimulation in a few cases.

It should be noted that the position of the tuberculum sellae in relation to the orbitofrontal white matter is uncertain. The space between the caudate and the nucleus accumbens and the orbitofrontal gray matter is narrow, and an autopsy case has been reported in which the lesion entered the orbitofrontal gray matter in several locations.[31] More rigorous techniques can be developed through the use of modern imaging techniques.

Surgical Results

In a series of 30 subcaudate tractotomies, we noted one postoperative, small intracerebral hematoma beneath the frontal burr hole. This hematoma did not require operative evacuation and did not result in a lasting neurologic deficit.

FIGURE 102-1 A 54-year-old patient who had a subcaudate tractotomy in September 1991. *A,* The target as determined by bony landmarks on a lateral x-ray study. *B,* The position of the anterior cerebral arteries as seen on a sagittal magnetic resonance imaging (MRI) scan. *C,* The lesion as seen on a sagittal MRI, T1-weighted image, 6 months after the stereotactic procedure. *D,* The same lesion as seen on an axial T2-weighted MRI, 1 day after the stereotactic procedure.

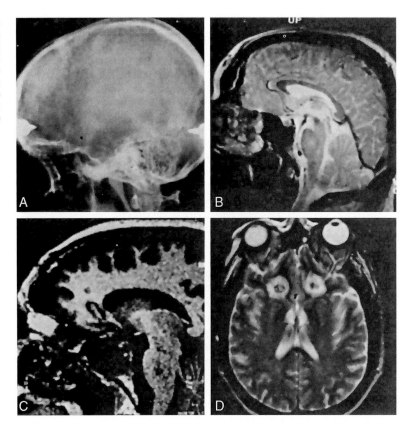

Psychiatric Results

We reviewed 21 successive surgical cases from the first 11 years of activity of the review board on NMD. Twelve patients had a bifrontal stereotactic subcaudate tractotomy,[32] and nine patients underwent a progressive leukocoagulation[33] in the paracingular and orbitofrontal areas. The mean age of the group (12 females and 9 males) was 43 years (range, 27 to 65 years). Follow-up data were available for 16 of the 21 cases; at follow-up 3 patients had died, 1 from suicide and 2 of natural causes. Follow-up results were obtained an average of 7 years (range, 2 to 9 years) after surgery.

To assess the psychiatric status of the OCD patients who underwent surgery, a questionnaire was mailed during the follow-up period to these surgical patients and their therapists. Specific questions concerning the target symptoms (obsessions, compulsions, anxiety, and depressive mood) were asked on a 6-point scoring scale, ranging from "the problem is over" (1 point) to "the problem is worse" (6 points). As for the target symptoms, a positive evolution was reported by the patients and their therapists. The overall obsessive-compulsive symptomatology score dropped from 5/6 to 3.5/6 at follow-up, an improvement of 26.5% according to the surgical patients. The evaluation of the therapists is more impressive: their scores dropped from 5.5 to 3 at follow-up, an improvement of 41%. The difference between patient scores before surgery and at follow-up was statistically significant for the target symptoms obsessions and anxiety. In the therapist scores, the level of statistical significance was reached for the four target symptoms compulsions,

obsessions, anxiety, and depression. Given the previously existing, unyielding resistance of these cases to therapeutic improvements and the long-standing duration of disabling symptoms, the results of these surgical procedures are important and noteworthy.

The same follow-up study was made of seven OCD patients who had refused psychosurgery even though a positive recommendation for surgery had been given by the review board. In contrast with the findings in the patients who had undergone surgery, those patients who had not undergone surgery did not show any significant improvement in the target symptoms over a 1-year period, as reported by themselves and their therapists. A detailed statistical analysis of the scores of this patient group who refused psychosurgery revealed that any changes in the various scores failed to reach a statistical significance for all the target symptoms (compulsions, obsessions, anxiety, and depression).

Our major clinical findings and observations for the OCD patients who had undergone surgery can be summarized as follows:

- In a patient with positive symptomatic evolution, the improvement in anxiety and mood usually precedes that in obsessional or compulsive symptoms. The change in the latter symptoms is generally delayed (up to several months), and a direct influence of stereotactic surgery on this performative aspect of behavior is generally not observed. Some researchers like Sachdev and colleagues[34] state that the improvement in obsessive-compulsive symptoms (i.e., 38%) was independent of the changes in anxiety and depression scores, arguing for a specific antiobsessional effect of surgery.

- Early somatic side effects are mainly a transient confusional state due to local cerebral edema and can be visualized by MRI. This confusional state persists for a few days or weeks and, in our experience, is linked to positive long-term results. Infrequently, we also notice ataxia, oral dyskinesia, and transient urinary incontinence.

- In comparison with the patient's preoperative condition, we often note that after surgery, the patient exhibits a greater sensitivity to anxiolytic and antidepressant drugs; that is, most could not tolerate postoperatively the high doses or combination of drugs they had been taking preoperatively. It may be that psychosurgery influences the sensitivity of the central nervous system to these drugs. Similar observations have been made in patients with bipolar affective disorder after stereotactic subcaudate tractotomy. Lovett and Shaw[35] reported that in five patients (of a total of nine), drugs that were ineffective before subcaudate tractotomy appeared to become effective subsequently.

- After surgery, some patients responded favorably to previously ineffective psychotherapeutic procedures. The improvement of the anxiety level may play a key role here, and we recommend restarting intensive psychological and behavior therapy after surgery.

- Transient unwanted behavioral problems or changes of personality traits were observed as greater impulsiveness, being more "extroverted," as well as reduced reactivity and apathy. For this reason, we are cautious about recommending surgery in a patient who presents with a personality disorder with a low threshold of acting out, such as cluster B of the personality disorders defined by the *DSM-IV*.[18] The organic personality disorder or postleukotomy syndrome does not occur with the actual stereotactic techniques. The symptom of disinhibited behavior can be transiently present after surgery. In our follow-up study, patients who underwent surgery reported greater assertiveness or vitality, improved social behavior, and a larger capacity to experience internal feelings and express emotions. Lovett and Shaw[35] reported that even in bipolar affective disorders, hypomanic episodes have been more sensitive to subcaudate tractotomy than depressive episodes, and that they have either stopped or occurred in a very attenuated form.

- Delayed somatic side effects include grand mal seizures occurring several years after the operation. Among our 21 patients who underwent surgery, this adverse effect occurred in 3 patients, but 2 of them had only one seizure after alcohol abuse.

- All patients in our series underwent extensive psychological testing before surgery and at least 6 months after psychosurgery. The tests applied were Wechsler's Adult Intelligence Scale, the Minnesota Multiphasic Personality Inventory, the modified work learning test, and the Grassi, Hooper, and Bourdon Wiersma tests. Comparison of test results obtained before and after surgery failed to reveal any significant deterioration in psychological functioning. In some patients, an improvement in IQ was noted; it was considered a result of decreased anxiety or diminished intrusion of obsessive-compulsive hindrance during the test procedure. Psychological test evidence of changes in personality as well as neuropsychological deficits could not be verified. These findings are in accordance with neuropsychological outcome studies from psychosurgery in OCD, which showed mainly subnormal performances on the Wisconsin Card Sorting Test but no deficit in memory or intellectual functions.[36,37]

NEUROMODULATION PROCEDURES

Because lesioning procedures and their possible side effects are irreversible, it was logical to find out, in analogy with what has been done for Parkinson's disease and intractable pain, whether electrical stimulation of a brain structure whose destruction may ameliorate certain symptoms of a given psychiatric disorder might produce the same beneficial effects. The disease and the target chosen for stimulation were based on the long-term results of the Karolinska group in OCD with anterior capsulotomy. In 29 patients (thermocapsulotomy, $n = 19$; gamma knife capsulotomy, $n = 10$) both psychiatric and MRI follow-up data (median, 8.4 years) were available. A right-sided anatomically defined lesion was identified in all successfully treated patients. The common topographic denominator was situated in the approximate middle of the anterior limb of the internal capsule on the plane parallel to the commisura anterior–commisura posterior line at the level of the foramen of Monro and 4 mm above on the plane defined by the internal cerebral vein. This region was unaffected in patients with poor outcome. On the left side, no particular lesion topography was associated with clinical outcome.[38]

In 1999, it was shown that bilateral DBS of the anterior limb of the internal capsule in a target that was identical to the one targeted in capsulotomy could induce relevant beneficial effects in OCD, which suggested that long-term stimulation might be useful in the management of treatment-resistant forms of this psychiatric disorder.[39] This preliminary finding was confirmed in a single case-based design of three patients with a follow-up period of 33, 33, and 39 months, respectively, in which clinical and rigorous scientific practice were combined to document changes in emotions, behavior, personality traits, and executive functions during DBS treatment.[40] In the same issue of *Acta Psychiatrica Scandinavica* in which the previous mentioned results were published, there is an editorial with the title "Psychosurgery for Obsessive-Compulsive Disorder—Concerns Remain."[41] As far as DBS for OCD is concerned, the guest editor questioned whether the effects of DBS are fully reversible and observed that the physiologic mechanisms underlying the beneficial effect of DBS are not well understood and may be extremely complex and referred to the experience of DBS in Parkinson's disease in which declines in working memory, speed of mental processing, coordination, phonemic fluency, long-term consolidation of verbal material, encoding of visuospatial material, and frontal behavior discontrol in the subgroup of elderly patients had been observed.

In 2003 another OCD case report was published with 1-year follow-up from a different center in which a marked improvement was noted in the OCD symptomatology and general psychosocial functioning with stimulation of the anterior limb of the capsula interna.[42] This report was followed by an editorial[43] that, after having evoked the lack of enthusiasm of physicians or the general public for neurosurgical procedures to treat psychiatric disorders, argues that a larger trial to test the usefulness of DBS in patients with intractable OCD is appropriate.

Although a specific identified brain abnormality has not been determined, there is growing evidence for a neurobiologic basis for OCD. Abnormalities in frontal lobe and basal ganglia function in OCD patients have led to hypotheses about a dysfunction in the neurocircuits that connect those two regions.[44,45] The fibers of these frontostriatalpallidal loops are believed to pass through the anterior limb of the internal capsule, the target of capsulotomy.[24]

In 2003 the long-term results of DBS of the anterior limb of the capsula interna in four patients with OCD were reported.[46] The follow-up periods were 31, 26, 24, and 21 months, respectively. Figure 102-2 shows the position of the electrodes, and Figure 102-3 shows the clinical results of these four patients. fMRI studies of patient 4 are shown in Figure 102-4, and Figure 102-5 shows digital substraction analysis performed with positron emission tomography (PET) data in patients 1, 2, and 3.

According to the neuroimaging data, the electrical stimulation–induced activation was highest in a midline focus within the pons. Near the electrode tip, stimulation-related activity was found in the left and right striata. Weaker activation was observed in the right frontal cortex, in the superior and middle temporal gyrus, and in the left and right striata, bilaterally. Digital substraction analysis performed with postoperative and preoperative positron computed scans showed a marked decrease in frontal metabolism after 3 months of stimulation (see Fig. 102-5). It should be noted that PET studies in patients with OCD symptoms have consistently shown increased [^{18}F] 2-fluoro-2-desoxy-D-glucose uptake in the prefrontal cortex.[48] An increased glucose metabolism was also found in the caudate nucleus.

The amplitude of the electrical current (i.e., 4 to 10.5 V with impedance approximately 700 O, pulse width 210 seconds, frequency 100 Hz) necessary to obtain clinically relevant effects in the patients in Figure 102-2 is high, and as a consequence the batteries of the implanted stimulation device need to be replaced every 5 to 12 months in all four patients, which of course is a problem. We guess that other structures, near the anterior limb of the capsula interna, may be a better target than the anterior limb of the capsula interna for neurostimulation procedures in OCD. The nucleus accumbens might be such a structure.

The nucleus accumbens is situated just ventral of the anterior limb of the capsula interna (Fig. 102-6). Neuroanatomists consider the nucleus accumbens as a gateway for limbic structures to reach the motor system.[50] The nucleus accumbens is a part of a loop that includes

connections between the prefrontal cortex and subcortical structures that comprise the striatum and thalamus and is also an important interface in the translation of relevant environmental stimuli into an adaptive motor response.[51]

FUTURE PROSPECTS

Despite several justified criticisms toward psychosurgery or NMD, we must observe that it never disappeared totally as a treatment modality for some selected psychiatric disorders when all other reasonable treatments had failed.

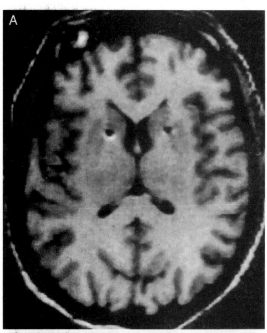

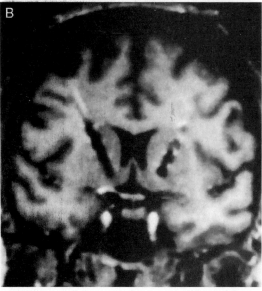

FIGURE 102-2 Axial (*A*) and coronal (*B*) T1-weighted magnetic resonance imaging studies of patient 3 showing the stimulating electrodes in the anterior limbs of the internal capsules. (From Nuttin BJ, Gabriels LA, Cosyns PR, et al: Long-term electrical capsular stimulation in patients with obsessive-compulsive disorder. Neurosurgery 52:1263–1274, 2003.)

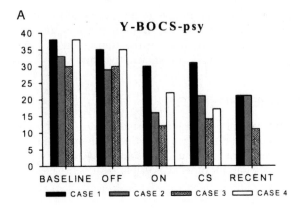

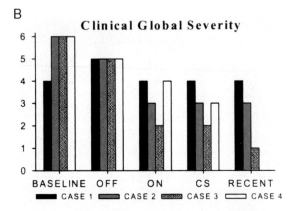

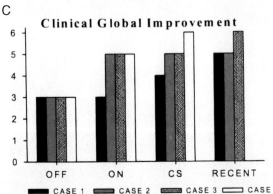

FIGURE 102-3 Bar graphs showing the effects of capsular stimulation on psychiatrist-rated Y-BOCS, CGS, and CGI scores. Y-BOCS (*A*) and CGS (*B*) scores of patients 1, 2, 3, and 4 are shown at presurgical baseline (*BASELINE*), in the stimulator-on condition (*ON*), and in the stimulator-off condition (*OFF*) of the crossover design, after 6 months of continuous stimulation, after the end of the crossover design phase (CS), and the patients' most recent scores in the stimulator-on condition (*RECENT*) (i.e., after 24 months in the trial for patient 2 and after 21 months in the trial for patient 3). Patient 3 refused to have the electrode switched off. Just before changing the electrode because of a dead battery, a Y-BOCS score was obtained. *C,* CGI ratings with reference to presurgical baseline levels of the same patients. Recent data for patient 1 are after capsulotomy. Y-BOCS score definitions: 0–7, subclinical; 8–15, mild; 16–23, moderate; 24–31, severe; 32–40, extremely severe. CGS score definitions: 0, no illness; 1, minimal; 2, mild; 3, moderate; 4, moderate–severe; 5, severe; 6, very severe. CGI score definitions: 1, much worse; 2, minimally worse; 3, no change; 4, minimally improved; 5, much improved; 6, very much improved. (From Nuttin BJ, Gabriels LA, Cosyns PR, et al: Long-term electrical capsular stimulation in patients with obsessive-compulsive disorder. Neurosurgery 52:1263–1274, 2003.)

Among the medical advances that explain the recent resurgence of interest in NMD we note:

- The actual stereotactic neurosurgical interventions have proven to be safe, highly reliable, and effective.
- The intervention is practiced in few well-known centers (1) where neurosurgeons and psychiatrists work closely and (2) with a review board for the ethical considerations and the monitoring of inclusion-exclusion guidelines.
- Advances into the neurobiology of OCD led to the development of new neuroanatomic models and insights into the working of the prefrontal cortex and basal ganglia.

The further development in apparatus technology and neurosurgical techniques, and the recent research with animal models for psychiatric disorders, open potential therapeutic perspectives and a growing understanding of brain functioning.

Transcranial Magnetic Stimulation

Rapid transcranial magnetic stimulation (rTMS) was first performed in a preliminary controlled study as a probe of prefrontal cortex involvement in OCD.[52] The data indicated a significant and selective reduction in compulsive urges after right prefrontal rTMS, while this was not the case after left prefrontal stimulation. Much information on rTMS and OCD can be found in the report of Greenberg and colleagues.[53]

Chronic Intrathecal Infusion of Drugs

It also has been shown that thyrotropin-releasing hormone (TRH) has direct effects on the central nervous system that are independent of pituitary or thyroid stimulation, and it is suggested that TRH may be relevant in the treatment of mood disorders. The blood-brain barrier for TRH is poor, but it has been shown in a small sample of refractory depressed patients that administration of TRH intrathecally by standard lumbar puncture induces a rapid improvement in mood and suicidality.[54] One strategy to administer TRH or eventually other agents is the use of surgically implanted pumps that deliver these drugs from an externally accessible reservoir to the lumbar cerebrospinal fluid at a programmable and adjustable rate.

Animal Research Models for Psychiatric Disorders

In OCD, stimulation of the capsula interna or nearby brain structures can alleviate some symptoms and signs, but consumption of electricity is high to obtain this effect. In order to find a better target, an animal model has been used and rats were tested for spontaneous alternation behavior in a T-maze and the effects of electrical stimulation and lesion of the nucleus accumbens in different conditions. Spontaneous alternation behavior is the natural tendency of most species to successively explore both arms of a T-maze alternatively. It could be shown that both the electrical stimulation and lesion in the nucleus accumbens decreased the alternation behavior of rats in a T-maze after administration of 8-OH-DPAT.[55] Alternation behavior of

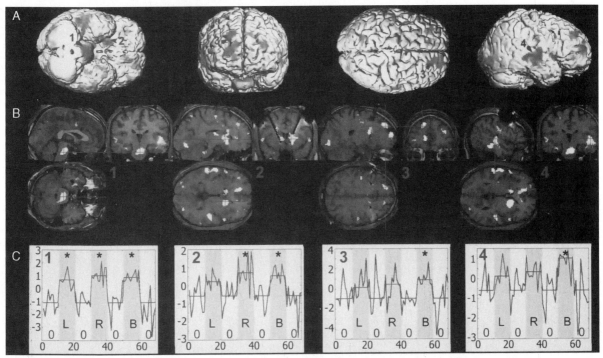

FIGURE 102-4   fMRI studies showing cortical and subcortical activation in patient 4 when brain activity is subtracted during the stimulation-off condition from brain activity shown during the stimulation-on condition, superimposed onto surface reconstructions (*A*) and sections of the patient's brain (*B*). Regions are labeled as follows: the midline focus in the pons (1), the striatum (2), the focus in the right frontal cortex (3), and the left superior temporal gyrus (4). In the brain sections, the left hemisphere is shown on the right or at the bottom. *C,* Percentage fMRI signal change (*blue line*) and statistically modeled signal change (*red line*) during left (*L*), right (*R*), simultaneous (*B*), and no stimulation (*0*) in the four labeled regions. Conditions for which stimulation versus no stimulation was significant ($p < 0.05$ corrected for multiple comparisons) are indicated by asterisks. (See Color Plate.) (From Nuttin BJ, Gabriels LA, Cosyns PR, et al: Long-term electrical capsular stimulation in patients with obsessive-compulsive disorder. Neurosurgery 52:1263–1274, 2003.)

FIGURE 102-5   Digital subtraction analysis was performed with [^{18}F]2-fluoro-2-desoxy-D-glucose positron computed tomographic (PET) images before electrode implantation and after 3 months in the stimulation-on condition for patients 1 (*upper*), 2 (*middle*), and 3 (*lower*). The magnetic resonance imaging (MRI) scan and the preoperative and postoperative PET images were coregistered by using an automated algorithm[47] and were subtracted after normalization for global counts. Only the voxels (color) in the postoperative PET scan with decreased glucose metabolism of more than 2 standard deviations are combined with the coregistered MRI scan (patients 1 and 3) or with the preoperative PET scan (patient 2). The coregistered MRI scan and the preoperative PET scan are displayed in gray scale. Red represents the strongest after reduction in glucose metabolism. The left hemisphere is shown in the images in the right column. (See Color Plate.) (From Nuttin BJ, Gabriels LA, Cosyns PR, et al: Long-term electrical capsular stimulation in patients with obsessive-compulsive disorder. Neurosurgery 52:1263–1274, 2003.)

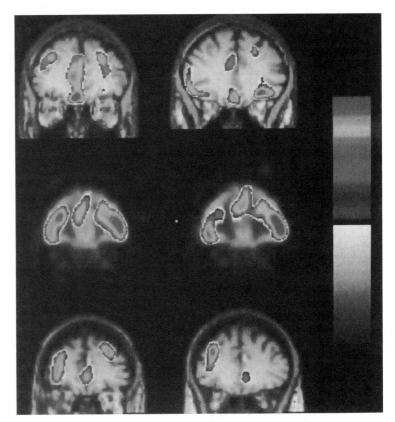

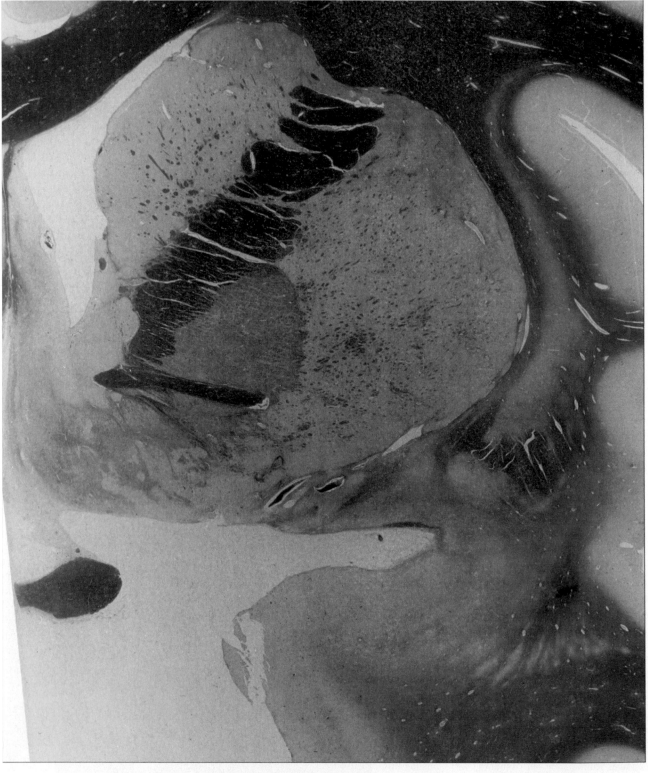

		AcM	accumbens n., medial part	CdM	medial caudate nucleus	ex	extreme capsule
		aco	anterior commissure, olfactory limb	CdV	ventral caudate nucleus	FLV	frontal horn of lateral ventricle
		aic	anterior limb of internal capsule	CG	cingulate gyrus	FOp	frontal operculum
		AMPO	anterior medial preoptic nucleus	cir	circular insular sulcus	FPu	putaminal fundus region
		bcc	body of the corpus callosum	CoCl	compact insular claustrum	GTI	great terminal island
		BSTC	bed nucleus of the stria terminalis, central division	DB	nucleus of the diagonal band	HDB	horizontal limb of the diagonal band
				DiCl	diffuse insular claustrum	IG	insular gyrus
		BSTL	bed nucleus of the stria terminalis, lateral division	DPe	dorsal periventricular hypothalamic nucleus	ilf	inferior longitudinal fasciculus
						Li	limen insulae
ac	anterior commissure	BSTM	bed nucleus of the stria terminalis, medial division	ec	external capsule	lml	external medullary lamina of the globus pallidus
AcCL	accumbens n., centrolateral part			EGP	external globus pallidus		
AcCM	accumbens n., centromedial part	CdL	lateral caudate nucleus	Ent	entorhinal cortex	lo	laterao olfactory tract

FIGURE 102-6 Atlas of the human brain developed by Jürgen K. May, Joseph Assheuer, and George Paxinos.[49] *Left,* Myelin-stained coronal section. *Right,* Corresponding schematic sections. The brain cut is perpendicular to the intercommissural line (ac-pc); the accompanying diagram is of the same size and defines position, extent, and relationship of nuclei and pathways. Section 20 is situated as indicated in the right upper corner, 1.3 mm in front of the midpoint of ac. (From Mai JK, Assheuer J, Paxinos G: Atlas of the Human Brain, 2nd ed. Philadelphia: Elsevier, 2004.)

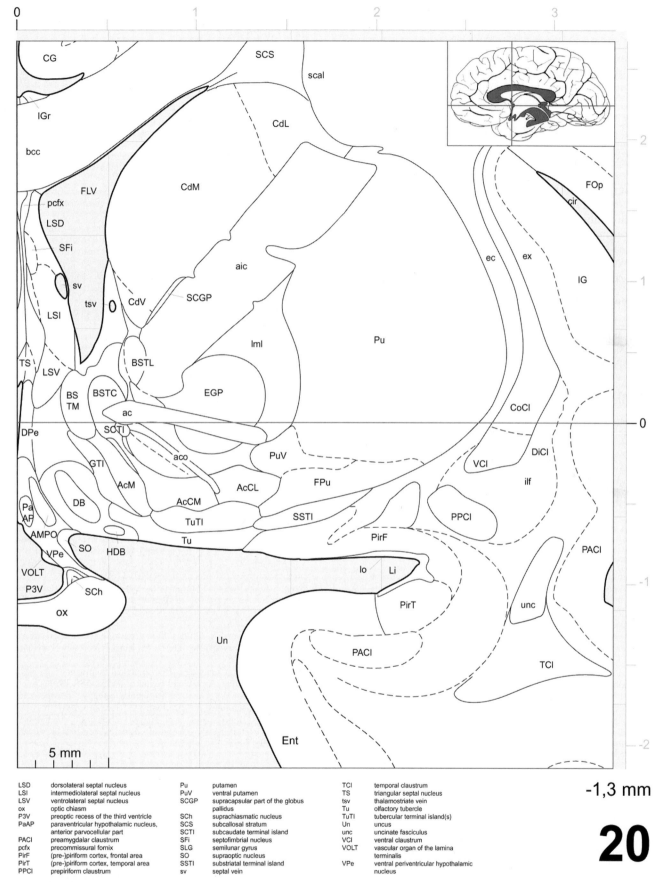

LSD	dorsolateral septal nucleus	Pu	putamen	TCl	temporal claustrum
LSI	intermediolateral septal nucleus	PuV	ventral putamen	TS	triangular septal nucleus
LSV	ventrolateral septal nucleus	SCGP	supracapsular part of the globus	tsv	thalamostriate vein
ox	optic chiasm		pallidus	Tu	olfactory tubercle
P3V	preoptic recess of the third ventricle	SCh	suprachiasmatic nucleus	TuTl	tubercular terminal island(s)
PaAP	paraventricular hypothalamic nucleus,	SCS	subcallosal stratum	Un	uncus
	anterior parvocellular part	SCTI	subcaudate terminal island	unc	uncinate fasciculus
PACl	preamygdalar claustrum	SFi	septofimbrial nucleus	VCl	ventral claustrum
pcfx	precommissural fornix	SLG	semilunar gyrus	VOLT	vascular organ of the lamina
PirF	(pre-)piriform cortex, frontal area	SO	supraoptic nucleus		terminalis
PirT	(pre-)piriform cortex, temporal area	SSTI	substriatal terminal island	VPe	ventral periventricular hypothalamic
PPCl	prepiriform claustrum	sv	septal vein		nucleus

−1,3 mm

20

FIGURE 102-6 Cont'd

rats in a T-maze after administration of the selective serotonin 1A receptor agonist 8-OH-DPAT is considered to model the compulsive and repetitive behavior of patients suffering from OCD.[56]

Another example concerns anorexia nervosa. One validated animal model for this disorder is the activity-based model. Normal rats that are allowed to eat 1 hour per day in ad libitum quantities will eat sufficiently to maintain or even increase their body weight. In contrast, rats that have access to a running wheel and are kept under the same feeding conditions will spontaneously restrict their food intake and will develop hyperactivity, resulting in a marked weight loss. If this feeding conditions continues, the emaciation often results in high mortality rates.[57] How is this behavior influenced by stimulation of certain brain structures such as the nucleus accumbens? This type of research may eventually pave the way for better treatment modalities such as DBS for patients with severe and intractable anorexia nervosa.

Acknowledgments

The authors are indebted to the Members of the Belgian Review Board of Neurosurgery for Mental Disorders and the Members of the OCD-DBS Collaborative Group, especially Bart Nuttin (Leuven, Belgium) and Loes Gabriels (Antwerp, Belgium).

REFERENCES

1. Cosyns P, Caemaert J, Haaijman W, et al: Functional stereotactic neurosurgery for psychiatric disorders: An experience in Belgium and The Netherlands. Adv Techn Stand Neurosurg 21:241–279, 1994.
2. Biver F, Goldman S, François A, et al: Changes in metabolism of cerebral glucose after stereotactic leukotomy for refractory obsessive-compulsive disorder: A case report. J Neurol Neurosurg Psychiatry 58:502–505, 1995.
3. Sachdev P, Sachdev J: Sixty years of psychosurgery: Its present status and its future. Aust N Z J Psychiatry 31:457–464, 1997.
4. Zohar J: Treatment of obsessive compulsive disorder: Algorithms for pharmacotherapy. Int J Psychiatry Clin Pract 1(Suppl):17–23, 1997.
5. Pato MT, Pato CN: Obsessive-compulsive disorder in adults. In Pato MT, Steketee G (eds): OCD across the Life Cycle. Washington, DC: American Psychiatric Press, 1997, pp 29–55.
6. Kelly D: Psychosurgery and the limbic system. Postgrad Med J 49:825–833, 1973.
7. Lippitz B, Mindus P, Meyerson B, et al: Lesion topography and outcome after thermocapsulotomy and gamma knife capsulotomy for obsessive-compulsive disorder: Relevance of the right hemisphere. Neurosurgery 44:452–460, 1999.
8. Malhi GS, Bartlett JR: Depression: A role for neurosurgery? Br J Neurosurg 14(5):415–423, 2000.
9. Ruck C, Andréewitch S, Flyckt K, et al: Capsulotomy for refractory anxiety disorders: Long-term follow-up of 26 patients. Am J Psychiatry 160(3):513–521, 2003.
10. Morgan JF, Crisp AH: Use of Leucotomy for Intractable Anorexia Nervosa: A Long-Term Follow-Up Study. New York: Wiley, 2000, pp 249–258.
11. Comité Consultatif National d'Ethique: Avis n° 71 sur "La Neuro-chirurgie fonctionnelle d'affections psychiatriques sévères." Cah CCNE 32:3–21, 2002.
12. Kim ML, Lee TK, Choi CR, et al: Review of long-term results of stereotactic psychosurgery. Neurol Med Chir (Tokyo) 42:365–371, 2002.
13. Dieckman G, Schneider-Joonietz B, Schneider H: Psychiatric and neuropsychological findings after stereotactic hypothalamotomy, in cases of extreme sexual aggressivity. Acta Neurochir Suppl 44:163–166, 1988.
14. Merskey H: Ethical aspects of the physical manipulation of the brain. In Bloch S, Chodoff P (eds): Psychiatric Ethics, 2nd ed. Oxford, UK: Oxford Medical Publications, 1991, pp 185–214.
15. Ramamurthi B: Stereotactic operation in behaviour disorders: Amygdalatomy and hypothalamotomy. Acta Neurochir Suppl 44:152–157, 1988.
16. Sano K, Mayanagi Y: Posteromedial hypothalamotomy in the treatment of violent, aggressive behaviour. Acta Neurochir Suppl 44:145–151, 1988.
17. Ballantine H, Giriunas I: Treatment of intractable psychiatric illness and chronic pain by stereotactic cingulotomy. In Schmidek H, Sweet WH (eds): Operative Neurosurgical Techniques, vol II. New York: Grune & Stratton, 1988, pp 1069–1075.
18. American Psychiatric Association: Diagnostic and Statistical Manual of Mental Disorders, 4th ed. Washington, DC: American Psychiatric Association, 1994.
19. Rezai AR, Rasmussen SA, Greenberg BD (eds): Surgery for Psychiatric Disorders. In Neurosurgery Clinics of North America 14(2):325, 2003.
20. Bridges PK, Bartlett JR, Hale AS, et al: Psychosurgery: Stereotactic subcaudate tractotomy: An indispensable treatment. Br J Psychiatry 165:599–611, 1994.
21. Mindus P, Rauch SL, Nyman H, et al: Capsulotomy and cingulotomy as treatments for malignant obsessive compulsive disorder: An update. In Zohar J, Marazzati D, Olivier B (eds): Current Insights in Obsessive Compulsive Disorder. Wiley, 1994, pp 245–276.
22. Nuttin B, Gybels J, Cosyns P, et al: The OCD-DBS Collaborative Group: Deep brain stimulation for psychiatric disorders [Letter]. Neurosurgery 51:519, 2002.
23. Hay P, Sachdev P: The present status of psychosurgery in Australia and New-Zealand. Med J Aust 157:17–19, 1992.
24. Knight GC: The orbital cortex as an objective in the surgical treatment of mental illness: The results of 450 cases of open operation and the development of the stereotactic approach. Br J Surg 2:114–124, 1964.
25. Scoville WB: Selective cortical undercutting as a means of modifying and studying frontal lobe function in man: Preliminary report on 43 operative cases. J Neurosurg 6:65–75, 1949.
26. Newcombe RL: Landmarks for lesions in the substantia innominata. In Hitchcock ER, Laitinen LV, Vaernet K (eds): Psychosurgery. Springfield, IL: Charles C Thomas, 1972, pp 289–290.
27. Le Gros Clark WE, Meyer M: Anatomical relationships between the cerebral cortex and the hypothalamus. Br Med Bull 6:341–344, 1950.
28. Glees P, Cole J, Whitty WM, et al: The effects of lesions in the cingular gyrus and adjacent areas in monkeys. J Neurol Neurosurg Psychiatry 13:178–190, 1950.
29. Le Gros Clark WE: The connexions of the frontal lobe of the brain. Lancet 1:353–356, 1948.
30. Knight GC: Further observations from an experience of 660 cases of stereotactic tractotomy. Postgrad Med J 49:845–854, 1973.
31. van Manen J, van Veelen CWM: Experiences in psycho-surgery in the Netherlands. Acta Neurochir Suppl 44:167–169, 1988.
32. Knight GC: Bifrontal stereotaxic tractotomy in the substantia innominata: An experience of 450 cases. In Hitchcock ER, Laitinen LV, Vaernet K (eds): Psychosurgery. Springfield, IL: Charles C Thomas, 1972, pp 267–277.
33. Crow HJ, Cooper R, Philips DG: Controlled multifocal frontal leucotomy for psychiatric illness. J Neurol Neurosurg Psychiatry 24:353–360, 1961.
34. Sachdev P, Hay P, Cumming S: Psychosurgical treatment of obsessive-compulsive disorder. Arch Gen Psychiatry 49:582–583, 1992.
35. Lovett L, Shaw D: Outcome in bipolar affective disorder after stereotactic tractotomy. Br J Psychiatry 151:113–116, 1987.
36. Cumming S, Hay P, Lee T, et al: Neuropsychological outcome from psychosurgery for obsessive-compulsive disorder. Aust N Z J Psychiatry 29:293–298, 1995.
37. Irle E, Exner C, Thielen K, et al: Obsessive-compulsive disorder and ventromedial frontal lesions: Clinical and neuropsychological findings. Am J Psychiatry 155:255–263, 1998.
38. Lippitz BE, Mindus P, Meyerson BA, et al: Lesion topography and outcome after thermocapsulotomy or gamma knife capsulotomy for obsessive compulsive disorder: Relevance of the right hemisphere. Neurosurgery 44:452–460, 1999.
39. Nuttin B, Cosyns P, Demeulemeester H, et al: Electrical stimulation in anterior limbs of internal capsules in patients with obsessive-compulsive disorder. Lancet 354:1526, 1999.
40. Gabriels L, Cosyns P, Nuttin B, et al: Deep brain stimulation for treatment-refractory obsessive-compulsive disorder: Psychopathological and neuropsychological outcome in three cases. Acta Psychiatr Scand 107:275–282, 2003.

41. Bejerot S: Psychosurgery for obsessive-compulsive disorder—Concerns remain. Acta Psychiatr Scand 107:241–243, 2003.

42. Anderson D, Ahmed A: Treatment of patients with intractable obsessive-compulsive disorder with anterior capsular stimulation. J Neurosurg 98:1104–1108, 2003.

43. Canterbury RJ: Deep brain stimulation for obsessive-compulsive disorder. J Neurosurg 98:941–942, 2003.

44. Rauch SL: Neuroimaging and neurocircuitry models pertaining to the neurosurgical treatment of psychiatric disorders. Neurosurg Clin N Am 14:213–223, 2003.

45. Greenberg BD, Murphy DL, Rasmussen SA: Neuroanatomically based approaches to obsessive-compulsive disorder, Neurosurgery and transcranial magnetic stimulation. Psychiatr Clin N Am 23:671–686, 2000.

46. Nuttin BJ, Gabriels LA, Cosyns PR, et al: Long-term electrical capsular stimulation in patients with obsessive-compulsive disorder. Neurosurgery 52:1263–1274, 2003.

47. Maes F, Collignon A, Vandermeulen D, et al: Multimodality image registration by maximization of mutual information. IEEE Trans Med Imaging 16:187–198, 1997.

48. Baxter LR: Brain imaging as a tool in establishing a theory of brain pathology in obsessive-compulsive disorder. J Clin Psychiatry 51(Suppl):22–26, 1990.

49. May JK, Assheuer J, Paxinos G: Atlas of the Human Brain, 2nd ed. Philadelphia: Elsevier, 2004.

50. Groenewegen HJ, Wright CI, Beijer AVJ: The nucleus accumbens: Gateway for limbic structures to reach the motor system? Prog Brain Res 107:485–511, 1996.

51. Zahn DS: An integrative neuroanatomical perspective on some subcortical substrates of adaptive responding with emphasis on the nucleus accumbens. Neurosci Biobehav Rev 24:85–105, 2000.

52. Greenberg BD, George MS, Martin JD, et al: Effect of prefrontal repetitive transcranial magnetic stimulation in obsessive disorder: A preliminary study. Am J Psychiatry 154:867–869, 1997.

53. Greenberg BD, Murphy DL, Rasmussen SA: Neuroanatomically based approaches to obsessive-compulsive disorder, neurosurgery and transcranial magnetic stimulation. Psychiatr Clin N Am 23:671–686, 2000.

54. Marangell LB, George MS, Callahan AM, et al: Effects of intrathecal thyrotropin-releasing hormone (Protirelin) in refractory depressed patients. Arch Gen Psychiatry 54:214–222, 1997.

55. van Kuyck K, Demeulemeester H, Feys H, et al: Effects of electrical stimulation or lesion in nucleus accumbens on the behaviour of rats in a T-maze after administration of 8-OH-DPAT or vehicle. Behav Brain Res 140:165–173, 2003.

56. Yadin E, Friedman E, Bridger WH: Spontaneous alternation behaviour: An animal model for obsessive-compulsive disorder. Pharmacol Biochem Behav 40:311–315, 1991.

57. Routtenberg A: "Self-starvation" of rats living in activity-wheels: Adaptation-effects. J Compr Physiol Psychol 66:234–238, 1968.

103 Cingulotomy for Intractable Psychiatric Illness

G. REES COSGROVE

The modern therapeutic approach to most psychiatric disease involves a combination of well-supervised psychotherapy, pharmacotherapy, and, in some instances, electroconvulsive therapy. Despite these treatment methods, many patients fail to respond adequately and remain severely disabled. In these patients, surgical intervention might be considered appropriate if the therapeutic result and overall level of functioning could be improved.

Psychosurgery was first proposed by the Portuguese neurologist Moniz[1]; his initial work involved alcohol injections into the white matter of the frontal lobes of institutionalized patients. This early experience first received cautious support in 1936 but was rapidly adopted, culminating in Moniz being awarded the Nobel Prize for Medicine in 1949. One of the most enthusiastic proponents of this new therapy was Freeman[2] in the United States, who championed prefrontal lobotomy first by bilateral coronal sectioning of the frontal lobes via burr holes and later by a transorbital approach. These early surgical techniques were crude and associated with major morbidity and mortality as high as 10%. Complications included severe cognitive impairment, personality changes, intracranial hemorrhage, and seizures.[3] The patients were believed to be "no longer distressed by their mental conflicts but also seem to have little capacity for any emotional experience." Standard intelligence quotient (IQ) tests revealed no significant postoperative deficits, and Freeman along with other practitioners of the day considered the side effects acceptable.

Surgery for intractable psychiatric illness became widely accepted and was used for a variety of diagnoses, including major affective disorders, obsessive-compulsive disease (OCD), and schizophrenia. Between the years 1942 and 1954, more than 10,000 cases in England and Wales and more than 18,000 cases in the United States were performed.[3] Despite or possibly because of such widespread and at times indiscriminate use, the field of psychosurgery has gone through cycles of acceptance and rejection that have always been emotionally charged.

In 1941, there was much controversy among neurologists, neurosurgeons, and psychiatrists with reservations regarding the scientific, ethical, and technical aspects of psychosurgery. This controversy drove efforts toward more rigorous clinical trials with a goal to reduce lesion size and direct lesions anatomically to specific brain regions. With the introduction of stereotactic techniques in 1947, methods for accurate lesioning of cortical and subcortical structures were available, and numerous target areas were identified. Fulton[4] was the first to suggest that the anterior cingulum would be an appropriate target for psychosurgical intervention, and cingulotomy was initially carried out as an open procedure.[5,6] Foltz and

White[7] reported their experience with stereotactic cingulotomy for intractable pain and noted the best results were in patients with concurrent anxiety-depressive states. Ballantine and colleagues[8] subsequently demonstrated the safety and effectiveness of cingulotomy in a large number of patients, and it has been the surgical procedure of choice in North America over the last 3 decades. In Europe, alternative targets were being used, and Knight[9] reported his experience with subcaudate tractotomy in 1964; Bingley and colleagues,[10] with anterior capsulotomy in 1972; and Kelley and colleagues,[11] with limbic leucotomy in 1973.

At the same time that surgical techniques became safer and lesion size became more discrete, psychotropic drugs were introduced that offered a safe alternative therapy and new hope. Chlorpromazine became available for use in the United States as an antipsychotic in 1954, and approval of major antidepressant medications soon followed. There was a sudden and dramatic decrease in the demand for surgical intervention.

Currently the accepted therapeutic approach to most psychiatric disease involves a combination of well-supervised psychotherapy, pharmacotherapy, and electroconvulsive therapy. Despite these modern treatment methods, many patients fail to respond adequately and remain severely disabled. In these patients, surgical intervention might still be considered appropriate if the therapeutic result and overall level of functioning could be improved. Although understanding of the anatomy and physiology has expanded and surgical ability to place discrete precise lesions with stereotactic techniques has evolved, the debate and controversy in this area continue.

ANATOMIC AND PHYSIOLOGIC BASIS FOR CINGULOTOMY

In 1937, Papez[12] published his paper entitled "A Proposed Mechanism of Emotion," in which he postulated that a reverberating circuit in the brain might be responsible for emotion, anxiety, and memory. The anatomic components of this circuit consisted of the hypothalamus, septal area, hippocampus, mammillary bodies, anterior thalamic nuclei, cingulate gyri, and their interconnections. This rudimentary limbic system was subsequently expanded to include paralimbic structures, including orbitofrontal, insular and anterior temporal cortices, the amygdala, and dorsomedial thalamic nuclei.[13] The hypothalamus, a central component in this system, controls autonomic function, and these functions in humans are often accompanied by subjective experiences and behavioral patterns. Stimulation of the hypothalamus in animals produces autonomic, endocrine, and complex motor effects, which supports the idea that the hypothalamus integrates and coordinates the behavioral expression of emotional states.[14,15] The neural outflow from the hypothalamus can be modulated by cortical and brain stem inputs, and the limbic system represents a direct conduit to the hypothalamus. Neocortical areas are connected to the limbic system proper by paralimbic structures.[16] The limbic system appears strategically situated to interconnect visceral and somatic stimuli with higher cortical functions and in this way may "add emotional coloring to the psychic process."[12]

Although the exact neuroanatomic and neurochemical basis of emotion in health and disease remains undefined, there is evidence that the limbic system and its interconnections with the basal ganglia and forebrain play a central role in the pathophysiology of psychiatric disorders. Electrical stimulation of specific areas within the limbic system (i.e., the anterior cingulum) has been shown in humans to alter autonomic responses and anxiety levels[17,18] and can cause movements in awake patients that resemble compulsive actions.[19] Neuroimaging studies also implicate a circuit composed of orbitofrontal cortex, striatum, thalamus, and anterior cingulate cortex in the pathophysiology of OCD. Abnormalities of glucose metabolism have been found in the caudate nucleus, orbitofrontal cortex, and cingulum in patients with OCD on positron emission tomography (PET).[20,21] Specialized PET images taken of patients during obsessive states reveal uniform hypermetabolism in the caudate nucleus, anterior cingulum, midfrontal cortex, and left thalamus, all structures connected with the limbic system.[22] Anatomic imaging with magnetic resonance imaging (MRI) has suggested focal abnormalities in these striatal areas[23] and smaller caudate nuclei in patients with OCD.[24] Similarly, PET studies have shown that reduced glucose metabolism in the lateral frontal cortex is a correlate of the depressive state in certain patients.[25]

The clinical observation that many patients with Sydenham's chorea and Tourette's syndrome have OCD and that 20% of patients with OCD have motor tics has prompted some authors to implicate a common pathophysiologic mechanism for movement disorders and OCD.[26] The frontal-striatal-pallidothalamic connections that have been well characterized for the control of motor function may explain some features of OCD. Modell and associates[27] postulate that this network has two components: an orbitofrontal-thalamic loop mediated by the excitatory neurotransmitter glutamate and an orbitofrontal-striatal-thalamic loop mediated by various transmitters, including glutamate, dopamine, serotonin, γ-aminobutyric acid, and glutamate. In this model, overactivity of the orbitofrontal-thalamic loop gives rise to obsessive-compulsive behavior.

Neurochemical models suggest that affective and anxiety disorders may be mediated via monoaminergic systems. In particular, the serotoninergic system has received emphasis with respect to OCD. Because of the diffuse nature of the monoaminergic projections and their role as neuromodulators, however, these models are not particularly instructive in terms of the functional neuroanatomy relevant to different neurosurgical treatments as they are currently used. Although the exact neuroanatomic and neurochemical mechanisms underlying depression, OCD, and other anxiety disorders remain unclear, it is intuitively appealing to believe that these psychiatric disorders might reflect a final common pathway of limbic dysregulation. Contemporary neurobiologic models of anxiety and affective disorders have also emphasized the fundamental role of the limbic system and its related structures.[27–29] In fact, all psychosurgical procedures have been directed at some component within this system, and some authors prefer the term limbic system surgery to psychosurgery.

PATIENT SELECTION

Only patients with severe, chronic, disabling, and treatment-refractory psychiatric illness should be considered for cingulotomy. The severity of the patient's illness must be manifest in terms of subjective distress and a decrement in psychosocial functioning. Chronicity refers to the enduring nature of the illness and in some cases may be less important than severity. The illness must also be refractory to systematic trials of pharmacologic, psychologic, and, when appropriate, electroconvulsive therapy before considering neurosurgical intervention.

Initially, cingulotomy was used for a variety of psychiatric diagnoses, and any patient with a severe psychiatric illness was once considered a candidate for surgical intervention. The indications for psychosurgery are now more restrictive. Currently the major psychiatric diagnostic groups as defined by the *Diagnostic and Statistical Manual, 3rd edition, revised* (DSM-III-R)[30] that might benefit from cingulotomy are: (1) chronic anxiety states, including OCD, and (2) major affective disorder (i.e., major depression or bipolar disorder). In many instances, patients present with mixed disorders combining symptoms of anxiety, depression, and OCD, and these patients remain candidates for surgery. Schizophrenia is not currently considered an indication for cingulotomy. A history of personality disorder, substance abuse, or other axis II symptoms is often a relative contraindication to surgery. Appropriate selection of patients for surgery is a major issue and remains the primary responsibility of the psychiatrist, guided by the informed and expert opinions of the other members of the psychosurgical team.

To determine that the psychiatric illness is refractory to treatment despite appropriate care, all patients must be referred by the treating psychiatrist. The referring psychiatrist must demonstrate an ongoing commitment to the patient and the evaluation process and must agree to be responsible for postoperative management. Detailed questionnaires that document the extent and severity of the illness as well as a thorough account of the diagnostic and therapeutic history must be provided by the psychiatrist. The specifics of pharmacologic trials should include the agents used, dose, duration, response, and reason for discontinuation for any suboptimal trial. Adequate trials of electroconvulsive therapy or behavioral therapy when clinically appropriate must also be demonstrated.

The patient and the family must agree to participate completely in the evaluation process as well as the postoperative psychiatric treatment program. In general, only adult patients (>18 years old) who are able to render informed consent and who express a genuine desire and commitment to proceed with cingulotomy are accepted.

If the patient meets the aforementioned criteria, at Massachusetts General Hospital, they then undergo a more detailed presurgical screening evaluation by a multidisciplinary Cingulotomy Assessment Committee consisting of three psychiatrists, two neurosurgeons, a neurologist, a nurse, and a secretary. Thorough review of the medical record is carried out to ensure that the illness is refractory to an exhaustive array of conventional therapies. The Massachusetts General Hospital evaluation also includes an electroencephalogram, brain MRI scan, neuropsychologic testing, and independently conducted clinical examinations by a psychiatrist, neurologist, and neurosurgeon in the outpatient setting. An electrocardiogram and appropriate blood tests are obtained to assess medical risks and to exclude organic causes for mental status abnormalities. Validated clinical research instruments are used to quantify psychiatric symptom severity, such as a Yale-Brown Obsessive Compulsive Scale (YBOCS) score of greater than 20 for OCD or a Beck Depression Inventory (BDI) score greater than 30 for affective disorders. Disability may be reflected by a Global Assessment of Function (GAF) score of less than 50.

There must be unanimous agreement that the patient satisfies selection criteria, that the surgery is indicated, and that the requirements for informed consent are fulfilled. A family member or close relative must also understand the evaluation process; understand the indications for, risks of, and alternatives to cingulotomy; and agree to be available to provide emotional support for the patient during the hospitalization.

SURGICAL TECHNIQUE

Cingulotomy was initially performed using ventriculography, but over the past several years this has been replaced by MRI-guided stereotactic techniques. This scanning allows for more accurate placement of the lesions and direct visualization of individual differences in cingulate and ventricular anatomy.

Stereotactic Frame Application

Beginning at midnight on the day before surgery, the patient is allowed nothing by mouth except for his or her usual medications. One hour before arrival in the operative suite, administration of droperidol (Inapsine) 5 mg intramuscularly and diazepam (Valium) 10 mg orally successfully sedates even the most anxious patient. On arrival in the operating room, a peripheral intravenous line is inserted, and additional intravenous sedation is administered as needed. An MRI-compatible Cosman-Roberts-Wells stereotactic head ring (Radionics, Inc., Burlington, MA) is applied to the patient's head after infiltration of the pin insertion sites with local anesthesia (1% lidocaine with 1:200,000 epinephrine). Pin sites are chosen so that the head ring lies well below the target plane. Placement of the frame is facilitated by use of an adjustable Velcro strap, which avoids the use of painful ear bars. The ring should be applied as symmetrically as possible, without rotation or tilt.

Target Acquisition

After attachment of an appropriate MRI-compatible stereotactic localizer, the entire assembly is secured to the MRI couch mount adaptor to keep the patient and stereotactic apparatus immobilized. First, a T1-weighted midsagittal MRI scan (TR 300 milliseconds; TE 17 milliseconds) is obtained as a reference to identify the cingulate gyri bilaterally, approximate the location of burr holes, and plan the electrode trajectory. Next, oblique coronal sections (4-mm thickness and 1-mm intervals) are obtained parallel to the proposed electrode trajectory, spanning the entire anterior cingulate gyri and the frontal horns of the lateral ventricles. Target coordinates are calculated for a point in the anterior cingulate gyrus 2 to 2.5 cm posterior to the tip of the frontal horn, 7 mm from the midline, and 1 to 2 mm above the roof of the lateral ventricle bilaterally (Fig. 103-1). Additional target points can be calculated 14 mm from the midline at the same vertical and anteroposterior positions, bilaterally to ensure that all of the cingulate bundle is interrupted. After successful target calculation, the patient is returned to the operating room.

Anesthesia and Patient Positioning

The patient's pulse, blood pressure, oxygen saturation, and electrocardiogram are continuously monitored so long as the patient is in the operating room. Although the procedure is performed under local anesthesia, the patient is heavily sedated to minimize patient discomfort and anxiety. Oxygen is administered by nasal cannula, but Foley catheterization and unnecessary external lines are avoided.

The patient is placed in a semireclining position on the operating table with the head positioned low enough to prevent air embolism. The stereotactic frame is then secured to the operating table using the Mayfield-Kees adaptor to ensure that the neck is in a neutral, comfortable position. The scalp is shaved in the frontal region along the coronal suture and scrubbed with soap solution and alcohol. The patient's head and stereotactic ring are then covered with a sterile plastic cover. No additional draping is generally necessary. Sterile basins are positioned for surgical instruments on the right and lesioning electrode on the left. A broad-spectrum antibiotic is administered intravenously before the skin incision is made.

Lesioning

After the Cosman-Roberts-Wells arc-ring assembly is placed over the patient's head and secured to the head ring, a limited bicoronal scalp incision is made after infiltration of local anesthesia (lidocaine 1% with 1:200,000 epinephrine). Burr holes are placed bilaterally just anterior to the coronal suture and 1.5 cm from the midline. A hand-held Hudson perforator is preferred over pneumatic-powered drills to minimize patient anxiety. After bipolar cauterization, the dura is opened, and an entrance point is chosen that avoids cortical vessels. A standard thermocoagulation electrode (Radionics, Inc., Burlington, MA) with a 10-mm uninsulated tip is inserted to the target coordinates and heated to 85°C for 90 seconds. After adequate cooling, the electrode is then withdrawn 10 mm, and a second lesion is made, using the same lesion parameters. This results in a lesion of approximately 2 cm in vertical height and 8 to 10 mm in diameter in the anterior cingulum (Fig. 103-2). To ensure complete interruption of the cingulate bundle at the target

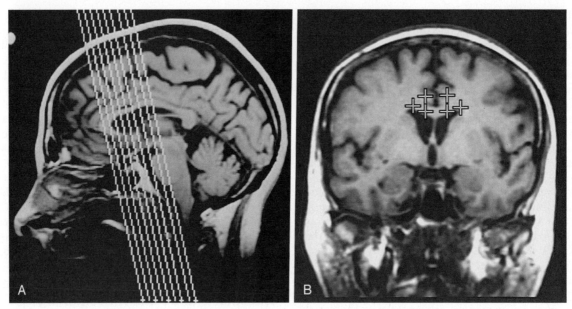

FIGURE 103-1 T1-weighted midsagittal stereotactic images demonstrating coronal oblique scans through the anterior cingulate region (*A*); coronal images approximately 2 to 2.5 cm posterior to the tip of the frontal horns of the lateral ventricles (*B*).

site, a third lesion can be placed more laterally over the roof of the lateral ventricle using the same lesioning technique. The procedure is then performed in an identical fashion on the opposite side. The burr holes are filled with Gelfoam sponge and bone dust, and the scalp incision is closed in layers. A sterile dressing is applied, and the stereotactic frame is removed with antibiotic cream applied to the pin sites in the scalp.

POSTOPERATIVE CARE

The patient is initially observed in the recovery room until fully awake then transferred to the neurosurgical ward.

Standard postoperative observation is carried out for the early detection and management of complications. A postoperative MRI scan is obtained to document lesion placement and to rule out perioperative complications. Mild oral analgesics are all that is generally required postoperatively. Occasionally the acute effects of cingulotomy in combination with high doses of psychotropic medication may cause mild drowsiness, but most patients are maintained on their preoperative drug regimen. Minor symptoms of headache, low-grade fever, and nausea are common after cingulotomy, as with all stereotactic procedures, but generally last less than 24 to 48 hours. Transient unsteady gait, dizziness, confusion, urinary retention,

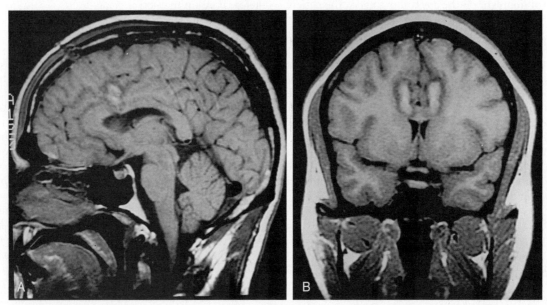

FIGURE 103-2 T1-weighted MRI scans of the cingulotomy lesions seen 24 hours postoperatively in the sagittal (*A*) and coronal (*B*) views.

and isolated seizures can occur but are generally mild and self-limited.

Psychiatric patients require careful, long-term psychiatric management to readjust their medications (often to lower doses) and proceed with other conventional therapies, such as psychotherapy and electroconvulsive therapy, which are often more effective postoperatively. Cingulotomy is not considered as curative but rather as an adjunct to optimal psychiatric treatment. The support of family members or close friends is essential to the successful management of postcingulotomy patients. They provide emotional support for the patient and can alert the psychiatrist to any abnormal behavior or symptoms postoperatively. About half of the patients require a repeat cingulotomy. Reoperation and enlargement of the cingulotomy lesion is considered if there has been no or unsatisfactory response to the initial cingulotomy after 3 to 6 months. Multiple cingulotomies can be performed safely after adequate time has elapsed between procedures (Fig. 103-3). Repeat lesions can be made anterior or posterior to the initial lesion but not more than 2.5 cm posterior to the tip of the frontal horn to avoid injury to the premotor area. Occasionally a third cingulotomy can be considered if the results of the initial two procedures were unsatisfactory or only temporary. In these situations, we generally recommend converting the cingulotomy to a limbic leucotomy.

SURGICAL RESULTS

Although many patients experience an immediate reduction in anxiety, there is generally a delay to the onset of beneficial effect on depression and obsessive-compulsive symptoms. This latency has been observed by many centers and may suggest that the beneficial effects are related not only to interruption of neural pathways but also to reorganization

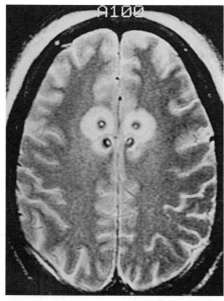

FIGURE 103-3 T2-weighted MRI scans of a patient who has undergone repeat cingulotomy demonstrating both the acute (<48 hours) and chronic (>6 months) lesions in the axial view. The acute lesion has significantly more perilesional edema and mass effect.

of neural pathways after injury. This latency may be as long as 6 to 12 weeks and must be clearly explained to the patient and referring psychiatrist. If there has been no response to the initial cingulotomy after 3 to 6 months, reoperation and enlargement of the cingulotomy lesion is considered.

The results of bilateral cingulotomy in 198 patients suffering from a variety of psychiatric disorders were reported retrospectively by Ballantine and colleagues in 1987 (see reference 8). This cohort came from a larger group of 696 cingulotomies in 465 patients, of whom 273 were operated on for psychiatric disease. Adequate follow-up data were available on 198 of 273 patients and included questionnaires, review of clinical records, and outpatient visits. The psychiatric diagnosis was reclassified retrospectively with newer DSM-III criteria, and a seven-point clinical rating scale of outcome was used. This scale defined postoperative results as follows: 5, normal and on no treatment; 4, functionally normal but requiring medication or psychotherapy; 3, much improved; 2, slight improvement; 1, no change; 0, worse; or S, suicide. Any patient with a postoperative result of 3 (much improved) or better was considered a successful outcome. The outcome was rated by the referring clinicians and is open to rater bias but still has some validity. With a mean follow-up of 8.6 years, 64% of patients with severe affective disorder and 56% of patients with OCD were found to have experienced worthwhile improvement. In 14 patients suffering from nonobsessive anxiety disorders, 79% were found to be functionally normal or have shown marked improvement. Overall, 62% of all patients operated on had a successful outcome. No improvement or patients being worse after surgery was observed in 12%, but most of these cases were in the schizophrenic, personality disorders, or miscellaneous diagnostic categories. Most of the depressed patients (83%) were suicidal, and 9% of patients committed suicide during the follow-up period. This annual suicide rate postcingulotomy of 1%, however, is less than the expected average annual suicide rate for severely depressed patients.[31] Using the identical outcome measures employed by Ballantine,[8] a more modern retrospective study of MRI-guided stereotactic cingulotomy yielded similar success rates underscoring the positive bias that occurs with subjective outcome rating scales.[32] Patients with affective disorders seem to respond better than those with OCD, and approximately 40% of patients require more than one procedure.

A more detailed retrospective study evaluating cingulotomy in 33 patients with refractory OCD using unbiased observers has also been reported. Outcome was rated using validated research tools, including the Massachusetts General Hospital Visual Analog Assessment scale, Maudsley Obsessional Compulsive Inventory, YBOCS, Clinical Global Improvement (CGI), and BDI by unbiased observers. This study demonstrated that, using strict criteria for defining a successful outcome, at least 25% to 30% of patients benefited substantially from cingulotomy.[33]

A prospective long-term follow-up study of 18 patients who underwent cingulotomy for intractable OCD has also been completed.[34] Preoperative evaluation included Structured Clinical Interview for DSM-III-R Diagnosis (SCID) for Axis I disorders and the Structured Interview for Diagnosis of Personality Disorders-Revised (SIDP-R) for Axis II disorders. Administration of a YBOCS, YBOCS symptoms checklist, CGI, and BDI were undertaken before surgery by unbiased observers in all patients. Follow-up evaluation was carried out every 6 months by personal or telephone interview with administration of a YBOCS, Massachusetts General Hospital Visual Analog Assessment scale, CGI, BDI, Sickness Impact Profile (SIP), and SAFTEE, a tool used in psychopharmacologic medication studies that identifies side effects and adverse outcome. A successful outcome (responder) was acknowledged only if the patient had a greater than 35% improvement on YBOCS and a CGI of 1 or 2. Patients who had a greater than 35% improvement on YBOCS or a CGI of 1 or 2 were considered possible responders. Five patients (28%) met these conservative criteria as treatment responders, and two others (11%) were considered possible responders. Overall the entire group improved significantly in terms of functional status, and no significant adverse effects were encountered. The value of this study is that it is the first to demonstrate in a prospective manner that cingulotomy is effective as measured by standard psychiatric rating scales and unbiased independent observers. No significant adverse effects were encountered.

Although cingulotomy appears effective in a proportion of severely affected patients, it must also be proven to be a safe procedure with minimal morbidity and few side effects. In more than 800 cingulotomies performed at the Massachusetts General Hospital since 1962, there have been no deaths and no infections. Two acute subdural hematomas occurred early on in the series secondary to laceration of a cortical artery at the time of introduction of ventricular needles, but only one patient suffered permanent neurologic impairment.[35] Early postoperative seizures have been seen in 1% of patients and are generally easily controlled with anticonvulsant medication. Headache and mild temperature elevation postoperatively are common, and temporary urinary dysfunction can occur occasionally.

An independent analysis of 34 patients who underwent cingulotomy demonstrated no significant behavioral or intellectual deficits as a result of the cingulate lesions themselves.[36] The only clear-cut neurologic deficit demonstrated was a deterioration of performance on the Taylor Complex Figure Test in patients older than 40 years of age. A comparison of preoperative and postoperative Wechsler IQ scores demonstrated significant gains postoperatively. This improvement was greatest in patients with chronic pain and depression but negligible in those with the diagnosis of schizophrenia.

DISCUSSION

Cingulotomy, capsulotomy, subcaudate tractotomy, and limbic leucotomy are the most common psychosurgical procedures performed today, but with currently available data it is impossible to determine whether there is one optimal surgical technique or strategy. Many obstacles prevent a direct comparison of results across centers. These obstacles include diagnostic inaccuracies, nonstandardized presurgical evaluation tools, center bias, and varied outcome assessment scales. In virtually all published reports, however, some modification of the Pippard Postoperative Rating Scale[37] or

equivalent has been used to determine clinical outcome. The Pippard Scale rates outcome in five categories:

A. Symptom-free
B. Much improved, some symptoms remaining but no additional treatment necessary
C. Slightly improved
D. Unchanged
E. Worse

If categories A and B are considered satisfactory outcomes, in patients with OCD, subcaudate tractotomy was effective in 50%, cingulotomy in 56%, limbic leucotomy in 61%, and capsulotomy in 67%. In patients with major affective disorder, subcaudate tractotomy was effective in 68%, cingulotomy in 65%, limbic leucotomy in 78%, and capsulotomy in 55%.

Kullberg[38] attempted to compare cingulotomy and capsulotomy in the treatment of 26 patients in a randomized fashion. Six of 13 capsulotomy patients and 3 of 13 cingulotomy patients were better, but transient deterioration in mental status was much more marked after capsulotomy than after cingulotomy. Fodstad and co-workers[39] reported a similar experience but studied only four patients in total. Two prospective studies were compared in an attempt to evaluate the efficacy of cingulotomy and capsulotomy in OCD.[40] Using the best available research methods and well-accepted rating scales of disease and outcome, exhaustive preoperative and postoperative evaluations were carried out. Of the capsulotomy patients, 45% had clear-cut improvement, and in cingulotomy patients, 39% were improved. Side effects from the procedure were more evident after capsulotomy.

Based on these methods of comparison, the clinical superiority of any one procedure is not convincing, even though many centers claim advantages for their specific surgical intervention. No matter which structure in the limbic system is chosen for ablation, the clinical outcome appears similar. All procedures seem to be well tolerated with minimal side effects or complications when applied with the modern stereotactic techniques. Cingulotomy is the treatment of choice in the United States, whereas in Europe, capsulotomy and limbic leucotomy are more prevalent. All procedures appear roughly equivalent from a therapeutic standpoint, but in terms of unwanted side effects, cingulotomy appears to be the safest of all procedures currently performed.

Regardless of the choice of procedure, surgical failures should be investigated, and if the lesion size or location is suboptimal, consideration should be given to a repeat procedure. In 5 of the 24 patients in the series by Mindus and Nyman,[41] a significant correlation was found between neuroradiologic ranking of a target site and the psychiatric outcome, suggesting that the site and extent of lesion may be important influences on outcome. Repeat surgery in capsulotomy patients has been reported as high as 20%.[38] At least 45% of patients undergoing cingulotomy require repeat operation, with good results being salvaged in half.[32,34] The exact size or volume of tissue required for an effective outcome at each of the target sites has yet to be determined.

Although controversy exists regarding the exact choice of surgical procedure, there is unanimous agreement that the presurgical evaluation should be performed by committed multidisciplinary teams with expertise and experience in the surgical treatment of psychiatric illness. Accurate diagnosis based on the DSM-III-R classification scheme is encouraged, and prospective trials using standardized clinical instruments with long-term follow-up are needed. Comparisons of preoperative and postoperative functional status in addition to target psychiatric symptoms remain important parameters in characterizing outcome. All centers with experience emphasize the importance of rehabilitation postoperatively and the need for ongoing psychiatric follow-up. The operation is not a panacea and should be considered as only one aspect in the overall management of these patients.

Psychosurgery in the past has unquestionably been misapplied and remains controversial even today. The interpretation of data in the field of psychosurgery remains a target for personal, professional, and ethical bias. Responsible centers that continued to perform surgery of this nature after its decline reported success rates of 60% to 70%. Today, many of these same centers using more rigorous measures of outcome report success rates of 30% to 40%. This kind of success rate is hardly dramatic, but if an experimental add-on pharmacotherapeutic agent was introduced that produced a 30% to 40% response rate in a group of treatment-refractory OCD or depression patients, it would be embraced as a wonderful new therapy. The patients undergoing surgery for psychiatric indications are desperately ill, and their lives are severely impaired. Under these circumstances, it may be acceptable to offer surgery in the hopes of salvaging a life, even if the intervention might risk subtle neuropsychologic or personality changes.

CONCLUSIONS

Cingulotomy can be helpful in certain patients with severe, disabling, and treatment-refractory psychiatric disease, including major affective disorders, OCD, and chronic anxiety states. It should be performed only by an expert multidisciplinary team with experience in these disorders. Cingulotomy should be considered as one part of an entire treatment plan and must be followed by an appropriate psychiatric rehabilitation program. Many patients are greatly improved after surgery, and the complications and side effects are few. Cingulotomy remains an important therapeutic option for disabling psychiatric disease and is probably underused.

REFERENCES

1. Moniz E: Prefrontal leucotomy in the treatment of mental disorders. Am J Psychiatry 93:1379–1385, 1937.
2. Freeman W, Watts JW: Psychosurgery: Intelligence, Emotion and Social Behavior following Prefrontal Lobotomy for Mental Disorders. Springfield, IL: Charles C Thomas, 1942.
3. Tooth JC, Newton MP: Leucotomy in England and Wales 1942–1954: Reports on Public Health and Medical Subjects No. 104. London: Her Majesty's Stationary Office, 1961.
4. Fulton JE: Frontal Lobotomy and Affective Behavior: A Neurophysiological Analysis. New York: WW Norton, 1951.
5. Le Beau J: Anterior cingulectomy in man. J Neurosurg 11:268–276, 1954.
6. Whitty CWM, Duffield JE, Tow PM, et al: Anterior cingulectomy in the treatment of mental disease. Lancet 1:475–481, 1952.
7. Foltz EL, White LE Jr: Pain relief by frontal cingulotomy. J Neurosurg 19:89–94, 1962.
8. Ballantine HT, Bouckoms AJ, Thomas EK, et al: Treatment of psychiatric illness by stereotactic cingulotomy. Biol Psychiatry 22:807–819, 1987.
9. Knight GC: The orbital cortex as an objective in the surgical treatment of mental illness: The development of the stereotactic approach. Br J Surg 51:114–124, 1964.
10. Bingley T, Leksell L, Meyerson B, Rylander G: Long term results of stereotactic anterior capsulotomy in chronic obsessive-compulsive neurosis. In Sweet, WH (ed): Neurosurgical Treatment in Psychiatry, Pain and Epilepsy. Baltimore: University Park Press, 1977, pp 287–299.
11. Kelley D, Richardson A, Mitchell-Heggs N: Stereotactic limbic leucotomy: Neurophysiologic aspects and operator technique. Br J Psychiatry 123:133–140, 1973.
12. Papez JW: A proposed mechanism of emotion. Arch Neurol Psychiatry 38:725–743, 1937.
13. McLean PD: Some psychiatric implications of physiologic studies on the frontotemporal portion of limbic system. Electroencephalogr Clin Neurophysiol 4:407–418, 1952.
14. Ranson SW: The hypothalamus: Its significance for visceral innervation and emotional expression. Trans Coll Physicians Phila [Series IV] 2:222–242, 1934.
15. Hess WR: Diencephalon: Autonomic and Extrapyramidal Functions. New York: Grune & Stratton, 1954.
16. Mesulam M-M: Patterns in behavioral neuroanatomy: Association areas, the limbic system, and hemispheric specialization. In Mesulam M-M (ed): Principles of Behavioral Neurology. Philadelphia: FA Davis, 1985, pp 1–70.
17. Kelley D: The limbic system, sex and emotions. In Anxiety and Emotions: Physiological Basis and Treatment. Springfield, IL: Charles C Thomas, 1980, pp 197–300.
18. Laitinen LV: Emotional responses to subcortical electrical stimulation in psychiatric patients. Clin Neurol Neurosurg 81:148–157, 1979.
19. Talairach J, Bancaud J, Geier S: The cingulate gyrus and human behaviour. Electroencephalogr Clin Neurophysiol 34:45–52, 1973.
20. Baxter LR, Jr, Schwartz JM, Bergman KS, et al: Caudate glucose metabolic rate changes with both drug and behavior therapy for obsessive compulsive disorder. Arch Gen Psychiatry 49:681–689, 1992.
21. Rauch SL, Jenike MA: Neurobiological models of obsessive compulsive disorder. Psychosomatics 34:20–32, 1993.
22. Rauch SL, Jenike MA, Alpert NM, et al: Regional cerebral blood flow measured during symptom provocation in obsessive-compulsive disorder using ^{15}O-labelled CO_2 and positron emission tomography. Arch Gen Psychiatry 51:62–70, 1994.
23. Weilburg JB, Mesulam MM, Weintraub S, et al: Focal striatal abnormalities in a patient with obsessive compulsive disorder. Arch Neurol 46:233–236, 1989.
24. Luxenberg JS, Swedo SE, Flament MF, et al: Neuroanatomical abnormalities in obsessive compulsive disorder detected with a quantitative x-ray computed tomography. Am J Psychiatry 145:1089–1093, 1988.
25. Baxter LR, Schwartz JM, Phelps ME, et al: Reduction of prefrontal glucose metabolism common to three types of depression. Arch Gen Psychiatry 46:243–250, 1989.
26. Green RC, Pitman RK: Tourette syndrome and obsessive-compulsive disorder. In Jenike MA, Baer L, Minichiello WE (eds): Obsessive-Compulsive Disorders: Theory and Management. Littleton, MA: PSG Publishing, 1986, pp 147–164.
27. Modell J, Mountz J, Curtis G, et al: Neurophysiologic dysfunction in basal ganglia/limbic striatal and thalamocortical circuits as a pathogenetic mechanism of obsessive compulsive disorder. J Neuropsychiatry 1:27–36, 1989.
28. Gorman JM, Lieboritz MR, Fyer AJ, et al: A neuroanatomical hypothesis for panic disorder. Am J Psychiatry 146:148–161, 1989.
29. Nauta WJN: Connections of the frontal lobe with the limbic system. In Laitinen LV, Livingston KE (eds): Surgical Approaches in Psychiatry, Proceedings of the 3rd International Congress of Psychosurgery. Cambridge, England: Medical and Technical Publishing, 1973, pp 303–314.
30. American Psychiatric Association: Diagnostic and Statistical Manual of Mental Disorders, 3rd ed, revised. Washington, DC: American Psychiatric Association, 1987.
31. Pokorney AD: Prediction of suicide in psychiatric patients. Arch Gen Psychiatry 40:249–257, 1983.
32. Spangler W, Cosgrove GR, Ballantine HT, et al: MR-guided stereotactic cingulotomy for intractable psychiatric disease. Neurosurgery 38:1071–1078, 1996.
33. Jenike MA, Baer L, Ballantine HT, et al: Cingulotomy for refractory obsessive compulsive disorder: A long term follow-up of 33 patients. Arch Gen Psychiatry 48:548–555, 1991.

34. Baer L, Rauch SL, Ballantine HT, et al: Cingulotomy for intractable obsessive-compulsive disorder: A prospective long-term follow-up of 18 patients. Arch Gen Psychiatry 52:384–392, 1995.

35. Ballantine HT, Giriunas IE: Treatment of intractable psychiatric illness and chronic pain by stereotactic cingulotomy. In Schmidek HH, Sweet WH (eds): Operative Neurosurgical Techniques, vol 2, 1st ed. New York: Grune & Stratton, 1982, pp 1069–1075.

36. Corkin S, Twitchell TE, Sullivan EV: Safety and efficacy of cingulotomy for pain and psychiatric disorders. In Hitchcock ER, Ballantine HT, Myerson BA (eds): Modern Concepts in Psychiatric Surgery. Amsterdam: Elsevier, 1979, pp 253–272.

37. Pippard J: Rostral leucotomy: A report on 240 cases personally followed up after one and one half to five years. J Ment Sci 101:756–773, 1955.

38. Kullberg G: Differences in effect of capsulotomy and cingulotomy. In Sweet WH, Obrador S, Martin-Rodriguez JG (eds): Neurosurgical Treatment in Psychiatry, Pain and Epilepsy. Baltimore: University Park Press, 1977, pp 301–308.

39. Fodstad H, Strandman E, Karlsson B, et al: Treatment of obsessive compulsive states with stereotactic anterior capsulotomy or cingulotomy. Acta Neurochir (Wien) 62:1–23, 1982.

40. Mindus P, Rasmussen SA, Lindquist C: Neurosurgical treatment of obsessive-compulsive disorder: Implications of understanding frontal lobe function. J Neuropsychiatry Clin Neurosci 6:467–477, 1994.

41. Mindus P, Nyman H: Normalization of personality characteristics in patients with incapacitating anxiety disorders after capsulotomy. Acta Psychiatr Scand 83:283–291, 1991.

104 Microvascular Decompression Surgery for Hemifacial Spasm

ANTHONY M. KAUFMANN and MARSHALL F. WILKINSON

Hemifacial spasm (HFS) is a cranial nerve rhizopathy caused by vascular compression on the proximal facial nerve root. While the condition is not painful or life threatening, its physical, psychological, and social consequences can be significantly disabling. When the diagnosis is recognized, patients usually request treatment, and may choose between repeated botulinum toxin (Botox) injections or potentially curative surgery. The microvascular decompression (MVD) procedure is often the preferred choice, provided it can be performed with a high rate of success and minimal complication risk.

CLINICAL CHARACTERISTICS

HFS is a syndrome of unilateral involuntary twitching and contractions of facial muscles. The prevalence is approximately 10 per 100,000 population, with a 2:1 female predominance.[1] The mean age of onset is 45 to 55 years, with rare occurrences in childhood or infancy.[2,3] There are few reports of bilateral (asynchronous)[4] or familial[5,6] HFS. Typically the disease begins with relatively minor and intermittent twitching of the upper and/or lower eyelids. The spasms then progress in frequency, severity, and extent. There is usually sequential advance from the orbicularis oculi to buccal, orbicularis oris, mentalis, and platysma muscles. The frontalis muscle is rarely involved. A small subset of patients with HFS have spasms that begin in the lower face, with subsequent rostral progression, referred to as atypical hemifacial spasm.[7] In advanced or severe HFS, spasms of the orbicularis oculi muscles may lead to forceful eye closure (Fig. 104-1). Patients may also experience sustained contractions of the affected facial muscles, tonus phenomenon, lasting seconds or minutes. While the rate of progression is variable, severe pan-hemifacial involvement develops over an average of 8 years. Spontaneous disease cure is exceptionally rare.

Few patients experience remissions of HFS, and only at the mild and early stages of the disease. Spasms usually occur frequently or continuously throughout the day, and diminish or disappear during sleep. Spasms occur spontaneously, but are often induced by voluntary facial movements, talking, smiling, laughing, or crying. Stress, anxiety, self-consciousness, and fatigue are also common aggravating factors. A positional component is sometimes described, such that the spasms may increase or decrease with certain head positions. Alleviating factors are rare, although some patients may temporarily diminish spasms with an effort to relax the face. Between episodes of visible spasms, patients may describe an underlying sensation of facial tightening,

tension, or fine movements. Some also experience low-pitched tinnitus or clicks, heard in the ipsilateral ear. These auditory symptoms are likely related to abnormal activity of the stapedius muscle, innervated by the facial nerve.[8] There are, however, no alterations of taste (chorda tympany) or autonomic symptoms of tearing or nasal discharge such as may be seen in migrainous neuralgia (cluster headache). A small subgroup of patients with HFS have concurrent trigeminal neuralgia. Cushing coined the term *painful tic convulsif* to describe this double cranial nerve hyperactivity disorder[9] that may be caused by neurovascular compression of both the trigeminal and facial nerves.[10,11] Others have used the same term to describe the combination of HFS and geniculate neuralgia, also relieved with MVD of the facial nerve (including nervus intermedius).[12] A rare combination of trigeminal neuralgia, HFS, and glossopharyngeal neuralgia has also been described and similarly treated.[13,14]

The diagnosis of HFS is established on the basis of appropriate history, observation of characteristic involuntary involvement of ipsilateral muscles of facial expression, and absence of confounding neurologic complaints or deficits.

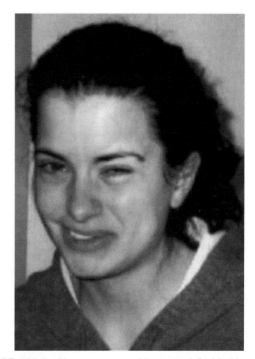

FIGURE 104-1 Young woman with severe left-sided hemifacial spasm.

A careful neurologic examination, however, may uncover at least a subtle weakness of ipsilateral facial muscles, especially in patients with advanced or severe HFS. Testing of facial strength often induces spasms or tonus phenomenon, and provides an opportunity to observe the extent and severity of muscle involvement. Other disorders of unilateral abnormal facial movements are usually clearly discernible from HFS. These include synkinesis seen following facial nerve injury recovery, myokymia related to central disorders such as multiple sclerosis and brain stem gliomas, habit tic, and focal seizures. We have rarely found it necessary to employ electrophysiologic investigations to establish or confirm the diagnosis of HFS. If examined, a needle electrode electromyogram (EMG) will demonstrate prominent paroxysmal discharges (20 to 400/second) in the affected muscles, and sometimes short bursts of activity between symptomatic spasms.[15] The blink reflex may demonstrate abnormal spread into other facial muscles on the ipsilateral side.[16–19] The characteristic abnormal motor response or "lateral spread" can also be evaluated in conscious patients using surface electrodes, but is more effectively utilized as an intraoperative monitoring technique, as described below.

Routine use of diagnostic imaging studies is also not necessary to establish or confirm the diagnosis of HFS. While the culprit neurovascular compression can sometimes be visualized on standard computed tomographic (CT) scans or magnetic resonance images (MRIs), a "negative" report does not invalidate the diagnosis or etiologic cause (Fig. 104-2). Some specialized MRI sequences can identify the vessel contact on the facial root exit zone with a reasonably high degree of sensitivity and specificity.[17,20–27] The culprit vessel, however, may be a small artery or even a vein, not visible with any diagnostic imaging techniques. Therefore, we do not use preoperative imaging to screen patients for surgical eligibility, but rather to rule out concurrent pathology (e.g., tumors) that may rarely be encountered in patients with HFS.[28–34]

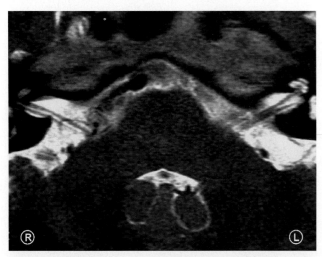

FIGURE 104-2   Magnetic resonance image prior to microvascular decompression (MVD) for left-sided hemifacial spasm (HFS) disclosed prominent neurovascular compression only on the contralateral asymptomatic side. This patient developed contralateral HFS 2 years later, indicating a potential period of latency between the occurrence of neurovascular compression and the development of HFS. MVD operations successfully alleviated HFS on both sides.

ETIOLOGY

HFS is a cranial nerve hyperactivity disorder analogous to trigeminal neuralgia and glossopharyngeal neuralgia, caused by pulsatile neurovascular contact on the root exit/entry zone.[35] This concept has evolved since the first observations made by Dandy in the 1920s and 1930s during posterior fossa operations he pioneered for the partial sectioning of trigeminal nerve root for the treatment of trigeminal neuralgia.[36] Without the aid of a microscope for magnification or illumination, he found neurovascular compression in 45% of 215 cases and postulated this to be the cause of trigeminal neuralgia.[37] Although he did not extrapolate these observations to HFS, Dandy stated, "In many instances the nerve is grooved or bent by the artery. This I believe is the cause of *tic douloureux*."[38]

Others had also suggested that vascular compression may be a cause of HFS.[39,40] In the 1950s, Gardner recognized vascular compression in the region of the trigeminal nerve root entry zone in patients with trigeminal neuralgia,[41,42] and vascular contact on the distal facial nerve root in a patient with HFS treated with intentional nerve injury.[43] In 1962, Gardner and Sava reported a series of 19 patients with HFS who underwent similar surgery.[44] In seven patients they found a close relationship between the facial nerve and the anterior inferior cerebellar artery that was separated with placement of a Gelfoam sponge. While they noted the common association between such normal vessels and the distal facial nerve root, they did not make reference to vascular contacts in the region of the facial root exit zone.

The current concept of neurovascular compression as a cause of trigeminal neuralgia, HFS, and glossopharyngeal neuralgia stems from pioneering work by Jannetta. He and Rand developed a transtentorial retrogasserian rhizotomy technique for the treatment of trigeminal neuralgia, introducing the use of an operating microscope for this purpose.[45] In five consecutive operations, they found branches of the superior cerebellar artery compressing the trigeminal nerve root. Jannetta also noted no similar compression in 56 cadaver dissections or during suboccipital craniectomies for other indications. He postulated the etiology of trigeminal neuralgia to be pulsatile neurovascular compression on the proximal portion of the nerve root, where central myelin extends several millimeters beyond the brain stem origin before transitioning to peripheral myelin at the Obersteiner-Redlich zone. Regarding the role for MVD surgery, Jannetta wrote in 1967, "This possibly definitive procedure, namely, release of the artery without nerve section, is planned in a future series of patients."[46]

However, prior to performing any MVD for trigeminal neuralgia, Jannetta extrapolated this neurovascular compression hypothesis to HFS, after appreciating the analogous features of both diseases. The first microvascular decompression surgery was performed in 1966, for a patient with HFS. A prominent pontomedullary vein compressing the facial root exit zone was the culprit. This was coagulated and divided, and the patient has remained spasm free for more than 30 years.[35] In 1970, Jannetta published a series of seven MVD operations for HFS, where he had found neurovascular compression on the nerve root exit zone in all cases.[47] Similar findings, and high rate of disease cure, were reported in subsequent larger series[48–50] and by other surgeons who adopted MVD surgery as a treatment for HFS.[51]

NEUROPHYSIOLOGY

In a paper titled "Concerning the Mechanism of Trigeminal Neuralgia and Hemifacial Spasm" Gardner postulated, "Both are expressions of an unstable and reversible pathophysiologic state caused by a mild compression of the nerve root which permits transaxonal excitation while not interfering with axonal conduction."[52] This hypothesis implicating a peripheral mechanism of ephaptic transmission was widely accepted and expanded on, as summarized by Wilkins,[53] and continues to have advocates.[19,54-56] However, Ferguson was the first to note that such "cross-talk" between facial nerve axons was not sufficient to explain the symptoms and signs of HFS.[57] It now appears that a central pathophysiological mechanism exists, involving an induced and potentially reversible hyperexcitability within the facial motor nucleus. This likely develops in response to aberrant or altered neural input, generated by the pulsatile vascular compression upon the facial nerve root that is invariably found in HFS.[58] Neurophysiologic evidence for this concept includes studies of the abnormal muscle response in HFS known as lateral spread, as well as F waves and facial motor-evoked potentials.

Lateral spread is produced by electrical stimulation of one branch of the facial nerve, resulting in EMG response in facial musculature innervated by different nerve branches.[59] When one facial branch is stimulated (e.g., temporal), the passive cable properties of axons propagate the stimulus pulse in two directions: (1) orthodromically, resulting in the normal muscle stimulation (i.e., frontalis), and (2) antidromically, toward the central nervous system. In HFS, this antidromic stimulus pulse is "redirected" at some point along the nerve, and produces an orthodromic pulse in neighboring facial nerve axons that stimulate other facial muscles (e.g., mentalis). The transmission times involved in the lateral spread response can be determined with intraoperative recordings, and indicate that the antidromic impulses are redirected within the central nervous system (Fig. 104-3). If a peripheral mechanism or ephaptic signaling were responsible, then the latency for the lateral spread response should equal the sum of:

1. The latency of a stimulus pulse delivered to facial nerve branch and recorded at the site of vascular compression; and
2. The latency from direct facial root stimulation at the site of vascular compression and the resulting muscle depolarization.

However, the sum of these latencies consistently falls short of the actual lateral spread latency by approximately 2 msec,[58-60] a finding we have corroborated during surgery for HFS. The additional 2 msec likely represents the signal transmission times of central projections and processing within the facial motor nucleus, and argues in favor of a potentially reversible central pathophysiology.[61] Successful alleviation of the culprit neurovascular compression typically results in prompt reduction or elimination of the lateral spread response, and is a strong predicator of HFS cure.[58,61-65]

An additional line of inquiry utilizing F-wave analysis provides further evidence of hyperexcitability of the facial motor neuron pool in HFS. An F wave is produced when a motor axon is stimulated at supramaximal intensity.

The orthodromic stimulus pulse results in muscle depolarization (M wave). The antidromic stimulus pulse travels to the motor neuron cell bodies in the central nervous system. In conditions of abnormal excitability, this strong depolarizing pulse will then redepolarize the axon hillock, resulting in a weak orthodromic wave along the same axon, back to the muscle producing the F wave.[66] Ishikawa and colleagues have shown that F waves are exaggerated in patients with HFS and are alleviated concurrently with the disappearance of lateral spread following MVD.[67-69]

Recently, we have introduced facial motor-evoked potentials (fMEPs) as another neurophysiologic technique to study HFS during MVD surgery. In a series of eight consecutive patients, we found that the fMEPs on the spasm side were of larger amplitude and duration when compared with the nonspasm side or with patient controls with trigeminal neuralgia. Others have made similar observations.[70,71] But perhaps more interesting were the dynamic changes in the fMEPs we found during MVD. The "exaggerated" fMEPs reverted to normal levels similar to the nonspasm side concurrently with the elimination of the lateral spread responses (Fig. 104-4). These fMEP observations are consistent with the hypothesis that the facial motor neuron pool is hyperexcitable prior to decompression of the nerve. Furthermore, the vascular compression of the nerve root provides a triggering signal for plastic changes within the facial nucleus. Removal of the peripheral pulsatile irritation results in a correction of the central pathophysiology, with subsequent reduction and cure of HFS.

MANAGEMENT OPTIONS

HFS can be disabling and many patients report troubling physical, social, and psychological consequences of the disease. Spasms of the eyelid are distracting, and contractions of the orbicularis oculi lead to eye closure that interferes with binocular vision. The intermittent or continuous facial distortions are potentially embarrassing, and are aggravated by speaking, anxiety, and the stress caused by self-consciousness. It is therefore not surprising that many sufferers attempt to avoid or minimize social situations. This may lead to dramatic lifestyle changes to careers and relationships. It is also clear that that not all sufferers are equally affected by similar degrees of disease severity. We administered two standardized evaluations of social anxiety symptoms to 97 nonselected patients with HFS, 85% of whom were receiving serial Botox injections. There was a wide range of scores on both the Social Interaction Anxiety Scale (SIAS) and Social Phobia Scale (SPS).[72] The 48 patients who elected to undergo MVD surgery had significantly higher levels of distress and social anxiety. As one would expect, the SAIS and SPS scores normalized after successful surgery and HFS cure (Fig. 104-5). Management decisions, therefore, must be made by patients based on their own personal experience of disease significance and a reasonable appraisal of the treatment options.

Medical treatment of HFS can be offered, although rarely provides satisfactory alleviation of spasms. Small series with short durations of follow-up have reported modest benefit with carbamazepine, baclofen, clonazepam, orphenadrine, or gabapenfin.[73-78] Early surgical treatments

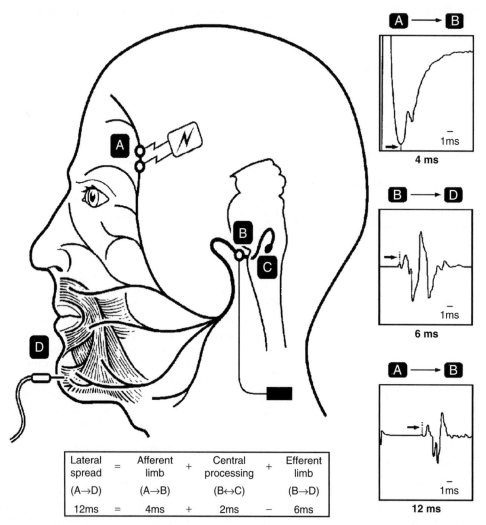

Lateral spread	=	Afferent limb	+	Central processing	+	Efferent limb
(A→D)		(A→B)		(B↔C)		(B→D)
12ms	=	4ms	+	2ms	−	6ms

FIGURE 104-3 Neurophysiology of hemifacial spasm. The lateral spread response is evoked by electrical stimulation of the temporal branch of the facial nerve at A and is recorded as an electromyographic response of the mentalis muscle at D. The latency of this response can be partitioned into three components: A→B, an antidromic signal elicited from the stimulation site of the facial nerve branch and recorded at the site of neurovascular compression on the facial root exit zone (REZ); B↔C, central projections between the REZ and putatively hyperactive/hyperexcitable facial nucleus that have not been directly measured; and B→D, the orthodromic transmission from direct stimulation of the REZ and recorded as an electromyographic response at the mentalis muscle. The box inserts show intraoperative recordings of these responses and their measured latencies. The summation equation demonstrates that the lateral spread response is composed of the postulated three components and provides evidence of a central pathophysiology in hemifacial spasm.

were directed at denervation of the affected facial musculature, by injury of the facial nerve root, trunk, or peripheral branches.[53] While even relatively light injury or nerve manipulation may provide immediate relief, the predictable consequence is some degree of facial weakness. Analogous to rhizotomy for trigeminal neuralgia, the more severe or permanent the facial nerve injury, the more effective and long lasting the reduction of HFS, but at the expense of a greater degree of facial paresis. Furthermore, the abnormal involuntary facial movements usually recur, even with extreme measures such as complete facial trunk division combined with facial-hypoglossal nerve anastomosis.[79] The use of these destructive surgical interventions has now been replaced by the two principal treatment options of serial Botox injections or MVD surgery.[80]

Intramuscular injection of commercially available Botox has become widely employed for a variety of indications.

Its application in HFS was introduced in the 1980s[81,82] and received U.S. Food and Drug Administration approval in 1989. It has been adopted as the treatment of choice by many movement disorder neurologists and ophthalmologists. The drug produces a chemodenervation by irreversibly blocking the presynaptic acetylcholine release at the neuromuscular junction. The aim of each treatment is to reduce the excessive muscle activity without producing significant functional weakness. This is relatively titratable on the basis of volume and number of sites injected. Botox provides temporary relief, although muscle strength and spasms recover over 2 to 4 months as new presynaptic exocytotic mechanisms are regenerated. Advocates for serial Botox injections for HFS point out that the treatment is relatively noninvasive, safe, and 90% "effective."[83–85] Effectiveness is loosely defined as the patients' report of (temporary) spasm reduction and their willingness to return regularly for repeat injections.

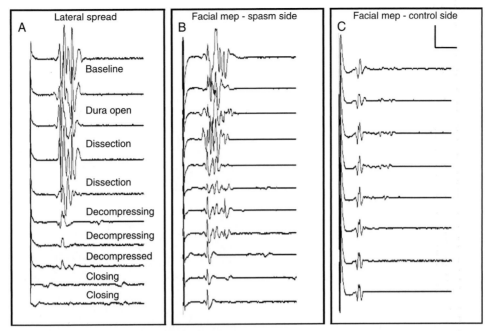

FIGURE 104-4   Lateral spread and facial motor-evoked potentials (fMEP) during microvascular decompression (MVD) for hemifacial spasm. *A,* The lateral spread response from the right mentalis at the start of surgery (baseline) through to completion (closing) during a typical MVD procedure. *B* and *C,* The fMEP measured at the mentalis muscles following electrical stimulation of the contralateral scalp. There was concurrent reduction and elimination of the abnormal muscle responses, as well as lateral spread and ipsilateral fMEP hyperexcitability, as the culprit neurovascular compression was alleviated. Contralateral fMEP served as a control and remained stable. (Vertical bar denotes 25 μV and horizontal bar 10 msec.)

Serial Botox injections are most effective for control of relatively minor twitching of the eyelid or orbicularis oculi muscles. However, the balance between adequate spasm reduction and avoidance of deforming facial weakness is more difficult to achieve when spasms become more severe and extend to the larger buccal and orbicularis oris muscles.[86,87] Transient side effects and minor complications are frequent, although major complications are rare. Botox injections do not appear to slow or halt the progression of HFS, because the underlying neurovascular compression and central hyperactivity of the facial nucleus persist. Patients relying on Botox treatments are therefore committed to three or four injection sessions annually for life, and likely with diminishing satisfaction.

MVD surgery, also known as the Jannetta procedure, is the only means to potentially cure HFS. Appropriate surgical candidates include those without medical contraindications, who have determined that their own disease-related disability is significant enough to consider an operation. There is no absolute exclusion based on age alone, and a trial of serial Botox injections is not a prerequisite before considering MVD. Favorable MVD surgery results have been reported from several centers. Complete or major reduction (greater than 75%) of HFS should be achieved in over 80% of patients, with over 90% of these cured.[51] The most likely neurologic complications of permanent postoperative hearing loss or facial weakness should occur in less than 5%. Other major complications are rare, and the mortality rate with MVD is 0.3% for the estimated 1500 surgeries performed annually in the United States.[88] Even better outcome and safety results may be routinely achieved

at specialized centers with large case loads and among neurosurgeons with MVD surgery experience (see Outcomes section). We have found that the majority of patients prefer the treatment option of MVD over serial Botox injections, provided such favorable outcomes can be reliably achieved.[89]

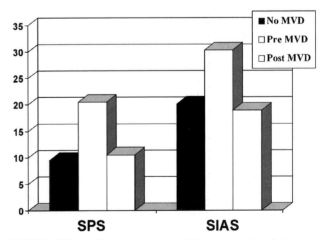

FIGURE 104-5   Disease-related social stress and anxiety were assessed in 97 patients with hemifacial spasm using the Social Interaction Anxiety Scale (SIAS) and Social Phobia Scale (SPS). The majority of these patients were receiving serial Botox injections (85%) when MVD surgery was offered at our center. Significant differences were seen between the 49 patients who declined microvascular decompression (MVD) (*black*) and the 48 who elected MVD (*white*) (*p* < .05 nonpaired *t*-test). Postoperative scores at 3 to 6 months were significantly lower (*p* < .05, paired *t*-test).

SURGICAL TECHNIQUE

Opening and Approach

We have performed over 400 MVD surgeries, including 115 for HFS, using the lateral decubitus position with the surgeon seated behind the head. A subaxillary roll is placed to alleviate pressure on the contralateral brachial plexus, and additional padding is secured under the ulnar and common peroneal nerves on the dependent side. Adjustable bolsters and tape secure the patient, with attention to avoiding excessive traction on the ipsilateral brachial plexus. The knees are slightly bent and positioned in direct alignment such that the lumbar region is perpendicular to the floor. This facilitates cerebrospinal fluid (CSF) drainage by intraoperative lumbar puncture for rare cases that this is desired. A three-pin clamp is applied, and the head is drawn posteriorly while the chin is flexed. A space of two fingerbreadths should be maintained between the chin and thyroid cartilage to avoid excessive flexion and kinking of the endotracheal tube. Additional adjustments include a 10- to 15-degree drop of the vertex and 5 to 10 degrees of contralateral rotation to bring the retrosigmoid space toward a horizontal plane. We routinely administer perioperative antibiotics and antiemetics prior to making the skin incision but do not routinely use mannitol, hyperventilation, or anticonvulsants.

The surgical exposure is planned to provide maximal access to the most anterior-inferior aspect of the retrosigmoid space, at the junction of the posterior fossa floor and distal sigmoid sinus. The mastoid tip extends approximately 2 mm caudal to the posterior fossa floor. The digastric groove and posterior edge of the mastoid process parallels the underlining sigmoid sinus. A straight line drawn between the lateral canthus, root of zygoma, and inion approximates the inferior edge of the transverse sinus (Fig. 104-6). A 4- to 6-cm incision is marked 1 cm behind the mastoid process, after parting the hair or performing a limited shave (Fig. 104-7A). The incision is carried down through successive layers, and a single self-retaining retractor is placed to maintain the exposure. The occipital artery and lesser occipital nerve are often encountered and may sometimes be preserved after dissection. The subperiosteal plane is extended with monopolar cautery. Superiorly, the suboccipital muscle origin at the lateral aspect of the nuchal line is elevated. Inferiorly, the opening should extend to the inferior edge of the occipital squamous bone. One must be aware of the potential to encounter an ectatic extracranial vertebral artery loop and avoid its inadvertent injury. The posterior aspect of the mastoid process and digastric groove are cleared. Emissary veins coursing anterolaterally through bone toward the sigmoid sinus are readily controlled with wax, after their bony opening is cleared of soft tissue.

A retrosigmoid craniectomy of 1 × 2 to 2 × 3 cm is fashioned with a high-speed pneumatic burr and 3- to 5-mm angulated rongeurs. The occipital squamous bone is removed inferiorly until the floor is seen end-on, although the superior extent of the craniectomy need not extend to the transverse sinus. The posterior edge of the sigmoid sinus is clearly visualized up to and including its junction with the posterior fossa floor (Fig. 104-7B). Compromise in the anterolateral or inferior extent of exposure severely limits the angle of surgical approach to the facial root exit zone.

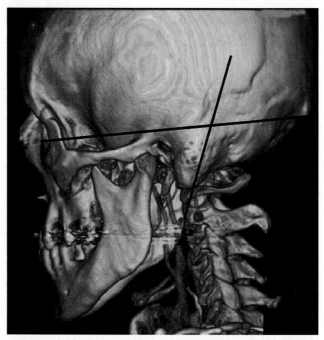

FIGURE 104-6 Bone landmarks for planning a retrosigmoid craniectomy. The horizontal line connecting the lateral canthus root to the zygoma and to the inion approximates the location of the distal transverse sinus, while the vertical line along the mastoid process approximates the sigmoid sinus. The mastoid tip projects below the posterior fossa floor.

Such a shortcoming of the opening may lead to an inadequate surgical exposure, compensation with excessive cerebellar retraction, or both. Conversely, overzealous bone removal posteromedially does not enhance visualization of the target structures, but does expose the cerebellum to increased risk for mechanical injury from impact or excessive retraction. The mastoid air cells are often entered and are sealed with a thin wall of bone wax to prevent entry of irrigation fluid, blood, or CSF. Prior to opening dura, the soft-tissue self-retaining retractor is loosened one or two notches, reducing unnecessary tissue stretch and postoperative incisional pain.

Dura opening should take full advantage of the anterior-inferior extent of the craniectomy exposure. A C-shaped incision reflected over the sigmoid sinus is usually sufficient, although this may be extended into a Y shape with a caudal leaflet reflected inferiorly. CSF may spontaneously drain from the subdural space, resulting in "relaxation" of the cerebellum and opening a surgical corridor to the deeper arachnoid cisterns. This CSF release may be facilitated by gentle downward pressure on the cerebellum. In younger patients, little or no subdural CSF may escape at this early stage and the cerebellum herniates uncomfortably through the dural opening (another reason to limit the craniectomy size). Contusion or laceration of the cerebellum is avoided by maintaining the cerebellum beneath the dura with gentle compression. The anesthesiologist is asked to confirm normal ventilation pressures and end-tidal carbon dioxide levels. In rare cases, spinal CSF drainage by an intraoperative lumbar puncture may be employed to reduce intracranial volume. However, it is usually most effective to

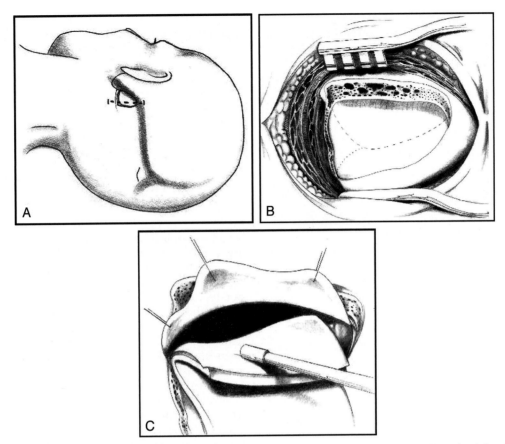

FIGURE 104-7 Approach used in microvascular decompression for hemifacial spasm. *A,* The head is positioned to bring the retrosigmoid region toward a horizontal plane. The incision is traced approximately one fingerbreadth behind the mastoid process. *B,* The retrosigmoid craniectomy extends to the posterior fossa floor, seen end on, and anterolaterally until the edge of the sigmoid sinuses is clearly exposed. The C-shaped dura flap is reflected anteriorly, and an additional Y extension may be added if necessary. *C,* The initial intradural approach is directed inferolaterally, to elevate the cerebellum and access the deep arachnoid cisterns. We use a cottonoid-latex "slider" that advances easily over the moistened brain surface. (© Jon Stepaniuk)

bring the microscope into use, gently retract the cerebellum a few millimeters, and open the deep arachnoid cisterns as described below.

The operating microscope is directed inferolaterally, and exposure is advanced over the anterior-inferior aspect of the cerebellum (Fig. 104-7C). Retraction is applied by suction and bayonet over the 0.5 × 3 inch cottonoid and latex sheet "slider" (Fig. 104-8). The cerebellum is elevated a couple of millimeters from the posterior fossa floor. This exposes bulging arachnoid of the deep cistern, which is opened to release the CSF and further "deflates" the cerebellum. Excessive retraction at this stage may avulse the inferior cerebellar bridging vein and result in brisk bleeding. This vein should therefore be identified, coagulated, and divided with care to recognize the coalesced cervical rootlets of the accessory nerve coursing over the dura. The cerebellum is then retracted at a 45-degree angle to both the petrous bone and posterior fossa floor, with gentle outward elevation from the lower cranial nerves. The approach is then advanced with sharp dissection of the arachnoid membrane overlying cranial nerves IX through XI that arise from the posterolateral sulcus of the medulla (Fig. 104-9A). The proximal facial nerve root may now come into view, although usually remains obscured by the cerebellum. While further exposure can be gained with forceful retraction, this will

unnecessarily compress the cerebellum and stretch the vestibulocochlear nerve. Instead, attention is directly rostrally, and arachnoid that is tethering the cerebellar flocculus and vestibulocochlear nerve is sharply dissected and released (Fig. 104-9B). This opens a wider corridor to the more proximal nerve roots and brain stem origin, with minimal retraction required.

The facial nerve root originates at the lateral aspect of the pontomedullary sulcus at the supraolivary faucet, a couple of millimeters rostral to the glossopharyngeal root entry zone. It melds with the anterior-inferior surface of the pons, before detaching and crossing the subarachnoid space toward the porus acousticus. The facial "root exit zone" refers to the portion of nerve that maintains the central oligodendrocyte-derived myelin. It extends from the root exit point to a couple of millimeters beyond the detachment point, and then transitions to peripheral Schwann cell–derived myelin.[90] Immediately lateral to the facial nerve lies the vestibulocochlear nerve, choroid plexus, and flocculus. The facial root exit zone is most effectively visualized through an infrafloccular approach, with retraction lifting the cerebellum rostrally and minimizing stretch of the vestibulocochlear nerve. We often complete the early stages of the surgery without using the self-retaining retractor, and rely on gentle pressure applied to the cottonoid-latex slider

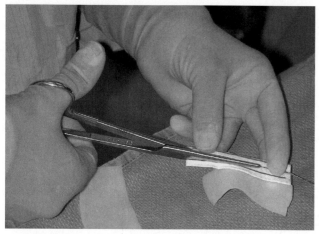

FIGURE 104-8   All cerebellar retraction is applied over a cottonoid-latex slider. These are prepared by cutting matching lengths of cottonoid strips and latex from surgical gloves or penrose drains. When moistened, these advance smoothly over the brain surface and help avoid contusion or laceration from the retractor or instruments.

with the suction shaft. Final visualization of the facial root exit zone, however, is usually facilitated with a tapered retractor blade (3-mm) elevating the flocculus and choroid plexus (Fig. 104-9C).

Intradural bleeding should be a rare event during MVD surgery, and is most likely to result from inadvertent disruption of a bridging vein coursing from the cerebellum to dural sinuses. Appropriate anticipation of these veins, careful dissection, and thorough coagulation before sectioning is essential. Occasionally venous bleeding may erupt from an unseen source "around the corner." This may lead to complete obscuration of the surgical field and may be complicated by swelling of the cerebellum. Similar bleeding and swelling may occur if the patient lightens from anesthetic and coughs or strains, a situation we have encountered in six MVD surgeries. Should this occur, sharp instruments, including the brain retractor, are removed. Gentle retraction of the cerebellum should be maintained with the cottonoid-latex slider. The intradural space is then thoroughly irrigated, and over several minutes the swelling subsides. The venous bleeding often spontaneously stops, and if not, thorough exploration may identify the culprit vein. This may be directly coagulated or gently tamponaded under direct visualization; blind packing should be avoided.

Decompression

There is a common close relationship between the distal facial and vestibulocochlear nerves with branches of the anterior-inferior cerebellar artery. These are not typically of concern during MVD for HFS. Attention instead must be directed to the facial root exit zone, where culprit neurovascular compression is found in nearly all cases. Severe distortion of the distal facial nerve root is responsible in less than 2%.[91,92] The most common culprit vessels are elongated loops of the anterior-inferior cerebellar artery or posterior-inferior cerebellar artery, which impinge directly against the facial nerve root emerging from the anterior-inferior pons. The goal of MVD surgery is to reorient the axis of the offending vascular loop(s), rather than simply

place a "cushion" between the nerve and vessel. Arachnoid that is tethering the vessels is divided, although the apex of the loop may remain firmly positioned against the nerve. Decompression is therefore more easily achieved by beginning the vessel mobilization proximal and/or distal to the point of maximal compression. Care must be taken to identify and preserve any perforator vessels coursing from the cerebellar arteries to the brain stem or cranial nerves. These may limit the extent of vessel mobilization, although they rarely impose an insurmountable obstacle. Shredded Teflon felt implants are placed to maintain the vessels in new orientation, such that pulsations are no longer directed against the nerve root (Fig. 104-10).

We have exclusively used shredded Teflon felt implants for MVD surgery. These are inert and do not incite any significant inflammatory reaction. When viewed at reoperation months or years later, we have been impressed that the shredded Teflon felt lifts quite easily from the surrounding structures. Conversely, nonshredded Teflon felt should not be used, as we have observed this to densely "scar" against the dura and neurovascular structures. The implants are prepared at the time of surgery by teasing fibers from Teflon felt with a toothed forceps or hemostat clamp. The fibers are rolled between moistened fingers to form tight cigar-shaped implants of various sizes (Fig. 104-11). A fine bayonetted forceps is used to deliver these implants, and angulated microdissectors aid in adjusting their positions. The final decompression typically employs 3 to 10 shredded Teflon felt implants. Each should contribute to the repositioning of the offending vessel(s) and/or securing the positioning of other implants, without producing distortion of the cranial nerves or kinking of vessels. It should be recalled that HFS is caused by pulsatile neurovascular compression on the nerve root, rather than static contact with a tumor or implant material.

An ectatic vertebral artery is implicated in about one fourth of HFS cases. This is evident on preoperative diagnostic imaging, and may produce severe distortion of the cranial nerves and brain stem (Fig. 104-12). A variety of techniques to mobilize and reposition the ectatic vertebral artery have been described, including the use of various "slings" secured to dura.[93-97] However, a stepwise approach to repositioning the large artery using shredded Teflon felt implants is usually effective and is our preferred technique. In these cases, the initial view of the facial root exit zone is obscured by the ectatic loop that cannot easily be elevated into full view. Attention should first be directed to the more proximal vertebral artery. Working between rootlets of the vagus and glossopharyngeal nerves, the vessel is elevated ventrally off the medulla and shredded Teflon implants are placed to maintain the new position. The distal posterior-inferior cerebellar artery is usually encountered here, as it descends around the lateral medulla and courses between lower cranial nerve rootlets. This vessel will often also contribute to the facial nerve compression and should therefore be elevated with the vertebral artery. As the shredded Teflon felt implants are sequentially added, the apex of the large loop gradually moves away from the facial nerve root exit zone. Further mobilization can now readily be achieved with additional placement of large shredded Teflon felt implants distally between the ectatic vertebral artery and pons. Prior to covering the root exit zone itself, additional neurovascular

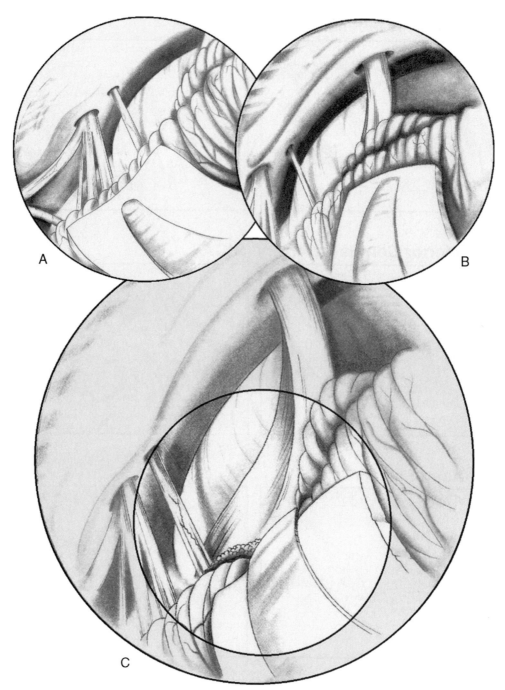

FIGURE 104-9   Exposure of the facial root exit zone (REZ) is achieved in three stages. *A,* Initial approach is inferolaterally to elevate the cerebellum from the lower cranial nerves IX–XI. An inferior cerebellar bridging vein is typically present and may be easily avulsed. We usually coagulate and divide this, cautious not to injure the accessory nerve (cervical portion) that courses nearby over the dura. Sharp dissection of arachnoid is coupled with rostral and outward retraction of the cerebellum to provide a view of the upper medulla. More cephalad view of the facial REZ, however, will usually be restricted by arachnoid tethering of the vestibulocochlear nerve and flocculus. *B,* This should be released to avoid traction on the delicate cranial nerves and potential hearing loss. There will usually be vessels associated with the distal cisternal portions of cranial nerves VII and VIII. These are rarely implicated as culprits in hemifacial spasm and only require attention if they restrict mobilization of the cerebellum. *C,* Visualization of the facial REZ is achieved by an infrafloccular approach, elevating the cerebellum perpendicular to the vestibulocochlear nerve, rather than applying direct lateral retraction. Neurovascular compression from one or more culprit vessels may occur anywhere along the REZ that extends from the pontomedullary sulcus to a couple of millimeters beyond the detachment point from the pons. Typical neurovascular compression scenarios are shown in Figure 104-10. (© Jon Stepaniuk)

Anterior-Inferior Cerebellar Artery (AICA)

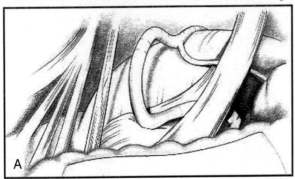 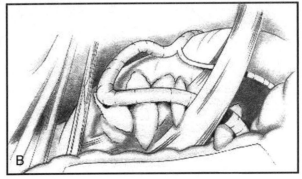

Posterior-Inferior Cerebellar Artery (PICA)

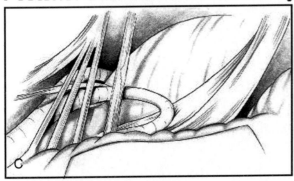 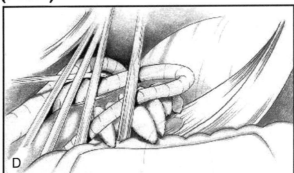

Ectatic Vertebral Artery

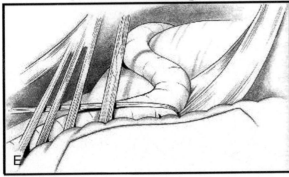 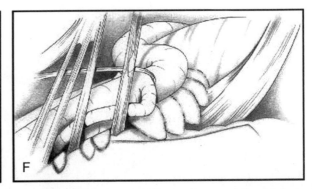

FIGURE 104-10   Neurovascular compression in hemifacial spasm is usually related to the cerebellar arteries or ectatic vertebral artery impinging on the root exit zone (REZ). Multiple vessel contacts are not uncommon and should all be alleviated. The most prominent vessel contact is usually an arterial loop tightly apposed against the facial REZ. After wide arachnoid dissection, vessel mobilization is initiated away from the point of maximal compression. A series of shredded Teflon felt implants are sequentially placed to maintain the apex of the vessel loop in a new orientation, rather than simply provide a cushion. Special care is required to avoid injury or distortion of the delicate perforating arteries or cranial nerves. (© Jon Stepaniuk)

compression should be sought and is usually found. The posterior-inferior cerebellar artery, its origin identified by crossing hypoglossal nerve rootlets, as well as any length or loop of the anterior-inferior cerebellar artery contacting the proximal facial nerve, should also be elevated prior to the placement of the final shredded Teflon felt implants (see Fig. 104-10E and F).

In rare cases, the pontine surface of the root exit zone is free from significant neurovascular contacts. In two cases we found the culprit vessel impinging on the root exit point, at the pontomedullary sulcus. In another two cases, similar pathology was seen in combination with more typical neurovascular compression. This most proximal portion of the root exit zone may be difficult to visualize, and may require approach between glossopharyngeal and vagus nerve rootlets. We occasionally have found it helpful to use a small angulated mirror, while others have used angled endoscopes.[98,99] In all cases it is important to visualize the entire course of the facial root exit zone and associated vasculature.

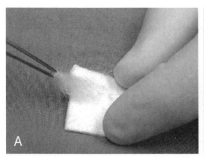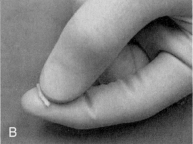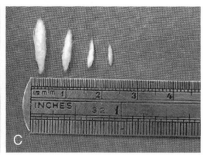

FIGURE 104-11   Shredded Teflon felt implants are prepared at the time of surgery. Fibers are grasped with forceps or a hemostat and rolled between moistened fingers to form implants of various sizes.

The vast majority of neurovascular compression causing HFS is related to arteries impinging on the ventral-caudal aspect of the root exit zone. It is not clear whether this area is particularly susceptible to the pulsatile irritation or simply more prone to neurovascular impingement due to its anatomic configuration. Culprit vessels may occasionally be situated against the dorsorostral aspect of the facial nerve root as it detaches from the pons. Such compression is most common in patients with atypical HFS, and should also be alleviated whenever present.[7,100] We typically do not address simple venous contacts that parallel the facial nerve or its root exit zone. In four cases, however, we found a prominent brain stem vein coursing across the facial root exit zone, and this was the only culprit in two cases. In the first case we mobilized the vein off the nerve, before coagulating and dividing it. A successful decompression was completed, although the patient suffered a facial palsy with moderate recovery. In the more recent cases, we carefully avoided manipulation of the portion of vein adherent to the facial nerve, and instead coagulated and divided the vein on either side of the nerve, but still produced a temporary facial weakness in one case.

In rare cases when no significant neurovascular contacts are evident on the facial root exit zone, attention should be directed to the more distal facial nerve. We have encountered this scenario in two cases. The distal facial nerves were severely distorted and kinked by an unusual relationship with the anterior-inferior cerebellar arteries. In both cases, the apex of the vessel loop was relatively fixed by a prominent labyrinthine branch. Nevertheless, it was possible to mobilize the facial nerve around the vessel loop, and maintain a more relaxed course with the placement of the Teflon felt implants, successfully curing the HFS. It has also been rare to encounter associated pathologies during MVD for HFS. We have seen this twice in over 115 surgeries; a previously irradiated acoustic neuroma and an unruptured aneurysm of the posterior-inferior cerebellar artery origin. In both cases, concurrent neurovascular compression on the facial nerve root exit zone was identified and alleviated, resulting in a cure of HFS.

Closing

Meticulous hemostasis is confirmed prior to closure. We no longer request a Valsalva maneuver, as this may stimulate premature emergence from anesthesia and coughing by the patient who is not pharmalogically paralyzed. A watertight closure is facilitated by keeping the dura moist throughout surgery. We accomplish this by tucking saline-soaked Gelfoam behind the reflected dural flap. The edges of bone are again sealed with wax, taking care not to "stuff" the air cells. We routinely reconstruct the small craniectomy defect

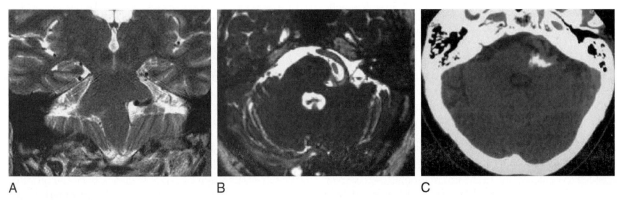

FIGURE 104-12   Neurovascular compression in hemifacial spasm caused by an ectatic vertebral artery and associated vessels. Preoperative magnetic resonance image discloses a severe compression and distortion of the ipsilateral pontomedullary region, as well as an underlying artery branch (*A* and *B*). Following microvascular decompression, the postoperative computed tomography scan shows the radiodense shredded Teflon felt implants and the ectatic vertebral artery (and associated vessels) that have been mobilized off the brain stem and facial root exit zone.

with a cranioplasty of methylmethacrylate, without need for any rigid fixation. The soft tissues are closed in multiple layers, including an absorbable skin suture, and antibacterial ointment is applied in lieu of a bandage. Patients are then observed in a neurosurgical step-down unit or intensive care unit overnight, maintaining close attention to any alteration of vital signs or neurologic assessments. In over 400 MVD surgeries we have performed, one patient (with trigeminal neuralgia) developed a major postoperative complication.[101] This person deteriorated into coma 6 hours following MVD and required ventricular drain placement and surgical decompression of a cerebellar venous infarct. Although her recovery was excellent, this experience highlights the need for close observation the first day following surgery.

INTRAOPERATIVE MONITORING

The structures most susceptible to intraoperative injury during MVD for HFS are cranial nerves VI through XII, and especially the cochlear and facial nerves. A thorough appreciation for their normal course and neurovascular relationships facilitates safe surgical navigation and maneuvering. The gentle and atraumatic microsurgical technique that effectively avoids cranial nerve injury also minimizes the risk for cerebellar or vascular injury. Attention to minimizing measurable neurophysiological changes during MVD surgery has been associated with complication avoidance.[51,102-104] In the next sections we describe the intraoperative monitoring techniques routinely used during all our MVD surgeries.

Brain Stem Auditory Evoked Responses

The cochlear nerve is particularly sensitive to even minor degrees of manipulation and stretching.[105] The axons of this nerve are invested with the central oligodendrocyte-derived myelin throughout its cisternal course. Furthermore, the cochlear nerve separates into multiple tiny filaments that traverse the lamina cribrosa at the fundus of the internal auditory canal, where they may be torn with minor degrees of traction.[106,107] The monitoring of brain stem auditory evoked potentials (BAEPs) aids in the preservation of hearing by alerting the surgeon of alterations in cochlear nerve function that may be reversed before any permanent injury develops. The BAEP uses auditory stimuli and measures the transduction of sound into a series of bioelectric waveforms, labeled I to V. As the transduction process ascends bilaterally within the brain stem, the latency and amplitude of the largest standing wave (usually wave V) is measured against the baseline response. The BAEP is an averaged response to auditory clicks delivered at 11.1 Hz, comprising 500 sweeps over a total of 45 seconds. Nerve status can also be based on a shorter recording when artifacts (e.g., bipolar coagulation) are contaminating the average.

Recording leads for the BAEP are placed at A1 and A2 and referenced to Cz according to the international 10–20 system. Standard tube phones with foam inserts are used to deliver the auditory stimuli: rarefaction clicks ipsilaterally and white noise contralaterally. All electrode wires are incorporated into a braid primarily for reducing electrical noise, but a single bundle of leads are also less obtrusive and easier

to manage. It is time well spent to anticipate and eliminate potential points of contact with surgical personnel, who can produce bumping artifacts or act as antennae by leaning against leads and transmitting noise into the recordings. Keeping all recording leads together in a braided "cable" also allows for quick trouble shooting if the leads are in too close a proximity to other sources of noise (e.g., fluid warmers). Wires such as electrocardiographic leads may also attract and transmit unwanted ambient signals into the neuromonitoring system, so contact between these should also be carefully avoided.

The ipsilateral wave V is typically the largest amplitude wave of the BAEP and is generally the wave observed throughout a surgical procedure. However, the responses can become obscured or altered by spurious signals included in the average or by rapidly developing changes in nerve function. Trying to obtain a "clean" average may require several precious minutes, by which time irreversible nerve damage may have occurred. Our solution is to look to the ipsilateral wave III that should mirror changes in wave V (unless there is damage to the brain stem pathway between the neural generators of III and V). We can also refer to the contralateral wave V that is also generated by the ipsilateral auditory stimulus but is usually not contaminated by "bumping" artifacts because the recording leads are on the opposite side and protected from incidental contact. If the ipsilateral wave V becomes indistinct, an astute monitoring person can quickly confirm the legitimacy by looking at the contralateral response, which is obtained simultaneously. If the contralateral wave also has become unreadable, then the response probably reflects a physiological "event."

Figure 104-13 shows the morphology of the BAEP and the dynamic changes that can occur during a typical MVD operation. It is common to see a small (0.3-msec) increased latency of wave V at the early stages of intracranial dissection. Changes of less than 1 msec are generally acceptable, although any increased latency should alert the surgeon of possible unnecessary cochlear nerve traction or stress, which can usually be alleviated with an alteration of surgical technique. If BAEP latency increases beyond 1 msec, the cause should be identified and corrected. This may be suboptimal or excessive retraction, arachnoid tethers between the flocculus and cochlear nerve, vascular compression, or direct mechanical pressure by the retractor or instruments. BAEPs delayed beyond 1.5 to 2.0 msec are associated with increased risk of hearing loss.[103] In 4% of our cases, we have seen BAEP changes reach or exceed 2 msec (Fig. 104-14). If such delays occur, we typically cease further dissection and remove the retraction, irrigate the intracranial field with warm saline, and wait for responses to return toward normal, usually within a couple of minutes. BAEP should be monitored until surgery is complete, as dramatic loss of BAEP may rarely occur during closure, likely related to shift of neurovascular structures as CSF reaccumulates. Immediate reexploration may identify and correct an offending neurovascular conflict with the cochlear nerve.[108] We have found that constant feedback from the monitoring team provides tremendously valuable information during MVD. Although guarantees of hearing preservation cannot be made, we have had sufficient confidence to agree to perform MVD surgeries for three patients with severe HFS and contralateral deafness, successfully without complication.

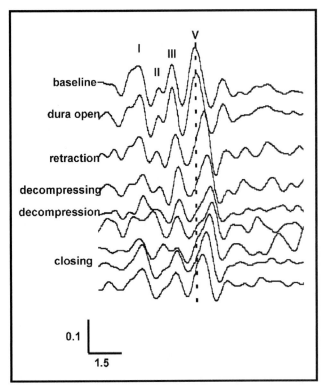

FIGURE 104-13 A series of averaged brain stem auditory evoked potentials (BAEPs) obtained in response to ipsilateral rarefaction clicks during microvascular decompression (MVD) for hemifacial spasm (HFS). Peaks of the BAEP waves are designated with roman numerals as shown. The vertical line running through each sweep indicates the latency of wave V at baseline. Note the horizontal shift of wave V during the procedure. The maximum latency change of 0.7 msec is the average we encounter during MVD for HFS. (Vertical scale bar is in microvolts and horizontal scale in milliseconds.)

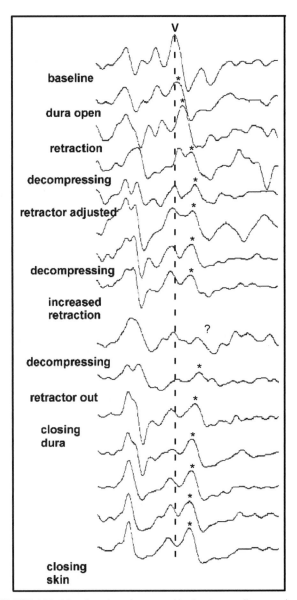

FIGURE 104-14 A series of averaged brain stem auditory evoked potentials (BAEPs) during microvascular decompression for hemifacial spasm where the response transiently disappeared. In the trace labeled "increased retraction," wave V (∗) disappears into the background noise. This series of averages shows the deformation and subsequent loss of wave V during periods of cochlear nerve stress or traction. Surgical alterations were made to facilitate recovery of the response and prevent permanent hearing loss.

Attention to minimizing and correcting changes of BAEP latency guide the surgeon in adopting a gentle approach. This not only helps prevent cochlear nerve damage and hearing loss, but also reduces the risk for other mechanical or retractor-related injuries.

Lateral Spread EMG

As described earlier, lateral spread is an evoked EMG response to the electrical stimulation of one facial nerve branch recorded in a facial muscle innervated by a different branch. The first step in monitoring lateral spread is consultation with the anesthetist to ensure that neuromuscular blockade is short acting and used only for intubation. We apply all of the electrodes once the patient is asleep, and our preference is to use needle electrodes. These are secured to the patient using waterproof tape (face) or staples (scalp). Bipolar EMG recordings from the orbicularis oculi, orbicularis oris, and the mentalis muscles are performed throughout the procedure. A ground electrode is usually placed in the contralateral trapezius, mainly for convenience, although we also have used the forehead (FPz) with similar effect. As for BAEPs, electrode wires are braided together and directed toward the amplifier inputs in a manner that minimizes contact with surgical personnel. The recorded signals are fed through an audio amplifier so that the surgical team can hear the EMG activity. The amplifier gain is

adjusted to give between 0.5 to 1 mV full deflection, and filter settings are usually 100 to 3000 Ω. Evaluating lateral spread is easiest when there is no spontaneous activity from the facial musculature. Although occasionally observed, spontaneous activity is typically of much lower amplitude than the lateral spread response; large-amplitude spontaneous twitches are rarely encountered in the anesthetized patient.

To elicit the lateral spread response, we typically stimulate the temporal branch of the facial nerve and monitor the EMG response from the orbicularis oculi, orbicularis oris, and mentalis muscles. We have used both subdermal needle and surface "patch" electrodes to deliver the stimulus and find either are adequate for the task. We use a constant current stimulation of 2 to 30 mA delivered at 1 Hz with 0.2 msec pulse width. The lateral spread amplitude has been 10.4 to 255 μV (85.7 ± 64.9 μV), and latency 9.8 to 17.8 msec (12.5 ± 2.2 msec). Occasionally the lateral spread response is inconsistently evoked using a stimulus frequency of 1 Hz. In these circumstances, increasing the stimulus frequency and not necessarily the amplitude can usually provoke adequate lateral spread responses, assuming that neuromuscular blockade or misplaced stimulating electrodes are not the cause. It has been our experience that stimulation of the temporal branch results in the most consistent lateral spread responses, particularly from the oris and mentalis muscles. Interestingly, applying the stimuli to the mandibular branch is not nearly as efficacious, and the directionality of the lateral spread remains an interesting physiologic question.

Lateral spread is usually immediately reduced or eliminated with MVD of the facial nerve root, demonstrating the plasticity of the abnormal neural activity (Fig. 104-4). Several groups have strongly advocated the importance of observing lateral spread and its subsequent abolition as an indicator of sufficient decompression of the facial nerve.[58,61–65] There is, however, a small incidence of false-negative and false-positive results when relying on lateral spread as a prediction of HFS cure.[109–111] Our experience with observing lateral spread can be generally condensed into two outcomes: lateral spread was completely abolished upon decompression of the facial nerve; or lateral spread was significantly reduced but persisted despite thoroughly decompressing all sources of neurovascular contact. In less than 5% of cases is the lateral spread response not present or not reduced with MVD. As always, the best guide to achieving success in MVD surgery is to thoroughly explore the entire course of the facial nerve root exit zone, alleviating all arterial contacts and venous compression, rather than being distracted by incidental and usually irrelevant neurovascular contacts at the distal facial nerve root. Nevertheless, monitoring of lateral spread is quite a reliable neurophysiological technique to indicate whether the culprit vessel(s) have been adequately mobilized, and we encourage its routine use in MVD for HFS.

Facial Motor-Evoked Potentials

As mentioned earlier, we have recently included fMEPs in our neuromonitoring regimen. We use the Cadwell CV-2 stimulator with the "polarity switch" option that permits selective motor cortex stimulation from both sides of the scalp. Subdermal electrodes are positioned at C3 and C4 (10-20 system) and serve as the stimulating leads. We find that producing consistent fMEPs is relatively easy using a single pulse (150 to 200 μsec) and amplitudes between 90 and 220 V. Figure 104-4 illustrates a typical result for bilateral fMEPs and lateral spread responses during the course of an MVD for HFS. The temporal effects between lateral spread and the ipsilateral fMEP responses are remarkably similar and consistent as described earlier (see Neurophysiology section). In our initial eight patients monitored with both lateral spread and fMEPs, we found that fMEP duration decreased from 18.1 ± 1.2 msec to 7.7 ± 0.7 msec and amplitudes from 246.7 ± 70.4 μV to 66.8 ± 27.5 μV ($p < .03$) on completion of the MVD. These changes were concurrent with the elimination of lateral spread in seven of eight

patients and 50% reduction in the other. The fMEP also serves as a continuous monitor of facial nerve integrity, although further experience is required to validate its sensitivity and reliability in predicting and influencing outcome of MVD surgery.

Free Running Electromyography

The goal of MVD surgery is atraumatic alleviation of vascular contacts, and intraoperative monitoring is an essential guide in achieving this aim. Audio amplification of the EMG signal is a helpful feature to gauge the response of the facial nerve during surgery. Inadvertent contact with the facial nerve by instruments or placement of shredded Teflon implants may generate a short burst of high-frequency EMG responses (greater than 50 Hz). These responses are rarely neurotonic in nature, but should still be avoided using careful microsurgical technique. Conversely, prolonged high-pitched, high-frequency responses of up to 200 Hz are sometimes referred to as "mosquito buzzes" or "injury potentials" and probably indicate a compromise of nerve membrane integrity. This is a classic early warning feature and should be brought to the attention of the surgeon immediately so that further nerve irritation or injury can be avoided.

In addition to facial nerve monitoring we also use EMG monitoring of the glossopharyngeal and vagus cranial nerves under particular circumstances. This may be most valuable when an ectatic vertebral artery will require mobilization. Surgical irritation, impact, or stretch on these lower cranial nerves is assessed as described for the facial nerve. EMG monitoring of the glossopharyngeal nerve can be accomplished by insertion of needle electrodes into the ipsilateral soft palate. For vagus nerve we use either percutaneous insertion of needles into the cricothyroid membrane or a commercially available laryngeal surface electrode (Neurovision Medical, Ventura, CA). Our preference is the latter, which easily attaches to the endotracheal tube prior to intubation. The correct placement of the recording electrode can be confirmed by intraoperative stimulation of the corresponding nerves using a hand-held stimulator.

POSTOPERATIVE COURSE AND OUTCOMES

Approximately half of the patients are ambulatory and eating well on the first postoperative day, and may be discharged within 24 to 48 hours. The other half of patients have moderate to severe headaches and nausea that typically subsides over a couple of days. The average length of stay is 3.5 days. As soon as postoperative fatigue and intermittent headaches resolve, usually over 2 to 8 weeks, patients may resume a full level of activity and employment. A common complaint is fullness of the ipsilateral ear with some "watery" distortion of hearing, related to fluid within the mastoid air cells. This also typically resolves in a few weeks. At the time of hospital discharge, patients should also be advised of potential delayed complications such as CSF leak from the incision, nose, or nasopharynx, wound infection, and meningitis (aseptic or bacterial). We also warn our patients of the small chance of developing a delayed-onset facial nerve palsy that typically resolves spontaneously without recurrence of HFS.[112] This has been encountered in 5% of our patients, occurring 7 to 14 days following the operation. In all but one case, there had been severe facial nerve compression by an ectatic vertebral artery, and the situation is analogous to delayed Bell's palsy sometimes seen after a resection of an acoustic neuroma. The postoperative course of hemifacial spasm is variable.[113,114] Approximately one third to one half of the patients have immediate and permanent relief from spasms. Others have a gradual reduction of spasms over 2 to 3 months, and rarely as long as 1 year. Patients should be warned that spasms are often immediately reduced after surgery, but may return to baseline in the first few days (often after discharge) and then gradually disappear.

Lovely summarized results from 20 series of MVD for HFS published between 1980 and 1996, including 10 to 648 patients each (2095 total).[51] The success rate was 85.8%, ranging from 79% to 100%. Excellent results (i.e., cure) occurred in most patients, with fewer than 10% having good results (i.e., marked improvement). In the largest of these series, Barker and colleagues presented Jannetta's 20-year experience (1972 to 1992).[48] Culprit neurovascular compression was found in all cases; the posterior-inferior cerebellar artery was most commonly involved (68.2%), followed by the anterior-inferior cerebellar artery (35.3%) and vertebral artery (23.9%). Veins were also treated in 20.4%, but were the sole culprit in only 2.9%. Kaplan-Meier methods showed excellent results in 84% and good results (greater than 75% spasm reduction) in 7% at 10 years following first MVD. There were no operative deaths, and occurrence of brain stem infarct (0.2%), cerebellar hematoma (0.3%), or bacterial meningitis (0.6%) were rare. Combined with permanent postoperative hearing loss (3.2%) or facial weakness (3.4%), these major complications occurred in less than 8% of patients. Similar results have been reported in more recent series with over 100 patients.[21,101,115–117] Our own series of MVD for HFS is summarized in Table 104-1.

In the review by Lovely, the rate of major complications ranged between 3.3% and 79%, with 8 of 20 series reporting rates over 10%. Success and morbidity rates do vary between centers and surgeons.[118] A recent study estimated that 1500 MVD surgeries are performed annually in the United States, including approximately 300 for HFS. Neurosurgeons performing these operations had a wide range of ongoing experience, with a median annual case load of three; 29% performed only one operation per year and only 1% performed more than 29 operations per year.[88] While surgical mortality was uncommon, morbidity rates were lower at high-volume centers with high-volume surgeons. In our own study of MVD surgery at two Canadian centers, there were significant differences in outcome, complications, and patient satisfaction (3.5 vs. 9.5 of 10, $p < .5$), that also corresponded to differences in surgeon volume of experience. Several other reports have highlighted the correlation between the surgical experience and better outcomes from MVD, and have also credited the routine use of intraoperative monitoring with greater success and reduced complications rates.[102,104,116,117,119]

Minor complications of MVD surgery are reported in 5.3% to 46.3% of patients.[51] Our own results are tabulated in Table 104-1 and include transient postoperative neurologic deficits and surgical complications without

TABLE 104-1 ▪ First Microvascular Decompression Surgeries for 115 Patients with Hemifacial Spasm

Preoperative History	
Female gender	58%
Age at onset	45 ± 12 yr (19–75 yr)
Preoperative duration	8 ± 6 yr (1–30 yr)
Age at surgery	53 ± 12 yr (19–85 yr)
Prior Botox injections	64%
Outcome (%)	
Excellent (98%–100% spasm free)	84%
Good (>75% spasm reduction)	7%
Fail (<75% spasm reduction)	9%
Complications (no. of patients)	
Major	
Death	0
Stroke	0
Hematoma	0
Bacterial meningitis	0
Permanent facial weakness (mild–moderate)	2
Permanent hearing loss (complete)	1
Transient	
Immediate facial weakness	4
Delayed-onset facial weakness	6
Aseptic meningitis	5
Cerebrospinal fluid leak	2
Tinnitus	3
Balance difficulty	4
Wound infection	1
Dysphagia	2

long-term sequelae. The most common and troubling of these in our experience has been the delayed onset of chemical or aseptic meningitis. Barker and colleagues noted this following 16% of their 782 operations for hemifacial spasm.[48] In our own series, 5% of patients have required readmission for investigations to rule out the rare case of bacterial meningitis and to institute treatment of intravenous fluids and corticosteroids. Most patients recover within 1 to 2 weeks and resume full activity within 2 to 3 months postoperatively.

The vast majority of MVD procedures should result in HFS cure or major spasm alleviation. Most failures are evident within the first 12 to 24 months after surgery.[51,120] There are three possible reasons why MVD may fail to cure HFS: (1) the central pathophysiologic state of hyperactivity or hyperexcitability is not fully reversible in a small subset of patients; (2) a recurrence of neurovascular compression by a previously treated culprit vessel or a new culprit vessel; or (3) an incomplete or inadequate MVD of the facial nerve root. Although HFS often subsides gradually after successful MVD, we advocate re-exploration if there is no improvement within 3 months or significant persisting spasms at 9 to 12 months. Redo MVD in this situation has a 50% chance of curing HFS, although one may find the culprit neurovascular compression had been adequately alleviated at the first surgery.[48,119] We and others have seen better results following redo MVD when the prior surgery was done elsewhere. Barker and colleagues noted that among 57 such patients, reoperation results were excellent in 73%, good in

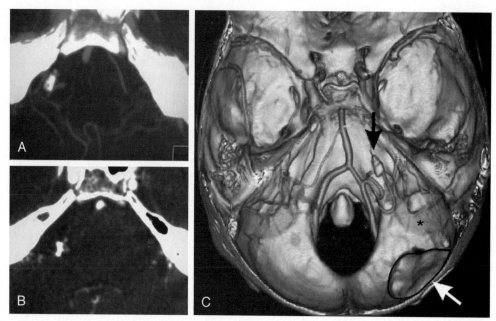

FIGURE 104-15 Preoperative computed tomography (CT) scans of the patient referred for redo microvascular decompression (MVD) after initial surgery failed to alleviate hemifacial spasm (HFS). Axial CT images (*A* and *B*) show radiodense implant material situated distal and rostral to the facial root exit zone (REZ) and culprit neurovascular compression remaining. The 3-dimensional reconstruction (*C*) shows the implant material (*black arrow*) situated rostral to a distal loop of the posterior-inferior cerebellar artery. The retromastoid craniectomy (*white arrow*) did not extend anterolaterally to the sigmoid sinus (*) and therefore would have limited the neurosurgeon's view to the facial REZ. Subsequent redo MVD was performed, with the extension of the craniectomy to the sigmoid sinus. The culprit neurovascular compression was alleviated and HFS cured.

13%, and failed in 14%. In our own experience, we have found persisting neurovascular contact on the facial root exit zone that had not been previously alleviated. In some of these cases, the root exit zone had apparently not been exposed at the prior surgery, while in others the implant material of solid Teflon felt or sponge materials was positioned distally on the facial nerve and produced difficult adhesions requiring a tedious dissection. In most of these cases we found the original craniectomy had not extended to the sigmoid sinus and posterior fossa floor. This explained, at least in part, why the root exit zone had not been adequately explored and decompressed (Fig. 104-15).

SUMMARY

HFS is a potentially disabling cranial rhizopathy caused by pulsatile neurovascular compression on the facial nerve, usually at the root exit zone. The neurosurgical techniques employed in the MVD operation provide the potential to cure this disease. The risks for surgical complications should be minimal, especially when neurophysiologic monitoring is used as an intraoperative aid. Although alternative treatment option of lifelong repeated Botox injections should be presented to all patients, MVD is often preferred when the favorable surgical outcomes can be reliably achieved.

Acknowledgments

We thank Mrs. C. J. Byrnes and Ms. Heather Long for their assistance in the preparation of this manuscript.

REFERENCES

1. Auger RG, Whisnant JP: Hemifacial spasm in Rochester and Olmsted County, Minnesota, 1960–1984. Arch Neurol 47:1233–1234, 1990.
2. Chang JW, Chang JH, Park YG, et al: Microvascular decompression of the facial nerve for hemifacial spasm in youth. Childs Nerv Syst 17:309–312, 2001.
3. Levy EI, Resnick DK, Jannetta PJ, et al: Pediatric hemifacial spasm: The efficacy of microvascular decompression. Pediatr Neurosurg 27:238–241, 1997.
4. Tan EK, Jankovic J: Bilateral hemifacial spasm: A report of 5 cases and a literature review. Mov Disord 14:345–349, 1999.
5. Carter JB, Patrinely JR, Jankovic J, et al: Familial hemifacial spasm. Arch Ophthalmol 108:249–250, 1990.
6. Coad JE, Wirtschafter JD, Haines SJ, et al: Familial hemifacial spasm associated with arterial compression of the facial nerve. J Neurosurg 74:290–296, 1991.
7. Jannetta PJ: Hemifacial spasm. In Samii M, Jannetta PJ (eds): The Cranial Nerves: Anatomy, Pathology, Pathophysiology, Diagnosis, and Treatment. Berlin: Springer-Verlag, 1981, pp 484–493.
8. Diamant H, Enfors B, Wiberg A: Facial spasm: With special reference to the chordoma tympani function and operative treatment. Laryngoscope 77:350–358, 1967.
9. Cushing H: The major trigeminal neuralgias and their surgical treatment based on experiments with 332 Gasserian operations. Am J Med Sci 160:157–184, 1920.
10. Cook BR, Jannetta PJ: Tic convulsif: Results in 11 cases treated with microvascular decompression of the fifth and seventh cranial nerves. J Neurosurg 61:949–951, 1984.
11. Maurice-Williams RS: Tic convulsif: The association of trigeminal neuralgia and hemifacial spasm. Postgrad Med J 49:742–745, 1973.
12. Yeh H, Tew JM Jr: Tic convulsif, the combination of geniculate neuralgia and hemifacial spasm relieved by vascular decompression. Neurology 34:682–684, 1984.
13. Kobata H, Kondo A, Iwasaki K, et al: Combined hyperactive dysfunction syndrome of the cranial nerves: Trigeminal neuralgia, hemifacial spasm, and glossopharyngeal neuralgia: 11-year experience and review. Neurosurgery 43:1351–1361, 1998.

14. Platania N, Nicoletti GF, Barbagallo G, et al: Concurrent trigeminal and glossopharyngeal neuralgia, hemifacial spasm and hypertension by neurovascular compression: Case report. J Neurosurg Sci 41:303–307, 1997.
15. Hjorth RJ, Willison RG: The electromyogram in facial myokymia and hemifacial spasm. J Neurol Sci 20:117–126, 1973.
16. Auger RG: Hemifacial spasm: Clinical and electrophysiologic observations. Neurology 29:1261–1272, 1979.
17. Eekhof JL, Aramideh M, Speelman JD, et al: Blink reflexes and lateral spreading in patients with synkinesia after Bell's palsy and in hemifacial spasm. Eur Neurol 43:141–146, 2000.
18. Nielsen VK: Pathophysiology of hemifacial spasm. I: Ephaptic transmission and ectopic excitation. Neurology 34:418–426, 1984.
19. Nielsen VK: Electrophysiology of hemifacial spasm. In May M (ed): The Facial Nerve. New York: Thieme, 1986, pp 487–497.
20. Arbab AS, Nishiyama Y, Aoki S, et al: Simultaneous display of MRA and MPR in detecting vascular compression for trigeminal neuralgia or hemifacial spasm: Comparison with oblique sagittal views of MRI. Eur Radiol 10:1056–1060, 2000.
21. Chung SS, Chang JW, Kim SH, et al: Microvascular decompression of the facial nerve for the treatment of hemifacial spasm: Preoperative magnetic resonance imaging related to clinical outcomes. Acta Neurochir (Wien) 142:901–906, 2000.
22. Fukuda H, Ishikawa M, Okumura R: Demonstration of neurovascular compression in trigeminal neuralgia and hemifacial spasm with magnetic resonance imaging: Comparison with surgical findings in 60 consecutive cases. Surg Neurol 59:93–99, 2003.
23. Girard N, Poncet M, Caces F, et al: Three-dimensional MRI of hemifacial spasm with surgical correlation. Neuroradiology 39:46–51, 1997.
24. Ho SL, Cheng PW, Wong WC, et al: A case-controlled MRI/MRA study of neurovascular contact in hemifacial spasm. Neurology 53:2132–2139, 1999.
25. Nagaseki Y, Horikoshi T, Omata T, et al: Postoperative oblique sagittal MR imaging of microvascular decompression for hemifacial spasm. Acta Neurochir (Wien) 141:737–742, 1999.
26. Nagaseki Y, Omata T, Ueno T, et al: Prediction of vertebral artery compression in patients with hemifacial spasm using oblique sagittal MR imaging. Acta Neurochir (Wien) 140:565–571, 1998.
27. Yamamoto S, Ryu H, Tanaka T, et al: Usefulness of high-resolution magnetic resonance cisternography in patients with hemifacial spasm. Acta Otolaryngol Suppl 542:54–57, 2000.
28. Digre K, Corbett JJ: Hemifacial spasm: Differential diagnosis, mechanism, and treatment. In Jankovic J, Tolosa E (eds): Advances in Neurology. New York: Raven, 1988, pp 151–176.
29. Galvez-Jimenez N, Hanson MR, Desai M: Unusual causes of hemifacial spasm. Semin Neurol 21:75–83, 2001.
30. Iwai Y, Yamanaka K, Nakajima H: Hemifacial spasm due to cerebellopontine angle meningiomas—two case reports. Neurol Med Chir (Tokyo) 41:87–89, 2001.
31. Ruggieri RM, Manfre L, Calbucci F, et al: Therapeutic considerations in cerebellopontine angle lipomas inducing hemifacial spasm. Neurol Sci 21:329–331, 2000.
32. Samii M, Matthies C: Acoustic neurinomas associated with vascular compression syndromes. Acta Neurochir (Wien) 134:148–154, 1995.
33. Sprik CWJD: Hemifacial spasm due to intracranial tumor: An international survey of botulinum toxin investigators. Ophthalmology 95:1042–1045, 1988.
34. Zappia JJ, Wiet RJ, Chouhan A, et al: Pitfalls in the diagnosis of hemifacial spasm. Laryngoscope 107:461–465, 1997.
35. Jannetta PJ, Resnick D: Cranial rhizopathies. In Youmans JR (ed): Neurological Surgery: A Comprehensive Guide to the Diagnosis and Management of Neurosurgical Problems, 4th ed, vol 5. Philadelphia: WB Saunders, 1996, pp 3563–3574.
36. Dandy WE: An operation for the cure of tic douloureux: Partial section of the sensory root at the pons. Arch Surg 18:687–734, 1929.
37. Dandy WE: Concerning the cause of trigeminal neuralgia. Am J Surg 24:447–453, 1934.
38. Dandy WE: Surgery of the Brain. In Lewis DDW, Walters W (eds): Lewis's Practice of Surgery. Hagerstown, MD: Prior, 1948, pp 167–187.
39. Campbell E, Keedy C: Hemifacial spasm: A note on the etiology in two cases. J Neurosurg 4:342–347, 1947.
40. Laine ENP: Hemispasme facial gueri par intervention sur las fossa posterieure. Rev Neurol (Paris) 80:38–40, 1948.
41. Gardner WJ: Response of trigeminal neuralgia to "decompression" of sensory root: Discussion of cause of trigeminal neuralgia. JAMA 170:1773–1776, 1959.
42. Gardner WJ, Pinto JP: The Taarnhjo operation: Relief of trigemina neuralgia without numbness. Clev Clin Q 20:364–367, 1953.
43. Gardner WJ: Five year cure of hemifacial spasm. Clev Clin Q 27:219–221, 1960.
44. Gardner WJ, Sava GA: Hemifacial spasm: A reversible pathophysiological state. J Neurosurg 19:240–247, 1962.
45. Jannetta PJ, Rand RW: Transtentorial retrogasserian rhizotomy in trigeminal neuralgia by microneurosurgical technique. Bull Los Angeles Neurol Soc 31:93–99, 1966.
46. Jannetta PJ: Arterial compression of the trigeminal nerve at the pons in patients with trigeminal neuralgia. J Neurosurg 26:159–162, 1967.
47. Jannetta PJ: Microsurgical exploration and decompression of the facial nerve in hemifacial spasm. Curr Top Surg Res 2:217–220, 1970.
48. Barker FG, Jannetta PJ, Bisonette DJ, et al: Microvascular decompression for hemifacial spasm. J Neurosurg 82:201–210, 1995.
49. Jannetta PJ, Abbasy M, Maroon JC, et al: Aetiology and definitive microsurgical treatment of hemifacial spasm. J Neurosurg 47:321–328, 1977.
50. Jannetta PJ: Outcome after microvascular decompression for typical trigeminal neuralgia, hemifacial spasm, tinnitus, disabling positional vertigo, and glossopharyngeal neuralgia (honored guest lecture). Clin Neurosurg 44:331–383, 1997.
51. Lovely T: Efficacy and complications of microvascular decompression: A review. Neurosurg Q 8:92–106, 1998.
52. Gardner WJ: Concerning the mechanism of trigeminal neuralgia and hemifacial spasm. J Neurosurg 19:947–958, 1962.
53. Wilkins RH: Hemifacial spasm: A review. Surg Neurol 36:251–277, 1991.
54. Neilsen VK: Electrophysiology of the facial nerve in hemifacial spasm: Ectopic/ephaptic excitation. Muscle Nerve 8:545–555, 1985.
55. Tankere F, Maisonobe T, Lamas G, et al: Electrophysiological determination of the site involved in generating abnormal muscle responses in hemifacial spasm. Muscle Nerve 21:1013–1018, 1998.
56. Yamashita S, Kawaguchi T, Fukuda M, et al: Lateral spread response elicited by double stimulation in patients with hemifacial spasm. Muscle Nerve 25:845–849, 2002.
57. Ferguson JH: Hemifacial spasm and the facial nucleus. Ann Neurol 4:97–103, 1978.
58. Moller AR, Jannetta PJ: Physiological abnormalities in hemifacial spasm studies during microvascular decompression operations. Exp Neurol 93:584–600, 1986.
59. Moller AR, Jannetta PJ: On the origin of synkinesis in hemifacial spasm: Results of intracranial recordings. J Neurosurg 61:569–576, 1984.
60. Moller AR: Cranial nerve dysfunction syndromes: Pathophysiology of microvascular compression. In Barrow DL (ed): Surgery of the Cranial Nerves of the Posterior Fossa. Chicago: American Association of Neurological Surgeons, 1993, pp 131–154.
61. Moller AR, Jannetta PJ: Microvascular decompression hemifacial spasm: Intraoperative electrophysiological observations. Neurosurgery 16:612–618, 1985.
62. Haines SJ, Torres F: Intraoperative monitoring of facial nerve during decompression surgery for hemifacial spasm. J Neurosurg 74:254–257, 1991.
63. Harper CM: AAEM Case Report #21: Hemifacial spasm: Preoperative diagnosis and intraoperative management. Muscle Nerve 14:213–218, 1991.
64. Moller AR: Evoked Potential in Intraoperative Monitoring. Baltimore: Williams & Wilkins, 1988.
65. Moller AR, Jannetta PJ: Monitoring facial EMG responses during microvascular decompression operations for hemifacial spasm. J Neurosurg 66:681–685, 1987.
66. Kimura J: Electrodiagnosis in Diseases of Nerve and Muscle, 3rd ed. Oxford, UK: Oxford University Press, 2001.
67. Ishikawa M, Ohira T, Namiki J, et al: Electrophysiological investigation of hemifacial spasm after microvascular decompression: F waves of the facial muscles, blink reflexes, and abnormal muscle responses. J Neurosurg 86:654–661, 1997.
68. Ishikawa M, Namiki J, Takase M, et al: Effect of repetitive stimulation on lateral spread and F-waves in hemifacial spasm. J Neurol Sci 142:99–106, 1996.
69. Ishikawa M, Ohira T, Namiki J, et al: Abnormal muscle response (lateral spread) and F-wave in patients with hemifacial spasm. J Neurol Sci 137:109–116, 1996.

70. Kojima A, Ohira T, Takase M, et al: Long-latency response to transcranial magnetic stimulation in patients with hemifacial spasm. Electroencephalogr Clin Neurophysiol 109:285–289, 1998.

71. Kotterba S, Tegenthoff M, Malin JP: Hemifacial spasm or somatoform disorder—postexcitatory inhibition after transcranial magnetic cortical stimulation as a diagnostic tool. Acta Neurol Scand 101:305–310, 2000.

72. Mattick RP, Clark JC: Development and validation of measures of social phobia scrutiny feat and social interaction anxiety. Psychiatr Clin North Am 24:643–659, 1998.

73. Alexander GE, Moses H: Carbamazepine for hemifacial spasm. Neurology 32:286–287, 1982.

74. Bandini F, Mazzella L: Gabapentin as treatment for hemifacial spasm. Eur Neurol 42:49–51, 1999.

75. Daniele O, Caravaglios G, Marchini C, et al: Gabapentin in the treatment of hemifacial spasm. Acta Neurol Scand 104:110–112, 2001.

76. Herzberg L: Management of hemifacial spasm with clonazepam. Neurology 35:1676–1677, 1985.

77. Hughes EC, Brackman DE, Weinstein RC: Seventh nerve spasm: Effect of modification of cholinergic balance. Otolaryngol Head Neck Surg 88:491–499, 1980.

78. Sandyk R, Gillman MA: Baclofen in hemifacial spasm. Int J Neurosci 33:261–264, 1987.

79. Iansek R, Harrison MJG, Andrew J: Hypoglossal-facial nerve anastomosis: A clinical and electrophysiological follow-up. J Neurosurg Psychiatry 49:588–590, 1986.

80. Iwakuma T, Matosumoto A, Nakamura N: Hemifacial spasm: Comparison of three different operative procedures in 110 patients. J Neurosurg 57:753–756, 1982.

81. Fruch BR, Musch DC: Treatment of facial spasms with botulinum toxin. Ophthalmology 93:917–923, 1986.

82. Kraft SP, Lang AE: Cranial dystonia, blepharospasm and hemifacial spasm: Clinical features and treatment including the use of botulinum toxin. Can Med Assoc J 139:837–844, 1988.

83. Defazio G, Abbruzzese G, Girlanda P, et al: Botulinum toxin A treatment for primary hemifacial spasm: A 10-year multicenter study. Arch Neurol 59:418–420, 2002.

84. Hsiung GY, Das SK, Ranawaya R, et al: Long-term efficacy of botulinum toxin A in treatment of various movement disorders over a 10-year period. Mov Disord 17:1288–1293, 2002.

85. Taylor JDN, Kraft SP, Kazdan MS, et al: Treatment of blepharospasm and hemifacial spasm with botulinum A toxin: A Canadian multicentre study. Can J Ophthalmol 26:133–138, 2003.

86. Kaufmann AM, Ranawaya R, Lye T, et al: Hemifacial spasm natural history and treatment [Abstract]. Can J Neurol Sci 26(Suppl):26, 1999.

87. Snir M, Weinberger D, Bourla D, et al: Quantitative changes in botulinum toxin A treatment over time in patients with essential blepharospasm and idiopathic hemifacial spasm. Am J Ophthalmol 136:99–105, 2003.

88. Kalkanis SN, Eskandar EN, Carter BS, et al: Microvascular decompression surgery in the United States, 1996 to 2000: Mortality rates, morbidity rates, and the effects of hospital and surgeon volumes. Neurosurgery 52:1251–1261, 2003.

89. Kaufmann AM, Krawetz P, Hobson D, et al: Management variations for hemifacial spasm [Abstract]. J Neurosurg 92:549, 2000.

90. Tomii M, Onoue H, Yasue M, et al: Microscopic measurement of the facial nerve root exit zone from central glial myelin to peripheral Schwann cell myelin. J Neurosurg 99:121–124, 2003.

91. Fukuda M, Kameyama S, Honda Y, et al: Hemifacial spasm resulting from facial nerve compression near the internal acoustic meatus—case report. Neurol Med Chir (Tokyo) 37:771–774, 1997.

92. Ryu H, Yamamoto S, Sugiyama K, et al: Hemifacial spasm caused by vascular compression of the distal portion of the facial nerve: Report of seven cases. J Neurosurg 88:605–609, 1998.

93. Bejjani GK, Sekhar LN: Repositioning of the vertebral artery as treatment for neurovascular compression syndromes: Technical note. J Neurosurg 86:728–732, 1997.

94. Fukushima T: Posterior fossa microvascular decompression in the management of hemifacial spasm and trigeminal neuralgia. No Shinkei Geka 10:1257–1261, 1982.

95. Kyoshima K, Watanabe A, Toba Y, et al: Anchoring method for hemifacial spasm associated with vertebral artery: Technical note. Neurosurgery 45:1487–1491, 1999.

96. Rawlinson JN, Coakham HB: The treatment of hemifacial spasm by sling retraction. Br J Neurosurg 2:173–178, 1988.

97. Shigeno T, Kumai J, Endo M, et al: Snare technique of vascular transposition for microvascular decompression—technical note. Neurol Med Chir (Tokyo) 42:184–189, 2002.

98. Badr-El-Dine M, El Garem HF, Talaat AM, et al: Endoscopically assisted minimally invasive microvascular decompression of hemifacial spasm. Otol Neurol 23:122–128, 2002.

99. Magnan J, Caces F, Locatelli P, et al: Hemifacial spasm: Endoscopic vascular decompression. Otolaryngol Head Neck Surg 117:308–314, 1997.

100. Ryu H, Yamamoto S, Miyamoto T: Atypical hemifacial spasm. Acta Neurochir (Wien) 140:1173–1176, 1998.

101. Kaufmann AM: Results with the Jannetta procedure [Abstract]. Can J Neurol Sci 30:I04, 2003.

102. McLaughlin MR, Jannetta PJ, Clyde BL, et al: Microvascular decompression of cranial nerves: Lessons learned after 4400 operations. J Neurosurg 90:1–8, 1999.

103. Moller AR, Moller MB: Does intraoperative monitoring of auditory evoked potentials reduce incidence of hearing loss as a complication of microvascular decompression of cranial nerves? Neurosurgery 24:257–263, 1989.

104. Wilkinson M, Chan S, Kozey-Rodgers M, et al: Routine intra-operative monitoring improves neurological outcome [Abstract]. Can J Neurol Sci 30:I07, 2003.

105. Sekiya T, Moller AR, Janetta PJ: Pathophysiological mechanisms of intraoperative and postoperative hearing deficits in cerebellopontine angle surgery: An experimental study. Neurochirurgie (Wien) 81:142–151, 1986.

106. Sekiya T, Moller AR: Avulsion rupture of the internal auditory artery during operations in the cerebellopontine angle manipulations: An electrophysiological and morphological study in dogs. Neurosurgery 21:631–637, 1987.

107. Sekiya T, Moller AR: Effects of cerebellar retractions on the cochlear nerve: An experimental study on rhesus monkeys. Neurochirurgie (Wien) 90:45–52, 1988.

108. Wahlig JB, Kaufmann A, Balzer J, et al: Intraoperative loss of auditory function relieved by microvascular decompression of the cochlear nerve. Can J Neurol Sci 26:44–47, 1999.

109. Isu T, Kamada K, Mabuchi S, et al: Intra-operative monitoring by facial electromyographic responses during microvascular decompression surgery for hemifacial spasm. Acta Neurochir (Wien) 138:19–23, 1996.

110. Jakob J, Mooij MD, Mustafa MK, et al: Hemifacial spasm: Intraoperative electromyographic monitoring as a guide for microvascular decompression. Neurology 49:1365–1371, 2001.

111. Kiya N, Banner U, Yamauchi K, et al: Monitoring of facial evoked EMG for hemifacial spasm: A critical analysis of its prognostic value. Acta Neurochir (Wien) 143:365–368, 2001.

112. Lovely TJ, Getch CC, Jannetta PJ: Delayed facial weakness after microvascular decompression of cranial nerve VII. Surg Neurol 50:449–452, 1998.

113. Ishikawa M, Nakanishi T, Takamiya Y, et al: Delayed resolution of residual hemifacial spasm after microvascular decompression operations. Neurosurgery 49:847–854, 2001.

114. Shin JC, Chung UH, Kim YC, et al: Prospective study of microvascular decompression in hemifacial spasm. Neurosurgery 40:730–734, 1997.

115. Goto Y, Matsushima T, Natori Y, et al: Delayed effects of the microvascular decompression on hemifacial spasm: A retrospective study of 131 consecutive operated cases. Neurol Res 24:296–300, 2002.

116. Kondo A: Follow-up results of microvascular decompression in trigeminal neuralgia and hemifacial spasm. Neurosurgery 40:46–51, 1997.

117. Samii M, Gunther T, Iaconetta G, et al: Microvascular decompression to treat hemifacial spasm: Long-term results for a consecutive series of 143 patients. Neurosurgery 50:712–719, 2002.

118. Sweet WH, Poletti CE: Complications of precutaneous rhizotomy and microvascular decompression operations for facial pain. In Schmidek HH, Sweet WH (eds): Operative Neurosurgery Techniques: Indications, Methods, and Results, 2nd ed. Orlando: Grune & Stratton, 1988, pp 1139–1143.

119. Piatt JH Jr, Wilkins RH: Treatment of tic douloureux and hemifacial spasm by posterior fossa exploration: Therapeutic implications of various neurovascular relationships. Neurosurgery 14:462–471, 1984.

120. Payne TD, Tew JM: Recurrence of hemifacial spasm after microvascular decompression. Neurosurgery 38:686–691, 2003.

Current Management of Cervical Dystonia

JEFFREY E. ARLE and THOMAS N. WARD

Cervical dystonia, a term now preferred to *spasmodic torticollis* or *torticollis* is the most common form of focal dystonia (Table 105-1). This condition affects more than 50,000 people in the United States alone.[1,2] Cervical involvement is part of a spectrum within the larger picture of generalized dystonia, although it is unusual for adult patients to progress from cervical dystonia to a more generalized form. This chapter delineates most aspects of the medical and surgical management of this often severely disabling disorder.

NEUROLOGIC ASSESSMENT AND MANAGEMENT

Dystonia is a neurologic condition characterized by prolonged, sustained muscle contractions that result in abnormal body positions or twisting movements and may be associated with repetitive movements such as tremor.[3,4]

Dystonias are classified in various ways: by age of onset, by etiology, by genetics, or by which part(s) of the body are affected. When affecting one body part, it is called a focal dystonia.[5] Cervical dystonia is the most common focal dystonia, but may also occur clinically as part of a more widespread dystonia, which results in abnormal positions of the head and neck. Most cases of cervical dystonia are idiopathic, although a careful history often reveals a familial occurrence of other movement disorders, including other

dystonias such as writer's cramp or tremor. The superimposed head tremor that occurs in some cases may be either a dystonic tremor or essential tremor, which is often comorbid with cervical dystonia.[4]

Secondary cervical dystonia is relatively uncommon. Although an underlying etiology is unlikely to be found, a careful neurologic evaluation is appropriate to look for other etiologies of torticollis (see Table 105-1). The more common secondary forms of cervical dystonia are either post-traumatic or due to dopamine-blocking medications such as metoclopramide and neuroleptic agents.[5]

Specific inquiry needs to be made about medications, toxic exposures, occupational history, and head/neck/upper extremity trauma. Psychiatric history is important; while psychogenic dystonia is uncommon, it does occasionally occur. More importantly, such a history might lead one to suspect exposure to neuroleptics, or to the possibility of a neurologic condition that can manifest as psychiatric illness, such as Huntington's disease or lupus.

Features to assess during the interview and examination include the position of the head/neck/shoulders, any associated movements such as tremor, and the presence of a geste antagoniste. The presence of such sensory tricks as touching the chin or placing the occiput against the wall to restore normal posture has been thought to be pathognomonic of dystonia. Occupational history, history of medication use, history of trauma, and family history should be explored in detail.[1] Beyond the history and examination, ancillary testing such as magnetic resonance imaging of the brain and cervical spine are useful.

TREATMENT

Until recently, treatment with various oral medications was the initial form of therapy for this disorder. Anticholinergic agents (e.g., trihexyphenidyl), benzodiazepines, baclofen, and dopaminergic agents have all been tried and retain some utility, especially as adjunct therapy.[2] Significant side effects limit their efficacy. These agents may be tried as initial therapy, especially in mild/responsive cases, or used in addition to treatment with botulinum toxin and/or surgery (see below).

Botulinum toxin injections have become the mainstay in the treatment of cervical dystonia.[5] The concept of utilizing this potent biologic agent as a medical therapy was pioneered by Drs. Alan Scott and Edward Schantz.[6] During the 1980s, the therapeutic use of botulinum toxin was studied extensively for many conditions, especially cervical dystonia. By 1990 it was demonstrated to be highly effective and safe,[7] and U.S. Food and Drug Administration approval has been granted for treatment of this condition both with types A (Botox) and B (Myobloc, known in Europe as Neurobloc). The various preparations of toxin are not interchangeable and dosing must be individualized. The advantages of using this form of treatment are that the clinical effects remain largely local, and doses can be adjusted both in terms of where the injections are placed and the size of the dose. Side effects are generally mild, predictable, and temporary.[4] This therapy should be administered by physicians experienced in the use of this agent and by those who are able to adjust therapy and manage side effects.

Botulinum toxin works in dystonia by causing a reversible chemical denervation. The toxin is taken up by cholinergic nerve endings and prevents the release of acetylcholine, causing a temporary chemical denervation. For type A, clinical weakness may begin to manifest by the first or second day after injection, and maximal clinical effects usually occur in less than 2 weeks. The duration of benefit typically averages 3 months.[8]

There are various injection strategies that have been used to treat cervical dystonia with botulinum toxin. The key to successful management involves selecting which muscles to inject and at what dose of toxin, thereby to weaken them appropriately. If the pattern of torticollis strongly suggests which muscles are involved based on clinical inspection/examination, then an injection strategy may be made on clinical grounds (Table 105-2).[9] Should clinical assessment alone yield an unsatisfactory response, electromyographic (EMG) assessment may help disclose which muscles, including deeper muscles, are involved, and to what extent. There is some controversy as to whether initial use of EMG assessment and guidance provides superior results.[4,10]

Candidates for this therapy are of most any age, although contractures will not respond. Contraindications include pregnancy, concurrent use of other drugs that impair neuromuscular transmission such as aminoglycosides, and neuromuscular disorders such as myasthenia gravis and Lambert-Eaton syndrome.[4] Side effects are generally mild and temporary and include excessive weakness, dysphagia, and dry mouth (particularly with type B toxin). Dysphagia is a common complaint of patients with cervical dystonia even prior to treatment, and specific inquiry regarding this problem needs to be made at the initial assessment.[11] When dysphagia

occurs due to or exacerbated by botulinum toxin therapy, it seems to be more likely with higher doses of toxin, especially when given anteriorly in the neck, such as the sternocleidomastoid (SCM) muscles. It has been shown that the distance to the pharyngeal muscles is shorter with injections into the SCM. Women, presumably due to smaller neck circumferences, may be at higher risk. Borodic has given useful suggestions to limit this complication, such as limiting dosing of Botox to less than 100 units in the SCM.[12]

Botulinum toxin therapy for cervical dystonia is successful for the majority of patients who receive it, and pain, which is a frequent associated problem, often responds to this therapy as well. Injections can be repeated every several months depending on need. Occasional patients do not respond well to these agents. These "primary nonresponders" are not fully understood, although suboptimal injection strategy and insufficient dosing are invoked as explanations. Another clinical problem, secondary nonresponse (loss of response), may also occur. Some individuals produce neutralizing antibodies that render subsequent toxin therapy ineffective. There are several ways of assessing patients for the presence of these antibodies. Repeated high doses of botulinum toxin with inadequate intervals between treatment sessions are thought to explain these occurrences. Patients who have become unresponsive to one antigenic type of toxin may be candidates for therapy with another type.[4,13]

Botulinum toxin therapy may be used as initial treatment for cervical dystonia, or after drug therapy or surgical treatment. Conversely, drug therapy may be added if the response to botulinum toxin is inadequate. Patients who have not achieved an adequate response to drugs and/or botulinum toxin may be candidates for surgical evaluation.

NEUROSURGICAL OPTIONS AND TECHNIQUES

As Bertrand noted on this subject in a previous edition of this book, the great majority of patients with cervical dystonia have symptoms that resolve during sleep, are not psychogenic, can be initiated by a single trauma, are exacerbated by emotion, and overall have few instances of complete and persisting remission (less than 5%). Despite advances in medical control using botulinum toxin, up to 20% of patients become resistant to these agents, have no

---

TABLE 105-2 ▪ Initial Clinical Injection Strategy

Position	Muscle(s) Involved	Dose Range (Botox) (Approximate)
Pure rotation of head	Contralateral SCM	20–100 units
Head turned, face down	Contralateral SCM, ipsilateral splenius capitis, splenius cervicis, trapezius	20–100 units in SCM 100–150 units
Head turned, face up	Ipsilateral SCM, ipsilateral splenius capitis, splenius cervicis, trapezius	20–100 units 100–150 units
Retrocollis	Bilateral posterior cervical muscle groups (splenius capitis, splenius cervicis, trapezius)	40–120 units per side
Shoulder elevation	Ipsilateral levator scapulae, ipsilateral trapezius	20–60 units

Typical maximal dose of Botox per session for CD is 250 units.
Adapted from Borodic GE, Mills L, Joseph M: Botulinum A toxin for the treatment of adult-onset spasmodic torticollis. Plast Reconstr Surg 87(2): 285–289, 1991.

beneficial effect from the injections, or have other adverse side effects.[14] These patients, if their dystonia is severe enough, may become candidates for surgical intervention.

Surgical treatments for cervical dystonia have been attempted since at least the 17th century beginning with sectioning of the sternocleidomastoid muscle by Minnius, a German physician, in 1641.[15] Sectioning of either the spinal accessory nerve (Buyalsky, 1850) or the first three anterior cervical roots has also been described in early surgical treatises.[16,17] Not only do such references suggest that invasive treatments have been tried for several centuries, but also that cervical dystonia as a disorder has been recognized as such for at least as long, although the term *dystonia* itself is credited to Oppenheim from a description in 1911.[18] Despite the array of sectioning, denervating, stimulating, or ablating techniques that have been tried, cervical dystonia remains a complex disorder without a perfect treatment. Some of the still-employed surgical techniques from the more recent past as well as more current applications of deep brain stimulation (DBS) and ablation will be reviewed here with an emphasis on these more recent developments.

An excellent critical review was provided by Lang,[19] who examined the complications and outcome data from the literature, concluding that, in general, poor controls, inadequate follow-up, poor characterization of pre- and postoperative deficits, and lack of randomized, blinded, and/or prospective studies significantly hamper the ability to decide whether or not most of the surgical techniques are beneficial and justify any attendant morbidity. Complication rates with these procedures can be significant. Moreover, determining the best methods of assessing outcomes in dystonia with either medical or surgical management remains a subject of debate, not because there aren't particular scales to use, but as in Parkinson's disease, there is not yet a consensus as to which aspects of dystonia might truly contribute to quality of life versus merely the focal motor change.[20–22]

Cervical dystonia is now almost universally managed by injections of botulinum toxin.[23,24] Usually, type A toxin is used initially, but over the previous 10 to 15 years other subtypes (e.g., B or F) have been tried.[25] An early summary of the development of botulinum toxin for widespread clinical use can be found in the reports of Schantz and Johnson and specifically for this indication in those of Poewe and Wissel and Giladi and colleagues, among others.[6,23,26] Large series suggest that the rate of achieving benefit with botulinum toxin alone is high and the complication rate is quite low.[8,26–29] As noted earlier, selective injections using data as to which muscles are involved by EMG, and judicious dosing, can be most beneficial and is, in many ways, a more attractive option than performing surgical selective denervation procedures.

Although bilateral neck injections can cause dysphagia and, rarely, require intubation for airway protection, the downside of botulinum toxin treatments is almost exclusively that they need to be repeated on a fairly regular basis. Some patients, however, may see relief of symptoms for several years after a single injection as opposed to receiving injections every 3 to 6 months.[30] Overall, patients who initially respond to botulinum toxin injections but then become resistant (presumably from antibody development) have better outcomes from more invasive denervation procedures.[31–33] Newer subtypes of the toxin are being

evaluated to supplement the initial botulinum toxin type A failures,[34] and many failures from botulinum toxin may be avoided by using toxin with different protein load characteristics[35] where antibodies may be less likely to develop.

Failures with botulinum toxin treatments have been managed more often over the previous two decades with selective denervation procedures than with any other surgical procedure.[33,36–41] Dandy had sought to develop and refine this approach over 70 years ago.[42] It should be noted, however, as with most instances of historical prominence, there are others who now in retrospect lend appropriate context to what is remembered many years later. In this case, McKenzie reported on sectioning the spinal accessory and upper cervical nerves through an intradural approach 6 years prior to Dandy's report.[43] Moreover, McKenzie was modifying a report by Taylor in 1915,[44] who had described posterior rhizotomies of the upper four cervical roots for spasmodic torticollis. Dandy felt a more peripheral approach was perhaps less morbid. Finney and Hughson described the intradural approach as "unnecessarily dangerous."[45] However, as Bertrand pointed out, their extradural sectioning without the selective data provided by EMG could not have been significantly different functionally from the rhizotomies they had criticized.[46]

Before the more recent versions of selective nerve sectioning, anterior rhizotomies were the mainstay of treatment, although long-term follow-up was sparsely studied other than anecdotally, and the rate of swallowing or sensory deficits postoperatively is now considered unacceptably high.[19] It is still unclear whether a significant long-term (greater than 5-year) benefit occurs with the more selective denervation techniques. Although Ford and co-workers examined 16 patients with 5-year follow-up, Cohen-Gadol and colleagues examined 162 patients at 3 months and then 130 of those at an average of 3.5 years.[39,41] By collapsing average numbers from the Cohen-Gadol analysis, it appears that approximately 50% of these patients had good to excellent results maintained over 3.5 years, whereas Ford and colleagues concluded that only about a third of their patients improved over 5 years and the average improvement was 30%. Braun and Richter studied 155 patients over 13 years, but with an average follow-up period of only 32.8 months.[33] Good to excellent results were seen in just under 50% of their patients as well, and there was an 11% recurrence rate. Meyer reported on 30 patients, with an average of 26 months of follow-up.[40] Taira and Hori reported on 30 patients who underwent a modified denervation procedure and were compared with 20 patients who underwent the more classic (Bertrand-type) denervation.[47] Their approach involved intradural ventral rhizotomies of C1 and C2 and extradural sectioning of the C3–6 posterior rami along with contralateral peripheral sectioning of the spinal accessory nerve. Sensory loss in the C2 distribution in their modified technique was significantly diminished, as was blood loss. Another thoughtful review of the earlier and more recent rhizotomy literature has been provided by Villavicencio and Friedman, who themselves reported over 80% good to excellent results in 58 patients over a year after surgery from anterior cervical nerve root and selective spinal accessory nerve sectioning.[48] One patient, however, died from pneumonia after having swallowing difficulties from the surgery, two patients had cervical subluxations following the procedures, and another developed a transient myelopathy postoperatively. Krauss and co-workers. also used intradural sectioning and extradural sectioning in a review of 46 patients who had been medically refractory.[38] An advantage of their study was that average follow-up was 6.5 years. Their outcomes showed that only 33% of patients were excellent or notably improved by surgery.

Among older, less well-documented studies assessing myotomy or myectomy, microvascular decompressions without nerve sectioning, and various combinations of C1 through C6 rhizotomies, 70% to 90% of patients are reported as having good to excellent results.[46,49–51] More recent, better-documented studies typically find that 30% to 40% have good or excellent results. Bertrand's more recent publication reviewed his experience with 260 cases of medically refractory cervical dystonia treated with selective denervation (but 26 having a central ablative procedure as well), involving the posterior rami between C1 and C6 as determined by the degree of each individual component of the torticollis. Of these patients, 40% had total relief of abnormal movements and another 48% had very good results with some residual abnormal movements.[37]

A summary of muscles typically involved in rotational torticollis, anterocollis, retrocollis, or laterocollis and, in particular, capturing the essence of how to think about the problem overall can be found in this passage from Bertrand[37]:

The unqualified statement that spasmodic torticollis is a bilateral disease, which dates back to the days before electromyography, has been detrimental to the evolution of its surgical management and has led to the impression that antagonist muscles on either side are usually involved. On the contrary, in a classic case of rotational torticollis without anterocollis or retrocollis, spontaneous abnormal discharges can be found in the sternocleidomastoid on one side and the posterior cervical group, especially the splenius, on the other. The contralateral antagonist muscles do not participate or may even be inhibited. Rarely, the contralateral semispinalis may contribute to rotation, but the trapezius is never involved. When the patient attempts to turn against the abnormal movements, the affected antagonist muscles may discharge instead of relax. In retrocollis, the extensors on either side, which are then synergists, evidently discharge simultaneously, whereas in laterocollis, the muscles that participate are all on the same side, for instance, the posterior cervical group with the ipsilateral sternocleidomastoid and possibly the trapezius and levator scapulae. In most instances, a combination of movements occurs, such as rotation with extension or flexion or inclination, so that the muscles that seem involved must be carefully verified because combinations vary from one patient to another. Flexion with inclination of the head to the left and rotation to the right may be caused by involvement of the left sternocleidomastoid and the ipsilateral semispinalis, whereas rotation to the right with slight inclination and extension of the occiput to the right suggests involvement of the left sternocleidomastoid combined mostly with the right splenius. In lateroretrocollis, if extension is pronounced, the contralateral semispinalis may be involved. Rarely, the sternomastoid contralateral to the movement may be discharging in an attempt to reduce the movement. Also, if muscle involvement is more diffuse, a tremor might persist

after surgery. However, large movements evidently cannot occur unless the antagonists are relaxed. Unfortunately, the false impression of bilaterality has led to the use of indiscriminate bilateral symmetric denervation, such as bilateral rhizotomy, thus suppressing normal uninvolved muscles necessary for normal posture and movements (Bertrand, 1995, pp 1649–1650).

Stereotactic ablations have been tried both for other forms of dystonia and specifically for cervical dystonia. Complications from this procedure include fatal or debilitating hemorrhage, although a small hemorrhage near the tip of the ablating electrode may serve to contribute to the desired lesion rather than compromising the outcome in some instances. Bertrand noted, after reviewing 117 cases for the International Congress on Neurological Surgery in 1985, that he had begun treating patients with "spasmodic torticollis" or adult-onset dystonia dominated by cervical involvement using either thalamotomy or pallidotomy followed by selective denervation procedures. However, after several years, he abandoned the central ablative procedures in favor of peripheral denervation first, as he found that correcting the more severe abnormal movements "often sufficed."[46]

In the early 1950s, pallidotomy was attempted with some success, but throughout the 1960s this procedure was largely displaced by thalamotomy.[52,53] Two studies were also reported with lesions in part of the ansa lenicularis to interrupt part of the frontal capsular head-turning pathways.[54,55] Review of the efficacy of these lesions over 20 years indicate that some benefit can be achieved with them in many

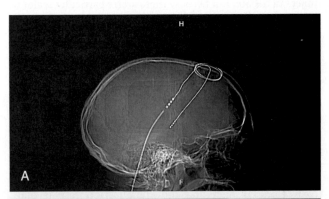
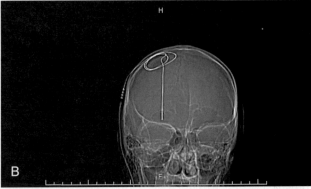

FIGURE 105-1 *A,* Lateral skull x-ray showing the implanted deep brain stimulating electrode and connecting wire placed in the globus pallidus pars interna for dystonia. *B,* Anteroposterior skull x-ray in the same patient.

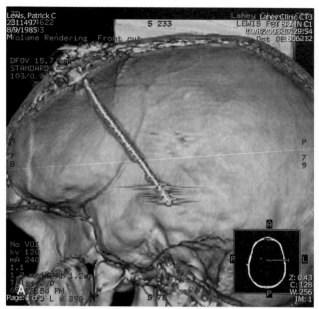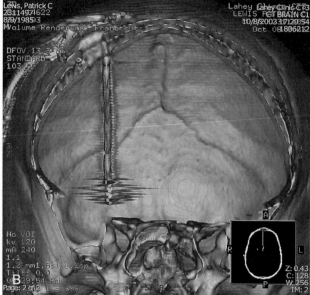

FIGURE 105-2 *A,* Lateral three-dimensional reconstruction magnetic resonance scan in the place of the deep brain stimulation electrode in the globus pallidus pars interna for dystonia. *B,* An anteroposterior reconstruction in the same patient.

hyperkinetic disorders including cervical dystonia but that bilateral ablations are likely to produce unwanted deficits (e.g., dysarthria). Such conclusions are supported by the analyses of Tasker, who reviewed the results of almost 1000 patients who underwent thalamotomy for dystonia.[56] Most cases were not for cervical dystonia, but the procedure is the same as that used for cervical dystonia and the conclusions regarding complication rates are consistent.

During an ablative procedure, recordings and stimulation are often performed prior to lesioning. This enables surgeons to appreciate that stimulation, particularly at higher frequencies, can alleviate tremor, rigidity, and bradykinesia. Because of its similarities to lesions in effect, stimulation was tried in the thalamus, globus pallidus, and subthalamic nucleus for both essential tremor and Parkinson's disease with success. More recently, high-frequency stimulation has been tried in generalized dystonias (DYT-1 positive or negative, or secondary generalized dystonias) as well as in cervical dystonia. The advantages of stimulation versus ablation are reversibility, avoidance of bilateral deficits, and programmability. The drawbacks with the current stimulation devices are a somewhat higher infection rate and the need for battery changes. Several studies involving DBS treatment for dystonia have been reported.[57–60] Mundinger tried DBS for cervical dystonia and reported his results in seven patients in 1977.[61–63] His target was in the subthalamic nucleus and included parts of H1 and H2 in the region of the ansa and zona incerta. Krauss and colleagues reported an experience with eight patients with severe cervical dystonias who were refractory to medical management. In three of the eight there was a severe cervical myelopathy, a result of the chronic cervical motion and abnormal posturing. These patients underwent DBS in the globus pallidus pars interna (GPi) bilaterally. After a mean of 20 months of stimulation, these patients demonstrated improvements in their severity, disability, and pain scores of 63%, 69%, and 50%.

The overall mean amplitude used was 3.8 V, higher than a typical value needed to treat Parkinson's patients. All three patients with cervical myelopathy subsequently underwent cervical decompression after placement of the DBS electrodes[38] (Figs. 105-1 and 105-2).

CONCLUSIONS

Cervical dystonia is a disease eminently treatable with botulinum toxin in the majority of cases. However, when this approach is not helpful, either selective denervation with or without central ablation unilaterally or DBS (particularly for bilateral interventions) should be considered. Procedures in the GPi or possibly the subthalamic nucleus are the most efficacious. Because DBS has a very low (less than 3%) morbidity rate and is reversible, programmable, and can be used bilaterally, it would seem to be the option of choice currently when medical treatments fail.

REFERENCES

1. Consky ES, Lang AE: Clinical assessments of patients with cervical dystonia. In Jankovic J, Hallett M (eds): Therapy with Botulinum Toxin. New York: Marcel Decker, 1994, p 2172.
2. Velickovic M, Benabou R, Brin MF: Cervical dystonia pathophysiology and treatment options. Drugs 61(13):1921–1943, 2001.
3. Jankovic J, Fahn S: Dystonic disorders. In Jankovic J, Tolosa E (eds): Parkinson's Disease and Movement Disorders, 3rd ed. Baltimore: Williams & Wilkins, 1998, pp 513–551.
4. Lou J-S, Jankovic J: Essential tremor: Clinical correlates in 350 patients. Neurology 41:234–238, 1991.
5. Tintner R, Jankovic J: Botulinum toxin for the treatment of cervical dystonia. Expert Opin Pharmacother 2(12):1985–1994, 2001.
6. Schantz EJ, Johnson EA: Botulinum toxin: The story of its development for the treatment of human disease. Perspect Biol Med 40(4):317–327, 1997.
7. The Therapeutics and Technology Assessment Subcommittee of the American Academy of Neurology. Assessment: The clinical usefulness of botulinum toxin-A in treating neurologic disorders. Neurology 40:1332–1336, 1990.

8. Greene P, Kang U, Fahn S, et al: Double-blind, placebo-controlled trial of botulinum toxin injections for the treatment of spasmodic torticollis. Neurology 40:1213–1218, 1990.

9. Borodic GE, Mills L, Joseph M: Botulinum A toxin for the treatment of adult-onset spasmodic torticollis. Plast Reconstr Surg 87(2):285–289, 1991.

10. Comella CL, Buchman AS, Tanner CM, et al: Botulinum toxin injection for spasmodic torticollis: Increased magnitude of benefit with electromyographic assistance. Neurology 42:878–882, 1992.

11. Comella CL, Tanner CM, DeFoor-Hill L, Smith C: Dysphagia after botulinum toxin injections for spasmodic torticollis: Clinical and radiologic findings. Neurology 42:1307–1310, 1992.

12. Borodic GE, Joseph M, Fay L, et al: Botulinum A toxin for the treatment of spasmodic torticollis: Dysphagia and regional toxin spread. Head Neck 12:392–398, 1990.

13. Jankovic J, Schwartz K: Response and immunoresistance to botulinum toxin injections. Neurology 45:1743–1746, 1995.

14. Adler CH, Kumar R: Pharmacological and surgical options for the treatment of cervical dystonia. Neurology 55(12 Suppl 5):9–14, 2000.

15. Putnam TJ, Herz E, Glaser GH: Spasmodic torticollis. Arch Neurol Psych 61:240–247, 1949.

16. Aziz T, Yianni J: Recent advances in the surgical treatment of dystonia. ACNR 2(3):14–15, 2002.

17. Keen WW: A new operation for spasmodic wry neck: Namely, division or exsection of the nerves supplying the posterior rotator muscles of the head. Ann Surg 13:44–47, 1891.

18. Oppenheim H: Uber Eine Eigenartige Krampfkrankheit des Kindlichen und Jugenlichen Alters. Neurol Centralbl 30:1090–1107, 1911.

19. Lang AE: Surgical treatment of dystonia. Dystonia 3. Adv Neurol 78, 1998.

20. Lindeboom R, de Haan RJ, Aramideh M, et al: Treatment outcomes in cervical dystonia: A clinimetric study [Review]. Mov Disord 11(4):371–376, 1996.

21. Tarsy D: Comparison of clinical rating scales in treatment of cervical dystonia with botulinum toxin. Mov Disord 12(1):100–102, 1997.

22. Lindeboom R, Brans JW, Aramideh M, et al: Treatment of cervical dystonia: A comparison of measures for outcome assessment. Mov Disord 13(4):706–712, 1998.

23. Poewe W, Wissel J: Use of botulinum toxin in the treatment of cervical dystonia [Review]. Baillieres Clin Neurol 2(1):179–185, 1993.

24. Poewe W, Deuschl G, Nebe A, et al: What is the optimal dose of botulinum toxin A in the treatment of cervical dystonia? Results of a double-blind, placebo-controlled, dose ranging study using Dysport— German Dystonia Study Group. J Neurol Neurosurg Psychiatry 64(1):13–17, 1998.

25. Greene P, Fahn S: Use of botulinum toxin type F injections to treat torticollis in patients with immunity to botulinum toxin type A. Mov Disord 8:479–483, 1993.

26. Giladi N, Meer J, Kidan C, et al: Interventional neurology: Botulinum toxin as a potent symptomatic treatment in neurology. Isr J Med Sci 30(11):816–819, 1994.

27. Borgmann R: Treatment of spasmodic torticollis with botulinum toxin type A—A five year experience [Norwegian]. Tidsskr Nor Laegeforen 117(13):1889–1891, 1997.

28. Kwan MC, Ko KF, Chan TP, Chan YW: Treatment of dystonia with botulinum A toxin: A retrospective study of 170 patients. Hong Kong Med J 4(3):279–282, 1998.

29. Naumann M, Yakovleff A, Durif F, BOTOX Cervical Dystonia Prospective Study Group: A randomized, double-masked, crossover comparison of the efficacy and safety of botulinum toxin type A produced from the original bulk toxin source and current bulk toxin source for the treatment of cervical dystonia. J Neurol 249(1):57–63, 2002.

30. Giladi N, Meer J, Kidan H, Honigman S: Long-term remission of idiopathic cervical dystonia after treatment with botulinum toxin. Eur Neurol 44(3):144–146, 2000.

31. Braun V, Richter HP, Schroder JM: Selective peripheral denervation for spasmodic torticollis: Is the outcome predictable? J Neurol 242(8):504–507, 1995.

32. Braun V, Mayer M, Antoniadis G, et al: Reconstruction of the spinal accessory nerve with an anastomosis to the dorsal C3 branch: Technical note. Neurosurgery 38(1):208–210, 1996.

33. Braun V, Richter HP: Selective peripheral denervation for spasmodic torticollis: 13 year experience with 155 patients. J Neurosurg 97 (2 Suppl):207–212, 2002.

34. Dressler D, Bigalke H, Benecke R: Botulinum toxin type B in antibody-induced botulinum toxin type A therapy failure. J Neurol 250(8):967–969, 2003.

35. Jankovic J, Vuong KD, Ahsan J: Comparison of efficacy and immunogenicity of original versus current botulinum toxin in cervical dystonia. Neurology 60(7):1186–1188, 2003.

36. Arce C, Russo L: Selective peripheral denervation: A surgical alternative in the treatment for spasmodic torticollis: Review of fifty-five patients. Mov Disord 7:128, 1992.

37. Bertrand CM: Selective peripheral denervation for spasmodic torticollis: Surgical technique, results, and observations in 260 cases. Surg Neurol 40(2):96–103, 1993.

38. Krauss JK, Loher TJ, Pohle T, et al: Pallidal deep brain stimulation in patients with cervical dystonia and severe cervical dyskinesias with cervical myelopathy. J Neurol Neurosurg Psychiatry 72:249–256, 2002.

39. Ford B, Louis ED, Greene P, Fahn S: Outcome of selective ramisectomy for botulinum toxin resistant torticollis. J Neurol Neurosurg Psychiatry 65(4):472–478, 1998.

40. Meyer CH: Outcome of selective peripheral denervation for cervical dystonia. Stereotact Funct Neurosurg 77(1–4):44–47, 2001.

41. Cohen-Gadol AA, Ahlskog JE, Matsumoto JY, et al: Selective Peripheral denervation for the treatment of intractable spasmodic torticollis: Experience with 168 patients at the Mayo Clinic. J Neurosurg 98(6):1247–1254, 2003.

42. Dandy WE: Operation for Treatment of Spasmodic Torticollis. Arch Surg 20:1021–1032, 1930.

43. McKenzie KG: Intrameningeal division of the spinal accessory and roots of the upper cervical nerves for the treatment of spasmodic torticollis. Surg Gynecol Obstet 39:5–10, 1924.

44. Taylor AS: Operation for relief of spasmodic torticollis. In Johnson (ed): Operative Therapeutics, vol 1. New York: Appleton-Century-Crofts, 1915, pp 525–612.

45. Finney JMT, Hughson W: Spasmodic torticollis. Ann Surg 81:255–269, 1925.

46. Bertrand CM: Surgical management of spasmodic torticollis and adult-onset dystonia. In Schmidek HH, Sweet WH (eds): Operative Neurosurgical Techniques, 3rd ed, vol 2. Philadelphia: WB Saunders, pp 1649–1659.

47. Taira T, Hori T: Peripheral neurotomy for torticollis: A new approach. Stereotact Funct Neurosurg 77(1–4):40–43, 2001.

48. Villavicencio AT, Friedman AH: Intradural rhizotomy for the treatment of torticollis, dystonias. In Gildenberg PL, Tasker RR (eds): Textbook of Stereotactic and Functional Neurosurgery. 1998, pp 1039–1051.

49. Hamby WB, Schiffer S: Spasmodic torticollis: Results after cervical rhizotomy in 50 cases. J Neurosurg 31:323–326, 1969.

50. Jho HD, Jannetta PJ: Spasmodic torticollis treated with microvascular decompression of the spinal accessory nerve and the brainstem. J Neurosurg 70:312A, 1989.

51. Chen X, Ma A, Liang J, et al: Selective denervation and resection of cervical muscles in the treatment of spasmodic torticollis: Long-term follow-up results in 207 cases. Stereotact Funct Neurosurg 75(2–3):96–102, 2000.

52. Cooper IS: Results of 1,000 consecutive basal ganglia operations for parkinsonism. Ann Intern Med 52:483–499, 1960.

53. Mundinger F, Riechert T: Die stereotaktischen Hirnoperationen zur Behandlung extrapyramidaler Bewengungsstörungen (Parkinsonismus und Hyperkinesen) und ihre Resultate. Fortschr Neurol Psychiatr 31:1–66, 1963.

54. Mazars G, Merienne L: Surgical treatment of spastic torticolloisand associated dyskinesias by interruption of cortico-capsular head-turning pathways. Excerpta Med Int Congress Series 293:18, 1974.

55. Stejskal L, Vladyka V, Tomanek Z: Surgical possibilities for alleviation of axial dyskinesias—Comparison with forced movements of the head and eyes. Appl Neurophysiol 44:320–329, 1981.

56. Tasker RR: Surgical treatment of the dystonias. In Gildenberg PL, Tasker RR (eds): Textbook of Stereotactic and Functional Neurosurgery. New York: McGraw-Hill, 1998, pp 1015–1032.

57. Coubes P, Roubertie A, Vayssiere N, et al: Treatment of DYT-1-generalised dystonia by stimulation of the internal globus pallidus. Lancet 355:2220–2221, 2000.

58. Vercuiel L, Pollak P, Fraix V, et al: Deep brain stimulation in the treatment of severe dystonia. J Neurol 248:695–700, 2001.

59. Parkin S, Aziz T, Gregory R, Bain P: Bilateral internal globus pallidus stimulation for the treatment of spasmodic torticollis. Mov Disord 16:489–493, 2001.

60. Krauss JK, Toups EG, Jankovic J, Grossman RG: Symptomatic and functional outcome of surgical treatment of cervical dystonia. J Neurol Neurosurg Psychiatry 63(5):642–648, 1997.

61. Bechtereva NP, Bondartchuk AN, Smirnov VM, et al: Therapeutic electrostimulations of deep brain structures. Vopr Neirokhir 1:7–12, 1972.

62. Bechtereva NP, Bondartchuk AN, Smirnov VM: Method of electrostimulation of the deep brain structures in treatment of some chronic diseases. Confin Neurol 37:136–140, 1975.

63. Mundinger F: New stereotactic treatment of spasmodic torticollis with a brain stimulation system [German]. Med Klin 72(46):1982–1986, 1977.

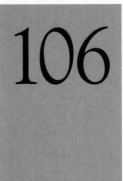

106 Retrogasserian Glycerol Rhizolysis in Trigeminal Neuralgia

BENGT LINDEROTH and STEN HÅKANSON

INTRODUCTION

Many patients with trigeminal neuralgia (TN) are elderly, often with concurrent diseases, and therefore there is a constant search for appropriate therapeutic methods with low surgical risk, little impact on facial sensibility, and the ability to be performed under local anesthesia. Glycerol rhizolysis, the procedure described in this chapter, is such a method. The availability of a method that can be used even in medically infirm patients may also widen the indications for surgical treatment, because the usual regimen with carbamazepine, other anticonvulsants, or baclofen is known to cause severe side effects in many patients. These problems apply particularly to patients with paroxysmal facial pain associated with multiple sclerosis (MS).

HISTORY

The discovery of the beneficial effects of glycerol in patients with TN was purely accidental. During the course of development of a procedure for producing lesions in the gasserian ganglion in patients with TN in the 1970s, in which the Leksell gamma knife in Stockholm was to be used, x-ray contrast medium (metrizamide) and glycerol were tried as vehicles for a radiopaque metal dust (tantalum powder). The tantalum powder was to be introduced into the retroganglionic cistern as a permanent marker to constitute a visible target for the subsequent stereotactic calculations.[1,2] Glycerol was chosen as the vehicle because, being the base for triglyceride formation in the body, it was presumed to be harmless, and its viscosity would ensure that the tantalum suspension was maintained long enough for the powder to be deposited in the trigeminal cistern. In fact, glycerol had been used earlier in the treatment of TN as a vehicle for the highly neurolytic phenol,[3] which was used for percutaneous treatment of TN at that time. It was noted that merely injecting the glycerol and tantalum dust mixture in patients abolished paroxysmal pain before the gamma knife procedure. On the basis of these observations, Håkanson developed the technique for treating TN by glycerol injection into the trigeminal cistern. The first series of patients was presented in 1981,[4] and the method was then rapidly adopted in many neurosurgical centers.

Over the years, many series of patients treated using Håkanson's procedure, or some variation of the original method, have been reported. The results from different series have been highly variable. In many centers the outcome has been quite satisfactory,[5-9] and glycerol rhizolysis has continued to be the method of choice, particularly for elderly and infirm patients. In other services, the results have been so discouraging (Siegfried, 1985, and Rhoton, 1985, unpublished results, both cited in Sweet[10]; Price, 1985, unpublished results, cited in Sweet[11] and Fujimaki and colleagues[12]) that some neurosurgeons have entirely abandoned the procedure.

In this chapter, beginning with a description of the mechanisms behind the beneficial effects of glycerol, the possible reasons for these discrepancies are examined and a standard procedure to ensure maximum efficacy and safety is described.

PROBABLE MECHANISMS OF ACTION OF GLYCEROL

Retrogasserian glycerol rhizolysis is thus a purely empirical method, the beneficial effects of glycerol having been discovered accidentally. There has been much debate about the putative mechanisms behind the effects of glycerol on paroxysmal pain. It is evident from the side effects (e.g., hypesthesia) that the substance is neurolytic in the concentrations used for injection.

An important issue is whether the neurolytic effect is selective for a certain fiber spectrum. From clinical observations, it is clear that the trigger mechanism for the pain paroxysms is activated by tactile stimulation and impulse propagation in large myelinated fibers.

Morphologic Effects of Glycerol

Glycerol is a trivalent alcohol normally present in human tissue, where it forms the skeleton of the triglycerides, among other functions.[13,14] Glycerol readily penetrates cell membranes and seems to possess distinct cryoprotective properties beneficial to cells. Its toxicity is low, and comparatively high doses must be injected systemically or intrathecally to induce toxic effects.[15,16] Glycerol's neurolytic action is thought to be due to its hypertonicity, a condition known to injure nerve fibers, especially thin, unmyelinated, and myelinated fibers.[17] Although the myelin sheath of the coarse fibers gives some transitory protection from this effect, length of exposure, neuron type, and the presence of previous demyelination may be important determinants of the vulnerability of individual fibers. For example, with longer exposures, Robertson[18] and Pal and colleagues[19] observed that myelinated fibers were particularly vulnerable, and the degree of damage positively correlated with fiber diameter.

Studies on isolated animal nerve fibers show morphologic changes after exposure to glycerol. These consist of disruption of the tight junction between the Schwann cells and the axolemma, without damage to the axon proper.[20] Bathing the fibers in glycerol initially causes the axons to shrink, with a return to basal volume after equilibration of the substance over the cell membranes. With transfer to iso-osmotic conditions, the fibers swell markedly before returning to their normal volume. Thus, marked structural changes are observed with glycerol administration, but the conduction properties of the treated nerve axons remain intact.[20]

After intraneural and perineural injection of glycerol, Håkanson[21] and Rengachary and associates[22] observed axolysis with marked myelin sheath swelling. The coarse myelinated fibers sustained the most severe damage, whereas the small-diameter myelinated and unmyelinated fibers are relatively well preserved.[19] In contrast, Bremerich and Reisert[23] found only slight histomorphologic changes after glycerol injection in the region of the foramen ovale in the rat in their long-term (180 days) comparative study of axonal damage after injection of glycerol, phenol-glycerol, and saline. A more recent study in dogs submitted to glycerol injection into one trigeminal ganglion[24] demonstrated axonolysis both in myelinated as well as in nonmyelinated fibers.

The damage following glycerol injection into a cavity with isotonic body fluid is probably considerably less severe. However, Lunsford and associates[9] observed extensive areas of myelin degradation and axonal swelling in cats subjected to retrogasserian glycerol injections 4 to 6 weeks earlier.

The site of glycerol effects has been specifically studied by Stajcic,[25] who injected ³H-labeled glycerol into peripheral branches of the maxillary nerve and in the infraorbital canal of rats. The amount of radioactivity detected in the nerve distal to the foramen rotundum, as well as in the ipsilateral and contralateral gasserian ganglion, was less than 0.1% in all specimens. The author concluded that a retrograde transport mechanism behind the effect is improbable and that the beneficial effect of glycerol occurs at the site of injection.

There is as yet no publication of an autopsy series of patients with TN treated by retrogasserian glycerol rhizolysis. Sweet[11] provides an anecdotal description of a patient undergoing a retrogasserian glycerol injection of the extreme volume of 1.5 mL, with subsequent development of anesthesia dolorosa. At a posterior fossa craniotomy "many months" later, the trigeminal rootlets were markedly atrophic.

Neurophysiologic Changes after Glycerol Application

It is likely that the change in osmolarity causes the damage to nerve axons, and the morphologic changes seem to be minimized by a gradual alteration in the osmolarity (e.g., by slowly instilling and removing glycerol from the compartment housing the axons). The functional consequences of glycerol application to normal and damaged nervous tissue are known only fragmentarily, but there are a few observations that might apply to the clinical use of the substance.

Burchiel and Russel[26] studied the effect of glycerol on normal and damaged nerves in a rat neuroma model. The neuromas, produced by sectioning of the saphenous nerve, were mechanosensitive and discharged both spontaneously and in response to light manipulation. These researchers found evidence supporting the view that glycerol exerts its major action on the large-diameter fibers. Exposure of the injured nerve to glycerol induced a short episode of increased spontaneous firing in the nerve, a response shown to originate from the myelinated fibers.

The observation by Rappaport and associates[27] that glycerol injected into neuromas was more effective than alcohol in decreasing autotomy in rats suggests that autotomy may be related to unpleasant "ticlike" paresthesias. The therapeutic mechanism, according to these investigators, could be suppression of ectopic impulse barrage from the neuroma.

Sweet and co-workers[28] found that glycerol injected into the trigeminal cistern of patients abolished the late components (corresponding to A-delta and C fibers) of trigeminal root potentials recorded with electric stimulation of the surface of the cheek. These recordings were made only minutes after the injection, and therefore do not permit conclusions concerning long-term effects.

Hellstrand and colleagues (unpublished data; see Håkanson[21]) studied the effects of glycerol both on isolated frog nerve and on trigeminal root fibers after cisternal injection in the cat. They observed a severe reduction of the evoked potentials with glycerol but a nearly total restoration after rinsing the compartment with saline. This recoverability probably has a bearing on the clinical effects and must be taken into account when interpreting the short-term observations of Sweet and associates[28] referred to previously. Based on the knowledge that glycerol requires at least 30 minutes to equilibrate across a membrane of a living cell and according to the aforementioned experimental observations, evacuation of the glycerol from the cistern after a short time (e.g., 5 to 20 minutes[10,29,30]) might induce more severe damage, especially to fine fiber systems, than a slow unloading by diffusion into the subarachnoid space.

Longer-term observations of trigeminal evoked potentials have been reported by Bennett and Lunsford,[31] who investigated patients before and 6 weeks after trigeminal glycerol rhizolysis. They confirmed the earlier findings of Bennett and Jannetta[32] that thresholds were elevated and evoked potentials had a markedly increased latency on the affected side compared with the healthy one. An additional, unexpected finding was that these aberrations were "normalized" after glycerol rhizolysis. Because partially demyelinated fibers are known to conduct with a slower velocity and at a lower rate,[33,34] they interpreted this finding to indicate that glycerol selectively attacked partially damaged trigeminal axons and, after their elimination, the evoked trigeminal potentials appeared "normalized."

Further long-term observations were supplied by Lunsford and colleagues,[9] who noted the clearest changes in trigeminal evoked potentials in cats in the large-diameter myelinated fibers, with additional changes noted as late as 6 weeks after the injection.

Quantitative sensory testing using von Frey hairs, mechanical pulses, and the Marstock technique[35] also corroborates the notion that glycerol acts mainly on the large myelinated fiber spectrum.[36] Eide and Stubhaug[37] examined thresholds for tactile and temperature stimuli in patients with TN before and after glycerol rhizolysis. They found evidence that pain relief after glycerol treatment involved normalization of previously abnormal temporal summation phenomena with little accompanying sensory loss. Kumar and associates[38] found postinjection quantitative abnormalities of the blink reflex that correlated with sensory impairment.

Thus experimental and clinical observations indicate that the effects of glycerol may be due to its hyperosmolarity and that the rate of alteration of osmolarity is critical for the effect. Furthermore, there are indications that the effect is exerted through actions on large myelinated fibers, notably those with previous damage to the myelin sheath, thereby possibly affecting the "trigger mechanism" for pain paroxysm. Glycerol may also downregulate central neuronal hyperexcitability, often without signs of significant additional nerve damage.[37]

INDICATIONS

The main indication for glycerol rhizolysis remains classic idiopathic TN. Common reasons for progressing to surgical treatment include deficient control of paroxysms in spite of an adequate pharmaceutical regimen, severe medication side effects, development of drug allergy or intolerance, and signs of hepatic malfunction ascribed to medication.

Paroxysmal facial pain in MS is another prime indication. The initial outcome in this group of patients is as satisfactory as for idiopathic TN, but the long-term results are, as with other available methods, less encouraging. This is further discussed below.

Patients with signs of deafferentation should, in principle, not be submitted to a neurolytic procedure. However, many patients with TN previously treated by other methods display signs of neural damage, such as hypesthesia, allodynia, hyperalgesia, and some degree of continuous deafferentation pain. Such patients should be accepted for treatment only if a paroxysmal pain component is dominant and after careful evaluation of sensory deficits. If such patients are accepted for glycerol rhizolysis, the procedure should be carried out with the utmost care, using only a small amount of glycerol.

The same considerations also apply to the use of glycerol rhizolysis in atypical facial pain/painful trigeminal neuropathy. In general, the method is not indicated in these cases. Only when a dominant paroxysmal component is present and the signs of deafferentation are slight may the method be considered. Both neurosurgeon and patient should be aware that the procedure might aggravate the deafferentation and therefore the constant neuropathic pain.

Preoperative Evaluation

The preoperative evaluation should be focused on the presence of typical signs of TN, previous treatments, the pharmaceutical regimen, the presence of sensory deficits, constant pain components, and ipsilateral hearing loss. Because we recommend the use of contrast medium injection in all cases, intolerance to iodine and previous adverse reactions to contrast medium should be determined. A magnetic resonance imaging study, or a computed tomography scan with and without contrast injection, should be performed before surgery. The surgeon must evaluate the patient before the procedure to individualize premedication and describe the details of the procedure to the patient to ensure good cooperation during its performance. Most patients tolerate the procedure well in local anesthesia with adequate premedication and with only slight sedation (see Technique section), but very anxious patients may require general anesthesia.

TECHNIQUE

The original technique of Håkanson has been subject to many modifications by various neurosurgeons. These variations encompass the type of anesthesia selected, general or local; patient position and fluoroscopic projection; whether cisternography is performed; other modes of localization of the needle tip (electric stimulation; reactions to drop-by-drop injection of glycerol); the dose of glycerol used; instillation of glycerol in one step or as minute volumes in an incremental fashion, with intermittent sensory testing; trials to empty the cistern after attaining a satisfactory effect according to perioperative testing; and how long the patient is kept sitting with the head flexed after completion of the procedure.

Some of these modifications have resulted in less satisfactory results.[10,12,29,39] We consider retrogasserian glycerol rhizolysis to be an anatomically oriented method aimed at graded lesioning of fibers in a certain locus. Thus the localization procedure should also be anatomic and the treatment should be meticulously performed, using the smallest possible volume of pure, sterile glycerol considered to be effective in each case.

The procedure as it is currently performed at the Department of Neurosurgery, Karolinska University Hospital, Stockholm, is described in this section.

Anesthesia and Sedation

Until the late 1990s, retrogasserian glycerol rhizolysis was performed with the patient awake and premedicated approximately 45 minutes before the start of the session with 5 to 10 mg of subcutaneous morphine hydrochloride-scopolamine and 2.5 mg of intramuscular droperidol. The doses were adjusted according to the age and condition of the patient. In some cases, 0.5 mg of atropine was given intravenously immediately before the procedure to prevent bradycardia during needle insertion. An intravenous line with slow infusion of Ringer's solution is maintained during and for some hours after the session.

Our current protocol involves sedation with intravenous propofol using a syringe-pump. No intubation is required and oxygen is supplied via a nasal catheter. Usually a low oral dose of benzodiazepine is used 1 hour preoperatively. The legs are wrapped or compression stockings applied to counteract blood pressure decrease in the semisitting position. General anesthesia and endotracheal intubation are used only in the particularly anxious patient. If used, it is important that the anesthesia be terminated with the patient in the sitting position with his or her head flexed according to the surgeon's instructions.

The skin at the point of needle insertion and the underlying soft tissue is infiltrated with local lidocaine 0.5%.

Positioning

Since the mid-1990s, a modified dentist's operating chair has been used in the surgical theater in conjunction with a standard C-arm fluoroscopic image intensifier with image-storing capacity, which provides sufficient picture quality for the clinical procedure.

In most cases, fluoroscopy with lateral projection is used when the cistern is punctured. Further guidance is obtained by switching to the anteroposterior projection. In difficult cases in which entering the proper part of the oval foramen is a problem, the patient's head may be extended and rotated 15 to 20 degrees from the affected side, and the fluoroscopy arm tilted to give an axial-oblique projection of the skull base including the foramen ovale. With some older equipment, it might be difficult to readily identify the proper foramen on the fluoroscopy monitor. If one needle has already penetrated the foramen, the identification should be easy, and a new needle can readily be inserted in the desired (often medial) part of the foramen.

Anatomic Landmarks and Important Structures

The trigeminal cistern is punctured by the anterior percutaneous route through the foramen ovale, as described by Härtel.[40] After local anesthesia, a 22-gauge lumbar cannula (outer diameter 0.7 mm; length 90 mm) is inserted from a point approximately 3 to 4 cm lateral to the corner of the mouth. The trajectory is aimed at a point that lies, in the lateral view, approximately 0.5 cm anterior to the anterior margin of the mandibular joint, and in the anteroposterior view, toward the medial margin of the pupil with the eyeball in the neutral position. There are several landmarks that may be used for reaching the foramen ovale,[41,42] but in most cases these two coordinates are sufficient.

Often, it is wise to direct the needle to touch the medial wall of the foramen. The needle is then withdrawn a short distance, redirected a few millimeters more lateral and introduced through the medial part of the foramen. Intermittent fluoroscopy is used during these maneuvers.

When the needle penetrates the foramen, the patient may experience a brief episode of pain due to penetration of V3 and the semilunar ganglion. As a rule, the cannula should not reach beyond the clival contour as seen on the orthogonal lateral projection.

When the tip of the cannula is located inside the arachnoid of the trigeminal cistern, there should be a spontaneous exit of cerebrospinal fluid (CSF). Because the location of the trigeminal ganglion and cistern can vary in relation to the landmarks of the skull base, a contrast injection must be performed to ascertain the correct site for glycerol injection. However, spontaneous CSF drainage is not sufficient for accepting the location as intracisternal.

Trigeminal Cisternography

The technique we use is essentially the same as that described by Håkanson,[43] although estimation of the cisternal volume is of less importance for deciding what volume of glycerol to inject. The contrast medium must be water soluble, with high radiographic attenuation and low toxicity, and must have a higher specific gravity than CSF. The contrast medium used since 1986 is iohexol (300 mg iodine/mL).[44] Approximately 0.3 to 0.6 mL is injected with the patient sitting with his or her head slightly flexed to retain as much of the medium in the cistern as possible. If intermittent fluoroscopy is used during injection, the position of the needle tip may be estimated immediately, but it should always be confirmed by radiography in both the lateral and anteroposterior projections. The typical appearance of the trigeminal cistern is illustrated in Figure 106-1. Ideally, the sensory root filaments (and sometimes the motor portion) should be visualized by lateral cisternography, leaving no doubt about the intracisternal position of the tip. The typical 45-degree medial tilt of the cistern should be seen from the anteroposterior view (Fig. 106-1B). The appearance of the cistern may vary considerably between patients, and it is essential that the surgeon be familiar with this anatomy. Furthermore, there is a subdural-extracisternal compartment in Meckel's cave that may be injected with contrast medium (Fig. 106-2). This usually happens when contrast medium is injected without prior spontaneous CSF drainage, or if the needle is dislodged from the intracisternal position during injection.

Specific Difficulties

Spontaneous CSF drainage from the needle does not guarantee an intracisternal tip location. In fact, if the cannula is placed a few millimeters too lateral, the tip may be located in the subtemporal subarachnoid space, and a brisk flow of CSF will still be produced. Subsequent cisternography solves this problem (Fig. 106-3A), which shows the proximity of the cisternal and subtemporal subarachnoid compartments in the anteroposterior projection. Figure 106-3B and C illustrate a pure subtemporal contrast injection. Our strategy in this case is to leave the first needle in place and to introduce a second needle using the first one for guidance (Fig. 106-4A and B). It cannot be overemphasized that spontaneous CSF drainage is required before contrast injection. If, in such a case, the contrast medium is injected without fulfilling this requirement, the glycerol may be deposited in the extra-arachnoid, subdural compartment (see Fig. 106-2).

Another problem may arise if the patient's head is not adequately tilted forward during the injection, because the contrast medium then flows out the porus trigemini and escapes to the posterior fossa, with insufficient cisternal filling to confirm the correct position of the needle tip (Fig. 106-5). This situation may also result in an underestimation of the cisternal volume.

Contrast Evacuation

When the intracisternal position of the tip has been confirmed, the syringe is gently removed from the cannula and the contrast medium permitted to flow out of it in a drop-by-drop fashion. We usually evacuate the cistern by tilting the patient to the supine position. If it is difficult to evacuate all contrast medium from the bottom of the cistern to permit the glycerol to reach the lowest root fibers (see later), the patient can be placed in the Trendelenburg position for a few minutes, a maneuver that permits the contrast medium to drain to the posterior fossa. Furthermore, the cistern may be flushed with 2 to 3 mL of sterile saline until the control radiograph indicates that the cistern is emptied. Some of

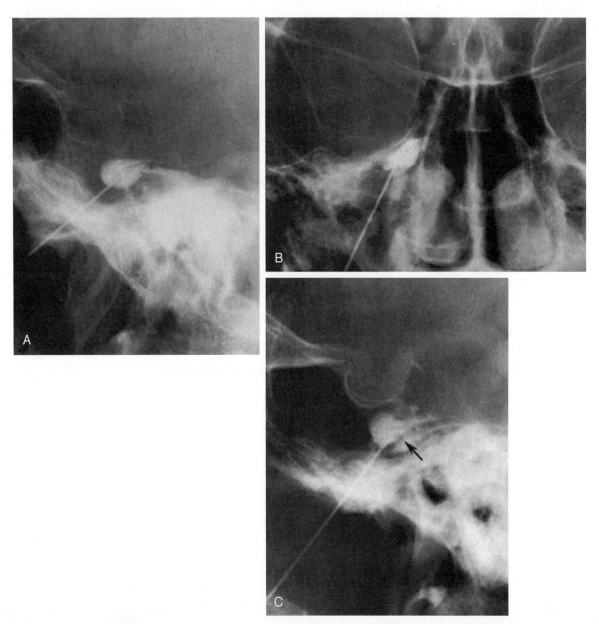

FIGURE 106-1   The typical appearance of the trigeminal cistern filled with contrast medium in the lateral (*A*) and anteroposterior projections (*B*). Note the root fibers (*A*) that give the cistern its striped texture. In the lateral projection (*C*), there is also sparing of contrast, which indicates the position of the trigeminal motor root (*arrow*).

the less satisfactory results are probably due to failure to empty the cistern properly.[12,39]

Glycerol Injection

Glycerol injection should always be performed with the patient in the sitting position to minimize extracisternal spillover. The glycerol should be anhydrous (greater than 99.5%) and sterile, and should be injected slowly from a 1-mL syringe. In general, 0.18 to 0.30 mL is sufficient, and the usual dose ranges from 0.22 to 0.28 mL (present average, 0.26 mL). When the neuralgia encompasses all three branches with multiple trigger points, a somewhat larger volume is used. Injection exceeding 0.35 mL is discouraged because of the risk for postoperative sensory deficits. Furthermore, inability to demonstrate an adequate

intracisternal needle tip position precludes a subsequent glycerol injection.

Branch Selectivity

If it is desired to inject glycerol selectively into one or more trigeminal branches, one of the following four maneuvers can be used.

First, the volume of glycerol can be varied to fill more or less of the cistern. When the trigeminal cistern has been emptied entirely after contrast injection, the amount of glycerol injected partly determines which branches will be influenced. With the head of the patient only slightly flexed, a small volume of glycerol (i.e., 0.15 to 0.2 mL) is deposited at the bottom of the cistern and mainly affects the fibers of the third and second branches. Increasing the

FIGURE 106-2 Schematic picture of the different compartments in Meckel's cave. The arachnoid is drawn with a *wavy line*. Note the sites (*) where extracisternal deposits of contrast medium and glycerol may be performed. (From Pauser G, Gerstenbrand F, Gross D [eds]: Gesichtsschmerz, Schmerzstudien Z. New York: Verlag, 1979.)

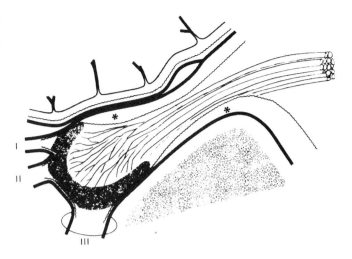

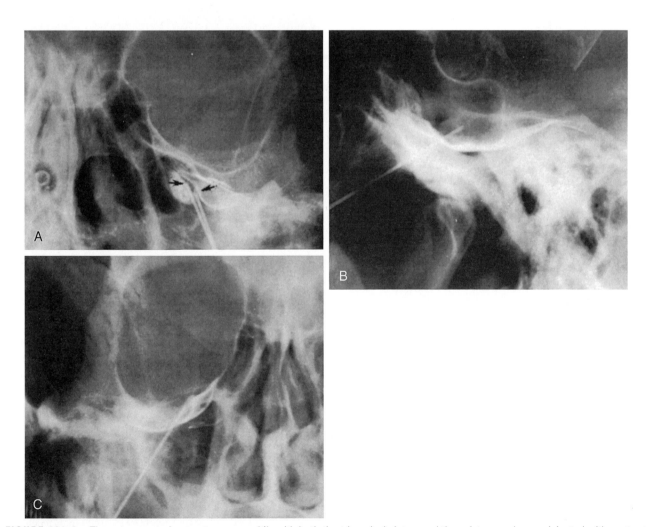

FIGURE 106-3 The anteroposterior roentgenogram (*A*), with both the trigeminal cistern and the subtemporal space injected with contrast medium, illustrates the proximity of these two compartments. Medially, the contrast-filled cistern (*arrow*) is seen barely pierced in its lateral margin by one of the needles. Injection of contrast medium through the lateral needle yielded a filling of the subtemporal space (*arrow*) instead. The lateral roentgenogram (*B*), shows a pure subtemporal contrast injection. *C*, Subtemporal outflow of contrast medium in the anteroposterior projection is shown. No contrast filling of the cistern was obtained, although exit of cerebrospinal fluid from the needle was noted.

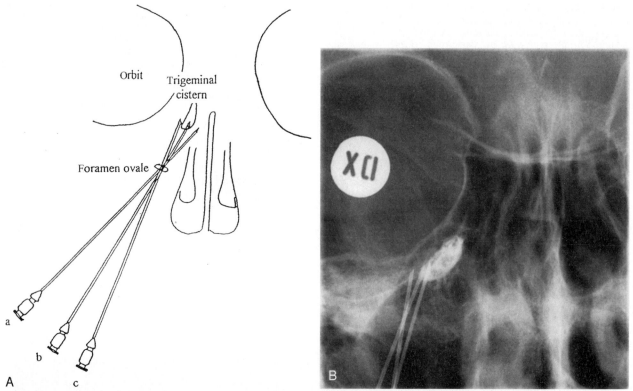

FIGURE 106-4 The schematic figure (*A*) illustrates that because the foramen ovale is a fulcrum point, the needle entry site determines the intracranial destination of the needle tip. A too lateral puncture site produces a medial tip position. An entry that is too medial results in placement of the needle lateral to the trigeminal cistern (c). A puncture site that is too lateral produces a medial tip position (a). The adequate entry is shown by the track (b). (From Jho HD, Lunsford LD: Percutaneous retrogasserian glycerol rhizotomy. Neurosurg Clin North Am 8:63–74, 1997.) *B*, The anteroposterior roentgenogram demonstrates the penetration of the foramen with three needles. Contrast injection via the most medial, only, produces cistern filling.

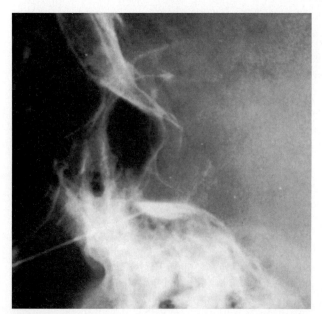

FIGURE 106-5 During contrast injection, the patient's head should be tilted forward to prevent immediate contrast flow to the posterior fossa. In this case, the positioning of the head was not adequate, and some contrast escaped to the posterior fossa, which is the reason why the filling of the cistern was only partial.

amount of glycerol causes additional rhizolysis in the two upper portions.

Second, contrast medium may be left at the bottom of the cistern to protect the third branch. Both contrast agents have a specific gravity exceeding that of pure glycerol (with 300 mg iodine/mL, iohexol = 1.345 g/L; compared with glycerol = 1.242 g/L and CSF = 1.007 g/L). This implies that these substances, when deposited in the same compartment, replace the original CSF contents and are layered with the contrast medium at the bottom and the glycerol on top of that.

With the head slightly flexed and a little contrast medium remaining at the bottom of the cistern, thus protecting the fibers of the third branch, glycerol may be gently injected to form a layer floating on the contrast medium. Rhizolysis will then engage mainly the upper two branches.

When treating a patient with third branch neuralgia, no contrast medium is allowed to remain in the cistern for the glycerol injection.

Third, the position of the needle tip is partly indicative of which branch will be most affected. The tip of the cannula should preferentially be positioned in the part of the cistern traversed by the root fibers to be treated. This means that for treatment of third branch neuralgia, the optimal position is in the lower part of the cistern, whereas a first or second branch neuralgia is best treated using a tip site in the upper portion.

During or immediately after injection of glycerol, the patient experiences strong paresthesias, or sometimes even pain in one or more of the divisions of the trigeminal nerve. This is an indication that the substance has been deposited inside the cistern and is affecting the closest root fibers. Proper placement of the needle seems especially important for reinjections when adhesions inside the cistern may be present and partially prevent the glycerol from settling to the bottom.

Finally, the position of the patient's head during and after the injection also produces some selectivity. The patient should be sitting in the upright position during the injection. For first branch neuralgia, the head should be maximally flexed (i.e., approximately 40 degrees) and should be kept in approximately that position for 1 hour after the injection. For second branch treatment, flexion should be approximately 25 degrees, and for the third branch, the head should be slightly tilted laterally toward the affected side, but kept upright in the anteroposterior plane.[5]

The selectivity obtained by varying the head position has been studied by Bergenheim and colleagues,[45,46] who found a highly selective effect of this maneuver with regard to the ophthalmic branch, but less selectivity for the two lower branches.

Immediately before glycerol injection, the free flow of CSF from the needle should be checked to ascertain a persisting intracisternal tip position. Dislocation is not unusual, especially if the full length of the needle had to be used and the patient moves his or her cheek.

In certain cases, a longer needle has to be used to reach the cistern proper. Often, thin needles (outer diameter 0.7 mm) of adequate length are not readily available in the hospital and have to be ordered separately. We discourage the use of thicker needles because it makes the procedure more painful, theoretically causes more mechanical damage to the ganglion, and makes the estimation of injected volume of glycerol more difficult.

Finally, when the tip of the needle is placed posteriorly in the cistern close to its clival passage, the injection might cause pain projected to the eye, which is why such a position should be avoided. It is also possible that corneal complications are related to injections in this area.

Permanent Marking of Cistern

A permanent marking of the cistern is recommended and can easily be achieved with a mix of glycerol and sterile radiopaque tantalum dust (Merck, Haar, Germany; grain size less than 0.042 mm). Approximately 0.5 g of tantalum is mixed with 2 mL of glycerol and the suspension is then used for injection to outline the bottom of the cistern (Fig. 106-6). This is of considerable help as a guide if reinjections are needed. With certain requirements fulfilled, permanent marking may replace the need for renewed cisternography. The tantalum marking is clearly visible on radiography years after the injection. There are no indications that the metal dust causes inadvertent effects or otherwise influences the results of the treatment.

Special Considerations for Repeated Injection

Incomplete pain relief after the initial injection seems in most cases to be the result of technical problems during

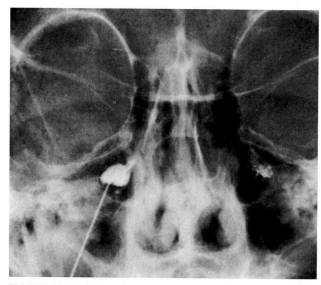

FIGURE 106-6 The trigeminal cistern on the patient's left side is permanently marked by tantalum dust, which lines the arachnoid of the bottom and walls of the cistern (anteroposterior view). The right cistern has been punctured and injected with contrast medium. After marking of the cistern with tantalum, the puncture and glycerol injection may be carried out without the intervening cisternography.

the procedure. Reinjections should not be performed within 3 to 4 weeks after the initial trial to allow late responders to emerge. Before reinjection, facial sensibility is carefully examined, and if sensory impairment is found, the reinjection should be performed with a minimal amount of glycerol. Alternatively, a nondestructive procedure should be considered in these patients.

When trigeminal cisternography is performed after one or more intracisternal glycerol injections, a less satisfactory outlining of the cistern sometimes is obtained, probably due to adhesions within the cistern induced by the glycerol or contrast medium.[47] The situation seems to be the same regardless of whether tantalum has been added.

If the cistern has been properly marked by tantalum dust during the initial injection and the marking is clearly visible during fluoroscopy, reinjection may be very simple and fast. When the position of the tip of the cannula is within the cistern according to radiography in the lateral and at least two anteroposterior projections at different angles, spontaneous drainage of CSF through the needle confirms an intracisternal tip position. However, if there is no exit of CSF through the cannula, cisternography with positive contrast should be performed.

Because of the cisternal adhesions, images on repeat cisternography may differ from the initial cisternography films. This also points to the advantage of placing the needle tip in the part of the cistern housing the root fibers to be treated because the glycerol might become trapped by fibrotic strands, preventing it from reaching the bottom of the cistern.

In contrast to our experience and the observations of Rappaport and Gomori,[47] Lunsford[48] noted no abnormalities of the cistern in patients undergoing repeated glycerol injections.

Postoperative Management

After injection, the patient should remain seated upright in bed with his or her head in the selected position for an hour. There is no convincing evidence that extending the time of controlled head positioning increases the therapeutic effect. However, there are indications that shortening the period of fiber exposure to glycerol by actively evacuating it from the cistern may cause more extensive and less well-controlled rhizolysis.[10,45] Sweet[10,30] reported that if first branch sensory loss appears, leaving the glycerol in the cistern for 12 minutes or more may result in persistent corneal anesthesia. Hence, he recommended evacuation of the glycerol from the cistern within 10 minutes after the onset of first branch analgesia.

The latency for relief from neuralgia varies. Approximately half of the patients report that their paroxysms disappear immediately after the glycerol injection. In the remaining group, there may be occasional spells during the first postoperative day and sometimes for periods of up to 5 days, after which the neuralgia fades away. Even longer latencies of up to 3 weeks have been reported.[48] In younger patients, the procedure may be performed on an outpatient basis. In elderly or weak patients or following general anesthesia, hospital stay overnight is usually required.

Facial sensibility should be examined on the first postoperative day and after 3 months. Patients are encouraged to report fevers, ulcers in the vicinity of the mouth, rash, eye problems, or any adverse effects that might be due to the treatment. A telephone report to the surgeon about the treatment effects is due 10 days after surgery.

The pharmaceutical regimen for the neuralgia is usually tapered off during 7 to 10 days after a successful injection. If high doses of carbamazepine have been used, we usually decrease the daily intake by 100 mg every second day.

If several drugs are used, the patient is provided with a schema for gradual decrease of pharmacotherapy after discharge from the hospital.

RESULTS

Outcomes are reviewed with respect to initial and long-term relief from the paroxysmal pain, rate of recurrence, and various complications such as sensory disturbances recorded, herpes eruptions, and postoperative meningitis of the aseptic and bacterial types. Some of the major series are examined, and relevant data are given in tables and text.

Evaluation of Different Series

A major problem in the evaluation of results from different series is the variation in technique. Different methods have been used by different authors to determine an intracisternal needle position before glycerol injection. Strategies vary from that recommended—use of cisternography,[6,7,48,49] drop-by-drop incremental glycerol injection, and perioperative recording of sensory response[5,8,50]—to use of electric stimulation in the same way as is done in selective thermocoagulation.[28,29]

In some series, cisternography is not used,[8,50,51] in some only in conjunction with treatment of first branch neuralgia, and in others only when there is no spontaneous CSF outflow through the cannula.[52] The extent to which cisternography is used in the series reviewed is shown in Table 106-1. In our experience, there is a relationship between the quality of the cisternography, the adequacy of needle placement, and the treatment outcome.

A very important factor is the amount of glycerol used. Sometimes the range of volumes is not explicit, and in several series it far exceeds the original recommendations.[8,12,53,54]

TABLE 106-1 ■ Results of Glycerol Rhizolysis*

Authors	No. of Patients	With Cisternography (%)	Pain Free after First Injection (%)	Total Pain Free at Follow-up (%)
Håkanson[49] (1983)	100	100	>96[†]	>75
Lunsford[48] (1985)	62	100	>74[†]	>66
Arias[5] (1986)	100	50	>95[†]	>95
Beck et al[63] (1986)	58	31	>67[†]	>72
Dieckmann et al[7] (1987)	252	100	>91[†]	>85
Saini[51] (1987)	550	0	>76[†]	>17
Burchiel[39] (1988)	46	100	>80[†]	>53
Young[8] (1988)	162	Some	>90[†]	>78
Waltz et al[74] (1989)	200	100	>73[†]	>74
Fujimaki et al[12] (1990)	122	100	>80[†]	>26
North et al[50] (1990)	85	0	>90[†]	>50
Ischia et al[54] (1990)	112	100	>92[†]	>71
Steiger[52] (1991)	122	100	>84[†]	>59
Slettebø et al[55] (1993)	60	100	>93[†]	>50
Bergenheim and Hariz[56] (1995)	99	100	>97[†]	>76
Jho and Lunsford[42] (1997)	523	100	>90[†]	>55
Blomstedt and Bergenheim[58] (2002)	139	100	>95[†]	50
Febles et al[57] (2003)	30	100	‡	66

*Outcomes of 18 major studies. Number of patients, use of cisternography for ascertaining intracisternal injection, percentage of patients with initial pain relief after first injection, and percentage of patients pain free (including reinjections) at follow-up are given.

[†]Most failures previously treated by destructive method; otherwise 96%.

‡Not reported.

TABLE 106-2 ▪ **Pain Recurrence after Glycerol Rhizolysis***

Authors	No. of Patients	Early Recurrence (<2 yr, %)	Late Recurrence (>2 yr, %)	Range of Follow-up
Håkanson[49] (1983)	100	~26	~43	5–10 yr
Lunsford[48] (1985)	62	~21	~†	3–28 mo
Arias[5] (1986)	100	~2	~10[†]	2–3 yr
Beck et al[63] (1986)	58	~11	~†	2–40 mo
Dieckmann et al[7] (1987)	252	~11	~37[†]	2–5 yr
Saini[51] (1987)	550	~41	~92[†]	1–6 yr
Burchiel[39] (1988)	46	~47	~75[†]	3–44 mo
Young[8] (1988)	162	~11	~34[†]	6–67 mo
Waltz et al[74] (1989)	200	~23	~25[†]	25–64 mo
Fujimaki et al[12] (1990)	122	~45	~72[†]	38–54 mo
North et al[50] (1990)	85	~40	~55[†]	6–54 mo
Ischia et al[54] (1990)	112	~20	~26[†]	1–5 yr
Steiger[52] (1991)	122	~30	~41[†]	1–96 mo
Slettebø et al[55] (1993)	60	~27	~55[†]	4.5–9 yr
Bergenheim and Hariz[56] (1995)	99	~33 (1 yr)	~†	12 mo
Jho and Lunsford[42] (1997)	523	~13	~†	11 yr
Blomstedt and Bergenheim[58] (2002)	139	~35	~45	Up to 11 yr
Febles et al[57] (2003)	30	†	33	Median 33.5 mo

*Percentage of patients in each series with early recurrence (within 2 years) after treatment and late (cumulative) recurrence (after 2 years). Follow-up range is also indicated.
†Not reported.

This has to be taken into account when interpreting the data (ranges of volumes of glycerol used are given later; see Table 106-3).

A third factor of major importance for the outcome is whether the patient has been subjected to some other destructive procedure before (or after) the glycerol rhizolysis and if information about this is given in the reports. This is of critical importance with regard to the estimation of sensory disturbances after the procedure, and it also has an impact on deciding the volume of glycerol to use in a specific case.

In some series, patients with diagnoses other than classic TN are included. It is often impossible to determine this from the results. This is of course most important when judging the outcome, because the results, as described later, in other facial pain conditions often are inferior to those in classic tic.

Short- and Long-Term Results

The outcomes in 18 major series with long-term follow-up periods encompassing more than 2700 patients are given in Table 106-1. Cisternography was used routinely for all patients in only 13 of the series.[7,12,39,42,48,49,52–58]

The percentage of patients experiencing relief from paroxysmal facial pain within 2 weeks varies in the different series from 67% to 97%. There is no clear association between the mere use of cisternography and success rate for either immediate or long-term outcomes. This finding may seem remarkable in light of the experiences of the current authors, but it may also point to large differences in the accuracy of the cisternographic procedure.

The follow-up periods in these series range from a few months to more than 10 years. The recurrence rates are difficult to estimate correctly because of the differences in techniques of reporting, statistics, and so forth. More recently, however, Kaplan-Meier analysis has been used by several researchers,[39,50,52,54] facilitating the interpretation of recurrences.

The recurrence rate in relation to length of follow-up is reviewed in Table 106-2. Within roughly 2 years of treatment, between 2% and 50% of patients with a successful initial outcome experience recurrent pain. This large variation obviously casts doubt on both the technical performance of the procedure and the follow-up methodology. It is difficult to evaluate how many of the patients have been reinjected, and if these cases are included in the final results.

The original Stockholm series of 100 patients was followed between 5 and 10 years (mean, 5 years, 4 months). At the last follow-up, 53% were still pain free after the first injection. Twenty-two patients had at that time been reinjected with glycerol and, in total, 75% of patients from the entire series were pain free, and an additional 23% had only mild pain easily controlled by a pharmaceutical regimen.[36] The average volume of glycerol injected in this series was 0.21 mL.

The average risk of recurrence within 2 years is approximately 20%, and the rate of late reappearance of symptoms (within 5 to 10 years) approaches 50%. Nevertheless, because injection can be repeated and carries little risk for the patient, most of the patients (more than 75%) may be maintained pain free by a small number of reinjections (Table 106-1). By comparison, Jannetta[59] found an 80% rate of permanent pain relief in most series of microvascular decompression, 10% with some pain, and a 10% failure rate.

Two reports of major series of patients with TN treated by glycerol rhizolysis have been presented by Spaziante and colleagues[60] and Lunsford and Duma.[61] The two series comprise 191 and 480 patients, respectively. The follow-up periods are as long as 10 years. The percentage of patients pain free immediately after treatment was 93% in the series of Spaziante and associates[60]; long-term follow-up showed that 77%[60] and 75%[61] of patients were pain free. No patients with anesthesia dolorosa were observed, but mild hypesthesia was found in 46% and 20%, respectively.

Both teams of researchers concluded that glycerol rhizolysis is a mildly neurodestructive procedure indicated as the first choice[60] in elderly patients, those with MS, and in patients in whom other procedures, including microvascular decompression, have been unsuccessful.[61]

A 1997 report of the Pittsburgh series by Jho and Lunsford[42] showed that of their large group of 523 patients, 90% were immediately pain free and 55% stayed pain free at follow-up (which extended to more than 10 years). The highest figures for patients initially pain free are those of Håkanson[4] (96%) and Bergenheim and Hariz[56] (97%).

Side Effects and Complications

Glycerol rhizolysis in the hands of an experienced and careful neurosurgeon should not result in serious complications. A fatal myocardial infarction has been reported[42,61,62] in the recovery room after the procedure. Because glycerol rhizolysis is used in patients of advanced age and sometimes with severe disabilities, the number of severe complications is remarkably low. Other serious complications relate to the attempts to penetrate the foramen ovale with a needle (e.g., intracranial hemorrhage) rather than glycerol instillation per se.[11]

The most feared consequence of neurolytic procedures, postoperative anesthesia dolorosa, is rarely observed after glycerol rhizolysis. An exception to this is the rather heterogeneous series of 552 cases by Saini,[51] in which rhizolysis was performed without cisternography or some other technique to confirm the localization of the needle tip before glycerol injection. In this series, the number of patients with anesthesia dolorosa amounted to 26 (5%).

Furthermore, 16 patients (3%) had signs of disturbance of third branch motor function. This malfunction resolved within 3 to 4 months after injection. Transient masseter weakness has also been described by others.[53,54] Otherwise, only single cases with transitory cranial nerve dysfunction after glycerol rhizolysis have been reported. Some of these are reviewed by Sweet.[11]

A recent review of 260 consecutive procedures performed in 139 patients between 1986 and 1987 reported a fairly high frequency of perioperative side effects.[58] In this series there occurred both a variety of intraoperative technical obstacles, severe vasovagal responses, and even cardiac arrest. In total, complications or side effects occurred in 67.3% of procedures. The side effects and complications are detailed in Tables 106-3 and 106-4. This series evidently encompasses learning curves for several surgeons. Penetration of the foramina of Versalius (0.8%) and spinosum (0.4%) occurred, as did buccal penetration (1.5%). Actually, three patients (1.2%) reported a postoperative ipsilateral decrease of hearing ability. Arterial bleeding occurred in 0.4%, while venous blood from the needle occurred in 3.5%.

Postoperative Facial Sensory Disturbance

A disturbance of facial sensibility is not uncommon after the procedure but usually lasts for a few hours to 1 to 2 weeks. This is not tabulated as a side effect. The following discussion focuses on persistent alterations in sensory function or perception in the trigeminal area: (1) postoperative hypesthesia, slight or severe; and (2) the presence of dysesthesia or allodynia. Paresthesias that are not unpleasant are not included.

TABLE 106-3 ▪ Sensory Complications after Glycerol Rhizolysis*

Authors	No. of Patients	Volume of Glycerol (mL)	Slight Hypesthesia (%)	Severe Hypesthesia (%)	Dysesthesia (%)
Håkanson[49] (1983)	100	0.2–0.3	60	0	0
Lunsford[48] (1985)	62	0.15–0.25[†]	21[†]	0	3[‡]
Arias[5] (1986)	100	0.1–0.4	13	0	0
Beck et al[63] (1986)	58	0.2–0.4	17	2	0
Dieckmann et al[7] (1987)	252	0.15–0.4	20	1	2
Saini[51] (1987)	550	0.2–0.3	**	5[§]	11
Burchiel[39] (1988)	46	0.15–?	72	7	13
Young[8] (1988)	162	0.15–0.55	72	12	3
Waltz et al[74] (1989)	200	0.2–0.6	37	7	2
Fujimaki et al[12] (1990)	122	0.3–0.5	63	29	26
North et al[50] (1990)	85	0.3–0.4	4	2[¶]	4[¶]
Ischia et al[54] (1990)	112	0.4–0.5	32	0	3
Steiger[52] (1991)	122	0.2–0.35[†]	53[†]	**	13
Slettebø et al[55] (1993)	60	0.15–0.70	35[§]	3[§]	13
Bergenheim and Hariz[56] (1995)	99	0.20–0.35	42	6	5
Jho and Lunsford[42] (1997)	523	0.20–0.50	32	6[†]	2
Blomstedt and Bergenheim[58] (2002)	139	0.13–0.35	47.3	45.5	22.7
Febles et al[57] (2003)	30	**	53	13	**

*Percentage of different types of sensory disturbance in each series. Range of glycerol volumes used is also indicated. In several series, it cannot readily be judged in sensory disturbances recorded after glycerol treatment were already present before the procedure. Furthermore, other destructive procedures may have been subsequently used without specific notice.
[†]Many with previous or additional destructive procedures.
[‡]After herpes reactivation.
[§]Only cases with previous destructive procedures.
[¶]Transient.
**Not reported.

TABLE 106-4 ▪ Infectious Complications after Glycerol Rhizolysis*

Authors	No. of Patients	Herpes Reactivation (%)	Aseptic Meningitis (%)	Bacterial Meningitis (%)
Håkanson[49] (1983)	100	50	0	0
Lunsford[48] (1985)	62	13	3	0
Arias[5] (1986)	100	10	2	0
Beck et al[63] (1986)	58	9	4	0
Dieckmann et al[7] (1987)	252	77	1	1
Saini[51] (1987)	550	3	†	†
Burchiel[39] (1988)	46	5	2	2
Young[8] (1988)	162	38	0	1
Waltz et al[74] (1989)	200	†	7	1
Fujimaki et al[12] (1990)	122	†	†	†
North et al[50] (1990)	85	†	†	†
Ischia et al[54] (1990)	112	†	†	†
Steiger[52] (1991)	122	†	0	0
Slettebø et al[55] (1993)	60	†	1.6	†
Bergenheim and Hariz[56] (1995)	99	†	†	†
Jho and Lunsford[42] (1997)	523	37	0.6	†
Blomstedt and Bergenheim[58] (2002)	139	3.8	1.5	1.5
Febles et al[57] (2003)	30	†	†	†

*Percentage of cases in each series with herpes simplex reactivation, aseptic meningitis, and bacterial meningitis.
†Not reported.

Hypesthesia

Serious sensory disturbance (e.g., anesthesia dolorosa) is rare after glycerol rhizolysis. However, transitory facial hypesthesia is a common phenomenon (up to 70%) after the procedure. The complaints usually vanish 3 to 6 months after the operation.[5,8,36,53]

The frequency of slight hypesthesia persisting for longer periods is variable between different series (see Table 106-3). In some series, only a small percentage of patients experience this,[5,50] but in others more than two thirds present with hypesthesia at follow-up.[8,39]

More severe hypesthesia and anesthesia is rare (see Table 106-3). There is only one series with a figure approaching 30%.[12] This is of course unacceptable, and the clinicians consequently abandoned the procedure. The figures from the series of Saini,[51] Burchiel,[39] Young,[8] Waltz and associates,[53] Bergenheim and Hariz,[56] and Jho and Lunsford[42] must also be considered high (5% to 12%). There are at least four possible explanations for this outcome: (1) some of these patients may have had other previous or subsequent destructive procedures; (2) there may have been technical difficulties during the procedure; (3) the volume of glycerol injected may have been too large; and (4) previous procedures may have produced cistern obliteration by fibrosis.[42,47,48] Sweet[11] described a case in which 1.5 mL of glycerol was injected in 0.1-mL increments, resulting in anesthesia dolorosa. When properly performed, the incidence of severe sensory disturbances with glycerol rhizolysis should be low (less than 1%).[7,36,48,49,61]

Dysesthesia

Dysesthesia (allodynia), spontaneous or touch-evoked unpleasant sensations, should occur rarely and mostly transiently after glycerol rhizolysis. The incidence is between 0 and 4% (see Table 106-3). However, Fujimaki and associates,[12] Burchiel,[39] Steiger,[52] Saini,[51] and Slettebø and colleagues[55] report dysesthesia with frequencies between 11%

and 26%. One major cause of this side effect is a previous neurodestructive procedure with a sensory disturbance not specifically recorded before the glycerol rhizolysis. Some patients may also have had procedure-induced herpes eruptions resulting in this condition,[48] although this has not been observed by us. Whatever the reason, these figures are high, and dysesthesias should not be present in more than 2% of previously untreated patients with TN treated by glycerol rhizolysis.[5,7,42,48,49,53,63]

Infectious Side Effects

Serious infectious complications after retrogasserian glycerol rhizolysis are rare. However, reactivation of latent viral infections of neural tissue (notably herpes simplex type 1) seems more common than expected (see Table 106-4).

Herpes Activation

The activation of latent herpes simplex infections is a phenomenon encountered intermittently in neurologic surgery.[64] Table 106-4 indicates the incidence of herpes simplex activation after glycerol injection. The incidence varied among different series from 3% to 77% for postoperative viral infections and this probably also largely reflects variations in accuracy of follow-up. Perioral and gingival ulcers presenting during the first week after treatment are common, but more serious outbreaks are rare. The mouth ulcers usually require no specific therapy.

Aseptic Meningitis

High fever, nuchal rigidity, and CSF pleocytosis presenting 24 to 36 hours after the procedure may indicate a meningeal reaction to an agent introduced into the trigeminal cistern. CSF cultures are usually negative. Patients presenting with these symptoms should be treated with high-dose intravenous antibiotics. When negative CSF cultures are reported, the antibiotics are discontinued. These patients usually recover completely within a few days without any sequelae.

Steroids may shorten the condition's course.[48] Patients who experienced this adverse reaction after a previous treatment have undergone repeat injections with intravenous corticosteroid prophylaxis without any problems.

Aseptic meningitis appears with a frequency of 0% to 7% (see Table 106-4).

The etiology of this reaction is obscure, although contrast agents, glycerol, tantalum dust,[48] and the extent of manipulation or number of ganglion penetrations are suspects. Some investigators report diminished frequency of reactions after reducing the amount of contrast medium.[53] In the Stockholm series, the frequency was 2% during the metrizamide era. Since this contrast medium was exchanged for iohexol in January 1986, we have had very few cases of aseptic meningitis. The plausibility of contrast medium as the causative agent is also supported by Arias,[5] who presented a series of 100 patients of whom approximately 50% were treated without preliminary contrast medium injection. In the group subjected to contrast injection, two patients presented with aseptic meningitis, whereas no case was found in the other group. However, aseptic meningeal reactions are observed after other manipulations of the trigeminal root as well.[59]

Bacterial Meningitis

Bacterial meningitis after percutaneous puncture of Meckel's cave is rare.[36,65] The most common bacterial agents are those colonizing the upper respiratory tract.[66] The most likely cause is inadvertent (and often unrecognized) penetration of the oral cavity mucosa. The frequency of bacterial meningitis after glycerol rhizolysis is between 0% and 2% (see Table 106-4). The frequency in the Stockholm series remains at maximally 0.5% and seems related to the extent of manipulation during the procedure. All patients have recovered without serious sequelae after antibiotic treatment.

SPECIAL CONSIDERATIONS IN PATIENTS WITH MULTIPLE SCLEROSIS

The paroxysmal facial pain in patients with MS may be clinically identical to that of classic TN. Therefore, all methods used for symptomatic treatment of TN, except microvascular decompression, also may be used in MS. TN is present in approximately 1% to 2% of patients with an established diagnosis of MS.[67-69] In different series of TN, the prevalence of MS seems to range from 2% to 4%, but incidences of up to 8% have been reported.[70,71] Furthermore, the occurrence of bilateral facial pain is not uncommon in MS (see Fig. 106-6), but is extremely rare in idiopathic TN.

The initial success rate is approximately equal for idiopathic TN and for TN in MS, whichever therapeutic method is used,[71] but the late results differ considerably between the two. The recurrence rate of TN is much higher in association with MS. Dieckmann and colleagues[7] and Linderoth and Håkanson[71] reported a recurrence rate of more than 40% at a 2-year follow-up; the recurrence rate in classic TN was approximately 11% during the same period in Dieckmann and colleagues' series. After longer follow-up periods (8 to 79 months after injection), Linderoth and Håkanson[71] reported over 60% recurrent tics in the MS group, whereas the recurrence rate for the entire TN group (approximately 300 patients) was 38%.

Elevated recurrence rates after treatment of TN in MS have also been observed with selective thermocoagulation. Broggi and Franzini[72] reported a 40% recurrence rate among patients with MS after thermorhizotomy compared with 9% in a series of patients without MS. This finding could not be corroborated by Brisman,[73] who found no significant difference in recurrence rates between 16 MS cases and 219 non-MS cases.

The low tolerance of patients with MS to pharmacologic agents, both in form of carbamazepine and as anesthesia and sedation, merits specific comment. Linderoth and Håkanson[71] reported that more than 90% of their patients with MS and TN complained of adverse medication effects. The symptoms in the MS group were often an aggravation of preexisting symptoms. Thirty-eight percent of the patients with MS had to discontinue carbamazepine because of such symptoms. After glycerol treatment, 82% of the patients previously on carbamazepine were able to terminate it.

We believe that paroxysmal facial pain in MS should be liberally treated by glycerol rhizolysis to save the patient from the incapacitating side effects of a heavy drug regimen. Patients with MS are often disabled, weak, and considered at risk from general anesthesia; a method that does not require general anesthesia is therefore recommended.

GLYCEROL RHIZOLYSIS IN THE TREATMENT OF OTHER TYPES OF FACIAL PAIN

In painful trigeminal neuropathy (previously called atypical facial pain), a paroxysmal component may exist in addition to the continuous neuropathic pain. The etiology varies (e.g., trauma, infection, postoperative, tumor, idiopathic) but includes previous treatment for TN. We agree with Dieckmann and colleagues,[6] Waltz and associates,[74] Lunsford and Apfelbaum,[62] Rappaport,[75] and Rappaport and Gomori[47] that glycerol rhizolysis is contraindicated in most such cases and may aggravate a preexisting neuropathy. The sole exception is when the paroxysmal component completely dominates the clinical picture, diminishing the quality of life for the patient, and where the sensory disturbance is minimal. In such a case, a small amount of glycerol could be injected (0.15 mL). If complete pain relief is obtained (duration at least 3 months), a second injection may be performed using a somewhat larger glycerol volume.

Severe, intractable cluster headache (migraneous neuralgia, Horton's syndrome) has also been treated by ipsilateral glycerol injection into the trigeminal cistern[50,74,76] (G. Sundbärj, personal communication, 1988). The outcome has been partial, and transitory relief from symptoms has been achieved only in some of the patients, comparable with that obtained by other manipulations of the trigeminal system.[80] However, one long-term follow-up study of 18 patients, followed during an average 5.2 years, demonstrated that 83% of the patients obtained immediate relief, the frequency of attacks decreased markedly, and the condition recurred in only 39% during the study period.[76] Thus, glycerol therapy in cluster headache may offer some relief in chronic cases of moderate severity, but in patients with extreme pain, periorbital edema, and so on, glycerol treatment injection does not provide adequate symptom alleviation. Instead, chronic hypothalamic DBS has recently proven effective in selected cases.[77]

Glycerol rhizotomy has furthermore been reported to provide relief from the paroxysmal pain component in selected cases of SUNCT (short-lasting, unilateral, neuralgiform hemicrania with conjunctival injection and tearing),[78] although negative outcomes of surgical therapies in this condition also have been published.[79]

RETROGASSERIAN GLYCEROL RHIZOLYSIS VERSUS OTHER OPERATIVE TREATMENTS FOR TRIGEMINAL NEURALGIA

Glycerol rhizolysis is an inexpensive, seemingly simple procedure that must be meticulously performed by an experienced surgeon to obtain satisfactory results. The major indication remains typical idiopathic TN, particularly in the elderly, weak, or infirm. If a young patient chooses to undergo glycerol rhizolysis in place of a microvascular decompression, he or she may do so. However, if this patient has a relatively rapid recurrence, he or she should be urged to accept the open procedure instead.

In most cases, it should be possible to affect all the trigeminal branches with some selectivity; the most problematic might be the mandibular branch. With careful technique it should be possible to perform rhizolysis in that branch as well. In some patients subjected to several reinjections, adhesions inside the cistern may impede the glycerol from reaching the lowermost fibers. In such cases, selective thermocoagulation—or trigeminal nerve compression with a balloon—may be considered.

In our opinion, microvascular decompression in young patients without MS and glycerol treatment in elderly or weak patients are the methods of choice in classic TN.

CONCLUSION

Trigeminal glycerol rhizolysis should be offered to healthy patients in their eighth decade or older with classic TN, as well as to somatically fragile patients and those with MS. It also is an option in younger patients reluctant to undergo major surgery. With meticulous technique, the method is well tolerated by patients, can be performed with the patient under local anesthesia or under slight sedation only, and carries little risk for severe side effects. The recurrence rate, although usually slightly higher than that with microvascular decompression, compares well with other percutaneous methods, particularly in view of the low risk of severe postoperative sensory disturbance.

REFERENCES

1. Leksell L: Trigeminusneuralgi: Några neurofysiologiska aspekter och en ny behandlingsmetod. Lakartidningen 68:5145–5158, 1971.
2. Håkanson S, Leksell L: Stereotactic radiosurgery in trigeminal neuralgia. In Pauser G, Gerstenbrand F, Gross D (eds): Gesichtsschmerz: Schmerzstudien 2. New York: Gustav Fischer Verlag, 1979.
3. Jefferson A: Trigeminal root and ganglion injections using phenol in glycerine for relief of trigeminal neuralgia. J Neurol Neurosurg Psychiatry 26:345–352, 1963.
4. Håkanson S: Trigeminal neuralgia treated by the injection of glycerol into the trigeminal cistern. Neurosurgery 9:638–646, 1981.
5. Arias MJ: Percutaneous retrogasserian glycerol rhizotomy for trigeminal neuralgia: A prospective study of 100 cases. J Neurosurg 65:32–36, 1986.
6. Dieckmann G, Veras G, Sogabe K: Retrogasserian glycerol injection or percutaneous stimulation in the treatment of typical and atypical trigeminal pain. Neurol Res 9:48–49, 1987.
7. Dieckmann G, Bockermann V, Heyer C, et al: Five-and-a-half years experience with percutaneous retrogasserian glycerol rhizotomy in treatment of trigeminal neuralgia. Appl Neurophysiol 50:401–413, 1987.
8. Young RF: Glycerol rhizolysis for treatment of trigeminal neuralgia. J Neurosurg 69:39–45, 1988.
9. Lunsford LD, Bennett MH, Martinez AJ: Experimental trigeminal glycerol injection: Electrophysiologic and morphologic effects. Arch Neurol 42:146–149, 1985.
10. Sweet WH: Glycerol rhizotomy. In Youmans JR (ed): Neurological Surgery, 3rd ed. Philadelphia: WB Saunders, 1990, pp 3908–3921.
11. Sweet WH: Faciocephalic pain. In Apuzzo MLJ (ed): Brain Surgery: Complication Avoidance and Management. New York: Churchill Livingstone, 1993, pp 2053–2083.
12. Fujimaki T, Fukushima T, Miyazaki S: Percutaneous retrogasserian glycerol injection in the management of trigeminal neuralgia: Long-term follow-up results. J Neurosurg 73:212–216, 1990.
13. Bunge RP: Myelin degeneration in tissue culture. Neurosci Res Progr Bull 9:496–498, 1971.
14. Dulhunty AF, Gage PW: Differential effects of glycerol treatment on membrane capacity and excitation-contraction coupling in toad sartorius fibers. J Physiol (Lond) 234:373–408, 1973.
15. Diechmann D: Glycerol-effects upon rabbits and rats. Indust Med 2:5–6, 1941.
16. Baxter BW, Schacherl U: Experimental studies on the morphological changes produced by intrathecal phenol. CMAJ 86:1200, 1962.
17. King JS, Jewett DL, Sundberg HR: Differential blockade of cat dorsal root C-fibers by various chloride solutions. J Neurosurg 36:569–583, 1972.
18. Robertson JD: Structural alterations in nerve fibers produced by hypotonic and hypertonic solutions. J Biophys Biochem Cytol 4:349–364, 1958.
19. Pal HK, Dinda AK, Roy S, Banerji AK: Acute effect of anhydrous glycerol on peripheral nerve: An experimental study. Br Neurosurg 3:463–470, 1989.
20. Freeman AR, Reuben JP, Brandt PW, Grundfest H: Osmometrically determined characteristics of the cell membrane of squid and lobster giant axons. J Gen Physiol 50:423–445, 1966.
21. Håkanson S: Trigeminal Neuralgia Treated by Retrogasserian Injection of Glycerol. Published dissertation. Stockholm: Karolinska Institute, 1982.
22. Rengachary SS, Watanabe IS, Singer P, Bopp WJ: Effect of glycerol on peripheral nerve: An experimental study. Neurosurgery 13:681–688, 1983.
23. Bremerich A, Reisert I: Die perineurale Leitungsblockade mit Glycerin und Phenol-Glycerin: Eine histomorphologisch-morphometrische Studie. Dtsch Zahnartzl Z 46:825–827, 1991.
24. Isik N, Pamir MN, Benli K, et al: Experimental trigeminal glycerol injection in dogs: Histopathological evaluation by light and electron microscopy. Stereotact Funct Neurosurg 79(2):94–106, 2002.
25. Stajcic Z: Evidence that the site of action of glycerol in relieving tic douloureux is its actual site of application. Dtsch Zahnartztl Z 45:44–46, 1990.
26. Burchiel KJ, Russell LC: Glycerol neurolysis: Neurophysiological effects of topical glycerol application on rat saphenous nerve. J Neurosurg 63:784–788, 1985.
27. Rappaport ZH, Seltzer Z, Zagzag D: The effect of glycerol on autotomy: An experimental model of neuralgia pain. Pain 26:85–91, 1986.
28. Sweet WH, Poletti CE, Macon JB: Treatment of trigeminal neuralgia and other facial pains by retrogasserian injection of glycerol. Neurosurgery 9:647–653, 1981.
29. Sweet WH, Poletti CE: Problems with retrogasserian glycerol in the treatment of trigeminal neuralgia. Appl Neurophysiol 48:252–257, 1985.
30. Sweet WH: Retrogasserian glycerol injection as treatment for trigeminal neuralgia. In Schmidek HH, Sweet WH (eds): Operative Neurosurgical Techniques, 2nd ed. New York: Grune & Stratton, 1988, pp 1129–1137.
31. Bennett MH, Lunsford LD: Percutaneous retrogasserian glycerol rhizotomy for tic douloureux. II: Results and implications of trigeminal evoked potentials studies. Neurosurgery 14:431–435, 1984.
32. Bennett MH, Jannetta PJ: Evoked potentials in trigeminal neuralgia. Neurosurgery 13:242–247, 1983.

33. Raminsky M, Sears TA: Internodal conduction in undissected demyelinated nerve fibers. J Physiol 227:323–350, 1972.

34. Waxman SG, Brill MH: Conduction through demyelinated plaque in multiple sclerosis: Computer simulations of facilitation by short internodes. J Neurol Neurosurg Psychiatry 69:39–45, 1978.

35. Fruhstorfer H, Lindblom U, Schmidt WG: Method for quantitative estimation of thermal thresholds in patients. J Neurol Neurosurg Psychiatry 39:1071–1075, 1976.

36. Håkanson S: Surgical treatment: Retrogasserian glycerol injection. In Fromm GH, Sessle BJ (eds): Trigeminal Neuralgia: Current Concepts Regarding Pathogenesis and Treatment. Boston: Butterworth-Heinemann, 1991, pp 185–204.

37. Eide PK, Stubhaug A: Sensory perception in patients with trigeminal neuralgia: Effects of percutaneous retrogasserian glycerol rhizotomy. Stereotact Funct Neurosurg 68:207–211, 1997.

38. Kumar R, Mahapatra AK, Dash HH: The blink reflex before and after percutaneous glycerol rhizotomy in patients with trigeminal neuralgia: A prospective study of 28 patients. Acta Neurochir (Wien) 137:85–88, 1995.

39. Burchiel KJ: Percutaneons retrogasserian glycerol rhizolysis in the management of trigeminal neuralgia. J Neurosurg 69:361–366, 1988.

40. Härtel F: Die Leitungsanästhesie und Injectionsbehandlung des Ganglion Gasseri und der Trigeminusstämme. Arch Klin Chir 100: 193–292, 1912.

41. Nugent GR, Berry B: Trigeminal neuralgia treated by differential percutaneous radiofrequency coagulation of the gasserian ganglion. J Neurosurg 40:517–523, 1974.

42. Jho HD, Lunsford LD: Percutaneous retrogasserian glycerol rhizotomy. Neurosurg Clin North Am 8:63–74, 1997.

43. Håkanson S: Transoval trigeminal cisternography. Surg Neurol 10:137–144, 1978.

44. Shaw DD, Bach-Gansmo T, Dahlström K: Iohexol: Summary of North American and European clinical trials in adult lumbar, thoracic and cervical myelography with a new nonionic contrast medium. Invest Radiol 20(Suppl):44–50, 1985.

45. Bergenheim AT, Hariz MI, Laitinen LV: Selectivity of retrogasserian glycerol rhizotomy in the treatment of trigeminal neuralgia. Stereotact Funct Neurosurg 56:159–165, 1991.

46. Bergenheim AT, Hariz MI, Laitinen LV: Retrogasserian glycerol rhizotomy and its selectivity in the treatment of trigeminal neuralgia. Acta Neurochir (Wein) 58(Suppl):174–177, 1993.

47. Rappaport ZH, Gomori JM: Recurrent trigeminal cistern glycerol injections for tic douloureux. Acta Neurochir (Wien) 90:31–34, 1988.

48. Lunsford LD: Trigeminal neuralgia: Treatment by glycerol rhizotomy. In Wilkins RH, Rengachary SS (eds): Neurosurgery, vol 3. New York: McGraw-Hill, 1985, pp 2351–2356.

49. Håkanson S: Retrogasserian glycerol injection as treatment of tic douloureux. Adv Pain Res Ther 5:927–933, 1983.

50. North RB, Kidd DH, Piantadosi S, Carson BS: Percutaneous retrogasserian glycerol rhizotomy. J Neurosurg 72:851–856, 1990.

51. Saini SS: Retrogasserian anhydrous glycerol injection therapy in trigeminal neuralgia: Observations in 552 patients. J Neurol Neurosurg Psychiatry 50:1536–1538, 1987.

52. Steiger HJ: Prognostic factors in the treatment of trigeminal neuralgia: Analysis of a differential therapeutic approach. Acta Neurochir (Wien) 113:11–17, 1991.

53. Waltz TA, Dalessio DJ, Ott KH, et al: Trigeminal cistern glycerol injections for facial pain. Headache 25:354–357, 1985.

54. Ischia S, Luzzani A, Polati E: Retrogasserian glycerol injection: A retrospective study of 112 patients. Clin J Pain 6:291–296, 1990.

55. Slettebø H, Hirschberg H, Lindegaard K-F: Long-term results after percutaneous retrogasserian glycerol rhizotomy in patients with trigeminal neuralgia. Acta Neurochir (Wien) 117:231–235, 1993.

56. Bergenheim AT, Hariz MI: Influence of previous treatment on outcome after glycerol rhizotomy for trigeminal neuralgia. Neurosurgery 36:303–310, 1995.

57. Febles C, Werner-Wasik M, Rosenwasser RH, et al: A comparison of treatment outcomes with gamma knife radiosurgery versus glycerol rhizotomy in the management of trigeminal neuralgia. Int J Radiat Oncol Biol Phys 57(2 Suppl):253, 2003.

58. Blomstedt PC, Bergenheim AT: Technical difficulties and perioperative complications of retrogasserian glycerol rhizotomy for trigeminal neuralgia. Stereotact Funct Neurosurgery 79:168–181, 2002.

59. Jannetta PJ: Surgical treatment: Microvascular decompression. In Fromm GH, Sessle BJ (eds): Trigeminal Neuralgia: Current Concepts Regarding Pathogenesis and Treatment. Boston: Butterworth-Heinemann, 1991, pp 145–157.

60. Spaziante R, Cappabianca P, Graziussi G, et al: Percutaneous retrogasserian glycerol rhizolysis for treatment of trigeminal neuralgia: Results in 191 patients [Abstract]. Acta Neurochir (Wien) 117:97, 1992.

61. Lunsford LD, Duma CH: Percutaneous retrogasserian glycerol rhizotomy: A ten-year experience [Abstract]. Acta Neurochir (Wien) 117:97, 1992.

62. Lunsford LD, Apfelbaum RI: Choice of surgical therapeutical modalities for treatment of trigeminal neuralgia: Microvascular decompression, percutaneous retrogasserian thermal or glycerol rhizotomy. Clin Neurosurg 32:319–333, 1985.

63. Beck DW, Olson JJ, Urig EJ: Percutaneous retrogasserian glycerol rhizotomy for treatment of trigeminal neuralgia. J Neurosurg 65:28–31, 1986.

64. Nabors MW, Francis CK, Kobrine AI: Reactivation of herpesvirus in neurosurgical patients. Neurosurgery 19:599–603, 1986.

65. Nugent GR: Surgical treatment: Radiofrequency gangliolysis and rhizotomy. In Fromm GH, Sessle BJ (eds): Trigeminal Neuralgia: Current Concepts Regarding Pathogenesis and Treatment. Boston: Butterworth-Heinemann, 1991, pp 159–184.

66. Aspevall O, Hillebrant E, Linderoth B, Rylander M: Meningitis due to *Gemella hemolysans* after neurosurgical treatment of trigeminal neuralgia. Scand J Infect Dis 23:503–505, 1991.

67. Rushton JG, Olafson RA: Trigeminal neuralgia associated with multiple sclerosis. Arch Neurol 13:383–386, 1965.

68. Brett DC, Ferguson GG, Ebers GC, Paty DW: Percutaneous trigeminal rhizotomy: Treatment of trigeminal neuralgia secondary to multiple sclerosis. Arch Neurol 39:219–221, 1982.

69. Jensen TS, Rasmussen P, Reske-Nielsen E: Association of trigeminal neuralgia with multiple sclerosis: Clinical and pathological features. Acta Neurol Scand 65:182–189, 1982.

70. Chakravorty BG: Association of trigeminal neuralgia with multiple sclerosis. Arch Neurol 14:95–99, 1966.

71. Linderoth B, Håkanson S: Paroxysmal facial pain in disseminated sclerosis treated by retrogasserian glycerol injection. Acta Neurol Scand 80:341–346, 1989.

72. Broggi G, Franzini A: Radiofrequency trigeminal rhizotomy in treatment of symptomatic non-neoplastic facial pain. J Neurosurg 57:483–486, 1982.

73. Brisman R: Trigeminal neuralgia and multiple sclerosis. Arch Neurol 44:379–380, 1987.

74. Waltz TA, Dalessio DJ, Copeland B, Abbott G: Percutaneous injection of glycerol for the treatment of trigeminal neuralgia. Clin J Pain 5:195–198, 1989.

75. Rappaport ZH: Percutaneous retrogasserian glycerol injection for trigeminal neuralgia: One year follow-up. Pain Clin 1:57–61, 1986.

76. Pieper DR, Dickerson J, Hassenbuch SJ: Percutaneous retrogasserian glycerol rhizolysis for treatment of chronic intractable cluster headaches: Long-term results. Neurosurgery 46(2):363–370, 2000.

77. Franzini A, Ferroli P, Leone M, Broggi G: Stimulation of the posterior hypothalamus for treatment of chronic intractable cluster headaches: First reported series. Neurosurgery 52(5):1095–1099, 2003.

78. Hannerz J, Linderoth B: Neurosurgical treatment of short-lasting, unilateral, neuralgiform hemicrania with conjunctival injection and tearing. Br J Neurosurgery 16(1):55–58, 2002.

79. Black DF, Dodick DW: Two cases of medically and surgically intractable SUNCT: A reason for caution and argument for a central mechanism. Cephalalgia 22(3):201–204, 2002.

80. Ekbom K, Lindgren L, Nilsson BY, et al: Retro-gasserian glycerol injection in the treatment of chronic cluster headache. Cephalalgia 7:21–27, 1987.

107 Gamma Knife Radiosurgery for Trigeminal Neuralgia

RONALD BRISMAN

INTRODUCTION

Trigeminal neuralgia refers to brief, paroxysmal, trigeminally distributed face pain that is usually unilateral and is triggered by light touch about the face, such as talking, eating, or brushing the teeth. It can be caused by a tortuous blood vessel, tumor, vascular malformation, or demyelinating plaque. Sometimes, no apparent cause can be determined. GKRS can provide successful treatment regardless of the cause or the patient's medical condition.

HISTORY

In 1971, Lars Leksell[1] reported two patients with typical tic douloureux (trigeminal neuralgia) who were operated on in 1953 with stereotaxic radiosurgery exposing the trigeminal ganglion and root to a single heavy dose of ionizing radiation. Complete relief was obtained without any loss of facial sensation, and the patients remained free of pain for a follow-up period of 18 years. In 1977, Håkanson and Leksell[2] reported 50 patients with typical trigeminal neuralgia who were treated during the preceding 5 years with the Leksell gamma radiation unit. The majority experienced complete or partial relief with no appreciable sensory loss or other adverse effects.

INDICATIONS FOR GAMMA KNIFE RADIOSURGERY

As neurosurgical procedures (GKRS) to treat trigeminal neuralgia have become less invasive and safer, the indications for their use have become less restrictive. Medications such as carbamazepine (Tegretol) and/or oxcarbazepine (Trileptal) are highly effective and should be tried before any neurosurgical intervention. Medicines, however, do not continue to work for many patients because they either no longer relieve pain or cause adverse side effects. For these patients, neurosurgical procedures such as GKRS are indicated. Patients do not need to wait for agonizing pain or spend much of their lives impaired by high-dose, multiple pharmacotherapy.

METHODS

Gamma Knife

Almost all stereotactic radiosurgery used for treatment of trigeminal neuralgia has been done with the gamma knife, where the energy source is derived from decaying ^{60}Co. A 4-mm collimator is used to deliver one isocenter to the cisternal part of the trigeminal nerve near the pons. Two isocenters have been used with treatment of a longer segment of the trigeminal nerve. However, a randomized study has shown that better pain relief does not occur from two isocenters, which may result in added dysesthesias.[3] Isocenter doses are usually from 70 to 90 Gy, as doses less than 70 Gy have been shown to be less effective.[4] Anywhere from the 20% to 50% isodose line is placed near the surface of the pons. When higher doses are used, the isocenter is usually placed further away from the pons.

The Author's Gamma Knife Radiosurgery Series

Between May 1998 and December 2003, the author has done 518 GKRS procedures for trigeminal neuralgia; 422 GKRS procedures were done on 359 patients with essential trigeminal neuralgia (no tumor, arteriovenous malformation, or multiple sclerosis), 78 GKRS procedures on 56 patients with multiple sclerosis, 18 GKRS procedures on 14 patients with tumor, and 3 GKRS procedures on 2 patients with arteriovenous malformations.

Patients with essential trigeminal neuralgia were treated with 75 to 76.8 Gy as the maximal dose. A single isocenter was given to the cisternal trigeminal nerve with a 4-mm collimator. It was placed so that usually the 40% to 50% isodose line touched the outer surface of the pons and was centered on the trigeminal nerve as seen on axial, coronal, and sagittal views (Fig. 107-1). The Elekta Model B gamma knife unit (Elekta Instruments, Inc., Atlanta, GA) was used on all patients.

On August 24, 2000, the output factor was increased from 0.85 to 0.87. Of the initial 181 GKRS procedures for essential trigeminal neuralgia, a true maximal dose of 76.8 Gy was given. On subsequent patients, a true maximal dose of 75 Gy was used.

At the time of GKRS, T1-weighted, axial, 1-mm thick magnetic resonance imaging (MRI) scans were obtained through the area of the trigeminal nerve at its exit from the brain stem, often without and then after injection of 15 mL gadolinium diethylenetriamine pentaacetic acid (3-dimensional gradient echo acquisition in steady state, 20-degree flip angle, TR 30 milliseconds, TE 7 milliseconds, matrix 256×256, 1 excitation, 28 frames, and 24-cm field of view) (see Fig. 107-1).

Patients with pacemakers who could not undergo MRI were imaged with computed tomography, usually without and with 75 mL intravenous contrast (Omnipaque, 300 mgI/mL [iohexol], Amersham Health) through the

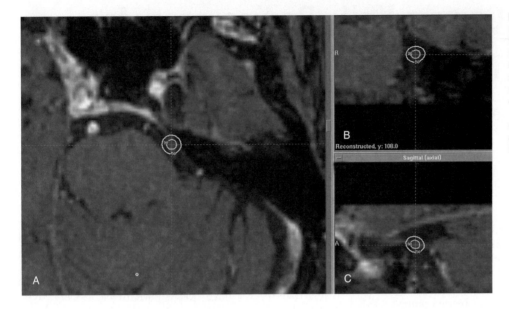

FIGURE 107-1   Left trigeminal neuralgia. One 4-mm isocenter is placed on the cisternal trigeminal nerve so that the 40% to 50% isodose line touches the surface of the pons. Magnetic resonance imaging, T1 with contrast: *A*, axial; *B*, coronal; *C*, sagittal views. The central circle is the 90% isodose line and the outer circle is the 50% isodose line.

trigeminal nerve with no angulation of the gantry, sequential scans, 1-mm-thick sections, no spacing, 2 seconds for each scan, and soft-tissue imaging. More recently, we have done computed tomography scanning after subarachnoid contrast and find that it is helpful in improving the imaging of the trigeminal nerve in those who cannot undergo MRI (Fig. 107-2).[5]

Some patients are claustrophobic and very fearful of the MRI. These patients require sedation with either oral (lorazepam [Ativan] 0.5 to 2 mg), intravenous (midazolam [Versed] 1 to 3 mg), or other anxiolytic medications and appropriate monitoring.

Patients who are anticoagulated can undergo GKRS. However, if the anticoagulation can be safely stopped before GKRS, this is preferable.

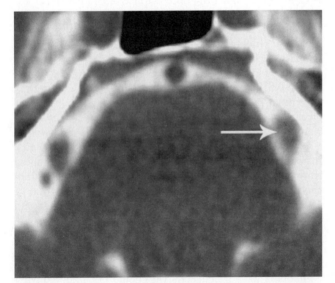

FIGURE 107-2   Computed tomography scanning after subarachnoid contrast at time of gamma knife radiosurgery. The trigeminal nerve is clearly seen as an oval hypointense area (*arrow*). The patient has a pacemaker and left trigeminal neuralgia.

Patients who have a cerebellopontine angle mass, such as a tumor or arteriovenous malformation and trigeminal neuralgia can undergo GKRS either to the tumor itself (if it is smaller than 3 cm in maximum diameter) or to the trigeminal nerve.[6]

Patients with multiple sclerosis and trigeminal neuralgia can be treated with GKRS directed at the cisternal trigeminal nerve, similarly to the way that one would treat essential trigeminal neuralgia. However, because patients with multiple sclerosis and trigeminal neuralgia respond less well than those with essential trigeminal neuralgia, the author has recently been treating multiple sclerosis trigeminal neuralgia patients with a maximal dose of 85 Gy.

Linear Accelerator

Recently, the results of radiosurgery for treatment of trigeminal neuralgia with a radiosurgery system that is not gamma knife have been reported by one center.[7,8] This is linear accelerator (LINAC) radiosurgery that was done on a "dedicated" LINAC system (Novalis; BrainLAB, Heimstetten, Germany) that was designed exclusively for stereotactic radiation, specifically to treat central nervous system targets. In one report, there were 41 patients with essential trigeminal neuralgia who received from 70 to 90 Gy to the isocenter with either a 5- or 7.5-mm collimator.[7] The second report, which includes many of the same patients, reviewed 25 patients with essential trigeminal neuralgia who were treated with 90 Gy with a 5-mm collimator.[8]

RESULTS

Pain Relief

Gamma Knife

GKRS for trigeminal neuralgia has been done throughout the world on more than 12,560 patients as of June 2003 (source: Leksell Gamma Knife Society). A number of

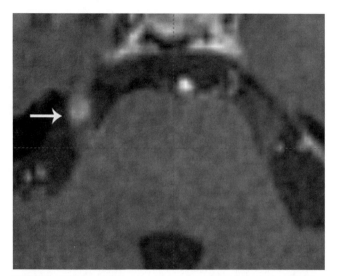

FIGURE 107-3 Magnetic resonance imaging with contrast 7 months after gamma knife radiosurgery shows an area of enhancement (*arrow*) of the right trigeminal nerve where the radiation was given.

publications involving several hundred patients have confirmed the safety and efficacy of this technique. After approximately 2 years of follow-up (mean, 19.8 months; median, 2 years, 3 years, and 24 months), pain relief was 50% or more in 66%, complete in 40%, no pain no medicines in 55%, and 90% or more in 56%, respectively.[9–12] Results for selected groups were much better. For those who had not undergone previous surgery, there was complete pain relief in 70.4%[11] and no pain no medicines in 67%,[10] and for those with typical trigeminal neuralgia and no previous surgery, initial pain relief was achieved in 95.5% with recurrence in only 3.3%.[9] There is usually a delay between GKRS and pain relief with a median time of 3 weeks (range, 1 day to 20 weeks) to complete pain relief[10] or 2 (±5.1) months.[11]

MRI with contrast done several months after the GKRS often shows an area of contrast enhancement in the trigeminal nerve where the radiation was delivered (Fig. 107-3).

The Author's Gamma Knife Radiosurgery Series

In the author's series of GKRS for trigeminal neuralgia, 329 patients with trigeminal neuralgia without tumor or multiple sclerosis have been followed for at least 6 months (or until reoperation); 60.8% were female and age was 70 years (median) and 68 (mean) at the time of GKRS; 290 patients had typical trigeminal neuralgia symptoms, whereas 39 had an atypical component, usually some constant pain as well as the paroxysmal triggered pain; 192 (58%) patients had no neurosurgical procedure before the GKRS, whereas 137 (42%) patients had at least one previous procedure; 172 patients had no pre-GKRS surgery and no atypical features. Pain relief achieved is seen in Table 107-1.

Linear Accelerator

Results of LINAC radiosurgery for trigeminal neuralgia reveal that at last follow-up (mean follow-up, 23 months) for 41 patients with trigeminal neuralgia without tumor or multiple sclerosis treated with a mean of 83 Gy at the isocenter, greater than 50% pain relief was sustained in 12 (62.3%) patients at 1 year.[7] At last follow-up of 25 patients treated with 90 Gy and followed for a median of 18 months, 17 (68%) maintained 50% or better pain relief.[8]

Factors That Influence Pain Relief

Although radiation doses less than 70 Gy were shown to be less likely to cause relief,[4] the effects of increasing the dose beyond 70 Gy have not been clearly established.[4,10] Nevertheless, there is a definite suggestion that higher doses, such as 90 Gy, may result in better relief than 70 Gy.[13,14] Actual doses greater than 90 Gy may have been used in some studies in which the published data may have been based on old output factors. The onset of pain relief is also faster (median, 3 weeks) when higher doses are used such as 90 Gy in all patients[13] with a median of 3 weeks (90 Gy in 44% of patients, the rest received 70 or 80 Gy in one or two isocenters)[10] than in patients treated with a lower dose, with a median of 2 months (0.9% with 90 Gy, 94.5% with 70 to 85 Gy).[11] Because higher doses are more likely to cause

TABLE 107-1 ▪ Pain Relief after Gamma Knife Radiosurgery (75–76.8 Gy)

	All Patients				Typical TN, No Prior OR Last Follow-up
	6	24	48	Last Follow-up	
Time after GKRS (mo)					
Range	0.5–10.4	0.5–33.3	0.8–55.0	0.5–62.0	0.5–61.9
Median	5.9	24.1	47.9	24.1	24.0
Mean	6.2	21.3	35.7	26.3	25.5
No. of patients	318	241	116	329	172
98%–100% relief, no pain, no meds	119 (37.4)*	85 (35.3)	45 (38.8)	100 (30.4)	60 (34.9)
≥90% relief, no pain, slight meds, or slight pain ± meds	41 (12.9)	54 (22.4)	13 (11.2)	68 (20.7)	42 (24.4)
75%–89% relief	76 (23.9)	12 (5.0)	5 (4.3)	26 (7.9)	10 (5.8)
50%–74% relief	20 (6.3)	9 (3.7)	3 (2.6)	17 (5.2)	11 (6.4)
<50% relief	38 (11.9)	17 (7.1)	5 (4.3)	28 (8.5)	10 (5.8)
Reoperate	24 (7.5)	64 (26.6)	45 (38.8)	90 (27.4)	39 (22.7)

*Percentage of patients is listed in parentheses.
GKRS, gamma knife radiosurgery; TN, trigeminal neuralgia.

dysesthesias,[13,14] the author recommends that maximal doses be in the range of 75 to 85 Gy for most patients.

Other factors may result in improved pain relief. Patients who had no previous surgery for trigeminal neuralgia and were found on high-resolution MRI to have contact between a blood vessel and the trigeminal nerve were more likely to have pain relief than those without such contact.[12] Patients in whom the isocenter was placed closer to the brain stem (so that the ≥20% isodose line treated ≥20 mm³ of the brain stem) also did better than those with the same maximal dose, in whom the isocenter was placed farther away.[15]

Factors that lessen but do not preclude the chance of pain relief after GKRS are multiple sclerosis,[16] atypical features,[9,11] and previous surgery.[9–11,16]

There are methodologic factors that may explain some of the differences noted in the results of series of patients treated for trigeminal neuralgia. These include variations in methods of data collection, criteria for pain relief (percentage, qualitative descriptors, or use of medicines) and the interval at which results are obtained.

Complications

Gamma Knife

The main complication that occurs occasionally from GKRS results from trigeminal dysfunction, which may cause impaired facial sensation and dysesthesias. These occur in 2.7%, 9.2%, 10.2%, 12%, and 16.7% of patients, respectively.[9–13] Higher doses of radiation are more likely to cause dysesthesias, and doses of 90 Gy may cause bothersome dysesthesias in 16.7%[13] or 32%[14] of patients. Also important is the duration of follow-up, as dysesthesias may take up to 19 months (median, 8 months) to develop.[11] There are no reports of trigeminal motor weakness, keratitis, or extratrigeminal complications after GKRS for trigeminal neuralgia.

In one series of 42 patients who were treated with at least a maximum of 90 Gy (possibly higher because of an old output factor), 4 patients developed impairment of taste sensation.[13]

In another series of 41 patients treated with 80 Gy, 3 patients complained of a dry feeling around their conjunctiva, and their corneal reflexes were diminished or absent.[17] No other abnormalities of the cornea and conjunctiva were found on ophthalmologic examination. The facial numbness in two of these patients gradually improved during the 14-month follow-up period. This dry eye syndrome was more likely to occur in patients who had an irradiated volume of brain stem receiving more than 12 Gy that exceeded 28 mm³.

The Author's Gamma Knife Radiosurgery Series

Two hundred seventeen patients without recurrence requiring another operation after GKRS for trigeminal neuralgia completed a questionnaire that graded any new numbness or dysesthesias post-GKRS on a scale of 0 to 10 in which 10 is the most bothersome. Dysesthesia scores of more than 5 occurred in 3 of 144 (2%) of patients who had no neurosurgical procedure for trigeminal neuralgia before the GKRS and in 4 of 77 (5%) of those who had a previous procedure; some of these patients had their dysesthesias caused by the initial denervating procedure, which was not GKRS. There were no other complications.

Linear Accelerator

Of 25 patients treated with LINAC with 90 Gy for essential trigeminal neuralgia, 32% developed mild facial numbness, but none developed painful numbness or anesthesia dolorosa; 12% developed subjective decreased but not absent corneal sensation.[8]

REPEAT GAMMA KNIFE RADIOSURGERY

A second GKRS can be done for patients with recurrent trigeminal neuralgia after an initial GKRS. The results of a second GKRS were similar to those of an initial GKRS.[18] Maximal doses of 35 to 120 Gy have been given for a second GKRS.[18–21] Although results from relatively few patients have been reported, there is a suggestion that better pain relief and more dysesthesias are seen with higher doses.[19] The only complications have been dysesthesias, which are uncommon when low doses (40 Gy) are used. Significant new dysesthesias (score greater than 5 on a scale of 0 to 10) developed in two of 45 patients (4.4%).[19] Patients who have never had a neurosurgical procedure before their first GKRS are more likely to respond to a second GKRS than those who had a previous procedure.[19]

The author prefers to wait at least 6 months from the time of an initial GKRS before offering a second one and has usually treated with 40 Gy as the maximum dose but has subsequently increased the dose of radiation at time of a second GKRS to 50 Gy. There is no clear evidence as to exactly where the isocenter should be placed for a second GKRS. The author has tried to minimize brain stem radiation so that if the 40% to 50% isodose line was placed on the surface of the pons at the time of the first GKRS, then at the second GKRS, we would place an approximately 20% isodose line on the pontine surface.

PATIENT MANAGEMENT

There are a number of factors that should be considered when planning a neurosurgical treatment for patients with trigeminal neuralgia and deciding which procedure (GKRS, percutaneous procedures, or microvascular decompression [MVD]) to do. These include the patient's age, medical condition, division of pain, severity of pain, presence of multiple sclerosis, hearing impairment, history of other procedures, and tolerance for risk.

GKRS is a very attractive option for patients with trigeminal neuralgia because it relieves pain in most patients and has the lowest complication rate. It is particularly attractive for older patients or those with significant medical illness. It can be done safely, not only for patients who have never had a previous procedure but also for those who have had other neurosurgical interventions.

Percutaneous procedures, such as radiofrequency electrocoagulation,[22] glycerol rhizolysis,[23] and balloon microcompression,[24] are a little more invasive than GKRS. The percutaneous procedures are more likely to cause dysesthesias and corneal denervation, especially if GKRS is done with 75 Gy rather than higher doses. Motor trigeminal impairment, although usually temporary, occurs not infrequently with radiofrequency electrocoagulation and balloon microcompression. More heavy intravenous sedation is usually required for the percutaneous procedures. Although GKRS can be done for patients with trigeminal neuralgia and multiple sclerosis, percutaneous techniques are especially attractive for these patients.

MVD is the most invasive procedure for trigeminal neuralgia, although it can be done safely on most patients.[25] Younger patients with vascular compression seen on thin-section MRI are often good candidates. Thin-section (1 mm thick) MRI, T1-weighted images without and with contrast, and T2 pictures can often show vascular contact with the trigeminal nerve. Such contact was seen in 59%[12] or 67%[26] of patients with trigeminal neuralgia who had not undergone previous surgery. Sometimes (23.8% of patients with trigeminal neuralgia) no contact is seen and sometimes (17.1%) another vessel is close but not clearly touching the trigeminal nerve.[12] Occasionally, one can see a small area of demyelination in the dorsolateral pons in patients who do not carry a definite clinical diagnosis of multiple sclerosis. This pontine lesion may be the cause of the trigeminal neuralgia and is more likely to be seen when there is no definite vessel in contact with the trigeminal nerve. Although even thin-section MRI is not an exact indicator of the true anatomic relationships, patients who do not have vessel-nerve contact on such MRI are less likely to have it seen in the operating room.[27] GKRS can relieve pain whether or not there is vascular contact seen on the MRI. The author is less eager to recommend MVD when high-resolution MRI clearly shows no vessel near the trigeminal nerve or when pontine demyelination is visualized.

Although the likelihood of pain relief after GKRS can be similar to that achieved with MVD, higher doses of radiation, such as 90 Gy, are needed to accomplish this. With these doses, dysesthesias will be more likely. With lower doses of radiation, such as 75 Gy, recurrent pain may be more likely, but dysesthesias will occur less often.

GKRS can treat pain in any of the three divisions of the trigeminal nerve. The treatment is the same, regardless of which division is affected. The very low risk of corneal denervation is particularly attractive, even for first division pain. Corneal denervation is more likely from radiofrequency electrocoagulation, especially if a first division lesion is attempted. Neither balloon microcompression nor MVD is likely to cause corneal denervation, both of which, like GKRS, can successfully treat pain regardless of the trigeminal division affected.

There is usually a delay of a few weeks before GKRS achieves pain relief. Sometimes patients have acute and severely disabling pain that prevents them from eating and needs to be relieved quickly. Usually, immediate relief from agonizing pain can be achieved with adjustment of medications or a local anesthetic, and dehydration can be prevented with intravenous fluids. In those rare circumstances when acute relief of pain cannot be achieved by lesser means, neurosurgical procedures such as percutaneous denervation or MVD, which can provide immediate relief, would be preferable to GKRS.

Hearing loss on the side of trigeminal neuralgia may occur after MVD and may be permanent if there is cochlear damage or temporary from fluid passing through mastoid air cells into the middle ear. Hearing loss can also occur from percutaneous techniques, such as radiofrequency electrocoagulation and balloon microcompression, and from fluid in the middle ear secondary to motor trigeminal dysfunction, which impairs

function of the eustachian tube. This hearing loss is usually temporary, but it can take several months for motor trigeminal dysfunction to reverse itself. Patients who have contralateral hearing impairment may be particularly disabled if they then lose hearing on the other side. Hearing impairment does not occur with GKRS.

Other procedures done in the past may influence the choice of a procedure for recurrent trigeminal neuralgia. Patients with recurrent trigeminal neuralgia after an initial GKRS can have a second GKRS, a percutaneous procedure, or MVD. Few data are available on the success and safety of a third GKRS if pain recurs after a second GKRS. Although the risks of an initial MVD are greater than the risks of the other procedures, the risks of a second MVD are much greater than the risks of an initial MVD.[25]

Patient preferences vary, and these are important factors to be considered in deciding on a neurosurgical procedure. How willing is the patient to accept the possibility of recurrence of pain, dysesthesias, or the complications, sometimes severe, associated with MVD?

CONCLUSIONS

GKRS is a safe and effective method for treating trigeminal neuralgia. There are fewer complications with GKRS than the other neurosurgical procedures. Recurrent pain can be treated with either a repeat GKRS or one of the other neurosurgical options.

The one small series of patients treated with LINAC suggests that this method may also be safe and effective for trigeminal neuralgia, but more patients followed for a longer time are needed to confirm this.

REFERENCES

1. Leksell L: Stereotaxic radiosurgery in trigeminal neuralgia. Acta Chir Scand 37:311–314, 1971.
2. Håkanson S, Leksell L: Stereotactic gamma radiation in trigeminal neuralgia [abstract]. Excerpta Med Int Congr Series 418:57, 1977.
3. Flickinger JC, Pollock BE, Kondziolka D, et al: Does increased nerve length within the treatment volume improve trigeminal neuralgia radiosurgery? A prospective double-blind, randomized study. Int J Radiat Oncol Biol Phys 51:449–454, 2001.
4. Kondziolka D, Lunsford LD, Flickinger JC, et al: Stereotactic radiosurgery for trigeminal neuralgia: A multiinstitutional study using the gamma unit. J Neurosurg 84:940–945, 1996.
5. Worthington C, Hutson K, Boulware R, et al: Computerized tomography cisternography of the trigeminal nerve for stereotactic radiosurgery: Case report. J Neurosurg 93(Suppl 3):169–171, 2000.
6. Regis J, Metellus P, Dufour H, et al: Long-term outcome after gamma knife surgery for secondary trigeminal neuralgia. J Neurosurg 95:199–205, 2001.
7. Smith ZA, DeSalles AAF, Frighetto L, et al: Dedicated linear accelerator radiosurgery for the treatment of trigeminal neuralgia. J Neurosurg 99:511–526, 2003.
8. Goss BW, Frighetto L, DeSalles AAF, et al: Linear accelerator radiosurgery using 90 Gray for essential trigeminal neuralgia: Results and dose volume histogram analysis. Neurosurgery 53:823–830, 2003.
9. Young RF, Vermeulen S, Posewitz A: Gamma knife radiosurgery for the treatment of trigeminal neuralgia. Stereotact Funct Neurosurg 70(Suppl 1):192–199, 1998.
10. Pollock BE, Phuong LK, Gorman DA, et al: Stereotactic radiosurgery for idiopathic trigeminal neuralgia. J Neurosurg 97:347–353, 2002.
11. Maesawa S, Salame C, Flickinger JC, et al: Clinical outcomes after stereotactic radiosurgery for idiopathic trigeminal neuralgia. J Neurosurg 94:14–20, 2001.
12. Brisman R, Khandji AG, Mooij RBM: Trigeminal nerve-blood vessel relationship as revealed by high-resolution magnetic resonance imaging and its effect on pain relief after gamma knife radiosurgery for trigeminal neuralgia. Neurosurgery 50:1261–1267, 2002.

13. Nicol B, Regine WF, Courtney C, et al: Gamma knife radiosurgery using 90 Gy for trigeminal neuralgia. J Neurosurg 93(Suppl 3):152–154, 2000.

14. Pollock BE, Phuong LK, Foote RL, et al: High-dose trigeminal neuralgia radiosurgery associated with increased risk of trigeminal nerve dysfunction. Neurosurgery 49:58–64, 2001.

15. Brisman R, Mooij R: Gamma knife radiosurgery for trigeminal neuralgia: Dose-volume histograms of the brainstem and trigeminal nerve. J Neurosurg 93(Suppl 3):155–158, 2000.

16. Brisman R: Gamma knife radiosurgery for primary management for trigeminal neuralgia. J Neurosurg 3(Suppl 3):159–161, 2000.

17. Matsuda S, Serizawa T, Sato M, et al: Gamma knife radiosurgery for trigeminal neuralgia: The dry-eye complication. J Neurosurg 97 (Suppl 5):525–528, 2002.

18. Hasegawa T, Kondziolka D, Spiro R, et al: Repeat radiosurgery for refractory trigeminal neuralgia. Neurosurgery 50:494–500, 2002.

19. Brisman R: Repeat gamma knife radiosurgery for trigeminal neuralgia. Stereotact Funct Neurosurg 81:43–49, 2003.

20. Pollock BE, Foote RL, Stafford SL, et al: Results of repeated gamma knife radiosurgery for medically unresponsive trigeminal neuralgia. J Neurosurg 93(Suppl 3):162–164, 2000.

21. Shetter AG, Rogers CL, Fiedler PF, et al: Gamma knife radiosurgery for recurrent trigeminal neuralgia. J Neurosurg 97(Suppl 5):536–538, 2002.

22. Sweet WH, Wepsic JG: Controlled thermocoagulation of trigeminal ganglion and rootlets for differential destruction of pain fibers. 1: Trigeminal neuralgia. J Neurosurg 40:143–156, 1974.

23. Håkanson S: Trigeminal neuralgia treated by the injection of glycerol into the trigeminal cistern. Neurosurgery 9:638–646, 1981.

24. Lichtor T, Mullan JF: A 10-year follow-up review of percutaneous microcompression of the trigeminal ganglion. J Neurosurg 72:49–54, 1990.

25. Barker FGI, Jannetta PJ, Bissonette DJ, et al: The long-term outcome of microvascular decompression for trigeminal neuralgia. N Engl J Med 334:1077–1083, 1996.

26. Jawahar A, Kondziolka D, Kanal E, et al: Imaging the trigeminal nerve and pons before and after surgical intervention for trigeminal neuralgia. Neurosurgery 48:101–110, 2001.

27. Chang JW, Chang JH, Park YG, et al: Microvascular decompression in trigeminal neuralgia: A correlation of three-dimensional time-of-flight magnetic resonance angiography and surgical findings. Stereotact Funct Neurosurg 74:167–174, 2000.

108 Percutaneous Stereotactic Rhizotomy in the Treatment of Intractable Facial Pain

CHAD J. MORGAN and JOHN M. TEW, JR.

HISTORICAL PERSPECTIVE AND OVERVIEW

The field of neurosurgery has a rich history of technological innovations, of which percutaneous stereotactic rhizotomy for trigeminal neuralgia claims a unique longevity. In fact, there have been only two major modifications to the technique since its original description by Kirschner in 1932.[1] The first and most substantial advance was made in 1969 when White and Sweet[2] refined the procedure with the use of the following: a short-acting anesthetic agent that permits the patient to awake rapidly for sensory testing during the operation; electrical stimulation for precise localization; a reliable radiofrequency current for production of the lesion; and temperature monitoring for precise control of lesion configuration. The next innovation made by the Tew, van Loveren, and Keller group included both the introduction of the Tew curved-tip electrode[3] (Radionics, Burlington, MA, U.S.A.) and the modification of the technique for cannulization of the foramen of ovale using image-guided fluoroscopy.[4] The curved-tip electrode enabled precise targeting of the trigeminal root and ganglion and reduced the need for frequent repositioning of the cannula. Without substantive modification since, percutaneous radiofrequency rhizotomy for trigeminal neuralgia has proven to be invaluable with high rates of success, acceptable durability, a respected safety profile, and a high level of patient satisfaction.

The differential thermocoagulation of trigeminal rootlets forms the theoretical basis for percutaneous radiofrequency rhizotomy. Supported by the studies of Letcher and Goldring[5] and others,[6,7] this concept proposes that the compound action potentials of A-delta and C fibers (nociceptive fibers) in a nerve are blocked at a lower temperature than are the compound action potentials of larger A-alpha and A-beta fibers that carry tactile sensations. Although physiologic studies have demonstrated the temperature-dependent selective destruction of A-delta and C fibers, some histologic studies have not documented this selective destruction of fibers after thermocoagulation.[8] Nevertheless, clinical observations in humans show the selective preservation of touch perception after radiofrequency trigeminal neurolysis. This discrepancy may be explained by the nonquantitative nature of histologic studies in which a single destroyed A-beta fiber can be more conspicuous than the destruction of 10 C fibers.

These historical references offer a perspective for today's neurosurgeons who are expected to lead a multidisciplinary team that can offer medical and surgical treatments directed to meet the needs of each patient who suffers with trigeminal neuralgia. The surgeon's skills should include the performance of microvascular decompression, percutaneous stereotactic techniques, and radiosurgery. In this chapter, we share our experience with percutaneous stereotactic rhizotomy using thermal ablation and seek to facilitate the understanding of a remarkably gratifying procedure.

INDICATIONS AND PATIENT SELECTION

Fundamentally, the diagnosis of typical trigeminal neuralgia must be established before any treatment paradigm is selected. We define the disorder by the following five criteria: (1) paroxysmal sharp and shooting pain that is characterized by exacerbations and remissions, (2) pain that follows the distribution of the trigeminal nerve, (3) a normal neurologic examination that includes no significant loss of facial sensation, (4) magnetic resonance imaging (MRI) of the brain that demonstrates neither mass lesions nor demyelinating plaques, and (5) pain that is induced by cutaneous stimulation.

All patients with trigeminal neuralgia preferentially undergo a trial of medical therapy using antiepileptic medication (typically carbamazepine). Failure or intolerance of this first-line treatment leads to the use of alternative medications such as gabapentin, baclofen, and phenytoin. Among those patients treated medically, long-tem relief fails in about 75% because of either pain recurrence or the development of toxic adverse effects. These patients are ultimately deemed to be surgical candidates.

When surgery is considered, we ask that patients and their families read and listen to an explanation of the surgical procedures and alternative methods of treatment currently proven to control trigeminal neuralgia as well as consult with others who have undergone surgical treatment for trigeminal neuralgia. These tactics aid to reinforce the patient's understanding of the procedures and provide an appreciation of possible undesirable sensory effects. Our policy is to let informed patients make their own decisions regarding the mode of treatment.

On the basis of our experience and a review of the literature, we conclude the following. First, percutaneous techniques and posterior fossa exploration offer advantages

1519

and disadvantages. Second, radiofrequency rhizotomy is the procedure of choice for older patients (older than 65 years) undergoing their first surgical treatment. Third, microvascular decompression of cranial nerve V is recommended for healthy patients who have isolated pain in the first ophthalmic trigeminal division or in all three trigeminal divisions, and patients who desire no sensory deficit.[9]

CANNULIZATION, STIMULATION, AND LESION PRODUCTION

In this section, the senior author describes his experience performing more than 2400 percutaneous stereotactic rhizotomies. We believe the three key steps to the procedure include (1) cannulization of the foramen ovale and the trigeminal cistern, (2) stimulation for pain reproduction and determination of intensity threshold, and (3) generation of an effective partial sensory lesion. To this end, we first review the nuances related to the successful cannulization of the foramen ovale and trigeminal cistern. Secondly, we discuss the subtleties of stimulation that allow for superior lesion production. Finally, we provide an algorithm that allows for the generation of an effective partial sensory lesion. This three-step approach to percutaneous radiofrequency ablation of the trigeminal nerve has proven safe and effective in more than 95% of patients.

Step 1: Cannulation of the Foramen Ovale

The procedure begins by administration of 0.4 mg of intramuscular atropine to reduce oral secretions and prevent bradycardia. The patient is positioned supine on the fluoroscopic table with the head in the neutral position. Next, Hartel's anatomic landmarks are plotted on the face as a point beneath the medial aspect of the pupil, a point 3 cm

anterior to the external auditory meatus, and a point 2.5 cm lateral to the oral commissure (Fig. 108-1A and B).[10] The first two points provide the rostral/caudal and medial/lateral trajectories for the penetration of the foramen ovale, and the third point is where the needle penetrates the skin of the jaw. After the affected cheek is prepared with Betadine (Purdue-Frederick, Norwalk, CT, U.S.A.), the patient is anesthetized with an intravenous injection of 30 to 50 mg of methohexital. A 21-gauge spinal needle placed in the deltoid subcutaneous tissue acts as a reference electrode.

Before cannulization of the foramen, an understanding of the skull base anatomy and its anatomic variants is essential (Fig. 108-2). Aberrant placement of the cannula can result in unintended neurovascular injuries. Use of lateral fluoroscopic imaging will aid in avoiding the following: cannulization of the inferior orbital fissure (IOF) anterosuperiorly or the jugular foramen posteroinferiorly, or intracranial placement of the cannula through aberrant foramina (e.g., foramen of Vesalius, which lies anteromedial to the foramen ovale, or innominate canal of Arnold, which lies posterior to the foramen ovale). Pulsatile blood flow through the cannula indicates penetration of the internal carotid artery (ICA). Puncture of the ICA can occur in three locations: at the proximal C2 segment at the carotid canal, the C3 segment with the electrode passing through the cartilage of the foramen lacerum, and the cavernous (C4) segment (Fig. 108-3). This third type of penetration was described by Rish,[11] who noted that an anteromedial electrode passing through the foramen ovale can penetrate the C4 segment of the ICA. If ICA penetration occurs, the cannula is withdrawn promptly, manual pressure is applied over the posterior pharyngeal space, the procedure is discontinued, and the patient is allowed 24 to 48 hours for convalesce. Ischemic complications, such as hemiparesis, and carotid-cavernous fistula have resulted from puncture of the ICA.[11] Generally, arterial punctures are minimized by

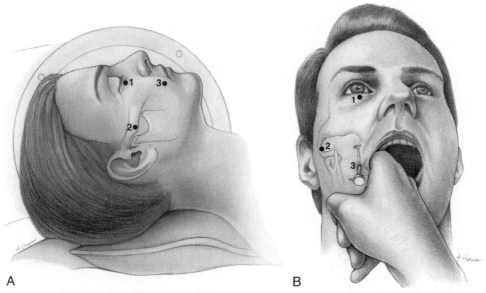

FIGURE 108-1 Hartel's anatomic landmarks for access to the foramen of ovale. *A,* Shows a point 3 cm anterior to the external auditory meatus (1), a point beneath the medial aspect of the pupil (2), and a point 2.5 cm lateral to the oral commissure (3). *B,* The target is the foramen, at the intersection of the three planes. The surgeon's finger guides placement to the lateral pterygoid wing. (Printed with permission from the Mayfield Clinic.)

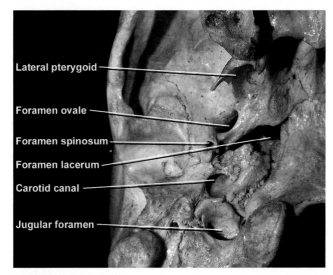

FIGURE 108-2   Skull base anatomy important to the successful execution of percutaneous stereotactic rhizotomy. (Printed with permission from the Mayfield Clinic.)

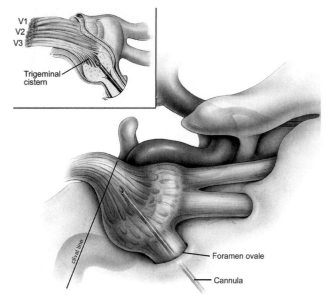

FIGURE 108-4   Optimal cannula placement through the foramen ovale into the trigeminal cistern located retrogasserian. The resting point of the tip should be approximated by the clival line. (Printed with permission from the Mayfield Clinic.)

refraining from broad angular readjustments of the electrode and diligent attempts to avoid trajectories that are either posterolateral or posteromedial to the foramen of ovale; such trajectories jeopardize the carotid canal and foramen lacerum, respectively.

The primary goal of the cannulization step is the penetration of the medial portion of the foramen ovale and placement of the electrode's tip in the retrogasserian rootlets (Fig. 108-4). Using Hartel's landmarks, we advocate either the direct penetration technique or the sequential palpation in which the surgeon processes the cannula down the smooth surface of the infratemporal fossa toward the superior-medial aspect of the foramen (Fig. 108-5). If the cannula enters the posterolateral aspect of the foramen,

it may elude the trigeminal cistern and not contact the trigeminal ganglion within its dural investment. Additionally, as the electrode is advanced, it may not reach the maxillary or ophthalmic divisions of the rootlet.

Once anesthetized, an oral airway inserted between the molars prevents the patient from involuntarily biting the surgeon's finger that guides the cannula. The index finger of a gloved hand is placed inside the patient's cheek just inferior and lateral to the lateral pterygoid wing. A standard 100-mm, 20-gauge cannulated needle is then directed from a point 2.5 cm lateral to the orbital commissure toward the

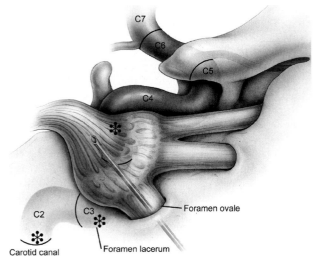

FIGURE 108-3   Relationship of the cannula tip to the segments of the internal carotid artery (ICA). Potential puncture sites (∗) include the C2 segment via the carotid canal, the C3 segment at the lacerum segment, and the C4 segment medial to the trigeminal ganglion within the cavernous sinus. (Printed with permission from the Mayfield Clinic.)

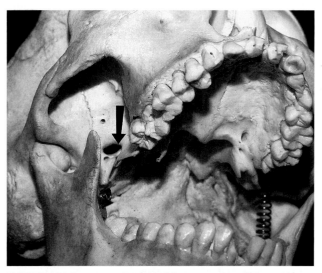

FIGURE 108-5   View of the skull base anatomy. Oriented in the trajectory taken by the cannula aimed at the right foramen ovale via Hartel's landmarks. The surgeon can sequentially walk down the infratemporal fossa (*arrow*) to the superomedial aspect of the foramen of ovale. (Printed with permission from the Mayfield Clinic.)

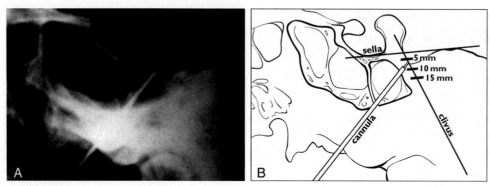

FIGURE 108-6   Electrode trajectory. *A,* Lateral radiograph. *B,* Shows ideal trajectory 5 to 10 mm below the floor of the sella turcica at the clival line. (Printed with permission from the Mayfield Clinic.)

medial portion of the foramen ovale. Although placement is by freehand manipulation, fluoroscopic visualization is important to assist localization. Use of the image intensifier in the lateral plane effectively localizes the needle.[4] Entrance of the cannula into the foramen is signaled by a wince and a brief contraction of the masseter muscle, indicating contact with the mandibular sensory and motor fibers. Before the cannula is advanced any further, a lateral fluoroscopic image is obtained to confirm proper placement in the foramen ovale (Fig. 108-6). Fluoroscopy allows targeting a point of the lateral projection of the clivus, which is 5 to 10 mm below the floor of the sella (Fig. 108-3). Difficulty penetrating the foramen ovale should cause pause and a return to a fundamental principle: namely, the safest approach to the foramen ovale is a trajectory that begins anteromedially to the foramen. In this manner, the surgeon can sequentially palpate, using the cannula along the smooth surface of the infratemporal fossa, and enter the superior medial aspect of the foramen. This technique allows the electrode to enter the trigeminal cistern and sequentially contact each of the three divisions of the trigeminal root. Furthermore, targeting the anteromedial portion of the foramen ovale reduces the risks associated with probing alternative portions of the skull base and lowers the incidence of hematoma due to venous or arterial hemorrhage.

Proper positioning of the cannula within the trigeminal cistern allows free flow of cerebrospinal fluid through the cannula in most patients, except for those few who have undergone previous surgical procedures or chemical injection. However, egress of cerebrospinal fluid does not ensure that the cannula lies in the proper position (retrogasserian). Cerebrospinal fluid can also be obtained either from the infratemporal subarachnoid space if the needle is too deep or from the region distal to the gasserian ganglion if the dural subarachnoid sleeve extends beyond the rootlets. Fluoroscopy must ascertain that the trajectory does not either project anterior to the sella where the cannula may penetrate the IOF or lie too low on the clivus (greater than 15 mm) where entry into the jugular foramen may occur.

Step 2: Stimulation of the Trigeminal Nerve

After penetration of the foramen of ovale, the electrode is passed through the cannula. Subtle adjustments made in the position of the electrode tip allow for precise stimulation of the division of the trigeminal root. When making these adjustments and generating stimuli, the surgeon should meet two important objectives. The first objective is the precise reproduction of the patient's trigeminal pain pattern. An appropriate stimulus will effectively replicate the patient's pain and lessen the likelihood of lesions in adjacent divisions. The key to precise stimulation is principally related to electrode tip placement (as described below). The second objective focuses on a determination of intensity threshold required to reproduce the patient's typical pain, thus providing the neurosurgeon with insight about the duration and temperature required to generate an effective partial sensory lesion. Below is a guide for translation of a stimulus threshold into an initial lesion.

Targeted stimulation begins with the manipulation of the electrode's tip in two dimensions as viewed on lateral fluoroscopy: the relationship of the electrode tip to the profile of the clivus and the curvature of the electrode's tip. When the tip rests at the level of the clivus, a stimulating pulse typically elicits paresthesias in the maxillary division rootlets. Advancement beyond the clival profile moves the electrode into the territory of the ophthalmic division rootlets, while withdrawal of the needle from the level of the clivus targets the mandibular division rootlets (Fig. 108-7). The electrode's tip should not be advanced more than 10 mm deep to the profile of the clivus because the tip can contact the abducens nerve in this region. Sometimes the needle must be redirected more anteromedially to bring the tip closer to the posterior clinoid process for closer contact with the ophthalmic division. If the globe moves during stimulation, the cannula is too near the cranial nerves (CNs) in the cavernous sinus or perhaps near the brain stem. Stimulus-evoked facial contractions indicate that the electrode is either too deep, inclined too low on the clivus, or the stimulation level is too high. A lesion should not be made if there is any indication of motor CN III, IV, VI, or VII activity or arterial bleeding.

After this initial placement and understanding of clival relationships, the axial rotation of the curved electrode permits a secondary form of targeting. Precise anatomic localization within the sensory root is aided by this maneuverability. The curved electrode tip is a coil spring that carries a thermocouple, stimulator, and lesion-generating probe. When the electrode is fully inserted into the cannula, the curved tip extends 5 mm beyond the end of the cannula and

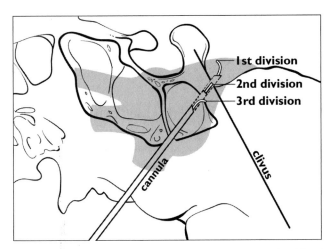

FIGURE 108-7 Composite illustration shows the relationship of the trigeminal rootlets to the clivus. When the electrode tip is proximal to the clivus, the third division is stimulated. When superimposed on the clivus, the second division is stimulated. Once beyond the clivus, the first division fibers are stimulated. (Printed with permission from the Mayfield Clinic.)

TABLE 108-1 ▪ Proposed Paradigm to Convert a Stimulus to an Initial Lesion

Stimulation Intensity (mV)	Probe Temperature (°C)	Duration of Lesion (sec)
<0.3	60	60
0.3–0.4	65	60
0.4–0.8	70	60
0.8–1.0	75	60
>1.0	Abort and reposition electrode	

Printed with permission from the Mayfield Clinic.

projects 3 mm perpendicular to the long axis of the electrode. Insulation of the cannula with polytetrafluoroethylene allows only the extruded portion of the electrode (0 to 5 mm) to be conductive. Rotation of the electrode can occur through a 360-degree axis for stimulation and lesion production. However, final placement of the electrode's tip is determined by the patient's response to electrical stimulation. A tip projecting cephalad or medial provides better access to the fibers of the ophthalmic division, whereas the caudal or lateral projection should enable contact with the mandibular fibers (see Fig. 108-7). Additionally, if the electrode contacts the motor root and elicits stimulation of the masseter or pterygoid muscles, the electrode can be rotated laterally to reduce the incidence of a lesion that may result in a trigeminal motor paresis.

Several general principles apply to satisfy the first objective of reproducing the patient's exact pain profile. A square-wave current of 100 to 400 mV at 50 Hz and 1-msec duration typically reproduces the paroxysmal bouts of pain that are reminiscent of trigeminal neuralgia. Stimulation at higher voltage (500 to 1000 mV) may be required in patients who have had previous intracranial rhizotomy or repeated alcohol injections. Alternatively, stimulation can be achieved with mild heat (less than 50°C). The evoked response not only localizes but reliably indicates the probe temperature required for lesion production. Consequently, the threshold current responsible for eliciting pain can be translated into a temperature and duration for the initial lesion, thus fulfilling the second objective. Specifically, the sensitivity of the nerve to a stimulus can be used to extrapolate an effective partial sensory lesion. Our paradigm for conversion of a stimulus threshold to an initial lesion is found in Table 108-1.

Step 3: Lesion Production

Generation of a lesion with dense hypalgesia in the primarily affected division(s) provides sufficient longevity yet limits the morbidity associated with more dense lesions. We believe that the ease of the procedure allows for additional

treatments in patients with recurring pain, and this dense hypalgesia provides clinical effectiveness and high patient acceptance.

With the information gained during stimulation, additional intravenous anesthetic is administered and a preliminary lesion is produced. The geometry of the lesions varies with the medium. Reproducible lesions are 5 × 5 × 4 mm, are eccentric, and are oriented toward the curve of the electrode. The electrode tip measures 0.5 mm in diameter. A thermocouple sensor located at the tip of the electrode provides calibration accuracy of ±2°C over a range of 30°C to 100°C. A facial flush (secondary to antidromic release of vasodilatory neuropeptides, such as substance P and calcitonin gene–related peptide), usually appears at this point and helps to localize the region of the nerve root undergoing thermal destruction.[12–14]

Next the patient is permitted to fully awaken, and careful sensory testing of the face is conducted. Repeat lesions are produced until the desired effect is achieved. After an initial lesion is produced as guided by our paradigm, subsequent lesions of 60- to 90-second duration are made by increasing the temperature 5°C with each sequential lesion. When analgesia is approached, great care is exercised to avoid overshooting the desired result, which includes preservation of the sense of touch. After production of a partial lesion, completion of the lesion is frequently possible without the use of additional anesthetic agent and with constant sensory testing that allows for fine control of the level of denervation. This tactic is particularly valuable when it is imperative to avoid analgesia and to preserve cranial sensitivity (as for a V1 lesion).

After the desired degree of sensory loss has been achieved, the patient is observed for an additional 15 minutes to determine whether a fixed lesion has been produced. If the examination indicates a stable level of hypalgesia, the distribution and degree of deficit are documented by careful sensory testing. The function of the masseter, pterygoid, facial, and ocular muscles is also recorded. The patient is then returned to the hospital room and is observed for 4 hours. During this period, the patient and family are informed of the requisite eye care, chewing exercises, and the consequences of facial hypalgesia. Anticonvulsant medications are sequentially tapered before their discontinuation.

RESULTS

We have treated more than 2400 patients with trigeminal neuralgia by percutaneous radiofrequency trigeminal rhizotomy.

We used the straight electrode in the initial 700 cases and the curved-tip electrode in all subsequent cases with some modification of tactics and technique. Of the first 1200 patients treated, mean age was 57 years (range, 10 to 95 years) at onset and 65 years (range, 25 to 97 years) at the time of surgery. Trigeminal neuralgia had been present for a mean of 8 years, and was characterized by increasingly severe episodes of paroxysmal pain and progressively shorter periods of remission. Thirty-five percent of patients had undergone a previous operation, including nerve avulsion, alcohol injection subtotal rhizotomy, ganglionectomy, microvascular decompression, or percutaneous rhizotomy. About one third of the patients had an unnecessary dental extraction or manipulation after onset of trigeminal neuralgia. In 4% of patients, the disorder developed immediately after dental extraction. In 4% of patients, multiple sclerosis was the presumed cause of the trigeminal neuralgia. The incidence of bilateral involvement was 18% in patients with multiple sclerosis and 5% in patients without multiple sclerosis.

Of these initial 1200 patients, 93% reported excellent or good results after percutaneous stereotactic rhizotomy (mean follow-up of 9 years; range, 1 to 21 years). In our prospective study of 154 patients who were followed for 15 years, 95% rated the outcome of percutaneous radiofrequency trigeminal rhizotomy as excellent or good.[15]

Recurrence of Trigeminal Neuralgia

In a retrospective study of 1200 patients followed for a mean of 9 years (range, 1 to 21 years), pain recurred in 20% of patients, including pain recurrence that was minor and required no medication in 5%; moderate pain that was well controlled with medication in 5%; and severe pain that required a surgical procedure in the remaining 10%.[9] In a prospective study of 154 patients followed for 15 years, the Kaplan-Meier analysis estimated a 25% pain recurrence rate at 15 years with recurrences occurring early: 15% within 5 years, 7% within 5 to 10 years, and 3% within 10 to 15 years.[15] Pain recurrence correlated directly with the degree of sensory loss: 60% of patients with mild hypalgesia had pain recurrence compared with 25% of patients with dense hypalgesia and 20% of patients with analgesia (see Figs. 108-7 and 108-8). The median pain-free survival rate was 32 months for patients with mild hypalgesia and more than 15 years for those with analgesia or dense hypalgesia.

Adverse Effects

Sensory

All patients experience some degree of numbness in the face after a successful radiofrequency thermocoagulation procedure. Troublesome numbness and paresthesias as a result of the inherent sensory deficit proved to be the most consistent adverse effect with both the straight and curved electrode techniques. The incidence of this adverse effect has decreased with the curved electrode[9]; our initial 1200 patients had an overall 3% incidence for major paresthesias (Table 108-2). Seventeen percent of the patients described an intermittent crawling, burning, or itching sensation that did not require treatment. These paresthesias

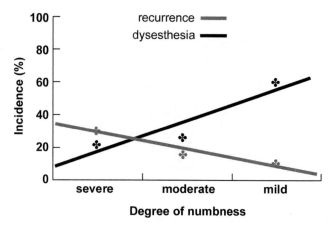

FIGURE 108-8 Recurrence rates (15-year follow-up) in 154 patients. Trigeminal neuralgia and dysesthesias as a function of the extent of initial numbness; notice the elevated incidence of pain recurrence in patients with a lesser extent of numbness. (Printed with permission from the Mayfield Clinic.)

usually diminished with time, and, interestingly, the more active and mentally alert patients reported fewer disturbances of sensation. A constant, severe dysesthesia in an anesthetic or analgesic zone (anesthesia dolorosa) rarely occurred with the straight electrode, and occurred in only one patient with the curved electrode. Tactics to reduce dysesthesia include testing sensations continuously during lesion production, asking the patient whether numbness is tolerable during the procedure, quantifying rather than qualifying numbness, and stopping lesion production when pain during thermocoagulation is no longer felt.

Ocular

Corneal analgesia developed in 6% of patients; this complication was reduced with the use of the curved electrode (see Table 108-2). Neurogenic keratitis developed in 2% of patients. Within this group, 30% had corneal analgesia rather than anesthesia, thus indicating that touch perception did not necessarily protect against corneal ulceration. However, early ophthalmologic care allowed resolution of the corneal abrasions in all patients. Application of a soft contact lens, meticulous eye care, and occasional tarsorrhaphy prevented permanent visual loss.

Transient diplopia occurred in 1% of patients. The most commonly injured nerves in order of frequency were the abducens nerves located in the lateral dural wall of the cavernous sinus, trochlear nerve, and oculomotor nerve. The most persistent diplopia lasted 4 months, and all occurrences resolved spontaneously.

Motor Paresis

Paresis of muscles innervated by the motor root of the trigeminal nerve occurred in 16% of patients. The motor root lies medial to the ganglion and may be avoided by lateral rotation of the curved electrode if stimulation produces contraction of the masseter or pterygoid. Thus the incidence of immediate postoperative muscle paresis was reduced from 24% to 7% by use of the more mobile curved electrode (see Table 108-2). In most cases, the deficit was partial and transient.

TABLE 108-2 ▪ **Complications in 1200 Patients after Percutaneous Radiofrequency Rhizotomy (Including Those Undergoing Multiple Percutaneous Radiofrequency Rhizotomies)**

	Patients (%)		
Complication	**Curved Electrode (500 Cases)**	**Straight Electrode (700 Cases)**	**Total (1200 Cases)**
Dysesthesia	11	27	20
Minor	9	22	17
Major	2	5	3
Anesthesia dolorosa	0.2	1.6	1
Absent corneal reflex	3	8	6
With V1 pain	8	20	15
With V2 pain	2	8	5
With V3 pain	0.3	2	1
Keratitis	0.6	4	2
Masseter/pterygoid weakness*	7	24	16
Diplopia*	0.5	2	1.2
Oculomotor			0.1
Trochlear			0.5
Abducens			0.6
Meningitis			0.2
Carotid-cavernous fistula			0.1
Intracranial hemorrhage			0
Death			0

*Nearly all trigeminal motor root and extraocular nerve palsies represented axonotmesis and resolved within 6 to 12 months.

Herpes Simplex

Lesions of herpes simplex were noted in 3% of patients. This figure is undoubtedly low because most patients were not examined more than 48 hours after surgery.

DISCUSSION

When contemplating the most appropriate surgical intervention for a particular patient with trigeminal neuralgia, the advantages and disadvantages of the three primary treatment modalities must be considered. Each technique—percutaneous (thermal ablation, glycerol injection, and balloon compression), microvascular decompression, and stereotactic radiosurgery—possesses certain attributes and limitations. Additionally, peripheral neurectomy of any of the three peripheral branches of the trigeminal nerve must still be considered an option by all surgeons who treat this condition. In evaluating each technique, one should consider the rates of paresthesias and dysesthesias, incidence of unintended trigeminal deficits, longevity of the effect, length of time from procedure until effectiveness, and morbidities specifically inherent to the procedure. In this manner, neurosurgeons can tailor an approach for each patient.

The most troublesome adverse effect after percutaneous thermal ablation is sensory paresthesias. The documented ability of the curved electrode tip to directly contact the involved sensory fibers allows the production of a more selective lesion than that produced by a straight electrode, thus enabling the reduction of undesirable sensory effects. We recommend a lesion that produces dense hypalgesia in the primarily involved trigeminal division. Our early enthusiasm to prevent pain recurrence by creation of a dense sensory lesion in the face has been replaced by a strategy to produce a reduced sensory lesion. Although the incidence

of pain recurrence may increase, we believe that the ease of repeating the procedure justifies the creation of partial sensory lesions in an effort to reduce undesirable side effects (e.g., dysesthesia, corneal sensation). Based on our experience, a lesion of dense hypalgesia is associated with a 25% risk of pain recurrence over 15 years and a 15% risk of dysesthesia, which is usually minor and does not require treatment.[15] In our review of the literature of series that included more than 100 patients reported from 1989 to 2003,[16-29] percutaneous radiofrequency rhizotomy was effective in controlling pain associated with trigeminal neuralgia, had minimal morbidity, and demonstrated acceptable rates of recurrence (Table 108-3). Furthermore, the radiofrequency rhizotomy procedure can easily be repeated with neither higher complication rates nor reduction in efficacy.

Alternative percutaneous techniques, such as retrogasserian glycerol injection or balloon compression, have not been detailed as thoroughly in the literature. Glycerol rhizotomy has theoretical appeal as a mechanism to relieve pain without sensory loss. However, data suggest that this technique is destructive and requires sensory denervation to avoid a high rate of recurrence.[30] Table 108-4 summarizes the results of several large series of patients treated with glycerol rhizotomy.[30-41] Dysesthesia, which was once hoped to be eliminated with this technique, still constitutes a major complication in most series. Although this technique appears to preserve the motor rootlets and the corneal reflex, the recurrence rates in some series have been prohibitively high. Symptoms of chemical meningitis occasionally constitute a major perioperative morbidity.[42]

Retrogasserian balloon compression is likewise a destructive procedure that can cause dysesthesia and facial numbness. Table 108-5 summarizes the results of several large series of patients treated with this procedure.[16,17,43-49] Because balloon compression boasts a relative preservation

TABLE 108-3 ▪ **Results of Percutaneous Stereotactic Radiofrequency Rhizotomy in Series (Since 1989) of at least 100 Patients**

Series	No. of Patients (n)	Follow-up (yr)	Long-Term Pain Relief	Significant Dysesthesia	Corneal Analgesia	Trigeminal Motor Weakness	Cranial Nerve Palsy	PO Morbidity	Severe PO Morbidity or Mortality
								Percentage (%)	
Fraioli et al[16]	533	6.5	89	NR	3	3	0.2	0.2	0
Frank and Fabrizi[17]	700	>3	75	NR	1	8	0.1	0.1	0
Miserocchi et al[18]	111	1–7	80	6.3	2	NR	0	0	0
Broggi et al[19]	1000	9	78	6.5	17	10	0.5	0.5	0
Sweet[20]	702	5.5	63	9	9	65	0.4	0.5	0
Ischia et al[21]	124	3.7	67	6	2	3	4	NR	NR
Nugent[22]	1070	9	73	6.5	3.5	26	0.2	0.5	0.2
Zakrzewska and Thomas[23]	265	3.8	71	8	9	NR	NR	NR	0
Tew and Taha[24]	1200	9	79	4	6	16	1	1.3	0
Oturai et al[25]	185	1–16 (avg 8)	51	4	NR	NR	NR	NR	NR
Spendel et al[26]	182	0.5–10	95	NR	NR	NR	NR	NR	NR
Mathews and Scrivani[27]	258	1–6.5 (avg 3)	74	8	2.3	28.8	0	0	0
Kanpolat et al[28]	1600	1–5	75	1.8	5.7	4.1	0.13	1.6	0
Tronnier et al[29]	316	14	25	0.9	0	NR	0.8	NR	0.8

Printed with permission from the Mayfield Clinic.
  avg, average; NR, not reported; PO, postoperative.

of small myelinated and unmyelinated fibers, this procedure may have a role in treating patients with pain of the first trigeminal division (V1) who require preservation of the corneal reflex. However, similar results can be achieved by supraorbital and supratrochlear neurectomy. The relatively high incidence of carotid-cavernous fistula formation in one series[43] probably was related to the large size of the needle (14 gauge) used. Anecdotal reports of death and other complications after rhizotomy have created concerns about the use of clinical rhizotomy and balloon compression procedures.

Among the open intracranial procedures for trigeminal neuralgia, posterior fossa exploration of the trigeminal rootlets for microvascular decompression and open partial rhizotomy are most often performed. Transtemporal decompression is rarely performed because of the association with high rates of recurrence and complications.[50] Microvascular decompression usually relieves trigeminal neuralgia and boasts a recurrence rate equal to that of percutaneous rhizotomy.[51–59] In a study of 1155 patients who underwent microvascular decompression during a 20-year period (median follow-up, 6.2 years), Barker and co-workers found most postoperative recurrences occurred

TABLE 108-4 ▪ **Results of Glycerol Rhizotomy in Series of at least ~100 Patients Since 1989**

Series	No. of Patients (n)	Follow-up (yr)	Long-Term Pain Relief	Significant Dysesthesia	Corneal Analgesia	Trigeminal Motor Weakness	Cranial Nerve Palsy	PO Morbidity	Severe PO Morbidity or Mortality
								Percentage (%)	
Bergenheim et al[30]	99	1	64	7	5	0	0	0	0
Young[31]	162	0.5–5.5	63	3	2	0	0	0.6	0
Waltz et al[32]	200	—	55	2	NR	NR	0	NR	NR
Fujimaki et al[33]	122	4.5	22	13	0	0	0	0	0
Ischia et al[34]	112	3.5	73	3	8	0	0	0	0
De La Porte et al[35]	120	—	NR	0	2.5	0	NR	0	0
Steiger[36]	122	5	41	13	16	4	0	0	0.8
Cappabianca et al[37]	191	1–7	70	0	10	6	0	6	NR
Jho and Lunsford[38]	523	0.5–11	46	2	0	0	0	0	0
Hananson and Linderoth[39]	100	5.4	57	0	0	0	0	0	0
Jho and Lunsford[40]	365	11	77	2	0	NR	NR	0.6 (aseptic meningitis)	1
Erdem and Alkan[41]	157	4	62	8.9	NR	NR	NR	NR	NR

Printed with permission from the Mayfield Clinic.
  NR, not reported; PO, postoperative.

TABLE 108-5 ▪ Results of Balloon Compression in Reported Series with at least 100 Patients

Series	No. of Patients (n)	Follow-up (yr)	Long-Term Pain Relief	Significant Dysesthesia	Corneal Analgesia	Trigeminal Motor Weakness	Cranial Nerve Palsy	PO Morbidity	Severe Morbidity or Mortality
				Percentage (%)					
Fraioli et al[16]	159	3.5	81	7.6	NR	3	0	0	0
Frank and Fabrizi[17]	212	<3	75	0	0	9	0.9	1.8	0
Lichtor and Mullan[43]	100	1–10	78	4	0	0	0	2	0
Lobato et al[44]	144	0.5–4.5	83	3	0	12	2.8	4.8	0
Addenneibi et al[45]	200	4.2	68	10.6	3	7	0	NR	0.5
Brown and Gouda[46]	141	2	68	6	0	0	0	5	0
Correa and Teixeira[47]	158	5	70–80	15	0	33	1.9	1.3 (meningitis)	0
Skirving and Dan[48]	496	10.7	68	3.8	0	3.4	1.6	0	0
Chen and Lee[49]	127	2	91	3.3	NR	NR	1.6	3.9	0

Printed with permission from the Mayfield Clinic.
NR, not reported; PO, postoperative.

within the first 2 years after surgery; 30% of the patients experienced a recurrence during the study period.[56] Ten years after the procedure, the rate of facial pain recurrence was less than 1% per year. Therefore, this procedure provides an attractive alternative, particularly in young patients, because the technique virtually eliminates troublesome numbness. However, posterior fossa exploration is associated with higher mortality and morbidity rates than with any percutaneous technique. We are mindful that trigeminal neuralgia is a benign condition and posterior fossa exploration should be considered carefully in patients who have significant risk factors for craniotomy (e.g., physiologic age older than 65 years or poor medical condition). When discussing the option of microvascular decompression with patients, it is advisable to state that a definite compression of the trigeminal nerve may be absent during posterior fossa exploration (estimated 15% in cumulative series).[9] In some centers, these patients may undergo a partial trigeminal rhizotomy, a procedure that carries at least the same risk for dysesthesia as a percutaneous procedure. However, we no longer perform surgical rhizotomy because the percutaneous procedure is considerably more accurate and less morbid in our experience.

Stereotactic radiosurgery is the newest addition to the neurosurgeon's armamentarium. Although this modality should be discussed with each patient, two aspects deserving of consideration were highlighted in a literature review by Lopez and colleagues.[60] First, the technique typically requires 1 to 2 months to achieve effective pain relief. In a population of patients with such debilitating pain, this interval of time may prove unfavorable. Secondly, despite a favorable side effect and complication profile, the actuarial outcome data for stereotactic radiosurgery is decidedly less favorable when compared with most percutaneous techniques.

Overall, microvascular decompression and percutaneous radiofrequency rhizotomy have comparable rates of pain relief, which are highest among the available procedures. Conversely, glycerol rhizotomy and radiosurgery have the highest rates of pain persistence or recurrence. All percutaneous procedures are associated with dysesthesia, while balloon compression

carries the highest risk for postoperative motor trigeminal weakness. Radiofrequency rhizotomy has the highest risk for postoperative loss of corneal sensations after surgery for V1 pain. Microvascular decompression carries the highest risk for postoperative hearing loss and perioperative morbidity and mortality.

Given all of the above data, our institution continues to rely primarily on percutaneous radiofrequency rhizotomy and microvascular decompression. Radiofrequency rhizotomy is the procedure of choice for most elderly patients undergoing first surgical treatment. Compared with posterior fossa exploration, all percutaneous techniques have lower incidences of hearing loss, facial palsy, intracranial complications, perioperative morbidity, and mortality. Among the percutaneous techniques, we believe radiofrequency rhizotomy affords the most selective and graded lesion, and can be easily repeated in those patients who experience recurrent facial pain. Microvascular decompression is recommended for healthy patients who have isolated pain in the first ophthalmic trigeminal division or in all three trigeminal divisions, and for patients who desire no sensory deficit. Patients treated by microvascular decompression may enjoy long pain relief without troublesome numbness. In those patients with recurrent pain following a microvascular decompression, we prefer to employ radiofrequency rhizotomy as the secondary technique. Because the comparison of cumulative data for different surgical procedures may not reflect the expected outcome, the surgeon should be flexible enough to offer the best procedure for each patient, guided by personal experience and the preference of the patient.

SUMMARY

Percutaneous rhizotomy of the trigeminal nerve via thermal ablation is a safe and elegant procedure when performed by experienced neurosurgeons. Treatment of this benign disorder demands use of such a procedure that is associated with low morbidity and negligible mortality. If patients experience a recurrence, a repeat percutaneous radiofrequency rhizotomy does not pose a significant problem because the procedure is easily repeated. Therefore, higher recurrence rates are acceptable to reduce the risk for denervation paresthesias and dysesthesias.

REFERENCES

1. Kirschner M: Elektrocoagulation des ganglion gasseri. Zentralbl Chir 47:28–41, 1932.
2. White JC, Sweet WH: Pain and the Neurosurgeon. Springfield, IL: Charles C Thomas, 1969, pp 594–621.
3. van Loveren H, Tew JM, Keller JT, Nurre MA: A 10-year experience in the treatment of trigeminal neuralgia: A comparison of percutaneous stereotaxic rhizotomy and posterior fossa exploration. J Neurosurg 57: 757–764, 1982.
4. Tew JM Jr, Keller JT, Williams DS: Application of stereotactic principles to the treatment of trigeminal neuralgia. Appl Neurophysiol 41:146–156, 1978.
5. Letcher FS, Goldring S: The effect of radiofrequency current and heat on peripheral nerve action potential in the cat. J Neurosurg 29:42–47, 1968.
6. Brodkey JS, Miyazaki Y, Ervin FR, et al: Reversible heat lesions with radiofrequency current. J Neurosurg 21:49–53, 1964.
7. Frigyesi T, Siegried J, Groggi G: The selective vulnerability of evoked potentials in the trigeminal sensory root to graded thermocoagulation. Exp Neurol 49:11–21, 1975.
8. Smith HP, McWhorter JM, Chalia VR: Radiofrequency neurolysis in a clinical model: Neuropathological correlation. J Neurosurg 55: 246–253, 1981.
9. Taha JM, Tew JM Jr: Comparison of surgical treatments for trigeminal neuralgia: Reevaluation of radiofrequency rhizotomy. Neurosurgery 38:865–871, 1996.
10. Hartel F: Uber die intracranielle injektionen behandlung der trigeminus-neuralgie. Med Klin 10:582, 1914.
11. Rish BL: Cerebrovascular accident after percutaneous thermocoagulation of the trigeminal ganglion. J Neurosurg 44:376–377, 1976.
12. Gonzalez G, Onofrio BM, Kerr FW: Vasodilator system of the face. J Neurosurg 42:696–703, 1975.
13. Goadsby P, Edvinsson L, Ekman R: Release of vasoactive peptides in the extracerebral circulation of humans and the cat during activation of the trigeminovascular system. Ann Neurol 23:193–196, 1988.
14. Tran Dinh Y, Thurel C, Cunin G, et al: Cerebral vasodilation after the thermocoagulation of the trigeminal ganglion in humans. Neurosurgery 31:658–663, 1992.
15. Taha JM, Tew JM Jr: A prospective 15-year follow-up of 154 consecutive patients with trigeminal neuralgia treated by percutaneous stereotactic radiofrequency thermal rhizotomy. J Neurosurg 83:989–993, 1995.
16. Fraioli B, Esposito V, Guidetti B, et al: Treatment of trigeminal neuralgia by thermocoagulation, glycerolization, and percutaneous compression of the gasserian ganglion and/or retrogasserian rootlets: Long-term results and therapeutic protocol. Neurosurgery 24:239–245, 1989.
17. Frank F, Fabrizi A: Percutaneous treatment of trigeminal neuralgia. Acta Neurochir (Wien) 97:128–130, 1989.
18. Miserocchi M, Cabrini G, Motti E, et al: Percutaneous selective thermorhizotomy in the treatment of essential trigeminal neuralgia. J Neurosurg Sci 33:179–183, 1989.
19. Broggi G, Franzini A, Lasio G, et al: Long-term results of percutaneous retrogasserian thermorhizotomy for "essential" trigeminal neuralgia: Considerations in 1000 patients. Neurosurgery 26:783–787, 1990.
20. Sweet WH: Treatment of trigeminal neuralgia by percutaneous rhizotomy. In Youmans J (ed): Neurological Surgery. Philadelphia: WB Saunders, 1990, pp 3888–3921.
21. Ischia S, Luzzani A, Polati E, et al: Percutaneous controlled thermocoagulation in the treatment of trigeminal neuralgia. Clin J Pain 6:96–104, 1990.
22. Nugent RG: Surgical treatment: Radiofrequency gangliolysis and rhizotomy. In Fromm GH, Sessle BJ (eds): Trigeminal Neuralgia: Current Concepts Regarding Pathogenesis and Treatment. Stoneham, MA: Butterworth-Heinemann, 1991, pp 159–184.
23. Zakrzewska J, Thomas D: Patient's assessment of outcome after three surgical procedures in the management of trigeminal neuralgia. Acta Neurochir (Wien) 122:225–230, 1993.
24. Tew JM Jr, Taha JM: Percutaneous rhizotomy in the treatment of intractable facial pain (trigeminal, glossopharyngeal, and vagal nerves). In Schmidek HH, Sweet WH (eds): Operative Neurosurgical Techniques, 3rd ed. Philadelphia: WB Saunders, 1995, pp 1469–1484.
25. Oturai AB, Jensen K, Eriksen J, Madsen F: Neurosurgery for trigeminal neuralgia: Comparison of alcohol block, neurectomy, and radiofrequency coagulation. Clin J Pain 12:311–315, 1996.
26. Spendel MC, Deinsberger R, Lanner G: Operative treatment of trigeminal neuralgia. Stereotact Funct Neurosurg 68:187–189, 1997.
27. Mathews ES, Scrivani SJ: Percutaneous stereotactic radiofrequency thermal rhizotomy for the treatment of trigeminal neuralgia. Mt Sinai J Med 67:288–299, 2000.
28. Kanpolat Y, Savas A, Bekar A, Berk C: Percutaneous controlled radiofrequency trigeminal rhizotomy for the treatment of idiopathic trigeminal neuralgia: 25-year experience with 1,600 patients. Neurosurgery 48:524–532, 2001.
29. Tronnier VM, Rasche D, Hamer J, et al: Treatment of idiopathic trigeminal neuralgia: Comparison of long-term outcome after radiofrequency rhizotomy and microvascular decompression. Neurosurgery 48:1261–1267, 2001.
30. Bergenheim A, Hariz M, Laitinen L, et al: Relation between sensory disturbance and outcome after retrogasserian glycerol rhizotomy. Acta Neurochir (Wien) 111:114–118, 1991.
31. Young R: Glycerol rhizolysis for the treatment of trigeminal neuralgia. J Neurosurg 69:39–45, 1988.
32. Waltz T, Dalessio D, Copeland B, et al: Percutaneous injection of glycerol for the treatment of trigeminal neuralgia. Clin J Pain 5:195–198, 1989.
33. Fujimaki T, Fukushima T, Miyazaki S: Percutaneous retrogasserian glycerol injection in the management of trigeminal neuralgia: Long-term follow-up results. J Neurosurg 73:212–216, 1990.
34. Ischia S, Luzzani A, Polati E: Retrogasserian glycerol injection: A retrospective study of 112 patients. Clin J Pain 6:291–296, 1990.
35. De La Porte C, Verlooy J, Veeck G, et al: Consequences and complications of glycerol injection in the cavum of Meckel: A series of 120 consecutive injections. Stereotact Funct Neurosurg 54–55:73–75, 1990.
36. Steiger H: Prognostic factors in the treatment of trigeminal neuralgia: Analysis of a differential therapeutic approach. Acta Neurochir (Wien) 113:11–17, 1991.
37. Cappabianca P, Spaziante R, Graziussi G, et al: Percutaneous retrogasserian glycerol rhizolysis for treatment of trigeminal neuralgia: Technique and results in 191 patients. J Neurosurg Sci 39:37–45, 1995.
38. Jho HD, Lunsford LD: Percutaneous retrogasserian glycerol rhizotomy. Neurosurg Clin N Am 8:63–74, 1997.
39. Hakanson S, Linderoth B: Injection of glycerol into the gasserian cistern for treatment of trigeminal neuralgia. In Gildenberg P, Tasker R (eds): Textbook of Stereotactic and Functional Neurosurgery. New York: McGraw-Hill, 1998, pp 1697–1706.
40. Jho HD, Lunsford LD: Percutaneous retrogasserian glycerol rhizotomy: Current techniques and results. Neurosurg Clin N Am 8:63–64, 1997.
41. Erdem E, Alkan A: Peripheral glycerol injections in the treatment of idiopathic trigeminal neuralgia: Retrospective analysis of 157 cases. J Oral Maxillofac Surg 59:1176–1180, 2001.
42. Sweet WH: The treatment of trigeminal neuralgia (tic douloureux): Current concepts. N Engl J Med 315:174–177, 1986.
43. Lichtor T, Mullan J: A 10-year follow-up review of percutaneous microcompression of the trigeminal ganglion. J Neurosurg 72:49–54, 1990.
44. Lobato R, Rivas J, Sarabina R, Lamas E: Percutaneous microcompression of the gasserian ganglion for trigeminal neuralgia. J Neurosurg 72:546–553, 1990.
45. Addennebi B, Mahfouf L, Nedjahi T: Long-term results of percutaneous compression of the gasserian ganglion in trigeminal neuralgia. Stereotact Funct Neurosurg 68:190–195, 1997.
46. Brown J, Gouda J: Percutaneous balloon compression of the trigeminal nerve. Neurosurg Clin N Am 8:53–62, 1997.
47. Correa CF, Teixeira MJ: Balloon compression of the gasserian ganglion for the treatment of trigeminal neuralgia. Stereotact Funct Neurosurg 71:83–89, 1998.
48. Skirving DJ, Dan NG: A 20-year review of percutaneous balloon compression of the trigeminal ganglion. J Neurosurg 94:913–917, 2001.

49. Chen JF, Lee ST: Comparison of percutaneous trigeminal ganglion compression and microvascular decompression for the management of trigeminal neuralgia. Clin Neurol Neurosurg 105:203–208, 2003.
50. Svien HS, Love JG: Results of decompression operation for trigeminal neuralgia four years plus after operation. J Neurosurg 16:653–655, 1959.
51. Bederson J, Wilson C: Evaluation of microvascular decompression and partial sensory rhizotomy in 252 cases of trigeminal neuralgia. J Neurosurg 71:359–367, 1989.
52. Sindou M, Amrani F, Mertens P: Microsurgical vascular decompression in trigeminal neuralgia: Comparison of 2 technical modalities and physiopathologic deductions: A study of 120 cases. Neurochirurgie 36:16–25, 1990.
53. Klun B: Microvascular decompression and partial sensory rhizotomy in the treatment of trigeminal neuralgia: Personal experience with 220 patients. Neurosurgery 30:49–52, 1992.
54. Cutbush K, Atkinson R: Treatment of trigeminal neuralgia by posterior fossa microvascular decompression. Aust N Z J Surg 64:173–176, 1994.
55. Mendoza N, Illingworth R: Trigeminal neuralgia treated by microvascular decompression: A long-term follow-up study. Br J Neurosurg 9:13–19, 1995.
56. Barker F, Jannetta P, Bissonette D, et al: The long-term outcome of microvascular decompression for trigeminal neuralgia. N Engl J Med 334:1077–1083, 1996.
57. Kondo A: Follow-up results of microvascular decompression in trigeminal neuralgia and hemifacial spasm. Neurosurgery 40:46–51, 1997.
58. Lee KH, Chang JW, Park YG, et al: Microvascular decompression and percutaneous rhizotomy in trigeminal neuralgia. Stereotact Funct Neurosurg 68:196–199, 1997.
59. Pagura J, Rabello J, De Lima W: Microvascular decompression for trigeminal neuralgia. In Gildenberg P, Tasker R (eds): Textbook of Stereotactic and Functional Neurosurgery. New York: McGraw-Hill, 1996, pp 1715–1721.
60. Lopez BC, Hamlyn PJ, Zakrzewska JM: Systematic review of ablative neurosurgical techniques for the treatment of trigeminal neuralgia. Neurosurgery 54:973–983, 2004.

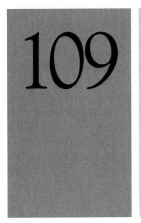

109 Neurovascular Decompression in Surgical Disorders of Cranial Nerves V, VII, IX, and X

RUSSELL R. LONSER and RONALD I. APFELBAUM

INTRODUCTION

The compression of specific cranial nerves at their entrance to or exit from the brain stem has been linked to a number of clinical conditions. Tic douloureux or trigeminal neuralgia is the most common, and perhaps the best described and investigated, of these cranial nerve disorders. Dandy[1] was the first to observe, in 1932, that vascular compression of the trigeminal nerve in the posterior fossa might be the cause of tic douloureux. Similarly, Gardner and Sava[2] later described vascular compression of the seventh cranial nerve in more than half the patients on whom they operated via the posterior fossa for hemifacial spasm, the motor equivalent of trigeminal neuralgia. However, it was not until Jannetta[3] applied the operating microscope to the systematic study of these problems that the truly remarkable incidence of pathologic vascular compression of cranial nerves at their entry to or exit from the brain stem was appreciated. Based on his findings, Jannetta devised an operative technique (microvascular decompression) to displace these vessels from the affected nerve without sacrificing neural integrity.[3,4] This technique has been used to relieve the specific cranial nerve syndromes successfully in the majority of patients treated. This chapter discusses the individual cranial nerve vascular compressive syndromes and the decompression techniques that can be used in treating them.

FIFTH CRANIAL NERVE

Clinical Presentation

Trigeminal neuralgia is characterized by a stereotypical clinical syndrome. Patients with trigeminal neuralgia exhibit brief, intense paroxysms of pain confined to one or more divisions of the trigeminal nerve. These attacks are usually triggered by light cutaneous stimuli within the trigeminal territory. The pain typically is described as an intense stabbing or electric shock sensation that patients frequently describe by rapidly flinging open their hands to indicate the paroxysmal nature of the jolts of pain. The pain is often more pronounced during the day, and many patients are pain free or have markedly fewer episodes at night. The most common areas of involvement are in the second and third trigeminal divisions, specifically anteriorly and in the region of the mouth. Because the mouth is a common site of symptoms, patients may undergo unnecessary dental surgery without achieving relief before the diagnosis of trigeminal neuralgia is made. Patients classically guard their faces, refuse to be touched, and avoid shaving, washing, applying makeup, chewing, and brushing their teeth because any of these actions may provoke an attack. Over time, patients will frequently report an increase in the number of attacks, reduction of pain-free periods, and occasionally sensory disturbances in the involved trigeminal distributions(s).[4,5]

Differential Diagnosis

Trigeminal neuralgia is occasionally the presenting complaint of a patient with multiple sclerosis. Trigeminal neuralgia occurs in 1% to 3% of patients afflicted with multiple sclerosis. Similarly, 2% to 4% patients with trigeminal neuralgia eventually are found to have multiple sclerosis.[6] The clinical picture and site of the pathologic process (the root entry zone of the nerve) appear to be identical in patients with idiopathic trigeminal neuralgia and those with multiple sclerosis. However, in multiple sclerosis, the cause of neuralgia is intrinsic demyelination of the nerve, which is not due to extrinsic vascular compression. Subsequently, microvascular decompression will not benefit patients with multiple sclerosis, and a neural destructive procedure should be used to treat medically refractory cases.

A history of sustained facial pain that is not paroxysmal must be questioned carefully. Patients sometimes describe frequent repetitive jabs of pain as one prolonged attack. This does not preclude the diagnosis of trigeminal neuralgia. However, slowly developing pain that builds in intensity, lasts for variable periods of time (often hours to days), and then subsides is not characteristic of trigeminal neuralgia. The most common mistake in the diagnosis of trigeminal neuralgia, in our experience, has been mislabeling patients who have chronic cluster syndrome. This and other atypical facial pain syndromes will not respond to surgical decompressive procedures.

Various other conditions must be considered in the differential diagnosis of trigeminal neuralgia. These include herpes zoster (postherpetic neuralgia), dental disease, orbital disease, temporomandibular dysfunction, and temporal arteritis, as well as post-traumatic neuralgias. None of these typically presents with the classic lancinating paroxysmal pain of trigeminal neuralgia. Once the clinical diagnosis of trigeminal neuralgia is made, magnetic resonance imaging (MRI) should be performed to rule out demyelinating disease, infection, inflammatory processes, vascular malformations, and neoplasms.

Medical Therapy

After the diagnosis of trigeminal neuralgia is made, a trial of 100 mg carbamazepine given twice daily is initiated. The dose is increased by 100 mg every other day until pain control is achieved or toxicity develops. Patients are instructed to take this medication on a full stomach and to have monthly hematologic studies performed so that toxicity can be detected early. In this manner, good control of the pain can be achieved in the majority of patients.[7,8] Patients who are allergic or intolerant to carbamazepine can be treated with phenytoin, oxcarbazepine, clonazepam, or baclofen. Although gabapentin is frequently promoted for this indication, no studies have been reported showing its efficacy, and it has rarely proven useful in our clinical experience. Surgery is reserved for patients whose pain is refractory to medical treatment or who develop medication-related side effects.

Indications

If the patient meets the typical clinical picture and fails medical therapy, surgical treatment options include microvascular decompression, selective percutaneous lesioning (with radiofrequency thermal coagulation or glycerol chemoneurolysis), or stereotactic radiosurgery of the trigeminal nerve. It is our practice to explain the relative benefits and risks of the surgical treatment options and assist the patient in choosing among these procedures (Table 109-1). We believe that microvascular decompression is the procedure of choice for the treatment of trigeminal neuralgia in otherwise healthy and relatively young (generally younger than 70 years old) patients.[9]

Preoperative Evaluation

We perform high-resolution MRI of the posterior fossa before treatment to reveal any unrecognized neoplasms, infectious causes, inflammatory processes, demyelinating plaques, or vascular malformations. We rarely obtain cerebral angiograms because the information obtained by routine angiography is not helpful enough to warrant the small but inherent risk associated with arteriography.

Anesthetic Considerations

During the operation, the patient should be chemically paralyzed and under controlled ventilation for two reasons: first, this minimizes motion in the field, which is greatly magnified by the operating microscope, and second, it prevents the patient from developing a gasp reflex should a small amount of air embolization occur. This reflex occurs with only a tiny entrainment of air and can rapidly result in massive air embolism.

To detect air embolization, a Doppler precordial detector and an end-tidal carbon dioxide monitor are used because they can detect even minute amounts of air. This detection allows the anesthesiologist to raise the venous pressure and prevent further entrainment of air, avoiding massive air embolization. The effectiveness of these methods of intravenous air detection is such that we have abandoned the use of central venous pressure catheters for this type of surgery. The central venous pressure catheter was originally inserted to allow the aspiration of air trapped in the right atrium. Small amounts of air, however, do not sequester in the atrium but pass through the heart into the pulmonary circulation. If detected at its earliest stages, raising the venous pressure to prevent further entrainment is sufficient.

When the patient is positioned in a sitting position, positive end-expiratory pressure, although not routinely employed, can be used to raise the venous pressure almost to the level of the head, creating the physiologic equivalent of having the patient supine. This approach should prevent any air entrainment and add a further margin of safety. The level of venous pressure can be adjusted to avoid significantly raising intracranial venous pressure with its associated increase in intracranial pressure.

If the patient is placed in a lateral decubitus position, the risk of air embolism is less but not fully obviated so similar monitoring is probably warranted. As with all neurosurgical anesthesia, it is desirable for the patient to have as smooth an induction as possible; it is even more important that the termination of anesthesia be effected in such a manner that the patient is allowed to awaken gradually and not buck on the endotracheal tube.

TABLE 109-1 ▪ **Relative Benefits of Percutaneous Trigeminal Neurolysis, Radiosurgical Trigeminal Neurolysis, and Microvascular Decompression of the Trigeminal Nerve for the Treatment of Trigeminal Neuralgia**

Procedure	Benefits	Drawbacks
Percutaneous trigeminal neurolysis	Safe, well tolerated despite age or infirmity Brief or no hospitalization Easily repeated if necessary	Treats symptoms, not cause Destructive, permanently alters facial sensation Risk of corneal anesthesia Dysesthetic sequelae can be severe Increased recurrence with passage of time
Stereotactic radiosurgery	Safe, well tolerated despite age or infirmity No hospitalization	Treats symptoms, not cause Delayed therapeutic response Risk of corneal anesthesia Increased recurrence with passage of time Limited therapeutic data
Microvascular decompression	Spares nerve, nondestructive No numbness No dysesthesia No corneal anesthesia Treats apparent cause, may be curative	General anesthesia required Craniectomy required Increased risk of serious and lethal complications Should be limited to healthy, relatively young (<65–70 yr) patients

Positioning

Although the patient can be positioned in either a sitting position or the lateral decubitus position for microvascular decompressive procedures, we use the sitting position for this procedure because it can be easily achieved in patients of any physiognomy and produces a relaxed operative field with the intracranial structures in their normal anatomic relationships. Moreover, it offers advantages for the anesthesiologist in that it avoids chest compression, allows good ventilation, and provides good access to the patient. In this position, cerebrospinal fluid and irrigant do not pool but flow out of the wound. Bleeding can be irrigated from the wound, minimizing the use of suction during the operation. This aspect is critical because of the potential risk of inadvertent injury to cranial nerves, other neural structures, or small blood vessels with suctioning.

We achieve the sitting position using a pin-fixation head holder for rigid fixation of the skull. The patient's head is rotated 15 to 30 degrees to the ipsilateral side. The head is flexed gently to provide ample room for placing one or two fingers beneath the patient's chin (Fig. 109-1). The elevation (or angle) of the back of the table is such that the patient is actually in a semisitting or slouched position, although higher elevation of the back rest may be necessary in the older patient with a less flexible neck.

Operative Procedure

After the patient is satisfactorily anesthetized and positioned, the operative table is angled an additional 15 to 20 degrees to the ipsilateral side so that the surgeon approaches the patient at an angle of approximately 45 degrees from the midline. The hair is shaved only from the posterior quadrant of the head on the affected side, and sterile preparation and draping is performed. The incision is vertical and located 3 to 5 mm medial to the mastoid notch (Fig. 109-2). We use a linear incision approximately 8 cm in length that is centered two thirds above and one third below the mastoid notch (see Fig. 109-2).

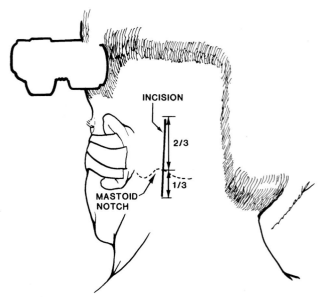

FIGURE 109-2 Placement of the incision for microvascular decompression of the fifth, seventh, and ninth cranial nerves. For decompression of the fifth cranial nerve, the incision (*solid line*) is positioned as shown so that two thirds of the length is above the level of the mastoid notch. For decompression of cranial nerves VII and IX, the incision is placed slightly lower so that one half of the length is above the level of the mastoid notch. (From Apfelbaum RI: Microvascular decompression of the trigeminal nerve. In Wilson CB (ed): Neurosurgical Procedures: Personal Approaches to Classic Operations. Baltimore: Williams & Wilkins, 1992, pp 137–155.)

To reduce scalp bleeding, the scalp is routinely infiltrated with 0.5% lidocaine with epinephrine (1:200,000). After incision of the skin, hemostasis is achieved with Dandy clamps secured to the drapes with elastic bands. Electrocautery is used to divide the occipital muscle mass down to the occipital bone. The anastomosis between the occipital and posterior auricular branches of the external carotid artery is often encountered with this exposure and divided. The muscle mass is then stripped from the posterior surface of the occipital bone. Care must be taken not to strip too far laterally because this determines the exposure once the self-retaining retractor is placed. Bridging emissary veins are coagulated, and their openings in the bone are sealed with bone wax. A Valsalva maneuver at this point can confirm hemostasis.

A modified Weitlaner retractor (Apfelbaum retractor) that serves as the base for a self-retaining brain retractor (Codman & Shurtleff, Inc., Raynham, MA) is then placed within the wound (Fig. 109-3). The retractor is secured by placing a gauze sponge through the loops of the handle and clipping it to the drape above the patient's head to provide good three-point fixation and achieve adequate stability for the retractor arm (see Fig. 109-3). Several burr holes are made and enlarged into a circular craniectomy (2.5 to 3 cm) (Fig. 109-4). The craniectomy should extend superiorly to the transverse sinus and laterally to expose the sigmoid sinus. The lateral extension of the bony opening often carries the craniectomy over mastoid air cells, which are thoroughly waxed at the completion of the craniectomy. Care is taken to displace the dura as the rongeuring proceeds to avoid entering the dura or venous sinuses.

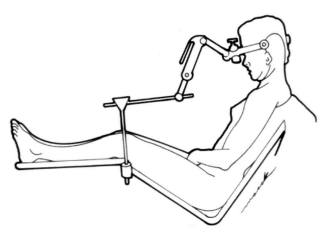

FIGURE 109-1 Lateral view of patient positioning on the operating table. (From Apfelbaum RI: Microvascular decompression of the trigeminal nerve. In Wilson CB (ed): Neurosurgical Procedures: Personal Approaches to Classic Operations. Baltimore: Williams & Wilkins, 1992, pp 137–155.)

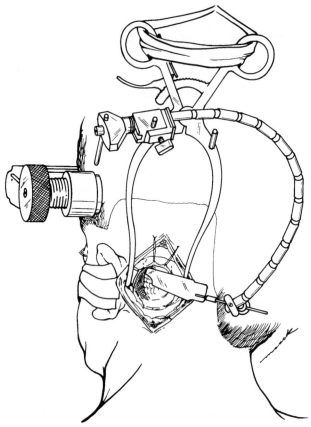

FIGURE 109-3 Position of the self-retaining retractor. Fixation of the retractor base to the drapes via an encircling gauze sponge provides a firm three-point fixation. The notched blade of the retractor serves to protect cranial nerves VII and VIII. (From Apfelbaum RI: Microvascular decompression of the trigeminal nerve. In Wilson CB (ed): Neurosurgical Procedures: Personal Approaches to Classic Operations. Baltimore: Williams & Wilkins, 1992, pp 137–155.)

Bridging veins may also be encountered and must be coagulated.

The dura then is opened in an inverted L-shaped manner 3 to 5 mm parallel to the sigmoid and transverse sinuses (see Fig. 109-4). The dura can be further opened in a T shape at the superior corner if increased exposure is needed. The dura is then secured with tenting sutures superiorly and laterally to retract the sinuses slightly and complete the exposure.

Occasionally, adhesions or bridging vessels are encountered along the superior posterior margin of the cerebellum along the transverse sinus. These must be divided sharply to free the cerebellum. A flexible retractor arm is then placed on the retractor base. This retractor arm should be positioned so that a gentle arch is formed and sharp kinks and bends are avoided (see Fig. 109-3). Its tension is adjusted so that it remains in any position in which it is placed but can be readily moved without undue force. A specially shaped retractor blade that has an elongated finger at its superior margin (Codman & Shurtleff, Inc.) is used (see Fig. 109-3). The purpose of the finger is to allow deeper retraction in the vicinity of the trigeminal nerve, while avoiding deep retraction and potential injury to the seventh and eighth cranial nerves. A narrow retractor blade could achieve the same depth of exposure superiorly but might penetrate into the cerebellum. Once the retractor blade is in place, the superior lateral margin of the cerebellum is retracted in a medial-to-inferomedial direction and the operating microscope is brought into use.

Before placing the microscope, an armrest is brought into position. This is a Mayo stand, modified as suggested by Malis, with the top removed and replaced with a 6 × 18 in. piece of metal. This metal sheet is padded, covered with a plastic sheet, and then covered with sterile drapes. Its height can be independently adjusted from the operating table to provide adequate support for the surgeon's arms.

Our standard procedure is to set up the operating microscope with the left-sided stereoscopic binocular observer tube for the surgical assistant. The scrub nurse is positioned on the surgeon's right. This positioning is used for all cases regardless of whether the exposure is on the right or left side of the patient. It allows for a standardized operative setup with excellent access between the surgeon and the nurse.

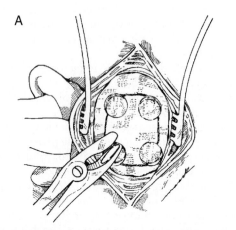
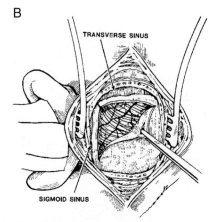

FIGURE 109-4 *A,* Placement of initial burr holes and rongeuring of the base to create a circular craniectomy. *B,* Dural incision for a left-sided approach showing the L-shaped dural incision. The exposure afforded by the dural opening can be expanded by expanding the opening in a T shape at the corner of the opening. Note that the transverse and sigmoid sinuses are exposed by the craniectomy. (From Apfelbaum RI: Microvascular decompression of the trigeminal nerve. In Wilson CB (ed): Neurosurgical Procedures: Personal Approaches to Classic Operations. Baltimore: Williams & Wilkins, 1992, pp 137–155.)

With the microscope in place, the cerebellum is gently retracted further medially. The approach should be angled as sharply as necessary to visualize the cerebellar surface. Adhesions and small bridging vessels are lysed as the cerebellum is retracted. Once the lateral extent of the cerebellum is visualized, the angle of approach is changed to follow the petrous bone anteriorly. McLaughlin and colleagues[10] refer to this change as "turning the corner" and emphasize the necessity of doing this under direct vision. At this point, the petrosal vein can be identified. This vein frequently is encountered two thirds of the way from the dura to the trigeminal nerve, but great variability exists, and it may be absent or positioned very close to the nerve. It often consists of two channels that form a Y-shaped bifurcation just before entering the dura. To permit adequate retraction and deeper dissection, the petrosal vein may need to be coagulated and divided sharply.

Once the petrosal vein has been identified and addressed, the retractor blade can be advanced. This is done while keeping the retractor blade close to the tentorium, which should be relatively horizontal in the operative field (variations in this view can be corrected with the use of the Trendelenburg control of the operating table). By advancing over the superior surface of the cerebellum, the surgeon can avoid the seventh and eighth nerves. It is not necessary to open the arachnoid around them. This approach exposes the arachnoid overlying the trigeminal nerve. If any bleeding is encountered while retracting the cerebellum, a dorsal bridging vein from the cerebellum to the tentorium may have been torn. Removing the retractor and depressing the cerebellum slightly will allow inspection of this area and control of this problem before proceeding. This tear is an infrequent occurrence, but the surgeon must be aware of its possibility. When possible, we first open the arachnoid about the petrosal vein to inspect the trigeminal nerve. This approach allows detection of compressing veins whose removal by petrosal vein resection would lead to the erroneous assumption of a negative exploration. Such inspection also provides the possibility of preserving a portion of the petrosal system, while still allowing adequate access to the trigeminal nerve. Preservation of part or all of the petrosal venous system is desirable in terms of reducing risk of venous cerebellar infarction.

The arachnoid overlying the fifth nerve is then opened sharply and widely to expose this area. This opening may be difficult because of the depth at which the work is being done and because of the narrow exposure. In some cases, the arachnoid is quite thin and translucent and can be easily punctured and teased free; in other cases, it is thick and opaque and must be sharply dissected. A great deal of care must be taken to avoid tugging on underlying structures. The trigeminal nerve is usually easily identified at this point, and the neurovascular relationships at the brain stem then can be identified.

The site of pathology is typically at the brain stem, and vessels impinging distally on the nerve are not usually the cause of the problem. The typical situation involves the superior cerebellar artery looping down in front of the nerve and emerging from the nerve dorsally at the point where the nerve exits the brain stem (Fig. 109-5). Opening the arachnoid widely allows a full inspection of the entire circumference of the nerve at the brain stem. The first vessel seen may not be the only vascular channel involved in the neurovascular compression because in a significant number of cases, multiple vessels have been encountered. It is also necessary to open the arachnoid anterior to the nerve to allow proper placement of the prosthesis.

The fourth nerve is a thin, delicate structure in the arachnoid above the fifth nerve and usually just below the tentorium. One of the reasons that sharp rather than blunt dissection of the arachnoid is recommended is that great care must be taken to avoid injuring this nerve. In addition, care must be taken in the dissection of this arachnoid to avoid injuring small vascular channels traversing the subarachnoid space.

The Jannetta microsurgical instruments (V. Mueller & Co., Chicago, IL), Rhoton dissectors (V. Mueller & Co.), or Apfelbaum dissectors (Integra Life Sciences Corp., Plainsboro, NJ) are of sufficient length and properly fashioned to allow adequate vision throughout the operation. Various microsurgical scissors including the Kurze left and right pistol-grip scissors (V. Mueller & Co.) as well as straight and angled bayoneted microscissors are also employed. Once the arachnoid is opened fully and the area inspected completely, the exact nature of the compression can be determined. A microdental mirror (warmed in hot saline to reduce fogging) may be useful in inspecting the region anterior to the nerve. This trigeminal nerve exposure is carried out directly over the seventh and eighth nerves (see Fig. 109-5). The presence of these nerves must be kept in mind to avoid traumatizing them during the dissection or while inserting or removing instruments. The arterial loops that are found are then carefully dissected free of the trigeminal nerve.

When the superior cerebellar artery is the problem, the intent is to elevate it to a horizontal rather than vertical orientation and to displace it upward and away from the nerve (see Fig. 109-5). This elongated vessel may have small branches going to the brain stem. Normally, these branches do not present a problem in the elevation of the vessel as long as their position is kept in mind. Venous channels above or below the nerve are dissected away from the nerve and are coagulated and divided. The coagulation of these vessels is facilitated by the use of small up-and-down angled bipolar forceps that prevent the spread of current to the adjacent neural structures. In the case of vessels compressing the nerve inferiorly, they must be displaced further inferiorly away from the nerve. In all cases, it is important to avoid kinking the arterial channels as they are repositioned.

To secure these vessels free of the nerve, a small prosthesis is inserted between the artery and the nerve (see Fig. 109-5). For this purpose, we use either Ivalon or shredded polytetrafluoroethylene (Teflon) felt. Ivalon, a synthetic polyvinyl formyl alcohol foam sponge material (Unipoint Industries, High Point, NC) has been safely used as a biologic implant for more than 30 years. This material comes packed in formalin and must be washed carefully to remove all traces of preservative. It can then be cut into small blocks and autoclaved. Before its use, Ivalon must be soaked for approximately 10 minutes in a saline solution to rehydrate it and allow it to become soft and pliable. A small block of the material is then carved to fit between the artery and the nerve. We usually fashion the block into a saddle-shaped

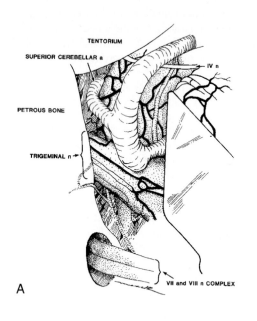

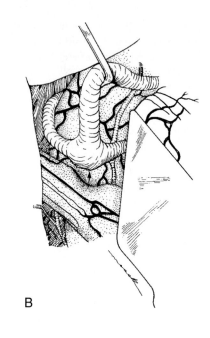

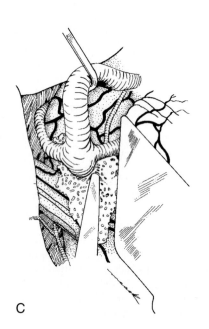

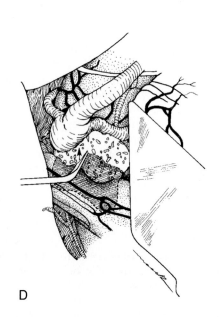

FIGURE 109-5   *A,* Schematic view of a left trigeminal nerve decompression. The superior cerebellar artery is compressing the superior edge of the trigeminal nerve. *B,* Elevation of the superior cerebellar artery reveals indentation and grooving by the artery. *C,* Ivalon is gently worked in between the nerve and compressing artery. *D,* The Ivalon is placed between the artery and the nerve so that the thrust of the arterial force is now directed away from the underlying nerve. (From Apfelbaum RI: Microvascular decompression of the trigeminal nerve. In Wilson CB (ed): Neurosurgical Procedures: Personal Approaches to Classic Operations. Baltimore: Williams & Wilkins, 1992, pp 137–155.)

structure so that it fits completely over the nerve. This structure effectively alters the arterial force vectors and creates a satisfactory decompression. In the case of a vessel inferior to the nerve, a similar type of sponge with a longer posterior element is fashioned, and this posterior element is inserted inferior to the nerve between the artery and the vein.

Shredded Teflon felt is another suitable prosthetic material and is particularly useful when the perineural subarachnoid space is narrow. The felt is shredded by grasping and tearing it with two hemostats to create a soft prosthesis resembling

a cotton ball. It is gently interposed between the nerve and artery in a large enough quantity to ensure a decent decompression. The Teflon felt is somewhat easier to place than Ivalon. A slightly higher risk of an aseptic meningeal reaction (headache and sterile cerebrospinal fluid pleocytosis) may occur with Teflon; the reaction is self-limited but may nevertheless prolong recovery time.

On several occasions, we have created a sling using a partial thickness of the tentorium that was looped down around the vessel and reattached to the tentorium with a small suture. This was effective when the subarachnoid space was too cramped to place Ivalon without adding compression to the nerve but was technically much more difficult than inserting the sponge prosthesis. If venous channels alone are encountered, no prosthesis is required and the channels are coagulated and divided. Coagulation alone shrinks them, which increases the tension on the nerve and allows for potential recanalization so the coagulated vessels should always be divided. Tumors can also be the sole cause of neural compression or found displacing a vessel against the nerve.

After decompression, if visible spasm is produced in vessels by the surgical manipulation, topical papaverine applied to a very small piece of Gelfoam is placed on the vessel for a few minutes to reverse the spasm. The operative field is then irrigated, and the retractor is removed. The cerebellum should be inspected at this point to be sure that there is no surface bleeding. We routinely place a piece of Gelfoam over the surface of the cerebellum and then effect a watertight dural closure using continuous and interrupted 4-0 braided sutures. A watertight closure minimizes the chance of a subsequent cerebrospinal fluid leak. We then place the rongeured bone fragments and drilling slurry wrapped in Gelfoam sponge into the craniectomy defect to provide a matrix for new bone formation and improved cosmesis. Wound closure then is effected in layers using various grade resorbable sutures followed by a running nylon skin suture. A small light surgical dressing is then applied.

Postoperative Considerations

Patients are nursed in the semisitting position for the first 24 hours and are observed carefully for any alterations in neural function or signs of pressure in the posterior fossa, resulting from cerebellar swelling or hematoma. Patients are allowed out of bed and begin oral intake on the first postoperative day. The urinary catheter is removed at that time, and intravenous fluids are discontinued as soon as the patient is able to achieve an adequate oral intake. The surgical dressing is removed on the second postoperative day.

Many patients have a postoperative headache. We routinely prescribe mild narcotic analgesics (codeine). The headache usually subsides within the first 2 days but may occasionally persist for several weeks. Most patients recover rapidly from this procedure and are ready for discharge by the third to fifth postoperative day. The majority of patients prefer a week at home for additional convalescence. During that time, their activities are not restricted, and they are encouraged to increase their activity gradually.

Operative Results

Compression of the trigeminal nerve was found in 450 of 466 patients (97%) (Table 109-2). In 380 (82%) patients, an artery was found compressing the nerve, most frequently the superior cerebellar artery (Table 109-3). In six cases (1.2%), an artery associated with a cerebellopontine angle tumor was found compressing the fifth cranial nerve (see Table 109-2).

Generally, our clinical results of this procedure correspond well with those of Janetta as reported by Barker and colleagues.[4] Most patients awaken from anesthesia without tic pain, but some continue to have postoperative pain for a few days or weeks (Table 109-4). This pain is less than that present immediately before surgery and will gradually taper off.

TABLE 109-2 ▪ Operative Findings in 466 Consecutive Patients Undergoing Microvascular Decompression for Trigeminal Neuralgia

Operative Finding	No. of Patients
Arterial channels (alone, with veins, or AVM)	374
Venous channels alone	65
Tumor (with artery, 6; without artery, 6)	12
Negative	15
Total	466

AVM, arteriovenous malformation.

Carbamazepine or phenytoin may be restarted for tic pain relief if necessary, and then slowly tapered over a few weeks. In long-term follow-up (mean, 77 months) of 466 consecutive patients operated on over more than 20 years (Table 109-5), the pain has been completely controlled with or without medication in 373 (81%) of patients. Five percent of these patients have had an occasional jab of pain but have not required any medication. An additional group of 63 (14%) patients have required medication for full pain control after surgery. Before surgery, all these patients had pain that was uncontrolled with maximal medical therapy. Although they have not experienced a perfect result, this group of patients has been greatly benefited by the procedure. Eighty-eight (18%) patients have experienced severe recurrences during this long follow-up period that have been refractory to medical therapy. These instances are failures of the procedure and have necessitated an additional, usually destructive procedure to achieve relief.

Complications

The complications in our series are presented in Table 109-6. Five deaths have occurred in this series, emphasizing the need for careful patient selection and screening. Cerebellar hemorrhagic infarction resulted in three deaths. We believe that this potentially lethal complication can be limited by minimizing the number of veins sacrificed at surgery. The most common type of complication is cranial nerve palsy. Fourth nerve palsy represents the most frequent of these and occurred in 16 (4%) patients. In all these cases, the diplopia has subsided over time (a few weeks to several months). Facial nerve palsy has occurred in six (1%) patients and hearing loss in

TABLE 109-3 ▪ Compressive Artery Found at Surgery in 466 Patients Undergoing Microvascular Decompression for Trigeminal Neuralgia

Artery Found	No. of Patients (%)
SCA	305 (80)
SCA and AICA	36 (9)
AICA	31 (8)
Basilar	6 (2)
Trigeminal	1 (0.2)
Unnamed	1 (0.2)
Total	380 (100)

AICA, anterior inferior cerebellar artery; SCA, superior cerebellar artery.

TABLE 109-4 ■ **Initial Results of 466 Patients Treated with Microvascular Decompression for Trigeminal Neuralgia**

Result	No. of Patients (%)
Complete relief	423 (91)
Immediate	366 (79)
At discharge	27 (6)
After discharge	30 (6)
Pain reduced	30 (6)
With medication	23 (5)
With additional surgery	7 (1.5)
Pain not relieved	8 (2)
Died	5 (1)

14 (3%) patients. The facial nerve palsies have been self-limited and resulted in good to satisfactory recovery in all but one case. Hearing loss was mild in five (1%) patients and severe in nine (2%) patients. Patients who develop a hearing loss usually do not recover their hearing, although one of our patients did. This type of hearing loss must be distinguished from modest decreases in hearing that many patients experience immediately postoperatively because of fluid behind the eardrum (presumably tracking in through the mastoid area). This is a benign, self-limited process that clears spontaneously within a few weeks.

Occasionally, patients will experience nonpainful, twinge-like feelings in the face that are often described as a "zippy" sensation. It is not painful but often produces great anxiety in the patients who fear that it portends the return of their pain. These feelings are frequent in our experience. They usually subside with the passage of time and do not appear to indicate a potential return to pain.

Conclusions

The Jannetta microvascular procedure, as detailed here, has proven to be an effective means of treating trigeminal neuralgia in most patients by treating the apparent cause of the problem rather than merely the symptoms. It offers the major advantage of sparing neural function and avoiding anesthesia dolorosa, other dysesthetic sensations, or facial sensory losses such as corneal anesthesia, but it carries with it a small risk of serious sequelae, including death.[4,9,11] Although small but not insignificant risks are associated with this procedure, we believe that microvascular decompression remains the treatment of choice for trigeminal neuralgia.

TABLE 109-5 ■ **Long-Term Results of 466 Patients Treated with Microvascular Decompression for Trigeminal Neuralgia**

Result	No. of Patients (%)
No recurrence	289 (62)
Mild pain, no medication required	21 (5)
Pain medically controlled	63 (14)
Severe pain not controlled medically	88 (18)
Died	5 (1)
Total	466 (100)

TABLE 109-6 ■ **Complications Noted in Series of Microvascular Decompression (*N* = 466)**

Complication	No. of Patients (%)
Died	5 (1)
Cerebellar infarction	6 (1)
Supratentorial infarction	3 (0.6)
Brain stem infarction	1 (0.2)
Focal seizures	5 (1)
Cranial nerve dysfunction	
Fourth nerve palsy (transient)	18 (4)
Sixth nerve palsy (transient)	2 (0.4)
Seventh nerve palsy (permanent)	5 (1)
Seventh nerve palsy (transient)	1 (0.2)
Eighth nerve palsy	14 (3)
Facial numbness	19 (4)
Dizziness, disequilibrium, ataxia	15 (3)

SEVENTH CRANIAL NERVE

Clinical Presentation

The motor analogue of trigeminal neuralgia is hemifacial spasm, which is caused by vascular compression of the seventh cranial nerve. This disorder is less frequent than trigeminal neuralgia. We typically see five cases of trigeminal neuralgia for each case of hemifacial spasm. Females are more frequently affected than males (3:2 ratio). Although rare reports of this disorder in children exist, it is typically an adult disorder with a mean age at onset of 45 years.[12]

Patients with this condition have repetitive, painless paroxysmal twitching of the facial muscles. Classically, this disorder starts with the muscles around the eyes and progresses slowly and insidiously to involve the middle and lower facial musculature. In severe cases, the spasm spreads to involve both the corrugator muscle of the forehead and the platysma muscle on the anterior neck. At times, severe sustained contractures lasting for several seconds, the so-called tonus phenomenon, will occur. The patient cannot voluntarily relax, so the contractures result in a grotesque disfigurement with forced closure of the eye and a tight grimace of the mouth.

Hemifacial spasm is often misdiagnosed as an emotional problem because, like many neurologic problems, it becomes worse during periods of emotional stress. The symptoms can have a profound influence on an individual's life by altering self-image, affecting relationships with others, and seriously altering career potential. Later, as the disease progresses, the repetitive frequent eye closures may alter an individual's ability to read or drive a car safely. Moreover, mild facial motor weakness may be noted between spasms and hearing may be moderately impaired.

Electromyography can be used to help establish the diagnosis of hemifacial spasm. Electromyographic studies in cases of hemifacial spasm characteristically reveal 5 to 20 rhythmically occurring burst discharges per second, along with individual discharges and longer-lasting bursts. The rate of discharge of the latter may be as high as 150 to 250 per second.[13] These findings are pathognomic for hemifacial spasm and can help resolve any uncertainty about the diagnosis.

Differential Diagnosis

The differential diagnosis of this condition includes several entities. Emotional and nervous tics differ from hemifacial spasm in their multifocal presentation, involving multiple muscles that are innervated by various nervous territories rather than being confined solely to the territory of a unilateral facial nerve. Blepharospasm is a bilateral forced contracture of the musculature about the eye. It differs from hemifacial spasm in its bilateral nature and involvement of only the musculature about the eye rather than a steady progression down the face. It appears to have a totally different cause and is not thought to respond to this type of surgery.

More closely mimicking hemifacial spasm are the synkinetic movements that may occur after aberrant regeneration of the facial nerve after Bell's palsy. A history of antecedent Bell's palsy with these movements developing on regeneration of the nerve will be most helpful in excluding it. Synkinetic movements develop with regeneration of the nerve and not as a late finding some time after adequate recovery from Bell's palsy. Facial myokymia also must be considered in the differential. These undulating wormlike movements associated with intrinsic brain stem pathology have a distinct and diagnostic electromyographic pattern. The association of other cranial nerve defects may also help to clarify this diagnosis.

Medical Therapy

In contrast to trigeminal neuralgia, no medical treatment has been effective in relieving this problem permanently. Some success has been obtained with the injection of botulinum toxin into affected muscles. The effect is frequently limited and requires repeated injections. Concern also exists about the cumulative toxicity of repeated botulinum injections.

Indications

Patients who are in reasonably good health and are generally younger than 70 years of age are potential surgical candidates. Alternative options that have been used for the treatment of hemifacial spasm include (1) selective neurotomy, (2) distal nerve avulsion, and (3) facial nerve sectioning with or without anastomosis to the hypoglossal or spinal accessory nerve. Selective neurotomy and distal nerve avulsion result in incomplete improvement and are associated with recurrence and facial nerve palsy. Partial division of the facial nerve, although immediately effective, frequently results in recurrence of symptoms that coincides with regeneration of the sectioned facial nerve. Repeated sectioning of the facial nerve after progression or recurrence results in additional neural destruction that eventually causes a permanent facial palsy. In an attempt to avoid recurrence after sectioning, some authors have attempted seventh nerve sectioning with subsequent anastomosis to either the spinal accessory or hypoglossal nerve in an effort to prevent distal facial nerve regeneration. This technique does not always prevent distal regeneration and recurrence and can result in tongue atrophy and facial paralysis. Because of these problems, we believe that the treatment of choice for hemifacial spasm is microvascular decompression the seventh cranial nerve.

Preoperative Considerations

Once the diagnosis of hemifacial spasm is established by clinical and electrical evaluation, high-resolution MRI of the posterior fossa with and without contrast material should be obtained. Neoplasm, inflammation, infection, and nonneoplastic structural lesions that are revealed by thin-cut MRI studies should be treated accordingly. As in trigeminal neuralgia, the absence of a visualizable vascular loop on imaging does not rule out such a lesion. Preoperative and anesthetic considerations as well as patient positioning are identical to that described previously for trigeminal neuralgia. Intraoperative monitoring of the seventh (electromyography) and eighth (brain stem auditory evoked responses) cranial nerves is useful during this procedure.[14,15]

Operative Procedure

The incision is positioned so that one half of the incision length is above the level of the mastoid notch (see Fig. 109-2). The exposure of the occipital bone and the craniectomy then are performed as detailed previously. Similar to trigeminal nerve microvascular decompression, the craniectomy is extended laterally to expose the sigmoid sinus. Vertically, the craniectomy (see Fig. 109-4) is extended superiorly to just below the transverse sinus and inferiorly to the floor of the posterior fossa. At this point, the bone is usually fairly thin and curves to extend almost straight away from the surgeon. It is important to not leave a lip on this area that will prevent the free egress of cerebrospinal fluid. The dura is opened in an L-shaped or reverse L-shaped manner 3 to 5 mm parallel to the sigmoid sinus and the floor of the posterior fossa fairly close to these structures and, if necessary, it can be further opened in a T shape. The dural edges are then secured with tenting sutures to widen the exposure.

The same type of self-retaining retractor system is used, but the retractor blade is arced from side to side and tapers in width (Aesculap Inc., Center Valley, PA). This retractor is placed beneath the cerebellum, and the cerebellum is elevated at its inferior lateral margin. The operating microscope, configured exactly as previously described, is brought into use at this juncture. Under magnified vision, the cerebellum is gently elevated. It is important that the cerebellum is elevated by retracting upward on it rather than retracting it from lateral to medial. The latter may cause traction injuries to the seventh and eighth nerves. A cottonoid strip is then placed along the medial inferior edge of the intradural exposure and acts as a wick to facilitate the drainage of cerebrospinal fluid and prevent it from welling up in the operative field. With elevation of the cerebellum, the retractor can be advanced anteriorly under direct vision until the spinal part of the eleventh cranial nerve comes into view. The arachnoid at this area is opened sharply, which allows further elevation of the cerebellum and exposure of the remaining nerves of the jugular foramen (Fig. 109-6). Occasionally, minute bridging veins will have to be coagulated and divided to effect this exposure. Once the ninth cranial nerve, which is usually slightly separated from the tenth and eleventh nerves, is identified, the exposure is carried medially by sequentially dividing the arachnoid (using sharp dissection) between the ninth nerve and the cerebellum.

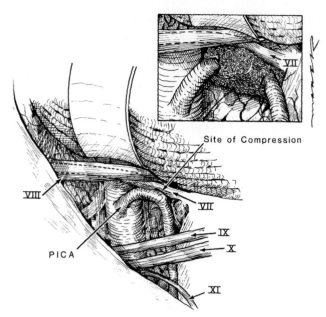

FIGURE 109-6 Microvascular decompression for hemifacial spasm. The retractor is elevating the cerebellum, exposing the posterior inferior cerebellar artery (PICA), which compresses the root exit zone of the facial nerve (VII). The inset shows the vessel displaced posteriorly and inferiorly away from the nerve by shredded Teflon felt.

TABLE 109-7 ▪ Operative Findings in 73 Consecutive Patients Undergoing Microvascular Decompression for Treatment of Hemifacial Spasm

Cause of Seventh Nerve Compression	No. of Patients (%)
Loop of AICA	29 (40)
Loop of PICA	22 (30)
Vertebral artery at AICA origin	7 (10)
Vertebral artery at PICA origin	4 (5)
Vertebral artery exclusively	4 (5)
AICA and PICA	3 (4)
Vein	2 (3)
Aneurysm	1 (1)
Bone exotosis	1 (1)
Total	73 (100)

AICA, anterior inferior cerebellar artery; PICA, posterior inferior cerebellar artery.

No attempt is made at this point to identify the seventh and eighth nerves at the porus acusticus (although they often may be in view). They are not followed from the porus acusticus medially to the brain stem because this increases the risk of injury to the eighth nerve. Rather the dissection is carried out just above the ninth nerve, and by sharply dividing the arachnoid, the cerebellum is gently elevated. Proceeding laterally to medially in this manner, the choroid plexus emanating from the lateral recess of the fourth ventricle will soon come into view. Its elevation will expose the root entry zone of the seventh and eighth nerves at the brain stem.

Two techniques are helpful at this point: (1) the operating table is rotated forward using the Trendelenburg control to increase the exposure superiorly toward the seventh and eighth nerves and to minimize the retraction that is necessary and (2) the retractor blade is replaced with a blade that has an elongated process in its center (Codman & Shurtleff, Inc.). This finger-like protrusion can be advanced up under the choroid plexus to elevate it and improve the visualization. This is a difficult area in which to work comfortably. With the patient's head flexed and the table tilted forward, the facial nerve will be visible in front of the eighth nerve with its origin slightly inferior. We use a facial nerve stimulator to confirm localization. The facial nerve usually has a slightly gray coloration compared with the pure white appearance of the eighth nerve. The individual components of the eighth nerve normally are not appreciated as separate nerves but rather run together as a compact bundle.

The site of cross-compression is found in this region where the seventh nerve leaves the brain stem. Several different vessels have been encountered in our experience (Table 109-7). The anterior inferior cerebellar artery may loop up against the nerve and then continue either laterally or inferiorly. The posterior inferior cerebellar artery likewise can loop up to compress this area before taking a more inferior

course. An ectatic vertebral artery can sometimes cause the same problem. On one occasion, an indentation of the nerve was noted but no definite vascular channel was found. On closer inspection, an exostotic protuberance from the floor of the posterior fossa was noted, and when the retractor was released, it could be seen that this protuberance mated with the indentation on the nerve. In this instance, the protuberance was removed with a high-speed diamond drill to effect relief.

When a vessel is encountered, it must be carefully dissected free of the nerve and placed in such a way that relieves the pressure on the nerve, while not kinking or compromising the vessel. Small tethering branches to the brain stem often limit the degree of displacement that can be achieved. One must always be aware of the possible presence of small branches along the medial side of the vessel going to the brain stem, especially at the apex of loops. After carefully dissecting the vessel free of the nerve and using the utmost care not to manipulate either the seventh or eighth nerves, an Ivalon sponge prosthesis is fashioned to fit between the two. This sponge often takes on a complicated shape because of the limited access in this area and the necessity of accommodating a number of different structures. We try to interdigitate the prosthesis between the vessels and often fashion protuberances on it to fit within the loops of the vessel to help anchor it in place. Alternatively, shredded Teflon felt is softer and easier to manipulate. It may be less likely to compress the adjacent nerves and also less likely to compromise the vessel and its branches. The Teflon felt should be shredded to a cotton-ball-like consistency (see Fig. 109-6) because it provides inadequate cushioning and is easily displaced when employed in sheet form. Absorbable materials, such as a Gelfoam sponge, should be avoided because the vessel may return to its compressive position against the nerve on absorption. Similarly, muscle, which is attractive because it is easy to insert, has led to recurrences as the muscle atrophied under the continued arterial pulsations and allowed the artery and nerve to come into contact once more.

Once a satisfactory decompression of the nerve is achieved, spasm is lysed with topical papaverine, the area is irrigated, and the retractor is removed, while the effects of this maneuver on the vascular anatomy are carefully observed.

Closure and postoperative care are identical to those used in treating patients with trigeminal neuralgia nerve decompression.

Operative Results

In 73 consecutive cases, a cause of compression was identified in each situation. No negative explorations were encountered (see Table 109-7). The most common cause of arterial compression was the anterior inferior cerebellar artery (40%), followed by the posterior inferior cerebellar artery (30%) (see Table 109-7).

Generally, our clinical results are similar to those of Barker and colleagues[16] and Samii and colleagues.[17] In our series, hemifacial spasm was relieved in all patients after microvascular decompression (Table 109-8). Sixty-seven patients (92%) had good (six patients [8%]) or complete (61 patients [84%]) relief of spasm on long-term follow-up (mean follow-up, 8.8 years). All patients who had long-term follow-up (70 patients [96%]) had a greater than 50% reduction in twitches (see Table 109-8).

Eighteen patients (25%) had recurrence of symptoms. Twelve patients had mild recurrences (less than 50% of preoperative level), and 10 of these resolved spontaneously. Three patients had moderate recurrences (50% of preoperative symptom level) and one resolved spontaneously, but the others worsened significantly. Three patients had a significant (equivalent to preoperative symptom level) return of symptoms and one of these resolved spontaneously. We reoperated on one of the patients who had a significant return of symptoms at 5 months. Re-exploration revealed an unsatisfactory positioning of the prosthesis. The prosthesis was replaced, resulting in full resolution of his facial spasm after surgery.

Complications

Most complications resulted in transient neurologic deficits or dysfunction (Table 109-9). Transient problems included facial weakness ($n = 11$), focal seizures ($n = 2$), and supratentorial stroke ($n = 1$). The transient facial weakness began in six patients 1 week after surgery. Three of these patients had trace weakness that could only be detected with careful examination. Of the other three patients, one developed moderate and two developed severe facial weakness that resolved over 2 to 6 months. Two patients had new-onset focal seizures at 1 and 6 months postoperatively. One patient

TABLE 109-8 ▪ The Long-Term Results (Mean Follow-up, 8.8 years) of the 73 Consecutive Patients Undergoing Microvascular Decompression for Hemifacial Spasm

Result	No. of Patients (%)
Excellent (complete resolution of symptoms)	61 (84)
Good (rare residual twitches)	6 (8)
Fair (50% reduction in twitches)	3 (4)
Poor (return of preoperative symptoms)	0 (0)
Unavailable	3 (4)
Total	73 (100)

TABLE 109-9 ▪ Complications in 73 Consecutive Patients Undergoing Microvascular Decompression of the Seventh Cranial Nerve for Hemifacial Spasm

Complication	No. of Patients (%)
Permanent	
Brain stem stroke (quadriplegia)	1 (2)
Unilateral hearing loss	2 (3)
Transient	
Facial weakness	
Trace	8 (11)
Moderate	1 (1)
Severe	2 (3)
Focal seizure	2 (3)
Supratentorial stroke	1 (1)

had a supratentorial stroke and recovered completely. Three complications resulted in permanent deficits (see Table 109-9) including quadriplegia secondary to a brain stem infarct (one patient) and moderate hearing loss (two patients).

Conclusions

Microvascular decompression as applied to the treatment of hemifacial spasm offers even more convincing results than those obtained in the treatment of trigeminal neuralgia because of both the lack of efficacious alternative forms of therapy and the very visible and graphic effects of the surgical procedure. This procedure carries a small but significant risk of serious sequelae. It is a more difficult procedure than the decompression of the trigeminal nerve, and its potential benefits must be weighed carefully in this nonlethal, painless condition.

FIFTH AND SEVENTH CRANIAL NERVES

Cushing[18] described a few patients with the combined clinical picture of trigeminal neuralgia and hemifacial spasm, a condition that he termed *tic convulsif*. In patients who appear to have features of both trigeminal neuralgia and hemifacial spasm, it is appropriate to explore the root entry zone of both the fifth and seventh cranial nerves.[19] Although vascular channels compressing on both nerves should be anticipated, it is conceivable that only one nerve will be affected because of anomalous innervation. It is always the safest course to explore both nerves.

NINTH CRANIAL NERVE

Clinical Presentation

Glossopharyngeal neuralgia is a condition that is analogous to trigeminal neuralgia occurring in the ninth cranial nerve territory. The incidence of these two disorders differs greatly with glossopharyngeal neuralgia being much less common than trigeminal neuralgia. Females are more commonly affected than males (2:1).[20] The onset of symptoms is typically between the ages of 40 and 60 years, with a peak incidence in the fifth decade.[20]

This disorder has been classified into two groups based on the origin of pain. Patients with the tympanic form have pain that starts in the region of the ear and radiates to the throat, whereas patients with the oropharyngeal form have pain that begins in the throat and radiates to the ear. Despite differences in the origin of pain, patients classically describe the pain as a paroxysmal shooting, stabbing, or lancinating. Both sides of the face and throat are equally affected.[20] Consistent with the close anatomic proximity of the vagal system, cases in which paroxysms have been associated with bradycardia, syncope, and occasionally asystole have been reported. The paroxysms are frequently triggered by swallowing cold beverages but can be precipitated by yawning, talking, chewing, coughing, sneezing, or touching in the region of the tragus. These episodic attacks often occur in clusters that last from days to months and frequently relapse.

The diagnosis of glossopharyngeal neuralgia can be confirmed by the application of topical cocaine (10%) to the patient's trigger zone. Patients with glossopharyngeal neuralgia will typically report immediate relief from the painful paroxysms, as well as prevention of retriggering with stimulation for 1 to 2 hours after the administration of the anesthetic.

Differential Diagnosis

A classic history and topical cocaine testing frequently make diagnosis of this disorder straightforward. In some instances, the diagnosis is not clear and other disorders must be considered. Trigeminal neuralgia (particularly involving the third division) can mimic many of the symptoms of glossopharyngeal neuralgia or occur concurrently with it. The paroxysmal nature of cluster headaches can sometimes be confused with glossopharyngeal neuralgia. The pain from superior laryngeal nerve neuralgia can also be mistaken for glossopharyngeal neuralgia.

Medical Therapy

Medical therapy for this disorder is similar to that of trigeminal neuralgia. Initially, control of symptoms should be attempted with carbamazepine with appropriate laboratory and clinical monitoring (see "Medical Therapy" under "Trigeminal Neuralgia"). Failure of carbamazepine therapy should prompt trials with other agents as outlined in the "Medical Therapy" section under "Trigeminal Neuralgia."

Indications

Once the diagnosis of glossopharyngeal neuralgia is established and other underlying structural or inflammatory causes are ruled out, medical therapy should be instituted as outlined above. Microvascular decompression is indicated in patients who are refractory to medical therapy. Patients selected for surgery should be in good medical condition and are generally younger than 70 years of age.

Preoperative Considerations

After a diagnosis of glossopharyngeal neuralgia, the underlying cause of the condition should be sought. High-resolution MRI with and without contrast material through the posterior fossa is used to determine whether the neuralgia is the result of neoplasm, infection, inflammation, vascular malformation, or other lesion. Each lesion should be treated accordingly.

Surgical options other than microvascular decompression for the treatment of glossopharyngeal neuralgia include (1) percutaneous thermal rhizotomy of the glossopharyngeal at the jugular foramen, (2) extracranial sectioning of branches of the glossopharyngeal nerve, (3) intracranial sectioning of the glossopharyngeal nerve, and (4) sectioning of the upper vagal nerve rootlets. The nonspecific nature of percutaneous rhizotomy of the glossopharyngeal nerve can provide relief from pain but not infrequently results in permanent dysphagia and hoarseness. Extracranial sectioning of the glossopharyngeal or vagal nerve for neuralgia may provide immediate relief but is associated with recurrence of symptoms. Intracranial sectioning of the glossopharyngeal nerve and at times the upper fibers of the vagus nerve has been successful at relieving glossopharyngeal neuralgia. It is usually well tolerated but can result in vocal cord paralysis, diminished gag reflex, and dysphagia. Microvascular decompression can be used to avoid these difficulties and provide a permanent solution to the symptoms associated with glossopharyngeal neuralgia.

The anesthesia and positioning for microvascular decompression of the ninth cranial nerve are the same as for seventh nerve decompression.

Operative Procedure

As in surgery on the seventh cranial nerve, the incision is positioned so that one half of the incision length is above the level of the mastoid notch. The operative exposure is the same as the one detailed for the seventh cranial nerve with the modification that the root entry zone of the ninth cranial nerve is inspected and decompressed. This exposure is accomplished by following the superior surface of the ninth nerve back to the brain stem and then visualizing this area, working between the seventh and eighth nerves above and the ninth nerve below or between the ninth and tenth nerves. When decompression cannot be achieved, sectioning of cranial nerve IX and the upper fascicles of cranial nerve X can provide good relief.

Operative Results

Because of the rare occurrence of this disorder, few large series with long-term follow-up have evaluated the efficacy of microvascular decompression for glossopharyngeal neuralgia.[20–22] In 2002, Patel and colleagues[20] reported the efficacy of microvascular decompression for glossopharyngeal neuralgia in 217 patients. This study found that immediately after surgery, 67% of patients had complete relief and an additional 25% had partial relief for an immediate postoperative success rate of 92%. Fifty-eight percent of the 50 patients with long-term follow-up (mean follow-up, 4 years) had complete relief of symptoms, 18% had partial relief (minimum of 4-point improvement on a continuous pain scale, with or without medications), and 24% had a lack of substantial improvement. Moreover, this study found that isolated throat pain was a positive predictor of operative success.

Complications

In the series reported by Patel and colleagues,[20] the rates of various complications were broken down into quartiles of approximately 50 patients over the time period extending from 1973 to 2000. Various complications including intracranial hematoma (rate of 0% to 5.8% over quartiles), brain stem infarction (0% to 4.1%), ninth/tenth cranial nerve palsy (0% to 4.2%), eighth/other cranial nerve palsy (0% to 4.2%), cerebrospinal fluid leak (1.5% to 5.8%), operative-related death (0% to 5.8%), and dysphagia (0% to 4.2%) were observed.

Conclusions

Microvascular decompression for the treatment of glossopharyngeal neuralgia provides similar results to those obtained in the treatment of trigeminal neuralgia. This procedure carries the obvious risks inherent to the regional anatomy. For these reasons, this procedure should only be undertaken in patients with a well-established diagnosis of glossopharyngeal neuralgia that is incapacitating and refractory to medical therapy. When decompression cannot be achieved, sectioning of cranial nerve IX and the upper few fascicles of cranial nerve X can provide good relief.

REFERENCES

1. Dandy W: The treatment of trigeminal neuralgia by the cerebellar route. Ann Surg 96:787–795, 1932.
2. Gardner W, Sava G: Hemifacial spasm—a reversible pathophysiologic state. J Neurosurg 19:240–247, 1962.
3. Jannetta PJ: Arterial compression of the trigeminal nerve at the pons in patients with trigeminal neuralgia. J Neurosurg 26(Suppl):159–162, 1967.
4. Barker FG 2nd, Jannetta PJ, Bissonnette DJ, et al: The long-term outcome of microvascular decompression for trigeminal neuralgia. N Engl J Med 334:1077–1083, 1996.
5. Burchiel KJ, Slavin KV: On the natural history of trigeminal neuralgia. Neurosurgery 46:152–155, 2000.
6. Jensen TS, Rasmussen P, Reske-Nielsen E: Association of trigeminal neuralgia with multiple sclerosis: Clinical and pathologic features. Acta Neurol Scand 65:182–189, 1982.
7. Campbell FG, Graham JG, Zilkha KJ: Clinical trial of carbazepine (Tegretol) in trigeminal neuralgia. J Neurol Neurosurg Psychiatry 29:265–267, 1966.
8. Rockliff BW, Davis EH: Controlled sequential trials of carbamazepine in trigeminal neuralgia. Arch Neurol 15:129–136, 1966.
9. Apfelbaum RI: Neurovascular decompression: The procedure of choice? Clin Neurosurg 46:473–498, 2000.
10. McLaughlin MR, Jannetta PJ, Clyde BL, et al: Microvascular decompression of cranial nerves: Lessons learned after 4400 operations. J Neurosurg 90:1–8, 1999.
11. Kalkanis SN, Eskander EN, Carter BS, et al: Microvascular decompression surgery in the United States, 1996 to 2000: Mortality rates, morbidity rates, and the effects of hospital and surgeon volumes. Neurosurgery 52:1251–1262, 2003.
12. Digre K, Corbett JJ: Hemifacial spasm: Differential diagnosis, mechanism, and treatment. Adv Neurol 49:151–176, 1988.
13. Magun R, Esslen E: Electromyographic study of reinnervated muscle and of hemifacial spasm. Am J Phys Med Rehabil 38:79–86, 1959.
14. Mooij JJA, Mustafa MK, van Weerden TW: Hemifacial spasm: Intraoperative electromyographic monitoring as a guide for microvascular decompression. Neurosurgery 49:1365–1371, 2001.
15. Polo G, Fischer C, Sindou MP, et al: Brainstem auditory evoked potential monitoring during microvascular decompression for hemifacial spasm: Intraoperative brainstem auditory evoked potential changes and warning values to prevent hearing loss—prospective study in a consecutive series of 84 patients. Neurosurgery 54:97–106, 2004.
16. Barker FG 2nd, Jannetta PJ, Bissonette DJ, et al: Microvascular decompression for hemifacial spasm. J Neurosurg 82:201–210, 1995.
17. Samii M, Gunther T, Iaconetta G, et al: Microvascular decompression to treat hemifacial spasm: Long-term results for a consecutive series of 143 patients. Neurosurgery 50:712–719, 2002.
18. Cushing H: The major trigeminal neuralgias and their surgical treatment based on experiences with 332 gasserian operations. Am J Med Sci 160:157–184, 1920.
19. Cook BR, Jannetta PJ: Tic convulsif: Results in 11 cases treated with microvascular decompression of the fifth and seventh cranial nerves. J Neurosurg 61:949–951, 1984.
20. Patel A, Kassam A, Horowitz M, et al: Microvascular decompression in the management of glossopharyngeal neuralgia: Analysis of 217 cases. Neurosurgery 50:705–711, 2002.
21. Kondo A: Follow-up results of using microvascular decompression for treatment of glossopharyngeal neuralgia. J Neurosurg 88:221–225, 1998.
22. Resnick DK, Jannetta PJ, Bissonnette D, et al: Microvascular decompression for glossopharyngeal neuralgia. Neurosurgery 36:64–69, 1995.

110 Spinal Cord Stimulation and Intraspinal Infusions for Pain*

GILBERT J. FANCIULLO and PERRY A. BALL

SPINAL CORD STIMULATION

Introduction and General Selection Criteria

The first clinical report of spinal cord stimulation (SCS) was published in 1967.[1] Since then, the use of implantable devices for the management of chronic pain has become well established in the United States, Europe, and Australia. Electrical stimulation of the spinal cord has proven efficacy for the relief of pain in patients with arachnoiditis, PVOD, peripheral nerve injury, complex regional pain syndrome, angina pectoris, and radiculopathy and pain of spinal origin.

Indications for SCS device implantation are not always clear. Experienced clinicians can be found debating the relative efficacy of implantation for specific diseases or in unique and complex patients. Despite the absence of randomized, controlled trials in many cases to prove the efficacy of SCS for specific conditions, strong recommendations for most patients can be made because the results of multiple observational studies can be considered overwhelming for major conditions.

General indications for SCS implantation can be applied to all potential candidates. It is usually accepted, but not proven, that patients who have objective findings related to their pain complaint will have better outcomes after implantation than patients who do not have such evidence. A clear exception to this rule is patients with complex regional pain syndrome (CRPS) for whom there is often not objective evidence of their pain complaint but who have been reported to respond well to SCS.[2]

Patients who have clear non-SCS surgical options with a good probability of success for relief of their pain should undergo the definitive surgical procedure rather than treatment with an implantable device. For example, a patient with an L5 radiculopathy and a magnetic resonance imaging scan that shows a herniated nucleus pulposis that compresses the L5 nerve root should be treated with a discectomy rather than implantation of an SCS system.

Implantation, although a relatively low morbidity procedure, is a surgical procedure, and less invasive or dangerous alternative treatments should be exhausted before consideration of implantation of these devices. These include physical medicine approaches, psychological approaches, anesthesia procedural approaches such as epidural steroid injections, and pharmacologic approaches. A trial with and failure to respond to oral opioid therapy before consideration for implantation of an SCS device is controversial, and there are no data to help with this decision. Variables include physician and patient preferences, history of substance abuse, patient tolerance, the type of pain, and family concerns, among others.

A psychiatric or psychological evaluation should be obtained before implantation. Patient outcome may depend on confounding coexisting psychiatric comorbidity. It is extremely important to assess patients for psychiatric disorders including substance abuse, pain disorder, somatization disorder, depression, factitious disorder, malingering, and personality disorder. Psychiatric comorbidity is a controversial and difficult topic to resolve. The presence of one or more of these disorders should not exclude the patient entirely from consideration for implantation but should be a strong vector in the decision-making process.

The final general indication for implantation is response to a trial of SCS. A survey of academic pain centers in the United States reveals that all respondents indicated that trials are done before implantation.[3] The average duration of a trial for spinal cord stimulation is 6.6 days. Two programs report that trials for SCS are done on the day of implantation in the operating room. Although some practitioners may believe that this is an inadequate trial, there is no evidence to compare duration of trial and outcome for SCS. There is general consensus that a trial of approximately 1 week with good pain relief is the best predictor of success with subsequent implantation.

Patient selection remains the biggest source of error in implantable therapies. There is no equation to define how to take into account the effects of ongoing litigation, history of substance abuse, unrecognized psychological disease, lack of employment, lack of a support system at home, disruptive sleeping patterns, abuse of medication, poor or good coping skills, cultural variables, family history of chronic pain, and so on. In addition, there will still be placebo responders to such dramatic interventions as an SCS implant.

Cost-effectiveness analysis of SCS versus best medical and conventional treatment for chronic pain shows that the cumulative 5-year costs for SCS were $29,123 per patient compared with $38,029 for patients treated with conventional methods.[4] In addition, 15% of patients on SCS returned to work compared with none of the patients in the conventional care group. A lifetime cost analysis of SCS versus costs and outcomes before SCS in patients with CRPS showed not only decreased pain and improved quality of life but a savings of $60,000 per patient.[5] Similar outcomes were obtained when comparing patients treated for intractable angina pectoris with and without SCS.[6,7]

Mechanism of Action and Device Characteristics

Transcutaneous electrical nerve stimulators are believed to reduce pain by stimulating large myelinated afferent

---

*See also Chapter 155, "Spinal Cord Stimulation for Chronic Pain."

nociceptive fibers in the periphery. This increase in large-fiber activity theoretically stimulates inhibitory interneurons in the substantia gelatinosa, thereby "closing the gate" on the transmission of painful information carried on small fibers. The first SCS implantation was performed based on this theory. This theory has been criticized based on the facts that only chronic, and not acute pain, is reduced by SCS; SCS works for neuropathic pain but not consistently for somatic pain (except for ischemic pain in peripheral vascular disease and angina pectoris, which cannot be characterized as neuropathic); paresthesias must overlap the painful area; several minutes are required before pain is suppressed; weeks of stimulation may be needed to reach maximal pain relief; and relief may outlast stimulation by long periods of time.[8] Pain relief cannot be explained based solely on the "gate control theory" of pain. The mechanism of action of SCS is unclear. Some support can be found for 10 different specific mechanisms or proposed mechanisms of action, and the reader is referred for further discussion to a recent review by Oakley and Prager.[8]

Neurochemical data suggest that SCS may reduce dorsal horn neuronal hyperexcitability. SCS induces dorsal horn release of γ-aminobutyric acid, substance P, serotonin, glycine, and adenosine while inhibiting the release of glutamate and aspartate. Evidence of a neurochemical mechanism of action is limited but suggestive. Neurophysiologic evidence suggests that SCS can cause suppression of wide dynamic range A-beta fibers normally responsive to mechanical, chemical, and thermal stimulation. In animal models with dorsal horn lesions, these effects are not suppressed. In addition, if the spinal cord is transected above the level of effective SCS, the effect of SCS is reduced. These experiments suggest that the dorsal columns may mediate the effect and that supraspinal mechanisms may be necessary to see an analgesic effect of SCS. Animal experiments also show the involvement of the anterior pretectal nucleus, which is an origin of descending pain inhibitory pathways.

SCS, either directly or indirectly, alters autonomic activity. These observations may be due to stimulation of release of vasoactive substances in the central or peripheral nervous system. Attempts to isolate the autonomic nervous system effects as a direct consequence of SCS and a definitive mechanism of action have been contradictory, and it is an oversimplification and inaccurate to ascribe nociceptive, antianginal, or anti-ischemic effects of SCS to an alteration in autonomic nervous system activity alone.

In summary, although information assisting understanding of SCS mechanism of action is accumulating, the precise mechanism of action seems to be complex and may vary depending on the clinical condition for which the device was placed. A single, simple, unifying mechanism of action of SCS is not evident at this time.

Improvement of equipment has increased efficacy and decreased the complication rates for implanted SCS systems. Complication rates have declined to approximately 8%, and reoperation rates may be as low as 4%.[9] Early SCS systems employed a single monopolar electrode that connected to a percutaneous externalized power source. The standard of care today involves implanted electrodes that are typically quadripolar but that can have dual octapolar electrodes. The number of potentially usable electrode combinations in a dual octapolar system is in the tens of millions. Programming of such a stimulator has not evolved to a point where one can

select from among all these combinations, but supporters contend that the large numbers of possible combinations, the closer proximity of electrodes, and the longer area of possible coverage improve the success rate and quality of relief.

The typical implanted electrode array is a quadripolar array. Each electrode can be programmed as either "on" or "off" or as an anode or a cathode. In using a quadripolar system, there are approximately 50 potentially usable combinations. The power systems are either via an implanted generator with a battery or an implanted device with a radiofrequency-coupled receiver transducer system. Implanted generators need to be replaced approximately every 3 to 7 years, whereas the receiver transducer does not have to be replaced. Patients with receiver transducer systems must wear an external device pasted to the skin to receive paresthesia.

A complete description and comparison of electrodes, generators, programming options, and devices can be found at the following Web sites:

http://www.medtronic.com/ physician/physician.html
http://www.ans-medical.com/physicians/index.html
http://www.advancedbionics.com

Indications and Specific Selection Criteria

The most common indication for SCS in the United States is for back or neck radiculopathic pain. Patients presenting with conditions such as lumbar or cervical radiculopathy, postlaminectomy syndrome, spondylolisthesis, spondylosis, or even persistent and refractory axial low back pain of uncertain etiology may respond to treatment with SCS and should be assessed. Topography of pain that is amenable to overlap by paresthesia of the spinal cord stimulating device is a requirement for successful treatment.[10] Radicular patterns tend to be more easily obtained than axial patterns, and for this reason, patients with pain predominantly in the extremities may be better candidates than patients with predominantly axial symptoms. This should not exclude a trial in an otherwise good candidate who has primarily axial symptoms. Although it is technically more difficult to obtain coverage of patients with predominantly axial back or neck pain, newer, more compact electrodes with multiple arrays sometimes placed bilaterally and triangularly might be useful in providing relief to patients with axial pain, and these arrays should be considered. Long-lasting relief is a reasonable goal. A large series of patients with follow-up of 2 to 20 years demonstrated that 52% of patients continued to have a 50% reduction in pain.[11] The authors noted that even among patients who did not claim a 50% reduction of pain, most patients continued to use their devices.

The evidence of efficacy of SCS for back and neck pain is not lacking. A literature review was performed on studies of patients with SCS for chronic leg and back pain and included all relevant articles identified through MEDLINE search from 1966 through 1994.[12] Fifty-nine percent of patients reported in these studies had greater than 50% pain relief at a time between 1 and 45 months after surgery. These authors noted the lack of a randomized trial at that time. Subsequent to this, a prospective, randomized comparison of SCS and reoperation in patients with persistent radicular pain with or without low back pain after lumbosacral spine surgery was conducted.[13] The primary outcome measure of this study was frequency of crossover to the alternative procedure. This study showed a statistically significant advantage of SCS over reoperation. A literature review on SCS for chronic pain of spinal origin was conducted by North and Wetzel,[9] who concluded that SCS is a valuable treatment option, particularly for patients with chronic pain of predominantly neuropathic origin and a topographic distribution involving predominantly the extremities. Efficacy may be better for spontaneous than for evoked pain.[14]

Pain associated with spinal cord injury has been treated with SCS. Most authors report satisfactory responses in a smaller percentage of their patients ranging between 20% and 40%.[15] Case reports supporting the use of SCS for whiplash and idiopathic acute transverse myelitis have been published.[16,17] Sindou and colleagues[18] reported the predictive value of somatosensory evoked potentials assessing neural conduction in the dorsal columns. These authors suggest that if central conduction time is abolished or significantly altered, then the success rate of SCS is dramatically less than in patients with normal preoperative central conduction times.

The usefulness of SCS for the treatment of postherpetic neuralgia has recently been described. A prospective case series involving 28 patients with either acute herpes zoster or postherpetic neuralgia were studied over 29 months. Eighty-two percent of patients with intractable pain for longer than 2 years had a median decrease in their visual analogue scale score from 9 to 1 (0 to 10 scale) as well as improvement in their pain disability index. Four patients with acute herpes zoster had prompt and dramatic improvement in their pain symptoms.[19]

The treatment of PVOD with SCS is the most common indication for this modality in Europe. For no other indication is the early evidence of efficacy more compelling and yet SCS for PVOD is not a common treatment in the United States. One study reported 37 patients receiving adequate pain relief after a trial in 41 patients with end-stage peripheral vascular disease.[20] Seventy-eight percent of patients reported substantial pain relief at a mean follow-up of 25 months. Another investigator reported the results of SCS in 20 patients with ischemic rest pain and ulcers.[21] Eighteen of 20 patients in this study had immediate relief of pain after electrical stimulation. These authors also reported improved skin nutritional flow leading to healing of ulcers of moderate size and increased salvage of feet with limb-threatening ischemia at 2-year follow-up. They report an increase in capillary density and an increase in red blood cell velocity and peak red blood cell velocity after arterial occlusion by intravital capillary microscopy.

More recently, SCS has been investigated by the European Peripheral Vascular Disease Outcome Study.[22] Patients with nonreconstructable critical leg ischemia showed increased limb survival when compared with patients receiving usual treatment without SCS as well as improved pain relief. Patients with transcutaneous oxygen pressure measurement of 10 to 30 mm Hg before SCS trial or if less than 10 mm Hg, an improvement to 20 mm Hg or more during the SCS trial received an implant. Limb amputations were 20% at 12 months in the SCS group compared with 46% in the matched no SCS group. These and other authors suggest the routine use of transcutaneous oxygen pressure both before and during the trial phase as a predictor of success.[23] A useful predictor of success in patients with diabetes with PVOD is

the absence of autonomic neuropathy.[24] Twenty-five of 28 patients with autonomic neuropathy failed SCS treatment, whereas all 32 patients without autonomic neuropathy had successful outcomes.

Evidence exists of the efficacy of SCS in severe Raynaud's phenomenon[25] and Buerger's disease.[26] SCS has shown remarkable effectiveness and should be considered as a treatment for patients with severe PVOD that is not amenable to surgical intervention.

Despite the lack of an identifiable objective lesion, SCS appears to be quite effective for treatment of CRPS. One report retrospectively reviewed experience with SCS and found 12 patients with CRPS who were followed up for an average of 41 months after implantation.[27] Eight of these patients reported excellent pain relief, and four patients reported good pain relief. Another study looked at 18 patients with CRPS.[28] Fourteen patients had a successful trial and subsequently had their systems internalized. Follow-up varied from 4 to 14 months. Six of 14 patients had good pain relief. Five had moderate pain relief. One had minimal and three had no pain relief. Of note is that pain relief was limited to the body parts covered by the paresthesia.

In a randomized trial comparing SCS plus physical therapy with physical therapy alone in 54 patients with CRPS, the SCS group had a mean reduction in pain of 2.4 cm (on a 1- to 10-cm scale) compared with an increase of 0.2 cm in the physical therapy alone group.[2] Health-related quality of life also improved in the SCS group, but, interestingly, there was no difference between the groups in functional status.

A recent report has demonstrated that response to sympathetic blockade can be predictive of a better outcome from SCS for patients with CRPS.[29] Thirteen of 13 patients with a positive response to sympathetic blockade had pain relief during the trial period, and 87% had greater than a 50% reduction in pain at 9 months. Only 3 of 10 patients with a negative response to sympathetic blockade had good relief and went on to permanent implantation, and only 33% had a 50% reduction in pain at 9 months.

It appears that at this time there are very good data to support the use of SCS for the treatment of CRPS if it is possible to obtain paresthesia coverage that overlaps the painful area.

The treatment of postamputation phantom or residual limb pain with SCS is still a controversial area. Contradictory reports for this and for brachial plexus avulsion injury pain exist, and it is not possible to make definitive recommendations for treating or not treating phantom limb or brachial plexus avulsion injury pain with SCS based on these data.

A large body of data supports the use of SCS for intractable angina pectoris. The complexity and implications of severe coronary artery disease as an indication for SCS requires discussion. The first published report of the use of SCS for angina was in 1987.[30] These investigators described 10 patients with intractable angina in whom SCS devices were implanted, which led to a decrease in the frequency and severity of angina and a major reduction in the use of antianginal medications. Other investigators followed with a report on 10 patients and added bicycle ergometry as a measure of exercise tolerance and showed an increase in work capacity, increased time to angina, decrease in recovery time, and a decrease in the magnitude of ST-segment depression associated with angina.[31] By 1991, it was shown that reductions in angina attacks continued over 9 months, and a persistence in increase in rate-pressure product (a measure of the ability of the heart to do work).[32] Between 1993 and 1994, results of a randomized, prospective study demonstrated improved exercise capacity, improved quality of life, and a decrease in ischemic episodes as measured by Holter monitor.[33-35] Complications were few and of a technical nature, and a surgical algorithm that did not involve a trial before implantation was described. It has been shown that SCS does not conceal myocardial infarction that may occur in patients with implanted devices.[36] A decrease in hospital admissions for patients with implanted SCS devices compared with a control group has been demonstrated.[37] In 80% of patients, the beneficial effect has been reported to last 1 year, and in 60%, improvement in exercise capacity and quality of life lasted as long as 5 years.[38-40] There are no data showing harmful or nontherapeutic effects of SCS for angina. The use of SCS may be beneficial even in critically ill patients. Janfaza and colleagues[41] reported the 6-week survival in such a patient, whereas other investigators have reported an effect insufficient to overcome the severity of ischemic disease, albeit relief of ischemic symptoms, until death occurred.[42]

A prospective, randomized trial of SCS versus coronary artery bypass grafting in 104 patients with severe angina, increased surgical risk, and no prognostic benefits from revascularization demonstrated long-lasting improvement in quality of life and comparable survival and symptom control in both groups.[43] Benefit after discontinuation of SCS has been shown for as long as 4 weeks after discontinuation.[44] No difference in anginal complaints, nitroglycerin intake, ischemia, or heart rate variability was shown. SCS has been shown to decrease hospitalization in patients with angina,[45] and there is evidence that modern SCS devices are compatible with modern pacemaking devices.[46,47]

Description of Technique

In our practice, patients who meet selection criteria are instructed not to eat or drink anything after midnight the night before their implantation trial. They are instructed to continue their nonsteroidal antiinflammatory drugs, but care is taken to discontinue other anticoagulants or platelet inhibitors for proper durations of time. The procedure is done in two stages. Both the trial phase (phase 1) and the generator implantation phase (phase 2) are done in the operating room with an anesthesiologist present. The trial phase or phase 1 involves either the placement of a percutaneous cylindrical electrode or a paddle-type electrode placed via minilaminectomy. The electrodes are either removed after a period of trial stimulation or are attached to a connecting cable during phase 1 allowing the electrode to remain under the skin entirely. In this case, the connecting cable can be removed and the electrode attached to a new sterile cable during phase 2.

Patients with chronic pain may have central changes that amplify painful signals. It is necessary to have the patient awake and able to answer questions appropriately to assess the location of paresthesia during the trial phase. Patients may require laminectomy for placement of a paddle-type electrode in the thoracic or cervical region. Patients with chronic pain often have multiple comorbidities, particularly patients with PVOD or intractable angina pectoris. These factors create an anesthetic challenge and require a preoperative consultation between surgeon and anesthesiologist to define goals and needs. Our typical anesthetic involves intravenous fentanyl and midazolam for analgesia, anxiolysis, and amnesia and propofol for sedation. The propofol can be turned off, and the patient awakened for questioning regarding paresthesia topography at appropriate intervals. We also use large volumes of local anesthetic, typically 0.5% lidocaine without epinephrine. A dose of 4 mg/kg (56 mL for a 70-kg person) can be safely administered even as a single dose and more can be administered after an hour or two. Another option is intravenous remifentanil plus local anesthetic, but this requires an anesthesiologist experienced in the use of this drug because the therapeutic window is often so narrow. Despite the best efforts of experienced practitioners, the implanter should be prepared for oversedation and the need for airway control during the procedure or suboptimal ability to describe the paresthesia topography. The patient should be advised that this is a possibility and that if it occurs, the electrode can still be placed without paresthesia guidance but success rate might be reduced. The patient should also be educated about information needs that will occur intraoperatively before getting to the operating room. A recent report describes the successful implantation of an SCS device in 19 of 19 patients undergoing laminectomy with 12.5 to 20 mg bupivacaine intrathecal spinal anesthesia.[48] In all patients with spinals and anesthesia throughout the surgical procedure, SCS paresthesia was readily appreciated by the patients.

There is no description of the absolute need for alertness and ability to communicate during surgery. It is generally accepted that, due to uncertainty about anatomic and physiologic overlap, simply placing the lead at the proper anatomic location will not reliably produce a paresthesia that will be effective in reducing pain. There are published case series in which successful implantation has been done under general anesthesia.[49]

A retrospective, nonrandomized review of surgical experience concluded that patients with flat electrodes placed via laminectomy had better pain relief that was longer lasting than patients who had percutaneously placed cylindrical electrodes.[49] A prospective, randomized, controlled trial has recently shown that electrode arrays implanted via laminectomy had lower amplitude requirements and better patient ratings of paresthesia coverage.[50] The decision as to whether to place a flat electrode via minilaminectomy or a percutaneously-placed cylindrical electrode is a controversial and emotionally charged issue because anesthesiologists, who place most of these devices, use a percutaneous approach and many neurosurgeons place leads via laminectomy. To further complicate matters, anesthesiologists should not place leads via laminotomy because they do not have the training, experience, or ability to manage complications and many pain specialist anesthesiologists derive substantial income from placing SCS devices. Additionally, other specialists such as physiatrists and neurologists are receiving training and are eligible for board certification in pain medicine and are implanting cylindrical leads. At this time, there is no overwhelming evidence of the advantage of placing electrodes via a laminectomy compared with percutaneously placed leads, but there is at least one compelling study.[50]

For percutaneous placement of a cylindrical electrode, the procedure is as follows. Patients are placed prone on a

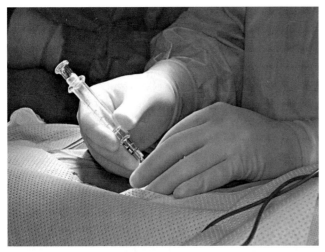

FIGURE 110-1 Intraoperative identification of the epidural space using a loss of resistance to air technique in preparation for placement of a percutaneous cylindrical electrode.

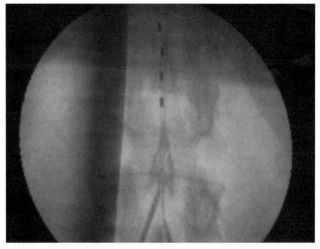

FIGURE 110-3 Quadripolar electrode being advanced under fluoroscopic guidance within the epidural space. Note the angle between the two most cephalad leads enabling steering of the electrode.

fluoroscopy table in the operating room and prepared for a surgical procedure that can last hours. We do not place a Foley catheter. Standard surgical preparation is done after identifying important landmarks fluoroscopically and marking the skin to identify them. The skin and subcutaneous tissue are anesthetized with local anesthetic before insertion of the 15-gauge epidural needle. The epidural space is identified using a loss of resistance to air or saline technique (Fig. 110-1). For a patient with an L5 radiculopathic pain pattern, the epidural space is entered at approximately T12–L1, at which point the cylindrical electrode is advanced through the needle and positioned using fluoroscopic guidance to the desired level at approximately T9–10, at which time trial stimulation is carried out (Figs 110-2 and 110-3). For placement of a device for stimulation of the upper extremity, entry is made at T1–3 with the electrode tip to arrive at C3–4 approximately. The target site for the electrode tip for a patient with angina is approximately T4–5. For a unilateral syndrome, the electrode should be positioned approximately 3 mm ipsilaterally

off midline. The electrode can be directed and "steered" using an angled stylet. Once the target anatomic site is reached, the electrode is anchored and attached to a temporary screening cable and a trial screener. The awakened patient is then questioned about the presence or absence and location of paresthesia coverage. Parameters that are available for adjustment include amplitude and pulse width and frequency, the same as with an implanted generator.

Once good paresthesia overlap to pain topography is obtained, the electrode is disconnected from the cable. A 5-cm vertical incision over the site of epidural needle placement is made. The subcutaneous tissue is undermined at the level of the lumbodorsal or supraspinous fascia, the epidural needle is carefully removed along with the electrode stylet, and the lead is anchored using an anchoring device that will prevent the electrode from migrating (Fig. 110-4). The electrode is attached to a percutaneous extension lead, and a tunneling device is used to exit the skin at a site approximately 10 cm lateral to the incision. The electrode in placed within

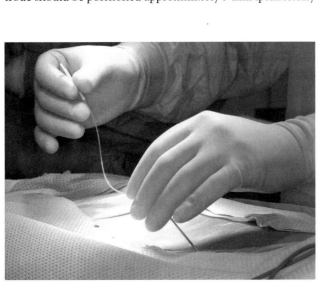

FIGURE 110-2 Advancement of cylindrical electrode through an epidural needle. Note that steering the electrode is possible by rotating the stylet hub of the electrode.

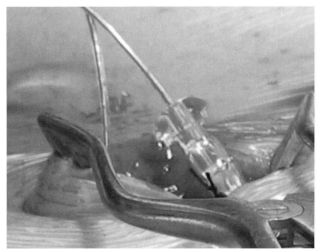

FIGURE 110-4 The cylindrical electrode is anchored within an undermined incision extending to the dorsolumbar fascia.

the incision with only the temporary connecting cable externalized. This allows the electrode to remain beneath the skin throughout the entire trial period. Care should be taken to avoid contact of the electrocautery device with the electrode. A defect in the electrode could result in a line of continuity between the externalized lead and the epidural space. If the patient has a successful trial, then it is necessary only to remove the extension lead, and the electrode, which has already been positioned and has not been exposed to a contaminated external environment, can remain in place. The skin and subcutaneous tissue are closed with interrupted Vicryl sutures and skin staples.

Placement of a paddle-type electrode or flat lead is done via a standard laminotomy procedure. The electrode is placed in the epidural space using the same anatomic targets as described for cylindrical electrode placement. A dual laminotomy is sometimes required to properly position the electrode.[51] Paresthesia overlap with topography of pain should be tested with the awake patient intraoperatively. The electrode cable is anchored to fascia, and the electrode is attached to a temporary percutaneous connecting wire as described previously.

At the conclusion of the phase 1 of implantation, the procedure is the same for both percutaneous and flat electrode management. The percutaneous connecting cable is attached to a trial screener, and the patient is screened at home for 4 to 7 days. When the patient returns, he or she is questioned about success of pain reduction. A general rule of thumb is that a reduction in pain of 50% or more is necessary to proceed to phase 2, but there are many exceptions and a careful assessment by the implanting surgeon is required for proper decision making. For patients with intractable angina pectoris, a reduction in the frequency, intensity, and duration of anginal episodes should be documented.

For phase 2, the patient is taken to the operating room and under local anesthesia with monitored anesthesiology care; the electrode and cable are removed if the trial was not successful. Patients who have had a successful trial will have their incision reopened, and the generator will be implanted in the buttock. A site selected below the belt line and cephalad enough to allow comfortable sitting should be selected. Generators can be implanted in a variety of anatomic sites including the abdomen, lateral thorax, and subclavicular and subaxillary space.

After local anesthetic infiltration, a horizontal incision is made in the skin planes large enough to enable placement of the generator. The pocket is created by sharp and blunt dissection and is made at a depth no greater than 2 cm to enable easy programming transcutaneously.

A tunneling tool is used to connect the midline incision to the pocket, and the extension wire is threaded through the tunnel. The system is connected, and the incisions are approximated in two layers using 3-0 Vicryl sutures for the deeper tissues and staples for skin closure. Familiarity with all the equipment is necessary before proceeding to the operating room.

Intraoperative problems peculiar to SCS implantation include an inability to properly position the electrode in the epidural space, inability to obtain paresthesia overlap of the painful area, and unanticipated events. We have described the inability to thread a percutaneous catheter in a patient with unidentified epidural lipomatosis.[52] The catheter was readily placed under direct vision after laminotomy. We use a dual laminotomy technique in those cases in which a proper anatomic position cannot be achieved through a single laminotomy to enable proper anatomic and physiologic positioning of a flat electrode and have estimated that unanticipated anatomic complications occur as often as 18% of the time in revision flat electrode placements.[51] Finally, it is uncommon, but it is sometimes impossible to obtain satisfactory paresthesia overlap of the painful area, particularly with angina pectoris and axial low back or neck pain, despite an unimpeded ability to manipulate the electrode(s). Even distal extremity paresthesia coverage can sometimes be impossible to obtain for unproven but theorized reasons such as epidural scarring or any impediment to the flow of electricity to and into the spinal cord.

Complications and Troubleshooting

Possible problems and complications of spinal cord stimulating devices have been well described. North and colleagues[11] had no major morbidity or mortality in their series of 320 patients undergoing implantation over 20 years. Their incidence of surgical wound infections, all superficial, was 5%, and they all cleared promptly with the removal of hardware and a short course of antibiotics, permitting a second implantation. They had a 7% failure rate manifested by fracture of the electrode or insulation failure; 5% of their systems failed because of a defect in the radiofrequency receiver.

There are case reports of cord compression due to hematoma, and these have mostly followed laminectomy rather than percutaneous implantation. Transient and reversible neurologic deficit have also rarely been reported. Radicular muscle twitches have rarely been reported, and there is one death reported due to pulmonary embolism. Prolonged and exaggerated postoperative pain has been reported, and the reason for this complication is not clear. Erosion through the skin of implanted materials has occurred, particularly in cachectic ill patients. The complication rates have continued to decrease with refinement of equipment and surgical technique and should be expected to continue to decrease. Late failure has also been reported.

There is a steady decrease in the success of pain relief over many years after implantation. Early failure may represent a defect in our ability to carefully screen these patients before implantation.

Patients should have a near-normal prothrombin time before proceeding with implantation. Patients with thrombocytopenia should be transfused with platelets before implantation. These patients should be carefully monitored for symptoms of acute epidural hematoma, and if these symptoms occur, they should be treated as a neurosurgical emergency.

All patients in our practice received a single preoperative dose of prophylactic antibiotic. The most common infectious agents were *Staphylococcus aureus* and *Staphylococcus epidermidis*. Pocket seromas are a self-limiting complication and usually will resolve within 2 months. Patients should be reassured, and only very occasionally is it necessary to aspirate these fluid collections. If there are signs of infection, the fluid can be aspirated and sent for Gram stain and culture and sensitivity.

A visible collection of fluid found subcutaneously under the back wound may represent a cerebrospinal fluid hygroma, especially if a known subarachnoid puncture occurred during electrode placement. These are self-limiting complications that have no clinical consequence. If there is a cerebrospinal fluid leak through the incision, the surgical wound should be taken down and resutured. For persistent postdural puncture headaches, a blood patch can be done. This should be done under fluoroscopic guidance to ensure no damage to the implanted electrode. Infected hygromas necessitate removal of the entire system.

Patients will present after successful implantation with complaints about their systems. Complaints can include a lack of stimulation, intermittent stimulation, a change in stimulation pattern, undesirable sensations, or inadequate pain relief. The most common solution is a simple reprogramming. A decrease in postoperative swelling or slight lead migration may account for many of the above problems and careful, thoughtful reprogramming can solve most of these difficulties. A lack of stimulation can indicate a dead battery, which will be evident with reprogramming but can also represent an open circuit. Measuring individual electrode impedances, palpation, and radiography can all help make this assessment. Fluid within a connector can cause intermittent stimulation as well as simply a loose connection. Palpation and impedance measurement can help identify the source of the problem. Burning at the pocket or lead-extension junction can indicate electrical leakage. A change in stimulation pattern can indicate lead migration. Insufficient relief can indicate disease progression or patient expectations that may have been too high.

If the source of the problem can be identified easily, then a directed surgical solution can be planned. For example, a patient with burning at the lead–connecting cable junction and lack of stimulation with abnormal impedances can have the lead–connecting cable junction site explored and repaired. Unfortunately, there are times when the precise site of malfunction is not clear and a surgical plan is necessary. The lead–connecting cable junction is a common malfunction site, and a good surgical plan would be to explore this junction first. If no abnormality such as fluid within the boot is evident, then the lead can be disconnected from the cable and the lead tested with alligator clips intraoperatively. If the lead is the source of the problem, it can be replaced. If it is not, then the system should be reconnected and retested in the operating room. If the system is still not functioning properly, then the generator–connecting cable incision can be opened and the connecting cable lead can be tested with alligator clips. The connecting cable can be replaced if indicated and if the lead–connecting cable complex is working but the generator connecting cable–lead complex is not, the generator should be replaced. The entire system should be explored if necessary, and the system should be functional by the time the patient leaves the operating room, even if the entire system needs to be replaced. There are three pieces of equipment that can potentially malfunction, and each piece can be isolated and tested. The intact and repaired system should be tested before leaving the operating room.

Generator life span is variable and depends on programming parameters and patient preferences for use. A patient who uses the device 24 hours per day at a voltage of 9 V with a high frequency may deplete an implanted battery in less than a year, whereas a patient with low voltage and frequency who uses the device 4 hours per day may obtain a decade of life from his or her battery. The former patient should probably be implanted with a radiofrequency transducer rather than a battery. Some implanters favor transducers for all their patients, citing no need for battery replacement as a valid reason. Many if not most patients will prefer the convenience of not needing a rubber donut on their skin with a portable power supply.

Summary

SCS is the most useful new tool in the armamentarium combating chronic pain to emerge in more than a decade. Its use is supported not only by overwhelming case series but by well-controlled clinical trials. The precise niche for SCS in the management of angina pectoris, PVOD, and even chronic low back and neck pain is still developing in the paradigm of care for patients with chronic pain. Future vectors of care and usefulness include discovering the role of different drugs when used in combination with SCS. Subeffective doses of gabapentin and pregabalin when combined with subeffective levels of SCS have been shown to be effective in reducing neuropathic pain.[53] Patients with neuropathic pain effectively treated with SCS have been shown in a double-blind, randomized study to respond to carbamazepine but not to sustained-release morphine when their SCS devices were turned off and they were "switched" to a painful state.[54]

Other areas under investigation include an automated, patient-interactive SCS adjustment device, which has been shown to provide better paresthesia overlap of painful regions, better analgesia, and longer battery life.[55] Better methods of obtaining axial paresthesia coverage, electrode placement under the arch of C1 and C2 for use in atypical facial pain, nerve root SCS cannulation, chemical augmentation with intrathecally administered drugs, sacral root stimulation for urinary incontinence, and improvements in systems and equipment all may add to the success of SCS as a therapeutic, nondestructive, reversible, and minimally invasive analgesic tool.[56]

INTRASPINAL INFUSION SYSTEMS

Introduction and General Selection Criteria

Intraspinal administration of opioids has been shown to be useful in patients who have not responded to other therapies or who have excessive side effects with other routes of administration. It is most useful and has proven efficacy when used for patients with cancer pain who develop unmanageable side effects to the high doses of opioids sometimes necessary to control pain or intractable pain states.[57-63] Success in treating nonmalignant chronic pain with intraspinal opioids has not been confirmed to the same extent but is commonly employed.[64,65] As with SCS, patient selection is likely to be the key predictor of success, but identifiable preimplantation variables have not yet been definitively identified. Negative predictors of success have been suggested to include major psychopathology, active mood disorders, dementia, severe anxiety, addictive disease, and severe social or economic stressors.

Patients whose pain does not respond to opioids may benefit from the addition of other drugs to their intraspinal regimen. Drugs reportedly used include local anesthetics, clonidine, baclofen, and opioids.[3,66] Local anesthetics, clonidine, and baclofen are typically used in combination with opioids and, except for clonidine, may not be useful as analgesics when administered alone. A recent review investigated clinical practices via an Internet-based survey and described drugs and combinations of drugs used by practitioners.[67] Drugs and combinations are shown in Figure 110-5.

The general indications for implantation of an analgesic infusion system are the same as for SCS. A trial with a single intraspinal injection or continuous infusion should be conducted before implantation.

Drug Selection and Systems

The use of neuraxial morphine through a continuous infusion pump as an effective treatment for pain of malignant origin has been well documented.[57–63] Morphine, hydromorphone, bupivacaine, baclofen, clonidine, sufentanil, ketamine, ropivacaine, fentanyl, meperidine, tetracaine, and experimental agents are used in academic pain centers in the United States.[3] The use of spinally administered drugs in the noncancer pain group is more complex. The indication for this therapy is very simply opioid-responsive pain in patients unable to tolerate alternate routes of administration or in whom alternate routes of administration are ineffective. The complexity arises when considering the impact of social, psychological, physical, financial, and emotional factors. Further complicating the issue is the impact of ongoing litigation, disability, and substance abuse, which are so prevalent in our society.

In a blinded, placebo-controlled study conducted in Australia, less than one third of patients using oral opioids for nonmalignant pain were found to have opioid-responsive pain on intrathecal testing.[68] Furthermore, these patients were significantly more distressed by testing with a battery of psychometric tools including the Beck Depression Inventory,

Pain Self Efficacy Questionnaire, and other measures of catastrophe and disability. These data are consistent with a recent report that showed that 40% of patients treated with opioids in two major academic pain centers exhibited aberrant behaviors that could be construed as drug seeking or had urine toxicology results inconsistent with reported use of drugs.[69] These studies underscore the complexities and difficulties inherent in treating patients with noncancer chronic pain.

Other problems in attempting to define efficacy in this group include the fact that there are only case series reporting the efficacy of intraspinal opioids in patients with nonmalignant pain and not the same overwhelming evidence of efficacy as exists for SCS. There are no studies with a control group comparison. There are few accurate descriptions of the incidence of continued use of supplemental oral opioids in patients receiving neuraxial opioids. Patients have not been stratified into etiologies of pain. Measurement of outcomes is largely unsatisfactory in all published studies. An expert panel recently produced an evidence-based review of the literature on intrathecal drug delivery, and their conclusion was that further study is warranted.[70]

It has been suggested that there are not enough data at this time to warrant the use of intraspinal opioids for nonmalignant pain. The real truth likely is that there are criteria that can be applied to select patients with specific painful conditions who are likely to respond to intraspinal opioid therapy. Patients with chronic pain are a heterogeneous, not a homogeneous, group. These conditions and criteria need to be defined.

The literature addressing the efficacy of intraspinal opioids for the relief of pain has continued to expand since 1980 when Bromage and colleagues[71] showed clearly that narcotics administered epidurally were capable of providing profound postoperative analgesia. Although postoperative and other short-term catheters for acute pain can be placed epidurally, catheters placed for cancer or long-term chronic pain conditions should be placed intrathecally. Catheter migration

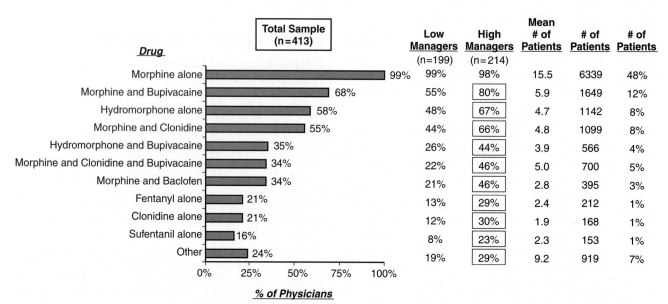

FIGURE 110-5 Drugs used by high (more than 15 patients being managed) and low (fewer than 15 patients being managed) managers of patients with analgesic infusion systems. (From Hassenbusch SJ, Portenoy RK: Current practices in intraspinal therapy—a survey of clinical trends and decision making. J Pain Symptom Manage 20:S4–S11, 2000.)

from the epidural to intrathecal space has been reported and can result in massive overdose and diffusion conditions across the dura/arachnoid membrane and can be affected by conditions such as carcinomatous meningitis or other inflammatory conditions, which can result in severe pain from a decrease in drug reaching the intrathecal space. For these reasons, catheters for implanted devices will typically be placed in the subarachnoid space.

Advantages of implanted systems include a decreased incidence of infection compared with percutaneous systems, increased patient comfort, and greater patient convenience.

One model of care is to use an implanted system in patients with a life expectancy of greater than 3 months and to use an externalized percutaneous system in other patients.

The gold standard infusate for opioids administered via an implanted intraspinal device is morphine. Drug selection is a complex issue requiring knowledge and experience. Clinical guidelines for drug selection are shown in Figure 110-6, and physiologic guidelines are outlined in Table 110-1.[72] Morphine can be maximally concentrated to approximately 50 mg/mL and is commercially available at a concentration of 25 mg/mL. Hydromorphone is commonly used in spinally

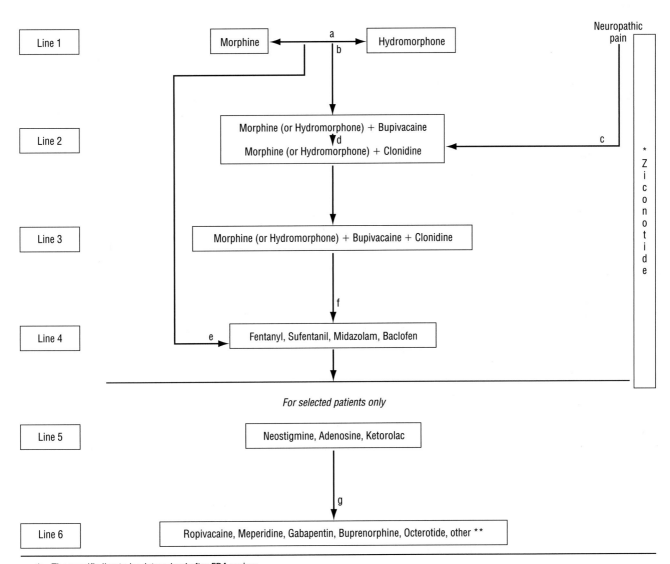

*   The specific line to be determined after FDA review
** Potential spinal analgesics: Methadone, Oxymorphone, NMDA antagonists

a. If side effects occur, switch to other opioid.
b. If maximum dosage is reached without adequate analgesia, add adjuvant medication (Line 2).
c. If patient has neuropathic pain, consider starting with opioid monotherapy (morphine or hydromorphone) or, in selected patients with pure or predominant neuropathic pain, consider opioid plus adjuvant medication (bupivacaine or clonidine), (Line 2).
d. Some of the panel advocated the use of bupivacaine first because of concern about clonidine-induced hypotension.
e. If side effects or lack of analgesia on second first-line opioid, may switch to fentanyl (Line 4).
f. There are limited preclinical data and limited clinical experience; therefore, extreme caution in the use of these agents should be considered.
g. There are insufficient preclinical data and limited clinical experience; therefore, extreme caution in the use of these agents should be considered.

FIGURE 110-6   Clinical guidelines for drug selection for intraspinal infusion. (From Hassenbusch SJ, Portenoy RK, Cousins M, et al: Polyanalgesic consensus conference 2003: An update on the management of pain by intraspinal drug delivery—report of an expert panel. J Pain Symptom Manage 27(6):546–563, 2004.)

TABLE 110-1 ▪ Physiologic Effects of Drugs Commonly Administered Intrathecally via an Analgesic Infusion System

	Motor Weakness	Decreased RR	Hypotension	Urinary Retention	Analgesia
Opioids	0	+	0	+	+
Clonidine	0	0	+	0	+
Baclofen	+	0	0	+	0
Local anesthetics	+	0	+	+	+

administered opioid infusion devices and is available in a concentration of 10 mg/mL. Clinicians can mix either morphine or hydromorphone (or another opioid) with bupivacaine in an attempt to manage severe neuropathic or somatic incident pain. Unfortunately, the maximal concentration of available bupivacaine is 40 mg/mL, limited by solubility, which may necessitate refilling the devices as often as monthly. The limiting factor is the size of the pump reservoir, which is only 18 mL in available programmable devices. Patients receiving bupivacaine infusion in their implanted devices often need to have refills on a monthly basis, whereas patients receiving opioid alone will usually require refills only every 90 days. Stability data for morphine in implanted pumps ensure stability for only 90 days.

Clonidine has been approved by the U.S. Food and Drug Administration for intraspinal delivery and is useful in managing refractory neuropathic pain, as are the local anesthetics. The limitation again with clonidine is a concentration factor requiring frequent refills of implantable devices when this agent is used. Clonidine is commercially available in a 100-μg/mL concentration, and patients will frequently require this amount and more on a daily basis. Compounding pharmacies can often provide much more potent concentrations limited only by solubility. There is evidence of synergy when the combination of clonidine and opioid is used as well as when opioid and bupivacaine are used together. Some practitioners use triple analgesic intraspinal therapy, particularly in patients with cancer, and combinations of morphine, bupivacaine, and clonidine are employed.

Baclofen is an extremely useful agent in the treatment of refractory spasticity. Sufentanil, fentanyl, ketamine, and meperidine are also reportedly used in implanted devices, but, again, there are no safety or efficacy data for these agents in these devices.

Both programmable and continuous flow rate devices are available for implantation in the United States. Programmable devices offer the advantage of the ability to change doses by adjusting flow rates. Continuous infusion devices require refilling with a different drug concentration to alter doses. Continuous infusion devices are not substantially less expensive than programmable devices, although they are available with larger reservoirs for drug and may enable longer refill intervals.

Trial, Implantation, and Complications

Before permanent implantation, it is generally accepted that a trial for responsiveness and tolerability is mandatory. Trials can be done by continuous infusion or bolus injection, with patients as inpatients or outpatients, and with drug administered epidurally or intrathecally for as short a period of time as

1 day, a single intrathecal bolus, or as long as 60 days. A recent comparison of a single intrathecal bolus of morphine versus as long as 4 days of continuous epidural infusion of morphine showed no difference in outcome.[73] Whatever the method or rationale for a trial, it is imperative that the trial be adequate to satisfy the physician's assessment of potential efficacy and tolerability. An arbitrary reduction in pain that has been selected by most practitioners is a 50% reduction in pain. This degree of reduction is necessary to define a trial sufficient to demonstrate the efficacy of an opioid.

The implantation procedure is done in the operating room with an anesthesiologist present to monitor the patient. Before moving the patient to the operating room, the patient is examined, and, while the patient is standing, the skin is marked at the site where the pump pocket will be placed. This should be below the costal margin and above the belt line if possible.

The patient is then carefully positioned laterally on the operating table so that the pump pocket side of the abdomen is up, and the patient is prepped such that the surgical team will have access to both the abdomen and the back where the catheter is to be inserted. Patients are administered antibiotic prophylaxis, usually with cefazolin, and sedation. The patient should preferably be awake enough to report pain should the placement needle touch a nerve root or spinal cord.

The procedure is well described by an experienced group of implanters attempting to reach a consensus on the best technique, with special attention to a low technical complication rate.[74] Complications addressed included catheter dislodgment and migration, fracture, kink or occlusion, cut or puncture, disconnect, and leak.

Other complications related to drug infusion devices have been described by Krames.[75] Surgical complications include bleeding, infection, pump pocket seroma, cerebrospinal fluid leak, cerebrospinal fluid hygroma, postdural puncture headache, and improper pocket placement. Catheter tip fibroma formation has been reported and is discussed further. Catheter tip epidermoid tumors can occur if epidermal cell are delivered into the subarachnoid space when accessing via the epidural needle. A small skin incision with a scalpel blade is necessary before inserting the epidural needle to prevent this complication.

The prevalence of catheter tip inflammatory masses or fibromas is a topic of controversy and importance. Although initially thought to be a rare occurrence, the prevalence may be as high as 1%. Spinal cord compression and permanent neurologic injury has been reported. The formation of these tumors is thought to be a direct response to opioid infusion and has been reported with both morphine and hydromorphone at the full range of doses. The occurrences are not limited to just high-dose infusions. There have been no reports of inflammatory catheter tip masses with infusions of baclofen alone or bupivacaine alone, but there is a report of occurrence with a bupivacaine/morphine infusion. The policy at Dartmouth Hitchcock Medical Center is to obtain an annual screening computed tomography scan to identify the catheter tip and fine-cut magnetic resonance imaging at the catheter tip level to assess for the presence of a mass. There are reports in the literature of spontaneous regression of masses when infusions are stopped, but if neurologic injury has occurred, consensus exists that they should be excised.

Catheter tip fibromas and epidermoid tumors may require excision and explantation of the catheter. Patients with increased pain or new neurologic deficits occurring some time after implantation should undergo magnetic resonance imaging to identify these treatable complications.

Mechanical problems include catheter kinking, catheter obstruction, catheter dislodgment, catheter disconnection, pump failure, and pump battery depletion. The first indication of a mechanical problem is an increase in the patient's pain. This has to be distinguished from development of tolerance or progression of disease. Pharmacologic complications include opioid-induced nausea and vomiting, urinary retention, pruritus, or inadequate analgesia. Nausea and vomiting, urinary retention, and pruritus should have been identified during the trial, but occasionally they will occur when increasing doses in an attempt to treat tolerance or control pain. These symptoms can be pharmacologically managed most of the time. If they cannot be managed, then a change to a different opioid can be attempted. Tolerance can also be managed by the addition of another agent such as a local anesthetic or clonidine.

It is imperative to follow careful technique when refilling these devices. The recommended technique for a programmable device is to expose the pump and surrounding areas completely and to cleanse with Betadine three times. A sterile fenestrated drape is then placed over the pump access site. Sterile gloves are used by the practitioner. The pump is palpated, and the desired access port is carefully identified. Templates can be used to aid in identifying these sites. A 22-gauge Huber (noncoring) needle is used to access the center port. Once accessed, the pump should be gently aspirated and the remaining fluid removed. The amount of fluid aspirated from the pump should reflect the amount described on interrogation of the pump by the programming computer in a programmable device. Five milliliters of refill solution should then be gently injected into the pump. Five milliliters should then be aspirated out, confirming the intrapump needle position.

The volume of solution representing the capacity of the pump should then be injected. The pump can then be reprogrammed to reflect the full reservoir volume. It is imperative that all these steps be followed when refilling the device. It is possible for even the most experienced practitioner to instill fluid subcutaneously. Occasionally, a thick fibrous capsule can form around implanted pumps, particularly pumps without the Dacron pouch, and passing the Huber needle through the fibrous capsule can feel the same as passing the needle through the rubber access port.

For a more thorough and recent review of neuraxial medication delivery including a literature review, indications, comparison of techniques, comparison of different types of pumps, and a synopsis of troubleshooting, the reader is referred to Prager.[76]

SUMMARY

Spinal cord stimulation and the use of intraspinal infusion systems for cancer and chronic pain are efficacious, cost effective, and integral tools in the armamentarium of anyone treating cancer or chronic pain. Patient selection, improvement in systems, increased safety, and the development of new drugs are targets for future work.

REFERENCES

1. Shealy CN, Mortimer JT, Reswick J: Electrical inhibition of pain by stimulation of the dorsal column: Preliminary clinical reports. Anesth Analg 46:489–491, 1967.
2. Kemler MA, Barandse GAN, van Kleef M, et al: Spinal cord stimulation in patients with chronic reflex sympathetic dystrophy. N Engl J Med 343:618–624, 2000.
3. Fanciullo GF, Rose RJ, Lunt PG, et al: The state of implantable pain therapies in the United States: A nationwide survey of academic teaching programs. Anesth Analg 88:1311–1316, 1999.
4. Kumar K, Malik S, Demeria D: Treatment of chronic pain with spinal cord stimulation versus alternative therapies: Cost-effectiveness analysis. Neurosurgery 51:106–116, 2002.
5. Kemler MA, Furnee CA: Economic evaluation of spinal cord stimulation for chronic reflex sympathetic dystrophy. Neurology 59:1203–1209, 2002.
6. Merry AF, Smith WM, Anderson DJ, et al: Cost-effectiveness of spinal cord stimulation in patients with intractable angina. N Z Med J 114:179–181, 2001.
7. Andrell P, Ekre, Eliasson T, et al: Cost-effectiveness of spinal cord stimulation versus coronary artery bypass grafting in patients with severe angina pectoris—long term results from the ESBY Study. Cardiology 99:20–24, 2003.
8. Oakley JC, Prager JP: Spinal cord stimulation: Mechanism of action. Spine 27:2574–2583, 2002.
9. North RB, Wetzel FT: Spinal cord stimulation for chronic pain of spinal origin: A valuable tong term solution. Spine 27:2584–2591, 2002.
10. Kumar K, Nath R, Wyant GN: Treatment of chronic by epidural spinal cord stimulation: A ten year experience. J Neurosurg 75:402–407, 1991.
11. North RB, Kidd DH, Zahuhurak M, et al: Spinal cord stimulation for chronic intractable pain: Experience over two decades. Neurosurgery 32:384–395, 1993.
12. Turner JA, Loeser JD, Bell KG: Spinal cord stimulation for chronic low back pain: A systematic literature synthesis. Neurosurgery 37:1088–1095, 1995.
13. North RB, Kidd David H, Lee MS, et al: A prospective, randomized study of spinal cord stimulation versus reoperation for failed back surgery syndrome: Initial results. Stereotact Funct Neurosurg 62:267–272, 1994.
14. Kim SH, Tasker RR, Oh MY: Spinal cord stimulation for nonspecific limb pain versus neuropathic pain and spontaneous versus evoked pain. Neurosurgery 48:1056–1065, 2001.
15. Canavero S, Bonicalzi V: Spinal cord stimulation for central pain. Pain 103:225–228, 2003.
16. Kirvela OA, Kotilainen E: Successful treatment of whiplash-type injury induced severe pain syndrome with epidural stimulation: A case report. Pain 80:441–443, 1999.
17. Laffey JG, Murphy D, Regan J, O'Keefe D: Efficacy of spinal cord stimulation for neuropathic pain following idiopathic acute transverse myelitis: A case report. Clin Neurol Neurosurg 101:125–127, 1999.
18. Sindou MP, Mertens P, Bendavid U, et al: Predictive value for somatosensory evoked potentials for long-lasting pain relief after spinal cord stimulation: Practical use for patient selection. Neurosurgery 52:1374–1384, 2003.
19. Harke H, Gretenkort P, Ladleif HU, et al: Spinal cord stimulation in postherpetic neuralgia and in acute herpes zoster pain. Anesth Analg 94:694–700, 2002.
20. Broseta J, Barbera J, De Vera JA, et al: Spinal cord stimulation in peripheral arterial disease: A cooperative study. J Neurosurg 64:71–80, 1986.

21. Jacobs MJ, Jorning PJ, Beckers RC, et al: Foot salvage and improvement of microvascular blood flow as a result of epidural spinal cord electrical stimulation. J Back Surg 12:354–360, 1990.

22. Amann W, Berg P, Gersbach P, et al: Spinal cord stimulation in the treatment of non-reconstructable stable critical leg ischemia: Results of the European peripheral vascular disease outcome study. Eur J Vasc Endovasc Surg 26:280–286, 2003.

23. Petrakis E, Sciacca V: Prospective study of transcutaneous oxygen tension measurement in the testing period of spinal cord stimulation in diabetic patients with critical lower limb ischemia. Int Angiol 19:18–25, 2000.

24. Petrakis E, Sciacca V: Does autonomic neuropathy influence spinal cord stimulation therapy success in diabetic patients with critical lower limb ischemia? Surg Neurol 53:182–189, 2000.

25. Neuhauser B, Perkmann R, Klingler PJ, et al: Clinical and objective data on spinal cord stimulation for the treatment of severe Raynaud's phenomenon. Am Surg 67:1096–1097, 2001.

26. Chierichetti F, Mambrini S, Bagliani, Odero A: Treatment of Buerger's disease with electrical spinal cord stimulation. Angiology 53:341–347, 2002.

27. Kumar K, Nath RK, Toth C: Spinal cord stimulation is effective in the management of reflex sympathetic dystrophy. Neurosurgery 40:503–509, 1997.

28. Barolat G, Schwartzman R, Woo R: Epidural spinal cord stimulation in the management of reflex sympathetic dystrophy. Stereotact Funct Neurosurg 53:29–39, 1989.

29. Hord ED, Cohen SP, Cosgrove GR, et al: The predictive value of sympathetic block for the success of spinal cord stimulation. Neurosurgery 53:626–633, 2003.

30. Murphy DF, Giles KE: Dorsal column stimulation for pain relief from intractable angina pectoris. Pain 28:365–368, 1987.

31. Mannheimer C, Augustinsson LE, Carlsson CA, et al: Epidural spinal electrical stimulation in severe angina pectoris. Br Heart J 59:56–61, 1988.

32. Gonzalez-Darder JM, Canela P, Martinez VG: High cervical spinal cord stimulation for unstable angina pectoris. Stereotact Funct Neurosurg 56:20–27, 1991.

33. de Jongste MJL, Staal MJ: Preliminary results of a randomized study on the clinical efficacy of spinal cord stimulation for refractory severe angina pectoris. Acta Neurochir Suppl 58:161–164, 1993.

34. de Jongste MJL, Haaksma J, Hautvast RWM, et al: Effects of spinal cord stimulation on myocardial ischaemia during daily life in patients with severe coronary artery disease. Br Heart J 71:413–418, 1994.

35. de Jongste MJL, Nagelkerke D, Hooyschuur CM: Stimulation characteristics, complications, and efficacy of spinal cord stimulation systems in patients with refractory angina. Pacing Clin Electrophysiol 17:1751–1760, 1994.

36. Anderson C, Hole P, Oxhoj H: Does pain relief with spinal cord stimulation for angina conceal myocardial infarction? Br Heart J 71:419–421, 1994.

37. Anderson C, Hole P, Oxhoj H: Spinal cord stimulation as a pain treatment for angina pectoris. Pain Clinic 8:333–339, 1995.

38. De Jongst MJL, Hautvast RWM, Hillege H, et al: Efficacy of spinal cord stimulation as an adjuvant therapy for intractable angina pectoris: A prospective randomized clinical study. J Am Coll Cardiol 23:1592–1597, 1994.

39. Bagger JP, Jensen BS, Johannsen G: Long-term outcome of spinal electrical stimulation in patients with refractory chest pain. Clin Cardiol 21:286–288, 1998.

40. Sanderson JE, Brooksby P, Waterhouse D, et al: Epidural spinal electrical stimulation for severe angina: A study of effects on symptoms, exercise tolerance and degree of ischemia. Eur Heart J 13:628–633, 1992.

41. Janfaza DR, Michna E, Pisini JV, Ross EL: Bedside implantation of a trial spinal cord stimulator for intractable anginal pain. Anesth Analg 87:1242–1244, 1998.

42. Fanciullo GJ, Robb JF, Rose RJ, Sanders JH: Spinal cord stimulation for intractable angina pectoris. Anesth Analg 89:305–306, 1999.

43. Ekre O, Eliasson T, Norrsell H, et al: Long-term effects of spinal cord stimulation and coronary artery bypass grafting on quality of life and survival in the ESBY study. Eur Heart J 23:1938–1945, 2002.

44. Jessurun GAJ, de Jongste MJL, Hautvast RWM, et al: Clinical follow-up after cessation of chronic electrical neuromodulation in patients with severe coronary artery disease: A prospective randomized controlled study on putative involvement of sympathetic activity. Pacing Clin Electrophysiol 22:1432–1439, 1999.

45. Murray S, Carson KGS, Ewings PD, et al: Spinal cord stimulation significantly decreases the need for acute hospital admission for chest pain in patients wit refractory angina pectoris. Heart 82:89–92, 1999.

46. Romano M, Brusa S, Grieco A, et al: Efficacy and safety of permanent cardiac DDD pacing with contemporaneous double spinal cord stimulation. Pacing Clin Electrophysiol 1:465–467, 1998.

47. Iyer R, Gnanadurai TV, Forsey P: Management of cardiac pacemaker in a patient with spinal cord stimulator implant. Pain 74:333–335, 1998.

48. Lind G, Meyerson BA, Winter J, Linderoth B: Implantation of laminotomy electrodes for spinal cord stimulation in spinal anesthesia with intraoperative dorsal column activation. Neurosurgery 53:1150–1154, 2003.

49. Villavicencio AT, Leveque JC, Rubin L, et al: Laminectomy versus percutaneous electrode placement for spinal cord stimulation. Neurosurgery 46:399–406, 2000.

50. North RT, Kidd DH, Olin JC, Sieracki JM: Spinal cord stimulation electrode design: Prospective, randomized, controlled trial comparing percutaneous and laminectomy electrodes—part I: Technical outcomes. Neurosurgery 51:381–384, 2002.

51. Ball PA, Fanciullo GJ: Pont de dolor: A dual laminotomy technique for placing and securing an electrode in the epidural space and comments about anatomic variation that may complicate spinal cord stimulation electrode placement. Neuromodulation 6:92–94, 2003.

52. Huraibi HA, Phillips J, Rose, et al: Intrathecal baclofen pump implantation complicated by epidural lipomatosis. Anesth Analg 91:429–431, 2000.

53. Wallin J, Cui J, Yakhnitsa V, et al: Gabapentin and pregabalin suppress tactile allodynia and potentiate spinal cord stimulation in a model of neuropathy. Eur J Pain 6:261–272, 2002.

54. Harke H, Gretenkort P, Ladleif H, et al: The response of neuropathic pain and pain in complex regional pain syndrome I to carbamazepine and sustained-release morphine in patients pretreated with spinal cord stimulation: A double-blinded randomized study. Anesth Analg 92:488–495, 2001.

55. North RB, Calkins S, Campbell DS, et al: Automated, patient-interactive, spinal cord stimulator adjustment: A randomized controlled trial. Neurosurgery 52:572–580, 2003.

56. Barolat G, Sharon AD: Future trends in spinal cords stimulation. Neurol Res 22:279–284, 2000.

57. Krames ES, Gershow J, Glassberg A, et al: Continuous infusion of spinally administered narcotics for the relief of pain due to malignant disorders. Cancer 56:696–702, 1985.

58. Shetter AG, Hadley MN, Wilkinson E: Administration of intraspinal morphine sulphate for the treatment of intractable cancer pain. Neurosurgery 18:740–747, 1986.

59. Van Dongen RTW, Crul BJP, De Bock M: Long-term intrathecal infusion of morphine and morphine/bupivacaine mixtures in the treatment of cancer pain: A retrospective analysis of 51 cases. Pain 55:119–123, 1993.

60. Coombs DW, Saunders RL, Gaylor M, et al: Epidural narcotic infusion and reservoir: Implantation technique and efficacy. Anesthesiology 56:469–473, 1982.

61. Andersen PE, Cohen JI, Everts EC, et al: Intrathecal narcotics for relief of pain from head and neck cancer. Arch Otolaryngol Head Neck Surg 117:1277–1280, 1991.

62. Hassenbusch SJ, Prem PK, Magdinec M, et al: Constant infusion of morphine for intractable cancer pain using an implanted pump. J Neurosurg 73:405–409, 1990.

63. Krames ES, Gershow J, Glassberg A, et al: Continuous infusion of spinally administered narcotics for the relief of pain due to malignant disorders. Cancer 56:696–702, 1985.

64. Magora F, Olshwang D, Eimerl D, et al: Observations on extradural morphine analgesia in various pain conditions. Br J Anaesth 52:247–252, 1980.

65. Winkelmuller M, Winkelmuller W: Long term effects of continuous intrathecal opioid treatment in chronic pain of nonmalignant etiology. J Neurosurg 85:458–467, 1996.

66. Coombs DW, Saunders MD, Lechance BS, et al: Intrathecal morphine tolerance: Use of intrathecal clonidine, DADLE, and intraventricular morphine. Anesthesiology 62:358–363, 1985.

67. Portenoy RK, Hassenbusch SJ: Current practices in intraspinal therapy—a survey of clinical trends and decision making. J Pain Sympt Manage 20:S4–S11, 2000.

68. Malloy A, Muir A, Sharp T, et al: Intrathecal testing with morphine in patients requiring regular opioids for analgesia. Negative responders were significantly more distressed and disabled than positive responders.

In Abstracts, 8th World Congress on Pain. Seattle, IASP Press, 1996, pp 391–392.

69. Katz NK, Sherburne S, Beach M, et al: Behavioral monitoring and urine toxicology testing in patients receiving long-term opioid therapy. Anesth Analg 97:1097–1102, 2003.

70. Bennett G, Serafini M, Burchiel KJ, et al: Evidence-based review of the literature on intrathecal delivery of pain medicine. J Pain Sympt Manage 20:S12–S36, 2000.

71. Bromage PR, Camporesi E, Chestnut D: Epidural narcotics for postoperative analgesia. Anesth Analg 59:473–480, 1980.

72. Bennett G, Burchiel K, Buchser, et al: Clinical guidelines for intraspinal infusion: Report of an expert panel. J Pain Sympt Manage 20:S37–S43, 2000.

73. Anderson VC, Burchiel KJ, Cooke B: A prospective randomized trial of intrathecal injection vs. epidural infusion in the selection of patients for continuous intrathecal opioid therapy. Neuromodulation 6:142–152, 2003.

74. Follett KA, Burchiel K, Deer T, et al: Prevention of intrathecal drug delivery catheter-related complications. Neuromodulation 6:32–41, 2003.

75. Krames ES: Intrathecal Infusional Therapies for Intractable Pain; Patient Management Guidelines. Minneapolis: Medtronic Neurological, 1991.

76. Prager JP: Neuraxial medication delivery: The development and maturity of a concept for treating chronic pain of spinal origin. Spine 27:2593–2605, 2002.

111 Open Cordotomy and Medullary Tractotomy

CHARLES E. POLETTI

OPEN CORDOTOMY

Indications

General Indications: Cancer Pain below T5

We have become progressively inclined to perform cordotomy operations only on patients suffering from medically intractable cancer pain whose longevity appears limited to less than 3 years. This decision has grown from the relatively high incidence of failures 1 to 2 years after cordotomy operations and the increasing late frequency of postcordotomy painful dysesthesias. The significant instance of unavoidable complications—including motor weakness and bladder and sexual dysfunction—is a further argument against using the operation, especially bilaterally, in patients with benign disease.

Accordingly, we have been reluctant to perform cordotomies in patients with peripheral nerve or spinal cord injuries, herpetic neuralgia, or chronic calcific pancreatitis, no matter how severely afflicted. With selected cancer patients, however, the operation often relieves suffering and obviates excessive use of narcotics. For these patients, the operation should be a priority option. If delayed too long, the operation may not arrest or reverse extensive suffering and debilitation. For patients with markedly limited life spans, a percutaneous cordotomy is often selected.

The use of cordotomy is further limited by progressive decreases in the level of analgesia during the first 6 months after the operation. Often, within 3 postoperative weeks, the level has fallen three to six segments, and at 6 months, the level may have lowered a total of six to eight segments. Thus most surgeons agree that even with high cervical cordotomies many patients may have no significant hypalgesia above T2–T3. After a T2–T3 thoracic cordotomy, the level of significant permanent hypalgesia or analgesia usually is about T10. Consequently, one can usually count on a year of analgesia six to eight levels below the operation. A further consideration to make before performing the cordotomy is that often, during these postoperative 6 months in which the level of analgesia is falling, the cancer is progressing to higher levels.

More important than determining the site of the referred pain is localizing the cancerous lesion that produces the pain. For instance, one of our patients with prostatic cancer and severe, deep lateral flank pain on the right side appeared to be a good candidate for unilateral open thoracic cordotomy until total-body computed tomography (CT) revealed a single metastasis eroding the right half of the T12 vertebra. On further direct questioning, the patient finally admitted to pain in the corresponding left lateral flank. In this case, unilateral cordotomy was no longer an option.

We believe that each cordotomy operation should be individually designed primarily on the basis of the location of the cancerous lesion producing the pain.

Unilateral Somatic Cancer: Unilateral Cordotomy

Unilateral cordotomies are most effective for cancer that is not invading the viscera and for cancer that is located away from the midline and at or below the lower cervical region. Thus excellent potential candidates are patients with cancer confined to the legs, the hips, the lateral retroperitoneal pelvic and abdominal space, the chest wall (e.g., breast cancer and Pancoast's tumor), and perhaps the lower brachial plexus. For disease below T8, we select a T2 unilateral thoracic cordotomy, which carries a lower risk than cervical cordotomy.

For cancer of the arms, as for that of the neck, nasopharynx, or face, a medullary tractotomy is worth considering instead of cordotomy, although the operative mortality and incidence of postoperative dysesthesias are slightly higher. An open C2–C3 cordotomy combined with a C2, C3, and C4 dorsal rhizotomy may relieve severe pain in the brachial plexus, upper extremity, shoulder, and neck.[1] We favor open C2–C3 cordotomy, occasionally combined with rhizotomy, over a C1–C2 percutaneous cordotomy, because of the marked anatomic variations at C1–C2 and the belief that consistently more complete, uncomplicated lesions with higher permanent levels of analgesia can be obtained using our open technique at C2–C3.

Unilateral Visceral Pain: Bilateral Cordotomy

In general, whenever a significant component of the pain is caused by disease invading the viscera, bilateral deep cordotomies are required for satisfactory relief of suffering. Often, the visceral pain from extensive cancer of the pancreas, intestine, colon, rectum, cervix, or uterus, and especially the stomach and esophagus, may be mediated by splanchnic nerves entering the spinal cord as high as T1. Many of these visceral nociceptive afferents do not cross to the other side of the spinal cord. Accordingly, in these patients, the best chance of satisfactory results rests with the highest bilateral cervical cordotomy advisable (i.e., C1–C2 percutaneous or C2–C3 open cordotomy combined with an open contralateral C5–C6 cordotomy).

Paramedian, Midline, and Bilateral Cancer: Bilateral Cordotomy

Whenever the cancer is close to the midline, unilateral cordotomy has a high probability of not securing prolonged relief. Affected patients often become aware of severe contralateral pain shortly after surgery. Accordingly, it should

1559

be emphasized that even for paramedian cancers, it is wise to perform a bilateral cordotomy.

When bilateral cordotomies are indicated, an open cordotomy is performed at two levels rather than a unilateral percutaneous cordotomy followed by an open operation.

Alternatives to Bilateral Cordotomy

Whenever open bilateral cordotomies are indicated, one should seriously consider various alternative operations that are available: a midline myelotomy operation may have a higher chance of relieving bilateral pain in the arms, shoulders, and neck as well as pain from bilateral visceral or extensive midline disease. In addition, midline myelotomies, compared with bilateral cordotomies, have a significantly lower incidence of later postcordotomy dysesthesias and bladder dysfunction, sleep apnea, and motor weakness.

Hitchcock[2,3] and Schvarcz[4-6] independently have pioneered central medullary myelotomies for high bilateral disease using stereotactic techniques. These appear promising but require special expertise.

My colleagues and I[7] have developed a technically simple nondestructive operation for intractable cancer pain in which a spinal epidural catheter is implanted for long-term administration of morphine. Using three administration systems, we demonstrated for the first time that direct spinal narcotics can be used for effective, long-term pain relief.

Consideration of Anatomy and Variations

Spinal Cord

The goal of anterolateral cordotomy is to create a lesion in fibers ascending in the spinothalamic tract (STT) that carry nociceptive input from one side of the body caudal to the level of the lesion. Marked anatomic variations of the spinal cord, however, frequently impede optimal transection of the STT. Four major areas of anatomic variation that concern the surgeon are: (1) the course of the STT, (2) the course of the corticospinal tract (CST), (3) the position of the dentate insertion, and (4) the width of the spinal cord. Thus, in cordotomy as in aneurysm surgery, the individual patient's anatomy must be identified or analyzed. It may often be necessary to perform a variation of the standard operation to maximize the probability of satisfactory results.

Spinothalamic Tract

In some persons, the STT does not appear to decussate at all. In these patients, a standard anterolateral cordotomy produces ipsilateral analgesia. Fortunately, these cases are rare. Most patients, however, probably have a number of uncrossed nociceptive fibers; perhaps these permit the recovery of pain after cordotomy. In particular, the nociceptive fibers mediating visceral pain in many cases do not decussate fully but instead ascend on both sides of the spinal cord. This should encourage the surgeon to perform bilateral cordotomies when visceral pain is thought to be significant.

Normally, the vast majority of the nociceptive fibers do decussate, following two predictable patterns. In the first pattern, the "sacral" fibers are positioned most posterolaterally and superficially. The more rostral fibers from the lumbar, thoracic, and cervical regions ascend to assume their course more anteromedially and deeply (Fig. 111-1). The sacral fibers may lie immediately anterior to the base of the normally positioned dentate (see Fig. 111-1). The cordotomy lesion therefore should first reach as far dorsally as the equator of the spinal cord, usually at the base of the dentate insertion. In some patients, beginning the lesion 1 to 2 mm anterior to this point results in sparing of the sacral fibers.

A second relatively predictable pattern reflects the observation that pain from the superficial part of the body is relayed by fibers close to the surface of the spinal cord. Progressively deeper are the fibers mediating the sense of temperature, deep pain, and finally visceral pain (see Fig. 111-1). Accordingly, the lesion must extend deep to the anterolateral surface of the cord, especially in patients with visceral disease. In most patients, a depth of 5 mm is required, even in the cervical region.

Perhaps most important, the lesion should include the medial and anterior portion of the anterior quadrant. It is often in this portion of the spinal cord that fibers from the anterior commissure ascend five to six segments or more before extending far enough laterally to assume their "classic" position in the "lateral" STT. In contrast, fibers from the dorsal horn appear to cross to the anterior commissure almost immediately (i.e., at the same level or at most within one to two segments). Yet these same fibers may then ascend for five to eight segments before "crossing" fully to form the lateral STT. Thus the "anterior" STT in humans consists of ascending fibers gradually coursing laterally to form the lateral STT.

Accordingly, a lesion in the lateral anterior quadrant, albeit deep, may produce analgesia extending rostrally only eight or more segments below the lesion. In contrast, a lesion of the anterior quadrant extending to the midline sometimes produces analgesia to within one segment of the lesion. Thus, especially in cervical cordotomies for which a primary goal is a high permanent level of analgesia, we recommend extending the lesion at least 1 to 2 mm anterior to the most medially exiting fibers of the ventral root (i.e., within 1 to 2.5 mm of the anterior spinal artery) (see Fig. 111-7). A lesion extending only as far anteriorly as the ventral root may yield a satisfactory level of analgesia in only 80% of patients. In fact, the technique described next usually permits a lesion of the entire anterior quadrant extending immediately to the midline anterior pial septum and anterior spinal artery. We think that this lesion produces the highest level of analgesia feasible—usually within two and occasionally within one segment.

Corticospinal Tract

Rarely, the CST does not decussate at all. Instead, it descends uncrossed in the anterolateral quadrant of the cord. In these rare patients, an anterolateral cordotomy would be expected to produce contralateral plegia because these aberrant tracts are thought to finally cross near the segment of their termination on the lower motor neuron. In addition, the data of Yakovlev and Rakic[8] indicate that these abnormal patterns of the CST are probably more common than is believed. It seems reasonable to assume that there may be associated abnormalities or displacements of the normally adjacent STT.

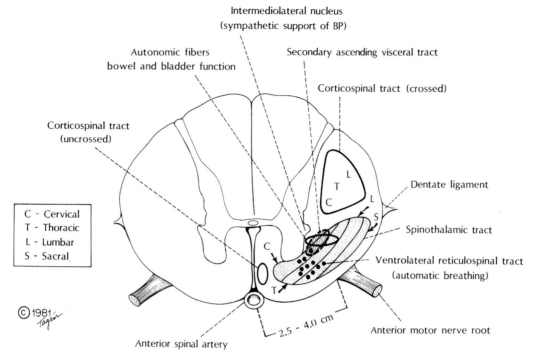

FIGURE 111-1 The spinal cord at T3 with the axon tracts relevant to making lesions of the spinothalamic tract (STT). Just dorsal to the equator of the cord is the descending corticospinal tract (CST). The lesion should start about 1 mm anterior to the anterior limit of the CST. The entire STT is shown, including the anterior and lateral components. It should be emphasized that intermingled within the STT fibers are other ascending and descending tracts. Of necessity, these must be lesioned to obtain a complete lesion of the STT. These tracts intermingled at least in part with the STT include the ventrolateral reticulospinal tract, which is responsible for nonvoluntary breathing, the descending autonomic fibers for bladder and bowel sphincter control, the ascending visceral tract, and sympathetic fibers just anterolateral to their origin in the intermediolateral nucleus. In the anteromedial aspect of the cord is the uncrossed CST adjacent to the midline septum and the anterior spinal artery. Note also that the distance from the medial-most exiting motor rootlet to the anterior spinal artery and midline varies from 2 to 3.5 mm. (Copyright © 1981 by Edith Tagrin.)

Commonly, however, even in normal patients, the decussating pyramidal fibers are not fully crossed and back into the posterior aspect of the cord until the caudal half of C2. Accordingly, we are inclined to perform our cervical cordotomies at C3. A C4–C5 level of analgesia, as discussed previously, may still be feasible if the lesion is extended to the midline. Clearly, when the decussation is abnormally low, careful stimulation and monitoring—even at C3—is necessary to avoid a lesion of the CST.

Dentate Insertion

The dentate ligament is formed by the joining of components of the ventral and dorsal spinal cord pia. Usually, these components join to form the dentate at the equator of the cord, just anterior to the anterior extent of the CST and just posterior to the posterior extent of the sacral fibers of the STT. In a number of cases, however, as Sweet[9] has noted, the dentate origin may form anterior or posterior to this equatorial line. When it is anterior to its most common position, a lesion beginning at the dentate and extending anteriorly may not transect nociceptive fibers from the sacrum. In cases of a posterior dentate, a lesion beginning just anterior to the dentate clearly has a high probability of producing an ipsilateral motor deficit. Accordingly, the lesion should begin at the equator of the cord, irrespective of the position of the dentate. Because the equator of the rotated cord is difficult to judge, we again stress physiologic stimulation and monitoring, preferably with the patient awake.

Spinal Cord Width

The width of the spinal cord appears to vary as well, in both the thoracic and cervical regions, especially in patients with advanced cancer. In one of our patients, for instance, extensive pelvic cancer invaded the lumbosacral plexus bilaterally, producing significant sensory deficits and virtual paraplegia. In this patient, the spinal cord at T2 under the microscope measured a total width of 5.2 mm. Obviously, it would have been injudicious to try to cut the anterior quadrant to a depth of 4 to 5 mm, especially because at the time we were still using a cordotomy knife, not a blunt instrument capable of palpating the anterior midline septum adjacent to the anterior spinal artery. Accordingly, we recommend measuring the width of the spinal cord in each case and using that specific dimension to determine the approximate depth of the lesion.

Preoperative Procedures

Preparations and Special Instruments

All patients are advised of the complications of cordotomy operations. When awakening the patient during the operation (wake-up anesthesia) appears appropriate, both the surgeon and the anesthesiologist discuss the details and alternatives with the patient. If there is any suspicion of impaired pulmonary function contralateral to the planned lesion, a comprehensive series of pulmonary function tests are performed. When motion of the contralateral hemidiaphragm is impaired, a unilateral cervical cordotomy may trigger fatal postoperative respiratory complications by interrupting the exclusively ipsilateral descending projections of the ventrolateral reticulospinal tract (see Fig. 111-1). The patient is wrapped with woven elastic bandages from the toes to the thigh to minimize the resulting operation-induced orthostatic hypotension; this is especially important when bilateral lesions are planned.

Electrophysiologic Monitoring Equipment

Because of the marked potential variability in the location within the spinal cord of both the lateral STT and the CST, we conclude that intraoperative electrophysiologic stimulation of the spinal cord combined with dorsal column–evoked responses and electromyelographic recording is useful. So as both to stimulate in the anterior quadrant to identify the STT in the awakened patient and later to stimulate while the lesion is being made (to warn of nearby CST fibers), we use a 45-degree Jacobsen ball that is insulated except over the distal half of the ball and at the end of the handle. A standard stimulator is attached to the uninsulated end of the handle, preferably a stimulator that is capable of constant current stimulation at 2 to 100 Hz. For measuring dorsal column potentials evoked by peroneal or median nerve stimulation, we use a Nicolet signal averager with bipolar epidural recording electrodes. This technique is described elsewhere.[10]

Especially when wake-up anesthesia is not used, we monitor CST function by stimulating as the lesion is being made while looking for motor responses and elicited electromyographic recordings distally. A small dental mirror on a malleable shaft is used to visualize the anterior spinal artery while the lesion is being made.

Operative Procedures

Anesthesia

With the improved techniques of wake-up anesthesia supplemented by local infiltration of the wound, we have discontinued the use of only local anesthetics for cordotomy operations. Wake-up anesthesia allows identification of the SST by stimulation, monitoring of bilateral motor function as the lesion is being made, and testing of the extent of the induced sensory deficit before it is too late to enlarge the lesion.

A third technique, in which the patient is awake after the initial cordotomy incision has been made, has also been described.[11] With this technique, segmental analgesia (C4 to T8) is produced by blocking the dorsal roots using a single injection of epidural bupivacaine. Because normal spinal cord function is preserved and the T2 laminectomy is easily tolerated, the patient remains fully awake and cooperative for testing sensory and motor function distal to T8 after the cordotomy lesions are produced.

The operative technique described here is designed especially to maximize the probability of obtaining an optimal lesion without subjecting the patient to being awake during surgery. The goal in this technique is making as large a lesion as feasible in the anterior quadrant without transecting the CST. The lesion extends dorsally to within

1 to 2 mm of the CST, medially to the midline anterior septum, and all the way anteriorly and anterolaterally. If there is a dominant variant of the CST in the anteromedial aspect of the spinal cord, it is identified by the stimulus at the top of the Jacobsen ball. As a result, our last seven patients have undergone surgery under continuous general anesthesia and all have had an initial contralateral distal hemianalgesia rising to within two segments of the complete anterior quadrant cordotomy without any detectable motor weakness.

Position

For unilateral cordotomy with wake-up anesthesia, the patient can be placed in the swimmer's position, with the thorax rotated 45 degrees up from horizontal. With the spinal cord rotated 45 degrees, the operating microscope can be focused almost vertically and the cord can be viewed from a transverse direction. When bilateral lesions are anticipated or when wake-up anesthesia is not employed, the patient should be placed prone. Especially for cervical cordotomies, the head is placed in a neutral position to decrease tethering of the cord, which may occur with too much flexion. For cervical operations, the head is held in a three-pin headrest, whereas during upper thoracic operations, the head is allowed to rest on a doughnut headrest. The fully bandaged legs should be elevated on blankets and the table set in moderate reverse Trendelenburg position. With the patient in this position, a decrease in blood pressure after bilateral lesions are made will indicate, as noted by Sindou (personal communication, 1981), that the depth and dorsal extent of the lesion are satisfactory.

Unilateral Cordotomy Procedure

A relatively long skin incision is made to provide wide lateral retraction of the skin and paraspinal muscles. This affords a view from a lateral angle of the anterior quadrant of the rotated cord.

For unilateral upper thoracic lesions, the T2 and T3 laminae are exposed, whereas bilateral upper thoracic lesions call for exposure of the laminae of T2, T3, and T4. A complete laminectomy is performed, extending fully laterally on the side of the planned lesion. Next, the yellow ligament above and below the laminectomy is removed, exposing the inferior edge of the rostral lamina and the superior edge of the caudal lamina. The bipolar electrodes for recording evoked potentials from bilateral peroneal nerve stimulation are inserted in the midline epidural space rostrally and caudally (Fig. 111-2).

The dura is then opened in a semicircular fashion, extending far enough laterally to allow direct visualization of the contralateral side of the spinal cord (Fig. 111-3). This permits exact measurement of the width of the spinal cord. The microscope is brought into the field. The arachnoid is opened for optimal visualization. The width of the cord is measured precisely under the microscope, and a piece of bone wax is used to mark half of the cord width from the tip of the Jacobsen ball. This measurement will be used during transection to gauge the depth of cordotomy and to allow the tip of the Jacobsen ball to reach the midline. Once the cord width has been measured, the arachnoid opening is extended laterally over the dentate ligament.

Traction of the dorsal or ventral roots during rotation of the cord may result in painful postoperative dysesthesias.

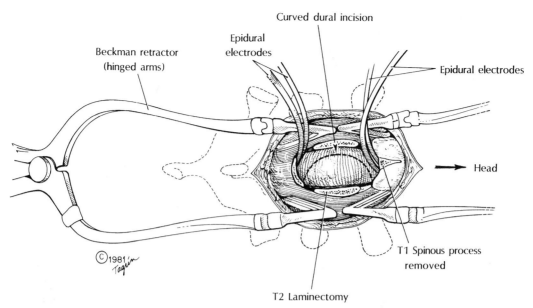

FIGURE 111-2 The spinous processes of T1, T2, and T3 are exposed. The T1 and T2 processes are removed. A complete bilateral laminectomy at T2 is shown extending far laterally on the side of the lesion. The rostral and caudal yellow ligaments are excised. The bipolar epidural electrodes are then inserted in the midline rostrally and caudally for recording sensory evoked potentials from bilateral peroneal stimulation. The projected dural incision is shown by the *dotted line*. (Copyright © 1981 by Edith Tagrin.)

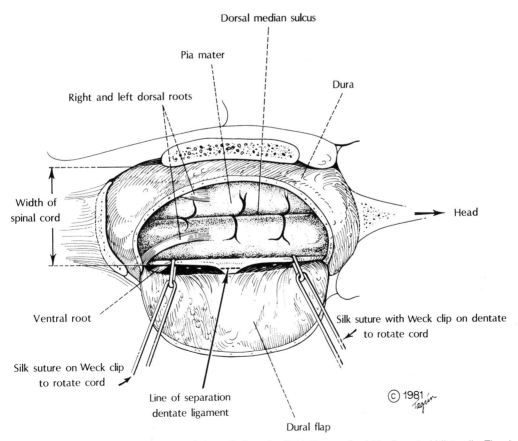

FIGURE 111-3 The dura is opened. The microscope is brought into the field. The arachnoid is dissected bilaterally. The dura is retracted contralaterally to permit direct measurement of the width of the spinal cord. Weck clips with silk sutures are applied to the dentate as shown. The arachnoid around the dorsal roots is dissected, freeing the roots to their exit point. (Copyright © 1981 by Edith Tagrin.)

The dorsal rootlets should therefore be freed from the cord to their point of exit or to the limit of the exposure. If necessary, the dorsal root should be cut to facilitate rotation rather than risk a traction injury with postoperative hyperesthesia. As previously mentioned, in cervical cordotomies, White and Sweet[1] suggest performing bilateral rhizotomies of the three accessible dorsal roots to raise the level of analgesia and to decrease the postoperative incisional pain. Other workers have found that rhizotomies do not improve the results of cordotomy.[12]

With the roots freed or cut, the cord is then rotated 45 degrees. To rotate the cord, a 4-0 silk suture is placed in two Weck clips, which are in turn placed on the dentate ligament (Fig. 111-4; see also Fig. 111-3). The silk sutures are then used to put traction on the Weck clips and the dentate for rotating the cord. If the patient is under local anesthesia and experiences pain as the cord is rotated, the dorsal root should be cut. Alternatively, cerebrospinal fluid should be aspirated and a small cottonoid soaked in 10% cocaine should be applied selectively to the posterior roots. If the root is sufficiently mobilized beforehand, however, pain during rotation is rarely elicited. With careful microsurgical dissection, the intact dentate insertion usually is strong enough to rotate the cord. If not, traction can be applied directly on the anterior root to rotate the cord. One should not be afraid to rotate the cord too far. If the anterior spinal artery along the anterior midline cannot be satisfactorily viewed, the dentate above and below the level of interest can be cut, permitting the cord to be rotated as much as 90 degrees. Electrophysiologic monitoring electrodes offer additional safety, but we have not found their use to be mandatory if these techniques are followed as described.

Once the cord is rotated 45 degrees, a small dental mirror on a malleable handle can be used to visualize the exact course of the anterior spinal artery in the anterior midline septum and the medial limit of the exit of the ventral rootlets (Fig. 111-5; see also Fig. 111-4). At the most avascular part of the exposed anterior quadrant, the tip of a No. 11 blade is inserted into the equator of the spinal cord. As noted, this is usually located immediately under the dentate insertion. The exact site of the dentate attachment can be established by observation and blunt palpation on the dentate insertion in a dorsoventral manner.

Microsurgical scissors are placed in the small hole made in the pia by the No. 11 blade (see Fig. 111-4). Only the pia arachnoid is then cut with the microscissors around the anterior quadrant of the cord. Cutting the pia with sharp scissors decreases the chance of avulsing the dentate attachment. Small pial vessels may be cauterized with bipolar microforceps. We incise the pia to a point 2 mm anterior to the medial-most exit of the ventral root, which should be at least 1 mm from the anterior spinal artery. An advantage of making the pial cut initially, before the lesion in the tracts, is that the natural shape of the cord is subsequently preserved while the instrument is being inserted. Cutting the pia with a knife tends to distort the anatomy of the cord, making an accurate lesion difficult and placing indirect traction on adjacent vascular and neural structures.

With the incision in the pia, the cord is ready for cordotomy. Clearly, in making the spinal cord lesion, the two principal cautions are to avoid transecting the CST and to avoid damage to the anterior spinal artery and its main branches. The CST is particularly vulnerable to damage during cordotomy procedures, and as mentioned previously,

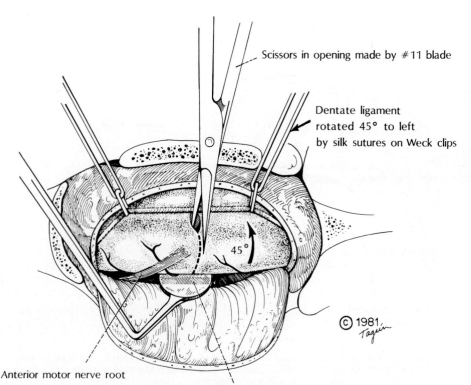

Scissors in opening made by #11 blade

Dentate ligament rotated 45° to left by silk sutures on Weck clips

45°

© 1981 Tagrin

Anterior motor nerve root

Anterior spinal artery reflected in dental mirror

FIGURE 111-4 The lateral attachment to the dentate ligament has been cut. Traction is applied on the silk sutures attached by Weck clips to the dentate until the cord is rotated 45 degrees. A small dental mirror is placed ventrolaterally to permit visualization of the anterior midline septum and the course of the anterior spinal artery. The microscissors are placed into the hole made in the pia just anterior to the equator of the cord. These are used to cut the pia arachnoid around the anterior quadrant to within 1 to 2 mm of the anterior midline septum. This is usually about 2 mm anterior to the medial-most exiting ventral rootlet. (Copyright © 1981 by Edith Tagrin.)

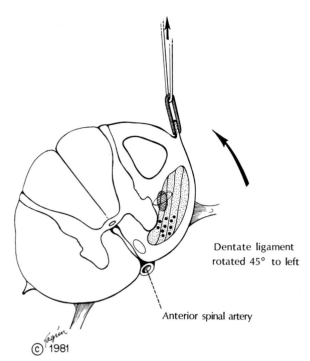

FIGURE 111-5 The orientation of the relevant tracts within the cord once it has been rotated 45 degrees. (Copyright © 1981 by Edith Tagrin.)

Dentate ligament rotated 45° to left

Anterior spinal artery

© 1981

anatomic variations limit the surgeon's ability to execute an adequate lesion without the possibility of damaging the motor system.

Our operative technique for making the lesion is unique in that it involves the use of a blunt Jacobsen ball to stimulate simultaneously while making the lesion. The stimulator is attached to the end of the handle of the Jacobsen ball instrument. A ground electrode is inserted in the paraspinal muscles. Stimulation parameters are set for 1-millisecond pulses delivered at 1.5 V. Such a stimulus elicits responses in the CST with motion in the ipsilateral arm or leg in the asleep, unparalyzed patient when the ball tip approaches within 1 mm of the CST. The blunt-tipped instrument permits safe traverse of the anterolateral cord all the way to the medial septum while the proximity of the instrument to the CST dorsally is concurrently monitored by looking for stimulation-evoked motor responses. Although the Jacobsen ball is a blunt instrument, it does not distort the very soft tissue of the cord. It has been our experience, particularly with midline myelotomies, that the Jacobsen ball is fully satisfactory for transecting spinal cord tracts.

The Jacobsen ball is inserted at the equator of the cord at the dorsal-most limit of the pial opening and is directed into the transverse axis of the cord until the bone wax indicates that the ball is halfway across the width of the cord. Because the spinal cord has been rotated 45 degrees, the tip of the Jacobsen ball is also angled 45 degrees. Thus, during this initial motion, the shaft of the instrument is held vertically (Fig. 111-6A, B). Usually, the transverse diameter of the cord in the upper thoracic region is approximately 10 mm, so initially an incision to a depth of approximately 5 mm is indicated. In the cervical region, the cord may be as wide as 16 mm, in which case an incision to 8 mm is permissible. As mentioned previously, however, the size of

the cord may vary. We have seen a cord width as small as 5.2 mm in the thoracic region, presumably because of atrophy of the dorsal columns and descending CSTs. In that particular case, it was necessary to insert the ball to only 2.5 mm so as to place the lesion at the center of the cord.

As the ball passes near the gray matter of the anterior horn, an ipsilateral trapezius contraction may be obtained during cervical cordotomy and contraction of intercostal muscles may be obtained during thoracic cordotomy. The presence of distal ipsilateral motor responses indicates that the stimulating Jacobsen ball is too close to the descending CST and must be directed more anteriorly. Redirection of the ball is most commonly necessary when one is working in the cervical region, where the motor fibers may not be exclusively dorsal to the equator of the cord. Once the ball is in the center of the cord (see Fig. 111-6B), it is drawn directly anteriorly along the palpable medial septum to the anteromedial corner of the anterior quadrant. The ball is then drawn laterally along the pia for about 1 to 2 mm until it exits from the cord at the most anteromedial extent of the pial incision (Fig. 111-7).

The ball should be drawn flush against the pia of the midline septum and the anterior quadrant. The pia is firm and can be readily palpated safely from inside the cord with the Jacobsen ball. There may be marked anatomic variation in the anteromedial portion of the anterior quadrant with a large, uncrossed CST. Should this be the case, one would expect contralateral motor responses in this region from the Jacobsen ball. We have not yet encountered such a case. Should this occur, it seems prudent to skirt this tract when making the first lesion. The ball tip of the Jacobsen instrument usually can be seen as it comes out of the pia, but if not there is usually ample room to insert the mirror to see exactly where the ball exits. If it exits as planned, there is a high probability that the lesion is satisfactory.

It is important, as shown in Figure 111-7, to make the lesion as close as possible to the midline septum. This is especially important in the cervical region, where recently crossed fibers may lie close to the septum for many levels before assuming a more lateral and dorsal position. Hardy and colleagues[13] think that an incision extending to the midline can raise the level of resulting analgesia virtually to the level of the lesion.

Selective cervical cordotomies (i.e., partial lesions of the anterolateral quadrant) are not recommended for two reasons: first, cancer may spread to wider areas, and second, the topologic distribution of the STT does not appear to be sufficiently specific for reliable results.

It should be stressed that in the cervical region, the anterior spinal artery is usually 4.5 to 5 mm from the center of the exit zone of the anterior nerve root. A lesion 2 mm from the midline will still be 2.5 to 3 mm away from the center of the exiting ventral root. Except for the danger of entry into the anterior spinal artery, there does not appear to be any disadvantage to making an incision in the medial anterior quadrant as well. We have not seen a case of contralateral motor weakness caused by transection of the uncrossed descending motor tracts.

In summary, when making the initial lesion, the surgeon should attempt to transect virtually the entire anterior quadrant of the cord from the equator anteriorly, extending to the midline.

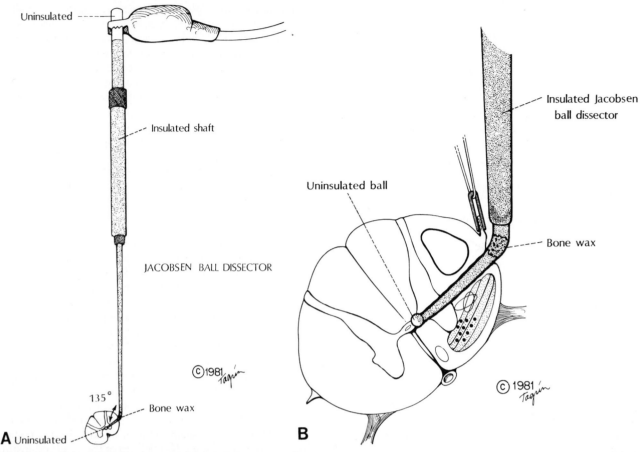

FIGURE 111-6 *A,* The 45-degree Jacobsen ball tip has been inserted just anterior to the equator of the cord and, while stimulating, is slowly advanced in the transverse axis of the cord until the tip reaches the midline (i.e., until the distal part of the bone wax marker on the tip is flush against the lateral aspect of the cord). The tip should pass far enough dorsally to include the intermediolateral nucleus, and all the tracts depicted in Figure 111-1 except for the crossed CST. *B,* An enlarged view of the Jacobsen ball instrument after the initial insertion. Note that the distal half of the Jacobsen ball is uninsulated. If this ball passes closer than 1 mm to the CST during its insertion into the cord, ipsilateral motor responses will be elicited. In this case, the ball should be redirected more anteriorly. From this position, the ball is then slowly directed 90 degrees anteriorly, palpating the midline septum. (Copyright © 1981 by Edith Tagrin.)

After the initial cordotomy lesion has been made, the patient may be awakened to test the extent of the resulting analgesia as well as the integrity of motor function. Before the patient is awakened, lidocaine should be injected profusely into the paraspinal muscles. When the patient wakes, pain may originate from traction on a dorsal root. This can be blocked with lidocaine or cocaine.

With the patient awake, it is advisable to test for deep visceral pain as well as for pinprick perception. This is especially important for patients in whom a significant portion of disease lies in deep structures of the pelvis. Both legs should also be tested for motor strength because the pyramidal tracts may not be crossed, in which case the contralateral limbs may be supplied by the spinal tract in the anterior medial quadrant with the lesion.

If the level of analgesia is not cephalad enough, the lesion should be extended medially and anteriorly to include fibers adjacent to the anterior midline septum. A lesion resulting in a level of analgesia that is not sufficiently caudal (e.g., sparing the perineum and sacral distribution) should be extended closer to the equator and thus closer to the crossed CST. The initial cordotomy lesion can be further extended with the patient awake because transection of the

STT is not perceived as a painful stimulus. This arrangement permits functional monitoring of the motor system as well while the lesion is being extended.

Upon achievement of a satisfactory distribution of analgesia, the patient is reanesthetized for closure. The Weck clips on the dentate are cut free, the cord is allowed to return to normal position, and the wound is closed.

Bilateral Cordotomy Procedure

Bilateral high cervical cordotomies are not performed because of the high risk of sleep apnea and other complications. If bilateral analgesia is necessary, a percutaneous or open cordotomy can be performed unilaterally at C2 or C3, with a contralateral cordotomy at C5–C6 performed by the posterior or anterior approach through the C5–C6 disc space. Usually, when contralateral analgesia at a high level is not mandatory, a percutaneous cordotomy is performed at C2 on one side followed by a contralateral open thoracic cordotomy at T2 or T3.

When a lower bilateral level of analgesia is satisfactory, a bilateral operation should be performed in one stage in the upper thoracic region, with one lesion at T2 and the other contralateral at T4. For this operation, the laminae

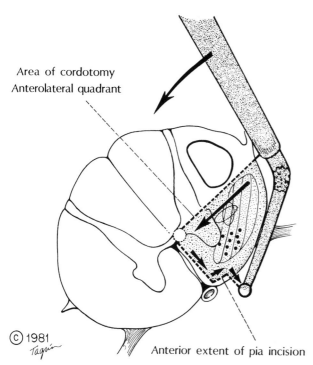

Area of cordotomy
Anterolateral quadrant

© 1981
Tagrin

Anterior extent of pia incision

FIGURE 111-7 The tip of the Jacobsen ball has been brought 90 degrees anteriorly, palpating the midline septum until the pia on the anterior aspect of the cord is felt. The ball is then drawn laterally along the pia until it exits from the cord at the medial-most extent of the pial incision previously made with the microscissors. (Copyright © 1981 by Edith Tagrin.)

at T2 and T4 are each removed as well as the spinous process of T3. The rest of the procedure is as described for unilateral cordotomy. If a previous unilateral cordotomy has been performed at T3 and it later becomes evident that a contralateral lesion is indicated, the second lesion can be made at the lower margin of T1 as early as 5 to 7 days postoperatively.

Postoperative Precautions

Sleep Apnea

After C2–C3 cordotomies, the patient should be placed in the intensive care recovery room, especially because of the danger of sleep apnea. When sent back to the floor, the patient should be monitored continuously with an apnea alarm, and tidal volume should be checked periodically. The nursing staff must be alert to the possible need for prompt respiratory assistance. The potential for sleep apnea may persist for a week postoperatively, after which these precautions can be relaxed. If sleep apnea occurs after a unilateral cervical cordotomy, the patient virtually always recovers after an adequate period of assisted support.

Weakness

At the first sign of postoperative motor weakness, we administer high-dose steroids and maintain the blood pressure, if necessary, to prevent any hypotension.

Hypotension

When bilateral lesions are made, the blood pressure must be monitored as the patient begins to mobilize—raising the

head off the bed, dangling the feet, and walking. Toe-to-groin woven elastic bandage wraps can be used, along with fluid loading and antihypotensive drugs as needed. The decrease in blood pressure—even with bilateral lesions—as well as orthostatic hypotension gradually clears and is a problem only if unrecognized. A single episode of severe hypotension may compromise the blood supply significantly, particularly that to the upper thoracic cord. This ischemia may extend the lesion to the adjacent CST.

Urinary Retention

If a Foley catheter has been placed before a bilateral procedure, a cystometrogram should be obtained several days postoperatively before the catheter is removed.

Operative Results

The incidence of postoperative pain relief in 3 months varies from 54% to 90%, with the average being 75%.[1,14–18] After 18 months, the rate of relief falls to approximately 50%, where it remains for several years. It is generally agreed that the incidence of pain relief is greater in those patients with postoperative paresis and sphincter disturbance, suggesting a direct relation between the degree of pain relief and the extent of the lesion.

A T3 cordotomy, according to Taren and colleagues,[19] should be expected to produce a postoperative sensory level up to T4–T5, including postoperative loss of superficial pain, temperature, deep pain, visceral pain, and itch. The permanent level, however, usually settles at T7 to T10. Grant and Wood[20] report an average permanent level of analgesia or hypalgesia only up to T5 after cervical cordotomy.

In some of our cases, satisfactory and persisting relief of pain is achieved without superficial cutaneous analgesia. This dissociation between pain relief and cutaneous analgesia is common in midline myelotomies and characterizes certain thalamic lesions. Although the neurophysiologic explanation is not clear for the spinal cord, we propose that two fiber systems are involved: in addition to the STT carrying acute pain perception, there also may be a midline multineuronal ascending system in the central gray matter of the spinal cord. This latter system may modulate the ability to suppress chronic pain.

Operative Failures and Recurrence of Pain

Operative Failures

The most common causes of failure to achieve satisfactory analgesia after cordotomy are as follows:

1. Failure to cut close enough to the equator of the cord, sparing the sacral representation in the spinal cord.
2. Failure to cut deep in the anterior quadrant, producing a satisfactory level of cutaneous analgesia without adequate relief of deep and visceral pain. Accordingly, to make sure the deep fibers carrying deep somatic visceral pain have been severed, one should test these fibers intraoperatively with wake-up anesthesia. A satisfactory test for visceral pain is inflation of a Foley balloon within the bladder.

3. Insufficient extension of the lesion anteriorly and medially, resulting in a level of analgesia many segments below the level of the cordotomy.
4. Failure to cut the anterior quadrant decisively, producing an incomplete lesion with limited and patchy analgesia.
5. Performing a unilateral cordotomy when a bilateral procedure was indicated.
6. Subsequent spread of the cancer above the level of analgesia. If such spread is anticipated, the initial cordotomy should be higher.
7. Anatomic variability of the spinal cord, resulting in an unsatisfactory lesion.

Recurrence of Pain with Fading of Analgesia

If the level of analgesia falls and islands of recovered nociception occur within a few days postoperatively, the spinothalamic fibers in the periphery of the lesion have probably been bruised but not severed. The first postoperative drop in analgesic level may be caused by recovery from direct injury by the operation, and the drop during the first week may be the result of recovery from edema and swelling. This process may explain the two- to five-segment drop in the analgesic level during the first 2 postoperative weeks.

In an excellent review of long-term follow-up of patients undergoing cordotomy, Grant and Wood[20] found that both islands and large areas of sensation returned even within a few months. It is conceivable that this recovery of pain perception is caused by collateral regeneration of new synaptic terminals[5] in short-chain internuncial neurons taking over the previous function of the long STT. White[21] found that 4 years after cordotomy, 54% of patients who had undergone cordotomy had recovered pain perception; subsequent higher anterolateral cordotomies generally proved unsuccessful in reinstituting analgesia.

In addition to the hypothesis of collateral sprouting, long-term fading of postcordotomy analgesia may be explained by altered synaptic and membrane excitability in preexisting, potentially alternative nociceptive pathways. Indeed, in addition to first-order neurons ascending to medullary nuclei from the posterior columns, other neurons send efferent projections from the segmental gray matter. These may be partially responsible for conducting impulses concerned with the abnormal reference of pain. Partial support for this alternative pathway lies in the fact that stimulation of the dorsal column during midline myelotomy is often reported as painful by the awake patient.

Another hypothesis explaining the return of pain perception is that intrasegmental polysynaptic complexes form from collaterals of the crossing STT fibers. These may separate near the midline from the crossing STT fibers ascending in the spinal periaqueductal central gray matter to the reticular formation. Support for this hypothesis lies in the fact that relief of pain is experienced after midline commissural myelotomy or central myelotomy often not associated with cutaneous analgesia.

Accordingly, we think that postcordotomy recovery of pain perception is less probably caused by spinal cord or thalamic axonal sprouting than by altered transsynaptic excitability in preexisting, potentially alternative nociceptive pathways.

Operative Complications

Mortality

The mortality rate in published series varies from 3% to 21%.[1,14–16] It is higher for unilateral cordotomies in the cervical region involving malignant disease and still higher for bilateral cervical cordotomies. The postoperative mortality clearly is higher in cancer patients than in patients with benign disease.

Respiratory Complications

Some authors indicate that respiratory complications are the most serious concern in high cervical cordotomies. In the past, sleep apnea has been a common cause of death. Voluntary control of respiration is mediated by the CST, but subconscious ipsilateral respiratory movements are controlled by pathways descending deep in the centrolateral part of the spinal cord. This descending unilateral respiratory pathway is called the ventrolateral reticulospinal tract. Its fibers are, at least in part, intermingled with the fibers of the lateral STT (see Fig. 111-1). Unilateral destruction of this pathway results in little functional respiratory loss unless contralateral respiratory function is poor. Accordingly, even for unilateral C2–C3 cordotomies, the function of the contralateral diaphragm should be evaluated preoperatively. Bilateral lesions clearly produce a high incidence of sleep apnea and death.

Postcordotomy Hypotension

Intraoperatively, there may be a sudden drop in blood pressure immediately after a cordotomy lesion has been made. Sindou (personal communication, 1981) makes the point that such a drop in pressure signifies that the lesions have been made deep enough and far enough dorsally to ensure transection of the fibers carrying visceral pain. In unilateral thoracic cordotomies, this drop is moderate and evanescent. The blood pressure usually returns to normal level by the end of wound closure. With bilateral lesions, the drop may be marked and protracted, lasting well into the postoperative period.

Blood pressure is maintained by spinal sympathetic pathways that descend partially intermingled with the ascending STT (see Fig. 111-1). Stimulation of these fibers elevates the blood pressure and the pressure within the bladder.[22] Unlike respiratory complications, blood pressure drop is seldom a cause of death or serious morbidity unless the patient is in a sitting position when the drop occurs.

As noted, hypotension in the postoperative period may produce ischemia, especially in the thoracic region, thus enlarging the surgical lesion and causing a new motor deficit.

Motor Weakness

Assuming that the CST has a relatively normal anatomy, the two principal causes of ipsilateral motor weakness after cordotomy are a lesion extending too far posteriorly, which damages the crossed CST, and an extension too far anteromedially, which damages the anterior spinal artery with resulting ischemia. A third possible mechanism is borderline ischemia accentuated by intraoperative or postoperative hypotension. That the upper thoracic cord is especially susceptible to such ischemic damage may explain why there is a higher incidence of paresis after thoracic cordotomy than after the cervical procedure.

The literature indicates that the incidence of paresis or paralysis after unilateral cordotomy varies from 0% to 11%.[15,16,23] Whereas the incidence after bilateral cordotomies can run as high as 24% (see reference 16). The incidence of permanent motor deficits is clearly much higher in bilateral lesions. We believe that the implementation of stimulation techniques as described decreases the incidence of paresis.

Bladder Dysfunction

Urinary bladder dysfunction after cordotomy is common. After unilateral cordotomy, this complication is relatively uncommon (0 to 8%).[1,15,23] The disturbance usually lasts only a few days and responds well to medical management. After bilateral cordotomies, either cervical or thoracic, the incidence of urinary dysfunction is much higher and its duration is often permanent.

When a cordotomy is done for sacral pain, sphincter disturbances are particularly likely. Nathan and Smith,[24,25] having studied the physiology of micturition and defecation, concluded that both the descending and the ascending fibers responding to distention and the desire to relax sphincters are assembled in a narrow band almost crossing the equator of the cord opposite the central canal. Figure 111-1 clearly shows the high risk of bowel and bladder disturbance if a bilateral cordotomy is performed for sacral pain with the incision made close to the equator.

Sexual Dysfunction

Sweet[9] claims that the fibers involved in sexual sensation and function lie so close to those for pain (see Fig. 111-1) that sexual function is almost always impaired after unilateral cordotomy and is permanently impaired after bilateral cordotomy. Taren and colleagues[19] report that after section of the anterolateral tracts, erection and ejaculation may still occur but sexual sensation at the moment of orgasm is lost. Sexual potency does not seem to be disturbed with unilateral cordotomy but is almost always lost after the bilateral procedure.

Dysesthesias

The abnormal sensations that may arise immediately after cordotomy, or as long as months after the operation, are sometimes divided into two groups: referred sensations and dysesthesias. Postoperatively, soreness of the skin and pain with girdle distribution may develop at or above the level of the lesion. This usually persists only for a few weeks and may be related to undue traction of the dorsal roots when the cord was rotated.

Referred sensations may be elicited by stimulation within the analgesic area in approximately 25% of patients. These sensations may be felt by the patient as noxious; they are poorly localized and often referred contralaterally. After bilateral cordotomy, the sensations may be referred to an area above the level of analgesia as well as to areas of escape within the analgesic zone.

More serious are the severe, constant, painful dysesthesias referred to levels below the cordotomy. Their onset is usually delayed, occurring with increasing frequency as the postoperative period lengthens. Postcordotomy dysesthesias become a serious problem in approximately 6% of patients after 2 to 3 years. As noted, cordotomy at a higher level is not effective.

MEDULLARY TRACTOTOMY

Anatomic Basis

The primary nociceptive afferents from cranial nerves V, VII, IX, and X all descend in the medulla adjacent to each other, forming the descending cranial nociceptive tract (DCNT). Nature, apparently in a degree of consideration for patients in pain and unparalleled in its design of the central nervous system, permits the neurosurgeon to interrupt virtually all orofacial primary nociceptive afferents by means of a single small ipsilateral lesion in the lateral dorsal medulla. Orofacial nociceptive cranial afferents, whether they enter via cranial nerves V, VII, IX, or X, all descend in a compact tract, traveling caudally in the dorsolateral aspect of the medulla. At the level of the obex, this tract is bounded dorsally by the nucleus cuneatus and ventrally by the contralateral ascending STT. The most superficial fibers of the tract, however, do not lie on the surface of the brain stem but are covered by the external arcuate fibers. (These fibers, important for coordination, arise from cells in the nucleus cuneatus accessorius and project to the cerebellum.)

The DCNT is 2 to 2.5 mm deep, its ventral margin being formed by the spinal trigeminal nucleus caudalis. In addition, the topographic localization of the fibers within the tract is distinct: descending in the most ventral portion of the descending trigeminal tract are fibers from the first trigeminal division. Immediately ventral to these fibers are the exiting motor fibers of cranial nerve XI. In turn, just ventral to these exiting motor fibers of cranial nerve XI, are the ascending fibers of the contralateral STT. Dorsal to the descending nociceptive fibers of the first trigeminal division are the fibers from the second trigeminal division, with the fibers from the third trigeminal division next. In turn, just dorsal to these nociceptive fibers of the trigeminal third division, are the primary nociceptive fibers from cranial nerve VII's nervus intermedius and, most dorsally, the descending nociceptive fibers of nerves IX and X. Finally, just dorsal to the descending nociceptive fibers of nerve X, are the ascending ipsilateral proprioceptive fibers immediately next to the nucleus cuneatus.

Accordingly, a surgical lesion made from the dorsal limit of the ascending contralateral STT (i.e., at the line demarcated by the exiting motor rootlets of cranial nerve XI) dorsally to the ventral limit of nucleus cuneatus transects first the nociceptive fibers from V1, followed by those from V2, V3, VII, IX, and X. If the lesion extends too far ventrally it will transect fibers from the contralateral STT; if too far dorsally, it will transect fibers entering the nucleus cuneatus.[1] In order to sever all the fibers from each nerve, one must extend the lesion to a depth of 3 to 3.5 mm. Making such a lesion necessarily transects the overlying external arcuate fibers as well. Interrupting these fibers accounts for the postoperative truncal and gait ataxia.

Rowbotham, in 1938, was the first to take advantage of this configuration of the descending trigeminal nociceptive tract by successfully performing a trigeminal medullary tractotomy in a patient suffering from severe migrainous neuralgia involving the distribution of the first trigeminal division. It was not until 1942, however, that, on the basis of clinical observations and interpretations of Cajal's neuroanatomic drawings, Sweet recognized that the spinal descending nociceptive tract included not only nociceptive fibers descending from the trigeminal nerve but nociceptive fibers descending from the seventh nervus intermedius and nerves IX and X. On the basis of these observations, Sweet demonstrated in 1945 that a single, slightly larger lesion in the dorsolateral medulla could interrupt virtually all primary nociceptive fibers from ipsilateral orofacial regions.

This medullary tractotomy of the DCNT, made dorsal to the exiting roots of nerve XI, should be distinguished from a medullary tractotomy of the contralateral ascending STT, made just ventral to the exiting roots of nerve XI. This operation, first performed by J. C. White, can be used to obtain contralateral analgesia to a dermatomal level as high as C2. Such a medullary tractotomy appears to be particularly appropriate for patients suffering from cancer invading the contralateral brachial plexus.

Indications

Even with the advent of intraventricular morphine, we think there continues to be an occasional patient in whom a unilateral lesion of the DCNT is the best available treatment. In our experience, these patients are most likely to be suffering from a slow-growing, indolent cancer affecting only one side of the face and oropharynx. Rarely, a patient suffers from extremely severe periodic migrainous neuralgia that is unresponsive to conservative regimens and for which retrogasserian trigeminal rhizotomy has failed. In these patients suffering from severe periodic migrainous neuralgia, occasionally an avulsion of the greater and lesser superficial petrosal nerve has also already been made, especially in patients with marked autonomic changes: tearing, unilateral hyperhidrosis, hemicranial flush, and nasal mucosal engorgement.

Another possible operation for patients suffering from periodic migrainous neuralgia has been to section the primary nociceptive afferents in the twelfth nervus intermedius as well as the nociceptive fibers entering nerve IX and the rostral rootlets of nerve X. As shown by Bischoff's meticulous microdissections, however, all pain fibers entering the seventh to eighth nerve root entry zone are, in fact, not confined to the discrete nervus intermedius. Not only may afferent nociceptive fibers course among the efferent motor fibers of nerve VII, but they may travel within the afferents of the body of nerve VIII. Accordingly, in patients with severe, acute disseminated periodic migrainous neuralgia, a lesion of the DCNT may be indicated. Patients with periodic migrainous neuralgia whose symptoms are confined to V1 and V2, as is typically the case, and whose neuralgia is unresponsive to caffeine-ergotamine therapy and all other medical regimens are almost certainly candidates first for a percutaneous retrogasserian trigeminal rhizotomy. Therefore, it is only patients who experience a recrudescence of pain after this initial surgical procedure or spread of pain to nontrigeminal distributions who may be candidates for lesions of the DCNT.

An advantage of a DCNT tractotomy over a rhizotomy of V1 and V2 is that the tractotomy produces analgesia without anesthesia and, invariably, when made at the rostrocaudal level of the obex, preserves corneal sensation. Because the midline portion of the dura and the posterior fossa is innervated by afferent pain fibers entering the seventh to eighth nerve complex, and nerves IX and X, it is also an advantage of the tractotomy to denervate these structures in patients with periodic migrainous neuralgia referred to the deep occipital region.

Operative Procedure

Instrumentation

The only special instrument used, in addition to the standard microneurosurgical array, is the Jacobsen ball dissector described previously for use in open cordotomy. If the patient is awake, the tip of the ball can be stimulated to determine physiologically when the lesion has extended ventrally past V1 fibers into the fibers of the contralateral STT, thus helping to determine the ventral limit of the V1 descending pain fibers. Similarly, the tip of the Jacobsen ball may be used to record evoked responses obtained by stimulating the dorsal column afferents from the median nerve. The sudden appearance of large evoked responses obtained by median nerve stimulation should indicate the approximation of the tip of the Jacobsen ball to the ascending dorsal fibers in the nucleus cuneatus, because the lesion is extended rostrally from V3 through VII, IX, and X fibers reaching the nucleus cuneatus.

Anesthesia

One can use either sustained general anesthesia or wake-up anesthesia. Satisfactory wake-up anesthesia, however, may be difficult after a prolonged exposure of the posterior fossa, especially when this is combined with a C1–C2 laminectomy in patients in whom a dorsal rhizotomy of C1 and C2 is also desired. Accordingly, Sweet,[9] on several occasions, has performed the suboccipital and upper cervical exposure in one operation and then performed a second stage in which the wound was merely reopened and the dura opened; the patient was promptly awakened after the initial lesion in the DCNT was made. With this technique, the patient may be fully satisfactorily awakened and extubated for detailed sensory testing. The patient is then put back to sleep briefly using intravenous methohexital sodium to make any required enlargement of the lesion. In our last two cases, however, both with extremely severe periodic migrainous neuralgia, I have preferred to use sustained general anesthesia and the techniques described here to obtain a fully satisfactory DCNT tractotomy.

Patient Position and Operative Technique

The patient is placed in a position halfway between lateral and prone with the head turned 45 degrees to the floor. The side of the anticipated tractotomy is placed upward (i.e., for a right-sided lesion). The patient is placed with the left shoulder on the table and the nose turned down to the left toward the floor. The head of the bed is elevated 20 to 30 degrees and the patient's head flexed forward, bringing the chin to within two fingerbreadths of the sternum.

The head is held in this position with a three-point skeletal fixation headrest.

A vertical midline incision is made from the low occipital region down to the upper cervical region. The incision is extended caudally in patients in whom a concomitant dorsal rhizotomy of C1, C2, and C3 is planned. A craniectomy in the middle and low suboccipital region is made in the midline and slightly more to the side of the lesion. If only a tractotomy is planned, laminectomy of C1 is not necessary. The dura is opened with an incision begun over the cerebellum and cerebellar tonsil on the side of the anticipated lesion. The incision is then carried down to the midline at the cervicomedullary junction and caudally at least to the level of C1—farther if rhizotomy is planned.

The microscope is then brought into the field and angled rostrally toward the inferior limit of the fourth ventricle. Retractors are placed on either side and are used to retract the cerebellar tonsils dorsolaterally until the obex is seen directly. The vermis does not have to be split. The cerebellar tonsil is then retracted further on the side of the anticipated lesion. (As noted, this is the cerebellar tonsil on the upper side, in that the patient has been positioned so that the side of the lesion is upward.)

A lesion of the DCNT may be made as far as 10 mm rostral to the obex, as advocated by Kunc, or at 2 mm below the obex, as we advocate. The more rostral tractotomy tends to make a slightly denser lesion for persons with severe cancer pain; however, it also produces more incoordination and ataxia. (The more rostral lesion interrupts more nociceptive fibers from cranial nerves VII, IX, and X but also transects more external arcuate fibers.) Using microsurgical techniques, we have been satisfied with the density of our lesions made 2 mm caudal to the obex.

The lesion is made in a plane transverse to the brain stem on the lateral dorsal side of the medulla, extending ventrally and dorsally. The line of demarcation between the most ventral descending fibers of V1 and the most dorsal fibers of the contralateral STT is clearly defined on the surface of the medulla by the point of exit of the roots of cranial nerve XI. Accordingly, the cerebellar tip should be retracted so as to visualize at least one emerging rootlet of nerve XI rostral and another rootlet caudal to the anticipated transverse level of the lesion. These may be stimulated, even in the asleep patient, to be sure they represent motor fibers of nerve XI. A line is drawn between these two exiting rootlets, and that line marks the ventral extent of the lesion. Dorsally, the distinct prominences of the nucleus gracilis, adjacent to the obex, and farther laterally of the nucleus cuneatus can be seen. The lateral extent of the surface presentation of the eminence of the nucleus cuneatus should mark the dorsomedial extent of the projected incision. Any small surface blood vessels can be teased to either side of the projected incision or gently cauterized.

The incision is begun by using the No. 11 blade to make a very small opening in the pia-arachnoid at the lateral extent of the eminence of the nucleus cuneatus. The microsurgical scissors are then used to incise the pia-arachnoid, going laterally and anteriorly until the incision reaches the line drawn between the two exiting rootlets of nerve XI. At this point, if the patient has been awakened, the nerves to be cut may be stimulated by mechanical pressure, as characterizes the sensitivity of these primary nociceptive afferents.

Both Kunc and Sweet have used needles or sharp nerve hooks to stimulate either the fibers of the DCNT or the proprioceptive fibers ascending to the nucleus cuneatus. The patient may refer the sensations to a very focal area, permitting discrimination among V1, V2, and V3 descending fibers. When the fibers of the nucleus cuneatus are stimulated mechanically, sensations are referred to the ipsilateral arm, neck, and back of the head. (Proprioceptive fibers from the lower portions of the body ascend to the nucleus gracilis.)

If the patient is awake, the lesion is extended ventrally until there is some nociceptive sensory loss in the contralateral distal lower extremity. The lesion is extended dorsomedially until there is some reference of sensation to the ipsilateral dorsal columns. The lesion should be made to a depth of only 3 mm. This is done in the current technique by putting a small piece of bone wax 3 mm up the shaft of the Jacobsen ball and then inserting the instrument only to that depth dorsally. As in the anterior quadrant of the spinal cord, there is little resistance even to the relatively blunt tip of the Jacobsen ball. Similarly, scarcely any bleeding occurs with this complete DCNT tractotomy. We recommend that the lesion extend ventrally at least partially into the contralateral STT and dorsally into the ascending proprioceptive fibers to enhance the probability of a complete lasting lesion of the DCNT, because the initial lesion tends to fade in the postoperative period.

Currently, as mentioned, we are relying on these microsurgical techniques to make the tractotomy lesion with the patient under sustained general anesthesia. Additional guidance should be available in the future through advanced electrophysiologic techniques.

A medullary tractotomy of the contralateral ascending STT uses the same position and exposure, although the incision begins just ventral to the exiting rootlets of nerve XI and extends more ventrally.[1,26]

Complications, Side Effects, Results, and Thoughts for the Future

Clearly, this DCNT tractotomy is a major operative procedure carrying mortality and morbidity greater than those of percutaneous trigeminal rhizotomy or percutaneous glossopharyngeal rhizotomy. The worst side effect is the inevitable degree of difficulty in walking produced by this lesion. In the immediate postoperative period, patients almost invariably suffer from incoordination and lateral pulsion. As noted, this is less the case for lesions made caudal to the level of the obex. Usually by 1 month after the operation, the degree of incoordination has cleared sufficiently for patients in most occupations to have normal function. Dysesthesias as occur with spinal lesions of the STT have not been a consistent problem with lesions of the DCNT.

The degree of pain relief tends to be commensurate with the extent of the analgesia produced by the lesion. Thus, lesions producing lasting analgesia throughout the distribution of the cranial nerves have a high probability of relieving pain of either cancerous or migrainous origin. Including a dorsal rhizotomy of C1, C2, and C3 improves results in patients whose migrainous neuralgia is not confined to orofacial regions. It is of interest that the pain of periodic migrainous neuralgia is eliminated by the DCNT tractotomy, whereas the autonomic symptoms, which are characteristic of periodic migrainous neuralgia, may often persist. In several of our patients with extremely severe periodic migrainous neuralgia who were suicidal despite intensive medical and psychiatric therapy and in whom radiofrequency failed, trigeminal lesions have been markedly relieved by a DCNT tractotomy. As noted, orofacial cutaneous and mucosal and corneal touch sensation is functionally preserved.

REFERENCES

1. White JC, Sweet WH: Pain and the Neurosurgeon. Springfield, IL: Charles C Thomas, 1969, pp 69, 629.
2. Hitchcock ER: Stereotactic myelotomy. Proc R Soc Med 67:771, 1964.
3. Hitchcock ER: Stereotactic cervical myelotomy. J Neurol Neurosurg Psychiatry 33:224, 1970.
4. Schvarcz JR: Stereotactic extralemniscal myelotomy. J Neurol Neurosurg Psychiatry 39:53, 1976.
5. Schvarcz JR: Functional exploration of the spinomedullary junction. Acta Neurochir (Wien) 24 (Suppl):179, 1977.
6. Schvarcz JR: Spinal cord stereotactic techniques: Trigeminal nucleotomy and extralemniscal myelotomy. Appl Neurophysiol 41:99, 1978.
7. Poletti CE, Cohen AM, Todd DP, et al: Clinical pain relieved by long-term epidural morphine: Two case reports with permanent indwelling systems for self-administration. J Neurosurg 55:581, 1981.
8. Yakovlev PL, Rakic P: Patterns of decussation of bulbar pyramidal tracts on two sides of the spinal cord. Trans Am Neurol Assoc 91:366, 1966.
9. Sweet WH: Recent observations pertinent to improving anterolateral cordotomy. Clin Neurosurg 23:80, 1976.
10. Macon JB, Poletti CE: Conducted somatosensory evoked potentials during spinal surgery. 1: Technical aspects. J Neurosurg 57:354, 1982.
11. Cowie RA, Hitchcock ER: The late results of anterolateral cordotomy for pain relief. Acta Neurochir (Wien) 64:39, 1982.
12. Granert VP, Sunder-Plassmann MS: Ergebnisse der zerikalen Chordotomie mit und ohne Rhizotomie bei konservitiv Therapie resistenten Schmerzen im Schulter-Arm Bereich. Zentralbl Neurochir 46:267, 1985.
13. Hardy D, LeClereq TA, Mercky F: Microsurgical selective cordotomy by the anterior approach. In Handa H (ed): Microsurgery: International Symposium on Microsurgery. Baltimore: University Park Press, 1973.
14. Brihaye J, Retif J: Comparison of the results obtained by anterolateral cordotomy at the dorsal level and at the cervical level. Neurochirurgie 7:258, 1961.
15. Diemath HE, Heppner F, Walker AE: Anterolateral cordotomy for relief of pain. Postgrad Med J 29:485, 1961.
16. Nathan PW: Results of anterolateral cordotomy for pain in cancer. J Neurol Neurosurg Psychiatry 26:353, 1963.
17. Dautenhahn D, Reynolds A, Darby R, et al: Thoracic epidural analgesia for open cordotomy. Anesth Analg 63:1036, 1984.
18. Jack T, Lloyd J: Long-term efficacy of surgical cordotomy in intractable nonmalignant pain. Ann R Coll Surg Engl 97:102, 1983.
19. Taren DA, Kahn EA, Humphrey T: The surgery of pain. In Kahn EA, Crosby EC, Schneider RC, et al (eds): Correlative Neurosurgery. Springfield, IL: Charles C Thomas, 1969.
20. Grant FC, Wood FA: Experiences with cordotomy. Clin Neurosurg 5:38, 1957.
21. White JC: Anterolateral cordotomy: Its effectiveness in relieving pain of nonmalignant disease. Neurochirurgica 6:83, 1963.
22. Kerr FW, Alexander S: Descending autonomic pathways in the spinal cord. Arch Neurol 10:249, 1964.
23. McKissock W: Second International Congress of Neurological Surgeons: International Congress Series No. 36 E27. Amsterdam: Excerpta Medica, 1961.
24. Nathan PW, Smith MC: Spinal pathways subserving defecation and sensation from the lower bowel. J Neurol Neurosurg Psychiatry 16:245, 1953.
25. Nathan PW, Smith MC: The centrifugal pathway for micturition within the spinal cord. J Neurol Neurosurg Psychiatry 21:177, 1958.
26. Poletti CE, Ojemann RG: Stereo Atlas of Operative Microneurosurgery. Reel 19, View 3, 1985, pp 264–265.

112 Microsurgical DREZotomy

MARC P. SINDOU

In the 1960s, a large number of anatomic and physiologic investigations of the spinal cord drew attention to the dorsal root entry zone (DREZ) as the first level of modulation for pain sensation.[1] These studies convinced the author to consider the DREZ as a possible target for pain surgery and, in 1972, to undertake anatomic studies and preliminary surgical trials in humans to determine whether a destructive procedure at this level was feasible and effective.[2]

The first DREZ operation was performed in March 1972 at the Neurological Institute Pierre Wertheimer in Lyon, France, on a patient with Pancoast's syndrome; microsurgical techniques were used to create a destructive lesion in the ventrolateral region of the DREZ. In that same year, several other patients with cancer pain underwent DREZ lesions. These initial results were encouraging, and within the next 2 years, the procedure was used in patients with neuropathic pain syndromes associated with paraplegia in December 1972, amputation in July 1973, and brachial plexus avulsion in January 1974.

RATIONALE

By definition, the DREZ is an entity that includes the central portion of the dorsal rootlet, Lissauer's tract, and layers I to V of the dorsal horn of the spinal cord where the afferent fibers synapse with the cells of the sensory pathways, especially the spinoreticulothalamic tract[2] (Fig. 112-1).

Dorsal Rootlets

Depending on the level of the spinal cord, each dorsal root divides into 4 to 10 rootlets that are 0.25 to 1.5 mm in diameter. Each rootlet is a distinct anatomic/functional entity, that is, a root in miniature. Anatomic studies[2,3] revealed a spatial segregation of afferent fibers in the DREZ according to their sizes and destinations (Figs. 112-2 and 112-3), and because of this, the lateral regrouping of the fine fibers allows them to be preferentially interrupted without destruction of the large fibers.

Whether all nociceptive fibers reach the spinal cord through the dorsal roots is unclear. Anatomic and electrophysiologic studies in animals showed that approximately 30% of the fibers in the ventral roots were afferent C axons originating from the dorsal root ganglion cells and projecting into the dorsal horn. These findings, which challenge the Bell-Magendie law, have been clarified. Most (but not all) of the central root afferents do not enter the cord through the lamina cribrosa of the ventral root but instead make a U turn to reach the dorsal horn via the dorsal root.[4]

Lissauer's Tract

Lissauer's tract is situated dorsolateral to the dorsal horn and comprises (1) a medial part, which the small afferents enter and where they trifurcate to reach the dorsal horn, either directly or through a two-metamere ascending or descending pathway, and (2) a lateral part, through which a large number of longitudinal endogenous propriospinal fibers interconnect different levels of the substantia gelatinosa. Lissauer's tract plays an important role in the intersegmental modulation of the nociceptive afferents.[5] Its medial part transmits the excitatory effects of each dorsal root to the adjacent segments, and its lateral part conveys the inhibitory influences of the substantia gelatinosa into the neighboring metameres.[6] Selective destruction of the medial part of Lissauer's tract's should cause a reduction in the regional excitability of the nociceptive afferents.

Dorsal Horn

Most of the fine nociceptive afferents enter the dorsal horn through the medial part of Lissauer's tract and the dorsal

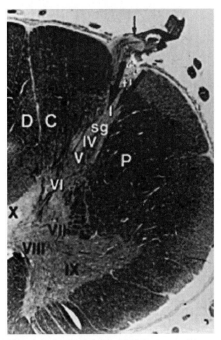

FIGURE 112-1 Rexed's lamination (I to IX). Transverse hemisection of the spinal cord (at the lower cervical level) with myelin stained by Luxol-fuschine shows the myelinated rootlet afferents that reach the dorsal column. DC, dorsal column; P, pyramidal tract; sg, substantia gelatinosa; tl, Lissauer's tract. The *small arrow* designates the pial ring of the dorsal rootlet (diameter, 1 mm). The *large arrows* show the MDT target.

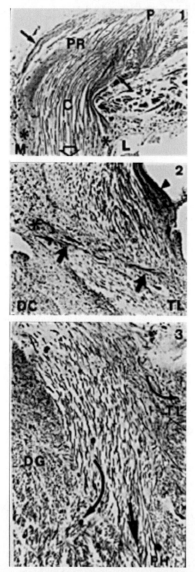

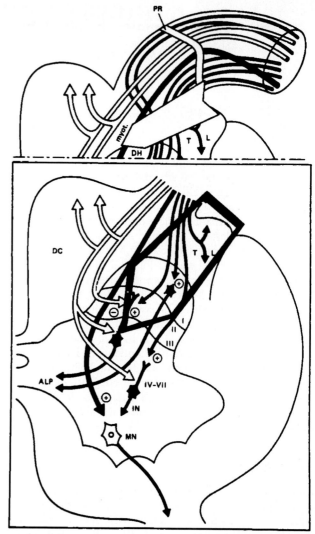

FIGURE 112-2 Course of nerve fibers at the dorsal root entry zone (DREZ) in humans. The diameter of the cervical rootlets chosen as examples is 1 mm. Axons are stained by the Bodian method. *1,* Longitudinal section before entry into the spinal cord. At the peripheral segment (P), the large and small fibers have no particular organization. Just before the pial ring (PR), the small fibers reach the rootlet surface (*arrows*), mainly in the lateral region (L). In the central segment (C), the small fibers are arranged in two bundles (*asterisks*) located on either side of the large fibers. *2,* Longitudinal section at the entry into the spinal cord. The large fibers constitute the center of the rootlet and run toward the dorsal column (DC). The small fibers form two bundles. One is lateral (*triangle*); the other is medial (*asterisk*). The medial portion runs obliquely across the rootlet (*arrows*) to reach Lissauer's tract (TL). Thus, most of the small fibers are regrouped at the lateral region of the DREZ. *3,* Longitudinal section of the rootlet with its afferent endings in the spinal cord. The large lemniscal fibers (*thick curved arrow*) are grouped medially to enter the dorsal column (DC). The large myotatic fibers (*straight arrow*) penetrate deeper into the posterior horn (PH) to reach the ventral horn. The small nociceptive fibers (*thin curved arrow*) are regrouped laterally to enter TL. (From Sindou M: Étude de la jonction radiculomédullaire postérieure: La radicellotomie postérieure sélective dans la chirurgie de la douleur. M.D. Thesis, Université Claude-Bernard, Lyon, 1972.)

FIGURE 112-3 Schematic representation of the dorsal root entry zone (DREZ) area and the target of microsurgical DREZotomy (MDT). *Upper part:* Each rootlet can be divided (owing to the transition of its glial support) into a peripheral segment and a central segment. The transition between the two segments is at the pial ring (PR), which is located approximately 1 mm outside the penetration of the rootlet into the dorsolateral sulcus. Peripherally, the fibers are mixed together. As they approach the PR, the fine fibers (considered nociceptive) more toward the rootlet surfaces. In the central segment, they group in the ventrolateral portion of the DREZ and enter the dorsal horn (DH) through Lissauer's tract (TL). The large myotatic fibers (myot.) are situated in the middle of the DREZ, whereas the large lemniscal fibers are located dorsomedially. *Lower part:* Schematic data on DH circuitry. Note the monosynaptic excitatory arc reflex, the lemniscal influence on a DH cell and an interneuron (IN), the fine fiber excitatory input onto DH cells, and the IN, the origins in layer I and IV to VII of the anterolateral pathways (ALP), and the projection of the IN onto the motor neuron (MN). DC, dorsal column. Rexed's laminae are marked from I to VI. The MDT (*arrowhead*) cuts most of the fine and myotatic fibers and enters the medial (excitatory) portion of the LT and the apex of the DH. It should preserve most lemniscal presynaptic fibers, the lateral (inhibitory) portion of TL, and most of the DH. (From Sindou M: Étude de la jonction radiculomédullaire postérieure: La radicellotomie postérieure sélective dans la chirurgie de la douleur. M.D. Thesis, Université Claude-Bernard, Lyon, 1972.)

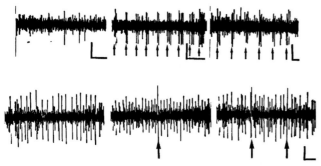

FIGURE 112-4 Dorsal horn microelectrode recordings in humans. The electrode was a floating tungsten-glass microelectrode, implanted intraoperatively by free-hand under the operative microscope approximately 5 mm in depth (i.e., in laminae IV to VI). *Upper trace:* Normal activity. Recordings in a nondeafferented dorsal horn at the lumbosacral level (patient with spasticity). *Left:* Almost no spontaneous activity (three spikes at random). *Middle:* Spike burst discharges (*arrows*) evoked by regular light tactile stimulation of the corresponding dermatome. *Right,* Spike burst discharges evoked by electrical stimulation of the corresponding peripheral nerve. *Lower trace,* Deafferentation hyperactivity. Recordings in the L5 cord segment of a patient with pain due to a traumatic section of the hemicauda equina from root L4 to S4. *Left:* Spontaneous activity of the recorded unit: continuous, regular, high-frequency discharge. *Middle:* The unit during light tactile stimulation of the L4 to S1 dermatomas (*arrow*). *Right:* During electrical stimulation of the tibial nerve (the *arrows* are two consecutive stimuli). Note the continuous regular discharge that remains unaltered. The *vertical bars* are 50 µV; the horizontal bars are 100 msec.) (From Jeanmonod D, Sindou M, Magnin M, Baudet M: Intraoperative unit recordings in the human dorsal horn with a simplified floating microelectrode. Electroencephalogr Clin Neurophysiol 80:477–489, 1991.)

aspect of the substantia gelatinosa. Ramon y Cajal's[7] recurrent collaterals of the large lemniscal fibers approach the dorsal horn through the ventral aspect of the substantia gelatinosa.[8,9] Because the dendrites of some of the spinoreticulothalamic cells make synaptic connections with the primary afferents inside the substantia gelatinosa layers, the substantia gelatinosa exerts a strong segmental modulating effect on nociceptive input. When the large lemniscal afferents within peripheral nerves or dorsal roots are altered, a reduction in the inhibitory control of the dorsal horn occurs.[1] This situation presumably results in excessive firing of the dorsal horn neurons (Fig. 112-4). This phenomenon, thought to be at the origin of deafferentation pain, has been identified in patients by electrophysiologic recordings[10–13] and has been reproduced in animal experiments.[14–16] Destruction of these hyperactive neurons should suppress the nociceptive impulses generated in the spinoreticulothalamic pathways. Pain-generating neurotransmitters should also be favorably modified by destruction of the dorsal horn apex neurons.[17]

PRINCIPLES OF DREZOTOMY

DREZotomy consists of a longitudinal opening incision of the dorsolateral sulcus, performed ventrolaterally at the entrance of the rootlets into the sulcus, and of microbipolar coagulations, performed inside the sulcus, down to the apex of the dorsal horn, continuously along all the spinal cord segments selected for surgery. The lesion, which penetrates the lateral part of the DREZ and the medial part of Lissauer's tract, extends to the apex of the dorsal horn, which can be

recognized by its brown-gray color. The average lesion is 2 to 3 mm deep, is made at a 35-degree angle medially and ventrally, and is presumed to destroy preferentially the nociceptive fibers grouped in the lateral bundle of the dorsal rootlets and the excitatory medial part of Lissauer's tract. The upper layers of the dorsal horn (I to V layers of Rexed's classification) are also destroyed if microbipolar coagulations are performed inside the dorsal horn. The procedure is presumed to (partially) preserve the inhibitory structures of the DREZ (i.e., the lemniscal fibers reaching the dorsal horn and the substantia gelatinosa propriospinal interconnecting fibers running through the lateral part of Lissauer's tract [Fig. 112-5]). The method, called microsurgical DREZotomy (MDT), was conceived to prevent complete abolition of tactile and proprioceptive sensations and to avoid deafferentation phenomena.[2,18] The depth and extent of the lesion depend on the degree of the desired therapeutic effect and on the preoperative sensory and functional status of the patient.

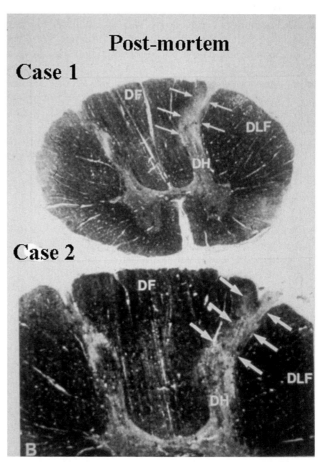

FIGURE 112-5 Postmortem histopathologic examination of the spinal cord after microsurgical DREZotomy. Transverse section of the spinal cord at the lower cervical level (C7–8), with myelin stained by Luxol-fuschine, in two different patients who died 3 months (*A*) and 45 days (*B*) after a microsurgical DREZotomy procedure performed for an advanced Pancoast's syndrome, on left side in both patients. DF, dorsal funiculus; DLF, dorsal lateral funiculus; DH, dorsal horn. Notice the postoperative changes in the dorsal root entry and the uppermost layers of the dorsal horn, on the left side between the *white arrows*.

SURGICAL ANATOMY

Working in the DREZ requires knowledge of the regional anatomy. Details of this anatomy have been given in previous publications.[19,20]

Dorsal Roots

Poorly individualized on leaving the ganglion, the rootlets separate approximately 1 cm before they penetrate the dorsolateral sulcus. They remain joined, however, by fine leptomeningeal membranes, which are easily separated with microdissection. The dorsal roots, which have a mostly symmetrical distribution, show different types of division and penetration of their rootlets according to their spinal cord level:

1. The posterior element of C1 (1 mm in diameter) exists in 80% of cases.
2. The superior cervical roots (C2–4) divide into an average of four rootlets, which are approximately 0.75 mm in diameter and are well separated from one another. Each rootlet has a cylindrical type of penetration.
3. The inferior cervical roots (C5–8) usually divide into six rootlets with a diameter of 1.5 mm. They are juxtaposed against one another. They also have a cylindrical type of penetration.
4. The thoracic roots divide into an average of five small-diameter rootlets (approximately 0.25 mm) and are widely spaced. Penetration is filiform or ribbon shaped.
5. The superior lumbar roots (L1–3) divide into 8 to 10 well-grouped rootlets. Often, each rootlet subdivides further into several small secondary filiform rootlets with diameters of less than 0.25 mm. They penetrate the sulcus separately. This type of penetration is called filiform penetration.
6. The lumbosacral roots (L4–S3) usually divide into seven rootlets that are approximately 1.5 mm in diameter. At entry into the spinal cord, they are often imbricated. Penetration is usually cylindrical.
7. The sacrococcygeal roots (S4–Co), often adherent to the filum terminale, usually divide into three slender rootlets with diameters of less than 0.25 mm. Penetration is filiform. Sometimes coccygeal nerve bundles are included in the fibrous sheath of the filum.

Before it deeply penetrates into the spinal cord, a rootlet sometimes takes a subpial course that is superficial to but three fourths embedded in the spinal cord tissue. This course can run as long as 1 mm along the dorsolateral sulcus, and such a segment cannot be dissected, as is frequently the case in the lower part of the cord, where the rootlets are obliquely oriented.

Dorsal Horn

The angulation of the DREZ lesion is determined by the axis of the dorsal horn in relation to the sagittal plane crossing the dorsolateral sulcus. According to 82 measurements performed by Young (personal communication, 1991, and unpublished data, 1990), the mean DREZ angle is at

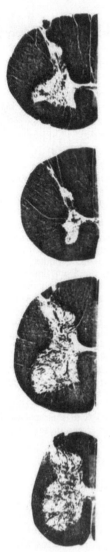

FIGURE 112-6 Variations of shape, width, and depth of the dorsal root entry zone area according to the spinal cord level. From top to bottom: C7, T5, L4, and S3.

30 degrees at C6, 26 degrees at T4, 37 degrees at T12, and 36 degrees at L3. The site and extent of the DREZ lesion are also determined by the shape, width, and depth of Lissauer's tract and the dorsal horn,[21] as is shown in Figure 112-6.

INDICATIONS

Pain Due to Malignancies

Good candidates are patients with a long life expectancy, general conditions compatible with open surgery, and topographically limited pain caused by well-localized lesions. Pancoast-Tobias syndrome at the thoracic apex is typically good indication for MDT[22]; the procedure is generally performed from C7 to T2. For more extended cervicothoracic cancers, percutaneous computed tomography–guided, open high cervical anterolateral cordotomy or stereotactic spinothalamic tractomy is preferable. Other good indications for MDT are painful conditions caused by circumscribed malignant invasions of the thorax, abdominal wall, or perineal floor and also pain due to limited neoplastic involvement of lumbosacral roots, plexuses, or both. Because extensive DREZ operations at the lumbar and/or sacral segments would inevitably result in leg hypotonia and/or sphincter disturbances, for pain below the waist in patients who are able to walk, the procedure should be indicated only if it is limited. For perineal pain, midline myelotomy can be an alternative. Intrathecal morphine is the technique of choice for advanced widespread pelvic cancers.

In our personal series, a good result (i.e., withdrawal of narcotics) was obtained by MDT in 87% of 49 patients operated on at the cervical or cervicothoracic level and in 78% of 38 patients who underwent surgery at the lumbar or sacral level for well-localized cancers. Survival time ranged from 1 month to 4 years (average, 14 months). Postoperative infection occurred in two patients, and in two patients, surgery was considered to have precipitated death.

Although restricted to a small number of patients among all those affected with pain due to malignancies, MDT is a valuable recourse for patients with topographically limited painful cancers.

Neuropathic Pain

Pain after Brachial Plexus Avulsion

All authors experienced in pain surgery and using DREZ procedures, whatever their modality, agree that DREZ operations are effective for pain developing after brachial plexus avulsion.[23–32] We do not limit the DREZ lesion to the avulsed segments but extend it to the adjacent remaining roots, especially if their level corresponds with the painful territory. Special care must be taken not to damage the adjacent dorsal column and pyramidal tract, especially when the cord is anatomically modified by the injury.

The long-term results in our series (Table 112-1) are concordant with those of the literature (Table 112-2).[24,26,27,29–31,33,38]

The group at Duke University reported a success rate of 54% in a series of 39 patients operated on with the radiofrequency (RF) thermocoagulation technique.[27] The Queen Square group in London, in their series of 44 patients treated also with thermocoagulation, obtained a 68% success rate.[28,29] Rath and colleagues[30] in Germany reported a 61% success rate in their 13 patients and Samii and colleagues,[31] also from Germany, reported a success rate of 63% in their important series of 47 patients also treated with RF thermocoagulation. Dreval[24] reported a 87% rate of success in his series of 127 patients in whom the DREZ lesions were performed using a special small ultrasonic probe.

Analysis of the literature concerning postoperative complications with RF or laser DREZ procedures for brachial plexus avulsion revealed (more or less severe) corticospinal and/or dorsal column deficits in 0% to 10% of the patients with laser DREZ and in as many as 50% of the patients with the RF technique, according to the reviewed series; there were fewer complications and side effects with MDT.[39] This seems to be due to the better accuracy and selectivity in the lesioning process with the microsurgical technique; with this method, the lesion is performed under magnified direct vision of the microscope and through an opening of the dorsolateral sulcus itself.

Pain after Spinal Cord or Cauda Equina Lesions

Most patients who underwent DREZ surgery for spinal cord or cauda equina lesions were patients with spinal injury (Table 112-3).[30,39–45] According to the author's experience,[45] MDT is effective only in patients whose pain had a radiculometameric distribution, that is, the pain corresponding with the level and extent of the spinal cord lesions (see Table 112-3). This pain was called segmental pain. In contrast, pain in the territory below the lesion, especially in the perineosacral area, is generally not influenced, even if DREZ surgery is performed

---

TABLE 112-1 ▪ **Author's Series of Microsurgical DREZotomy for Brachial Plexus Avulsion**

I. Results on Pain

No. of Patients	Follow-up	Excellent Relief (>75%) (= No Treatment)	Good Relief (>50%) (= Pain Controlled)*	Poor Relief (<50%)
55	On discharge	54 (98%)		1 (2%)
55	At 1 yr	39 (71%)	13 (23.6%)	3 (5.4%)
		94.6%		
55 (followed long term)	1–27 yr (average, 6 yr)	21 (38%) 69%	17 (31%)	17 (31%)

II. Complications and Side Effects (55 Patients)
Mortality: Nil
Local complications
  Cerebrospinal fluid fistula: 1 (transient)
  Meningitis: 2 (cured by antibiotics)
  Cervicalgias: slight (no need of antalgics)
Neurologic complications
  Ataxia in homolateral lower limb: mild, 4; severe, 2
  Motor deficit in homolateral lower limb: mild, 1
  Urogenital disturbances: 1
Neurologic side effects (persistent)
  Decrease in sensation in homolateral upper thorax: mild, 5; pronounced, 2
  Dysesthesias in homolateral upper limb: mild, 2
  New sensory deficit in homolateral upper limb: mild, 3; pronounced, 2

*Pain controlled with additional medications at moderate doses.

TABLE 112-2 ▪ Review of the Literature: Surgery in the Dorsal Root Entry Zone for Brachial Plexus Avulsion

Authors (Year)	Technique	No. of Patients	Pain Duration, Range (Mean)	Follow-up, Range (Mean)	Results				Complications		
					100%	75%	50%	25%	Motor	Sensory	Other
Nashold and Ostdahl (1979)[33]	RF-Th	18	1–24 yr (5.8 yr)	1–4 yr (1.8 yr)	55.6%	16.7%		27.7%	50%	72.2%	
Thiebault et al (1988)[34]	RF-Th	18		(6 yr)	83%	17%		0%	5.6%	38.9%	Cerebrospinal fluid: 2 patients; New pain: 5.3%
Ishijima et al (1988)[35]	RF-Th	19	—	(1.7 yr)	82.2%	17.8%		0%	62%		
Friedman et al (1988)[27]	RF-Th	39		1–10 yr	54%	13%		33%	40%	40%	
Young (1990)[36]	RF-Th, CO_2 laser	18 4		1–5 yr (4 yr)	RF 75% Laser 50%		RF 25% Laser 50%		RF, 6%; laser, 10%	RF, 3%; laser, 5%	Myelopathy: 1.3%; Urinary disturbance: 1.3%
Kumagai et al (1992)[37]	RF-Th	7	2–25 yr (10.8 yr)	2–25 yr (4.2 yr)	28.5%	14.3%	57.2%		14.2%	71.4%	New pain: 28.5%
Dreval (1993)[24]	Ultrasonic probe	124		(4 yr)		87%		13%	10%	15%	New pain: 10%
Thomas and Kitchen (1994)[29]	RF-Th	44	1–30 yr (7.3 yr)	1–12 yr (5 yr)	68%		11%	21%	22% (18%)p	18% (9%)p	
Rath et al (1996)[30]	RF-Th	14		3–12 yr (6.2 yr)	62%		15%	23%	43%		Death: 1 patient
Samii et al (2001)[31]	RF-Th	47	0.5–40 yr	2–18 yr		63%	37%		14% (5%)p		Subdural hematoma: 2 patients
Prestor (2001)[38]	Microsurgery	21	0.5–27 yr (7.7 yr)	2–10 yr (5.6 yr)	47.6%	33.3%	14.3%	4.8%	4.7%	14%	
Sindou et al (2005)[26]	Microsurgery	55	1–42 yr (9 yr)	1–27 (6 yr)	38%	31%	31%		1.8%	3.6%	Meningitis: 2 patients

RF-Th, radiofrequency thermocoagulation; p, permanent.

TABLE 112-3 ▪ Review of the Literature: Long-Term Results of Surgery in the Dorsal Root Entry Zone for Spinal Cord Injury

Author (Year)	Technique	No. of Patients	Good results (= Pain Relief >75%)	(Range) Mean Follow-up
Nashold and Bullit (1981)[40]	Radiofrequency	13	54%	(5 mo–3 yr)
Friedman and Nashold (1986)[41]	Radiofrequency	56	50%	(6 mo–5 yr)
Young (1990)[36]	Radiofrequency or CO_2 laser	20	55%	(3–5 yr)
Sampson et al (1995)[42]	Radiofrequency	39	54%	(1 wk–12 yr) 3 yr
Rath et al (1996)[30]	Radiofrequency	22	55%	(10 mo–13 yr) 5 yr
Spaic et al (1999)[44]	Microsurgery	6	100%	(7 mo–1 yr) 9 mo
Sindou et al (2001)[45]	Microsurgery	44	Segmental 68% Below lesion 0%	(1–20 yr) 7 yr

at the lower medullary segments. This is particularly true when the pain consists of a permanent burning sensation and is located in an infralesional, totally anesthetic area. Therefore, MDT must be reserved for pain syndromes related to the injured medullary segments and the adjacent ones if modified by consecutive pathologic processes (e.g., cavitation, gliosis, arachnoiditis).

Of paramount importance, in patients with incomplete paraplegia, DREZ lesions must be performed not too deeply and extensively to avoid additional neurologic deficits. On the contrary, in patients with complete motor and sensory deficits below the lesion, MDT can be done extensively on the selected segments.

In our series, because most of the trauma patients did not have complete treatment of their vertebral fracture at the time of the injury, MDT was preceded by a long dissection of the dura from the surrounding epidural fibrosis, a delicate freeing of the cord and roots from adhesive arachnoiditis and eventual residual bone fragments occupying the intradural space. This preparatory approach was performed as the first step of the whole operation in approximately half of the patients. In the other half, because exposure was particularly long and bloody, especially due to the necessity of removing the metallic rods, the approach was the first part of a two-staged operation, the second stage being done approximately 1 week later.

The best indications for DREZ surgery are the same as those for cordectomy (i.e., traumatic lesions of the spine below T10 with the complete functional interruption of the conus medullaris, especially when the pain is located in the legs rather than in the perineum).

Pain caused by lesions of cauda equina can also be favorably influenced by MDT performed on the corresponding spinal cord segments.

Postherpetic Pain

Results of surgery in the DREZ for postherpetic pain have been reported by a few groups.[30,46] In our experience, only superficial pain located in the affected dermatomes was significantly improved, especially when of the allodynic type. The permanent (burning or aching) deep component is rather unrelieved; it can even be aggravated, with the patient complaining of additional constrictive sensations after the operation.

At the operation, identification of the roots corresponding with the herpetic lesions is difficult. The observation

of an atrophy and a grayish color in the concerned root(s) can be helpful.

When the thoracic spinal cord is the target, because at this particular level the dorsal horn is narrow and deeply situated as shown in Figure 112-6, encroachment of the corticospinal tract laterally and of the dorsal column medially might happen if DREZ surgery is not prudently performed.

Before deciding on DREZotomy in patients with postherpetic neuralgia, one must be cautious. Although no death or postoperative neurologic complication occurred in our series of 10 patient, it is necessary to stress the possible vital risks in these patients, most patients being aged and psychologically impaired.

Pain Resulting from Peripheral Nerve Lesions

When pain resulting from peripheral nerve injuries is not relieved by transcutaneous neurostimulation or spinal cord stimulation, MDT may be considered. This group of patients with pain consisted of 42 patients in our series. From this experience, we conclude that MDT is indicated when the predominant component of pain is of the paroxysmal type (electrical flashing pain) and/or corresponds with allodynia/hyperalgesia or both. Good results can also be achieved in severe post-traumatic causalgic syndromes with disabling hyperpathia (i.e., complex regional pain syndromes, type II). The pain and the vasomotor disturbances can be favorably influenced. In patients without neurologic deficit, the DREZ lesion must not be too extensive in length and depth so that the tactile and proprioceptive sensory capacities can be (at least partially) retained and uncomfortable paresthesias avoided.

MDT can be also considered for severe occipital neuralgia. Surgery is performed at the C2–3 spinal cord segments. At this level, the procedure is easy through a C2 hemilaminectomy. The results in the author's three such cases were good. In the series of 11 cases published by Dubuisson,[47] the effects of the operation were also good.

After limb amputation, two main types of pain, which may coexist, can be encountered: pain in the phantom limb and pain in the stump. If spinal cord stimulation fails, DREZ surgery may be considered. Phantom limb pain is generally relieved when rootlets are found avulsed. Pain in the stump is inconstantly influenced; better results are obtained when the pain is of the paroxysmal and/or allodynic type. The newly developed precentral (motor) cortex stimulation seems to be promising for pain after amputation,[48,49] so that it will be tried first.

Hyperspastic States

Because muscular tone was diminished in the operated territories after MDT performed for the treatment of pain,[2,50] the procedure was applied as early as 1973 for harmful spasticity.[51,52] The antispastic effects can be explained by the fact that MDT interrupts the afferent components of the myotatic (monosynaptic) and the nociceptive (polysynaptic) reflexes and so deprives the somatosensory relays of the dorsal horn of most of their excitatory inputs.

Our series consists of three groups of patients: (1) Forty-five patients, mostly hemiplegic, underwent MDT at the cervical level for hyperspasticity in the upper limb. MDT was performed from C5 to T1 segments through a C3–7 hemilaminectomy. (2) One hundred fifty-one patients had MDT at the lumbosacral level for excessive spasticity complicating severe paraplegic states such as those observed in patients with multiple sclerosis. MDT was performed bilaterally through a T11 to L2 laminectomy from L2 down to S2 and additionally down to S5 when there was a hyperactive neurogenic bladder with urine leakage around the catheter. (3) Fifteen patients underwent MDT at the sacral (S2–3 or S2–4) level for hyperactive neurogenic bladder.

Forty-two of the 45 patients with harmful spasticity in the upper limb had associated pain. Eighty of the 151 patients with paraplegia had pain mostly as a result of spasms or contractures.

The cord levels related to the undesirable spasticity were identified by studying the muscle responses to bipolar electrical stimulation of the ventral and dorsal roots. The motor threshold for stimulation of ventral roots was one third that of the threshold for dorsal roots. The technical procedure was as follows. The ventrolateral aspect of the DREZ was exposed so that the microsurgical lesions could be performed in the dorsolateral sulcus, 2 to 3 mm deep and at a 35-degree angle (for cervical) or 45-degree angle (for lumbosacral) levels, all along the selected segments of the spinal cord (detailed description in "Surgical Technique"). Intraoperative neurophysiologic monitoring was used to help identify cord levels and quantify the extent of MDT (see "Intraoperative Neurophysiologic Monitoring").

Results have been detailed elsewhere.[53–56] Only a brief summary is given here. Follow-up ranged from 2 to 25 years (average, 9 years). For patients with paraplegia, a useful effect on lower limbs (i.e., a lasting decrease in tone allowing easy passive mobilization) was obtained in 87% of the patients. Bladder capacity was significantly improved in 85%; the patients who improved were those in whom the detrusor was not irreversibly fibrotic. For patients with hemiplegia with harmful spasticity in the upper limb, a good effect was obtained in 78%. The effect on the upper limb was significant and lasting, only at the level of the shoulder and elbow, allowing the reappearance of some voluntary movements when hidden behind hypertonia. The effect was much less beneficial at the level of the wrist and fingers, so that additional peripheral neurotomies, together with orthopedic surgery, were often required.

MDT constantly produced a decrease in sensation in the operated territories: mild in 40%, marked in 40%, and severe in 20%. When present, pain was durably relieved in 88% in both groups.

Based on that experience, the indications for hyperspastic states can be summarized as follows:

1. The hyperspastic hemiplegic upper limb can benefit from MDT when spasticity predominates in the shoulder and elbow. Wrist and fingers are less favorably influenced, especially when there are irreducible contractures and deformities in flexion and/or poor motor function in the extensors; in the latter eventuality, peripheral neurotomies together with tendon surgery may be preferred.
2. For lower limbs, because MDT generally has a dramatic effect on tone, surgical indications must be restricted to patients with paraplegia with severe disability and inability to walk. MDT is indicated if patients cannot be installed comfortably in a wheelchair or are exposed to pressure sores in bed, especially if additional pain resulting from spasms, contractures, and/or neurotrophic disturbances is present. Intrathecal baclofen therapy is an alternative to MDT.
3. MDT can be indicated to treat neurogenic bladder when there is no voluntary micturition and if there are uninhibited detrusor contractions resulting in voiding around the catheter or in between intermittent self-catheterization.

SURGICAL TECHNIQUE

Surgery is performed with the patient under general anesthesia, with an initial short-lasting curarization to allow intraoperative observation of motor responses to bipolar electrical stimulation of the nerve roots. Stimulated ventral roots have a motor threshold at least three times lower than that of dorsal roots. Standard microsurgical techniques are used with 10 to 25 times magnification. Special microinstruments for MDT have been made by Leibinger-Fischer (Freiburg, Germany) (Fig. 112-7).

Operative Procedure at the Cervical Level

The prone position with the head and neck flexed in the Concorde position has the advantage of avoiding brain collapse caused by cerebrospinal fluid depletion. The head is fixed with a three-pin headholder. The level of laminectomy is determined after identification of the prominent spinous process of C2 by palpation. For unilateral DREZ surgery, a hemilaminectomy, generally from C4 to C7, with preservation of the spinous processes, allows sufficient exposure of the posterolateral aspect of the cervical spinal cord segments that correspond with the upper limb innervation, that is, the rootlets of C5 to T1.

When roots are present, the dura and arachnoid are opened longitudinally. Then the exposed roots are dissected free by separating the tiny arachnoid filaments that bind them to each other, to the arachnoid sheath, and to the cord pia mater. The radicular vessels are preserved. Each ventral and dorsal root from C4 to T1 is electrically stimulated at the level of its corresponding foramen to identify precisely its muscular innervation and its functional value.

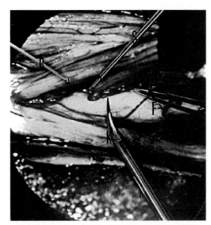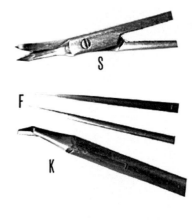

FIGURE 112-7   Technical principles of microsurgical DREZotomy (MDT) and necessary instruments. Exposure of the dorsolateral aspect of the conus medullaris on the left side. The rootlets of the selected dorsal roots are retracted dorsomedially and held with a (specially designed) ball-tip microsucker (B), which is used as a small hook, to gain access to the ventrolateral part of the dorsal root entry zone. After division with curved sharp microscissors (S) of the fine arachnoidal filaments that stick the rootlets together with the pia mater, the main arteries running along the dorsolateral sulcus are dissected and preserved, while the smaller ones are coagulated with a pair of sharp bipolar micro-forceps (F). Then, the incision is performed using a microknife (K), made with a small piece of razor blade inserted in the striated jaws of a curved razor blade holder (K). On average, the cut is a 35-degree angle descending to a depth of 2 to 3 mm. The surgical lesion is completed by performing microcoagulations under direct magnified vision (at a low intensity) inside the incision, down to the apex of the dorsal horn. These microcoagulations are made by means of the special sharp bipolar forceps (F), which is insulated except at the tip over 5 mm and graduated every millimeter.

Stimulated ventral roots have a motor threshold at least three times lower than that of dorsal roots. Responses are in the diaphragm for C4 (the response is palpable below the lower ribs), in the shoulder abductors for C5, in the elbow flexors for C6, in the elbow and wrist extensors for C7, and in the muscles intrinsic of the hand for C8 and T1.

Microsurgical lesions are performed at the selected levels, that is, those that correspond with the pain territory. The technique is summarized and illustrated in Figure 112-8. The incision is made with a microknife (razor blade in a blade holder or ophthalmologic microscalpel). Then microcoagulations are made in a "chain" (i.e., dotted) manner. Each microcoagulation is performed under direct magnified vision by short-duration (a few seconds), low-intensity bipolar electrocoagulation, with a specially designed sharp bipolar forceps incremented in millimeters. The depth and extent of the lesion depend on the desired therapeutic effect and the preoperative status of the limb.

If the laxity of the root is sufficient, the incision is performed continuously in the dorsolateral sulcus, ventro-laterally along all the rootlets of the targeted root, thus accomplishing a sulcomyelotomy. If not, a partial ventrolateral section is made successively on each rootlet of the root after the surgeon has isolated each one by separating the tiny arachnoid membranes that hold them together.

In brachial plexus avulsion (Fig. 112-9), an hemi-laminectomy with preservation of the spinous processes is performed ipsilateral to the avulsion according to the cord segments injured. As an example, for total plexus avul-sion, hemilaminectomy has to extend from C3 to C7. Dura is longitudinally opened and sustained laterally with sutures. Arachnoid opening may be difficult due to intense arachnoiditis with strong adhesions to the cord. Pseudomeningoceles with fragile membranes in place of dural sheaths are frequent at the level(s) of the avulsed segment(s). Under the operative microscope, the anatomic

aspect of all rootlets, whether ventral or dorsal, is carefully checked; rootlets can be normal, atrophic, or partially or totally avulsed. The functional status of the remaining rootlets is studied by observing muscular responses to their direct electrical stimulation. Dissection of the neural structures is often hard to achieve because of scar tissue adhering to the cord and the remaining rootlets. The cord may be dramatically atrophic and/or distorted. Atrophy and/or gliotic changes at the level of the avulsed roots can make identification of the dorsolateral sulcus difficult. In such cases, it is necessary to start exposure of the sulcus from the remaining root above and below the avulsed segments. The presence of tiny radicular vessels that enter the cord helps to determine the site of the sulcus. Yellow areas corresponding with old hemorrhages on the surface of the cord and/or microcavities in the depth of the sulcus and/or gliotic tissue within the dorsal horn provide guid-ance for tracing the dorsolateral sulcomyelotomy. When the sulcus is difficult to find, intraoperative monitoring of the dorsal column somatosensory evoked potentials evoked by stimulation of the homolateral tibial nerve is especially helpful.

The extent in length of DREZotomy is primarily estab-lished based on pain localization. Pain topography generally corresponds not only with the extent of the avulsed segments but also, although to a lesser degree, to the altered (i.e., atrophic, grayish, gliotic) adjacent rootlets. Therefore, DREZ surgery has to be conducted not only to the avulsed segments of the cord but also to the adjacent remaining roots, espe-cially if altered. After incision of the dorsolateral sulcus with a microknife, 2 mm in depth and oriented at an approxi-mately 35-degree angle ventrally and medially in the axis of the dorsal horn, dotted microcoagulations are performed inside the dorsal horn down to approximately the fifth layer (i.e., 3 mm in depth). The microcoagulations are made under magnified vision with a specially designed, sharp,

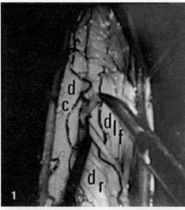

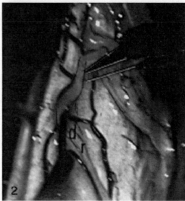

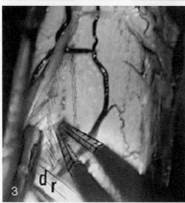

FIGURE 112-8 Microsurgical DREZotomy (MDT) technique at the cervical level. Exposure of the right dorsolateral aspect of the cervical cord at C6. *1*, The rootlets of the selected dorsal root (dr) are displaced dorsally and medially with a hook or a microsucker to obtain access to the ventrolateral aspect of the dorsal root entry zone in the dorsolateral sulcus. Using microscissors, the arachnoid adhesions are cut between the cord and the dorsal rootlets. dc, dorsal cord; dlf, dorsolateral funiculus. *2*, After having coagulated exclusively the tiny pial vessels, an incision of 2 mm in depth at 35 degrees ventrally and medially is made with a microknife in the lateral border of the dorsolateral sulcus. *3*, Then microcoagulations are performed down to the apex of the dorsal horn using a sharp graduated bipolar microforceps.

graduated bipolar forceps on both edges of the dorsolateral sulcus and inside the dorsal horn, to a depth of at least 3 mm from the surface of the cord. They have to be well located inside the dorsal horn in between the cuneate fasciculus on the medial side and the corticospinal tract on the lateral side to avoid neurologic deficits.

Operative Procedure at the Lumbosacral Level

When roots are present, the patient is positioned prone on thoracic and iliac supports and the head placed 20 cm lower than the level of the surgical wound to minimize the intraoperative loss of cerebrospinal fluid. The desired vertebral level is identified by palpation of the spinous processes or, if this is difficult, by lateral radiographic study that includes the S1 vertebra. Interspinous levels identified by a needle can then be marked with a nontoxic dye (methylene blue). A laminectomy, either bilateral or unilateral according to pain topography, is performed from T11 to L1 (or L2). The dura and arachnoid are opened longitudinally, and the filum terminale is isolated. Identification of roots is performed by electrical stimulation.

The L1 and L2 roots are easily identified at their penetration into their respective dural sheaths. Stimulation of L2 produces a response of the iliopsoas and adductor muscles. Identification of L3 to L5 is difficult for many reasons: (1) the exit through their respective dural sheaths is caudal to the exposure, (2) the dorsal rootlets enter the sulcus along an uninterrupted line, (3) the ventral roots are hidden in front of the dentate ligament, and (4) the motor responses in the leg to stimulation of the roots are difficult to observe intraoperatively because of the patient's prone position. Stimulation of L3 produces a preferential response in the adductors and quadriceps, of L4 in quadriceps, and of L5 in the anterior tibialis. Stimulation of the S1 dorsal root produces a motor response of the gastrocnemius-soleus group that can be confirmed later by repeatedly checking the Achilles ankle reflex before, during, and after MDT. Stimulation of the S2 to S4 dorsal roots (or better, directly, the corresponding spinal cord segments at the DREZ) can be assessed by recording of the motor vesical or anal response by use of cystomanometry, rectomanometry, or electromyography of the anal sphincter (or simply with a finger into the rectum). Because neurophysiologic investigations are time consuming to perform in the operating room, we have found that measurements at the conus medullaris can be sufficient in patients who already have severe preoperative impairment of their vesicoanal functions. These measurements, based on human postmortem anatomic studies, have shown that the landmark between the S1 and S2 segments is situated approximately 30 mm above the exit from the conus of the tiny coccygeal root.[2,20]

MDT at the lumbosacral levels follows the same principles as those at the cervical level. The technique is summarized and illustrated in Figure 112-10. At the lumbosacral level, MDT is difficult and possibly dangerous because of the rich vasculature of the conus. The dorsolateral spinal artery courses along the dorsolateral sulcus. Its diameter is 0.1 to 0.5 mm, and it is fed by the posterior radicular arteries and joins caudally with the descending anterior branch of the Adamkiewicz artery through the conus medullaris anastomotic loop of Lazorthes. This artery must be preserved by being freed from the sulcus.

Conus Medullaris and/or Cauda Equina Injury

In conus medullaris and/or cauda equina injury, surgery must be performed on the cord segments corresponding with the lesion, that is to the so-called segmental pain

FIGURE 112-9 Microsurgical DREZotomy (MDT) technique at the cervical level for C6 to T1 Brachial plexus avulsion on left side. *Upper and lower left:* T2-weighted magnetic resonance imaging shows pseudomeningoceles at the lower cervical spine on left side. *Upper right:* Operative view shows entire cervical spinal root freed from arachnoiditis by microsurgical dissection. The C5 dorsal root remains present but damaged with rootlets stuck together by focal arachnoiditis. Segments from C6 down to T1 on the left side are absent due to total avulsion. Left dorsolateral sulcus can be identified. *Lower right:* Operative view shows MDT on the C6 avulsed segment; incision into the DLS has been made with the microknife and dotted microcoagulations inside the sulcus made with the sharp bipolar microforceps.

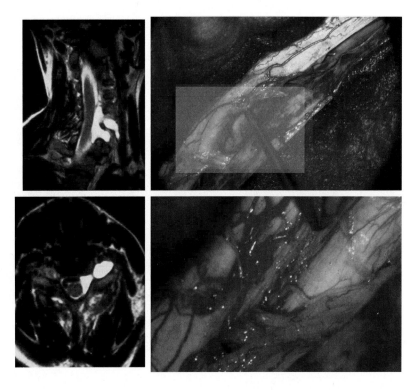

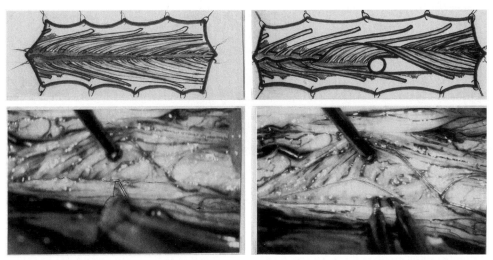

FIGURE 112-10 Microsurgical DREZotomy technique at the lumbosacral level. *Top left:* Exposure of the conus medullaris through a T11 to L1 laminectomy. *Top right:* Approach of the dorsolateral sulcus. For doing so, the dorsal rootlets of the selected roots are displaced dorsally and medially to obtain proper access to ventrolateral aspect of the dorsal root entry zone (DREZ). *Bottom left:* Operative view: The selected dorsal roots are retracted dorsomedially and held with a specially designed ball-tip microsucker used as a small hook to gain access to the ventrolateral part of the DREZ. After division of the fine arachnoidal filaments sticking the rootlets together with the pia mater with curved, sharp microscissors (not shown), the main arteries running along the dorsolateral sulcus are dissected and preserved, and the smaller ones are coagulated with a sharp bipolar microforceps (not shown). Then, a continuous incision is performed using a microknife, made with a small piece of razor blade inserted in the striated jaws of a curved razor blade holder. The cut is on average at a 45-degree angle and to a depth of 2 mm. *Bottom right:* Operative view: The surgical lesion is completed by doing microcoagulations under direct magnified vision, at a low intensity, inside the dorsolateral sulcomyelotomy down to the apex of the dorsal horn. These microcoagulations are made all along the segments of the cord selected to be operated on using a special sharp bipolar forceps, insulated except at the tip over 5 mm and graduated every millimeter.

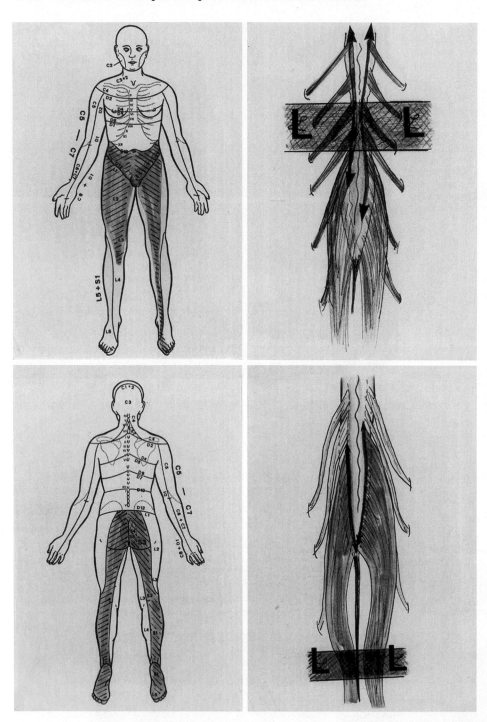

FIGURE 112-11   *Top:* Microsurgical DREZotomy (MDT) performed bilaterally in a patient with a spinal cord injury in the conus medullaris at the segments (*lines with double arrows*) corresponding with the "segmental pain" territories (*hatched dermatomes*). L-L, level of the responsible lesion in the spinal cord [patient with paraplegia].) *Bottom:* MDT performed bilaterally in the conus medullaris at the segments (*lines with double arrows*) corresponding with the pain territories (*hatched dermatomes*) in a patient with a cauda equina injury. L-L, level of the responsible lesion in the cauda equina.

(Figs. 112-11 and 112-12). A majority of patients with a conus medullaris lesion have plurisegmental damage; therefore, a large number of segments must be operated on. For cauda equina lesions, MDT must be restricted to the medullary segments corresponding with the injured roots.

The most frequent pathologic alterations due to spinal cord injuries have been well summarized by Nashold (personal communication):

> *Blunt injury to a segment of the spinal cord by a spinal dislocation results in a relatively localized spinal cord injury, whereas a gunshot wound may produce an injury that involves numerous segments above and below the injury.*

> *The initial insult is followed by central hemorrhage. After the hemorrhage resolves, small microcysts may form larger necrotic cavities (which can be seen on the MRI-Scan). As a result of the spinal injury, not only the spinal cord is damaged, but also the adjacent tissues including the dorsal and ventral roots and the arachnoidal tissue. The arachnoidal scarring at the site of the spinal injury may be enough to tether the cord.*

In most patients, the microsurgical procedure is preceded by a long dissection of the dura from the surrounding epidural fibrosis and a delicate dissection of the cord and the roots from adherent arachnoiditis. In patients with spinal fractures

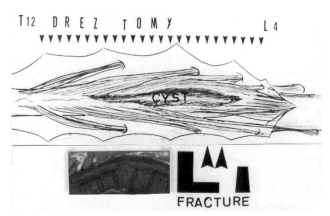

FIGURE 112-12 Patient with paraplegia with a spinal cord injury at the conus medullaris level (L1 fracture), with segmental pain in both legs (*hatched dermatomes*). Microsurgical DREZotomy (MDT) will be performed bilaterally in the corresponding conus medullaris segments (*lines with double arrows*). Drawing illustrates the intraoperative findings: necrotic cyst and gliosis in the segments of the conus medullaris corresponding with the vertebral fracture (L1 level). MDT was performed on both sides in the T12 to L4 spinal cord segments.

not previously completely operated, one must start with liberation of the neural structures from residual bone fragments occupying the intrarachidian space and even sometimes the intradural space. This preparatory approach may be long and bloody; in that eventuality, it is better to perform the first stage of the operation in a separate setting, followed by MDT 2 weeks later.

Intraoperative Neurophysiologic Monitoring (Fig. 112-13)

Surface somatosensory evoked potential recordings of dorsal root presynaptic potentials and dorsal horn postsynaptic potentials can be useful for identification of the spinal cord segments. Potentials have a maximal intensity at C6–7

and C8 for stimulation of the median and ulnar nerves, respectively, and at L5 to S2 and S2 to S4 for stimulation of the tibial nerve and the dorsal nerve of the penis (or clitoris), respectively.[57–59]

Recordings of surface somatosensory evoked potentials can also be helpful to monitor the surgical lesion itself. The dorsal column potentials can be monitored for checking the integrity of the ascending dorsal column fibers, especially when the dorsolateral sulcus is not clearly marked (as is frequent in [brachial] root avulsion). The dorsal horn potentials can be monitored to follow the extent and depth of MDT, particularly when good sensory functions are present before surgery.

In addition, unitary spikes generated in dorsal horn neurons are interesting to record during DREZotomy to evince abnormal activities.[11–13,60] These microelectrode recordings can be correlated to microdialysis studies of neurotransmitters.[17,61] Those electrophysiologic microrecordings and chemical microdialysis analyses are at present more for research than for practical use.

SUMMARY OF OTHER DREZ LESION PROCEDURES

In September 1974, Nashold and colleagues[62] started to develop DREZ lesions using the RF hermocoagulation as the lesion maker in the substantia gelatinosa of the dorsal horn first and later in the whole DREZ,[33,63] especially for pain resulting from brachial plexus avulsion. More recently, DREZ procedures were performed with the use of the laser by Levy and colleagues[64] and Powers and colleagues,[23] and with the use of an ultrasound probe by Kandel and colleagues[65] and Dreval,[24] also for pain caused by brachial plexus avulsion.

These various technical modalities, which are theoretically all directed to the DREZ, do not have exactly the same anatomic target and consequently the same sensory effects. (1) The RF thermocoagulation procedure is performed with an electrode implanted through the pia mater into the dorsal

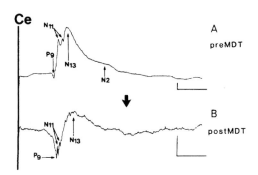

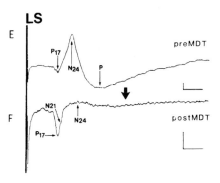

FIGURE 112-13 Effects of microsurgical DREZotomy (MDT) on the evoked electrospinogram. Recordings from the surface of the dorsal column, medially to the dorsal root entry zone at the C7 cervical (Ce) and the L5 lumbosacral (LS) segments, ipsilateral to the stimulation of the median and the tibial nerves, respectively, before (preMDT) and after (postMDT). The initial positive event P9 (for cervical) (P17 for lumbosacral) corresponds with the far-field compound potential originating in the proximal part of the brachial (lumbosacral) plexus. The small and sharp negative peaks N 11 (N21) correspond with near-field presynaptic successive axonal events, probably generated in the proximal portion of the dorsal root, the dorsal funiculus, and the large-diameter afferent collaterals to the dorsal horn. After MDT, all these presynaptic potentials remain unchanged. The large, slow, negative wave N13 (N24) corresponds with the postsynaptic activation of the dorsal horn by group I and II peripheral afferent fibers of the median (tibial) nerves. They are diminished after MDT (in the order of two thirds). The later negative, slow wave N2 (just visible in the cervical recording) corresponds with postsynaptic dorsal horn activity consecutive to the activation of group II and III afferent fibers. N2 is suppressed after MDT. (From Jeanmonod D, Sindou M, Mauguiere F: The human cervical and lumbosacral evoked electrospinogram: Intraoperative spinal cord surface recordings. Electroencephalogr Clin Neurophysiol 80:473–475, 1991.)

horn; the coagulation involves the whole dorsal horn and has an ovoid shape. (2) DREZ lesions made with the laser, mostly the carbon dioxide laser, are more superficial and have a V shape; they are often accompanied by small infarcts because of the coagulation of the vessels located at the DREZ. (3) The ultrasonic DREZ procedure had been almost exclusively used for brachial plexus avulsion pain; it has the particularity to evacuate the spongy and gliotic tissue situated in the dorsal horn apex. All these methods destroy the entire DREZ and dorsal horn structures; they do not allow preservation of sensory functions in the operated areas if present preoperatively.

CONCLUSION

Provided that selection of patients is rigorous, MDT can achieve good pain relief in some well-defined intractable painful syndromes. Adequate indications need a solid comprehension of pain mechanisms by the surgeon. Accurate surgery implies good knowledge of the radicular innervation (not only of the superficial but also of the deep structures of

the body) as well as of the surgical anatomy of the spinal cord and roots. Good training in microsurgery is required.

MDT is capable of sparing, more or less, lemniscal fibers in the operated segments, which can be useful in patients who still retain some functions in the painful territories. The distinctive feature of MDT is that it is performed at the junction of the peripheral and central parts of the somatosensory system. If done in a selective way, this position allows destruction of specific components of this system as a result of the spatial segregation and acts on gating mechanisms by influencing their modulatory activity to make it inhibitory. Electrophysiologic recordings, postoperative clinical examination, and postmortem anatomic studies in four personal cases support the notion that the action of MDT is due not only to a massive destruction of the DREZ area but also, at least in part, to a "retuning" of the dorsal horn.

After a total experience of operating on 452 patients in our department since 1972 for severe chronic pain, the author concludes that indications are as follows:

1. Cancer pain that is limited in extent (such as in Pancoast-Tobias syndrome).

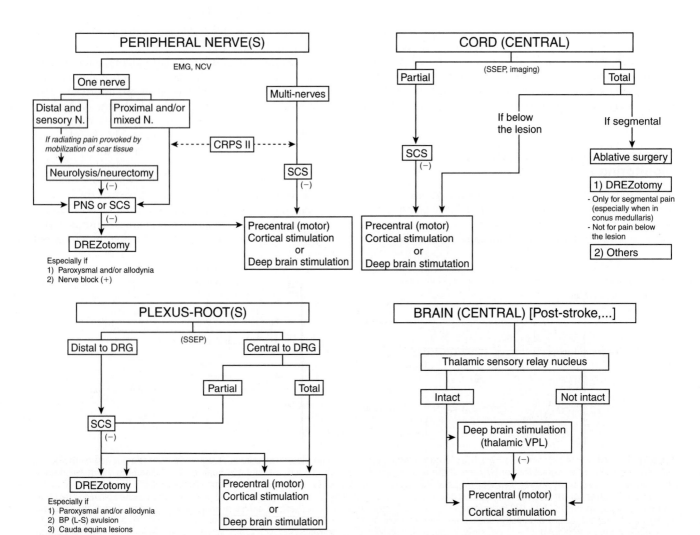

FIGURE 112-14 Algorithms for neuropathic pain, originating from lesions of peripheral nerves (*upper left*), plexus roots distal and central to ganglion (*lower left*), spinal cord (*upper right*), and brain (*lower right*). BP, brachial plexus; CRPS, complex regional pain syndrome; DREZ, dorsal root entry zone; DRG, dorsal root ganglion; EMG, electromyography; L-S, lumbo-sacral; NCV, nerve conduction velocity; PNS, peripheral nerve stimulation; SCS, spinal cord stimulation; SSEP, somatosensory evoked potentials; VPL, ventro-postero-lateral.

Paraplegia with Hyperspasticity

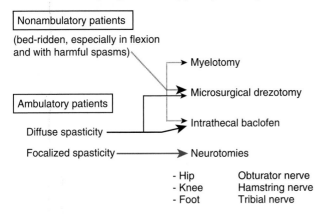

Hemiplegia with Hyperspasticity

Upper limb

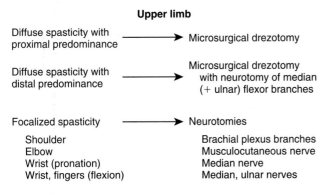

Hemiplegia with Hyperspasticity

Lower limb

Spastic foot	→	**Neurotomy of tibial nerve**

Equinus	→	Triceps surae
Varus	→	Posterior tibialis
Flesion of the toes	→	Flexor fascicles

FIGURE 112-15 Algorithms for disabling hyperspasticity in patients with paraplegia and hemiplegia.

2. Persistent neuropathic pain resulting from brachial plexus injuries, especially those with avulsion, and spinal cord lesions, but only for pain corresponding with segmental lesions. Pain below the lesion is not favorably influenced. Segmental pain caused by lesions in the conus medullaris and the cauda equina is most often significantly relieved. Pain resulting from cauda equina lesions can also be an indication. Peripheral nerve injuries, amputation, and herpes zoster, when the predominant component of pain is of the paroxysmal type and/or corresponds with (provoked) allodynia/hyperalgesia.

3. Disabling hyperspasticity, especially when accompanied by pain.

Surgery in the DREZ must be considered within the frame of all the methods belonging to the armamentarium

of pain surgery[66–68] (Fig. 112-14) or hyperspastic focalized states[69,70] (Fig. 112-15).

REFERENCES

1. Melzack R, Wall PD: Pain mechanism: A new theory. Science 150:971–979, 1965.
2. Sindou M: Etude de la jonction radiculo-médullaire postérieure: La radicellotomie postérieure sélective dans la chirurgie de la douleur. M.D. Thesis, Université Claude-Bernard, Lyon, 1972.
3. Sindou M, Quoex C, Baleydier C: Fiber organization at the posterior spinal cord-rootlet junction in man. J Comp Neurol 153:15–26, 1974.
4. Willis WD: Pain System. Basel: Karger, 1985.
5. Rand R: Further observations on Lissauer's tractolysis. Neurochirurgica 3:151–168, 1960.
6. Denny-Brown D, Kirk EJ, Yanagisawa N: The tract of Lissauer in relation to sensory transmission in the dorsal horn of spinal cord in the macaque monkey. J Comp Neurol 151:175–200, 1973.
7. Ramon y Cajal S: Histologie du Systéme Nerveux, vol 1. Paris: Maloine, 1901.
8. Szentagothai J: Neuronal and synaptic arrangement in the substantia gelatinosa. J Comp Neurol 122:219–239, 1964.
9. Wall PD: Presynaptic control of impulses at the first central synapse in the cutaneous pathway. In Eccles JC, Schadé JP (eds): Physiology of Spinal Neurons. Amsterdam: Elsevier, 1964, pp 92–118.
10. Loeser JD, Ward AA Jr, White LE Jr: Chronic deafferentation of human spinal cord neurons. J Neurosurg 29:48–50, 1968.
11. Jeanmonod D, Sindou M, Magnin M, et al: Intra-operative unit recordings in the human dorsal horn with a simplified floating microelectrode. Electroencephalogr Clin Neurophysiol 72:450–454, 1989.
12. Guenot M, Hupe JM, Mertens P, et al: New type of microelectrode for obtaining unitary recordings in the human spinal cord. J Neurosurg 91:25–32, 1999.
13. Guenot M, Bullier J, Rospars J, et al: Single-unit analysis of the spinal dorsal horn in patients with neuropathic pain. J Clin Neurophysiol 20:142–150, 2003.
14. Loeser JD, Ward AA Jr, White LE Jr: Some effects of deafferentation of neurons. J Neurosurg 17:629–636, 1967.
15. Albe-Fessard D, Lombard MC: Use of an animal model to evaluate the origin of and protection against deafferentation pain. In Bonica JJ, Lindblom V, Iggo A (eds): Advances in Pain Research and Therapy, vol 5. New York: Raven Press, 1983, pp 691–700.
16. Guenot M, Bullier J, Sindou M: Clinical and electrophysiological expression of deafferentation pain alleviated by dorsal root entry zone lesions in rats. J Neurosurg 97:1402–1409, 2002.
17. Mertens P, Ghaemmaghami C, Bert L, et al: Microdialysis study of amino-acid neurotransmitters in the spinal dorsal horn of patients undergoing microsurgical dorsal root entry zone lesioning. J Neurosurg 94:165–173, 2001.
18. Jeanmonod D, Sindou M: Somatosensory function following dorsal root entry zone lesions in patients with neurogenic pain or spasticity. J Neurosurg 74:916–932, 1991.
19. Sindou M, Fischer G, Mansuy L: Posterior spinal rhizotomy and selective posterior rhizidotomy. In Krayenbühl H, Maspes PE, Sweet WH (eds): Progress in Neurological Surgery, vol 7. Basel: Karger, 1976, pp 201–250.
20. Sindou M, Goutelle A: Surgical posterior rhizotomies for the treatment of pain. In Krayenbühl H (ed): Advances and Technical Standards in Neurosurgery, vol 10. Vienna: Springer-Verlag, 1983, pp 147–185.
21. Mertens P, Guénot M, Hermier M, et al: Radiologic anatomy of the spinal dorsal horn at the cervical level (anatomy-MRI correlations). Surg Radiol Anat 22:81–88, 2000.
22. Sindou M, Lapras C: Neurosurgical treatment of pain in the Pancoast-Tobias syndrome: Selective posterior rhizotomy and open antero-lateral C2-cordotomy. In Bonica JJ, Ventafrida V, Pagni CA (eds): Advances in Pain Research and Therapy, vol 4. New York: Raven Press, 1982, pp 199–209.
23. Powers SK, Adams JE, Edwards SB, et al: Pain relief from dorsal root entry zone lesions made with argon and carbon dioxide microsurgical lasers. J Neurosurg 61:841–847, 1984.
24. Dreval ON: Ultrasonic DREZ-operations for treatment of pain due to brachial plexus avulsion. Acta Neurochir (Wien) 122:76–81, 1993.
25. Emery E, Blondet E, Mertens P, et al: Microsurgical DREZotomy for pain due to brachial plexus avulsion: Long-term results in a series of 37 patients. Stereotactic Funct Neurosurg 68:155–160, 1997.

26. Sindou M, Blondet E, Emery E, et al: Microsurgical DREZotomy for pain due to brachial plexus avulsion: 1) clinical features 2) intraoperative anatomical findings and 3) long-term results, in a series of 55 patients J Neurosurg 102:1018–1028, 2005.

27. Friedman AH, Nashold BS, Bronec PR: Dorsal root entry zone lesions for the treatment of brachial plexus avulsion injuries: A follow-up study. J Neurosurg 22:369–373, 1988.

28. Thomas DGT, Jones ST: Dorsal root entry zone lesions in brachial plexus avulsion. Neurosurgery 15:966–968, 1984.

29. Thomas DGT, Kitchen ND: Long-term follow-up of dorsal root entry zone lesions in brachial plexus avulsion. J Neurol Neurosurg Psychiatry 57:737–738, 1994.

30. Rath SA, Braun V, Soliman N, et al: Results of DREZ-coagulations for pain related to plexus lesions, spinal cord injuries and post-herpetic neuralgia. Acta Neurochir (Wien) 138:364–369, 1996.

31. Samii M, Bear-Henney S, Ludemann W, et al: Treatment of refractory pain after brachial plexus avulsion with dorsal root entry zone lesions. Neurosurgery 48:1269–1277, 2001.

32. Moringlane JR, Samii M: Thermocoagulation of the substantia gelatinosa for the treatment of pain. Neurol Res 6:79–80, 1984.

33. Nashold BS, Ostdahl PH: Dorsal root entry zone lesions for pain relief. J Neurosurg 51:59–69, 1979.

34. Thiebault JB, Bruxelle J, Thurel C, et al: Pain in avulsion lesions of the brachial plexus: Relief by dorsal horn lesions. In Brunelli G (ed): Textbook of Microsurgery. Paris: Masson, 1988, pp 817–819.

35. Ishijima B, Shimoji K, Shimizu H, et al: Lesions of spinal and trigeminal dorsal root entry zone for deafferentation pain. Appl Neurophysiol 50:175–187, 1988.

36. Young RF: Clinical experience with radio-frequency and laser DREZ lesions. J Neurosurg 72:715–720, 1990.

37. Kumagai Y, Shimoji K, Honma T, et al: Problems related to dorsal root entry zone lesions. Acta Neurochir (Wien) 115:71–78, 1992.

38. Prestor B: Microsurgical junctional DREZ-coagulation for treatment of deafferentation pain syndromes. Surg Neurol 56:259–265, 2001.

39. Sindou M, Daher A: Spinal cord ablation procedures for pain. In Dubner A, Gebbart GF, Bond MR (eds): Proceedings of the Fifth World Congress on Pain. Amsterdam: Elsevier, 1988, pp 477–495.

40. Nashold BS, Bullitt E: DREZ-lesions to control central pain in paraplegics. J Neurosurg 55:414–419, 1981.

41. Friedman AH, Nashold BS: DREZ lesions for relief of pain related to spinal cord injury. J Neurosurg 65:465–469, 1986.

42. Sampson JH, Cashman RE, Nashold BS, et al: Dorsal root entry zone lesions for intractable pain after lesions to the conus medullaris and cauda equina. J Neurosurg 82:28–34, 1995.

43. Sindou M: Microsurgical DREZotomy (MDT) for pain, spasticity and hyperactive bladder: A 20 year experience. Acta Neurochir (Wien) 137:1–5, 1995.

44. Spaic M, Petkovic S, Tadic R, et al: Drez-surgery on conus medullaris (after failed implantation of vascular omental graft) for treating chronic pain due to spine (gunshot) injuries. Acta Neurochir (Wien) 141:1309–1312, 1999.

45. Sindou M, Mertens P, Wael M: Microsurgical DREZotomy for pain due to spinal cord and/or cauda equina injuries: Long-term results in a series of 44 patients. Pain 92:159–171, 2001.

46. Friedman AH, Nashold BS, Ovelmen-Levitt J: Drez-lesions for the treatment of post-herpetic neuralgia. J Neurosurg 60:1258–1261, 1984.

47. Dubuisson D: Treatment of occipital neuralgia by partial posterior rhizotomy at C1-3. J Neurosurg 82:581–586, 1995.

48. Tsubokawa T, Katayama Y, Yamamoto T, et al: Chronic motor cortex stimulation for the treatment of central pain. Acta Neurochir Suppl 52:137–139, 1991.

49. Mertens P, Nuti C, Sindou M, et al: Precentral cortex stimulation for the treatment of central neuropathic pain. Stereotatic Funct Neurosurg 73:122–125, 1999.

50. Sindou M, Fischer G, Goutelle A, et al: La radicellotomie postérieure sélective: Premiers résultats dans la chirurgie de la douleur. Neurochirurgie 20:391–408, 1974.

51. Sindou M, Fisher G, Goutelle A, et al: La radicellotomie postérieure sélective dans le traitement des spasticités. Rev Neurol 130:201–215, 1974.

52. Sindou M, Millet MF, Mortamais J, et al: Results of selective posterior rhizotomy in the treatment of painful and spastic paraplegia secondary to multiple sclerosis. Appl Neurophysiol 45:335–340, 1982.

53. Sindou M, Abdennebi B, Sharkey P: Microsurgical selective procedures in the peripheral nerves and the posterior root-spinal cord junction for spasticity. Appl Neurophysiol 48:97–104, 1985.

54. Sindou M, Mifsud JJ, Boisson D, et al: Selective posterior rhizotomy in the dorsal root entry zone for treatment of hyperspasticity and pain in the hemiplegic upper limb. Neurosurgery 18:587–595, 1986.

55. Sindou M, Jeanmonod D: Microsurgical DREZ-tomy for the treatment of spasticity and pain in the lower limbs. Neurosurgery 24:655–670, 1989.

56. Sindou M, Jeanmonod D, Mertens P: Surgery in the DREZ: Microsurgical DREZotomy for treatment of spasticity. In Sindou M, Abbott R, Keravel Y (eds): Neurosurgery for Spasticity. Wien: Springer-Verlag, 1991, pp 165–182.

57. Jeanmonod D, Sindou M, Mauguière F: The human cervical and lumbo-sacral evoked electrospinogram: Data from intra-operative spinal cord surface recordings. Electroencephalogr Clin Neurophysiol 80:477–489, 1991.

58. Turano G, Sindou M, Mauguière F: SCEP monitoring during spinal surgery for pain and spasticity. In Dimitrijevic MR, Halter JA (eds): Atlas of Human Spinal Cord Evoked Potentials. Boston: Butterworth-Heinemann, 1995, pp 107–122.

59. Sindou M, Turano G, Pantieri R, et al: Intraoperative monitoring of spinal cord SEPs, during microsurgical DREZotomy (MDT) for pain, spasticity and hyperactive bladder. Stereotact Funct Neurosurg 62:164–170, 1994.

60. Guenot M, Hupe JM, Mertens P, et al: Microelectrode recordings during microsurgical DREZotomy [abstract]. Stereotact Funct Neurosurg 67:56, 1996–1997.

61. Mertens P, Ghaemmaghami C, Perret-Liaudet A, et al: In vivo amino-acids concentrations in human dorsal horn studied by microdialysis during DREZotomy: Methodology and preliminary results [abstract]. Stereotact Funct Neurosurg 67:58, 1996–1997.

62. Nashold BS, Urban B, Zorub DS: Phantom pain relief by focal destruction of substantia gelatinosa of Rolando. In Bonica JJ, Albe-Fessard D (eds): Advances in Pain Research and Therapy, vol. 1. New York: Raven Press, 1976, pp 959–963.

63. Nashold BS: Modification of DREZ lesion technique [letter]. J Neurosurg 55:1012, 1981.

64. Levy WJ, Nutkiewicz A, Ditmore M, Watts C: Laser induced dorsal root entry zone lesions for pain control: Report of three cases. J Neurosurg 59:884–886, 1983.

65. Kandel EL, Ogleznev KJA, Dreval ON: Destruction of posterior root entry zone as a method for treating chronic pain in traumatic injury to the brachial plexus. Vopr Neurochir 6:20–27, 1987.

66. Gybels JM, Tasker RR: Central neurosurgery. In Wall PD, Melzack R (eds): Textbook of Pain, 4th ed. Edinburgh: Churchill Livingstone, 1999, pp 1307–1338.

67. Sindou M, Mertens P, Garcia-Larrea L: Surgical procedures for neuropathic pain. Neurosurg Q 11:45–65, 2001.

68. Burchiel KJ: Surgical Management of Pain. New-York/Stuttgart: Thieme, 2002.

69. Sindou M, Abbott R, Keravel Y: Neurosurgery for Spasticity. Wien: Springer-Verlag, 1991.

70. Decq P, Mertens P: La neurochirurgie de la spasticité. Neurochirurgie. Paris: Masson, 2003.

Surgical Management of Infections

113 Suppurative Intracranial Infections

HENRY H. SCHMIDEK

PYOGENIC BRAIN ABSCESS

Pyogenic brain abscess is a focal collection of pus within the brain. This condition has been the subject of discussion and of surgical treatment for hundreds of years. Among the earliest accounts of brain abscess was that of Fabricius Hildanus, approximately 400 years ago, who recommended trephination of the skull and drainage of the pus. Morgagni added to knowledge 300 years ago by relating some intracranial infections to an otogenic source. Dupuytren 150 years ago described the case of a soldier who had sustained a compound fracture of the skull and developed a hemiplegia several years later. The wound was opened, the dura incised, and a cannula placed through the brain. After this was done, an abscess was drained, and the patient recovered.

In 1876, Macewen[1] made his first definite and localizing diagnosis of brain abscess in an 11-year-old child who had fallen 2 weeks earlier and was in an obtunded and febrile condition with right-sided seizures. Macewen localized the lesion to the left third frontal convolution. Surgery was recommended but rejected by the family. At postmortem examination, the abscess was visible and was in the left frontal lobe. In 1881, Macewen performed his first operation for brain abscess and in 1893 published the results of his treatment of 94 patients with intracranial infections. Among the 94 cases were 5 surgically treated epidural abscesses; all 5 of these patients recovered. There were 25 patients with one or more brain abscesses; 19 of these 25 patients were operated on, and 18 recovered. The 19 patients treated surgically had a total of 22 brain abscesses evacuated, 21 successfully, in an era antedating antibiotics and accurate radiologic diagnosis.[1]

Drainage remained the preferred mode of treatment of brain abscesses for many years and was then followed by marsupialization of the lesion. This technique involves excising a small area of brain over the abscess, opening the abscess, and suturing the capsule to the dura. The abscess cavity is packed and gradually allowed to collapse and heal on itself. Sargent was first to regard excision of an abscess as the treatment of choice for thick-walled abscesses.[2] He used this approach in six patients, all of whom recovered. Although advances in microbiologic techniques, imaging of the central nervous system (CNS), antimicrobial agents, and neurosurgical methods have resulted in progressive diagnostic and therapeutic improvements, the management of intracranial suppurations is still associated with a significant morbidity and mortality rate.

Pathogenesis and Bacteriology

Pyogenic abscesses of the brain are uncommon lesions largely because of the brain's natural resistance to infection, a property mediated by its abundant vascular supply and the relative impermeability of the blood-brain barrier. The incidence of brain abscess is approximately 4 cases per 1 million, with men in their 20s and 30s predominating.[3] Peak ages vary, however, depending on predisposing influences; pediatric cases peak between the ages of 4 and 7, and a substantial minority of these children have congenital heart disease.[3] The overall occurrence of brain abscess does not appear to have changed significantly in the antibiotic era, and an active neurosurgical service in a hospital in a developed country can expect to see 4 to 10 cases annually.[4]

Pyogenic brain abscess formation is initiated when bacteria gain entry into cerebral tissues with trauma, contiguous spread from a suppurative focus, or hematogenous dissemination from a distant infection. The cause is cryptogenic in 15% to 20% of cases.[5] Abscesses secondary to spread from a contiguous focus of infection, such as paranasal sinusitis, otitis media, mastoiditis, and dental infection, account for 40% to 60% of cases.[6,7] These lesions are usually solitary, and their distribution in the brain reflects the predisposing lesion (Table 113-1). Seeding of the brain probably occurs via the valveless emissary veins draining the contiguous areas. Middle ear infections, usually chronic otitis media or chronic mastoiditis, can lead to temporal lobe or cerebellar abscesses by direct spread via the tegmen tympani or by translabyrinthine spread. Paranasal sinusitis can lead to frontal or temporal lobe abscesses by retrograde thrombophlebitis of the diploic veins. Frontal sinus infection can also lead to frontal lobe brain abscess when complicated by osteomyelitis of the frontal bone of the skull with dehiscence of the posterior table.

Penetrating cranial trauma is a well-described though relatively infrequent cause of pyogenic brain abscess, accounting for fewer than 10% of these infections.[6–8] The incidence of brain abscess was 3% in one large series of combat-acquired injuries from the Vietnam War, with most occurring in the setting of gunshot wounds to the head and retained bone fragments.[9] The interval from the time of injury to diagnosis may be considerably delayed, averaging nearly 4 months in one study.[8] A distinctive form of post-traumatic brain abscess that occurs largely in young children results from penetrating injuries of the orbital region and, less commonly, other areas of the skull from pencil tips, wooden sticks, wooden toys, and lawn darts.[10] The interval from injury to clinical presentation may extend

TABLE 113-1 ■ **Predisposing Lesions, Intracranial Location, and Bacteriology of Pyogenic Brain Abscess**

Predisposing Lesion	Intracranial Location	Predicted Bacteriology
Frontoethmoidal sinusitis	Frontal lobe	Aerobic and anaerobic streptococci, *Bacteroides* species, Enterobacteriaceae, *Haemophilus* species, *Staphylococcus aureus*, *Fusobacterium* species
Sphenoidal sinusitis	Frontal or temporal lobe	Same as in frontoethmoidal disease
Otitis media, mastoiditis	Temporal lobe or cerebellum	Aerobic and anaerobic streptococci, *Bacteroides fragilis*, Enterobacteriaceae, *Pseudomonas aeruginosa*
Dental sepsis	Frontal lobe	Polymicrobial *Bacteroides* species, *Streptococcus* species, *Fusobacterium* species
Penetrating trauma	Related to site of wound	*S. aureus*, *Clostridium species*, *Bacillus species*, Enterobacteriaceae
Postoperative	Related to site of surgery	*Staphylococcus epidermidis*, *S. aureus*, Enterobacteriaceae, *P. aeruginosa*, *Propionibacterium* species
Congenital heart disease	Multiple abscesses most commonly in distribution of middle cerebral artery	Viridans, anaerobic, and microaerophilic streptococci, *Haemophilus* species
Infective endocarditis	Same as in congenital heart disease	Streptococci, *S. aureus*
Pulmonary infection: lung abscess, empyema	Same as in congenital heart disease	Polymicrobial *Bacteroides* species, *Streptococcus species*, *Fusobacterium* species
Intra-abdominal infection	Same as in congenital heart disease	*Streptococcus species*, *B. fragilis*, Enterobacteriaceae

from days to years. Treatment, as in other penetrating cranial injuries, involves early surgical débridement.[11]

Brain abscesses are infrequent sequelae of neurosurgery, complicating approximately 0.1% of clean neurosurgical procedures.[5] The relative contribution of previous intracranial surgery or craniotomy as predisposing causes of pyogenic brain abscesses appears to be increasing.[12] Microorganisms, introduced at the time of surgery, infect the wound or bone flap and form an intracranial focus of suppuration by contiguous spread. Recently two reports have been published on infection following endovascular treatment of intracranial aneurysm. In one such case,[13] a 70-year-old female developed an intracranial abscess secondary to a Guglielme detachable coil (GDC) embolization of a giant right internal carotid artery aneurysm. The abscess was demonstrated by computed tomography (CT), and *Staphylococcus aureus* was cultured from the cerebrospinal fluid (CSF) and blood. The abscess was successfully treated with antibiotics. In another such case, a 55-year-old woman developed meningitis and a brain abscess surrounding a giant aneurysm treated with a GDC 3.5 years earlier. In this case the GDC acted as a colonizing foreign body, resulting in an abscess with *Salmonella* group D. Four weeks before treatment the patient had an infective illness with this organism.[14]

Hematogenous dissemination or metastatic seeding from a distant primary site of infection accounts for approximately 25% of brain abscesses.[4,6,7] These lesions are usually located in the distribution of the middle cerebral artery, tend to occur at the corticomedullary junction where capillary flow is slowest, and are frequently multiple and multiloculated.[5] Recognized sources of metastatic seeding include pulmonary lesions, such as arteriovenous fistulas,[15] often occurring with hereditary hemorrhagic telangiectasia[16]; infective endocarditis, rarely complicated by macroscopic brain abscess (<1%) but with microabscesses found at autopsy in 4%[17]; and deep-seated infections, such as osteomyelitis, pulmonary empyema, pelvic infections, and intra-abdominal infections. An increasingly important problem occurs in intravenous drug users with infected

valvular vegetations supplying emboli resulting in cerebral infarction, cerebral hemorrhage, brain abscess formation, and spinal epidural abscesses. Of note is that this population is prone to toxin-mediated diseases (tetanus and botulism), with the inoculation of these agents at injection sites.[18] Pyogenic brain abscess is a well-described though infrequent complication of esophageal dilation of caustic strictures and endoscopic sclerosis of varices, procedures that produce a transient bacteremia.[5,19,20] In general, however, transient bacteremia is unlikely to result in brain abscess in the absence of breaches of the blood-brain barrier or predisposing cerebral lesions, such as previous stroke or primary or metastatic neoplasms.[21,22]

Cerebral abscess complicates cyanotic congenital heart disease in 2% to 6% of cases,[5] and cyanotic congenital heart disease is a leading underlying cause of pediatric brain abscess, accounting for 6% to 50% of cases.[21] Tetralogy of Fallot and transposition of the great vessels underlie most cases, although any cardiac defect that results in significant right-to-left shunting appears to increase the risk. The pathogenesis probably involves increased blood viscosity as a result of chronic hypoxemia (due to right-to-left shunting), leading to areas of microinfarction within the brain that act as nidi for infection. The mortality from pyogenic brain abscess in this setting is high.

Intrasellar, brain stem, basal ganglia, and thalamic abscesses are rare.[5] Intrasellar abscesses generally occur in the setting of preexisting pituitary or sellar lesions, such as adenomas, craniopharyngiomas, Rathke's cleft cysts or, rarely, as a complication of transsphenoidal surgery.[23,24] These lesions may also occur as a result of intrasellar extension from sphenoid sinusitis. Abscesses of the brain stem are generally hematogenous in origin and may extend longitudinally over several levels of the brain stem.[21]

Cerebellar and temporal lobe abscesses are usually the result of contiguous spread from chronic otitis media or chronic mastoiditis.[25] The incidence of these lesions appears to have decreased over the past decades, probably as a result of improvements in the management of pediatric ear infections. The attempt to control otogenic infections with multiple courses of antibiotics, however, has led to some otologists and primary care physicians no longer considering the possibility of an inadequately controlled infectious process extending intracranially. We have seen several cases in which patients have presented in extremis after months of antimicrobial therapy and days to weeks of progressive headache in whom the symptoms were not appreciated or investigated.

The bacteria producing pyogenic brain abscess have changed over the past 50 years (see Table 113-1). Although previous reports emphasized the role of *S. aureus* and aerobic streptococci,[5] more recent studies reveal that anaerobic bacteria (including anaerobic streptococci) and Enterobacteriaceae have become more significant causes of brain abscess.[4] Multiple organisms, usually mixed aerobes and anaerobes, are seen in 30% to 60% of cases.[3,5] Negative cultures that had previously characterized a significant minority of brain abscess series have declined as a result of earlier diagnosis (and less empirical antimicrobial therapy) and improved bacteriologic culture techniques.[3]

The bacteriology of brain abscesses is determined by the pathogenesis of the lesion and the intracranial location of the primary infection (see Table 113-1). *Staphylococcus aureus* still accounts for 10% to 15% of cases, generally in the setting of trauma; streptococci are involved in nearly two thirds of cases, with *Streptococcus intermedius* having a particular predilection for causing focal suppurative infections.[5] The most common bacterial causes of acute pyogenic meningitis (*Streptococcus pneumoniae*, *Haemophilus influenzae*, *Neisseria meningitidis*) are rarely associated with brain abscess.[5,26]

Anaerobes are implicated in most brain abscesses, either as single pathogens or as a part of a polymicrobial infection.[27,28] *Bacteroides*, *Prevotella*, and *Fusobacterium* species account for most nonstreptococcal isolates.[5] Other bacterial species may be cultivated from brain abscesses in various clinical settings: *Clostridium* species, in association with an underlying malignancy or hemolytic-uremic syndrome[29]; *Propionibacterium acnes* in the postneurosurgical patient[30]; *Bacillus* species; *Listeria monocytogenes*, commonly a cause of meningitis or meningoencephalitis but rarely a cause of brain abscess; *Salmonella* species, associated with intracerebral hematoma.[5] Brain abscess in the neonatal period has a distinctive bacteriologic profile, with most of these lesions caused by *Proteus* species and *Citrobacter diversus*.[31] In contrast to meningitis caused by other pathogens, neonatal meningitis caused by these organisms is complicated by brain abscess in 40% to 75% of cases, so that early CT evaluation of neonates with meningitis or bacteremia caused by *Proteus* or *Citrobacter* species is recommended.[21]

The neuropathologic events that underlie brain abscess formation have been studied using α-streptococci in a canine model and found to correlate with CT scan findings.[32] A series of histopathologic stages has been described that appear to parallel the evolution of CT findings in human brain abscesses.[32,33] Early cerebritis (days 1–3) is a poorly circumscribed lesion characterized by acute inflammation and cerebral edema associated with bacterial invasion. Later (days 4–9), the zone of cerebritis expands, and necrosis develops with pus forming at the center of the lesion. CT scanning reveals some ring enhancement with diffusion of contrast material into the necrotic center. The early capsule

stage (days 10–13) demonstrates the establishment and maturation of a well-formed collagenous capsule associated with a reduction in the degree of cerebritis and some regression in the local edema. At the late capsule stage (day 14 and beyond), there is the continued maturation of a thick capsule with extracapsular gliosis and dense ring enhancement with little contrast diffusion on CT scan.

Capsule formation and ring enhancement on imaging studies are generally thinner and less complete on the ventricular side of the abscess.[33] This situation is probably related to the relatively poor vascularity of the deep white matter and reduced migration of fibroblasts into the area. This thinner area of capsule predisposes to ventricular rupture of the abscess.

The nature of the infecting organism influences encapsulation. Models using *Bacteroides* species show delayed capsule formation with multiple daughter abscesses suggesting incomplete containment of the infection,[12] whereas *S. aureus* experimental abscesses were larger, demonstrated delayed healing, and were associated with marked extracapsular abnormalities.[34] The route of infection also appears to affect capsule formation: abscesses resulting from hematogenous spread tend to have less extensive encapsulation than those arising from a contiguous focus of infection.[5] This situation is probably the result of microinfarcted areas of the brain arising from metastatic emboli leading to tissue hypoxia, impaired angiogenesis, and impeded fibroblast migration. Host variables also contribute to encapsulation. For example, in a canine model of brain abscess, immunosuppression with prednisone and azathioprine before bacterial inoculation leads to delayed histopathologic evolution with incomplete encapsulation as assessed by the diffusion of contrast media into the necrotic center of the lesion on CT imaging.[35]

Clinical Presentation

Most patients with pyogenic brain abscess have symptoms for less than 2 weeks, although the disease can present in an indolent fashion.[3] The presenting features of brain abscess depend on the size and intracranial location of the lesions, the virulence of the infecting agents, the immunologic status of the host, and the cerebral edema caused by the expanding intracranial mass lesion. The classic triad of fever, headache, and focal neurologic deficit is present in less than 50% of cases.[5] Headache, usually dull and poorly localized, is present in more than 70% of cases and is so nonspecific as to be a potential cause of diagnostic delays.[6,7,21] Sudden worsening of a preexisting headache in a patient with a brain abscess, especially if accompanied by the acute onset of meningeal signs, suggests either herniation or intraventricular rupture of the abscess.[21]

Fever occurs in 35% to 50% of adults[6,7,21] and is more common in children.[5] Symptoms and signs related to any underlying disease (e.g., paranasal sinusitis or otitis media), if present, may aid in the diagnosis. Altered levels of consciousness are often present.[6] Focal neurologic signs depend on the location of the lesions within the brain and the extent of cerebral edema[3]: frontal and parietal lobe abscesses are commonly associated with hemiparesis and aphasia, temporal lobe presentations may include aphasia or visual field disturbances, intrasellar lesions tend to mimic pituitary tumors, and cerebellar abscesses often present with ataxia and nystagmus.[25] Seizures occur in 25% to 35% of cases.[5] Patients present with multiple brain abscesses in approximately 10% of cases.[36]

Diagnosis

A moderate peripheral leukocytosis and elevated erythrocyte sedimentation rates are found in most patients with brain abscesses; however, blood cultures are rarely (~10%) positive.[6] Despite this fact, it is advisable to perform blood cultures on presentation (and before antimicrobial therapy). Lumbar puncture in the setting of brain abscess with mass effect is strongly contraindicated and rarely provides useful clinical information. The best opportunity to obtain a specific microbiologic diagnosis is at the time of surgery. Consultation and coordination of efforts between neurosurgeons and infectious disease specialists are crucial to ensure that the appropriate specimens are obtained and that cultures of abscess material are optimally handled and processed to enhance the chances of identifying the pathogen(s).

The usefulness of the broad range bacterial ribosomal DNA polymerase chain reaction (PCR) method combined with DNA sequencing has been used to examine pus and tissue from neurosurgical patients with suspected meningitis, brain abscess, spondylitis, or spinal epidural abscess. In one study, bacterial 23S ribosomal DNA was positive in 9 of 14 pus samples from patients with brain abscess or subdural empyemas; 8 of 14 were also positive on bacterial culture. In six patients with brain abscesses, bacteria were detected by both PCR and on bacterial culture. In one brain abscess, the sequencing identified several bacterial species. In three patients with intracranial infections, the specimens were positive by PCR but negative by culture. In eight patients, specimens were taken while the patients were on antibiotic therapy for a mean duration of 5.3 days; in three of these cases the causative bacteria could still be identified by PCR alone, even after intensive parenteral antibiotic therapy. In one case of *Mycoplasma hominis*, the organism was promptly identified by PCR alone whereas standard methods require prolonged culturing of the specimen.[37]

The locations of brain abscesses often indicate their origin: frontal lobe abscesses often arise from the paranasal sinuses or facial sepsis, temporal and cerebellar abscesses often have an otogenic origin, and parietal and occipital lesions often arise by the hematogenous spread of infection or after a neurosurgical procedure.

Computed tomography scan is excellent for the diagnosis of brain abscess, anatomic localization of the lesion, and evaluation of cerebral edema. Its value in the identification of cerebritis is improved by a delayed contrast-enhanced scanning technique.[21] The contrast-enhanced CT appearance of brain abscess is a hypodense lesion surrounded by ring enhancement with a variable peripheral zone of cerebral edema; dense ring enhancement is not a constant feature of abscesses but depends on the maturity of the lesion.

Although the sensitivity of CT scanning for brain abscess is 95% to 99%, the specificity is compromised by the inability of this modality to distinguish reliably brain abscess from metastatic tumor or some vascular lesions.[4,38] Indium-111-labeled leukocyte scanning may be used to complement CT scanning. Radiolabeled leukocytes accumulate in foci of active inflammation, enhancing the chances of distinguishing abscess from metastasis in inconclusive cases. In several small series, this technique has shown a high degree of diagnostic accuracy.[39,40]

Magnetic resonance imaging (MRI) provides imaging detail and resolution superior to CT scanning. MRI appears to be more sensitive than CT in detecting early cerebritis. Contrast-enhanced MRI has some distinct advantages over contrast-enhanced CT scanning: it is more accurate in delineating the extent of central liquefaction necrosis of the abscess; it has better sensitivity for early satellite lesions; it can detect extraparenchymal extension of the abscess (such as subdural empyema) earlier because the purulent material is hyperintense relative to CSF (as opposed to an isodense appearance on CT scan); in addition, it lacks bone artifact.[4,5] However, since the contrast-enhanced MRI reveals ring enhancement of a brain abscess that is similar to the enhancement seen in cystic or necrotic high-grade glioma or metastasis, it may be impossible to differentiate between these lesions. Recent publications suggest that diffusion weighted image (DWI) and apparent diffusion coefficient (ADC) calculations can help identify brain abscesses. Desbarats and colleagues[41] are able to identify a threshold ADC value of 1.10×10^{-3} mm^2/second below which a lesion can be classified as an abscess with a specificity of 100%. These low ADC values are attributable to the high viscosity of pus, which curtails the diffusion of water.

The application of proton magnetic resonance (MR) spectroscopy to the analysis of intracranial ring-enhancing lesions has also been reported. This technique detects the end products of bacterial metabolism: acetate, succinate, pyruvate, valine, leucine, and isoleucine are at high concentrations in pyogenic brain abscesses and have either not been detected or are at very low concentrations in cystic brain tumors.[42,43] Using this technology, it has been possible to distinguish some bacterial infectious lesions from neoplastic ones.[44-47] It does not apply to cases of parasitic abscesses (hydatid cyst), toxoplasmic abscesses, and cryptococcommas. In fungal abscesses, the amino acids are at low concentrations. At present it is thus impossible to differentiate between toxoplasmosis and lymphoma by MR spectroscopy in patients with HIV/AIDS.[43] It has also been suggested that response to treatment may be followed by demonstrating serial changes in spectral metabolite patterns.[47] In an analysis of 24 such patients with proton magnetic resonance spectroscopy, Dev and colleagues[47] found that lactate and amino acids were noted in the spectra of all patients regardless of the timing of spectroscopy relative to combined medical and surgical therapy. Acetate and pyruvate consistently disappeared after 1 week of combined therapy, suggesting that the proton magnetic resonance spectroscopy spectral patterns are specific for pyogenic brain abscess, and the change in these patterns is potentially useful in monitoring response to treatment.

Positron emission tomography (PET) has been used preoperatively to evaluate CNS mass lesions. In a recent study of the uptake of fludeoxyglucose F 18 (FDG) and [11C]methionine (11C-Met) tracers were used in brain abscess before treatment. The area showing an increased uptake of 11C-Met corresponds to the enhanced area on CT and MRI. After treatment, the area of lesions is smaller on

CT and MRI, and the PET studies also show decreased uptake. The mechanism of ^{11}C-Met uptake in the inflammatory area is thought to be not only a higher metabolic rate and active transport of amino acids, but also disruption of the blood-brain barrier. The mechanism of FDG uptake is also related to the degree of the inflammatory response and the increased density of inflammatory cells in the brain abscess. PET is useful both in detecting the inflammatory lesion and assessing the response to antibiotic therapy.[42]

Treatment

The optimal management of pyogenic brain abscess requires close collaboration among the neurosurgeon, radiologist, and infectious disease specialist. Although the precise therapeutic course may vary according to the specific clinical setting, the usual treatment combines antimicrobial therapy, serial imaging studies, and surgical drainage. In the absence of randomized, controlled clinical trials, the treatment of brain abscess derives largely from retrospective studies, case reports, experimental pharmacologic data, and clinical experience.

Systemic antimicrobial therapy is generally adjunctive to surgical treatment and is used to arrest the spread of infection within the CNS and to eradicate microscopic foci of infection not amenable to surgical drainage. The choice of antimicrobial therapy in brain abscess depends on the predicted source of the infection, the host setting, and the pharmacodynamics of the drugs.[49] The predisposing lesion or source of the abscess tends to predict the bacteriology of the lesion, which, in turn, determines the initial antimicrobial regimen (see Table 113-1). The initial empirical drug regimens and dosages are based on the presumptive underlying lesions (Table 113-2). Because it is usually necessary to start antimicrobial therapy before culture data are available, the initial antibiotic regimen is often changed as the pathogens are characterized.

The antiinfective agents needed to treat brain abscesses must be active against the pathogens and be capable of penetrating into the abscess cavity and achieving high levels in the abscess pus. CSF concentrations of drugs do not necessarily reflect the concentrations within the abscess cavity. Several studies have addressed the issue of antimicrobial penetration into abscess pus and found that penicillin G at high doses, metronidazole, trimethoprim-sulfamethoxazole, and chloramphenicol achieve therapeutic concentrations within abscess fluid.[50,51] Metronidazole attains such high levels in abscess fluid (34 to 42 μg/mL) that it is considered to be an important component of most regimens when anaerobes are potentially involved.[50] It must be used in combination with an agent active against microaerophilic streptococci (e.g., penicillin), because these organisms are frequent contributors to polymicrobial infection (see Table 113-1) and are resistant to metronidazole. Clindamycin, aminoglycosides, and first-generation cephalosporins penetrate abscess fluid poorly. Limited data are available on vancomycin and nafcillin (see Table 113-2).[5] Direct instillation of antimicrobial agents into the abscess cavity is probably unnecessary because agents are available that penetrate adequately when given systemically in high doses.[50,51]

Despite the dearth of data concerning the pharmacodynamics and clinical efficacy of newer antimicrobials in pyogenic brain abscess, these agents may have a role. Experimental evidence supports the potential utility of ceftriaxone, ceftazidime, and other third-generation cephalosporins as well as quinolones (e.g., ciprofloxacin), monobactams (e.g., aztreonam), and carbapenems (e.g., imipenem) in the management of these infections,[21] although imipenem and quinolones have a propensity to lower seizure thresholds.

The duration of antimicrobial therapy for brain abscess depends, to a large extent, on the adequacy of surgical drainage and the antimicrobial susceptibility profiles of the infecting organisms. In most cases, a 6- to 8-week course of antimicrobial therapy is recommended, with abscess resolution monitored by serial imaging studies. Complete resolution of the abscess and abnormal contrast enhancement may take 3 to 4 months. A residual area of contrast enhancement may persist for more than 6 months, and in a small percentage of these patients, the abscess recurs.

The role of corticosteroids remains controversial. Several experimental models have demonstrated that these agents

TABLE 113-2 ▪ **Empirical Antimicrobial Therapy of Suppurative Intracranial Infection Based on Predisposing Lesion**

Predisposing Lesion	Antimicrobial Therapy*
Frontoethmoidal sinusitis	Nafcillin (2 g q4hr) + metronidazole (500 mg q6hr) + ceftriaxone (2 g q12hr)
Sphenoidal sinusitis	Same as in frontoethmoidal disease
Otitis meida, mastoiditis	Penicillin G (18–24 mU/day divided into 6–12 doses or by continuous infusion) + metronidazole (500 mg q6hr) + ceftazidime (2 g q8hr)
Dental sepsis	Penicillin G (18–24 mU/day divided into 6–12 doses or by continuous infusion) + metronidazole (500 mg q6hr)
Penetrating trauma	Vancomycin (1 g q12hr) + metronidazole (500 mg q6hr) + ceftazidime (2 g q8hr)
Postoperative	Vancomycin (1 g q12hr) + ceftazidime (2 g q8hr)
Congenital heart disease	Same as in frontoethmoidal disease
Infective endocarditis	Nafcillin (2 g q4hr) + ceftriaxone (2 g q12hr)
Pulmonary infection: lung abscess, empyema	Same as in frontoethmoidal disease
Cryptogenic source	Nafcillin (2 g q4hr) + metronidazole (500 mg q6hr) + ceftazidime (2 g q8hr)

*Suggested initial empirical therapy may require modification once specific microbiologic data become available; dosing may require adjustment in patients with underlying renal or hepatic disease. All agents are to be given intravenously. An infectious disease consultation is advisable.

diminish antimicrobial entry into the CNS, reduce the elimination of viable organisms from the abscess cavity, and inhibit an effective, ring-enhancing, host inflammatory response.[4,5,52] In a rat model of brain abscess, a delay in encapsulation of the lesion occurs, but no differences in outcome occur with the use of steroids.[53] Limited retrospective clinical series yield conflicting data; some fail to reveal significant differences in outcome with the use of steroids,[6,54] whereas others have shown a worse outcome with their use.[55] The preponderance of evidence appears to weigh against the routine use of these agents as adjunctive therapy for brain abscess except when signs of increased intracranial pressure secondary to marked cerebral edema are present. In these cases, emergency drainage of the abscess is crucial, but treatment of an associated severe degree of cerebral edema mandates the use of steroids in high doses (e.g., dexamethasone 10 mg every 6 hours), tapered as the clinical condition and serial imaging improve.[21]

Anticonvulsants are used for the treatment and prophylaxis of seizures in these patients. We generally recommend perioperative use of these agents and their continuation after surgery, particularly in patients with seizures during their illness. The decision for long-term use depends on neurologic evaluation after the abscess has resolved.[21]

The nonoperative management of pyogenic brain abscess occurs in the setting of the neurologically stable patient with cerebritis; severe concomitant medical conditions that greatly increase the surgical risk; the presence of multiple abscesses in a surgically inaccessible, dominant, or disparate location; or the presence of multiple small abscesses.[4,5,56–59] Although this approach may be useful in these situations, the lack of diagnostic specimens requires empirical antimicrobial therapy that necessarily involves several agents with their combined attendant toxicities for an extended period of time without the potential for narrowing the regimen. Additionally, the time to the resolution of lesions may be prolonged, with the possibility of serious sequelae, because the lesion may continue to expand and may rupture into the ventricle. The decision to treat such lesions empirically with antimicrobials alone probably necessitates a longer duration of parenteral therapy (e.g., 12 weeks) and frequent imaging until resolution of radiographic abnormalities is achieved.

SURGICAL MANAGEMENT OF BRAIN ABSCESS

Surgery is of diagnostic and therapeutic value. Most abscesses larger than 2.5 cm cannot be cured without surgery. Surgical intervention allows not only pathologic diagnosis and a precise bacteriologic profile on which to base antiinfective therapy, but also reduction of mass effect, which improves the local microenvironment for antimicrobial activity by the removal of necrotic material. Various types of surgical procedures have been used in the management of brain abscess; however, the current state of the art involves image-guided stereotactic aspiration and irrigation of the cavity with antibiotic solution, or stereotactic endoscopic aspiration and irrigation. Numerous reports support these approaches, which share the advantages of precise localization, a minimal craniotomy, and the application to treating multiple lesions.[60–64] Some have suggested a trend toward a

lower incidence of seizures and other sequelae in those treated by aspiration as opposed to excision.[5] Image-guided stereotactic aspiration is a modality accurate to within a few millimeters with a diagnostic yield of 95%, is associated with transient morbidity only in 5%, and is highly effective in the definitive drainage of abscesses.[5,65]

Stereotactic image-guided craniotomy for complete abscess excision is useful in certain settings: multiloculated abscesses; failure of resolution after several aspirations; some posterior fossa lesions; some fungal abscesses; post-traumatic abscesses with retained bone fragments or foreign bodies[9]; and gas-containing abscesses, usually signifying the presence of an associated CSF fistula.[66]

Under emergent conditions or in the absence of the necessary equipment, aspiration of brain abscesses can be performed in the CT scanner. The CT scan is used to localize the lesion; scalp markers identify the approximate abscess location, size, and depth from the surface; and the biopsy needle is advanced, under CT guidance, into the abscess cavity. This technique has an accuracy of 4 to 5 mm and can be useful in these circumstances.[21,67]

Stereotactic drainage of several abscesses can usually be accomplished; a combination of several concurrent drainage procedures and prolonged medical therapy is effective.[68] In cerebellar abscess associated with edema, mass effect, and impending or actual obstructive hydrocephalus, image-guided craniotomy is favored to excise the lesion, relieve the mass effect on the brain stem, and reduce the chances of recurrence. Treatment of brain stem abscess is stereotactic drainage followed by prolonged antimicrobial therapy.

The clinical course of a patient with a pyogenic brain abscess is unpredictable; in 50% of patients with metastatic abscesses, death occurs within 5 to 14 days of symptoms. The management of these lesions is always an urgent problem and in many cases requires an emergent response. During the stage of cerebritis, antimicrobials are used with serial neurologic examinations and imaging studies to guide therapy. In most other settings, however, surgical intervention is undertaken. In the obtunded patient with a severe neurologic deficit and an encapsulated lesion, surgery for diagnosis and decompression is carried out emergently. The technique of surgical excision of a brain abscess that has failed to respond to aspiration and antimicrobial therapy or is in a particularly dangerous location (e.g., the posterior fossa) is analogous to the removal of any other brain tumor and should be carried out under frameless stereotactic guidance.

The intraventricular rupture of a brain abscess occurs with the progressive growth of the lesion. As the pus increases, the abscess expands toward the ventricle and may rupture, resulting in the sudden, catastrophic deterioration of the patient. The diagnosis is confirmed by presence of hydrocephalus and enhancement of the ventricular walls. Immediate ventricular drainage, intraventricular instillation of antibiotics, evacuation of the remaining abscess, and systemic antibiotic therapy are still associated with a management mortality rate of greater than 80%.[69,70]

Prognosis

The mortality from brain abscess has declined markedly over the past 30 years. Alderson and colleagues[71] noted a decrease in overall mortality from 42% in the 5-year period

1964 through 1968 to 10% during the 5-year period 1974 through 1978. Others have observed similar trends with even further reductions in mortality, 4% in 47 cases during the period 1981 through 1986.[55] The most significant influence in the improved outcome has been CT or MRI, allowing rapid diagnosis, surgical localization, and detection of postoperative complications.[38] In addition, microbiologic advancements have led to enhanced isolation and identification of anaerobes as causal agents, allowing for targeted therapy. More effective antimicrobials against gram-negative and anaerobic organisms and image-guided stereotactic surgery have also contributed considerably to the management outcomes. Despite these advances, the most important predictor of outcome is the patient's neurologic status at the time of presentation; mortality is highest in those with an altered consciousness[5,55] and rapid progression.[54]

When patients with several abscesses are properly managed, their survival rates are comparable to those with solitary lesions.[58] Long-term neurologic sequelae are common in survivors, occurring in 30% to 50% of cases.[5,54] Seizures and hydrocephalus are common residua. Seizures occur in about 10% of cases during the acute illness, and the subsequent incidence of seizures ranges from 35% to 75%, often starting years after the diagnosis.[72]

OSTEOMYELITIS OF THE SKULL

Osteomyelitis of the skull usually results from the contiguous spread of infection from a paranasal sinusitis, otogenic infection, or odontogenic infection, or after penetrating cranial trauma or craniotomy. Osteomyelitis of the frontal bone, subperiosteal abscess, and acute frontal sinusitis (Pott's puffy tumor) can spread via scalp veins and thrombophlebitis of the dural sinuses and veins.[73] Odontogenic infections can lead to osteomyelitis of the alveolar ridge of the mandible. Malignant otitis externa is a necrotizing osteomyelitis of the skull base caused by *Pseudomonas aeruginosa* and occurring largely in diabetics. The predisposing lesions generally predict the site of bone infection and the expected bacteriology of the infecting organisms (see Table 113-1).

Osteomyelitis arising from paranasal sinusitis presents with the findings of the underlying process (nasal discharge, localized pain and tenderness over the affected sinus, headache, localized edema, and, inconsistently, fever). Postoperative or post-traumatic osteomyelitis presents with findings referable to the site of the wound.

An elevated erythrocyte sedimentation rate is diagnostically helpful and provides a useful marker to monitor the efficacy of therapy using serial determinations. Blood cultures are obtained before initiating therapy. Aspiration of the incision and bone biopsy provide the definitive diagnostic tests; however, radiographic techniques are crucial to establish the extent of the process and provide a baseline for follow-up during treatment. MRI is extremely sensitive to signal changes in the marrow cavity and provides excellent detail of the skull base. It is the procedure of choice in investigating malignant otitis externa. Gallium-67-labeled and ^{111}In-labeled white blood cell scans are fairly sensitive, albeit nonspecific tests whose usage appears to be during the follow-up period. Single photon emission computed tomography (SPECT) technology enhances the monitoring

of therapy.[74] The treatment of cranial osteomyelitis is often surgical débridement, removal of infected bone flaps, and 4 to 6 weeks of parenteral antibiotic therapy. In addition, in cases arising from the sinuses or auditory canal, surgical débridement needs to be carried out by the otologist. The optimal management of acute infected bone flaps requires a combination of surgical débridement and at least 4 weeks of antimicrobial therapy.[75] Removal of the flap is usually necessary.

CRANIAL EPIDURAL ABSCESS AND SUBDURAL EMPYEMA

Cranial epidural and subdural empyema are usually seen after neurosurgical procedures or intracranial extension of otogenic disease.[76] Subdural empyema is also seen as a complication of meningitis, especially in children. In this situation, a loculated collection of pus develops and produces seizures, focal deficits, or altered consciousness. This lesion is identified when investigating a patient whose meningitis has atypical features. The intracranial infection may include brain abscess, with the patient presenting with meningitis, a brain abscess, and a subdural empyema.

Cranial epidural abscess arises between the skull and the dura in association with paranasal sinusitis, cranial osteomyelitis, or trauma or after surgery. Hlavin and colleagues,[77] in a retrospective study of 41 patients with subdural and epidural empyemas, report a change in the epidemiologic characteristics of these infections so that although sinusitis and otitis media were the predominant causes in this series, one or more previous craniotomies had been performed in two thirds of the patients, and the other causes accounted for one third of cases. In addition, this population was different from prior series in that a greater percentage of gram-negative aerobic bacteria were isolated. In an autopsy series, 80% of cases of cranial epidural abscess had evidence of an associated subdural abscess.[78] Purulent meningitis complicates 10% to 20% of subdural empyemas. The bacteriology of these lesions is analogous to that of brain abscess (see Table 113-1). Generally, the epidural abscess is an indolent lesion that presents with fever, headache, and neurologic signs. Untreated, this parameningeal focus can extend intracranially and involve the dural venous sinuses resulting in a septic thrombophlebitis. Gradenigo's syndrome is a specific presentation of temporal petrous apex infection characterized by ipsilateral facial pain and abducens palsy. CT and MRI demonstrate a hypodense, enhancing lesion. Treatment for the epidural abscess is either by burr hole drainage, or craniotomy with instillation of antibiotics combined with systemic antibiotic therapy.

The subdural space allows for the easy communication of infection to almost all parts of the brain's surface. Microbes gain access to the subdural space after traversing the epidural space and along diploic veins. Most subdural empyemas are located over the cerebral convexities, but they have also been identified infratentorially, between the hemispheres adjacent to the falx, and on the tentorium.[78] They may also occur bilaterally. The organisms producing these lesions are the same as those producing brain abscess and other intracranial infections (see Table 113-1). In contrast to the epidural infection, the clinical presentation of a subdural empyema is often fulminant, with an acute febrile illness followed by rapid neurologic deterioration.[79] The median time from the onset of symptoms to diagnosis is 4 days. Imaging studies demonstrate a crescent-shaped hypodense mass lesion on the surface of the brain, along the falx, or along the tentorium. The appearance is analogous to the subdural hematoma, and occasionally a preexisting subdural hematoma may become infected, blurring these diagnoses. Treatment consists of drainage of the purulent material, débridement of necrotic tissues, and high doses of systemic antibiotics (see Table 113-2). We treat these lesions by carefully delineating their extent with computer-guided technology and centering a minicraniotomy over the lesion. This procedure involves removing a 5-cm disc of bone overlying the lesion, evacuating the lesion, inspecting the subdural space adequately, and placing a catheter in the space for drainage and irrigation over the several days after surgery. This tactic represents a compromise between burr hole drainage and standard craniotomy and facilitates complete removal of pus beyond the bony edges often of loculated collections. Parenteral antibiotics are continued for 6 to 8 weeks, and serial radiographic studies are performed to identify adequacy of drainage. The development of new, often bilateral collections of pus has been found especially in association with abscesses secondary to rhinogenic causes. One report attributes this to ongoing seeding of pathogens from a septic thrombophlebitis into the subdural space. The mortality associated with this condition is 10% to 20% in most series, and more than half of surviving patients have neurologic residua.[77,80-85]

REFERENCES

1. Macewen M: Pyogenic Infection Diseases of the Brain and Spinal Cord: Meningitis, Abscess of Brain, Infective Sinus Thrombosis. Glasgow: James MacIehose & Sons, 1893.
2. Northfield DWC: The Surgery of the Central Nervous System: A Textbook for Postgraduate Students. Oxford: Blackwell Scientific Publications, 1973, pp 429–466.
3. Kaplan K: Brain abscess. Med Clin North Am 69:345–360, 1985.
4. Wispelwey B, Dacey RG Jr, Scheld WM: Brain abscess. In Scheld WM, Whitley RJ, Durack DT (eds): Infections of the Central Nervous System. New York: Raven Press, 1991, pp 457–486.
5. Wispelwey B, Scheld WM: Brain abscess. In Mandell GL, Bennett JE, Dolin R (eds): Principles and Practice of Infectious Diseases, 4th ed. New York: Churchill Livingstone, 1995, pp 887–900.
6. Chun HC, Johnson JD, Hofstetter M, et al: Brain abscess: A study of 45 consecutive cases. Medicine 65:415–431, 1986.
7. Yang S-Y: Brain abscess: A review of 400 cases. J Neurosurg 55:794–799, 1981.
8. Patir R, Sood S, Bhatia R: Post-traumatic brain abscess: Experience of 36 patients. Br J Neurosurg 9:29–35, 1995.
9. Rish BL, Caveness WF, Dillon JD, et al: Analysis of brain abscess after penetrating craniocerebral injuries in Vietnam. Neurosurgery 9:535–541, 1981.
10. Miller CF II, Brodkey JS, Colombi BJ: The danger of intracranial wood. Surg Neurol 7:95–103, 1977.
11. Shih TY, Kuo YL: Development of intracranial complications following transoral stab wounds in children: Report of two cases. Pediatr Neurosurg 37:35–37, 2002.
12. Osenbach RK, Loftus CM: Diagnosis and management of brain abscess. Neurosurg Clin N Am 3:403–420, 1992.
13. Jenkinson MD, Javadpour M, Nixon T, Warnke P: Intracerebral abscess formation following embolisation of an internal carotid artery aneurysm using Guglielmi detachable coils. Acta Neurochir (Wien) 145:703–706, 2003.
14. Kirollos RW, Bosma JJ, Radhakrishan J, Pigott TD: Endovascularly treated cerebral aneurysm using Guglielmi detachable coils acting as nidus for brain abscess formation secondary to Salmonella bacteremia: Case report. Neurosurgery 51:234–237, 2002.
15. Finkelstein R, Engel A, Simri W: Brain abscess: The lung connection. J Intern Med 240:33–36, 1996.
16. Press OW, Ramsey PG: Central nervous system infections associated with hereditary hemorrhagic telangiectasia. Am J Med 77:86–92, 1984.
17. Pruitt AA, Rubin RH, Karchmer AW, et al: Neurologic complications of bacterial endocarditis. Medicine 57:329–343, 1978.
18. Tunkel AR, Pradhan SK: Cerebral nervous system infections in injection drug users. Infect Dis Clin North Am 19:589–605, 2002.
19. Algoed L, Boon P, De Vos M, et al: Brain abscess after esophageal dilatation for stenosis. Clin Neurol Neurosurg 94:169–172, 1992.
20. Appignani A, Trizzino V: A case of brain abscess as complication of esophageal dilation for caustic stenosis. Eur J Pediatr Surg 7:42–43, 1997.
21. Mathisen GE, Johnson JP: Brain abscess. Clin Infect Dis 25:763–781, 1997.
22. Chen S-T, Tang L-M, Ro L-S: Brain abscess as a complication of stroke. Stroke 26:696–698, 1995.
23. Wolansky LJ, Gallagher JD, Heary RF, et al: MRI of pituitary abscess: Two cases and review of the literature. Neuroradiology 39:499–503, 1997.
24. Henegar MM, Koby MB, Silbergeld DL, et al: Intrasellar abscess following transsphenoidal surgery. Surg Neurol 45:183–188, 1996.
25. Shaw MDM, Russell JA: Cerebellar abscess: A review of 47 cases. J Neurol Neurosurg Psychiatry 38:429–435, 1975.
26. Grigoriadis E, Gold WL: Pyogenic brain abscess caused by Streptococcus pneumoniae: Case report and review. Clin Infect Dis 25:1108–1112, 1997.
27. Brook I: Bacteriology of intracranial abscess in children. J Neurosurg 54:484–488, 1981.
28. Sofianou D, Selviarides P, Sofianos E, et al: Etiological agents and predisposing factors of intracranial abscesses in a Greek university hospital. Infection 24:144–146, 1996.
29. Cheng Y-T, Huang C-T, Leu HS, et al: Central nervous system infection due to Clostridium septicum: A case report and review of the literature. Infection 25:171–174, 1997.
30. Berenson CS, Bia FJ: Propionibacterium acnes causes postoperative brain abscesses unassociated with foreign bodies: Case reports. Neurosurgery 25:130–134, 1989.
31. Renier D, Flandin C, Hirsch E, et al: Brain abscesses in neonates: A study of 30 cases. J Neurosurg 69:877–882, 1988.
32. Britt RH, Enzmann DR, Yeager AS: Neuropathological and computerized tomographic findings in experimental brain abscess. J Neurosurg 55:590–603, 1981.
33. Britt RH, Enzmann DR: Clinical stages of human brain abscesses on serial CT scans after contrast infusion: Computerized tomographic, neuropathological, and clinical correlations. J Neurosurg 59:972–989, 1983.
34. Enzmann DR, Britt RH, Obana WG, et al: Experimental Staphylococcus aureus brain abscess. AJNR Am J Neuroradiol 7:395–402, 1986.
35. Obana WG, Britt RH, Placone RC, et al: Experimental brain abscess development in the chronically immunosuppressed host: Computerized tomographic and neuropathological correlations. J Neurosurg 65:382–391, 1986.
36. Sharma BS, Khosla VK, Kak VK, et al: Multiple pyogenic brain abscesses. Acta Neurochir (Wien) 133:36–43, 1995.
37. Kupila L, Rantakokko-Jalava K, Javala J, et al: Aetiological diagnosis of brain abscess and spinal infections: Application of broad range bacterial polymerase chain reaction analysis. J Neurol Neurosurg Psychiatry 74:728–733, 2003.
38. Miller ES, Dias PS, Uttley D: CT scanning in the management of intracranial abscess: A review of 100 cases. Br J Neurosurg 2:439–446, 1988.
39. Palestro CJ, Swyer AJ, Kim CK, et al: Role of In-111 labeled leukocyte scintigraphy in the diagnosis of intracerebral lesions. Clin Nucl Med 16:305–308, 1991.
40. Bellotti C, Aragno MG, Medina M, et al: Differential diagnosis of CT-hypodense cranial lesions with indium-111-oxine-labeled leukocytes. J Neurosurg 64:750–753, 1986.
41. Desbarats LN, Herlidou S, deMarco G, et al: Differential MRI diagnosis between brain abscesses and necrotic or cystic brain tumors using the apparent diffusion coefficient and normalized diffusion-weighted images. Magn Res Imaging 21:645–650, 2003.
42. Bowen BC: Proton MR spectroscopy and the ring-enhancing lesion. AJNR Am J Neuroradiol 19:589–590, 1989.
43. Grand S, Passaro G, Ziegler A, et al: Necrotic tumor versus brain abscess: Importance of amino acids detected at 1H-MR spectroscopy—initial results. Radiology 213:785–793, 1999.

44. Grand S, Lai ES, Esteve F, et al: In vivo ^{1}H MRS of brain abscesses versus necrotic brain tumors. Neurology 47:846–848, 1996.

45. Martinez-Perez I, Moreno A, Alonso J, et al: Diagnosis of brain abscess by magnetic resonance spectroscopy: Report of two cases. J Neurosurg 86:708–713, 1997.

46. Kim SH, Chang K-H, Song IC, et al: Brain abscess and brain tumor: Discrimination with in vivo H-1 MR spectroscopy. Radiology 204:239–245, 1997.

47. Dev R, Gupta RK, Poptani H, et al: Role of in vivo proton magnetic resonance spectroscopy in the diagnosis and management of brain abscesses. Neurosurgery 42:37–43, 1998.

48. Tsuyuguch N, Sunada I, Ohata K, et al: Evaluation of treatment effects in brain abscess with positron emission tomography: Comparison of fluorine-18-fluorodeoxyglucose and carbon-11-methionine. Ann Nucl Med 17:47–51, 2003.

49. Artenstein AW, Kim JH: Antimicrobials for use in neurosurgical patients. In Wilkins RH, Rengachary SS (eds): Neurosurgery, 2nd ed. New York: McGraw-Hill, 1996, pp 3269–3283.

50. Black P, Graybill JR, Charache P: Penetration of brain abscess by systemically administered antibiotics. J Neurosurg 38:705–709, 1973.

51. Everett ED, Strausbaugh LJ: Antimicrobial agents and the central nervous system. Neurosurgery 6:691–714, 1980.

52. Quartey GRC, Johnston JA, Rozdilsky B: Decadron in the treatment of cerebral abscess: An experimental study. J Neurosurg 45:301–310, 1976.

53. Schroeder KA, McKeever PE, Schaberg DR, et al: Effect of dexamethasone on experimental brain abscess. J Neurosurg 66:264–269, 1987.

54. Seydoux C, Francioli P: Bacterial brain abscesses: Factors influencing mortality and sequelae. Clin Infect Dis 15:394–401, 1992.

55. Mampalam TJ, Rosenblum ML: Trends in the management of bacterial brain abscesses: A review of 102 cases over 17 years. Neurosurgery 23:451–458, 1988.

56. Boom WH, Tuazon CU: Successful treatment of multiple brain abscesses with antibiotics alone. Rev Infect Dis 7:189–199, 1985.

57. Rousseaux M, Lesoin F, Destee A, et al: Developments in the treatment and prognosis of multiple cerebral abscesses. Neurosurgery 16:304–308, 1985.

58. Mamelak AN, Mampalam TJ, Obana WG, et al: Improved management of multiple brain abscesses: A combined surgical and medical approach. Neurosurgery 36:76–86, 1995.

59. Adachi J, Uki J, Kazumoto K, et al: Diagnosis of brainstem abscess in the cerebritis stage by magnetic resonance imaging—case report. Neurol Med Chir (Tokyo) 35:467–470, 1995.

60. Chacko AG, Chandy MJ: Diagnostic and staged stereotactic aspiration of multiple bihemispheric pyogenic brain abscess. Surg Neurol 48:278–282, 1997.

61. Skrap M, Melatini A, Vassallo A, Sidoti C: Stereotactic aspiration and drainage of brain abscesses: Experience with 9 cases. Minim Invasive Neurosurg 39:108–112, 1996.

62. Bavetta S, Paterakis M, Srivatsa SR, Garvan N: Brainstem abscess: Preoperative MRI appearance and survival following stereotactic aspiration. J Neurosurg Sci 40:139–143, 1996.

63. Hellwig D, Bauer BL, Dauch WA: Endoscopic stereotactic treatment of brain abscesses. Acta Neurochir Suppl 61:102–105, 1994.

64. Fritsch M, Manwaring KH: Endoscopic treatment of brain abscess in children. Minim Invasive Neurosurg 40:103–106, 1997.

65. Shahzadi S, Lozano AM, Bernstein M, et al: Stereotactic management of bacterial brain abscesses. Can J Neurol Sci 23:34–39, 1996.

66. Young RF, Frazee J: Gas within intracranial abscess cavities: An indication for surgical excision. Ann Neurol 16:35–39, 1984.

67. Boviatis EJ, Kouyialis AT, et al: CT-guided stereotactic aspiration of brain abscess. Neurosurg Rev 26:206–209, 2003.

68. Dyste GN, Hitchon PW, Menezes AH, et al: Stereotaxic surgery in the treatment of multiple brain abscesses. J Neurosurg 69:188–194, 1988.

69. Isono W, Wakabayashi Y, Nakano T, et al: Treatment of brain abscess with ventricular rupture—three case reports. Neurol Med Chir (Tokyo) 37:630–636, 1997.

70. Zeidman SM, Geisler FH, Olivi A: Intraventricular rupture of purulent brain abscess: Case report. Neurosurgery 36:189–193, 1995.

71. Alderson D, Strong AJ, Ingham HR, et al: Fifteen-year review of the mortality of brain abscess. Neurosurgery 8:1–6, 1981.

72. Legg NJ, Gupta PC, Scott DF: Epilepsy following cerebral abscess: A clinical and EEG study of 70 patients. Brain 96:259–268, 1973.

73. Malone DG, O'Boynick PL, Ziegler DK, et al: Osteomyelitis of the skull base. Neurosurgery 30:426–431, 1992.

74. Seabold JE, Simonson TM, Weber PC, et al: Cranial osteomyelitis: Diagnosis and follow-up with In-111 white blood cell and Tc-99 methylene diphosphonate bone SPECT, CT, and MR imaging. Radiology 196:779–788, 1995.

75. Blomstedt GC: Craniotomy infections. Neurosurg Clin N Am 3:375–385, 1992.

76. Townsend GC, Scheld WM: Infections of the central nervous system. Adv Intern Med 43:403–447, 1998.

77. Hlavin ML, Kaminski HJ, Fenstermaker RA, et al: Intracranial suppuration: A modern decade of postoperative subdural empyema and epidural abscess. Neurosurgery 34:974–981, 1994.

78. Krauss WE, McCormick PC: Infections of the dural spaces. Neurosurg Clin N Am 3:421–433, 1992.

79. Dill SR, Cobbs CG, McDonald CK: Subdural empyema: Analysis of 32 cases and review. Clin Infect Dis 20:372–386, 1995.

80. Feuerman T, Wackym PA, Gade GF, et al: Craniotomy improves outcome in subdural empyema. Surg Neurol 32:105–110, 1989.

81. Miller ES, Dias PS, Utley D: Management of subdural empyema: A series of 24 cases. J Neurol Neurosurg Psychiatry 50:1415–1418, 1987.

82. Keet PC: Cranial intradural abscess management of 641 patients during the 35 years from 1952–1986. Br J Neurosurg 4:273–278, 1990.

83. Erdem H, Ozkan U, Devecioglu C, et al: Treatment of subdural empyema by burr hole. Isr J Med Sci 32:542–544, 1996.

84. Remy C, Grand S, Lai ES, et al: ^{1}HMRS of human brain abscesses in vivo and in vitro. Magn Reson Med 34:508–514, 1995.

85. Natoo N, Nadvi SS, Gouws E, van Dellen JR: Craniotomy improves outcomes for cranial subdural empyemas: Computed tomography-era experience with 699 patients. Neurosurgery 49:872–877, 2001.

114 Considerations of Infections after Craniotomy

GÖRAN C. BLOMSTEDT

Infection almost nullified surgical eminence before the 20th century and still claims a heavy toll after surgery. Meticulous hygiene is crucial for success in surgery, a truism that slowly spread in Western medicine in the 19th century. Cleansing was, however, recognized in ancient medicine: The word *hygiene* stems from Hygieia, the daughter of Aesculapius (latinization of Askleipos, 500 BC). In this chapter, aspects of central nervous system (CNS) infection, types of infection after craniotomy, their avoidance, and their treatment are considered. Shunt infections are not discussed in this chapter. Nonspecific problems, such as urinary tract infection, pneumonia, and bedsore, are not addressed.

INCIDENCE

Infection rates after craniotomy as reported during the 20th century are shown in Table 114-1.[1–24] Such percentages, however, must be looked on with skepticism, given the great variation in obtaining and conducting data. The most reliable data are obtained in connection with research projects, in which an investigator, using strictly specified criteria, scrutinizes all patient records, completed with questionnaires after discharge. Inclusion criteria, detection methods, and cohort base may vary (e.g., number of operations, number of patients operated on, number of patients discharged, or number of patients admitted) from study to study. A continuous infection register run by a hygienist, though not as reliable, is more useful for practical purposes because it allows detection of changes from year to year and even from month to month; for comparison between hospitals, it is of less value. The register is important in keeping track of bacterial strains and resistance patterns with special reference to highly resistant strains, such as methicillin-resistant *Staphylococcus aureus* and vancomycin-resistant *Enterococcus*.

VARIABLES AFFECTING INFECTION RATE

Infection rates fell sharply after the introduction of antisepsis and asepsis, but complete eradication of infections seems impossible to achieve. Human defense mechanisms usually have the edge over bacteria that are always present in the environment, and infection occurs as a result of a faltering balance between defenses, bacterial quantity, and bacterial virulence. Defenses are weakened with age, poor physical or mental condition, devitalized tissue, and foreign bodies. The quantity of bacterial contamination increases with large surgical fields, with reoperation, with long operating times, with inadequate aseptic technique, and with poor ventilation of the operating room.[25] Efforts to pinpoint single influences predisposing to infection are rarely convincing: isolation of one particular variable may be possible in laboratory conditions but is nearly always unreliable in a clinical situation; the impact of most variables is so small that extremely large groups are required to show statistical significance. Many recommendations are difficult to prove—for example, that a shunt operation should be done as the first procedure in the morning, that only a minimum of traffic should be allowed in the operating room, and that infected patients should be operated on as the last procedure of the day. In fact, most measures usually turn out to be nonsignificant when singled out. An example of this was a study showing that shaving the scalp before craniotomy is not necessary.[26] Most hospitals have their own routines, and although they differ, one may be just as good as the other. Nonetheless, it is probably advantageous to have a fairly rigorous scheme to be followed by all and taught to newcomers, the central issue being to minimize contamination.

TABLE 114-1 ▪ Infections after Craniotomy*

Author, Year	Percentage
von Eiselsberg and Ranzi,[1] 1913	12
Tooth,[2] 1913	12
Olivecrona,[3] 1934	15
Cushing and Eisenhardt,[4] 1938	2
Cairns,[5] 1939	2
Woodhall et al,[6] 1949	1
Wright,[7] 1966	6
Skultety and Nishioka,[8] 1966	2
Balch,[9] 1967	5
Green et al,[10] 1974	3
Chou and Erickson,[11] 1976	3
Cruse,[12] 1977	2
Quadery et al,[13] 1977	6
Chan and Thompson,[14] 1984	7
Jomin et al,[15] 1984	3
Vlahov et al,[16] 1984	7
Blomstedt,[17] 1985	8
Tenney et al,[18] 1985	4
van Ek et al,[19] 1986	8
Rasmussen et al,[20] 1990	6
Gaillard and Gilsbach,[21] 1991	9
Mindermann et al,[22] 1993	9
NNIS,[23] 1996	1
Korinek,[24] 1997	4

*When the article deals with prophylactic antibiotics, the infection rate for the group without antibiotics is given in this table. All figures are rounded to the nearest full number.

POSTOPERATIVE CEREBROSPINAL FLUID LEAK

Cerebrospinal fluid (CSF) leak after surgery and operation in a patient with a concurrent, non-CNS infection are, according to a retrospective study by Mollman and Haines[25] on 9202 neurosurgical patients, influences that increase the risk of infection. In a retrospective study by Blomstedt[17] of 1039 intracranial procedures (shunts excluded), postoperative CSF leak was also found to be the only highly significant risk factor: of 15 patients with a CSF leak, 6 developed infection versus 54 patients among 1024 patients without a CSF leak ($p = 0.0002$, Fischer's exact test). Every effort should be made to avoid CSF leak and to seal the leak if it occurs. If the dura cannot be completely closed, dural repair can usually be done with tissue obtained within the operating field, such as periosteum or fascia or, when big patches are required, fascia lata. Fat is quite efficient, especially for drilled-out cavities in the pneumatized bone. Fibrin glue may resorb too quickly to allow natural membranes to form, but is helpful for fixation of the patch.[27] Fear of human immunodeficiency virus, bovine spongiform encephalitis, and Creuzfeldt-Jakob disease has reduced the use of dura obtained from animals or cadavers.[101] This risk has been reduced considerably by preparing completely acellular material from animal membranes.[28] Several convenient artificial dural substitutes are available, but such nonvascularized material always runs the risk of contamination.[29] Biodegradable dural substitutes[30,31] offer the advantage that bacteria adhering to the material will over time lose their safe haven.

If CSF leak occurs after surgery, lumbar taps or draining may be helpful. Lumbar drainage lowers the CSF pressure, thus reducing the flow of CSF and allowing the fistula to scar. CSF drainage may cause retrograde flow through the fistula leading to pneumocephalus—a phenomenon more common in spontaneous than in postoperative CSF leak—which increases the risk of infection. In such cases early surgical repair is advisable. Persistent CSF leak may also be due to low levels of factor XIII.[32] In difficult cases, especially after repeated operations and radiotherapy, a microvascular tissue transplant may be necessary to seal the leak. If possible a locally harvested piece of muscle, with the vasculature intact, is convenient,[33] but a piece of anterior serratus muscle and its vessels can often be anastomosed to the superficial temporal artery and vein. Hydroxyapatite, a moldable bone substitute, is suitable for cranioplasty and has been used to seal defects in the skull base.[102]

Perioperative corticosteroids are widely used in connection with craniotomies to reduce postoperative brain swelling. These agents may have a negative effect on the healing of dura mater and arachnoid.[34]

The value of prophylactic antimicrobials with a CSF leak is controversial.[35] If one decides to use an antimicrobial in these circumstances, an agent is selected that is effective against the organisms that are most likely to be in the affected area (e.g., if leaking through the nose, the flora of the upper respiratory tract, such as *Diplococcus pneumoniae* and *Haemophilus influenzae*,[36] or if leaking through the skin, *Staphylococcus epidermidis*, *S. aureus*, and *Propionibacterium acnes*).[17] A CSF fistula substantially increases the risk of intracranial infection, and antimicrobial prophylaxis seems justified. In cases of CSF rhinorrhea, I use an oral penicillin, which covers most bacteria in the nose but causes few problems with resistance. In CSF leak through the skin, I use a first-generation cephalosporin.

PROPHYLACTIC ANTIMICROBIALS IN CRANIOTOMY

The value of antimicrobial prophylaxis in clean craniotomy is well documented in several controlled studies,[21,22,37-44] although other studies do not support the prophylactic use of antimicrobials in this situation.[24,45] The negative effects of antimicrobial prophylaxis are possible induction of resistant organisms, inadvertent slackening of aseptic discipline, idiosyncratic reactions to the drug, and expense of the drug. Because the recommended regimen involves a single perioperative dose, only the issue of aseptic techniques and the rare idiosyncratic reaction are relevant. Because the prophylaxis is targeted at the most likely organisms, an antimicrobial with a fairly narrow spectrum can be selected. Most investigators use a second- or third-generation cephalosporin, vancomycin, or fusidic acid. In my study, I chose vancomycin for prophylactic use for three reasons: (1) At the time, bone flap infection was the commonest infection in the department (Table 114-2), and vancomycin covered

---

TABLE 114-2 ▪ Infections after 1039 Intracranial Procedures*

	Suprat.	Infrat.	Translab.	Transsph.	Burr Hole	Ventric.	All
Superficial wound	13	1					14
Bone flap	29						29
Bacterial meningitis	5	3	2		1		11
Intracranial abscess	3		2		1		6
General sepsis	3				1		4
% Total infections	**53**	**4**	**4**		**3**		**64**
	9	4	100	0	2	0	6
Aseptic meningitis	19	9			3	1	13
Total procedures	**622**	**101**	**4**	**41**	**182**	**89**	**1039**

Infrat., infratentorial or suboccipital craniotomy; Suprat., supratentorial craniotomy; Translab., translabyrinthine approach; Transsph., transsphenoidal approach; Ventric., ventricular drainage.

*Shunt infection, urinary tract infection, and pneumonia not included.

Data from Blomstedt GC: Infections in neurosurgery: A retrospective study of 1143 patients and 1517 operations. Acta Neurochir (Wien) 78:81–90, 1985.

well the probable organisms staphylococci and *P. acnes*; (2) vancomycin was used sparingly; (3) resistance against vancomycin was extremely rare. The institution of routine vancomycin prophylaxis in all craniotomies brought about a substantial reduction in bone flap infections.[40] Vancomycin must be infused slowly to avoid flushing, the so-called red man's syndrome.[46,103] There is no antimicrobial agent that can be recommended universally. Each neurosurgical department must identify the specific types of infections it most frequently encounters, the infection rate (prophylactic antimicrobial treatment is recommended if it is >3%) and the bacteria that are most likely involved; moreover, the routines must be changed from time to time as circumstances change.

POSTCRANIOTOMY INFECTIONS

Infections after craniotomy can be divided into those within the CNS (e.g., meningitis and cerebral and subdural abscesses) and those outside the CNS (e.g., superficial wound and bone flap infections). These infections may spread from one compartment to the other, but different infections are to a large extent caused by different bacteria.

Central Nervous System Defenses against Infections

Bacteria do not readily cross the blood-brain barrier and blood-CSF barrier, but when these defenses are breached, the CSF is ill equipped to mount an efficient defense against bacteria. Such a defense requires high-affinity or type-specific antibodies. The complement system reacts with the antigen-bacteria complex to induce lysis, and opsonins combine with bacteria and bacterial fragments and render them susceptible for phagocytosis by polymorphonuclear cells. Normal CSF contains low concentrations of specific antibodies, complement, and opsonic proteins, or none, and polymorphonuclear cells are slow to reach the site of infection. If bacteria multiply rapidly, the opsonin supply can quickly be exhausted. Antimicrobial therapy, especially with a bacteriostatic antimicrobial, falls short in the absence of an efficient host response. The opsonic capacity seems to correlate with the leukocyte count of the infected CSF. A vigorous inflammatory response aids in the fight against infection by increasing penetration of opsonic protein and polymorphonuclear cells, but inflammation also causes cortical damage.

Most bacterial species (e.g., *Pneumococcus*, *Haemophilus*, *Meningococcus*, *Klebsiella*) that commonly cause meningitis possess a capsule that hampers opsonization, which in this situation is important for bacterial virulence. In contrast, the unencapsulated *S. aureus* rarely causes meningitis but frequently causes bacteremia, which the encapsulated bacteria rarely do.[47–52]

Antimicrobial Penetration into Cerebrospinal Fluid

Several conditions limit antimicrobial penetration into the CSF. The capillary bed of the choroid plexus and the meninges is nonfenestrated, and all organic compounds must pass through a lipid membrane. The lipid solubility of the antimicrobial agent is a variable in penetration. Ionization of the antimicrobial is another variable: the more ionized, the less lipid soluble. The pKa of penicillin G is 2.6, and at physiologic pH, the degree of ionization is high. The pH in plasma is normally 7.4 and in CSF 7.3, and the pH gradient between plasma and CSF favors outflux of lipid-soluble antimicrobials from the CSF. In purulent meningitis, acid metabolites lower the pH of CSF, which increases this gradient and reduces antimicrobial penetration. Other mechanisms associated with meningeal inflammation increase penetration into the CSF severalfold. A high degree of antimicrobial protein binding also reduces CSF penetration, as do high-molecular-weight and complex molecular structure. In addition, there are active bidirectional transport mechanisms for antimicrobials.[53–59]

Bacterial Meningitis

Postoperative bacterial meningitis is not common, but it is potentially lethal. External CSF drainage devices are commonly used in the intensive care unit and are risk factors for meningitis (odds ratio, 21.8; $p = 0.001$), as are extended antimicrobial treatment and infections elsewhere in the body.[60–62] Staphylococci do not cause spontaneous meningitis but produce postoperative meningitis, as do the gram-negative bacilli.[17,36,63–65] A fever is common in the postoperative period. If the temperature is very high, persistently high, rising, or fluctuating, particularly with a rising C-reactive protein, stiff neck, deteriorating consciousness, new neurologic symptoms, or a CSF fistula, meningitis should be suspected. If the level of consciousness is altered, a computed tomography (CT) scan is done before lumbar puncture. The CSF leukocyte criteria for postoperative meningitis is 100×10^6 cells/L with a minimum of 50% polymorphonuclear cells, or 400×10^6 cells/L regardless of the polymorphonuclear percentage.[66] The CSF glucose test is of little value in making the diagnosis of postoperative meningitis. Because the CSF cultures require 2 to 3 days, an elevated CSF cell count is used to decide the initial line of treatment.[36] Gram stain may show bacteria and may aid in the selection of antibiotics. Antibodies against bacterial substances, such as *Enterobacter* common antigen and teichoic acid, have not been useful. Determination of the probable route of infection helps in selecting the appropriate antimicrobial agent: airway bacteria (e.g., *Diplococcus pneumoniae*, *H. influenzae*, and streptococci) can be expected with a CSF leak through the ear or the nose, whereas staphylococci and gram-negative bacilli are more likely to be present if the leak comes through the skin.[17,36,67–69]

When one cannot identify a specific bacterial agent, the third-generation cephalosporins are good first-time antimicrobials,[70,71] although resistance may render them ineffective when most needed.[72–75] Intrathecal or intraventricular administration of some antimicrobials is possible if good antibiotic penetration into the CSF is not achieved by other routes. The aminoglycosides, in particular, have been successfully used, as has vancomycin. Cloxacillin, cephalosporins, and even penicillin have been used in this context, but the latter two may cause seizures, particularly when intrathecally administered.[76–79] The new antimicrobials, however, have made intrathecal and intraventricular administration unnecessary in most cases. The third-generation cephalosporins have a broad spectrum and a good effect at low concentrations and are suitable for infections in the CNS. The third-generation cephalosporins are fairly interchangeable, but cefotaxime and ceftizoxime have a slight edge against staphylococci, whereas ceftazidime and ceftriaxone may have an edge against *Pseudomonas*. Cefotaxime may penetrate the CNS slightly better than ceftriaxone. Ampicillin has become more useful when combined with sulbactam, a β-lactamase inhibitor. Aztreonam, a monocyclic β-lactam antimicrobial, penetrates well into the CSF and is a potent alternative in gram-negative meningitis, when the cephalosporins, penicillins, or aminoglycosides fail. It can be combined with antimicrobials against staphylococci and anaerobic bacteria.[80] The fluoroquinolones penetrate well into the CSF and are so well absorbed from the intestines that intravenous administration does not offer any advantage over oral administration.[81,82] Ofloxacin has a better effect against staphylococci, whereas ciprofloxacin is more potent against *Pseudomonas*.[83] Teicoplanin is a comparatively new antimicrobial, effective against aerobic and anaerobic gram-positive bacteria even when they are resistant against most other antimicrobials. This agent is not active against gram-negative bacilli and does not readily penetrate into the CNS in the absence of meningitis.

Antimicrobials are potent drugs but will remain so only if used cautiously; when the bacterium is known, a narrow-spectrum antimicrobial is preferred, and new-generation antimicrobials should be avoided unless they offer a clear advantage.

Postoperative Aseptic Meningitis

Most articles about aseptic meningitis refer to viral meningitis, an entity different from the postoperative aseptic meningitis discussed here. Reliable tests to distinguish between postoperative aseptic and bacterial meningitis are not available; only bacterial culture can help distinguish between the two.[66,84] When the bacterial culture is negative, the probable diagnosis is aseptic meningitis, yet there is a reluctance to trust a negative culture because a poorly treated bacterial meningitis may be fatal.[85] In one study on postoperative meningitis, all patients with the CSF leukocyte count indicating meningitis were started on antimicrobial treatment, and on the second or third day, when the cultures were available, those with negative cultures were assigned to a group on continued treatment or to a group in which antibiotic treatment was discontinued. No difference was found between the groups.[66] For the last decade, my routine for patients with meningitis has been to stop antimicrobial treatment if the cultures are negative. No randomized study is available to establish the value of corticosteroids in the treatment of postoperative aseptic meningitis, although Carmel and associates[86] suggest that corticosteroids may have a beneficial effect.

Postoperative Subdural and Brain Abscess

Postoperative brain abscess is uncommon, and when brain abscess developing after craniotomy is compared with patients with brain abscess of other origin, those who had undergone craniotomy were notable for older age, lack of fever,

evidence of wound infection, frequent false-negative CT scan, and a high percentage of gram-negative aerobic organisms or skin flora as pathogens.[24,87] In a study of 2941 patients who had undergone clean craniotomy, 39 patients developed intracranial abscess or empyema within 3 months of surgery. Of those, 14 had been operated on for a malignant glioma.[88] Subdural empyemas are sometimes connected with bone flap infection and sometimes with wound infection after burr hole evacuation of chronic subdural hematomas. In a retrospective study of postoperative infections, there were six abscesses after 1039 intracranial procedures: five subdural and one intracerebral (see Table 114-2).[17] The elapsed time from operation to the diagnosis of the abscess had a mean of 31 days. One patient had concomitant meningitis, one a bone flap infection, and one a superficial wound infection. Three of these patients died, one of these possibly as a result of this complication. One abscess was found at autopsy.

The diagnosis may be difficult because postoperative CT changes or tumor recurrence may mimic infections, but repeated CT scans and the clinical picture usually show progression. Diffusion-weighted magnetic resonance imaging may be beneficial for differentiating between the two.[89] Laboratory parameters, such as C-reactive protein or CSF leukocyte count, are not necessarily altered.[88,90] The treatment follows the same principles as with spontaneous abscesses[91]: antimicrobial treatment may suffice if the abscess is small, but surgical evacuation is usually necessary. Extirpation of an intracerebral abscess is sometimes preferred but may be more complicated than for spontaneous abscesses resulting from postoperative changes. The bacteria found in the study mentioned earlier[17] were *S. epidermidis*, *S. aureus*, and *P. acnes* (i.e., bacteria typical for wound and bone flap infection). The antimicrobial treatment should be adjusted when the culture is available, but because a brain abscess does not usually cause a meningeal reaction, drug penetration may be much less than in meningitis. A third-generation cephalosporin is a good first-line drug.

Superficial Postoperative Cranial Wound Infection

A superficial wound infection in the head has the potential to spread to the bone flap and to the meninges, and therefore these infections are of great concern.[68] To avoid wound infection, one must be punctilious in closing the wound: no devitalized tissue should be allowed, wound apposition should be meticulous, and the sutures should be slack enough to allow for normal wound swelling. Superficial infections do not readily spread to the meninges if the dura is intact, but the dura is often not watertight, and a CSF collection is often seen underneath the skin. In noninfected cases, spinal drainage can keep the persistently refilling subcutaneous space collapsed to allow the skin to adhere to the skull. With a skin infection, this drainage may promote spread of infection to the intradural space.

If there is frank CSF leak through the skin, a couple of stitches usually seals off the fistula, but suturing an infected skin or sealing the fistula may aggravate the infection and cause the fistula to grow. Instead, it may be necessary to reopen the wound, repair the dura, and, if possible, débride the wound. Difficult cases may require a vascularized flap to withstand the infection and adhere to the surrounding tissue. Lavish use of antimicrobials should generally be condemned, but the danger of the spread of infection from superficial to deeper layers after craniotomy is serious enough to warrant their use on clinical suspicion alone until bacterial cultures are available. For early detection of surgical wound infection, a plastic intravenous catheter can be inserted daily into the most inflamed part of the wound, then rolled across a blood agar plate. In the report on this technique, more than 15 colonies arising from near the tip of the catheter correlated with the occurrence of subsequent infection.[92] Patients in relatively poor condition who would in the past have been beyond neurosurgical treatment, are now treated; therefore, a prolonged stay in the intensive care unit is common. A combination of this and abundant use of antibiotics cause selection of the bacterial flora. Bacteria such as *Acinetobacter* may become endemic in such environments. Finding the reservoir requires diligence and, to identify specific species, special methods such as amplified ribosomal DNA restriction analysis.[93]

Postoperative Bone Flap Infection

In craniotomy, the bone is disconnected from the skull, devascularized, and devitalized. This process reduces the bone's natural resistance to infection and hampers antimicrobials from reaching the infectious focus. A bone flap infection may cause high fever, local suppuration, or a stubborn fistula. The standard treatment is removal of the infected bone flap, with cranioplasty months later.[94,95] Various artificial bone substitutes are on the market, and here too biodegradable alternatives have become available.[96] Repeated local débridement with long-term antimicrobial treatment may make bone removal unnecessary.[97] Chou and Erickson[11] used closed suction irrigation with topical antibiotics to save 50% of infected bone flaps. Some surgeons advocate leaving the bone flap attached to a muscle pedicle to preserve blood flow and resistance to infection; however, in a study comparing free with pedicled bone flaps, there was no difference in the rate of infection, but fewer pedicled bone flaps ultimately had to be removed.[20] My personal preference is a free bone flap, removed using meticulous no-touch technique and kept in a jar away from the surgical field until replaced. Releasing the muscle from the bone obviates freeing the temporal muscle from the skin flap and allows one to divide the muscle only posteriorly, and a broader base may leave the temporal muscle healthier.

Prophylactic antimicrobials are indicated in a craniotomy with a bone flap. This operation creates a devascularized body with reduced resistance against infection, and after a randomized study in my department, I routinely use one intraoperative dose of vancomycin in all craniotomies.[40] Vancomycin was chosen because of its narrow bacterial spectrum, which targets most bacteria causing bone flap infection: *S. aureus*, *S. epidermidis*, and *P. acnes*.[17,95–100] In a series of 2425 craniotomies in my department after the introduction of vancomycin prophylaxis, there were 15 bone flap infections (0.6%). This result compares (see Table 114-2) with a previous series with 29 bone flap infections after 622 supratentorial craniotomies (4.7%). Of the 15 patients in the latter series, 5 were prone to

circumstances reducing the effect of the antibiotic prophylaxis: two patients had open traumatic wounds, one was mentally debilitated and scraped his wound, one had to have his wound resutured due to unsatisfactory closure, and one underwent two craniotomies for trauma within 2 days, the vancomycin being neglected in the second operation.

CONCLUSIONS

The CNS is relatively well protected against invasion by infective agents, but when invasion does occur the defenses are relatively poor. Penetration of antimicrobial agents into the CNS varies from agent to agent but is usually lower than in the blood. These special circumstances have been discussed.

Postcraniotomy infections may occur in the CNS as meningitis or brain abscess or outside the CNS as a superficial wound infection or bone flap infection. The incidence on a neurosurgical service should not exceed 5%, but comparison between hospitals may be misleading: the figures depend on how the information is collected and on how the percentage is calculated. CSF leak increases the risk of infection and should be painstakingly avoided or promptly addressed if it occurs. The high risk of meningitis justifies antimicrobial prophylaxis in this situation. The choice of antimicrobial agent should be based on the bacteria that are most likely to be present; these differ if the CSF leak is through the nose or through the skin. Intraoperative antimicrobial prophylaxis in craniotomy is recommended because of the increased infection susceptibility of the free bone flap. The bone flap is devascularized tissue and, as is the case with foreign bodies, infection usually leads to its surgical removal. Superficial wound infection should be avoided through meticulous handling of the tissue and exact apposition without undue tension.

REFERENCES

1. von Eiselsberg AF, Ranzi E: Über die chirurgische Behandlung der Hirn und Ruckenmarkstumoren. Arch Klin Chir 102:309–478, 1913.
2. Tooth HH: The treatment of tumours of the brain, and the indications for operations. Trans 1st Cong Med London 8:203–299, 1913.
3. Olivecrona H: Die Parasagittalen Meningeome. Leipzig: Georg Thieme, 1934, pp 141–143.
4. Cushing H, Eisenhardt L: Meningiomas, Their Classification, Regional Behaviour, Life History, and Surgical End Results. Springfield, IL: Charles C Thomas, 1938, pp 733–734.
5. Cairns H: Bacterial infections during intracranial operations. Lancet 1:1193–1198, 1939.
6. Woodhall B, Neill RG, Dratz HM: Ultraviolet radiation as an adjunct in the control of post-operative neurosurgical infection. Ann Surg 129:820–825, 1949.
7. Wright RL: Postoperative Craniotomy Infections. Springfield, IL: Charles C Thomas, 1966.
8. Skultety FM, Nishioka H: Report on the cooperative study of intracranial aneurysms and subarachnoid hemorrhage: Section VIII, part 2. The results of intracranial surgery in the treatment of aneurysms. J Neurosurg 25:783–704, 1966.
9. Balch RE: Wound infection complicating neurosurgical procedures. J Neurosurg 26:41–44, 1967.
10. Green JR, Kanshepolsky J, Turkian B: Incidence and significance of central nervous system infection in neurosurgical patients. Adv Neurol 6:223–228, 1974.
11. Chou SN, Erickson DL: Craniotomy infections. Clin Neurosurg 23:357–362, 1976.
12. Cruse PJE: Infection surveillance. South Med J 70:48, 1977.
13. Quadery LA, Medley AV, Miles J: Factors affecting the incidence of wound infection in neurosurgery. Acta Neurochir (Wien) 39:133–141, 1977.

14. Chan RC, Thompson GB: Morbidity, mortality, and quality of life following surgery for intracranial meningioma. J Neurosurg 60:52–60, 1984.
15. Jomin M, Lesoin F, Lozes G: 500 ruptured and operated intracranial arterial aneurysm. Surg Neurol 21:13–18, 1984.
16. Vlahov D, Montgomery E, Tenney JH, et al: Neurosurgical wound infections: Methodological and clinical factors affecting calculations of infection rates. J Neurosurg Nurs 16:128–133, 1984.
17. Blomstedt GC: Infections in neurosurgery: A retrospective study of 1143 patients and 1517 operations. Acta Neurochir (Wien) 78:81–90, 1985.
18. Tenney JH, Vlahov D, Salcman M, et al: Wide variation in risk of wound infection following clean neurosurgery: Implications for perioperative antibiotic prophylaxis. J Neurosurg 62:243–247, 1985.
19. van Ek B, Bakker FP, van Dulken H, Dijkmans BA: Infections after craniotomy: A retrospective study. J Infect 12:105–109, 1986.
20. Rasmussen S, Ohrstrom JK, Westergaard L, Kosteljanetz M: Postoperative infections of osteoplastic compared with free bone flaps. Br J Neurosurg 4:493–495, 1990.
21. Gaillard T, Gilsbach JM: Intra-operative antibiotic prophylaxis in neurosurgery: A prospective, randomized, controlled study on cefotiam. Acta Neurochir (Wien) 113:103–109, 1991.
22. Mindermann T, Zimmerli W, Gratzl O: Randomized placebo-controlled trial of single-dose antibiotic prophylaxis with fusidic acid in neurosurgery. Acta Neurochir (Wien) 121:9–11, 1993.
23. National Nosocomial Infections Surveillance (NNIS) report, data summary from October 1986–April 1996, issued May 1996. A report from the National Nosocomial Infections Surveillance (NNIS) System. Am J Infect Control 24:380–388, 1996.
24. Korinek AM: Risk factors for neurosurgical site infections after craniotomy: A prospective multicenter study of 2944 patients. Neurosurgery 41:1073–1081, 1997.
25. Mollman HD, Haines SJ: Risk factors for postoperative neurosurgical wound infection: A case control study. J Neurosurg 64:902–906, 1986.
26. Lamas R, Picallos J, Pereira J, et al: Cranial Procedures without shaving. A 1-year experience at the Hospital Sao Joao [in Spanish]. Neurocirugia (Asturias, Spain) 14:140–143, 2003.
27. Kassam A, Horowitz M, Carrau R, et al: Use of Tisseel fibrin sealant in neurosurgical procedures: Incidence of cerebrospinal fluid leaks and cost-benefit analysis in a retrospective study. Neurosurgery 52:1102–1105, 2003.
28. Maher CO, Anderson RE, McClelland RL, et al: Evaluation of a novel propylene oxide-treated collagen material as a dural substitute. J Neurosurg 99:1070–1087, 2003.
29. Jallo GI, Koslow M, Hanna BA, et al: Propionibacterium as a cause of postneurosurgical infection in patients with dural allografts: Report of three cases. Neurosurgery 44:1138–1141, 1999.
30. Reddy M, Schoggl A, Reddy B, et al: A clinical study of a fibrinogen-based collagen fleece for dural repair in neurosurgery. Acta Neurochir (Wien) 144:265–269, 2002.
31. von Wild KR: Examination of the safety and efficacy of an absorbable dura mater substitute (Dura Patch) in normal applications in neurosurgery. Surg Neurol 52:418–424, 1999.
32. Kawamura A, Tamaki N, Yonezawa K, et al: Effect of factor XIII on intractable CSF leakage after a transpetrosal-approach operation: A case report. No Shinkei Geka 25:53–56, 1997.
33. Saint-Cyr M, Nikolis A, Moumdjian R, et al: Paraspinous muscle flaps for the treatment and prevention of cerebrospinal fluid fistulas in neurosurgery. Spine 28:86–92, 2003.
34. Marion DW, Janetta PJ: Use of perioperative steroids with microvascular decompression operations. Neurosurgery 22:353–357, 1988.
35. Clemenza JW, Kaltman SI, Diamond DL: Craniofacial trauma and cerebrospinal fluid leakage: A retrospective clinical study. J Oral Maxillofac Surg 53:1004–1007, 1995.
36. Kaufman BA, Tunkel AR, Pryor JC, Dacey RG Jr: Meningitis in the neurosurgical patient. Infect Dis Clin North Am 4:677–701, 1990.
37. Geraghty J, Feely M: Antibiotic prophylaxis in neurosurgery: A randomized controlled trial. J Neurosurg 60:724–726, 1984.
38. Shapiro M, Wald U, Simchen E, et al: Randomized clinical trial of intraoperative antimicrobial prophylaxis of infection after neurosurgical procedures. J Hosp Infect 8:283–295, 1986.
39. Young RF, Lawner PM: Perioperative antibiotic prophylaxis for the prevention of postoperative neurosurgical infections: A randomized clinical trial. J Neurosurg 66:701–706, 1987.
40. Blomstedt GC, Kytta J: Results of a randomized trial of vancomycin prophylaxis in craniotomy. J Neurosurg 69:216–220, 1988.
41. van Ek B, Dijkmans BA, van Dulken H, van Furth R: Antibiotic prophylaxis in craniotomy: A prospective double-blind placebo-controlled study. Scand J Infect Dis 20:633–639, 1988.
42. Winkler D, Rehn H, Freckmann N, et al: Clinical efficacy of perioperative antimicrobial prophylaxis in neurosurgery: A prospective randomized study involving 159 patients. Chemotherapy 35:304–312, 1989.
43. van Ek B, Dijkmans BA, van Dulken H, et al: Effect of cloxacillin prophylaxis on the bacterial flora of craniotomy wounds. Scand J Infect Dis 22:345–352, 1990.
44. van Ek B, Dijkmans BA, van Dulken H, et al: Clinical, bacteriological and cost-saving effects of antibiotic prophylaxis in craniotomy. Ned Tijdschr Geneeskd 136:16–20, 1992.
45. Rocca B, Mallet MN, Scemama F, et al: Perioperative remote infections in neurosurgery: Role of antibiotic prophylaxis [in French]. Presse Med 21:2037–2040, 1992.
46. Garrelts JC, Peterie JD: Vancomycin and the "red man's syndrome." N Engl J Med 312:245, 1985.
47. Simberkoff MS, Moldover NH, Rahal JJ Jr: Absence of detectable bactericidal and opsonic activities in normal and infected human cerebrospinal fluids: A regional host defense deficiency. J Lab Clin Med 95:362–372, 1980.
48. Waldvogel FA: Pathophysiological mechanisms in pyogenic infection: Two examples—pleural empyema and acute bacterial meningitis. In Majno G, Cotran RS, Kaufman N (eds): Current Topics in Inflammation and Infection. Baltimore: Williams & Wilkins, 1982, pp 115–122.
49. Zwahlen A, Nydegger UE, Vaudaux P, et al: Complement-mediated opsonic activity in normal and infected human cerebrospinal fluid: Early response during bacterial meningitis. J Infect Dis 145:635–646, 1982.
50. Bernhardt LL, Simberkoff MS, Rahal JJ Jr: Deficient cerebrospinal fluid opsonization in experimental Escherichia coli meningitis. Infect Immun 32:411–413, 1981.
51. Giampaolo C, Scheld M, Boyd J, et al: Leukocyte and bacterial inter-relationship in experimental meningitis. Ann Neurol 9:328–333, 1981.
52. Tofte RW, Peterson PK, Youngki K, et al: Opsonic activity of normal human cerebrospinal fluid for selected bacterial species. Infect Immunol 26:1093–1098, 1979.
53. Norrby R: A review of the penetration of antibiotics into CSF and its clinical significance. Scand J Infect Dis 14(Suppl):296–309, 1978.
54. Sande MA, Sherertz RJ, Zak O, et al: Factors influencing the penetration of antimicrobial agents into the cerebrospinal fluid of experimental animals. Scand J Infect Dis 14(Suppl):160–163, 1978.
55. Bergman T: Kinetics of tissue penetration. Scand J Infect Dis 14(Suppl):36–46, 1978.
56. Craig WA, Welling PG: Protein binding of antimicrobials: Clinical pharmacokinetics and therapeutic implications. Clin Pharmacokinet 2:252–278, 1977.
57. Fishman RA: Blood-brain and CSF barriers to penicillin and related organic acids. Arch Neurol 15:113–124, 1966.
58. Schanker LS: Passage of drugs into and out of the central nervous system. Antimicrob Agents Chemother 5:1044–1050, 1965.
59. Spector R, Levy P: The transport of gentamicin in the choroid plexus and cerebrospinal fluid. J Pharmacol Exp Ther 194:82–88, 1975.
60. Parodi S, Lechner A, Osih R, et al: Nosocomial Enterobacter meningitis: Risk factors, management, and treatment outcomes. Clin Infect Dis 37:159–166, 2003.
61. Huang CR, Lu CH, Chang WN: Adult Enterobacter meningitis: A high incidence of coinfection with other pathogens and frequent association with neurosurgical procedures. Infection 29:75–79, 2001.
62. Lozier AP, Sciacca RR, Romagnoli MF, Connolly ES Jr: Ventriculostomy-related infections: A critical review of the literature. Neurosurgery 51:170–182, 2002.
63. Dureux J, Voiriot P, Auque J, et al: Bases of antibiotherapy in neuromeningeal infections. Neurochirurgie 34:72–82, 1988.
64. Fong IW, Ranalli P: Staphylococcus aureus meningitis. QJM 53:289–299, 1984.
65. Mancebo J, Domingo P, Blanch L, et al: Postneurosurgical and spontaneous gram-negative bacillary meningitis in adults. Scand J Infect Dis 18:533–538, 1986.
66. Blomstedt GC: Postoperative aseptic meningitis. Acta Neurochir (Wien) 89:112–116, 1987.
67. Bryce GE, Nedzelski JM, Rowed DW, et al: Cerebrospinal fluid leaks and meningitis in acoustic neuroma surgery. Otolaryngol Head Neck Surg 107:81–87, 1991.

68. Chauveau D, Schlemmer B, Jedynak CP, et al: Postneurosurgical purulent meningitis: 31 cases. Presse Med 16:295–298, 1987.

69. Moore GF, Nissen AJ, Yonkers AJ: Potential complications of unrecognized cerebrospinal fluid leaks secondary to mastoid surgery. Am J Otol 5:317–323, 1984.

70. May T, Weber M, Gerard A, et al: Treatment of post-traumatic and post-neurosurgical bacterial meningitis with ceftriaxone alone or in combination with fosfomycin. Pathol Biol (Paris) 35:839–842, 1987.

71. Stahl JP, Croize J, Baud A, et al: Treatment of neurosurgical bacterial meningitis using the combination of ceftriaxone-fosfomycin. Pathol Biol (Paris) 34:479–482, 1986.

72. Brun-Buisson C, Philippon A, Ansquer M, et al: Transferable enzymatic resistance to third-generation cephalosporins during nosocomial outbreak of multiresistant *Klebsiella pneumoniae*. Lancet 2:302–306, 1987.

73. Sanders WE, Sanders CC: Inducible β-lactamases: Clinical and epidemiological implications for use of newer cephalosporins. Rev Infect Dis 10:830–838, 1988.

74. Parker RH, Park S: Safety of cefotaxime and other beta-lactam antibiotics. J Antimicrob Chemother 14(Suppl B):331–335, 1984.

75. de Lalla F, Privitera G, Ortisi G, et al: Third generation cephalosporins as a risk factor for *Clostridium difficile*–associated disease: A four-year survey in a general hospital. J Antimicrob Chemother 23:623–631, 1989.

76. Donauer E, Drumm G, Moringlane J, et al: Intrathecal administration of netilmicin in gentamicin-resistant ventriculitis. Acta Neurochir (Wien) 86:83–88, 1987.

77. Gump DW: Vancomycin for treatment of bacterial meningitis. Rev Infect Dis 3(Suppl):289–292, 1981.

78. Quintiliani R: The intrathecal and intraventricular administration of antibiotics in central nervous system infections. Conn Med 34:321–326, 1970.

79. Macfarlane DE, Baum-Thureen P, Crandon I: *Flavobacterium odoratum* ventriculitis treated with intraventricular cefotaxime. J Infect 11:233–238, 1985.

80. Sykes RB, Bonner DP: Aztreonam: The first monobactam. Am J Med 78(Suppl 2A):2–10, 1985.

81. Wise R, Lister T, McNulty CAM, et al: The comparative pharmacokinetics of five quinolones. J Antimicrob Chemother 18(Suppl D):71–81, 1986.

82. Wolff M, Reginer P, Daldoss C, et al: Penetration of pefloxacin into cerebrospinal fluid of patients with meningitis. Antimicrob Agents Chemother 26:289–291, 1984.

83. Wolfson JS, Hooper DC: The fluoroquinolones: Structures, mechanisms of action and resistance, and spectra of activity in vitro. Antimicrob Agent Chemother 28:581–586, 1985.

84. Brown EM: Infections in neurosurgery: Using laboratory data to plan optimal treatment strategies. Drugs 62:909–913, 2002.

85. Ross D, Rosegay H, Pons V: Differentiation of aseptic and bacterial meningitis in postoperative neurosurgical patients. J Neurosurg 69:669–674, 1988.

86. Carmel PW, Fraser RAR, Stein BM: Aseptic meningitis following posterior fossa surgery in children. J Neurosurg 41:44–48, 1974.

87. Hlavin ML, Kaminski HJ, Fenstermaker RA, White RJ: Intracranial suppuration: A modern decade of postoperative subdural empyema and epidural abscess. Neurosurgery 34:974–980, 1994.

88. Vogelsang JP, Wehe A, Markakis E: Postoperative intracranial abscess: Clinical aspects in the differential diagnosis to early recurrence of malignant glioma. Clin Neurol Neurosurg 100:11–14, 1998.

89. Guzman R, Barth A, Lovblad K-O, et al: Use of diffusion-weighted magnetic resonance imaging in differentiating purulent brain processes from cystic brain tumors. J Neurosurg 97:1101–1107, 2002.

90. Rousseaux M, Lesoin F, Clarisse J, et al: Postoperative abscesses and empyemas: A propos of 13 cases. Neurochirurgie 32:304–310, 1986.

91. Bidzinski J, Koszewski W: The value of different methods of treatment of brain abscess in the CT era. Acta Neurochir (Wien) 105:117–120, 1990.

92. Yip AW, Yuen KY, Seto WH, et al: A new semiquantitative culture method for early detection of surgical incisional wound infection. J Infect Dis 161:972–981, 1990.

93. Chandra R, Kapil A, Sharma P, et al: Identification of *Acinetobacter* species isolated from clinical specimens by amplified ribosomal DNA restriction analysis. Ind J Med Res 116:1–4, 2002.

94. Bullit E, Lehman RAW: Osteomyelitis of the skull. Surg Neurol 11:163–166, 1979.

95. Haines SJ, Chou SN: Infections of the scalp and osteomyelitis of the skull. In Wilkins RH, Rengachary SS (eds): Neurosurgery. New York: McGraw-Hill, 1985, pp 1964–1967.

96. Stendel R, Krischek B, Pietila TA: Biodegradable implants in neurosurgery. Acta Neurochir (Wien) 143:237–243, 2001.

97. Bruce JN, Bruce SS: Preservation of bone flaps in patients with postcraniotomy infections. J Neurosurg 98:1203–1207, 2003.

98. Sande MA, Mandell GL: Antimicrobial agents: Miscellaneous antimicrobial agents. In Goodman LS, Gilman A (eds): Goodman and Gilman's The Pharmacological Basis of Therapeutics. New York: Macmillan, 1980, p 1231.

99. Collignon PJ, Munro R, Sorrell TC: *Propionibacterium acnes* infection in neurosurgical patients: Experience with high-dose penicillin therapy. Med J Aust 145:408–410, 1986.

100. Schwalbe RS, Stapleton JT, Gilligan PH: Emergence of vancomycin resistance in coagulase-negative staphylococci. N Engl J Med 316:927–931, 1987.

101. Christenson JC, Pavia AT, Seskin K, et al: Meningitis due to *Ochrobactrum anthropi*: An emerging nosocomial pathogen: A report of 3 cases. Pediatr Neurosurg 27:218–221, 1997.

102. Ross DA, Marentette LJ, Thompson BG, et al: Use of hydroxyapatite bone cement to prevent cerebrospinal fluid leakage through the frontal sinus: Technical report. Neurosurgery 45:401–403, 1999.

103. Wilson CB: Ceftizoxime versus vancomycin and gentamicin in neurosurgical prophylaxis: A randomized, prospective, blinded clinical study. Neurosurgery 33:416–422, 1993.

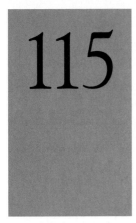

115 Neurosurgical Management of HIV-Related Focal Brain Lesions

E. THOMAS CHAPPELL and BARTON L. GUTHRIE

EPIDEMIOLOGY

The Centers for Disease Control and Prevention (CDC) currently reports that approximately 1 million people in the United States are immunopositive for the human immunodeficiency virus (HIV). To date, 774,467 cases of acquired immunodeficiency syndrome (AIDS) have been reported to the CDC, and only about 360,000 of those people are still alive.[1] Central nervous system (CNS) symptoms occur in 30% to 50% of AIDS cases, and as many as 90% have evidence of CNS disease at autopsy.[2-4] Approximately 10% of AIDS patients have focal CNS lesions that might serve as a target for a stereotactic biopsy.[2,5] One third of these patients will not have had prior manifestations of AIDS when they are referred for biopsy.

Intracranial disease is second only to pulmonary disease as a cause of morbidity and mortality in patients with AIDS.[6] Of the approximately 10% of patients with focal lesions in the brain, 30% to 70% have *Toxoplasma gondii* abscesses, and another 15% to 30% have primary or metastatic CNS lymphoma.[2,5-9] The remaining 20% include a myriad of bacterial (e.g., *Listeria, Escherichia coli*), fungal (e.g., *Cryptococcus, Aspergillus*), and viral (e.g., HIV, herpes, cytomegalovirus [CMV]) processes that can present as focal lesions on computed tomography (CT) or magnetic resonance imaging (MRI) of the brain.[2,5,9] Even the often diffuse virus-related process of progressive multifocal leukoencephalopathy (PML) frequently presents as a focal lesion.[8,9] Moreover, HIV-positive patients are also apparently susceptible to the same diseases as the HIV-negative population and, therefore, can have the usual primary and secondary brain tumors,[2,4,8] as well as the vascular (hemorrhage and infarction) lesions that occur in the brains of AIDS patients and the 4% to 20% of biopsies from which no definite diagnosis can be made. A comprehensive list of causes of focal brain lesions in HIV-positive patients is provided in Table 115-1. Furthermore, a few patients with AIDS have several CNS lesions of more than one etiology.[5]

PATIENT CONSIDERATIONS

Despite incubation periods of up to, and possibly greater than, 10 years as well as recent advances in treatment, AIDS remains an imminently fatal disease.[10-13] The CNS has now been identified as one of the reservoirs for HIV that makes its eradication from the body elusive, despite highly effective therapies.[14,15] Nonetheless, potentially effective therapies exist for approximately 90% of the identifiable causes of CNS

disease in patients with AIDS.[2] This fact suggests the usefulness of brain biopsy in the diagnosis and treatment of AIDS patients with focal brain disease. Since stereotactic biopsy is diagnostic in up to 96% of AIDS cases,[7] and since almost all treatable AIDS-related focal brain lesions do not require resection, there is virtually no need for an open procedure, except in rare cases of impending herniation due to mass effect. Furthermore, stereotactic biopsy is a low-risk procedure,[9] even in severely medically compromised patients (e.g., many of those with AIDS), because it can usually be performed with the patient under local anesthesia.[8] In most cases, a need for definitive diagnosis and low risk to the patient are persuasive in the decision to undertake an invasive diagnostic procedure. On the other hand, the communicable and fatal nature of HIV greatly compounds

---

TABLE 115-1 ▪ Etiologies of Focal Cerebral Lesions in HIV-Positive Patients

Infectious	Noninfectious
Parasites	***Neoplastic***
Toxoplasma gondii	Lymphoma (primary and
Cysticercosis	secondary)
Fungi	Kaposi's sarcoma
Cryptococcus	Glioma
Candida	Metastatic carcinoma
Histoplasma	Other*
Coccidiodies	***Vascular***
Aspergillus	Infarcts
Mucor	Hemorrhage
Mycobacteria	***Nondiagnostic***
Bacteria	
Escherichia coli	
Listeria	
Nocardia	
Salmonella	
Spirochetes	
Viruses	
Cytomegalovirus	
Herpesviruses	
Varicella zoster	
Papovavirus	

*There is no reason to believe that HIV-positive patients are not susceptible to the same neoplastic brain diseases as the rest of the population.

Modified from Levy RM, Bresdesen DE, Rosenblum ML: Neurological manifestations of the acquired immunodeficiency syndrome (AIDS): Experience at UCSF and review of the literature. J Neurosurg 62:475–495,1985.

this issue and raises the questions of risk to those performing the procedure and whether or not accurate diagnosis and treatment have an effect on outcome. Questions such as these have inherent ethical overtones, but some, possibly tenuous, scientific data on these issues are available to help in the decision-making process. Fortunately, the reduced incidence of opportunistic infections as a result of modern antiviral strategies has limited the surgeon's exposure to such complex considerations.[16,17]

RISK TO SURGEONS OPERATING ON HIV-POSITIVE PATIENTS

Solid data regarding the risk to surgeons who operate on patients who are HIV positive will never be available for several reasons. First, there is no way to be absolutely certain what other risk factors a given surgeon who contracts the virus might have and no way to be certain what operating mishaps, if any, can lead to transmission of the virus. In addition, more controversial issues, such as privacy, have an effect on the reporting of such data. Notwithstanding these issues, a few relatively scientific attempts at quantifying the risk of seroconversion (becoming HIV positive) in surgeons have been reported.[18,19] Schiff, for example, formulated a mathematical model for estimating a given surgeon's cumulative lifetime risk.[18] The model accounts for seroprevalence in the patient population; the inoculation rate, roughly based on surgical subspecialty; and the estimated probability of infection for a given procedural mishap. One survey estimated a greater than 6% 30-year risk in the 10% of surgeons considered at highest risk.[19] Even if estimates of a surgeon's risk of contracting HIV are of questionable accuracy, existing evidence raises the possibility of some risk, and any risk of contracting a fatal disease must be considered.

PREOPERATIVE EVALUATION

Radiographic

Accurate diagnosis and effective therapy for focal cerebral lesions in HIV-positive patients may not significantly alter the eventual outcome[20]; given even the slightest risk of disease transmission during an invasive procedure, the question arises whether the diagnosis can be made noninvasively. Although radiologists have reported an ability to make some diagnoses confidently on routine neuroimaging studies (CT and MRI), the consensus has been that the definitive diagnosis must be made histologically.[17] Dina, for example, found that if a mass in the brain of an HIV-positive patient enhanced, was unifocal, exhibited subependymal spread on CT or MRI, and was hyperdense on CT without contrast, it was never toxoplasmosis in his series of patients. However, he still recommended that these lesions undergo biopsy.[21] Since then other investigators have delineated a wider spectrum of CT and MRI findings for lymphoma, cautioning against confident radiographic diagnoses.[22] Some authors have suggested that metabolic imaging (positron-emission tomography [PET] and single photon emission computed tomography [SPECT]) make it possible to distinguish between malignant and nonmalignant lesions.[23,24] In fact, ^{201}Tl SPECT is more than 90% accurate in distinguishing between tumor and infection.[25] Moreover, it is accurate in distinguishing lymphoma from other focal lesions.[26] Despite eloquent attempts to characterize the various brain lesions seen on neuroimaging studies in HIV-positive patients, no constellation of findings is 100% diagnostic of any of the numerous disease entities.[27] Moreover, the possibility of numerous etiologies for several brain lesions cannot be ignored in these patients (Fig. 115-1).

Empirical Therapy

At best, neuroimaging is suggestive in the diagnosis of AIDS-related brain lesions. This does not mean, however, that one should proceed directly to brain biopsy. As noted earlier, most focal brain lesions in HIV-positive patients are *T. gondii* abscesses, which generally resolve when the patient is treated with adequate doses of sulfadiazine (or clindamycin) and pyrimethamine (anti-*Toxoplasma* therapy).[28,29] Rosenblum and associates thus proposed that stable HIV-positive patients with several lesions on MRI receive 2 to 3 weeks of empirical anti-*Toxoplasma* therapy.[30] If follow-up

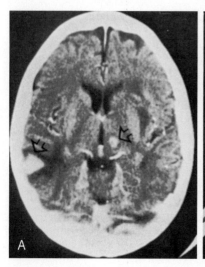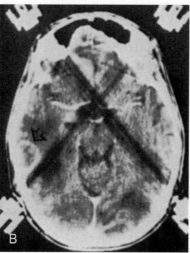

FIGURE 115-1   Contrast-enhanced CT scan of a 24-year-old man with AIDS. *A,* These lesions (*arrows*) improved and then stabilized after 1 year of anti-*Toxoplasma* therapy. *B,* After his symptoms recurred 1 year later, the patient had this scan, which revealed a new enhancing mass on the left. Biopsies of these lesions determined that those on the right side were due to toxoplasmosis, as expected, and the lesions on the left side were determined to be lymphoma.

images and physical examination fail to show improvement, these authors then recommend biopsy. This regimen appears prudent, and, although 40% of patients cannot tolerate the therapy, leading to inadequate treatment and often to biopsy, the incidence of toxoplasmosis in biopsy series is decreasing.[8,9] The algorithm should probably be extended to include any HIV-positive patient with one or more contrast-enhancing lesions on CT, because cerebral toxoplasmosis is not always multifocal.[8] In addition, deterioration in a patient who is on anti-*Toxoplasma* medications may warrant early biopsy. In short, a presumptive diagnosis of cerebral toxoplasmosis can be given confidently to an HIV-positive patient whose brain lesions resolve after administration of anti-*Toxoplasma* drugs. This regimen eliminates the need for biopsy in a population of patients who can tolerate the therapy and have no focal cerebral lesions of another etiology. However, radiographic evidence of improvement can be complicated by the concomitant administration of steroids, because some lesions improve with the administration of dexamethasone or prednisone (lymphoma, in particular).

Laboratory Evaluation

Rosenblum and colleagues[30] also suggested that in the absence of mass effect, cerebrospinal fluid (CSF) should be evaluated in HIV-positive patients with focal brain lesions. However, sensitivity and specificity for most causes of HIV-related focal lesions is less than optimal.[21,29,31–33] Only a few patients with lymphoma have abnormal CSF cytology, for example.[21,32] However, Epstein-Barr virus (EBV) may be a marker in the CSF for primary CNS lymphoma (PCNSL). The assay for EBV in the CSF requires gene amplification (polymerase chain reaction [PCR]).[34,35] Furthermore, although the CSF is always abnormal in toxoplasmosis patients, the findings are nonspecific.[29] In serologic tests (whether on the blood or the CSF), as expected, antibody titers are unreliable in immunocompromised patients.

Polymerase Chain Reaction

In recent years, the analysis of CSF in patients with HIV disease has been revolutionized by the advent of the PCR technique, reducing the need for brain biopsy.[16,36] Even minute amounts of DNA from various viral and bacterial particles can be detected in the CSF using PCR. JC virus (JCV, associated with PML), herpes simplex virus (HSV), varicella zoster virus (VZV), CMV, EBV (associated with PCNSL), *T. gondii*, and *Mycobacterium tuberculosis* have been detected in the CSF of HIV-positive patients. Threshold levels for detection of many of these antigens have now been defined.[37] Furthermore, the technique may be used in certain cases to monitor the efficacy of treatment or the progression of disease.[38,39] Antinori and associates analyzed the CSF for EBV, JCV, and *T. gondii* by PCR in 66 of 136 HIV patients with CNS lesions. Patients in whom anti-*Toxoplasma* therapy had failed also underwent stereotactic biopsy. These investigators found that if EBV DNA or *T. gondii* DNA tests were positive, the probability of PCNSL or toxoplasmic encephalitis, respectively, exceeded 0.96.[40] On the other hand, the absence of *T. gondii* DNA positivity in the CNS does not rule out the diagnosis of toxoplasmic encephalitis.[40,41] The same is true of bacteriologic examination of the CSF for tuberculosis.[42] Others report less sensitivity.[43]

More recently, Portolani and colleagues reported data that cast doubt on the role of EBV in HIV-related CNS disease.[44] Nonetheless, lumbar puncture may now provide enough diagnostic certainty to treat a patient without a histologic evaluation of tissue obtained by biopsy.

SURGERY

If unable to make a confident diagnosis by noninvasive or minimally invasive means for an HIV-positive patient who has a focal cerebral lesion that has not responded to anti-*Toxoplasma* therapy, the primary physician must ask a surgeon to consider biopsy. Such a measure is taken if the clinician and the patient and ultimately the surgeon agree that the risk of achieving a definitive diagnosis is outweighed by the potential for improving outcome. The authors reported their experience in the management of HIV-related focal brain lesions in an attempt to define the role of brain biopsy[8] and developed an algorithm that minimizes unnecessary risk to patients and surgeons. Decision making and the application of such an algorithm can now be further refined by the use of PCR analysis of the CSF.

Surgical Technique

Computed tomography–guided stereotaxis was used for all patients in the series. Single- or double-dose administration of intravenous contrast material with and without delayed image acquisition was used. De La Paz and Enzmann suggested that a double-dose delayed contrast CT provides the best results,[45] but MRI is still more sensitive and possibly more specific in the differential diagnosis of HIV-related brain lesions.[25,27,45,46] If a compatible stereotactic system is available, MRI guidance is a suitable alternative to CT. The efficacy of an ultrasound-guided technique merits its inclusion as a suitable alternative as well.[33] However, this procedure involves a more involved surgical opening and thus possibly an increased risk to the surgeon and the patient. The availability of frameless stereotactic systems allows the minimal invasion of a "twist-drill" or "burr hole" procedure without the discomfort of headframe application.

In most cases, intravenous sedation with "monitored anesthetic care" provides adequate anesthesia. General anesthesia is used at the patient's request, if it can be tolerated. The incidence of operative complications is low, but it may be prudent to monitor patients overnight in an intensive care setting.[9]

General criteria for biopsy have included the presence of an intracranial lesion that is identifiable on CT or MRI, failure of enhancing lesions to improve after at least 1 week of anti-*Toxoplasma* therapy, or a CT or MRI appearance that is highly uncharacteristic of toxoplasmosis. Finally, the patient must be able to tolerate the procedure without significant risk.

If several lesions are present, either the most accessible cerebral lesion in the least eloquent brain or a lesion not responding to therapy is selected. In general, specimens are taken from only one lesion, but the occasional case may warrant targeting more than one lesion (see Fig. 115-1).

TABLE 115-2 ▪ Characteristics of Patients Undergoing Stereotatic Biopsy of HIV-Related Cerebral Lesions at George Washington University Medical Center (November 1988 to October 1990, n = 25)

Characteristic	Number
Male	24
Homosexual	21
IVDA	2
Haitian	1
Female	1 (IVDA)
Age	Mean, 36 yr: range, 21–53 yr
Known to have AIDS before biopsy*	13 (for a median of 34 mo)
CNS lesion prompted diagnosis of AIDS	10
Karnofsky Performance Score	65 (range, 40–100)
Median follow-up[†]	8 wk
Dead	17
Lost of follow-up	1

AIDS, acquired immunodeficiency syndrome; CNS, central nervous system; HIV, human immunodeficiency virus; IVDA, intravenous drug abuser.

*Information lacking on two patients.

[†]Skewed by the large number of patients who died rapidly.

Target sites are chosen at the center of nonenhancing or homogeneously enhancing lesions and at the hyperdense border of ring-enhancing lesions.

Specimens are given to the pathologist for intraoperative smear cytology and frozen-section histology as needed. This process is repeated until diagnostic or clearly abnormal tissue is acquired. One or more additional specimens are sent for routine histology and transmission electron microscopy. A gram stain and bacterial, viral, and fungal cultures and stains are obtained. Levy and colleagues[7] reported that the diagnostic efficacy of brain biopsy in HIV-related brain lesions can be elevated to 96% through the use of these and various immunohistochemical techniques performed on at least six tissue samples.

Results

The records of 25 HIV-positive patients who were consecutively referred for biopsy of cerebral lesions at the George Washington University (GWU) Medical Center (Washington, DC) between November 1988 and October 1990 were reviewed. The preoperative characteristics of these 25 patients are shown in Table 115-2. It is notable that 13 of the 25 had been seropositive for HIV for a median of 34 months, and these people were diagnosed with AIDS before presenting for brain biopsy. In the 10 other patients for whom this information was available, the cerebral lesion precipitated the initial presentation for treatment and the diagnosis of AIDS. As shown in Table 115-3, this distinction had great bearing on the median survival after biopsy in these patients. The patients who had previous AIDS-related disease had a considerably shorter survival time than did those who were found to be HIV-positive at the time of presentation for biopsy (6 vs. 37 weeks). Of the 13 patients with AIDS before their biopsy, 9 had lymphoma. Conversely, all patients with lymphoma had AIDS before their procedure.

A listing of the biopsy diagnoses is also provided in Table 115-3. The relatively low incidence of toxoplasmosis, the single case of a low-grade glioma (not generally considered an HIV-related lesion), and the fact that five of the biopsies provided abnormal, but nondiagnostic, tissue are facts worth noting. Also of particular interest is that more than half of the lesions that enhanced on CT were lymphoma, and PML was the only diagnosis made from nonenhancing lesions. In fact, whether or not a lesion enhanced on CT correlated well with whether or not the biopsy affected the patient's therapy (Table 115-4). Of the 25 target lesions, 16 enhanced with contrast, and therapy was modified in 11 of 16 on the basis of the biopsy results. Of those 11, 10 were tumors (9 lymphomas, 1 low-grade astrocytoma) and the other was an HSV infection (Fig. 115-2). These patients were either receiving anti-*Toxoplasma* therapy or awaiting a treatment plan at the time of their biopsy; thus, the results led to more appropriate therapy. The remaining five patients with contrast-enhancing lesions included two with incompletely treated

TABLE 115-3 ▪ Results of Stereotactic Biopsy of HIV-Related Cerebral Lesions at GWU Medical Center (November 1988 to October 1990, n = 25)

Diagnosis	(%)	Contrast Enhancing (No.)	Contrast Negative (No.)	KPS (median)	Median Survival (weeks)	CNS First (unknown)*	Previous AIDS (No.)
Lymphoma	36	9	–	70	6	–	9
PML	24	–	6	60	18	4 (1)	1
Toxoplasmosis	8	2	–	80	37	1 (1)	–
Low-grade glioma	4	1	–	80	74	1	–
Herpes cerebritis	4	1	–	90	8	1	–
Cryptococcoma	4	1	–	50	1	–	1
Nondiagnostic	20	2 (12.5%)	3 (33%)	55	17	3	2
Total	100	16	9	NA	NA	10 (2)	13
				Median survival (weeks)	37	6	

KPS, karnofsky Performance score; NA, Not applicable; PML, progressive multifocal leukoencephalopathy.

*It is unknown from our data whether these patients had a CNS lesion first.

TABLE 115-4 ▪ Computed Tomographic Appearance versus Impact of Biopsy on Subsequent Treatment

	Contract Enhancing (No.)	None Enhancing (No.)
Changed treatment	11	0
Confirmed treatment in progress	3	0
No help with treatment	2 (12.5%)	9 (100%)

toxoplasmosis and one with a cryptococcal abscess who had suffered recurrent cryptococcal meningitis. Appropriate treatment was confirmed in these three patients. Two (12.5%) of the 16 contrast-enhancing targets yielded abnormal, but nondiagnostic, tissue at biopsy; thus the procedure had no impact on their treatment. In short, 87.5% of the patients with contrast-enhancing lesions obtained a diagnosis from their biopsy that modified or confirmed their therapy.

On the other hand, the patients with nonenhancing lesions experienced no therapeutic benefit from their biopsy. The abnormal tissue was nondiagnostic in one third of these cases, and the remainder had PML, for which no effective therapy exists (see Table 115-3). Only one patient suffered a complication of the procedure when a small hemorrhage with edema occurred at the operative site, leaving him somnolent for approximately 24 hours.

DISCUSSION

Several aspects of these data affect the surgeon's role in HIV-related cerebral disease. First, toxoplasmosis is the cause of CNS mass lesions in 25% to 70% of cases in most

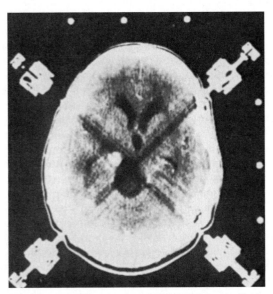

FIGURE 115-2 A CT scan of a patient with herpex simplex viral cerebritis as an example of how even viral encephalitides can present as lesions for biopsy.

large series,[2,5-7] whereas it occurred in only 2 of the 25 patients reported on here (8%, see Table 115-3). This is probably a result of the approach to CNS masses in AIDS patients outlined by Rosenblum and co-workers[30] and adopted by many practitioners who treat patients with AIDS. In general, patients with contrast-enhancing lesions on CT scans are treated for at least 7 to 10 days with anti-*Toxoplasma* therapy as tolerated. If follow-up CT scans reveal an unsatisfactory response, or a patient with a recent or current Karnofsky Performance Scale (KPS) of 70 or better deteriorates further (or fails to improve), the patient may be a candidate for biopsy. During this study, approximately 40 patients were treated at our institution for HIV-related focal cerebral lesions that were not referred for biopsy. About 20 of these had toxoplasmosis that responded to therapy, or the patients died during treatment. However, the remainder were treated empirically on the basis of presumptive (usually radiographic) diagnosis, or they were not treated on the basis of their clinical condition or the lack of an effective therapy (13 with presumed lymphoma and seven with presumed PML). This result suggests a tendency on the part of the referring physicians to weigh heavily the potential for poor outcome in AIDS patients with CNS lesions against the potential benefit of having an accurate tissue diagnosis to guide appropriate therapy.

In a more recent retrospective review, Nicolato and associates also performed stereotaxic biopsies on 25 patients with AIDS. Of the 25 patients, 19 came to biopsy after receiving empirical anti-*Toxoplasma* regimens, and the results led to a change in therapy in 90%. In addition, six patients had PML, three of which were being treated inappropriately; however, none of these lesions enhanced on double-dose contrast CT. This reflects a similar experience to that of the authors. However, there is no mention of patient outcome, how long the patients had suffered from AIDS before biopsy, or how many patients with contrast-enhancing lesions responded to empirical anti-*Toxoplasma* therapy.[47]

Lymphoma

Outcome for AIDS-related cerebral lymphoma, for instance, may further justify a conservative tendency. Patients without AIDS who are treated aggressively for CNS lymphoma may survive a median of 13.5 months, whereas AIDS patients with CNS lymphoma invariably suffer a fulminant course and die within 3 months.[48,49] This effect occurs whether or not the patients are treated and whether or not their lesions respond to therapy.[33] However, a more recent review found that HIV-positive patients with CNS lymphoma who were treated aggressively with external beam irradiation and chemotherapy survived a median of around 4 to 6 months as opposed to only 1 month if not treated.[48,50] Although scant data are available to document this, many clinicians who treat large numbers of HIV-positive patients suggest that recent advances in the treatment of HIV disease may make HIV patients with CNS lymphoma more like those without HIV with regard to survival after treatment. One author has even reported on a small number of patients who survived around 3 years after aggressive treatment of their HIV-related CNS lymphoma when they also received the most effective antiviral regimen currently available.[51]

The data presented earlier were gathered before these recent advances. However, they suggest that patients with AIDS who develop lymphoma do so late in the course of their disease and usually die of systemic disease or of other AIDS-related diseases (all nine lymphoma patients had AIDS before their biopsy). In fact, despite accurate diagnosis and a full course of low-dose radiation therapy (20 to 30 Gy) in six of nine of the patients with lymphoma, the median survival was only 6 weeks (see Table 115-3) (the other three patients could not tolerate or refused radiation therapy or died before treatment could be completed). Moreover, all nine patients were treated for toxoplasmosis until their biopsy findings led to a change in therapy. Furthermore, the authors have observed that patients with exceedingly low CD4 cell counts in the blood (<100 cells/μL) are more likely to have lymphoma. Conversely, those with CD4 counts above 100 cells/μL rarely have lymphoma. One set of investigators has documented an increased risk for PCNSL in HIV patients with CD4 counts less than 50 cells/μL.[52] These facts raise at least two questions about AIDS patients with a contrast-enhancing lesion: Should the physician adopt an aggressive approach and should the physician treat empirically for toxoplasmosis or perform a biopsy immediately and treat accordingly? The answers may depend on the stage of the patient's disease and his or her wishes after being informed of the prognosis and in light of their current and recent clinical condition.

Efficacy of Stereotactic Biopsy

Stereotactic biopsy provides an accurate diagnosis in approximately 95% of cases.[47,53,54] A percentage of nondiagnostic biopsies as high as that (20%) in the series reported on earlier can be greatly improved if the appropriate techniques are employed.[7,55] As mentioned, these techniques have been clearly outlined by Levy and associates.[7] Immunohistochemical techniques and special stains were not routinely used in the series noted earlier, which may account for the relatively high nondiagnostic rate. However, three of the diagnoses were made by transmission electron microscopy. The small risk of not achieving a diagnosis should be considered in the decision of whether or not brain biopsy should be recommended to a patient with an AIDS-related brain lesion.

Proposed Treatment Algorithm

Based on the data presented earlier, empirical anti-*Toxoplasma* therapy appears to be indicated for contrast-enhancing cerebral lesions in recently diagnosed HIV-positive patients. If the patient deteriorates or there is no improvement on follow-up CT, or if CSF analysis using PCR for the most likely etiologic entities suggests otherwise, or if the CD4 count is less than 100, biopsy should be considered. However, in patients with longstanding disease and contrast-enhancing lesions for whom an aggressive approach is selected, immediate biopsy may be warranted, unless CSF analysis, CD4 count, and SPECT scanning provide a sufficient level of confidence in the diagnosis. The high incidence of lymphoma in the later stages of AIDS and the fact that many other potentially treatable etiologies are reported to cause contrast-enhancing lesions

in the brains of AIDS patients both indicate such an approach.

The role of biopsy in AIDS patients with nonenhancing brain lesions is less clear. Brain biopsy seldom contributes to the therapy in these patients, but it may provide prognostic information and may be required by future experimental treatment protocols. However, the presence of JCV DNA in the CSF of these patients may be sufficient information. Accordingly, we have implemented the algorithm in Figure 115-3 to help determine when a biopsy should be performed in AIDS patients with cerebral lesions for whom an informed decision is made to treat the lesion aggressively. It is still not clear whether or not an aggressive approach using the proposed algorithm will improve outcome in AIDS-related brain disease or decrease the number of unnecessary biopsies and increase the yield of treatable diagnoses. Real proof of improved outcome would require a randomized controlled trial, which is not readily accomplished.

Aggressive versus Conservative Approach

Unfortunately, the question remains whether or not the risk of obtaining an accurate diagnosis is outweighed by the potential for improved survival. Accurate diagnosis, and thus appropriate therapy, can be made with absolute certainty only by obtaining tissue samples from AIDS-related brain lesions. However, patients whose lesions do not enhance on CT are apparently much less likely to have a treatable disease (our data imply they most often have PML). Patients with longstanding AIDS and contrast-enhancing lesions of the brain probably have lymphoma. Although most of these patients do poorly even with appropriate therapy, an earlier diagnosis and aggressive therapy in patients with a recent or current KPS of 70 or more may provide some survival benefit or, at least, useful information with regard to a treatment plan. This is especially true if current therapies for HIV disease are capable restoring the patients' immune systems. Moreover, patients who are recently or simultaneously found to be HIV-positive with cerebral lesions that enhance on CT but do not respond to anti-*Toxoplasma* treatment generally survive longer and thus might benefit from earlier targeted treatment for their cerebral disease. However, even under the best circumstances, survival is not likely to exceed a few months. PCR analysis of the CSF and CD4 count, and ^{201}Tl SPECT in some patients may provide sufficient diagnostic data for a treatment decision. Holloway and Mushlin undertook decision analysis to compare the treatment strategies of biopsy and no biopsy in patients with HIV disease in whom 2 weeks of anti-*Toxoplasma* treatment failed. They included diagnostic yield of biopsy, operative mortality, and life expectancy of lymphoma (treated and untreated). The life expectancy of the patients who had a biopsy was only 31 days greater than the 67 days predicted for those who did not have biopsies.[20] Patients, referring physicians, and surgical consultants could consider this type of information when making a decision regarding diagnosis and treatment of patients with HIV-related brain lesions.

With regard to the treatment of lymphoma, there is yet another consultant whose opinion must be held in highest regard. Most radiation oncologists are reticent, and rightly

FIGURE 115-3 A proposed treatment algorithm defining the role of stereotactic biopsy in patients with AIDS who have cerebral lesions based on the data presented. dx, diagnosis; EBV, Epstein-Barr virus; JCV, JC virus; KPS, Karnofsky Performance Score.

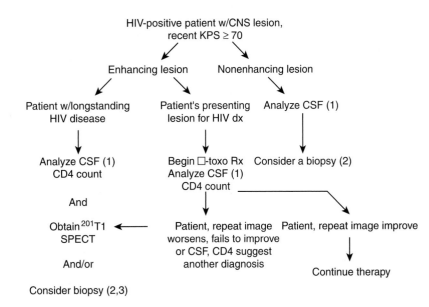

(1) Refers to PCR testing for *Toxoplasma gondii*, EBV, JCV, and possibly other etiologies as indicated.
(2) Decision making remains in the hands of the clinicians and the patient. Each case must be considered individually, balancing the risks and benefits of any diagnostic or treatment modality.
(3) The decision to biopsy and treat patients late in the course of their disease with presumed lymphoma must have included an honest discussion of the side effects of therapy and the limited average survival benefit.

so, to irradiate the brain empirically and, therefore, insist on a tissue diagnosis before prescribing radiation therapy. However, as data such as those reported here accumulated in the early days of the treatment of HIV-related brain disease, some radiation oncologists began to empirically irradiate the brains of HIV patients with CNS lesions that had not responded to toxoplasmosis therapy and were highly characteristic of primary cerebral lymphomas. However, when some of the data on these patients were analyzed, it appeared that the efficacy of such an approach might have been diminished by errors in diagnosis. Consequently, most radiation therapists, when currently faced with a request to treat CNS lesions in an HIV patient in whom toxoplasmosis therapy has failed, require that a tissue diagnosis be obtained before administering radiation therapy.[56,57] One commentator has even expressed concerns about a "catch-22"[58] in this regard. He is concerned that, because in the absence of a tissue diagnosis oncologists cannot be certain that all members of a treatment group have the same diagnosis, they are thus reluctant to develop and implement aggressive treatment regimens directed at the specific diagnosis. At the same time, if the neurosurgeon is reticent to perform a biopsy in the belief that the patient will probably suffer a poor outcome because of a lack of effective therapies, then the diagnoses required for proper treatment analyses are not available to the oncologist. This is yet another quandary in the decision-making process, and it might be solved by consultants and primary caregivers working together to develop treatment protocols, and then analyzing them carefully for their efficacy.

Ethics

A certainly fatal communicable disease such as AIDS raises yet another issue in the decision-making process peculiar to such a unique circumstance, that is, whether or not the risk to the surgeon and staff should be included in the formula. Medical ethicists have addressed the issue of physicians' obligations to treat patients with AIDS, and most feel that it is unethical for a physician to refuse to treat such patients simply because they have the disease.[59,60] There are, however, certain "limiting factors," not the least of which is "excessive risk." As noted earlier, accurately calculating the risk of a particular surgeon performing a particular procedure on an AIDS patient is not feasible. Nonetheless, if the formula and data outlined by Schiff[18] are applied to stereotactic biopsy, an estimated range can be derived. Assuming an injury rate of one significant injury per 50 biopsies (with a seroprevalence of 100%), 25 AIDS biopsies per year, and 30 years of practice, the probability of contracting HIV for a surgeon performing stereotactic brain biopsies on HIV-positive patients is 0.0075. By no one's standards does this constitute excessive risk. Even this is probably an overestimate considering that inoculation during a stereotactic biopsy is extremely improbable, especially if a percutaneous technique (as opposed to a burr hole) is used. Performance of the procedure by one surgeon and one surgical technician exchanging virtually all blunt instruments (except needles for local anesthetic and a scalpel for scalp puncture) on a Mayo stand minimizes the chance of a significant injury. In addition, the procedure is practically bloodless, and the use of a biooclusive drape further reduces exposure.

The only other potentially acceptable limiting variable to a physician's obligation to treat a patient with AIDS is the issue of "questionable benefit."[56] If no reasonable chance exists that the patient will benefit from the procedure, then the physician is under no obligation to treat. In fact, the physician is obliged not to treat.

This chapter is intended to assist the physician in the complex decision of whether or not to offer brain biopsy to a given patient who presents with an HIV-related brain lesion. That each case be evaluated on an individual basis is implied, and a suggested treatment algorithm is provided should a case warrant aggressive management. To reiterate, recently diagnosed HIV-positive patients with contrast-enhancing lesions warrant a course of anti-*Toxoplasma* therapy, and biopsy might be considered if this therapy fails. Patients with longstanding disease but with a KPS of 70 or more and contrast-enhancing lesions will probably benefit from accurate diagnosis and treatment of their cerebral disease. If the lesion is nonenhancing, the decision becomes more difficult, but in the authors' experience, biopsy of these lesions is seldom helpful. The prospective efficacy of this approach remains to be quantified. Related ethical issues cannot be ignored. However, with the available information in hand, the authors hope that the patient, the referring physician, and the surgical consultant can make the best decision in each case.

REFERENCES

1. Centers for Disease Control and Prevention National AIDS Hotline: as of October 1, 2003. Available at www.ashastd.org/nah/
2. So YT, Beckstead JH, Davis RL: Primary central nervous system lymphoma in acquired immune deficiency syndrome: A clinical and pathological study. Ann Neurol 20:566–572, 1986.
3. De Girlami U, Smith TW, Hienin D, Hauw JJ: Neuropathology of the acquired immunodeficiency syndrome. Arch Pathol Lab Med 114:643–655, 1990.
4. Kanzer MD: Neuropathology of AIDS. Crit Rev Neurobiol 5:313–362, 1990.
5. Levy RM, Bresdesen DE, Rosenblum ML: Neurological manifestations of the acquired immunodeficiency syndrome (AIDS): Experience at UCSF and review of the literature. J Neurosurg 62:475–495, 1985.
6. Loneragan R, Doust BD, Walker J: Neuroradiological manifestation of the acquired immunodeficiency syndrome. Australas Radiol 34:32–39, 1990.
7. Levy RM, Russell E, Yungbluth M, et al: The efficacy of image-guided stereotactic brain biopsy in neurologically symptomatic acquired immunodeficiency syndrome patients. Neurosurgery 30:186–190, 1992.
8. Chappell ET, Guthrie BL, Orenstein J: The role of stereotactic biopsy in the management of HIV-related focal brain lesions. Neurosurgery 30:825–829, 1992.
9. Apuzzo MJ, Chandrasoma PT, Cohen D, et al: Computed imaging stereotaxy: Experience and perspective related to 500 procedures applied to brain masses. Neurosurgery 20:930–937, 1987.
10. Falloon J: Current therapy for HIV infection and its complications. Postgrad Med 91:115–132, 1992.
11. Broder S (moderator): Antiretroviral therapy in AIDS. Ann Intern Med 113:604–618, 1990.
12. Kuo JM, Taylor JM, Detels R: Estimating the AIDS incubation period from a prevalent cohort. Am J Epidemiol 133:1050–1057, 1991.
13. Salzberg AM, Dolins SL, Salzberg C: HIV incubation times. Lancet 2:66, 1989.
14. Kolson DL: Neuropathogenesis of central nervous system HIV-1 infection. Clin Lab Med 22:703–717, 2002.
15. Lambotte O, Deiva K, Tardieu M: HIV-1 persistence, viral reservoir, and the central nervous system in the HAART era. Brain Pathol 13:95–103, 2003.
16. Roullet E: Opportunistic infections of the central nervous system during HIV-1 infection (emphasis on cytomegalovirus disease). J Neurol 246:237–243, 1999.
17. Vago L, Bonetto S, Nebuloni M, et al: Pathological findings in the central nervous system of AIDS patients on assumed antiretroviral therapeutic regimens: Retrospective study of 1597 autopsies. AIDS 16:1925–1928, 2002.
18. Schiff SJ: A surgeon's risk of AIDS. J Neurosurg 73:651–660, 1990.
19. Lowenfels AB, Wormser GP, Jain R: Frequency of puncture injuries in surgeons and estimated risk of HIV infection. Arch Surg 124:1284, 1989.
20. Holloway RG, Mushlin AI: Intracranial mass lesions in acquired immunodeficiency syndrome: Using decision analysis to determine the effectiveness of stereotactic brain biopsy. Neurology 46:1010–1015, 1996.
21. Dina T: Primary central nervous system lymphoma versus toxoplasmosis in AIDS. Radiology 179:823–828, 1991.
22. Thurnher MM, Rieger A, Kleibl-Popov C, et al: Primary central nervous system lymphoma in AIDS: A wider spectrum of CT and MRI findings. Neuroradiology 43:29–35, 2001.
23. O'Malley JP, Ziessman HA, Kumar PN, et al: Diagnosis of intracranial lymphoma in patients with AIDS: Value of SPECT. AJR Am J Roentgenol 163:417–421, 1994.
24. Hoffman JM, Waskin HA, Schifter T, et al: FDG-PET in differentiating lymphoma from non-malignant CNS lesions in patients with AIDS. J Nucl Med 34:567–575, 1993.
25. Rodriguez WL, Ramirez-Ronda CH: CNS involvement in AIDS patients as seen with CT and MR: A review. Bol Asoc Med P R 83:548–551, 1991.
26. Skiest DJ, Erdman W, Chang WE, et al: SPECT thallium-201 combined with *Toxoplasma* serology for the presumptive diagnosis of focal central nervous system mass lesions in patients with AIDS. J Infect 40:274–281, 2000.
27. Kupfer MC, Chi-Shing Z, Colletti PM, et al: MRI evaluation of AIDS-related encephalopathy: Toxoplasmosis vs. lymphoma. Magn Reson Imaging 8:51–56, 1990.
28. Mariuz PR, Luft BJ: Toxoplasmic encephalitis. AIDS Clin Rev 1:105–130, 1992.
29. Pons VG, Jacobs RA, Hollander H, et al: Nonviral infections of the central nervous system in patients with acquired immunodeficiency syndrome. In Rosenblum ML, Levy RM, Bresdesen DE (eds): AIDS and the Nervous System. New York: Raven Press, 1988, pp 263–284.
30. Rosenblum ML, Levy RM, Bresdesen DE: Algorithms for the treatment of AIDS patients with neurologic disease. In Rosenblum ML, Levy RM, Bresdesen E (eds): AIDS and the Central Nervous System. New York: Raven Press, 1988, pp 389–396.
31. Remick SC, Diamond C, Migliozzi JA, et al: Primary central nervous system lymphoma in patients with and without the acquired immune deficiency syndrome: A retrospective analysis and review of the literature. Medicine (Baltimore) 69:345–360, 1990.
32. So YT, Chaoucoir A, Davis RL, et al: Neoplasms of the central nervous system in acquired immunodeficiency syndrome. In Rosenblum ML, Levy RM, Bresdesen DE (eds): AIDS and the Central Nervous System. New York: Raven Press, 1988, pp 285–300.
33. Rosenblum ML, Levy RM, Bresdesen DE (eds): AIDS and the Nervous System. New York: Raven Press, 1988.
34. Cinque P, Brytting M, Vago L, et al: Epstein-Barr virus DNA in CSF from patients with AIDS-related primary lymphoma of the CNS. Lancet 342:398–401, 1993.
35. MacMahon E, Glass JD, Hayward SF, et al: Epstein-Barr virus: A tumor marker for primary central nervous system lymphoma [abstract]. Blood 78S:399, 1991.
36. Cinque P, Bossolasco S, Bestetti A, et al: Molecular studies of cerebrospinal fluid in human immunodeficiency virus type 1–associated opportunistic central nervous system diseases—an update. J Neurovirol 8(Suppl 2):122–128, 2002.
37. Tachikawa N, Goto M, Hoshino Y, et al: Detection of *Toxoplasma gondii*, Epstein-Barr virus, and JC virus DNAs in the cerebrospinal fluid in acquired immunodeficiency syndrome patients with focal central nervous system complications. Intern Med 38:556–562, 1999.
38. Antinori A, Cingolani A, De Luca A, et al: Epstein-Barr virus in monitoring the response to therapy of acquired immunodeficiency syndrome–related primary central nervous system lymphoma. Ann Neurol 45:259–261, 1999.
39. Lazzarin A, Castagna A, Cavalli G, et al: Cerebrospinal fluid beta 2-microglobulin in AIDS related central nervous system involvement. J Clin Lab Immunol 38:175–186, 1992.
40. Antinori A, Ammassari A, De Luca A, et al: Diagnosis of AIDS-related focal brain lesions: A decision-making analysis based on clinical and neuroradiologic characteristics combined with polymerase chain reaction assays in CSF. Neurology 48:687–694, 1997.
41. d'Arminio Monforte A, Cinque P, Vago L, et al: A comparison of brain biopsy and CSF-PCR in the diagnosis of CNS lesions in AIDS patients. J Neurol 244:35–39, 1997.
42. Kurisaki H: Central nervous system tuberculosis with and without HIV infection—clinical, neuroimaging, and neuropathological study [in Japanese] Rinsho Shinkeigaku 40:209–217, 2000.
43. Cingolani A, De Luca A, Larocca LM, et al: Minimally invasive diagnosis of acquired immunodeficiency syndrome–related primary central nervous system lymphoma. J Natl Cancer Inst 90:364–369, 1998.

44. Portolani M, Cermelli C, Meacci M, et al: Epstein-Barr virus DNA in the cerebrospinal fluid of patients with human immunodeficiency virus infection and central nervous system disorders. New Microbiol 22:369–374, 1999.

45. De La Paz R, Enzmann D: Neuroradiology of acquired immunodeficiency syndrome. In Rosenblum ML, Levy RM, Bredesen E (eds): AIDS and the Central Nervous System. New York: Raven Press, 1988, pp 121–154.

46. Rauch RA, Bazan C III, Jinkins JR: Imaging of infections of the central nervous system. Curr Opin Radiol 4:43–51, 1992.

47. Nicolato A, Gerosa M, Piovan E, et al: Computerized tomography and magnetic resonance guided stereotactic brain biopsy in nonimmuno-compromised and AIDS patients. Surg Neurol 48:267–277, 1997.

48. Baumgartner JE, Rachlin JR, Beckstead JH, et al: Primary central nervous system lymphomas: Natural history and response to radiation therapy in 55 patients with acquired immunodeficiency syndrome. J Neurosurg 73:206–211, 1990.

49. Hochberg FH, Miller DC: Primary central nervous system lymphoma. J Neurosurg 68:835–853, 1988.

50. Chamberlain MC, Kormanik PA: AIDS-related central nervous system lymphomas. J Neurooncol 43:269–276, 1999.

51. Hoffman C, Tabrizian S, Wolf E, et al: Survival of AIDS patients with primary central nervous system lymphoma is dramatically improved by HAART-induced immune recovery. AIDS 15:2119–2127, 2001.

52. Pluda JM, Venzon DJ, Tosato G, et al: Parameters affecting the development of non-Hodgkin's lymphoma in patients with severe human immunodeficiency virus infection receiving antiretroviral therapy. J Clin Oncol 11:1099–1107, 1993.

53. Friedman WA, Sceats DJ, Blake RN, Ballinger WE: The incidence of unexpected pathological findings in an image-guided biopsy series: A review of 100 consecutive cases. Neurosurgery 25:180–184, 1989.

54. Kaufman HK, Catalano LW: Diagnostic brain biopsy: A series of 50 cases and a review. Neurosurgery 4:129–136, 1979.

55. Zimmer C, Daeschlein G, Patt S, Weigel K: Strategy for diagnosis of Toxoplasma gondii in stereotactic brain biopsies. Stereotact Funct Neurosurg 56:66–75, 1991.

56. So YT, Beckstead JH, Davis RL: Primary central nervous system lymphoma in acquired immune deficiency syndrome: A clinical and pathological study. Ann Neurol 20:566–572, 1986.

57. Donahue BR, Sullian JW, Cooper JS: Additional experience with empiric radiotherapy for presumed human immunodeficiency virus–associated primary CNS lymphoma. Cancer 75:328–332, 1995.

58. Corn BW, Trock JT, Curran WJ Jr: Management of primary central nervous system lymphoma for the patient with acquired immunodeficiency syndrome: Confronting a clinical catch-22. Cancer 76:163–166, 1995.

59. Emanuel EJ: Do physicians have an obligation to treat patients with AIDS? N Engl J Med 318:1686–1690, 1988.

60. Zuger A, Miles SH: Physicians, AIDS, and occupational risk. JAMA 258:1924, 1987.

116

Surgical Management of Tuberculous Infections of the Nervous System

RANA PATIR, RAVI BHATIA, and PRAKASH NARAIN TANDON

Infection of the central nervous system (CNS) by *Mycobacterium tuberculosis* is invariably secondary to a primary focus elsewhere in the body. The avium, bovine, and atypical mycobacteria are rarely isolated from the nonimmunocompromised host. The primary site is usually pulmonary, bone, and gastrointestinal tract; genitourinary sites are less common. The incidence of CNS tuberculosis is a reflection of the overall incidence of tuberculosis in a population. Worldwide, tuberculosis has remained through the centuries and is still a leading cause of mortality from a single infectious disease.[1] Every year, an estimated 7.1 million new cases (of all forms) and 2.6 million deaths occur in Third World countries alone.[2] The incidence of the disease, which had declined dramatically in developed countries and to a great extent in Third World countries because of newer antituberculous drugs, has again increased with the advent of the acquired immunodeficiency syndrome (AIDS),[3–8] emergence of drug-resistant strains of tuberculosis, widespread intravenous drug abuse, and continuing poverty.[9] Tuberculosis has ceased to be a disease of quaint historical interest even in countries like the United States,[10] where the average decline of 5% per year in the tuberculosis case rate plateaued, and from 1986 there has been an increase in the number of reported cases to 2.6%.[6] Pitchenick and colleagues[7] reported that tuberculosis affected 61.4% of Haitians with AIDS. Chaisson and colleagues[8] found that of 287 cases of tuberculosis in a San Francisco population that excluded Asians, 12% had AIDS. In Britain, the incidence of CNS tuberculosis has again increased in areas with large immigrant populations.[11]

Tuberculosis of the nervous system, which merits the attention of a neurosurgeon, occurs in several forms, and more than one form may be present in the same individual (Table 116-1). This chapter deals only with tuberculomas, tuberculous meningitis (TBM), and spinal arachnoiditis. Pott's disease of the spine and tubercular encephalopathy are extensively described in orthopedic and neurologic texts.

TUBERCULOMAS

Incidence

The incidence of tuberculomas in India, which comprised 20% to 30% of all intracranial space-occupying lesions in the 1950s and 1960s, has declined since 1980.[12–15] Although tuberculosis is widely prevalent in Nigeria, only 15 cases of tuberculomas were detected in a 5-year period.[16]

Misdiagnosis was ruled out because a postmortem analysis of all patients dying of intracranial space-occupying lesions showed no cases of tuberculoma. Similarly, in Taiwan, where CNS tuberculosis is common,[17] tuberculomas constituted only 1% of all intracranial mass lesions. A combined series from several neurosurgical centers in Japan showed an incidence of only 2.6%.[18] Tuberculomas are increasingly reported in industrialized nations and account for 1% to 2% of all intracranial lesions.[19–25]

Location

Tuberculomas can occur at any site in the brain (Table 116-2). Unusual sites of tuberculomas include dura mater,[23,26] subdural space, orbital fissure, intraventricular, brain stem,[24,27–29] pituitary gland,[30–33] and hypothalamus.[34] Spinal intramedullary tuberculomas are rare,[35–40] and compared with 128 intracranial lesions, we have treated only five such cases.

Pathologic Features

The typical tuberculoma is a solid, well-defined, avascular mass with multiple nubbins extending into and compressing the surrounding brain. Typically, it is creamy white on the surface and has a pale yellow, often gritty caseating central core with a crenated margin. It has a firm gliotic capsule that at times has a pinkish appearance, which is usually referred to as the mature form of tuberculoma.[41] The immature form consists of multiple small tubercles, some with caseating or liquefied centers dispersed within an

TABLE 116-1 ■ **Tuberculosis of the Nervous System**

Anatomic Area	Manifestation
Intracranial tuberculosis	
Parenchymal	Tuberculoma
	Abscess
	Tubercular encephalopathy
Meningeal	Chronic meningitis
Calvarial	Osteomyelitis
Spinal tuberculosis	
Vertebral	Pott's disease of the spine
Meningeal	Arachnoiditis
Parenchymal	Tuberculoma

TABLE 116-2 ▪ Location of Intracranial Tuberculomas*

Location	Incidence (No.)
Supratentorial	
Parietal	28
Frontal	26
Temporal	15
Basal ganglia or thalamus	4
Sellar or suprasellar	4
Orbital fissure	1
Total	78
Infratentorial	
Cerebellum	44
Cerebellopontine angle	3
Tentorium	1
Brain stem	2
Total	50

*Depending on the location of the major component of the lesion; 128 surgically verfied cases from 1975 to 1992, All India Institue of Medical Sciences Hospital, New Delhi.

edematous brain. Severe edema, possibly caused by an allergic response,[41] may surround these tubercles. Tuberculomas vary in size from 1.5 to 8 cm. Giant tuberculomas can occupy an entire cerebral hemisphere,[42] and many adhere to the dura. The dural attachment can be very tenuous or so firm that the tumor resembles a meningioma.

Microscopically, the central zone of caseous necrosis is surrounded by tuberculous granulation tissue consisting of epithelioid cells, Langerhans' giant cells, and some lymphocytes, polymorphonuclear leukocytes, and plasma cells (Fig. 116-1). Acid-fast bacilli, although sparse, are usually present in both these layers. The brain surrounding a tuberculoma may show degenerated nerve fibers and nerve cells, thrombosed vessels, and, occasionally, swollen astrocytes and oligodendroglial cells. The changes in the small vessels can lead to microhemorrhages or microinfarcts, and these areas may coalesce.[43] Smaller satellite tuberculomas may surround the main mass.

Tuberculomas can take several unusual forms,[44,45] representing the spectrum of inflammatory reaction: (1) incipient tuberculoma, which may appear as an irregular, fleshy,

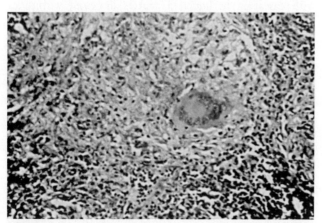

FIGURE 116-1 A photomicrograph of a typical tuberculoma with Langerhans' giant cells, epithelioid cells, and lymphocytes. Hematoxylin and eosin stain, magnification ×100.

gray cortical mass with associated meningeal tuberculomatosis or even grapelike clusters of tuberculoma along cerebral vessels; (2) subdural cyst overlying an intracerebral tuberculoma; (3) cystic tuberculoma; (4) tubercular abscess; (5) extensive edematous encephalopathy without a tuberculoma; (6) severe cerebral edema with a small, "inconsequential" tuberculoma; and (7) rarely, tuberculoma that has spread transdurally to the calvarium.

Tuberculosis is a classic example of a disease the resistance to which is mediated by cellular immunity. The nature of the immunologic compromise in AIDS, with its major effect on cellular immunity, increases host susceptibility to tuberculosis and abscess formation. Chronic inflammatory granulomas seen in immunocompetent patients are less common in patients with AIDS.[46] Organisms belonging to the *Mycobacterium avium-intracellulare* complex are the most common cause of systemic bacterial infection in patients with AIDS and have been demonstrated in 50% of such patients coming to autopsy.[47] Tubercular abscess is a distinct entity from a tuberculoma with central liquefaction. The abscess has a wall of chronic inflammatory cells without tubercular granulomas, and the "pus" contains a large number of acid-fast bacilli.

The liquefaction produced by hydrolytic enzymes released from brain tissue is thought to allow tubercle bacilli to proliferate, leading to abscess formation. Enzyme inhibitors from dead bacilli and necrotic tissue in caseous material have been reported to prevent liquefaction in tuberculous lesions.[48] The vessels in the reactive border zone of tuberculomas show marked proliferation of the basement membrane into several concentric layers associated with fragmentation. This basement membrane, consisting mainly of glycoproteins, may act as a newly formed antigen, initiating a cellular antibody reaction that results in vasculitis and brain damage.[49]

Radhakrishnan and colleagues[50] demonstrated immunohistochemically mycobacterial antigens in the paraffin section of 10 intracranial tuberculous granulomas, none of which demonstrated acid-fast bacilli. In 14 specimens of granulomatous lesions of nontubercular etiology, immunohistochemical stains were negative for mycobacterial antigens. Similarly, polymerase chain reaction assay using DNA extracted from formalin-fixed, paraffin-embedded materials can help differentiate tuberculomas from other granulomas.[51]

Clinical Features

Both sexes are equally affected.[41,52] In our series, there were 66 men and 62 women. Tuberculosis is a disease of the young; 70% of patients are younger than 30 years of age. Tuberculomas are uncommon in children younger than 4 years of age, although we have treated a 9-month-old infant with multiple tuberculomas.

The signs and symptoms of tuberculomas resemble those of other intracranial space-occupying lesions. As they enlarge gradually, the clinical picture is one of a slowly progressive lesion, although in at least 50% of patients, the symptoms are of less than 6 months' duration. Features helpful in distinguishing tuberculomas from other brain tumors are constitutional symptoms, such as weight loss, fever, or malaise; a history of active or known tuberculosis elsewhere in the body; close contact with a patient with an open case of tuberculosis; a high frequency of seizures even in association with a cerebellar lesion; a positive result on the Mantoux test; and a increased sedimentation rate. Infants and young children may have an enlarging head. The clinical diagnosis is often presumptive because in endemic areas, extracranial tuberculosis may coexist with a brain tumor. Pyrexia is variable and may not be present in more than 20% to 25% of patients,[52] and the Mantoux test result may be negative.[41] The clinical course may uncommonly show spontaneous remissions and relapses.[27] Clinical evidence of an active focus of tuberculosis, such as the lungs and lymph glands, may be present in only 33% of patients[41] and in approximately 10% of close relatives. Rare signs include scalp swelling, cerebrospinal fluid (CSF) rhinorrhea, features of a pituitary tumor,[30–33] unilateral proptosis, and trigeminal neuralgia.[41] The clinical picture may be confusing when multiple lesions are present. For instance, a 33-year-old woman presented with behavioral problems, homonymous hemianopsia, hemiparesis, and signs of a partial Brown-Séquard syndrome. On magnetic resonance imaging (MRI), she proved to have multiple tuberculomas in the brain and spinal cord. The diagnosis was established on a cervical lymph node biopsy and response to antituberculous drugs. Intramedullary tuberculomas with no evidence of extracranial tuberculosis are clinically indistinguishable from intramedullary tumors; the diagnosis may be suspected on MRI and is usually established at surgery.

Extrapulmonary manifestations, particularly CNS involvement, is frequently seen in patients with AIDS.[9,53] Seizures, headaches, and an altered mental state are common presentations, but fever is often absent. The infection is usually a reactivation of latent tuberculosis.[54]

The clinical setting of a rare but well-described paradoxical response to antituberculous drugs[9,55–59] has been reviewed by Hejazi and Hassler.[57] Most of these patients were young adults in whom inoperable intracranial tuberculomas located in high-risk regions had developed while they were receiving adequate antitubercular therapy. Frequently, intracranial tuberculomas develop or enlarge at a stage when systemic tuberculosis is responding to therapy. In this group of patients, associated TBM was a common feature. In TBM, symptoms of increased intracranial pressure (ICP) and development of focal neurologic signs, such as motor weakness, cerebellar signs, field defects, visual compromise, and behavioral problems in children, necessitate a search for expanding tuberculomas.

Radiographic Features

An abnormal chest radiograph is a pointer to the diagnosis of a tuberculoma.[60–64] The presence of calcification on conventional radiography is seldom conclusive, with the striking exceptions of the Inuit (Eskimos) and North American Indians, in whom nearly 60% of tuberculomas are known to have calcifications.[47] Calcification does not indicate an inactive lesion.[36] Calcification occurs in fewer than 6% of tuberculomas and is rarely extensive or dense.[42] Cerebral angiography invariably reveals an avascular mass, although surface tuberculomas adherent to the dura may show some peripheral vascularity.[42,64] An associated vascular spasm may be seen that is ascribed to tuberculous vasculitis.[62]

These angiographic findings may also be seen on magnetic resonance angiography.

Computed Tomography and Magnetic Resonance Imaging

Before the advent of computed tomography (CT), the diagnosis of an intracranial tuberculoma was established only by biopsy or after excision. With CT scanning, lesions as small as 1.5 cm in diameter can be fairly accurately identified. These small lesions, which exist without clinical evidence of elevated pressure, were excluded from earlier statistics that were based on surgical material. Reviews from South Africa,[65] India,[61,66,67] Hong Kong,[68] Great Britain,[69] Saudi Arabia,[63] and the United States[70] have pointed out that most tuberculomas are similar in appearance (Figs. 116-2 and 116-3).

The CT scan image of a tuberculoma is characterized by (1) a lesion that appears isodense with the brain or slightly hyperdense and enhances strongly with contrast, revealing a dense, unbroken ring of enhancement; (2) in some cases, an enhancing disc or nodular mass with a regular or irregular margin; and (3) combinations of rings and discs, which may coalesce. Uncommonly, tuberculomas may present as a nonenhancing lesion or even a strongly enhancing lesion that is indistinguishable from a meningioma. Welchman[65] noted that tuberculomas in which the CT characteristics differed from those with ring enhancement were not surrounded by brain parenchyma. He further described the target sign, wherein a central focus of calcification and occasional enhancement is surrounded by a peripheral ring of contrast enhancement (Fig. 116-4). The target sign is not specific for CNS tuberculosis and may lead to an erroneous diagnosis of tuberculosis.[71]

Multiplicity is common in CT scans of patients with tuberculomas. Bhargava and Tandon[60,61] found that 50% to 60% of cases may demonstrate multiple lesions.

Microtuberculomas

The CT scan also picks up small lesions less than 1.5 cm in size, disclike or ring shaped, single or multiple, with slightly increased attenuation that enhances with contrast, and surrounded by disproportionately extensive low-attenuating white matter edema. Bhargava and Tandon[61] labeled them *microtuberculomas*. Careful review of these cases suggests that not all those lesions are tuberculous in etiology. Indian neurologists and neurosurgeons encounter these lesions frequently in children and young adults, but reports have come from other countries as well. The patients usually present with focal epilepsy and no neurologic deficit. Although some of these cases are definitely tuberculomas, as proved by biopsy, others result from a variety of causes.[72–80]

Goulatia and colleagues[75] suggested that edema and increased vascular permeability due to seizures may be responsible for the CT appearance. Chandy and colleagues[73,74] found cysticercosis as the most common cause, and Ahuja and colleagues[72] noted that 12 of their 38 patients were seropositive for cysticercosis and two were seropositive for tuberculosis. On CT scan, tubercular lesions tend to be larger than 20 mm, more frequently irregular in outline, with a midline shift. *Cysticercus* cysts, in contrast, tend to be smaller than 20 mm, with a regular outline and no midline shift.[78] Obviously, it is not possible to arrive at a definitive

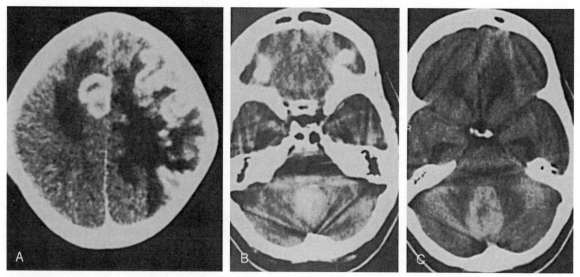

FIGURE 116-2   *A,* A contrast-enhanced computed tomography (CT) scan shows multiple rings and discs surrounded by areas of low attenuation, indicating edema characteristic of tuberculosis. *B* and *C,* Not all tuberculomas are typical. The contrast-enhanced CT scan of a 40-year-old female patient who presented with increased pressure and ataxia and who had bilateral cerebellar signs shows a high attenuating midline posterior fossa lesion, which was thought to be a glioma preoperatively and later proved to be a tuberculoma on histology.

etiologic diagnosis of these lesions. When first seen, they could represent tuberculomas, abscesses, *Cysticercus* granulomas, focal meningoencephalitis, astrocytomas, or metastases. A prospective study of the predictive value of CT diagnosis of intracranial tuberculosis concluded that "although the sensitivity of CT in the diagnosis of intracranial tuberculomas is 100%, and its specificity is 85.7%, the positive predictive value is only 33%." The low positive predictive value of making a diagnosis of intracranial tuberculosis based on CT alone has been cited as reason for obtaining histologic confirmation by open or stereotactic biopsy.[79] Nearly 30% to 40% of these lesions may regress,

either spontaneously or as a result of anticonvulsant drugs alone (Fig. 116-5).

Magnetic Resonance Imaging

On T1-weighted MRI, the granulomas show a slightly hyperintense rim surrounded by a complete or partial rim of slight hypointensity and central isointensity or mixed isointensity and hypointensity. On T2-weighted images, granulomas are hypointense or hyperintense. This hyperintense signal on T2-weighted images made lesions stand out even when there was only minimal central liquefaction.[81] On comparing MRI signal intensities with histologic results,

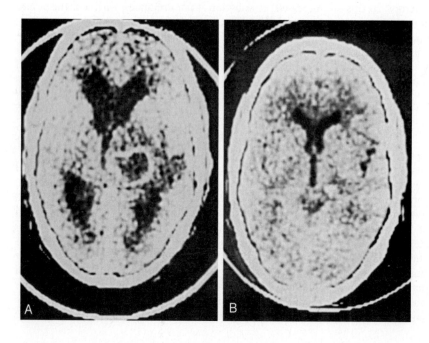

FIGURE 116-3 This patient, who had undergone a kidney transplantation and was on regular immunosuppressants, developed hemiparesis over a 10-day period. *A,* A contrast-enhanced scan shows a large ring-shaped lesion in the right thalamus. Stereotactic aspiration of pus revealed *Mycobacterium tuberculosis.* The patient improved rapidly on medical therapy. *B,* A repeat scan shows almost complete resolution of the lesion.

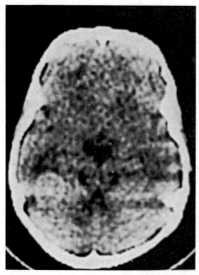

FIGURE 116-4 A contrast-enhanced scan of a 7-year-old girl with elevated intracranial pressure and cerebellar signs shows the target sign of a tuberculoma.

Kim and colleagues[82] noted that the hyperintense and hypointense rims on T1-weighted images corresponded to layers of collagenous fibers and inflammatory cellular infiltrate, respectively, whereas the central zone consisted of caseation necrosis and cellular infiltrate. T2-weighted images did not discriminate between the various layers. Gupta and colleagues[83] found that granulomas that consisted predominantly of macrophages and gliosis were hypointense on T2-weighted images. This characteristic hypointensity of intraparenchymal tuberculomas is not found in most other space-occupying lesions.[25] When the histologic pattern was one of marked cellular infiltration, with minimal gliosis, the appearance was hyperintense on T2-weighted images. In vivo proton magnetic resonance spectroscopy in hypointense lesions shows a marked increase in lipids compared with

normal brain parenchyma[84,85] (Figs. 116-6 to 116-8). Although the course of tuberculosis is more fulminant in the patient with AIDS, the imaging findings are similar to those in nonimmunosuppressed patients.[86]

Spinal intramedullary tuberculomas appear isointense or hypointense on T1-weighted images, and on T2-weighted images, the lesion is isointense, hypointense, or hyperintense, surrounded by a ring of hyperintensity because of the edema that commonly accompanies these lesions. On contrast enhancement, there is rim or nodular enhancement (Fig. 116-9).

Tuberculosis of the pituitary gland is rare, and clues to a tubercular etiology include intense contrast enhancement, meningeal enhancement, and a thick pituitary stalk.[31,32] Pachymeningeal tuberculosis typically is isointense on T1-weighted images and isointense to hypointense on T2-weighted images.[23,26]

Medical Treatment

Antituberculous Drugs

The drugs usually prescribed nearly always belong to a group of six antibiotics known to be effective in the treatment of extracranial tuberculosis (Table 116-3). The first-line agents most commonly used are isoniazid, rifampicin (rifampin), and pyrazinamide, all of which are bactericidal. Ethambutol, a bacteriostatic drug, or streptomycin in children too young to be monitored for visual acuity, is included in the initial treatment regimen if there is a possibility of drug resistance.[87]

The optimal duration of treatment is not definite because, apart from early trials with streptomycin,[88] there is only one controlled trial in the treatment of intracranial tuberculomas or TBM. Rajeswari and colleagues[89] tested the efficacy of a short-course chemotherapy in the treatment of brain tuberculoma in 108 patients and concluded that a 9-month course was effective. This is in marked contrast to the treatment of pulmonary tuberculosis, which is based on data obtained from well-controlled trials. However, at present,

FIGURE 116-5 A contrast-enhanced computed tomography scan of a patient who had right focal motor seizures shows (A) a disklike lesion with disproportionate surrounding low attenuation, which has disappeared 2 months later (B) on anticonvulsant therapy alone.

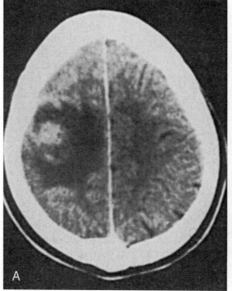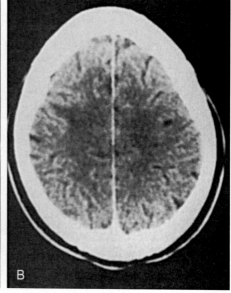

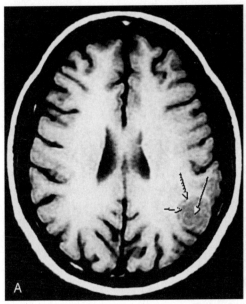 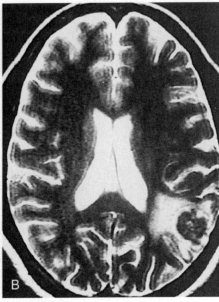

FIGURE 116-6 A magnetic resonance imaging scan of a tuberculoma shows on T1-weighted images, a slightly hyperintense rim (gliosis) surrounded by a complete or partial rim of slight hypointensity (inflammatory cellular infiltrate) and central isointensity, or mixed isointensity and hypointensity (caseation necrosis and cellular infiltrate) (A). B, On T2-weighted images, the granuloma was hypointense (predominantly consisted of paramagnetic free radicals in the macrophages and gliosis). This characteristic hypointensity of intraparenchymal tuberculomas is not found in most other space-occupying lesions. Lesions may be hyperintense as well on T2-weighted images when the histology is of marked cellular infiltration with minimal gliosis.

three or four drugs are administered for the initial 3 or 4 months, and two drugs for an additional 14 to 16 months.[9,52,70,87] Occasionally, drug treatment may have to be prescribed in larger doses for 18 months to 3 years for symptomatic intracranial tuberculomas developing during treatment of TBM.[90,91]

Transient disturbance in liver function is often observed in patients taking a combination of isoniazid and rifampicin. This needs to be monitored at regular intervals. The incidence of serious liver disturbance appears to be higher in Asians.[69] Pyridoxine (10 mg/day) is invariably added to prevent peripheral neuropathy due to isoniazid.

Most intracranial tuberculomas resolve with medical therapy.[52,65–69] The clinical and radiographic improvement

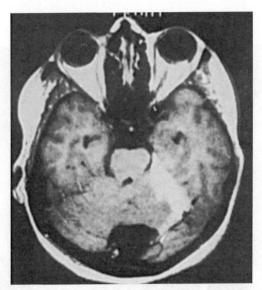

FIGURE 116-7 This magnetic resonance imaging scan of a 25-year-old woman who had headache and seizures for 5 months has an atypical appearance. At surgery, the lesion was confirmed as a tentorial tuberculoma.

is a result of the reduction in the size of the tuberculoma and the perilesional edema. Regardless of their size, lesions usually start to regress after 4 to 6 weeks, and most tuberculomas resolve within 12 to 14 months of treatment. In approximately one third of cases, telltale evidence of the lesion consists of an area of calcification, or sometimes just a speck of low attenuation.[52] Some ring lesions change their character and become disklike or nodular on treatment. In general, patients with increased ICP are slower to respond than those with seizures alone.

Medical treatment may occasionally result in liquefaction of the center of the lesion without any reduction in size.[29] In some patients, the tuberculoma may either show no change or actually increase in size on antituberculous drugs (see earlier).[19,57,59,92] Tuberculomas seem to enlarge and compress the surrounding brain without causing the destruction usually associated with a malignant tumor; as a result, they can resolve with minimal residual deficits.

Drug Resistance

Drug resistance of M. tuberculosis has been recognized since the early days of streptomycin therapy. The current threat is the emergence and spread of strains resistant to isoniazid or rifampicin, making chemotherapy with these agents ineffective. The mechanism is by chromosomal mutation with emergence of resistant clones on the backdrop of inadequate drug therapy. The incidence of acquired multidrug resistance (i.e., resistance to both isoniazid and rifampicin) ranges from 0% to 48%, with low rates in most regions of the world.[93,94] A high rate was reported from New York City.[95] A subsequent report of a decline in the prevalence of drug resistance in the New York study[96] highlights the effectiveness of a strong tuberculosis program and the need for continuous surveillance of drug resistance.[97]

Patients with organisms resistant to rifampicin and isoniazid have a high rate of treatment failure. Patients with human immunodeficiency virus infections not only are more prone to tuberculosis, they are more susceptible to

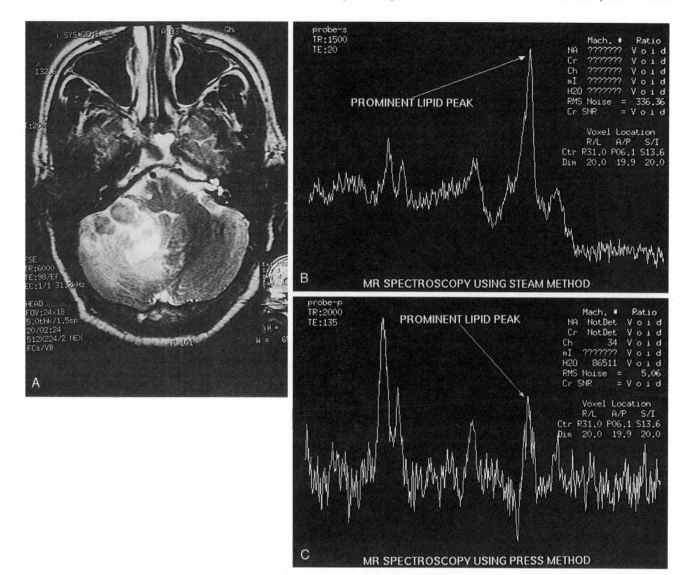

FIGURE 116-8   *A,* This axial T2-weighted image shows a conglomerate of closely opposed lesions with edema of surrounding white matter with mass effect. *B* and *C,* In vivo proton magnetic resonance spectroscopy of the hypointense lesions shows a characteristic lipid peak on stimulated echo acquisition mode (STEAM) and point resolved spectroscopy sequence (PRESS).

drug-resistant tuberculosis.[98–100] Such patients require a longer duration of therapy and may still die of tuberculosis despite optimal treatment.[100]

Corticosteroids are used in the presence of elevated ICP or severe cerebral edema as noted on CT scans. Treatment is seldom prolonged beyond 2 to 3 weeks, during which the corticosteroid therapy can produce dramatic improvement in the patient's clinical state. Occasionally, patients require steroids for a much longer period.

Anticonvulsant Medications

The high incidence of seizures with tuberculomas mandates the routine use of anticonvulsants. The drugs used are phenytoin or carbamazepine, adjusted in dose according to serum levels of the anticonvulsant. Patients taking phenytoin and isoniazid may acquire phenytoin toxicity because high levels of isoniazid in the serum can block metabolism of the anticonvulsant.

Surgery

A tuberculoma that severely elevates ICP and threatens life or vision merits emergent surgical excision. With the exception of these lesions, most neurosurgeons familiar with tuberculomas restrict surgical intervention to (1) patients who do not respond clinically or radiographically to antituberculous drugs; (2) patients whose diagnosis is in doubt, such as those with an atypical CT or MRI scan of the lesion; and (3) patients with obstructive hydrocephalus.

Complete excision of tuberculomas is usually reserved for smaller lesions in noneloquent areas of the brain. Larger lesions require subtotal excision when they cause pressure-related symptoms; rarely is complete removal necessary. An insistence on total excision at the cost of an undesirable neurologic deficit is to be discouraged. In cases of multiple tuberculomas, only the largest mass need be decompressed.

An appropriate craniotomy or craniectomy is performed over the site of the lesion. Perioperative ultrasonography

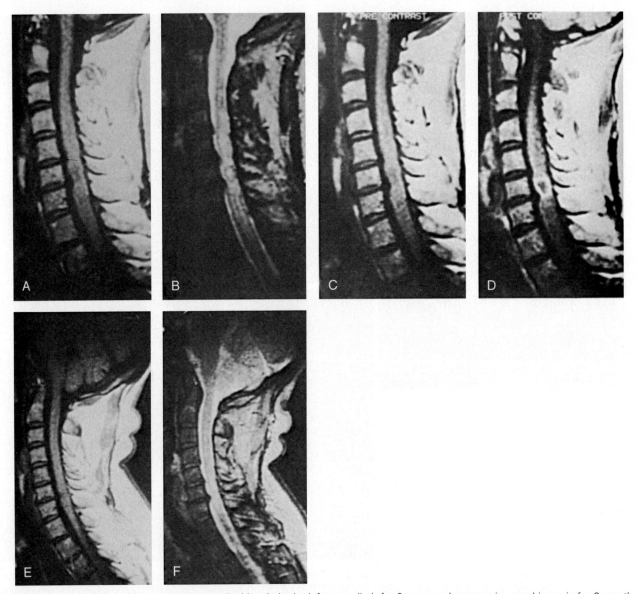

FIGURE 116-9   A 50-year-old woman presented with pain in the left upper limb for 2 years and progressive quadriparesis for 6 months. *A* and *B,* The T1-weighted image shows an intramedullary rounded hyperintense lesion at the C6 level, which is hyperintense with a thin rim of hypointensity around it on the T2-weighted image. The surrounding cord is swollen and edematous. *C* and *D,* The gadolinium–diethylene triamine pentaacetic acid–enhanced image highlights the lesion. *E* and *F,* The patient was put on antituberculous drugs, and 3 months later, a repeat magnetic resonance imaging scan shows resolution of the lesion.

TABLE 116-3 ▪ Antituberculous Drugs

Drug	Dosage	Contraindications	Side Effects
Isoniazid	Oral/intramuscular 300 mg/day (3–10 mg/kg)	Drug-induced liver disease	Peripheral neuritis, psychosis, optic neuritis, occasionally lupus syndrome, convulsions
Rifampicin	Oral 450–600 mg/day (10 mg/kg)	Jaundice, pregnancy	Liver toxicity, gastrointestinal symptoms, rarely shock, respiratory collapse
Ethambutol	Oral (15 mg/kg)	Optic neuritis	Optic neuritis, color blindness, peripheral neuritis
Pyrazinamide	Oral (20–30 mg/kg)	Liver damage	Hepatitis
Streptomycin	Intramuscular 1 g/day (20–25 mg/kg)	Pregnancy	Ototoxicity, renal damage

and image guidance are useful for accurate localization of small, deep-seated lesions. A clear plane of cleavage[41,42,64] exists between the firm, avascular tuberculoma and the edematous brain. The edema is usually not as pronounced as that associated with metastatic deposits. Tuberculous lesions are often on the cortical surface and adherent to the overlying dura. Although dural adhesions are usually separable with ease, the dural attachment at times can be extremely vascular, resembling that of meningiomas.[42] After the tumor surface is identified, it is removed piecemeal from within the confines of the granuloma. The ultrasonic aspirator is a useful aid in decompression. En bloc removal is indicated only for small lesions. Where the center is liquefied or necrotic, aspiration of the contents is sufficient; no attempt should be made to excise the capsule. Subcortical lesions are approached through a small corticectomy with preservation of as many vessels as possible. Parts of the tuberculoma adherent to major vessels, venous sinus, or brain stem are left in situ. The practice of frontal and temporal lobectomy or excision of edematous brain is seldom necessary to achieve decompression. Antitubercular chemotherapy is mandatory even after a complete excision of a tuberculoma.

After several months' administration of antituberculous drugs, the lesion may be tough in consistency and resistant to curetting. If surgical exploration is undertaken for an atypical lesion and a tuberculoma is encountered, minimal surgical manipulation is advised.

CT- or MRI-guided stereotactic biopsy and aspiration is the preferred mode of diagnosis and treatment for (1) deep-seated lesions, such as those in the thalamus or basal ganglia, and (2) tubercular abscesses or tuberculomas with a liquefied center that can be readily decompressed by this method. Atypical lesions also merit a stereotactic instead of an open biopsy. We prefer to use the Leksell frame and the Backlund biopsy kit for such procedures. Bhatia and colleagues[66] described 15 tuberculomas of the basal ganglia and thalamus. Two of the 15 lesions were stereotactically aspirated, yielding pus that showed acid-fast bacilli on the smear that were confirmed as M. tuberculosis on culture. Although the first patient, who had earlier received a kidney transplant, improved remarkably, the second patient was left with a residual hemiparesis (see Fig. 116-3). Although stereotactic biopsy can be quite safe,[28,101] because of cost considerations, a trial with antituberculous therapy is a worthwhile alternative in patients with strong circumstantial evidence of tubercular etiology, reserving surgery only for those lesions that continue to grow in spite of antituberculous drugs.[102] Stereotactic biopsy may also be a procedure of choice for patients with so-called single, small lesions, described earlier, if they fail to resolve on antiepileptic therapy. We have some reservations regarding the safety of biopsy of brain stem lesions, which can be extremely firm.

Chiasmal decompression may be indicated for a suprasellar tuberculoma developing during treatment for TBM. Brain stem tuberculomas are a rarity and seldom require surgical decompression; they may be sampled for biopsy specimen if the diagnosis is in doubt.[28]

A ventriculoperitoneal shunt may be required for a tuberculoma that causes hydrocephalus, resulting either from obstruction of the CSF pathway or from associated TBM. Tuberculomas of the pituitary gland are very rare lesions.[30-33]

We have operated on four such patients, none of whom was diagnosed before surgery. These were all solitary lesions, and three of them were operated on through the transsphenoidal route and one through the subfrontal route. Three patients made a good recovery but required long-term thyroid supplements; the fourth patient died after a stormy postoperative period. He contracted diabetes insipidus, hypothermia, and hypotension.

Results

Initial reports of mortality ranged from 10% to 27% for intracranial tuberculomas, but the results have improved dramatically since then. Harder and colleagues[63] reported no deaths in 20 cases, although two patients were lost to follow-up. In our experience of 50 consecutive cases,[52] one patient died in the hospital and one died 2 years after treatment, probably as a result of infection with a drug-resistant organism. Both of these patients had multiple tuberculomas and markedly elevated ICP. Numerous reports have been published of patients with deep-seated, inaccessible lesions and lesions in the brain stem who have had excellent recoveries.

TUBERCULOUS MENINGITIS

TBM is an uncommon condition in most technologically advanced countries, but it is a major cause of morbidity and mortality in countries where pulmonary tuberculosis is still common. TBM is a disease of childhood whose highest incidence is in the first 3 years of life. It is uncommon before the age of 6 months and is rare before the age of 3 months.[103] More recently, an increasing incidence in adults has been reported, not only in technologically advanced countries[104] but in countries like India. In our experience, adults account for 50% of all patients.

The major neurosurgical interest in TBM is the occurrence of hydrocephalus, tuberculomas, and, rarely, chiasmal and spinal arachnoiditis. In the acute stage, increased ICP is related to the general inflammatory process, increased CSF proteins, and impaired CSF absorption. Radioisotope studies show no obvious obstruction to the CSF flow in the acute stage.[105,106] When the disease becomes subacute or chronic, the inflammatory basal exudates extend along small proliferating blood vessels into the brain substance, leading to a border zone encephalitis associated with diffuse or focal ischemic changes due to vasculitis. Larger vessels, commonly the internal carotid artery siphon, its bifurcation, proximal segments of the middle cerebral artery, and sometimes the anterior cerebral artery, may get involved, leading to occlusion and infarction. The affected artery shows changes of periarteritis, massive subintimal fibrosis with narrowing or obstruction.[107,108]

Hydrocephalus is almost invariable in children who survive for more than 4 to 6 weeks and is most often caused by blockage of the basal cisterns and the sylvian fissures by tubercular exudate. In more chronic phases, hydrocephalus is caused by vascular adhesive arachnoiditis. In some cases, hydrocephalus may be caused by obstruction at the outlet of the fourth ventricle, and less commonly by obstruction at the level of the aqueduct, either as a result of circumferential narrowing of the brain stem by exudates or of an intraluminal tuberculoma. Obstruction of CSF circulation in TBM often occurs at multiple sites.[103] TBM may rarely be followed by the development of syringomyelia despite appropriate chemotherapy.[109]

As the disease becomes more chronic, the exudates become firm and organized. The clinical evidence of meningitis disappears, leaving behind thickened, localized, hard, fibrotic leptomeninges that may form a plaquelike cover over the cerebral hemispheres, posterior fossa, foramen magnum, or spinal cord. The disease, although localized, is still active and can cause progressive symptoms.[105] This condition is increasingly being recognized as a manifestation of CNS tuberculosis[23,26] and must be differentiated from idiopathic hypertrophic pachymeningitis.

Problems of Diagnosis

In many patients, the diagnosis of TBM still poses considerable difficulties. Examination of CSF is often inconclusive, tubercle bacilli being found on direct smears in no more than 10% to 15% of initial samples. A notable exception was the report of Kennedy and Fallon,[104] who isolated M. tuberculosis in 83% of 52 patients. The gold standard in the diagnosis of tuberculosis remains culturing in a Lowenstein-Jensen medium, the BACTEC radiometric system, a mycobacterial growth indicator tube, or luciferase reporter mycobacteriophage assays. The main limitation is the time taken for culture (2 to 6 weeks). As an alternative to bacteriologic methods, several newer techniques have been used to diagnose tuberculosis that are much faster. These include nucleic acid amplification methods and serologic tests.

Serologic tests include enzyme-linked immunosorbent assay to detect M. tuberculosis antigen 5,[110-112] the 38-kD antigen,[110] antigen 60 immunoglobulin G,[113] and lipoarabinomannan antigen.[111,114,115] In general, serologic tests for human immunodeficiency virus–related tuberculosis are disappointing.[110,114] Although specificity is very high, no single test gives 100% sensitivity. Future research is being directed toward identifying the best possible combination of antigens for the serodiagnosis of tuberculosis or a combination of serodiagnosis and polymerase chain reaction to improve sensitivity.[116]

On the whole, the clinical validity of nucleic acid amplification methods to detect M. tuberculosis remains controversial because, although the tests are rapid and sensitive, they remain inferior to culture with regard to sensitivity and specificity.[117-120] In specific clinical situations such as nonpurulent meningitis diagnosed based on cytology and biochemistry of CSF, in which the immediate diagnosis of tuberculosis is essential, such methods are used, overriding considerations of cost and sensitivity. When nucleic amplification results are negative, the test has to be repeated with a fresh specimen or with material obtained from fluid culture systems after 1 to 2 weeks of incubation to maximize the sensitivity. In tropical countries, CSF cultures tend to be less sensitive than nucleic acid amplification methods. Nguyen and colleagues[121] from Vietnam reported on 99 cases of confirmed or probable TBM based on clinical features of TBM and response to antitubercular treatment. They found that PCR had a sensitivity of 32%, culture 17%, and microscopy 1%. The Indian story has been similar, with positive culture rates of approximately 15% in the best of circumstances.[122,123]

To arrive at an early diagnosis of a disease in which any delay involves higher mortality and morbidity, Ahuja and colleagues[123] defined a set of criteria based on clinical features, CSF examination, CT findings, and the presence of extraneural tuberculosis. Seventy-six patients suspected of having tubercular meningitis were divided into definite, highly probable, probable, and possible tubercular meningitis categories based on the criteria. The validity of the criteria was tested using information from bacterial isolation, PCR test for tuberculosis, response to therapy, and autopsy. Ninety-one percent of the patients with highly probable and 66% with probable tuberculosis improved on antituberculosis therapy.

Advances in the use of nucleic acid amplification techniques for evaluating drug resistance need mention.[118,124] Molecular data are available for rifampicin, streptomycin, and isoniazid, but genetic data for other first-line drugs and for second-line drugs are not available. Mutations identified in the gene encoding the RNA polymerase B subunit (rpoB) directly confer rifampicin resistance to M. tuberculosis. The genetic resistance mechanism to isoniazid is more complicated and appears to be based on more than one molecular variant. Although identifying strains resistant to rifampicin is possible with the existing level of molecular technology, until details of genes conferring resistance are known for all first-line drugs, growth-dependent methods will remain the gold standard for determining drug susceptibility.

Imaging

Computed Tomography

Although normal scan results may be seen in the early stages of TBM, the following features may be demonstrable in the course of the illness: exudates in the basal cisterns or sylvian fissures, hydrocephalus, infarcts, tuberculomas, gyral and meningeal enhancement, and edema in the white matter.[1,125-128] The exudate enhancement is irregular and is unlike the sharply defined enhancement of circulating blood in normal vessels in the fissures and cisterns. Hydrocephalus is seen in more than one third of cases in the first scan and becomes more frequent as the disease progresses.[9,129]

In most cases, associated periventricular lucency indicates transependymal CSF flow caused by elevated ICP and is therefore an important sign of impending deterioration. Bullock and Van Dellen[126] pointed out that in TBM, periventricular lucency is likely to be a result of spread of the inflammatory process, making it an unreliable sign of elevated intraventricular pressure.

Magnetic Resonance Imaging

No consistent or characteristic signal abnormality attributed to meningeal inflammation or basal cistern exudate has been described. When hydrocephalus is present, long TR images show any associated interstitial accumulation of CSF as bilateral, rather uniform periventricular areas of increased intensity. MRI is more sensitive in demonstrating early infarcts than is CT[130] (Fig. 116-10).

Medical Treatment

There is evidence that bacille Calmette-Guérin vaccination offers some protection against tubercular meningitis.[131,132] Once meningitis is established, drug therapy similar to that

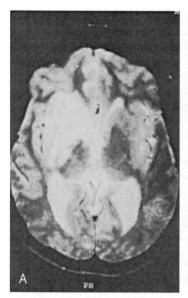 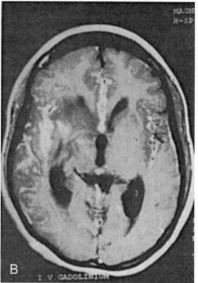 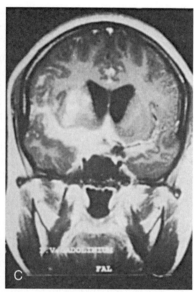

FIGURE 116-10 A 20-year-old woman with tubercular meningitis and left hemiparesis. *A,* The axial T2-weighted image (TR/TE = 2200/90) shows focal areas of infarction involving the striatum, the head of the caudate, and the internal capsule. *B* and *C,* Gadolinium–diethylene triamine pentaacetic acid–enhanced T1-weighted axial and coronal images (TR/TE = 600/15) demonstrate enhancing exudates in the interhemispheric and sylvian fissures, which are more marked on the right side. Note also the enhancement of the leptomeninges over the surface of the brain.

for tuberculomas is initiated (see Table 116-3). Short-course chemotherapy is well established for treatment of pulmonary tuberculosis but not for extrapulmonary disease. Goel and colleagues[133] reviewed 35 cases of TBM in which chemotherapy was given for periods of less than 2 years. Short-term therapy was associated with recrudescence of TBM and, in some cases, with the development of deep cerebral infarcts and permanent neurologic deficit.

In a critical reappraisal of the literature on adjunctive corticosteroid therapy in tuberculosis, Dooley and colleagues[134] concluded steroids did not reduce the efficacy of adequate antimycobacterial therapy and appeared to offer significant short- and long-term benefits in TBM. Several randomized trials of steroids in tubercular meningitis have appeared in the literature. In the first prospective, randomized, controlled trial of dexamethasone in tubercular meningitis, Kumarvelu and associates[135] concluded that dexamethasone appeared to be a useful adjunct, especially in patients with severe disease. A similar prospective, randomized, controlled trial of steroids in TBM in 141 consecutive children concluded that the survival rate and intellectual outcome were significantly better with steroids. There was enhanced resolution of basal exudates and tuberculomas on serial CT scanning. However, ICP and the incidence of basal ganglia infarction remained unchanged.[136] In a randomized, double-blind trial involving 59 adults with TBM, prednisolone was not found to be beneficial in patients with poor neurologic status, increased ICP, and cranial nerve palsies.[137]

Anticonvulsants are a desirable part of the drug therapy because of the high incidence of seizures in tubercular meningitis. The treatment protocol for long-term anti-convulsant therapy in children advocated by Patwari and colleagues[138] depends on the clinical and electroencephalo-graphic or scan characteristics suggestive of an abnormal focus resulting in secondary epilepsy. All children with focal seizures and those with generalized tonic-clonic seizures and tonic spasms manifesting more than once during hospitalization or associated with abnormal CT or electro-encephalographic findings were given long-term anti-convulsants. Children without seizures and those with generalized tonic-clonic seizures before hospitalization or not more than one seizure during the first week of hospitalization and without abnormal CT or electroencephalographic findings were not given long-term anticonvulsants. In the absence of anticonvulsants, seizures occurred in less than 10% of children in the first 3 months. However, close follow-up is essential, especially when anticonvulsant therapy has been withheld.

Surgery

Sir Hugh Cairns[139] first advocated ventricular decompression during the acute stage of TBM. Since then, numerous procedures have been tried, and reports have conclusively documented the efficacy of ventriculoatrial or ventriculo-peritoneal shunts for this condition.[128,139–142] The fear of spreading tubercle bacilli through the shunt is unfounded. Hydrocephalus may resolve with medical treatment alone; however, surgical diversion of CSF is indicated when hydro-cephalus is associated with symptomatic elevated ICP.

Ventriculoperitoneal shunts usually are preferred to ventriculoatrial shunts because of the numerous vascular complications associated with the latter. After a shunt is inserted, a progressive reduction in size of the ventricles occurs, but the ventricles may not return to normal size.[125] A low-pressure shunt appears to be best suited to these patients. Infrequently, separate shunts are required for each lateral ventricle if a CSF block is present at the level of Monro's foramen. Alternatively, an endoscopic interven-triculostomy eliminates the need for two ventricular ends. Loculations within ventricles could similarly be fenestrated to reduce the number of shunts required. Where the obstruction is at the aqueduct or the fourth ventricular outlet on imaging, it is tempting to perform a third ventriculostomy, but the surgeon must keep in mind that CSF frequently is obstructed at multiple sites, and bypassing one obstruction may simply uncover another.

Rarely, optochiasmal arachnoiditis may be responsible for the development of visual deterioration and may indicate a need for decompression of the optic nerves and chiasm.[92] Cerebral tuberculomas can develop insidiously during treatment of TBM,[55–59] and the patient may die as a result of elevated ICP. These tuberculomas tend to occur in deep structures, making surgical access difficult and hazardous. Steroids may be of help during the crisis.[57]

Results

The prognosis of TBM depends on the delay in treatment, the patient's level of consciousness, the presence and degree of exudates, and the presence of hydrocephalus and cerebral infarcts.[125,142–145] After tubercular meningitis, there is frequent marked, generalized impairment of cognitive and motor development.[146] Palur and colleagues[142] reviewed 114 patients with TBM and hydrocephalus who underwent shunt surgery. During a long-term follow-up period ranging from 6 months to 13 years (mean, 45.6 months), the mortality rate was 20% for patients in grade I (headache, vomiting, fever, and neck stiffness with normal sensorium and no neurologic deficit), 34.7% for patients in grade II (normal sensorium, neurologic deficit present), 51.9% for patients in grade III (altered sensorium but easily arousable with or without dense neurologic deficit), and 100% for patients in grade IV (deeply comatose, decerebrate, or decorticate posturing). Only grade at the time of admission was statistically significant in determining the final outcome ($P < 0.001$). The other factors studied included age at admission, duration of altered sensorium, CSF cell count at initial examination, CSF protein level at initial examination, number of shunt revisions required, and necessity of bilateral shunts. Early shunt surgery is advocated for patients in grades I and II. For patients in grade III, surgery may be performed either without a trial of external ventricular drainage or when an improvement in sensorium occurs after such a trial. All patients in grade IV should undergo external ventricular drainage, and only those who show a significant change in their neurologic status within 24 to 48 hours of drainage should undergo shunt surgery.

TUBERCULOUS SPINAL ARACHNOIDITIS

Tuberculous spinal arachnoiditis usually occurs as a result of a spread of meningitis from within the cranium either during the course of treatment, while the disease is still active, or after a variable period of months to years after the disease has "burnt out."[147,148] Sometimes the disease may start primarily in the spinal meninges because of rupture into the subarachnoid space of a superficial spinal tuberculoma.[149,150] Rarely, the disease occurs as a result of a direct transdural spread in caries spine.[151]

The maximal involvement is in the thoracic and thoracolumbar region, with longitudinal extensions ranging from a few segments to the entire cord. The disease is more marked posterior to the cord, and it may be difficult to distinguish the meninges from the cord. The meninges may become thickened and hard, whereas the cord is atrophied, soft, and edematous, with one or more visible tuberculomas on the surface. As the exudates organize, the spinal cord or roots get entrapped, producing a myeloradiculopathy.[152]

Clinical Features

The appearance of root pain, weakness of the lower limbs, and sphincter disturbances in a patient with tubercular meningitis suggests the diagnosis of an evolving spinal arachnoiditis. Examination reveals a mixture of upper and lower motor neuron signs with patchy sensory deficits.

Imaging

Tuberculous arachnoiditis on myelography shows an irregular thecal sac, nodularity, and thickening of the nerve roots with clumping of the roots to each other and the thecal sac, and CSF block. These findings are reflected on MRI scans. In addition, there are CSF loculations and an increase in CSF intensity on T1-weighted images, leading to loss of cord-CSF interface or a shaggy outline. Cord involvement is seen in more than 80% of cases in the form of increased intensity on T2-weighted images and cord cavitation (Fig. 116-11). With contrast, there is meningeal enhancement in 80%,

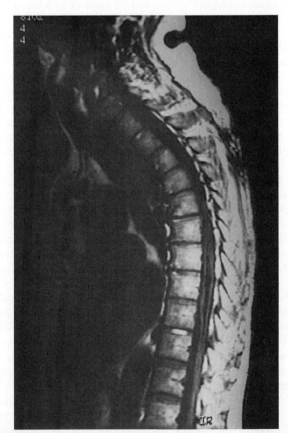

FIGURE 116-11 A case of tubercular spinal arachnoiditis in which the patient continued to deteriorate neurologically, even after completion of antitubercular treatment due to a developing syringomyelia.

although enhancement of the roots and cord is less frequently seen. Associated findings of tuberculous spondylitis, basal exudate, and intracranial granulomas are additional clues to the diagnosis.[153–155]

Treatment

It is generally accepted that steroids are a useful adjunct in treating patients threatened with paraplegia. Intrathecal steroids may help in further resolution of the exudate. Satish Chandra[156] have advocated intrathecal hyaluronidase to lyse the adhesions. Recurrence is common, and available treatments are not very effective. The outcome of surgical intervention is quite unpredictable, and it may be offered as a treatment option if the diagnosis is in doubt, in localized lesions, or if imaging suggests a cyst at the expected clinical level.

Acknowledgments

The authors thank D. C. Aggarwal, New Delhi, for providing Figures 116-7, 116-9, and 116-10, and Drs. Harsh Mahajan, Sandeep Kawlra, and Arun Mahajan, from GMR Institute of Imaging and Research, New Delhi, for Figures 116-6, 116-8, and 116-11.

REFERENCES

1. Bloom BR, Murray JL: Tuberculosis: Commentary on a re-emergent killer. Science 257:1055–1064, 1992.
2. Murray CJL: World tuberculosis burden. Lancet 335:1043–1044, 1990.
3. Slutkin G, Leowski J, Mann J: Tuberculosis and AIDS: The effect of the AIDS epidemic on the tuberculosis problem and tuberculosis programmes. Bull Int Union Tuberc Lung Dis 63:21–24, 1988.
4. Schurmann D, Nightingale SD, Bergmann F, Ruf B: Tuberculosis and HIV infection: A review. Infection 25:274–280, 1997.
5. Lesprit P, Zagdanski AM, de La Blanchardiere A, et al: Cerebral tuberculosis in patients with the acquired immunodeficiency syndrome (AIDS): Report of 6 cases and review. Medicine (Baltimore) 76:423–431, 1997.
6. Centers for Disease Control and Prevention: Tuberculosis final data: United States 1986. MMWR Morb Mortal Wkly Rep 36:817–820, 1988.
7. Pitchenick AE, Cole C, Russel B, et al: Tuberculosis, atypical mycobacteriosis and the acquired immuno-deficiency syndrome among Haitian and non Haitian patients in South Florida. Ann Intern Med 101:641–645, 1984.
8. Chaisson RE, Sheeter GE, Thever CP, Rutherford GW: Tuberculosis patients with the acquired immuno-deficiency syndrome, clinical features, response to therapy and survival. Am Rev Respir Dis 136:570–574, 1987.
9. Teoh R, Humphries MJ: Tuberculous meningitis. In Lambert HP (ed): Infections of the Central Nervous System. Philadelphia: BC Decker, 1991, p 189.
10. Davidson PT: Tuberculosis: New views of an old issue. N Engl J Med 312:1514–1515, 1985.
11. Tang LM, Swash M: Tuberculosis of the nervous system: A modern problem. J R Soc Med 78:429–432, 1985.
12. Lalitha VS, Dastur DK: Tuberculosis of the central nervous system. II: Brain tuberculomas vis-à-vis intracranial space-occupying lesions, 1953-1978. Neurol India 28:202–206, 1980.
13. Mathai KV, Chandy J: Tuberculous infection of the nervous system. Clin Neurosurg 14:145–177, 1966.
14. Ramamurthi B, Ramamurthi R, Vasudevan MC, et al: The changing face of tuberculomas. Ann Acad Med 22:852–855, 1993.
15. Tandon PN: Nervous system tuberculomas and their surgical management. Neurol Infect Epidemiol 1:109–117, 1996.
16. Ohaegbulam SC, Amuta J, Saddeqi N: Tuberculoma of the central nervous system in eastern Nigeria. Tubercle 60:163–166, 1979.
17. Tang LM, Chee CY, Cheng SY, et al: Neurological complications of tuberculous meningitis. In Sixth Asian and Oceanian Congress of Neurology Abstracts. Amsterdam: Excerpta Medica, 1983, pp 93–94.
18. Katsura S, Suzuki J, Wada T: A statistical study of brain tumors in the neurosurgical clinics of Japan. J Neurosurg 16:570–580, 1959.
19. Chambers ST, Hendrickse WA, Record C, et al: Paradoxical expansion of intracranial tuberculomas during chemotherapy. Lancet 1:181–184, 1984.
20. Anderson JM, MacMillan JJ: Intracranial tuberculoma: An increasing problem in Britain. J Neurol Neurosurg Psychiatry 38:194–201, 1975.
21. Lehrer H, Venkatesh B, Girolamo R, et al: Tuberculoma of the brain (revisited). AJR Am J Roentgenol 118:594–600, 1973.
22. Gropper MR, Schulder M, Sharan AD, Cho ES: Central nervous system tuberculosis: Medical management and surgical indications. Surg Neurol 44:378–384, 1995.
23. Parney IF, Johnson ES, Allen PB: "Idiopathic" cranial hypertrophic pachymeningitis responsive to antituberculous therapy: Case report. Neurosurgery 41:965–971, 1997.
24. Gropper MR, Schulder M, Duran HL, Wolansky L: Cerebral tuberculosis with expansion into brainstem tuberculoma: Report of two cases. J Neurosurg 81:927–931, 1994.
25. Kioumehr F, Dadsetan MR, Rooholamini SA, Au A: Central nervous system tuberculosis: MRI. Neuroradiology 36:93–96, 1994.
26. Goyal M, Sharma A, Mishra NK, et al: Imaging appearance of pachymeningeal tuberculosis. AJR Am J Roentgenol 169:1421–1424, 1997.
27. Mahanta A, Kalra L, Maheshwari MC, et al: Brain stem tuberculoma: An unusual presentation. J Neurol 227:249–253, 1982.
28. Rajshekhar V, Chandy MJ: Tuberculomas presenting as isolated intrinsic brainstem masses. Br J Neurosurg 11:127–133, 1997.
29. Pandya SK, Desai AD, Dastur HM: Caseative liquefaction within brain stem tuberculoma under drug therapy with simultaneous regression of cerebral tuberculomas. Neurol India 30:121–128, 1982.
30. Choudhary C, Mehta VS, Roy S: Tuberculoma of anterior pituitary: A case report. Neurol India 34:341–344, 1986.
31. Ashkan K, Papadopoulos MC, Casey AT, et al: Hypophyseal tuberculoma: Report of two cases. Acta Neurochir (Wien) 139:523–525, 1997.
32. Ranjan A, Chandy MJ: Intrasellar tuberculoma. Br J Neurosurg 8:179–185, 1994.
33. Brooks PH, Dumlao JS, Bronsky D, Waldstein SS: Hypophysial tuberculoma with hypopituitarism. Am J Med 54:777–781, 1973.
34. Indira B, Panigrahi MK, Vajramani G, et al: Tuberculoma of the hypothalamic region as a rare cause of hypopituitarism: A case report. Surg Neurol 45:347–350, 1996.
35. Jena A, Banerji AK, Tripathi RP, et al: Demonstration of intramedullary tuberculomas by magnetic resonance imaging: A report of two cases. Br J Radiol 64:555–558, 1991.
36. Rhoton EL, Ballinger WE Jr, Quisling R, Sypert GW: Intramedullary spinal tuberculoma. Neurosurgery 22:733–736, 1988.
37. Sanchez Pernaute R, Berciano J, Rebollo M, Pascual J: Intramedullary tuberculoma of the spinal cord with syringomyelia. Neuroradiology 38(suppl 1):105–106, 1996.
38. Gupta VK, Sharma BS, Khosla V: Intramedullary tuberculoma: Report of two cases with MRI findings. Surg Neurol 44:241–243, 1995.
39. Hanci M, Sarioglu AC, Uzan M, et al: Intramedullary tuberculous abscess: A case report. Spine 21:766–769, 1996.
40. Citow JS, Ammirati M: Intramedullary tuberculoma of the spinal cord: Case report. Neurosurgery 35:327–330, 1994.
41. Dastur HM: Tuberculoma. In Vinken PJ, Bruyn GW (eds): Handbook of Clinical Neurology, vol. 18. New York: Elsevier, 1975, pp 413–426.
42. Ramamurthi B, Varadarajan MG: Diagnosis of tuberculomas of the brain. J Neurosurg 18:1–7, 1961.
43. Dastur DK: Neurosurgically relevant aspects of pathology and pathogenesis of intracranial and intraspinal tuberculosis. Neurosurg Rev 6:103–110, 1983.
44. Sinh G, Pandya SK, Dastur DK: Pathogenesis of unusual intracranial tuberculomas and tuberculous space-occupying lesions. J Neurosurg 29:149–159, 1968.
45. Sandhyamani S, Roy S, Bhatia R: Tuberculous brain abscess. Acta Neurochir (Wien) 59:247–256, 1981.
46. Farrar DJ, Flanigan TP, Gordon NM, et al: Tuberculous brain abscess in a patient with HIV infection: Case report and review. Am J Med 102:297–301, 1997.
47. Armstrong FB, Edwards AM: Intracranial tuberculoma in native races of Canada, with special reference to symptomatic epilepsy and neurologic features. CMAJ 89:56–65, 1963.
48. Dannenberg AM Jr, Sugimoto M: Liquefaction of caseous foci in tuberculosis. Am Rev Respir Dis 113:257–259, 1976.

49. Dastur DK, Dave UP: Further observations on the fine structure of blood vessels in neurotuberculosis: Possible significance of vasculitis with proliferated basement membranes. Adv Neurol 20:577–589, 1978.

50. Radhakrishnan VV, Mathai A, Radhakrishnan NS: Immunohistochemical demonstration of mycobacterial antigen in intracranial tuberculoma. Indian J Exp Biol 29:641–644, 1991.

51. Osaki M, Adachi H, Gomyo Y, et al: Detection of mycobacterial DNA in formalin-fixed, paraffin-embedded tissue specimens by duplex polymerase chain reaction: Application to histopathological diagnosis. Mod Pathol 10:78–83, 1997.

52. Tandon PN, Bhargava S: Effect of medical treatment on intracranial tuberculoma: A CT study. Tubercle 66:85–97, 1985.

53. Martinez Vazquez C, Bordon J, Rodriguez Gonzalez A, et al: Cerebral tuberculoma: A comparative study in patients with and without HIV infection. Infection 23:149–153, 1995.

54. Bishberg E, Sunderam G, Reichman LB, Kapila R: Central nervous system tuberculosis with the acquired immunodeficiency syndrome and its related complex. Ann Intern Med 105:210–213, 1986.

55. Alame T, Keller K, Michel O, Sergysels R: Hyperthermia occurring with paradoxical development of cerebral tuberculomas. Respiration 63:381–383, 1996.

56. Borah NC, Maheshwari MC, Mishra NK, et al: Appearance of tuberculoma during the course of TB meningitis. J Neurol 231:269–270, 1984.

57. Hejazi N, Hassler W: Multiple intracranial tuberculomas with atypical response to tuberculostatic chemotherapy. Infection 25:233–239, 1997.

58. Lebas J, Malkin JE, Coquin Y, et al: Cerebral tuberculomas developing during treatment of tuberculous meningitis. Lancet 2:84, 1980.

59. Malik GM, Mubarik M, Basu JA, et al: Paradoxical expansion of cerebral tuberculomas during therapy for Pott's spine. J R Soc Med 89:643–644, 1996.

60. Bhargava S, Tandon PN: Intracranial tuberculomas: A CT study. Br J Radiol 53:935–945, 1980.

61. Bhargava S, Tandon PN: CNS tuberculosis: Lessons learned from CT studies. Neurol India 28:207–212, 1980.

62. Dastur HM, Desai AD: A comparative study of brain tuberculomas and gliomas based upon 107 case records of each. Brain 88:375–396, 1965.

63. Harder E, Al-Kawl MZ, Carney P: Intracranial tuberculomas: Conservative management. Am J Med 74:570–576, 1983.

64. Tandon PN, Pathak SN: Tuberculosis of the central nervous system. In Spillane JD (ed): Tropical Neurology. London: Oxford University Press, 1973, pp 51–62.

65. Welchman JM: Computerized tomography of intracranial tuberculoma. Clin Radiol 30:567–573, 1979.

66. Bhatia R, Tandon PN, Misra NK: Inflammatory lesions of the basal ganglia and thalamus: Review of twenty-one cases. Neurosurgery 19:983–988, 1986.

67. Vengsarkar US, Pisipaty RP, Parekh B, et al: Intracranial tuberculoma and the CT scan. J Neurosurg 64:568–574, 1986.

68. Teoh R, Humphries MJ, Hoare RD, O'Mahony G: Clinical correlation of CT changes in 64 Chinese patients with tuberculous meningitis. J Neurol 236:48–51, 1989.

69. Traub M, Colchester ACF, Kingsley DP, Swash M: Tuberculosis of the central nervous system. Q J Med 53:81–100, 1984.

70. Mayers MM, Kaufman DM, Miller MH: Recent cases of intracranial tuberculomas. Neurology 28:256–260, 1978.

71. Bargallo J, Berenguer J, Garcia Barrionuevo J, et al: The "target sign": Is it a specific sign of CNS tuberculoma? Neuroradiology 38:547–550, 1996.

72. Ahuja GK, Behari M, Prasad K, et al: Disappearing CT lesions in epilepsy: Is tuberculosis or cysticercosis the cause? J Neurol Neurosurg Psychiatry 52:915–916, 1989.

73. Chandy MJ, Rajsekhar VR, Ghosh S, et al: Single small enhancing CT lesions in Indian patients with epilepsy: Clinical radiological and pathological considerations. J Neurol Neurosurg Psychiatry 54:702–705, 1991.

74. Chandy MJ, Rajshekhar V, Prakash S, et al: Cysticercosis causing single small CT lesions in Indian patients with epilepsy. Lancet 1:390–391, 1989.

75. Goulatia RK, Verma A, Mishra NK, Ahuja GK: Disappearing CT lesions in epilepsy. Epilepsia 28:523–527, 1987.

76. Rajshekhar V: Etiology and management of single small CT lesion in patients with seizures: Understanding a controversy. Acta Neurol Scand 84:465–470, 1991.

77. Rajshekhar V, Chandy MJ: Validation of diagnostic criteria for solitary cerebral cysticercus granuloma in patients presenting with seizures. Acta Neurol Scand 96:76–81, 1997.

78. Rajshekhar V, Haran RP, Prakash GS, Chandy MJ: Differentiating solitary small cysticercus granuloma and tuberculomas in patients with epilepsy: Clinical and computerised tomographic criteria. J Neurosurg 78:402–407, 1993.

79. Selvapandian S, Rajshekhar V, Chandy MJ, Idikula J: Predictive value of computer tomography-based diagnosis of intracranial tuberculomas. Neurosurgery 35:845–850, 1994.

80. Wadia RS, Makhale CN, Kelkar AV, Grant KB: Focal epilepsy in India with special reference to lesions showing ring or disc-like enhancement on contrast computed tomography. J Neurol Neurosurg Psychiatry 50:1298–1301, 1987.

81. Gupta RK, Jena A, Singh AK, et al: Role of magnetic resonance (MR) in the diagnosis and management of intracranial tuberculoma. Clin Radiol 41:120–127, 1990.

82. Kim TK, Chang KH, Kim CJ, et al: Intracranial tuberculoma: Comparison of MR with pathologic findings. AJNR Am J Neuroradiol 16:1903–1908, 1995.

83. Gupta RK, Pandey R, Khan EM, et al: Intracranial tuberculomas: MRI signal intensity correlation with histopathology and localised proton spectroscopy. Magn Reson Imaging 11:443–449, 1993.

84. Gupta RK, Poptani H, Kohli A, et al: In vivo localized proton magnetic resonance spectroscopy of intracranial tuberculomas. Indian J Med Res 101:19–24, 1995.

85. Gupta RK, Roy R, Dev R, et al: Finger printing of *Mycobacterium tuberculosis* in patients with intracranial tuberculomas by using in vivo, ex vivo, and in vitro magnetic resonance spectroscopy. Magn Reson Med 36:829–833, 1996.

86. Villoria MF, Fortea F, Moreno S, et al: MR imaging and CT of central nervous system tuberculosis in the patient with AIDS. Radiol Clin North Am 33:805–820, 1995.

87. Bass JB Jr, Farer LS, Hopewell PC, et al: Treatment tuberculosis infection in adults and children: American Thoracic Society and The Centers for Disease Control and Prevention. Am J Respir Crit Care Med 149:1359–1374, 1994.

88. Medical Research Council (Streptomycin in Tuberculosis Trials Committee): Streptomycin treatment of tuberculous meningitis. Lancet 1:582–596, 1948.

89. Rajeswari R, Sivasubramanian S, Balambal R, et al: A controlled clinical trial of short-course chemotherapy for tuberculoma of the brain. Tuber Lung Dis 76:311–317, 1995.

90. Lees AJ, MacLeod AF, Marshall J: Cerebral tuberculomas developing during treatment of tuberculosis meningitis. Lancet 1:1208–1211, 1980.

91. Teoh R, Humphries MJ, O'Mahony G: Symptomatic intracranial tuberculoma developing during treatment of tuberculosis: A report of 10 patients and review of the literature. Q J Med 241:449–460, 1987.

92. Teoh R, Poon W, Humphries MJ, O'Mahony G: Suprasellar tuberculoma developing during treatment of tuberculous meningitis requiring urgent surgical decompression. J Neurol 235:321–322, 1988.

93. Cohn DI, Bustreo F, Raviglione MC: Drug resistant tuberculosis: Review of the worldwide situation and the WHO/IUATLD global surveillance project. Clin Infect Dis 24(suppl 1):121–130, 1997.

94. Paramasivan CN: An overview of drug resistant tuberculosis in India. Indian J Tuberc 45:73–81, 1998.

95. Frieden TR, Sterling T, Pablos-Mendez A, et al: The emergence of drug resistant tuberculosis in New York City. N Engl J Med 328:521–526, 1993.

96. Fujiwara PI, Cook SV, Rutherford CM, et al: Continuing survey of drug resistance tuberculosis, New York City, April 1994. Arch Intern Med 157:531–536, 1997.

97. WHO Global Tuberculosis Programme and IUATLD: Guidelines for surveillance of drug resistance in tuberculosis. WHO/TB/96 216. Geneva: World Health Organization, 1997.

98. Angarano G, Carbonara D, Costa D: Drug resistance of *Mycobacterium tuberculosis* strains isolated from HIV-infected Italian patients: Preliminary report from a multicentric study. The Italian Tuberculosis Drug Resistance Study Group. Microbiologica 18:69–72, 1995.

99. Kim SJ, Hong YP: Drug resistance of *Mycobacterium tuberculosis* in Korea. Tuber Lung Dis 73:219–224, 1992.

100. Pablos-Mendez A, Sterling T, Freiden TR: The relationship between delayed or incomplete treatment and all-cause mortality in patients with tuberculosis. JAMA 276:1223–1228, 1996.

101. Rajshekhar V, Chandy MJ: CT-guided stereotactic surgery in the management of intracranial tuberculomas. Br J Neurosurg 7:665–671, 1993.

102. Ramamurthi B, Ramamurthi R, Vasudevan MC, Sridhar K: The changing face of tuberculomas. Ann Acad Med Singapore 22:852–855, 1993.

103. Tandon PN, Bhatia R, Bhargava S: Tuberculous meningitis. In Vinken PK, Bruyn GW, Klawans HL (eds): Handbook of Clinical Neurology, vol. 8. Amsterdam: Elsevier, 1988, pp 195–226.

104. Kennedy DH, Fallon RJ: Tuberculous meningitis. JAMA 241:264–268, 1984.

105. Suwanwela E: Complications of tuberculous meningitis. Proc Aust Assoc Neurol 3:493–495, 1968.

106. Tandon PN, Rao MAP, Banerji AK, et al: Isotope scanning of the cerebrospinal fluid pathways in tubercular meningitis. J Neurol Sci 25:401–413, 1975.

107. Dastur DK, Manghani DK, Udani PM: Pathology and pathogenetic mechanisms in neurotuberculosis. Radiol Clin North Am 33:733–752, 1995.

108. Dastur DK, Wadia NH: Spinal meningitis with radiculomyelopathy: Part II. J Neurol Sci 8:261–297, 1969.

109. Fehlings MG, Bernstein M: Syringomyelia as a complication of tuberculous meningitis. Can J Neurol Sci 19:84–87, 1992.

110. Bothamley GH: Serological diagnosis of tuberculosis. Eur Respir J Suppl 20:676–688, 1995.

111. Gupta S, Bhatia R, Datta KK: Serodiagnosis of tuberculosis. J Commun Dis 27:208–214, 1995.

112. Radhakrishnan VV, Mathai A: Enzyme-linked immunosorbent assay to detect *Mycobacterium tuberculosis* antigen 5 and antimycobacterial antibody in cerebrospinal fluid of patients with tubercular meningitis. J Clin Lab Anal 5:233–237, 1991.

113. Thakur A, Mandal A: Usefulness of ELISA using antigen A60 in serodiagnosis of neurotuberculosis. J Commun Dis 28:8–14, 1996.

114. Ratanasuwan W, Kreiss JK, Nolan CM, et al: Evaluation of the MycoDot test for the diagnosis of tuberculosis in HIV seropositive and seronegative patients. Int J Tuberc Lung Dis 1:259–264,1997.

115. Park SC, Lee BI, Cho SN, et al: Diagnosis of tuberculous meningitis by detection of immunoglobulin G antibodies to purified protein derivative and lipoarabinomannan antigen in cerebrospinal fluid. Tuber Lung Dis 74:317–322, 1993.

116. Miorner H, Sjobring U, Nayak P, Chandramuki A: Diagnosis of tuberculous meningitis: A comparative analysis of 3 immunoassays, an immune complex assay and the polymerase chain reaction. Tuber Lung Dis 76:381–386, 1995.

117. Forbes BA: Critical assessment of gene amplification approaches on the diagnosis of tuberculosis. Immunol Invest 26:105–116, 1997.

118. Roth A, Schaberg T, Mauch H: Molecular diagnosis of tuberculosis: Current clinical validity and future perspectives. Eur Respir J 10:1877–1891, 1997.

119. Shankar P, Manjunath N, Mohan KK, et al: Rapid diagnosis of tuberculous meningitis by polymerase chain reaction. Lancet 337:5–7, 1991.

120. A new diagnostic test for tuberculous meningitis [editorial]. Tubercle 66:157, 1985.

121. Nguyen LN, Kox LF, Pham LD, et al: The potential contribution of the polymerase chain reaction to the diagnosis of tuberculous meningitis. Arch Neurol 53:771–776, 1996.

122. Selvakumar N, Vanajakumar, Thilothammal N, Paramasivan CN: Isolation of *Mycobacterium tuberculosis* from cerebrospinal fluid by the centrifugation and filtration methods. Indian J Med Res 103:250–252, 1996.

123. Ahuja GK, Mohan KK, Prasad K, Behari M: Diagnostic criteria for tuberculous meningitis and their validation. Tuber Lung Dis 75:149–152, 1994.

124. Pretorius GS, Sirgel FA, Schaaf HS, et al: Rifampicin resistance in *Mycobacterium tuberculosis*: Rapid detection and implications in chemotherapy. S Afr Med J 86:50–55, 1996.

125. Bhargava S, Gupta AK, Tandon PN: Tuberculous meningitis: A CT study. Br J Radiol 55:189–196, 1982.

126. Bullock MRR, Van Dellen JR: The role of cerebrospinal fluid shunting in tuberculous meningitis. Surg Neurol 18:274–276, 1982.

127. Kingsley DPE, Hendrickse WA, Kendall BE, et al: Tuberculous meningitis: Role of CT in management and prognosis. J Neurol Neurosurg Psychiatry 50:30–36, 1987.

128. Upadhyaya P, Bhargava S, Sundaram KP, et al: Hydrocephalus caused by tuberculous meningitis: Clinical picture, CT findings, and results of shunt surgery. Z Kinderchir 38:76–79, 1983.

129. Patwari AK, Aneja S, Ravi RN, et al: Convulsions in tuberculous meningitis. J Trop Pediatr 42:91–97, 1996.

130. Brown BC, Post MJD: Intracranial infections. In Atlas SW (ed): Magnetic Resonance Imaging of the Brain and Spine. New York: Raven Press, 1991, pp 520–523.

131. Zodpey SP, Maldhure BR, Shrikhande SN, Tiwari RR: Effectiveness of bacillus of Calmette-Guerin (BCG) vaccination against tuberculous meningitis: A case-control study. J Indian Med Assoc 94:338–340, 1996.

132. Rodrigues LC, Diwan VK, Wheeler JG: Protective effect of BCG against tuberculous meningitis and miliary tuberculosis: A meta-analysis. Int J Epidemiol 22:1154–1158, 1993.

133. Goel A, Pandya SK, Satoskar AR: Whither short course chemotherapy meningitis? Neurosurgery 27:418–421, 1990.

134. Dooley DP, Carpenter JL, Rademacher S: Adjunctive corticosteroid therapy for tuberculosis: A critical reappraisal of the literature. Clin Infect Dis 25:872–887, 1997.

135. Kumarvelu S, Prasad K, Khosla A, et al: Randomised controlled trial of dexamethasone in tuberculous meningitis. Tuber Lung Dis 75:203–207, 1994.

136. Schoeman JF, Van Zyl LE, Laubscher JA, Donald PR: Effect of corticosteroids on intracranial pressure, computed tomographic findings, and clinical outcome in young children with tuberculous meningitis. Pediatrics 99:226–231, 1997.

137. Chotmongkol V, Jitpimolmard S, Thavornpitak Y: Corticosteroid in tuberculous meningitis. J Med Assoc Thai 79:83–90, 1996.

138. Patwari AK, Aneja S, Chandra D, Singhal PK: Long-term anticonvulsant therapy in tuberculous meningitis: A four-year follow-up. J Trop Pediatr 42:98–103, 1996.

139. Cairns H: Neurosurgical methods in the treatment of tuberculous meningitis with a note on some of the unusual manifestations of the disease. Arch Dis Child 26:373–386, 1951.

140. Bhagwati SN: Ventriculoatrial shunts in tuberculous meningitis with hydrocephalus. J Neurosurg 35:309–313, 1971.

141. Bullock MRR, Welchman JM: Diagnostic and prognostic features of tuberculous meningitis on CT scanning. J Neurol Neurosurg Psychiatry 45:1098–1101, 1982.

142. Palur R, Rajshekhar V, Chandy MJ, et al: Shunt surgery for hydrocephalus in tuberculous meningitis: A long-term follow up study. J Neurosurg 74:64–69, 1991.

143. Kent SJ, Crowe SM, Yung A, et al: Tuberculous meningitis: A 30-year review. Clin Infect Dis 17:87–94, 1993.

144. Misra UK, Kalita J, Srivastava M, Mandal SK: Prognosis of tuberculous meningitis: A multivariate analysis. J Neurol Sci 137:57–61, 1996.

145. Verdon R, Chevret S, Laissy JP, Wolff M: Tuberculous meningitis in adults: Review of 48 cases. Clin Infect Dis 22:982–988, 1996.

146. Schoeman CJ, Herbst J, Nienkemper DC: The effect of tuberculous meningitis on the cognitive and motor development of children. S Afr Med J 87:70–72, 1997.

147. Rao BD, Subrahmanyam MV: Spinal cord complications of tuberculous meningitis. Neurol India 10:62, 1962.

148. Tandon PN, Misra RN, Singh B: Post meningitic spinal arachnoiditis. Bull All India Inst Med Sci 2:88–96, 1968.

149. Bawa TS, Wahi PL: Spinal tuberculous meningitis. J Ind Med Assoc 37:449–452, 1961.

150. Harbitz F: Tuberculosis of the spinal cord with peculiar changes. JAMA 78:330–331, 1922.

151. Garceau GJ, Brady TA: Pott's paraplegia. J Bone Joint Surg Am 32:87–96, 1950.

152. Wadia NH, Dastur DK: Spinal meningitis with radiculomyelopathy. Part 1: Clinical and radiological features. J Neurol Sci 8:239–260, 1969.

153. Gupta RK, Gupta S, Kumar S, et al: MRI in intraspinal tuberculosis. Neuroradiology 36:39–43, 1994.

154. Kumar A, Montanera W, Willinsky R, et al: MR features of tuberculous arachnoiditis. J Comput Assist Tomogr 17:127–130, 1993.

155. Sharma A, Goyal M, Mishra NK, et al: MR imaging of tubercular spinal arachnoiditis. AJR Am J Roentgenol 168:807–812, 1997.

156. Gourie-Devi M, Satish Chandra P: Hyaluronidase as an adjuvant in the management of tuberculous spinal arachnoiditis. J Neurol Sci 102:105–111, 1991.

117 Surgical Management of Fungal Infections of the Central Nervous System

REWATI RAMAN SHARMA, SANTOSH D. LAD, SANJAY J. PAWAR, NIHAL T. GURUSINGHE, SANAT N. BHAGWATI, and ASHOK K. MAHAPATRA

INTRODUCTION

Surgical infections of the nervous central system present with protean clinical manifestations, difficult diagnostic dilemmas, and special therapeutic challenges. The nervous system may be infected by bacterial (most common), viral (common), parasitic-protozoal (less common), and fungal (uncommon or rare) organisms. Fungi are common in our environment, but only few are pathogenic. In general, the fungi are organisms of low pathogenicity, emerging as opportunistic organisms thriving in a compromised host. Fungal infection may involve the craniospinal axis, meningeal coverings, cerebrospinal fluid (CSF), the brain, and the spinal cord separately or in various combinations. Although fungal infections (mycoses) of the central nervous system (CNS) are uncommon, the wide spectrum of neurologic manifestations of fungal infections in the CNS is of particular importance to neurosurgeons.[1-16] Therefore, the diagnosis of CNS fungal infection should be considered in appropriate clinical settings.

A greater awareness, an early diagnosis, and an appropriate management strategy provide some hope of lowering the morbidity and mortality.

HISTORICAL ASPECTS

Common fungal infections are relatively benign; serious ones are rare. There are morphologic similarities in various fungi, which create difficulty in differentiating these structurally complex forms.[1-17] In 1905, Van Hanseman had probably first demonstrated cryptococcus in spinal fluid, although cerebral cryptococcosis was initially described by Busse in 1894.[7] Oppe in 1897 reported the first case of cerebral aspergillosis in humans due to extension of fungal infection from sphenoid sinusitis.[2,14,17] Zenker, in Germany in 1861, described a lesion in the brain, which may have been caused by *Candida*.[2,17] However, Smith and Sano were the first to report a case of *Candida* meningitis in 1933.[14,17] Various postmortem studies have established that candidiasis is a more common CNS fungal infection than aspergillosis, zygomycosis, or cryptococcosis. Gonyea[17] reported three patients with blastomycosis meningitis in 1978 without extracranial infection, and Ophuls was first to report a coccidioidal brain lesion in 1905.[2] In 1952, Binford reported a case of cerebral abscess due to *Cladosporium*.[17]

Histoplasmosis was first described by Darling in 1906 in a patient with disseminated granulomatous infection. Histiocytes were studded with *Histoplasma capsulatum*.[18]

Gilchrist[19] described blastomycosis in 1894 and had successfully grown the organism in culture. Coccidiomycosis was described by Alejandro Dosadas and Robert Wernicke in 1892. However, Ophuls was the first to describe coccidioidal meningitis in 1905. Paracoccidioidomycosis was first described in 1908 by Adolf Lutz in Brazil. Kurchenmeister in 1855 described the first case of human *Zygomycetes* infection, and Gregory in 1943 described rhino cerebral zygomycosis.[9] Nocard in 1988 reported an aerobic acid-fast actinomycete in cattle that was called *Nocardia farcinica* by Trevisan in 1889. However, Eppinger is credited with the reporting of the first case of metastatic cerebral nocardial abscess with pulmonary nocardiosis.[20,21] Cases of CNS fungal infections with occasional improvement after evacuation of a cerebral abscess or removal of a granulomatous lesion were only sporadically reported before the era of antifungal drugs.

Antifungal chemotherapy began in 1903 with the successful use of potassium iodide for the treatment of sporotrichosis.[22] The first useful polyene drug, nystatin, in 1953, and a second polyene drug, amphotericin B, in 1956, were introduced.[8-28] Amphotericin B remains the standard against which other antifungal drugs are compared.[22,27] Other important antifungal drugs discovered are flucytosine (5-fluorocytosine in 1964) and the azole drugs (1970s): miconazole (1978), ketoconazole (1981), fluconazole (1990), and itraconazole (1992).[22-34] To reduce the toxicity of amphotericin B, liposomal amphotericin B or its combination with lipids has been introduced.[25,28,33] Fungal infections in the CNS have been recognized for more than 100 years; however, until the antifungal agent amphotericin B was discovered, the fungal infections were regarded as nearly impossible to treat effectively.

CLASSIFICATION AND EPIDEMIOLOGY

The phylum Thallophyta includes certain plants (cells contain chlorophyll and therefore synthesize their own food) and fungi (organisms devoid of chlorophyll are therefore saprophytic).[7] Fungi are ubiquitous microorganisms that may be unicellular or filamentous. The latter produces branching hyphae, which grow only at the apex. The enzymes produced by the complex fungal cell wall break down proteins, carbohydrates, and other macromolecules. The resultant micromolecules are taken up by the cells or hyphae to maintain their life processes.[16] Among 1 million known fungal species, 200 species are pathogenic to humans and only 20 fungal species produce invasive systemic infections including CNS disorders.

Fungi are classified as follows: pseudomycetes/yeasts (*Blastomycetes, Candida, Coccidioides, Cryptococcus, Histoplasma, Paracoccidioides, Sporotrichum*), septate mycetes (*Aspergillus, Cephalosporium, Cladosporium, Diplorhinotrichum, Hormodendrum, Paecilomyces, Penicillium*), and nonseptate mycetes (*Absidia, Basidiobolus, Cunninghamella Mortierella, Mucor, Rhizopus*).[2,4,7,16]

The dimorphic fungi such as *Coccidioides, Histoplasma, Sporotrichum, Paracoccidioides,* and *Blastomycetes* grow in mycelial units at 25°C (filamentous in nature), and convert to a yeast form (spherules) at normal body temperature in humans. Encapsulated yeast, *Cryptococcus neoformans,* maintains its morphology in normal human tissues and in nature similar to various septate and nonseptate mycetes. *Nocardia* and *Actinomyces,* although not true fungi, they are fungus-like bacteria that produce CNS lesions that mimic fungal infections and are therefore included in this chapter.

Prevalence, Dispersion, and Infection (Table 117-1)

Fungal infections are not notifiable diseases and precise information on their prevalence throughout the world is not available.[2,4,16] However, most fungal infections are not geographically restricted. Fungi are abundant in the environment including soil and vegetation. A little moisture and organic matter such as dead plant or animal material are all that are required for their growth. They have long been recognized as agents of spoilage and destruction. Although only few mycotic diseases are exclusively tropical, some of them are predominant in regions where they find ideal climatic conditions for their development. In addition, poverty, poor working conditions, and the habit of walking barefoot provide additional conditions for the spread of mycoses.

Fungal spores are common in the air, which is the medium for their dispersion. Humans acquire infection by inhalation of airborne spores, by implantation of viable fungal elements through cutaneous puncture wounds, by ingestion, by contagion from infected animals, or from organisms already present as commensals. Most human mycoses are confined to lining surfaces such as the skin, lungs, gastrointestinal tract, and female genitalia and do not involve deep parenchymal organs.[15] The common superficial mycoses are dermatophytosis (tinea pedis, tinea corporis, and tinea capitis), candidiasis (cutaneous, oropharyngeal, and vaginal), *Malassezia* infections (pityriasis versicolor, seborrheic dermatitis, and folliculitis), black and white piedra, and *Scytalidium* infections. The common subcutaneous mycoses are mycetoma, chromoblastomycosis, phaeohyphomycosis, and sporotrichosis. In the category of systemic mycoses, endemic respiratory mycoses include histoplasmosis, blastomycosis, coccidioidomycosis, paracoccidioidomycosis, and *Penicillium marneffei* mycosis, whereas common systemic opportunistic mycoses are caused by candidiasis, aspergillosis, cryptococcosis, and mucormycosis. Fungi that can cause deep systemic mycoses can also infect the nervous system. CNS fungal infections are usually secondary to hematogenous dissemination from a focus elsewhere in the body, most often pulmonary or intestinal or from other extracranial sites including prosthetic heart valves. Fungal infections in the brain are invariably secondary to infections elsewhere in the body; however, the site of entry may remain unrecognized and cases have been reported in which the only evidence of fungal infection was in the CNS.[17]

Routes of Dissemination

Candida organisms may be endogenous, inhibiting the digestive tract and vagina.[34-45] *Aspergillus*[46-61] and *Zygomycetes*[62-71] organisms colonize and infect the structures adjacent to the cranial cavity, such as the sinuses, nasopharynx, middle ear cavities, and mastoid air cells. Histoplasmosis[72-75] and cryptococcosis[76-81] spread by the bloodstream to the CNS, meninges, or parameningeal structures from a primary often subclinical pulmonary focus, and only rarely does the organism reach the CNS after direct inoculation after trauma, surgery, or lumbar puncture. Colonization of artificial prostheses, implants, and other devices such as intravenous or arterial lines, peritoneal dialysis catheters, or ventriculoperitoneal, ventriculoatrial, or external ventricular drainage systems by *Candida* is becoming increasingly common.[14,16,33,43,80-84]

Host Susceptibility and Fungal Virulence (see Table 117-1)

All fungi may be considered as potential pathogens, when normal defenses are compromised. The establishment of infection depends on the host defenses, route of fungal exposure, the size of the inoculum, and the virulence of the organism. The presentation for a given organism is fairly consistent regardless of the underlying host immune status. However, the immune status of the host does preselect certain organisms. Fungi, which produce systemic infection, fall into two major groups: pathogenic fungi and opportunistic fungi.[2-17] In general, pathogenic fungi infect both the normal host and individuals with reduced host defenses, whereas opportunistic fungi infect mainly the immunocompromised patients. Pathogenic fungi are usually yeasts capable of establishing life-threatening CNS mycotic infections (i.e., coccidioidomycosis, histoplasmosis, blastomycosis, sporotrichosis, and paracoccidioidomycosis). Cryptococcosis is found in equal numbers of otherwise healthy persons and immunosuppressed patients. Many opportunistic fungal infections develop almost exclusively in the immunosuppressed population. Septate mycetes (*Aspergillus*), nonseptate mycetes (*Zygomycetes*), and yeasts (*Cryptococcus* and *Candida* mycetes) are mainly opportunistic fungi. However, it must be realized that the distinction between pathogenic and opportunistic fungi is not absolute.

CNS fungal infections have been increasing in frequency in the past decade due to many factors, that is, growing number of immunocompromised patients who survive for a long time, widespread use of immunosuppressive drugs, a large aging population with an increased number of

TABLE 117-1 ▪ Fungal Infections Affecting the Central Nervous System

Fungal Genera	Classification — Species	Disease	Distribution and Habitat	Source and Modes of Dispersion and Infection Spread	Special Predisposing or Risk Factors	Pathogenic or Opportunistic	Portal or Entry	Primary Focus	Route of Dissemination
Pseudohyphae									
Candida (most common)	Candida albicans	Candidiasis	Worldwide commensal in GI tract, external genitalia, skin	Endogenously, contagion	Immunoincompetent states	Opportunistic	Mucosal invasion	Oroesophageal region, vagina	Hematogenous
Histoplasma (common)	Histoplasma capsulatum	Histoplasmosis	Worldwide, common in central and east U.S.	Soil; chicken, bird, and bat excreta Contamination of dust, inhalation	Immunoincompetent states, infants and young children and middle age	Pathogenic	Respiratory tract, GI tract, skin	Lungs, reticuloendo-thelial system	Hematogenous, lymphatic
Blastomyces (uncommon)	Blastomyces dermatitidis	Blastomycosis	North America, Africa	Soil, decaying wood, dogs, inhalation	Farmers; immunoincompetent states	Pathogenic	Skin, lungs	Lungs	Hematogenous
Coccidioides (less common)	Coccidioides immitis	Coccidioido-mycosis	Geographically restricted, mainly in southwest U.S., Mexico, South America	Contaminated soil, rodents, inhalation	Farmers	Pathogenic and opportunistic	Respiratory tract	Lungs	Hematogenous
Paracoccidioides (infrequent)	Blastomyces brasiliensis	Paracoccidioido-mycosis	South and Central America	Vegetation, soil inhalation	Farmers and people in rural area	Pathogenic	Naso-oropharyn-geal mucosa	Lungs	Hematogenous, lymphatic
Sporotrichum (infrequent)	Sporotrichum schenckii	Sporotrichosis	Central and South America, U.S., Japan, disappeared from Europe	Soil and plant inhalation	Farmers	Pathogenic	Cutaneous or pulmonary inoculation	Musculoskeletal tissue, mucosa, viscera	Hematogenous
Cryptococcus (very common)	Cryptococcus neoformans var. neoformans, C. neoformans var. gritti	Cryptococcosis	Worldwide, frequent in Europe	Soil and wood, bird excreta, fruit juices, milk	Immunocom-promised states; Immunoincom-petent states	Opportunistic and pathogenic	Respiratory tract	Lungs	Hematogenous
Septate Hyphae									
Aspergillus (very common)	Aspergillus fumigatus, Aspergillus niger, Aspergillus flavus	Aspergillosis	Worldwide	Soil, plants, and decaying matter	Immunocom-promised states	Opportunistic	Paranasal sinuses, respiratory tract, skin, orbit	Respiratory tract, lungs or GI tract, orbit, ear, nose, and throat	Hematogenous, lymphatic

(Continued)

TABLE 117-1 ▪ Fungal Infections Affecting the Central Nervous System—Cont'd

Fungal Genera	Classification		Distribution and Habitat	Source and Modes of Dispersion and Infection Spread	Special Predisposing or Risk Factors	Pathogenic or Opportunistic	Portal or Entry	Primary Focus	Route of Dissemination
	Species	Disease							
Cladosporium	*Cladosporium tricoides (bantianum)*	Chromoblasto-mycosis	Worldwide, more common in tropics	Soil and vegetation, decaying plants	Immunoincompe-tent (more common) and immunocompro-mised (less common) farmers; field, forest, and barefoot workers	Pathogenic or opportu-nistic	Skin	Skin	Hematogenous
Allescheria (rare)	*Allescheria boydii*	Allesheriosis (monosporiosis)	Worldwide	Soil, water	Immunocom-promised	Opportunistic	Skin, mucous membrane	Respiratory system	Hematogenous
Nonseptate Hyphae									
Phycomycetes Zygomycetes Mucoraceae Common *Rhizopus Mucor Absidia Cunninghamella* Uncommon *Saksenaea Mortierella Basidiobolus Conidiobolus*	*Rhizopus arrhizus Rhizopus oryzae*	Phycomycosis, zygomycosis (frequent), mucormycosis	Ubiquitous saprophytes	Manure, soil, decaying bread and fruits, normal nose and throat flora in 2% of patients	Immunocom-promised host: diabetic ketoacidosis, intravenous drug abuse, organ transplantation, immunosuppres-sive therapy, hematologic malignancies, corticosteroids, antibiotics, cytotoxic drugs, and AIDS	Opportunistic or pathogenic	Skin, paranasal sinuses, and nasopharynx	Rhinosino-orbital region, pulmonary system, GI tract, and skin	Direct invasion, hematogenous
Fungus-like Bacteria *Actinomyces*									
Nocardia	*Nocardia asteroides, Nocardia brasiliensis*	Nocardiosis	Worldwide	Soil and decaying vegetation	Immunoin-competent or immunocom-promised host: cytotoxic drugs or steroids	Pathogenic and opportu-nistic	Skin and lungs	Pulmonary or cutaneous	Hematogenous
Actinomyces	*Actinomyces israelii*	Actinomycosis	Worldwide	Normal inhabitant of the mouth and gut (not found free in nature)	Oral trauma, gingival infection, lung disease, bowel perforation	Pathogenic	Mouth and gut	Cervicofacial (most common), pulmonary, and abdominal	Direct invasion, hematogenous

AIDS, acquired immunodeficiency syndrome; GI, gastrointestinal.

malignancies (lymphoma and leukemia, especially when associated with leukopenia/granulocytopenia [*Candida* and *Aspergillus*]), the spread of acquired immunodeficiency syndrome, poorly controlled diabetes mellitus (zygomycosis), and renal and other transplant recipients requiring prolonged immunosuppression.[2,4,7,10,16,17]

CLINICOPATHOLOGIC SYNDROMES

Small numbers of fungi are yeasts made up of colonies of simple single cells. These yeast cells are of oval or elongate shape and reproduce by budding. Most fungi are molds that are made up of tubular branching chain of cells (hyphae). A colony of hyphae is called a mycelium. Some fungi such as *Candida* organisms take on an intermediate form (pseudomycetes) between yeasts and hyphae.

Fungi produce diseases due to their allergenicity, toxigenicity, pathogenicity, and neurotoxicity, but CNS mycoses are essentially due to serious infective processes.[16] Fungi infecting the CNS are found in three major morphologic forms with distinct clinicopathologic syndromes.[4,7,10]

1. Leptomeningitis (acute and chronic) is mainly produced by small pure yeasts (pseudomycetes) as large as 20 μm in diameter (blastomycosis, cryptococcosis, and histoplasmosis). Because of their small size, these fungi gain access to the cerebral microcirculation from which they infect the subarachnoid spaces.
2. Cerebral abscesses are produced by larger pseudomycetes (candidiasis). These intermediate-sized fungi occlude cerebral arterioles and result in adjacent tissue necrosis that rapidly converts to microabscesses. Persistence of infection causes granulomatous inflammatory reaction in adjacent leptomeninges, neural parenchyma, or both.
3. Very large branched septate (aspergillosis) or nonseptate mycetes (zygomycosis) produces cerebral infarction. These fungi mainly obstruct the intermediate- and large-sized cerebral arteries and invade the vessel wall causing cerebral arterial thrombosis and associated cerebral infarction. The evolving hemorrhagic cerebral infarcts may convert to septic infarcts with associated cerebritis and abscesses.

CLINICAL SPECTRUM OF CENTRAL NERVOUS SYSTEM FUNGAL INFECTIONS (Table 117-2)

In fungal infections (mycoses), the organism can invade tissues without an underlying predisposition (pathogenic fungi), but many of the common systemic mycoses affect patients with abnormalities in structure, immunity, and metabolism (opportunistic fungi).

The involvement of the CNS in fungal infection may be disseminated (cryptococcosis, coccidioidomycosis), focal (aspergillosis), or multifocal (candidiasis). Due to their protean manifestations in various clinical settings, CNS fungal infections present a difficult diagnostic and therapeutic challenge to neurosurgeons. Because these organisms are uncommon and often manifest in an indolent fashion,

diagnosis tends to be difficult and at times altogether missed. Expected mortality rates are high under the best circumstances, even with rapid diagnosis, aggressive medical therapy, and operative approach. The clinicopathologic findings and results of a combined series of verified cases of fungal and fungus-like bacterial (pathologic actinomycetic) infections of the CNS are presented from four major institutions where one of the authors (R.R.S.) either had worked (KEM Hospital, Bombay, India, and Royal Preston Hospital, Preston, Lancs, United Kingdom) or is working (Khoula Hospital, Muscat, Oman) or is associated with other (Bombay Hospital and Medical Research Centre, Mumbai, India) authors (Table 117-3).

Pseudomycetes Causing Infections of the Central Nervous System

Candidiasis, histoplasmosis, blastomycosis, coccidioidomycosis, paracoccidioidomycosis, sporotrichosis, and cryptococcosis are more frequently found compared with other pseudomycetes causing CNS infections.

Candidiasis

Clinical risks associated with invasive candidiasis are well recognized. In autopsy studies, the most common cerebral mycosis is caused by candidiasis.[2–17] Candidiasis commonly presents as thrush in the oral cavity or vagina, and, less commonly, skin and visceral organs are involved.[38] *Candida* organisms are found worldwide. Their pseudohyphae are associated with 2- to 3-μm spherical or oval blastospores. Candidiasis arises when the balance between *Candida* species and the host is altered in favor of the yeast.[45] *Candida albicans* originally infects the gastrointestinal tract (oral cavity and esophagus) after antibiotic treatment, then invades submucosal blood vessels, and finally disseminates hematogenously to the CNS. Organisms also reach CNS via colonization of ventricular drains, shunt tubing, and central venous lines.[14,16,33,43,82–84]

NEUROPATHOLOGY

In the CNS, fungus invades small blood vessels causing thrombosis and infarction. Disseminated granulomatous lesions may be scattered throughout the meninges and brain, causing meningitis or focal encephalitis.[4,7,16] Candidal meningitis can occur spontaneously as a complication of disseminated candidiasis or as a complication of an infected wound or ventriculostomies via direct inoculation of the organism into the CNS.[43] At autopsy, gross lesions may not be apparent. Microscopically multiple microabscesses and microgranulomas in the distribution of anterior and middle cerebral vessels are found.[4,7,16] The abscesses are composed of neutrophils, lymphocytes, and macrophages that evolve to a granuloma after a week. On histology, they are faintly basophilic when stained with hematoxylin and eosin (H&E) but are intensely stained with periodic acid–Schiff (PAS) and methenamine silver reaction.[4,7,9,11,12]

CLINICAL SYMPTOMATOLOGY

The clinical symptomatology of CNS candidiasis is that of low-grade meningitis.[39,44] A marked basal infiltration may cause multiple cranial nerve palsies and deterioration in the

TABLE 117-2 ■ Clinical Spectrum of Fungal Infections Affecting the Central Nervous System

Fungi	Fungal Characteristics	Special Features in Pathogenesis	Clinical Presentations	Diagnosis	Treatment	Prognosis of CNS Infections
Pseudohyphae						
Candida	True yeast; reproduce by budding cells 3–8 μm or filamentous	Occlude and invade small blood vessels causing thrombosis and infarction; focal encephalitis and meningitis	Meningitis, hydrocephalus, cerebral abscess, granulomas	CSF (from tubes or drains) studies, cultured from CSF or blood, chest film, immunologic tests, neuroimaging	Removal of the source of infection, correction of immunocompromised state, amphotericin B ± flucytosine, neurosurgical intervention as indicated	Poor; good with treatment
Histoplasma	True yeast; reproduce by budding cells 2–5 μm or filamentous	Gain access to cerebral microcirculation to infect subarachnoid spaces and causes chronic inflammation of basal meninges	Diffuse leptomeningitis, discrete granuloma (intraparenchymal), arteritis (granulomatous), miliary granulomas, chorioretinitis	CSF study, culture from CSF, peripheral blood smears, bone marrow examination, complement fixation test, neuroimaging	Amphotericin B, sulfonamides, arsenical and antimony compounds, neurosurgical intervention as indicated	Poor
Blastomyces	Dimorphic true yeast spherical cell 8–15 μg; multiplies by a single bud	Lack of neurotropism, meningeal inflammation, fibropurulent exudate, fibrosis; granulomatous reaction to suppurative reaction in brain meninges and bone	Meningitis: pachymeningitis, leptomeningitis, meningoencephalitis, brain abscesses, extradural abscesses, granulomas	CSF studies, culture, biopsy of granuloma, serologic tests, neuroimaging	Amphotericin B, neurosurgical intervention as indicated	Poor; good with treatment
Coccidioides	Dimorphic hyphae in nature and spherules in tissues (30–60 μm) filled with endospores (2–5 μm)	Chronic inflammation; a range of chronic granulomatous reaction; granulomatous with or without meningitis	Chronic meningitis, hydrocephalus, granuloma, abscesses, spinal cord compression	CSF examination, peripheral WBC counts (eosinophilia), serum precipitin test; skull films, punched-out lesions, neuroimaging	Amphotericin B (IV and intrathecal), ketoconazole, neurosurgical intervention as indicated	Poor; guarded with treament
Paracoccidioides	Dimorphic multiple thin necked buds arise from a single yeast cell 10–20 μm	Inflammatory response with a lymphohistiocytic infiltrate with granulomas, leptomeningeal fibrosis	Basal granulomatous leptomeningitis, obstructive hydrocephalus, granuloma, intraspinal or intracranial pseudotumorous granuloma	CSF study, chest film, neuroimaging, histology	Amphotericin B, sulfonamides + trimethoprim, neurosurgical intervention	Guarded
Sporotrichum (rare)	Dimorphic branching septate hyphae, spherical cells 2–6 μm	Meningeal, cerebral, and spinal inflammation resulting in granulomatous microabscesses	Chronic meningitis, microabscesses, paraplegia, quadriplegia, radiculopathy	CSF study, chest film, MRI or CT scans, histology	Amphotericin B, flucytosine, neurosurgical intervention	Guarded
Cryptococcus	Spherical budding yeast cell 5–20 μm	Exudative granulomatous meningeal inflammation causing thickening and opacity	Basal meningitis with hydrocephalus or cranial nerve deficits, intraparenchymal cysts, rarely granulomas	CSF study, smear examination (India ink showing mucoid capsule), MRI or CT scans	Amphotericin B, flucytosine, neurosurgical intervention	Fatal; extremely poor; guarded with treatment
Septate Hyphae						
Aspergillus (common)	Branching septate hyphae (3–12 μm), hyphal	Highly angiotropic vascular invasion with thrombosis,	Stroke; focal deficits; hemorrhagic infarcts;	Biopsy, culture CSF, immunologic tests,	Neurosurgical intervention, treatment of predisposing	Poor

Organism	Morphology	Pathology/Features	Clinical features	Diagnosis	Treatment	Prognosis
	branching forms acute angle in the direction of main hyphae, conidia 2–3 µm	inflammatory response causes cerebritis; septic infarcts with associated abscesses; SAH owing to mycotic aneurysms	occlusion of ICA, MCA, ACA; abscess; meningitis, arachnoiditis; granuloma; aspergilloma; spinal cord compression	neuroimaging	factors, amphotericin B + flucytosine	Poor
Cladosporium (rare)	Pigmented fungi (brown), septate slender hyphae (2–3 µm)	Frontal lobe commonly affected, single or multiple intraparenchymatous abscesses	Unilocular or multilocular cerebral abscess, meningitis and ventriculitis, causing hydrocephalus, granulomas (rarely)	Biopsy, CSF study, CT or MRI scans	Neurosurgical intervention	Poor
Allescheria (rare)	Septate hyphal rounded chlamydospores	Extravascular or intravascular invasion	Meningoencephalitis, microabscesses, hemorrhagic infarcts with leptomeningitis	Histology, culture, sputum examination, CSF examination, neuroimaging	Dapsone (diamino/diphenylsufone), miconazole, itraconazole, ketoconazole, neurosurgical intervention	
Nonseptate Hyphae						
Mucoraceae	Filaments (or stolons) from which rootlike rhizoids grow; hyphae 6–15 µm in diameter, 200 µm in length. From rhizoids, sprouts (sporangiospores) bearing sacs (sporangia) develop (characteristic hyphae are diagnostic)	Highly angiotropic, direct invasion of ICA causing thrombosis; direct invasion of frontal lobes (basal regions); hemorrhage from infarcted brain in deep gray matter and mycotic aneurysm; grow in the vessel wall, meninges, brain parenchyma	Ophthalmoplegia; focal deficits, i.e., hemiplegia from ICA occlusion or hemorrhage; frontal lobe abscess; cavernous sinus thrombosis; meningitis	High index in high-risk patients; ENT examination; CSF examination, hemorrhage; biopsy, nasal or sinus material or brain; serologic tests, antigen and antibodies in CSF; neuroimaging	Control of risk factors, amphotericin B; radical ENT and neurosurgical intervention	High mortality
Fungus-like Bacteria—Actinomycetes						
Nocardia	Beaded branching filaments aerobic gram-positive 2 µm thick; reproduced by fragmentation of the partially acid-fast hyphae	Thick yellow-green purulent exudate in cerebral abscess with poor encapsulation, meningitis unusual	Cerebral abscess, meningitis, osteomyelitis with extradural abscess	Examination of pus, biopsy, MRI or CT scan, chest film	Neurosurgical intervention, antibiotics (sulfonamides) + trimethoprim, erythromycin, fusidate, amikacin	Favorable
Actinomyces	Anaerobic gram-positive long filamentous branches terminating in eosinophilic clubs, sulfur granules	Cerebral abscess; epidural, subdural empyema; osteomyelitis; granuloma (unusual)	Intracranial abscesses, granuloma, craniospinal osteomyelitis	Granules in unstained and filaments in Gram stains in microscopic examination of pus and infected tissue, skull and spinal films (soap-bubble vertebra), neuroimaging	ENT or neurosurgical intervention; antibiotics, penicillin in high doses	Favorable

ACA, anterior cerebral artery; CNS, central nervous system; CSF cerebrospinal fluid; CT, computed tomography; ENT, ear, nose, and throat; ICA, internal carotid artery; IV, intravenous; MCA, middle cerebral artery; MRI, magnetic resonance imaging; SAH, subarachnoid hemorrhage; WBC, white blood count.

TABLE 117-3 ■ Clinicopathological Summary of the Combined Series* of Fungal and Fungus-like Bacterial Infections of the Central Nervous System

Serial No.	Clinical Characteristics	I. Pseudomycetes			II. Septate Mycetes			III. Nonseptate Mycetes	IV. Fungus-like Bacteria: Actinomycetes	
		Candidiasis	Blastomycosis	Coccidioidomycosis	Cryptococcosis	Aspergillosis	Cladosporiosis	Zygomycosis (Mucormycosis)	Nocardiosis	Actinomycosis
1	No. of cases	10	6	2	21	67	6	45	3	10
2	Sex: M/F ratio	6M/4F	3M/3F	2M	14M/7F	46M/21F	6M	29M/16F	3M	5M/5F
3	Average age (yr)	28	32	36	34	30	30	32	24	30
4	Predominant clinical syndromes†									
	(i) Meningitis/Ventriculitis	6	(2)	(2)	21	(10)	(1)	(13)	(3)	(1)
	(ii) Encephalitis	1	—	(1)	(13)	(16)	—	(11)	(2)	—
	(iii) Increased ICP									
	a. Hydrocephalus	(1)	—	(1)	(4)	(5)	(1)	(3)	—	—
	b. Abscess	2(1)	(1)	1(1)	—	6(1)	1(5)	4	2(1)	(3)
	c. Granulomas	—	6	1(1)	(2)	28(2)	5	4	—	9
	d. Cysts	—	—	—	(13)	2	—	4	—	—
	e. Co-existing tumors	—	—	—	—	—	—	2	—	—
	(iv) Orbito-rhino cerebral or craniofacial syndrome	(1)	(2)	—	—	(18)	—	(17)	(2)	9
	(v) Acute cerebrovascular events									
	a. Vasculitis	—	—	—	—	(20)	(1)	(32)	—	—
	b. ICA thrombosis	—	—	—	—	9(5)	(2)	8(17)	—	—
	c. Basilar thrombosis	—	—	—	—	(2)	—	(2)	—	—
	d. SAH	—	(1)	—	—	(1)	(5)	(1)	—	(1)
	e. Mycotic aneurysms	—	—	—	—	2(2)	—	(2)	—	(1)
	f. Hemorrhagic infarction	—	(1)	—	—	15(6)	—	26(2)	(1)	—
	(vi) Spinal syndrome	1	—	—	—	5 (granuloma)	—	—	—	1
	(vii) Craniospinal osteomyelitis	(1)	—	—	—	—	—	—	(1)	1
5	Appropriate surgical intervention, culture, CSF study, biospy	8	6	2	7	49	4	20	3	10
6	Diagnosis only at autopsy	2	—	—	14	18	2	25	—	—
7	Reconfirmation of antemortem diagnosis at autopsy (no. of cases)	2	1	1	3	9	—	1	—	—
8	Total no. of deaths	6	1	1	17	43	5	39	1	1
9	Mortality (%)	60	16.66	50	80	64	83.5	86.66	33.33	10
10	Overall prognosis	Poor	Good	Poor	Extremely poor	Poor	Extremely poor	Extremely poor	Poor	Good

*Khoula Hospital, Muscat, Sultanate of Oman (1986–Dec 2003); King Edward Memorial Hospital Bombay, India (1965–1995) and Royal Preston Hospital, Preston-Lancs, UK (1978–July 1998) and Bombay Hospital, Mumbai, India (1990–2002).

†Numbers without parentheses denote cases with primary clinical presentation. Numbers with parentheses denote secondary feature of the clinical presentation besides other primary features in presentation.

M, male; F, female.

level of consciousness, and frequently with hydrocephalus.[38,45] Spinal candidiasis is rare and can involve the vertebral body[35,36] and or the disc space[42] by hematogenous spread in patients with candidal sepsis. It may occur by local invasion and as a postoperative complication of spinal surgery. Persistent low back pain is a common complaint; however, 50% of cases may have significant neurologic deficits. Neuroimaging studies show nonspecific spondylitis and discitis. Among 10 cases of CNS candidiasis in our series, 6 patients presented with meningitis, 1 with encephalitis/cerebritis, 2 with cerebral abscesses (treated with aspirations), and the remaining 1 patient with upper cervical cord syndrome (diffuse cord changes at autopsy) associated with cervicovertebral osteomyelitis and discitis. One patient with meningitis had a cerebral abscess in addition, which was successfully drained by computed tomography (CT)-guided stereotactic surgery with good outcome (Fig. 117-1).

DIAGNOSIS

Diagnosis should be suspected in patients with external ventricular drains or blocked shunts. CSF examination including cultures should be routine. The CSF may show pleocytosis, with either neutrophils or lymphocytes predominating, and glucose is often low. Serial serum examinations (double diffusion, counter immunoelectrophoresis, immunofluorescence, and latex agglutination tests) are helpful. Funduscopic examination through a dilated pupil is invaluable in detecting endophthalmitis before permanent loss of vision occurs. Bone or disc biopsy, histology, and culture principally make the diagnosis of spinal candidiasis.[3,7,16]

The magnetic resonance imaging (MRI) in fungal spinal osteomyelitis usually shows hypointensity of the vertebral bodies on T1-weighted images with enhancement on contrast administration. There is a lack of hyperintensity within the discs on T2-weighted images with preservation of the intranuclear cleft, which is in contrast with pyogenic

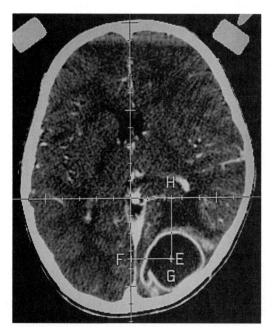

FIGURE 117-1   A computed tomography scan of the brain with a stereotactic frame shows a thick-walled, ring-enhancing candidal abscess in the left occipital region.

osteomyelitis in which the disc may be hyperintense with loss of intranuclear cleft on T2-weighted images.[85]

TREATMENT

Removal of infected artifacts, correction of underlying predisposing risk factors, neurosurgical intervention for cerebral abscesses, and amphotericin B with or without flucytosine form the mainstay of treatment. Amphotericin B, flucytosine, fluconazole, miconazole, and ketoconazole have been used successfully in spinal candidiasis. Decompressive surgery is required in patients with significant compressive spinal lesions. If there is evidence of pus collection on spinal MRI, then preoperative image-guided aspiration to prove the fungal nature of the lesion should be followed by preoperative antifungal medications, and then surgical débridement and fixation should be carried out with a full postoperative course of antifungal medications, which has achieved good results in many cases.[86] Fluconazole (with amphotericin B in initial phases) for a period of 3 to 6 months postoperatively may lead to the healing of fungal osteomyelitis with osseous consolidation.[87]

Histoplasmosis

Histoplasmosis is present throughout the world. It is the most frequently observed pulmonary mycotic infection in the eastern and central United States, whereas in Europe, its incidence is low. It is known to invade the reticuloendothelial system.[2,4,7,11,12,16] Lesions are found in the spleen, liver, and lymph nodes in addition to the lungs. CNS involvement is rare. The causative organism (2- to 5-µm yeast) is *H. capsulatum*, a dimorphic fungus. It is commonly found in soil. Organisms are inhaled with dust contaminated by chicken, bird, or bat excreta. The primary focus is formed in the lungs, where it becomes calcified, but it may occur in mouth, gastrointestinal tract, or skin. In immunocompetent individuals, CNS histoplasmosis is extremely rare,[72] but many patients with CNS involvement are immunocompromised by burns, antibiotics, steroids, and acquired immunodeficiency syndrome.[4,74] Even though approximately 25% of the U.S. population have positive histoplasmin skin tests, CNS involvement is rare.[16] Hematogenous dissemination may spread to the CNS. Neurologic involvement occurs in 10% to 20% of patients with disseminated histoplasmosis.

NEUROPATHOLOGY

Involvement of the CNS in histoplasmosis occurs in less than 1% of all patients with active histoplasmosis and includes diffuse leptomeningitis, discrete granuloma, periventricular granulomata, parenchymal granulomatosis, choroid plexus granulomata, and granulomatous arteritis.[4,7,11,16,74,75] In diffuse basilar leptomeningitis, there are thickening of the leptomeninges and thick yellow exudate with miliary granulomas along the blood vessels. In chronic cases, meningeal fibrosis with hydrocephalus develops. Meningitis is proportionally less prominent in histoplasmosis than in cryptococcosis and coccidioidomycosis. Histoplasmosis granulomas mimic sarcoidosis and other fungal or tubercular mass lesions consisting of central noncaseating granulomas or small caseous areas surrounded by macrophages, lymphocytes, plasma cells, and Langhans' giant cells. It is well demonstrated with PAS. In sections stained with H&E, shrinkage of the organisms produces a halo and gives the impression of a capsule.[7] Methenamine silver stain demonstrates macrophages packed with organisms, reactive gliosis, and fibrosis.

CLINICAL SYMPTOMATOLOGY

There are two peaks of incidence: in early childhood and in middle age.[75] Four forms are described: leptomeningitis, cerebritis, military granulomas, and spinal cord lesions. Leptomeningitis is common, whereas other CNS lesions in histoplasmosis are rare. The condition usually presents as chronic meningitis with or without hydrocephalus. Mass lesions are rare (Fig. 117-2), and occasionally chorioretinitis is seen. The skull and vertebrae may be involved by osteomyelitis with secondary spinal cord compression, especially with *Histoplasma duboisii*.[3,75]

DIAGNOSIS

Clinicians should maintain a high index of suspicion of patients who are from any area endemic for histoplasmosis. Definite diagnosis is made by demonstration of the organism by culture of sputum, CSF, and serum or by histology.[72-75] Complement fixation, agar gel, diffusion test, and radioimmunoassay (urine or serum) are helpful. Biopsy provides a more definitive answer. The CSF is usually under pressure and shows moderate pleocytosis of as many as 300 cells/mm³, which are more often mononuclear than polymorphonuclear in type. Protein is elevated, the glucose level is somewhat reduced, and the organism is cultured from the CSF samples in approximately 50% of cases. Peripheral blood smear and bone marrow examination may yield an early diagnosis. MRI shows enhanced mass lesions in the brain. On T1-weighted images, *Histoplasma* lesions appear as hypointense rims with surrounding edema on T2-weighted images. CT scans show ring-enhancing lesions.

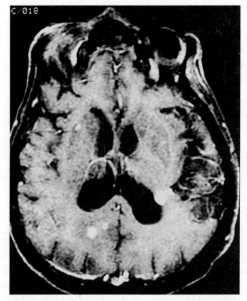

FIGURE 117-2 A postcontrast T1-weighted axial image of the brain demonstrates multiple homogeneously enhancing histoplasmosis granulomas. (Courtesy of Carl W. Hardin, MD, and J. Randy Jinkins, MD.)

TREATMENT

Untreated CNS histoplasmosis is nearly always fatal. Long-term treatment with amphotericin B and neurosurgical intervention, if needed, are required. In patients with infected shunts, initiation of antifungal therapy and removal of the shunt result in improvement.

Blastomycosis (North American Blastomycosis)

It is endemic in the southeastern regions of the United States and widely reported in Africa.[15,16,40] The causative agent, *Blastomyces dermatitidis*, is found in the soil, may have a natural reservoir in dogs, and has worldwide distribution. The fungus is a spherical cell 8- to 15-μm in diameter that multiplies by a single bud that is attached to the parent cell by a broad base. Blastomycosis is mainly a granulomatous (blastomycomas) disease that begins as a pulmonary lesion. The yeasts are phagocytized by pulmonary macrophages that may disseminate to produce secondary lesions in the skin, bone, and genitourinary system, but the CNS rarely becomes involved. In agricultural workers, the primary focus is in the lungs or skin.[15-17,40] Hematogenous spread of infection to the CNS occurs rarely (5%). Blastomycosis is rare even in immunocompromised patients and those with acquired immunodeficiency syndrome.[4,7,16] It is indeed an uncommon mycotic infection that rarely involves the CNS as compared with histoplasmosis and coccidioidomycosis.[88-94]

NEUROPATHOLOGY

The primary CNS blastomycosis is extremely rare, whereas secondary CNS involvement occurs in 3% to 33% of disseminated blastomycosis. Typically, cerebral blastomycosis produces leptomeningitis, meningoencephalitis, brain abscesses, dural abscesses, and adjacent granulomas. Grossly, two fifths of cases present with chronic leptomeningitis, one third with granulomas and abscesses, and one fourth with spinal epidural granulomas and abscesses. Epidural abscesses may occur secondary to craniovertebral osteomyelitis. Fibrosis in subarachnoid spaces can cause hydrocephalus.[92,93] Abscesses may be extradural, subdural, or intraparenchymatous. No region in the CNS or peripheral nervous system is immune. It may be focal or disseminated basal leptomeningitis with fibrinopurulent exudate that can block subarachnoid spaces causing hydrocephalus. Pachymeningitis may result. Histologic features elicit a mixed granulomatous and suppurative reaction. The center of an abscess contains caseous necrotic material with cells (lymphocytes, neutrophils, plasma cells, macrophages, Langhans' giant cells) and organisms. H&E unstained wet preparation, PAS, and methenamine silver stains demonstrate the organism. Bone and vertebral disc destruction with paraspinal abscess closely simulate tuberculous disease of the spine.[3,40,89,91,94]

CLINICAL SYMPTOMATOLOGY

CNS blastomycosis presents with headaches and neck stiffness; intracranial blastomycotic abscesses or granulomas result in increased intracranial pressure with or without localized signs.[88,92,93] Eventually these patients develop convulsions, mental deterioration, confusion, and lethargy. Plain CT scan may show iso- or hyperattenuating lesions. However, small solitary lesions show homogeneous enhancement on CT scanning with surrounding edema.

Slightly larger lesions may show ring-enhancing lesions with surrounding edema. In our series, all six patients with CNS blastomycosis had presented with signs and symptoms of increased intracranial pressure mainly due to granulomas. Motor impairment, cranial nerve palsies, and visual symptoms were also encountered in varying degrees. One patient had rhino-orbital blastomycosis, and another case had blasto-mycosis of the mastoid sinus. The initial clinical impression in four cases was a progressive space-occupying lesion and in two cases, a space-occupying lesion with meningeal signs. Neurosurgical intervention based on intraparenchymatous lesions, as seen on CT scans, had resulted in a good outcome in five patients with histologic diagnosis of blastomycotic granuloma. One patient died who had postmortem evidence of meningitis, subarachnoid hemorrhage, cerebral abscess, and cerebral infarction in addition to a cerebral granuloma. Blastomycosis in African countries commonly affects the thoracic spine, ribs, and sternum by direct extension from the lungs.[89,91,94] Osteomyelitis and discitis are associated with paraspinal abscess formation.[3,91] Clinical and radiographic features are similar to those of tuberculosis with which it sometimes coexists.[3]

DIAGNOSIS

Diagnosis is established by biopsy, cultures, CSF examination, and serologic tests (complement fixation test and double immunodiffusion test). CSF shows a predominantly lympho-cytic picture with cell counts of more than $1000/mm^3$, markedly elevated proteins, and reduced sugar. The CSF pressure is increased. Vertebral biopsy and culture establish the diagnosis of spinal blastomycosis.

TREATMENT

Antifungal drugs (amphotericin B, 2-hydroxystilbamidine, ketoconazole, fluconazole) are very effective, and neurosur-gical intervention for cerebral abscesses, granulomas, and hydrocephalus and spinal decompressive and stabilization procedures may be required if significant neurologic compro-mise is present. The prognosis is, however, poor if untreated but much better with an appropriate management.

Coccidioidomycosis (Modeling Valley Fever)

Coccidioidomycosis is caused by *Coccidioides immitis*, which is probably the most virulent of the fungi causing human mycoses, accounting for approximately 100,000 cases per year in the United States with 70 to 80 deaths annually.[95–98]

It is a geographically restricted mycosis, which includes regions of semiarid climate. Its distribution corresponds to areas where warm temperature and dry conditions exist. It is endemic in the southwestern United States (especially in San Joaquin Valley and Arizona where 85% of the population is skin test positive), Mexico, and South America, particularly Argentina and Paraguay.[99,100] Both mycelia and spores are carried a considerable distance by wind or transported by rodents. The causative organism *C. immitis* is a nonbudding spherical structure measuring 20 to 70 µm in diameter with a double refractile capsule. Mature forms are filled with numerous (two to five) small endospores. *C. immitis* is a dimorphic fungus producing hyphae and arthrospores in its saprophytic (soil) environment and spherules (sporangia) in infected tissues. Pulmonary infection is contracted by inhala-tion of the airborne arthroconidia in immunocompetent

or immunocompromised individuals. Most infections are self-limited. Approximately two thirds of cases of pulmonary infections are asymptomatic, whereas one third of cases develop mild to severe pulmonary disorders. However, most patients recover and develop strong specific immunity against infection.[101–103] The fungus is therefore considered both a pathogen and an opportunist. Hematogenous spread to the CNS occurs in approximately 50% of cases as a terminal event.[4,16]

NEUROPATHOLOGY

Meningeal inflammation results in accumulation of exudate, opacification of leptomeninges, and obliteration of sulci with caseous granulomatous nodules at the base of the brain and in the cervical region.[4,7,16,97,100] Extensive fibrosis causes obstructive hydrocephalus. Invasion of blood vessels leads to multiple aneurysms.[97] Unusually large granulomatous lesions and frank abscesses can occur in the brain or spinal cord parenchyma. The microscopic picture mimics tubercu-lous meningitis. Meningeal fibrosis, granulomas (organisms surrounded by epithelioid cells, giant cells, lymphocytes, and plasma cells), small abscesses with caseous necrosis, and vascular invasion are seen. On H&E stain, coccidioides are basophilic and are well demonstrated with methenamine silver stain.

CLINICAL SYMPTOMATOLOGY

CNS coccidioidomycosis presents as acute, subacute, or chronic symptomatic meningitis, transient focal deficits (aphasia and hemiparesis), confusion, restlessness, and depression. Multiple cranial nerve palsies, increased intracranial pressure, and hydrocephalus occur as complica-tions of basal meningitis and/or a mass lesion.[95,99–103] Donor-related coccidioidomycosis in organ transplant recipients has also been described. In our series, there was one fatal case of CNS coccidioidomycosis in which the patient had presented with signs of increased intracranial pressure, mul-tiple cranial nerve palsies, and rapidly progressive sensori-motor impairment in the limbs. MRI studies showed evidence of leptomeningitis, intraparenchymatous brain stem granulomatous lesions, and hydrocephalus (Figs. 117-3 and 117-4). Another patient with a nonfatal case of cere-bral granulomas and leptomeningitis underwent biopsy and was then treated with antifungal medications. Myelopathy may result due to adhesive meningitis or a mass lesion or an extradural abscess associated with vertebral osteomyelitis. Spinal coccidioidomycosis may present as acute or chronic spondylitis in the thoracic and lumbar regions, especially in cases of disseminated coccidioidomycosis.[3,96] Apart from vertebral bodies, the pedicles, transverse processes, laminae, spinous processes, and contiguous ribs may be affected; however, intervertebral discs are relatively spared. It usually presents as progressive spinal cord compression.[3,96,100] Paraspinal masses and sinuses are commonly seen, and rarely meningitis may occur with fatal outcome.

DIAGNOSIS

CSF is usually under increased pressure but occasionally shows evidence of a spinal block. A raised protein level, reduced glucose level, and persistent pleocytosis may be pres-ent, and the organisms can be recognized in wet preparations of the CSF. A high index of suspicion, increased erythrocyte

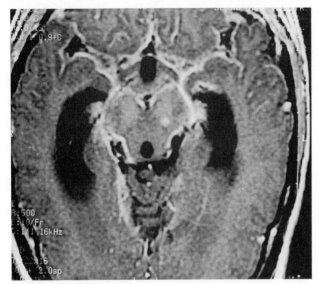

FIGURE 117-3 A postcontrast axial T1-weighted magnetic resonance imaging scan shows marked enhancement around the brain stem and basal cisterns due to coccidioidomycotic leptomeningitis with dilated temporal horns and an enlarged aqueduct suggestive of hydrocephalus. There is an enhancing round hyperintensity in the left tegmentum that is suggestive of a granuloma. (Courtesy of Sanjeev D. Athale, MD.)

sedimentation rate, chest radiograph (calcified nodes), craniospinal bone lesions, and CT/MRI scans of the cerebrospinal axis (mass lesion, hydrocephalus) form the mainstay of investigations. Osteomyelitis of the skull or vertebrae may be visible on the plain radiograph. Osteomyelitis may also present as causing punched-out lesions on the skull radiographs and an underlying abscess on CT/MRI studies. Radiolucent vertebral lesions devoid of surrounding sclerosis

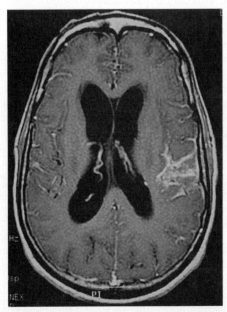

FIGURE 117-4 A postcontrast axial T1-weighted magnetic resonance imaging scan shows marked enhancement in the left superolateral cerebral sulci and adjoining dural surface in coccidioidomycosis meningitis. There is enlargement of both lateral ventricles. (Courtesy of Sanjeev D. Athale, MD.)

in early cases, whereas dense sclerotic vertebrae with normal disc spaces in the late stages are features seen on plain radiographs. However, bone changes and paraspinal lesions are well delineated on CT/MRI studies. The differential diagnosis includes multiple myeloma, sarcoidosis, histiocytosis, and metastases. It is unusual for coccidioidomycosis to present as a solitary bone lesion, which may mimic a primary bone tumor. Fine needle aspiration biopsy helps to differentiate between inflammatory and neoplastic processes involving bone by acquiring material for cytologic studies and cultures.[101]

TREATMENT

Intravenous amphotericin B is the most promising drug with intrathecal administration via lumbar puncture or a subcutaneous reservoir in seriously ill or deteriorating cases. When a localized mass lesion is causing compression of the brain/spinal cord, then appropriate neurosurgical intervention is carried out. Intrathecal azoles have been used. Coccidioidomycosis osteomyelitis remains a rare but difficult disease to treat with a lifelong risk of recurrence. Spinal decompression and stabilization, where indicated, may be required along with antifungal drugs (amphotericin B/ketoconazole).[3,4,15,16,96,100]

A combined medical and surgical approach has been shown to be effective, but medical therapy alone with intravenous amphotericin B followed by suppressive azole therapy may be effective in only selected patients.

Paracoccidioidomycosis (South American Blastomycosis)

This is a chronic progressive granulomatous disease primarily spreading from external nares to the lungs and to local lymph nodes.[104–108] It is present from Mexico to Argentina and in South American countries (Brazil, Venezuela, and Colombia).[4,7,16] It is especially endemic in South America and Mexico and is caused by *Paracoccidioides brasiliensis*, a dimorphic fungus. Multiple thick-walled buds arise from a single yeast. The organism lives in the soil or vegetation, and farmers are more affected. Lesions of the mucous membranes, especially of the mouth, nasal passages, pharynx, and lungs, are the primary foci in previously healthy patients. Disseminated disease involves many organs including the liver, spleen, and bones. The anatomoclinical manifestations of the disease have been classified as follows: tegumentary forms (mucocutaneous), lymphoid forms, visceral forms, and mixed forms.

NEUROPATHOLOGY

CNS involvement occurs in approximately one eighth of cases of systemic paracoccidioidomycosis. It is far more common in males than females. Systemic symptoms predominate in one half of cases and neurologic manifestations in one fifth of cases, whereas the rest of the cases present with combined symptomatology. Epilepsy is the most frequent neurologic presentation (50% of cases).

Three main types of pathologic CNS lesions are seen: (1) granulomas (South American blastomycoma/paracoccidioidomycoma [most common]), (2) meningitis with or without hydrocephalus (uncommon), and (3) an abscess (rare).[2,4,10–12,16,105–108] The pseudotumors or granulomas may be intraparenchymatous (common) or meningeal (uncommon). They may occur in the dura with clinical characteristics of meningiomas.[105,106,108] Leptomeningitis is typically basal granulomatous meningitis. The spread to the brain parenchyma occurs through the Virchow-Robin spaces, especially at the level of the hypothalamus and the lateral cerebral fissures. Granulomas are formed by epithelioid cells (Langhans' giant cells) and lymphohistiocytic inflammatory infiltrate. Nodules may resemble tubercles.

DIAGNOSIS

The diagnosis of systemic paracoccidioidomycosis is made by the demonstration of the *P. brasiliensis* organisms or a positive serology (double immunodiffusion), and the diagnosis of neuroparacoccidioidomycosis is made by means of a definitive CNS biopsy.

Routine H&E, PAS, and methenamine silver stains demonstrate the organisms very well. Organisms can also be demonstrated under polarized light as bright green rings when stained with picrosirius. *P. brasiliensis* may be seen on a 10% potassium hydroxide preparation of the infected fluid or sputum. On CT scans, granulomas are characterized by hypo-attenuating images with annular or nodular enhancement.

TREATMENT

Surgical excision of the mass lesions together with therapy with amphotericin B (drug of choice) offers the best chance of a good outcome. Sulfonamides, sulfamethoxazole, trimethoprim, and ketoconazole are also helpful. Sulfamethoxazole/trimethoprim is one of the best combinations for a good outcome. Therapy may also consist of long-term administration of itraconazole. Early diagnosis and adequate therapy may prevent extensive tissue destruction. Long-term follow-up is mandatory. Clinical improvement may be accompanied by diminishing *P. brasiliensis* antigen and antibody titers in cases of neuroparacoccidioidomycosis.[104–112]

Sporotrichosis

Sporotrichosis is caused by *Sporotrichum schenkii*, which is found in the soil and on the plants.[4,7,16] Domestic cats may be an important carrier of agents of sporotrichosis to humans.[113–115]

The organism is a gram-positive cigar-shaped body with occasional budding. In culture, branching septate hyphae bear conidia laterally or in groups. The conidia are ovoid to spherical and are 2 to 6 μm in size. It is a chronic benign infection involving the skin, mucous membranes, muscles, bones, and viscera resulting from direct inoculation. CNS infections occasionally result from direct traumatic implantation of the organisms and rarely from hematogenous spread causing meningitis and cerebritis.

NEUROPATHOLOGY

Cerebral sporotrichosis shows features of chronic meningitis, microabscesses, and granulomas.[4,16] Microscopically, widespread cortical granulomatous microabscesses in the brain, spinal cord, or spinal nerve rootlets are seen.

CLINICAL SYMPTOMATOLOGY

Meningitis presents as chronic occipital headaches and dizziness. Cerebral involvement results in transient episodes of aphasia, limb weakness, and visual disturbances progressing to lethargy and coma. Spinal involvement causes quadriplegia, paraplegia, and radicular pains.

DIAGNOSIS

The CSF shows pleocytosis, mostly lymphocytes (300 cells/mm³), a moderately increased protein level, and a reduced sugar level.

TREATMENT

Patients are treated with amphotericin B and flucytosine and neurosurgical interventions where indicated. Cutaneous and lymphocutaneous sporotrichosis may respond to ketoconazole and potassium iodide therapies.

Cryptococcosis (European Blastomycosis)

Cryptococcosis is one of the most common CNS fungal infections in immunocompromised patients.[116–121] It is ubiquitous but more common in Europe.[16] It is a generalized systemic visceral mycosis affecting previously healthy people[46]; however, in 50% of cases, it has been reported in immunocompromised subjects, children, and middle-age and elderly males.[22] Pigeon breeders are at special risk. The causative agent *C. neoformans* is spherical budding capsulated yeast (5 to 20 μm) (Fig. 117-5). It is found in soil and wood contaminated with bird excreta. It has been isolated from fruit juices and milk. *C. neoformans* var. *neoformans* causes disease in immunocompromised and *C. neoformans* var. *gattii* in immunocompetent hosts.[4] The portal of entry is the respiratory system. The primary focus lies in the lungs from where secondary systemic dissemination occurs via hematogenous spread. There is a strong neurotropic tendency to involve the meninges and brain.[76–81,108]

NEUROPATHOLOGY

The leptomeninges become infiltrated, thickened, and opaque (Fig. 117-6).[2,6,15,16,108] The Virchow-Robin spaces around penetrating vessels are distended with organisms (Fig. 117-7).[4,16] Granulomatous lesions can be found in the cerebral or spinal parenchyma. Spinal arachnoiditis may also be present. Chronic fibrosing leptomeningitis may cause hydrocephalus. Less commonly intraparenchymatous

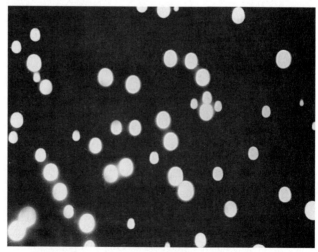

FIGURE 117-5 India ink preparation of the cerebrospinal fluid shows the mucoid capsule of the cryptococcal spherules.

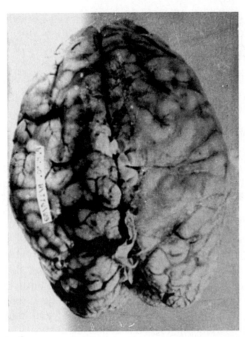

FIGURE 117-6 An autopsy specimen of cryptococcal meningitis shows slimy material on the cerebral surface in the right parietal region. This material fills the cortical sulci and covers the gyri.

cysts are seen (basal ganglionic regions), related to exuberant mucinous capsular material produced by the proliferating cryptococci.[5,76,80,97] Rarely fungi aggregate in an inflammatory lesion and produce small or large granulomas (cryptococcomas or torulomas) in the meninges, parenchyma, ependymal surfaces, or choroid plexuses.

Microscopic examination shows three types of tissue reactions: (1) disseminated leptomeningitis, (2) granulomas, and (3) intraparenchymal cysts.[2,4,16,78,108] In meningitis, there is minimal inflammatory response. The capsule of the fungus seems to impede inflammation by masking surface antigen. Inflammatory response consists of lymphocytes (mainly), plasma cells, eosinophils, fibroblasts, and multinucleated giant cells (studded with cryptococci).[4,7,108] Glial reaction and associated cerebral edema are minimal. Granulomas are more rarely late tissue reactions mimicking tubercles. They are composed of fibroblasts, giant cells (with fungal organisms), and necrotic areas. Multiple intraparenchymal cysts related to exuberant capsular material produced by the proliferating cryptococci create honeycomb cystic cerebral changes, especially in the basal ganglia. No membrane or capsule surrounds these cysts, which are well delineated from the surrounding tissue.[7,108,116,117] The inflammatory response (macrophages with fungi and giant cells) around these cystic lesions is minimal. In our series, all 21 patients had presented with meningitis, and at autopsy, 17 cases of meningitis were confirmed in the form of thickened hazy meninges with a characteristic slimy exudate over the superolateral surface and base of the brain. Among the secondary features, only three patients had multiple granulomas in the cerebral hemispheres and hypothalamus, and in the brain stem as well in two of these three patients. Tiny cryptococcal cysts in the brain parenchyma containing plasma-like coagulated material were seen in 13 cases, and multiple areas of cystic degeneration destroying the brain parenchyma extensively and containing cryptococci in 13 cases (Fig. 117-8). In one case, multiple areas of demyelination with coexisting cerebral edema were noted, and in four cases, dilated ventricles were noted. In two biopsy specimens, a granuloma consisted of inflammatory granulation tissue with foreign body giant cells and cryptococci.

CLINICAL PRESENTATION

CNS cryptococcosis commonly presents with nonspecific manifestations. Initially, patients usually present with headaches, nausea, vomiting, visual impairment, and papilledema, and later neck stiffness develops followed by fever, personality changes, seizures, deterioration in sensorium, cranial nerve palsies, and hydrocephalus.[5,79] In many patients, there are no physical signs. Periods of remission and relapse are noted. Cryptococcomas may produce focal signs that remain unchanged for months. Acute fatal meningitis in cryptococcosis is extremely rare.[4,5] In our series, all 21 patients with CNS cryptococcosis had presented with signs and

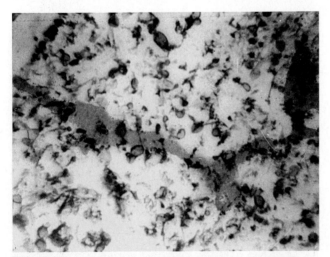

FIGURE 117-7 A section of a gross pathologic specimen in cerebral cryptococcosis shows extensive involvement of the brain matter by multiple cystic cavities that represent enlarged Virchow-Robin spaces.

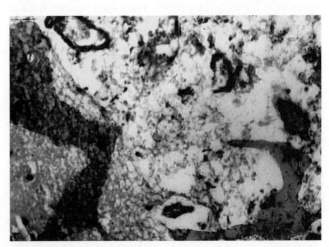

FIGURE 117-8 A section of a gross pathologic specimen in cerebral cryptococcosis shows multiple whitish granulomas and multiple intraparenchymatous cysts.

symptoms of meningitis with increased intracranial pressure. Fever, headache, and vomiting were the most common presenting symptoms. Altered sensorium, cranial nerve palsies, and visual symptoms were seen in six patients, and fatal meningitis in two. Spinal cryptococcal arachnoiditis may present with progressive myelopathy or myeloradiculopathy.[76–81,108]

DIAGNOSIS

Because the fungal capsule is transparent, the CSF remains clear, although xanthochromic and under high pressure. The cell count may go as high as 100 cells/mm^3 (mainly lymphocytes and polymorphs). The sugar and chloride levels are reduced, and total protein level may be elevated. Because the fungal capsule is transparent on routine microscopy, India ink–prepared CSF can demonstrate a mucoid capsule. Organisms can be seen in tissues with PAS and methenamine silver stains.[4,7,16] On mucicarmine and Alcian blue stains, the fungal capsule is well demonstrated. However, routinely, CNS cryptococcosis is diagnosed by positive cryptococcal antigen titer and India ink stain from CSF. Chest radiograph (pulmonary lesion) and CT/MRI brain scans (brain edema, hydrocephalus, basal meningitis, granuloma, and intraparenchymal cysts) are helpful (Figs. 117-9 and 117-10). The most common pattern of CNS cryptococcosis is ventricular dilation on CT and Virchow-Robin space dilation on MRI. MRI is more sensitive in detecting CNS cryptococcal infection such as Virchow-Robin space dilation and leptomeningeal enhancement. There is no significant pattern difference between immunocompromised and nonimmunocompromised patients with CNS cryptococcosis.[117] CSF culture should be done at 30°C for 5 days. This organism can be isolated in 95% of cryptococcal meningitis. Positive latex agglutination test with

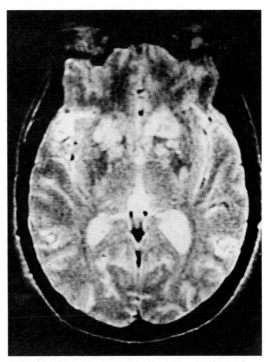

FIGURE 117-10 An axial T2-weighted conventional spin echo image shows scattered, small multiple hyperintense foci in both basal ganglia that are suggestive of enlarged Virchow-Robin spaces in cerebral cryptococcosis. (Courtesy of J. Randy Jinkins, MD.)

increasing serum titers of polysaccharide capsular antigen is of prognostic value.

TREATMENT

Untreated cryptococcal meningitis is generally fatal. Early aggressive therapy with combined amphotericin B and flucytosine offers the best chance for a cure. Alternatively, a 6-week course of amphotericin B followed with maintenance oral fluconazole gives good results. Granulomas, cysts, and hydrocephalus are treated on their own merits. Predisposing factors should be corrected. Failure of treatment raises the possibility of an underlying medical disorder such as acquired immunodeficiency syndrome. Patients receiving treatment before CNS complications should have a good prognosis.

Septate Hyphae Causing Infections of the Central Nervous System

Aspergillosis, chromoblastomycosis (cladosporiosis), and pseudallescheriasis are more frequent causes of CNS fungal infections as compared with other septate hyphal fungi and are therefore considered here.

Aspergillosis

The majority of cases of aspergillosis are reported from countries with a temperate climate where constant exposure to the high spore content of pathogenic *Aspergillus* species is present in the moldy work environment. Several species of *Aspergillus* can cause CNS infection, but most cases are due to *Aspergillus fumigatus*, *Aspergillus niger*, *Aspergillus flavus*, and *Aspergillus oxyzae*.[13,58] These are saprophytic

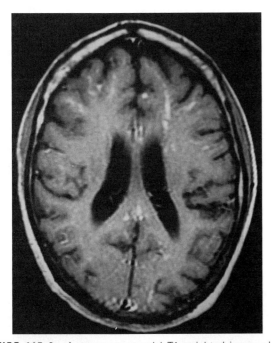

FIGURE 117-9 A postcontrast axial T1-weighted image shows small multiple enhancing areas in the white matter in both cerebral hemispheres that represent foci of cryptococcal infection. (Courtesy of J. Randy Jinkins, MD.)

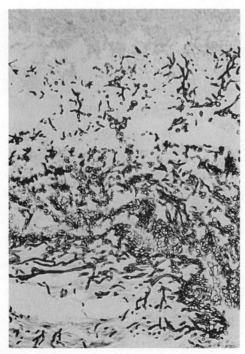

FIGURE 117-11   A photomicrograph (Grocott ×200) shows the septate hyphae (*Aspergillus*) invading the vascular wall. This is more pronounced at the periphery of the vessel wall.

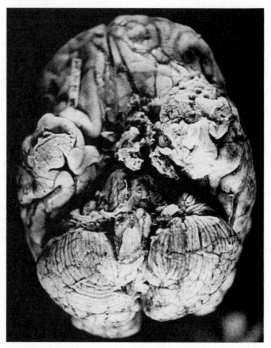

FIGURE 117-12   Basal view of the brain shows an optic chiasmal *Aspergillus* granuloma with extension into the left sylvian fissure and inferior surface of the temporal lobe.

opportunistic ubiquitous fungi found in soil, plants, and decaying matter and consist of branching septate hyphae varying from 4 to 12 μm in width (Fig. 117-11). They have a worldwide distribution. The primary portal of entry for *Aspergillus* organisms is the respiratory tract. Infection reaches the brain either directly from the nasal sinuses via vascular channels or is blood-borne from the lungs and gastrointestinal tract.[46–61] The infection may also be airborne, contaminating the operative field during a neurosurgical procedure.[13]

NEUROPATHOLOGY

In most cases, the CNS aspergillosis is of sinocranial origin, in which skull base syndromes are the presenting features. The primary focus usually lies in the paranasal sinuses. Chronic mycoses of the paranasal sinuses result in orbital, cranial, and intracranial (extradural, dural, and intradural) fungal lesions.[118–122] *Aspergillus* has a marked tendency to invade arteries and veins (angiotropic), producing a necrotizing angiitis, secondary thrombosis, and hemorrhage.[2,4,7,16,58] The onset of cerebral aspergillosis is heralded by acute manifestations of focal neurologic deficits in the anterior and middle cerebral arterial distributions.[2,4,7,46–61] In our series, 28 patients had granulomas causing neurologic deficits, 9 patients had primary presentation as internal carotid artery (ICA) thrombosis with rhinosinoaspergillosis, and in 7 other patients, ICA/basilar artery thrombosis was an associated feature. However, 15 patients presented with an acute stroke due to hemorrhagic infarction, and in 6 other cases, infarction developed during the course of management. The evolving hemorrhagic infarcts may convert to septic infarcts with associated cerebritis and abscesses. The fungal hyphae are found in large-, intermediate-, and small-sized blood vessels with invasion through

vascular walls into the adjacent tissue; invasion in the reverse direction can also occur.[7] Purulent lesions may be chronic and have a tendency for fibrosis and granuloma formation (Figs. 117-12 and 117-13). Microscopically, the most striking feature is the intensity of the vascular invasion with thrombosis, as was seen in our 20 cases of vasculitis; in 14 cases as ICA, middle cerebral artery, and anterior cerebral artery thrombosis; and in 2 cases as basilar thrombosis.

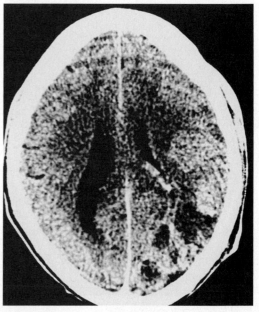

FIGURE 117-13   A contrast computed tomography scan shows multiple faintly ring-enhancing *Aspergillus* abscesses in the left occipital region.

In purulent lesions (a total of seven cases in our series), the pus is seen in the center of the abscesses with abundant polymorphs at the periphery. Granulomas consist of lymphocytes, plasma cells, and fungal hyphae as seen in 28 cases in the present study.

CLINICAL PRESENTATION

Aspergillosis should be considered in cases manifesting with acute onset of focal neurologic deficits due to a suspected vascular or space-occupying lesion, especially in immunocompromised hosts.[2,7,48,50,58,123,124] In patients with paranasal sinus disease, orbital extension with proptosis, ocular palsies, visual deterioration, and chemosis may occur.[48,58] Van Landeghem and colleagues[122] reported an interesting rare fatal case of cerebral aspergilloma located in the midbrain causing aqueductal stenosis and obstructive hydrocephalus. In Muscat, 44 cases of rhinosino aspergillosis were treated in the ear, nose, and throat department, and 9 of these had orbitorhinosinocerebral syndrome. There were nine other cases of orbitorhinosinocerebral syndrome in this series. The symptomatologies frequently encountered are headache, vomiting, convulsions, hemiparesis, fever, cranial nerve deficits, papilledema, and coma. In our series, most of the patients with CNS aspergillosis presented with signs and symptoms of an intracranial space-occupying lesion with increased intracranial pressure. Altered sensorium, acute stroke, hemiparesis/monoparesis, fever, visual symptoms, cranial nerve palsies, and progressive motor and sensory impairment of varying degree in the limbs were the most commonly encountered symptoms. Only a few patients were suspected of meningitis. Among our seven patients with cerebral aspergillus abscess, four died, and in three cases, aspiration with or without craniotomy resulted in a successful outcome (see Fig. 117-13). Features typical of meningitis and subarachnoid hemorrhage due to mycotic aneurysms may manifest.[125,126] We encountered two fatal cases of mycotic peripheral aneurysm of middle cerebral artery branch, and in two other cases of aspergillosis, mycotic aneurysm of ICA territory were noted at autopsy. Interestingly, in two fatal cases with primary brain tumor (glioblastoma multiforme in one and anaplastic astrocytoma in the other), aspergillosis was coexisting within the tumor mass. Spinal aspergillosis may present as lumbago and/or sciatica.[47,49,51,57,60,61] The spinal cord invasion may occur. Vertebral body involvement is common and paradural granulomas frequent.[54] We had five cases of spinal extradural granulomas, for which surgery was performed successfully, with one patient dying after long-term follow-up. Paraspinal abscesses are rare due to aspergillosis.

DIAGNOSIS

Aspergillosis is diagnosed by direct examination and culture. Spinal fluid pleocytosis (600 cells/mm³) and moderately elevated CSF proteins are present, but CSF sugar is usually normal. Organisms are rarely found in the CSF. Organisms are faintly visible with H&E and PAS stains; however, most are readily seen with methenamine silver stain. Plain radiographs, CT/MRI (Figs. 117-14 to 117-18), angiography (Figs. 117-19 to 117-21), and serial serologic tests (i.e., double diffusion counterimmunoelectrophoresis, immunofluorescence, enzyme-linked immunosorbent assay) significantly help in making a diagnosis. In spinal aspergillosis,

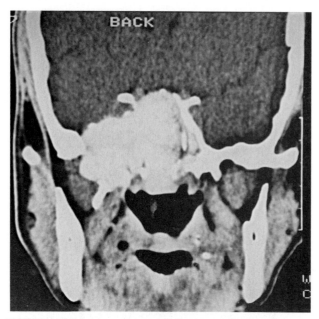

FIGURE 117-14 A contrast coronal computed tomography scan shows an opacified sphenoid sinus with a large enhancing *Aspergillus* granuloma that is eroding the skull base and extends to the left middle cranial fossa.

image-guided aspirations, vertebral biopsy, histologic examination, and culture establish the diagnosis.[3,4,7,9,16]

TREATMENT

Aggressive neurosurgical intervention for surgical removal of *Aspergillus* abscesses, granulomas, and focally infarcted brain and correction of underlying risk factors and amphotericin B combined with flucytosine and treatment of the

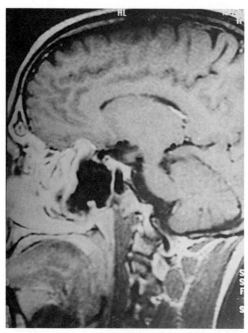

FIGURE 117-15 A right parasagittal postcontrast T1-weighted image shows enhancement of the sphenoid sinus mucosa with marked enhancement around the internal carotid artery but preserved flow void signals.

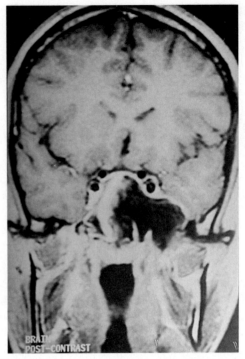

FIGURE 117-16 A coronal postcontrast T1-weighted image shows enhancement of the sphenoid sinus mucosa with flow void signals in both internal carotid arteries suggestive of normal flow in a case of *Aspergillus* sinusitis.

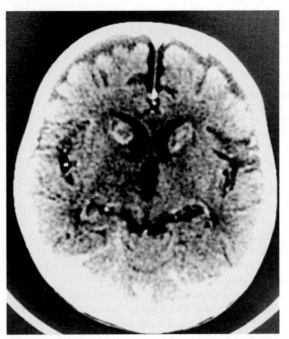

FIGURE 117-18 A postcontrast axial computed tomography brain scan in a case of cerebral aspergillosis shows ring enhancement in the head of both caudate nuclei that is suggestive of subacute infarctions. (Courtesy of Sanjeev D. Athale, MD.)

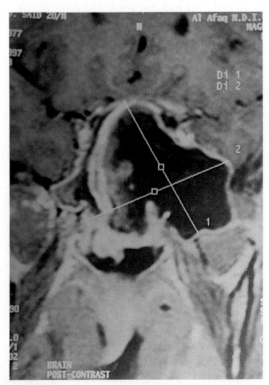

FIGURE 117-17 A coronal postcontrast T1-weighted image shows hyperintense *Aspergillus* sphenoid sinusitis with enhancement of the dura mater in the right middle cranial fossa.

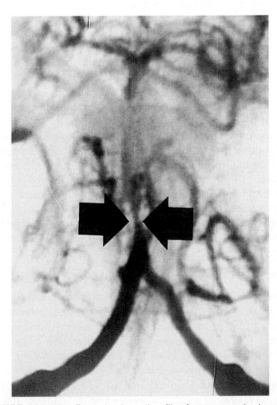

FIGURE 117-19 Frontal subtraction film from a vertebral arteriogram illustrates the extreme narrowing of the basilar artery (*arrows*) due to severe granulomatous *Aspergillus* meningitis. (Courtesy of J. Randy Jinkins, MD.)

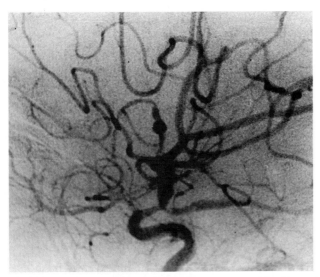

FIGURE 117-20 Lateral subtraction film from a right internal carotid arteriogram illustrates the supraclinoid internal carotid narrowing, the fusiform aneurysmal dilatation of the posterior cerebral artery originating from the internal carotid, aneurysmal dilatation of the middle cerebral stem, and the peripheral saccular aneurysm of one of the middle cerebral branches in a case of *Aspergillus* arteritis. (Courtesy of J. Randy Jinkins, MD.)

source of infection should form the mainstay of the management. After extensive intracranial surgery, the residual aspergillosis may be treated with a high dose of itraconazole (880 mg/day for 4 months followed by 400 mg/day for 5 months). The high dose of itraconazole is approximately 16 mg/kg/day for adults.[119] In spinal aspergillosis, aggressive antifungal therapy with amphotericin B is the primary treatment; however, flucytosine, itraconazole, miconazole, and sulfamethoxazole have been effective. Significant compressive myelopathy or myeloradiculopathy may warrant surgical decompression. Cases of spinal lesion with adhesive arachnoiditis have been reported. However, the prognosis of the CNS aspergillosis still remains poor.

Chromoblastomycosis (Phaeohyphomycosis): Cladosporiosis

This is a rare chronic subcutaneous mycosis presenting as a verrucoid colored or crusted cutaneous lesion.[4] It results when thorns or sharp vegetation inoculates the fungus into the subcutaneous tissue, especially in the lower extremity.[127–133] It is caused by many different pigmented fungi (i.e., *Cladosporium, Hormodendrum,* and *Phialophora*).[7,16,129] Many isolated case reports of this rare cerebral mycosis have been published.[134–138] Cladosporiosis is the most frequent mycosis of this group. *Cladosporium trichoioides* (var. *bantianum*) is most frequently isolated from a brain abscess.[130] It is saprophytic in soil and decaying vegetables and affects barefoot workers and farmers. It is considered a pathogen, but cases have been recorded in association with immunosuppressive treatment. Hyphae of *C. trichoioides* are slender, 2 to 3 μm in thickness, and septation occurs every 3 to 15 μm. Single-cell conidia are 3 to 4 μm in thickness. Cerebral chromoblastomycosis arises from a nonneural infected site (cutaneous and respiratory system) and spreads hematogenously to the brain.

NEUROPATHOLOGY

Any part of the brain may be involved; however, frontal lobes are the most common sites of *Cladosporium* infection. Typically, they produce intraparenchymatous abscesses associated with acute and chronic inflammatory changes with focal multinucleated giant cells.[2,4,7,16,128–130] These multilocular abscesses can extend into the subarachnoid spaces or toward cerebral ventricles, resulting in leptomeningitis and ventriculitis (Fig. 117-22). Interestingly, the CNS may be the only site of infection and meningitis may be the sole presentation. Brain abscesses (uni- or

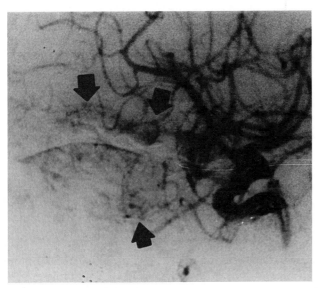

FIGURE 117-21 A lateral right carotid angiogram shows a mild blush of the invasive *Aspergillus* granuloma in the capsular region. (Courtesy of T. Beydoun, MD, and J. Randy Jinkins, MD.)

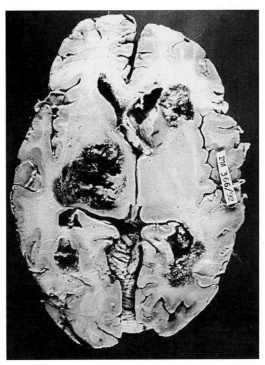

FIGURE 117-22 A gross autopsy section shows multiple *Cladosporium* cerebral abscesses.

multilocular) are commonly seen. Granulomatous reaction is rare and in many cases very minimal. Microscopically, a primary intraparenchymatous abscess consists of lymphocytes, polymorphs, histiocytes, giant cells, and the fungus with surrounding fibrosis and reactive gliosis. In our autopsy cases of cladosporiosis, all five cases showed blackish/brownish granulated tissue at the base of the brain and multiple areas of acute suppurative breakdown with areas of hemorrhage. Abscesses were multiple and scattered in different parts of the brain, and in one surviving patient, the abscess was single and localized to the occipital lobe. Associated meningitis was present in one case and hydrocephalus in other.

Histologic examination in four cases showed multiple areas of acute parenchymal necrosis and mixed inflammatory cells consisting of lymphocytes, polymorphs, multinucleated foreign body giant cells, and fungal elements. The structure of a chronic granuloma in the pons was seen in one case. In another case, there was associated granulomatous leptomeningitis. Blood vessel invasion by fungus and thrombosis was seen in two cases.

CLINICAL PRESENTATIONS

Most cases of cerebral phaeohyphomycosis have been reported among immunocompetent patients and less commonly in transplant recipients.[134-138] Headache, vomiting, convulsions, altered sensorium with fever, and increased intracranial pressure due to mass effect of cerebral lesions were present in our six cases. The clinical impression was of an intracranial space-occupying lesion in five cases, and an intracranial abscess in one case. Focal neurologic deficits, increased intracranial pressure, and CT/MRI evidence of brain granulomas, basal meningitis, haemorrhages, and abscesses are main presenting cliniconeuroimaging features.

DIAGNOSIS

The characteristic brown color of the fungi is recognized macroscopically.[4,16,129,132] However, pigment may not be apparent in preparations stained with PAS and methenamine silver, and therefore unstained preparations are more helpful. The *Cladosporium* organism is brown in cultures and tissue lesions. Biopsy specimens of the abscess wall and culture of the pus are diagnostic.

TREATMENT

Surgical therapy in combination with chemotherapy with itraconazole is recommended. Surgical removal of the cerebral abscesses is undertaken wherever possible. None of the antifungal drugs are very effective in these infections. High-dose itraconazole treatment and flucytosine are effective in some cases in combination with amphotericin B. The overall prognosis is poor.

Pseudallescheriasis (Monosporiosis): Allescheriasis and Scedosporiasis

Pseudallescheriasis or allescheriasis is a rare cerebral mycosis affecting mainly immunocompromised hosts.[7] It is the single most common cause of mycetoma in the United States.[4,139,140] The fungus *Pseudallescheria boydii* occurs in tissues as septate hyphae. It is a saprophyte having a worldwide distribution and is found in soil and water. The organism gains access to the tissues through the skin. The primary focus is in the skin or respiratory system and hematogenous

spread occurs to the CNS. Pseudallescheriasis is usually commonly associated with chronic bronchitis, emphysema, and sarcoidosis. The fungus grows as a mold within tissues causing necrosis and abscess formation.[4]

Systemic scedosporiasis due to the anamorph or asexual form, *Scedosporium apiospermum* (*P. boydii*) has become an important cause of an opportunistic mycosis, especially in patients undergoing high-risk hematopoietic stem cell transplantation.[141-143] A case of rapidly progressive cerebellar hyalohyphomycosis due to *S. apiospermum* in an allogeneic marrow graft recipient receiving treatment for severe graft versus host disease was reported by Safdar and colleagues.[143]

A rare fatal case of multiple true mycotic aneurysms in a child with a brain abscess due to *P. boydii* was reported by Messori and colleagues.[142]

NEUROPATHOLOGY

Typically, mass lesions resulting from pseudallescheriasis are hemorrhagic infarcts with associated leptomeningitis.[4,7,16,140] These hemorrhagic infarcts may be converted to cerebral abscesses. However, pseudallescheriasis is a rare cause of multiple brain abscesses or meningitis. In the wall of the abscess, there are numerous hyphae and rounded chlamydospores. Intravascular hyphae, a hallmark of aspergillosis, may also be found in pseudallescheriasis.

CLINICAL PRESENTATION

Patients may present with headaches, vomiting, neck stiffness, focal neurologic deficits, and signs of increased intracranial pressure. Sudden appearance of gross neurologic deficits in patients with cerebral infarction portends a poor prognosis.

DIAGNOSIS

CSF examination may show septate hyphae. However, demonstration of hyphae in tissue and culture are required for the diagnosis of pseudallescheriasis. CT/MR scans show nonspecific findings of brain abscess and/or hemorrhagic infarcts.

TREATMENT

Cerebral abscesses require neurosurgical intervention. Intravenous azole drugs (miconazole, itraconazole, or ketoconazole) are recommended, although Dapsone (diaminodiphenylsulfone) has also been used in this fungal infection.

Nonseptate Hyphae Causing Infections of the Nervous System: Phycomycosis, Zygomycosis, and Mucormycosis

Phycomycosis also encompasses zygomycosis in its broader group.[7,144] The term zygomycosis includes entorhinomucormycosis and mucormycosis.[4,7,144] The former is a tropical infection of subcutaneous tissue or paranasal sinuses caused by species of *Basidiobolus* and *Conidiobolus* after trauma-related implantation. The principal family causing CNS zygomycosis is Mucoraceae (mucormycosis has three main genera: *Rhizopus*, *Mucor*, and *Absidia*).[62-67] *Rhizopus arrhizus* and *Rhizopus oryzae* are responsible for 95% of cases. The other members of this group, *Saksenaea* and *Mortierella*, usually result in extra-CNS mycosis. The organisms are ubiquitous and are found in soil, manure, and decaying vegetation, and are frequently airborne. Mucormycosis occurs initially in the rhinosino-orbital region, respiratory system, gastrointestinal tract, and skin.[2,4,7,10,16,65,144,145] The CNS mucormycosis results either from direct invasion or hematogenous spread of nonseptate irregular hyphae with right-angle branches measuring 6 to 15 μm in diameter and 200 μm in length.[146–148] From hyphae, root-like rhizoids grow. From rhizoids, sporangiospore-bearing sporangia develop that contain brown spores (7 μm). Although these organisms are considered opportunistic, CNS mucormycosis has been described in previously healthy individuals.[149–153] It is widely found in the United States and often associated with diabetic ketoacidosis, intravenous drug abuse, renal transplantation, malignancy, and steroid therapy.[146–148] Mucormycosis ranks as the fourth most common CNS fungal infection in immunocompromised hosts, surpassed in frequency only by candidiasis, aspergillosis, and cryptococcosis. Six clinical syndromes have been described: cutaneous, pulmonary, gastrointestinal, rhinocerebral, cerebral, and disseminated. Pulmonary, rhinocerebral, and cerebral forms are common.[149–153] It may also present with endophthalmitis with a fatal outcome.[149]

In its rhinocerebral form,[62,144,145] the infection develops initially in the nasal mucosa, which becomes swollen and dark red-brown. Subsequent invasion of the antrum, periorbital region, adjacent orbital arteries, and ICAs may occur. The frontal lobes are involved by direct venous invasion through the orbital plate. When brain involvement results from hematogenous dissemination from pulmonary, gastrointestinal, or cutaneous sites, commonly thrombosis of the ICA and/or cavernous sinuses occurs with associated hemorrhagic infarction in deep basal ganglionic structures.[64,68,153]

NEUROPATHOLOGY

The fungus excites a mixed inflammatory response.[65] The hyphae occlude and penetrate vascular walls causing thrombosis and associated infarction.[16] Acute and chronic cerebritis are present. Hemorrhage into the infarcted brain or from mycotic aneurysms is typical.[2,4,7,16] These highly angiotropic fungi invade the walls of the vessels in the brain and meninges. Predominantly neutrophilic response and multinucleate giant cells are seen on microscopic examination. Granulomas are not typically seen. Mucor has a strong tendency to proliferate along and through the vascular structures producing arteritis with formation of aneurysms, pseudoaneurysms, vascular occlusion, and cerebral infarction.[64,68,153] In our series, the brain was examined in 33 cases at autopsy. Multiple hemorrhagic infarctions (Figs. 117-23 and 117-24) were seen in 28 cases, meningeal exudate in 13 cases, localized brain abscess in 4 cases, and marked cerebral edema in most cases. Areas of suppurative necrosis with hemorrhage in different parts of the brain were commonly noted. A complete thrombosis of one or more blood vessels of the circle of Willis could be seen in 8 patients, whereas partial occlusion was noted in 19 other cases, and mycotic aneurysms in 2 cases. Interestingly, in two patients with primary brain tumors (one malignant astrocytoma and one primary CNS lymphoma), mucormycosis was present within the brain tumor, which was operated on via stereotactic surgery. Surgical biopsy specimen showed four cases with typical features of a granuloma with fungal hyphae.

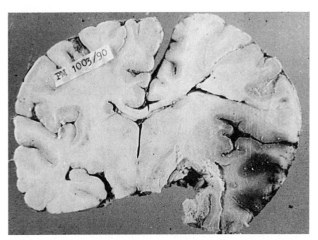

FIGURE 117-23 Coronal slice of a gross autopsy specimen of cerebral mucormycosis shows a left temporal hemorrhagic infarct with evidence of subarachnoid hemorrhage in the left sylvian fissure.

CLINICAL SYMPTOMS

Phycomycotic fungal infections of the CNS are rare and remain challenging problems occurring mostly in immunocompromised individuals with protean clinical manifestations, an unpredictable course, and unfavorable outcome in many cases despite aggressive neurosurgical interventions and recent antifungal drugs. Orbitorhinocerebral mucormycosis is a potentially lethal opportunistic fungal infection with rapid progression and high mortality. It occurs less commonly in an apparently normal host.[153]

In rhinocerebral mucormycosis, the pace of the illness is rapid with periorbital pain, nasal discharge, proptosis, chemosis, progressive visual loss, ophthalmoplegia with loss of sensation over the forehead, retro-orbital venous obstruction (cavernous sinus thrombosis), and involvement of the ICA producing contralateral hemiplegia (occlusive or hemorrhagic stroke).[65,144,145] In the present study, among 45 cases of

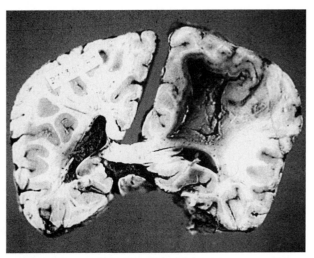

FIGURE 117-24 A coronal section (autopsy) shows a hemorrhagic mucormycotic cerebral infarct in the left parietal region, causing mass effect.

cerebral mucormycosis, there were 17 cases with orbitorhinocerebral syndrome. Among 34 cases presenting as acute stroke, in 26 cases an acute hemorrhagic infarct and in 8 cases complete ICA thrombosis/occlusions were noted. In another 17 cases, varying grades of ICA occlusion and in 2 cases basilar thrombosis were demonstrated at autopsy. Eight patients presented with a subacute space-occupying lesion and four with cerebral abscesses, and in four cases, granuloma with abscess formation was noted. There were two cases of a true zygomycotic fungal aneurysm, and in one case only subarachnoid hemorrhage was detected. In three patients, some degree of hydrocephalus was seen. The nasal passages and nasopharynx may show black areas of the mucosa and underlying bone. Frontal lobe abscess and infarct may result. Headaches, neck stiffness, convulsions, and hydrocephalus may result from initial meningeal involvement, and, later, the vascular invasion results in acute focal neurologic deficits (i.e., aphasia, hemiplegia, disorientation, and altered sensorium).[16,65] Once intracranial infection is established, the clinical course is acute in onset, with a rapid fulminating course resulting in high mortality within a few days.[4,153]

DIAGNOSIS

Biopsy of the necrotic material or mucosa and examination of the black nasal discharge are pathognomonic. The CSF is under normal pressure but may be hemorrhagic, with leukocytosis-increased proteins and sugar contents depending on the predisposing risk factors. Organisms are well shown with H&E, PAS, and methenamine silver stains. The fungi grow rapidly on Sabouraud's agar filling a Petri dish with a fluffy white growth in 2 to 3 days, which turns to dark brown by spores. Features on the CT scan of nasopharyngeal mucormycosis include opacification and bony destruction of the paranasal sinuses, orbital extension from the ethmoid sinuses producing proptosis and chemosis, and obliteration of the nasopharyngeal tissue planes. When this virulent fungus spreads intracranially, low attenuating abnormalities are noted on the CT scans, particularly in the anterior cranial fossa but may be in any part of the brain (Fig. 117-25). These regions show mass effect and contrast enhancement. Mucor may also cause large vessel obstruction and thereby cerebral infarction[64,65,68,69] (Figs. 117-26 and 117-27) and abscess formation (Fig. 117-28).

On CT scanning, nonenhancing, hypoattenuating lesions may represent areas of infarction or cerebritis. There may be homogeneous or peripheral enhancement. Thrombosis of the cavernous sinus causes nonenhancement of the sinuses. On MRI, hyperintense secretions are seen in the paranasal sinuses, with hyperintense thickening of the nasal mucosa on long TR images. A mixed picture of cerebritis and cerebral infarction as a hyperintense lesion is well outlined on proton density and T2-weighted images, especially in the frontotemporobasal regions. Flow void is absent in cases of carotid or basilar artery and cavernous sinus thrombosis. In such cases, mixed-signal inflammatory tissue is seen replacing the usual carotid flow void.[152]

Fairley and colleagues[150] reported survival and long-term follow-up of a case of orbitorhinocerebral mucormycosis in an immunocompetent patient after extensive orbital exenteration and débridement of involved adjacent structures along with liposomal amphotericin.

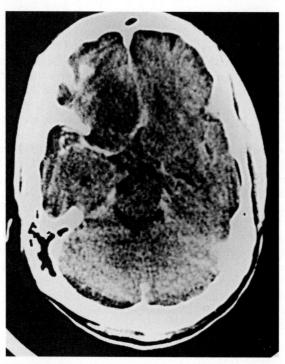

FIGURE 117-25 A contrast computed tomography brain scan shows a hypoattenuating cerebral infarct in the right basofrontal region with leptomeningeal enhancement in a case of cerebral mucormycosis.

TREATMENT

Control of risk factors, especially diabetes, is an important measure.[4,16,65] Amphotericin B, trimethoprim, and sulfamethoxazole are used. Early aggressive investigations including biopsies should be undertaken. Intensive treatment with amphotericin B is effective, but penetration of the drug is poor due to vascular occlusions and local gangrene of the bone. Radical surgical procedures to the orbit and sinuses reduce the infective mass but are major undertakings in ill patients. Irrigation of paranasal sinuses with antifungal

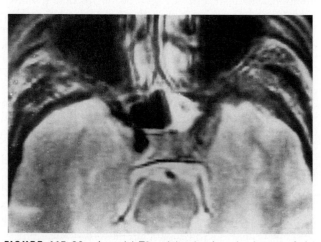

FIGURE 117-26 An axial T2-weighted spin echo image of the brain shows evidence of left ethmoid and sphenoid sinusitis with absent flow void in the left internal carotid artery in a case of mucormycosis. Normal flow void is seen in the right internal carotid artery. (Courtesy of J. Randy Jinkins, MD.)

agents should be performed. Even though the prognosis of this infection is usually poor, aggressive surgical extirpation combined with antifungal agents have helped. Exenteration may be required. Intravenous amphotericin B is of great value.[150] The maximal tolerated dose is given until progression is halted. The drug is continued for 10 to 12 weeks. Fifty percent of craniofacial infection may be cured, but survival of patients with cerebral, gastrointestinal, or disseminated mucormycosis is rare, and this virulent fungus causes death within few weeks if untreated. A team approach to management is recommended for early appropriate surgery and systemic antifungal agents.

Fungus-like Bacteria: Actinomycetes Causing Infections of the Nervous System

Actinomycetes are bacteria with narrow branched vegetative cells that superficially resemble fungi. The common ones belong to *Nocardia* (aerobic) and *Actinomyces* (anaerobic) species.

Nocardiosis

Nocardiosis has a worldwide distribution. *Nocardia* are thin (less than 1 μm thick), gram-positive aerobes with branching filaments; they are focally acid fast. *Nocardia asteroides* causes most human infections (90%), but *Nocardia brasiliensis* is also a pathogen (7%), particularly found in Central and South America.[154–157] *Nocardia otitidis-caviarum* very rarely (3%) causes nocardiosis. Approximately 1000 cases are reported in the United States each year. *Nocardia* are ubiquitous and common in soil and decaying vege-tation. Primary infection is pulmonary or cutaneous or is a chronic granulomatous disease of the bone.[155] It may develop in immunocompetent or immunocompromised hosts (receiving steroids or cytotoxic drugs or having pulmonary alveolar proteinosis, sarcoidosis, ulcerative colitis, or intestinal lipodystrophy).[158–161] There is hematogenous spread to the CNS.

NEUROPATHOLOGY

Nocardia organisms produce multiloculated solitary or multiple brain abscesses that are poorly encapsulated.[4,7,16] Central thick exudate is yellowish green in color. Meningitis infrequently coexists with parenchymal abscesses. An atypical case of a nocardial abscess of the choroid plexus has been reported by Mogilner and colleagues.[159] CNS granulomas are extremely rare in nocardiosis. Involvement of cranial or vertebral bones can cause osteomyelitis with secondary extradural abscesses. Microabscesses in the CNS are surrounded by dark red margins and contain neutrophils, mononuclear cells, liquefactive necrosis, reactive gliosis, and fibrosis. Chronic granulomatous changes when present adjacent to an abscess may show occasional giant cells.[2,4,7,16,117] Durmaz and colleagues[158] reported a case of multiple nocardial abscesses of the cerebrum, cerebellum, and spinal cord.

CLINICAL PRESENTATION

Nocardiosis affects men more than women (2 to 3:1) in their fourth through sixth decades of life. Nocardiosis occurs in three primary clinical syndromes: cutaneous, subcutaneous, and pulmonary (75% cases). The brain is the

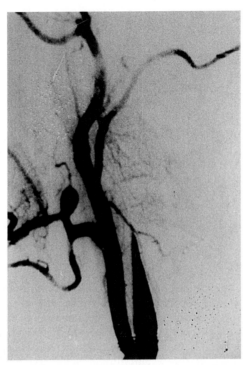

FIGURE 117-27 A left common carotid artery angiogram (lateral projection) shows a tapering occlusion of the internal carotid artery, indicating a subacute event in a case of mucormycosis. (Courtesy of J. Randy Jinkins, MD.)

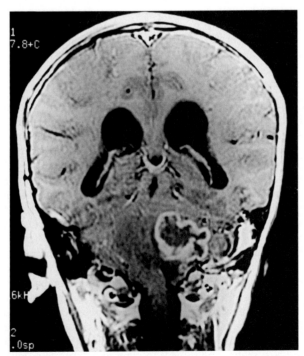

FIGURE 117-28 A coronal postcontrast T1-weighted image shows a thick-walled, ring-enhancing lesion in the left cerebellopontine angle cistern that is displacing the hypointense edematous brain stem to the opposite side. (Courtesy of Sanjeev D. Athale, MD.)

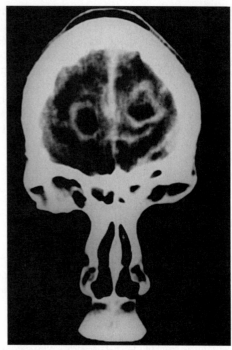

FIGURE 117-29 A contrast computed tomography scan shows two ring-enhancing abscesses, one in each frontal lobe with right frontal sinusitis. (Courtesy of Sanjeev D. Athale, MD.)

most common secondary site (25% cases). A brain abscess is far more common than meningitis.

These patients usually have a rapidly progressive clinical course with focal neurologic deficits depending on the location of the brain abscesses. Increased intracranial pressure may develop. Rupture of the abscess into subarachnoid spaces causes purulent meningitis. One of our patients with cerebral nocardiosis presented with frontal sinusitis, cranial osteomyelitis, extradural abscess, and bifrontal multiple intraparenchymatous abscesses in the frontal lobes (Fig. 117-29). Surgical excision of the abscesses was performed, but the patient died and no autopsy was performed. Our second patient with nocardiosis received a renal transplant and had a pulmonary lesion. He developed multiple cerebral abscesses that were aspirated stereotactically; the patient was then treated successfully with appropriate long-term drug therapy. Our third patient had a frontal sinus infection that was treated with antibiotics. He developed a frontal brain abscess that was aspirated stereotactically, and the diagnosis of nocardiosis was established. Aggressive management of the sinusitis and cerebral abscess resulted in a cure.

Spinal cord compression after vertebral osteomyelitis and intramedullary spinal abscess may rarely occur in nocardiosis.[154,156,157] Spinal nocardiosis occurs commonly in cervical and thoracic regions. It develops by hematogenous spread from a pulmonary focus and presents as localized pain, radiculopathy, or myelopathy. Intramedullary spinal cord abscess has been described. Vertebral bodies are commonly involved, and paraspinal abscess may be present.[154,156,157]

DIAGNOSIS

CSF shows few abnormalities unless meningitis coexists with the abscesses. The organism is difficult to culture, and multiple lumbar punctures may fail to isolate it. CSF findings

are nonspecific. CT and MRI scanning show ring enhancement in nocardial cerebral abscesses after administration of contrast material. In cases of intraventricular rupture of nocardial brain abscess, fluid-attenuated inversion recovery MRI may reveal a clear hyperintense component in the ventricle and a niveau formation inside the intracerebral lesion indicating intraventricular rupture of the brain abscess.[160] CT demonstrates hypoattenuating, contrast-enhancing lesions with surrounding edema. Indium 111–labeled leukocyte scanning may differentiate abscesses from neoplasms. The diagnosis depends mainly on obtaining specimens of pus from the lesions, usually at craniotomy or burr hole biopsy. These organisms are seen well on Gram or methenamine silver stain rather than H&E sections. It is easily cultured on Sabouraud's or beef infusion glucose agar in 1 to 4 weeks.

TREATMENT

Surgical drainage is often necessary, and at times, excision is appropriate. In contrast to actinomycosis, nocardiosis tends to be penicillin resistant. Recommended treatment is sulfamethoxazole with trimethoprim, 4 to 8 g/day in divided doses for 6 to 12 months. In allergic patients, clindamycin, minocycline, erythromycin, fusidic acid, and amikacin, depending on sensitivity testing, should be used. The progress is best monitored by CT/MRI scanning in appropriate settings and the general state of the patient. Mortality in disseminated nocardiosis approaches 80%. Abscess management (aspiration/excision) and appropriate chemotherapy form the basis of treatment. Although most cases of spinal nocardiosis can be managed with medical therapy (sulfonamides, trimethoprim, ampicillin, tetracycline, aminoglycosides, erythromycin, rifampicin, and cycloserine), surgery may be required in patients with spinal cord and or nerve root compression. Syringomyelia may occur as a delayed complication of treatment for nocardial brain abscess.[161] Neuronocardiosis is associated with significant morbidity and mortality rates.

Actinomycosis

CNS actinomycosis is a rare disease most frequently forming cerebral abscesses and infrequently granulomatous lesions.[162,163] Actinomycosis is worldwide in distribution.

Actinomyces israelii and less frequently *Actinomyces bovis* usually produce most human infections.[164] *A. israelii* is a normal inhabitant of the mouth and gut and is not found free in nature. It requires devitalized tissue to provide an anaerobic environment for growth.[165–167] The portal of entry is the damaged mucosal lining. Actinomycosis is a chronic suppurative and granulomatous infection characterized by multiloculated sulfur granules. The sulfur granules consist of thin (<1 μm), branching gram-positive actinomycetic filaments in matted tangles. The disease has three primary forms: cervicofacial (mandible), pulmonary, and abdominal (ileocecal region). CNS involvement occurs in 2% to 5% of all cases by direct tissue invasion or hematogenous dissemination.[168,169] The organism is uninhibited by the tissue planes and spreads to contiguous structures without difficulty.

The risk factors are dental pathology, intrauterine device, alcohol abuse, and Rendu-Osler-Weber disease.[162]

FIGURE 117-30 A contrast computed tomography brain scan shows a mixed-attenuation lesion in the left parietal region that is suggestive of a coexisting abscess with a large granuloma in a case of cerebral actinomycosis.

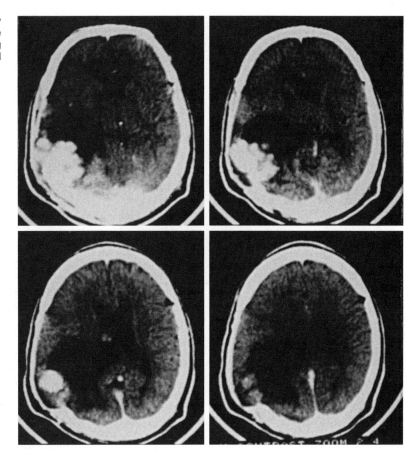

NEUROPATHOLOGY

Clinicopathologically, actinomycosis is characterized by draining sinuses, extensive fibrosis, and pus-filled microabscesses containing multilobulated sulfur granules.

The most common form of CNS actinomycosis is intracerebral abscess.[164–169] The abscess is typically a single, thick-walled, multilobulated lesion. In cervicofacial actinomycosis, the meninges are invaded, causing epidural and subdural empyemas associated with cranial osteomyelitis. Involvement of the spine in pulmonary actinomycosis occurs as a result of contiguous spread of infection with the production of osteomyelitis and epidural abscess.[166–169] Microscopically, actinomycotic abscesses have central liquefactive necrosis, neutrophils, mononuclear cells, granulation tissue, fibrosis, and bacterial filaments. Lymphocytes, plasma cells, and monocytes are present in the abscesses with multinucleated giant cells. Granulomas are usually not seen.[168]

CLINICAL SYMPTOMS

Intracranial actinomycotic abscess commonly presents with progressive symptoms and signs of increased intracranial pressure and focal neurologic deficits appropriate to the location.[168] Meningitis is rare and granulomas are unusual.[167,168] Cranial or spinal osteomyelitis with paradural abscesses may result.[165] The infection runs a relentless course over many years with destruction of contiguous bone and soft tissues. Nine patients with craniofacial actinomycosis with cerebral complications were seen at Khoula Hospital, Muscat.

These patients were treated with multiple courses of antibiotics. All patients had osteomyelitis and intracranial granulomas, and in three cases, cerebral abscesses were associated with granulomas (Fig. 117-30). In eight cases, the cranial spread was seen by contiguity from the scalp (Figs. 117-31 and 117-32) and the face, whereas one patient had an extradural granuloma after dental extraction.

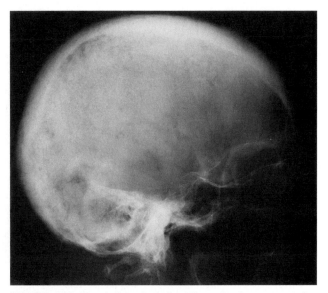

FIGURE 117-31 A lateral skull radiograph shows extensive cranial osteomyelitis in a case of craniocerebral actinomycosis.

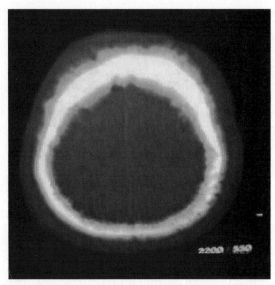

FIGURE 117-32 A bone window cranial computed tomography scan shows extensive irregular sawtooth appearance of the outer and inner tables of the skull due to actinomycotic osteomyelitis.

With neurosurgical management and medication, eight patients are asymptomatic, and one died due to extensive subarachnoid hemorrhage. In this case, no autopsy was performed.

Spinal actinomycosis (Fig. 117-33) results from direct extension from a pulmonary or abdominal actinomycotic focus and involves vertebral bodies, related ribs, pedicles, laminae, and spinous processes; however, intervertebral discs are spared in actinomycosis.[166,169] The anterior vertebral body surface may show a sawtooth appearance. Paraspinal abscess and pus-draining sinuses are common, whereas spinal cord compression is rare. One of our patients had craniocervical actinomycosis with marked swelling of the cervical soft tissues and destruction of the occipital bone and posterior elements of the upper cervical spine. She was diagnosed by biopsy and treated with long-term medical therapy. There was no spinal instability.

DIAGNOSIS

A high index of suspicion is needed in patients who have history of dental extraction, appendectomy, or pulmonary infection. Involvement of the jaw may show painless swelling, woody induration, and sinus tracts that discharge pus intermittently.[168] The diagnosis requires demonstration of sulfur granules (which are actually tightly clumped colonies of the causative agent *A. israelii*) present in the pus in the draining sinus or in biopsy sections. Similar to actinomycosis, sulfur granules may be seen in infection with other actinomycetes (i.e., maduromycosis).[7] Gram stain shows positive long branching filaments and on H&E sections and basophilic filaments terminating in eosinophilic clubs. Plain skull radiographs may demonstrate osteomyelitis or sinusitis.[169] Soap bubble vertebrae (areas of rarefaction in active and areas of sclerosis in long-standing infection) may be seen on spinal radiographs.[3] CT brain scan usually demonstrates a solitary thick-walled ring-enhancing abscess with surrounding edema. Granulomas are seen as slightly hyperattenuating lesions with contrast enhancement. MRI with gadolinium–diethylenetriamine pentaacetic acid enhancement shows an irregularly enhancing mass lesion mimicking a mass lesion such as a meningioma.[163] MRI reveals extensive involvement of the neighboring dura, falx, and subdural spaces in cases of craniospinal osteomyelitis and epidural/subdural empyema. The organism grows on microaerophilic or anaerobic cultures. CSF studies tend to be normal or nonspecific.

TREATMENT

It includes the surgical aspiration or excision of intracranial infection.[168] Large doses of penicillin (at least 10 to 20 million U/day) given over a period of 3 to 4 months. Ofloxacin, rifampicin, tetracycline, and lincomycin are used in patients allergic to penicillin. Penicillin may effect a cure in spinal actinomycosis; however, surgical drainage, spinal decompression, and stabilization procedures may have to be undertaken when indicated. Because of optimal therapy, the prognosis is far better than that for true fungal infections. In some cases, a complete resolution of the

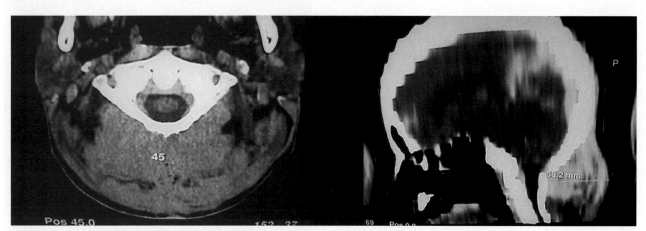

FIGURE 117-33 An axial computed tomography scan at the level of atlas shows a sawtooth appearance of posterior elements of the atlas and extensive involvement with swelling of the posterior paraspinal muscles and soft tissues, which is well seen in a sagittal reconstruction in a case of craniospinal actinomycosis.

infection may be achieved by means of surgical treatment and prolonged antibiotic therapy.

Management of Central Nervous System Fungal Infections

The following are the principal aims of management of recognized CNS fungal infections: (1) correction of underlying pathogenic risk factors, (2) removal of the source of infection, (3) neurosurgical interventions to deal with cerebrospinal fungal infections in or around the craniovertebral cavity, and (4) institution of effective antifungal drugs.

A high clinical index of suspicion is vital in diagnosing CNS fungal infections. Once diagnosed, the aforementioned aims need to be fulfilled. First, effective control of the pathogenic risk factors (i.e., immunosuppression, neutropenia, diabetes, ketoacidosis, and conditions requiring steroid use) is of paramount importance. Second, the source of fungal infection should be removed whenever possible (i.e., removal of drains, shunt systems, intravenous access lines, radical surgical procedures to the orbit and paranasal sinuses, irrigation of aerated sinus cavities with antifungal drugs). Third, appropriate neurosurgical interventions must be performed judiciously whenever indicated in various clinical syndromes (discussed later). Fourth, use of appropriate antifungal drug therapy.

CLINICAL SYNDROMES OF THE CENTRAL NERVOUS SYSTEM FUNGAL INFECTIONS

The following clinical syndromes are commonly encountered in CNS fungal infections and should be recognized and managed accordingly.

Meningeal Syndrome

It is commonly seen in cryptococcosis, candidiasis, and coccidioidomycosis.[16,17,39,100,108] Tuberculous meningitis must be ruled out and fungal infection detected by careful CSF studies (routine Gram stain, India ink preparation, detection of fungal capsular antigen, complement fixation test for CSF antibody to the fungus, and culture). In our combined series, 6 patients with CNS candidiasis and 21 patients with CNS cryptococcosis had presented with a meningeal syndrome; however, meningitis as a secondary feature was coexisting with other manifestations in cases of blastomycosis, coccidioidomycosis (Fig. 117-34), aspergillosis, *Cladosporium* infection, zygomycosis, nocardial infection, and actinomycosis (see Table 117-3). Intravenous drug therapy alone is generally successful in treating cryptococcal (amphotericin B + flucytosine) and *Candida* (amphotericin B) meningitis. Coccidioidal meningitis is a chronic infection that also requires intraventricular or intrathecal (cisternal/lumbar route) administration of amphotericin B for successful outcome.[16,22] Patients presenting with chronic leptomeningitis due to blastomycosis and histoplasmosis are treated with amphotericin B and fluconazole because the azole drugs (itraconazole and ketoconazole) have poor CSF penetration but are recommended as primary drugs for non-meningeal systemic blastomycosis and histoplasmosis.[7,22,24,27]

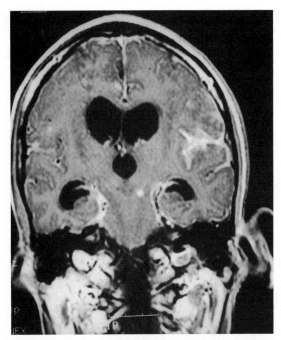

FIGURE 117-34 A coronal contrast-enhanced T1-weighted magnetic resonance image in a case of coccidioidomycotic brain stem granuloma shows extensive leptomeningeal hyperintensity in the basal as well as superolateral cerebral surfaces signifying chronic leptomeningitis with fibrosis and causing secondary communicating panventricular hydrocephalus.

Encephalitis/Cerebritis

Fungal infection of the brain parenchyma is usually associated with meningeal involvement. The process ranges from diffuse inflammation to multiple focal lesions. Superficial cortical and subcortical lesions as well as deep-seated basal ganglionic and thalamic lesions are best diagnosed stereotactically and in patients with extracraniospinal mycosis with ultrasound-guided tissue sampling. In the present series, one patient with CNS candidiasis initially had encephalitis (Fig. 117-35) and later multiple cerebral abscesses developed. Encephalitis was mainly seen as a coexisting feature in our cases of CNS coccidioidomycosis, cryptococcosis, aspergillosis, zygomycosis, and nocardiosis (see Table 117-3). Management includes débridement of infected and devitalized tissue, control of underlying disease, and systemic amphotericin B (or lysosomal amphotericin B) and/or flucytosine. Candidiasis and mucormycosis exemplify diffuse fungal encephalitis in immunocompromised hosts with a poor outcome.[4,16,45,65]

Increased Intracranial Pressure

An acute or subacute increase in intracranial pressure may be due to hydrocephalus and/or space-occupying lesions (abscesses, granulomas, cysts, and coexisting brain tumors).

Symptomatic Hydrocephalus: Meningitis/Ventriculitis

Symptomatic hydrocephalus develops secondary to arachnoid scarring, particularly in the basal regions, or obstruction within the ventricular system (Fig. 117-36). In these cases,

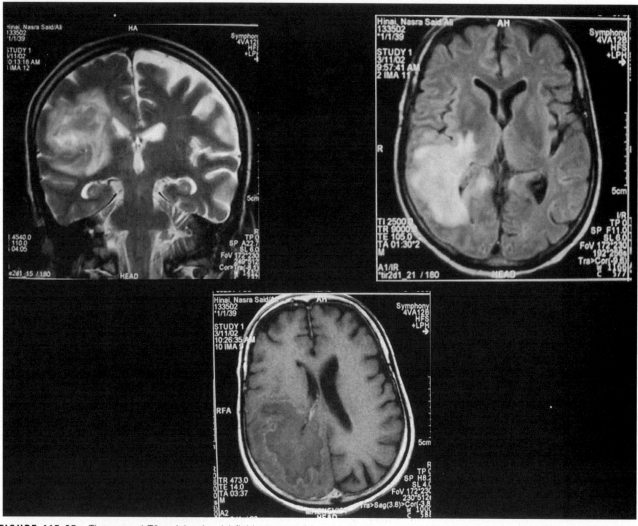

FIGURE 117-35   The coronal T2-weighted, axial fluid-attenuated inversion recovery (FLAIR) and axial T1-weighted magnetic resonance images show an irregular, large, slightly hypointense subcortical parieto-occipital lesion on T1-weighted image that became slightly hyperintense on T2-weighted image and better defined on the FLAIR image in a case of candidal encephalitis cerebritis.

CSF shunting may be necessary. Ventriculoperitoneal shunt, unilateral or bilateral, may be required to relieve increased intracranial pressure. In our series, hydrocephalus as a secondary phenomenon was seen in 15 patients and was managed with ventricular tapping and/or ventriculoperitoneal shunt surgery when indicated. Interestingly, cryptococcal meningitis or meningoencephalitis may appear as pseudotumor cerebri with slit ventricles requiring bilateral subtemporal decompression. However, an unusually high incidence of shunt obstruction due to fungal organisms and the additional risk of introducing fungal infection intraperitoneally have been reported.[4,16,82–84]

Fungal Abscesses

Candidiasis, aspergillosis, cladosporiosis, mucormycosis, and fungus-like bacterial diseases (nocardiosis [Fig. 117-37] and actinomycosis) commonly produce CNS fungal abscesses.[41,45,70,96,130] Because fungal organisms disseminate hematogenously from an extracranial site of infection, they cause multiple areas of infection within the brain. Initially, meningoencephalitis occurs with vasculitis-thrombosis, and

later, hemorrhagic cerebral infarction develops and then an abscess forms. Abscess-forming organisms may progress in a fulminant fashion leading rapidly to death. Extremely preterm neonates and neonates with predisposing conditions such as congenital or acquired immunodeficiency are at high risk of systemic fungal infections. Abscess formation in the brain is a severe complication and occurs in 70% of neonates with systemic fungal infection. Sonography can be used to diagnose abscesses in the brain in these patients. Candidal abscesses are small, multiple, round, hypoechoic lesions with echogenic rims in both brain hemispheres, whereas aspergillotic abscesses may be a few large echogenic areas in periventricular locations. In our series, 16 patients presented with cerebral abscesses, and in another 13 cases, brain abscess was associated with other presenting clinical entities. Initially, stereotactic (or ultrasound-guided) drainage is indicated for most solitary or multiple fungal abscesses followed by appropriate drug therapy and later excision of the abscess whenever possible. The progress of the treatment is best monitored by neuroimaging (CT/MRI scans) and the general state of the patient.

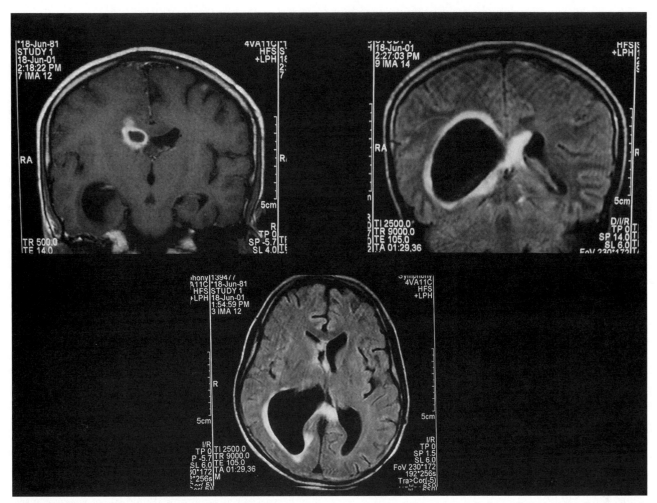

FIGURE 117-36   The coronal and axial T1-weighted magnetic resonance images (of a stereotactically confirmed and well-treated case of subcortical mucormycotic granuloma) show hyperintense ependymal lining and subependymal and septal regions signifying unilateral ventriculitis with a trapped ventricle causing unilateral lateral ventricular hydrocephalus due to blockage of Monro's foramen.

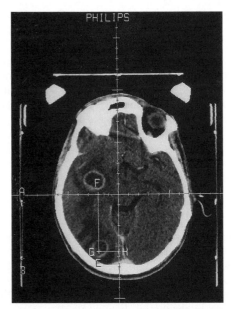

FIGURE 117-37   A computed tomography scan of the brain with a stereotactic frame shows right temporal and occipital intra-parenchymatous nocardial abscesses managed successfully with stereotactic aspirations and medical therapy.

Central Nervous System Fungal Granulomas

CNS fungal granulomas are commonly produced by aspergillosis, histoplasma, blastomycosis, paracoccidioidomycosis, cryptococcosis, and fungus-like bacterial lesions (actinomycosis).[2,4,7,55,65,166,167] There were 53 cases of CNS fungal granulomas in our series (Figs. 117-38 and 117-39), and in 5 other cases, granulomas were the secondary features. Surgical excision was performed when indicated. Infective masses should be surgically removed whenever possible in the first instance. Fungal granulomas resemble tuberculomas except that they have a more fibrous consistency. They often need to be cut with a knife or scissors because they resist curetting. The clear plane of cleavage seen with tuberculomas or meningiomas is not present and adherence to the dura is firmer. Unlike tuberculomas, a fungal granuloma should be completely excised whenever possible and then followed by appropriate drug therapy.

Intraparenchymal Cerebral Cysts

Intraparenchymal cerebral cysts (Figs. 117-40 to 117-42), especially in the basal ganglia, may sometimes develop into cryptococcosis,[4,7,16,108] which may require stereotactic

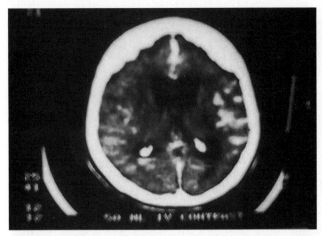

FIGURE 117-38 The contrast-enhanced axial computed tomography scan lights up multiple small leptomeningeal and cortical granulomas with irregularity and thickening of the cranial bones in a case of craniocerebral actinomycosis.

or ultrasound-guided drainage. In the present series, there were 13 cases of intraparenchymal (basal ganglionic-thalamus) cysts as a secondary feature in cryptococcosis. However, none of the cysts needed surgical aspiration.

Fungal Infections Coexisting with Brain Tumors (Figs. 117-43 and 117-44)

Cerebrospinal or craniospinal tumors may harbor fungal infections. In such cases, mycosis thrives within the cellular matrix of the intraparenchymal tumors. In our series, there were four cases of mycoses associated with brain tumors. In two cases, aspergillosis was coexisted with cerebral gliomas

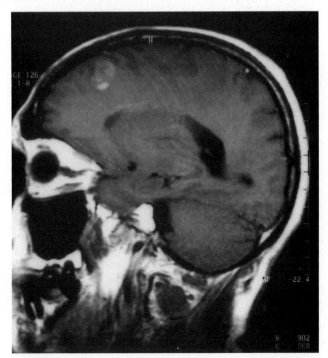

FIGURE 117-39 A sagittal T1-weighted magnetic resonance scan shows a frontal subcortical hyperintense aspergilloma with an isointense irregular center.

(one case of glioblastoma multiforme and one case of malignant astrocytoma). Both these patients were operated on via stereotactic surgery. Initially in the postoperative period, these patients were clinically well; however, 72 hours later, they suddenly worsened in sensorium, and repeat CT scans showed extensive cerebral edema and cerebral infarction with a fatal outcome. In two other cases, mucormycosis was coexisting with brain tumors (in one case astrocytoma and in one case malignant CNS lymphoma). Both of these patients were operated on via stereotactic trephine craniotomy, and the lesions were excised. Delayed ependymitis and unilateral hydrocephalus due to blockage of Monro's foramen developed in a patient with mucormycosis. He was referred to the oncology department in another hospital after insertion of the Ommaya reservoir. The second patient with lymphoma was also referred to the oncology department in another hospital. Both these patients succumbed within 4 months after surgery. In our experience, mycoses coexisting within the malignant brain tumors have a very poor prognosis.

Orbitorhinocerebral Syndrome

Fungal infections involving the nasal cavities, paranasal sinuses, orbit, cranial bones, and mandible may be the source of intracranial infection[144–148] (Fig. 117-45). Aspergillosis and zygomycosis are more commonly associated with rhinocerebral syndrome. In our combined series, 49 cases of cerebral mycosis secondary to rhinosino-orbital or craniofacial syndrome were noted. During the same period, 44 cases of fungal rhinosino-orbital syndrome without cerebral involvement were managed in our ear, nose, and throat department. Nasal discharge and facial or periorbital pain may be the initial symptoms. Proptosis, progressive visual loss, sensory impairment in ophthalmic division of the trigeminal nerve, chemosis progressing to ophthalmoplegia, blindness, periorbital, and facial swelling may occur. Diabetic ketoacidosis is the most common predisposing factor. Later, ipsilateral carotid occlusion results in a contralateral hemiplegia and ipsilateral blindness. Upward extension of infection via the orbital plate may result in a frontal lobe abscess. Control of diabetes, radical surgical procedures to the orbit and paranasal sinuses, neurosurgical intervention for intracranial infection, and aggressive antifungal drug therapy including irrigation of aerated paranasal sinuses with antifungal agents are needed. Excision of necrotic tissue and drainage of paranasal sinuses are indicated in these patients. Actinomycosis and nocardiasis may also result in cranial osteomyelitis, as seen in our eight cases and produce secondary intracranial infection and therefore require appropriate drug therapy and surgery.

Acute Cerebrovascular Events

CNS fungal infection may present as a sudden cerebrovascular event due to cerebral fungal arteritis causing occlusion, mainly ICAs and its branches, as well as due to fungal aneurysms causing subarachnoid hemorrhage (Fig. 117-46). One of our cases had presented with subarachnoid hemorrhage with intracerebral hematoma due to a mycotic aneurysm of the middle cerebral artery branch, which was excised with a good outcome. Another case had a typical

FIGURE117-40 Axial T1-weighted plain and contrast-enhanced images and a T2-weighted axial image show multiple tiny areas of hyperintensity, especially in the basal ganglia and mild meningeal enhancement in a case of cryptococcal meningitis at the time of diagnosis.

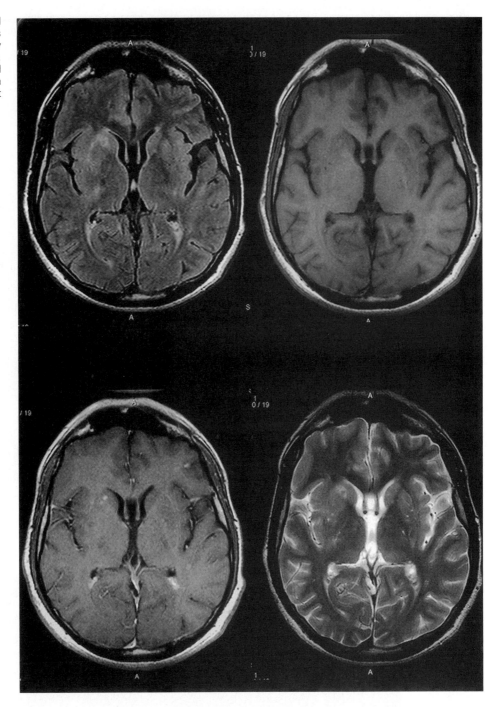

presentation of SAH due to an anterior communicating artery aneurysm. This patient had a rebleed and died. No autopsy was performed. Four other cases of mycotic aneurysms were diagnosed at autopsy. Aspergillosis and zygomycosis mainly obstruct the large- and intermediate-sized cerebral arteries.[58,64,68] The hyphae invade the vessel walls, causing cerebral arterial thrombosis, cerebral infarction, and cerebritis. The evolving hemorrhagic infarcts may convert into septic infarcts. In cases of cerebral fungal arteritis in which direct surgery is inappropriate, reliance has to be placed on the antifungal antibiotics and supportive therapy. Seventeen cases in our series primarily presented as ICA thrombosis, whereas in other 24 cases, ICA thrombosis and

in 4 cases, basilar artery thrombosis were noted as secondary features in association with other presenting primary syndromes. Fungal aneurysms commonly present with severe sudden subarachnoid hemorrhage, which is usually fatal in most cases. The rarity of fungal aneurysm is obvious, as only approximately 40 cases have been described in the literature.[170,171] Aspergillus is the most common causative organism of cerebral fungal aneurysm but uncommonly *Penicillium, Coccidioides, Zygomycetes,* and other fungi may cause single or multiple aneurysms.[37,125,147,170,171] The warning symptoms or signs are absent in most cases, and therefore the disease progresses rapidly and is quite lethal, as in our cases. If an aneurysm is recognized, it should be excised

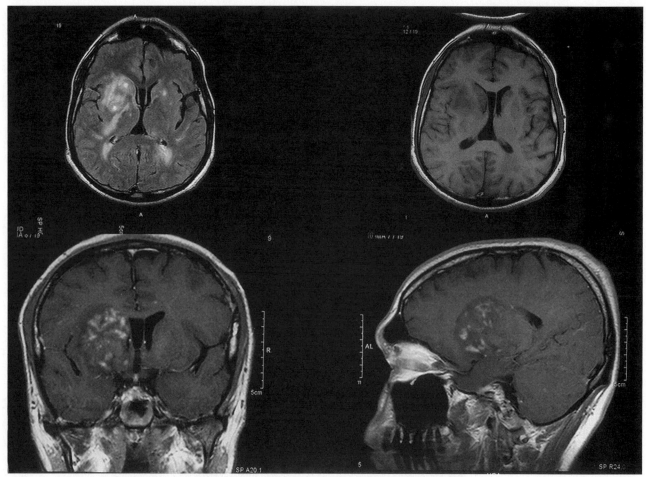

FIGURE 117-41 T1-weighted axial fluid-attenuated inversion recovery and conventional images and coronal and sagittal images show scattered small multiple hyperintense foci (dilated Virchow-Robin spaces: intraparenchymal cerebral cysts) with intense cerebral edema and some meningeal hyperintensity at the time of acute stroke in a case of cryptococcal meningitis. No surgical intervention was needed.

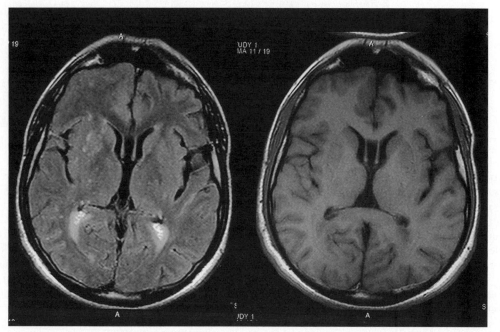

FIGURE 117-42 T1-weighted contrast-enhanced and plain axial magnetic resonance scans after clinical recovery on medical therapy show resolution of many intraparenchymal cryptococcal basal ganglionic cysts and resolution of cerebral edema.

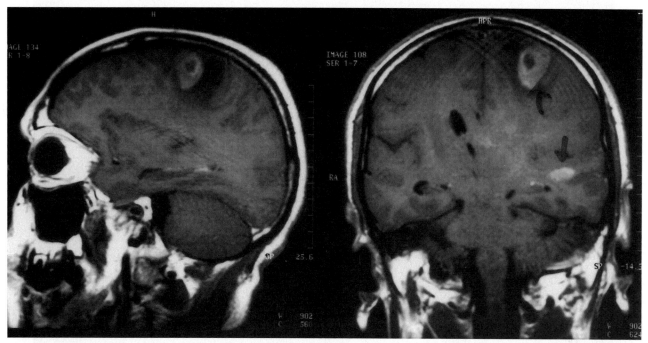

FIGURE 117-43   The T1-weighted magnetic resonance images show multiple hyperintense corticosubcortical white matter lesions in the left hemisphere: one lesion with a small hypointensity in the center located in the posterior part of the middle frontal gyrus (glioma with *Aspergillus* fungal infection) and an another homogeneously hyperintense lesion in the superior temporal gyrus (granuloma) in a patient with malignant astrocytoma.

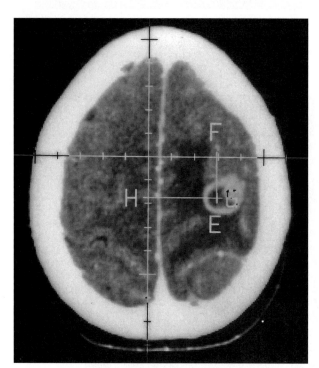

FIGURE 117-44   A computed tomography brain scan with a stereotactic frame shows an irregular thick-walled, ring-enhancing coexisting mucormycotic lesion within malignant astrocytoma.

whenever possible. However, in general, the outlook is dim for these patients with CNS fungal infections presenting with acute cerebrovascular events.

Spinal Fungal Infections

Spinal fungal lesions causing compressive myelopathy are exceedingly rare. However, they may present as intramedullary lesions, spinal arachnoiditis, paradural infections, and vertebral osteomyelitis. Commonly coccidioidomycosis,[96] blastomycosis,[91] histoplasmosis,[75] aspergillosis[51] (five cases of extradural granulomas in our series), rarely candidiasis[35] (one case in our study), and exceptionally cryptococcosis[3,108] (spinal intramedullary lesion) may present with spinal symptomatology. Fungus-like bacteria (*A. israelii* and *N. asteroides*) also rarely present with spinal lesions.[124,169] One of our patients had extensive craniocervical actinomycosis and was treated effectively with medications. Approximately 100 cases of spinal actinomycosis and fewer than a dozen cases of spinal nocardiosis have been reported in the literature. Plain radiographs show osteomyelitis. Nonspecific findings of spondylitis, paraspinal abscesses, and granulomas on CT/MRI scans are seen (Fig. 117-47). Vertebral biopsy, histologic examination, pus culture, and examination establish the diagnosis. Antifungal drugs and neurosurgical intervention for paraspinal abscesses, spinal granulomas, and vertebral lesions are needed. Spinal decompressive and stabilization procedures may be required in patients with compressive myelopathy and myeloradiculopathy. The prognosis is, however, poor.

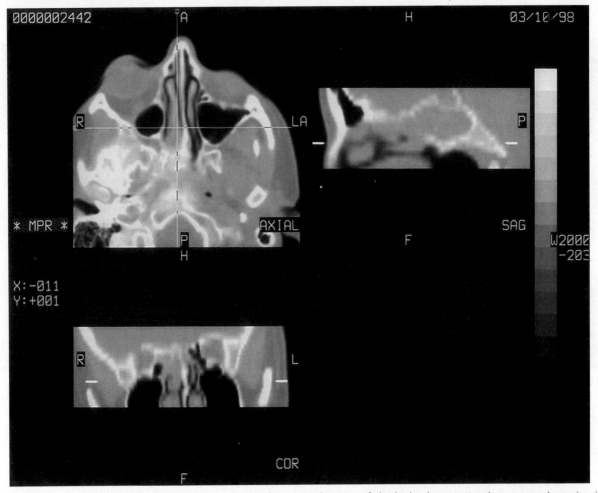

FIGURE 117-45 Orbitorhinocerebral syndrome. A computed tomography scan of the brain shows extensive paranasal pansinusitis in a case of orbitorhinocerebral syndrome due to aspergillosis.

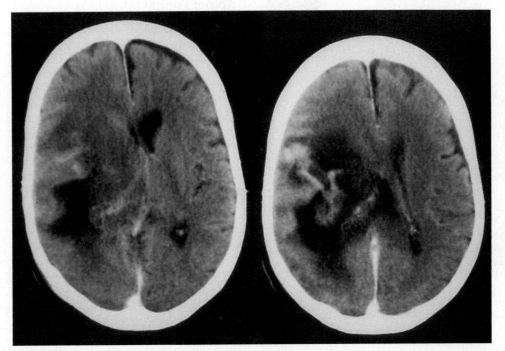

FIGURE 117-46 Acute cerebrovascular events. A computed tomography (CT) brain scan (*left*) shows a right basal ganglionic infarct with mass effect causing compression of the right lateral ventricle and subfalcine herniation. After acute worsening in sensorium, a repeat CT scan (*right*) showed an acute bleed in the territory of middle cerebral artery, which was due to a peripheral mycotic aneurysm.

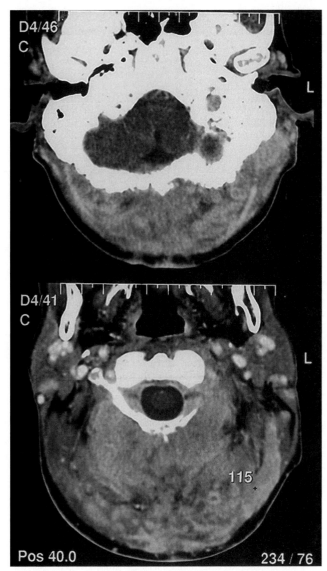

FIGURE 117-47   Spinal fungal infections. A contrast-enhanced computed tomography scan of the craniocervical junction and upper cervical spine (axis) shows extensive erosive craniospinal osteomyelitis with a large mixed-attenuation lesion in the posterior cervical region, especially the laminae and facets.

ANTIFUNGAL CHEMOTHERAPY

Antifungal therapy has advanced rapidly in the past few years, and it is more likely that the recommendations for chemotherapy of CNS fungal infection may be changed in the near future as our understanding of fungal infections improves and new antifungal drugs are discovered.[22,172]

Currently, two groups of drugs are used: one group of drugs is produced by various organisms (amphotericin B) and the other group consists of synthetic preparations (flucytosine and azoles).[22–34]

Amphotericin B

Amphotericin A and B are isolated by-products from a fermentation process of *Streptomyces nodosus*, a soil actinomycete.[22] Amphotericin B is useful in human fungal infections. It binds to ergosterol in the fungal cell membrane and causes increased membrane permeability, leakage of cell components, and cell death. Drug auto-oxidation may also cause cell damage. Amphotericin B is poorly absorbed orally, with less than 5% bioavailability, necessitating intravenous administration as a colloidal suspension with sodium deoxycholate. Because it precipitates in normal saline, it must be given in solution with 5% dextrose in water. Peak levels occur during the first hour of a 4- to 6-hour infusion, with high levels persisting for 6 to 8 hours. Hepatic or renal failure and hemodialysis do not affect drug clearance.[24–28] High concentrations are found in the liver, spleen, kidneys, and lungs. Interestingly, in adults, CSF concentration is 2% to 4% of the serum concentrations. Initial half-life is 12 to 18 hours, and late-phase half-life is approximately 15 days. It is a first-line drug active against *Candida*, *Cryptococcus*, *Aspergillus*, Mucorales organisms, among others and as a second or alternative drug active against blastomycosis, histoplasmosis, and coccidioidomycosis. However, *Candida lusitaniae*, *Trichosporon beigelli*, and *P. boydii* are usually resistant to amphotericin B.[22]

An intravenous test dose of 1 mg or 0.1 mg/kg infused over 30 minutes to rule out anaphylaxis (occurring in 1% of cases) is recommended. The dose is increased from 0.25 mg/kg to 1.0 to 1.5 mg/kg as a once-daily intravenous infusion given over 2 to 4 hours. Fever and chills are noted in 50% of cases, and therefore premedication with diphenhydramine, meperidine, or hydrocortisone should be instituted. Nephrotoxicity occurs early in the course of treatment, generally within the first 2 weeks and usually is reversible in 80% of cases. Symptomatic and biochemical abnormalities are treated per indications.

Liposomal Amphotericin B

Encapsulating amphotericin B into liposomal vesicles or binding of amphotericin B to other lipid carriers is reported to result in a significant reduction in toxicity and possibly an increased therapeutic index of the drug.[25] Three formulations are AmBisome, Amphocil (amphotericin B colloidal dispersion, ABCD), and amphotericin B lipid complex (ABLC, Abelcet).[22,25,28] These preparations accumulate in the reticuloendothelial system and have low nephrotoxicity in patients with life-threatening mycoses. At present, these compounds are used only in cases of intolerance to or failure of conventional amphotericin B therapy. ABLC is used in invasive aspergillosis in as high a dose as 7 mg/kg/day. Liposomal amphotericin B appears to be safe, effective, and well tolerated in very low-birth-weight infants as well.[22,25] Their main uses at present are for treatment of invasive aspergillosis, *Fusarium* infection, and mucormycosis.

Flucytosine

5-Fluorocytosine or flucytosine is a chlorine analogue of cytosine. It is useful in combination with amphotericin B in the management of deep mycoses (i.e., candidiasis, cryptococcosis, and chromoblastomycosis).[22,27,30,34] Absorption from the gut is rapid and complete. Spinal fluid concentrations reach as high as 75% of serum concentration. The dose is 50 to 150 mg/kg/day given orally at 6-hour intervals. Ninety percent of the drug is excreted unchanged in urine. Hepatic and renal toxicity and myelotoxicity are less frequent. The drug is readily cleared with hemodialysis and peritoneal dialysis. In approximately 65% cases, diarrhea, nausea, and vomiting are common side effects, which are treated symptomatically. The 2-hour postdose levels are usually maintained between 50 and 70 μm/mL. The levels above 100 μm/mL are associated with a higher incidence of myelosuppression and enterocolitis. It is contraindicated in pregnancy because of its teratogenic effects in rats.[22]

Azoles

These drugs interfere with the biosynthesis of sterols and fungal cell membrane lipids, thereby causing an increased permeability and cellular damage. Ketoconazole, although less expensive as a long-term therapy, is less well tolerated and has more toxic effects than either fluconazole or itraconazole. However, these three drugs are effective alternatives to amphotericin B and flucytosine for selected systemic mycoses: blastomycosis, coccidioidomycosis, and histoplasmosis.[22,26,32,34] Itraconazole in sporotrichosis and aspergillosis and fluconazole in cryptococcal and coccidioidal meningitis and candidiasis are very effective. Ketoconazole penetrates CSF poorly, especially CSF of non-inflamed meninges. Fluconazole appears to be superior to amphotericin B for maintenance therapy in cryptococcal meningitis in patients with acquired immunodeficiency syndrome. To improve efficacy, reduce side effects, and decrease duration of therapy, the antifungal drug combinations are used such as amphotericin B and flucytosine in systemic candidiasis and cryptococcal meningitis.[22]

SUMMARY

Fungal and pathologic actinomycetic infections of the CNS result in significant mortality and morbidity, even in successfully treated patients. Greater awareness of their protean clinical manifestations, diverse neuropathologic features, unpredictable neurosurgical complications, and difficult diagnostic and therapeutic challenges are of paramount importance in the appropriate management of such uncommon cases. A high index of suspicion in a high-risk patient is needed. A significant proportion of cases requires only medical management. Even with current antifungal drugs, however, when CNS complications ensue, an appropriate and timely neurosurgical intervention is mandatory.

Acknowledgments

We express our sincere gratitude to all the past and present members of the neurosciences and ear, nose, and throat departments at these four institutions who were directly or indirectly involved in the overall medical and operative management of these patients. The authors are especially grateful to J. Randi Jinkins, MD, FACR, Associate Professor, Director of Neuroradiology, Department of Radiology, The University of Texas Health Science Center at San Antonio, and Sanjeev Athale, MD (member American Association of Neuroradiology), Neuroradiologist, Department of Radiology at Khoula Hospital, Muscat, Oman, for their guidance and assistance in the literature and in providing neurodiagnostic material. The authors thank Mazin Al-Khaburi, FRCS, Head of the Ear, Nose, and Throat Department and his colleagues at Al Nahda Hospital, Muscat, Oman, not only for providing clinical statistics of rhinosino-orbital syndromes but for help at every stage.

REFERENCES

1. Bauserman SC, Schochet SS, Jr: Bacterial, fungal and parasitic diseases of the central nervous system. In Nelson JS, Parisi JE, Schochet SS, Jr (eds): Principles and Practice of Neuropathology. London: Mosby, 1993, pp 42–74.
2. Bazan C, Rinaldi MG, Rauch RR, Jinkins R: Fungal infections of the brain. Neuroimag Clin N Am 1:57–88, 1991.
3. Carey ME: Infections of the Spine and Spinal cord: In Youmans JR (ed): Youmans Neurological Surgery, vol. 5, 4th ed. Philadelphia: WB Saunders, 1996, pp 3270–3304.
4. Chimelli L, Mahler-Araujo MB: Fungal infections. Brain Pathol 7:613–627, 1997.
5. Friedman AH, Bullitt E: Fungal infections. In Wilkins RH, Rengachary SS (eds) Neurosurgery. New York: McGraw-Hill, 1985, pp 2002–2010.
6. Jorgensen JH, Rinaldi MG: A Clinicians Directory of Bacteria and Fungi. Indianapolis: Eli Lilly, 1987, pp 70–72.
7. Kirkpatrick JB: Neurologic infections due to bacteria, fungi and parasites. In Davis RL, Robertson DM (eds): Textbook of Neuropathology, 2nd ed. Baltimore: Williams & Wilkins, 1991, pp 719–803.
8. Mori T, Ebe T: Analysis of cases of central nervous system fungal infections reported in Japan between January 1979 and June 1989. Int Med 31:174–179, 1992.
9. Rippon JW: Medical Mycology: The Pathogenic Fungi and the Pathogenic Actinomycetes. Philadelphia: WB Saunders, 1988.
10. Salaki JS, Louria DB, Chmel H: Fungal and yeast infections of the central nervous system. Medicine (Baltimore) 63:103–132, 1984.
11. Scaravilli F: Parasitic and fungal infections of the nervous system. In Adams JH, Corsellis JAN, Duchen LW (eds): Greenfield's Neuropathology. London: Edward Arnold, 1984, pp 304–337.
12. Scaravilli F: Parasitic and fungal infections of the nervous system. In Hume-Adams JH, Corsellis JAN, Duchen LW (eds) Greenfield's Neuropathology. London: Edward Arnold, 1992, pp 400–446.
13. Sharma RR, Gurusinghe NT, Lynch PG: Cerebral infarction due to *Aspergillus* arteritis following glioma surgery. Br J Neurosurg 6:485–490, 1992.
14. Sunde N: Fungal infections: In Palmar JD (ed): Manual of Neurosurgery. New York: Churchill Livingstone, 1996, pp 896–898.
15. Walsh TJ, Gonzalez C, Lymon CA, et al: Invasive fungal infections in children: Recent advances in diagnosis and treatment. Adv Pediatr Infect Dis 11:187–290, 1996.
16. Wiles CM, Mackenzie DWR: Fungal diseases of the central nervous system. In Kennedy PGE, Johnson RT (eds): Infections of the Nervous System. London: Butterworths, 1987, pp 93–117.
17. Gonyea EF: The spectrum of primary blastomycotic meningitis: A review of central nervous system blastomycosis. Ann Neurol 3:26–39, 1978.
18. Darling TS: A protozoan general infection producing pseudotubercles in the lungs and focal necrosis in the liver, spleen and lymph nodes. JAMA 46:1283–1285, 1906.
19. Gilchrist TC: Protozoan dermatitis. J Cutan Genet Dis 12:496–499, 1894.
20. Kissane JM (eds): Anderson's Pathology. St. Louis: CV Mosby, 1990.
21. Wood M, Anderson M (eds): Neurological Infections. Philadelphia: WB Saunders, 1988.
22. Al-Mohsen I, Hughes WT: Systemic antifungal therapy: Past, present and future. Ann Saudi Med 18:28–38, 1997.
23. Bell WE: Treatment of fungal infection of the central nervous system. Ann Neurol 9:417–422, 1981.
24. Camarata PJ, Dunn DL, Farney AC, et al: Continuous intracavitary administration of amphotericin-B as an adjunct in the treatment of *Aspergillus* brain abscess: Case report and review of the literature. Neurosurgery 31:575–579, 1992.
25. De Marie S: Liposomal and lipid-based formulations of amphotericin-B. Leukemia 10(Suppl 2):93–96, 1996.
26. Goodpasture HC, Hershberger RE, Barnett AM, Peteric JD: Treatment of central nervous system fungal infections with ketoconazole. Arch Intern Med 145:879–880, 1985.
27. Graybill JR: The future of antifungal therapy. Clin Infect Dis 22 (Suppl 2):166–178, 1996.
28. Hiemenz JW, Walsh TJ: Lipid formulations of amphotericin-B: Recent progress and future direction. Clin Infect Dis 22(Suppl 2):133–144, 1996.

29. Joly V, Aubry P, Ndayiragide A, et al: Randomized comparison of amphotericin-B deoxycholate dissolved in dextrose or intralipid for treatment of AIDS-associated cryptococcal meningitis. Clin Infect Dis 23:556–562, 1996.
30. Medoff G, Brajtburg J, Kobayashi GS: Antifungal agents useful in therapy of systemic fungal infections. Am Rev Pharmacol Toxicol 23:303–330, 1983.
31. Slavoski LA, Tunkel AR: Therapy of fungal meningitis. Clin Neuropathol 18:95–112, 1995.
32. Van de Velde VJ, Van Peer AP, Heykants JJ, et al: Effect of food on the pharmacokinetics of a new hydroxy propyl-beta-cyclodextrin formulation of itraconazole. Pharmacotherapy 16:424–428, 1996.
33. Walsh TJ, Hiemenz JW, Anaissie E: Recent progress and current problems in treatment of invasive fungal infections in neutropenic patients. Infect Dis Clin North Am 10:365–400, 1996.
34. Walsh TJ, Peter J, McGough DA, et al: Activities of amphotericin-B and antifungal azoles alone and in combination against *Pseudoallescheria boydii*. Antimicrob Agents Chemother 39:1361–1364, 1995.
35. Almekinders LE, Greene WB: Vertebral *Candida* infections: A case report and review of the literature. Clin Orthop 267:174–178, 1991.
36. Friedman BC, Simon GL: Candida vertebral osteomyelitis. Report of three cases and a review of the literature. Diagn Microbiol Infect Dis 8:31–36, 1987.
37. Goldman JA, Fleischer AS, Leifer W, et al: *Candida albicans* mycotic aneurysms associated with systemic lupus erythematosus. Neurosurgery 4:325–328, 1979.
38. Hostetter MK: New insights into *Candida* infections. Adv Pediatr 209–230, 1996.
39. Nguyen MH, Yu VL: Meningitis caused by *Candida* species: An emergency problem in neurosurgical patients. Clin Infect Dis 21:323–327, 1995.
40. Osmund JD, Schweitzer G, Dunbar JM, et al: Blastomycosis of the spine with paraplegia. S Afr Med J 45:431–434, 1971.
41. Parker JC, Mc Closkey JJ, Lee RS: The emergence of candidiosis: The dominant postmortem cerebral candidosis. Am J Clin Pathol 70:31–38, 1978.
42. Pennisi AK, Davis DO, Wiesel S, et al: CT appearance of *Candida* diskitis. J Comput Assist Tomogr 9:1050–1054, 1985.
43. Sanchez-Portocarrero JM, Martin-Rabadan P, Saldana CJ, Pareza-Cecilia E: *Candida* cerebrospinal fluid shunt infection: Report of two new cases and review of the literature. Diagn Microbiol Infect Dis 20:33–40, 1994.
44. Sugarman B, Massanari RM: *Candida* meningitis in patients with CSF shunts. Arch Neurol 37:180–181, 1980.
45. Tventen L: Candidiasis. In Vinken PJ, Bruyn GW, Klawans H (eds): Handbook of Clinical Neurology: Infections of the Nervous System, vol. 35. Amsterdam: Elsevier North-Holland, 1978, pp 413–442.
46. Artico M, Pastore FS, Polosa M, et al: Intracerebral *Aspergillus* abscess: Case report and review of the literature. Neurosurg Rev 20:135–138, 1997.
47. Byrd B, Weiner MH, McGee ZA: *Aspergillus* spinal epidural abscess. JAMA 248:3138–3139, 1982.
48. Casey AT, Wilkeins P, Uttley D: Aspergillosis infection in neurosurgical practice. Br J Neurosurg 8:31–39, 1994.
49. Chee YC, Poh SC: *Aspergillus* epidural abscess in a patient with obstructive airway disease. Postgrad Med J 59:43–45, 1983.
50. Deshpande DH, Desai AP, Dastur HM: Aspergillosis of the central nervous system. Neurol India 23:167–175, 1975.
51. D'Hoore K, Hoogmartens M: Vertebral aspergillosis: A case report and review of the literature. Acta Orthop Belg 59:306–314, 1993.
52. Freely M, Steinberg M: *Aspergillus* infection complicating transsphenoidal yttrium-90 pituitary implant: Report of two cases. J Neurosurg 46:530–532, 1977.
53. Galassi E, Pozzati E, Poppi M, Vinci A: Cerebral aspergillosis following intracranial surgery: Case report. J Neurosurg 49:308–311, 1978.
54. Gupta R, Singh AK, Bishnu P, Malhotra V: Intracranial *Aspergillus* granuloma simulating meningioma on MR imaging. J Comput Assist Tomogr 14:467–469, 1990.
55. Haran RP, Chandy MJ: Intracranial *Aspergillus* granuloma. Br J Neurosurg 7:383–388, 1993.
56. Jinkins JR, Siqueira E, Al-Kawi MZ: Cranial manifestations of aspergillosis. Neuroradiology 29:181–185, 1987.
57. Mawk JR, Erickson DL, Chou SN, et al: *Aspergillus* infections of the lumbar disc spaces. J Neurosurg 58:270–274, 1983.
58. Savaria-Gomez J: Aspergillosis of the central nervous system. In Vinken PJ, Bruyn GW, Klawans H (eds): Handbook of Clinical Neurology: Infections of the Nervous System, vol. 35, Amsterdam: Elsevier North Holland, 1978, pp 395–400.
59. Schwartz S, Thiel E: Clinical presentation of invasive aspergillosis. Mycoses 40(Suppl 2):21–24, 1997.
60. Seth NK, Varkey B, Wagner D: Spinal cord *Aspergillus* invasion: Complication of an aspergilloma. Am J Clin Pathol 84:763–769, 1985.
61. Wagner DK, Varkey B, Seth NK, et al: Epidural abscess, vertebral destruction and paraplegia caused by extending infection from an aspergilloma. Am J Med 78:518–522, 1985.
62. Bhattacharya AK, Deshpande AR, Nayak SR, et al: Rhinocerebral mucormycosis: An unusual case presentation. J Laryngol 106:48–49, 1992.
63. Bichile LS, Abhyankar SC, Hase NK: Chronic mucormycosis manifesting as hydrocephalus. J Neurol Neurosurg Psychiatry 48:1188, 1985.
64. Carpenter DF, Brubaker LH, Powell RO, et al: Phycomycotic thrombosis of the basilar artery. Neurology 18:807–812, 1968.
65. Dehmy P: Phycomycosis (mucormycosis): In Vinken PJ, Bruyn GW (eds): Infections of the Nervous System. Part III. Handbook of Clinical Neurology, vol. 35. Amsterdam: North Holland, 1978, pp 541–556.
66. Escobar A, Del Brutto OH: Multiple brain abscesses from isolated cerebral mucormycosis. J Neurol Neurosurg Psychiatry 53:431–433, 1990.
67. Hopkins RJ, Rothman M, Fiore A, Goldblum SE: Cerebral mucormycosis associated with intravenous drug use: Three case reports and review. Clin Infect Dis 19:1133–1137, 1994.
68. Martin FP, Lukeman JM, Ranson RF, et al: Mucormycosis of the central nervous system associated with thrombosis of the internal carotid artery. J Paediatr 44:437–442, 1954.
69. Parfrey NA: Improved diagnosis and prognosis of mucormycosis. Medicine (Baltimore) 65:113–123, 1986.
70. Pierce PF, Jr, Solomon SL, Kaufman L, et al: *Zygomycetes* brain abscesses in narcotic addicts with serological diagnosis. JAMA 248:2881–2882, 1982.
71. Price DL, Wolpow ER, Richardson EP: Intracranial phycomycosis: A clinicopathological and radiological study. J Neurol Sci 14:359–375, 1971.
72. Goodwin RA, Loyd JE, Des Prez RM: Histoplasmosis in normal hosts. Medicine (Baltimore) 60:231–236, 1981.
73. Vakili ST, Eble JN, Richmond BD, et al: Cerebral histoplasmoma. J Neurosurg 59:332–336, 1983.
74. Weidenheim KM, Nelson SJ, Kure K, et al: Unusual patterns of histoplasma capsulatum meningitis and progressive multifocal leukoencephalopathy in a patient with the acquired immunodeficiency virus. Hum Pathol 23:581–586, 1992.
75. Wheat LJ, Batteiger BE, Sathapatayavangs B: *Histoplasma capsulatum* infections of the central nervous system: A clinical review. Medicine (Baltimore) 69:244–260, 1990.
76. Al-Soub H: Bilateral visual loss due to cryptococcal meningitis. Ann Saudi Med 16:84–86, 1996.
77. Blackie JD, Danta G, Sorrell T, Collignon P: Ophthalmological complications of cryptococcal meningitis. Clin Exp Neurol 21:263–270, 1985.
78. Chan KH, Mann KS, Yue CP: Neurosurgical aspects of cerebral cryptococcosis. Neurosurgery 25:44–47, 1989.
79. Diamond RD: Cryptococcus neoformans. In Mandell GL, Bennett JE, Dolin R (eds): Principles and Practice of Infectious Diseases. New York: Churchill Livingstone, 1995, pp 2331–2339.
80. Diamond RD, Bennett JE: Prognostic factors in cryptococcal meningitis: A study in 111 cases. Ann Intern Med 80:176–181, 1974.
81. Mitchell DH, Sorrell TC, Allworth AM, et al: Cryptococcal disease of the CNS in immunocompetent hosts: Influence of cryptococcal variety on clinical manifestations and outcome. Clin Infect Dis 20:611–616, 1995.
82. Chiou CC, Wong TT, Lin HH: Fungal infections of ventriculoperitoneal shunts in children. Clin Infect Dis 19:1049–1053, 1994.
83. Tang LM: Ventriculoperitoneal shunt in cryptococcal meningitis with hydrocephalus. Surg Neurol 33:314–319, 1990.
84. Yadav SS, Perfect J, Friedman AH: Successful treatment of cryptococcal ventriculoatrial shunt infection with systemic therapy alone. Neurosurgery 23:372–373, 1988.
85. Williams RL, Fukui MB, Meltzer CC, et al: Fungal spinal osteomyelitis in the immunocompromised patients: MR findings in three cases. Am J Neuroradiol 20:381–385, 1999.
86. EL-Zaatari MM, Hulten K, Fares Y, et al: Successful treatment of *Candida albicans* osteomyelitis of the spine with fluconazole and surgical debridement: Case report. J Chemother 14:627–630, 2002.

87. Rosler-Meier D, Brunner-La Rocca HP, Senn P, Schlumpf U: *Candida albicans* spondylitis: Successful treatment with fluconazole: Two case reports. Schweiz Reindsch Med Prax 85:520–525, 1996.

88. Bradsher RW: Blastomycosis. Clin Infect Dis 14(Suppl 1):582–590, 1992.

89. Detrisac DA, Harding WG, Greiner A, et al: Vertebral North American blastomycosis. Surg Neurol 13:311, 1980.

90. Frean J, Blumberg L, Woolf M: Disseminated blastomycosis masquerading as tuberculosis. J Infect 26:203–206, 1993.

91. Krarup C, Davis CH, Symon L: Spinal blastomycosis: Case report. J Neurol Neurosurg Psychiatry 47:217–218, 1984.

92. Leers WD: North American Blastomycosis. In Vinken PJ, Bruyn GW, Klawans H (eds): Handbook of Clinical Neurology: Infections of the Nervous System, vol. 35. Amsterdam: Elsevier North Holland, 1978, pp 401–411.

93. Roos KL, Bryan JP, Maggio WW, et al: Intracranial blastomycoma. Medicine (Baltimore) 66:224–235, 1987.

94. Titrud LA: Blastomycosis of the cervical spine. Minn Med 58:729–732, 1975.

95. Deresinski SC, Stevens DA: Coccidioidomycosis in compromised host. Experience at Stanford University Hospital. Medicine (Baltimore) 54:377–395, 1974.

96. Deresinski SC: Coccidioidomycosis of bone and joints. In Stevens DA (ed): Coccidioidomycosis: A Text: New York: Plenum, 1980, pp 195–209.

97. Michel PS, Vinters HV: Coccidioidomycosis of the central nervous system: Neuropathological and vasculopathic manifestations and clinical correlates. Clin Infect Dis 20:400–405, 1995.

98. Nakazawa G, Lulu RE, Koo AH: Intracerebellar coccidioidal granuloma. AJNR Am J Neuroradiol 4:1243–1244, 1983.

99. Saviers ML: Disseminated coccidioidomycosis among Southwestern American Indians. Am Rev Respir Dis 109:602, 1974.

100. Sobel RA, Ellis WC, Nielsen SL, et al: Central nervous system coccidioidomycosis: A clinicopathological study of treatment with and without amphotericin-B. Hum Pathol 15:980–995, 1984.

101. Caraway NP, Fanning CV, Stewart JM, et al: Coccidioidomycosis osteomyelitis masquerading as a bone tumor: A report of 2 cases. Acta Cytol 47:777–782, 2003.

102. Holley K, Muldoon M, Tasker S: *Coccidioides immitis* osteomyelitis: A case series review. Orthopaedics 25:827–832, 2002.

103. Wright PW, Pappagianis D, Wilson M, et al: Donor related coccidioidomycosis in organ transplant recipient. Clin Infect Dis 37:1265–1269, 2003.

104. Colli B, Assirati J, Jr, Machado HR, et al: Intramedullary spinal cord paracoccidioidomycosis: Report of two cases. Arq Neuropsiquiatr 54:466–473, 1996.

105. Giraldo R, Restrepo A, Gutierrez F: Pathogenesis of paracoccidioidomycosis: A model based on the study of 46 patients. Mycopathologia 58:63–70, 1976.

106. Londero AT, Ramos CD: Paracoccidioidomycosis: A clinical and mycotic study of forty-one cases observed in Santa Maria, RS, Brazil. Medicine 52:771–775, 1972.

107. Minguetti G, Madalozzo LE: Paracoccidioidal granulomatosis of the brain. Arch Neurol 40:100–102, 1983.

108. Weenink HR, Bruyn GW: Cryptococcosis of the nervous system. In Vinken PJ, Bruyn GW (eds): Infections of the Central Nervous System Part III. Handbook of Clinical Neurology, vol. 35. Amsterdam: North Holland, 1978, pp 459–502.

109. de Almeida SM, Queiroz-Telles F, Teive HA, et al: Central nervous system paracoccidioidomycosis: Clinical features and laboratory findings. J Infect 48:193–198, 2004.

110. Forjaz MH, Fischman O, de Camargo ZP, et al: Paracoccidioidomycosis in Brazilian Indians of the Surui tribe: Clinical laboratory study of 2 cases. Rev Soc Bras Med Trop 32:571–575, 1999.

111. Godoy H, Reichart RA: Oral manifestations of paracoccidioidomycosis: Report of 21 cases from Argentina. Mycoses 46:412–417, 2003.

112. Villa LA, Tobon A, Restrepo A, et al: Central nervous system paracoccidioidomycosis: Report of a case successfully treated with itraconazole. Rev Inst Med Trop Sao Paulo 42:231–234, 2000.

113. Fleury RN, Taborda PR, Gupta AK, et al: Zoonotic sporotrichosis. Transmission to humans by infected domestic cat scratching: Report of four cases in San Paulo, Brazil. Int J Dermatol 40:318–322, 2001.

114. Naqvi SH, Becherer P, Gudipati S: Ketoconazole treatment of a family with zoonotic sporotrichosis. Scand J Infect Dis 25:543–545, 1993.

115. Rafal ES, Rasmussen JE: An unusual presentation of fixed cutaneous sporotrichosis: A case report and review of the literature. J Am Acad Dermatol 25:928–932, 1991.

116. Barenfanger J, Lawhorn J, Drake C: Nonvalue of culturing cerebrospinal fluid for fungi. J Clin Microbiol 42:236–238, 2004.

117. Cheng YC, Ling JF, Chang FC, et al: Radiological manifestations of cryptococcal infection in central nervous system. J Chin Med Assoc 66:19–26, 2003.

118. Choi MY, Bae IH, Lee JH, Lee SJ: Aspergillosis presenting as an optic neuritis. Korean J Ophthalmol 16:119–23, 2002.

119. Imai T, Yamamoto T, Tanaka S, et al: Successful treatment of cerebral aspergillosis with a high oral dose of itraconazole after excisional surgery. Intern Med 38:829–832, 1999.

120. Murthy JM, Sundaram C, Prasad VS, et al: Sino-cranial aspergillosis: A form of central nervous system aspergillosis in South India. Mycoses 44:141–145, 2001.

121. Sharma RR, Pawar SJ, Ravi RR, et al: A solitary primary *Aspergillus* brain abscess in an immunocompetent host: CT guided stereotaxy with an excellent outcome. Pan Arab J Neurosurg 6:62–65, 2002.

122. Van Landeghem FK, Stiller B, Lehmann TN, et al: Aqueductal stenosis and hydrocephalus in an infant due to *Aspergillus* infection. Clin Neuropathol 19:26–29, 2000.

123. Goodman ML, Coffey RJ: Stereotactic drainage of *Aspergillus* brain abscess with long term survival: Case report and review. Neurosurgery 24:96–99, 1989.

124. Nov AA, Cromwell LD: Computed tomography of neuroaxis aspergillosis. J Comput Assist Tomogr 9:413–415, 1984.

125. Chou SM, Chong YY, Kinkel R, et al: A proposed pathogenetic process in the formation of *Aspergillus* mycotic aneurysm in the central nervous system. Ann Acad Med Singapore 22(Suppl 3): 518–528, 1993.

126. Poitrowski WP, Pilz P, Chuang IH: Subarachnoid hemorrhage caused by a fungal aneurysm of the vertebral artery as a complication of intracranial aneurysm clipping. J Neurosurg 73:962–964, 1990.

127. Aviv JE, Lawson W, Boltone EJ, et al: Multiple intracranial mucocoeles associated with phaeohyphomycosis of the paranasal sinuses. Arch Otolaryngol Head Neck Surg 116:1210–1213, 1990.

128. Bennett JE, Bonner H, Janning AE, Lopez RI: Chronic meningitis caused by *Cladosporium trichoides*. Am J Clin Pathol 59:398–407, 1973.

129. Dixon DM, Walsh TJ, Merz WG, McGinnis MR: Infections due to *Xylophyta bantiana* (*Cladosporium trichoides*). Rev Infect Dis 11:515–525, 1989.

130. Goel A, Satoskar A, Desai AP, Pandya SK: Brain abscess caused by *Cladosporium trichoides*. Br J Neurosurg 6:591–593, 1992.

131. Kullu S, Onol B, Kustimor S, et al: Cerebral cladosporiosis. Surg Neurol 24:437–440, 1985.

132. McGinnis MR, Borelli D, Padhye AA, et al: Reclassification of *Cladosporium bantianum* in the genus *Xylophyta*. J Clin Microbiol 23:1148–1151, 1986.

133. Salem FA, Kannangara DW, Nachum R: Cerebral chromomycosis. Arch Neurol 40:173–174, 1983.

134. Hart AP, Sutton DA, McFeeley PJ, Kornfeld M: Cerebral phaeomycosis caused by a dermatiaceous scopulariopsis species. Clin Neuropathol 20:224–228, 2001.

135. Keyser A, Schmid FX, Linde HJ, et al: Disseminated *Cladophialophora bantiana* infarction in a heart transplant recipient. J Heart Lung Transplant 21:503–505, 2002.

136. Nobrega JP, Rosemberg S, Adami AM, et al: Fonsecaea Pedrosoi Cerebral phaeohyphomycosis ("chromoblastomycosis"): First human culture-proven case reported in Brazil. Rev Inst Med Trop Sao Paulo 45:217–220, 2003.

137. Trinth JV, Steinback WJ, Schell WA, et al: Cerebral phaeohyphomycosis in an immunodeficient child treated medically with combination antifungal therapy. Med Mycol 41:339–345, 2003.

138. Umabala P, Lakshmi V, Murthy AR, et al: Isolation of a *Nodulisporium* species from a case of cerebral phaeohyphomycosis. J Clin Microbiol 39:4213–4218, 2001.

139. Kershaw P, Freeman R, Templeton D, et al: *Pseudoallescheria boydii* infection of the central nervous system. Arch Neurol 47:470–472, 1990.

140. Selby R: Pachymeningitis secondary to *Allescheria boydii*: Case report. J Neurosurg 36:225–227, 1972.

141. Marcinkowski M, Bauer K, Stoltenburg-Didinger G, Versmold H: Fungal brain abscesses in neonates: Sonographic appearances and corresponding histopathologic findings. J Clin Ultrasound 29:417–421, 2001.

142. Messori A, Lanza C, DeNicola M, et al: Mycotic aneurysms as lethal complication of brain pseudoallescheriasis in a near-drowned child: A CT demonstration. AJNR Am J Neuroradiol 23:1697–1699, 2002.

143. Safdar A, Papadopoulos EB, Young JW: Breakthrough *Scedosporium apiospermum* (*Pseudoallescheria boydii*) brain abscess during therapy for invasive pulmonary aspergillosis following high risk allogenic hematopoietic stemcell transplantation: Scedosporiasis and recent advances in antifungal therapy. Transpl Infect Dis 4:212–217, 2002.

144. Ellis CJK, Daniel SE, Kennedy PG, et al: Rhino-orbital zygomycosis. J Neurol Neurosurg Psychiatry 48:455–458, 1985.

145. Hussain S, Salahudin N, Ahmad I, et al: Rhinocerebral invasive mycosis: Occurrence in immunocompetent individuals. Eur J Radiol 20:151–155, 1995.

146. Gupta SK, Manjunath-Prasad KS, Sharma BS, et al: Brain abscess in renal transplant recipients: Report of three cases. Surg Neurol 48:284–287, 1997.

147. Kikuchi K, Watanabe K, Sugawara A, et al: Multiple fungal aneurysms: Report of a rare case implicating steroids as predisposing factor. Surg Neurol 24:253–259, 1985.

148. Nampoory MR, Khan ZU, Johny KV, et al: Invasive fungal infections in renal transplant patients. J Infect 33:95–101, 1996.

149. Bhansali A, Sharma A, Kashyap A, et al: Mucor endophthalmitis. Acta Ophthalmol Scand 79:88–90, 2001.

150. Fairley C, Sullivan TJ, Bartley P, et al: Survival after rhino-orbital mucormycosis in an immunocompetent patient. Ophthalmology 107:555–558, 2000.

151. Georgopoulou S, Kounougeri E, Katsenos C, et al: Rhinocerebral mucormycosis in a patient with cirrhosis and chronic renal failure. Hepatogastroenterology 50:843–845, 2003.

152. Mathi M, Chaouir S, Amil T, et al: Rhino-orbito-cerebral mucormycosis. J Radiol 83:165–167, 2002.

153. Sharma RR, Pawar SJ, Delmendo A, et al: Fatal rhino-orbito-cerebral mucormycosis in an apparently normal host: Case report and literature review. J Clin Neurosci 8:583–586, 2001.

154. Laurin JM, Resnik CS, Wheeler D, et al: Vertebral osteomyelitis caused by *Nocardia asteroides*: Report and review of the literature. J Rheumatol 18:455–458, 1991.

155. Palmer DL, Harvey RL, Wheeler JK: Diagnosis and therapeutic considerations in *Nocardia asteroides* infection. Medicine (Baltimore) 53:391–401, 1974.

156. Peterson JM, Awad I, Ahmed M, et al: *Nocardia* osteomyelitis and epidural abscess in the nonimmunosuppressed host. Cleve Clin Q 50:453–459, 1983.

157. Siao P, McCabe P, Yagnik P: Nocardial spinal epidural abscess. Neurology 39:996, 1989.

158. Durmaz R, Atasoy MA, Durmaz G, et al: Multiple nocardial abscesses of cerebrum, cerebellum and spinal cord causing quadriplegia. Clin Neurol Neurosurg 103:59–62, 2001.

159. Mogilner A, Jallo GI, Zagzag D, Kelly PJ: *Nocardia* abscess of the choroids plexus: Clinical and pathological case report. Neurosurgery 43:949–952, 1998.

160. Oshiro S, Ohnishi H, Ohta M, Tsuchimochi H: Intraventricular rupture of *Nocardia* brain abscess—case report. Neurol Med Chir (Tokyo) 43:360–363, 2003.

161. Young WF: Syringomyelia presenting as a delayed complication of treatment for *Nocardia* brain abscess. Spinal Cord 38:265–269, 2000.

162. Benito Leon J, Munoz A, Leon PG, et al: Actinomycotic brain abscess. Neurologia 13:357–361, 1998.

163. Ushikoshi S, Koyanagi I, Hida K, et al: Spinal intrathecal actinomycosis: A case report. Surg Neurol 50:221–225, 1998.

164. Alday R, Lopez-Ferro MO, Fernandez-Guerrero M, et al: Spinal intrathecal empyema due to *Actinomyces israelii*. Acta Neurochir (Wien) 101:159–162, 1989.

165. Bolton CF, Ashenhurst EM: Actinomycosis of the brain. CMAJ 90:922–928, 1964.

166. David CV, Jayalakshmi P: Actinomycosis of the spine: Two case reports. Med J Malaysia 38:161–163, 1983.

167. Khosla VK, Banerjee AK, Chopra JS: Intracranial actinomycoma with osteomyelitis simulating meningioma: Case report. J Neurosurg 60:204–207, 1984.

168. Lad SD, Chandy MJ: Craniofacial actinomycosis. Br J Neurosurg 5:361–370, 1991.

169. Nolan RL, Ross JD, Chapman SW: Thoracic actinomycosis presenting as spinal cord compression. J Miss State Med Assoc 31:41–45, 1990.

170. Ahuja GK, Jain N, Vijayaraghavan M, Roy S: Cerebral mycotic aneurysm of fungal origin. J Neurosurg 49:107–110, 1978.

171. Hadley MN, Martin NA, Spetzler RF, Johnson PC: Multiple intracranial aneurysms due to *Coccidioides immitis* infection. J Neurosurg 66:453–456, 1987.

172. del Brutto OH: Central nervous system mycotic infections. Rev Neurol 30:447–459, 2000.

118 Neurosurgical Aspects of Neurocysticercosis

R. FRANCISCO ESCOBEDO,[†] ALFREDO GOMEZ-AVINA, and SALVADOR RUIZ-GONZALEZ

Most parasites that reach nervous tissue do so hematogenously. Considering the number of parasites that exist, it is surprising that so few cases of central nervous system (CNS) invasion occur. This relatively low incidence is probably the result of the protection afforded by the blood-brain barrier[1] and certain immunologic reactions that are not well understood.

The most important determinant of the incidence of parasitic diseases is the hygienic character of the environment. These diseases are seen more frequently in geographic areas in which sanitary control of the water supply, agricultural systems, and food handling is poor. A tropical climate also favors the development of some parasites, and these disorders have often been considered tropical diseases. Parasitic disorders, however, are being seen with increasing frequency in industrialized nations because of the migration of infected persons from endemic areas. Parasitic infections of the CNS have spread to groups and countries in which such diseases were previously rare.[2,3] Parasitic diseases affecting the CNS include amebiasis, malaria, coenurosis, echinococcosis, schistosomiasis, paragonimiasis, trichinosis, filariasis, angiostrongyliasis, *Toxocara canis* encephalitis, and gnathostomiasis. Most of these disorders are not treated surgically. The discussion in this chapter is restricted to cysticercosis, the most common of these disorders affecting the CNS, for which surgical treatment is indicated.[4]

CYSTICERCOSIS

Human cysticercosis results when a person serves as the intermediate host of *Taenia solium*, the porcine tapeworm; the larvae develop in various body tissues. The presence of the encysted larvae in the nervous tissue, its cavities, or its coverings constitutes the disease known as *neurocysticercosis*. The cysts are called *Cysticercus cellulosae*.[5]

T. solium infestation is endemic in Africa, Eastern Europe, Indonesia, parts of Asia (India and China), and several areas of Latin America. Cases occur sporadically in other parts of the world. The incidence varies according to the economic and social condition, as reflected in the level of hygiene of a region, with lower socioeconomic groups having a higher incidence of the disease.[1-7]

In endemic countries, 5% to 10% of all patients requiring surgery on the CNS are operated on for cysticercosis. These patients constitute approximately 25% of all adult patients operated on for increased intracranial pressure.[8]

Autopsy studies in general hospitals from endemic countries have shown an incidence of neurocysticercosis in the general population of 3% or 4% for either the active disease form or inactive sequelae. In most cases, the disease was asymptomatic.[9,10] At the Institute of Neurology and Neurosurgery in Mexico City, being a concentration center, approximately 10% of autopsies revealed neurocysticercosis.[11-13] This chapter is based on our experience in the management of approximately 1000 cases of neurocysticercosis.

PARASITE AND ACQUISITION OF INFECTION

In the usual cycle of transmission, only the pig harbors the larval stage of *T. solium*; humans acquire the adult tapeworm by eating undercooked pork. The larval infection is acquired through the ingestion of food contaminated with *T. solium* eggs, each of which contains an active embryo or oncosphere. The oncospheres are liberated by digestive juices. They then penetrate the wall of the small intestine and burrow into the vessels, from which they are carried to distant sites. The organisms lodge in various tissues, mainly muscle, skin, brain, and eye.[1-5]

PATHOPHYSIOLOGY

Once the embryos have arrived in the brain, they go through different biologic stages.

Encephalitic Stage

The encephalitic stage is the initial stage and is characterized by a focal inflammatory reaction with local brain edema that could produce symptoms such as headache and, in some cases, focal seizures.

Cystic Stage

If the parasites are not destroyed by the immune reaction, they grow and develop into larvae, or cysticerci, in 60 to 70 days. This is the most common form and the best known. The typical cysticerci have an ovoid form and are approximately 0.5 inch in diameter, consisting of a fragile membrane, fluid, and a scolex with suckers and hooks. The cysts can live in tissue for long periods of time.

Cysticerci most commonly lodge in the brain and skeletal muscle. The larvae vary in size from approximately 5 mm to approximately 5 cm. Cysticerci can lodge in the parenchyma of the brain (in approximately 60%), the subarachnoid space (meningobasal and cortical, in approximately 40%), the

---

[†]Deceased.

TABLE 118-1 ▪ Symptoms and Signs of Neurocysticercosis*

Focal effect
Mass effect
Inflammatory response
   On nervous tissue
   On meninges-arachnoid
   On vessels
Hydrocephalus caused by obstruction
   Of foramina
   Of aqueduct
   Of cisterns
   Of subarachnoid space

*All of these processes may coexist in the same patient.

ventricular system (in approximately 10%), mixed areas (in >50%), and the spine (in nearly 1%).

The location, number, and size of these lesions determine the clinical manifestations.[1,8,14] The manifestations are also the result of focal and mass effect and of the inflammatory response to the cysticerci in the nervous tissue, the meninges, or the vessels; the focal effect; the mass effect; and the effect of obstruction of the foramina, ventricular system, subarachnoid space, and cisterns of the brain.

Cysts can lodge in the ventricular system and cause an obstructive hydrocephalus, either because of the cysts themselves or because of the inflammatory response they incite. Endothelial proliferation can occur in the cerebral arteries and arterioles as a result of vasculitis, and the vessel may become occluded. These processes can coexist in the same patient (Table 118-1). The combination of these factors and the distribution of the lesions makes neurocysticercosis a pleomorphic disease. Except when acute massive exposure exists, symptoms appear only after a latent period of a few years because in most cases, viable cysts incite little inflammatory response from the host.[1,12,15] The number of cysts, the duration of the illness, the location of cerebral cysticerci, their enlargement, and the local inflammatory response that they provoke can lead to a clinical syndrome with focal neurologic manifestations, cranial nerve palsies, or a tumor-like presentation.

Racemose Form

When the membrane of the cyst continues growing and becomes distended or when a group of cysts develop together and are located at the deepest portions of the fissures or at the base of the brain in the subarachnoid space, they incite chronic meningitis and arachnoiditis, after which a communicating or noncommunicating hydrocephalus frequently develops.

Partially Degenerated Stage

The cyst partially degenerates, as a regular process of its natural history; the clear fluid content becomes jelly-like, and it is no longer viable.

Totally Degenerated Stage

Should the cysts degenerate, a lipocalcareous infiltration develops and becomes calcified, making the cysts easier

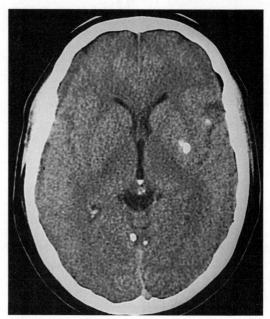

FIGURE 118-1   A noncontrast computed tomography scan shows multiple round calcifications.

to diagnose from computed tomography (CT) scan (Fig. 118-1).[6,14]

CLINICAL SIGNS AND SYMPTOMS

The clinical picture is not uniform and may be present in various forms that range from a benign self-limited disorder to a severe life-threatening condition.[4] The disease follows an idiosyncratic course, depending on the individual's immune response, the severity of infestation, the location of the cysts, and the size, site, and number of neurologic lesions. If the cysticerci are single or few in number and are lodged in a nonstrategic area of the brain, no signs of disease may be present, as has been seen in approximately 75% of the cases, according to necropsy series.[7–10] If large numbers of cysts are present or if they lodge in eloquent areas of the CNS, seizures, focal deficits, increased intracranial pressure secondary to mass effect or communicating and noncommunicating hydrocephalus, and meningitis may develop. Frequently, the predominating signs or symptoms change during the course of infection. Focal, jacksonian, or generalized seizures occur in 30% to 92% of patients, depending on the reported series. Headache is practically universal in patients with hydrocephalus. Nausea, vomiting, impaired vision, confusion, dizziness, and ataxia are also common manifestations of the disease. Papilledema and changes in mental status frequently occur in patients with hydrocephalus, and focal deficits are common in those with mass lesions.[12,13,16–19]

DIAGNOSIS

The diagnosis of neurocysticercosis is established by a combination of the clinical history, physical findings, signs, results of laboratory and immunologic tests, and CT scans or magnetic resonance imaging (MRI). The neurologic signs and symptoms are nonspecific, but the finding of multiple subcutaneous cysts strongly suggests the diagnosis. Epilepsy is the most common presentation of neurocysticercosis. Partial seizures with or without secondary generalization are typical.[20]

The most important clinical aspects that facilitate the diagnosis are as follows:

1. Knowledge of patient's country of origin and a history of exposure in an endemic zone
2. Late-onset seizures or partial epilepsy[19]
3. History of personal or family taeniasis
4. Neurologic symptoms, particularly if associated with increased intracranial pressure
5. Mental deterioration in a nonelderly patient
6. Presence of chronic, persistent headache

The cerebrospinal fluid (CSF) is usually abnormal and suggests chronic meningitis manifested as lymphocytic pleocytosis and, in some cases, CSF eosinophilia, decreased glucose level, and elevated protein level.[7,15] Immunologic testing of the CSF is useful in cysticercosis, in contrast to serologic testing, which is neither highly sensitive nor specific.[9] Although numerous tests are available, there are no standardized antigens or methods. *T. solium* antigen preparations identify cross-reactive antibodies in some patients with echinococcosis, schistosomiasis, or other cestode infections. Despite these drawbacks, however, detection of antibodies in a patient with a typical clinical appearance and compatible CT or MRI findings generally establishes the diagnosis.[13,21–23]

CT is the most useful study, and the findings are diagnostic in most cases. The appearance of cerebral cysticercosis on CT scans varies and depends on the stage of the disease: a hyperdense, nodular mass is seen in the encephalitic phase; hypodense, round lesions of varying sizes sometimes surrounded by an enhanced ring are seen when the lesion is cystic (Figs. 118-2 to 118-5). In later stages of the disease, the cysts may be calcified (Fig. 118-6). Some lesions can be seen on

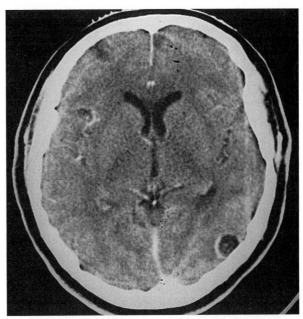

FIGURE 118-3 A contrast-enhanced computed tomography scan of the same patient as in Figure 118-2 shows the multiple parenchymal cysts as round lesions with a ring of enhancement.

CT scans only with contrast enhancement. The diagnosis is less certain when single lesions are present or radiographic findings are nonspecific, such as in hydrocephalus. Subarachnoid or intraventricular cysts are difficult to detect with CT scans, and a positive contrast medium (metrizamide) introduced into an obstructed lateral ventricle may be required to demonstrate them.[17–22,24–29]

MRI is also useful in making the diagnosis in most cases. The findings of cerebral cysticercosis on MRI vary according to the stage of the disease: a hyperintense, nodular mass highly surrounded by edema is seen in the encephalitic phase;

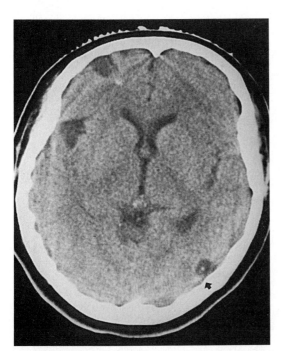

FIGURE 118-2 A noncontrast computed tomography scan shows multiple parenchymal cysts as hypodense round lesions. Scolex is visible as a small point in the interior of the parietal cyst (*black arrow*).

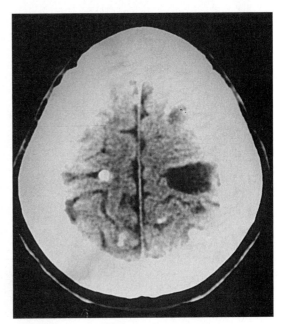

FIGURE 118-4 A computed tomography scan of a patient with a single large cyst and calcifications.

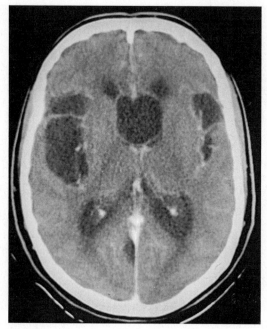

FIGURE 118-5   A computed tomography scan of a patient with the combined form of neurocysticercotic lesions: hydrocephalus, large cyst, racemose cyst, and intraventricular cyst.

hypointense, round lesions of varying sizes are seen during the cystic stage (Figs. 118-7 and 118-8); and not so hypointense, round cysts are seen during a partially degenerated phase (see Fig. 118-6). When gadolinium as contrast material is used, a ringlike enhancement can be seen at the wall membrane of the cyst, representing inflammatory reaction, and when T2-weighted MRI is performed, the surrounding edema is clearly demonstrated (Fig. 118-9). The calcified cysticerci are not well demonstrated on MRI. Subarachnoid and intraventricular cysts as well as hydrocephalus[21] are well shown in some cases (Fig. 118-10). In cases of suspected spinal neurocysticercosis, myelography and CT scans or MRI are recommended.[24–27]

PROGNOSIS

The prognosis of cysticercosis is variable and difficult to assess, and the course and tempo of the disease may change, partly because of differences between the individual's immunologic responses and by an increased inflammatory reaction in previously quiescent, viable cysts. Many patients with neurocysticercosis are asymptomatic; their disease is discovered incidentally on radiographic studies performed for other reasons, and they have a good prognosis. Another group of patients have minimal nonspecific complaints, such as headache or dizziness, and some others have major neurologic symptoms, such as seizures, increased intracranial pressure, focal neurologic signs, mental deterioration, or involvement of the cranial nerves that requires immediate investigation

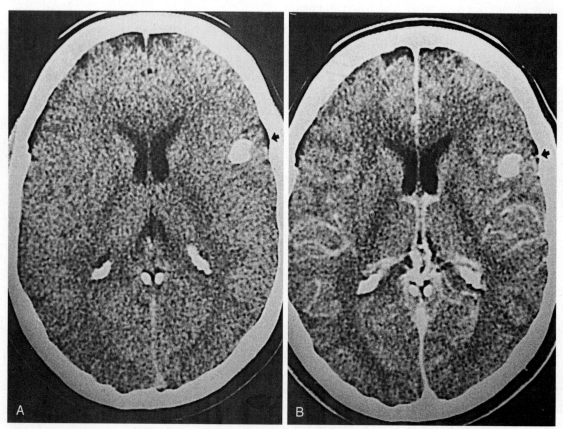

FIGURE 118-6   A computed tomography scan of a patient with a calcification (*arrow*). *A,* Without contrast; *B,* with contrast. Note that there is no enhancement of the calcification, or around it, corresponding to an inactive form.

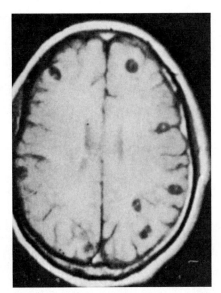

FIGURE 118-7 A magnetic resonance image shows multiple parenchymal cysts as round hypointense lesions. Scolex is visible as a small point in the interior of some cysts.

because they have a serious prognosis.[7,29–31] A review of 20,206 autopsies carried out at the General Hospital in Mexico City between 1953 and 1984 revealed 481 cases of neurocysticercosis (2.38%), of which only 189 (32.29%) were persons who actually died of neurocysticercosis, emphasizing the large number of asymptomatic or relatively benign cases of this disease.[7]

NATURAL HISTORY AND THERAPY

Therapeutic approaches must be selected for each patient according to the number, location, and stage of cysticerci and the degree of the inflammatory response raised by the host against the parasite.[4] Supportive therapy includes anticonvulsant medication and steroids; the latter have been reported to cause short-term and sometimes long-term symptomatic improvement.

Two antiparasitic drugs, praziquantel and albendazole, have been demonstrated to have a beneficial effect in parenchymal and cortical macroscopic viable cysts appearing on CT scans as hypodense images (Fig. 118-11) or hypointense images on MRI as well as in some subarachnoid, cisternal, or ventricular cysts.[4] These drugs interfere with the metabolism of the parasite and should be administered combined with steroids at the same time, to control the inflammatory process that appears in the surrounding nervous tissue when the parasites are going to die, but do not influence the calcified cysts, arachnoiditis, or hydrocephalus associated with the disease.[32–40]

Surgical therapy, either shunting procedures or focal extirpation as appropriate, is recommended for patients presenting fulminant signs of intracranial pressure resulting from hydrocephalus or large focal space-occupying lesions.[41,42]

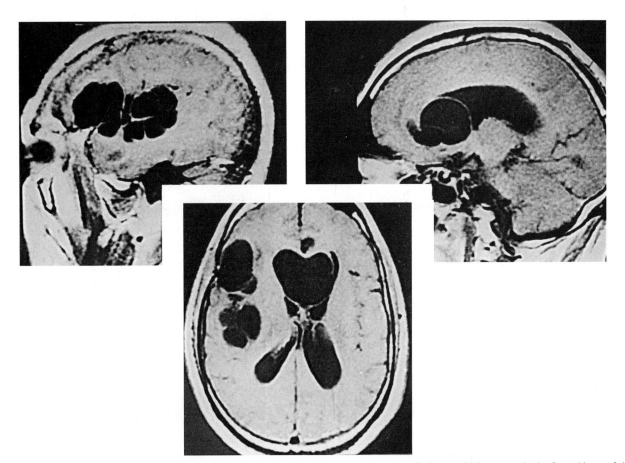

FIGURE 118-8 A magnetic resonance image from a patient with a giant cyst, a racemose lesion, and a large cyst in the frontal horn of the lateral ventricle.

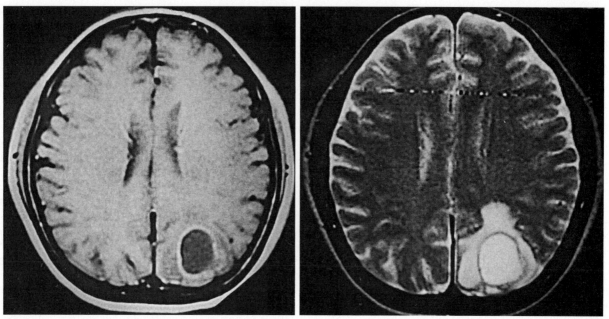

FIGURE 118-9   Magnetic resonance imaging (MRI) with gadolinium. On the left side, a ringlike enhancement is displayed; on the right side, a T2-weighted MRI scan is shown of the same patient in which the surrounding edema is clearly demonstrated.

The surgical approach in the treatment of neurocysticercosis depends on the number, size, and location of the cysticerci and the anatomic-pathologic characteristics of the infection. The following areas must be defined:

1. The number of cysts (single or multiple cysts)
2. The size of the cysts (>2 cm or <2 cm in diameter; is there a mass effect?)
3. The location of the cysts (in the parenchyma of the brain or spinal cord; in the subarachnoid space of the base, cisterns, or convexity; in the ventricles; in the subarachnoid space of the spine; or mixed types)
4. The biologic stage of the parasite (Fig. 118-12) (encephalitic stage, viable cyst with clear fluid content, racemose type of cyst, partially degenerated cyst with jelly-like content, or degenerated cyst that is calcified)
5. The secondary pathologic conditions produced in the CNS by the presence of the cysts (Fig. 118-13) (arachnoiditis-meningitis, ependymitis, vasculitis with or without ischemic sequelae,[43] or communicating or noncommunicating hydrocephalus)[31]

The surgical approach varies, depending on whether larvae are situated in brain or spinal cord parenchyma or are intraventricular, whether they are single or multiple, whether they are of the cellulosae or racemose variety, and whether they are located in the cortex or in the basal subarachnoid space or both, if there is a communicating or obstructive hydrocephalus, or if an adherent arachnoiditis or ependymitis is present. Most cases involve mixed types of the disease, calcified forms with parenchymatous cysts, cisternal cysts, basilar adhesive arachnoiditis, and hydrocephalus (Table 118-2).[8,31]

To optimize the outcome of these patients, the natural history of this disease must be clearly understood, and a good CT or MRI diagnosis must be made so that the best treatment can be selected. The different biologic stages produce different damage and different clinical pictures, and they demand different therapeutic approaches.

Acute Encephalitic Stage

In the acute encephalitic phase with local brain edema, if the parasites in the brain are single or few in number, the embryo could be destroyed and disappear, as could the brain edema in a few weeks (Fig. 118-14). If a great number of parasites arrive in the brain, however, which occurs mainly in young

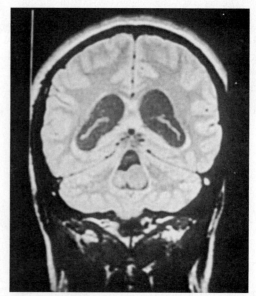

FIGURE 118-10   A magnetic resonance imaging scan in which two round lesions corresponding to cysticerci are shown in an enlarged fourth ventricle.

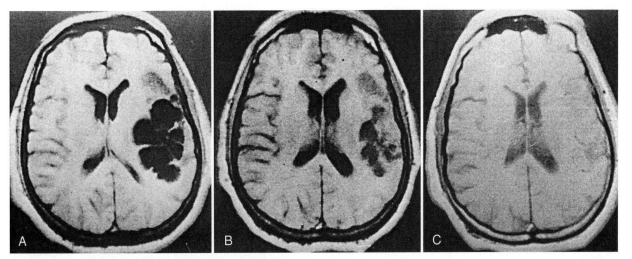

FIGURE 118-11 Magnetic resonance imaging before and after albendazole therapy. *A*, A large racemose cyst before treatment. *B*, The same cyst 11 days after treatment. Note the partial disappearance of the lesion and almost complete resolution (*C*) of the lesion 2 months after treatment.

people, the patients could have frequent seizures, and the clinical picture is complicated by severe increased intracranial pressure. The diagnosis in this stage can be confirmed with CT or MRI, which shows multiple nodular masses (Fig. 118-15).

The treatment should consist of steroids, antiparasitic agents, and anticonvulsants. Usually, in 6 or 8 weeks, the inflammatory process disappears, and the patient recovers. In some cases in which the number of parasites is high, the intracranial pressure reaches critical levels without ventricular dilatation, and medical therapy has been of little value, surgical decompression through large craniotomies may be required.

Cystic Stage

If the parasites are not destroyed, they grow and develop into the cystic stage, producing symptoms that vary according to the severity of the infection and the location and size of the cysts. In cases with no increased intracranial pressure, specific antiparasitic drugs (praziquantel or albendazole) combined with steroids should be used as the only treatment. Among this type of cyst, some cases require surgical treatment.

Single Cysts

Cysts in the brain that produce focal symptoms, such as reluctant partial seizures, could benefit from the extirpation of the cysticercus or cysticerci (Fig. 118-16).

Giant or Racemose Cysts

Giant or racemose cysts are cysts 2 cm or larger or racemose lesions presenting as a tumor-like mass that are predominantly localized in the parenchyma of the cerebral hemispheres or at a major cerebral sulcus, such as the sylvian fissure. These masses have the appearance of an enhancing, ringlike abscess or tumor 2 to 3 inches in diameter on CT or MRI. These lesions are treated by total excision. In cases of multiple cysts, in which one large cyst appears to be primarily responsible for a focal neurologic symptom or deficit, its removal is also indicated.

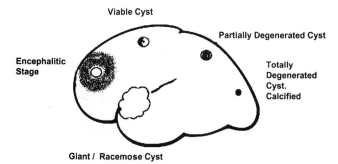

FIGURE 118-12 The biologic stage of neurocysticercosis.

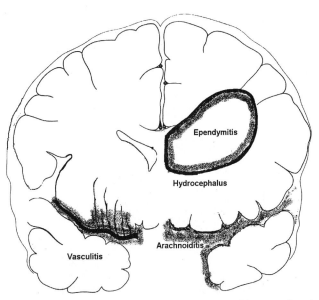

FIGURE 118-13 The secondary pathologic conditions produced by neurocysticercosis.

TABLE 118-2 ▪ **Indications for Surgical Treatment of Neurocysticercosis**

Cysts ≥ 2 cm producing focal symptoms or a mass effect
Severe increased intracranial pressure
Cysts obstructing ventricular channels
Hydrocephalus
Spinal cord compression

The surgical approach to parenchymal or subarachnoidal cysts should be through microsurgical dissection, in which attempts are made to separate the thin-walled cyst from the surrounding nervous tissue and vessels, permitting total excision. In some cases, the cyst can be extracted by aspiration or by traction with forceps. One of the reasons for failure in surgical results is the presence of inflammatory tissue that affects the wall vessels, producing vasculitis, which compromises local blood flow.

Nicely extirpating the cyst is possible, but in many cases, cleaning the area of the brain from the arachnoiditis and vasculitis is not easy. We have used a carbon dioxide laser, sharply focused and at low power, to dissect and separate these structures and to extirpate as much as possible the inflammatory tissue that usually surrounds the cysts and is adjacent to vessels and adherent to nervous tissue (Fig. 118-17).

The cyst wall often is so thin and delicate that there is always the danger that the cyst will tear during dissection and its fluid contents will spill into neighboring areas of the brain. Among 114 cases of cysts, corresponding to a studied group that were operated on, the membranes of the extracted cyst were torn in 69%. Even though this complication causes concern, we have not found the spillage of cyst contents to have subsequent deleterious consequences. In most cases, steroid therapy is maintained throughout the perioperative period. If a cyst is firmly attached to surrounding structures and cannot be totally removed, the cavity is marsupialized and

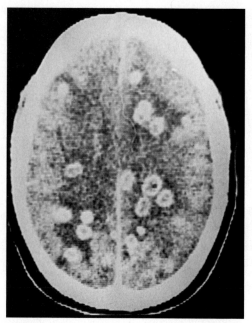

FIGURE 118-15   A contrast computed tomography scan of a patient with multiple nodular masses in the acute encephalitic stage. A severe inflammatory reaction is present.

left as open as possible so that it has a connection with the subarachnoid space.[31]

Ventricular Cysts

Cysts that migrate within the ventricular system can obstruct the foramen of Monro, the aqueduct of Sylvius, the fourth ventricle, or the cisterna magna. The larvae, when accessible, are removed to reestablish CSF flow. Because of the possibility of future inflammatory reactions to the cysts, the removal of all accessible ventricular cysts is recommended.

Although most patients have multiple intraventricular cysts, a sufficient number of patients have solitary cysts, the removal of which may be curative.[24,25] Cysts located in the lateral or third ventricle near the foramen of Monro are reached through a frontal craniotomy and a transcortical or a transcallosal approach. In these cases, the septum pellucidum should be fenestrated to ensure adequate bilateral ventricular drainage.

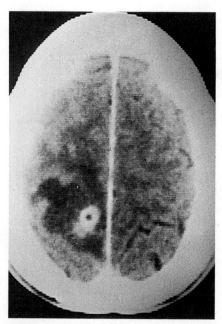

FIGURE 118-14   A contrast computed tomography scan of a patient with an active lesion in the acute encephalitic phase.

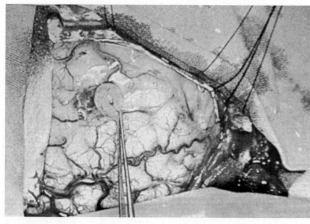

FIGURE 118-16   A cortical cyst is dissected and ready for excision.

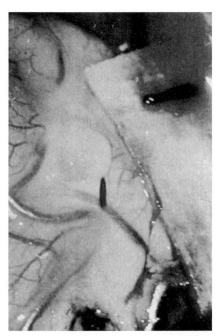

FIGURE 118-17   A cyst located in a brain fissure with an associated inflammatory reaction. This is a milky white process over the cortex and around the vessels. A thrombosed vessel is also visible in the field.

The tendency of intraventricular cysts to migrate may explain why so many tend to be found in the fourth ventricle. Imaging studies in these cases demonstrate the presence of the cysts or of a large fourth ventricle, which is sometimes disproportionately large compared with the rest of the ventricular system. This finding in a patient with cysticercosis is highly suggestive of an isolated ventricle or an intraventricular cyst.[25]

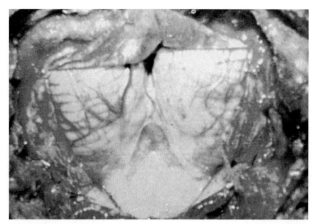

FIGURE 118-19   A cluster of cysts in the cisterna magna.

A posterior fossa approach is performed with a suboccipital craniotomy. A midline exposure permits excision of a cyst or cluster of cysts if they are at the cisterna. Many times, the cysts are blended in the middle of thick membranes, representing forms of chronic meningitis, and a creamy yellow material, representing the inflammatory response combined with dead parasites. The dissection and separation of these structures are extremely difficult (Figs. 118-18 and 118-19). Cystic masses can also be found in the cerebellopontine angle, in the lateral medullary recess, and even on the cerebellar hemispheres. When cysts are located within the fourth ventricle or the cerebral aqueduct, these areas are explored after the thickened tela choroidea is opened and both cerebellar tonsils are separated (Fig. 118-20). In some cases, dividing the inferior vermis is necessary before the cyst can be extracted by gentle aspiration or traction with flat-bladed forceps on the walls of a smooth cyst. This step can be supplemented by irrigation for hydraulic dissection and a Valsalva maneuver, which assists in exposing and delivering lesions from deep recesses that may

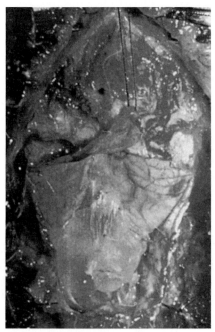

FIGURE 118-18   The suboccipital approach shows the cisterna containing several transparent cysts.

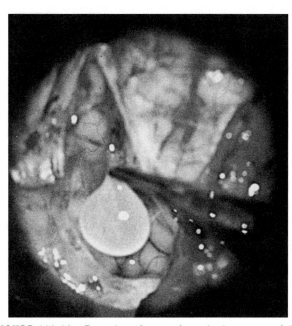

FIGURE 118-20   Extraction of a cyst from the lower part of the fourth ventricle.

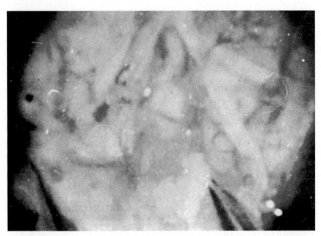

FIGURE 118-21 After the cyst has been removed from the cisterna and fourth ventricle, a creamy yellow inflammatory response (combined with dead parasites) is seen.

not have been previously suspected. These maneuvers often reestablish CSF flow. In some cases, injecting 30 or 40 mL of saline into the lateral ventricle pushes down cysts within the ventricular system and confirms the free flow of CSF (Fig. 118-21). If CSF flow is not reestablished by these measures, a shunt should be performed immediately or within a short period of time.[31,44,45] In cases of deep-seated cysts in the lateral ventricles, the posterior part of the third ventricle, or the lower areas of the hemispheres, the use of a stereotactic endoscopic system to introduce forceps, suction, or cannulas for the excision or draining of the cysts should be considered.[31,44-47]

Hydrocephalus

In cerebral cysticercosis, the cysts are usually multiple, and the inflammatory reaction is widely distributed; despite this, many of these intraventricular cysts are removable. Hydrocephalus or increased intracranial pressure, however, can persist as a result of ependymitis along the walls of the ventricle originating from the *frozen ventricle* that remains enlarged despite shunting; more frequent is ependymitis at the foramen of Monro or at the aqueduct of Sylvius or as a result of basilar adhesive arachnoiditis, which blocks the free circulation and absorption of CSF over the base or surface of the brain. In these cases, shunting CSF into the bloodstream or the peritoneal cavity is indicated. In most cases of neurocysticercosis, the CSF protein content is high, and the catheter eventually becomes occluded and requires revision. Of 448 hydrocephalic patients with neurocysticercosis in which CSF shunts were applied, systems became occluded and required revision in 42%; the occlusion was identified at the ventricular catheter in 65%, the distal catheter in 12%, in both catheters in 10%, and in an unknown place in 13%. Similar results were obtained with all types of shunt systems.[31]

Chiasmatic Cysts

Cysticerci located in the chiasmatic region can produce an inflammatory reaction and adhesive arachnoiditis that affects the optic nerves and chiasm from fibrotic entrapment in the arachnoidal sheaths.[9] These cases are difficult surgical problems because the chronic basilar adhesive meningitis forms a thick membrane that surrounds all the structures on the

ventral surface of the brain, including the brain stem. Cysts are often blended into this mass of adhesions. These membranes are firmly attached to the optic nerves, the optic chiasm, and the internal carotid arteries. Microsurgical dissection supplemented by bipolar coagulation and, in certain cases, carbon dioxide laser can decompress these structures and remove cysts.[30,31] The vascular damage (ischemia of the optic nerves) already established could remain without improvement.

Spinal Cysts

Cysticerci located in the spine result in symptoms that indicate injury to the spinal cord or the nerve roots. Myelography, CT, or MRI shows cysts or a block caused by arachnoiditis. In these cases, laminectomy should be performed, the dura opened, the cyst or cysts removed, and adherent membranes removed or freed up to free the neural structures. There is a report[48] of a patient with cervical intramedullary cysticercosis detected through MRI, who obtained complete resolution of the lesion, and progressive neurologic improvement after albendazole and steroid treatment.

Partially Degenerated Stage

When the partially degenerated stage is diagnosed through CT or MRI and is not associated with increased intracranial pressure, the treatment should be through specific antiparasitic drugs (albendazole or praziquantel) that, in most cases, favor the process of destruction of the cysts already initiated. Drugs that provide symptomatic relief, such as anticonvulsants or steroids, which control the inflammatory reaction, may be required.

Totally Degenerated Stage

When the cysts have totally degenerated and become calcified, similar to an inactive foreign body, no specific treatment is indicated except anticonvulsant drugs in cases of seizures. This is the most common form of cysticercosis found in an outpatient neurologic clinic.

CONCLUSION AND SUMMARY

Surgery is not indicated in all cases of neurocysticercosis, and when performed, it is not necessarily curative because multiple disseminated cysts cannot be treated surgically, and the arachnoidal adhesions and cerebral vasculitis and its sequelae may produce permanent neurologic complications. In selecting the surgical approach (Fig. 118-22), the surgeon should be aware of the possibility of an associated ependymitis and the potential for current or eventual outlet obstruction, despite the removal of a particular cysticercus. Direct surgical excision of one or a group of cystic lesions may be the primary therapy in most of these cases because the surgical approach treats symptomatic manifestations. Most surgical procedures are palliative. Surgery can partially and temporarily relieve increased intracranial pressure and, occasionally, the focal symptoms caused by a cortical or subcortical cysticercus, even though this is not the rule.[31,41-45] Although improvement occurs, other evidence of disease precludes the idea of curing the underlying disorder surgically. Experience with ventricular shunts indicates that

FIGURE 118-22   Different surgical approaches are used to treat neurocysticercosis.

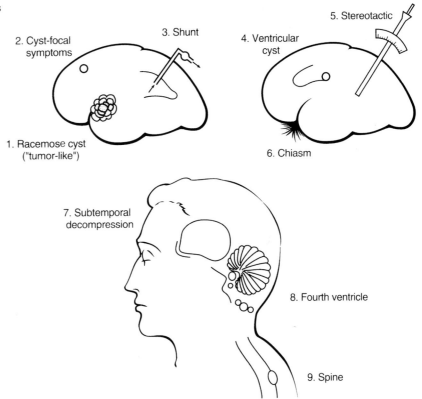

although they are effective for alleviating CSF blockage, the catheter eventually becomes occluded and requires revision.

In contrast to the complex problems and frustrations encountered with the mixed and disseminated forms of neurocysticercosis, removal of solitary intraventricular cysts is often followed by prompt improvement and excellent recovery. Such cysts are potentially curable. Sometimes a patient requires several staged surgical procedures. For instance, in some cases, a shunt followed by the direct excision of cysts in the fourth ventricle or at the sylvian fissure is required; other cases require primary excision of cystic lesions and secondary shunting (Fig. 118-23).

When planning the management of a patient with neurocysticercosis, the physician must bear in mind the great variability of the disease. The physician must also have a clearly defined diagnosis through CT or MRI of the biologic stage of the parasite as well as of the type, number, location, and size of the lesions and the extent of the brain damage, all of which determine the therapeutic option to be used, as follows:

1. Asymptomatic calcifications: no treatment
2. Symptomatic calcification, such as seizures: anticonvulsants
3. Increased intracranial pressure: surgery (CSF shunt, cyst excision, decompression)

FIGURE 118-23   Initial and long-term results in 519 cases of surgical neurocysticercosis. (From Escobedo F: Neurosurgical aspects of neurocysticercosis. In Schmidek H, Sweet W (eds): Operative Neurosurgical Techniques, 3rd ed. Philadelphia: WB Saunders, 1995, p 1714.)

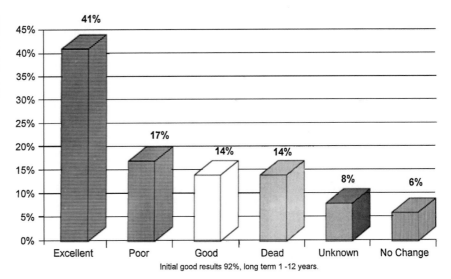

4. Focal neurologic symptoms associated with a cyst larger than 2 cm in diameter corresponding with the functional topography: surgery (excision)
5. Parenchymatous hypodense cysts on CT or hypointense cysts on MRI with or without scolex: antiparasitic drugs (albendazole, praziquantel)
6. Cases with severe inflammatory brain tissue reaction (on CT or MRI or in CSF), vasculitis, or both: steroids, in some cases combined with decompressive surgery and parasitic drugs (albendazole, praziquantel)
7. Spinal cysts: surgery (laminectomy, excision, decompression)

The surgical approach in the treatment of neurocysticercosis depends on the following:

1. Number, size, and location of the cysts
2. Biologic stage of the parasite
3. Presence of hydrocephalus
4. Inflammatory reaction of meninges, ependyma, and vessels with or without secondary ischemia
5. The surgical approach differs depending on the following factors:
   - Whether cysts are located in the parenchyma or in the ventricles
   - Whether cysts are located in the cortex, in the subarachnoid space of the base and cisterns, or in both
   - Whether cysts are in the presence of communicating or obstructive hydrocephalus or if adhesive arachnoiditis or ependymitis are present
   - Whether cysts are, as in most cases, mixed types of the disease, such as calcified forms with cysts, arachnoiditis, and hydrocephalus.

Acknowledgment

Some figures relating results in surgical procedures were obtained from the study by Dr. Pedro Penagos as his thesis at the Instituto Nacional de Neurología y Neurocirugía in Mexico City.

REFERENCES

1. Escobar A, Nieto D: Cysticercosis. In Minkler J (ed): Pathology of the Nervous System, Vol 3. New York: McGraw-Hill, 1972, pp 2507–2515.
2. Miller BL, Goldberg MA, Heiner D, et al: Cerebral cysticercosis: An overview. Bull Clin Neurosci 48:2, 1983.
3. Gardner B, Goldberg M, Douglas H, et al: The natural history of parenchymal CNS cysticercosis. Neurology 34(Suppl 1):90, 1984.
4. Sotelo J, Flisser A: Neurocysticercosis: Practical treatment guidelines disease management. CNS Drugs 7:17–25, 1997.
5. Willms K: Cestodes. In Gorbach S, Bartlett JG, Blacklow NR (eds): Infectious Diseases. Philadelphia: WB Saunders, 1992, pp 2021–2037.
6. Escobar A: The pathology of neurocysticercosis. In Palacios E, Rodriguez Carbajal J, Taveras J (eds): Cysticercosis of the Central Nervous System. Springfield, IL: Charles C Thomas, 1983, pp 27–54.
7. Willms K: Cestodes (tapeworms). In Gorbach SL, Bartlett JG, Blacklow NR (eds): Infectious Diseases, 2nd ed. Philadelphia: WB Saunders, 1998, pp 2481–2499.
8. Escobedo F, González-Mariscal G, Revuelta R, et al: Surgical treatment of cerebral cysticercosis. In Flisser A, Willms K, Lacletted P, Larralde C (eds): Cysticercosis: Present State of Knowledge and Perspectives. New York: Academic Press, 1982, pp 201–206.
9. Sotelo J: Neurocysticercosis. In Roos KL (ed): Central Nervous System Infectious Diseases and Therapy. New York: Marcel Dekker, 1997, pp 545–571.
10. Rabiela C, Ma T: Anatomopathological aspects of human brain cysticercosis. In Flisser A, Willms K, Laclette JP, Larralde C (eds):

Cysticercosis: Present State of Knowledge and Perspectives. New York: Academic Press, 1982, pp 179–200.
11. Del Brutto O, Santibañez R, Noboa C, et al: Epilepsy due to neurocysticercosis: Analysis of 203 patients. Neurology 42:389–392, 1992.
12. Escobedo F, García-Ramos G, Sotelo J: Parasitic disorders and epilepsy. In Nistico G, Di Perri R, Meinardi H (eds): Epilepsy: An Update on Research and Therapy. New York: Alan R Liss, 1983, pp 227–233.
13. Sotelo J, Guerrero V, Rubio F: Neurocysticercosis: A new classification based on active and inactive forms: A study of 753 cases. Arch Intern Med 145:442, 1985.
14. Itabashi HH: Pathology of CNS cysticercosis. Bull Clin Neurosci 48:6, 1983.
15. Gajdusek C: Introduction of Taenia solium into West New Guinea with a note on an epidemic of burns from cysticercus epilepsy in the Ekari people of the Wissel Lakes area. P N G Med J 21:329, 1978.
16. Feinberg W, Valdivia RF: Cysticercosis presenting as a subdural hematoma. Neurology 34:1112, 1984.
17. Salazar A, Sotelo J, Martínez H, et al: Differential diagnosis between ventriculitis and cyst of fourth ventricle in neurocysticercosis. J Neurosurg 59:660, 1983.
18. Wendy MG, Snodgrass RS: Intraparenchymal cerebral cysticercosis in children: A benign prognosis. Pediatr Neurol 1:151, 1985.
19. Medina M, Rosas E, Rubio DF, Sotelo J: Neurocysticercosis as the main cause of late-onset epilepsy in Mexico. Arch Intern Med 150:325, 1990.
20. Bittencourt PRM, Adamolekum B, Bharucha N, et al: Epilepsy in the tropics: II. Clinical presentations pathophysiology: Immunologic diagnosis, economics and therapy. Epilepsia 37:1128–1137, 1996.
21. Suss R, Maravilla KR, Thompson J: Magnetic resonance imaging of intracranial cysticercosis: Comparison with CT and anatomopathologic features. AJNR Am J Neuroradiol 7:235–242, 1986.
22. Ramos KM, Montoya RM, Padilla A, et al: Immunodiagnosis of neurocysticercosis. Arch Neurol 49:633–636, 1992.
23. García H, Martínez M, Gilman R: Diagnosis of cysticercosis in endemic regions. Lancet 338:549, 1991.
24. Rodríguez CJ, Palacios E, Azar-Kia B, et al: Radiology of cysticercosis of the central nervous system including computed tomography. Radiology 125:127, 1977.
25. Kerin D, Chi-Shing Z, Tsai F, et al: Transventricular migration of a cysticercal cyst during pneumoencephalography. Bull Clin Neurosci 48:61, 1983.
26. Kramer LD, Locke GE, Bird SE, Daryabagi J: Cerebral cysticercosis: Documentation of natural history with CT. Radiology 171:459–462, 1989.
27. Mehringer CM, Hieshima G, Grinnell VS, et al: Radiologic considerations in neurocysticercosis. Bull Clin Neurosci 48:24, 1983.
28. Rodríguez Carbajal J, Salgado P, Gutiérrez R, et al: The acute encephalitic phase on neurocysticercosis: Computed tomographic manifestations. AJNR Am J Neuroradiol 4:51, 1985.
29. Miller B: Spontaneous radiographic disappearance of cerebral cysticercosis: Three cases. Neurology 33:1377, 1983.
30. Escobedo F: Neurosurgical aspects of neurocysticercosis. In Schmidek H, Sweet W (eds): Operative Neurosurgical Techniques, 2nd ed. New York: Grune & Stratton, 1988, pp 93–100.
31. Escobedo F: Neurosurgical aspects of neurocysticercosis. In Schmidek H, Sweet W (eds): Operative Neurosurgical Techniques, 3rd ed. Philadelphia: WB Saunders, 1995, pp 1705–1715.
32. Robles C, Chavarría M: Un caso de cisticercosis cerebral curado me©dicamente. Gac Med Mex 116:65, 1980.
33. Botero D, Castaño S: Treatment of cysticercosis with praziquantel in Colombia. Am J Trop Med Hyg 31:811, 1982.
34. Lawner PM: Medical management of neurocysticercosis with praziquantel. Bull Clin Neurosci 48:102, 1983.
35. Kori SH, Olds R: PZQ therapy and NMR scans in cerebral cysticercosis. Neurology 34(Suppl 1):89, 1984.
36. Sotelo J, Escobedo F, Rodríguez Carbajal J, et al: Therapy of parenchymal brain cysticercosis with praziquantel. N Engl J Med 310:1001, 1984.
37. Sotelo J, Torres B, Rubio Donnadieu F, et al: Praziquantel in the treatment of neurocysticercosis: Long-term follow-up. Neurology 35:752, 1985.
38. Escobedo F, Penagos P, Rodríguez Carbajal J, et al: Albendazole therapy for neurocysticercosis. Arch Intern Med 147:738–741, 1987.
39. Vazquez V, Sotelo J: The course of seizures after treatment for cerebral cysticercosis. N Engl J Med 327:696–701, 1992.
40. Jung H, Hurtado M, Medina M, et al: Dexamethasone increases plasma levels of albendazole. J Neurol 237:279–280, 1990.

41. Escobedo F: Surgical treatment of neurocysticercosis. In Palacios E, Rodríguez Carbajal J, Taveras J (eds): Cysticercosis of the Central Nervous System. Springfield, IL: Charles C Thomas, 1983, pp 114–148.
42. Kramer L: Medical treatment of cysticercosis-ineffective. Arch Neurol 52:101–102, 1995.
43. Cantú C, Barinagarrementeria F: Cerebrovascular complications of neurocysticercosis. Arch Neurol 53:233–239, 1996.
44. Apuzzo MLJ, Dobkin WR, Chi-Shing Zee, et al: Surgical considerations in the treatment of intraventricular cysticercosis-an analysis of 45 cases. J Neurosurg 60:400, 1984.
45. Stern EW: Neurosurgical considerations of cysticercosis of the central nervous system. J Neurosurg 55:1040–1043, 1981.
46. Neal J: An endoscopic approach to cysticercosis cysts of the posterior third ventricle. Neurosurgery 36:1040–1043, 1995.
47. Seigel RS, Davis LE, Kaplan RJ, et al: CT-guided aspiration of a cysticercotic thalamic cyst. Bull Clin Neurosci 48:48, 1983.
48. Corral I, Quereda C, Moreno A, et al: Intramedullary cysticercosis cured with drug treatment. Spine 21:2284–2287, 1996.

119 Spinal Infections: Vertebral Osteomyelitis and Spinal Epidural Abscess

RICHARD K. OSENBACH and KENNETH LITTLE

INTRODUCTION

Spinal infection encompasses a spectrum of pathologic entities including intervertebral disc space infection, vertebral osteomyelitis (VO), spinal epidural abscess (SEA), spinal subdural empyema, and intramedullary spinal cord abscess. Although each may occur as a separate isolated process, they often occur in combination, especially spinal osteomyelitis and SEA. Disc space infection, VO, and SEA have become fairly common, whereas spinal subdural empyema and spinal cord abscess remain rare. Straightforward uncomplicated cases of vertebral body osteomyelitis and discitis often present insidiously and rarely require emergent neurosurgical intervention. In contrast, classic teaching has generally maintained that SEA represents a neurosurgical emergency. Indeed, there are clearly instances in which prompt diagnosis and urgent neurosurgical intervention are critical to preventing a neurologic catastrophe. Notwithstanding, despite traditional teaching, over the past decade, a progressive trend has been emerging toward nonoperative management of SEA in carefully selected patients with excellent outcomes.

This chapter reviews the diagnosis and management of intraspinal suppuration with the major emphasis on VO and SEA because these conditions are of greatest importance to neurosurgeons. In particular, the emerging role of contemporary neuroimaging techniques is discussed along with the current role of surgery, particularly in light of the more recent trend toward nonoperative management.

EPIDEMIOLOGY OF SPINAL INFECTION

Pyogenic infection of the vertebral column has traditionally been of little concern to neurosurgeons due to its relatively infrequent occurrence. However, the incidence of spinal infection in general has increased over the past two decades, particularly the incidence of VO and SEA. Indeed, a search of the literature from the past 20 years reveals well in excess of 200 publications on VO and SEA. Although now recognized as a distinct clinical entity of growing neurosurgical significance, it was not so long ago that SEA was regarded as a relatively rare condition. Although early series reported an incidence of only one case per 10,000 hospital admissions,[1] more recent reports have clearly demonstrated that the incidence of SEA is on the rise.[2–7] Danner and Hartman[2] noted a 15-fold increase in the incidence of SEA at New York Hospital between 1971 and 1982. During the 3-year period of 1980 to 1982, a case incidence of SEA of 2.8 per 10,000 hospital admissions was recorded compared with 0.18 cases per 10,000 admissions only 10 years earlier. Between 1983 and 1992, Rigamonti and colleagues[6] demonstrated more than a 10-fold increase in the incidence of SEA in the University of Maryland Medical System. During this 10-year period, 75 patients with a discharge diagnosis of SEA were identified among a total of 74,477 admissions, an incidence of 10 cases per 10,000 admissions. Indeed, similar observations have been made at other large institutions.

Among the reasons for this increase include the growth of an elderly population, many of whom have multiple chronic medical conditions, an overall increase in the number of individuals of any age with a chronic debilitating illness (e.g., diabetes, chronic renal failure), a rising incidence of intravenous (IV) drug abuse, increased use of indwelling IV catheters, and an increase in the number of transplant recipients and the use of immunosuppressive drugs in this population. The burgeoning number of complex spinal procedures using instrumentation and the increased use of percutaneous spinal studies and procedures (e.g., discography, epidural steroid injection, spinal cord stimulator implants, long-term epidural catheters for pain management) also have likely contributed to the increased rate of spinal infection. Indeed, the presence of a foreign body in or adjacent to the epidural space and/or introduction of organisms during invasive procedures provide the ideal environment for the development of spinal suppuration. The increased sophistication in neuroimaging techniques such as magnetic resonance imaging (MRI) has not only markedly enhanced the ability to detect these disorders but has allowed earlier diagnosis, thereby avoiding many of the complications that occur with delayed diagnosis. Finally, it is also possible that some perceived increases in incidence may even be related at least partially to referral patterns that tend to concentrate these patients in tertiary care facilities.

PATHOGENESIS AND PATHOPHYSIOLOGY

It has been noted that spontaneous disc space infection is more common in children, whereas pyogenic VO primarily affects adults.[8] This is in large measure related to the blood supply of the vertebral body and intervertebral disc. In children and adolescents, the intervertebral disc receives a direct blood supply through collateral blood vessels that arise from the penetrating nutrient arteries and then penetrate the vertebral end plates as well as from circumferential superficial metaphyseal arteries. By 15 to 20 years of age, these vessels shrink and undergo involution such that in adults there is no longer a direct vascular communication between the vertebral body and intervertebral disc. Consequently, in children, bacteremia usually produces a primary infection of the disc or discitis that most commonly presents as an acute systemic illness. The vertebral body usually becomes involved secondarily when the disc space infection erodes through the vertebral end plates. Due to the absence of a direct blood supply to the disc in adults, the pathogenesis of VO is different. In adults, blood-borne bacteria tend to lodge in the relatively avascular areas adjacent to the subchondral bone where blood flow is sluggish. Hematogenous seeding of the vertebral body can occur through direct arterial seeding by way of nutrient arteries derived from the posterior spinal, intercostal, and lumbar arteries. Alternatively, transient bacteremia from urinary sepsis or instrumentation of the urinary tract may lead to retrograde venous seeding through Batson's epidural venous plexus, which shares numerous connections with the pelvic veins.[9] Once the infection becomes established in the subchondral bone, the vertebral end plates are progressively eroded and destroyed, which allows the infection to secondarily involve the disc. Additionally, anastomoses from one metaphysis to another may allow infection to spread to one or more adjacent vertebral bodies.

VO can affect any level of the spinal axis, although the thoracic and lumbar regions seem to be most often involved. In the authors' series, 70% (28 of 40) of cases involved either the thoracic or lumbar spine[4] and in the series of McHenry and colleagues,[10] of 255 cases, 89% occurred in the thoracic or lumbar spine. Notwithstanding, involvement of the cervical spine is certainly not rare or even uncommon.[10] Rezai and colleagues[11] reported the cervical spine to be the most common site of involvement (44%) in their series of 57 patients. Moreover, spinal infections that occur in IV drug users appear to have some predilection to involve the cervical spine, especially in patients with infections due to *Pseudomonas aeruginosa*.[8]

Spinal epidural abscess can develop in three ways: (1) by direct extension from a contiguous site of infection such as VO, (2) by hematogenous seeding from a remote source of infection (e.g., subacute bacterial endocarditis, long bone osteomyelitis, pulmonary abscess), or (3) by direct contamination during invasive procedures such as spinal surgery, administration of an epidural anesthetic, computed tomography (CT)–guided needle biopsy, or lumbar puncture.[2,3,7,12]

The most common location for SEA is the thoracic spine, followed by the lumbosacral and cervical regions. Although SEA can occur spontaneously, it often develops as a complication of VO, and it is therefore not surprising that the distribution of SEA is similar to that seen in VO. In a large review of 738 patients with SEA collected from the literature, 72% were located in the thoracic or lumbar spine.[7] Danner and Hartman[2] reviewed 139 cases of SEA and found that 119 of 139 cases (86%) involved either the thoracic or lumbar spine; nearly 80% were located in the dorsal half of the spinal canal. Dandy[13] was the first to comment on the regional distribution of SEA. He observed that the majority of cases seemed to involve the thoracic spine and that most occurred dorsally within the spinal canal, and Dandy's early observations have indeed been recapitulated in most published series

of SEA.[2,3,5–7,12] The explanation for this is grounded in the anatomy of the epidural space that Dandy[13] so elegantly described. The spinal epidural space contains loose areolar tissue as well as numerous veins. It is limited to the dorsal aspect of the spinal canal; ventrally, the dura is tightly adherent to the posterior aspect of the vertebral bodies and their ligaments from the first cervical through the second sacral vertebrae. It is only caudal to S2 that the epidural space becomes circumferential, surrounding the dura on all sides.

Another important anatomic factor is the regional variation in the size or depth of the spinal epidural space. In the cervical region, it is more of a potential space that becomes more apparent at the cervicothoracic junction and then becomes[16] wider in a rostral-to-caudal direction, attaining a depth of 0.5 to 0.75 cm between T4 and T8. The space then tapers between approximately T11 and L2 and then again enlarges caudally to attain its greatest depth. The aforementioned anatomic factors account for the rostral-caudal distribution of SEA and the preference for spontaneous abscesses to occur in the dorsal epidural space. Posterior abscesses commonly occur spontaneously, the result of hematogenous seeding of the epidural space from a distant site of infection. Due to a lack of resistance to rostral-caudal spread, these collections not uncommonly extend over multiple vertebral segments and can occasionally involve nearly the entire spinal axis.[14,15] In contrast, longitudinal extension over multiple segments of ventral abscesses that develop secondarily as a complication of an adjacent vertebral body osteomyelitis is usually restricted by the adherence of the dura and is therefore uncommon.[4] However, because of adherence of the ventral dura, an anterior abscess is also more likely to penetrate the dura and lead to subdural empyema and/or spinal cord abscess.

Neurologic dysfunction is common in patients presenting with SEA. The mechanism by which neurologic deficit occurs in patients with SEA has been attributed to a variety of factors including mechanical compression of the neural elements, thrombosis of major arteries, and/or veins supplying and draining the cord, respectively, impairment of the intrinsic microcirculation of the cord, and infectious vasculitis.[2] Unfortunately, there is a paucity of correlative histopathologic data, thereby making it difficult to define the exact pathophysiology in many cases. Because SEA is a space-occupying lesion, it would be intuitive to suggest that mechanical compression should be the most obvious explanation for neurologic deficit. Indeed, mechanical compression is undoubtedly a contributory and often significant factor, but it alone does not adequately explain the profound deficit that frequently occurs in patients with SEA. Indeed, it is not uncommon for the degree of neurologic compromise to be out of proportion to the magnitude of spinal cord compression as demonstrated by imaging studies as well as observations made at the time of surgery.[2,3,12] In fact, in the series of Browder and Meyers[16] of SEA, autopsy evidence failed to reveal any physical deformation of the cord. On the other hand, Baker and colleagues[17] observed extensive destructive changes within the spinal cord that they believed could not be due to mechanical compression alone.

It has been hypothesized that there may be some type of vasculopathy or vascular mechanism to explain the precipitous onset of neurologic deficit in some cases of SEA, although evidence of this is inconsistent. Pathologic vascular changes including congestion and/or thrombosis of pial vessels, inflammation and thrombosis of small arteries and veins within the subarachnoid space, inflammatory infiltrates in the pia directly involving the walls of blood vessels, organized material within the lumen of the anterior spinal artery, and venous thrombosis and infarction of the cord have all been described. However, in some cases, no demonstrable changes involving either arteries or veins can be found.

Although vascular compromise is an attractive theory to explain spinal cord dysfunction in SEA, its validity is not universally accepted. Feldenzer and colleagues[18,19] used an animal model of SEA with *Staphylococcus aureus* as the etiologic agent and failed to find any gross or histopathologic evidence of vascular thrombosis or vasculitis. They concluded that spinal cord dysfunction in SEA is primarily related to compression rather than ischemia and further suggested that arterial and/or venous occlusion occurred only in advanced cases. If in fact these experimental findings accurately reflect those in humans, then it would certainly suggest that in the absence of irreversible spinal cord infarction, urgent surgical decompression *might* promote at least some degree of neurologic recovery. Because neither theory can be absolutely confirmed or refuted, the available evidence would therefore seem to indicate that the cause of spinal cord dysfunction in patients with SEA is likely multifactorial, with both mechanical compression and vascular factors playing a role.

RISKS FACTORS FOR VERTEBRAL OSTEOMYELITIS AND SPINAL EPIDURAL ABSCESS

A number of medical conditions represent risk factors for the development of spinal infection (Table 119-1). Diabetes mellitus has been cited as an important risk factor in patients with VO or SEA.[2–8,20] Approximately 15% of patients with SEA are diabetic.[7] Diabetes alters the host immune response, rendering patients more susceptible to infection, particularly to staphylococcal organisms. IV drug abuse has become

---

TABLE 119-1 ▪ Risk Factors and Medical Conditions Associated with Vertebral Osteomyelitis and Spinal Epidural Abscess

Medical Conditions
Diabetes mellitus
Intravenous drug use
Alcoholism
Malignancy
Chronic renal failure/dialysis
Degenerative spinal disorders

Infections
Soft tissue (e.g., wound infection, skin abscess)
Urosepsis
Pulmonary (e.g., pneumonia, abscess)
Dental/periodontal infection
Endocarditis
Septic arthritis

Invasive Procedures
Spinal surgery
Epidural injections (e.g., anesthesia, steroids, opiods)
Paravertebral injections
Discography
Vascular access procedures

---

increasingly associated with pyogenic spinal infection.[8] This particular population of individuals not only has an increased vulnerability to infection in general, but the practice of using contaminated needles in an often unsanitary environment significantly increases the risk of developing septicemia and bacterial endocarditis, factors that predispose to spinal infection. Chronic ethanol abuse has also been implicated as a risk factor for VO. However, the incidence of ethanol abuse in patients with VO or SEA is generally no higher and often lower than that in the general population, and, therefore, the role of alcohol may be affected by the patient population under consideration. In many cases, alcoholics consume diets deficient in protein that results in compromise of the immune system. It is speculative whether other factors such as poor personal hygiene or other sociologic characteristics play a role in this association. Other illnesses and factors that have been implicated as risk factors for spinal infection include malignancy, an alteration in immunity such as that seen in transplant recipients, and long-term steroid use. Interestingly, although the number of patients with acquired immune deficiency syndrome has steadily increased, there does not seem to have been a concomitant rise in the incidence of SEA in this subpopulation. It has been suggested that nonpenetrating trauma may predispose one to the development of spinal infection, but solid evidence of this association is lacking.

Both VO and SEA most commonly occur as a result of hematogenous seeding from a metastatic source of infection. If carefully sought, a definitive etiology for SEA can be found in 50% to 80% of patients.[2–8] The most common extraspinal sources include skin and/or soft-tissue foci, urinary or respiratory infections, sepsis, intra-abdominal abscess, subacute bacterial endocarditis, dental/periodontal infections, and septic arthritis. It has been suggested that as many as 60% of metastatic infections that occur in association with urosepsis affect the skeleton, with more than 80% affecting the spine. Subacute bacterial endocarditis has been associated with spinal infection, and it might naturally be expected that subacute bacterial endocarditis would be relatively common in patients with spinal infection. Surprisingly, this association was reported in only 1% of 854 patients with SEA.[7] The lack of subacute bacterial endocarditis as a more frequent cause of spinal infection perhaps is likely not due to the fact that subacute bacterial endocarditis does not result in spinal seeding but rather may reflect prompt diagnosis and treatment of subacute bacterial endocarditis with early eradication of a subclinical spinal infection. As noted previously, SEA may develop as a complication of VO. However, in the review by Reihaus and colleagues,[7] only 59 of 854 (7%) cases of SEA were associated with VO, a figure that seems surprisingly low. Finally, more than 20% of patients with SEA have undergone some type of invasive procedure. Although it might be intuitive to assume that spinal surgery would be a significant risk factor, in fact the incidence is quite low. Less than 3% of cases of SEA are preceded by an open surgical procedure on the spine.[7] Spinal infection is actually more common after nonsurgical invasive procedures such as epidural anesthesia, placement of epidural catheters for long-term spinal analgesia, and paravertebral injections.

MICOBIOLOGY OF VERTEBRAL OSTEOMYELITIS AND SPINAL EPIDURAL ABSCESS

There are numerous microorganisms capable of producing spinal infection, some rather uncommon.[8] Both VO and SEA are primarily bacterial infections. The pathogen(s) responsible depends on a number of factors including the etiology of infection and the immunologic status of the host. Fungal infections have been reported but usually occur in immunocompromised patients. Individual cases of parasitic infection have also been reported, but these tend to occur in certain geographic regions where parasitic infections are endemic. When adequate culture material is obtained and meticulous diligent microbiologic isolation techniques applied, a causative organism(s) can be identified in more than 90% of patients with spinal infection.[2–8,10] McHenry and colleagues[10] reported a 100% isolation rate in 255 patients with VO. Of 850 patients with SEA, a causative organism(s) was identified in 93% of cases.[7] Not surprisingly, the bacteriologic profiles of VO and SEA are relatively similar (Table 119-2). Gram-positive organisms are isolated in nearly two thirds of patients with VO but account for more than 80% of cases of SEA.[10] S. aureus is by far the most common pathogen, accounting for 56% of cases of VO but more than 75% of cases of SEA. S. aureus is implicated in the majority of cases secondary to skin and soft-tissue infections, in cases related to IV drug use, and infections that occur after spinal surgery.[10] S. aureus is also the most common organism encountered in cases occurring in young children. Gram-negative infections have been recognized with increasing frequency and for some reason seem to be more common in patients with VO than SEA.[7,10] Escherichia coli is responsible for approximately 47% to 54% of all gram-negative infections, although other gram-negative organisms such as Enterobacter sp., Proteus sp., and Pseudomonas sp. are not uncommonly found, with Pseudomonas appearing to be especially prominent in IV drug abusers.[8] In contrast to pyogenic brain abscess, anaerobic spinal infection is less common. Less than 10% of cases of VO and less than 1% of cases of SEA are caused by anaerobic bacteria. The incidence of tuberculous involvement of the spine mirrors that of tuberculosis in general. Although the incidence of tuberculous infection of the spine has sharply declined in this country, in some parts of the world, tuberculosis remains the most common cause of VO.

Effective treatment of VO or SEA obviously hinges on identification of the causative organism such that specific antibiotic therapy can be employed. Ideally, diagnostic cultures should come from the affected vertebral body and/or disc, from contiguous paravertebral tissues (i.e., psoas abscess), the epidural space, or from blood cultures.[8] Indeed, in the majority of cases, a diagnostic culture can usually be obtained from at least one of these sources. Multiple blood cultures should be obtained in all patients with suspected spinal infection. Blood cultures are positive in as many as 77% of patients with VO and may occasionally represent the only source from which the causative microorganism can be retrieved.[4,8,11] Cultures from other infectious foci suspected of being the source of infection should also be obtained and may in fact yield the organism responsible for the spinal infection. However, therapy should generally not be based entirely on cultures obtained from a remote extraspinal site because occasionally this may not represent the infecting organism.

Cultures from the vertebral body or intervertebral disc can usually be obtained relatively easily by CT-guided percutaneous aspiration/biopsy. The diagnostic yield of percutaneous aspiration varies from less than 50% to approximately 70%.[4,8,10,11] Ideally, antibiotics should be withheld until cultures have been obtained because this will obviously improve the chances of obtaining a positive culture. There may be multiple reasons that a particular biopsy is negative including the influence of antibiotic therapy, inaccurate needle placement, or inadequate specimens. However, the relative role of these factors is not clear in the literature. Consequently, if the initial percutaneous biopsy specimen fails to produce a diagnosis, strong consideration should be given to repeating the percutaneous biopsy a second and perhaps even a third time, especially in the absence of a positive blood culture. Every effort should be made to discontinue all antibiotics unless the patient is being treated for some other serious systemic infection. Indeed, a percutaneous procedure is less invasive and associated with less morbidity than an open surgical procedure, especially in patients with multiple underlying comorbidities. If multiple percutaneous biopsies fail to yield a diagnosis and blood cultures are negative but an obvious potential source of infection has been identified (e.g., urinary tract infection), then a decision must be made whether to perform an open surgical procedure or treat the patient based on the best available information, namely, a

---

TABLE 119-2 ▪ **Bacteriological Profile in Patients with Vertebral Osteomyelitis and Spinal Epidural Abscess**

Organism	Vertebral Osteomyelitis	Spinal Epidural Abscess
Total patients	356*	814[†]
Cultures negative	NS	61 (7.5%)
Gram-positive cocci	236 (66.3%)	679 (83.4%)
Staphylococci	201 (56.5%)	621 (76.3%)
Streptococci	35 (9.8%)	58 (7.1%)
Gram-negative organisms	89 (25%)	55 (6.7%)
Miscellaneous organisms	13 (3.7%)	19 (2.3%)
Anaerobes	10 (2.8%)	6 (0.7%)
Polymicrobial infection	26 (7.3%)	27 (3.3%)

*Percentages based on 358 episodes of in 356 patients (data from McHenry et al.[10] and Fischer et al.[20]).
   †Percentages based on 753 patients with positive cultures of a total of 814 patients (data from Reihaus et al.[7]).

positive culture from a remote source. This particular judgment must be made on a case-by-case basis taking into consideration the overall medical condition of the patient, the potential morbidity of an open surgical procedure, and the potential problems of long-term treatment with multiple empirical antibiotics. Therefore, if multiple attempts at percutaneous biopsy fail to produce a diagnostic culture, and there are no complicating factors such as spinal instability or progressive neurologic deficit, then it would seem reasonable to initiate antibiotics as long as there is positive blood culture or at the very least a positive culture from a concomitant site of infection. Although this approach may not be ideal, it may be perfectly reasonable depending on the individual situation. The patient should be carefully observed for a clinical response and/or a decrease in the erythrocyte sedimentation rate (ESR). If after several weeks of what should be appropriate therapy, there appears to be little or no response, antibiotics should be discontinued for at least 48 hours and an open procedure performed to obtain appropriate cultures.

CLINICAL PRESENTATION

Perhaps the most important aspect regarding the clinical presentation of patients with VO and SEA is its variability. Early findings can be subtle and may often be overshadowed by the presence of one or more underlying illnesses that may dominate the clinical picture. Consequently, the initial diagnosis in patients with VO or SEA is not infrequently erroneous.[7,8] In fact, in the review of Danner and Hartman,[2] the correct diagnosis was initially made in only 19 of 109 (17%) patients who eventually were found to have an SEA. Although the most mistaken diagnoses are meningitis and intervertebral disc prolapse, a whole host of both neurologic and nonneurologic diagnoses have been entertained.[7] Thus a high index of suspicion is required to make an early and accurate diagnosis and prevent the development of neurologic dysfunction.

The clinical course of both conditions is not uncommonly insidious in onset and relatively indolent but occasionally may be more acute and rapidly progressive. As discussed previously, uncomplicated VO tends to present as a more acute illness with systemic signs in children, whereas adults usually have a more chronic indolent course. The duration of symptoms ranges from as little as 1 week to as long as 8 months.[4,10,11] In general, most patients with uncomplicated VO experience symptoms on average for 1 to 2 months before the diagnosis is made, although the duration of symptoms may be significantly shorter in cases complicated by spinal instability or epidural abscess. Local spinal pain that is aggravated by motion along with exquisite spinal tenderness are almost uniformly present. As many as one third of patients with VO also relate a prominent radicular component.[4,10,11] Fever is present in 48% to 78% of patients at the time of diagnosis, although fever is often a manifestation of systemic infection. Examination of the spine universally reveals localized spinal tenderness, spasm of the paraspinous muscles, and limited range of motion. Delay in diagnosis can lead to neurologic complications related to secondary SEA and/or spinal instability in 25% to 50% of patients. Because the diagnosis is often initially missed, neurologic findings are seen in as many as 50% of patients at the time of diagnosis.[4] The incidence of neurologic deficit is not surprisingly greatest in patients with cervical or thoracic disease and significantly lower in patients with lumbar involvement.[4,10] Although neurologic deficit is most often due to compression of the spinal cord or cauda equina, motor deficits can also occur secondary to a paravertebral abscess affecting the lumbosacral plexus within the retroperitoneum.

The variability in clinical presentation of SEA is related to multiple of factors including the tempo of progression of the infection, the region of the spine involved, whether the infection is related to hematogenous seeding or extension of a local process, the host immune status, and the pathogenicity or virulence of the infectious agent.[8]

Heusner[1] provided the classic description of the clinical presentation of SEA, of four phases that generally evolve in sequence: (1) spinal pain; (2) radicular pain; (3) muscular weakness, sensory loss, sphincter dysfunction; and finally (4) complete paralysis. The rapidity with which one stage progresses to another in a given patient depends on the factors previously outlined. Progression from spinal and radicular pain to neurologic dysfunction tends to occur more rapidly with spontaneous abscesses that result from hematogenous seeding in which systemic manifestations are often a prominent part of the clinical picture. On the other hand, cases of SEA that result from local extension of adjacent VO usually evolve at a slower pace, often progressing over weeks or even months until the infection becomes clinically apparent.

Spinal pain is also universally present with SEA and like VO is associated with localized spinal tenderness to palpation or percussion. Once initiated, the pain becomes progressively more severe and intractable. More than 90% of patients develop radicular pain, which usually follows the onset of spinal pain by several days but in some cases may actually precede the onset of spinal pain. Depending on the level of spinal involvement, radicular pain may mimic a variety of other conditions including classic sciatica due to a herniated disc, an acute abdominal process, herpes zoster, or even myocardial infarction.[2,7] Fever that exceeds 38°C is present at some point during the course of the illness in 66% to 75% of patients, irrespective of whether the presentation is acute or chronic. In patients with a chronic clinical course, constitutional symptoms such as weight loss and malaise are not unusual. The presence of headache and/or nuchal rigidity may reflect the presence of a parameningeal reaction or in some cases frank meningitis. It must be cautioned that the characteristic features of SEA may not be prominent in children and the clinical picture may be dominated by nonspecific findings such as fever, malaise, irritability, headache, and vomiting.[21] Reluctance of the child to lie prone, irritability with movement, and rigidity of the spine may be the only clues to the diagnosis before the onset of neurologic deficit.

Unfortunately, the diagnosis of SEA is all too frequently made after the onset of neurologic dysfunction, which occurs in as many as 90% of patients in some clinical series.[7] As many as 75% of patients with SEA may have some degree of motor weakness, which may be unilateral or bilateral or involve a single extremity. Sensory loss is usually incomplete and may occur in a radicular pattern or present as a discrete sensory level. However, complete loss of all sensory modalities is associated with a very poor prognosis. The point at which neurologic dysfunction begins is especially critical because, once initiated, the time from onset of weakness to complete paralysis often is less than 24 hours and can occur in as little as 30 minutes, a feature of SEA that emphasizes the need for rapid diagnosis and emergent surgical intervention. Furthermore, the patient who presents with a chronic clinical course should not engender a feeling of complacency because these patients can also deteriorate rapidly.

The differential diagnosis includes other more common conditions that share some of the clinical features of epidural infection. Acute transverse myelitis, 8 to 20 times more common than SEA, should be part of the differential diagnosis in patients with back pain, fever, and progressive neurologic deficit.[2] Transverse myelitis customarily differs in that back pain is somewhat less prominent and the progression to maximal neurologic deficit is often more rapid than in SEA. Currently, the routine use of MRI in this setting should easily differentiate the two conditions. However, if MRI is unavailable, myelography will reveal a complete or partial block in patients with SEA but will be unremarkable in cases of transverse myelitis.

Metastatic neoplasms of the spine frequently invade the epidural space and may present a picture similar to a chronic epidural abscess. In particular, lymphoma may metastasize to the spine in as many as 5% of cases; fever and systemic manifestations, which are common with lymphoma, may further confuse the clinical picture. Spontaneous intraspinal hematomas can also occasionally occur and mimic the presentation of SEA.

LABORATORY FINDINGS

Generally speaking, routine laboratory investigation is for the most part nonspecific and is therefore not particularly helpful in establishing the diagnosis of spinal infection. As previously discussed, blood cultures are often positive in patients with spinal infection and should be obtained routinely, along with cultures from any other potential source of infection. Otherwise, elevation of the ESR (normal, 0 to 20 mm/hour), although nonspecific, is the most constant laboratory abnormality in patients with VO or SEA.[2–8] An elevated ESR is certainly not diagnostic of infection but can be helpful in supporting or perhaps more importantly excluding the diagnosis in the appropriate clinical setting. Mean values generally range between 40 and 145 mm/hour. Spinal infection would indeed be unusual in the presence of a completely normal ESR, but it should be noted that falsely low values can occur in patients with polycythemia or hyperproteinemia. The ESR is more valuable in monitoring the progress of therapy than in establishing a diagnosis. Typically, patients with VO receiving effective antibiotic therapy will demonstrate a consistent downward trend in the ESR as treatment progresses.[4] In a large series of patients successfully treated for VO, the ESR fell to two thirds (67%) of pretreatment values in all patients and to less than 50% of pretreatment values in the majority of patients by the completion of antibiotic treatment.[8] The ESR does not always return to normal even in successfully treated patients, but a declining trend should generally be observed, unless the ESR remains elevated due to the presence of some other inflammatory process. Furthermore, absolute values of the ESR must be interpreted with caution because despite successful therapy, the ESR may remain

elevated to varying degrees for as long as 6 months in as many as 75% of patients and does not in and of itself necessarily indicate treatment failure or dictate the need for further antibiotic therapy.

The peripheral white blood cell count is usually normal or only slightly elevated (10,000 to 13,000 mm³) in patients with uncomplicated VO or SEA and shows no significant trend with therapy.[4,8] Significant leukocytosis generally indicates an active systemic infection. There is considerable information in the older literature regarding cerebrospinal fluid (CSF) analysis, particularly in patients with SEA. The CSF usually shows evidence of a parameningeal process manifested by pleocytosis, elevated protein, and normal glucose. However, the CSF can also be entirely normal or reveal frank pus consistent with accompanying bacterial meningitis. However, because CSF analysis usually adds little information, lumbar puncture should be discouraged in patients with SEA, especially those with a dorsal lumbar abscess due to the risk of introducing bacteria into the CSF. If there are clinical features to suggest a meningitis and imaging studies show the lumbar region to be uninvolved, then CSF can be obtained safely. Alternatively, if the lumbar region is involved and a CSF sample is critical to instituting therapy for meningitis, CSF can be obtained in most patients by a radiographically guided C1–2 puncture.

RADIOGRAPHIC STUDIES

Imaging studies of the spine represent the cornerstone of diagnosis for both VO and SEA. A plain film examination of the spine should be performed in all patients with suspected VO or SEA. Plain radiographs are helpful in localizing the level and extent of the lesion and in assessing the extent of deformity, if present. Unfortunately, early in the course of VO, plain radiographs may be entirely normal and provide little or no clue to the diagnosis. The earliest finding on plain radiographs is narrowing of the intervertebral disc space, which occasionally can be seen as early as 2 weeks after the onset of symptoms but more frequently appears 6 to 8 weeks into the illness.[10,11,22,23] As the infection continues, there is progressive vertebral body destruction accompanied by a variable degree of paravertebral inflammatory reaction. In severe cases, there is sufficient destruction of the vertebral body that partial collapse and spinal instability occur. Sclerosis, new bone formation, and finally fusion occur late as the infection resolves and healing takes place. Fusion may not be evident radiographically for as long as 1 year, and in some cases may require 5 years. In patients who fail to achieve bony fusion, a fibrous union usually functions equally effectively. Unfortunately, the characteristic sequence of radiographic changes often lags well behind the clinical presentation and is frequently not helpful in establishing an early diagnosis.

CT has become an important imaging modality in the diagnosis of spinal infection in general and VO in particular. CT provides excellent detail of the bony anatomy and the paravertebral soft tissues. CT readily demonstrates the lytic destructive changes within the vertebral body as well as gas within the disc space or soft tissues (Fig. 119-1). The paravertebral soft-tissue swelling that accompanies osteomyelitis usually completely surrounds the spine ventrally, a feature that is often helpful in differentiating an infectious from a

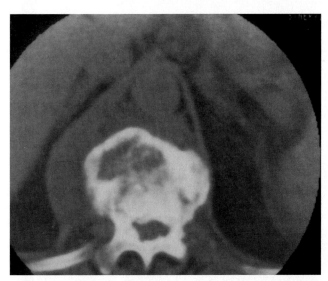

FIGURE 119-1 Axial computed tomography scan in a patient with vertebral osteomyelitis. Note the destructive changes of the vertebral body as well as the paravertebral soft-tissue reaction.

neoplastic process. In the latter, there is usually minimal to no soft-tissue reaction. Also, the bony changes produced by tumors may often involve the posterior elements, a finding that is uncommon in osteomyelitis.[4] Although identification of SEA has been reported using CT alone, it is generally thought that plain CT is not particularly sensitive for demonstrating SEA.[24] Now, given the availability of MRI, CT is probably most valuable in performing image-guided percutaneous biopsies of the vertebral body and paravertebral tissues to obtain culture material. It is also effective in performing aspiration of paravertebral abscesses. Image-guided CT biopsy has been shown to be safe and effective in obtaining diagnostic material at all levels of the spine.

MRI has become the single most important imaging modality in the evaluation of infectious and inflammatory diseases of the spine.[25–27] There are distinct advantages of MRI over other imaging modalities including its ability to perform multiplanar imaging and to directly visualize the paraspinal soft tissues and spinal cord as well as being noninvasive. Additionally, the abnormalities seen on MRI in patients with VO usually become apparent long before the findings that can be detected on plain radiographs. Modic and colleagues[25,26] described the classic MRI findings of VO. Typically, T1-weighted images reveal a confluent region of decreased signal intensity in the affected vertebral body with loss of delineation of the end plates from the intervertebral disc, whereas spin echo T2-weighted sequences reveal increased signal intensity in the disc and end plates along with loss of the normal internuclear cleft (Fig. 119-2). These changes mostly result from the increased water content of the tissue that occurs from the inflammatory process and associated tissue ischemia. The T1-weighted sequences primarily provide morphologic information (e.g., presence of SEA, paravertebral soft abnormalities); the T2-weighted images are more sensitive to the presence of increased water content within the bone or disc. There is often little or no soft-tissue contrast between the involved bone, interspace, and paravertebral and epidural soft tissues in which cases gradient echo

sequences may prove helpful. Administration of gadolinium often shows enhancement of the affected vertebral body and disc.

MRI has essentially supplanted CT myelography in the evaluation of patients with suspected SEA. Not only is MRI as sensitive as CT myelography, but the numerous advantages of MRI noted previously significantly expand the ability to differentiate SEA from other conditions included in the differential diagnosis including neoplastic disease, disc herniation, intraspinal hematoma, spinal cord infarction, syringomyelia, and transverse myelitis. In patients with a ventral abscess associated with VO, T1-weighted images typically demonstrate a soft-tissue mass with tapering edges at the rostral and caudal poles that displaces the thecal sac away from the posterior aspect of the vertebral body. Occasionally, the abscess may look indented by the confines of the posterior longitudinal ligament. Spontaneously occurring posterior abscesses have a greater tendency to extend over multiple spinal segments, and cases have been described with involvement of nearly the entire spinal axis. It has been suggested that it may be possible to differentiate frank pus from granulation tissue with MRI.[28] In the cases cited, more discrete areas of increased signal intensity on T2-weighted images were believed to correspond with liquid pus. Administration of gadolinium results in enhancement of chronic granulation tissue, but there is usually little to no enhancement of the abscess cavity itself. In the authors' experience, there has not been any consistent correlation between MRI findings and the consistency of the epidural infection. Practically, this differentiation may not be terribly important because both liquid pus and granulation tissue are equally capable of causing neural compression, and surgical decompression may be required regardless. Radionuclide imaging with technetium, gallium-67, and indium-111 may provide a valuable adjunct to diagnosis, particularly for VO, especially before changes on plain radiographs become evident. In cases of VO, technetium scans generally show a diffuse uptake of tracer in the region of infection (Fig. 119-3). Technetium scans have a fairly high sensitivity of approximately 90%, but a specificity of only 78% and an accuracy of 86%.[25] The probability of a positive study is increased with the duration of symptoms and in long-standing cases approaches 100%. However, false-negative scans do occur, particularly in children and elderly patients. Gallium scanning has a sensitivity roughly equivalent to that of technetium (89%), a specificity of 85%, and an accuracy of 86% in the diagnosis of spinal infection. Diagnostic accuracy can be improved to approximately 94% by combining technetium and gallium imaging. Indium-111 leukocyte labeling has proven helpful in the evaluation of soft-tissue infections as well as infections involving the appendicular skeleton. Unfortunately, indium scans have not been found to be particularly beneficial in the diagnosis of spinal infection. This may be due to the fact that many cases of VO are chronic by the time they come to clinical attention and the inflammatory response may have a paucity of leukocytes. Overall, the sensitivity of indium scans is only 17%, the specificity approximately 100%, and the accuracy 31%. Single photon emission tomography has also been shown to be a sensitive scintigraphic modality for the early detection of spondylitis, although the role of this modality has yet to be determined.[29]

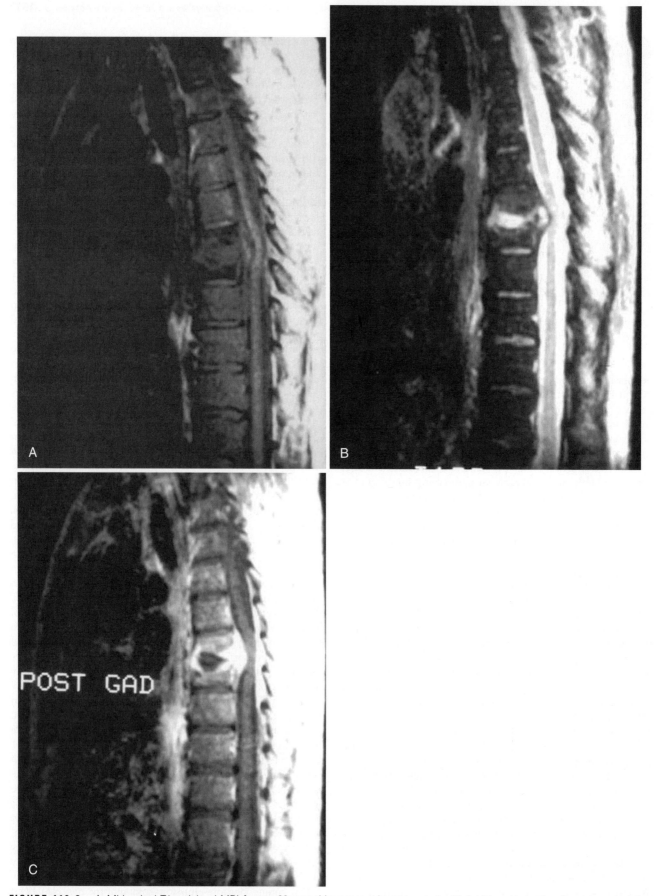

FIGURE 119-2 *A,* Midsagittal T1-weighted MRI from a 62-year-old woman who presented with midthoracic back pain and myelopathy. There is decreased signal intensity of the involved vertebral bodies. The spinal cord is draped over a ventral mass representing a combination of retropulsed bone and induration of the posterior longitudinal ligament. *B,* The T2-weighted sequence reveals increased signal intensity of the involved vertebral bodies, particularly of the intervertebral disc. After administration of gadolinium (*C*), there is enhancement within the vertebral body and the ventral epidural abscess is more clearly defined.

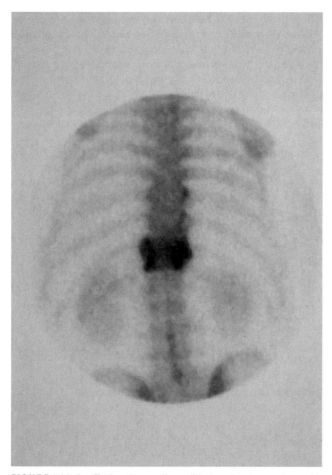

FIGURE 119-3 Technetium radionuclide imaging in a patient with vertebral osteomyelitis shows focal uptake of the radiotracer at the involved level.

MANAGEMENT OF VERTEBRAL OSTEOMYELITIS AND SPINAL EPIDURAL ABSCESS

The management of patients with VO and SEA is not uniform, and controversy exists regarding the role of surgery, the optimal surgical procedure, and the duration and route of antibiotic therapy. Although SEA was once considered exclusively a surgical disease, there has been a recent move toward nonsurgical treatment in selected patients.

Antibiotic Therapy

Antibiotic therapy represents one of the cornerstones of treatment of VO and SEA. Whenever possible, and particularly in the absence of any serious systemic infection, antibiotics should be withheld until cultures have been obtained. Institution of empirical antibiotics before obtaining cultures will considerably reduce the chances of recovering the offending organism and may unnecessarily commit the patient to long-term therapy with multiple agents rather than with a single agent directed toward the specific organism. However, if there are signs of rapid neurologic deterioration either due to the spinal infection itself or in unusual circumstance to secondary bacterial meningitis, and all cultures cannot be immediately obtained, the risk of a negative culture is far outweighed by the overwhelming requirement to begin immediate treatment for a life-threatening infection. In such cases, the choice of antibiotics should be made according to the most likely organism based on the presumed etiology of infection. Once the presence of spinal infection (VO or SEA) has been established and all appropriate cultures have been obtained, antibiotics should be initiated. Before culture results are available, empirical therapy should be broad spectrum including coverage of staphylococci, gram-negative organisms, and anaerobes.[8] A reasonable combination of agents might include vancomycin or nafcillin, a third-generation cephalosporin, and metronidazole. Once the organism(s) has been identified, therapy can be tailored specifically to the pathogen. In general, antibiotics should be used that are known to achieve therapeutic levels in the spine such that bacteriocidal levels can be achieved.

The dose, route, and duration of antibiotic therapy advocated by various investigators for the treatment of VO and SEA have been extremely variable.[2–8,10,11] Indeed, there are no prospective, randomized, controlled studies comparing various treatment regimens. For treatment of VO, some authors advocate 6 to 8 weeks of parenteral antibiotics only, whereas others propose 4 to 8 weeks of parenteral therapy followed by oral therapy of varying duration. In the review of Sapico and Montgomerie[8] of 162 patients with VO, 33% of patients who received no antibiotics either died or had prolonged morbidity related to their disease. Patients who received less than 4 weeks of parenteral therapy either failed treatment outright or relapsed significantly more often than those who received more than 4 weeks of parenteral antibiotics ($p < 0.05$ by χ^2 analysis). Consequently, for patients with uncomplicated VO, Sapico and Montgomerie[8] have advocated 8 weeks of IV antibiotics *without* further oral therapy as adequate treatment. In a long-term study of 253 patients with VO, McHenry and colleagues[10] also noted poor outcomes in patients treated for less than 4 weeks. Moreover, we noted no difference in symptomatic and neurologic outcomes or recurrent infection between patients treated for 8 weeks compared with those treated longer than 8 weeks.[4] Therefore, based on our own observations as well as those of others, the efficacy of complementary oral therapy at best remains unclear and is probably not necessary in most cases.

The duration of antibiotic therapy recommended in the literature for SEA has also been variable. However, most authors advocate at least a 4- to 6-week course of IV therapy.[6] In the presence of VO, the duration of IV therapy should be extended to 8 weeks.[4] Although some authors recommend additional oral therapy for as long as several months, the necessity or benefit of this practice is not clear.

Role of Immobilization

Spinal immobilization has traditionally played an integral role in the treatment of VO. It is clearly indicated in cases of documented or impending spinal instability. However, in the absence of overt spinal instability, the absolute need for and duration of immobilization is unclear. The main goal of immobilization in uncomplicated cases is to reduce pain and prevent postinfection spinal deformity, the risk of which is increased with involvement of two adjacent vertebral bodies or greater than 50% reduction in height of a single vertebral body. The senior author (R.O.) employs external immobilization in all patients with VO until pain is either gone or minimal. For infections of the thoracic or lumbar spine, a custom-molded acrylic orthosis is preferred, whereas in the cervical spine, the orthosis used depends on the level involved, the presence of instability, and whether the patient has undergone surgery.

Surgery for Vertebral Osteomyelitis

The role of surgery in uncomplicated cases of VO remains controversial. Many authors believe that uncomplicated cases can be effectively managed with antibiotics and immobilization with good outcomes and minimum morbidity. Others think that surgery has a more primary role in treatment, citing a lower incidence of postinfection spinal deformity, a reduction in recurrent infection, avoidance of neurologic deficit, and an earlier return to a functional capacity in support of their position. The major indications for surgery include the following: (1) to obtain a bacteriologic diagnosis when closed biopsy is deemed unsafe or when multiple adequately performed closed biopsies have been negative, blood cultures are negative, and no other source of infection is apparent; (2) when a significant abscess is present causing unremitting fever and systemic signs of sepsis; (3) in cases refractory to adequate nonoperative management in which the ESR remains markedly elevated or there is persistence of significant spinal pain; (4) in the presence of neurologic deficit due to spinal cord compression; and (5) in cases associated with significant vertebral body destruction and spinal deformity, especially in the cervical spine.[21,22]

Spinal deformity and instability occur in 2% to 28% of patients with VO, although not all kyphotic deformities result in neurologic compromise. In pyogenic disease, bony involvement usually includes the anterior and middle columns, and posterior column involvement is distinctly unusual in the absence of previous surgery. Spinal deformity begins with a loss of anterior column height and progresses to kyphosis. In very advanced cases, severe translational deformity and even complete dislocation may occur. Therefore, posterior decompressive procedures are usually contraindicated in this condition unless they are combined with circumferential reconstruction of the spine.[23] Indeed, in such instances, an unstabilized laminectomy will almost always exacerbate the problem (Fig. 119-4). The goal in such cases is to restore the integrity of the anterior column with a weight-bearing construct.[23] If in fact the posterior column is intact and deformity is limited to kyphosis or loss of lordosis, then an anterior-only reconstruction should be sufficient. However, if the posterior column is deficient from previous surgery, then both anterior and posterior reconstruction is necessary.

In most cases that come to surgery, at least one and usually both of the involved vertebrae have little viable structure left after débridement. This requires a two-level corpectomy/three-level discectomy to completely débride the diseased bone and to expose end plates that are strong enough to supportive a reconstructive strut.[23] Anterior column reconstruction can be performed using autologous iliac graft.[11,23] More recently, longitudinal titanium cages packed with cancellous iliac autograft or allograft have been used successfully at all levels of the spine.[23] In cases with posterior element integrity, the cages placed between

T7 and L4 can be stabilized with a rigid anterior device. Above T7, a single rod can be placed laterally and then supplemented with rigid double rods posteriorly. If L5 must be included in the construct, posterior segmental instrumentation should be applied to the sacrum. In the cervical spine, anterior buttress plates may be placed across the cage. If there is absence or loss of posterior element integrity, posterior instrumentation should be added to the anterior construct.[23]

It has been traditionally taught that instrumentation should be avoided in the presence of infection. Indeed, it is generally thought by many individuals that a foreign body may perpetuate the infection. However, over the past several years, an increasing number of authors have reported the successful use of instrumentation without sequelae as long as all obviously infected material has been removed[22,23] (Fig. 119-5). Indeed, reoperation for recurrence or removal of infected hardware would appear to be a relatively minor problem. Although the decision whether to use instrumentation in the presence of infection must be weighed case by case, there are two key features of the disease that would prompt consideration for spinal instrumentation: (1) whether the infectious process has destroyed bone to render the spine unstable under physiologic loading and (2) whether the surgical procedure itself has rendered the spine unstable.

Surgery for Spinal Epidural Abscess

Traditionally, the management of SEA has consisted of immediate surgery followed by antibiotic therapy of variable duration. Surgical management of SEA clearly has advantages. Most important is the ability to decompress compromised neural tissues, thereby preventing further neurologic deterioration. Devitalized tissue that acts as a nidus for infection can also be removed, allowing antibiotics to function more efficiently. Additionally, intraoperative cultures taken from the epidural space in some cases may be the only source from which the organism can be cultured. This can be extremely important in terms of choosing the appropriate antibiotic regimen.

The type of surgical procedure chosen obviously depends on the site of neural compression, the location within the spinal axis, and the overall medical condition of the patient. Under most circumstances, the procedure should be based on the site of maximal compression. For spontaneous abscesses that are located dorsally and not associated with VO, a laminectomy over the involved levels will generally provide adequate decompression (Fig. 119-6). In most cases, the abscess does not extend over more than three or four segments of the spine, and in such cases, laminectomy can easily be performed over the entire area of involvement. All purulent material should be removed through gentle suction and warm irrigation. In some patients with more chronic abscesses, there may be a significant component of granulation tissue that is often relatively adherent to the dura. If patience is exercised, this can be dissected free in most cases. It is usually better to leave a small amount of granulation on the dura than to risk a dural tear and contamination of the subarachnoid space. If all purulent material has been thoroughly removed, it is the authors' preference to perform primary closure of the wound without a drain because there is no evidence that leaving a drain will lessen the chance of recurrence.

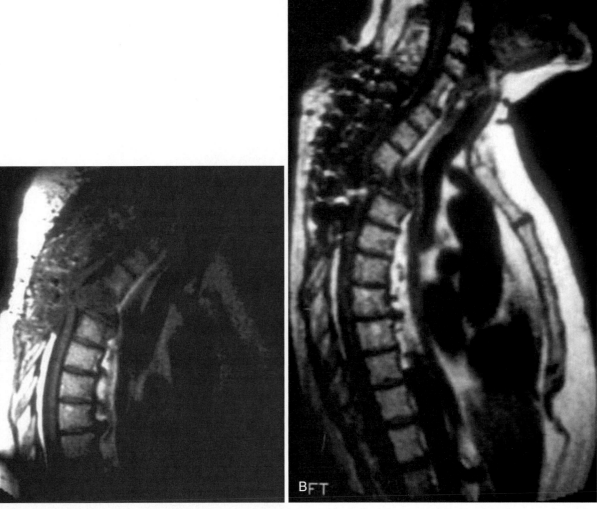

FIGURE 119-4   *A*, T1-weighted magnetic resonance image from a 67-year-old woman who presented with fever, thoracic pain, and mild lower extremity weakness. Note the extensive destruction of the vertebral body and the ventral epidural mass that displaces and deforms the cord. She underwent a laminectomy after which a decline in neurologic function was demonstrated. *B*, Postoperative magnetic resonance imaging demonstrates instability with retrolisthesis of the rostral vertebral body. She subsequently underwent further surgery for spinal stabilization with improvement in neurologic function.

Some patients occasionally develop an SEA that extends over many segments and in rare cases involves the entire spinal axis. In such cases, it is not feasible to perform a laminectomy over the entire spine. Schulz and colleagues[15] have described a minimally invasive technique for decompression of abscesses that extend over a long distance. The technique involves performing a one- or two-segment laminectomy at the most rostral and caudal levels of the abscess. A Fogarty No. 5 catheter can then be advanced into the epidural space until the balloon is visualized at the other laminectomy site. The balloon is inflated with 1 to 1.5 mL of air and then slowly and gently withdrawn until it reaches the insertion site, allowing purulent material to be "milked" from the epidural space. The procedure is then repeated until purulent material has been adequately removed. The authors have used this technique in two

patients and found that two passes of the inflated catheter were sufficient. Although this technique is attractive, it obviously must be used with delicacy and caution and its use should probably be limited to acute abscesses that consist primarily of liquid pus.

Percutaneous CT-guided aspiration has also been reported as a minimally invasive technique for drainage of SEA.[14,30,31] Percutaneous aspiration is a technique that in effect bridges the gap between open surgical treatment and nonoperative medical therapy and offers an alternative to surgery in selected patients. Percutaneous aspiration is effective only for posterior abscesses that primarily contain liquid pus. It is obviously contraindicated for ventral abscesses. The major obvious complication is inadvertent penetration of the dura with contamination of the CSF and development of meningitis. Although this technique has been used relatively

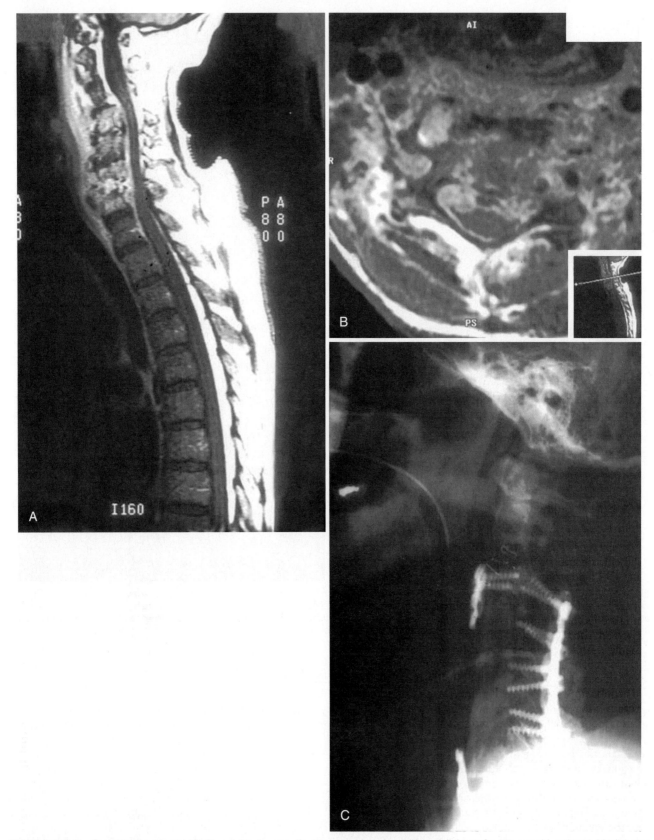

FIGURE 119-5 Sagittal (*A*) and axial (*B*) T1-weighted magnetic resonance imaging with gadolinium of a 54-year-old patient with diabetes who presented with a 2-week history of neck pain, fever, and quadriparesis. His erythrocyte sedimentation rate was 85 mm/hour. There is involvement of several vertebral bodies with cord compression due to an associated ventral epidural abscess. At surgery, the majority of the abscess consisted of granulation tissue with only a small amount of liquid pus that was completely removed. This patient was managed with a multilevel corpectomy and fusion with both anterior and posterior spinal instrumentation (*C*) without complications.

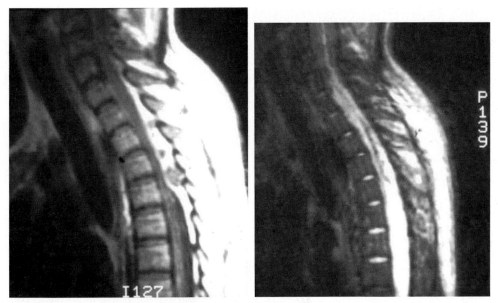

FIGURE 119-6   Mid-sagittal T1-weighted magnetic resonance imaging with gadolinium of a 22-year-old intravenous drug user who presented with fever, back pain, and paraparesis. This study demonstrates a spontaneous dorsally located epidural abscess extending over multiple levels. Note the absence of any changes associated with osteomyelitis. The patient underwent decompressive laminectomy and evacuation of a mostly liquid epidural abscess that grew *Pseudomonas aeruginosa*. After 8 weeks of intravenous antibiotics, she recovered full neurologic function.

infrequently, the success rate in terms of pain relief and resolution of the abscess appears to be good.

Although SEA has traditionally been considered a surgical disease, there has been an increasing tendency toward more conservative nonoperative treatment of this condition.[2,5,6,7,31,32] This approach is predicated on early identification of the organism such that specific antibiotic therapy can be initiated. The characteristics of patients with SEA for whom nonoperative therapy might be considered include (1) patients who are neurologically intact or have minimal neurologic findings, (2) patients in whom the surgical morbidity is unacceptable high, (3) patients with extensive spinal involvement, and (4) patients who have been paraplegic for more than 48 hours.[6] A more conservative approach

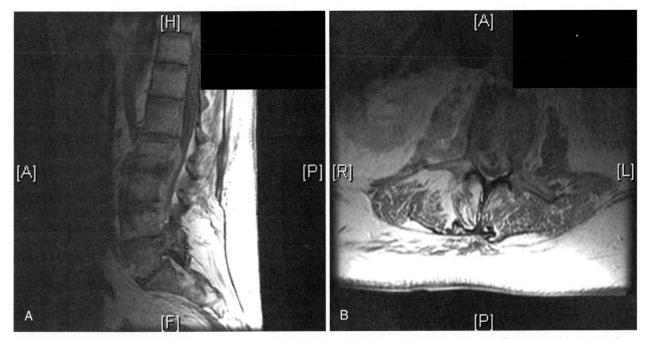

FIGURE 119-7   This 66-year-old morbidly obese woman with diabetes, hypertension, chronic renal insufficiency, and osteoporosis was transferred after being hospitalized for more than 8 weeks with spinal and abdominal pain. She presented with slightly less than antigravity function in the lower extremities that had been present and stable for the entire 8 weeks, and she was nonambulatory. Sagittal T1-weighted magnetic resonance imaging with gadolinium (A) shows changes consistent with osteomyelitis from L2 to L4. A ventral epidural abscess is well seen on the axial views (B).

(Continued)

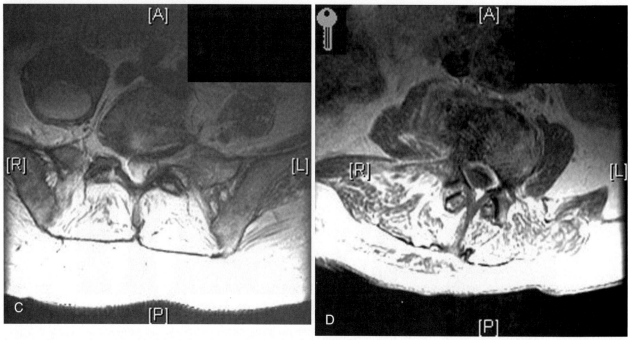

FIGURE 119-7 Cont'd There is also a large paravertebral abscess within the right psoas muscle. This abscess was drained using percutaneous computed tomography guidance; cultures revealed *Staphylococcus aureus*. Given her significant comorbidity and the fact that her condition had been stable for more than 2 months, she was treated nonoperatively with 12 weeks of intravenous antibiotics. She became asymptomatic, and her neurologic function slowly improved. One year after diagnosis and treatment, she is asymptomatic and has a normal neurologic examination. *D,* Magnetic resonance imaging at 1 year shows resolution of the ventral epidural mass that was initially present.

may be particularly applicable in patients with lumbar abscesses in whom the epidural space is relatively larger and the spinal cord has terminated (Fig. 119-7). However, these patients require vigilant monitoring because neurologic deterioration can still occur despite appropriate antibiotic therapy. Patients with cervical and thoracic abscesses generally merit more aggressive treatment given the smaller epidural space and the potential for greater neurologic deficit. Any sign of neurologic deficit should prompt one to abandon conservative therapy and proceed with surgical intervention.

OUTCOME

The ability to diagnose SEA in a timely fashion, coupled with improvements in antibiotics and surgical technique, has resulted in a steady decline in mortality rates. Between 1954 and 1980, the mortality rate from SEA decreased from 34% to 16%; between 1991 and 1997, the mortality rate remained constant at approximately 15%.[7] More recent reports have shown some improvement, but, unfortunately, despite the advances cited previously, the mortality rate in patients with SEA has remained unacceptably high.[6] Just more than 40% of patients with make a complete recovery. Approximately 45% of the patients who survive will be left with some degree of neurologic impairment; 16% have significant weakness or complete paralysis resulting in long-term disability.[7] The outcome in patients who survive depends primarily on the degree and duration of neurologic impairment at the time of diagnosis. Not surprisingly, patients with severe neurologic deficit have a much poorer prognosis than do patients who are neurologically intact.[6] Some authors have also pointed out that patients with a more chronic clinical course have a better prognosis than do patients who present with a rapid tempo. Based on the literature, it cannot be overstressed that the single most important factor in reducing mortality and permanent neurologic morbidity is early diagnosis and institution of treatment *before* the onset of any neurologic deficit.

REFERENCES

1. Heusner AP: Nontuberculous spinal epidural infections. N Engl J Med 239:845–854, 1948.
2. Danner RL, Hartman BJ: Update of spinal epidural abscess: 35 cases and review of the literature. Rev Infect Dis 9:265–274, 1987.
3. Hlavin ML, Kaminski HJ, Ross JS, et al: Spinal epidural abscess: A ten-year perspective. Neurosurgery 27:177–184, 1990.
4. Osenbach RK, Hitchon PW, Menezes AH: Diagnosis and management of pyogenic vertebral osteomyelitis in adults. Surg Neurol 33:266–275, 1990.
5. Sampath P, Rigamonti D: Spinal epidural abscess: A review of epidemiology, diagnosis, and treatment. J Spinal Disord 12:89–93, 1999.
6. Rigamonti D, Liem L, Sampath P, et al: Spinal epidural abscess: Contemporary trends in etiology, evaluation, and management. Surg Neurol 52:189–197, 1999.
7. Reihaus E, Waldbaur H, Seeling W: Spinal epidural abscess: A meta-analysis of 915 patients. Neurosurg Rev 232:175–204, 2000.
8. Sapico FL, Montgomerie JZ: Pyogenic vertebral osteomyelitis: Report of nine cases and review of the literature. Rev Infect Dis 1:754–776, 1979.
9. Batson OV: The function of the vertebral veins and their role in the spread of metastases. Ann Surg 112:138–149, 1940.
10. McHenry M, Easley K, Locker G: Vertebral osteomyelitis: long-term outcome for 253 patients from 7 Cleveland-area hospitals. Clin Infect Dis 34:1342–1350, 2002.
11. Rezai A, Woo H, Errico T, Cooper P: Contemporary management of spinal osteomyelitis. Neurosurgery 44:1018–1025, 1999.
12. Curling OD, Gower DJ, McWhorter JM: Changing concepts in spinal epidural abscess: A report of 29 cases. Neurosurgery 27:185–192, 1990.

13. Dandy WE: Abscess and inflammatory tumors in the spinal epidural space (so-called) pachymeningitis externa. Arch Surg 13:477–494, 1936.
14. Lyu R, Chen C, Tang L, Chen S: Spinal epidural abscess successfully treated with percutaneous, computed tomography-guided, aspiration and parenteral antibiotic therapy: Case report and review of the literature. Neurosurgery 51:509–512, 2002.
15. Schulz C, Comey C, Haid R: Pyogenic spinal epidural abscess: A minimally invasive technique for multisegmental decompression. J Spinal Disord 14:546–549, 2001.
16. Browder J, Meyers R: Pyogenic infections of the spinal epidural space: A consideration of the anatomic and physiologic pathology. Surgery 10:296–308, 1947.
17. Baker AS, Ojemann RG, Schwartz MN, et al: Spinal epidural abscess. N Engl J Med 293:463–468, 1975.
18. Feldenzer JA, McKeever PE, Schaberg DR, et al: Experimental spinal epidural abscess: A pathophysiological model in the rabbit. Neurosurgery 20:859–867, 1987.
19. Feldenzer JA, McKeever PE, Schaberg DR, et al: The pathogenesis of spinal epidural abscess; microangiographic studies in an experimental model. J Neurosurg 69:110–114, 1988.
20. Jimenez M, Colmenero J, Sanchez-Lora F, et al: Postoperative spondylodiskitis: Etiology, clinical findings, prognosis, and comparison with pyogenic spondylodiskitis. Clin Infect Dis 29:339–345, 1999.
20. Fischer EG, Greene CS, Winston KR: Spinal epidural abscess in children. Neurosurgery 9:257–260, 1981.
21. Levi A, Sonntag V: Pyogenic vertebral osteomyelitis. In Osenbach R, Zeidman S (eds): Infections in Neurological Surgery: Diagnosis and Management. Philadelphia: Lippincott–Raven, 1999, pp 257–264.
22. Cahill D, Abshire B: Pyogenic vertebral osteomyelitis. In Batjer H, Loftus C (eds): Textbook of Neurological Surgery: Principles and Practice. Philadelphia: Lippincott Williams & Wilkins, 2002.
23. Leys D, Lesoin F, Viaud C, et al: Decreased morbidity from acute bacterial spinal epidural abscesses using computed tomography and nonsurgical treatment in selected patients. Ann Neurol 17:350–355, 1985.
24. Smith A, Blaser S: MR of infectious and inflammatory diseases of the spine. Crit Rev Diagnc Imaging 32:165–189, 1991.
25. Modic M, Berino RE, Porter BA, et al: Imaging spinal osteomyelitis and epidural abscess with short T1 recovery (STIR). Am J Neuroradiol 9:563–564, 1988.
26. Modic MT, Feiglin DH, Piraino DW, et al: Vertebral osteomyelitis: Assessment using MR. Radiology 157:157–166, 1985.
27. Antuaco EJ, McConnell JR, Chadduck WM, et al: MR imaging of spinal epidural sepsis. AJNR Am J Neuroradiol 8:879–883, 1987.
28. Tzen K, Yen T, Yang R, et al: The role of ^{67}Ga in the early detection of spinal epidural abscesses. Nucl Med Commun 21:165–170, 2000.
29. Cwiekel W: Percutaneous drainage of abscess in psoas compartment and epidural space: Case report and review of the literature. Acta Radiol 32:159–161, 1991.
30. Tabo E, Okhuma Y, Kimura S, et al: Successful percutaneous drainage of epidural abscess with epidural needle and catheter. Anesthesiology 80:1393–1395, 1994.
31. Lu C, Chang W, Chen L, et al: Adult spinal epidural abscess: Clinical features and prognostic factors. Clin Neurol Neurosurg 104:306–310, 2002.
32. Tang H, Lin H, Liu Y, Li C: Spinal epidural abscess—experience with 46 patients and evaluation of prognostic factors. J Infect 45:76–81, 2002.

120 Primary Reconstruction for Spinal Infections

MAX C. LEE, JOHN MISLOW, and RICHARD G. FESSLER

INTRODUCTION

The recent resurgence of spinal infections, attributed to an increase in immunocompromised patients and antibiotic-resistant strains, has become a significant problem for most spine surgeons. Indications for operative intervention are not always clear. In addition, questions about timing and which procedure to use frequently arise. This chapter's purpose is to clarify the indications for surgical intervention in patients with spinal infections and discuss various options for their surgical stabilization.

BACKGROUND AND EPIDEMIOLOGY

Spinal infections may be divided into two groups: pyogenic and nonpyogenic. The culprit in pyogenic infections may be bacteria or mycobacteria, and in nonpyogenic infections, it may be fungi, yeast, or parasites.[1-5] Spinal pyogenic osteomyelitis represents 2% of all cases of osteomyelitis and 7% of osteomyelitis in adults. The spine represents the most common site of hematogenously acquired osteomyelitis.[6-12] Patients with spinal osteomyelitis have a mean age of 58 years and a 1.5:1 male-to-female ratio, although some studies demonstrate no male preponderance.[1] Risk factors were identified in 77% of cases, with 53% of patients having multiple risk factors (average of three risk factors per patient). Primary risk factors included diabetes mellitus (44%); extraspinal infection, especially urinary tract infections (33%); long-term steroid use (24%); malignancy (17%); and alcoholism (11%),[1,13] and additional risk factors were acquired immunodeficiency syndrome infection and chemotherapy treatment.

The presentation of spinal osteomyelitis may be insidious. The average time to diagnosis is more than 3 months except for intravenous drug abusers, who present with a more fulminant course (3 weeks to 3 months). Predominant localization is in the thoracic (52%) and lumbar (43%) spine.[13] Presenting symptoms are varied; 15% of patients with spinal osteomyelitis present with neurologic deficits, and of patients with tuberculous spondylitis, 50% to 75% present with a neurologic deficit.[14-17] Axial spinal pain was present in 95% of cases. Radicular pain varied from 20% to 65% of cases. Of the neurologic deficits that were identified in 74% of cases, significant weakness was present in 33% and paralysis in 8%. Mechanical instability may also occur, with deformities more prevalent in the thoracic spine and associated with a greater neurologic deficit (Frankel grades A to C). Mortality rates for this serious infection are reported at between 1% and 20%.

On diagnostic imaging, these patients display interesting features. Primary radiographic findings of discitis were identified in 45% (with associated spinal deformity in 33% of these) and primary radiographic findings of osteomyelitis were identified in 55% (associated spinal deformity in 55% of these). Osteolytic radiographic abnormality generally involves the vertebral end plates. These findings may be demonstrated on plain radiographs and computed tomography. In addition, magnetic resonance imaging is 96% sensitive and 92% specific, with an overall 94% accuracy of diagnosis. Characteristic magnetic resonance imaging findings are a confluent decreased signal of the disc and adjacent vertebral bodies with indiscernible margins on T1-weighted images.

In addition to physical examination and radiographic imaging, some laboratory investigations may shed light on the diagnosis. Blood cultures are positive for the causative organism in as many as 70% of cases.[3] An extraspinal source can be identified in 40% of cases. These sources may include infections of the urinary tract, pulmonary system, and integument. Needle biopsy of the lesion may be done under direct or radiographic imaging, with a diagnostic yield of 50% to 70%.

NEUROLOGIC AND MECHANICAL INSTABILITY

The neurosurgeon is consulted only 15% to 20% of the time (Figs. 120-1 and 120-2) in patients with spinal infections, and the majority of these consultations are for an open biopsy or because of neurologic deficit. The goal of treatment in these patients is the maximal preservation of neurologic function. This goal may be attained through aggressive decompression of neural tissue, parenteral antibiotics, and spinal stabilization. Other goals of surgical intervention include the prevention of sepsis through aggressive débridement of abscesses, which may lead to the permanent eradication of infection.

The surgical management of spinal infections is broad and can be divided into the management of potential neurologic threat and the management of mechanical instability. Determining the state of neurologic threat or mechanical instability assists with decisions about surgical approach and technique. Neurologic potential injury requires at least a neural decompression with or without spinal arthrodesis, while mechanical instability requires spinal arthrodesis. Whether to augment spinal arthrodesis with spinal fixation is determined by the degree of instability. In general, the correction of a spinal deformity or severe instability requires spinal fixation in the form of spinal instrumentation. Lesser degrees of instability may be improved by bed rest or rigid external bracing.

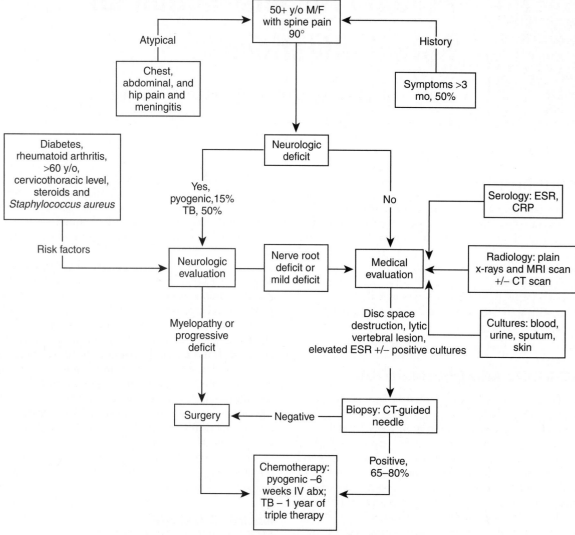

FIGURE 120-1   Algorithm for the evaluation of spinal osteomyelitis. abx, antibiotics; CRP, C-reactive protein; CT, computed tomography; ESR, erythrocyte sedimentation rate; IV, intravenous; M/F, male/female ratio; MRI, magnetic resonance imaging; TB, tuberculosis; y/o., years old.

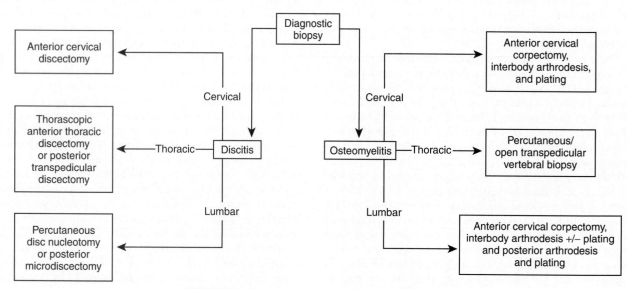

FIGURE 120-2   Surgical diagnostic biopsy alternatives.

In pyogenic discitis, interbody fusion usually occurs spontaneously. This fusion, however, may be accompanied by foraminal narrowing and kyphosis or listhesis. Because spinal osteomyelitis generally involves the vertebral body and adjacent disc spaces, an anterior surgical approach is used to allow direct access to the infectious focus for aggressive débridement. Aggressive anterior débridement is mandatory also for successful reconstruction. Posterior decompression and posterior access to anterior decompressions have led to spinal instability.

In tuberculous spondylitis, spontaneous fusion is not common, and progressive kyphotic deformity is common. This may lead to progressive neurologic deterioration. Although medical therapy continues to be the cornerstone of therapy, surgical intervention is commonly performed to optimize functional outcomes.[18]

CONTROVERSIES IN ARTHRODESIS

The question of whether to perform arthrodesis in the setting of spinal infections is controversial. Should vertebral reconstruction be performed primarily or delayed? If arthrodesis is required, should the graft be vascularized, autologous, or allograft? If instrumentation would augment spinal stabilization, should it be performed primarily or delayed? Does placement of instrumentation in a patient with an ongoing infection aggravate the patient's condition prohibitively? Here we present an attempt to answer some of these pressing questions.

Spinal Stabilization with Grafts

Autograft

Primary reconstruction using bone grafting and spinal instrumentation remains controversial in some cases; however, for spinal infections, indications are clear, for example, aggressive anterior débridement unambiguously requires spinal reconstruction to prevent deformity. Interbody arthrodesis is performed with the appropriate bone graft based on anatomy, biomechanics, and availability. Although use of interbody grafts remains controversial, it has been accepted for spinal osteomyelitis.[1,19,20] Autologous interbody bone grafting in the presence of active infection was first reported by Wiltberger in 1952 for chronic vertebral osteomyelitis and has been used safely ever since.[21–27] Although iliac crest bone grafts are preferred, vascularized rib grafts have been successfully used.[28,29]

Allograft

Fibula allografts have been shown to be effective in the cervical spine.[30,31] Ozdemir and colleagues[32] and Govender[33] attempt to address concerns regarding implantation of devitalized bone in an actively infected spine by assessing the efficacy of allograft fibular fusion and anterior spinal stabilization as an alternative treatment of tuberculous spondylitis. They each performed retrospective studies on patients with tuberculous spondylitis managed surgically with allograft and anterior stabilization. Appropriate chemotherapy was completed postoperatively, and patient radiographic and clinical follow-up was 1 to 3 years in duration. Of 28 patients, 26 completed the 3-year follow-up (two patients died of causes unrelated to surgery or infection). Ninety-six percent of the patients were evaluated as having bony fusion. One patient experienced instrument failure that was revised with no complications. No other clinically relevant complications were reported. Segmental correction was maintained successfully in all patients. Govender[33] reported fusion and remodeling in 33 patients and partial remodeling in 8 patients, with an overall correction of preoperative kyphosis in 42%. From these results, both Ozdemir and colleagues and Govender concluded that anterior spinal instrumentation and allograft are an effective method for the local control of segmental stability and kyphosis in tuberculous spondylitis and that surgeons should not refrain from allograft placement after radical débridement.

Titanium Cages

Titanium cages have gained wide acceptance in the field for their role in the reconstruction of the anterior column of patients without concomitant infection. Hee and colleagues[34] addressed the efficacy of using anterior titanium mesh cages and posterior instrumentation after anterior débridement in the surgical treatment of vertebral osteomyelitis. They performed a retrospective, single-center study of 21 consecutive patients undergoing débridement and instrumentation for vertebral osteomyelitis. Ten patients received supplemental posterior instrumentation, and five patients had reconstruction of the anterior column with titanium cages. Mean follow-up time was 67 months with wide variance (24 to 120 months). Greater improvement in sagittal alignment was noted for patients with titanium cages implanted ($p = 0.0009$) and for those with posterior instrumentation ($p = 0.005$) than for patients who did not receive either of these interventions. A trend toward fewer postoperative complications emerged for patients who had posterior stabilization with titanium cages. Hee and colleagues thus concluded that the use of posterior stabilization and titanium cages in the surgical treatment of vertebral osteomyelitis is safe and effective.

Liljenqvist and colleagues[35] address the question of whether expandable titanium cages are as effective as bone grafts in settings of spinal infection Liljenqvist and colleagues retrospectively examined 20 patients (6 cervical, 13 thoracic, 1 lumbar) who underwent a single-stage posterior instrumentation and anterior débridement and decompression, with placement of an expandable titanium cage filled with morselized autologous bone. Patients were followed for an average of 2 years. At the end of 2 years, no patients had experienced major complications or recurrent infections, and stability and neurologic function were restored in all patients. The authors conclude that titanium cages are as effective as allogenic bone grafts alone in the setting of spinal infection.

Other Methods

In addition, other methods for interbody fusion have been attempted in the setting of infection. The literature regarding the use of bone cement and methylmethacrylate is particularly scant. Rath and colleagues[36] inserted methylmethacrylate into the resection cavity in 2 of 43 patients. Of these two cases, a late infection recurrence occurred in one. Conversely, Carragee[37] reported a case augmented with bone cement with no recurrence of infection at

13 months postoperatively. Redfern and colleagues[38] reported six cases in which a metal rod was embedded in bone cement and implanted into the resection site with no recurrent infection and one case of delayed wound healing.

Primary Spinal Stabilization

Instrumentation Indications

Mechanical instability may depend on the natural history of the disease, presence of preoperative spinal deformity, and occurrence of iatrogenic segmental instability secondary either to surgical decompression or the pathologic tissue destruction. Spinal reconstruction for spinal infections should follow the same biomechanical recommendations as for trauma and tumor reconstruction with the appropriate use of bone grafting and spinal instrumentation. Several models have been developed to predict the best treatment plan (Figs. 120-3 to 120-5). Using the Denis model[39] for spinal thoracolumbar trauma, the appropriate surgical treatment plan can be determined for each spinal deformity. The combination of anterior and middle column failure warrants an anterior interbody reconstruction, with spinal instrumentation if necessary. Anterior and posterior column failure may warrant a posterior reconstruction with spinal instrumentation and interbody arthrodesis. Interbody arthrodesis specifically is required if short-segment posterior instrumentation is desired for the treatment of spinal deformity. Middle and posterior column failure warrants a posterior reconstruction with spinal instrumentation. Three-column failure warrants anterior and posterior reconstructions with spinal instrumentation.

The model of Kostuik and Errico[40] allows prediction of mechanical instability when no spinal deformity or neural compression exists. If débridement is performed, the compartments involved by the disease and the surgical disruption of compartments can predict postoperative instability. The surgical approach should minimize additive compartment disruption. Spinal reconstruction should be used to address the predictable postoperative instability. Also, if more than four compartments are involved or there is more than three fourths vertebral body involvement, there is a neurologic risk, especially if weight bearing is allowed, secondary to spinal instability and the predictable inability to resist compressive and flexion-compression forces. Spinal reconstruction should be considered in these selected cases if medically appropriate. If a medical condition prohibits surgical reconstruction, strict bed rest may be necessary until consolidation occurs during healing of the infection.

External Instrumentation

Jeanneret and Magerl[41] reported an alternative method of managing spinal osteomyelitis. They used percutaneous external spinal fixation for the treatment of osteomyelitis in 23 patients. The treatment consisted of percutaneous vertebral biopsy for bacteriologic diagnosis, installation of a suction and irrigation system into the intervertebral disc space, and posterior stabilization with an external fixator placed percutaneously. Two patients required anterior débridement and bone grafting because of progression of bone destruction. In eight patients, this treatment was used emergently and followed by an elective planned anterior débridement and interbody arthrodesis. In 12 patients, the infection healed without further treatment. Jeanneret and Magerl propose this procedure as an alternative option in selected high-risk patients.

Internal Instrumentation

The first surgical series of spinal instrumentation to stabilize the unstable spine secondary to spinal infections is that by Redfern and colleagues[38] published in 1988. Since then,

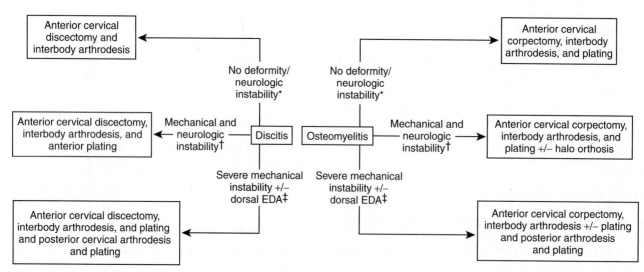

FIGURE 120-3   Surgical algorithm for cervical spine infections. EDA, epidural abscess.
*Neurologic instability: the risk of neurologic deterioration by the natural history of the disease; three to four compartments are involved based on the Kostuik and Errico model, generally of the vertebral body.
†Mechanical instability: the risk of painful spinal deformity by the natural history of the disease; three to four compartments are involved with associated spinal deformity.
‡Five or six compartments are involved with spinal deformity, or three or four compartments are involved requiring a posterior approach for drainage of the epidural abscess.

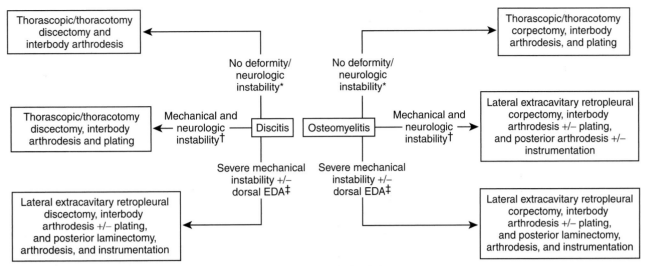

FIGURE 120-4 Surgical algorithm for thoracic spine infections. EDA, epidural abscess.
*Neurologic instability: the risk of neurologic deterioration by the natural history of the disease; three or four compartments are involved based on the Kostuik and Errico model, generally of the vertebral body.
†Mechanical instability: the risk of painful spinal deformity by the natural history of the disease; three or four compartments are involved with an associated spinal deformity.
‡Five or six compartments are involved with spinal deformity, or three or four compartments are involved requiring a posterior approach for drainage of the epidural abscess.

several publications have reported experience with spinal instrumentation for acute spinal pyogenic infections.[3,31,36,37,42–46] There are many published series and reports supporting the use of bone arthrodesis and spinal instrumentation for the reconstructive treatment of tuberculous spondylitis. Bone grafting and spinal instrumentation are well established for use in the reconstruction of tuberculous spondylitis.[17,33,44,47–52]

Przyblyski and Sharan[53] evaluated the efficacy of combining débridement, autograft, and instrumentation in patients who have failed medical management. A retrospective study was performed on 17 patients from 1996 to 1999, all of whom were diagnosed with pyogenic spondylitis. Patients underwent single-stage débridement, arthrodesis, and plating followed by 6 weeks of postoperative antibiotics. Mean follow-up was 30 months. All patients experienced significant postoperative reduction in pain as well as significant improvement of neurologic deficits and independent ambulation. The authors conclude from this study that single-stage débridement, arthrodesis, and internal fixation may be

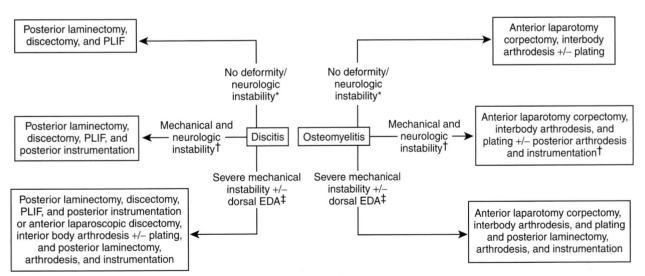

FIGURE 120-5 Surgical algorithm for lumbar spine infections. EDA, epidural abscess; PLIF, posterior lumbar interbody fusion.
*Neurologic instability: the risk of neurologic deterioration by the natural history of the disease; three or four compartments are involved based on the Kostuik and Errico model, generally of the vertebral body.
†Mechanical instability: the risk of painful spinal deformity by the natural history of the disease; three or four compartments are involved with an associated spinal deformity.
‡Five or six compartments are involved with spinal deformity, or three or four compartments are involved requiring a posterior approach for drainage of the epidural abscess.

used in active spinal infection without increased complications, provided that 6 weeks of appropriate antibiotics are completed postoperatively.

Dietze and colleagues[31] retrospectively reviewed 27 patients with spinal infections, 20 of whom required surgical débridement and reconstruction. Interbody grafts were placed in 18 patients (10 autologous, 8 allograft), and posterolateral onlay grafts were placed in 14 patients. Spinal instrumentation used in 15 patients (4 with anterior plating, 11 with posterior fixation). After an average follow-up period of 37 months, the authors demonstrated that primary arthrodesis and instrumentation can be performed in acute spinal infections.

Carragee[1] retrospectively reviewed 111 patients with pyogenic vertebral osteomyelitis. Forty-two patients underwent débridement and arthrodesis, and 14 patients also had instrumentation of the spine. None of the patients had any compromise of outcome.

To examine whether anterior instrumentation alone with radical débridement and fusion is an acceptable treatment, Benli and colleagues[54] performed a retrospective study of 63 patients (average age, 46.8 ± 13.4 years), all with tuberculous spondylitis. All patients underwent anterior radical débridement with anterior fusion and anterior instrumentation with an average follow-up of 50.9 ± 12.9 months. Local kyphosis was measured preoperatively, postoperatively, and at the last follow-up visit; vertebral collapse, destruction, abscess, and canal compromise were assessed with magnetic resonance imaging. Benli and colleagues reported that instrumentation corrected kyphotic deformity in 80% of all patients. Of 25 patients (39.7%) with neurologic symptoms, 20 (80%) experienced full recovery and 4 (16%) experienced partial recovery. The study notes one postoperative complication, a persistent infection that was resolved by an aggressive antibiotic regimen. The authors conclude that anterior reconstruction and instrumentation are a safe and effective method in the surgical treatment of tuberculosis spondylitis. Similarly, Hassan[52] demonstrates complete recovery of preoperative neurologic symptoms in 12 of 14 patients with anterior cervical débridement and fusion with a kyphosis correction from 21.6 degrees to 2.5 degrees at 38 months. Although some advocate anterior and posterior fixation, anterior instrumentation may be adequate for single-level spondylodiscitis.[45,55]

Most thoracic and lumbar spine cases (70%) were approached surgically with staged anterior and posterior approaches. Of cases treated with bone arthrodesis, 80% were augmented with spinal instrumentation. No spinal instrumentation was placed directly into infected bone. These surgical series represent aggressive management of advanced infections of the spine. Aggressive management includes complete surgical débridement of foci, spinal reconstruction with arthrodesis and instrumentation, and prolonged antibiotic therapy. Antibiotic therapy entails 1 to 3 months of parenteral antibiotics and 3 months of oral antibiotics based on culture identification and sensitivities. Neurologic improvement occurred in 73% of cases, with 27% improving one Frankel grade and 15% improving two Frankel grades. Bone fusion rates averaged across these series were 96%. Reconstruction failure occurred in 17.5%, of which 7.5% were attributed directly to spinal instrumentation complications. Of reconstruction failures, 7.5%

required reoperation, but not all cases of spinal instrumentation failure required reoperation. Half of the reoperations were secondary to bone arthrodesis complications. The total complication rate in these cases was 65%: 40% medical complications and 33% surgical complications. Of complications, 11.6% required reoperation, and there was a 5% deep wound infection incidence. The mortality rate in this high-risk population was 11.6%, exclusively attributed to medical complications of surgery and premorbid disease. Since then, others have also demonstrated good outcomes with anterior débridement and interbody fusion supplemented with posterior instrumentation.[32,56-58]

In contrast to staging the procedure, Chen and colleagues[59] demonstrated the adequacy of one-stage posterior decompression and instrumentation in patients with advanced spinal tuberculosis and poor general condition. This was demonstrated in a retrospective review of 12 patients with spinal tuberculosis and angular deformity of more than 25 degrees. They noted spontaneous bony fusion of the vertebrae in 75% at 1 year. In addition, they appreciated a posterior or posterolateral fusion in 92%. Faraj and Webb[43] also describe success with posterior instrumentation in the setting of pyogenic infections in a retrospective review of 31 patients.

Safran and colleagues[46] examined whether sequential or simultaneous anterioposterior reconstruction of infected lumbar spine is superior via a 10-patient retrospective study. Seven patients underwent same-day anterioposterior reconstruction; the remaining three underwent reconstruction on separate days. All 10 patients regained stability with no persistent infection in 24 months of follow-up. The authors concluded that combined and sequential decompression and stabilization were equally efficacious in setting of lumbar spine infection.

In poor surgical candidates with extensive posterior and anterior infective degeneration, the "360" fusion may fare better if surgery is split into two stages. Fukuta and colleagues[44] attempted to determine whether two-stage surgical treatment is as efficacious as a 360 fusion in very sick patients. The authors performed a retrospective study of eight patients between 1997 and 2001, all of whom were diagnosed with vertebral osteomyelitis and all of whom had significant systemic morbidities (diabetes mellitus, pneumonia, hypertension, end-stage renal disease). Patients underwent a two-stage instrumentation, first undergoing posterior instrumentation (with no contact with infected regions), then 13.9 ± 10.5 weeks recuperation with antibiotics, followed by anterior débridement and arthrodesis. At 9-month follow-up, patients' average pain level decreased from 7.3 to 2.6 of 10, neurologic states improved significantly, and radiographic images were consistent with stable fusion in all patients. Complications included two patients with posterior wound infections whose wounds were successfully closed. Wound infections are not surprising in light of the multiple comorbidities of the study's patient population. Fukuta and colleagues concluded that a two-stage treatment for pyogenic or tuberculous spondylitis provided satisfactory results and may be used in patients who are in poor general condition. The authors note that this treatment requires two exposures to general anesthesia, a serious consideration if patient has pulmonary insufficiency.

There are statements that instrumentation should not be used in the presence of active infection, but clear explanations are not provided. The use of spinal instrumentation may increase the potential for the development of postoperative infection.[60–62] Pathobiologic studies suggest multiple variables for induction of infection: foreign body–associated tissue damage, impairment of host defenses, bacterial trapping by fibrin, sequestration of bacteria in implant interstices, and generation of a biofilm on implant surfaces.[63–65] However, whether this prohibits the use of spinal instrumentation in the presence of infection is not entirely clear. Several reports of the treatment of infected spinal instrumentation without removal of the instrumentation and eradication of the infection exist.[66–69]

RECURRENT SPINAL INFECTION AFTER PRIMARY RECONSTRUCTION

Detailed follow-up data with antibiotic courses and time off antibiotics were limited.[66] Clinical follow-up was longer than 2 years in 15 of 20 cases (75%), with an average follow-up period after surgery of 37 months. Fourteen of 15 cases had an average follow-up off antibiotics of 32.4 months. There has been no documented recurrent spinal infection. One patient developed a new infectious focus 7 months off antibiotics in the hip joint without evidence of recurrent spinal infection and was treated with another course of prolonged antibiotics. Another case developed a deep wound infection 1 month postoperatively. This patient persisted with a generalized malaise and elevated sedimentation rate of 58 but no neurologic deficit and no radiographic evidence of persistent or recurrent osteomyelitis. There were three cases of multiple spinal foci of infection (15%). In all three cases, the second spinal focus responded minimally to appropriate medical therapy. Two of these cases required spinal reconstruction and are presented in this series. There was no case of a new second focus that developed after treatment of the primary focus. There were two cases of multiple contiguous levels (10%). Rath and colleagues[36] reported two recurrences after primary spinal reconstruction.

The time course of follow-up required to state successful eradication of osteomyelitis accurately is not well established. Studies suggest that 1 year may not be enough time because of reports of delayed infections more than 1 year postoperatively. In their study of adult osteomyelitis, Cierny and colleagues[70] found the indium scan to be positive in 87% at 1 year and 6% at 2 years. There were only two treatment failures beyond 1 year, however. The time off antibiotics in relation to this follow-up period has not been clearly addressed. The series of Dietze and colleagues[31] has follow-up periods of 37 months and 34 months off antibiotics, representing 75% of the cases.

REPRESENTATIVE CASES

Case 1

A 64-year-old white woman underwent lower gastrointestinal endoscopy without complications for workup of lower gastrointestinal bleeding. Several hours later, she became septic. Blood cultures were positive for *Proteus* organisms.

Parenteral antibiotics were given with stabilization of the clinical status. Three weeks after the septic event, the patient began to complain of neck pain. Over the next couple of days, the pain became more severe, and rapid weakness developed. Examination revealed paraspinous neck spasm with decreased range of motion and moderate tenderness with tracheal deviation. Neurologic examination revealed left triceps and hand 3/5 monoparesis with loss of the triceps reflex, and 3 to 4/5 paraparesis, including a neurogenic bladder. Radiographic studies showed C5 and C6 vertebral destruction based at the metaphysis, adjacent to the C5–6 disc. There was an associated angulation centered at the C5–6 disc. Magnetic resonance imaging showed osteomyelitic changes in the C5 and C6 vertebrae and associated prevertebral and ventral epidural abscesses. Axial imaging clearly showed posterior deflection and flattening of the cervical spinal cord (Fig. 120-6). The patient was treated emergently with an anterior transcervical approach, C5 and C6 complete corpectomies, and excision of necrotic debris. Drainage of the ventral epidural abscess restored spinal cord pulsations. A fibula allograft was used for interbody arthrodesis, and fixation with a Caspar plate using bicortical screw purchase into C4 and C7 was performed. The patient was kept in a hard cervical collar for 8 weeks. Intraoperative cultures were negative. The patient had received a 10-day course of antibiotics for the septic episode. The antibiotic ceftriaxone (Rocephin) was given, 1 g intravenously every 12 hours, for 6 weeks, followed by 3 months of oral ciprofloxacin, 500 mg twice daily. Over 6 weeks, the patient's neurologic examination returned to normal except for 4/5 left triceps weakness. Bladder function returned to normal. Radiographic studies showed good bone fusion (Fig. 120-7). After a follow-up period of 45.5 months, the patient was without evidence of a recurrence.

Case 2

A 61-year-old white woman with non-insulin-dependent diabetes mellitus and obesity presented with the subacute development of paraplegia and a history of chronic thoracic spine pain. Examination revealed a 2/5 paraplegia with loss of bowel and bladder function and bilateral Babinski's reflexes. No distinct sensory level could be determined. Radiographic evaluation showed multilevel thoracic spine involvement (T6, T7, and T8) with a ventral and lateral epidural abscess (Fig. 120-8). Her erythrocyte sedimentation rate was 122 with a white blood cell count of 12,100. She underwent emergent T6, T7, and T8 corpectomies and interbody arthrodesis with autologous rib grafts and posterior autologous onlay arthrodesis with segmental spinal instrumentation using a Texas Scottish Rite Hospital hook-rod construct from T3–10, performed through a lateral extracavitary retropleural approach. Intraoperative cultures were positive for *Staphylococcus aureus*. She was treated with 4 weeks of vancomycin, and then converted to oral dicloxacillin for 3 months. At 1-year follow-up, the patient's clinical examination improved to an independent ambulatory state using a cane with a 4/5 paraparesis and radiographic fusion (Fig. 120-9). An extended follow-up at 3 years revealed normal motor strength, but the patient still used a cane because of a mild proprioceptive deficit. No evidence of recurrent infection was present.

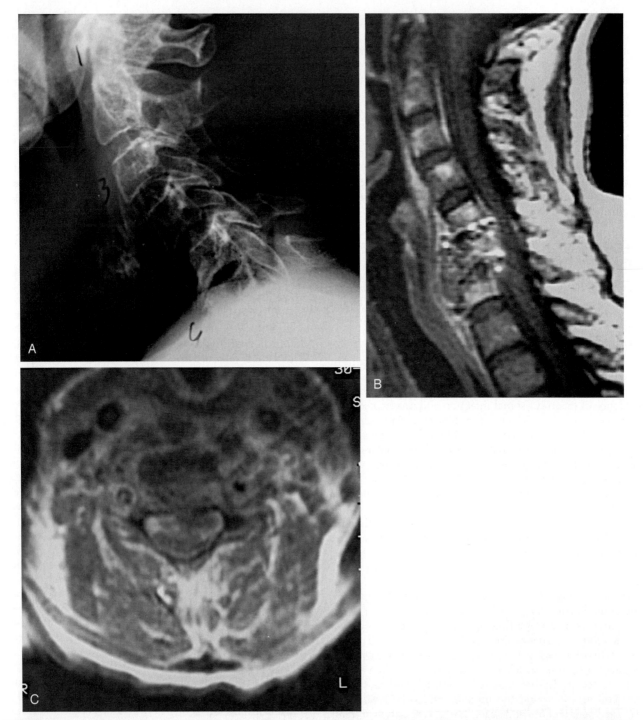

FIGURE 120-6   *A*, Preoperative plain lateral cervical spine radiograph shows the loss of C5–6 disc space height with sclerotic end plates and associated mild angulation. Not fully appreciated without the hot light is prevertebral soft-tissue swelling. Sagittal (*B*) and axial (*C*) gadolinium-enhanced T1-weighted images show loss of height, irregularity, and enhancement of the end plates of the C5–6 disc space. There is inhomogeneous uptake of gadolinium in the C5, C6, and C7 vertebral bodies with extensive involvement of the C6 body. This uptake suggests the possibility of osteomyelitis in these bodies, and one must be prepared for this possibility. However, this pattern may be a result of an inflammatory reaction secondary to the adjacent infection. The C7 body was not thought clinically to be involved at the time of surgery. Note the large prevertebral and ventral epidural abscesses with spinal cord flattening and compression.

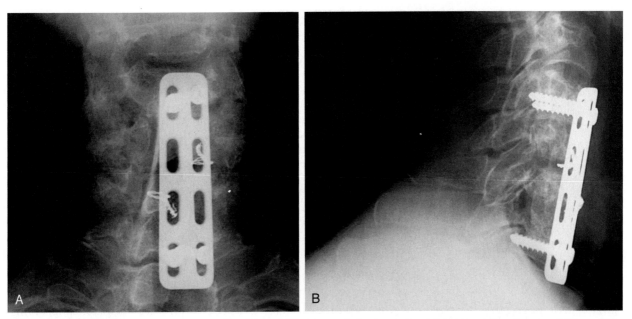

FIGURE 120-7 Postoperative anteroposterior (*A*) and lateral (*B*) plain cervical spine radiographs at 6 months show good incorporation of the autologous iliac crest interbody graft from C4 to C7. The Caspar plates remain in good position. There is no evidence of a recurrent infection at 15 months postoperatively.

Case 3

A 57-year-old white woman with steroid-dependent rheumatoid arthritis was admitted to the hospital for sepsis secondary to pyelonephritis. Blood cultures were positive for *S. aureus*, and parenteral antibiotics were begun. Over the next week, she developed progressive low back pain and severe left upper thigh radicular pain. Examination revealed diffuse marked lumbar back pain and bilateral positive straight leg raise. Neurologic examination revealed bilateral 4/5 foot drop, absent Achilles' reflexes, and bilateral

Babinski's reflexes. Radiographic studies showed L1 and L2 destructive changes based at the metaphysis adjacent to the L1–2 disc and increased end plate sclerosis and loss of disc space height at the L4–5 disc. There were associated bilateral iliopsoas muscular abscesses and L1–2 disc destruction and ventral granulation mass. The iliopsoas abscesses were drained percutaneously using a computed tomography–guided technique. Cultures were positive for *S. aureus*, and parenteral vancomycin was begun. She was stabilized medically and then underwent staged surgical procedures: first,

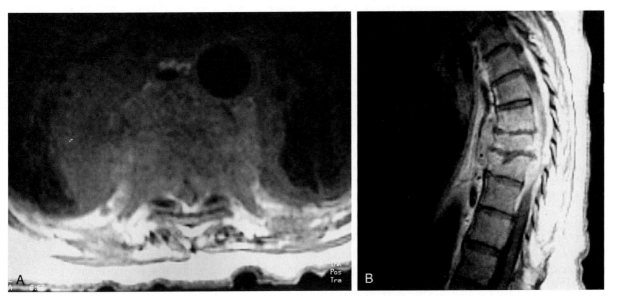

FIGURE 120-8 Preoperative axial (*A*) and sagittal (*B*) magnetic resonance imaging contrast-enhanced T1-weighted images. The sagittal image reveals multilevel thoracic spine involvement (T6, T7, and T8). There are an extensive ventral epidural abscess and an associated prevertebral abscess. The axial image shows the thecal sac distortion by the ventral epidural abscess.

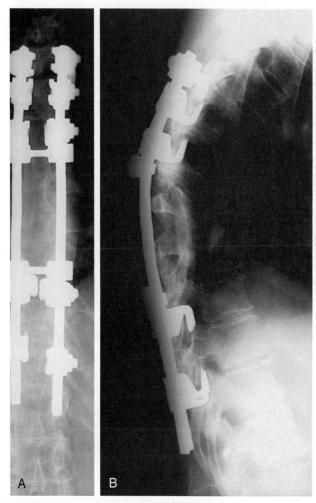

FIGURE 120-9 Postoperative anteroposterior (AP) (*A*) and lateral (*B*) plain radiographs at 1 year postoperatively. The AP view is of poor quality but reveals the intact spinal instrumentation construct. The lateral view, again, reveals the intact spinal instrumentation construct consisting of a T3-10 Texas Scottish Rite Hospital hook-rod construct. Also, note the hyperdensity overlaying the transverse processes between the first set of hooks. This density is a fused interposed autologous rib graft. The autologous rib graft, which is used for interbody arthrodesis, is also visualized and well incorporated.

a retroperitoneal approach for L1 and L2 corpectomies and humerus allograft interbody arthrodesis and 5 days later, a posterior T12–L3 onlay arthrodesis using autologous iliac crest bone graft and T12–L3 segmental fixation using Texas Scottish Rite Hospital pedicle screw and rod construct. Postoperatively, a clamshell orthosis was used during weight bearing for 3 months. Over 6 weeks, the patient regained full motor strength and return of her Achilles' reflexes.

The patient was treated with vancomycin, 1 g intravenously every 12 hours, for 3 months and placed on oral dicloxacillin, 500 mg orally every 6 hours. After 1 month of oral antibiotics (4 months postoperatively), she began to have increasing low back pain. Examination revealed new low back pain and loss of returned Achilles' reflexes. Motor strength was normal. Radiographic studies showed progressive

end plate sclerosis and loss of height at the L4–5 disc space and a persistent central disc bulge with granulation tissue. There was also another associated contiguous iliopsoas abscess on the left. The sedimentation rate, which had returned to normal, was again increased to 70. Another staged surgical procedure was performed: first, a retroperitoneal approach for a L3–4 discectomy and partial L4 corpectomy, evacuation of the adjacent iliopsoas abscess, and autologous tricortical iliac crest interbody arthrodesis and second, a posterior L3–S1 onlay arthrodesis using autologous iliac crest bone graft and L3–S1 segmental fixation using Texas Scottish Rite Hospital pedicle screw and rod construct incorporating the previous construct. Postoperatively, a clamshell orthosis was used during weight bearing for 3 months. Over 6 weeks, the patient had resolution of back pain and normal motor strength. She was treated with another 3 months of parenteral vancomycin followed by 3 months of oral dicloxacillin. The sedimentation rate returned to normal after 3 months. At 3 months, there was radiographic evidence of loosening of one of the sacral screws. At 6 months, this screw loosening was stable. The patient died in May 1994 from metastatic cancer. A workup for her cancer revealed no evidence of recurrent spinal infection (Fig. 120-10). Follow-up was 26 months after her last operation and 34 months after her first operation without evidence of a recurrence.

CONCLUSION

The neurosurgical goals for spinal infection remain unchanged: preservation of neurologic function, prevention of sepsis, eradication of infection, and spinal stabilization. Decompression of neural tissue, parenteral antibiotics, and spinal stabilization maximize the preservation of neurologic function. Aggressive débridement of abscesses and parenteral antibiotics maximize prevention of sepsis and eradication of infection. Spinal stabilization requires spinal immobilization and may require primary spinal reconstruction with bone arthrodesis and spinal instrumentation. The indications for spinal instrumentation should be specific and reserved for clear spinal instability. Reconstruction and instrumentation of the spine are acceptable during active spinal osteomyelitis, providing that débridement of diseased tissue is complete and an appropriate antibiotic therapy course is completed. Acceptable materials for reconstruction include autologous graft, allograft, and titanium cages. Anterior-posterior reconstruction can be performed as a single or staged procedure. Removal of instrumentation is generally unnecessary with the proper duration of antibiotics. However, this is not clearly answered within this study, and the possibility of delayed symptomatic cryptic infection of the instrumentation may still exist.[71]

Surgical decision making must take into account the total condition of the patient and the balance of the host defenses and the virulence of the pathogen. Selected cases may be at an increased risk of operative and postoperative complications. Thus, the patient, family, and medical team must all participate in the decision-making process. The successful outcome in these challenging patients comes from a team effort between the internist, infectious disease specialist, and spine surgeon.

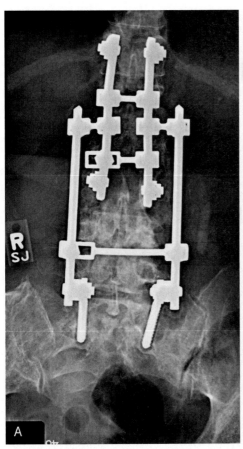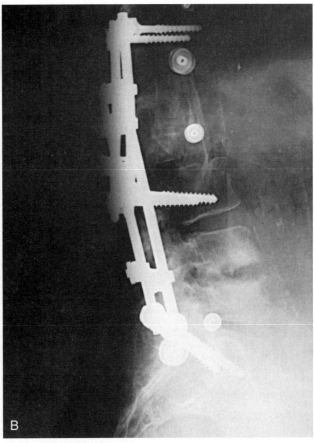

FIGURE 120-10 Postoperatively, after 1 week of oral antibiotics (completed 3 months of parenteral antibiotics), the patient had new low back pain; she had lost her Achilles' reflex and had an elevated erythrocyte sedimentation rate. The L4–5 discitis was thought to have become refractory to antibiotic treatment. A staged approach was performed to remove the disc and reconstruct the disc anteriorly with autologous iliac crest interbody arthrodesis and to fuse and fixate posteriorly with autologous iliac crest onlay arthrodesis and L3–S1 posterior segmental instrumentation, which was connected to the previous posterior construct. At the time of surgery, there was no evidence of recurrent infections at the previous L1–2 site or evidence of a deep wound infection involving the previous grafting and instrumentation. Anteroposterior (*A*) and lateral (*B*) plain lumbar radiographs at 2 years show the prior humerus T12–L3 interbody allograft with evidence of incorporation and the intact T12–L3 posterior segmental instrumentation. The new posterior segmental instrumentation is also shown to use sacral pedicle screw fixation and linkage to the previous construct to create a conjoined construct that fixates T12–S1. The L4–5 iliac crest interbody autograft cannot be well visualized. (From Dietze DD, Fessler RG, Jacob RP: Primary reconstruction for spinal infections. J Neurosurg 86:981–989, 1997.)

REFERENCES

1. Carragee EJ: Pyogenic vertebral osteomyelitis. J Bone Joint Surg Am 79:874–880, 1997.
2. Bridwell KH, Campbell JW, Barenkamp SJ: Surgical treatment of hematogenous vertebral *Aspergillus* osteomyelitis. Spine 15:281–285, 1990.
3. Nolla JM, Ariza N, Gomez-Vaquero C, et al: Spontaneous pyogenic vertebral osteomyelitis in nondrug users. Semin Arthritis Rheum 31:271–278, 2002.
4. van Ooij A, Beckers JM, Harpers MJ, Walenkamp GH: Surgical treatment of aspergillus spondylodiscitis. Eur Spine J 9:75–79, 2000.
5. Wrobel CJ, Chappell ET, Taylor W: Clinical presentation, radiological findings, and treatment results of coccidioidomycosis involving the spine: Report on 23 cases. J Neurosurg 95(1 Suppl):33–39, 2001.
6. Blumberg KD, Balderston RA: Presentation and treatment of pyogenic vertebral osteomyelitis. Semin Spine Surg 8:115–125, 1996.
7. Currier BL, Eismont FJ: Infections of the spine. In Rothman RH, Simeone FA (eds): The Spine. Philadelphia: WB Saunders, 1992, pp 1319–1380.
8. Kulowski J: Pyogenic osteomyelitis of the spine: An analysis and discussion of 102 cases. J Bone Joint Surg 18:343–364, 1936.
9. Lestini WF, Bell GR: Spinal infection: Patient evaluation. Semin Spine Surg 8:81–94, 1996.
10. Malawski SK, Lukawski S: Pyogenic infections of the spine. Clin Orthop 272:58–66, 1991.
11. Sapico FLM, Montgomerie JZM: Vertebral osteomyelitis: Report of nine cases and review of the literature. Infect Dis Clin North Am 4:539–550, 1990.
12. Waldvogel F, Medoff G, Swartz MN: Osteomyelitis: A review of clinical features, therapeutic considerations and unusual aspects. N Engl J Med 282:198–206, 1970.
13. Frankel H, Hancock DO, Hyslop G, et al: The value of postural reduction in the initial management of closed injuries of the spine with paraplegia and tetraplegia. Paraplegia 7:179–192, 1969.
14. Nussbaum ES, Rockswold GL, Bergman TA, et al: Spinal tuberculosis: A diagnostic and management challenge. J Neurosurg 83:243–247, 1995.
15. Rezai AR, Lee M, Cooper PR, et al: Modern management of spinal tuberculosis. Neurosurgery 36:87–98, 1995.
16. Garvey TA, Eismont EJ: Tuberculous and fungal osteomyelitis of the spine. Semin Spine Surg 8:126–141, 1996.
17. Moon M: Tuberculosis of the spine: Controversies and a new challenge. Spine 22:1791–1797, 1997.
18. Khoo LT, Mikawa K, Fessler RG: A surgical revisitation of Pott distemper of the spine. Spine J 3:130–145, 2003.
19. Calderone RR, Larsen JM: Overview and classification of spinal infections. Orthop Clin North Am 27:1–8, 1996.

20. Zeidman SM, Rhines L, Prakash S, et al: Spinal epidural abscess. Contemp Neurosurg 17:1–5, 1995.
21. Emery SE, Chan DP, Woodward HR: Treatment of hematogenous pyogenic vertebral osteomyelitis with anterior debridement and primary bone grafting. Spine 14:284–291, 1989.
22. Fang D, Cheung KM, Dos Remedios ID, et al: Pyogenic vertebral osteomyelitis: Treatment by anterior spinal debridement and fusion. J Spinal Disord 7:173–180, 1994.
23. Stone JL, Cybulski GR, Rodriguez J, et al: Anterior cervical debridement and strut-grafting for osteomyelitis of the cervical spine. J Neurosurg 70:879–883, 1989.
24. Wiltberger B: Resection of vertebral bodies and bone grafting for chronic osteomyelitis of the spine. J Bone Joint Surg Am 34:215–218, 1952.
25. Hodgson AR, Stock FE: Anterior spine fusion for the treatment of tuberculosis of the spine: The operative findings and results in the first one hundred cases. J Bone Joint Surg Am 42:295–310, 1960.
26. Kemp HBS, Jackson JW, Jeremiah JD, et al: Anterior fusion of the spine for infective lesions in adults. J Bone Joint Surg Br 55:715–734, 1973.
27. Kirkaldy-Willis WH, Thomas TG: Anterior approaches in the diagnosis and treatment of infections of the vertebral bodies. J Bone Joint Surg Am 47:87–110, 1965.
28. Bradford DS, Daher YH: Vascularized rib grafts for stabilisation of kyphosis.J Bone Joint Surg Br 68:357–361, 1986.
29. Louw JA: Spinal tuberculosis with neurological deficit: Treatment with anterior vascularised rib grafts, posterior osteotomies and fusion. J Bone Joint Surg Br 72:686–693, 1990.
30. Whitecloud TSI, LaRocca H: Fibular strut graft in reconstructive surgery of the cervical spine. Spine 1:33–43, 1976.
31. Dietze DD Jr, Fessler RG, Jacob RP: Primary reconstruction for spinal infections. J Neurosurg 86:981–989, 1997.
32. Ozdemir HM, Us AK, Ogun T: The role of anterior spinal instrumentation and allograft fibula for the treatment of Pott disease. Spine 28:474–479, 2003.
33. Govender S: The outcome of allografts and anterior instrumentation in spinal tuberculosis. Clin Orthop 398:60–66, 2002.
34. Hee HT, Majd ME, Holt RT, Pienkowski D: Better treatment of vertebral osteomyelitis using posterior stabilization and titanium mesh cages. J Spinal Disord Tech 15:149–156, 2002.
35. Liljenqvist U, Lerner T, Bullmann V, et al: Titanium cages in the surgical treatment of severe vertebral osteomyelitis. Eur Spine J 12:606–612, 2003.
36. Rath SA, Neff U, Schneider O, et al: Neurosurgical management of thoracic and lumbar vertebral osteomyelitis and discitis in adults: A review of 43 consecutive surgically treated patients. Neurosurgery 38:926–933, 1996.
37. Carragee E: Instrumentation of the infected and unstable spine: A review of 17 cases from the thoracic and lumbar spine with pyogenic infections. J Spinal Disord 10:317–324, 1997.
38. Redfern RM, Miles J, Banks AJ, et al: Stabilisation of the infected spine. J Neurol Neurosurg Psychiatry 51:803–807, 1988.
39. Dietz F: Spinal instability as defined by the three-column spine concept in acute spine trauma. Clin Orthop 189:65–67, 1984.
40. Kostuik JP, Erricoun J: Differential diagnosis and surgical treatment of metastatic spine tumors. In Frymoyer JW (ed): The Adult Spine: Principles and Practice. New York: Raven Press, 1991, pp 861–888.
41. Jeanneret B, Magerl F: Treatment of osteomyelitis of the spine using percutaneous suction/irrigation and percutaneous external spinal fixation. J Spinal Disord 7:185–205, 1994.
42. Dimar JR, Carreon LY, Glassman SD, et al: Treatment of pyogenic vertebral osteomyelitis with anterior debridement and fusion followed by delayed posterior spinal fusion. Spine 29:326–332, 2004.
43. Faraj AA, Webb JK: Spinal instrumentation for primary pyogenic infection report of 31 patients. Acta Orthop Belg 66:242–247, 2000.
44. Fukuta S, Miyamoto K, Masuda T, et al: Two-stage (posterior and anterior) surgical treatment using posterior spinal instrumentation for pyogenic and tuberculotic spondylitis. Spine 28:E302–E308, 2003.
45. Klockner C, Valencia R: Sagittal alignment after anterior debridement and fusion with or without additional posterior instrumentation in the treatment of pyogenic and tuberculous spondylodiscitis. Spine 28:1036–1042, 2003.

46. Safran O, Sagir S, Floman Y: Sequential or simultaneous, same-day anterior decompression and posterior stabilization in the management of vertebral osteomyelitis of the lumbar spine. Spine 23:1885–1890, 1998.
47. Osman G, Kumano K, Yalcin S, et al: A single stage posterior approach and rigid fixation for preventing kyphosis in the treatment of spinal tuberculosis. Spine 19:1039–1043, 1994.
48. Rajasekaran S, Soundarapandian S: Progression of kyphosis in tuberculosis of the spine treated by anterior arthrodesis. J Bone Joint Surg Am 71:1314–1323, 1989.
49. Al-Sebai MW, Al-Khawashki H, Al-Arabik, Khan, F: Operative treatment of progressive deformity in spinal tuberculosis. Int Orthop 25:322–325, 2001.
50. Chen WJ, Wu CC, Jung CH, Chen LH, et al: Combined anterior and posterior surgeries in the treatment of spinal tuberculous spondylitis. Clin Orthop 398:50–59, 2002.
51. Guven O: Posterior instrumentation and anterior interbody fusion for tuberculous kyphosis of dorsal and lumbar spines. Spine 21:1840–1841, 1996.
52. Hassan MG: Anterior plating for lower cervical spine tuberculosis. Int Orthop 27:73–77, 2003.
53. Przybylski GJ, Sharan AD: Single-stage autogenous bone grafting and internal fixation in the surgical management of pyogenic discitis and vertebral osteomyelitis. J Neurosurg 94(1 Suppl):1–7, 2001.
54. Benli IT, Acaroglu E, Akalin S, et al: Anterior radical debridement and anterior instrumentation in tuberculosis spondylitis. Eur Spine J 12:224–234, 2003.
55. Yilmaz C, Selek HY, Gurkan I, et al: Anterior instrumentation for the treatment of spinal tuberculosis. J Bone Joint Surg Am 81:1261–1267, 1999.
56. Moon MS, Woo YK, Loe KS, et al: Posterior instrumentation and anterior interbody fusion for tuberculous kyphosis of dorsal and lumbar spines. Spine 20:1910–1916, 1995.
57. Mukhtar AM, Farghaly MM, Ahmed SH: Surgical treatment of thoracic and lumbar tuberculosis by anterior interbody fusion and posterior instrumentation. Med Princ Pract 12:92–96, 2003.
58. Sundararaj GD, Behera S, Ravi V, et al: Role of posterior stabilisation in the management of tuberculosis of the dorsal and lumbar spine. J Bone Joint Surg Br 85:100–106, 2003.
59. Chen YC, Chang MC, Wang ST, et al: One-stage posterior surgery for treatment of advanced spinal tuberculosis. J Chin Med Assoc 66:411–417, 2003.
60. Micheli LJ, Hall JE: Complications in the management of adult spinal deformities. In Epps CH (ed): Complications in Orthopaedic Surgery. Philadelphia: Lippincott, 1986, pp 1227–1229.
61. Moe JH: Complications of scoliosis treatment. Clin Orthop 53:21–30, 1967.
62. Transfeldt EE, Lonstein JE: Wound infections in elective reconstructive spinal surgery. Orthop Trans 9:128–129, 1985.
63. Buret A, Ward KH, Olson ME, et al: An in vivo model to study the pathobiology of infectious biofilms on biomaterial surfaces. J Biomed Mater Res 25:865–874, 1991.
64. Dougherty SH: Pathobiology of infection in prosthetic devices. Rev Infect Dis 10:1102–1117, 1988.
65. Gristina AG, Naylor P, Myrvik Q: Infections from biomaterials and implants: A race for the surface. Med Prog Technol 14:205–224, 1988.
66. Dietze DD Jr, Haid RW Jr: Antibiotic-impregnated methylmethacrylate in treatment of infections with spinal instrumentation: Case report and technical note. Spine 17:981–987, 1992.
67. Glassman SD, Dimar JR, Puno RM, et al: Salvage of instrumental lumbar fusions complicated by surgical wound infection. Spine 21:2163–2169, 1996.
68. Levi AD, Dickman CA, Sonntag VK: Management of postoperative infections after spinal instrumentation. J Neurosurg 86:975–980, 1997.
69. Thalgott JS, Cotler HB, Sasso RC, et al: Postoperative infections in spinal implants: Classification and analysis—a multicenter study. Spine 16:981–984, 1991.
70. Cierny G, Pennick JJ Mader JT: A clinical staging system for adult osteomyelitis. Contemp Orthop 10:17–37, 1985.
71. Smith MM, Vasseur PB, Saunders HM: Bacterial growth associated with metallic implants in dogs. J Am Vet Med Assoc 195:765–767, 1989.

Section XVIII

Neurosurgical Management of Spinal Disorders

121 Craniovertebral Abnormalities and Their Neurosurgical Management

JOHN C. VAN GILDER and ARNOLD H. MENEZES

Craniovertebral junction abnormalities can be developmental, genetic, or acquired in origin.[1-4] To effectively treat these disorders when symptomatic, the clinician must have a knowledge of the embryology and the functional anatomy of the area. A myriad of abnormal neurologic findings may be present that are secondary to compression or ischemia of neural tissue. The surgical management of these disorders is dependent on precise identification of the underlying pathophysiologic condition as determined by appropriate radiologic studies. The operative treatment includes anterior and posterior approaches to the craniovertebral junction with and without bony fusion. Our experience with more than 2000 patients treated surgically who had neurologic symptoms from craniovertebral abnormalities is the basis for management of these complex disorders. The disorders can be classified as listed in Table 121-1.

HISTORY

Subsequent to the first description of spontaneous atlantoaxial dislocation in 1830 by Bell,[5] lesions of the cervicomedullary junction have emerged from being medical curiosities to being conditions that can be effectively managed. Except for acute dislocations, the treatment of occipitoatlantoaxial joint pathologic entities was marked with failure before the era of skeletal traction. Subsequently, it was apparent that most acute and chronic dislocations could be reduced even years after the initial injury.

The early operative procedures were posterior decompression of the cervicomedullary junction with and without fusion for stabilization. Posterior decompression in patients with irreducible ventral compression of neural tissue at the craniovertebral area is often associated with a high operative risk and a low incidence of improvement: most patients are unchanged or have increased neurologic deficit.[6]

More recently, transpalatine-transoral[1-4,7-13] and extrapharyngeal[14-18] ventral operations were described for fractures, tumors, congenital abnormalities, infection, and inflammatory conditions at the cervicomedullary junction. Stabilization of the atlantoaxial occipital joints usually has been performed by fusing of the spinal column posteriorly. No single anterior or posterior surgical procedure can be used for all patients with craniovertebral abnormalities: the operation or combination of operations must be selected on an individual basis to correct the pathologic process responsible for the neurologic deficit.[1-4,11,17]

EMBRYOLOGY AND ANATOMY

By definition, the craniovertebral junction includes the basiocciput, the foramen magnum, the atlas, and the axis vertebra. The occipital bone is formed by fusion of four sclerotomes. The proatlas is the most caudal of the sclerotomes and loses its identity in humans. The neural arch of the primitive proatlas divides into anterior and posterior segments.[20] The former gives rise to the occipital condyles, and the latter fuses with the atlas to help form its rostral articular facets. If the posterior segment of the proatlas remains

---

TABLE 121-1 ▪ Classification of Craniovertebral Junction Abnormalities

Developmental Anomalies of the Craniovertebral Junction

Malformations of Occipital Bone
Clivus segmentations
Remnants around foramen magnum
Basilar invagination
Condylar hypoplasia
Abnormal occipitoatlantal alignment

Malformations of Atlas
Failure of atlas segmentation from occiput (assimilation)
Atlantoaxial fusion
Aplasia of atlas arches

Malformations of Axis
Irregular atlantoaxial segmentation
Dens dysplasias
   Ossiculum terminale persistens
   Os odontoideum
   Hypoplasia-aplasia
Segmentation failure of C2–C3

Neural Dysgenesis

Genetic and Acquired Abnormalities of Craniovertebral Junction

Abnormalities at the Foramen Magnum
Basilar impression (secondary basilar invagination)
Foraminal stenosis
Traumatic occipitoatlantal dislocation
Os odontoideum
Tumors

Atlantoaxial Instability
Errors of metabolism
Down's syndrome
Infections
Inflammatory
Traumatic atlantoaxial dislocations
Miscellaneous

---

separate, the atlas has bipartite cranial articular facets, a rare anomaly that may result in horizontal instability of this joint. The proatlas also forms the dorsal portion of the C1 lateral masses and gives rise to the distal ossification center of the dens.[21]

The atlas is derived from the first cervical sclerotome as well as the proatlas. The body of the atlas as such disappears and gives origin to the dens. The anterior arch of the atlas has one center of ossification, although at times two centers may be present. The posterior arches of the atlas ossify by the age of 3 to 4 years.

The axis is developed from four primary ossification centers. The dens is formed by the C1 sclerotome, the two neural arches and the body of the axis are formed from the C2 sclerotomes, and the tip of the dens develops from the proatlas. The tip of the dens is fused with the body by the age of 12 years, and the remainder of the segments ossify and are fused by the age of 3 years.[21]

Dysgenesis of the odontoid process may encompass many congenital anomalies. Failure of the proatlas and the dens to fuse results in ossiculum terminale. Os odontoideum represents failure of the odontoid process and the axis body to fuse. Hypoplasia and agenesis of the dens is the result of developmental failure of the distal ossification centers. The common pathophysiology that produces neurologic deficit with agenesis or hypoplasia of the dens is instability between the first and second cervical vertebrae that results from incompetence of the cruciate ligament.

An occipital vertebra is a bony structure that is separate from the foramen magnum and incorporates the occipital condyles. The anterior arch may be partially or completely fused to the anterior margin of the foramen magnum, and the transverse process, if present, does not have a foramen for the vertebral artery. In contrast, an atloido-occipital fusion is characterized by ankylosis between the atlas and the skull base, usually with persistence of the normal joints. The transverse process of the atlas has foramina for the vertebral arteries.

The occipitoatlantoaxial joints are complex, both anatomically and kinematically.[22,23] Anatomically, two occipitoatlantal articulations exist. There are four atlantoaxial joints, with a common synovial lining between the dens and the anterior arch of the atlas, the dens, and the transverse ligament, and between the four lateral masses. The second cervical nerve passes through the capsule of each atlantoaxial joint.

The occipitoatlantoaxial joints provide for ante- and retroflexion, lateral flexion, or tilting and rotation. They thus function as a ball-and-socket joint. Flexion-extension and lateral bending occur at the occipitoatlantal joint, and flexion-extension and axial rotation occur at the atlantoaxial joint.

The lateral atlantoaxial joints have convex articular surfaces with a horizontal orientation. Because these convex surfaces are not exactly reciprocal, a telescoping effect occurs during rotation of the head. There is relatively limited movement of the atlantoaxial joint, and head-spine motion is basically between the occipital condyles and C2. Because of the intervening C1–C2 convex joint, potential exists for decreased stability at the craniovertebral junction with extension, flexion, and rotation. Hypermobility of the occipitoatlantal joint may progressively increase in patients with

congenital high cervical fusion, which may be the etiology of basilar invagination associated with the Klippel-Feil abnormality.[24]

The dens is approximated to the anterior arch of the atlas by the transverse ligament, which is anchored to the tubercle on the mesial aspect of each lateral mass of the atlas. This ligament is responsible for the stability of the atlantoaxial joint. The axis is connected to the occiput by (1) the alar ligaments that course obliquely upward from the posterior lateral surface of the dens to the anterior and medial surface of the occipital condyles; (2) the apical dens ligament, which continues from the medial aspect of the foramen magnum to the tip of the dens; (3) the tectorial membrane (an extension of the deep layer of the posterior longitudinal ligament); and (4) the cruciate ligament, which consists of the transverse ligament plus triangular ascending and descending slips to the anterior rim of the foramen magnum and the axis, respectively (Fig. 121-1A, B).

The development of the neck musculature is inadequate to supplement joint stability until the age of 8 years. Before this age, laxity of the ligamentous tissue permits excessive movement of the occipitoatlantoaxial articulations.[25,26] Forward gliding of the skull in relation to the spine occurs if hypoplastic occipital condyles are present. This is the mechanism for the development of neurologic deficit in children who have spondyloepiphyseal dysplasia, Conradi's syndrome, or Morquio's syndrome. These syndromes are often associated with ossiculum terminale.

The lymphatic drainage to the occipitoatlantoaxial joints is through retropharyngeal glands to the deep cervical lymphatic chain. In children, because the neck musculature is not fully developed, C1–C2 subluxation may develop secondary to nasopharyngeal infections.[27]

In the osseoligamentous destruction caused by rheumatoid arthritis, the synovial bursa and associated ligaments that surround the odontoid process are damaged and result in loss of stability.[28] Subluxation may occur secondary to the atlas moving anteriorly on the axis (caused by insufficiency of the cruciate ligament or fracture of the odontoid process), secondary to the atlas moving posteriorly on the axis (from erosion or fracture of the odontoid process), or by telescoping of the skull on the axis (from destruction of the axis lateral masses or apophyseal joints).[28] Chronic subluxation often results in ligamentous hypertrophy and the accumulation of granulation tissue behind the odontoid process from the hypertrophied soft tissue. Even though normal bone alignment is present on roentgenograms, there may be ventral compression of the cervicomedullary junction by soft tissue.

SIGNS AND SYMPTOMS

Cervicomedullary junction abnormalities produce a myriad of symptoms and signs, including myelopathy; brain stem, cranial nerve, and cervical root dysfunction; vascular insufficiency; or any combination of these.[1-4,11,29] An abnormal general appearance, usually concerning the neck, is seen with congenital abnormalities of the craniovertebral junction. The most common congenital anomaly, atloido-occipital fusion, has a high incidence of associated findings, consisting of low hairline, torticollis, short neck, and limitation of neck movement.[24] Similarly, the classic triad of shortening of the

FIGURE 121-1 The anatomic relationships of the bone and soft tissue in the midsagittal (*A*) and axial (*B*) planes of the craniovertebral junction.

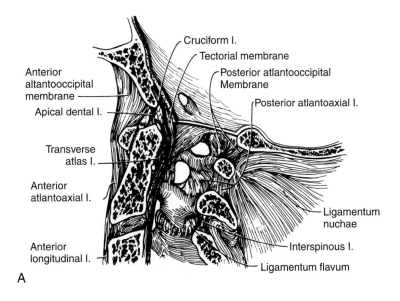

Anterior altantooccipital membrane

Apical dental I.

Transverse atlas I.

Anterior atlantoaxial I.

Anterior longitudinal I.

Cruciform I.

Tectorial membrane

Posterior atlantooccipital Membrane

Posterior atlantoaxial I.

Ligamentum nuchae

Interspinous I.

Ligamentum flavum

A

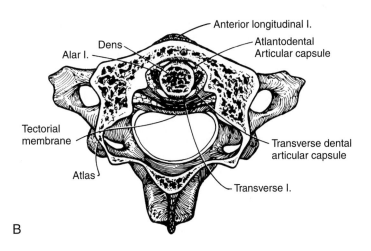

Anterior longitudinal I.

Dens

Alar I.

Atlantodental Articular capsule

Tectorial membrane

Transverse dental articular capsule

Atlas

Transverse I.

B

neck, low posterior hairline, and restriction of neck motion is described in the Klippel-Feil syndrome.[30]

Myelopathy was the most common neurologic deficit in our series, occurring in 98% of the patients. The initial symptoms, such as lack of physical endurance, may be subtle, particularly in younger patients. The severity of myelopathy is variable and may present as different degrees of weakness in the upper or lower extremities. False localizing signs were common, and motor deficits included monoparesis, hemiparesis, paraparesis, tetraparesis, and quadriparesis. A myelopathy mimicking the central cord syndrome was often present in patients with basilar invagination. The pathophysiology of motor myelopathy has been attributed to repetitive trauma on the pyramidal tracts secondary to chronic compression.[1,31] The false localizing signs have been attributed to stagnant hypoxia of the cervical spinal cord from venous stasis.[32]

Sensory abnormality is usually manifested by neurologic deficit relating to posterior column dysfunction. Hypalgesia that reflected spinal thalamic tract dysfunction was unusual, occurring in only 5% of patients, and is usually associated with severe paralysis. Bladder incontinence was unusual, the most common symptoms being urgency or hesitancy of urination.

Cervical root symptoms are usually manifested by suboccipital headaches in the sensory distribution of the greater occipital nerve. The dysesthesias are from irritation of the second cervical nerve as it traverses through the lateral atlantoaxial joint capsule.

Brain stem signs included nystagmus to lateral gaze, and downbeat nystagmus is not uncommon. This latter finding has been well documented in cervicomedullary pathologic conditions.[33] Respiratory arrest and sleep apnea were associated with both anterior and posterior compression of the cervicomedullary junction, and resolved in each after decompression. Dysfunction of the trigeminal, glossopharyngeal, vagus, accessory, and hypoglossal cranial nerves has been identified in our patient population, as have dysmetria, internuclear ophthalmoplegia, and facial diplegia. Tinnitus, diminished hearing, or both, were present in approximately 25% of the patients but were an infrequent complaint.

Symptoms attributed to vascular compromise included syncope, vertigo, episodic hemiparesis, altered level of consciousness, and transient loss of visual fields. These symptoms may be secondary to repetitive trauma of the spinal cord vessels or intermittent obstruction by angulation or stretching of the vertebral or anterior spinal arteries resulting from excessive mobility of an unstable atlantoaxial joint. Although several patients exhibited vascular symptoms, angiographic evidence of vascular compromise at the craniovertebral junction was rarely demonstrated.

DIAGNOSTIC INVESTIGATIONS

Several reference lines are used to evaluate plain roentgenograms in the assessment of the cervicobasilar relationships.[34] McRae's line measures the sagittal diameter of the foramen magnum from its anterior margin to its posterior margin (average, 35 mm). Towne's projection is useful for determining the transverse diameter of the foramen magnum (35 mm ± 4 mm). Chamberlain's line is a diagonal from the hard palate to the posterior margin of the foramen magnum (Fig. 121-2). The odontoid process should not extend more than one third of its length above this line. Wackenheim's clivus-canal line is drawn along the posterior surface of the clivus, and basilar invagination is present if this line is intersected by the odontoid process (see Fig. 121-2). Fishgold's digastric line is measured on the frontal projection and connects the digastric grooves. The line is normally 11 mm ± 4 mm above the atloido-occipital junction. The digastric line is the upper limit of position for the odontoid tip. Patients with abnormalities of the craniovertebral junction become symptomatic when the effective diameter of the spinal canal at the foramen magnum (from the posterior surface of the odontoid process to the posterior margin of the foramen magnum) is less than 19 mm.

Special radiologic procedures are necessary for the clarification of the etiology and pathophysiology of the craniovertebral abnormalities.[1-4] These examinations of the cervicomedullary junction include magnetic resonance imaging (MRI; Fig. 121-3A), computed tomography (CT), single- or 3-dimensional CT (see Fig. 121-3B), plain radiographs, and pluridirectional polytomography (see Fig. 121-14). These studies provide complementary information.

The most significant examination of the posterior fossa contents and spinal cord is provided by MRI, which demonstrates the medulla and cervical spinal cord with great clarity.

Abnormality in size and position of the cervicomedullary junction, abnormality of cerebellar tonsil position, and the presence or absence of hydromyelia are demonstrated without the use of ionizing radiation (see Fig. 121-3A). Contrast injection of the subarachnoid space before a CT study or polytomography is valuable for the correlation of a specific bone abnormality with change in the adjacent subarachnoid space. Diagnostic studies of the craniovertebral junction in the flexion-extension positions (with or without contrast material) can best be performed with plain radiographic studies or preferably MRI.

OPERATIVE TECHNIQUE

No single anterior or posterior surgical procedure can be used for all patients with occipitoatlantoaxial abnormalities. The operation or combination of operations for each patient must be selected based on a complete understanding of embryology, functional anatomy, pathophysiology, and investigative radiologic abnormalities as described in the previous sections.

The treatments of craniovertebral junction abnormalities can be divided into those for deformities that can be realigned and those for deformities that cannot be realigned (Fig. 121-4). Deformities that are reducible may require immobilization by bracing or posterior fusion. Deformities that are irreducible are divided into ventral and dorsal compression categories. In the former, the operative procedure is transoral or extrapharyngeal decompression, and in the latter, posterior decompression. No further surgery is necessary after decompression if the craniovertebral junction is stable. If instability is present, both ventral and posterior decompression require a posterior fusion for stability. All abnormalities can be classified into these six operative categories for treatment.[1-4]

Reducible Pathologic Condition: Requiring Immobilization Only

Approximately 5% of patients had reducible pathologic conditions that required immobilization only as their treatment. The most common etiologies of these deformities were posttraumatic atlantoaxial subluxations, cruciate ligament tears, and following neck or throat infections.

We have purposely omitted from this discussion odontoid and atlantoaxial fractures that require fixation only because the causes and treatment of these entities are well documented in the literature.[35,36] Although some reducible pathologic conditions can be realigned by positioning only, most require up to 15 lb of skeletal traction with Crutchfield tongs, Gardner-Wells tongs, or a halo ring.

The halo ring with pin fixation has the advantage over other traction devices in that changing the apparatus attached to the skull is unnecessary when the patient is placed in a body brace. An acrylic vest lined with lamb's wool is preferable, and lightweight metals or alloys have replaced the stainless-steel rings, pins, and vertical support bars. Metals such as aluminum, titanium, or graphic alloy do not distort CT or MRI scans of patients who are immobilized in such a brace. The halo brace fixation is preferred for stabilization of the craniovertebral junction because of its superiority over other methods of bracing in the rostral cervical spine.[37]

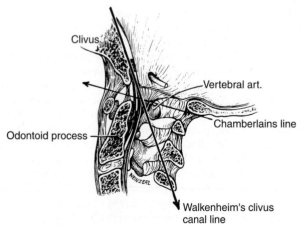

Clivus
Vertebral art.
Chamberlains line
Odontoid process
Walkenheim's clivus canal line

FIGURE 121-2 A midsagittal section of the craniovertebral junction illustrating Chamberlain's and Wackenheim's clivus-canal lines.

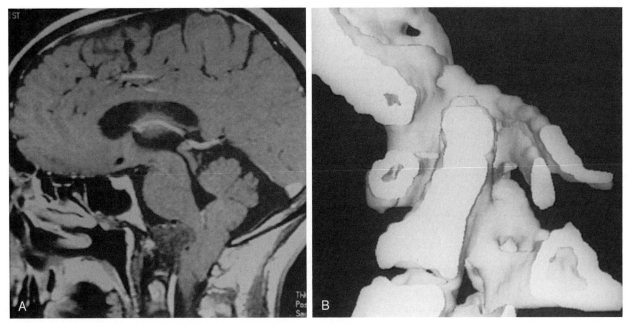

FIGURE 121-3 *A,* Midline sagittal T1-weighted MRI to illustrate a ventral chordoma. *B,* A 3-dimensional CT scan of basilar invagination at the craniovertebral junction.

Reducible Lesions: Posterior Cervical Fusion

Among the 34% of patients with reducible pathologic conditions, 88% had instability that required posterior cervical fusion (Table 121-2). Similar to those with reducible lesions requiring immobilization only, a few patients could be realigned with positioning only, but most required skeletal traction using either Gardner-Wells tongs or a halo ring apparatus. The traction is initiated at 7 lb, followed by a graded increase up to a maximum of 15 lb. Continuing traction for 7 to 14 days may be necessary to obtain satisfactory position before stabilization. Under certain pathologic conditions, we have not been successful in realigning the craniovertebral junction with cervical traction. These conditions include basilar invagination in which the tip of the odontoid process is 20 mm or more above the foramen magnum, fracture at the base of the dens, and complete separation of the atlas's posteroanterior arches.

Operative Technique

Before administration of anesthesia, the patient is intubated while awake by use of regional block and topical anesthesia to the pharynx and larynx. After intubation, the patient is positioned on the operating table in the prone position. The head is placed in the cerebellar headrest, with the clinician ensuring that no pressure is placed about the eyes. Skeletal traction is maintained throughout the operation at between 5 and 10 lb, which is sufficient to maintain satisfactory alignment of the cervicomedullary junction.

After the patient is positioned on the operating table, a lateral roentgenogram is obtained to confirm that proper occipitocervical alignment has been maintained. The neurologic examination is repeated to ensure that no significant change has occurred after positioning. The patient is then anesthetized. Pin fixation to the head is to be avoided in these patients because we have observed neurologic deterioration with pin fixation in patients who have an unstable spine.

FIGURE 121-4 Algorithm for treatment of craniocervical abnormalities.

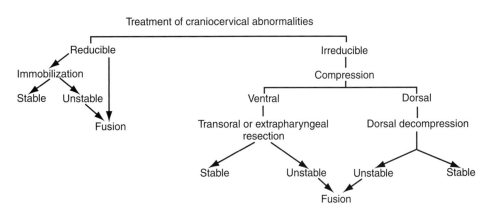

TABLE 121-2 ▪ **Surgical Treatment of Craniovertebral Anomalies**

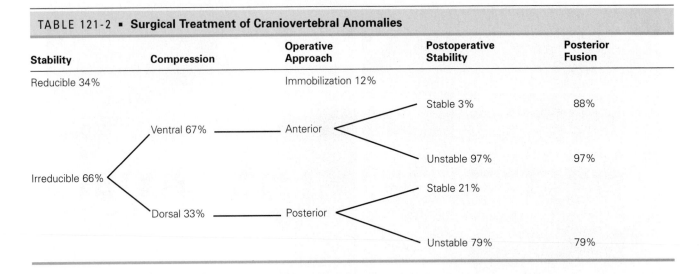

Stability	Compression	Operative Approach	Postoperative Stability	Posterior Fusion
Reducible 34%		Immobilization 12%		
Irreducible 66%	Ventral 67%	Anterior	Stable 3%	88%
			Unstable 97%	97%
	Dorsal 33%	Posterior	Stable 21%	
			Unstable 79%	79%

A midline incision is made from the inion to C4 down to the deep cervical fascia. The spinous processes are exposed by excision through the avascular ligamentum nuchae. With precautions taken to avoid excessive vertebral manipulation, a combination of cutting current and a two-periosteal-elevator technique (one elevator is used to retract the muscle, and the other is used for subperiosteal dissection) is used to dissect the paracervical musculature off the spinous processes and laminae in a subperiosteal plane. The suboccipital musculature is dissected from the squamous occipital bone in the subperiosteal plane by use of both cutting current and sharp-blunt dissection.

In patients with an unstable atlantoaxial articulation, fusion includes only the rostral two or three cervical vertebrae. In patients with occipitoatlantoaxial instability, the fusion includes the occiput in addition to the atlantoaxial vertebrae. A notch is placed inferiorly and superiorly on each lamina, and a hole is drilled through each side of the occipital bone lateral to the foramen magnum. Twisted 25- or 26-gauge stainless wire is placed under each lamina and through the occipital bones (Fig. 121-5). The twisted wire is prepared by bending the wire into two equal lengths, securing the bent

end into a hand drill, and grasping the free ends with needle holders. The wire is twisted by turning the drill and keeping equal tension on the free wire ends. This maneuver increases the tensile strength of the wire approximately 16 times. More recently, Songar cables have been substituted for twisted wire.[38] The advantage of these cables is that they are more pliable yet have equivalent strength when compared with the wire.

Bone donor sites are either the rib or iliac crest.[39] The bone graft is notched adjacent to the lamina, and a notch or a hole is placed in the rostral end for the occipital wire. The graft is secured to the opposing laminar surface, or the occipital bone, or both, by twisting the ends of the wires together (see Fig. 121-5). Bone chips can be placed along the fusion area for additional strength.

Patients are kept in skeletal traction for 3 to 7 days after surgery. Before ambulation they are immobilized in a halo brace and kept in the brace until the fusion is solid. The duration for immobilization is usually 3 to 4 months for atlantoaxial fusion and 6 to 12 months for occipitoatlantoaxial fusion. For the latter, less prolonged immobilization may result in nonunion, union in an abnormal position, or in

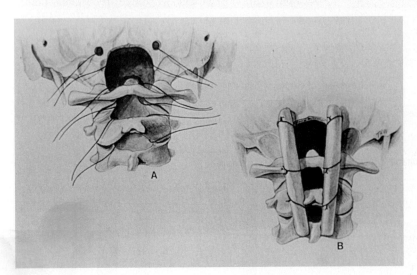

FIGURE 121-5 *A*, Placement of the twisted wire under the laminae and through the occipital bone. *B*, The bone graft is secured to the occiput and laminae by the wire.

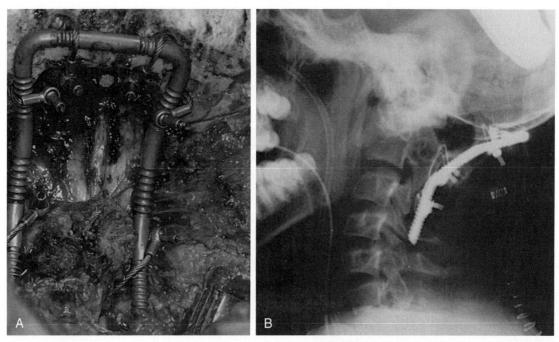

FIGURE 121-6 *A,* Intraoperative photograph to illustrate cables securing a titanium loop to the occiput and laminae of C1 and C2. *B,* Postoperative lateral roentgenogram showing the loop and bone fusion in place.

patients with rheumatoid arthritis, further cranial settling with subsequent increased neurologic deficit.

Occipitoatlantoaxial Posterior Fusion with Instrumentation

In severely disabled patients such as those with rheumatoid arthritis, immediate stabilization can be obtained by instrumentation. We previously had utilized acrylic and wire fixation.[40–42] Several instrumentation procedures have been introduced for occipitocervical and atlantoaxial fusion, including clamps, rods, and contoured loops.[43,44] The placement of instrumentation serves only for the immediate postoperative period until osseous fusion has occurred.[45]

We prefer using custom-contoured loop instrumentation to span the occiput and upper cervical spine. The use of titanium instrumentation and cables is preferred to allow for postoperative MRI.

The exposure is as previously described for rib graft fusion. The titanium loop is placed against the dorsal occipitocervical articulation, and the contour of the loop is custom fitted to the patient. Cables secure the loop at the points of fixation to the occiput as well as the dorsal aspects of the laminae from C1 to C3 (Fig. 121-6A). In most patients, the titanium cables can be cinched to 30 lb torque pressure (maximum) at the occiput and C2. At C1 and C3, the torque pressure is between 15 and 20 lb. Rib grafts are placed medial to the instrumentation so as to have contact with the bony surface of the occiput and laminae of the cervical spine (see Fig. 121-6B).

Posterior Atlantoaxial Transarticular Screw Fixation

Although atlantoaxial instability is traditionally treated with posterior arthrodesis using wiring and bone grafts, the transarticular screw fixation is useful in conditions such as previously failed operative fusion. This procedure, initially described by Magerl and Seemann, has become increasingly popular as a supplement to bone fusion.[46,47]

The patient is positioned with crown halo traction on the operating table, and lateral fluoroscopy is used throughout the procedure. After exposure of the C1–C2 facets, removal of their ligamentum flavum and cartilage from the joints, and exposure of the C2 root, the cortical bone of the inferior facet is penetrated at its posterior aspect 3 to 4 mm from the medial edge with a bone awl. A K wire is inserted and passed toward the anterior arch of C1, 10 degrees to the ventricle to ensure passage through the C2 pars interarticularis. A threaded tap is then inserted over the guidewire, and after removal a screw is then advanced over the guidewire. The screw is usually 40 to 46 mm in length and should be measured so that when fully inserted the head is positioned flush against the bone (Fig. 121-7). Screws that are misdirected can result in neurologic injury, inadequate fixation, vertebral artery injury, and damage to the pharynx.[48]

Posterior Decompression with and without Fusion

In those patients who had irreducible pathology, 33% had posterior compression. Subsequent to posterior decompression, 79% were unstable and required fusion (see Table 121-2).

The patient positioning on the operating table, the anesthesia induction technique, and the operative exposure of the spinous process and lamina are identical to the description outlined under posterior cervical fusion. A suboccipital craniectomy is performed that includes the posterior and lateral bone surrounding the foramen magnum. The laminae and spinous processes of C1 and C2 (and C3 if necessary) are removed in a rostrocaudal direction. The laminectomy should extend laterally to the medial portion of the facets.

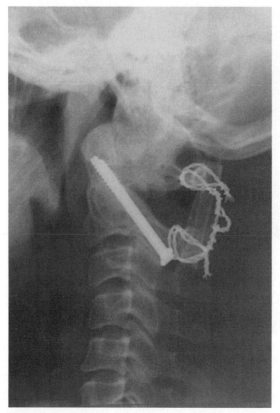

FIGURE 121-7   Lateral roentgenogram to illustrate placement of atlas-axis transarticular screws with bone fusion.

It is important to excise all compressive soft tissue, including the constricting dural band that is frequently present in the Chiari malformation at the level of the foramen magnum.

If stabilization is necessary after laminectomy is performed, lateral interfacet fusion is used. The muscles and capsular ligaments of the C1 and C2 posterior facets, or of the C3 posterior facets, are removed with cutting current, periosteal elevators, and curets. Holes are then drilled through the inferior facet into the interfacet joint of each vertebra. If the suboccipital bone is incorporated into the fusion, one or two holes are drilled on each side of the occipital bone lateral to the foramen magnum. A 25- or 26-gauge stainless-steel twisted wire is prepared as described in the previous section and is passed through the openings (Fig. 121-8A). Passing the wire through the interfacet joint is facilitated by spreading of the joint with a Freer elevator. Either rib- or split-thickness iliac bone is placed adjacent to the facets, or occiput, and is secured in place by the wires (see Fig. 121-8B). The postoperative management of the lateral fusion is identical to that described for the posterior fusion without laminectomy. The patient must remain in halo immobilization for 6 to 12 months after the procedure.

Instrument stabilization as previously described for posterior cervical fusion can be utilized by anchoring the metal loop with cables passing through the facets.

Transoral-Transpharyngeal Approach

The goal of the transoral-transpharyngeal operation is to correct ventral irreducible compression of the cervicomedullary junction. Sixty-seven percent of the irreducible cases have ventral compression of the craniomedullary junction and require an anterior approach for decompression (see Table 121-2). Pharyngeal and nasal cultures are obtained 3 days before the proposed surgery to treat any pathogenic flora present with antibiotics. If normal flora is present, no antibiotics are necessary. It is prudent to have the patient's nutritional status in the best condition possible before surgery.

The patient is placed supine on the operating table with 5 to 10 lb of skeletal traction to maintain alignment of the craniovertebral junction. The previously outlined techniques of intubation and administration of general anesthesia are used in this procedure. We had previously performed a tracheostomy in each patient to ensure an adequate airway postoperatively. With additional experience, we began using our current technique of inserting a malleable endotracheal tube and leaving it in place for 24 to 48 hours postoperatively, rendering tracheostomy unnecessary. A gauze packing may be used to occlude the pharynx to prevent blood leakage into the stomach.

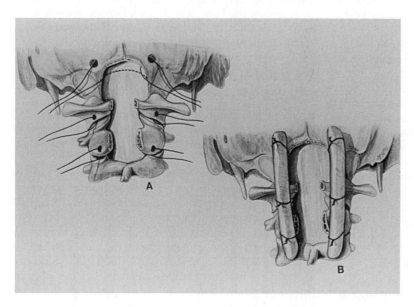

FIGURE 121-8   *A,* Placement of holes and wire through the occipital bone and the C1 and C2 inferior facets after a laminectomy. *B,* The bone graft is secured to the occiput and facets by wire.

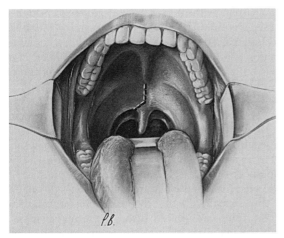

FIGURE 121-9 The midline incision in the soft palate (*broken line*).

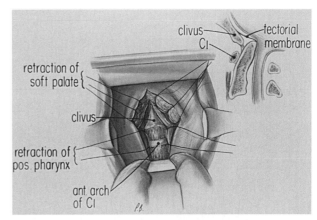

FIGURE 121-10 Exposure of the clivus, the atlas's anterior arch, and the odontoid process. Stay sutures retract the soft palate and pharynx. A corresponding midline sagittal drawing is shown in the upper right *inset*.

The mouth is kept open with a Dingman retractor, with placement of a rubber guard over the teeth. Self-retaining retractors are attached to the frame of this instrument to depress the tongue. The retraction on the tongue should be loosened intermittently during the operation to prevent lingual congestion.

The soft palate is infiltrated with 1% lidocaine (Xylocaine) with 1:200,000 epinephrine or normal saline, and a midline incision is made that extends from the hard palate and diverts from the midline at the base of the uvula (Fig. 121-9). This incision ensures minimal bleeding and unrestricted healing to the soft palate, because the palatine artery and its accompanying palatine nerve enter the soft palate laterally and terminate in the midline. Stay sutures for retraction are placed on the soft palate flaps to allow for maximal exposure through the pharynx to the caudal portion of the clivus. For situations in which surgery is necessary through the clivus or in patients with a foreshortened clivus and platybasia, the hard palate is exposed and the posterior 7 to 10 mm is resected. This allows high nasopharyngeal exposure without splitting the mandible or doing a median glossotomy.

The arch of the atlas and the caudal extent of the clivus can be palpated by the surgeon through the retropharyngeal musculature. A linear midline incision is made through the posterior pharyngeal wall to the anterior longitudinal ligament and its rostral extension, the atloido-occipital ligament. The retropharyngeal musculature is easily separated from these ligaments, and stay sutures or a self-retaining retractor is used to maintain lateral retraction of the muscle.

After exposure of the anterior longitudinal ligament, the operating microscope is used to provide magnification and a concentrated light source. The ligament is coagulated to reduce bleeding, and the anterior body of the axis, anterior arch of the atlas, and caudal anterior clivus are exposed in the subperiosteal plane by use of a periosteal elevator (Fig. 121-10). The ventral atlantoaxial articulation is separated, and the anterior atlas is removed with a 1.5-mm footplate, 45-degree-angled punch rongeur to expose the caudal odontoid process (Fig. 121-11). The apical ligament with its attachment to the caudal clivus is removed, and if the odontoid invagination is severe, resecting a portion of the caudal clivus may be necessary. If resection of the caudal clivus is required, the tissue posterior to the clivus must be carefully

separated from the bone because the dura can be easily penetrated, and troublesome bleeding may occur from the marginal sinus.

The surgeon should next identify the distal tip of the odontoid process by subperiosteal dissection of ligamentous tissue from its osseous ventral surface (Fig. 121-12). The bulk of the odontoid process is then removed with a steel cutting burr. A diamond burr is then substituted to remove the tip and the thin dorsal bony shell of the dens to avoid tearing the posterior soft tissue. We prefer to use a 45-degree-angled handpiece attachment to the drill to provide unrestricted visualization of the surgical field. After the posterior tissue plane at the odontoid tip is identified, the odontoid process and body of the axis are removed in a rostral-to-caudal direction for decompression of the cervicomedullary junction (Fig. 121-13).

In patients with rheumatoid arthritis and other inflammatory disorders, hypertrophy and thickening of the ligamentous tissue may be extensive. Adequate ventral decompression is not accomplished until this tissue is removed adjacent to the dura (see Fig. 121-13). After identification of the dural ligamentous plane rostrally, dissection of the granulation tissue is completed in a caudal direction by sharp and

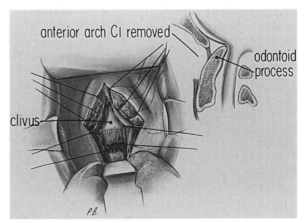

FIGURE 121-11 The operative area after excision of the C1 anterior arch with the apical ligament intact. A corresponding midline sagittal drawing is shown in the upper right *inset*.

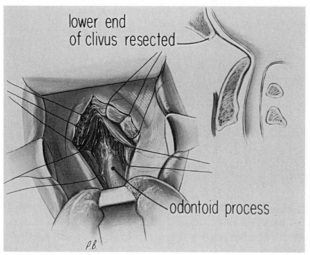

FIGURE 121-12 The operative area after excision of the apical ligament and caudal clivus, with exposure of the odontoid tip. A corresponding midline sagittal drawing is shown in the upper right *inset.*

blunt instrumentation. The surgeon can be assured that adequate cervicomedullary decompression has been accomplished when the pulsatile dura protrudes ventrally into the decompression site.

If the dura is torn or cerebrospinal fluid is identified, closure of the dura can be difficult.[49,50] In our experience, repair of the fistula can be accomplished by placing two or three layers of fascia over the rent. The fascia is harvested from the external oblique aponeurosis or fascia lata from the anterior lateral thigh. This fascia graft is reinforced with a fat pad before closure of the operative wound. In this situation, a lumbar cerebrospinal fluid drain is inserted and maintained for 7 to 10 days after surgery.

If a tumor such as a chordoma is encountered (see Fig. 121-3A), direct visualization of its extent is possible.[51]

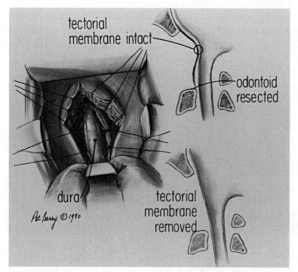

FIGURE 121-13 The operative area after the dens has been removed. The sagittal drawing (*upper right*) shows inadequate decompression secondary to a hypertrophied tectorial membrane. The sagittal drawing (*lower right*) demonstrates adequate decompression following removal of the ventral soft tissue.

Piecemeal removal is done without undue traction in case of dural penetration. In situations when an intradural lesion is encountered, a midline incision in the ventral dura is made beginning inferiorly and proceeding rostrally. If the circular sinus is prominent, the linear incision is converted into a cruciform one just caudal to the sinus to avoid troublesome bleeding. The tumor resection is facilitated by a previously placed spinal subarachnoid drain to relieve cerebrospinal fluid turgidity. When the intradural operation is completed, the dural leaves are approximated in as watertight a closure as possible. A fascia and fat graft is placed over the closure as previously described.

The pharyngeal musculature and aponeurosis are closed with interrupted 000 absorbable sutures in two layers. Mattress sutures are placed through the oral mucosa and include the muscle to ensure snug approximation. The soft palate tissue is approximated by closing of the mucosa with interrupted sutures on the ventral and dorsal surfaces. Preoperative and postoperative roentgenograms of basilar invagination and the odontoid resection are illustrated in Figure 121-14.

In children, the cruciate ligament and tectorial membrane should be preserved in addition to the periosteum of the dens; this measure will allow for new bone formation, and spontaneous ventral fusion has occurred in several of our cases. Similarly, spontaneous anterior bone fusion commonly occurs after posterior fusion in children.

After surgery, the patient is kept in 5 lb of skeletal traction. Intravenous fluids are continued for 5 to 6 days, followed by gradually increased feedings to a regular diet by the 10th to 12th day after surgery. It was initially felt that approximately 20% of patients demonstrated craniovertebral stability based on flexion-extension polytomes obtained 5 to 8 days postoperatively. Subsequently, the craniovertebral instability has been found to exceed 97%, and a posterior fusion is recommended following transoral surgery.

If intravenous antibiotics are used, they are discontinued 48 hours after surgery if the dura is intact. If the dura is violated and a fascial graft has been used for repair, intravenous antibiotics are continued for 14 days after surgery. If a tracheostomy is present, it is discontinued as soon as the patient's status permits.

Transcervical Extrapharyngeal Approach

The anterior retropharyngeal approach to the upper cervical spine has been described by several authors.[14-18] This approach provides anterior access to the neural elements from the clivus to the third cervical vertebra without entrance into the oral cavity and allows for a ventral fusion. The authors have used a variation of these procedures for the extrapharyngeal approach.[17]

The identical precautions are taken as previously described in the transoral procedure regarding anesthesia and intubation. The cervical incision is initiated behind the ear and extends over the mastoid process to 2 cm below the angle of the mandible toward the midline rostral to the hyoid bone. At the level of the omohyoid muscle, the incision is extended vertically over the sternomastoid muscle, converting the transverse incision into a T. The extent of this vertical limb depends on the level of cervical spine that is necessary to be exposed. After dissection through the

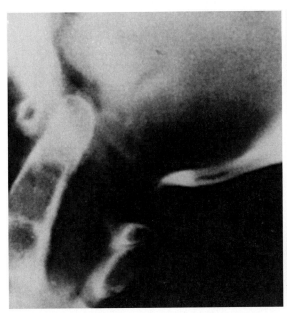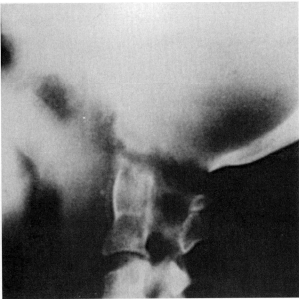

FIGURE 121-14 Preoperative lateral polytomogram to illustrate basilar invagination with air contrast medium (*left*). Note the congenital C2–C3 segmentation failure. The postoperative lateral polytomogram after resection of the odontoid (*right*).

subcutaneous tissue and platysma muscle, the inferior division of the facial nerve is identified and retracted. The dissection is continued anterior to the sternomastoid muscle and carotid sheath. The submandibular salivary gland is elevated, and if resection is done, it is important to ligate the salivary duct to prevent a fistula. The posterior belly of the digastric muscle is followed to its tendinous insertion and is transected after first transfixing it with a suture for subsequent reapproximation. The stylohyoid muscle is divided to allow medial retraction of the laryngopharynx. The hypoglossal nerve is identified in its path between the external and internal carotid arteries at the hyoid bone and mobilized superiorly, taking care to preserve the descendens hypoglossi branch. After entering the retropharyngeal space, the prevertebral fascia is vertically incised and the longus colli muscles exposed. These latter are detached from their medial origin to expose the anterior arch of the atlas and clivus. Orientation to the midline must be maintained at all times and care taken with retraction to prevent injury to the hypoglossal nerve as it emerges from the condylar foramen.

Anterior decompression is done using a high-speed drill, and the technique is similar to that described for the transoral operation. After decompression of the neural elements, bone fusion is completed using a tricorticate iliac crest graft or fibular or rib strut between the caudal clivus and vertebra.

Closure proceeds by first suturing the longus colli muscles in the midline and reapproximating the digastric tendon with 2-0 and 3-0 Nurulon suture, respectively. After the platysma muscle and skin closure, no drains are used.

The authors have used this procedure infrequently secondary to the increased risk of hypoglossal nerve injury and the difficulty in visualizing the deep midline structures at the craniocervical level. This approach is best suited for extradural pathology at the axis and subaxial level. A halo vest is placed on the third or fourth postoperative day and the stabilization maintained until bone fusion. If the pathologic process has made the spine unstable, the patient is kept in traction until posterior stabilization is achieved.

REFERENCES

1. VanGilder JC, Menezes AH, Dolan KD: Craniovertebral Junction Abnormalities. Mt. Kisco, NY: Futura Publishing Company, 1987.
2. Menezes AH, VanGilder JC: Platybasia, basilar invagination, and cranial settling. In Apuzzo MLJ (ed): Brain Surgery Complication, Avoidance and Management. New York: Churchill Livingstone, 1993, pp 2029–2049.
3. Menezes AH, VanGilder JC: Anomalies of the craniovertebral junction. In Youmans JR (ed): Neurological Surgery, 3rd ed. Philadelphia: WB Saunders, 1990, pp 1359–1420.
4. Menezes AH: Craniovertebral junction. In Albright AG, Pollack EF, Addison FD (eds): Principles and Practice of Pediatric Neurosurgery. New York: Thieme, 1999, pp 363–386.
5. Bell C: The Nervous System of the Human Body. London: Longman, Rees, Orme, Brown, & Green, 1830.
6. Dastur DK, Wadia NH, Desai AD, et al: Medullo-spinal compression due to atlanto-axial dislocation and sudden haematomyelia during decompression: Pathology, pathogenesis, and clinical correlations. Brain 88:897–924, 1965.
7. Menezes AH, VanGilder JC: Transoral-transpharyngeal approach to the anterior craniovertebral junction: 10 year experience of 72 patients. J Neurosurg 69:895–903, 1988.
8. Crockard HA, Calder I, Ransford AO: One stage transoral decompression and posterior fixation in rheumatoid atlanto-axial subluxation. J Bone Joint Surg Br 72:682–685, 1990.
9. Greenberg AD, Scoville WB, Davy LM: Transoral decompression of the atlantoaxial dislocation due to odontoid hyperplasia: Report of two cases. J Neurosurg 28:266–269, 1968.
10. DiLorenzo N: Transoral approach to extradural lesions of the lower clivus and upper cervical spine: An experience of 19 cases. Neurosurgery 24:37–42, 1989.
11. VanGilder JC, Menezes AH: Craniovertebral junction abnormalities. In Wilkins RH, Rengachery S (eds): Neurosurgery. New York: McGraw-Hill, 1996, pp 3587–3591.
12. Moore LJ, Schwartz HC: Median labiomandibular glossotomy for access to the cervical spine. J Oral Maxillofac Surg 43:909–912, 1985.
13. Hall JE, Denis F, Murray J: Exposure of the upper cervical spine for spinal decompression by a mandible and tongue splitting approach. J Bone Joint Surg Am 59:121–123, 1977.

14. DeAndraek JR, MacNab I: Anterior occipito-cervical fusion using an extra-pharyngeal exposure. J Bone Joint Surg Am 51:1621–1626, 1969.

15. McAfee PC, Bohlman HH, Riley LH, Jr, et al: The anterior retropharyngeal approach to the upper part of the cervical spine. J Bone Joint Surg Am 69:1371–1383, 1987.

16. Whitesides TE, Jr: Lateral retropharyngeal approach to the upper cervical spine. In Cervical Spine Research Society (eds): The Cervical Spine. Philadelphia: JB Lippincott, 1983, pp 517–527.

17. Menezes AH: Surgical approaches to the craniocervical junction. In Weinstein SL (ed.): The Pediatric Spine: Principles and Practice. New York: Raven Press, 1994, pp 1311–1327.

18. Kawashima M, Tanriover N, Rhoton AL, Jr, et al: Comparison of the far lateral and extreme lateral variants of the atlanto-occipital transarticular approach to the anterior extradural lesions of the craniovertebral junction. Neurosurgery 53:662–675, 2003.

19. Menezes AH, VanGilder JC, Clark C, et al: Odontoid upward migration in rheumatoid arthritis or "cranial settling." Analysis of 45 patients. J Neurosurg 63:500–509, 1985.

20. Ganguly DN, Roy KK: A study of the craniovertebral joint in the man. Anat Anz 114:433–452, 1964.

21. Bailey DK: The normal cervical spine in infants and children. Radiology 59:712–719, 1952.

22. Werne S: The craniovertebral joints. Acta Orthop Scand (Suppl 23):1–50, 1957.

23. White AA III, Panjabi MM: The clinical biomechanics of the occipitoatlantoaxial complex. Orthop Clin North Am 9:867–878, 1978.

24. Manaligod JM, Menezes AH, Bauman NM, et al: Cervical vertebral anomalies in patients with anomalies of the head and neck. Ann Otol Rhinol Laryngol 108:925–933, 1999.

25. Holmes JC, Hall JE: Fusion for instability and potential instability of the cervical spine in children and adolescents. Orthop Clin North Am 9:923–943, 1978.

26. Gilles RH, Bina M, Sotrel A: Infantile atlanto-occipital instability. The potential danger of extreme extension. Am J Dis Child 133:30–37, 1979.

27. Sullivan AW: Subluxation of the atlanto-axial joint. Sequel to inflammatory process in the neck. J Pediatr 35:451–464, 1949.

28. Clark CR, Menezes AH: Rheumatoid arthritis: Surgical considerations. In Rothman RH, Simeone FA, et al (eds): The Spine. Philadelphia: WB Saunders, 1999, pp 1281–1301.

29. Michie I, Clark M: Neurological syndromes associated with cervical and craniocervical anomalies. Arch Neurol 18:241–247, 1968.

30. Klippel M, Feil A: Un cas d'absence des vertebres cervicales avec cage thoracique remmtant jusqu'a la base du craine. Nouv Icon Soipetriene 25:223–228, 1912.

31. Menezes AH: Acquired abnormalities of the craniovertebral junction. In Winn HR (ed): Youman's Neurological Surgery. Philadelphia, WB Saunders, 2003, pp 4569–4585.

32. Taylor AR, Bymes DP: Foramen magnum and high cervical cord compression. Brain 97:473–480, 1974.

33. Cogan DG, Barrows LJ: Platybasia and Arnold-Chiari malformation. Arch Ophthalmol 52:13–29, 1954.

34. Dolan KD: Cervicobasilar relationships. Radiol Clin North Am 15:155–166, 1977.

35. Apuzzo MLJ, Heiden JS, Weiss MH, et al: Acute fractures of the odontoid process: An analysis of 45 cases. J Neurosurg 48:85–91, 1978.

36. Bohlman HH, Ducker TB, Levine AM, et al: Spine trauma in adults. In Rothman RH, Simeone FA (eds): The Spine, vol 2, 3rd ed. Philadelphia: WB Saunders, 1992, pp 973–1165.

37. Johnson RM, Hart DL, Simmons EF, et al: Cervical arthroses: A study comparing their effectiveness in restricting cervical motion in normal subjects. J Bone Joint Surg Am 59:332–339, 1977.

38. Menezes AH: Craniovertebral junction congenital abnormalities. In Kaye AH, Black P (ed): Operative Neurosurgery. London, Harcourt International, 2000, pp 1755–1770.

39. Sawin PD, Traynelis VC, Menezes AH: A comparative analysis of fusion rates and donor site morbidity for autogenic rib and iliac crest bone grafts in posterior cervical fusions. J Neurosurg 88:255–265, 1998.

40. Duff TA: Surgical stabilization of traumatic cervical spine dislocation using methyl methacrylate: Long term results in 26 patients. J Neurosurg 64:39–44, 1986.

41. Panjabi MM, Hopper W, White AA III, et al: Posterior spine stabilization with methyl methacrylate: Biochemical testing of a surgical specimen. Spine 2:241–247, 1977.

42. VanGilder JC, Menezes AH: Craniovertebral abnormalities and their neurosurgical management. In Schmidek HH, Sweet WH (eds): Operative Neurosurgical Techniques: Indications, Methods, and Results, 3rd ed. Philadelphia: WB Saunders, 1995.

43. Menezes AH: Posterior occipital C1–2 fusion. In Menezes AH, Sonntag VH (eds): Principles of Spinal Surgery. New York: McGraw Hill, 1996, pp 1051–1066.

44. Crockard HA, Pozo JL, Ransford AO, et al: Transoral decompression and posterior fusion for rheumatoid atlantoaxial subluxation. J Bone Joint Surg Br 68:350–356, 1986.

45. Coyne TJ, Fehlings MG, Wallace MC, et al: C1–2 posterior cervical fusion: Long term evaluation of results and efficacy. Neurosurgery 37:688–693, 1995.

46. Magerl F, Seemann PS: Stable posterior fusion of the atlas and axis by transarticular screw fixation. In Kehr P, Weidner A (eds): Cervical Spine. Berlin: Springer-Verlag, 1986, pp 322–332.

47. Dickman CA, Sonntag VKH: Posterior C1–2 transarticular screw fixation for atlantoaxial arthrodesis. Neurosurgery 43:275–279, 1998.

48. Wright NM, Lauryssen C: Vertebral artery injury in C1–2 transarticular screw fixation: Results of a survey of the AANS/CNS Section on Disorders of the Spine and Peripheral Nerves. J Neurosurg 88:634–640, 1998.

49. Guity A, Young PH: A new technique for closure of the dura following transsphenoidal and transclival operations. J Neurosurg 72:824–828, 1990.

50. Yamaura A, Makino H, Isobe K, et al: Repair of cerebrospinal fluid fistula following transoral transclival approach to a basilar aneurysm [Technical note]. J Neurosurg 50:834–836, 1979.

51. Menezes AH, Greenlee JDW: Transoral approach. In Chordomas and Chondrosarcomas of the Skull Base and Spine. New York, Thieme, 2003, pp 139–145.

122 Treatment of Odontoid Fractures

MAXWELL BOAKYE, PRAVEEN V. MUMMANENI,
GERALD E. RODTS, JR., and REGIS W. HAID, JR.

INTRODUCTION

Anderson and D'Alonzo classified odontoid fractures in to three types based on the location of the fracture line.[1] Type I fractures occur through the tip of the dens, type II through the base of the odontoid process, and type III fractures through the body of C2. In addition, a type IIA fracure has been described by Hadley and colleagues[2] and involves a comminution of the base of the odontoid process. Odontoid fractures may occur in isolation or in combination with fractures of the atlas.

Surgical Indications

There is considerable controversy regarding the management of odontoid fractures. In general, most type I fractures can be treated with a rigid collar,[1] and almost all type I and III fractures can be treated in halo fixation with excellent results.[3–6] Although halo fixation has been successfully used for treatment of acute type II fractures, the nonunion rates have been unacceptably high.[3] The American Association of Neurological Surgeons and Congress of Neurological Surgeons (AANS/CNS) Joint Section on Disorders of the Spine and Peripheral Nerves recently performed an extensive evidence-based review on the treatment of odontoid fractures.[7] Although there were insufficient type I data to recommend treatment standards, the study authors recommended surgical stabilization and fusion for the treatment of type II odontoid fractures in patients 50 years and older. External immobilization was considered as an option for initial management of all injuries. Surgical fixation was considered as an option in cases of dens displacement of 5 mm or more, comminution of the odontoid fracture (type IIA), or inability to achieve or maintain fracture alignment with external immobilization.

Surgical fixation avoids the morbidity associated with halo fixation (e.g., pin site infections, falls), particularly in the elderly population. Surgical fixation can be performed anteriorly or posteriorly. Options for posterior fixation include C1–C2 wiring techniques,[8] C1–C2 transarticular techniques,[9] or C1 lateral mass–C2 pedicle or C2 pars screw constructs.[10–12] Although posterior approaches have proven to be effective in the management of acute type II odontoid fractures, they usually require iliac crest bone graft (with associated graft harvest complications) and also lead to loss of C1–C2 axial rotation. C1–C2 wiring techniques as sole treatment are not recommended, because patients must be immobilized in a halo to achieve an acceptable fusion rate.[3]

As a result, our preference has been to use posterior fixation only in cases where the anterior odontoid fixation technique is contraindicated. The advantages of an anterior approach to C1–C2 stabilization include immediate stabilization via single screw placement,[12] absence of bone graft requirement, and no postoperative halo immobilization. In addition, anterior odontoid screw fixation is less technically demanding than C1–C2 transarticular screw placement.

Contraindications for Surgery

Anterior odontoid screw fixation is contraindicated in patients with osteoporosis or osteopenia, barrel chest from severe chronic obstructive pulmonary disease or emphysema, or with cervicothoracic kyphosis. In addition, we do not recommend odontoid screw fixation in patients with nonreducible fractures, nonunion longer than 3 months, oblique fractures oriented from anterior-inferior to posterior-superior, fractures with associated transverse ligament rupture, or fractures that need flexion for reduction. These patients are best treated with a posterior C1–C2 fixation technique.

Posterior C1–C2 transarticular fixation, on the other hand, is contraindicated in patients with thoracic kyphosis, aberrant or ectatic vertebral arteries, nonreducible subluxation, severely dysmorphic C1–C2 anatomy, or previous vertebral artery injury or occlusion.

Combination C1–C2 Fractures

Odontoid fractures often occur in combination with fractures of the atlas. Combination fractures of the atlas and odontoid are more likely to be associated with greater morbidity and mortality compared with isolated fractures of the atlas or axis alone.[13] The AANS/CNS Joint Section on Disorders of the Spine and Peripheral Nerves performed a detailed review of the literature on combination C1–C2 fractures. There were insufficient data to recommend treatment standards or guidelines for these fractures. External rigid immobilization can be used to successfully treat the majority of C1 and odontoid combination fractures.[13] Surgical fixation was recommended for fractures with an atlantodens interval of greater than 5 mm. Surgical stabilization can usually be accomplished using posterior C1–C2 stabilization, although there have been reports of successful treatment of these fractures using anterior odontoid screw fixation.[14] In the presence of posterior arch incompetence, posterior fixation can be accomplished using occipital cervical fixation or transarticular screw fixation[13] or C1 lateral mass–C2 pars screw fixation.

SURGICAL TECHNIQUES

The techniques of odontoid screw fixation, C1–C2 transarticular screw fixation, and C1 lateral mass–C2 pars construct are described in this section. For anterior odontoid screw fixation and posterior C1–C2 transarticular screw placement we prefer to use the Universal Cannulated Screw System

(Medtronic Sofamor Danek, Memphis, TN). For C1 lateral mass–C2 pars screw constructs, we prefer to use the Vertex system (Medtronic Sofamor Danek, Memphis, TN).

Technique of Anterior Odontoid Screw Fixation

Following fiberoptic intubation with in-line stabilization, the patient is positioned supine with neck extended under lateral fluoroscopy. The head is supported on a foam doughnut and taped to the table. A second fluoroscope is placed in the anteroposterior (AP) direction to obtain AP views in addition to the lateral views. A radiolucent mouth gag or rolled gauze is used to keep the mouth open for transoral AP views. This fluoroscopic configuration allows for simultaneous AP and lateral views during guidewire and screw placement.

A transverse incision is made at the level of the cricothyroid cartilage, and a standard Cloward-type approach to the C5–C6 prevertebral space is performed. The prevertebral fascial dissection is bluntly extended to the C2–C3 interspace. A self-retaining retractor is placed under the longus colli muscles at C5–C6 to maintain exposure. We prefer to use the Apfelbaum retractor set (Aesculap, San Franscisco, CA) for enhanced rostrocaudal exposure. The acutely angled superior blade is placed in the submandibular area and coupled caudally to the medial-lateral retractor. This creates an adequate working channel in the C2–C3 interspace. Alternatively, a METRx retractor tube (Medtronic Sofamor Danek) may be placed to provide a working channel for placement of the hardware.

Using biplanar fluoroscopy, a 2-mm threaded Kirschner wire (K wire) in a drill guide is anchored in the midline in the anteroinferior edge of C2 (Fig. 122-1). Before drilling, the K wire is impacted approximately 3 to 5 mm into the anteroinferior aspect of the C2 body. The 7-mm cannulated drill is then passed over the K wire and rotated by hand to cut a shallow groove in the C3 body and C2–C3 annulus. Under biplanar fluoroscopy, the K wire is drilled across the fracture line into the distal cortex at the tip of the dens. The K wire position should be constantly monitored on biplanar fluoroscopy. It is important not to start drilling too anteriorly or superiorly on the C2 body, because this frequently leads to a less than ideal trajectory. A nonoptimal trajectory can be corrected by drilling a new hole.

The K wire helps maintain fracture alignment before screw placement. The guide tube for the K wire is removed, and a cannulated drill bit is used to drill a pilot hole over the K wire. The length of the drilled hole can be measured using the cannulated depth gauge. A 4.0-mm self-tapping, partially threaded cannulated lag screw is then inserted over the K wire. The head of the screw is countersunk 2 mm into the C2 body (Fig. 122-2). The tip of the screw should engage the distal odontoid fragment. To obtain a lag effect, the screw threads should not cross the fracture line. Optimal screw placement is shown in Figure 122-3. The K wire is removed after confirmation of screw placement. Single-screw fixation provides excellent stabilization, and two screws provide no additional biomechanical advantage.[12] The neck can be manually flexed and extended to confirm immediate stability of screw placement and alignment.

An alternative technique for placing odontoid screws is recommended if there is persistent binding or shearing of

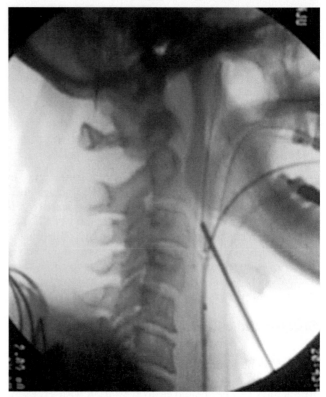

FIGURE 122-1 Lateral fluoroscopic image showing ideal K wire placement and trajectory. The ideal position of the guidewire is 3 to 5 mm below the anteroinferior edge of the C2 body. It is important to avoid starting drilling too anteriorly or superiorly on the C2 body, because this frequently leads to a less than ideal trajectory.

the K wire during drilling. In this "gliding hole technique" for placing solid odontoid screws, described by Sasso,[15] a 2.5-mm drill bit is used to drill the hole to the cortical tip of the dens. A 3.5-mm bit is then used to drill the hole up to the fracture line but not across it. The entire hole is

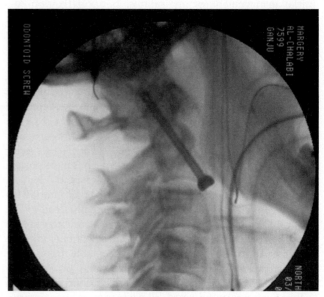

FIGURE 122-2 Lateral fluoroscope image showing cannulated screw placement after removal of guidewire. The head of the screw is slightly countersunk into the C2 body.

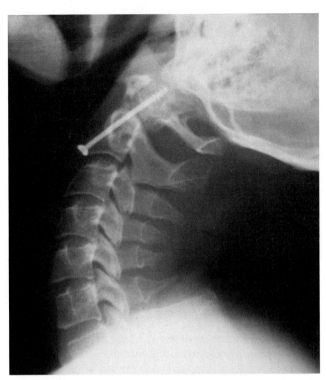

FIGURE 122-3 Lateral cervical radiograph showing optimal place-ment of a cannulated odontoid screw. The tip of the screw should engage the distal odontoid fragment. To obtain a lag effect, the screw threads should not cross the fracture line.

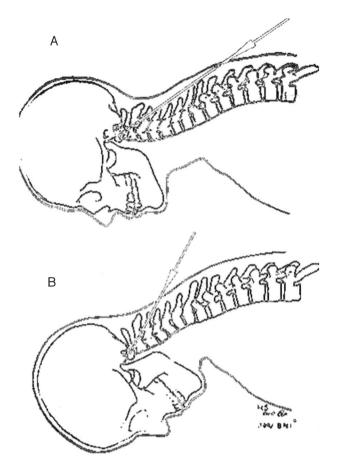

FIGURE 122-4 Drawing illustrating ideal head positioning for C1–C2 transarticular screw fixation. The neck should be neutral and head flexed in a "military tuck" position. This ensures posterior transla-tion and reduction and allows instruments to achieve the desired C1–C2 trajectory.

tapped with a 3.5-mm tap to the tip of the dens. A 3.5-mm fully threaded screw is then placed. This gliding hole tech-nique is also recommended in patients with high fractures where it may be difficult to place the threads of a lag screw above the fracture line.

We recently reviewed our long-term results of anterior odontoid screw fixation.[12] Twenty-six patients with acute type II odontoid fractures underwent single-screw anterior odontoid fixation. With a mean follow-up of 30 months, fusion was noted radiologically in 25 of 26 (96%) patients. One patient required postoperative external immobilization because of suboptimal screw position. Another patient required posterior fixation as a result of inadequate fracture reduction. There were no complications related to the surgical procedure.

Some authors have described curettage and débridement of old C2 fractures with subsequent odontoid screw fixation. However, we do not recommend odontoid screw fixation in old fractures. We prefer posterior fixation techniques instead.

Technique of Posterior C1–C2 Transarticular Screw Fixation

Following general anesthesia, the patient is positioned prone with the head secured in a three-point Mayfield headholder (OMI, Inc., Cincinnati, OH). The head is slightly flexed in the military tuck position, keeping the neck neutral (Fig. 122-4). This allows for posterior translation and reduc-tion and allows instruments to achieve the desired trajectory. The suboccipital area extending to the midthoracic area is prepped and draped. Lateral C-arm fluoroscopy is then used

to assess the cervical alignment and plan screw trajectory. The ideal placement for the drill guide is next determined. A long instrument is placed adjacent to the neck outside the incision, and the ideal trajectory is noted on C-arm fluoroscopy. The ideal trajectory should cross the C1–C2 joint and terminate at the anterior arch of C1. This also aids in identification of a good percutaneous entrance site to achieve the desired trajectory. This entry site gener-ally is approximately 2 cm lateral to the T1 spinous process. Following a midline incision, the posterior elements of C1–C3, the C2–C3 facet joint, and the C2 pars are exposed and identified. The superior and medial aspects of the C2 pars are palpated using a No. 4 Penfield, which is subse-quently used to gently displace the C2 root rostrally. Excessive bleeding can be minimized by avoiding dissection in the region of the lateral pars. Bipolar coagulation and hemostatic agents such as thrombin-soaked Gelfoam (UpJohn, PA) or Floseal (Baxter, CA) can be used to control bleeding. A 1-cm stab incision is placed at the T1 percuta-neous entry site. A guide tube is percutaneously advanced through the stab incision and docked at the C2 entry site (Fig. 122-5). The C2 entry site is located about 3 to 4 mm rostral and 3 to 4 mm lateral to the inferomedial edge of the C2–C3 facet joint. An awl or high-speed drill is used to create a small trough for the K wire entry site. Reduction of

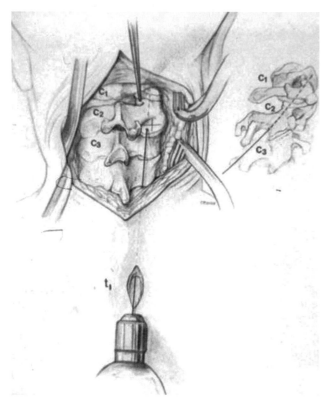

FIGURE 122-5   Drawing illustrating the percutaneous entrance site, the drill guide docking site, and the rostral mobilization of the C2 nerve.

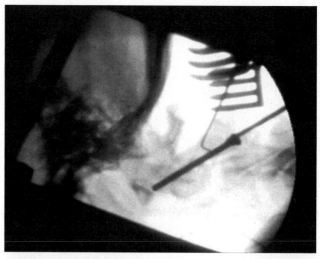

FIGURE 122-6   Lateral fluoroscopic image of a cannulated screw advanced over a K wire. The tip of the K wire and screw should ideally stop 3 to 4 mm posterior to the anterior C1 tubercle.

to pharyngeal soft tissue or injury to the hypoglossal nerve. Optimal screw placement is demonstrated in Figure 122-7. The technique is repeated on the contralateral side. To avoid delayed screw breakage, it is recommended to use 4.0-mm rather than 3.5-mm titanium cannulated screws.

C1–C2 subluxation must be performed before K wire drilling. This may be achieved using gentle C1–C2 manipulation under fluoroscopy or by first performing a posterior interspinous tension band construct. The K wire is drilled typically with a 5- to 15-degree medial angulation in the sagittal plane into the C2 pars, across the C1–C2 joint, aiming at the anterior tubercle of C1. More medial angulations risk violation of the spinal canal. The superior angle is guided by fluoroscopy. The tip of the K wire should ideally stop 3 to 4 mm posterior to the anterior C1-tubercle. Occasionally, the K wire can be observed traversing the C1–C2 joint. Often the surgeon will perceive changes in the drilling resistance as the K wire travels across the four cortical surfaces during drilling. These are the C2 entry cortex, the superior C2 articular surface, the inferior C1 articular cortex, and the anterior cortex of the C1 ring. Intermittent pulses with the drill rather than continuous drilling provide the surgeon with better proprioceptive feedback and control as the K wire is advanced. Following K wire placement, the cannulated drill bit is inserted over the wire and a pilot hole is drilled to the target point at the anterior tubercle of C1. To prevent K wire migration during drilling, an assistant can hold the K wire with a needle driver as the drill bit is advanced. The pilot hole is tapped over the K wire into the lateral mass of C1. After tapping, a fully threaded 4.0-mm screw is then placed over the K wire (Fig. 122-6).

The screw length can be easily measured directly from the drill or from the K wire. Screws are typically 34 to 44 mm in length. Longer screws may lead to a breach of the anterior cortical wall of the C1 lateral mass, causing injury

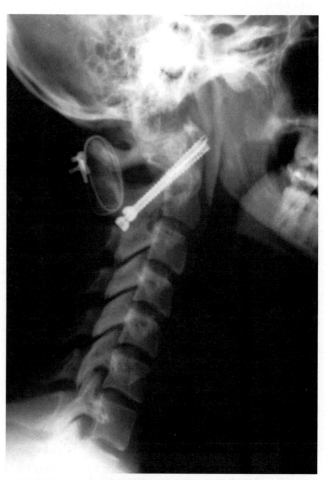

FIGURE 122-7   Lateral cervical radiograph showing optimal position of C1–C2 transarticular screws.

Following transartarticular screw fixation, a supplemental posterior tension band construct is placed. We prefer to use the Sonntag modification of the Gallie-type fusion with Atlas titanium cables (Medtronic Sofamor Danek) and tricortical iliac crest bone graft.[16] Supplemental posterior C1–C2 wire fixation provides added stability in flexion and extension.

In a recent review of our series, C1–C2 transartarticular screw fixation was performed in a series of 75 patients over a 6-year period, with a mean follow-up of 2.4 years.[9,17] Nine patients had unilateral screws placed. Patients were maintained in rigid external collars for a mean of 11 weeks. Five patients were placed in halo immobilization for a mean of 13 weeks. Fusion was noted in 72 (96%) patients. There were two cases of superficial wound infections (one at the graft site and one at the cervical incision site), which were successfully treated with antibiotics. Four patients had transient suboccipital hypesthesia. There were no vertebral artery injuries or screw breakages. All C1–C2 transartarticular screws were supplemented with a C1–C2 interspinous wiring construct.

Avoiding Vertebral Artery Injury

It is important to examine the preoperative magnetic resonance imaging scan and parasagittal computed tomography (CT) slices through the pars to comprehensively evaluate vertebral artery position and anatomy before attempting transartarticular screw placement. Abnormal vertebral artery anatomy precludes bilateral transartarticular screw placement in 18% of patients and unilateral screw placement in 3% of patients.[17,18] In such patients, alternative techniques such as C1 lateral mass screws–C2 pedicle or C2 pars screw constructs, as described by Harms and Melcher,[10] Fiore and colleagues,[19] and Mummaneni and co-workers,[11] should be utilized.

Vertebral artery injury typically occurs from lateral violations of C1–C2. If hemorrhage occurs after drilling, it is recommended to proceed with screw placement to tamponade the vessel, but avoid the procedure on the contralateral side. This avoids possible bilateral vertebral artery injury, which is likely to be fatal. Immediate postoperative angiogram should be obtained to assess for dissection and for possible vertebral artery occlusion. In such instances the surgeon should utilize alternative techniques such as C1–C2 wiring[16] for posterior stabilization.

Use of Neuronavigation

Sometimes it is helpful to use neuronavigation for surgical planning. We prefer to use the Stealth Station (Medtronic Sofamor Danek) for this purpose. Thin-slice CT scans from the occiput to C3 are obtained using a protocol specific for the Stealth Station system. Three-dimensional reconstruction views are obtained through the Stealth workstation. Transartarticular screws are then placed virtually on the 3-dimensional model. This useful exercise provides excellent preoperative visualization of the actual screw trajectory and confirms that a safe trajectory can be achieved with respect to the vertebral artery. Although neuronavigational assistance can be intraoperatively utilized, we have found regular C-arm fluoroscopy to be the most helpful for sagittal plane guidance during surgery.

Technique of C1 Lateral Mass Screw–C2 Pars/Pedicle Screw Fixation

The patient is positioned prone with the head immobilized in a Mayfield three-point headholder. The head is slightly flexed in a "military tuck" position to facilitate exposure of the C1–C2 area. The arms are tucked at the sides, and the shoulders are pulled caudally with tape. A midline incision is made extending from the inion to the C3 spinous process, and a subperiosteal exposure of the C1 posterior arch, the C2 lateral mass, and the C2–C3 facet joint is performed. Lateral dissection over the posterior arch of C1 is performed to expose the vertebral artery in the vertebral artery groove (sulcus arteriosus of C1). The C2 nerve root is identified and mobilized inferiorly. Bleeding from the perivertebral venous plexus can be controlled with bipolar coagulation and application of hemostatic agents such as Gelfoam or Floseal. The lateral mass of C1, inferior to the C1 arch, is exposed. Next the medial wall of the C1 lateral mass is palpated using a Penfield No. 4. This serves as the medial extent of screw placement. The medial aspect of the transverse foramen should be identified and serves as the lateral limit of screw placement. The entry point for screw placement is determined and prepared. The ideal point is 3 to 5 mm lateral to the medial wall of the C1 lateral mass, at the junction of the lateral mass and inferior aspect of the C1 arch (Fig. 122-8). A high-speed drill with a 3-mm round burr is used to remove a small portion of the inferior aspect of the C1 arch overlying the entry point. This creates a trough or recess for the screw head and rod or plate (Fig. 122-9). The vertebral artery and the C2 nerve root should be protected with Penfield dissectors during drilling, tapping, and placement of the screw. A 3-mm drill bit is used to drill a hole angulated about 10 degrees medially toward the anterior cortex of C1. The drill is aimed toward the anterior tubercle of C1 so as to penetrate the ventral cortex of the lateral mass midway between the superior and inferior facets of C1. The hole is tapped with a 3.5-mm tap, and a 4.0-mm C1 lateral mass screw is placed. Screw lengths are typically 32 to 38 mm; the screw head sits posterior to the C1 arch.

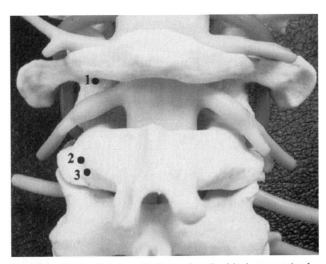

FIGURE 122-8 Spine model illustrating the ideal entry point for a C1 lateral mass screw. (1) Also shown are entry points for a C2 pedicle screw (2) and C2 pars screw (3).

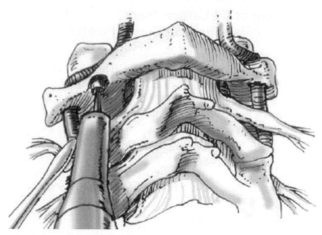

FIGURE 122-9 A high-speed drill with a 3-mm round burr is used to create a defect in the posterior inferior arch of C1. This creates a recess for the screw head.

We prefer the Vertex polyaxial screw rod system (Medtronic Sofamor Danek) for this technique.

C2 Pars Screw Placement

We have previously described our techniques of C2 pars or pedicle screw placement.[11,19,20] Following placement of a C1 lateral mass screw, a C2 pars or pedicle screw is then placed. The C2 pars is the portion of the C2 vertebra between the superior and inferior articular surfaces. The C2 pedicle is the portion of the C2 vertebra connecting the dorsal elements with the vertebral body. The C2 pars screw is placed using a starting point and in a trajectory similar to that of a C1–C2 transarticular screw, except that it is much shorter. The entry point is 3 mm rostral and 3 mm lateral to the medial C2–C3 facet joint. The screw follows a steep trajectory parallel to the C2 pars (often 40 degrees or more). We usually are able to achieve this trajectory by extending the incision down to C4 without using a percutaneous stab incision at T1. The C2 pars screw is placed with a 10-degree medial angulation. The typical screw length is 16 mm, which often stops short of the transverse foramen. Because this is a unicortical screw, we prefer to use a 4.0-mm-diameter screw, which affords increased purchase.

C2 Pedicle Screw Placement

As an alternative to C2 pars screws, screws can be placed in the C2 pedicle. The starting point for a C2 pedicle screw is typically 2 mm superior and 2 mm lateral to the starting point for the C2 pars screw described earlier (see Fig. 122-8). The screw is placed with 15 to 25 degrees of medial angulation and 20 degrees upward angulation. The hole is drilled with a 3-mm drill bit and tapped before screw placement. Following C2 screw placement, the C1–C2 screws are connected to rods and the connection is secured with locking cap screws. The completed construct is illustrated in Figure 122-10. The construct is then supplemented with a Sonntag wiring construct if the lamina of C1 and C2 are preserved. Otherwise arthrodesis is performed by careful decortication of the exposed surfaces of the C1–C2 joints by using a high-speed drill and packing cancellous iliac crest

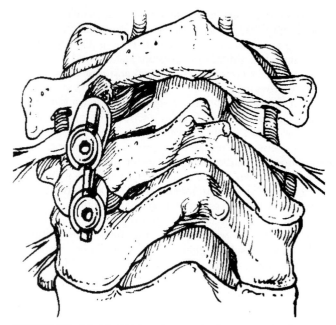

FIGURE 122-10 Final C1 lateral mass with C2 pars screw construct.

autograft over the joints. Since 1998 the construct has been used in a series of 25 patients with minimal complications.[11,19] We have not had any cases of hardware complications in more than 25 cases performed. We have had one case of pseudoarthrosis that has not required revision surgery.

CONCLUSIONS

In this chapter we presented an overview of the treatment of odontoid fractures based on current recommendations by the AANS/CNS Joint Section on Disorders of the Spine and Peripheral Nerves. In addition, we discussed the various surgical treatment options for odontoid fractures.

REFERENCES

1. Anderson LD, D'Alonzo RT: Fractures of the odontoid process of the axis. J Bone Joint Surg Am 56:1663–1674, 1974.
2. Hadley MN, Browner CM, Liu SS, et al: New subtype of acute odontoid fractures (type IIA). Neurosurgery 22:67–71, 1988.
3. Greene KA, Dickman CA, Marciano FF, et al: Acute axis fractures: Analysis of management and outcome in 340 consecutive cases. Spine 22:1843–1852, 1997.
4. Hadley MN, Browner C, Sonntag VK: Axis fractures: A comprehensive review of management and treatment in 107 cases. Neurosurgery 17:281–290, 1985.
5. Hadley MN, Dickman CA, Browner CM, et al: Acute axis fractures: A review of 229 cases. J Neurosurg 71:642–647, 1989.
6. Julien TD, Frankel B, Traynelis V, et al: Evidence-based analysis of odontoid fracture management. Neurosurg Focus 8: 2000.
7. Isolated fractures of the axis in adults. Neurosurgery 50:S125–S139, 2002.
8. Dickman CA, Sonntag VK, Papadopoulos SM, et al: The interspinous method of posterior atlantoaxial arthrodesis. J Neurosurg 74:190–198, 1991.
9. Haid RW, Jr: C1–C2 transarticular screw fixation: Technical aspects. Neurosurgery 49:71–74, 2001.
10. Harms J, Melcher RP: Posterior C1–C2 fusion with polyaxial screw and rod fixation. Spine 26:2467–2471, 2001.
11. Mummaneni PV, Haid RW, Jr, Traynelis VC, et al: Posterior cervical fixation using a new polyaxial screw and rod system: Techniques and surgical results. Neurosurg Focus 12: 2002.

12. Subach BR, Morone MA, Haid RW, Jr, et al: Management of acute odontoid fractures with single-screw anterior fixation. Neurosurgery 45:812–819, 1999.
13. Management of combination fractures of the atlas and axis in adults. Neurosurgery 50:S140–S147, 2002.
14. Guiot B, Fessler RG: Complex atlantoaxial fractures. J Neurosurg 91:139–143, 1999.
15. Sasso R: Anterior odontoid fixation, In Bradford DS, Zdeblick TA (eds): Master Techniques in Orthopedic Surgery. The Spine, 2nd ed. Philadelphia: Lippincott Williams & Wilkins, 2003, pp 79–86.
16. Dickman CA, Sonntag VK, Papadopoulos SM, et al: The interspinous method of posterior atlantoaxial arthrodesis. J Neurosurg 74:190–198, 1991.
17. Haid RW, Jr, Subach BR, McLaughlin MR, et al: C1–C2 transarticular screw fixation for atlantoaxial instability: A 6-year experience. Neurosurgery 49:65–68, 2001.
18. Paramore CG, Dickman CA, Sonntag VK: The anatomical suitability of the C1–2 complex for transarticular screw fixation. J Neurosurg 85:221–224, 1996.
19. Fiore A, Haid RW, Jr, Rodts GE, et al: Atlantal lateral mass screws for posterior spinal reconstruction. Technical note and case series. Neurosurg Focus 12: 2002.
20. Mummaneni PV, Haid RW, Jr, Fiore A, et al: Posterior fixation options for the C1–C2 complex: Wires, clamps, and screws. Contemp Neurosurg 25:1–8, 2003.

123 Surgical Management of Injuries of the Cervical Spine and Spinal Cord

VASILIOS A. ZERRIS, GERHARD M. FRIEHS, and PRAKASH SAMPATH

EPIDEMIOLOGY

The prevalence of spinal cord injury is estimated to be 906 cases per 1 million population, affecting approximately 250,000 individuals in the United States.[1] Each year, 5000 to 10,000 persons in the United States suffer spinal cord injury; 20 to 35 persons per 1 million survive until hospital admission.[1,2] Spinal cord injury occurs most frequently among men between 15 and 20 years of age.[3] The most common mechanisms of injury are motor vehicle accidents, falls, water sports accidents, and penetrating injuries resulting from gunshot or knife wounds. Approximately 60% of spinal injuries involve the cervical region, with the highest incidence of cervical spine injury occurring at the C5 and C6 levels.[3–5] Injuries to C3–T1 gradually decrease with age, whereas the incidence of fractures to C1 and C2 gradually rises because of odontoid fractures in the elderly.[6]

GUIDELINES

The literature related to spinal cord injury has been plagued by controversy.[7–9] In response, the American Association of Neurological Surgeons/Congress of Neurological Surgeons Joint Section on Disorders of the Spine and Peripheral Nerves in March 2002 published a set of guidelines intended to provide a scientifically based method for evaluating and treating acute cervical spine and cervical cord injuries. According to the quantity and quality of available data, recommendations were classified as standards, guidelines, or options. Of the 22 separate issues addressed, three qualified as standards.

The first two standards pertain to the radiographic evaluation of patients with cervical spine injury. Patients who are awake, alert, not intoxicated, without neck pain or tenderness, and with no associated significant systemic injuries do not require further radiographic evaluations. In patients who do not satisfy the foregoing requirements, a three-view cervical spine series should be the first imaging study.[10–12] This can be supplemented by computed tomography (CT) for areas that are suspect or that are not well visualized by plain film.[13] The third standard relates to the prophylaxis against deep venous thrombosis and thromboembolism.[14] In patients with severe motor deficits secondary to spinal cord injury, prophylactic treatment for thromboembolism should be initiated. Low-molecular-weight heparins, adjusted-dose heparin, and rotating beds, in combination with compression stockings or electrical stimulation, are all recommended strategies.

The remaining 19 guidelines and options are meant as diagnostic and treatment aids for the treating physician and should be tailored according to the individual needs of each patient. Two of the options address issues relating to pre-admission immobilization and transportation. Any patient with cervical spine injury or with adequate mechanism of injury should be immobilized at the scene of the injury.[14] A combination of backboard, supportive blocks, and rigid cervical collar may be used. Patients should be transported rapidly and carefully to the closest capable medical center.[15] Upon arrival at the medical facility the initial clinical examination tool used should be the American Spinal Injury Association international standards.[16–18] If the patient has a complete cervical spinal cord injury, a fracture through the foramen transversarium, vertebral subluxation, or signs/symptoms of posterior circulation ischemia, conventional angiography or magnetic resonance imaging (MRI) are valuable options to diagnose potential vertebral artery injuries.[19] Observation or initiation of heparin anticoagulation may be instituted depending on the severity of the vertebral artery injury and patient symptomatology. If the patient is diagnosed with acute spinal cord injury, he or she should be treated within an intensive care setting. This allows for optimization of his or her general medical condition, including nutritional support, and close monitoring of the patient's neurologic status.[20,21] Throughout initial patient resuscitation and inpatient treatment, every effort should be made to avoid a systolic blood pressure less than 90 mm Hg. A mean arterial pressure of 85 to 90 mm Hg is recommended for the first week following injury.[22] In patients with no additional rostral injury, early closed reduction of cervical spine fracture-dislocation injuries is an option.[23] In patients who cannot be neurologically assessed before, during, and after the reduction, or who undergo unsuccessful reduction, MRI should be used. In the pediatric population the guidelines and options for radiographic assessment of the patient are similar to the standards for radiographic assessment of adult patients. Assessment of need, choice of modality, and views depends on a large extent on the patient's neurologic and mental status as well as the type of injury.[24] Some of the literature suggests that advantageous treatment options for children might include thoracic elevation and occipital recess during immobilization in children 8 years of age or younger, halo immobilization of injuries at the C2 synchondrosis in children younger than 7 years of age, and consideration of operative treatment of isolated ligamentous injuries. In patients with spinal cord injury but no radiographic abnormality, careful multimodality radiographic evaluation, radiographic survey of the entire spinal column, external immobilization until ligamentous injury is ruled out, external immobilization for up to 3 months, and avoidance of heavy physical activity for up to 6 months may be beneficial options.[25] The guidelines also address the controversial issue of the administration of corticosteroids to patients with acute cervical spinal cord injury. When the initial and follow-up data of the National Acute Spinal Cord Injury Study (NASCIS-2) trial were presented, there was a significant paradigm shift in the pharmacologic treatment of patients with acute cervical spine injuries.[26,27] With time, several issues surrounding the methodology and validity of this trial were raised.[28–30] Despite these concerns, the medical-legal ramifications of the studies remained significant, and the majority of clinicians continued to use corticosteroid administration as part of the initial treatment. The guidelines offer an objective review of all available literature relating to this issue. Based on the available data, treatment with methylprednisolone for 24 to 48 hours cannot be regarded as a standard or guideline.[31] Rather, it should be considered a clinical option and the benefits should be weighed against the potential significant harmful side effects of systemic corticosteroid administration.[32,33]

INITIAL EVALUATION AND CARE

Cervical spine injury is estimated to occur in 3% of the patients who present to the emergency department.[1,5,34] Given the paucity of therapeutic modalities to induce spinal cord regeneration once injury has occurred, the primary goals of initial treatment in a patient with a suspected cervical spine injury are preservation of life, maintenance of neurologic function, prevention of secondary or further cord injury, and restoration of nerve and cord function where possible through decompression or traction, spinal stabilization, and early rehabilitation. The formation of regional spinal cord injury centers has tremendously influenced the outcomes of patients with cervical spine injuries.[35] These centers provide a multidisciplinary approach to emergency, medical, surgical, and rehabilitative care. This team approach has decreased the mortality of cervical cord injury significantly from 80% 50 years ago to less than 5% in more recent years.[36,37]

Initial management begins at the accident scene with personnel trained in the safe, expeditious evacuation of these patients to a hospital capable of providing definitive care.[38] The victim's head and neck must be immobilized until formal evaluation can rule out a fracture-dislocation. The evaluation should include inspection of the head and neck area—especially the forehead and occiput—for abrasions or contusions. Posterior nuchal tenderness is strongly suggestive of a spinal injury, as is any significant trauma at or above the level of the clavicle. Unconscious and uncooperative patients are a particularly difficult group

to evaluate. These patients, especially those involved in a high-impact injury, should all be assumed to have sustained a cervical spine injury until formally cleared by trained physicians.

Once a patient with a potential spinal injury is identified at an accident scene, respiratory and cardiovascular resuscitation should proceed with extreme caution. If the patient requires extrication, the entire spine should be kept immobilized, with the neck in a neutral position. Immobilizing the neck with a hard collar alone is usually inadequate and may need to be supplemented with sandbags around the neck. A Philadelphia halo immobilizer, if available, is a better orthosis. We do not advocate cervical traction without radiologic control, because this method may exacerbate a spinal deformity and worsen a neurologic deficit. If lifesaving resuscitative measures are necessary in the field, extreme care must be taken to minimize motion of the neck. Nasotracheal intubation may provide the least amount of motion.

Many effective and simple alternative methods of transportation of cervical spine injury patients have been identified, but because aspiration and shock are the major causes of morbidity and mortality, we advocate transporting patients in 10 to 30 degrees of Trendelenburg's position as a prophylactic measure when feasible. Optimally, victims with spinal cord injury should be moved by the log-rolling maneuver, which minimizes the chances of secondary neurologic injury.

Paramedics at the accident scene can provide valuable information by use of a standard neurologic assessment scheme. Assessment of motor and sensory levels can accurately pinpoint the level and nature of spinal cord or nerve injury. The motor level of a spinal cord injury is defined as the lowest level of significant motor function. A quick assessment of the patient's ability to breathe (diaphragmatic function) can be followed by a quick screening of the patient's ability to move his or her head and each of the extremities as well as the feet and toes. In the unconscious or impaired patient, proximal and distal motor response can be assessed in each extremity by use of noxious stimuli to ascertain gross motor function. In the alert patient, a systematic examination of the major motor groups of the upper and lower extremities, proceeding rostrally to caudally, provides baseline information for determination of improvement or deterioration (which, in certain cases, may necessitate a change in therapeutic management). At the accident scene, we advocate the grading of motor function as follows: 0 = no palpable contraction; 1 = strength sufficient to move the joint; 2 = strength against gravity; and 3 = full strength against resistance. More subtle grading scales are of no help in the field setting.[39]

EMERGENCY DEPARTMENT EVALUATION AND INTENSIVE MEDICAL MANAGEMENT

On arrival of the patient in an emergency department, resuscitation should proceed in the usual fashion with priority given to the establishment of an airway, providing adequate ventilation, and supporting the cardiovascular system. In a patient with suspected cervical spine injury, however, all resuscitative measures should attempt to maintain cervical immobilization and adequate spinal cord perfusion.[40]

Airway and Breathing Considerations

The establishment of a secure airway as well as the maintenance of adequate oxygenation and gas exchange can pose a significant problem in the patient with cervical spine injury, especially if the patient is unconscious or uncooperative.[39,41] In an awake patient with isolated spinal injury, it may be possible to secure the airway with a simple nasal trumpet or facemask. If endotracheal intubation is needed, it is imperative that this be performed with in-line traction of the cervical spine. Sometimes an awake, blind nasal intubation can be performed. Fiberoptic intubation is the safest form of endotracheal intubation and should be attempted when feasible and appropriate. Occasionally, in a patient in whom securing an airway is particularly difficult, it may be necessary to perform an emergent cricothyroidectomy. An alternative technique is to penetrate the cricothyroid membrane with a 14-gauge angiocatheter attached to a 5-mL syringe. These maneuvers can act to maintain adequate air exchange temporarily until a definitive tracheostomy can be performed under a more controlled setting.

Cardiovascular Considerations

Acute hypotension (shock) in the trauma setting can pose a diagnostic conundrum, especially in a patient with suspected cervical spinal cord injury. Spinal cord shock is believed to occur from massive loss of vasomotor tone secondary to neuronal injury and should be suspected if there is neurologic evidence of significant cord injury. Time-consuming diagnostic tests are often performed in lieu of a careful physical examination to determine if the cause of hemodynamic instability is hemorrhage or spinal cord injury–induced sympathectomy. The incidence of blunt intra-abdominal trauma in patients with cervical cord injury is low (7.6%), and these patients rarely require surgical repair to stop the hemorrhage.[42] Intra-abdominal injury as the cause of hemorrhagic shock in patients who suffer blunt trauma to the cervical cord usually occurs only in patients sustaining a major injury, such as pelvic-ring disruption, femoral fracture-dislocation, intrathoracic injury, and abdominal wall injury.[42] For patients without these associated injuries but with clinical signs of spinal shock, invasive diagnostic tests, such as diagnostic peritoneal lavage, needlessly delay appropriate management.

Rapid restoration of cardiac output and tissue perfusion is necessary during the acute phase of spinal cord injury.[43] This restoration can be achieved initially with aggressive fluid resuscitation. Because proper fluid resuscitation may be complicated by overload, invasive patient monitoring is usually necessary once the patient has left the emergency department. Aggressive hemodynamic monitoring includes pulmonary and peripheral arterial catheters. Pulmonary artery monitoring can be helpful in optimizing tissue perfusion by manipulating cardiac output and vascular reactivity. Optimal cardiac output is determined at the point at which the oxygen consumption plateaus in the face of rising oxygen delivery (and paralleled rising cardiac output). We achieve optimal cardiac output by fluid and vasoactive agent administration. Because constant measurement of

cardiac output (and oxygen delivery) and extraction is not feasible, optimal perfusion is arbitrarily set at a mean arterial pressure of at least 90 mm Hg. This value is calculated with the pulmonary artery catheter measurements and adjusted when other mean arterial pressure values correlate with optimal perfusion.

Experimental models demonstrate that elevating the blood pressure beyond normotensive levels improves spinal cord blood flow and improves outcome.[44,45] We commonly employ vasoactive agents to alter vascular reactivity. Dopamine and dobutamine are the most commonly used agents, although phenylephrine (Neo-Synephrine) can also be used in patients who develop tachycardia from higher levels of dopamine and dobutamine. Concomitant low-dose dopamine should be used with phenylephrine as a precaution against renal ischemia. Epinephrine has a small therapeutic window, which complicates the cardiovascular manipulation and limits its therapeutic index, particularly in the elderly or in those with underlying heart disease.

We generally provide hemodynamic manipulation for 5 days, based on edema formation peaking 48 to 72 hours after acute spinal cord injury: five days of therapy allows a 48-hour margin beyond this peak. Patients with more labile responses to vasoactive stimulation may require longer courses of therapy while being weaned off hemodynamic support.

The sympathectomy response and autonomic dysreflexia that can occur after spinal cord injury are important phenomena to recognize and treat.[41,43] These phenomena are generally thought to parallel the signs of complete neurologic injury in the spinal cord and are usually manifested by great lability in blood pressure and respiratory patterns. As a result, it may be necessary to alter vasoactive treatment to prevent hypertensive or hypotensive crisis. The pulmonary vasculature response is also altered in spinal cord injury and can lead to increased permeability of the capillary bed in the lungs. In our experience, neurogenic pulmonary edema is quite uncommon, but if unrecognized and left untreated, it can rapidly lead to adult respiratory distress syndrome. We advocate close monitoring of pulmonary status in the patient with spinal cord injury.

DIAGNOSTIC IMAGING OF THE CERVICAL SPINE

Imaging of the injured cervical spine has significantly evolved as a result of advances in neuroradiology. These different techniques are complementary, and their discriminate use is cost effective.

Plain Radiographs

Indications for cervical spine radiographs have generally included the following[46-48]:

1. A significant mechanism of injury
2. An unreliable history
3. An altered mental status
4. Complaint of neck pain or neurologic symptoms
5. A positive physical examination, including pain on palpation of the neck and neurologic signs

Cervical spine radiographs have been criticized as expensive, as being of low yield, and for causing unnecessary radiation exposure to the patient.[48,49] The need for balancing cost effectiveness and the risk of missing a cervical spine fracture has also received attention.[50] We believe, however, the threshold for obtaining a plain radiograph of the cervical spine should be low. A high index of suspicion should be maintained (especially in high-risk patients) to prevent the oversight of an unstable, occult cervical spine fracture with potentially devastating consequences.[42]

The simple cross-table, horizontal, lateral view radiographic study should be initially performed to exclude a fracture or significant soft-tissue injury. A high-quality, lateral cervical spine radiograph can be accurate in 70% to 90% of cases.[6,51] The cervical anteroposterior view should be the next radiograph performed. Though not as sensitive as the lateral view, anteroposterior films can provide valuable information about the alignment of the spine, the spinal canal, and the spacing of the pedicles. In a cooperative patient, visualization of the atlantoaxial articulation should be obtained with the open-mouth odontoid view. Although the sensitivity and accuracy of each view alone are inadequate, the sensitivity of the cervical spine series has been estimated at 93% and the accuracy at 84% in diagnosing fracture-dislocations.[6,51] An oblique view best depicts the uncinate processes, pedicles, inferior and superior facets, and laminae. The C7–T1 relationship may be determined in this view, which may negate the need for a swimmer's view.[52] In certain patients with no obvious abnormality on initial radiographs, lateral flexion-extension views may also be important to assess the integrity of the ligaments.

Computed Tomography

We routinely perform CT studies in patients with any abnormality on plain films, or those in whom lower cervical spine (C7–T1) anatomy cannot be appreciated, who are unconscious, who are uncooperative, or in whom clinical concerns for occult spinal injury are present.[53] The use of contiguous or overlapping thin sections with reformatting in different planes greatly increases the ability to demonstrate subtle fractures and intraspinal pathology not detected by plain radiographs (Fig. 123-1A and B).[54,55] Posterior arch fractures (Fig. 123-2), fractures and subluxations of the articular facets (Fig. 123-3), C1 and C2 fractures (Fig. 123-4), and intraspinal bone fragments (Fig. 123-5) are best visualized by CT. CT is also useful for the visualization of the craniocervical and cervicothoracic junctions, but there are certain pitfalls to the untrained eye that can lead to an errant diagnosis.[56] Using other modalities that complement CT is important. We also recommend CT with 2-dimensional reconstructions whenever possible, because this can detect jumped or perched facets in the absence of fracture and aid in assessing spinal alignment.

Magnetic Resonance Imaging

The development of MRI has revolutionized the ability to diagnose soft-tissue injury in and around the spinal cord. Although MRI is inferior to CT in assessing bony anatomy,

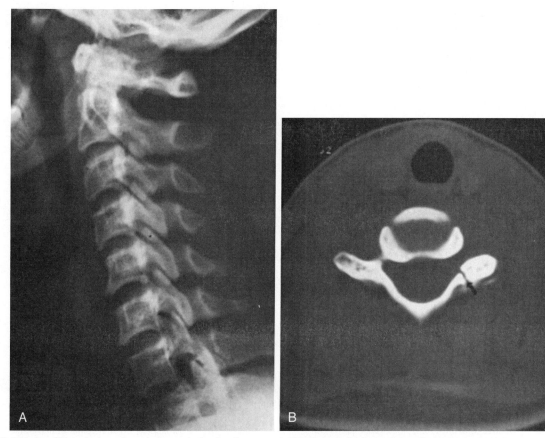

FIGURE 123-1   CT detection of a subtle cervical spine fracture. *A,* This lateral cervical spine radiograph obtained in a trauma patient with lower cervical pain is normal. *B,* A C7 left laminar-articular mass junction fracture is detected by CT (*arrow*).

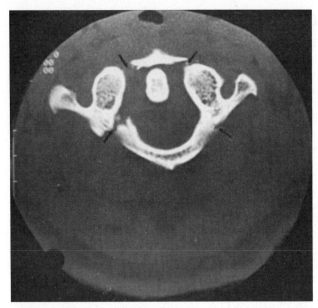

FIGURE 123-2   CT scan of a Jefferson fracture. The axial image reveals four-part fracture of C1 ring (*arrows*). Anterior arch fractures are not usually seen by radiography.

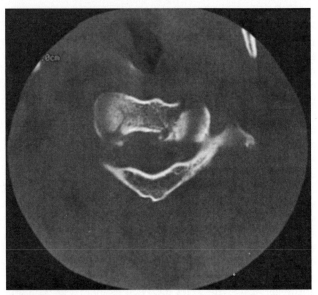

FIGURE 123-4   CT scan of a type III odontoid fracture. The axial image reveals comminution of C2 body and narrowing of spinal canal due to anterior displacement of C1 secondary to transverse alar ligament injury.

it is far superior in determining whether there is cervical disc herniation, ligamentous injury, epidural blood, or intraparenchymal spinal cord injury.[53,57–59] Our current MRI protocol includes the following sequences: (1) T1-weighted spin-echo sagittal images, (2) fast spin-echo T2-weighted sagittal images with fat suppression, (3) gradient-echo (small flip angle of 10 to 15 degrees) sagittal images, (4) 3-dimensional gradient-echo volumetric axial images, and (5) T1-weighted spin-echo axial images. This examination requires 25 to 30 minutes to perform, and most patients are immobilized in a rigid collar (Philadelphia Collar Company, Westville, NJ) with plastic fasteners for the MRI.[59–61]

Two cervical immobilization devices that permit acceptable MRI quality include a PMT halo cervical orthosis (PMT Corporation, Chanhassen, MN) and an MRI-compatible Bremer halo system (Bremer Medical Corporation, Jacksonville, FL). When cervical traction immobilization is required to maintain reduction, in-line cervical traction can be achieved with MRI-compatible graphite tongs and a series of nonferrous pulleys and water bags, or a Sokhoff board and plastic traction weights. Ventilatory support, if required, is provided by a Siemens SY-900 servoventilator

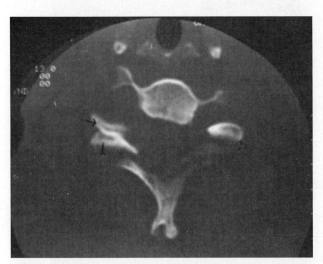

FIGURE 123-3   CT scan of a unilateral facet fracture. The axial image reveals dislocation of the right inferior facet (*arrow*) anterior to the superior facet (*arrowhead*) of the vertebral body below. Note diastasis of the contralateral left facetal joint (*open arrow*) and rotation of the vertebral body.

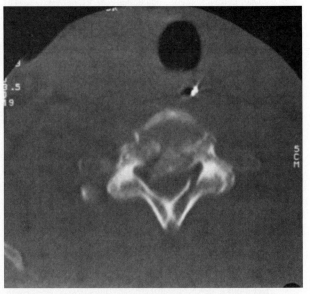

FIGURE 123-5   CT scan of a vertebral burst fracture. The axial image shows a markedly retropulsed posterior fragment from the C7 vertebral body encroaching on the spinal canal. A left laminar fracture is also seen.

(Siemens-Elema, Iselin, NJ) placed at least 1.2 meters from the magnet. A 12-foot, low-compliance pediatric circuit connects the ventilator to the patient's endotracheal tube. This system provides all standard modes of respiratory support without detectable deterioration in image quality.[61]

Although information derived from plain radiographs and CT is usually sufficient to diagnose the extent and severity of spinal column injury, we prefer to perform an MRI scan on any patient with incomplete neurologic deficit after cervical cord injury or in whom operative reduction and stabilization is being considered, provided that the patient is hemodynamically stable and has no contraindication to an MRI examination.[59] MRI can better assess the site and extent of spinal cord compression before reduction (e.g., an occult disc herniation) and is the preferred modality to detect root compression or avulsion within the intervertebral foramen. MRI can also help to clarify if a mechanical basis can explain a delayed increase of neurologic deficit or in cases in which a level of deficit does not correlate with the level of injury of the osseous spine. The limitations of plain radiographs and CT become particularly obvious in the patient with clinical evidence of spinal cord injury and no evidence of bone injury either on the plain radiographs or on the CT scan of the neck.[56,59,62]

Compression of the cervical spinal cord may result from dislocated vertebrae, displaced fragments (Fig. 123-6),

osteophytes, or ossification of the posterior longitudinal ligament. Fracture-dislocations are underdiagnosed by MRI, when compared with CT, in 50% of cases[63]; however, disc protrusions are more easily recognized by MRI than by CT (Fig. 123-7). In a series of 33 patients studied with both modalities, only 27% of disc protrusions seen on MRI were visualized by CT.[63] Epidural hematomas may develop acutely after trauma, in a delayed fashion, or after open or closed reduction of the spinal column (Fig. 123-8). The MRI appearance of a hematoma changes over time; an acute hematoma has a low signal on T2-weighted images because of intracellular deoxyhemoglobin and has a progressively increasing signal on T1-weighted images, as extracellular methemoglobin content increases.[60]

Even more dramatic is the difference between the abilities of CT and MRI to recognize direct cord injury (Figs. 123-9A, B and 123-10): in one study, MRI could identify such changes in 13 cases of cord injuries, compared with none visualized on CT.[63] MRI has proved particularly useful in demonstrating the structural changes associated with an acute central cord syndrome. In this situation, a hyperintense signal is seen within the parenchyma of the cervical spinal cord on gradient-echo MRI without features characteristic of hemorrhage in either T1-weighted or T2-weighted images.

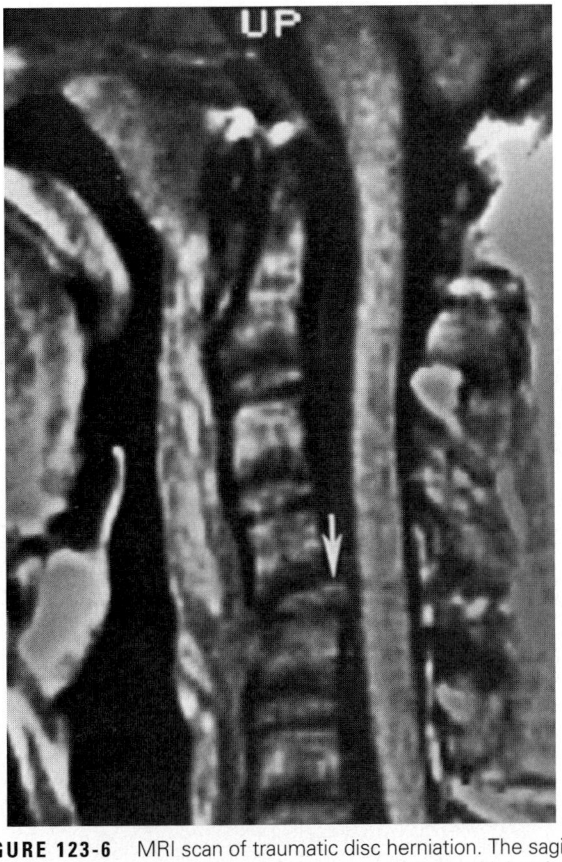

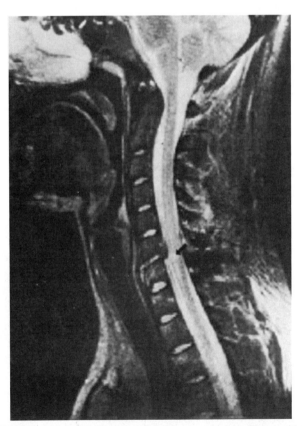

FIGURE 123-6 MRI scan of traumatic disc herniation. The sagittal T1-weighted image shows hyperflexion sprain at C4–C5 with herniation of the intervertebral disc (*white arrow*) at this level. The cord is not indented by the disc. (From Mirvis SE, Young JWR: Cervical spine trauma. In Mirvis SE, Young JWR [eds]: Imaging in Trauma and Critical Care. Baltimore: Williams & Wilkins, 1992, pp 291–379.)

FIGURE 123-7 MRI scan of cord compression. The sagittal T2-weighted image shows retropulsion of a posterior bone fragment from C6 impacting the cord. A contusion (bright signal) is observed in the cord adjacent to the fragment (*arrow*). The C6–C7 intervertebral disc is extruded anteriorly. Titanium posterior fixation allows follow-up MRI without significant artifact. (From Mirvis SE, Young JWR: Cervical spine trauma. In Mirvis SE, Young JWR [eds]: Imaging in Trauma and Critical Care. Baltimore: Williams & Wilkins, 1992, pp 291–379.)

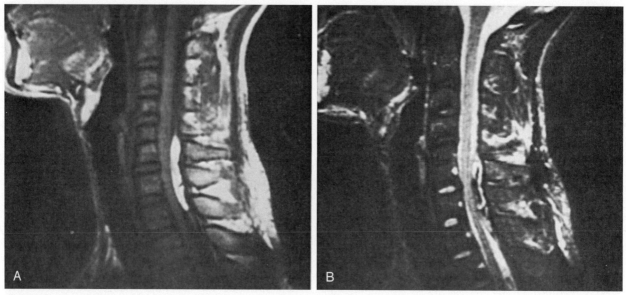

FIGURE 123-8   MRI scan of an epidural hematoma. *A,* T1-weighted MRI shows high signal intensity in the posterior epidural space at C5–C7 level. The spinal cord is compressed. *B,* T2-weighted sequence shows a low signal center compatible with intracellular hemoglobin, with a bright surrounding area compatible with extracellular methemoglobin. (From Mirvis SE, Young JWR: Cervical spine trauma. In Mirvis SE, Young JWR [eds]: Imaging in Trauma and Critical Care. Baltimore: Williams & Wilkins, 1992, pp 291–379.)

Pathologic correlation in necropsy specimens showed no evidence of blood within the cord parenchyma, but diffuse disruption of axons, especially within the lateral columns in the region occupied by the corticospinal tracts.[58,64,65] That more severe trauma, however, is likely to be accompanied by tissue destruction, mostly in the anterior horn area.[58]

The ability of MRI to image the spinal cord directly not only makes it a more sensitive diagnostic test, but also theoretically could enable it to provide important prognostic clues in the early phases of treatment. Limited evidence suggests that MRI scans obtained in the acute period provide information on the potential for recovery of neurologic function.[37]

This evidence has important ramifications because it may be possible to correlate the MRI pattern observed in the acute phase after injury with prognostic information.[66]

MRI is also useful in the demonstration of ligament injuries, which helps in establishing the mechanism of trauma in the course of evaluating damage to the spinal cord.[67] MRI demonstrates ligaments as regions of low signal intensity. Injured ligaments manifest increased signal on T2-weighted sequences because of edema, and disrupted ligaments demonstrate a discontinuity in the normal continuous low signal intensity of the ligament (Figs. 123-11 and 123-12).

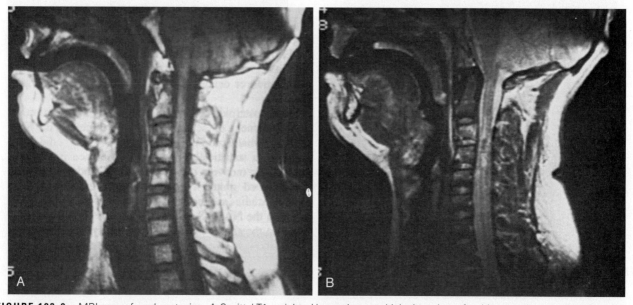

FIGURE 123-9   MRI scan of cord contusion. *A,* Sagittal T1-weighted image in a quadriplegia patient after blunt trauma reveals some widening of the spinal cord at C3 and C4. There is a C3 anterior compression fracture. *B,* On the T2-weighted sequence, there is a bright signal at C3–C4, with a central low signal suggestive of central blood and surrounding edema. C3 and C4 compression fractures are observed.

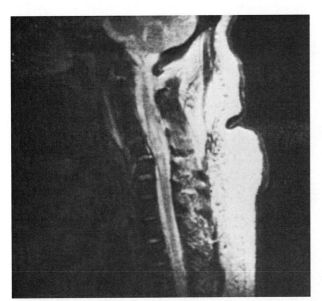

FIGURE 123-10   MRI scan of cord contusion. The sagittal T2-weighted image obtained in quadriplegic patient shows C4 on C5 anterior subluxation with stripping of the posterior longitudinal ligament from C3. A spindle-shaped region of increased signal spreads distally from the site of impact indicating edema. (From Mirvis SE, Young JWR: Cervical spine trauma. In Mirvis SE, Young JWR [eds]: Imaging in Trauma and Critical Care. Baltimore: Williams & Wilkins, 1992, pp 291–379.)

Cervical vascular injury may accompany blunt force injury to the neck. This type of injury can result in overstretching, excessive torsion, direct impact, or laceration of the major arteries, which can result in the absence of a flow void (spin echo) or of increased signal (gradient echo), indicating a vascular injury. Recently, MR angiography has been applied to the diagnosis of cervical vascular injuries (Fig. 123-13A to C).

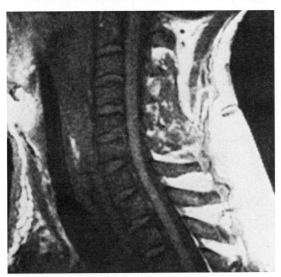

FIGURE 123-11   MRI scan of ligament disruption. The sagittal image shows loss of low signal stripe at C6–C7 (*arrow*) and widening of corresponding anterior disc space. The finding is compatible with hyperextension injury with anterior longitudinal ligament and anterior annulus fibrosus injury. (From Mirvis SE, Young JWR: Cervical spine trauma. In Mirvis SE, Young JWR [eds]: Imaging in Trauma and Critical Care. Baltimore: Williams & Wilkins, 1992, pp 291–379.)

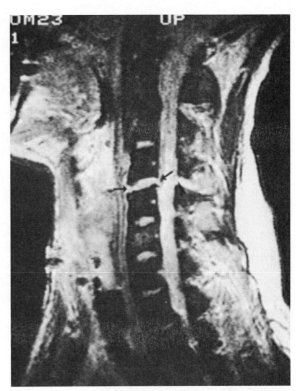

FIGURE 123-12   MRI scan of ligament injury. The sagittal T2-weighted gradient-echo image in an acutely quadriplegic patient shows complete disruption of the anterior and posterior longitudinal ligaments (*arrows*) as well as the posterior ligamentum flavum (*arrowhead*).

NONSURGICAL MANAGEMENT

The principles of nonsurgical management of cervical spine injury include pharmacologic therapy with maintenance of adequate spinal cord perfusion, realignment of the cervical spine with traction, and external orthotic devices for cervical immobilization.

Pharmacologic Treatment

The goal of medical treatment in acute spinal cord injury is to restore adequate spinal cord perfusion and oxygenation. This goal is accomplished by providing adequate volume replacement, atropine to treat bradycardia, and vasopressors to support the blood pressure if fluid resuscitation alone does not restore adequate tissue perfusion.

The degree of bradycardia occurring after cord injury may be aggravated by hypoxia and tracheal suctioning, which may trigger a vagal response not balanced by any sympathetic reflex. Early preventive treatment of gastric dilatation is also useful in the prevention of acute hypoxia resulting from poor ventilation or delayed hypoxia occurring after aspiration or sepsis.

Corticosteroids remain the cornerstone in the current medical treatment of acute spinal cord trauma. The original National Acute Spinal Cord Injury Study (NASCIS-1) did not demonstrate a statistically significant difference in the rates of neurologic recovery between naloxone-treated and methylprednisolone-treated groups of patients[68,69]; however, other data from animal studies suggest that the dose of methylprednisolone used in the NASCIS-1 study was below

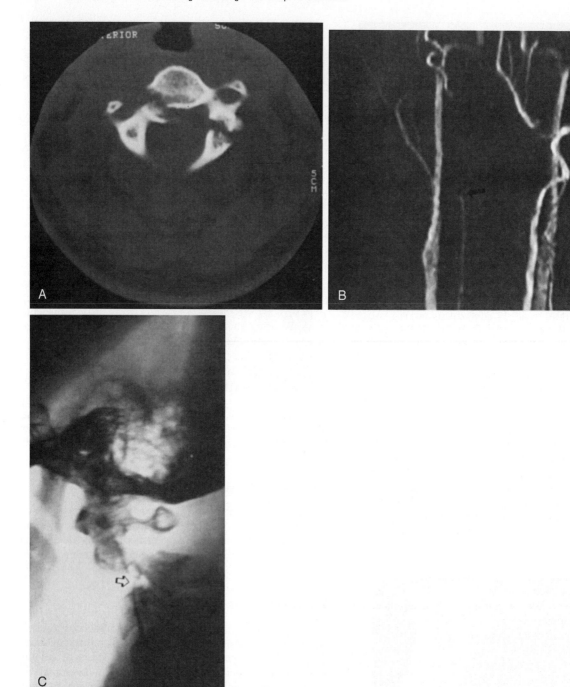

FIGURE 123-13 MR angiogram of cervical vascular injury. *A*, Axial CT image shows a hangman-type fracture at C2 extending into the right vertebral artery foramen. *B*, MR angiogram (2-dimensional, time-of-flight) shows complete occlusion of the right vertebral artery (*arrow*) at the C2 level. *C*, Lateral view of the neck from digital arteriogram confirms complete interruption of the vessel just below the fracture site (*open arrow*). The patient remained asymptomatic.

the theoretical therapeutic threshold.[44,70] The NASCIS-2 study was undertaken to study the effects of higher doses of methylprednisolone, and this study demonstrated that patients with acute spinal cord injury treated with methylprednisolone at higher doses have a better neurologic recovery than the control group if treated within the first 8 hours after the injury.[36] The 1-year follow-up study of NASCIS-2 confirmed that improvements in patients treated with high-dose methylprednisolone continued at 1 year.[71] The NASCIS-2 trial raises a considerable degree of skepticism about the value of naloxone in the management

of acute spinal cord injury and shows that frequently, encouraging results from animal data cannot be translated to humans.[72–77] The NASCIS-3 study was undertaken to compare the efficacy of methylprednisolone administered for 24 hours with methylprednisolone administered for 48 hours or tirilazad mesylate administered for 48 hours in patients with acute spinal cord injury.[78] Tirilazad was found to cause no improvement in neurologic recovery, but methylprednisolone did show modest improvement when initiated 3 to 8 hours after injury and then given for 48 hours.

Thyrotropin-releasing hormone improves neurologic outcome in experimental studies of cervical cord injury,[79,80] but no proof exists of its efficacy in humans in clinical trials.[45] Gangliosides have also been reported to enhance functional recovery of damaged neurons in animals.[81] Gangliosides, present in high concentrations in central nervous system cells, form a major component of the cell membrane. Initial clinical trials suggest that the use of gangliosides improves recovery of neurologic function after 1 year.[82–87] Currently, a large, multicenter study is under way to confirm on a larger scale the efficacy of these exciting new pharmacologic agents in acute spinal cord injury.[75,87,88]

Use of Orthotic Devices in Cervical Spine Trauma

Orthotic devices can be used as postoperative adjuncts, to reduce motion and promote the healing of disrupted osseous and ligamentous structures in nonsurgical patients, or as a treatment for the pain of muscle spasm.[89]

The selection of an orthotic device depends on the degree of immobilization desired. A comparison of different types of orthoses was done by Johnson and co-workers.[90–92] The cervical collar, the Philadelphia collar, the Yale brace, the sterno-occipitomandibular immobilization brace, and the halo vest were tested in flexion-extension and lateral bend as well as in axial rotation. This study concluded that the longer and stiffer devices offer better immobilization and that the nonhalo orthoses somewhat restrict flexion-extension and lateral bending but not rotation. The best, though by no means absolute, immobilization of the upper cervical spine is provided by the halo vest, whereas immobilization of the lower cervical spine is not provided adequately by any one orthosis, including the halo.[89,92]

The soft collar provides minimal immobilization, and we limit its use to the treatment of pain caused by muscle spasm after more serious osseous or ligamentous injuries have been ruled out. The Philadelphia collar provides greater immobilization and support than the soft collar, especially in flexion-extension movement. We often use the Philadelphia collar in the early postoperative course, after internal fixation. The Yale brace is used as a postoperative adjunct after some fixation procedures and provides better immobilization than the Philadelphia collar because it extends along the length of the sternum anteriorly and along the thoracic spine posteriorly.

The halo brace provides the most reliable control of motion, especially in the high cervical spine.[89,92] We use the halo brace extensively, especially in the nonoperative management of high cervical fractures. The halo vest, however, does not prevent motion in either the normal or the injured spine. Lateral radiographs taken with the patient in the supine and upright positions have shown evidence of intervertebral motion. At the noninjured level, the degree of motion can amount to 3.9 degrees of angulation, with the greatest motion occurring between occiput and C1 (see reference 93). At the injured level, sagittal plane angulation can average 7.0 degrees, and translation can average 1.7 mm between the two positions.[93] This information is the basis for obtaining supine and upright radiographs of the cervical spine after the application of the halo device. Furthermore, any observation of excessive motion should immediately suggest that an alternative method of treatment be considered.

Traction

Traction immobilizes the fracture and can reestablish normal spinal alignment; moreover, when it succeeds in reducing the fracture, traction helps provide initial decompression of the spinal cord. If traction does not succeed in reducing a fracture-subluxation within a reasonable period of time, operative reduction should be considered. The timing of surgery remains a controversial point. Some authors argue that early operation is associated with significant morbidity or, at best, is hazardous.[94] Others believe that early intervention is not associated with a higher incidence of complications.[95]

Closed reduction can be accomplished with either Gardner-Wells tongs (Codman, Raynham, MA) or MRI-compatible tongs (PMT) made of a graphite composite with titanium pins. Halo rings may be the appropriate track-reduction device when halo vest stabilization is used for a given fracture. The site for the Gardner-Wells tongs placement is determined primarily by one of three desired effects: straight in-line traction, as in burst or some chip fractures; flexion traction, for reduction of unilateral or bilateral locked facets; or the less likely extension traction, for flexion fractures with angulated retroluxations.

Traction pin placement should be below the equator of the skull, typically, 1.5 cm above the pinna. This placement is extremely important when higher weights are necessary to reduce bilaterally locked facets. The possible complications of a slipped pin include significant scalp laceration, skull fracture, and more importantly, neurologic deterioration from too rapid a resubluxation of the cervical spine. For straight in-line traction, tongs are placed on an auditory meatal line drawn from the inferior, external auditory meatus through the most anterosuperior edge of the pinna. Flexion traction is accomplished by placing Gardner-Wells pins 2 cm behind the anterior meatal line. This point is located directly above the mastoid process. The rate and speed in reducing locked facets, often with lower reduction weights, are significantly improved with this pin placement.

Because of the relatively low incidence of retroluxations, extension traction is less commonly employed. Extension via tong placement alone is possible but often requires anterior displacement of the shoulders when the commonly employed Stryker or Roto-Rest bed (Stryker, Kalamazoo, MI) is used. This displacement is required because the downward or extension direction of traction is mechanically limited by the integral traction configurations on these beds. Placement of the tongs anterior to the anterior meatal line should be limited to 1 cm; because of the much thinner squamous temporal bone, the risk of skull fracture and epidural hematoma increases, as does the patient's discomfort from temporalis muscle involvement.

The amount of weight permitted for closed reduction of the cervical spine is a matter of debate.[96–103] The initial weight for traction typically has been stated as 5 pounds per vertebra to the level of injury. Some centers limit the total weight to 10 pounds per vertebra. For example, a bilaterally locked facet at C5–C6 is limited to 50 pounds. Other centers have used weights of two thirds of the patient's body weight with success and without significant complication.[96,98,102] Others have used 140 pounds without any complications.[102] Distraction is the most common untoward result in closed reduction. Most often, distraction is not a complication, however, because some degree of distraction is required to reduce the jumped facet, and immediate reduction in weight usually reverses the distraction.

Radiologic guidance should be employed when closed reduction of the spine is attempted.[96,98,100,102] As much of the cervical spine as possible should be imaged during the reduction procedure; maximal imaging reduces the potential for distraction of an unrecognized injury. Evidence of distraction, particularly when heavier weights are used, must be identified as soon as possible. In most instances, standard plain film radiography is technically acceptable, but it may have some significant disadvantages. The first disadvantage is the additional radiation exposure. When a total of 100 pounds is used in 5-pound increments, with corresponding standard radiographs, 30 films can be taken. (With judicious use of fluoroscopy, however, the amount of radiation is diminished by nearly half.) The second disadvantage is the increased time and personnel required to perform standard radiography; a radiologic technician is not always available for a sequence of reduction films with each increase in weight. If the institution is busy when a patient with a cervical spine subluxation arrives, the amount of time between films and the total time of the reduction procedure are greatly increased. With the evidence that functional recovery may depend on rapid reduction, prolonged reductions requiring 8 to 12 hours are not consistent with diminution of further damage. Before the advent of closed reduction, when fluoroscopic guidance under neurosurgical control was used, longer reduction procedures were common. Presently, each 5-pound increase in weight is imaged. The end points of increasing weight are as follows:

1. Successful reduction, which is followed by a prompt decrease in weight, particularly in cases of high weight applied for bilaterally locked facets (postreduction maintenance weight for spine injury is typically 20 to 25 pounds)
2. New or increased neck pain or evidence of a worsening deficit
3. Unsuccessful reduction at weights of two thirds of the body weight
4. Exceeding a 4-hour limit for reduction

In cases of unsuccessful reduction, the weights are reduced to one third of the attempted weight, and muscle relaxants, typically diazepam, are administered.[39,98] Because diazepam is a respiratory depressant when given at higher doses, it must be used with caution in patients who develop pulmonary compromise as a result of the loss of intercostal muscle function. The sequence of increasing weight is then repeated to two thirds of the body weight.

If the reduction procedure is still unsuccessful, progression to medical paralysis after elective awake intubation is an option for the patient with a complete neurologic deficit. This procedure is performed after the weight is reduced—usually to approximately 25 pounds. The drawbacks to performing reductions under medical paralysis are the potential complications of the intubation and mechanical ventilation as well as the loss of the patient's response (i.e., pain) to the reduction or to the worsening clinical status. For these reasons, intubation paralysis is reserved for the functionally transected patient.

The 4-hour time limit for reduction is self-imposed: rapid reduction with the aid of fluoroscopy has improved the functional recovery in a small number of completely paralyzed patients. In the best scenario, the 4-hour time limit includes the total time elapsed from the time of injury. Delays in patient transfer significantly limit reduction attempts within an hour from the time of arrival. If all attempts at closed reduction are unsuccessful, expedient preparations should be made for open reduction and fusion.

SURGICAL MANAGEMENT

A cervical spine fracture-dislocation can be stabilized by various internal fixation techniques. The surgical approach (anterior, posterior, or combined) depends on the level of instability and the mechanism of injury. The goal of internal fixation is to immobilize the spine until a bony arthrodesis occurs, to reduce the deformity, to restore a stable spine, and to achieve neural decompression. Operative intervention in the unstable spine has the following advantages:

1. Providing the optimal mechanical environment for neurologic recovery[39,98]
2. Facilitating early mobilization and avoiding the adverse effects of prolonged bed rest
3. Creating the opportunity for an earlier start of the rehabilitation process

Arthrodesis from the Occiput to C3

Occipitocervical Dislocation

Occipitocervical dislocation is a highly unstable cervical spine injury that is frequently fatal and rarely presents in isolation. When sufficient rotational force is exerted between the occiput and C1 (atlas), however, a rotational dislocation can occur. These injuries can be quite difficult to diagnose without good-quality CT scans.[56] They should be treated aggressively because they can lead to potentially devastating outcomes.[104] We advocate immediate operative occiput to C2 or C3 fusion using either wire stabilization or plating.[105] In addition, we recommend postoperative halo bracing for 3 months.[106]

Jefferson's Fracture

Traumatic spondylolisthesis (bursting) of the ring of C1 caused by direct downward axial loading is a fracture that can best be appreciated on the open-mouth anteroposterior radiograph. Widening of the distance between the odontoid and lateral masses of C1 should prompt a CT scan with 2-dimensional reconstructions. Spence's rule states that the overhang from the lateral masses of C1 on each side should not exceed 6.9 mm. In general, isolated Jefferson's fractures rarely require internal fixation and are best managed with halo bracing until the fracture heals. A combination of Jefferson's fracture and odontoid fracture is not uncommon, however.[107] In this scenario, the traditional treatment is conservative bracing with a halo vest for 6 to 8 weeks followed by delayed posterior C1–C2 arthrodesis.[108] More contemporary management uses anterior internal fixation of the dens using an odontoid screw[109–111] or early C1–C2 posterior transarticular screws.[112–114]

Hangman's Fracture

Traumatic spondylolisthesis of the arch of C2 can lead to varying degrees of instability depending on the nature and severity of the injury. Classification of these fractures by Levine and Edwards[115] has aided optimal treatment. Type I fractures result from hyperextension and axial loading. They have no angulation and less than 3 mm of displacement. These are generally stable fractures and can usually be treated with collar bracing alone. Type II fractures occur secondary to severe flexion in addition to hyperextension and axial loading. On radiographs, there is significant angulation, significant displacement (>3 mm), or both. These fractures require closed reduction followed by immobilization with a halo vest. Type IIA hangman's fractures represent a special class in which there is minimal displacement but severe angulation of C2. This type of injury is caused by flexion-distraction and can sometimes be managed with gentle extension followed by halo vest immobilization for extended periods of time. Alternatively, these fractures may require open reduction followed by posterior internal fixation in an uncooperative or unreliable patient. Type III fractures are grossly unstable and require prompt recognition, because even minimal traction can lead to severe neurologic impairment. These are usually caused by flexion-compression injuries and involve bilateral facet dislocation in addition to fracture of the neural arch. Almost always, these fractures require open surgical reduction followed by internal fixation. Because of the incompetence of the neural arch of C2, it may be necessary to perform an occiput to C3 fusion or C2–C3 fusion with lateral mass plates.[106,115-118]

Atlantoaxial Instability

The ligamentous instability of the C1–C2 complex secondary to transverse ligament rupture may be corrected through either C1–C2 or occipital–C2 wiring and fusion, depending on the integrity of the arch of C1.[106,110,114,117,119-123] The primary indication for an occipitocervical fusion is gross occipitoatlantal joint instability or atlantoaxial instability in the absence of a structurally deficient posterior atlantal arch (Fig. 123-14A and B). Occipitoatlantal instability is most often associated with trauma, and treatment is directed toward reduction and stabilization by external fixation, followed by internal arthrodesis. Several methods have been advocated, including placing a simple inlay of bone graft using corticocancellous bone between the occiput and C2, wiring cancellous bone to the posterior arch of the atlas, or wiring the second cervical vertebra to the adjacent occiput through an adjacent occipital burr hole.[103,119,120,124] Other options include placing anatomically conforming occipitocervical loops fashioned from a Wisconsin or Luque rod or a large, threaded Steinmann pin with associated cancellous bone chips into the lateral gutters.[117] A standard 39-mm fragment T plate bent backward at its head-shaft junction and sewed to the occiput and the spinous process of C2 by fixation screws has also been described.[125] Commercially available occipitocervical precontoured plating systems can greatly ease instrumentation.

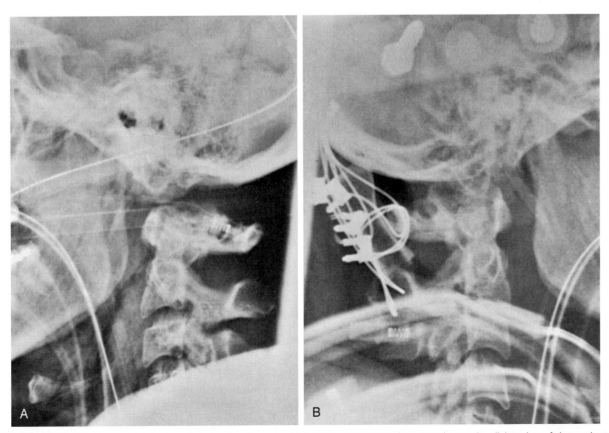

FIGURE 123-14 Atloido-occipital fusion. *A,* Lateral radiograph obtained in a trauma patient reveals anterior dislocation of the occiput and disarticulation of the occipital condyles in the atlas. *B,* Tension band wiring and bone graft span from the occiput, through posterior C1, and into the C2 spinous process to obtain fixation.

Odontoid Fractures

Fractures of the dens have been classified into three types: type I, involving the tip of the odontoid process, which is extremely uncommon; type II, which extends through the base of the odontoid process; and type III, which extends into the C2 body.[93] Odontoid fractures are best visualized radiographically by a combination of the open-mouth odontoid projection and the lateral projection. If nondisplaced, odontoid fractures may be difficult to appreciate by radiographs and might require tomography or CT. When CT is used, axial images must be closely spaced in 1.5- or 2-mm sections to avoid volume averaging a fracture within the CT slice. A high incidence of nonunion has been described with type II odontoid fractures that reaches nearly 100% when fractures remain displaced by more than 5 mm.[126] Type III fractures occur through the C2 body and generally proceed to good fusion with immobilization. Because of the rarity of type I dens fractures, these injuries have been more recently divided into high (type II) and low (type III) fractures.[93]

Numerous procedures have been described for atlantoaxial arthrodesis.[88,93,103,117,119,127–131] We favor a tricortical iliac crest graft wedged between the laminae of C1–C2. By use of a flexible-cable system[132] threaded beneath the arch of C1 for lamina-to-spinous process fusions, the cable is then passed through or otherwise anchored to the strut graft (Fig. 123-15).

A posterior atlantoaxial (transarticular) facet screw fixation approach has been described that allows for the placement of screws (3.5-mm diameter) through the C2 pedicle, across the C1–C2 facet, and into each lateral

mass of the atlas.[103,112–114,131,133,134] The atlas and axis become rigidly coupled, and when the articular surfaces of C1–C2 are prepared, a solid fusion across the facet joint is accomplished. Although some advocate an interspinous C1–C2 wiring and fusion in addition to transarticular fixation,[119] experience suggests that a high degree of fusion be achieved without halo immobilization or C1–C2 interspinous wiring.[123,135]

Anterior odontoid screw fixation is best reserved for patients with an acute type II odontoid fracture, an intact transverse ligament, or a subluxation greater than 6 mm or patients in whom posterior fractures of the C1 ring or C2 spinous process preclude posterior fusions (Fig. 123-16A and B).[93,103,109,111,129] Although numerous reasons have been given for an increased incidence of nonunion in type II odontoid fractures (including amount of displacement, direction of displacement, and patient age), the advantages of direct fixation are immediate stabilization, restoration of normal spine biomechanics, sparing of the normal rotation between C1 and C2, and no external arthrosis. The major limitations are the surgeon's inability to add bone graft to enhance fusion and the procedure's contraindication in transverse atlas ligament disruption.[111,121,129,136]

Anterior C1–C2, transarticular screw fixation is similar to odontoid screw fixation. Operative exposure is identical, intraoperative C-arm fluoroscopic visualization is necessary in the anteroposterior and lateral dimensions for the transarticular approach, and the facet joints are decorticated with an angled curet to enhance fusion.[93,110,111,129,137] The screws are placed into the C2 vertebral body in the groove between the body and the superior C2 facet. The angle of drilling is adjusted in a superolateral direction to allow for the passage of the drill through the lateral mass of C2, across the C1–C2 joint space, and into the lateral mass of C1. Either cortical or self-tapping cancellous screws may be used. In contrast to a transodontoid screw, the technique sacrifices all motion of C1–C2.[137]

C3–T1 Arthrodesis

There has been a tremendous shift in the treatment of cervical spine trauma with an increasing amount of attention being paid to anterior approaches to cervical arthrodesis. The contemporary management of cervical spine disease in its most basic form surmises that the cervical approach should be dictated by the predominant location of the pathology. This paradigm works well for many degenerative processes of the cervical spine, but it is wholly inadequate for the management of cervical spine trauma. In the injured cervical spine, many complicating factors, such as coexisting trauma, cardiovascular instability of the patient, long-term rehabilitative issues, and social issues, may preclude the use of a particular operative approach. In addition, the experience and preference of the surgeon, the availability of internal fixation devices, and the use of allograft versus autograft all have a critical role in determining the optimal approach. In some instances, it may be necessary to perform an anterior and a posterior procedure.

Because operative approach can be a complex decision, we advocate gathering as much radiographic information as possible before intervention. For example, a lower cervical spine facet fracture-dislocation can be stabilized using a simple posterior wiring technique, but an undiagnosed anterior

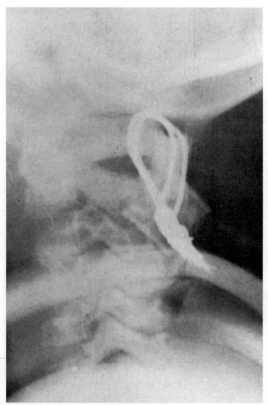

FIGURE 123-15   Lateral cervical radiograph showing C1–C2 wire and a bone graft posterior arthrodesis.

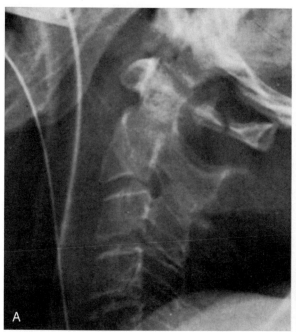 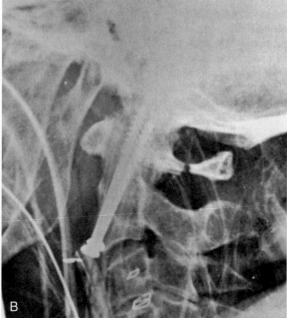

FIGURE 123-16   Anterior odontoid screw fixation. *A,* Lateral cervical radiograph in a trauma patient reveals a posteriorly displaced type III odontoid fracture and a posterior C1 ring fracture. *B,* Postoperative radiograph shows an anterior odontoid screw placement fixating fracture.

herniated disc may change the treatment protocol. Ideally, we obtain both CT and MRI studies whenever feasible.

Anterior Approaches

The anterior approach to the cervical spine has been advocated for the management of cervical spine injuries since 1961. Since that time, authors have advocated various anterior approaches to stabilize the cervical spine, including the use of metal plates and interbody fusions with iliac crest bone grafts or fibular strut grafts.[136,138–144] Several anterior plating systems have been advocated[136,139,140] that use osteosynthetic metal plates and instrumentation designed specifically for this technique.

In the presence of anterior and posterior column injury, anterior fusion without internal fixation may result in bone graft displacement, angulation across the unstable motion segment, or resubluxation.[136] Anterior plate fixation systems were developed to avoid such complications and to avoid the need for a combined anterior and posterior fusion or an anterior fusion followed by prolonged, external orthotic immobilization.

Anterior plates have been shown to be highly effective when vertebrectomies or discectomies are necessary to stabilize or decompress an unstable spine. These systems permit neural decompression and spinal fusion in a single-stage surgical procedure. We reserve the anterior approach for cases in which compromise of the canal anteriorly by bone or disc has been documented unequivocally along with posterior instability. Plating provides immediate stabilization, permitting the safe performance of all nursing maneuvers intended to reduce patient morbidity. It also provides early mobilization unencumbered by a halo vest.[136,139,140] Moreover, by temporarily reducing micromobility and holding the bone graft under compression (without migration), plating facilitates bone healing.

Many plating systems have been designed. The earlier anterior plating systems required bicortical engagement of

the bone screws for optimal plate fixation; the use of intra-operative fluoroscopy was preferred during the placement of these plates to minimize the risk of injury to the dura and spinal cord. With such precautions, these early anterior fixation systems quite effectively stabilized the traumatized spine.[139,145] In more recent years, anterior plating systems that are MRI compatible have become widely available.[95,136,140] These systems generally do not require bicortical engagement of the screws; potential complications to the spinal cord and the necessity of intraoperative fluoroscopy are avoided (Fig. 123-17). They also lock in a triangular fashion into a plate that resists pullout. The insertion of a second screw, a locking screw, into the head of the anchor screw expands the anchor screw head, forming a constrained construct. The locking screw compresses the anchor screw against the plate hole and locks the screws to the plate.[146] Similar to all anterior cervical operative procedures, recurrent laryngeal nerve injury, arterial injury, and esophageal injury are among the known complications, although they are rare.[136,141,142,146–148]

Posterior Approaches

With the rare exception of documented traumatic disc herniation, facet injuries should be approached posteriorly because the posterior ligamentous complex is disrupted by flexion, distraction, and rotational forces so that the only structure maintaining some integrity at this level is the anterior spinal ligamentous complex. Surgical intervention should not disrupt the intact structures and increase the instability and stress on a fixation construct.

Many surgical options are available for posterior stabilization,* but the interspinous process wiring and bone grafting approach proposed by Rogers in 1957 is the most commonly used. Interspinous wiring alone, even though

---

*References 96, 101, 105, 114, 119, 123, 128, 135, 137, 144, 149–154.

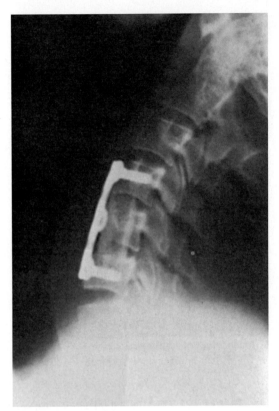

FIGURE 123-17 Synthes plate fixation. Postoperative study obtained with Synthes plate fixation anteriorly from C4 to C6 and interbody bone grafts in the intervertebral disc spaces.

it provides adequate stabilization against translational forces, may not provide stability against rotational forces. A bilateral facet-to-spinous process approach, with iliac bone graft fusion using a flexible-strand titanium cable system (Songer Cable System, Danek Medical, Memphis, TN) (Fig. 123-18), is an effective technique in stabilizing the cervical spine for bilateral locked facets.[112] If one or both facets are disrupted or if laminae or spinous processes are missing or incompetent, posterior cervical screw plates for the lateral masses are the preferred internal fixation devices (Fig. 123-19).[105,114,123,153,155] A contoured universal bone plate system (AME, Dallas, TX) has been designed for lateral mass fixation to restore the normal lordotic curvature of the cervical spine. Indications for this plating system include cervical subluxation without fracture, postlaminectomy instability, bilaminar and spinous process fractures precluding use of cable, recurrence of subluxation, or angulation despite halo immobilization.[114]

Appropriate techniques must be employed to prevent injury to the vertebral artery and nerve root during bicortical penetration necessary to ensure adequate screw fixation to the lateral masses. Roy-Camille and colleagues[154] and Margerl and Seemm[112] have described techniques for optimal screw insertion.[156] The most important principle is to angle the screw cephalad enough to be parallel to the facet and lateral enough to avoid root or vertebral artery injury. In addition, caution should be used when lateral mass screws are placed in C7 because of the transitional morphology of this vertebra. We advocate bone grafting into the facet joint at this level.

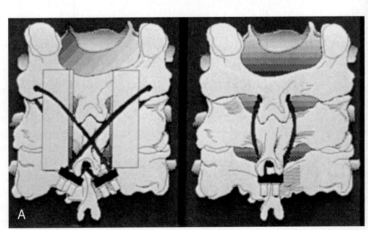

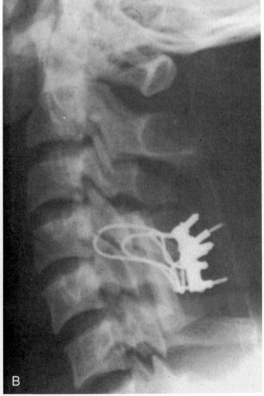

FIGURE 123-18 Facet-to-interspinous process posterior fixation. *A,* Schematic drawing of the facet-to-spinous process with the iliac bone graft fusion and interspinous fusion. *B,* Lateral radiograph showing the combined facet-to-spinous process and interspinous wiring.

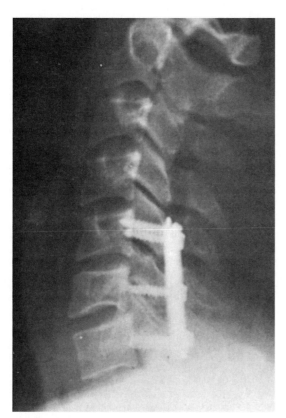

FIGURE 123-19 Posterior lateral mass fixation plating.

Interlaminar clamps (Halifax Clamp, Codman) can be used for cervical subluxation secondary to posterior ligamentous injury with minimal or no posterior body element fracture,[114,130,152,157] but they should be used judiciously in the presence of significant vertebral body injury. With great advances in posterior plating devices, interlaminar clamps have become less popular.

Many other cervical fixation techniques have been proposed. In general, sublaminar wiring to immobilize the cervical spine below C2 should be avoided. Blindly passing wire under the laminae can be hazardous because of the relatively small size of the canal in relation to the spinal cord. In addition, when the wire is passed under three laminae, the wire tends to bow anteriorly, compromising the neural canal and encroaching on the dura and spinal cord. Operative manipulation and tension adjustment of the stainless-steel wire used in such a fusion is often difficult, suboptimal, and subject to a degree of malleability. Methyl methacrylate with combinations of Kirschner pins, wire mesh, and sublaminous wiring has also been proposed as a form of cervical fixation.[139] The disadvantages of acrylic (i.e., it does not bind to bone, it weakens with time, and it remains as a permanent foreign body), however, probably outweigh its benefits in traumatic spine surgery.

Unilateral facet injuries have traditionally been treated with halo traction. With time, however, nonanatomic reduction and cervical translation can be associated with late pain and stiffness. We advocate operative decompression and fixation even with unilateral injuries, which offers the best chance for prevention of late spinal instability and pain from pseudarthrosis. We use an innovative construct

for unilateral injuries that involves a combination of bilateral and lateral mass plates in addition to a single interspinous cable wire.

SUMMARY

Despite great improvements in understanding of spinal cord injury and biomechanics of the cervical spine, and the development of better operative techniques, the morbidity and mortality of traumatic injuries of the cervical spine remain high.[2,158] The challenge for the future lies not so much with prevention of further injury to the cervical spine after injury as it does with spinal cord regeneration and restoration of function. Timely and appropriate stabilization of the cervical spine will always have a crucial role in the ultimate outcome of a spinal injury.

REFERENCES

1. DeVivo MJ, Fine PR, Maetz HM, Stover SL: Prevalence of spinal cord injury: A reestimation employing life table techniques. Arch Neurol 37:707–708, 1980.
2. DeVivo MJ, Rutt RD, Black KJ, et al: Trends in spinal cord injury demographics and treatment outcomes between 1973 and 1986 [published erratum appears in Arch Phys Med Rehabil 73:1146, 1992]. Arch Phys Med Rehabil 73:424–430, 1992.
3. Ryan MD, Henderson JJ: The epidemiology of fractures and fracture-dislocations of the cervical spine. Injury 23:38–40, 1992.
4. Meyer PR, Jr, Cybulski GR, Rusin JJ, Haak MH: Spinal cord injury. Neurol Clin 9:625–661, 1991.
5. Fine PR, Kuhlemeier KV, DeVivo MJ, Stover SL: Spinal cord injury: An epidemiologic perspective. Paraplegia 17:237–250, 1979.
6. Zeidman SM, Ducker TB, Raycroft J: Trends and complications in cervical spine surgery: 1989–1993. J Spinal Disord 10:523–526, 1997.
7. Bracken MB, Aldrich EF, Herr DL, et al: Clinical measurement, statistical analysis, and risk-benefit: Controversies from trials of spinal injury. J Trauma 48:558–561, 2000.
8. Coleman WP, Benzel D, Cahill DW, et al: A critical appraisal of the reporting of the National Acute Spinal Cord Injury Studies (II and III) of methylprednisolone in acute spinal cord injury. J Spinal Disord 13:185–199, 2000.
9. Hurlbert RJ: Methylprednisolone for acute spinal cord injury: An inappropriate standard of care. J Neurosurg 93:1–7, 2000.
10. Anonymous: Radiographic assessment of the cervical spine in symptomatic trauma patients. Neurosurgery 50:S36–S43, 2002.
11. Brohi K, Wilson-Macdonald J: Evaluation of unstable cervical spine injury: A 6-year experience. J Trauma 49:76–80, 2000.
12. Hoffman JR, Wolfson AB, Todd K, et al: Selective cervical spine radiography in blunt trauma: Methodology of the National Emergency X-Radiography Utilization Study (NEXUS). Ann Emerg Med 32:461–469, 1998.
13. Tan E, Schweitzer ME, Vaccaro L, et al: Is computed tomography of nonvisualized C7–T1 cost-effective? J Spinal Disord 12:472–476, 1999.
14. Anonymous: Deep venous thrombosis and thromboembolism in patients with cervical spinal cord injuries. Neurosurgery 50:S73–S80, 2002.
15. Anonymous: Radiographic assessment of the cervical spine in symptomatic trauma patients. Neurosurgery 50:S36–S43, 2002.
16. Anonymous: Clinical assessment after acute cervical spinal cord injury. Neurosurgery 50:S21–S29, 2002.
17. Kirshblum SC, Memmo P, Kim N, et al: Comparison of the revised 2000 American Spinal Injury Association classification standards with the 1996 guidelines. Am J Phys Med Rehabil 81:502–505, 2002.
18. Maynard FM, Jr, Bracken MB, Creasey G, et al: International Standards for Neurological and Functional Classification of Spinal Cord Injury. American Spinal Injury Association. Spinal Cord 35:266–274, 1997.
19. Anonymous: Management of vertebral artery injuries after nonpenetrating cervical trauma. Neurosurgery 50:S173–S178, 2002.
20. Anonymous: Management of acute spinal cord injuries in an intensive care unit or other monitored setting. Neurosurgery 50:S51–S57, 2002.

21. Anonymous: Nutritional support after spinal cord injury. Neurosurgery 50:S81–S84, 2002.

22. Anonymous: Blood pressure management after acute spinal cord injury. Neurosurgery 50:S58–S62, 2002.

23. Anonymous: Initial closed reduction of cervical spine fracture-dislocation injuries. Neurosurgery 50:S44–S50, 2002.

24. Anonymous: Management of pediatric cervical spine and spinal cord injuries. Neurosurgery 50:S85–S99, 2002.

25. Anonymous: Spinal cord injury without radiographic abnormality. Neurosurgery 50:S100–S104, 2002.

26. Bracken MB, Shepard MJ, Collins WF, Jr, et al: Methylprednisolone or naloxone treatment after acute spinal cord injury: 1-year follow-up data. Results of the Second National Acute Spinal Cord Injury Study. J Neurosurg 76:23–31, 1992.

27. Bracken MB, Shepard MJ, Collins WF, et al: A randomized, controlled trial of methylprednisolone or naloxone in the treatment of acute spinal-cord injury. Results of the Second National Acute Spinal Cord Injury Study. N Engl J Med 322:1405–1411, 1990.

28. Nesathurai S: The role of methylprednisolone in acute spinal cord injuries. J Trauma 51:421–423, 2001.

29. Nesathurai S: Steroids and spinal cord injury: Revisiting the NASCIS 2 and NASCIS 3 trials. J Trauma 45:1088–1093, 1998.

30. Short DJ, El Masry WS, Jones PW: High dose methylprednisolone in the management of acute spinal cord injury—a systematic review from a clinical perspective. Spinal Cord 38:273–286, 2000.

31. Anonymous: Pharmacological therapy after acute cervical spinal cord injury. Neurosurgery 50:S63–S72, 2002.

32. Wing PC, Nance P, Connell DG, et al: Risk of avascular necrosis following short term megadose methylprednisolone treatment. Spinal Cord 36:633–636, 1998.

33. Matsumoto T, Tamaki T, Kawakami M, et al: Early complications of high-dose methylprednisolone sodium succinate treatment in the follow-up of acute cervical spinal cord injury. Spine 26:426–430, 2001.

34. Fraser A, Edmonds-Seal J: Spinal cord injuries. Anesthesia 37:1084–1098, 1982.

35. Ducker TB: Treatment of spinal cord injuries. N Engl J Med 322:1459–1461, 1990.

36. Bracken MB, Shepard MJ, Collins WF, et al: A randomized, controlled trial of methylprednisolone or naloxone in the treatment of acute spinal-cord injury: Results of the Second National Acute Spinal Cord Injury Study [see Comments]. N Engl J Med 322:1405–1411, 1990.

37. Bracken MB: Methylprednisolone in the management of acute spinal cord injuries [Letter; comment]. Med J Aust 153:368, 1990.

38. Shatney CH: Initial resuscitation and assessment of patients with multisystem blunt trauma. South Med J 81:501–506, 1988.

39. Wolf AL: Initial management of brain- and spinal-cord-injured patients. Emerg Med Serv 18:35–41, 1989.

40. Vaccaro AR, An HS, Betz RR, et al: The management of acute spinal trauma: Prehospital and in-hospital emergency care. Instr Course Lect 46:113–125, 1997.

41. Porter SS: Anesthetic management of the patient with a spinal cord injury. Kans Med 89:299–304, 1988.

42. Albuquerque F, Wolf A, Dunham CM, et al: Frequency of intra-abdominal injury in cases of blunt trauma to the cervical spinal cord. J Spinal Disord 5:476–480, 1992.

43. Piepmeier JM, Lehmann KB, Lane JG: Cardiovascular instability following acute cervical spinal cord trauma. Cent Nerv Syst Trauma 2:153–160, 1985.

44. Arias MJ: Effect of naloxone on functional recovery after experimental spinal cord injury in the rat. Surg Neurol 23:440–442, 1985.

45. Arias MJ: Treatment of experimental spinal cord injury with TRH, naloxone, and dexamethasone. Surg Neurol 28:335–338, 1987.

46. Knopp RK: Evaluation of the cervical spine: Unresolved issues. Ann Emerg Med 16:819–820, 1987.

47. Ringenberg BJ, Fisher AK, Urdaneta LF, Midthun MA: Rational ordering of cervical spine radiographs following trauma. Ann Emerg Med 17:792–796, 1988.

48. Roth BJ, Martin RR, Foley K, et al: Roentgenographic evaluation of the cervical spine: A selective approach. Arch Surg 129:643–645, 1994.

49. Spain DA, Trooskin SZ, Flancbaum L, et al: The adequacy and cost effectiveness of routine resuscitation-area cervical-spine radiographs. Ann Emerg Med 19:276–278, 1990.

50. Mace SE: The unstable occult cervical spine fracture: A review. Am J Emerg Med 10:136–142, 1992.

51. Streitwieser DR, Knopp R, Wales LR, et al: Accuracy of standard radiographic views in detecting cervical spine fractures. Ann Emerg Med 12:538–542, 1983.

52. Murphey MD, Batnizky S, Batnizky JM: Diagnostic imaging of spinal trauma. Radiol Clin North Am 27:855–872, 1989.

53. Mirvis SE: Applications of magnetic resonance imaging and three-dimensional computed tomography in emergency medicine. Ann Emerg Med 18:1315–1321, 1989.

54. Keene JS, Goletz TH, Lilleas F: Diagnosis of vertebral fractures: A comparison of conventional radiography, conventional tomography, and computed axial tomography. J Bone Joint Surg Am 64:586–594, 1982.

55. Nunez DB, Jr, Quencer RM: The role of helical CT in the assessment of cervical spine injuries. AJR Am J Roentgenol 171:951–957, 1998.

56. Kowalski HM, Cohen WA, Cooper P, Wisoff JH: Pitfalls in the CT diagnosis of atlantoaxial rotary subluxations. AJR Am J Roentgenol 149:595–600, 1987.

57. Mirvis SE, Geisler FH, Jelinek JJ, et al: Acute cervical spine trauma: Evaluation with 1.5-T MR imaging. Radiology 166:807–816, 1988.

58. Martin D, Schoenen J, Lenelle J, et al: MRI-pathological correlations in acute traumatic central cord syndrome: Case report. Neuroradiology 34:262–266, 1992.

59. Benzel EC, Hart BL, Ball PA, et al: Magnetic resonance imaging for the evaluation of patients with occult cervical spine injury. J Neurosurg 85:824–829, 1996.

60. Mirvis SE, Wolf AL: MRI of acute cervical spine trauma. Appl Radiol 21:15–22, 1992.

61. Mirvis SE, Borg U, Belzberg H: MR imaging of ventilator-dependent patients: Preliminary experience. AJR Am J Roentgenol 149:845–846, 1987.

62. Pang D, Pollack IF: Spinal cord injury without radiographic abnormality in children—the SCIWORA syndrome. J Trauma 29:654–664, 1989.

63. Levitt MA, Flanders AE: Diagnostic capabilities of magnetic resonance imaging and computed tomography in acute cervical spinal column injury. Am J Emerg Med 9:131–135, 1991.

64. Quencer RM, Bunge RP, Egnor M, et al: Acute traumatic central cord syndrome: MRI-pathological correlations. Neuroradiology 34:85–94, 1992.

65. Quencer RM, Nunez D, Green BA: Controversies in imaging acute cervical spine trauma. AJNR Am J Neuroradiol 18:1866–1868, 1997.

66. Schaefer DM, Flanders AE, Osterholm JL: Prognostic significance of magnetic resonance imaging in the acute phase of cervical spine injury. J Neurosurg 76:218–223, 1992.

67. Harris JH, Yeakley JW: Hyperextension-dislocation of the cervical spine: Ligament injuries demonstrated by magnetic resonance imaging. J Bone Joint Surg Br 74:567–570, 1992.

68. Bracken MB, Shepard MJ, Hellenbrand KG, et al: Methylprednisolone and neurological function 1 year after spinal cord injury: Results of the National Acute Spinal Cord Injury Study. J Neurosurg 63:704–713, 1985.

69. Bracken MB, Collins WF, Freeman DF, et al: Efficacy of methylprednisolone in acute spinal cord injury. JAMA 251:45–52, 1984.

70. Benzel EC, Khare V, Fowler MR: Effects of naloxone and nalmefene in rat spinal cord injury induced by the ventral compression technique. J Spinal Disord 5:75–77, 1992.

71. Bracken MB, Shepard MJ, Collins WF, Jr, et al: Methylprednisolone or naloxone treatment after acute spinal cord injury: 1-year follow-up data: Results of the Second National Acute Spinal Cord Injury Study [see Comments]. J Neurosurg 76:23–31, 1992.

72. Bracken MB: Pharmacological treatment of acute spinal cord injury: Current status and future prospects. Paraplegia 30:102–107, 1992.

73. Bracken MB: Pharmacological treatment of acute spinal cord injury: Current status and future projects. J Emerg Med 11:43–48, 1993.

74. Bracken MB, Holford TR: Effects of timing of methylprednisolone or naloxone administration on recovery of segmental and long-tract neurological function in NASCIS 2 [see comments]. J Neurosurg 79:500–507, 1993.

75. Zeidman SM, Ling GS, Ducker TB, Ellenbogen RG: Clinical applications of pharmacologic therapies for spinal cord injury. J Spinal Disord 9:367–380, 1996.

76. Ducker TB, Zeidman SM: Spinal cord injury: Role of steroid therapy. Spine 19:2281–2287, 1994.

77. Ducker TB: Medical treatment in spinal cord injuries (Editorial). J Spinal Disord 9:381, 1996.

78. Bracken MB, Shepard MJ, Holford TR, et al: Administration of methylprednisolone for 24 or 48 hours or tirilazad mesylate for 48 hours in the treatment of acute spinal cord injury: Results of the Third National Acute Spinal Cord Injury Randomized Controlled Trial. JAMA 277:1597–1604, 1997.

79. Faden AI, Jacobs TP, Holaday JW: Thyrotropin-releasing hormone improves neurologic recovery after spinal trauma in cats. N Engl J Med 305:1063–1067, 1981.

80. Faden AI, Jacobs TP, Smith MT, Holaday JW: Comparison of thyrotropin-releasing hormone (TRH), naloxone, and dexamethasone treatments in experimental spinal injury. Neurology 33:673–678, 1983.

81. Geisler FH, Dorsey FC, Coleman WP: GM1 gangliosides in the treatment of spinal cord injury: Report of preliminary data analysis. Acta Neurobiol Exp (Wars) 50:515–521, 1990.

82. Geisler FH, Dorsey FC, Coleman WP: Recovery of motor function after spinal-cord injury—a randomized, placebo-controlled trial with GM-1 ganglioside [published erratum appears in N Engl J Med 325:1659–1660, 1991] [see comments]. N Engl J Med 324: 1829–1838, 1991.

83. Geisler FH, Dorsey FC, Coleman WP: Correction: Recovery of motor function after spinal-cord injury—a randomized, placebo-controlled trial with GM-1 ganglioside [Letter]. N Engl J Med 325:1659–1660, 1991.

84. Geisler FH, Dorsey FC, Coleman WP: GM-1 ganglioside in human spinal cord injury. J Neurotrauma 9:S407–S416, 1992.

85. Geisler FH, Dorsey FC, Coleman WP: Past and current clinical studies with GM-1 ganglioside in acute spinal cord injury. Ann Emerg Med 22:1041–1047, 1993.

86. Geisler FH: GM-1 ganglioside and motor recovery following human spinal cord injury. J Emerg Med 11:49–55, 1993.

87. Geisler FH: Clinical trials of pharmacotherapy for spinal cord injury. Ann NY Acad Sci 845:374–381, 1998.

88. Morris GF, Marshall LF: Recent advances in the management of spinal cord injury. West J Med 166:413–414, 1997.

89. Sears W, Fazl M: Prediction of stability of cervical spine fracture managed in the halo vest and indications for surgical intervention [see Comments]. J Neurosurg 72:426–432, 1990.

90. Johnson RM, Hart DL, Simmons EF, et al: Cervical orthoses: A study comparing their effectiveness in restricting cervical motion in normal subjects. J Bone Joint Surg Am 59:332–339, 1977.

91. Johnson RM, Hart DL, Owen JR, et al: The Yale cervical orthosis: An evaluation of its effectiveness in restricting cervical motion in normal subjects and a comparison with other cervical orthoses. Phys Ther 58:865–871, 1978.

92. Johnson RM, Owen JR, Hart DL, Callahan RA: Cervical orthoses: A guide to their selection and use. Clin Orthop 154:34–45, 1981.

93. Anderson LD, D'Alonzo RT: Fractures of the odontoid process of the axis. J Bone Joint Surg Am 56:1663–1674, 1974.

94. Marshall LF, Knowlton S, Garfin SR, et al: Deterioration following spinal cord injury: A multicenter study. J Neurosurg 66:400–404, 1987.

95. Levi L, Wolf A, Rigamonti D, et al: Anterior decompression in cervical spine trama: Does the timing of surgery affect the outcome? Neurosurgery 29:216–222, 1991.

96. Wolf A, Levi L, Mirvis S, et al: Operative management of bilateral facet dislocation. J Neurosurg 75:883–890, 1991.

97. Star AM, Jones AA, Cotler JM, et al: Immediate closed reduction of cervical spine dislocations using traction. Spine 15:1068–1072, 1990.

98. Sonntag VK, Hadley MN: Nonoperative management of cervical spine injuries. Clin Neurosurg 34:630–649, 1988.

99. Sabiston CP, Wing PC, Schweigel JF, et al: Closed reduction of dislocations of the lower cervical spine. J Trauma 28:832–835, 1988.

100. Maiman DJ, Barolat G, Larson SJ: Management of bilateral locked facets of the cervical spine. Neurosurgery 18:542–547, 1986.

101. Geisler FH: Acute management of acute cervical spinal cord injury. Md Med J 37:525–530, 1988.

102. Cotler JM, Herbison GJ, Nasuti JF, et al: Closed reduction of traumatic cervical spine dislocation using traction weights up to 140 pounds. Spine 18:386–390, 1993.

103. Abla AA, Park HC, Lee KC, et al: Upper cervical spine trauma. Surg Neurol 47:432–434, 1997.

104. Dickman CA, Papadopoulos SM, Sonntag VK, et al: Traumatic occipitoatlantal dislocations. J Spinal Disord 6:300–313, 1993.

105. Cooper PR, Cohen A, Rosiello A, Koslow M: Posterior stabilization of cervical spine fractures and subluxations using plates and screws. Neurosurgery 23:300–306, 1988.

106. McAfee PC, Cassidy JR, Davis RF, et al: Fusion of the occiput to the upper cervical spine: A review of 37 cases. Spine 16:S490–S494, 1991.

107. Deen HG, Tolchin S: Combination Jefferson fracture of C1 and type II odontoid fracture requiring surgery: Report of two cases. Neurosurgery 25:293–297, 1989.

108. Bucholz RD, Cheung KC: Halo vest versus spinal fusion for cervical injury: Evidence from an outcome study [see comments]. J Neurosurg 70:884–892, 1989.

109. Esses SI, Bednar DA: Screw fixation of odontoid fractures and nonunions. Spine 16:S483–S485, 1991.

110. Geisler FH, Cheng C, Poka A, Brumback RJ: Anterior screw fixation of posteriorly displaced type II odontoid fractures. Neurosurgery 25:30–38, 1989.

111. Apfelbaum RI: Anterior screw fixation for odontoid fractures: Disorders of the cervical spine. In Camins MB, O'Leary PF (eds): Disorders of the Cervical Spine. Baltimore: Williams & Wilkins, 1992, pp 603–608.

112. Margerl F, Seemm PS: Stable posterior fusion of the atlas and axis by transarticular screw fixation. In Kehr P, Werdner A (eds): Cervical Spine I. Berlin: Springer-Verlag, 1987, pp 322–327.

113. Montesano PX, Magerl F, Jacobs RR, et al: Translaminar facet joint screws. Orthopedics 11:1393–1397, 1988.

114. Cooper PR: Posterior stabilization of the cervical spine. Clin Neurosurg 40:286–320, 1993.

115. Levine AM, Edwards CC: The management of traumatic spondylolisthesis of the axis. J Bone Joint Surg Am 67:217–226, 1985.

116. Calatayud Maldonado V, Maiman DJ: Management of Hangman's fracture. Surg Neurol 47:326–327, 1997.

117. Dickman CA, Douglas R, Sonntag VK: Occipitocervical fusion: Posterior stabilization of the craniovertebral junction and upper cervical spine. BNI Q 6:2–14, 1990.

118. Jenkins LA, Capen DA, Zigler JE, et al: Cervical spine fusions for trauma: A long-term radiographic and clinical evaluation. Orthop Rev Nov(Supp):13–19, 1994.

119. Dickman CA, Sonntag VK, Papadopoulos SM, Hadley MN: The interspinous method of posterior atlantoaxial arthrodesis. J Neurosurg 74:190–198, 1991.

120. Dickman CA, Sonntag VK: Surgical management of atlantoaxial nonunions. J Neurosurg 83:248–253, 1995.

121. Dickman CA, Sonntag VK: Injuries involving the transverse atlantal ligament: Classification and treatment guidelines based upon experience with 39 injuries [Letter; Comment]. Neurosurgery 40:886–887, 1997.

122. Dickman CA, Greene KA, Sonntag VK: Injuries involving the transverse atlantal ligament: Classification and treatment guidelines based upon experience with 39 injuries [see Comments]. Neurosurgery 38:44–50, 1996.

123. Anderson PA, Henley MB, Grady MS, et al: Posterior cervical arthrodesis with AO reconstruction plates and bone graft. Spine 16:S72–S79, 1991.

124. Wertheim SB, Bohlman HH: Occipitocervical fusion: Indications, technique, and long-term results in thirteen patients. J Bone Joint Surg Am 69:833–836, 1987.

125. Heywood AWB, Learmonth ID, Thomas M: Internal fixation for occipitocervical fusion. J Bone Joint Surg Br 70:708–711, 1988.

126. Fujii E, Kobayashi K, Hirabayashi K: Treatment in fractures of the odontoid process. Spine 13:604–609, 1988.

127. Dickman CA, Crawford NR, Paramore CG: Biomechanical characteristics of C1–2 cable fixations. J Neurosurg 85:316–322, 1996.

128. Hardy RW, Jr: The posterior surgical approach to the cervical spine. Neuroimaging Clin North Am 5:481–490, 1995.

129. Montesano PX, Anderson PA, Schlehr F, et al: Odontoid fractures treated by anterior odontoid screw fixation. Spine 16:S33–S37, 1991.

130. Holness RO, Huestis WS, Howes WJ, Langille RA: Posterior stabilization with an interlaminar clamp in cervical injuries: Technical note and review of the long term experience with the method. Neurosurgery 14:318–322, 1984.

131. Paramore CG, Dickman CA, Sonntag VK: The anatomical suitability of the C1–2 complex for transarticular screw fixation. J Neurosurg 85:221–224, 1996.

132. Huhn SL, Wolf AL, Ecklund J: Posterior spinal osteosynthesis for cervical fracture/dislocation using a flexible multistrand cable system: Technical note. Neurosurgery 29:943–946, 1991.

133. Song GS, Theodore N, Dickman CA, Sonntag VK: Unilateral posterior atlantoaxial transarticular screw fixation. J Neurosurg 87:851–855, 1997.

134. Marcotte P, Dickman CA, Sonntag VK, et al: Posterior atlantoaxial facet screw fixation. J Neurosurg 79:234–237, 1993.

135. Halliday AL, Henderson BR, Hart BL, Benzel EC: The management of unilateral lateral mass/facet fractures of the subaxial cervical spine: The use of magnetic resonance imaging to predict instability. Spine 22:2614–2621, 1997.

136. Laus M, Zappoli FA, Alfonso C, et al: Anterior surgery in trauma of the cervical spine. Chir Organi Mov 82:97–104, 1997.

137. Dickman CA, Sonntag VKH, Marcotte PJ: Techniques of screw fixation of the cervical spine. BNI Q 8:9–26, 1992.

138. Cabanela ME, Ebersold MJ: Anterior plate stabilization for bursting teardrop fractures of the cervical spine. Spine 13:888–891, 1988.

139. Caspar W, Barbier DD, Klara PM: Anterior cervical fusion and Caspar plate stabilization for cervical trauma. Neurosurgery 25:491–502, 1989.

140. Connolly PJ, Esses SI, Kostuik JP: Anterior cervical fusion: Outcome analysis of patients fused with and without anterior cervical plates. J Spinal Disord 9:202–206, 1996.

141. Bishop RC, Moore KA, Hadley MN: Anterior cervical interbody fusion using autogeneic and allogeneic bone graft substrate: A prospective comparative analysis. J Neurosurg 85:206–210, 1996.

142. Kostuik JP, Connolly PJ, Esses SI, Suh P: Anterior cervical plate fixation with the titanium hollow screw plate system. Spine 18:1273–1278, 1993.

143. Randle MJ, Wolf A, Levi L, et al: The use of anterior Caspar plate fixation in acute cervical spine injury. Surg Neurol 36:181–189, 1991.

144. Cooper PR: Operative management of cervical spine injuries. Clin Neurosurg 34:650–674, 1988.

145. Oliveira JC: Anterior plate fixation of traumatic lesions of the lower cervical spine. Spine 12:323–329, 1987.

146. Suh PB, Kostuik JP, Esses SI: Anterior cervical plate fixation with the titanium hollow screw plate system. Spine 15:1079–1081, 1990.

147. Hamilton A, Webb JK: The role of anterior surgery for vertebral fractures with and without cord compression. Clin Orthop 300:79–89, 1994.

148. Barros Filho TE, Oliveira RP, Grave JM, Taricco MA: Corpectomy and anterior plating in cervical spine fractures with tetraplegia. Rev Paul Med 111:375–377, 1993.

149. An HS, Gordin R, Renner K: Anatomic considerations for plate-screw fixation of the cervical spine. Spine 16:S548–S551, 1991.

150. Geisler FH, Mirvis SE, Zrebeet H, Joslyn JN: Titanium wire internal fixation for stabilization of injury of the cervical spine: Clinical results and postoperative magnetic resonance imaging of the spinal cord. Neurosurgery 25:356–362, 1989.

151. Hadley MN, Fitzpatrick BC, Sonntag VK, Browner CM: Facet fracture-dislocation injuries of the cervical spine. Neurosurgery 30:661–666, 1992.

152. Holness RO: Halifax clamps for posterior cervical fusion [Letter; comment]. J Neurosurg 75:836–839, 1991.

153. Jones EL, Heller JG, Silcox DH, Hutton WC: Cervical pedicle screws versus lateral mass screws: Anatomic feasibility and biomechanical comparison. Spine 22:977–982, 1997.

154. Roy-Camille R, Saillant G, Mazel C: Internal fixation of the unstable cervical spine by posterior osteosynthesis with plates and screws. In Sherk NH (ed): The Cervical Spine. Philadelphia: JB Lippincott, 1989.

155. Cooper PR: The Axis Fixation System for posterior instrumentation of the cervical spine. Neurosurgery 39:612–614, 1996.

156. Heller JG, Carlson GD, Abitbol JJ, Garfin SR: Anatomic comparison of the Roy-Camille and Magerl techniques for screw placement in the lower cervical spine. Spine 16:S552–S557, 1991.

157. Holness RO, Huestis WS: Halifax interlaminar clamps [Letter]. Neurosurgery 23:127–128, 1988.

158. DeVivo MJ, Black KJ, Stover SL: Causes of death during the first 12 years after spinal cord injury. Arch Phys Med Rehabil 74:248–254, 1993.

124 Meningiomas of the Foramen Magnum

BERNARD GEORGE

The foramen magnum meningioma is one of the most challenging tumors to excise surgically because of its frequent implantation on the anterior margin of the foramen magnum and its involvement of many important structures, including the medulla, the vertebral arteries, and the lower cranial nerves. In one of the first reported cases of intracranial meningioma, the tumor was described as being located at the foramen magnum.[1] This case involved a 50-year-old woman with progressive paraplegia. When the patient died 5 months after the clinical presentation, an autopsy showed a nut-sized fibromeningioma on the inferior basal gutter. Included among other series of posterior fossa meningiomas are occasional cases of foramen magnum meningiomas[2–8] and series of foramen magnum tumors.[9–18] The first report of a foramen magnum meningioma approached surgically was published by Elsberg and Strauss in 1929.[19] This report was followed by those of Symonds and Meadows,[20] Salazkin,[21] Dodge and colleagues,[13] Arseni and Ionesco,[22] Stein and colleagues,[15] Krayenbuhl,[23] Zoltan,[24] and Guidetti and Spallone.[18] Recently surgery around the craniocervical junction has found a new interest with the developments of new surgical approaches.[25–28] Then better results of surgical treatment of foramen magnum meningiomas were reported.[28–32]

The exact limits of implantation of a foramen magnum meningioma have been debated. The location is generally agreed to be the margin of the occipital foramen with possible extension down to C2; however, reports describing upward extension and location of the border between the clivus and the foramen magnum vary among authors. Cushing and Eisenhardt[3] defined as foramen magnum meningiomas only those tumors located on the margin of the foramen magnum. Castellano and Ruggiero[6] included as foramen magnum meningiomas those lesions of the lower third of the clivus that do not involve the pons. Dany and colleagues[33] argued that clival tumors are lesions whose location is anterior to the basilar trunk. According to Guidetti and Spallone,[18] the designation of a foramen magnum tumor "should be confined to tumors extending symmetrically or asymmetrically into both posterior fossa and spinal canal as previously proposed by Arseni and Ionesco." The author

considers a foramen magnum meningioma as any meningioma with the main part of the dural attachment situated between the junction of the medial and lower third of the clivus for the upper limit and the superior aspect of the C2 laminae for the inferior limit. Consequently, the foramen magnum area includes anteriorly the lower third of the clivus, anterior arch of atlas, and odontoid process; laterally the jugular tubercle, occipital condyle, and lateral mass of atlas; and posteriorly the lower part of the occipital bone and posterior arch of atlas with the two first intervertebral spaces (C0-1 and C1-2).

The foramen magnum meningioma is a rare tumor. In 1953, Castellano and Ruggiero[6] published Olivecrona's series of posterior fossa meningiomas. This extensive series included only three foramen magnum tumors. In 1971, Lecuire and Dechaume[7] presented a French cooperative study of 240 cases of posterior fossa meningioma, which included 20 foramen magnum tumors. The Mayo Clinic series reported by Dodge and colleagues,[13] Yasuoka and colleagues,[16] and Meyer and colleagues[17] included 102 cases of foramen magnum tumors, with 78 meningiomas observed between 1924 and 1982. The French Cooperative Study[30] reported in 1993 includes 230 cases of foramen magnum tumors with 106 meningiomas collected over the 1982 to 1992 period. This study represents approximately one case of foramen magnum meningioma every 2 years per department. In the author's department, 206 cases of foramen magnum tumors, including 75 meningiomas, were treated over the past 20 years. Posterior fossa meningiomas account for approximately 2% of all intracranial tumors and 10% of all meningiomas.[3,5–7,23,30] According to Castellano and Ruggiero,[6] Lecuire and Dechaume,[7] and Meyer and colleagues,[17] foramen magnum meningiomas represent 4% to 10% of posterior fossa meningiomas. The foramen magnum is the least frequent site of a posterior fossa meningioma (Table 124-1). Other reports confirm these figures.[4,5,34,35] In a report by Yasargil and colleagues[8] on a series of posterior fossa meningiomas, 20 tumors were located on the clivus, 30 were located on the petrous bone, and three were located at the foramen magnum.

TABLE 124-1 ▪ Distribution Frequency of Posterior Fossa Meningiomas Including Tumors of the Foramen Magnum

Study	Foramen Magnum (%)	Clivus (%)	Convexity (%)	Tentorium (%)	Petrous Bone (%)
Castellano and Ruggiero[6] (71 patients)	4	11	10	30	42
Lecuire and Dechaume[7] (218 patients)	9	8	12	26	45

TABLE 124-2 ▪ Foramen Magnum Tumors in the French Cooperative Study and in the Author's Series

	French Cooperative Study, 1982–1992 (N = 230)	Author's Series, 1980–1997 (N = 143)
Meningioma	106	51
Neurinoma	49	33
Chordoma	28	18
Bone tumors	32	28
Miscellaneous tumors	15	13

Meningioma is the most common foramen magnum tumor. The meningioma-to-neurinoma ratio varies as follows in the different series reported here: 26:4 (Dodge and colleagues[13]), 78:23 (Meyer and colleagues[17]), 17:9 (Guidetti and Spallone[18]), and 75:36 in the series by the author's group. Other types of tumor at this site are less common and include chordomas and different types of bone and intradural tumors (Table 124-2).[17,28,36-39]

The sex distribution of the foramen magnum meningioma is similar to sex distributions of meningiomas at other locations. At least two thirds of patients are women in all series reviewed.[7,17,18] The author's series of 59 women and 16 men confirms these figures.

The patients' ages ranged from 12 to 81 years in the series by Meyer and colleagues[17] with an average age of 49 years. The average age in the author's series was 52 years (range, 14 to 76). The average interval from first symptom to diagnosis was 2.5 to 4 years in most series. Yasargil and colleagues[8] noticed that this interval is likely to be longer in men and in midline (clival) tumors. In the author's series, the interval ranged from 1 to 18 months (average, 9). This shorter interval is explained by the prompt use of computed tomography (CT) and magnetic resonance imaging (MRI) to investigate all cases.

CLINICAL SYMPTOMS

Many reports have emphasized the protean and misleading manifestations of foramen magnum tumors. In many reports, the discussion is devoted mainly to the possible confusion of this diagnosis with symptoms and signs produced by such entities as hydrocephalus, multiple sclerosis, cervical spondylosis, intramedullary tumor, syringomyelia, and carpal tunnel syndrome.[14,17,18,40] Similarly, some reports expressed concern about the explanation of some atypical symptoms, such as stereoanesthesia[41] and atrophy of intrinsic muscles of the hands, that are seen in association with foramen magnum meningioma.[14,16] Since the advent of CT and MRI, these concerns no longer represent major diagnostic problems. A more useful system of classification is now based on the severity of the patients' symptoms. The author uses the grading system proposed by Yasargil and colleagues[8]: grade I patients have a single symptom; grade II patients have mild or moderate symptoms; grade III patients have pronounced cranial nerve, brain stem, and cerebellar symptoms; and grade IV patients are bedridden.

The first symptoms are generally upper neck pain and posterior headaches with neck stiffness. Motor deficit and sensory disturbances are less frequent. At the time of diagnosis, motor and sensory deficits are observed in 53% and 42% of patients. Lower cranial nerve palsy is present in 30% of patients, and sphincter disturbances are present in 13%. The number of patients with severe symptoms, such as tetraplegia (11 cases), hemiplegia (five cases), and paraplegia (one case), is noteworthy. One patient was in a coma with an almost complete tetraplegia, and another patient with tetraplegia could remain sitting only because he stopped breathing at each attempt to lie down. Exceptional modalities of presentation have been reported, such as subarachnoid hemorrhage,[42,43] syringomyelia,[30,44-46] and incidental discovery.[30] During the 20 years of this series, there is a trend to more and more minor symptoms at the time of diagnosis. Over the past 5 years, 24 new patients were seen, but only two of them had a moderate motor deficit and two others had lower cranial nerves palsy. The remaining patients presented only neck pain and stiffness.

DIAGNOSTIC IMAGING

In all 75 of the cases from the author's group, the diagnosis of the foramen magnum tumor was established by CT scan; it was confirmed by air or contrast myelography in the first eight patients and by MRI in the remaining patients. CT is particularly helpful in identifying calcification within the tumor and bone modification at the site of origin of the meningioma, although these findings are not frequent in foramen magnum meningiomas.[47,48]

MRI complements CT by providing excellent definition of the tumor's relationship to the surrounding structures, particularly to the upper spinal cord and medulla and to the vertebral arteries.[17,49,50] In addition, MRI provides a good demonstration of the tumor's development in the three planes, coronal, sagittal, and horizontal, and, in many cases, can precisely delineate the extent of dural involvement because the dura involved by the meningioma can usually be differentiated from the normal dura. For these reasons, MRI has largely supplanted CT and myelography during diagnostic investigations. A diagnosis of an extramedullary tumor of the foramen magnum obtained through MRI is normally not doubted.

With the development of CT angiography and magnetic resonance angiography, most relevant information about the tumor and surrounding vessels can be obtained; the tumor size and location as well as the size, displacement, and main branches of the vertebral arteries are generally well demonstrated. Even the abnormal origin of the posterior inferior cerebellar artery, which may be at or below the level of the foramen magnum,[51-53] can be identified. Because the tumoral vascularity is generally well appreciated, angiography no longer has many indications. It is still useful only in cases for which embolization is contemplated (Fig. 124-1).

The preoperative workup is of utmost importance to plan the surgical strategy. Especially important is the definition of the tumoral location in relation to three elements (Table 124-3 and Fig. 124-2): the neuraxis, the vertebral artery, and the dura mater. A tumor may be anterior, lateral, or posterior to the neuraxis. An anterior tumor is attached on both sides of the anterior midline and displaces the neuraxis posteriorly. Anterior tumors enlarge the space in front of the neuraxis. To reach them, one has to turn the neuraxis around.

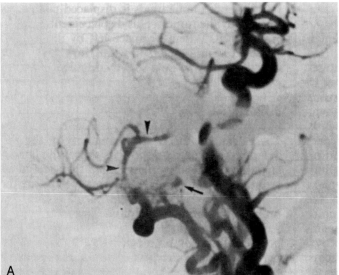
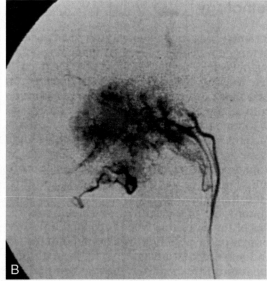
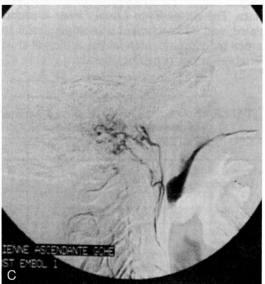

FIGURE 124-1 Arteriography. *A,* Posterior displacement of the vertebral artery (*arrowheads*) with a small radiated tumoral injection (*arrow*). (From George B, Dematons C, Cophignon J: Lateral approach to the anterior part of the foramen magnum. Surg Neurol 29:484–490, 1988. Copyright © 1988 by Elsevier Science Publishing Co., Inc.). *B,* Selective injection of the ascending pharyngeal artery with marked tumoral staining. *C,* Control after embolization of the ascending pharyngeal artery (the same patient as in *B*).

A lateral tumor is attached laterally to the anterior midline and displaces the neuraxis laterally. With a posterior approach, the neuraxis is already shifted laterally, facilitating the tumoral access. The difference between anterior and lateral tumors is well demonstrated by MRI midline sagittal views on which the continuity of the neuraxis is visible for the former, whereas it is not for the latter. Posterior tumors are attached posteriorly to the denticulate ligament.

Tumors may be located above, below, or on both sides of the vertebral artery. The surgical exposure has to be adjusted so that for tumors located above the vertebral artery, the bone resection is extended above the vertebral artery toward the occipital condyle and jugular tubercle. For tumors located below the vertebral artery, the bone resection is extended below this vessel toward the lateral mass of the atlas. In this case, the lower cranial nerves are always displaced superiorly and posteriorly. Consequently, in tumors situated below the

TABLE 124-3 ▪ Localization of Foramen Magnum Meningiomas in Regard to the Neuraxis, Dura Mater, and Vertebral Artery

	French Cooperative Study	Author's Series
Neuraxis		
Anterior	33	24
Lateral	59	26
Posterior	14	1
Dura mater		
Intradural	91	45
Extradural	4	2
Intradural and extradural	11	4
Vertebral artery		
Above	10	7
Below	51	23
Above and below	45	21

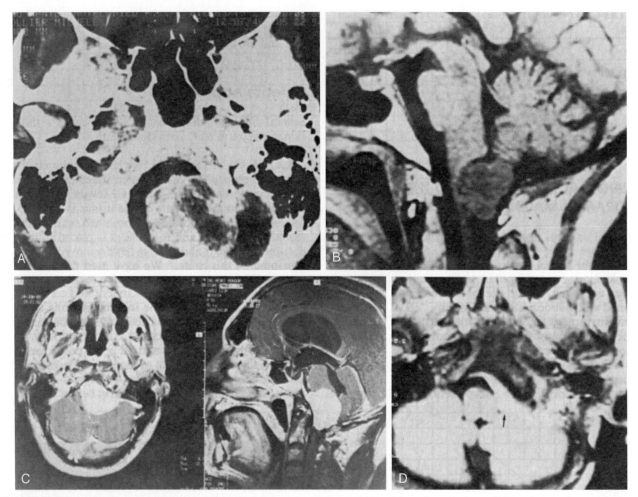

FIGURE 124-2   The type and localization of foramen magnum meningioma. *A,* Type I, lateral meningioma. *B,* Type I, posterior meningioma. *C,* Type I, lateral meningioma. *D,* Type II, en plaque meningioma.

vertebral artery, the nerves are to be searched at the superior pole of the tumor. Conversely, in tumors located above the vertebral artery, these nerves may be displaced in different ways; their location cannot be anticipated. Tumors that have developed on both sides of the vertebral artery raise the most difficult problems.

In regard to the dura mater, meningiomas are most commonly intradural; however, in a few cases, they may extend outside of the intradural space or even be entirely extradural.[30] These forms with extradural components usually exhibit invasive features into the bone, muscles, and even sheaths of nerves and vessels. Particular surgical approaches are necessary to expose their different compartments, and complete resection is generally impossible.

PATHOLOGY

Foramen magnum meningiomas are typically benign meningoepithelial or fibroblastic meningiomas.[15,16] Other types, such as anaplastic, angioblastic, and melanotic meningiomas, can also be observed at this level.[8,30,41,54,55] Psammomatous forms seem more frequent at the foramen magnum level than at other intracranial sites. They account for 54% in the author's series and for 58% in the French Cooperative Study (Table 124-4).

Macroscopically, the tumors differ according to their mode of implantation.[7] Type I is a tumor arising from a base of approximately 1 to 1.5 cm. This type of foramen magnum meningioma is most frequently encountered. The site of attachment may be quite wide because differentiation of the true insertion from a peripheral zone of firm adherence is often difficult. Most of the author's cases belonged to this type of wide, although limited, attachment. In six patients, the tumor's site of attachment was broad, and the tumor

TABLE 124-4 ▪ Histology of Foramen Magnum Meningiomas

	French Cooperative Study (*N* = 106)	Author's Series (*N* = 51)
Meningothelial	40	24
Fibroblastic	12	9
Transitional	19	7
Psamomma	19	6
Angioblastic	2	4
Hemangiopericytoma	3	1
Melanotic	1	—
Unknown	10	—
Psamomma bodies	56	26

TABLE 124-5 ▪ Sites of Attachment of Foramen Magnum Meningiomas

	Anterior	Lateral	Posterior
Dodge et al[13]	8	20	—
Stein et al[15]	1	21	3
Lecuire and Dechaume[7]	10	8	2
Guidetti and Spallone[18]	4	10	3
George et al	24	26	1

was of the en plaque type (type II). En plaque meningiomas in the posterior fossa extend into the petroclival and subtemporal areas.[2,4,7,8,35] In these six patients, the tumor extended from the foramen magnum to the petrous bone, foramen jugulare, and retropharyngeal space. The classic type I tumor mass is round or lobulated, and its attachment is mostly anterior in the foramen magnum or lateral at the site at which the vertebral artery penetrates the dura (Table 124-5; see Fig. 124-2).[3]

SURGICAL ANATOMY

To understand the regional anatomy of the foramen magnum, one needs to note its shape: The lateral walls are almost vertically oriented, and their rostral endings are at the jugular tubercles (Fig. 124-3). These tubercles are the only elements between the foramen jugulare and the upper limit of the foramen magnum. The foramen magnum seems to belong more to the spinal canal than to the posterior fossa.

Embryologically, the foramen magnum partly represents the first cervical vertebra and is defined as the enlarged upper part of the spinal canal (see Fig. 124-3B). The anterior and lateral walls are made of bony elements connected by strong ligaments. The natural openings that the surgeon may use are posterior. There is no intervertebral foramen at the first two interspaces because the joints are anterior, with the first two nerves merging posterior to the joints.

The vascularization of the foramen magnum dura mater is noteworthy, and many studies have addressed this subject.[56-60] The anterior dura is fed by the anterior meningeal artery, which is the third space branch of the vertebral artery. It anastomoses with a branch of the ascending pharyngeal artery passing through the condylar canal. The posterior meningeal artery, originating from the vertebral artery or the occipital artery, supplies the dura of the posterior part of the foramen magnum, and a mastoidal ramus from the occipital artery supplies the posterolateral part of the foramen magnum. All these arteries may supply a foramen magnum meningioma according to its extension. This vascular pattern is often not made obvious by standard arteriography, but it can be well visualized after selective catheterization injection of these vessels.[59] In highly vascular tumors, consideration should be given to preoperative embolization.[61]

TREATMENT

Surgery is the definitive form of treatment of foramen magnum meningioma except when it is contraindicated by major medical problems. Surgical treatment is particularly

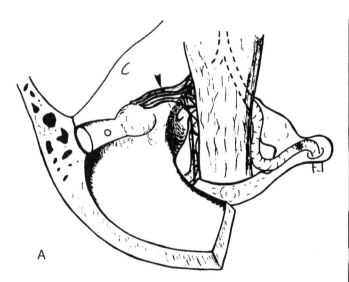
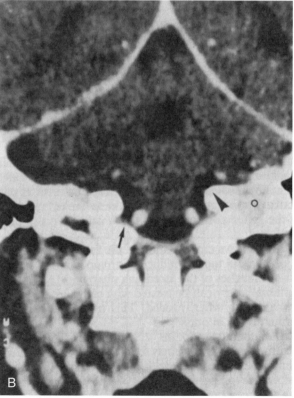

FIGURE 124-3 Anatomy. *A,* Relationships in the foramen magnum between the spinal cord, medulla, and vertebral artery (*asterisk*), cranial nerves IX, X, and XI (*arrowhead*), and sigmoid sinus (*circle*). *B,* Computed tomography scan in coronal view shows the lateral wall of the foramen magnum with the jugular tubercle (*arrowhead*), jugulare foramen (*circle*), and condylar canal with vertebral artery (*arrow*).

important for relieving the severe compression of the spinal cord and medulla, which is usually present.

Preoperative embolization of the tumor's blood supply is a useful tool for reducing intraoperative bleeding. Small branches of the ascending pharyngeal artery and vertebral artery can be treated with catheterization and embolization when needed. This technique was performed four times in the author's series.

Radiotherapy remains a controversial method of treatment of meningiomas for many authors, although some investigators report that it can reduce the rate of recurrence of partially removed meningiomas.[62–64] It has also been proposed as a preoperative measure to reduce vascularity in highly vascular meningiomas.[63–65] Even with radiosurgery, the risk of inducing a lesion of the adjacent neuraxis appears high because of the proximity of functionally important structures that have already been subjected to compression and surgical manipulation. Radiotherapy had been applied in one case of the author's series when a tumor recurred after surgery, but it did not stop the tumor growth, and the patient had to undergo reoperation.

Obstructive hydrocephalus may occur with these tumors. Because surgery involves opening the foramen magnum, it provides immediate relief of obstructive hydrocephalus, should such a condition be present. Dexamethasone (12 to 18 mg/day) is given to all surgical patients for 3 days preoperatively and postoperatively.

SURGICAL APPROACHES TO THE FORAMEN MAGNUM

Several surgical approaches to the foramen magnum have been used; some of these approaches are preferred for clival meningiomas: the transbasal approach,[66] the subtemporal preauricular infratemporal fossa approach,[67,68] and the middle fossa approach combined with suboccipital craniectomy.[69] The main problem in surgery for foramen magnum meningiomas is the prevention of injury to the neuraxis. Such prevention can be accomplished in two ways: anteriorly, in which case one cannot see the medulla, or posteriorly, in which case it is difficult to visualize the tumor. Because the anterior and posterior approaches have their limitations, they are now extended laterally to obtain best visualization of the neuraxis and the tumor.

Anterior Approaches

Several different anterior cervical approaches to the foramen magnum have been described.

Anterolateral Approach

The author's group has extensively used a lateral approach to the foramen magnum for hourglass neurinomas at the C1 and C2 levels.[28,39,70] In this approach, the intradural part of the meningioma is difficult to follow unless the procedure is combined with a suboccipital craniectomy and the patient is placed in lateral decubitus. Shucart and Kleriga[71] have removed a C1 meningioma by this route. The author has used this approach on the five patients with type II foramen magnum meningiomas with wide zones of attachment and cervical extension (Table 124-6). In this exposure, the incision is along the anterior edge of the sternocleidomastoid

TABLE 124-6 ■ Surgical Technique (Author's Series)

Localization	MPA	PLA	ALA	ALA + PLA
Anterior	1 ID	23 ID	—	—
Lateral	2 ID	18 ID	2 ED	3 ID–ED
Posterior	1 ID	1 ID–ED	—	—

ALA, anterolateral approach; ED, extradural; ID, intradural; MPA, midline posterior approach; PLA, posterolateral approach.

muscle, the mastoid process, and the occipital crest up to the midline. The transverse processes of C1 and C2 are exposed, passing between the external aspect of the internal jugular vein and the sternocleidomastoid muscle; the spinal accessory nerve is freed and retracted inferiorly before the vertebral artery is exposed with unroofing of the transverse foramen of C1. A laminectomy of C1 and craniectomy of the inferior and lateral parts of the occipital bone, including part of the mastoid process, are then performed.

This approach allows the sigmoid sinus to be exposed down to the foramen jugulare and the vertebral artery to be seen from C2 to its intracranial part. The approach is quite lateral to the spinal cord and medulla. The intradural space can be reached but through a narrow and deep surgical field unless the occipital condyle and lateral mass of the atlas are extensively drilled out. A better exposure is gained by using the lateral extension of the posterior approach. This posterolateral approach also has the advantage of providing more comfortable working conditions and better visualization of the neural structures. The anterolateral approach is essentially applied on extradural processes. In the case of a tumor with intradural and extradural components, the posterolateral and anterolateral approaches can be associated in the same or in two different stages, as the author did in three cases.

Transcervical Transclival Approach

Developed by Stevenson and colleagues[72] in 1966, the transcervical transclival approach provides an exposure affording a narrow space that is anterior to the foramen magnum. To widen the exposure, Guidetti and Spallone[18] dislocated the mandibular condyle. In this approach, the incision passes through the digastric and stylohyoid muscles. The prevertebral fascia is then separated from the pharyngeal fascia and is incised. The exposure is similar to that of the transoral-transclival approach, but it offers the advantage of not operating in a contaminated field (the mouth). The transcervical-transclival approach has been used by Guidetti and Spallone[18] in one foramen magnum meningioma that had earlier been partially removed by a posterior approach.

Transoral-Transclival Approach

Initially developed to correct spinal deformities at the cervicomedullary junction[73] and later to treat intradural lesions, such as aneurysms, the transoral-transclival approach[74,75] was used by Mullan and colleagues[76] to remove a clival sarcoma. In 1987, Miller and Crockard[77] reported using this approach in two patients with foramen magnum meningiomas. Although with this approach, work can proceed intradurally and the neuraxis is not situated between the surgeon and the tumor, the transoral route is associated with some specific technical problems. In both patients treated by Miller and Crockard, cerebrospinal leakage occurred. As discussed by Pasztor,[78] the transoral-transclival approach seems more suitable in the treatment of extradural lesions.

POSTERIOR APPROACH

The standard posterior approach involves a combination of an upper cervical laminectomy and a lower midline posterior fossa craniectomy. This procedure has been described previously.[7,8,18] With this approach, a postoperative worsening of the preoperative condition may occur, with tetraplegia or respiratory disturbances resulting from excessive manipulations of the medulla. Monitoring of somatosensory-evoked potential responses helps reduce this risk.

Posterolateral Approach (Posterior Approach with Lateral Enlargement)

The posterolateral approach provides a lateral extension to the standard posterior approach and is used to gain access to the anterior part of the foramen magnum (Figs. 124-4

and 124-5).[27,28,54] The patient may be placed in a supine, lateral, or sitting position. The author usually uses the sitting position with the patient placed in a G suit and the central venous pressure controlled for prevention of air embolism.[79] In any of these positions, the degree of neck flexion must be checked with great care. Excessive neck flexion can worsen the compression of the medulla. The head is kept straight, but the operating table is rotated to the opposite side. The choice of the side is based on the lateral extension of the tumor, or if the tumor is quite anterior and medial, surgery is performed on the side of the nondominant vertebral artery. In other cases, the right side is preferred by a right-handed surgeon, so that instruments are as remote as possible from the medulla.

In this exposure, the incision runs medially from C4 to the occipital protuberance, then curves laterally to the mastoid process on the chosen side. The occipital head of the sternocleidomastoid muscle is divided. The inferior part of the occipital bone and the laminae of C1 and C2 are exposed (see Fig. 124-4). This exposure is bilateral, but it extends far laterally on the chosen side. The posterior aspect of the

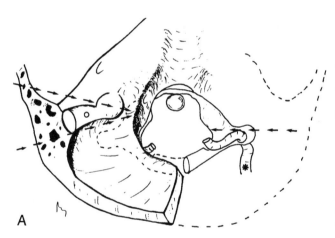

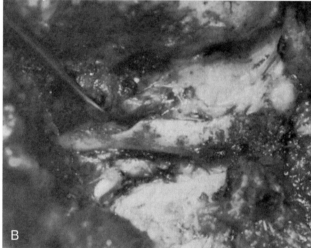

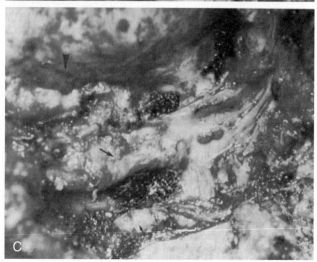

FIGURE 124-4 Surgical technique. *A,* Lateral enlargement of the posterior approach at the level of C1 (*right*) and of the foramen jugulare, with and without section of sigmoid sinus (*left*). (From George B, Dematons C, Cophignon J: Lateral approach to the anterior part of the foramen magnum. Surg Neurol 29:484–490, 1988. Copyright © 1988 by Elsevier Science Publishing Co., Inc.) *B,* Freeing of the vertebral artery above the arch of the atlas (*left side*). *C,* Lateral opening of the foramen magnum. Sigmoid sinus (*arrowhead*), vertebral artery (*large arrow*), and second cervical nerve (*small arrow*) are shown (the same case as in *B*).

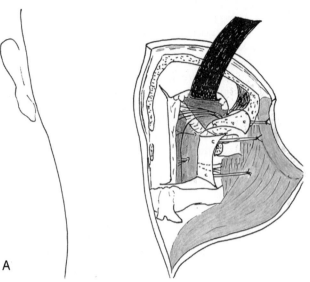 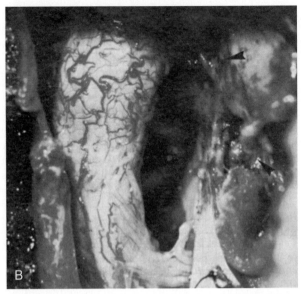

FIGURE 124-5 *A,* Scheme of the dural opening. *B,* Operative view after tumor removal. The vertebral artery is shown (*arrowhead*).

mastoid process and the transverse process of C1 are brought into view. The laminae of C1 and C2 are exposed subperiosteally; the second cervical root appears between C1 and C2. The surgeon can follow the second cervical root for at least 2 cm before it passes behind the vertebral artery. The lamina of the atlas is exposed, first along its inferior edge, then along its superior edge. The work progresses subperiosteally, and the superior aspect of the C1 lamina is exposed, which reveals the periosteal sheath of the vertebral artery. In this way, the vertebral artery and the venous plexus are not injured; both are left within this periosteal sheath.[70] The vertebral artery is freed from its groove on the atlas to the transverse foramen. The internal limit of this groove is indicated by an abrupt change in the height of the posterior aspect of the C1 lamina. At this point, the vertebral artery runs upward and internally to reach and pass through the dura. This portion is dissected, and the periosteal sheath up to the dura is preserved (see Fig. 124-4).

The craniectomy is performed and includes the inferior part of the occipital bone. It extends laterally with some mastoid resection when the sigmoid sinus has to be exposed down to the foramen jugulare. A laminectomy of C1 and C2 is then performed. It can be extended as far lateral as the occipital condyle and lateral mass of the atlas. In most cases, these bone structures can be preserved because working along the vertebral artery, which turns around them, gives sufficient access to tumors even anteriorly located. In the author's experience, for meningiomas, it was never necessary to drill more than one third of these bone elements. The approach to a foramen magnum meningioma must never be transcondylar. In some cases, the tumor extends toward the internal auditory canal and foramen jugulare. In such cases, the posterior half of the foramen jugulare wall is drilled out, which permits the sigmoid sinus to be divided. For anteriorly situated tumors, additional space may be gained by transposing the vertebral artery. This procedure involves unroofing the transverse foramen of C1 and mobilizing the vertebral artery inside its periosteal sheath medially and at the site of

its dural penetration. This last maneuver is best performed after opening the dura and then cutting the dura circumferentially around the artery. Opening and cutting of the dura are required in case of insertion around the vertebral artery dural penetration, as the author did in seven cases.

Laminectomy and craniectomy must extend beyond the posterior midline so as to avoid any compression of the spinal cord or medulla against the bone of the opposite side during manipulation of the tumor. The rostrocaudal extent of the lamina opening must span the tumor's limits for the same reason.

The dura is opened in the midline at the cervical level and in a V shape over the cerebellum (see Fig. 124-5A). Perpendicular cuts are made toward the vertebral artery and between C1 and C2. A small contralateral cut is made at the C1 level to decompress the neuraxis on the opposite side, while keeping the neuraxis covered and protected. If necessary, the sigmoid sinus may now be divided after its proximal ligation. The distal segment in the foramen jugulare is packed with oxidized cellulose. At this time, the vertebral artery may be freed from its dural ring.

The dentate ligament at the C1 and C2 level is divided to alleviate spinal cord compression. The C1 and occasionally C2 roots may be divided to help release the neuraxis and enlarge the tumoral access. They must be cut distal to their connection with the medullary root of the accessory nerve.

Dissection is carried out under the microscope, which is used after opening the dura and continues to be used until the dura is closed. En bloc removal of an anteriorly or anterolaterally located tumor is never advisable. The bulk of the tumor must first be removed with the ultrasonic aspirator, with the surgeon working toward the tumor's zone of attachment (see Fig. 124-5B). The best method involves making a large opening on the lateral aspect of the tumor, then progressing obliquely toward the dura; in this manner, a large triangular portion can be removed with most of the area of attachment exposed and coagulated. This procedure also allows some tumor to remain posteriorly to protect the anterolateral aspect of the medulla and spinal cord while the bulk of the tumor is removed. Later, this remaining portion of tumor, now devascularized, is resected. It is generally a good option to start debulking the tumor and coagulating the dural zone of attachment at the inferior part where the main vascular feeder (the anterior meningeal artery) reaches the tumor.

The neuraxis must be kept in place. No retraction is necessary even to reach the anterior midline and even to go beyond it. The space progressively given along the tumor resection is used to work in front of the neuraxis. The dura covering the neuraxis must not be folded laterally so as to keep intact the small connections with the arachnoid, which hold the neuraxis and prevent it from falling into the empty space. No cottonoid sponges have to be placed in the area anterior to the neuraxis (see Fig. 124-5).

Difficulties arise when the lower cranial nerves or the vertebral artery is embedded in the tumor. In all cases, the area of tumor attachment, or at least the superficial layer of dura at this site, is resected. This resection is not always possible around the site of vertebral artery dural penetration and at the foramen jugulare.

The dura is closed in a watertight fashion. If the mastoid cells have been opened, the mastoid cavity is filled with bone dust mixed with fibrin glue. It is then covered by a musculoaponeurotic flap fashioned from the deep aspect of the sternocleidomastoid muscle and sutured onto the dura.

RESULTS

The author's group has used the posterolateral approach in 70 patients; the anterolateral approach was preferred in the five cases with extradural and cervical extension. In three of these five cases, the lateral approach was combined with a posterolateral approach (see Table 124-6). In this series, the vertebral artery was transposed medially in four cases, and the sigmoid sinus was divided in four cases. The lateral access to the anterior aspect of the foramen magnum provided by the posterolateral approach has been sufficiently large to allow dissection in front of the spinal cord and medulla without manipulation of these structures. In all cases, the bone drilling was limited at the level of the occipital condyle and lateral mass of the atlas. No postoperative instability was observed.

For intradural tumor, complete resection (Simpson grades I and II) was achieved in 68 cases (96%) (Table 124-7). In most cases, the dural zone of insertion was removed. In four cases, the dura was only coagulated. In two cases, the resection was not complete. One patient underwent surgery through a too-limited posterolateral approach at the beginning of

the author's experience. The other patient was in critical condition with coma and tetraplegia. The resection of the anterior bilateral meningioma was deliberately incomplete, leaving a portion of the tumor on the opposite side of the approach. The intention was to realize a contralateral approach in a second stage after clinical recovery. The patient did not improve, however, and eventually died. Three other patients presented preoperatively with a severe tetraplegia with breathing difficulties; all of them recovered completely in a short time. All patients had a follow-up examination by CT and since 1982 by MRI at 1, 3, 6, and 10 years. No one case of recurrence was observed in these patients with intradural meningiomas.

The rate of resection in cases of meningioma with an extradural component is much lower because of the usually invasive feature of these forms of meningioma. A complete resection would have often required the sacrifice of the vertebral artery and the lower cranial nerves. In the author's series, the vertebral artery was divided and resected in two cases, but the lower cranial nerves were preserved in five of six cases. A complete resection was achieved only in three cases, whereas a subtotal removal was performed in the three others. Despite this fact, no recurrence has been observed in these extradural forms within 4 to 10 years of follow-up. One patient, however, died of the development of multiple meningiomas in the cervical spine and the cavernous sinus.

The clinical results (Table 124-8) in the author's series showed improvement with a lower postoperative than preoperative grade in 90% of the cases. No difference between anterior and lateral location was noted. In 94% of patients, the postoperative grade is 0, 1, or 2 (no to moderate symptoms). The clinical condition did not improve in only one patient, and three patients died. These three deaths were all observed at the beginning of the author's experience. One death was related to an air embolism at a time when prevention by G suit and hypervolemia was not available. Since then, no new case of air embolism has been observed, whereas all the posterolateral approaches (70 cases) were performed in the sitting position. The second death was due to a pulmonary embolism on the sixth postoperative day. The third death was in the already mentioned patient in poor condition preoperatively in whom tumor resection was intentionally incomplete. To these three deaths must be added the patient reported previously with multiple meningiomas and another who died 1 year postoperatively of an unrelated cause.

The surgical results reported in the literature for 161 foramen magnum tumors showed 13% mortality. Of these patients, 68% had good results, 10% had fair results, and 9% had poor results. Mortality of 5%, 11%, 11%, and 21% has been reported for these tumors by Meyer and colleagues,[17] Guidetti and Spallone,[18] Zoltan,[24] and Stein and colleagues.[15]

TABLE 124-7 ▪ Extent of Resection (Author's Series)

Localization	Complete	Subtotal	Partial
Anterior	22 ID	1 ID	1 ID
Lateral	2 ED, 1 ID–ED, 20 ID	3 ID–ED	—
Posterior	1 ID	—	—
Total	46	4	1

ED, extradural; ID, intradural.

TABLE 124-8 ▪ Postoperative Clinical Condition (Author's Series)

Localization	Improved	Stable	Worsened
Anterior	21	1	2
Lateral	25	—	1
Posterior	1	—	—
Total	47	1	3

Although the foramen magnum meningioma is a rare tumor, it is the most common and most severe of all tumors situated in the foramen magnum. In most cases, the lateral enlargement offered by the posterolateral approach permits exposure and complete removal of the tumor without manipulation of the upper spinal cord and medulla; however, surgical results still largely depend on the patient's preoperative condition. Early diagnosis is an important feature and is established using CT and MRI. These examinations must also precisely define the tumor location and its relation with the dura and vertebral artery so that the best surgical approach can be chosen. In every intradural form, the goal must be a complete resection with limited drilling of the occipital condyle and lateral mass of the atlas. This goal can be achieved in most cases with reduced morbidity and mortality.

REFERENCES

1. Hallopeau H: Note sur deux faits de tumeur du mésocéphale, 1874. Gazette Médicale 3:111–112, 1874.
2. Rasdolsky L: Zur Frage der Klinik der Meningeome der hinteren Schadelgrube. Z Ges Neurol Psychiat 156:211–244, 1936.
3. Cushing H, Eisenhardt L: Meningiomas: Their Classification, Regional Behavior, Life History and Surgical End Results. Springfield, IL: Charles C Thomas, 1938.
4. Petit-Dutaillis D, Daum S: Les méningiomes de la fosse postérieure: Premier mémoire. Rev Neurol 81:557–572, 1949.
5. Russell JR, Bucy PC: Meningiomas of the posterior fossa. Surg Gynecol Obstet 96:183–192, 1953.
6. Castellano F, Ruggiero G: Meningiomas of the posterior fossa. Acta Radiol (Stockh) 104(suppl):1–177, 1953.
7. Lecuire J, Dechaume JP: Les méningiomes de la fosse cérébrale postérieure. Neurochirurgie 17(suppl 2):1–146, 1971.
8. Yasargil MG, Mortara RW, Curcic M: Meningiomas of basal posterior cranial fossa. Adv Tech Stand 7:3–115, 1980.
9. Rhein JH: Tumor in the region of the foramen magnum. Arch Neurol Psychiatry 11:432–435, 1924.
10. Piehl MR, Reese HH, Steelman HF: The diagnostic problem of tumors at the foramen magnum. Dis Nerv Syst 11:67–76, 1950.
11. Riser M, Lazorthes G, Anduze-Archer H, et al: Des tumeurs craniorachidiennes (tumeurs du trou occipital). Rev Neurol 82:394–410, 1950.
12. Martin P, Kleyntjens F: Tumeurs sous-durales du trou occipital. Rev Neurol 82:313–334, 1950.
13. Dodge HW, Love TG, Gottlieb CA: Benign tumors at the foramen magnum. J Neurosurg 13:603–617, 1956.
14. Cohen L, Macrae D: Tumors in the region of the foramen. J Neurosurg 19:462–469, 1962.
15. Stein BM, Leeds NE, Taveras IM, Pool JL: Meningioma of the foramen. J Neurosurg 20:740–751, 1963.
16. Yasuoka S, Okazaki H, Daube JR, MacCarty CS: Foramen magnum tumors: Analysis of 57 cases of benign extramedullary tumors. J Neurosurg 49:828–838, 1978.
17. Meyer FB, Ebersold MJ, Reese DF: Benign tumors of the foramen magnum. J Neurosurg 61:136–142, 1924.
18. Guidetti B, Spallone A: Benign extramedullary tumors of the foramen magnum. Adv Tech Stand 16:83–120, 1988.
19. Elsberg CA, Strauss I: Tumors of the spinal cord which project into the posterior cranial fossa: Report of a case in which a growth was removed from the ventral and lateral aspects of the medulla oblongata and upper cervical cord. Arch Neurol Psychiatry 21:261–273, 1929.
20. Symonds CP, Meadows SP: Compression of the spinal cord in the neighbourhood of the foramen magnum. Brain 60:52–84, 1937.
21. Salazkin MA: Classification, clinical and diagnostic features of tumors extending through the foramen magnum. Vopr Neirochir 6:22–28, 1953.
22. Arseni C, Ionesco S: Contribution à l'étude des tumeurs situées au niveau du foramen magnum occipitale. Psychiatr Neurol Neurochir 63:170–183, 1960.
23. Krayenbuhl H: Special clinical features of the foramen magnum. Schweiz Arch Neurol Neurochir Psychiatry 112:205–218, 1973.
24. Zoltan L: Die Tumoren im foramen occipitale magnum. Acta Neurochir 30:217–225, 1974.
25. Al Mefty O, Borba LA, Aoki N, et al: The transcondylar approach to extradural nonneoplastic lesions of the craniovertebral junction. J Neurosurg 84:1–6, 1996.
26. Bertalanffy H, Seeger W: The dorsolateral, suboccipital, transcondylar approach to the lower clivus and anterior portion of the cranio-cervical junction. Neurosurgery 29:815–821, 1991.
27. George B, Dematons C, Cophignon J: Lateral approach to the anterior part of the foramen magnum. Surg Neurol 29:484–490, 1988.
28. George B, Lot G: Anterolateral and posterolateral approaches to the foramen magnum: Technical description and experience from 97 cases. Skull Base Surg 5:9–19, 1995.
29. Arnautovic KI, Al Mefty O, Husain M: Ventral foramen magnum meningiomas. J Neurosurg 92:71–80, 2000.
30. George B, Lot G, Velut S: Pathologie tumorale du foramen magnum. Neurochirurgie 39(suppl):1–89, 1993.
31. Pirotte B, David PH, Noterman J, et al: Lower clivus and foramen magnum anterolateral meningiomas: Surgical strategy. Neurol Res 20:577–584, 1998.
32. Sen CN, Sekhar LN: An extreme lateral approach to intradural lesions of the cervical spine and foramen magnum. Neurosurgery 27:197–204, 1990.
33. Dany A, Delcour J, Laine E: Les méningiomes du clivus. Neurochirurgie 9:249–277, 1963.
34. Tristan TA, Hodes PJ: Meningiomas of the posterior cranial fossa. Radiology 70:1–14, 1958.
35. Markham JW, Fager CA, Horrax G, Poppen JL: Meningiomas of the posterior fossa. AMA Arch Neurol Psychiatry 74:163–170, 1955.
36. Abrahamson I, Grossman M: Tumor of the upper cervical cord. Trans Am Neurol Assoc 47:149–168, 1921.
37. Aring CD: Lesions about the junction of medulla and spinal cord. JAMA 229:1879, 1974.
38. MacCarty CS, Lougheed LE, Brown JR: Unusual benign tumor at the foramen magnum: A report of a case. J Neurosurg 16:463–467, 1959.
39. George B, Lot G: Neurinomas of the first two cervical nerve roots: A series of 42 cases. Neurosurgery 82:917–923, 1995.
40. Abott KH: Foramen magnum and high cervical cord lesions simulating degenerative disease of the nervous system. Ohio State Med 46:645–651, 1950.
41. Rubinstein JE: Astereognosis associated with tumors in the region of the foramen magnum. Arch Neurol Psychiatry 39:1016–1032, 1938.
42. Hamer J: Meningioma of the foramen magnum presenting as subarachnoid hemorrhage and cerebellar hematoma. Neurochirurgia 22:169–172, 1979.
43. Scott G, Filizzlo F, Giuseppe S: Repeated subarachnoid hemorrhages from a cervical meningioma. J Neurosurg 66:779–781, 1987.
44. Hirata Y, Matsukado Y, Kaku M: Syringomyelia associated with a foramen magnum meningioma. Surg Neurol 23:291–294, 1985.
45. Harbitz F, Lossius I: Extramedullary tumour: Arachnitis fibrosa cystica et ossificans: Gliosis of the medulla. Acta Psychiatr Neurol 4:51–57, 1929.
46. Rhyner PA, Hudgins RJ, Edwards MSB, Brant-Zawadzki M: Magnetic resonance imaging of syringomyelia associated with an extramedullary spinal cord tumor: Case report. Neurosurgery 21:233–235, 1987.
47. New PFJ, Scott WR, Schnur JA, et al: Computed tomography with the EMI scanner in the diagnosis of primary and metastatic intracranial neoplasms. Radiology 114:75–87, 1975.
48. Thompson JLG: Computerized axial tomography in posterior fossa lesions. Clin Radiol 29:233–250, 1978.
49. Wagle VG, Villemure JG, Melanson D, et al: Diagnostic potential of magnetic resonance in cases of foramen magnum meningiomas. Neurosurgery 21:622–626, 1987.
50. Potts DG, Zimmerman RD: Nuclear magnetic resonance imaging of skull base lesions. Can J Neurol Sci 12:327–331, 1985.
51. Kim KS, Weinberg PE: Foramen magnum meningioma. Surg Neurol 17:287–289, 1982.
52. George B, Laurian C: The Vertebral Artery: Pathology and Surgery. Wien: Springer-Verlag, 1987.
53. Frankhauser H, Kamano S, Hanamura T, et al: Abnormal origin of the posterior inferior cerebellar artery. J Neurosurg 51:569–571, 1979.
54. George B, Lot G, Boissonnet H: Meningioma of the foramen magnum: A series of 40 cases. Surg Neurol 47:371–379, 1997.
55. Portugal JR, Alencar A, Brito Lira LC: Melanotic meningioma complicated by disseminated intravascular coagulation. Surg Neurol 21:275–281, 1984.
56. Wolff BS, Newman CM, Khilnani MT: The posterior inferior cerebellar artery on vertebral angiography. AJR Am J Roentgenol 87:322–337, 1962.

57. Dilenge D, David M: La branche méningée de l'arteïre vertébrale. Neurochirurgia (Stuttgart) 84:121–126, 1965.

58. Greitz T, Lauren T: The anterior meningeal branch of the vertebral artery. Acta Radiol Diagn 7:219–224, 1968.

59. Djindjian R, Merland JJ: Superselective arteriography of the external carotid artery. Heidelberg: Springer, 1978.

60. Salamon GM, Combalbert A, Raybaud C, Gonzalez J: An angiographic study of meningiomas of the posterior fossa. J Neurosurg 35:731–741, 1971.

61. Dilenge D, Calderon H: Catheterisme supersélectif et embolisation des pédicules artériels de deux méningiomes de la fosse postérieure. Neurochirurgie 22:711–720, 1976.

62. Bernstein M, Gutin PH: Interstitial irradiation of skull base tumours. Can J Neurol Sci 12:366–370, 1985.

63. Wara WM, Sheline GE, Newman H, et al: Radiation therapy of meningiomas. Am J Roentgenol Radium Ther Nucl Med 123:453–458, 1975.

64. Bouchard J: Radiation Therapy of Tumors and Diseases of the Nervous System. Philadelphia: Lea & Febiger, 1966.

65. Heppner F: Präoperative Bestrahlung gefäbreicher Hirngeschwülste. Radiol Austriaca 12:33–39, 1961.

66. Derome P: The transbasal approach to tumors invading the base of the skull. In Schmidek HH, Sweet WH (eds): Current Techniques in Operative Neurosurgery. New York: Grune & Stratton, 1977, pp 223–245.

67. Sekhar LN, Schramm VL, Jones NF: Subtemporal preauricular infratemporal fossa approach to large lateral and posterior cranial base neoplasms. J Neurosurg 67:488–499, 1987.

68. Hakuba A, Nishimura S, Jang BJ: A combined retro-auricular and preauricular transpetrosal-transtentorial approach to clivus meningiomas. Surg Neurol 30:108-116, 1988.

69. Sakaki S, Takeda S, Fujita H, Ohta S: An extended middle fossa approach combined with a suboccipital craniectomy to the base of the skull in the posterior fossa. Surg Neurol 28:245–252, 1987.

70. George B, Laurian C, Keravel Y, Cophignon J: Extradural and hour-glass cervical neurinomas: The vertebral artery problem. Neurosurgery 165:591–594, 1985.

71. Shucart WA, Kleriga E: Lateral approach to the upper cervical spine. Neurosurgery 6:278–281, 1980.

72. Stevenson GC, Stoney RJ, Perkins RK, Adams JE: A transcervical transclival approach to the ventral surface of the brain stem for removal of a clivus chordoma. J Neurosurg 64:544–551, 1966.

73. Southwick WO, Robinson RA: Surgical approaches to vertebral bodies in the cervical and lumbar regions. J Bone Joint Surg Am 39:631–644, 1957.

74. Fox H: Obliteration of midline vertebral aneurysm via basilar craniectomy. J Neurosurg 26:406–412, 1967.

75. Wissinger P, Danoff D, Wisiol LS, et al: Repair of aneurysm of the basilar artery by a transcervical approach: Case report. J Neurosurg 26:417–419, 1967.

76. Mullan S, Naunton R, Hekmat-Pana H, Vailati G: The use of an anterior approach to centrally placed tumors in the foramen magnum and vertebral column. J Neurosurg 24:536–543, 1966.

77. Miller E, Crockard A: Transoral transclival removal of anteriorly placed meningiomas of the foramen magnum. Neurosurgery 20:966–988, 1987.

78. Pasztor E: Transoral approach for epidural craniocervical pathological processes. Adv Tech Stand 12:126–170, 1985.

79. Schurando P, Payen D, Beloucif S, George B: Prevention of venous air embolism in neurosurgical sitting position by combination of lower body positive pressure and PEEP without fluid loading. Anesthesiology 69:3A, 1988.

125 Microsurgery of Syringomyelia and Syringomyelia Cord Syndrome

ULRICH BATZDORF

DEFINITION AND CLASSIFICATION

Syringomyelia is characterized by a cavity, a syrinx, existing within the spinal cord, the myelon. Current usage implies that the fluid-filled cyst within the spinal cord is of varying size, shape, and location; the fluid is clear, colorless, and either identical with, or closely resembling, cerebrospinal fluid (CSF). As commonly used, the term does not include cysts whose fluid is formed by intramedullary spinal cord tumors, such as ependymomas or hemangioblastomas, although such tumors may be associated with syringomyelic cavities.

Syringomyelia should be recognized as a condition that, with few exceptions, develops as an epiphenomenon of an underlying pathologic process. Our understanding of these relationships has been increased immensely since the introduction of magnetic resonance imaging (MRI) technology. MRI has also changed syringomyelia from being a relative neurologic rarity to an entity that every neurosurgeon may expect to see in his or her practice. Conditions associated with syringomyelia can be classified as shown in Table 125-1.

It is thought that syringobulbia represents the rare cephalad extension of a syringomyelic cavity into the brain stem. It appears to respond to the same surgical interventions that apply to syringomyelia due to abnormalities at the craniocervical junction.[1]

Focal widening of the central canal, although not infrequently designated as "syringomyelia" in current radiologists' reports, appears to be a distinct entity that in many instances is not progressive and does not require surgical therapy. These remnants of the normal central canal are not uncommon and are perhaps best designated as hydromyelic cavities. Typically they are fusiform in shape and perfectly round and central on axial images.[2]

ABNORMALITIES AT THE CRANIOCERVICAL JUNCTION

Most patients with syringomyelia due to abnormalities at the craniocervical junction have cerebellar tonsillar descent, which, for many years, collectively have been referred to as Chiari I malformation, or Arnold-Chiari malformation. These eponyms serve as a shorthand for a varied group of conditions, some even of different etiologies, that seem to share the characteristic of being associated with a comparatively small bony posterior fossa, certainly relative to volume of its content: the cerebellum and brain stem.[3,4]

Anatomic variants associated with a small posterior fossa volume are listed in Table 125-2.

In the face of the present trend toward minimal surgical intervention, it is important to distinguish these patients from those who have similar-appearing syringomyelia but without evident tonsillar descent. The assumption is made that all patients with syringomyelia have some impediment to the normal, nearly instantaneous equalization of CSF pressure above and below the foramen magnum. The cause of such impaired fluid dynamics is more apparent when the cerebellar tonsils project through the foramen magnum and act as a partial plug. When tonsil descent is not present, impaired CSF dynamics should be looked for and verified by other techniques such as cardiac-gated CSF flow studies at the craniocervical junction and, in rare instances, by myelography (Fig. 125-1).

Clinical Symptomatology and Signs

The clinical presentation of patients with syringomyelia due to abnormalities at the craniocervical junction has been described by many authors.[5–12] Symptoms fall into three major categories, the first two representing what might be called the Chiari syndrome.

1. Symptoms related to impaired CSF dynamics
2. Neurologic symptoms due to brain stem and cranial nerve involvement, that is, related to hindbrain descent
3. Spinal cord symptoms due to the syringomyelic cavity

Symptoms and Signs Related to Impaired Cerebrospinal Fluid Dynamics

Headache is the leading symptom in this category.[13,14] Characteristically, it is located at the base of the skull or upper neck posteriorly and is brought on by situations associated with a Valsalva maneuver, such as coughing, laughing, or straining. As such, the headaches are usually of brief duration, lasting only seconds or minutes, but they may have a prolonged "after ring" or may radiate into the occipital area, retromastoid area, or vertex. In some patients, similar headaches, at times associated with vertigo, are produced by neck extension. Rarely, these maneuvers may also produce transient visual obscuration. Papilledema is rarely seen, although retinal venous pulsations often cannot be recognized when the fundi are examined with the patient in the

---

TABLE 125-1 ▪ Common Conditions Associated with the Development of Syringomyelia

A. Syringomyelia related to abnormalities at the craniocervical junction
  1. Conditions associated with descent of the cerebellar tonsils (also referred to as hindbrain herniation and Chiari I malformation)
    a. Small posterior fossa
    b. Basilar invagination
    c. Os odontoideum
    d. Posterior fossa mass lesions, including arachnoid cysts
  2. Conditions associated with descent of the cerebellar tonsils and portions of the vermis, fourth ventricle, pons, and medulla (also referred to as Chiari II malformation) (Almost always associated with spina bifida and myelomeningocele)
  3. Conditions not associated with descent of the cerebellar tonsils
    a. Retained rhombic roof
    b. Vascularized membranes
    c. Inflammatory membranes
B. Syringomyelia related to abnormalities at the spinal level
  1. Post-traumatic lesions
    a. Not associated with spinal deformity
    b. Associated with evidence of major spinal trauma
    c. Associated with major post-traumatic spinal deformity that causes narrowing of the spinal canal
    d. Associated with previous intradural surgery
  2. Postinflammatory conditions
    a. Bacterial or fungal meningitis
    b. Chemical irritants (e.g., iophendylate [Pantopaque])
  3. Disc disease: spondylosis
  4. Tumors that have caused focal narrowing of the subarachnoid space (intradural or extradural neoplasms)
C. Conditions analogous to syringomyelia but outside the spinal cord
  1. Syringomyelia: an extension of syringomyelia into the pons
  2. Some basal ganglion cysts: an extension of syringomyelia
D. Conditions resembling syringomyelia but of unknown clinical siginificance
  Focal widening of the central canal of the spinal cord

---

sitting position. It is not uncommon for patients to realize in retrospect that such headaches, perhaps in milder form, have been present for many years.

The author is aware of only one fatality after a prolonged bout of coughing in a man who had previously been diagnosed as having hindbrain descent.

TABLE 125-2 ▪ Anatomic Variants and Other Conditions Associated with a Small Posterior Fossa

Posterior/dorsal
  Low insertion of torcular/tentorium
  Horizontally oriented occipital bone with shallow posterior fossa
  Thickened skull resulting from vitamin D–resistant rickets or other factors
  Thickened dura
  Space-occupying arachnoid cyst
Anterior/ventral
  Basilar invagination
  Os odontoideum

Neurologic Symptoms and Signs Due to Brain Stem and Cranial Nerve Involvement

It may not always be possible to distinguish symptoms due to hindbrain descent and compression of the (lower) brain stem by the cerebellar tonsils from those due to cranial nerve distortion, traction, or compression.[8,9] Syringobulbia, although rare, may be identifiable on MRI as a separate cause of similar symptoms.

Ocular symptoms may include the patient's awareness of nystagmoid eye motion, double vision, and transient visual obscurations. Facial paresthesias, dysesthesias, or numbness, usually unilateral, are not uncommon. Dizziness and vertigo are frequent complaints. Lower cranial nerve palsies may present as frequent episodes of aspiration, impaired coughing and swallowing, or alteration in the quality of the voice.

In the examination of these patients, it is important to note the cranial nerve abnormalities, and particularly to test for the gag reflex and posterior pharyngeal motor and sensory function.

Neurologic Symptoms and Signs Due to the Syringomyelic Cavity within the Spinal Cord

The intramedullary cyst is capable of both destroying and compressing neural tissue. As the cyst expands, it may do so in a somewhat asymmetrical fashion. The cyst may appear septated (at least on midsagittal MRI); in other instances, it may consist of two or more parallel cavities of equal or unequal rostrocaudal extent. Even when a cyst appears rounded on axial images, it may not be symmetrically situated with respect to spinal cord structures. As a result of these considerations, neurologic deficits are often asymmetrical and tend to involve one side more than the other.

1. Upper extremity weakness and atrophy, often involving the hand(s), are the result of anterior horn cell destruction.
2. Loss of pain and temperature sensation, often in a "cape" distribution over the shoulder(s), results from spinothalamic tract destruction or compression. Such loss of pain and temperature sensation may extend over the trunk and into one or both lower extremities. Classically (but not universally), position and vibratory sensations are preserved at fingers and toes, even when pain and temperature sensation is severely impaired.[15]
3. Dysesthetic pain, often in the distribution of part or all of the area of sensory loss, is presumed to result from destruction of the internuncial neurons in the intermediolateral cell columns.
4. Spasticity is most likely due to compression of the corticospinal tracts and most often involves the lower extremities.
5. Loss of sweating is due to interruption of autonomic pathways, presumably also in the intermediolateral cell column.
6. Loss of deep tendon reflexes results from interruption of the reflex arc and is commonly seen in the involved upper limb(s).

FIGURE 125-1 *A,* Cerebellar tonsillar descent in a 16-year-old patient with extensive syringomyelia. The patient was treated by durotomy and pericranial grafting. *B,* Syringomyelia in a 21-year-old patient who did not have cerebellar tonsillar descent but had a thick, very vascularized dura that was stitched back but not grafted because of extensive coagulation required for hemostasis.

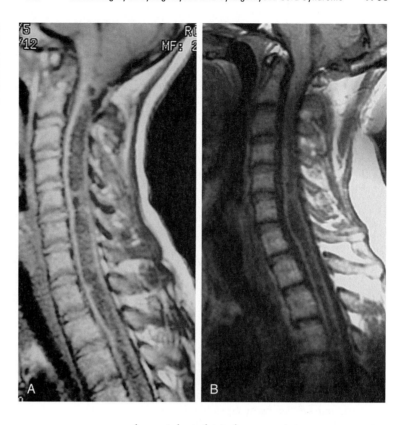

DIAGNOSTIC INVESTIGATION

MRI is the major diagnostic tool to investigate patients with suspected syringomyelia. The imaging criteria that define significant tonsil descent are not precise and are in a state of evolution; however, at present two criteria are applied to the appearance of the tonsils:

1. Descent of the cerebellar tonsils 5 mm below the foramen magnum is generally accepted as abnormal.[16]
2. Pointed or wedge-shaped rather than rounded tonsils are also considered abnormal.

Much controversy exists regarding the exact measurement that represents significant tonsil descent, and it would appear that some individuals have low-lying cerebellar tonsils, that is, with tips just below the inferior margin of the foramen magnum, without any clinical manifestations of the Chiari syndrome. There are, however, a few surgeons who now believe that even minimal tonsil descent may be symptomatic.[17] The evidence of this is largely based on relief of symptoms by decompressive surgery. Similarly, the presence of rounded tonsils does not *absolutely* exclude a significant abnormality at the craniocervical junction.

Cardiac-gated MRI has the capability of demonstrating "flow" in the form of pixels of different signal intensity reflecting motion of CSF behind the cerebellar tonsils, in front of the brain stem, and at the level of the foramen magnum as well as fluid motion within a syrinx cavity.[18,19] Demonstrating absence of flow of CSF behind the cerebellar tonsils is a means of confirming impairment in CSF circulation and is a factor helping to decide in favor of surgical intervention.

In patients with syringomyelia at any spinal level who did not show evidence of tonsillar descent on MRI and do not have a history of spinal trauma and whose history does not

present a clear etiologic basis (e.g., previous surgery, meningitis), it is important that the MR scan be repeated with ionic contrast material to exclude the presence of a tumor as the source of the cord cyst. When there is no explanation for the development of the syrinx cavity, it is recommended that myelography be performed using water-soluble contrast material, with careful observation for any point of even transient delay of flow of contrast. In the event that a complete block to upward flow of contrast from a lumbar injection is observed, contrast should also be injected via a lateral C1–2 puncture, so the extent of the subarachnoid block can be bracketed.

SURGERY FOR TREATMENT OF SYRINGOMYELIA

There are two general approaches to the surgical treatment of syringomyelia:

1. Decompression of the subarachnoid space, aimed at eliminating the mechanism responsible for syrinx formation
2. Shunting of fluid from the syrinx cavity

These approaches are discussed separately for both craniocervical junction–related abnormalities and for primary spinal forms of syringomyelia.

Surgery for Syringomyelia Related to Abnormalities at the Craniocervical Junction

Posterior Decompressive Procedures for Adult-type Abnormalities (Chiari I Malformation)

The surgical approach to dealing with syringomyelia related to abnormalities at the craniocervical junction is based on an attempt to eliminate the mechanism responsible for development and enlargement of the syringomyelic cavity. Our understanding of the pathophysiologic mechanism by which a syrinx cavity forms and expands is still far from complete. Entrance of fluid through the rostral end of a patent central canal, once thought to explain all syringomyelia,[20] applies to only a small number of patients. The concept currently believed to explain most cases of syringomyelia is that there is partial obstruction to the flow of CSF at the craniocervical junction.[21] The normal, nearly instantaneous equalization of pressure above and below the foramen magnum is impeded by the cerebellar tonsils, wedged into the foramen magnum alongside the cervical-medullary junction. An arachnoid membrane at the base of the brain or a retained rhombic roof would have a similar effect. Surgical therapy directed at improving flow of CSF at the craniocervical junction underlies many of the current surgical treatment approaches, although there is disagreement on how this is best accomplished.[1,22,23] There are also different theoretical explanations for the mechanism responsible for the reduction in syrinx size seen.

BONE REMOVAL

Suboccipital or posterior fossa decompression has long been used as part of the surgical treatment for syringomyelia related to abnormalities at the craniocervical junction. Although it may originally have been considered only a part of the exposure necessary to accomplish other maneuvers (such as plugging of the obex), it appears that removal of bone at the foramen magnum in itself relieves part of the compression of the subarachnoid space. The relative inelasticity of the dura in adults, however, makes enlargement of the foramen magnum alone insufficient therapy, and opening of the dura is an additional decompressive step employed by many surgeons, including the author.[22,24] Since restoration of normal CSF circulation at the craniocervical junction is the goal of the procedure, a relatively small suboccipital craniectomy, approximately 2.5 to 3.0 cm in width and approximately a similar measurement upward from the edge of the foramen magnum, is used by the author. Larger craniectomies followed by dural opening may result in ptosis of the cerebellum through the newly created defect.[25] Some surgeons recommend a much more extensive removal of bone overlying the posterior fossa, based on the premise that the posterior fossa is unusually small in patients with "Chiari malformation." The dura, however, is left intact when these larger decompressions are performed. The long-term outcome of this approach has not yet been assessed.

DURAL OPENING WITH OR WITHOUT CLOSURE

Most surgeons consider it essential to perform some type of maneuver applied to the dura to achieve adequate decompression at the craniocervical junction.[1,22,23] Dural decompression ranges from splitting the dura to leave only the inner of the two dural layers,[26] the assumption being that the remaining dura will stretch sufficiently over time so that the subarachnoid space is adequately opened. In young children, the dura appears to be more elastic. Other surgeons, including this author,[22] prefer to open the dura, usually in a Y-shaped manner, to allow a more complete and immediate enlargement of the subarachnoid space (Fig. 125-2). Leaving the underlying arachnoid intact can be technically

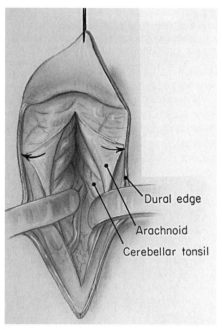

FIGURE 125-2   Exposure of cerebellar tonsils through a Y-shaped dural opening. The tonsils are held apart with retraction. (From Batzdorf U: Syringomyelia: Current Concepts in Diagnosis and Treatment. Baltimore: Williams & Wilkins, 1991, p 169.)

challenging, and durotomy is best performed under magnification. Coagulation of vessels within the leaves of the dura should also be performed with microcoagulation forceps to minimize the area of dural coagulation. It has been found that larger areas of coagulation lead to dural necrosis, which may result in suture pullout when a dural graft is placed. In a few patients, extensive vascular "lakes" have been encountered between the dural leaves. These have required extensive coagulation or suture coaptation of the dural leaves for hemostasis. In these patients, no attempt has been made to place a dural graft, and the "wide open" approach, recommended by Williams,[1] has been employed.

A firm "band" may be seen crossing the outer surface of the dura at the level of the craniocervical junction. It is believed that this represents the periosteal (pericranial) reflection at the edge of the foramen magnum. It can usually be elevated from the dura and amputated at the lateral edges of the decompression. Not infrequently prominent veins exist at the dural attachment of this "band."

Opinions differ regarding watertight dural closure after decompression. Some surgeons advocate leaving the dura open, with the arachnoid either intact[27] or open,[1] and have stitched the dural edge to the muscle wall of the surgical cavity to ensure that the dura remains widely patent. Complications of cerebellar ptosis through the dural opening with intact arachnoid have been encountered.[25] The author prefers to close the dura with autologous pericranium. Bovine pericardium and autologous fascia lata also seem to provide adequate closure and support. Synthetic materials such as polyglactin mesh may be partly resorbed and thus might encourage pseudomeningocele formation.[28] The suture line is challenged with a Valsalva maneuver. Application of fibrin glue, preferably constituted from autologous cryoprecipitate with thrombin and calcium, may enhance healing without CSF leakage.[29]

ARACHNOID

There is a general trend to leave the arachnoid intact once the dura has been opened.[23] This reduces or eliminates spillage of blood into the subarachnoid space. It is, however, arguable whether this approach is equally valid for all situations. When there are little tonsillar descent and no accompanying syringomyelia, leaving the arachnoid intact may well be acceptable. When there is significant tonsillar descent and syringomyelia is present, opening of the arachnoid with reduction of the tonsils appears necessary in some, if not all, patients if diminution of the syrinx cavity is to follow. Gradual ascent of the tonsils and rounding of wedge or "peg-shaped" tonsils have been described in hindbrain descent of differing etiologies,[23,30] but this is not universally seen when the arachnoid is left intact and the tonsils have descended significantly. The author opens the arachnoid in such patients and divides any accessible arachnoid bands. The edge of the retracted arachnoid is held against the dural edge with temporary metal (titanium) clips, facilitating dural closure in which the dural graft is sutured in such manner that the patient's dura and arachnoid are incorporated in the dural closure line (Fig. 125-3).

TONSIL REDUCTION

Reduction of the volume of the cerebellar tonsils has been practiced for many years. Subpial resection of the tonsils was advocated by Bertrand,[31] and other means of accomplishing reduction in size of the tonsils have also been employed.[5,20] The aim of this maneuver is to facilitate unrestricted outflow of CSF from the fourth ventricle. The author prefers the application of bipolar coagulation to the intact pial surface (Fig. 125-4) on the dorsal and medial surface of the cerebellar tonsils, care being taken to avoid close proximity to significant arterial vessels, in particular the posterior inferior cerebellar artery. In some patients, the cerebellar tonsils have become firm and gliotic so that the desired shrinkage with

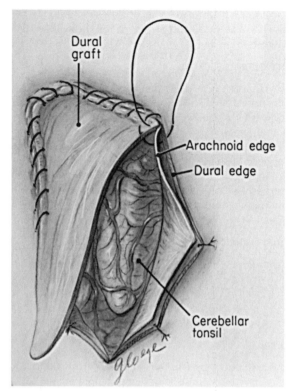

FIGURE 125-3 Suturing of dural graft with the suture incorporating the dura, arachnoid, and graft. (From Batzdorf U: Syringomyelia: Current Concepts in Diagnosis and Treatment. Baltimore: Williams & Wilkins, 1991, p 173.)

bipolar surface coagulation is not achieved, in which case subpial resection is performed with the ultrasonic aspirator. After hemostasis, the pia may be reapproximated with a fine proline suture, or the tonsillar pial envelope may be effectively compressed with a tantalum clip. Obex plugging procedures

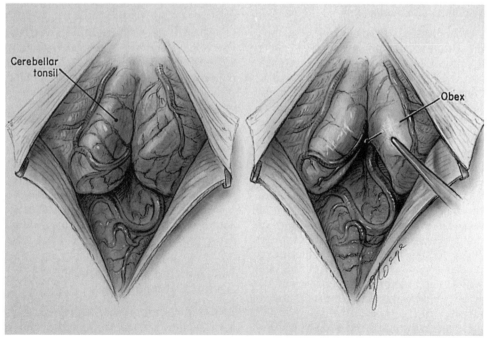

FIGURE 125-4 Bipolar coagulation of cerebellar tonsils. The medial and dorsal tips of the tonsils are touched with a low setting of bipolar current. (From Batzdorf U: Syringomyelia: Current Concepts in Diagnosis and Treatment. Baltimore: Williams & Wilkins, 1991, p 171.)

are no longer performed by most surgeons. Patency of the central canal at the obex is present in only a small percentage of patients.[32]

FOURTH VENTRICLE SHUNTING

In the situation in which the cerebellar tonsils are encased in dense arachnoid scar, elevating or separating the cerebellar tonsils is dangerous and may account for some of the poor outcomes observed by surgeons many years ago.[33] This type of CSF flow restriction can be managed by inserting a piece of shunt tubing into the fourth ventricle under ultrasound guidance[34,35] and placing the distal end of this internal shunt into the cervical subarachnoid space. The shunt tubing should be anchored with one or more fine sutures.

RETAINED RHOMBIC ROOF

Restriction of CSF outflow due to a membranous cover over the fourth ventricle outlets, first described by Gardner and Angel,[20] is only rarely encountered. Such membranes are divided under magnification with the edges held apart by fine suture to prevent reapproximation.

RESULTS

In a series of 36 patients evaluated by this author[5] after surgery, headache and spinal pain improved in 90% of patients manifesting these symptoms, spasticity was reduced in 64% of patients, extremity weakness showed some improvement in 59%, dysesthetic pain was somewhat relieved in approximately 58% of patients, whereas reduction in sensory deficit was seen in 30% of individuals. In a study of 133 patients, 80% of those treated with foramen magnum decompression alone remained free of symptoms.[36] Complications include increased neurologic deficit, respiratory problems, pseudomeningocele formation, and ptosis of the cerebellum.[10,37]

Posterior Decompression Procedure for Cerebellar Descent in Infants (Chiari II Malformation)

The more severe form of hindbrain descent seen in infants, particularly those with myelomeningocele, represents a different entity from the adult form of hindbrain descent.[38] The obstruction of the CSF pathways calls into play similar pathophysiologic mechanisms and may lead to the formation of a syringomyelic cavity. Characteristic features of the infantile form of hindbrain descent include more extensive descent of posterior fossa structures (the vermis, tonsils, fourth ventricle, and portions of the pons and medulla) below the foramen magnum, the common association with myelomeningocele, the presence of an unusually large foramen magnum, and the close application of cerebellar structures to the brain stem, making elevation or reduction of cerebellar tissue impossible. The possibility of rapid clinical deterioration is also a feature. The treatment of these infants is often more limited. Laminectomy sufficient to unroof the descended structures and dural opening are agreed to be essential steps. Controversy exists regarding the extent of any intradural manipulations: establishment of drainage from the fourth ventricle is desirable but not always possible.[39] At least in the past, obex plugging maneuvers were performed.[38,39] The dura is either closed[40] or left widely open.[41] If hydrocephalus is present, ventricular

shunting should be considered before the posterior fossa is approached.

RESULTS

Early operation is now believed to be associated with a good outcome in this high-risk group of patients. Of 15 patients treated at the Toronto Hospital for Sick Children,[41] 88% were reported to show a complete recovery after surgery.

Anterior Decompression Procedures for Anterior Encroachment on the Posterior Fossa due to Basilar Invagination and Os Odontoideum

This group of patients comprises a relatively small percentage of patients with anterior brain stem displacement and even compression. Cerebellar tonsillar descent, without or with syringomyelia, may be seen in this group of patients. The surgical treatment consists of transoral resection of the odontoid followed by posterior fusion procedure when instability exists or is anticipated. Menezes[10] described seven children in whom the procedure was successfully performed, with syrinx collapse seen in five of the seven patients. Anterior compressive problems are not limited to the pediatric population. In milder cases and in the absence of other bony abnormalities of the craniocervical junction, posterior decompression may suffice to relieve problems due to tonsillar descent.

Shunting of Syringomyelic Cavities

Drainage of syrinx cavities with a shunt tube has been practiced for many years. Shunting has been performed by several different approaches:

1. Shunting into the spinal subarachnoid space[42,43]
2. Shunting into the subarachnoid cistern of the posterior fossa[44]
3. Extracavitary shunting into the peritoneal[45] or pleural cavities[46]

The author's experience with the long-term benefits of shunting syringomyelic cysts has been disappointing.[47] The immediate response to shunting is often dramatic in terms of cyst collapse and with respect to resolution of some syrinx-related symptoms. However, the long-term failure and complication rate of shunting has been significant.[47,48] Most common among these is shunt obstruction, often the result of collapse of the walls of the syrinx cavity around the perforations of the shunt catheter, with subsequent ingrowth of glial tissue occluding the openings. Shunting is not helpful if there are separate longitudinal cavities. In the case of extracavitary shunts, tethering of the spinal cord by the shunt tubing may occur and may explain neurologic worsening in the face of seemingly adequate cyst drainage. Some surgeons[42,43] have reported better results with subarachnoid shunting. The author prefers to reserve shunting for situations in which decompressive techniques have failed or cannot be applied.

Microsurgery for Primary Spinal Syringomyelia

As for neurosurgical procedures directed at syringomyelia in association with abnormalities at the craniocervical junction, surgery for primary spinal syringomyelia involves either decompressive surgery or shunting.

Decompression Surgery

Scarring of the subarachnoid space producing at least partial obstruction to CSF flow may result from trauma, inflammation, and postoperative intradural arachnoid reaction. Narrowing of the subarachnoid space can also be produced by severe kyphotic spinal deformity and by intradural spinal cord tumors. Arachnoid cysts or diverticula may be associated with syringomyelia.

In investigating these patients, it is desirable to obtain a precise localization of the arachnoid scar with water-soluble contrast myelography. If a focal subarachnoid scar on the wall of a diverticulum can be identified in juxtaposition to the syrinx cavity (it would generally be rostral to the syrinx cavity), such a scar or web lends itself to resection. A focal scar is one extending only a few millimeters, possibly a centimeter, in width. Myelography from below and above will often provide a more accurate delineation of the scar than MRI. Inflammatory processes such as tuberculous or fungal meningitis result in widespread scarring of the subarachnoid space extending over many spinal segments, and surgical resection of such scar is not feasible.

The laminectomy used to approach the surgical resection of the scar should be centered over the area of the scar but extend both rostral and caudal to accommodate a dural graft.[36,49] The laminectomy defect should be as wide as possible without damaging the facet joints. Resection of scar should be performed with the operating microscope. The instillation of a drop of indigo carmine into the subarachnoid space rostral to the scar has been used to define the area of resection more precisely (Fig. 125-5). This should be done with a tuberculin syringe and very fine needle to avoid contamination of the entire field with blue dye. Very fine needle (26-gauge or smaller) aspiration of the syrinx cavity with a tuberculin syringe has also been used in a few patients to "jump start" the process of syrinx collapse.

The area of scar resection is bridged with a dural graft, which should extend at least half the distance of a spinal segment rostral and caudal to the point of resection. The choice of graft material is perhaps more limited than for suboccipital procedures. Bovine pericardium has been most commonly used by the author; autologous fascia lata, stripped of its fatty or areolar layer, also can be used except in patients with long-standing paraplegia in whom this fascia becomes atrophic. Tenting sutures, from graft to dorsal fascia or to adjacent muscle, have sometimes been used to prevent attachment of the graft to the spinal cord. Considerations similar to those detailed for post-traumatic scars apply to postsurgical scars, which are generally quite focal.

Williams,[21] consonant with his recommendation of leaving the posterior fossa dura and arachnoid open, also recommends leaving the spinal dura open and relying on the fascial closure to provide a watertight seal. To the author's knowledge, however, this approach is not widely imitated.

When the subarachnoid space is narrowed due to kyphotic deformity of the spine, dorsal decompression by the technique described above must be *preceded* by bony decompression of the kyphos and, if necessary, anterior fusion. Only after the decompressed spine has stabilized should dorsal intradural decompression be undertaken (Fig. 125-6).

Syrinx cavities that result from obstruction of the subarachnoid space by intradural tumors, such as hemangioblastomas, seldom require treatment beyond resection of the tumor.[50] The syrinx cavity will collapse once the tumor has been resected.

Shunting Procedures

Shunting of primary spinal syringomyelic cysts has also been widely employed[43,45,46,51,52]; however, every myelotomy performed for placement of a shunt catheter risks an increase in neurologic deficit. Cysts that develop after inflammatory lesions are often honeycombed, and the MRI scan may give the impression of a confluent cavity because the fine septa are beyond the limits of resolution. The author has had the experience of introducing a shunt into a finely honeycombed cavity of this type, and afterward there was a significant increase in neurologic deficit.

As is the case of syringomyelia related to abnormalities of the craniocervical junction, shunting of syrinx cavities of primary spinal etiology is reserved for situations in which other treatment options are not available or have failed.

POSTOPERATIVE CARE

Surgical procedures in which the dura and arachnoid are opened always involve the possibility of CSF leakage and meningitis. Patients who have undergone decompression procedures of the foramen magnum area are nursed in a 30-degree, head-elevated posture in the immediate postoperative period. After spinal decompressions, it is advisable to maintain patients flat in bed for the first 72 hours after surgery. In more delayed fashion, there is risk of pseudomeningocele formation. To reduce the risk of early breakdown of the dural closure, patients are advised to avoid heavy lifting and straining for an arbitrary period of 3 months. It is also recommended that patients take appropriate medications to avoid constipation, which might cause them to strain. For the same reason, it is recommended that patients take a cough suppressant medication if they develop a cough in the early

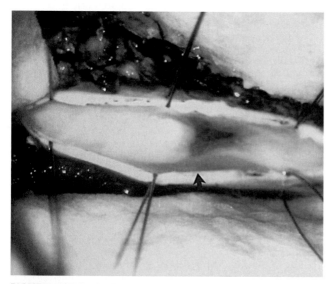

FIGURE 125-5 Indigo carmine injected proximal to a myelographically demonstrated arachnoid scar (*arrow*). The dye sharply outlines the area of scar impeding cerebrospinal fluid flow. The syrinx cavity was caudal to the scar.

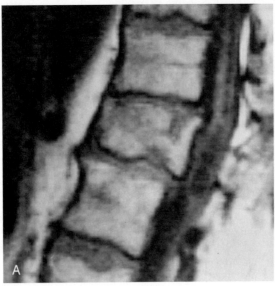 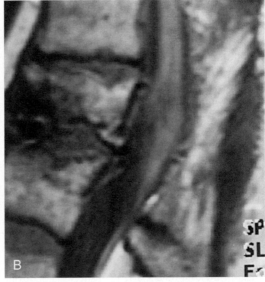

FIGURE 125-6   *A,* Post-traumatic syringomyelic cavity in a 44-year-old patient who sustained a fracture at L1 13 years earlier. *B,* Partial resolution of a syrinx cavity, associated with clinical improvement, after two-stage decompression. The first procedure was the anterior removal of the superior corner of the vertebral body of L1; the second stage, involving a laminectomy and placement of dural graft, was performed 3 months later.

weeks after surgery. It is assumed that the dural closure line is firm by the third month after surgery. If a fluid leak from the wound is apparent early after surgery, it is advisable to place a lumbar CSF drain for several days. It is the author's practice to obtain a baseline postoperative scan 3 months after surgery; scans obtained very soon after surgery are misleading because of the unavoidable signals from surgical trauma. Early scans are recommended only if there is an unexplained postoperative problem.

REFERENCES

1. Williams B: Surgery for hindbrain related syringomyelia. In Symon L, Calliauw L, Cohadon F, et al (eds): Advances and Technical Standards in Neurosurgery, vol. 20. New York: Springer-Verlag, 1993, pp 107–164.
2. Holly LT, Batzdorf U: Slitlike syrinx cavities: A persistent central canal. J Neurosurg 97:161–165, 2002.
3. Badie B, Mendoza D, Batzdorf U: Posterior fossa volume and response to suboccipital decompression in patients with Chiari I malformation. Neurosurgery 37:214–218, 1995.
4. Sahuquillo J, Rubio E, Poca M, et al: Posterior fossa reconstruction: A surgical technique for the treatment of Chiari I malformation and Chiari I/syringomyelia complex-preliminary results and magnetic resonance imaging quantitative assessment of hindbrain migration. Neurosurgery 35:874–885, 1994.
5. Batzdorf U: Syringomyelia, Chiari malformation and hydromyelia. In Youmans JR (ed): Neurological Surgery, vol. 2, 4th ed. Philadelphia: WB Saunders, 1996, pp 1090–1109.
6. Cahan LD, Bentson JR: Considerations in the diagnosis and treatment of syringomyelia and the Chiari malformation. J Neurosurg 57:24–31, 1982.
7. Carmel PW: The Chiari malformations and syringomyelia. In Hoffman HJ, Epstein F (eds): Disorders of the Developing Nervous System: Diagnosis and Treatment. Boston: Blackwell Scientific, 1986, pp 133–151.
8. Dyste GN, Menezes AH: Presentation and management of pediatric Chiari malformations without myelodysplasia. Neurosurgery 23:589–597, 1988.
9. Foster JB, Hudgson P: The clinical features of communicating syringomyelia. In Barnett HMJ, Foster JB, Hudgson P (eds): Syringomyelia. London: WB Saunders, 1973, pp 16–29.
10. Menezes AH: Chiari I malformations and hydromyelia. Pediatr Neurosurg 92:146–154, 1991.
11. Saez RJ, Onofrio BM, Yanagihara T: Experience with Arnold-Chiari malformation, 1960–1970. J Neurosurg 45:416–422, 1976.
12. Williams B: Syringomyelia. Neurosurg Clin N Am 1:653–685, 1990.
13. Nightingale S, Williams B: Hindbrain hernia headache. Lancet 1:731–734, 1987.
14. Williams B: Cough headache due to craniospinal pressure dissociation. Arch Neurol 37:226–230, 1980.
15. Oppenheim H: Lehrbuch der Nervenkrankheiten, 2nd ed. Berlin: Karger, 1898, pp 276–278.
16. Barkovich AJ, Wippold JF, Sherman JL, et al: Significance of cerebellar tonsillar position on MR. AJNR Am J Neuroradiol 7:795–799, 1986.
17. Grabb PA, Mapstone TB, Oakes WJ: Ventral brainstem compression in children and young adults with Chiari I malformations. Neurosurgery 44:520–528, 1999.
18. Armonda RA, Citrin CM, Foley KT, et al: Quantitative cine-mode MRI of Chiari I malformations: An analysis of CSF dynamics. Neurosurgery 35:214–224, 1994.
19. Enzmann DR: Imaging of syringomyelia. In Batzdorf U (ed): Syringomyelia: Current Concepts in Diagnosis and Treatment. Baltimore: Williams & Wilkins, 1991, pp 116–139.
20. Gardner WJ, Angel J: The mechanism of syringomyelia and its surgical correction. Clin Neurosurg 6:131–140, 1959.
21. Williams B: Progress in syringomyelia. Neurol Res 8:130–145, 1986.
22. Batzdorf U: Chiari I malformation with syringomyelia: Evaluation of surgical therapy by magnetic resonance imaging. J Neurosurg 68:726–730, 1988.
23. Oldfield EH, Muraszko K, Shawker TH, Patronas NJ: Pathophysiology of syringomyelia associated with Chiari I malformation of the cerebellar tonsils: Implications for diagnosis and treatment. J Neurosurg 80:3–15, 1994.
24. Halamandaris CG, Batzdorf U: Adult Chiari malformation. Contemp Neurosurg 11:1–6, 1989.
25. Duddy MJ, Williams B: Hindbrain migration after decompression for hindbrain hernia: A quantitative assessment using MRI. Br J Neurosurg 5:141–152, 1991.
26. Isu T, Sasaki H, Takamura H, et al: Foramen magnum decompression with removal of the outer layer of the dura as treatment for syringomyelia occurring with Chiari I malformation. Neurosurgery 33:845–850, 1993.
27. Lapras C, Guilburd JN, Patet JD: La malformation de Chiari type II. Neurochirurgie 34(Suppl 1):53–58, 1988.
28. Paré LS, Batzdorf U: Syringomyelia persistence after Chiari decompression as a result of pseudomeningocele formation: Implications for syrinx pathogenesis: Report of three cases. Neurosurgery 43:945–948, 1998.
29. Shaffrey CI, Spotnitz WD, Shaffrey ME, et al: Neurosurgical applications of fibrin glue: Augmentation of dural closure in 134 patients. Neurosurgery 26:207–210, 1990.

30. Payner T, Prenger E, Berger TS, et al: Acquired Chiari malformations: Incidence, diagnosis and management. Neurosurgery 34:429–434, 1994.
31. Bertrand G: Dynamic factors in the evolution of syringomyelia and syringobulbia. Clin Neurosurg 20:322–333, 1973.
32. West RJ, Williams B: Radiographic studies of the ventricles in syringomyelia. Neuroradiology 20:5–16, 1980.
33. Penfield W, Coburn DF: Arnold Chiari malformation and its operative treatment. Arch Neurol Psychiatry 40:328–336, 1938.
34. Hankinson J: Syringomyelia and the surgeon. In Williams D (ed): Modern Trends in Neurology, vol. 5. London: Butterworths, 1970, pp 127–148.
35. Peerless SJ, Durward QJ: Management of syringomyelia: A pathophysiological approach. Clin Neurosurg 30:531–576, 1983.
36. Klekamp J, Batzdorf U, Samii M: Die Wiederherstellung einer freien Liquorpassage als chirurgisches Behandlungsprinzip der Syringomyelie. Akt Neurol 23:68–74, 1996.
37. Williams B: A critical appraisal of posterior fossa surgery for communicating syringomyelia. Brain 101:223–250, 1978.
38. Carmel PW: Management of the Chiari malformation in childhood. Clin Neurosurg 30:385–406, 1983.
39. Hoffman HJ: Syringomyelia in childhood. In Batzdorf U (ed): Syringomyelia: Current Concepts in Diagnosis and Treatment. Baltimore: Williams & Wilkins, 1991, pp 151–162.
40. Vandertop WP, Asai A, Hoffman HJ, et al: Surgical decompression for symptomatic Chiari II malformation in neonates with myelomeningocele. J Neurosurg 77:541–544, 1992.
41. Park TS, Hoffman HS, Hendrick EB, et al: Experience with surgical decompression of the Arnold Chiari malformation in young infants with myelomeningocele. Neurosurgery 13:147–152, 1983.
42. Isu T, Iwasaki Y, Akino M, et al: Syringo-subarachnoid shunt for syringomyelia associated with Chiari malformation (type I). Acta Neurochir (Wien) 107:152–160, 1990.
43. Tator CH, Meguro K, Rowed DW: Favorable results with syringosubarachnoid shunts for treatment of syringomyelia. J Neurosurg 56:517–523, 1982.
44. Milhorat TH, Johnson WD, Miller JI, et al: Surgical treatment of syringomyelia based on magnetic resonance criteria. Neurosurgery 31:231–245, 1992.
45. Edgar RE: Surgical management of spinal cord cysts. Paraplegia 14:21–27, 1976.
46. Williams B, Page N: Surgical treatment of syringomyelia with syringopleural shunting. Br J Neurosurg 1:63–80, 1987.
47. Batzdorf U, Klekamp J, Johnson JP: A critical appraisal of syrinx cavity shunting procedures. J Neurosurg 89:382–388, 1998.
48. Sgouros S, Williams B: A critical appraisal of drainage in syringomyelia. J Neurosurg 82:1–10, 1995.
49. Klekamp J, Batzdorf U, Samii M, et al: Treatment of syringomyelia associated with arachnoid scarring caused by arachnoiditis or trauma. J Neurosurg 86:233–240, 1997.
50. Kaden B, Cedzich C, Schultheiss R, et al: Disappearance of syringomyelia following resection of extramedullary lesion. Acta Neurochir (Wien) 123:211–213, 1993.
51. Barbaro NM, Wilson CB, Gutin PH, et al: Surgical treatment of syringomyelia: Favorable results with syringoperitoneal shunting. J Neurosurg 61:531–538, 1984.
52. Suzuki M, Davis C, Symon L, et al: Syringo-peritoneal shunt for treatment of cord cavitation. J Neurol Neurosurgery Psychiatry 48:620–627, 1985.

SUGGESTED READINGS

Klekam J, Samii M: Syringomyelia: Diagnosis and Treatment. Berlin/Heidelberg/New York: Springer-Verlag, 2002.
Tamak N, Batzdorf U, Nagashima T (eds): Syringomyelia: Current Concepts in Pathogenesis and Management. Tokyo: Springer-Verlag, 2001.

126 Surgical Management of the Rheumatoid Cervical Spine

ROBIN A. JOHNSTON and JAMES M. BORTHWICK

In this chapter we describe the pathology, investigation, clinical presentation, and surgical management of patients with rheumatoid disease affecting the cervical spine. A variety of surgical techniques applicable to this condition are discussed, as is the decision-making process concerning surgical management. Outcome assessment and the variables associated with favorable and poor outcomes are considered.

Rheumatoid disease is a systemic condition that directly or indirectly affects almost every tissue in the body. The most important spinal effects occur in the cervical spine, which demonstrates inflammatory or erosive changes in a substantial proportion of patients with rheumatoid disease. Relatively few patients develop neurologic symptoms, although the effects of even a modest myelopathy superimposed on widespread arthropathy may have profound consequences on mobility and independence. Recognition and management of this subset of the rheumatoid population is evolving and improving the outlook for affected patients. The days of managing such patients with bed rest and cervical immobilization are long past, and the application of better surgical techniques for access, decompression, and stabilization has been enhanced through superior imaging of the cervical spine by magnetic resonance imaging (MRI) and computed tomography (CT). Surgical decision making is always made easier in the light of information concerning the natural history of the condition, and this information has highlighted the contrast between radiologic appearances and neurologic deficit. The issue of prophylactic surgical management is being addressed, but as yet there is no overall agreement on some fundamental aspects of surgical treatment, including choice of procedure. What is clear is that management should be tailored to meet individual patient needs. The greater part of the rheumatoid disease is managed by physicians with an increasing recognition that intervention by a spinal surgeon is more likely to be effective in the early stages of cervical spine involvement. Just as in other situations in spine surgery, the less the neurologic deficit, the more optimistic the prognosis after surgery.

A close liaison with medical colleagues in the management of rheumatoid disease is a prerequisite for good surgical decision making and for the development of effective, efficient management policies. The surgical skills required cross the barriers that previously separated neurosurgeons and orthopedic surgeons. Microsurgical access and decompression should be combined with fusion and fixation techniques to provide a comprehensive, modern management strategy. The argument for specialized practice in this type of spine surgery is compelling.

CLASSIFICATION AND PATHOLOGY

Rheumatoid disease affects 1% to 2% of the white population in the Western hemisphere, and females are affected considerably more frequently than males. The incidence of cervical spine involvement varies with the population studied, and estimates vary from 25% to 90%.[1–6] The rate of cervical spine involvement increases as the population studied nears the need for surgical treatment. Most sources agree that cervical spine involvement is present in more than 80% of patients who have had the condition for more than 10 years, indicating a correlation between the duration and severity of rheumatoid disease and involvement of the cervical spine.[2] The development of neurologic features is much less common and highlights the poor correlation between radiologic appearances and neurologic deficit.[4,7] Pellicci and colleagues[7] studied a population of patients in whom there was radiologic evidence of cervical spine involvement in 43% initially. Five years later, the incidence of radiologic involvement had increased to 70%. The severity of radiologic changes also increases with time as might be expected, although this does not necessarily presage the development of neurologic symptoms.

In clinical practice, the association and understanding that exist between the spine surgeon and the rheumatologist determine the level at which the screening procedure is set. The sheer numbers of patients dictate that it is impractical for spine surgeons to see all patients with radiologic involvement only. The clinical and radiologic screening sensitivity also vary according to local pressures and local practice, but accumulating evidence indicates that it must not be such that only patients with advanced myelopathy are seen by the spine surgeon.

By far the most commonly affected level is C1–C2, accounting for greater than 80% of all rheumatoid disease in the cervical spine. Subaxial involvement usually affects the upper cervical to midcervical segment and may occur in combination with C1 and C2 disease. No level is exempt, however, and the synovial joints are primarily affected by the pathologic process, which also attenuates the supporting vertebral ligaments and vertebral bone density. The term pannus refers to an inflammatory exudate overlying the lining layer of synovial cells within the joint, but its meaning has been expanded by common usage to include the inflammatory mass of fibrous tissue formed as a result of synovial joint degeneration.

Rheumatoid disease derives from a deranged immunologic state in which the primary target tissues are synovial joints, and in particular those of the distal limbs are most commonly affected. At the histologic level, the inflamed joint shows proliferation of synovial cells, hypervascularity, and infiltration by giant cells and lymphocytes reflecting the inflammatory nature of the condition. Destructive changes occur in the adjacent cartilage and subchondral bone and are seen in the early stage of any synovial joint affected by this condition. By the time a spinal surgeon becomes involved in management, the histologic changes have usually progressed to a more chronic level, and the erosion that occurs in the cartilage and bone together with infiltration and disruption of supporting ligaments ultimately leads to the anatomic destruction of the joint with subsequent malalignment. In the cervical spine, the periodontoid synovial joints are affected, and the overall process leads to loss of bone substance from the vertebra. At the C1–C2 level, the transverse atlantal ligament and the apical and alar ligaments are affected, as are the joints between the occipital condyles and the lateral masses of C1 and the corresponding atlantoaxial joints. Relapsing and remitting but ultimately progressive, this process leads to anatomic and functional degradation of the affected joint. This process may be asymmetric across any given joint surface and can lead to subluxation in any plane. In most cases, the spinal cord can accommodate and compensate for the gradually progressive malalignment, although eventually neurologic compromise may occur. The affected joints may remain mobile or may undergo fibrous or occasionally bony ankylosis. Eventually the joint tissues are destroyed, and the condition becomes locally inactive. In its wake, the process may leave a mass of tough, white fibrous tissue, the product of years, if not decades, of progressive joint destruction. This end-stage chronic inflammatory mass of tissue, frequently but incorrectly referred to as pannus, surrounds a tiny fragment of remaining odontoid bone, and the size of the fibrous mass may be such that it causes direct spinal cord compression, a feature that is not visible on plain x-ray examination (Fig. 126-1). O'Brien and colleagues[8] looked at the histologic appearances of the periodontoid inflammatory tissue and identified two distinct types. One type had recognizable synovial tissue with cellular elements of an inflammatory response. In older, more chronic cases the periodontoid tissue was hypocellular fibrous tissue.

Vertebral malalignment at C1–C2 is most commonly in a forward direction, with C1 moving forward on C2. Depending on the symmetry or local joint involvement, however, C1 may tilt laterally or even rotate on C2. Should the odontoid process and ligaments become grossly attenuated, C1 may slip posteriorly on C2.[9] Destruction of the atlanto-occipital and atlantoaxial joints leads to loss of height of the lateral masses of C1 with subsequent upward subluxation of the odontoid process through the foramen magnum. This condition is also referred to as vertical subluxation. In surgical planning, it is important that the direction of subluxation is clearly ascertained and its cause understood (Fig. 126-2). Fujiwara and colleagues[10,11] have looked longitudinally at groups of patients with cervical rheumatoid disease and made two main observations. The more profound the peripheral joint disease, the more likely was involvement of the cervical spine. Also they noted a trend in progression of C1–C2 malalignment from anterior

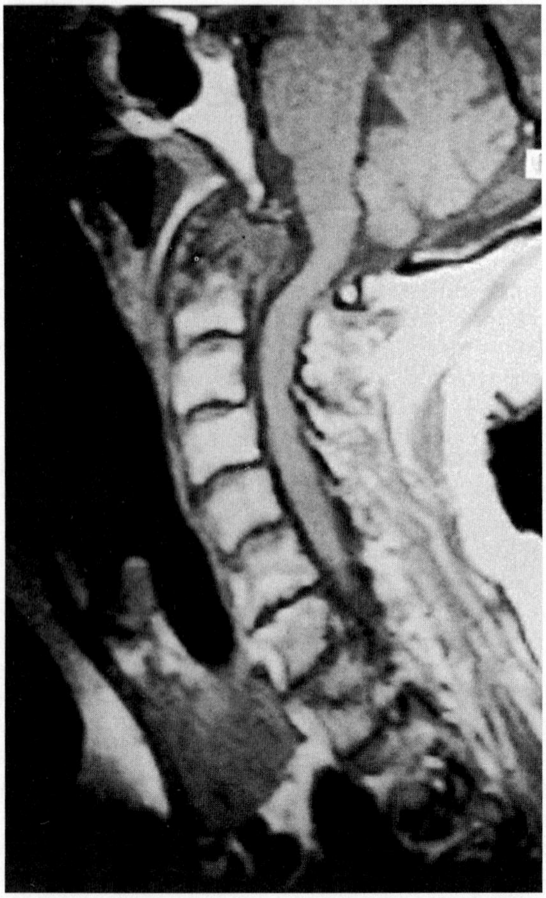

FIGURE 126-1 MRI scan showing erosion of the odontoid and replacement by chronic inflammatory tissue leading to compression and distortion of the spinal cord.

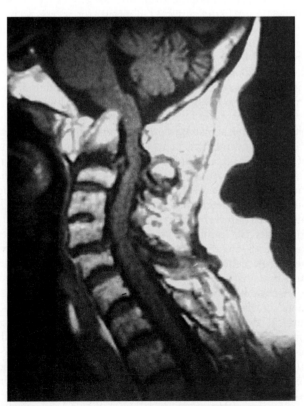

FIGURE 126-2 MRI scan of vertical translocation of the odontoid through the foramen magnum. This may be reducible.

atlantoaxial subluxation through combined anterior and vertical subluxation to vertical subluxation alone.

The pathologic process may leave the malaligned vertebrae in a fixed position, or they may retain mobility, which has the potential for causing neurologic damage through spinal cord or nerve root compression. This instability is rarely of the acute type, such as is associated with spine trauma, but is a more gradual process set against a background in which the normal everyday movements of the cervical spine probably cause repetitive microinjuries to the cord, which eventually accumulate to produce a clinical myelopathy. Ischemic cord changes are noted in a few reported autopsy cases and may be due to intermittent vascular compression or to purported rheumatoid vasculopathy, although the latter is disputed.[12–16]

No histologic features within the spinal cord are unique to rheumatoid disease. Examination of the affected spinal cord shows chromatolysis of the cell bodies with axonal destruction and retraction balls, but there is no inflammatory response within the blood vessels of the spinal cord. The neuronal destruction and fallout leading to spinal cord atrophy are probably the result of persistent compression or intermittent repetitive injury when the spinal canal has become compromised.

RADIOLOGIC INVESTIGATIONS

Initial screening of patients with cervical rheumatoid disease is carried out by plain x-ray examination, which is less sensitive in comparison with CT or MRI but is more accessible. Statistics on the radiologic incidence of cervical rheumatoid disease are compiled largely on the basis of plain x-ray examination, and one can speculate on different results if these investigations were to be carried out by more sophisticated imaging. Lateral cervical views taken in flexion and extension positions are necessary to give a true reflection of potential malalignment. Anterior subluxation may increase during flexion and reduce to almost normal during extension. Normal vertebral alignment does not necessarily correlate with the absence of spinal cord compression, especially at C1–C2, where there may be a large mass of fibrous or inflammatory tissue replacing or lying adjacent to the odontoid process. The odontoid itself is best seen by an open-mouth view, although this may be precluded by anky-losis of the temporomandibular joints. The standard mea-surement of 3 mm between the posterior margin of the anterior arch of the atlas and the odontoid process is misleading. What is relevant is the size of the spinal canal, and this may be compromised by soft tissue that remains unseen on plain x-ray examination. In addition, voluntary flexion of the cervical spine is often unconsciously limited by the patient, because of pain or because of an awareness that excessive flexion causes neurologic symptoms, perhaps only fleeting and vague at this stage.

Disintegration of the odontoid warns of possible posterior subluxation at C1–C2, and asymmetric involvement of the lateral joints suggests the possibility of either rotation or lateral displacement of C1 on C2. Vertical subluxation may be seen on plain views, although in some patients this may be difficult because of obscuring of the anatomic landmarks, including the odontoid tip, the posterior edge of the hard palate, and the posterior rim of the foramen magnum.

A variety of radiologic methods are available by which to determine the degree of upward movement of the odontoid process from plain radiographs, but these have been made superfluous by better imaging.[17]

The most common subaxial appearances are those pro-duced by forward subluxation of one vertebra on the vertebra below, often associated with loss of vertebral height and ero-sion of the end plates. This forward subluxation may give rise to the impressive staircase appearance in which it is impor-tant to determine whether or not the subluxation increases during flexion of the cervical spine. This process may occur at a single level or at multiple levels. Combinations of mobile and fixed subluxations can result in an increased cervical lordotic curve, a kyphotic cervical curve, or a double-curved cervical spine. The quality of bone tissue can also be crudely estimated by radiographs indicating poten-tial problems associated with surgical fixation and fusion.

Plain radiographs, though a useful and relatively inex-pensive means of screening the rheumatoid population, cannot provide the detailed information required for surgical decision making and planning. Potential surgical candidates require investigation by CT or MRI, both carried out in the flexion and extension positions.[17,18] There is much to recommend either of these investigations, and the selection of which (or both) is to be used is determined by availability, the quality of the imager, and personal preference. CT provides good definition of bone structure and malalignment, but it requires the use of intrathecal contrast material to appreciate soft tissues. Reformation of images in the sagittal and coronal planes is helpful for vertebral alignment and management. In modern-generation MRI, horizontal images are more informative than those of CT. Whichever method is selected, the surgeon needs to know (1) which vertebral levels are affected, (2) what type and degree of subluxation is present, (3) whether this subluxation is mobile or fixed, (4) whether there is spinal cord compres-sion, and (5) whether the cord compression reduces or increases with cervical movement (Figs. 126-3 and 126-4).

Software for 3-dimensional image reconstruction is now widely available, but in our personal experience, it has so far not proved to be of much value in operative planning. Occasionally, vertebral MR angiography is required when posterior circulation insufficiency is thought to contribute to the clinical presentation by compromise of one or another vertebral artery because of malalignment of C1–C2. With rotation and lateral displacement at C1–C2, it is important to be aware of the precise location of the ver-tebral arteries because these may present much closer to the midline than would otherwise be expected.

Not every patient who develops rheumatoid disease in the cervical spine progresses to develop myelopathy. Pellicci and co-workers[7] noted that although 80% of their patients demonstrated radiologic progression of rheumatoid disease, only 36% developed progressive neurologic symptoms. Other authors have noted an even lower incidence of neu-rologic deficit, with the range being quoted variously between 11% and 58%, which presumably reflects the pop-ulation studied as much as anything.[19–21]

The standard measurement of the anterior atlanto-dens interval (AADI) correlates poorly with the patient's clini-cal neurologic condition. It is not uncommon to be referred a patient with an AADI of 2 cm, only to find that the

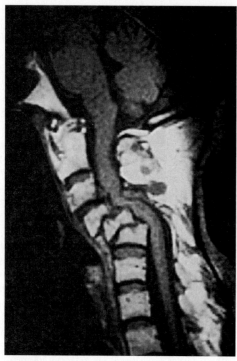

FIGURE 126-3   MRI scan of severe, fixed, kyphotic deformity due to subaxial rheumatoid disease.

patient is entirely free of neurologic symptoms and signs. The posterior atlanto-dens interval (PADI) is a much more relevant measurement, being the distance between the posterior cortex of the odontoid and the nearest point on the posterior arch of the atlas. This distance has been found to correlate statistically with the presence and severity of myelopathy.[22,23] This work concluded that the PADI is an important predictor of neurologic recovery after surgery in addition to preoperative neurologic state, and all patients who had a PADI of at least 14 mm made a satisfactory

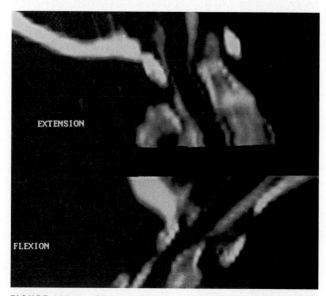

FIGURE 126-4   CT myelogram sagittal reconstructions of C0, C1, C2 levels in flexion and extension. Compression of the spinal cord is severe in flexion and only slightly relieved during extension.

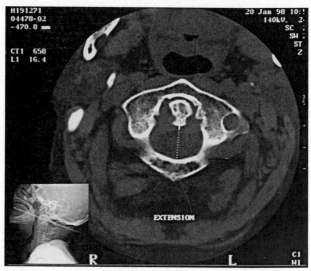

FIGURE 126-5   A CT image through C1–C2 in extension with measurement of the posterior atlanto-dens at 16.4 mm.

postoperative neurologic recovery. The smaller the PADI, the worse the postoperative prognosis. A PADI of 14 mm or less has a high likelihood of being associated with considerable neurologic deficit compared with the AADI, which is an unhelpful measurement. The PADI can easily be measured from a CT scan and the measurements carried out in flexion and extension (Figs. 126-5 and 126-6).

CLINICAL FEATURES AND PATIENT SELECTION

The earliest indication of cervical involvement is commonly midline spinal pain, sometimes referred into the trapezius regions or into the suboccipital area. The degree of radiologic involvement at this stage may be minor, and in this group of patients with minimal radiologic damage and relatively trivial symptoms, there is at present little further to do other

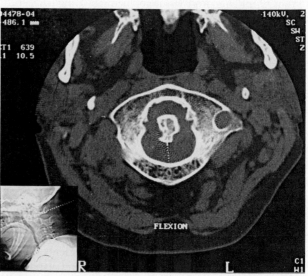

FIGURE 126-6   A CT image through C1–C2 in flexion with measurement of the posterior atlanto-dens at 10.5 mm.

than to recognize that the spine is involved and that deterioration may occur in the future. Symptomatic treatment is all that is needed. Attempts to establish prognostic markers to identify patients who are likely to deteriorate and develop cervical myelopathy have been of limited value. Patients with multiple and severe peripheral joint disease are more likely to have upper cervical spine involvement.[24] The use of sophisticated imaging techniques to measure cervical cord diameter may prove to be of more value. Dvorak and colleagues[3] observed that six of seven patients with a cord diameter of less than 6 mm in any position of the spine had signs of myelopathy. This unsurprising observation begs the question about whether other structural measurements of the cord, such as segmental volume or cross-sectional area, might be of predictive value in identifying patients who require intervention at a stage before the development of myelopathy. The same authors did not find any useful correlation between clinical myelopathy and motor-evoked potentials, although changes in the latter may precede the development of clinical signs. The search for prognostic indicators will continue, but it may be that, as with cervical degenerative disease, the natural course of the illness in individual cases is not predictable, at least in the early stages.[25]

In general, cervical rheumatoid myelopathy is usually present in patients who are more severely affected systemically, and this influences surgical morbidity and mortality. In particular, the presence of interstitial pulmonary disease is associated with reduced postsurgical survival.[26] There is evidence that, once established, rheumatoid cervical myelopathy progresses, although the rate of progression is variable and unpredictable—a situation similar to cervical degenerative myelopathy.[7] Among the earliest to note this were Marks and Sharp,[24] who found that 50% of their myelopathic patients died within 6 months of beginning nonoperative treatment. They noted also that not all of the deaths were directly related to neurologic causes, and many of their patients were already severely affected. This alarming observation probably contributed to the trend toward earlier and more aggressive surgical intervention.

Progressive myelopathy is the clearest indication for surgical intervention, but not all rheumatoid patients with myelopathy progress and deteriorate. Evidence is accumulating that better surgical results are obtained in patients who are less severely affected neurologically and systemically at the time of surgery. This evidence produces increasing pressure to perform surgical procedures at an earlier time, when a less complicated operation may suffice and when the general condition of the patient is more favorable. As the time of surgical intervention is increasingly pushed back, the question of preventive surgery becomes ever more large, although at present there is insufficient evidence to justify surgical intervention in patients without neurologic symptoms.

Sensory symptoms comprise paresthesia, numbness, and loss of proprioception in various combinations, usually involving the upper limbs. The patient may also give an indication of L'Hermitte's symptom, and these sensory manifestations are of prime importance in clinical diagnosis because motor weakness is considerably more difficult to determine in the presence of severe, widespread joint involvement. Grading muscle power using the standard Medical Research Council system is frequently difficult, often inaccurate, and sometimes impossible. Symptoms such as easy fatiguability or a general feeling of weakness, which is separate from the patient's appreciation of normal joint symptoms, may be early indications of muscle weakness. Careful attention to the history is important because neurologic examination can be of variable value. The presence of clearly exaggerated deep tendon reflexes confirms the diagnosis, but often these are unobtainable because of local joint destruction or replacement. Plantar responses, in particular, are rarely present for this reason. An exaggerated jaw reflex may indicate medullary compression as a result of vertical subluxation of the odontoid process, but this may be modified by temporomandibular joint disease. Hyperreflexia is taken as a sign of cord damage, but Floyd and associates[27] could not correlate this with the onset of weakness.

Rogers and colleagues[28] and Toolanen[29] have questioned the existence of cranial nerve deficits in patients with rheumatoid disease. In a series of 235 patients, nystagmus was present only in patients with coexistent Chiari type I malformation. Similarly, other cranial nerve symptoms, such as dysphonia and trigeminal sensory loss, may be explained on the basis of arytenoid joint involvement or upper cervical plexus radiculopathy. They suggest that a proprioceptive deficit indicating posterior column compression is important when deciding whether or not a posterior fixation should be carried out using the sublaminar wiring technique.

It is increasingly clear that preoperative clinical grading systems are useful for evaluating surgical treatment. Casey and co-workers[30] found that the highest mortality and morbidity occur in patients who fall into Ranawat grade IIIB (quadriparesis, unable to walk). More detailed classification of function and disability perhaps properly belongs with the primary rheumatologic specialties, but surgical outcome analysis on the basis of preoperative neurologic condition is increasingly relevant.

The second major indication for surgical treatment of patients with cervical involvement is intractable suboccipital pain. This pain is due to traction or compression or irritation of the C2 nerve root, most often associated with forward subluxation of C1 on C2. The patient complains of suboccipital pain radiating to the retromastoid region. This pain may present in a relatively sudden fashion related to neck posture or with a more continuous background pain interspersed with exacerbations. Pain is associated with abnormal alignment of C1 on C2 together with active synovitis, and if medical treatment fails to bring about relief, surgical stabilization has an excellent chance of achieving lasting pain resolution.

Preoperative evaluation can be difficult in patients with advanced rheumatoid disease and must take account of the systemic manifestations of the condition. These manifestations influence the degree of difficulty with which the procedure is carried out and have an effect on progress. The mental attitude of the patient is also important, and, despite the often prolonged history with repeated surgical intervention, these patients generally have a robust attitude. The degree of arthropathy may also influence the functional outcome, and in some advanced cases, even if the neurologic deficit can be reversed, the severity of joint involvement may preclude useful functional recovery. For these reasons, preoperative evaluation should not be undertaken by the spine surgeon alone but in consultation with the relevant associated specialties.

Evidence is accumulating that in patients in whom the neurologic deficit is severe (Ranawat grade IIIB, severe myelopathy, nonambulatory), the results of surgical intervention are poor with significantly higher complication and morbidity rates. In addition, many of these patients do not achieve any degree of independence and remain in care despite the surgery. In one series, only 15% of grade IIIB patients regained independent ambulation after surgery, although this result has to be set against a small series, which reported that 83% of similar-grade patients showed significant improvement. In patients at the grade IIIB level, spinal cord diameter and cross-sectional area are significantly smaller compared with patients in better grades, and their prognosis for recovery is significantly worse. Surgical intervention may be inappropriate for some of these patients.[30,31] Moskovich and colleagues[32] have suggested that in these severely affected patients bone grafting can be safely omitted from the stabilization procedure. They contend that a stable fibrous union may be adequate, and the morbidity of the surgery is reduced by omitted bone harvesting.

ANESTHETIC ASSESSMENT AND MANAGEMENT

Preoperative anesthetic assessment of a patient permits the anesthesiologist to decide if the patient's general condition will allow survival after surgical intervention with the minimum of morbidity not specifically related to the surgery performed. Optimizing the patient's medical condition before surgery may reduce morbidity and mortality.

An adequate medical history often gives the anesthesiologist a good overall impression of the patient's condition. Good exercise tolerance before a relatively rapid deterioration may indicate good cardiovascular and respiratory reserve. However, if the patient's condition has been deteriorating slowly over a period of years, it may be impossible to gauge these reserves. In some cases exercise tolerance may be good but the patient is limited by disease in other joints or the social circumstances in which he or she lives. Current drug therapy and the use of alcohol, tobacco, and other agents should be noted, as should any drug allergies, including antibiotics.

A full medical examination should pay particular attention to the cardiovascular and respiratory systems. Severe anemia or inadequate peripheral oxygenation may be observed and investigated as indicated. Endocarditis, myocarditis, pericarditis, pericardial effusions, coronary arteritis, and conduction defects may occur in rheumatoid disease. Aortitis and valvular involvement produce aortic insufficiency. A careful search for signs of left ventricular failure should be made.

A full blood count may indicate the presence and degree of anemia. It is rare to require the transfusion of patients before surgery, but because cross-matching of blood may be hampered by the presence of antibodies, the laboratory may require a considerable period of time to obtain the necessary amount of compatible blood. Estimation of blood urea and electrolytes gives a useful indication of renal function and

potassium status, particularly if the patient is on therapy for a cardiac condition. Electrocardiography and chest radiography are performed and consideration given to echocardiography. Pulmonary function tests to measure forced expiratory volume and forced vital capacity can indicate respiratory reserve.

Of particular interest to the anesthesiologist is the available access to the airway. There are two main groups of problems. In patients who have unstable cervical spines, manipulation of the head and neck is hazardous. In others who have fused cervical spines, such manipulation can be difficult or even impossible. In addition, temporomandibular joint disease may prevent the patient's mouth from opening to a sufficient degree to permit the insertion of a laryngoscope. The condition of the dentition may exacerbate the problem. A grossly deviated nasal septum or the presence of nasal polyps may impede access to the airway by the nasal route. Various tests are available to attempt to assess the degree of difficulty that may be anticipated in attempts to intubate the trachea. A review by Frerk,[33] in which the modified Mallampati test and the measurement of the thyromental distance were assessed, showed a high success rate in identifying patients with compromised airways. However, one must be aware that no method is foolproof.

ANESTHESIA

Patients whose cervical spines are stable and in whom it is anticipated that there is acceptable access to the airway may be anesthetized in a conventional manner. Premedication using a benzodiazepine such as temazepam is adequate unless the patient is in significant pain, in which case an analgesic may be indicated. Many patients and anesthesiologists are now finding the omission of premedicant drugs acceptable. Routine monitoring before anesthetic induction includes the electrocardiography, noninvasive arterial blood pressure measurement, pulse oximetry, capnography, and volatile anesthetic agent measurement. The use of a peripheral nerve stimulator will indicate when full muscular relaxation has been achieved. After preoxygenation, anesthesia is induced with a short-acting intravenous agent. Propofol is almost universal in Western medicine now, but others will achieve the same end. Neuromuscular blockade is achieved with vecuronium or the quicker but shorter lived rocuronium. Although succinylcholine chloride is still the fastest-acting agent, its painful side effects can be distressing for the patient. The trachea may then be intubated, usually by the oral route, and fixed to the patient with adhesive tape. Anesthesia can be maintained by ventilating the lungs with a volatile agent such as isoflurane or sevoflurane in either an oxygen–nitrous oxide or an oxygen-air mixture. The omission of nitrous oxide removes an analgesic agent and necessitates a higher concentration of volatile agent but may reduce the incidence of postoperative nausea and vomiting. Analgesia may be provided by an opioid such as morphine, but shorter-acting derivatives may also be of use. Nonsteroidal anti-inflammatory drugs provide good additional analgesia and have been shown to reduce the amount of postoperative opioid requirements. Diclofenac has proved to be effective, but there may be advantages in the use of Cox-2 anti-inflammatory drugs with their reduced effects on gastric mucosa and platelet function.

There would appear to be little benefit from the use of total intravenous anesthesia, but it is not contraindicated. Residual neuromuscular blockade is reversed at the end of the procedure and the trachea extubated when spontaneous ventilation is adequate and protective airway reflexes have returned.

It may be difficult or impossible to safely intubate patients with unstable or fused cervical spines by conventional methods. The use of the intubating fiberscope has made the management of these patients much easier and safer. The authors' preferred technique is to premedicate the patient with a drying agent such as glycopyrronium bromide and an oral benzodiazepine with good amnesic effects such as lorazepam. Intravenous sedation with target-controlled propofol allows verbal contact and cooperation to remain with the patient during tracheal intubation. Nasal intubation is preferable for transoral surgery because it provides an easier angle of access to the laryngeal inlet. To facilitate this procedure, the nasal mucosa is anesthetized with 10% cocaine applied with cotton wool pledgets and/or a proprietary preparation of 5% lidocaine and 0.5% phenylephrine. The posterior wall of the oropharynx may be anesthetized with a lidocaine spray. The nasal passages can be dilated and further anesthetized by inserting nasopharyngeal airways coated in lidocaine jelly, starting with a size 6.0-mm and increasing to a 7.0-mm or even 7.5-mm airway and leaving this in place for several minutes. The larynx may be anesthetized either by a cricothyroid puncture and injection of lidocaine or by a "spray as you go" technique through the fiberscope suction channel. The nasal airway is removed and the authors prefer to insert a reinforced tracheal tube into the pharynx before passing the fiberscope through the tube. This ensures that the tube will pass into the pharynx and usually points the fiberscope in the correct direction from the outset. The fiberscope is passed between the cords into the trachea and advanced so that the carina is visualized. The tracheal tube is then advanced over the fiberscope with a screwing action; when the anesthesiologist is sure of tracheal intubation, the fiberscope is removed and the tube secured to the face with adhesive tape. If the patient is to be prone for part of the procedure it may be wise to suture the tube to the nose. Other techniques using such instruments as the intubating laryngeal mask or light wands may be of use in some cases and tracheostomy may rarely be required. A nasogastric tube can be passed through the other nasal passage.

Anesthesia can be maintained using either an inhaled or intravenous technique. Although spontaneous respiration was utilized in the past to permit observation of continuing respiratory function, this is no longer necessary and controlled ventilation is preferred. Acute changes in arterial pressure as measured by an invasive technique occur before respiratory alteration if the brain stem is being compromised. Although blood loss is usually less than 300 mL, good venous access is advised. Central venous access is not necessary in the majority of patients but may benefit some individuals. If the surgeon considers that there is a high chance of breaching the dura, then it may be useful to insert a lumbar spinal cerebrospinal fluid (CSF) drain before the start of surgery but keep it closed until its use is required.

POSTOPERATIVE CARE

After surgery the patient is nursed in the intensive care unit and regains consciousness while receiving adequate sedation and analgesia. The stomach is kept empty with regular suction and free drainage of the nasogastric tube and the use of prokinetic drugs such as metoclopramide. Reducing the gastric pH with H_2 antagonists such as ranitidine may help reduce the risks of damage to the suture line should gastric regurgitation occur despite all attempts to prevent it. Respiratory support is gauged to maintain adequate gas exchange and can be reduced over a 24-hour period, when it would be hoped that the patient could be extubated. Occasionally temporary tongue swelling or pharyngeal dysfunction may delay extubation. Clear intravenous fluids provide hydration in the first 24 hours postoperatively, and peripheral intravenous nutrition can be given for 3 days until the surgeon feels it is appropriate to resume oral feeding.

SURGICAL ASSESSMENT

It is important to know the direction of subluxation and whether this is fixed or mobile. At the C1–C2 level, it must be clear whether the subluxation is anterior (the most common form), posterior, lateral, rotatory, or vertical. Anterior, vertical, and posterior subluxation may require an anterior surgical procedure in combination with the posterior approach, whereas the less common lateral and rotational subluxations usually require only posterior stabilization.

The site of cord compression may be anterior or posterior, or both, but it is crucial to know whether cord compression decreases when vertebral alignment is returned to normal. In most cases in which the subluxation is mobile, extension of the cervical spine reengages the cervical vertebrae in better alignment, and in a substantial percentage of cases this resolves the cord compression, indicating that posterior fixation and fusion in this position is sufficient. In some patients, even normal vertebral alignment is associated with soft-tissue compression of the spinal cord, indicating that direct decompression by an anterior approach may be necessary. In cases in which the subluxation is fixed, the site of cord compression is identified, and this indicates the direction of the primary decompression surgery (see Fig. 126-1). Once the route of access is clear and the means of decompression selected, consideration must be given to whether stabilization is required at the same operation. It has been shown that removal of the odontoid process leads to considerable instability in most if not all patients with cervical rheumatoid disease.[34] The early 1990s saw an increase in the use of transoral surgery for cervical rheumatoid disease. The purpose was to remove the odontoid and the chronic fibrous tissue mass compressing the spinal cord. The frequency of transoral surgery for cervical rheumatoid disease in most centers has decreased considerably over the past 5 years, presumably for a number of reasons including earlier diagnosis and referral. However, it is also becoming clear that the periodontoid fibrous tissue mass, which is essentially an attempt at stabilization equivalent to callus around a fracture, will resolve if the C1–C2 motion segment is fixed. This may therefore preclude the need for transoral decompression in many cases.[35,36]

When vertical odontoid subluxation occurs, the tip of the odontoid process rarely passes beyond the lower third of the clivus, whereas in congenital anomalies of this region extreme upward subluxation is possible. Access to the lower third of the clivus can be achieved through the transoral-transpharyngeal route. In some patients it may be possible to reduce the vertical subluxation using careful cervical traction over a period of days. If the subluxation reduces, the patient may be stabilized in the reduced position using occipitocervical fixation and fusion techniques. Placing patients with rheumatoid disease in a recumbent position in traction invites diverse medical complications but may be carried out successfully within an intensive care unit if necessary.

If the anterior transoral approach is to be used, the patient's ability to open the mouth sufficiently wide is relevant because ankylosis of the temporomandibular joints may severely curtail this. Normal mouth opening when the teeth are present is on the order of 60 mm (three fingerbreadths). Many rheumatoid patients are without teeth, which facilitates access, but unless the opening is at least 40 mm (two fingerbreadths), the surgical access and room for maneuvering is severely curtailed. Opening may be improved by prior surgical freeing of the temporomandibular joints, whereas other options include division of the mandible and longitudinal section of the tongue, although for rheumatoid disease these are very rarely necessary.

The position of the vertebral arteries should be recognized at the C1 level as they emerge from the vertebral artery canal and pass posteriorly across the superior surface of C1. In most cases, this position presents no problem for either anterior or posterior surgical access to C1. When C1 is rotated, however, and this is seen on CT scan, the arteries present closer to the midline than normal.

When the subaxial spine is involved, it is necessary to know how many and which levels are affected. A period of light cervical traction, usually no more than 48 hours, should provide radiologic evidence about the mobility and reducibility of subaxial subluxation if this is not already evident from flexion and extension radiographs. In addition, repeated clinical examination indicates whether or not the patient experiences neurologic improvement when the spine is more correctly aligned. In these patients, even relatively short periods of traction and immobility may generate complications, such as joint stiffness, venous thrombosis, respiratory infection, and skin necrosis.

C1–C2 subluxations and subaxial subluxation can occur simultaneously, raising the difficult question of which is the more relevant with respect to the neurologic symptoms. Often, with radiologic and clinical information, this is an easily solved problem, but there are instances when it is not clear which is the more important level of compression, and combined procedures may be indicated in these cases (Fig. 126-7).

SURGICAL TECHNIQUE

The primary aims of surgical treatment of the rheumatoid cervical spine are to relieve the neurologic symptoms (including pain) and prevent their recurrence. This outcome should be achieved at minimal general and neurologic risk to the patient, while preserving cervical spine mobility as far as possible. There are three main components to surgery of the spine: access, decompression, and stabilization.

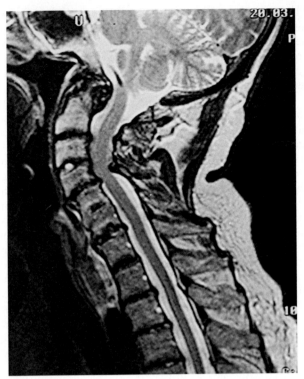

FIGURE 126-7 MRI scan showing coexisting periodontoid and subaxial rheumatoid disease.

Anterior Subaxial Access

The patient is positioned supine on the operating table with the shoulders, cervical spine, and occiput well supported. Care must be exercised to ensure that there are no involuntary or excessive movements of the cervical spine with the patient fully anesthetized. Positioning is initially best carried out with the patient still in a supportive external orthosis or in cervical traction. The operation may be carried out from either side, although most surgeons use the right side. The head is rotated approximately 15 degrees to the left, and anesthetic tubing is positioned so that it does not interfere with perioperative radiographs.

For most approaches to this region for cervical degenerative disease, an oblique incision crossing the medial border of the sternocleidomastoid is generally sufficient. The height of this incision depends on the level to be reached and on the morphology of the patient's neck. For rheumatoid disease, it is usual to require access to several levels, and for this purpose, an incision parallel to the medial border of sternocleidomastoid is preferable to a more horizontal incision. This incision is especially useful if stabilization is to be carried out across several vertebral segments. If access to the T1 vertebra is needed, this can be facilitated by section of the medial insertion of the sternocleidomastoid muscle approximately 1 cm above its insertion into the sternum and clavicle if necessary.

Dissection is carried through the tissue planes of the neck in a standard fashion using careful separation techniques with dissecting scissors, and the anterior cervical vertebral surface is palpated between the carotid sheath laterally and the pharynx and larynx medially.

Division of the omohyoid muscle is sometimes required, and occasionally it is necessary to divide the superior thyroid artery between ligatures. Care should be taken to preserve as far as possible the internal and external laryngeal branches of the vagus nerve, the latter crossing with the superior thyroid artery in most cases. The prevertebral fascia is identified, lifted, and divided with scissors to expose the anterior longitudinal ligament, discs, and vertebral bodies, which are bordered by the medial edges of the longus colli muscles.

At this stage, it is necessary to identify the correct vertebral level, and this is achieved using one or more spinal needles inserted a few millimeters into a vertebral disc, for the purposes of image intensifier identification. A small but important step at this point is to excise part of an identified disc using a knife, such that the needle can now be removed from the operative field, still leaving the disc clearly identified. Retractors are carefully hooked below the medial edge of the longus colli muscle on each side. Frequently, this involves electrocoagulation of venous vessels in this region. The upper and lower extremities of the affected vertebral segments are now clearly identified before proceeding to the decompression phase of the procedure.

Transoral Access

The transoral and transpharyngeal route provides direct, relatively uncomplicated access to the odontoid and periodontoid tissues, a procedure further facilitated if the patient has no teeth. This is a bacteriologically colonized surgical field and one in which it is unnecessary and probably impossible to achieve sterilization. The authors use a water-soluble iodine solution to gently swab the oral and pharyngeal tissues briefly before making the initial incision. A throat pack is inserted to prevent blood and iodine from reaching the stomach and causing retching or vomiting in the postoperative period.

The cervical spine should be slightly extended before this operation, and the patient may be placed in the lateral position as described by Crockard and colleagues[37] or in the fully supine position. The former permits combined anterior and posterior surgery to follow in sequence without necessitating breaking from the procedure, turning the patient, and again preparing the area. Personal preference dictates the position to be used. We prefer to place the patient in the supine position: the surgeon stands at the patient's head and is able to maneuver the microscope from side to side as required during the operation. The supine position permits the surgeon to work from the front facing the patient, from the head in the upside-down position, or from the right or left sides.

A ring retractor of the Crockard type or something similar permits access by retracting the tongue and holding the mouth open. Prolonged, excessive tongue retraction can rarely lead to postoperative macroglossia resulting from edema, and this risk may be lessened by easing the retractor for a few minutes every half hour. Additional specialized instrumentation includes soft palate and pharyngeal retractors.

The posterior wall of the pharynx can be easily palpated with the finger to identify the anterior tubercle of C1, which usually lies behind the soft palate. The latter may be retracted up and away toward the nasopharynx using specially designed retractors that fit onto the ring base. Alternatively, the soft palate may be divided for the greater part of its length but short of its insertion into the hard palate. The soft palate heals well if resutured carefully, but the junction of hard and soft palate is the area most at risk of wound breakdown. Division of the soft palate, if necessary, is done using fine-point cutting electrocautery, just to one side of the midline. The sides of the soft palate can now be retracted using pharyngeal retractors, and the posterior wall of the pharynx is exposed. This is divided in the midline for 2 cm above and below the anterior tubercle of C1.

Pharyngeal retractors are inserted, and the deep fibers of the constrictor muscle attached to the anterior arch of C1 and the anterior surface of the C2 body are gradually dissected laterally, allowing wider exposure. Once the clean bone has been exposed, the pharyngeal retractors are finally inserted, taking care to safely secure the armored endotracheal tube and the nasogastric tube lateral to the retractor feet, one on either side. The decompression phase of the procedure can now commence.

Posterior Access

For posterior access, usually exposure of the C0–C3 region, the patient is either in the fully prone position or is held laterally as described earlier. The cervical spine should be in a neutral or a slightly extended position in most cases. Cervical traction may or may not be used according to the circumstances. It is helpful and reassuring to have a radiograph of the spine in the immediate preoperative position. The slight degree of cervical extension produces skin folds, which are a nuisance in making and closing the surgical incision that runs from just below the inion as far down the cervical spine as necessary. The musculature is dissected bilaterally through the relatively avascular midline, although vessels of the subaxial plexus are encountered around the spinous process of C2, and the dissection is carried laterally to the facet joints on each side below C2–C3.

The suboccipital bone is gradually exposed bilaterally, approaching the foramen magnum with care. Fine-needle point electrocautery is an excellent method of accurate muscle dissection. The C1–foramen magnum level is exposed last, beginning in the midline with care initially to identify the posterior arch of C1. In some patients with rheumatoid disease, the posterior arch of C1 is narrow and thin, whereas in others, it may be located more anteriorly than normal, even in the slightly extended position of the cervical spine. The soft tissues of the atlanto-occipital space and the space between C1 and C2 may bulge posteriorly, indicating the degree of compression caused by the malalignment of C1. Care must be exercised not to disrupt the dura using electrocautery or sharp dissection, if this is preferred. The posterior arch of C1 is exposed bilaterally as far as the groove for the vertebral artery, which location is presaged by a collection of veins. If fixation is to include the C1 lateral masses, the vertebral artery can be mobilized subperiosteally and lifted clear of the upper surface of C1. When the subaxial lateral masses are to be used for fixation, dissection should not extend beyond the lateral edge of the mass, since this is unnecessary and will lead to venous hemorrhage.

Anterior Subaxial Decompression

The myelopathy caused by subaxial rheumatoid disease is often due to stepwise malalignment of the subaxial cervical spine. Reduction of this malalignment by traction may be sufficient in a few cases to bring about cord decompression. When the malalignment is mobile and easily reducible, the patient may be placed on the operating table in a reduced and acceptably aligned condition. In this situation, the decompression has, in effect, been achieved and can be further confirmed by image intensifier.

When the malalignment is fixed or cannot be reduced to a satisfactory degree, it is necessary to remove one or more of the vertebral bodies to obtain satisfactory cord decompression. If a fixed irreducible kyphos is present, this needs to be excised to provide the decompression, perhaps requiring removal of three or more vertebral bodies.

Decompression is begun by removing the intervertebral discs using a combination of a small-bladed knife, disc rongeurs, and small curved or angled curets. Once it has been established how many vertebrae and discs must be excised, the vertebral bodies can now be efficiently removed using a high-speed drill with a variety of burrs, which provide both end and side cutting when appropriate. This is best done using the operating microscope, especially as the posterior cortical plates are approached. These may be extensively thinned down using a cutting burr and finally flipped up using a blunt hook or fine bone punch. There are no osteophytes formed at levels affected by rheumatoid disease. The corpectomy is carried laterally to the medial edge of the uncovertebral joints, leaving a thin layer of lateral corticocancellous bone.

The ventral dura is exposed, and the edges of the bone resection are trimmed using either a small diamond-tipped burr or a thin-based micropunch. The cranial and caudal extremities are prepared to receive bone graft by thinning the central cartilaginous end plates to expose cancellous bone to interface with the graft.

Transoral Decompression

The anterior tubercle and arch of C1 are most easily removed using a high-speed drill with a cutting burr. Very occasionally odontoid removal is achievable without complete excision of the C1 anterior arch. Immediately posterior to the anterior tubercle and arch of C1 lies the synovial joint, which will be replaced by the fibrous product of chronic inflammation of the synovial membrane.[8] This tissue is pale in color, is tough in texture, and has to be removed to expose the anterior surface of the odontoid process. Removal of this fibrous tissue can be difficult but can be achieved using a KTP (potassium-titanyl-phosphate) laser, which is particularly useful for this purpose.

The odontoid process, or what remains of it, is as far as possible defined at its base, sides, and apex. The cortical bone may be of such poor quality that a blunt hook or similar instrument can easily be pushed through into the interior, which frequently is soft, poor-quality cancellous bone. The inflammatory tissue may replace part or all of the odontoid process or can separate it from the base of the C2 vertebra. Odontoid resection is achieved using a high-speed drill using cutting and diamond-tipped burrs. Care must be

exercised not to displace a mobile odontoid posteriorly toward the cord, especially if it is disconnected from the body of C2. The posterior cortex of the odontoid can be removed using a thin-based micropunch or a diamond-tipped burr. It is important to ensure that the odontoid apex has been removed, because it often remains attached to the apical and alar ligaments. If it is inadvertently left behind, the apex continues to cause cord compression. The resection is carried inferiorly to the body of C2, and in most cases this is sufficient to relieve bone compression.

When the odontoid has moved vertically because of collapse of the lateral masses of C1, it usually comes to lie posteriorly to the lower third of the clivus. In irreducible cases, the lower edge of the clivus is identified by dividing and dissecting laterally the overlying mucous membrane and the insertion of the anterior longitudinal ligament. The lower edge of the clivus, once exposed, can then be gradually removed using a drill or a thin-based micropunch. The lower third of the clivus can be reached and removed in this way to gain access to the odontoid lying posteriorly.

Odontoid removal exposes the remains of the transverse atlantal ligament and the remnants of the apical and alar ligaments. These may be markedly attenuated by the inflammatory process or even absent. Ligaments do not specifically have to be divided or removed, although this may happen during the course of the removal of posterior odontoid inflammatory tissue. This latter tissue, when present in bulk, may be the prime cause of cord compression, and its removal is crucial to the completion of a satisfactory decompression. Farther posteriorly lies the continuation of the posterior longitudinal ligament, the membrana tectoria. This can be identified and should be carefully opened into the extradural space. By this stage, it should become apparent that CSF pulsations are being transmitted into the newly decompressed operative field. Inadvertent opening of the dura is uncommon in rheumatoid disease, but should this happen a seal can be obtained using layers of fascia and muscle, with fibrin and thrombin tissue glue. A lumbar CSF drain is inserted as soon as the operation is finished if not already in position, and strong consideration is given to inserting a lumbar peritoneal CSF shunt 4 or 5 days later.

Closure of the pharyngeal wound is carried out in two layers, and we prefer to use a small round-bodied needle with an absorbable suture. Closely spaced individual sutures are placed through the constrictor muscles and finally through the mucous membrane and muscles. The soft palate, when divided, should be closed in three layers beginning posteriorly. The same type of suture material is preferred, and the deepest suture lifts muscle and posterior mucous membrane. The middle layer approximates the muscle of the soft palate, and the ventral layer approximates mucous membrane and muscle.

Posterior Decompression

It is unusual in the authors' experience for a posterior decompression to require more than the removal of the posterior arch of C1, although others report the use of cervical laminectomy and fusion for subaxial rheumatoid disease.[35,36,38] The need to remove the posterior arch of C1 is determined from preoperative imaging and confirmed at surgical exposure by the bulging tissues above and below a fixed anterior subluxation of C1. Passing any instrument below the posterior arch of C1 is difficult and dangerous in this situation. The posterior neural arch may be severely eroded by the disease process, but even so its removal should be carried out from the posterior surface rather than by passing instruments below the arch. High-speed drills and small fine-pointed bone nibblers are safest. The resection is carried laterally until the lateral surface of the dura is seen.

Anterior Subaxial Stabilization

The rheumatoid spine cannot be stabilized using an isolated Cloward's or Smith-Robinson type of fusion procedure. Anterior cervical fusion must be combined with anterior instrumentation, posterior fixation and fusion, or external orthotic support. It is preferable to use a Smith-Robinson technique to fuse a reducible malaligned cervical spine, because the cervical vertebrae frequently have lost height, making a multilevel Cloward's type of procedure difficult and more prone to local collapse and further angulation. The Smith-Robinson type of graft permits retention of much of the vertebral height and is more applicable for multilevel surgery. Alternatively, one or more vertebral bodies may be excised depending on the deformity and local conditions.

Bone strength and quality vary from just adequate to poor in rheumatoid disease and affect the bone fusion rate. The authors prefer to obtain bone grafts from the anterior iliac crest rather than using bank bone, xenografts, or fibular struts. Particularly in more severely affected patients, however, harvesting bone from the iliac crest or anywhere else adds to the morbidity of the procedure, and other options may be considered. The graft sites are carefully measured for depth, height, and width, and the bone grafts are tailored to size, being inserted with the use of cervical traction, which is then removed, producing a degree of compression to enhance bone fusion.

Anterior cervical plates are frequently used in cervical rheumatoid disease to enhance fusion. The two main choices are systems using cortical screws that penetrate the anterior and posterior cortical plates for better grip and a locking plate system using cancellous screws that do not penetrate the posterior cortical plate. These plates serve the purpose of securing the bone graft in position and add a degree of internal stability, which should enhance bone fusion. If bone quality is poor, the screws are easily dislodged and the plate may provide little or no stability. In patients in whom the bone quality is satisfactory, the use of these plates, in combination with an external orthosis, can be sufficient to obviate the need for additional posterior fixation.

In cases in which the malalignment is irreducible and several vertebral bodies have been removed, replacement by a single graft of corticocancellous bone is necessary. This graft is best obtained from the anterior iliac crest and tailored precisely for length, depth, and width. It is inserted under cervical traction, which is then released to generate compression force on the graft. The graft surfaces are prepared flat for a tight fit. In this situation, anterior plate instrumentation should be employed to secure the graft in position according to not only the individual circumstances but also and especially the bone quality. Dynamic cervical plates are available that permit a degree of telescoping to

occur, probably to the benefit of fusion, although more experience with these is necessary to demonstrate longer term benefits.

Posterior Stabilization

Most posterior stabilization procedures for cervical rheumatoid disease involve the occipital, C1, and C2 levels. After an odontoid resection, the C1–C2 complex is less stable, and in rheumatoid disease, posterior fixation and fusion is probably always indicated.[34] In many cases, a C1–C2 fixation is satisfactory, but in certain situations, it is necessary to include the suboccipital region. These situations include that in which the posterior arch of C1 is too attenuated by the disease to accept fixation, when a laminectomy of C1 has been carried out, and in the rare situation when there is an occipitialized or bifid C1 vertebra. When there is loss of lateral mass height and vertical subluxation of the odontoid, it is necessary to carry out an occipitocervical procedure. In a few cases, incorporation of the C1 lamina into the fixation may prove technically difficult or excessively risky, and the surgeon may opt for the safer alternative of an occipito–C2 fusion.

A simple onlay bone graft supported by an external orthosis is less frequently used now, and in most cases, some form of internal fixation is used to enhance bone fusion. A wide variety of devices are available for occipitocervical fusions, including the Ransford loop, which is a modification of the Luque system contoured to allow wiring of the suboccipital bone. This device provides rigid fixation, which may be extended as far down the cervical spine as necessary using sublaminar wire techniques. This system provides a more rigid fixation than simple wiring with bone graft and external orthosis, which is reported to carry a pseudarthrosis rate of 50%.[39-43] The technique described by Brattström and Granholm[44] using a combination of wire, bone graft, and methyl methacrylate is a simple and reasonably effective method of fusion, although its use has much declined in favor of more complex internal fixation arrangements, including shaped plates and transarticular screw fixation.[45] Introduced in the 1970s, the Brattstrom fixation is a simple procedure that has a reported bone fusion rate of about 70%.[46]

C1–C2 fusion procedures may comprise a wire fixation supplemented by bone grafting with external orthotic support. There are a wide variety of methods by which the wire can be configured, including the Gallie technique, the Brooks technique, and the method described by Roy-Camille. They involve the passage of sublaminar wires at C1, C2, or both, and this requires experience, great care, and appropriate instrumentation to prevent the wire from impinging the posterior surface of the spinal cord. The space available deep to the lamina is judged from preoperative imaging, and the presence of posterior column sensory loss suggests that this method should not be used in this situation.[28] The two main types of wire used are monofilament and multistranded cable wire, the latter of which is considerably more flexible while still incorporating high tensile strength. Passage of cable wire is greatly facilitated by its flexibility and is greatly preferred in the cervical spine. The passage of sublaminar wires at C2 and below is accomplished by initially removing part of the spinous processes and exposing the midline raphe between the flaval ligaments at the interspaces. The sublaminar space is carefully explored at each end with a blunt-ended, angled probe; the distance is assessed; and the wire is selected.

At all times, great care must be taken to prevent impaction on the spinal cord during passage and especially after the wires have been passed but are not yet secured in position, although this is more relevant to monofilament wire. Removal of strands of soft tissue and ligament at the site of insertion and site of extraction of the wire makes the task easier. With multistranded cable wire, a length of suture material can be passed initially and the flexible wire gently pulled through, or the fine wire leader may be used to guide the cable through the midline at the apex of the lamina. When the wires are in position and looped into the selected conformation, they are tightened around the bone graft. Cable wire should be tightened with the appropriate instrument and secured into position. Bone graft is obtained from the posterior iliac crest, fashioned to shape, and secured between the posterior arches of C1 and C2. Care must be taken to ensure that the graft does not compress the dural surface.

Other options for posterior fixation include laminar clamps and plate or rod systems incorporating lateral mass screws. As with anterior plates, posterior bone screws are highly dependent on bone quality and may not be suitable in many rheumatoid patients. In the subaxial cervical spine, adjacent levels may simply be wired together using a sublaminar technique, although it is not recommended that this be done over greater than two levels, because the wire curves within the spinal canal if more than two levels are fixed. Interspinous and interfacet wiring are possible but less secure means of internal fixation and rely heavily on external support.

Bone graft is applied to surfaces that have been carefully decorticated using a high-speed drill. The rate of bone fusion depends on many variables, including the rigidity of the internal and external fixation, and the more rigid methods of fixation are associated with higher bone fusion rates. The need for any form of bone grafting has been called into question, however. It is argued that bone fusion is unnecessary, and in frail patients especially, the duration and morbidity of the operation are reduced when no bone graft is harvested. It may be that fixation alone can provide sufficient stabilization in some patients. This is a stimulating challenge to accepted practice and one whose verification or otherwise should be made clear.[32]

High bone fusion rates are reported with the use of C1–C2 transarticular screw fixation, but it is a technique that requires careful preoperative assessment of the local vertebral anatomy. It is necessary to identify size and position of the vertebral artery canal at C2 with respect to the size of the pedicle. Encroachment of the vertebral artery canal by size or by position can preclude the use of C1–C2 transarticular screws. Other contraindications to this technique include incomplete reduction of C1–C2 subluxation or destruction of the C1 or C2 vertebrae such that the normal landmarks cannot be identified. Lateral screening by fluoroscopy is mandatory during the procedure, but screening in the anteroposterior direction is usually difficult and sometimes impossible. Some of the early series on this technique reported low complication rates, but a more recent series has

encountered a small but definite incidence of vascular and neurologic complications.[37,38,44-46] One report that specifically focused on patients with rheumatoid disease found that 10 of 76 screws that were inserted were subsequently found to be incorrectly positioned. This incorrect positioning was associated with a 50% chance of the other screw fracturing within a few weeks as a result of excessive loading. When malposition of one or another screw does occur, the use of a Halo orthotic support is recommended. Actual neurologic complications appear to be relatively infrequent, although vascular complications involving the vertebral artery must be considered. Some patients with abnormal C1–C2 anatomy do not lend themselves to this technique, and to this must be added an additional cohort of patients with pathologic conditions. If C1–C2 transarticular screw fixation is to be considered, careful preoperative imaging and assessment of local anatomy are necessary to decide whether or not the technique is feasible in an individual patient.[47-51]

Various forms of external orthosis exist, ranging from simple cervical collars of the clerical type to Philadelphia-style collars to the SOMI brace and Halo fixators. Each have different degrees of fixation that they impart to the cervical spine, and the appropriate device should be selected according to individual needs.

More recent technical advances include the use of minipolyaxial screws which can be used at every level from C1 to C7 inclusive. The polyaxial nature of the screw head means that the rods require less contouring and can be placed more medially than with older systems. The minipolyaxial screws can be inserted into the lateral masses of C1,[52] the pars of C2, the lateral masses of C3 to C7, or the pedicles of C7. Fluoroscopic control is recommended, particularly when fixing C1 and C2 vertebrae (Fig. 126-8).

Fixation to the occiput entails securing the rods to the occipital component, which in turn is usually fixed by screws to the suboccipital bone. A variety of devices and constructs are available, but the most secure fixation is probably to the

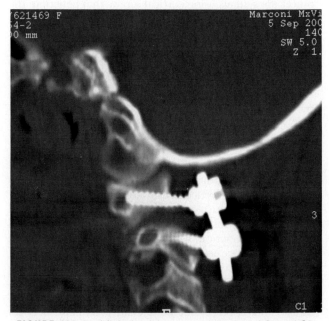

FIGURE 126-8 Minipolyaxial screw stabilization of C1 and C2.

midline suboccipital crest of dense cortical bone, particularly in rheumatoid patients. The thickness of this can be assessed on CT scan, being generally greater than 10 mm in contrast to the much thinner bone laterally. Other techniques include "inside-outside" bolts and a case report of occiput–axis screw fixation.[53,54] Occipitocervical fixation should be in the neutral position of about 45 degrees, although whether this angle is applicable to the rheumatoid population is not clear.[55]

OUTCOME: MORBIDITY AND COMPLICATIONS

Although rheumatoid arthritis is a systemic disease, the morbidity associated with surgery of the rheumatoid cervical spine is generally low.[37–39,41,56,57] Wound dehiscence and infection are perhaps the most common problems, but even these are infrequent. Postsurgical leakage of CSF after transoral surgery is a major potential problem that usually requires re-exploration and reclosure with CSF diversion. The use of fibrin and thrombin tissue glue with a lumbar CSF drain as soon as the leak is recognized during the operation provides an effective means of sealing the leak and reducing the risk of fatal meningitis, which brought the earliest transoral operations into disrepute.[58,59] Rheumatoid patients, more than other surgical patients, are prone to the complications of prolonged recumbency, including infections and venous thrombosis, but in addition they develop generalized joint stiffening that prolongs the recovery period. Early graduated mobilization is recommended, preferably within a unit experienced in surgery of patients with rheumatoid disease.

Bone fusion rates are lower in comparison with other conditions, but it may be that solid bone fusion is not necessary in every case. Perhaps a strong fibrous union is sufficient for posterior C1–C2 stabilization for root pain.[2,32]

Early postoperative mortality rates are generally reported in the range of 0% to 12%, although the cause of death is often not directly related to the surgical procedure.[38,41,57] Postoperative respiratory, cardiac, or other major system complications reflect the generally frail physical condition of these patients. Increased mortality rates are associated with patients in the more severe neurologic grades (Ranawat IIIA or IIIB). This association was noted by Zoma and colleagues[39] and reinforced by Casey and colleagues.[30] Santavirta and colleagues[2] observed that a higher mortality risk after surgery is associated with coincident cardiac disease and with vertical subluxation of the odontoid process greater than 3 mm. They also noted the tendency of patients classified in the worst neurologic grades to have a poor outcome and limited survival. Saway and colleagues[26] noted that the survival of postoperative patients is correlated with disease severity and, in particular, with presence of interstitial lung disease. This correlation was so strong that the role of cervical surgery at this stage should be carefully considered.

The neurologic gains can be considered either as therapeutic or prophylactic, depending on the clinical presentation. It is difficult to provide an overall estimate of neurologic improvement in this type of surgery, because many of the reported series offer a variety of patients, often small in number and using a variety of surgical procedures.[60] Case selection has a major influence on outcome and morbidity. Neurologic improvement after surgery occurred in about 40%

of patients in older series.[59,61–63] It is increasingly clear that patients who are more severely affected systemically and neurologically and those with complex combination forms of vertebral subluxation are likely to have a worse prognosis in terms of natural history and surgical treatment. The final common pathway that determines whether neurologic recovery occurs is the extent of spinal cord damage caused by the disease. The spinal cord diameter and cross-sectional area correlate with the clinical severity and clearly suggest that a spinal cord thus affected has less chance of recovery. In their study of 134 patients in Ranawat grades IIIA and IIIB, Casey and co-workers[30] compared the operative complication rates and early postsurgical morbidity rates in the two groups. The results were significantly worse in more severely affected patients (complication rate 42% vs. 24% and 1 month postoperative morbidity rate 17.7% vs. 8.9%). More importantly, functional outcome and pain relief after surgery was worse in grade IIIB patients, and these poor outcomes mirror the advanced state of neurologic dysfunction, spinal cord atrophy, and general physical debilitation in this group. Only 16% of patients at grade IIIB were able to walk after surgery.

Others report more optimistic results with these most severely affected patients.[31] Using simple posterior wiring techniques together with postoperative Hal fixation, Peppelman and colleagues[31] report an impressive 83% of patients in grade IIIB who showed at least one Ranawat grade of improvement. Such conflicting results point to the need for further data on the outcome and efficacy of surgery relating to the preoperative neurologic grade rather than focusing on finer technical aspects of metal fixation.

A posterior fusion procedure at C1–C2 for C2 root pain is associated with an excellent chance of producing successful pain relief, probably to a large extent regardless of which method is selected for fixation and fusion and probably whether or not bone fusion occurs.

The burgeoning interest and wealth of publication over the past 10 to 15 years concerning the surgical management of rheumatoid disease of the cervical spine reflects the important role surgery has to play in the overall management of these patients. This role is reasonably well defined against the background of the natural history of the condition and the likelihood of progressive myelopathy. The morbidity and mortality risks associated with surgery are becoming clear, and the greatest neurologic benefit is increasingly recognized to be associated with lesser grades of myelopathy. It is to be hoped that the next few years will deliver more accurate information on the outcome of surgical management through the reporting of series containing large numbers of well-identified patients having standardized surgical treatment.

CONCLUSIONS

The surgical management of patients with cervical rheumatoid disease not only presents a challenging combination of pathology, management, and decision making, but it also requires familiarity with a wide range of surgical fixation and fusion techniques. The diverse range of surgical procedures available should not detract from the overriding purpose of management, which is to bring about recovery from or prevent neurologic deficit and to restore spinal integrity.

It is probable that more than one surgical technique is safe and successful for a given type of cervical spine involvement. It is now possible to investigate thoroughly the vertebral abnormality and to select a surgical management protocol most appropriate to deal with that particular problem. Tailoring the procedure and management to individual requirement rather than applying a universal algorithm is likely to produce superior results.

As surgical management of this condition evolves, the variables that are associated with a poor outcome are being more clearly identified. Treating end-stage or advanced disease provides a severe surgical and anesthetic challenge. However, simpler, safer, and more effective procedures might be employed at earlier states in the disease process. The natural history of the condition is being elucidated, and one of the aims of any audit of this group of patients should be to identify those who are likely to deteriorate. Because of continuing uncertainty concerning this, the role of prophylactic cervical spine surgery remains unclear.

Acknowledgment

The authors acknowledge the contribution of Helen Wilson to the preparation and completion of this chapter.

REFERENCES

1. Stevens JC, Cartlidge NEF, Saunders M, et al: Atlanto-axial subluxation and cervical myelopathy in rheumatoid arthritis. Q J Med 159:391–408, 1971.
2. Santavirta S, Konttinen YT, Laasonen E, et al: Ten-year result of operation for rheumatoid cervical spine disorders. J Bone Joint Surg Br 73:116–120, 1991.
3. Dvorak J, Grob D, Baumgartner H, et al: Functional evaluation of the spinal cord by magnetic resonance imaging in patients with rheumatoid arthritis and instability of upper cervical spine. Spine 14:1057–1064, 1989.
4. Mathews JA: Atlanto-axial subluxation in rheumatoid arthritis. Ann Rheum Dis 33:526–531, 1974.
5. Bland JH: Rheumatoid arthritis of the cervical spine. J Rheumatol 3:319–341, 1974.
6. Corbett M, Dalton S, Young A, Silman A, Shipley M: Factors predicting death, survival and functional outcome in a prospective study of early rheumatoid disease over fifteen years. Br J Rheumatol 32:717–723, 1922.
7. Pellicci PM, Ranawat CS, Tsairis P, Bryan WJ: A prospective study of the progression of rheumatoid arthritis of the cervical spine. J Bone Joint Surg Am 63A:342–350, 1981.
8. O'Brien MF, Casey ATH, Crockard HA, Pringle J, Stevens JM: History of the craniocervical junction in chronic rheumatoid arthritis: A clinicopathologic analysis of 33 operative cases. Spine 27:2245–2254, 2002.
9. Santavirta S, Kankaanpaa U, Sandelin J, et al: Evaluation of patients with rheumatoid cervical spine. Scand J Rheumatol 16:9–16, 1987.
10. Fujiwara K, Owaki H, Fujimoto M, Yonenobu K, Achi T: A longterm follow up study of cervical lesions in rheumatoid arthritis. J Spine Dis 13:519–526, 2000.
11. Fujiwara K, Fujimoto M, Owaki H, et al: Cervical lesions related to the systemic progression in rheumatoid arthritis. Spine 23:2052–2056, 1998.
12. Manz HJ, Luessenhop AJ, Robertson DM: Cervical myelopathy due to atlantoaxial and subaxial subluxation in rheumatoid arthritis. Arch Pathol Lab Med 107:94–98, 1983.
13. Nakano KK, Schoene WC, Baker RA, Dawson DM: The cervical myelopathy associated with rheumatoid arthritis: Analysis of 32 patients with 2 postmortem cases. Ann Neurol 3:144–151, 1978.
14. Hughes JT: Spinal cord involvement by C4-C5 vertebral subluxation in rheumatoid arthritis: A description of 2 cases examined by necropsy. Ann Neurol 1:575–582, 1977.
15. Kudo H, Iwano K: Surgical treatment of subaxial cervical myelopathy in rheumatoid arthritis. J Bone Joint Surg 73B:474–480, 1991.
16. Crockard HA: Surgical management of cervical rheumatoid problems. Spine 20:2584–2590, 1995.
17. Bell GR, Stearns KL: Flexion-extension MRI of the upper rheumatoid cervical spine. Orthopaedics 14:969–974, 1991.
18. Krodel A, Refior HJ, Westermann S: The importance of functional magnetic resonance imaging in the planning of stabilizing operations on the cervical spine in rheumatoid patients. Arch Orthop Trauma Surg 109:30–33, 1989.
19. Oda T, Fujiwara K, Yonenobu K, Azuma B, Ochi T: Natural course of cervical spine lesions in rheumatoid arthritis. Spine 20:1128–1135, 1995.
20. Conaty JP, Mongan ES: Cervical fusion in rheumatoid arthritis. J Bone Joint Surg 63A:1218–1227, 1981.
21. Sherk HH: Atlantoaxial instability and acquired basilar invagination in rheumatoid arthritis. Orthop Clin North Am 9:1053–1063, 1978.
22. Kauppi M, Hakala M: Prevalence of cervical spine subluxations and dislocations in a community based rheumatoid arthritis population. Scand J Rheumatol 23:133–136, 1994.
23. Boden SD: Rheumatoid arthritis of the cervical spine. Surgical decision making based on predictors of paralysis and recovery. Spine 19:2275–2280, 1994.
24. Marks JS, Sharp J: Rheumatoid cervical myelopathy. Q J Med 199:307–319, 1981.
25. Dillin WH, Watkins RG: Clinical syndromes in cervical myelopathy. In Rothman RH, Simeone FA (eds): The Spine, 3rd ed. Philadelphia: WB Saunders, 1992, pp 560–564.
26. Saway PA, Blackburn WD, Halla JT, Alarcon GS: Clinical characteristics affecting survival in patients with rheumatoid arthritis undergoing cervical spine surgery: A controlled study. J Rheumatol 16:890–896, 1989.
27. Floyd AS, Learmonth ID, Mody G, Meyers OL: Atlanto-axial instability and neurologic indicators in rheumatoid arthritis. Clin Orthop 241:177–182, 1989.
28. Rogers MA, Crockard HA, Moskovich R, et al: Nystagmus and joint position sensation: Their importance in posterior occipitocervical fusion in rheumatoid arthritis. Presented at the 19th Annual Meeting, Cervical Spine Research Society, Philadelphia, December 1991.
29. Toolanen G: Cutaneous sensory impairment in rheumatoid atlanto-axial subluxation assessed quantitatively by electrical stimulation. Scand J Rheumatol 16:27–32, 1987.
30. Casey ATH, Crockard HA, Bland JM, et al: Surgery on the rheumatoid cervical spine for the non-ambulant myelopathic patient—too much, too late? Lancet 347:1004–1007, 1996.
31. Peppelman WC, Kaus DR, Donaldson MD, Agarwal A: Cervical spine surgery in rheumatoid arthritis: Improvement of neurologic deficit after cervical spine fusion. Spine 18:2375–2379, 1993.
32. Moskovich R, Crockard HA, Shott S, Ransford AO: Occipitocervical stabilization for myelopathy in patients with rheumatoid arthritis: Implications of not bone-grafting. J Bone Joint Surg Am 82A:349–365, 2000.
33. Frerk CM: Predicting difficulties in intubation. Anaesthesia 46:1005–1008, 1991.
34. Dickman CA, Locantro J, Fessler RG: The influence of transoral odontoid resection on stability of the craniovertebral junction. J Neurosurg 77:525–530, 1992.
35. Grob D, Wirsch R, Graver W, Sturzenegger J, Dvorak J: Atlantoaxial fusion and retrodental pannus in rheumatoid arthritis. Spine 22:1580–1583, 1997.
36. Bohlman HH: Point of view: Atlantoaxial fusion and retrodental pannus in rheumatoid arthritis. Spine 22:1584, 1997.
37. Crockard HA, Calder I, Ransford AO: One stage transoral decompression and posterior fixation in rheumatoid atlanto-axial subluxation. J Bone Joint Surg 72B:682–685, 1990.
38. Santavirta S, Konttinen YT, Laasonen E, et al: Ten year results of operation for rheumatoid cervical spine disorders. J Bone Joint Surg 73B:116–120, 1991.
39. Zoma A, Sturrock RD, Fisher WD, et al: Surgical stabilization of the rheumatoid cervical spine. J Bone Joint Surg 69B:8–12, 1987.
40. Wertheim SB, Bohlman HH: Occipitocervical fusion. J Bone Joint Surg 69A:833–836, 1987.
41. Ranawat CS, O'Leary P, Pellicci P, et al: Cervical spine fusion in rheumatoid arthritis. J Bone Joint Surg 61A:1003–1010, 1979.
42. Chan CP, Ngian KS, Cohen L: Posterior upper cervical fusion in rheumatoid arthritis. Spine 17:268–272, 1992.
43. Ferlic DC. Clayton ML, Leidholt JD, Gamble WE: Surgical treatment of the symptomatic unstable cervical spine in rheumatoid arthritis. J Bone Joint Surg 57A:349–354, 1975.

44. Brattström H, Granholm L: Atlanto-axial fusion in rheumatoid arthritis. Acta Orthop Scand 47:619–628, 1976.
45. Grob D, Dvorak J, Gschwend N, Froehlich M: Posterior occipitocervical fusion in rheumatoid arthritis. Arch Orthop Trauma Surg 110:38–44, 1990.
46. Grob D, Dvorak J, Panjabi MM, Antinnes JA: The role of plate and screw fixation in occipito-cervical fusion in rheumatoid arthritis. Spine 19:2545–2551, 1994.
47. Grob D, Jennaret B, Aebi M: Atlanto-axial fusion with transarticular screw fixation. J Bone Joint Surg 83B:972–976, 1991.
48. Casey ATH, Madawi AA, Veres R, Crockard HA: Is the technique of posterior transarticular screw fixation suitable for rheumatoid atlantoaxial subluxation? Br J Neurosurg 11:508–519, 1997.
49. Magerl F, Seeman PS: Stable posterior fusion of the atlas and axis by transarticular screw fixation. In Weidner PA (ed): Cervical Spine. New York: Springer-Verlag, 1991, pp 322–327.
50. Hanson PB, Montesano PX, Sharkey NA, Rauschning W: Anatomic and biomechanical assessment of transarticular screw fixation for atlantoaxial instability. Spine 16:1141–1145, 1991.
51. Madawi AA, Casey ATH, Solanki GA, Tuite G, Crockard HA: Radiological and anatomical evaluation of the atlantoaxial transarticular screw fixation technique. J Neurosurg 86:961–968, 1997.
52. Harms J, Melcher RP: Posterior C1-C2 fusion with polyaxial screw and rod fixation. Spine 26:2467–2471, 2001.
53. Sandhu FA, Pait TG, Benzel E, Henderson F: Occipitocervical fusion for rheumatoid arthritis using the inside-outside stabilization technique. Spine 28:414–419, 2003.
54. Dvorak MF, Fisher C, Boyd M, et al: Anterior occiput to axis screw fixation. Part 1: A case report, description of a new technique and anatomical feasibility analysis. Spine 28:E54–E60, 2003.
55. Phillips FM, Phillips CS, Wetzel FT, Gelinas C: Occipitocervical neutral position: Possible surgical implications. Spine 24:775–778, 1999.
56. Slatis P, Santavirta S, Sandelin J, Konttinen YT: Cranial subluxation of the odontoid process in rheumatoid arthritis. J Bone Joint Surg 71A:189–195, 1989.
57. Clark CR, Goetz DD, Menezes AH: Arthrodesis of the cervical spine in rheumatoid arthritis. J Bone Joint Surg 71A:381–392, 1989.
58. Hadley MN, Spetzler RF, Sonntag VKH: The transoral approach to the superior cervical spine. J Neurosurg 81:16–23, 1989.
59. Crockard HA: The transoral approach to the base of the brain and upper cervical cord. Ann R Coll Surg Engl 67:321–325, 1985.
60. Hamilton JD, Gordon M, McInnes IB, et al: Improved medical and surgical management of cervical spine disease in patients with rheumatoid arthritis over 10 years. Ann Rheum Dis 59:434–438, 2000.
61. Clark CR, Goetz DD, Menezes AH: Arthrodesis of the cervical spine in rheumatoid arthritis. J Bone Joint Surg 71A:381–392, 1989.
62. Slatis P, Santavirta S, Sandelin J: Cranial subluxation of the odontoid process in rheumatoid arthritis. J Bone Joint Surg 71A: 189–195, 1989.
63. Crockard HA, Essigman WK, Sevens JM, et al: Surgical treatment of cervical cord compression in rheumatoid arthritis. Ann Rheum Dis 44:809–816, 1985.

127 Cervicothoracic Ankylosing Spondylitis

WILLIAM H. SWEET[†]

HISTORY

Ankylosing spondylitis was first fully described by W. von Bechterew of St. Petersburg, Russia. His original accounts in 1892 in Russian, followed by papers in German in 1893 and 1897,[1–3] emphasize an increasing immobility of the entire spine as a result of ossification or calcification of all its joints and ligaments. The title of his first detailed publication was "Re Rigidity of the Vertebral Column and Its Deformity as a Special Form of Illness." The permanence of the skeletal insignias of the disease has permitted the discovery of such a skeleton in the third Egyptian dynasty circa 2980 to 2900 BC.

Connor describes a segment of skeleton (dated 169 AD) consisting of the ilium, sacrum, 5 lumbar and 10 thoracic vertebrae, and 3 right and 2 left ribs bound together by bone and replacing the ligaments.[4] The articulations were so effaced that they made one uniform continuous bone with, for example, no marks to suggest the former site of the apophyses. Boland[5] gave a fuller historical account, with references to seven probable descriptions of the disorder in the latter half of the 19th century.

GENERAL FEATURES

General features of ankylosing spondylitis have been given various designations: "fusion or rigidity of the vertebral column,"[3] "chronic ankylosing inflammation of the vertebral column and hip joints,"[6] "spondylosis rhizomélique,"[7] "chronic ankylosing rigidity of the vertebral column,"[8] and "chronic arthritis ankylopoetica of the vertebral column."[9] The British have been using the term *ankylosing spondylitis* for more than a half century, but in 1941, the American Rheumatic Association adopted the term *rheumatoid spondylitis*.[5] Its members gradually agreed that this disorder is distinct from rheumatoid arthritis, and in December 1963, they officially capitulated and also adopted the term *ankylosing spondylitis*.

Comprehensive accounts of the clinical features of the disorder have been provided by Boland[5] and by Wilkinson and Bywaters.[10] The latter work is based on 222 hospital patients seen during 16 years, 212 of whom were followed up. The male:female ratio was 4.4:1 in this series; other investigators note a male-to-female predominance as high as 10:1.[11] The first symptoms appeared before the age of 30 years in 64% of the cases and before the age of 40 in 89%. Close relatives of 6% definitely had the disorder. In 64%, the onset was in the sacroiliac joints or lumbar spine, giving rise to aching in the buttocks, nearly always radiating

into one or both upper thighs. In three others, the radiation of pain extended into the calf or heel, in contrast with that of a protruded disc, which usually extends into the full length of the sciatic distribution. At this stage, radiographs showed ankylosis mainly of the sacroiliac and lumbar articular joints. Joints in the limbs or higher in the spine were the sites of initial involvement in the remaining third of the cases, and corresponding differences existed in the reference of pain. Those with spinal onset often noted anomalous worsening of the pain after resting and relief after activity. Some not only were awakened by pain but had to arise during the night to "limber up" before going back to sleep. Heavy exertion, however, also brought on or worsened pain in some patients. The longer the duration of the disease was, the greater was the extent of spinal involvement. The areas affected included the cervical spine, the area of greatest vulnerability to trauma, in 50% of the cases, and hips, shoulders, or both in 39%. Chest expansion, impairment of which is often an early sign, was reduced to 5 cm or less in 96% and to less than half that in 62% of those with the disease for 20 years or more (normal, ≥7 cm). Despite ossification of the ligaments, varying degrees of osteoporosis are usually present in the bones. The spinal rigidity did not prevent 63% of patients from working after more than 20 years of illness.

Some American publications failed to discriminate this disorder from various spondylitises of inflammatory rheumatoid arthritis, and analyses of human leukocyte antigens (HLAs), and the biologic characteristics of the major histocompatibility complex revealed bewildering congeries of new arthritic entities. The absence of both subcutaneous rheumatic nodules and "rheumatoid factor" in the bloodstream provides at least a preliminary basis for the diagnosis of ankylosing spondylitis used in this analysis. In their 92 cases, Kinsella and colleagues[12] also noted normal blood levels of antinuclear factor and antithyroglobulin.

SPECIAL FEATURES THAT INCREASE THE RISK OF SURGERY

Because spinal fractures occur much more often in young, otherwise healthy adults than in older adults, surgeons may not bother to appraise intensively the general physical status of much older patients. Reduced chest expansion is an early and valuable sign of the disorder.[13] It typically involves so many systems[14] that a follow-up study of 836 such patients for an average of 13 years revealed a twofold increase in mortality rate for men over that of the general population.[15]

The disease may begin with bouts of intermittent fever, anorexia, weight loss, easy fatigability, and anemia. Based in part on biopsy results obtained in the early stages of the

[†]Deceased.

1793

disease from radiographically identified arthritis in the manubriosternal joint, Cruickshank[16] found an initial osteitis that started with villus hyperplasia of the synovium, edema and lymphocytes, plasma cells, histiocytes, and, at times, hemorrhage. Vascular fibrous granulation tissue may appear at the joint margins. Later, fibrous destruction, reactive sclerosis, and ankylosis predominate. A continuing vulnerability to an inflammatory process is suggested by bouts of acute anterior uveitis or iritis, usually unilateral, which occurs in 25%; such an attack may be the first symptom.[15]

An abnormal fibrotic process may appear at many sites. Thus, the aortic valvular cusps develop a fibrous thickening and focal medial necrosis leading to aortic regurgitation in 3%. Fibrous tissue may invade the atrioventricular bundle, causing conduction defects. Late in the disease, the fibrosis may involve both upper pulmonary lobes, causing cough, dyspnea, and even death of massive hemoptysis. This feature plus the immobility of the ribs may make full pulmonary function studies essential because approximately half of the deaths occurring after fractures of the cervical spine in these cases have pulmonary causes. In a few patients, a major proliferation of fibrous tissue occurs in the spinal canal, at times in the thoracic region, but more often in the cauda equina.

Another long-term consequence of this malady is systemic vascular degeneration. This degeneration may cause the increased mortality rate relative to that of the general population, which is fourfold for all gastrointestinal disease, especially ulcerative colitis and other inflammatory disease of the gastrointestinal tract. The increased risk is twofold for cerebrovascular disease and is 40% greater for other circulatory diseases.[15] Deposition of immunoglobulin, complement, and fibrinogen in the walls of small renal vessels has been shown to be an early pathologic change in the walls of such renal vessels in biopsy specimens of young patients with ankylosing spondylitis.[17] These changes probably account for the amyloidosis that causes uremic death in 6%.

The fact that the bone marrow is at special risk is evinced by the curious complications of radiotherapy formerly given to control pain. These problems were moderately to completely relieved in 88% of 20 patients at 6 months by doses not exceeding 2000 cGy to any one of four or five spinal fields irradiated in each patient.[10] However, a broad survey by the British Medical Research Council[18] revealed that of 100 deaths in such patients, 41 resulted from acute myelogenous leukemia and seven from aplastic anemia after radiotherapy. No deaths of leukemia or lymphoma were encountered in the 836 patients who were given no irradiation therapy and followed up an average of 13 years by Radford and colleagues.[15] The fragile character of the patients is further emphasized by the postoperative deaths of 13 of the 100 treated by spinal ostectomy or cup arthroplasty of the hip, procedures that were performed in an attempt to increase the patient's mobility.

There is a striking correlation between the B27 form of HLA and this disease; that is, it is present in only 5% to 8% of the white population as a whole but is found in 90% of this group with this form of spondylitis. This disease is 90 times more likely to occur in an HLA-B27–positive man than an HLA-B27–negative person. Similarly, a high incidence of HLA-B27 antigen exists in those with uveitis.[19]

The genetic material encoding structures responsible for the immune response related to histocompatibility is concentrated in a small region in the short arm of chromosome 6. This region, designated the major histocompatibility complex, codes for three classes of gene products, of which class I molecules are expressed on almost all cell surfaces. They consist of one heavy (molecular weight 4500) chain and one light (<12,000) polypeptide chain. These include three reduplicated gene loci for the three groups of HLAs designated A, B, and C.[19] The B27 marker is considered to be associated with disturbances in immune mechanisms that lead to susceptibility to rheumatic disease.[20]

Clearly, investigations to determine the presence of the often occult manifestations just described should, if feasible, precede surgery.

RADIOGRAPHIC FEATURES

Early radiographic changes are most likely to be seen in the pelvis and lumbar spine. Calcification at the ischial tuberosity at the origin of the hamstring muscles is illustrated in Figure 127-1, and "squaring" of the anterosuperior and anteroinferior corners of the lumbar vertebrae as seen in the lateral view is shown in Figure 127-2. The late radiographic characteristics of the various spondyloarthritides were summarized by Martel and Braunstein.[21] In the sagittal projections of the spine, a continuous vertical line of calcification joining the two rows of apophyseal joints gives rise to the typical "railway line" appearance (Fig. 127-3). In the same projection, an arc of calcification often forms a lateral boundary to the disc on each side and joins the two vertebral bodies. This is the "bamboo" type of ankylosis (Fig. 127-4). The complete calcified fusion of the intervertebral discs and the apophyseal joints usually involves the posterior longitudinal ligament but can also occur posterior to the spinal canal in the ligamenta flava and those between the spinous processes, thus uniting them. According to Cruickshank's[18] personal studies of biopsy samples from 25 patients and autopsy findings from 12, the anterior longitudinal ligaments do not share in this calcification.

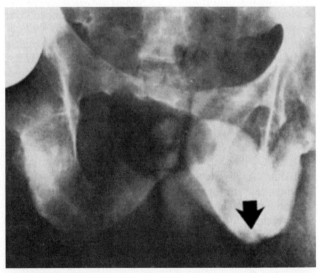

FIGURE 127-1 Early stage of a lesion with erosion and sclerosis at the enthesis of the hamstring muscles at the ischial tuberosities (*arrow*). (From Martel W, Braunstein EM: Spondyloarthritides. In Tavares J, Ferrucci JT [eds]: Radiology: Diagnosis-Imaging-Intervention, vol 5. Philadelphia: JB Lippincott, 1988, pp 2–5.)

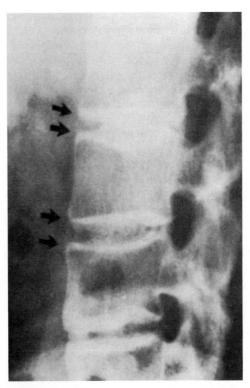

FIGURE 127-2 Early stage of a lesion with erosion of the anterior superior ligament and the anterior longitudinal ligament, leading to "squaring of these corners." (*Arrows* indicate minimal lesions.) (From Martel W, Braunstein EM: Spondyloarthritides. In Tavares J, Ferrucci JT [eds]: Radiology: Diagnosis-Imaging-Intervention, vol 5. Philadelphia: JB Lippincott, 1988, pp 2–5.)

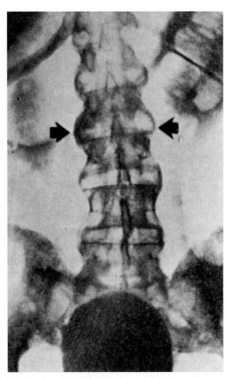

FIGURE 127-4 Late-stage bamboo spine created by calcified area covering the outer aspects of the lumbar intervertebral discs (*arrows*). (From Guttman L: Injuries of the Spine and Spinal Cord. Oxford: Blackwell Scientific, 1976, p 176.)

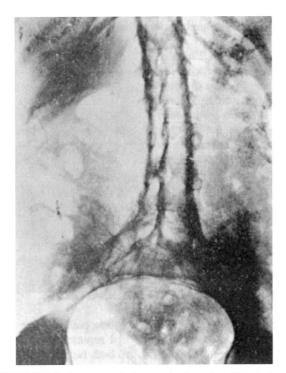

FIGURE 127-3 Late-stage "railway spine" produced by continuous lines of calcification including and connecting apophyseal joints with osteoporotic vertebral bodies. (From Guttman L: Injuries of the Spine and Spinal Cord. Oxford: Blackwell Scientific, 1976, p 176.)

However, in many cases, this ligament must have shared in the transverse disruption. This growth tends to convert the spinal column to a continuous calcified cylinder, as first described by Simmonds[22] in two postmortem specimens of the entire spine, which he macerated and then sawed into long, sagittal slices for analysis by photography and radiography. He also noted that the ribs were rigidly attached to the vertebrae and to each other by calcification at the joints and at the costotransverse and intertransverse ligaments and those between the costal tubercles, thereby accounting for the final gross reduction in inspiratory chest expansion. This extraordinary calcification is accompanied by osteoporosis of the bony vertebrae themselves. Such a spine proves prone to fracture with relatively minor trauma, especially in the cervical region. Numerous published reports have described ataxia of drunkenness leading to a fracture of the ankylosed cervical spine. These features also make the fractures hard to discern, and the kyphosis may interfere with magnetic resonance imaging and computed tomography scanning. This vulnerability extends throughout the involved spine, and many investigators have reported on more than one fractured vertebra that occurred after a single accident. Thus, in the 23 patients of Fox and colleagues,[23] 28 fractures were present. Several major disasters have ensued when the second fracture, usually lower and less symptomatic, is not recognized. For example, one of the Mayo Clinic patients became paraplegic when transferred from his bed to a gurney. An L1 fracture became displaced, and no recovery occurred after decompressive surgery and stabilization.[23] Sensory changes that might point to a second spinal lesion should be sought. As soon as feasible after the primary site of fracture has been stabilized and until normality of the rest of the spine has been demonstrated, the patient should be treated with the same scrupulous precautions as initially.

At times, all the calcification is so protective (and clouds the radiographic studies) that neither the patient nor the doctor even suspects fracture. Such events have been diagnosed only when a later, more serious fracture occurs, at times within hours after the patient has been discharged from the emergency department with a clean bill of health. In others, the transverse fracture is sufficiently incomplete that the wearing of a sturdy, supportive collar permits adequate stabilization until bony healing, usually rapid, occurs. Unfortunately, the fracture is more often of a peculiarly dangerous type in that the break is similar to that of a long bone, that is, it is roughly horizontal through the whole spinal column. This commonly produces major dangerous mobility of the upper or lower segment in any direction. Apparently, the tough elastic ligaments after fracture dislocation of an otherwise normal cervical spine tend to prevent distraction and gross horizontal displacements so that simple application of skull tongs and traction in a neutral direction in the long axis of the cervical spine nearly always provides the necessary stabilization in the presence of normal cervical ligaments. Moreover, such patients are likely to be able to rotate their head safely to a useful degree because that motion occurs at the C1–2 level.

However, in cervical ankylosing spondylitis, the usually transverse fracture also involves the calcified ligaments extending horizontally through all elements, front to back. Most of the fractures are actually through the calcified disc. Also, the upper segment may become distracted, or separated rostrocaudally to a startling degree, moving up and away from the lower segment and causing further trauma to the cord. This distraction is likely to be worsened by modest weights of the skeletal tong traction. The injury may become still worse when the mobile upper segment slides in any direction in the horizontal plane and causes intolerable pressure on the cord. Figure 127-5 illustrates the frightful sequence that may ensue.

MANAGEMENT LEADING TO DISASTER

Some of the special problems of these patients were graphically illustrated by one of the first reported cases, that of Abdi.[9] His 47-year-old patient had both hip joint and spinal ankylosis that progressed for more than 20 years to minimal motion at any level from C2 to the sacrum. In an effort to give him a little motion at the hip joints, an orthopedic surgeon manipulated them under general anesthesia. The right hip remained fixed, but the left hip became mobile. To the consternation of all concerned, the procedure also caused a total transverse fracture of the lumbar spine through the disc at L2–3, with a total permanent loss of all motor function below that level. At autopsy 71, 2 months later, a 2-cm diastases bridged by callus was found between the second and third lumbar vertebral bodies. Possibly because of uncertainty as to the vigor of the operative manipulation, the lesson from this well-studied and superbly described case largely escaped notice.

Perhaps because of the relative rarity of the disorder and the lack of disabling symptoms, despite decades of its known presence in most patients, many physicians are unaware of

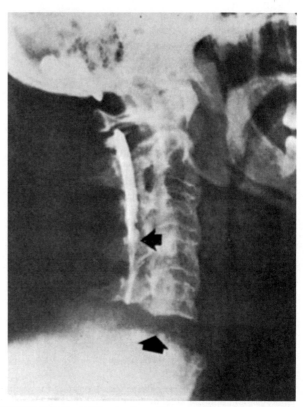

FIGURE 127-5 While drunk, a 49-year-old man fell to the floor, striking his head. He became quadriplegic at once owing to a total transverse lesion of the spinal cord at C6 from a total transverse fracture through the C5–6 disc with posterior displacement of the superior aspect of the cervical spine. Traction that was increased to 100 pounds by Gardner-Wells tongs did not reduce the fracture. A myelogram of a complete block at upper C4 (*small arrowhead*) with extreme distraction at the C5–6 disc (*large arrowhead*). At laminectomy, the cord was liquefied and necrotic opposite C5. Postoperatively, lesions ascended one segment permanently. (From Murray GC, Persellin RH: Cervical fracture complicating ankylosing spondylitis: A report of eight cases and review of the literature. Am J Med 70:1033–1041, 1981.)

the extraordinary propensity of the disorder to disable. Not until trauma abruptly strikes does the physician realize what a serious set of problems a patient can present. The known presence of ankylosing spondylitis should lead at once to the suspicion of fracture. One of my patients fell while drunk just before he got into bed. Over the next several days, an increasing weakness of his right upper limb was treated as radial nerve weakness of "a Saturday night palsy." The patient had thought it best not to mention that he had been so drunk that he fell, and, he added, "Besides, I didn't hurt myself when I fell." He progressed to quadriplegia and death. Some patients, such as the only one I saw as a medical student, had maintained enough bone and ligamentous continuity that a Thomas collar worn for several weeks maintained stability of the spine until rapid healing had occurred. Pain in an upper limb but no neurologic deficit led him and me to think that the whole episode was trivial.

Such experiences do not prepare the unwary for the following vicissitudes. Bohlman[24] reported that failure to diagnose significant spinal injury in his hospital's emergency department occurred in four of eight such patients; three returned later with quadriplegia. The fourth, given

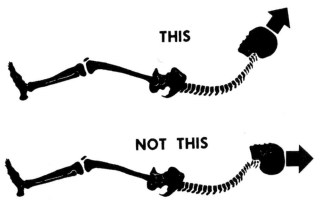

FIGURE 127-6 The proper line of traction in patients with major cervical kyphosis and fracture. The diagram illustrates why the horizontal position of a fracture at cervical kyphosis courts disaster. (From Young JS, Cheshire DJE, Pierce JA, et al: Cervical ankylosis with acute spinal cord injury. Paraplegia 15:133–146, 1978.)

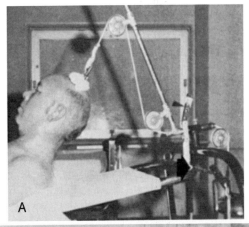

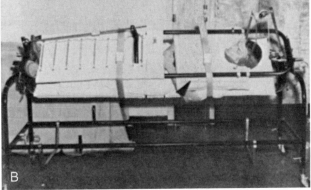

FIGURE 127-7 Proper line of traction in patients with major cervical kyphosis and fracture. *A*, Fracture through the body of C6 reduced by applying traction with the neck flexed 55 degrees from the horizontal patient supine. The device depicted permits turning a patient through 360 degrees while maintaining this constant angle. A metal outrigger to support the pulleys is attached to the front of the bed. *B*, The patient is being turned to show the board supporting the chest and shoulders. The flange (*arrow*) prevents sliding. (From Ackerman EA: Cervical fraction in flexion: A method of maintaining a constant angle prone or supine. J Bone Joint Surg 54:1114–1116, 1972.)

a tranquilizer before discharge in the emergency department, fell, became quadriplegic, and remained so. Figure 127-6 illustrates why placement of the head and upper neck in the same long axis as the body can kill the patient with a rigid cervical kyphosis. Ackerman[25] illustrated an apparatus that he developed to place the traction at a proper angle to maintain reduction of a fracture in a kyphotic cervical spine, and then to keep that essential angle while the patient was being rotated from a supine to a prone attitude and back again (Fig. 127-7).

Detwiler and colleagues[26] reported on a patient with a C7–T1 subluxation and a C6 compression fracture who had normal neurologic examination findings when he was first placed flat in a bed with a Philadelphia collar. The next day, an incomplete neurologic lesion abruptly developed at the T2 level; axial traction helped at first, but later, dyspnea proceeded to respiratory arrest and fatal anoxia.

The second patient in the study of Detwiler and colleagues experienced only neck pain after a fall. He was transported on the usual backboard; during transportation, his head was kept in a "neutral" position, neither flexed nor extended, a tactic continued in the hospital during examination and radiography. During this time, he became aware that flexion of his head helped, and extension toward the "neutral" position made his neck pain steadily worse. His medical attendants all assured him that they were well trained and knew they were doing the right thing; radiographic films showed a C5–6 dislocation, and examination now revealed a total transverse lesion at C5–6; the final result was death.[26]

Surin[27] described a special vacuum cushion into which the patient settles; it maintains the head in the proper degree of flexion during transport and examinations, and it appears to be of special value during computed tomography and magnetic resonance imaging as well as when the patient is in bed.

Osgood and colleagues[28] reported on a 47-year-old man whose spine was fused in marked flexion for 25 years. The patient had a through-and-through horizontal fracture at the C7 body, but posterior bony elements and ligaments remained fused. The patient was neurologically intact except for pain and numbness in the left arm. The patient refused skeletal traction and was placed in a Thomas collar.

One day later, the patient was neurologically normal. Then, the patient had tingling in the legs; 3 hours later, C6–7 quadriplegia developed. Bilateral fractures of C6–7 facets were present at the time of posterior decompression and fixation, and later, anterior fusion and stabilization were achieved and led to improvement in severe quadriparesis. The lesson learned was that the Thomas collar was inadequate, even though the fracture was initially incomplete.

Raine[29] reported on a 60-year-old woman who, 2 weeks after a fall, experienced neck pain. A fracture was found at approximately C6 or C7, with 30-degree forward angulation. Despite the support of a collar, lasting paraplegia resulted.

A 75-year-old man, the second patient in Raine's study, fell out of a wheelchair and sustained a C6 transverse fracture. The collar was not tolerated by the patient, although without it, attacks of tingling in all limbs, cyanosis, and loss of consciousness arose. Posterior fusion occurred, and death of respiratory failure occurred the next month.

Lemmen and Laing[30] reported on a drunk patient with urinary retention and mental confusion who was admitted to the hospital and gradually experienced motor but not sensory loss below C5. Radiographs showed a C5 body anterior to C6, for which tongs were applied. Radiographs taken the next day showed worse distraction of C5 on C6. Sudden respiratory arrest and death occurred after the patient was turned from the face-down to the face-up position. At autopsy, all ligaments connecting C5 to C6 were torn through completely.

Bohlman[24] reported that seven of eight patients with ankylosing spondylitis cervical spine injuries had neural loss. C6–7 injury caused subluxation and quadriplegia; tong traction was performed at once. The next day, death followed respiratory arrest while the patient was being turned during application of a Minerva jacket.

The second patient in Bohlman's study[24] had a C6–7 injury that caused subluxation and anterior cord syndrome. Tong traction was followed by greater leg weakness. The final result was that the patient was barely able to walk.

The third patient in Bohlman's study had C7–T1 subluxation and anterior cord syndrome. After laminectomy, the patient was left in tongs. Further dislocation occurred, and weakness worsened. Eventually, however, the patient made a full recovery.

Osgood and colleagues[28] reported on a patient who had an injury accompanied by a loud snap in the neck; quadriparesis occurred for 24 hours and then cleared. Nine days later, a C5–6 fracture was seen through both anterior and posterior elements. Tongs at 15 pounds were applied straight horizontally. More forward slipping of C5 on C6 occurred. The patient became rapidly and permanently quadriplegic.

Osgood and colleagues[31] reported on a 65-year-old man whose radiographs showed through-and-through fracture dislocations at both C7–T1 and T9–10. Flaccid quadriplegia from C5 was present with maldirected traction in tongs. The patient had multiple left rib fractures, left flail chest, and left pneumothorax. Autopsy revealed spinal cord C5–T2 fragmentation and marked instability at a T9–10 fracture. "Log rolling" the patient at autopsy from side to side by force applied to either shoulder caused 1- to 2-cm rotational and side-to-side dislocation of fracture margins. Epidural hemorrhage occurred at both sites.

Murray and Persellin[32] reported on a motor vehicle accident victim whose neurologic examination and radiographic study results showed the neck to be normal, but the zone below C6 was poorly seen. Repeat studies of the entire spine revealed the same result. "Electric shocks" occurred in the torso and all limbs when the patient's head was moved. Increased neck pain occurred on transfer to the bed, and motor and sensory deficits were present in both legs. CT showed a 90% anterior shift of C7 on T1. Tongs were applied and then a laminectomy was performed, after which tongs were continued. Proper alignment was not maintained. Episodes of decreased heart and respiratory rate occurred when the patient was turned on postoperative days 6, 9, and 10. Pneumonia ensued and then death.

Detwiler and colleagues[26] reduced a C6–7 subluxation by cervical flexion, but pain in this position led the patient to insist on change. Realignment in minimal extension led to total transverse cord lesion at T3; death soon followed.

In another patient in the study of Detwiler and colleagues,[26] aspiration occurred while this patient was in traction, despite a functioning nasogastric tube. Respiratory arrest occurred. Emergency intubation with the patient's neck extended led to a total transverse lesion at C5.

Distraction and hyperextension appeared on radiography. Death occurred soon after.[26] Clearly, tong traction has been failing because the lower and upper segments of the broken spinal column, once properly replaced, must not be allowed to move on each other. Traction tongs cannot ensure this immobility.

The extreme variability of these patients is further illustrated by case 3 of Woodruff and Dewing.[33] This 33-year-old man, who had been completely bedridden for a year, was being turned in a Stryker frame. His head was allowed to be unsupported for "a moment"; it promptly fell into extension, causing a painful snapping sensation in the neck. Although no new neurologic abnormalities were noted at once and his fracture through the C5–6 interspace was undisplaced, increasing dysphagia developed, and he died 3 days later.

INDICATIONS AND RESULTS OF OPEN OPERATION

In a review of all the published cases of this infrequent disorder that I could find in a language that I could read, I encountered seven articles[26,32,34–38] in which clear-cut indications for early open operation in a fractured ankylosed spondylitic cervical spine were enunciated. In each, a delayed or worsening neural loss occurred after the fracture or the spine was unstable or irreducible by traction. This stance was taken even by Hunter and Dubo,[35] whose summary of 64 such patients revealed that of those treated nonoperatively, 30% died, whereas 40% of those treated by open operation died.

I reviewed the reports on 108 patients whose fracture dislocation was between C3 and T1. Sixty-six of the patients initially were or became quadriplegic before operation. Of the 48 who did not undergo surgery, 8 became better, and 2 others were normal. Of the 18 treated by surgery, not 1 was better or normal. There were 38 patients whose cord lesions fell short of producing complete paralysis in the legs and in some of both upper limbs. Of the 24 such patients who did not have an operation, 72% became better or normal, whereas only 50% of 14 who did have an operation became better or normal. Although immobilized fracture sites tend to heal rapidly in these patients, internal fixation poses a great risk in these multiply diseased patients, and the autologous grafts or metal screws, bands, straps, or wires tend to loosen in their porotic bones.

TRACTION USING TONGS VERSUS HALO VEST

Practical directions of details of application of the halo vest are given by Young and colleagues.[39–41] Examples of the problems follow.

A 68-year-old man fell, and his forehead struck a table, causing nuchal and bilateral shoulder pain. After 4 days of bed rest, he had a mild bilateral sensorimotor loss while cranial tongs were maintaining the best possible alignment. However, a gradual increase in sensorimotor loss in all four limbs seemed beyond control. By 3 weeks after the injury, he had pneumonia, mental confusion, atrial fibrillation, dysphagia, and loss of bladder function. A halo vest was then applied, with gratifying improvement. In another month, he was at home and walking. By 13 weeks, the spine had fused at the fracture sites, and the halo was removed. At 18 months, the only anesthetic area was the right lateral thumb. Improved cervical alignment had been achieved during the healing process.

Surin[27] reported on a quadriplegic patient in whom tongs reduced a fracture, but it redislocated at once when the patient was placed in the halo vest. The fracture was kept reduced only by continuous traction near vertical on the halo ring until the fracture was healed. Unfortunately, the quadriplegia persisted.

In the second patient in Surin's study, the reduced fracture was "immobilized" in a halo vest; neurologic examination results remained normal. One week later, the patient became quadriplegic while sleeping. Traction on the halo ring was begun at once. Only slight anterior dislocation was present at the fracture. Full motor recovery occurred in 24 hours. Traction was needed for 8 weeks.

Surin points out that the vest component of the therapy does not fit the deformed thorax, and Hunter and Dubo,[35] Weinstein and colleagues,[36] and Surin[27] all described failures of the apparatus. In two of the patients for whom treatment failed, tetraplegia developed. However, these three groups of investigators and at least five others agree that the halo vest is the best approach currently available.[32,36,42–44]

Halo Vest

Although the halo vest accomplishes the desired objective of immobilization if the fit to the chest is tight enough, this chest compression is a major drawback because immobile ribs, pulmonary fibrosis, and pulmonary failure have been established as the most common cause of death in the disease.

The comprehensive 1992 report of Rowed[42] on 21 patients recommends against axial traction before placement of the halo vest. Of 11 patients treated conservatively, 7 were able to walk, work, or both, and 2 died, whereas only 2 of the 10 surgically treated patients became employable. However, the two groups are not really clinically comparable. I recommend the use of head and pelvic halos firmly fastened to each other as a relatively low-risk tactic to achieve stabilization after constantly monitored reduction of the fracture dislocation.

STRESS FRACTURES OR PSEUDARTHROSES

In one of the earlier descriptions of new or worsening pain and progressive bent-over posture, a chronic rheumatoid lesion was diagnosed. However, as more cases have been studied, it is apparent that much more frequently, so-called stress fractures or pseudarthroses may develop a few months to 20 years after ankylosing spondylitis occurs in any location from the atlantoaxial region[45] to the lower lumbar region.[46]

At the Mayo Clinic from 1984 to 1989,[23] a period during which high-quality computed tomography scans were in use, 23 patients with ankylosing spondylitis were seen. Investigators at this institution saw 16 stress fractures or pseudarthroses in 12 patients and 12 traumatic fractures in 11 patients, all between 33 and 71 years of age. In addition, six patients had neither fracture nor pseudarthroses, and their progressive kyphosis prevented them from seeing above

a specific horizontal view line. Fox and colleagues[23] report that in the presence of fractures or pseudarthroses associated with severe spinal instability but no neurologic deficit, they perform both an anterior and a posterior fusion. In patients with persisting pain related to the stress fracture, Marsh[46] concluded that the rigidity occurring at all other levels concentrates all movements at the fracture site. He seeks confirmation of the diagnosis of significant abnormality at this site by computed tomography and radionuclide imaging, to which magnetic resonance imaging could be added. Marsh goes on to say that internal fixation without bone grafting produces immediate pain relief by rapid fracture union. These stress fractures are more common in the lower spine.

EPIDURAL AND SUBDURAL HEMATOMAS

Although I found that only one subdural and 20 epidural hematomas in patients with ankylosing spondylitis were reported in the literature, many more may have been missed because of the difficulty in performing myelography on patients with deformed torsos and the immediate serious lesion of the cord produced by the direct trauma to it. A third reason for a higher incidence of epidural hemorrhage in the patient with ankylosing spondylitis was discovered by Schneider and colleagues,[47] who made the diagnosis based on the rapid deterioration in spinal cord function within a few hours of the injury in all three of their cases. The displaced fractured bone had direct access to the epidural space and poured blood into it in each case. The bleeding was so profuse that it was difficult to stop, even at operative exposure. Injury to the generous plexus of epidural veins was not the source of the bleeding. The hematoma at operation in one of their cases extended only to the C5, C6, and C7 levels and was only in the posterior half of the cord and only 4 mm thick, whereas at autopsy 14 days later, it extended from C2 to T5. The operative removal of the clot took place approximately 24 hours after the injury. The hematoma was removed from the other two patients approximately 12 hours after the trauma. Unfortunately, the clot in the third patient was 3 to 4 cm thick, surrounded the dura, and extended from C3 to C7; the patient died of pneumonia on the 14th postoperative day. At autopsy, no significant epidural clot was found. Only one patient, 58 years old with a 1.5-cm clot from C5 to T1, slowly made a full recovery.

Rowed[42] reported the high incidence of two epidural hematomas in 21 patients, one discovered at autopsy and the other in the course of removal of a herniated intervertebral disc. He also removed herniated discs from two other patients with ankylosing spondylitis; in all three cases, the discs were removed because they were causing spinal cord compression.

In six other patients, a full recovery was achieved. In three of the six, recovery followed removals that were performed within approximately 12 hours of injury.[48–50] In another patient, the progression of neural deficit took 36 hours to reach a not quite total transverse lesion, then remained constant another 48 hours, during which a lumbar puncture showed normal dynamics, cerebrospinal fluid protein, and cell count. Nevertheless, Lowrey[51] operated, and the patient recovered approximately 1 year later. The patient of Hissa and colleagues[52] had such a delayed onset and gradual worsening of his symptoms that a myelography was not performed until the sixth day after the injury. Myelography revealed a complete block at T2, leading to removal of an epidural hematoma from T2 to T7, followed by a slow but total recovery at 2 years. One of Bohlman's[24] four patients also eventually recovered completely after a laminectomy and removal of an unexpected large epidural hematoma and a period of worsened motor power. Each of the patients of Agnetti and colleagues,[53] Osgood and colleagues,[31] and Rowed[42] and three of the patients of Bohlman[24] died, respectively, at 1 month, 7 days, 1 day, 1 day, and 18 days. The diagnosis in each was made post mortem. In three patients,[26,34,54] laminectomy revealed the hematoma, the delay in the removal of which partially explains the major persisting neural sequelae.

A subdural hematoma was found in one patient,[55] in whom the neural deficit progressed so slowly to paraplegia that a myelogram was not obtained until 1 month after the injury. The partial block was diagnosed as an intradural extramedullary defect at T12–LI. The time to major recovery from the hematoma removal was not stated.

The hope of finding a hematoma, a ruptured disc, or a bony fragment compressing the cord should lead the physician to try to obtain some form of radiographic image. Pan and colleagues[56] reported the first demonstration by magnetic resonance imaging of a post-traumatic cervical spinal epidural hematoma, and Garza-Mercado[48] has followed with the more difficult task of securing such a study in a patient with cervical ankylosing spondylitis. The vacuum cushion of Surin[27] may help to maintain the proper position of head and neck during these studies.

The most urgent poorly solved problem is the maintenance of proper neck position for healing and in the optimal region for pulmonary prophylaxis. We are concentrating on a halo-pelvic apparatus.

Two carefully conceived papers from 1992 and 1993 present the two major divergent views on the place of laminectomy and internal stabilization, that of Fox and colleagues[23] is more aggressive than that of Rowed.[42]

OSTEOTOMY FOR CORRECTION OF DEFORMITY

Severe fixed hip flexion, lumbar spine flexion, thoracic kyphos, cervical spine flexion, or any combination of these can gradually distort the patient into a shape approaching a full circle. Although many patients continue to work despite grotesquely severe deformity, when the top of the patient's head is maintained perpendicular to the floor, chin on chest as the patient stands, then the patient cannot see ahead at all, and correction becomes a necessity. The cervical vertebrae are the most logical and the most hazardous of sites for the procedure. The orthopedic surgeon Simmons[57] has the largest experience in the United States in this field.

ATLANTOAXIAL SUBLUXATION

Atlantoaxial subluxation is an uncommon feature of ankylosing spondylitis. In the series of Wilkinson and Bywaters,[10] only one of 212 patients had atlantoaxial subluxation. Sharp and Purser[58] diagnosed this disorder in only 17 of the

approximately 1000 patients with spondylitis seen in their clinic. They described these cases, plus five others, in a remarkably detailed account of each patient, which the neurosurgeon would do well to study if he or she is to treat such a rare condition. The dislocation consists of forward movement of the anterior arch of the atlas away from the odontoid process of the axis. The movement occurs as a consequence of a tear or excessive stretching of the transverse ligament, which lies against the posterior surface of the dens and attaches to bony knobs on the medial aspect of the two lateral masses of the atlas. Failure of this ligament is much more common in rheumatoid arthritis than in ankylosing spondylitis and is related to inflammation of the associated synovial joints in this disorder. The diagnosis is made from a pair of lateral radiographs in maximal flexion and maximal extension. The principal symptom is pain in the upper cervical, suboccipital, and retrobulbar areas that is usually worsened by sudden movements or by a succession of these, as occurs during a ride on a bumpy road. Correction and stabilization of the displacement usually result in complete relief of symptoms.

Although intensive cervical muscle exercises, when prescribed, tend to worsen the symptoms, I have found no horror stories such as abound in the injuries to the rest of the cervical spine in ankylosing spondylitis. Radiographs show that the amount of the increased interval between the atlas and dens does not fully describe the problem in these patients. Of 19 cases of Sharp and Purser,[58] six had intervals that were essentially normal at 2 to 4 mm, and five had intervals that were moderately increased, measuring 5 to 7 mm. The remaining eight had intervals averaging 12 mm and ranging from 8 to 17 mm.

A marked degree of fixed forward tilt of the head can also be very painful. Thus, in one patient, the atlas-dens interval in maximal flexion was normal at 3 mm, and she also had 17 degrees of forward tilt and was essentially fixed at this angle, which was still in 15-degree flexion on maximal extension. She also maintained 10 degrees of rotation of her head to the left. Her intolerable pain was almost completely relieved by skull traction and was completely eliminated by occipitocervical fusion. In another patient, the head was fixed in a complete rotary dislocation of the atlas to the right. Most of the patients have some rotation and tilting of the head in addition to a fixed forward tilt. Only two of the 22 patients had a major neurologic deficit at the time that active treatment began, six had lesser deficits, and the rest were neurologically normal.

In many of the patients, the rarity of this feature of their ankylosing spondylitis led to a protracted delay in making the diagnosis. Sharp and Purser[58] found that the physician could at times make the diagnosis clinically. By pressing with the palm of one hand on the patient's forehead and the thumb of the other hand on the patient's C2 spinous process, the examiner could feel a backward sliding motion of the hand, which was best elicited by having the patient relax the neck in a semiflexed position.

One patient had no specific treatment because the diagnosis was not made until autopsy, although this final procedure did not occur until after a long illness that led to tetraplegia that the authors thought could have been postponed or arrested had the atlantoaxial dislocation been treated. In three others, this aspect of the disease required no treatment. Three others did reasonably well with merely a plastic or cardboard collar, but a fourth steadily worsened until his dislocation was reduced by skull traction and maintained by occipitocervical fusion. Skeletal traction followed by an autologous iliac bone graft for an occipitocervical fusion was carried out in nine patients of Sharp and Purser. Skull traction was continued preoperatively until no further reduction occurred and was continued during the fusion operation. In some cases, the traction was continued until the graft was united. Pain from the displacement was present in all nine cases and was completely relieved in all. Cord damage in five of the nine was mild to moderate in four patients, who recovered from it completely, and severe in one, in whom moderate improvement occurred. Two cases with a rotary subluxation of the atlas on axis were also helped substantially by specific modifications of the skeletal traction. In this disorder, symptoms are clearly amenable to major alleviation.

Acknowledgment

The author expresses his appreciation to the Neuro-Research Foundation for its assistance during the preparation of this manuscript.

REFERENCES

1. Bechterew W: Steifigkeit der Wirbelsäule und ihre Verkrümmung als besondere Erkrankungsform. Neurol Centralbl 12:426–434, 1893.
2. Bechterew W: Akinesia Algera. Neurol Centralbl 12:531–534, 1893.
3. Bechterew W: Von der Verwachsung oder Steifigkeit der Wirbelsäule. Dtsch Z Nervenheilk 11:327–337, 1897.
4. Connor B, cited by Blumberg BS: Arch Rheum 1:553, 1958.
5. Boland EW: Ankylosing spondylitis. In Hollander JE (ed): Arthritis and Allied Conditions. Philadelphia: Lea & Febiger, 1966, pp 633–655.
6. Strumpell A: Bemerkung über die chronische, ankylosierende Entzündung der Wirbelsäule und der Huftgelenke. Dtsch Z Nervenheilk 11:338–342, 1897.
7. Marie P: Sur la spondylose rhizomelique. Rev Med 8:285–315, 1898.
8. Fraenkel E: Über chronische ankylosierende Wirbelsäulenversteifung. Fortsch Geb Röntgenstr Nuklearmed Ergänzungsbd 7:62–90, 1903.
9. Abdi O: Über ein Fall von chronischer Arthritis Ankylopoetica der Wirbelsäule: Fraktur der Wirbelsäule und Quetschung der Cauda equina. Milt Hamburgischen Staatskrank Anst 4:57–74, 1904.
10. Wilkinson M, Bywaters EGL: Clinical features and course of ankylosing spondylitis. Am Rheum Dis 17:209–228, 1958.
11. Calin A, Fries JF: Striking prevalence of ankylosing spondylitis in "healthy" W27 positive males and females. N Engl J Med 293:835–839, 1975.
12. Kinsella TD, MacDonald FR, Johnson LG: Ankylosing spondylitis: A late re-evaluation of 92 cases. CMAJ 95:1–9, 1966.
13. Hart FD, Bogdanovitch A, Nichol WD: The thorax in ankylosing spondylitis. Ann Rheum Dis 9:116, 1950.
14. Calabro JJ: An appraisal of the medical and surgical management of ankylosing spondylitis. Clin Orthop 60:125–148, 1968.
15. Radford EP, Doll R, Smith PG: Mortality among patients with ankylosing spondylitis not given x-ray therapy. N Engl J Med 297:572–576, 1977.
16. Cruickshank B: Pathology of ankylosing spondylitis. Clin Orthop 74:43–58, 1971.
17. Linder E, Pasternack A: Immunofluorescence studies on kidney biopsies in ankylosing spondylitis. Acta Pathol Microbiol 78:517–525, 1970.
18. Cruickshank B: Pathology of ankylosing spondylitis. Bull Rheum Dis 10:211–214, 1960.
19. Solomon G, Winchester R: Immunogenetic aspects of inflammatory arthritis. In Taveras JM, Ferrucci JT (eds): Radiology: Diagnosis-Imaging-Intervention, vol 5. Philadelphia: JB Lippincott, 1988, pp 1–4.
20. Brewerton DA: HLA-B27 and the inheritance of susceptibility to rheumatic disease. Arthritis Rheum 19:656–668, 1976.
21. Martel W, Braunstein EM: Spondyloarthritides. In Taveras J, Ferrucci JT (eds): Radiology: Diagnosis-Imaging-Intervention, vol 5. Philadelphia: JB Lippincott, 1988, pp 1–5.
22. Simmonds M: Über Spondylitis deformans und ankylosierende Spondylitis. Fortschr Gebd Röntgenstr Nuklearmed Ergänzungsbd 7:51–62, 1903.
23. Fox MW, Onofrio BM, Kilgore JE: Neurological complications of ankylosing spondylitis. J Neurosurg 78:871–878, 1993.
24. Bohlman HH: Acute fractures and dislocations of the cervical spine. J Bone Joint Surg Am 61A:1119–1142, 1979.
25. Ackerman EA: Cervical traction in flexion: A method of maintaining constant angle prone or supine. J Bone Joint Surg Am 54:1114–1116, 1972.
26. Detwiler KN, Loftus CM, Menezes AH, et al: Management of cervical spine injuries in patients with ankylosing spondylitis. J Neurosurg 72:210–215, 1990.
27. Surin VV: Fractures of the cervical spine in patients with ankylosing spondylitis. Acta Orthop Scand 51:79–84, 1980.
28. Osgood C, Martin LG, Ackerman E: Fracture-dislocation of the cervical spine with ankylosing spondylitis. J Neurosurg 39:764–769, 1973.
29. Raine GET: Fractures of the cervical spine. Proc R Soc Med 63:657–658, 1970.
30. Lemmen LJ, Laing PG: Fracture of the cervical spine in patients with rheumatoid arthritis. J Neurosurg 16:542–550, 1959.
31. Osgood CP, Abbasy M, Mathews T: Multiple spine fractures in ankylosing spondylitis. J Trauma 15:163–166, 1975.
32. Murray GC, Persellin RH: Cervical fracture complicating ankylosing spondylitis: A report of eight cases and review of the literature. Am J Med 70:1033–1041, 1981.
33. Woodruff FP, Dewing SB: Fracture of the cervical spine patients with ankylosing spondylitis. Radiology 80:17–21, 1963.
34. Grisolia A, Bell RL, Peltier LF, et al: Fractures and dislocations of the spine complicating ankylosing spondylitis. J Bone Joint Surg Am 49:339–344, 1967.
35. Hunter T, Dubo H: Spinal fractures complicating ankylosing spondylitis. Ann Intern Med 88:546–549, 1978.
36. Weinstein PR, Karpman RR, Gall E, et al: Spinal cord injury, spinal fracture and spinal stenosis in ankylosing spondylitis. J Neurosurg 57:609–616, 1982.
37. Malik GM, Sanders JL: Surgical treatment of rheumatoid arthritis, ankylosing spondylitis, and Paget's disease with neurologic deficit. In Schmidek HH, Sweet WH (eds): Operative Neurosurgical Techniques: Indications, Methods and Results. Philadelphia: WB Saunders, 1988, pp 1295–1306.
38. Janda WE, Kelly PJ, Rhoton AL, et al: Fracture dislocation of the cervical part of the spinal column in patients with ankylosing spondylitis. Mayo Clin Proc 43:714–721, 1968.
39. Young R, Thomassen EH: Step by step procedure for applying the halo ring. Orthop Rev 3:62–64, 1974.
40. Young JS, Cheshire DJE, Pierce JA, et al: Cervical ankylosis with acute spinal cord injury. Paraplegia 15:133–146, 1977–1978.
41. Young R, Murphy DJ: Step by step procedure for applying the halo vest. Orthop Rev 4:33–36, 1975.
42. Rowed DW: Management of cervical spinal cord injury in ankylosing spondylitis: The intervertebral disc as a cause of cord compression. J Neurosurg 77:241–246, 1992.
43. Freeman LW: Ascending spinal paralysis: Case presentation. J Neurosurg 16:120–122, 1959.
44. Kiwerski J, Wieclawek H, Garwacka I: Fractures of the cervical spine in ankylosing spondylitis. Int Orthop 8:243–246, 1985.
45. Martel W, Page JW: Cervical vertebral erosions and subluxations in rheumatoid arthritis and ankylosing spondylitis. Arthritis Rheum 3:546–556, 1960.
46. Marsh CH: Internal fixation for stress fractures of the ankylosed spine. J R Soc Med 78:377–379, 1985.
47. Schneider RC, Cherry G, Pantek H: The syndrome of acute central cervical spinal cord injury. J Neurosurg 11:546–577, 1954.
48. Garza-Mercado R: Traumatic extradural hematoma of the cervical spine. Neurosurgery 24:410–414, 1989.
49. Pecker J, Javalet A, Le Menn G: Spondylarthrite ankylosante et paraplégie par hématorachis extra-dural traumatique. Presse Med 68:183–184, 1960.
50. Ver Brugghen A: Extradural spinal hemorrhage. Ann Surg 123:154–159, 1946.
51. Lowrey JJ: Spinal epidural hematomas: Experiences with three patients. J Neurosurg 16:508–513, 1959.
52. Hissa E, Boumphrey F, Bay J: Spinal epidural hematoma and ankylosing spondylitis. Clin Orthop 208:225–227, 1986.

53. Agnetti V, Monaco F, Mutani R: Post-convulsive spinal epidural haematoma in ankylosing spondylitis. Eur Neurol 18:230–233, 1979.
54. Fast A, Parikh S, Marin EL: Spine fractures in ankylosing spondylitis. Arch Phys Med Rehabil 67:595–597, 1986.
55. Sokoloff J, Coel MN, Ignelzi RJ: Spinal subdural hematoma. Radiology 120:116, 1976.
56. Pan G, Kulkarni M, MacDougall DJ, et al: Traumatic epidural hematoma of the cervical spine: Diagnosis with magnetic resonance imaging. J Neurosurg 68:798–801, 1988.
57. Simmons EH: The surgical correction of flexion deformity of the cervical spine in ankylosing spondylitis. In Sherk HH, Dunn EJ, Eismont FJ, et al (eds): The Cervical Spine, 2nd ed. Philadelphia: JB Lippincott, 1989, pp 573–598.
58. Sharp J, Purser DW: Spontaneous atlanto-axial dislocation in ankylosing spondylitis and rheumatoid arthritis. Ann Rheum Dis 20:47–77, 1961.

Cervicothoracic Ankylosing Spondylitis: Commentary

MICHAEL L. WOLAK

Dr. Sweet's chapter "Cervicothoracic Ankylosing Spondylitis" (AS) remains a classic. His clinical assessment, depicted through personal and reported experiences, highlights the importance of recognizing patients presenting with ankylosing disease. Perhaps the most important lesson relates to the potentially devastating consequences associated with failure to institute appropriate treatment options. Even with such an appreciation, significant challenges and risks remain in the management of patients with AS who present with function-limiting spinal deformity, fracture, or compromised neurologic function.

Spondyloarthropathies constitute a group of interrelated, chronic inflammatory rheumatic diseases estimated to occur in approximately 2% of the general population, with an overall male predominance.[1] Included within this disease category are AS, reactive (Reiter's) arthritis, psoriatic arthritis, and enteropathic arthritis. Multisystem involvement is seen in all the spondyloarthropathies. Each diagnostic subtype is variably associated with characteristic extra-articular manifestations, including inflammatory disease of the gastrointestinal, ocular, cardiac, and pulmonary organ systems.[2] Spondyloarthropathies are not associated with rheumatoid factor (i.e., seronegative) and show a strong association with the class I major histocompatibility complex allele HLA-B27. AS is considered the most common and prototypic seronegative spondyloarthropathy. The prevalence of AS in American and European whites is 0.1% to 0.2%, with considerable variance in disease prevalence seen among different ethnic and racial groups. Despite the fact that more than 90% of patients with AS are positive for HLA-B27 (normal, 4% to 8% in the white population), the disorder affects only 1% to 2% of individuals with this haplotype. Overall, 90% of individuals harboring the HLA-B27 allele do not develop AS, supporting the involvement of additional genetic and environmental factors that have yet to be clearly elucidated.[3,4]

AS has a predilection for joints of the axial skeleton, including sacroiliac, discovertebral, apophyseal, costovertebral, and paravertebral ligamentous structures. Sacroiliac joints are characteristically involved early in the disease, and the clinical diagnosis is often supported by radiographic evidence of sacroiliitis, the hallmark of AS. Inflammatory reactions involve subchondral granulation tissue that erodes involved joints, which are gradually replaced by fibrocartilage that becomes ossified. With long-standing disease, interosseous bridging and characteristic bony fusion (ankylosis) occurs. As the disease ascends the spinal column (spondylitis), there is primary involvement of the intervertebral discs and apophyseal joints that undergo inflammatory destruction that ultimately leads to ankylosis. The vertebral bodies are relatively unburdened of axial load, owing to a lack of gravitational forces that are borne predominantly by fused posterior elements and become square and osteoporotic. As the disease progresses, there is ossification and eventual destruction of the intervertebral discs, and bony fusion of the vertebral bodies ensues via vertical bony bridges (syndesmophytes). The progressive nature of the disease can lead to involvement of the entire axial skeleton and ligamentous support tissue, with spinal ankylosis producing severe deformity and immobility.

In extreme cases, normal lumbar lordosis is lost, the thoracic spine assumes an accentuated kyphosis and cervical motion is restricted with head fixation in a flexed position. Fixed flexion deformities in the cervical or cervicothoracic regions can lead to a "chin on chest" situation that severely restricts the forward vision and may interfere with mandibular function. Esophageal or tracheal kinking may provoke dysphagia or dyspnea, respectively. Nerve root (radiculopathy) and cord (myelopathy) compression may arise from flexion deformity or with atlantoaxial subluxation resulting from the weight of the head during constant flexion. The osteotomy is preferentially carried out at C7–T1 because spinal canal is relatively wide at this level, inadvertent damage to the C8 nerve root results in less detriment to hand function than damage to more rostral nerve roots, and the vertebral arteries pass anterior to the transverse process of C7.[5,6] Nonetheless, cervicothoracic osteotomy is a difficult procedure and the complication rate is high, in many instances involving quadriparesis, nerve root palsy, subluxation, and pseudarthrosis.

The risk of spinal fracture is significantly increased in AS, and the risk increases with disease progression.[7] The ankylosed spine has a reduced number of mobile segments, with varying degrees of osteoporosis often present. Therefore, forces applied to the spine must be absorbed by a rigid structure with a reduced dampening effect provided by a reduced number of functioning discs. The combination of immobile, porotic bone produces fracture patterns that differ from those typically seen in an otherwise normal spine. Fracture lines tend to involve the entire vertebral body and ossified ligaments in a transverse fashion. The fracture site opens with both extension and flexion, favoring nonunion and predisposing these lesions to translation and instability. Patients with known AS who have spinal trauma or neurologic complaints require urgent clinical and radiographic assessment.

Nondisplaced fractures are often difficult to identify by plain radiographs due to spinal osteoporosis and the already pathologic appearance of the ankylosed spine. However, in an era when the availability of advanced imaging modalities has become customary, it seems reasonable to suggest that a CT scan is indicated in every patient with AS who presents after trauma or with a neurologic complaint.

Fractures may occur with even the most trivial of injuries; case reports indicate that, in many incidences, there is no history of traumatic injury, and the fracture has been referred to as "autofracture."[8] Regardless of the ability to identify an isolated event, the incidence of neurologic deficit is high, requiring a low threshold of suspicion for spinal fracture in a patient with AS presenting with even subtle neurologic complaints. AS is most often encountered in the thoracolumbar spine, with approximately 30% of cases involving the cervical spine; the lower cervical spine is particularly prone to fractures.[9,10] Severe neurologic deficits occur in as many as 57% of cases, and mortality is double that of cervical fractures seen in the generally healthy population.[11] Contributing to the high morbidity and mortality associated with spinal fractures are systemic manifestations associated with AS. Stable fractures in neurologically intact patients can be managed conservatively via rigid immobilization with pseudarthrosis a possible complication, whereas those patients with immediate or progressive neurologic deficits require surgical decompression and fixation.

Proper conservative management with counseling, pharmacologic suppression of joint inflammation, and physical therapy to preserve axial joint function enables most patients with AS to lead relatively normal and productive lives. Surgical management only addresses the secondary mechanical consequences of disease progression, most often in the form of deformity, major instability, and their neurologic consequences. The major advances over recent years have not been so much in the surgical indications or approaches but in the technical progress that has made these procedures safer and allowed better stabilization, enabling earlier mobilization. Advances have been made in the quality and accessibility of diagnostic imaging, internal fixation devices, anesthesiology techniques and intraoperative neurophysiologic monitoring.[12]

REFERENCES

1. Braun J, Bollow M, Remlinger G, et al: Prevalence of spondylarthropathies in HLA-B27 positive and negative blood donors. Arthritis Rheum 41:58–67, 1998.
2. Taurog J, Arnett F, Khan M, et al: Seronegative spondyloarthropathies. In Klippel J, Weyand C, Wortmann R (eds): Primer on the Rheumatic Diseases, 11th ed. Atlanta: Arthritis Foundation, 1997, pp 180–195.
3. Sieper J, Braun J, Rudwaleit M, et al: Ankylosing spondylitis: An overview. Ann Rheum Dis 61(Suppl 3):iii8–iii18, 2002.
4. Olivieri I, van Tubergen A, Salvarani C, et al: Seronegative spondyloarthritides. Best Pract Res Clin Rheumatol 16:723–739, 2002.
5. Mehdian SM, Freeman BJ, Licina P: Cervical osteotomy for ankylosing spondylitis: An innovative variation on an existing technique. Eur Spine J 8:505–509, 1999.
6. Webb J, Sengupta D: Posterior cervicothoracic osteotomy. In Vaccarp A, Albert T (eds): Spine Surgery: Tricks of the Trade. New York: Thieme, 2003, p 35.
7. Olerud C, Frost A, Bring J: Spinal fractures in patients with ankylosing spondylitis. Eur Spine J 5:51–55, 1996.
8. Tait TJ, Barlow G, Iveson JM: Cervical spine fracture in ankylosing spondylitis: A case of 'auto-fracture.' Br J Rheumatol 37:467–468, 1998.
9. Harding JR, McCall IW, Park WM, et al: Fracture of the cervical spine in ankylosing spondylitis. Br J Radiol 58:3–7, 1985.
10. Alaranta H, Luoto S, Konttinen YT: Traumatic spinal cord injury as a complication to ankylosing spondylitis: An extended report. Clin Exp Rheumatol 20:66–68, 2002.
11. Murray GC, Persellin RH: Cervical fracture complicating ankylosing spondylitis: A report of eight cases and review of the literature. Am J Med 70:1033–1041, 1991.
12. Szpalski M, Gunzburg R: What are the advances for surgical therapy of inflammatory diseases of the spine? Best Pract Res Clin Rheumatol 16:141–154, 2002.

128 Ankylosing Spondylitis and Management of Spinal Complications

PATRICK W. HITCHON, AARON M. FROM, PAUL M. PELOSO, DILIP K. SENGUPTA, and ARNOLD H. MENEZES

THE SPONDYLOARTHROPATHIES IN RELATION TO COMMON JOINT DISORDERS

The spondyloarthropathies are a family of disorders thought to occur in approximately 1% to 2% of the white population. They include ankylosing spondylitis (AS), arthritis associated with inflammatory bowel disease (Crohn's and ulcerative colitis), reactive arthritis (Reiter's syndrome), and psoriatic arthritis. The seronegative spondyloarthropathies are so named due to the absence of rheumatoid factor in the serum. These disorders are distinguished by inflammation of the spine and sacroiliac structures, inflammation of peripheral joints, and associated features such as enthesitis, skin, eye, and gut abnormalities. Spinal inflammation is the hallmark of the spondyloarthropathies and is recognized as morning stiffness lasting more than 45 minutes, improvement with activity, and pain that is not relieved with rest. These people are typically forced out of bed by pain, feel best with continued low-grade activity, and generally feel better as the day progresses or after exercise. Noninflammatory or mechanical joint pain, by contrast, is better with rest and worsened with activity and typically causes most problems at the end of the work day.

The sacroiliac joints can be involved clinically and radiographically, presenting as buttock pain lasting 6 to 12 weeks, with morning stiffness. Peripheral arthritis tends to be in the lower extremities, with involvement of hips, knees, and ankles in an asymmetrical pattern, with associated joint effusions, although involvement of the upper extremities also occurs in wrists, elbows, and shoulders. Enthesitis is inflammation of the tissue connecting tendons and ligaments to the periosteum and is most often appreciated as pain, occasionally associated with swelling, around large muscle group insertions: the shoulders, the elbows, the knees, and around the Achilles' tendon and the plantar fascia. Dactylitis, or sausage digit, is a variant and presents as diffuse swelling of an entire finger or toe, which may resemble cellulitis.[1-3] Thus the following discussion is specific to the inflammatory spondyloarthropathies with spinal involvement, most typified by AS.

CLINICAL PRESENTATION AND DIAGNOSIS

The diagnosis of a spondyloarthritis should be suspected in all individuals younger than 40 years of age who have back pain for more than 3 months or recurrent episodes of low back pain who also have morning stiffness in their back lasting longer than 45 minutes that is predictably relieved with exercise.[4,5] Sacroiliac joint pain, presenting as buttock pain lasting for several weeks, asymmetrical lower limb joint swelling, dactylitis, and skin disease should be sought as they commonly coexist. Their presence should heighten the suspicion for a spondyloarthritis. Skin disease is typically a scaly, red rash, as is seen with psoriasis, keratodermia of the soles, or dyshydrosis of the palmar and plantar surfaces. Eye pain with redness and loss of vision characterizes uveitis. Often patients have a family history of AS, uveitis, psoriasis, or inflammatory bowel disease. Inflammatory bowel disease and inflammatory eye disease are the most common extraspinal features, whereas potentially serious heart, lung, and kidney involvement is rare.[1,6-23]

Physical examination reveals decreased spinal motion in all directions, although extension and lateral bending are most affected. Reduced chest expansion, measured at the fourth intercostal space, is a specific but late finding of AS. Enthesitis should be sought at the shoulders, elbows, knees, and feet.

Back pain lasting more than 3 months, with significant morning stiffness is sufficient reason to obtain radiographs of the sacroiliac joints and lumbar spine. The sacroiliac joint radiographs show areas of both erosion (widening) and sclerosis (narrowing). The lumbar spine can show erosions and sclerosis of the vertebral corners and, in time, calcification of the anterior longitudinal ligament. Radiographic changes can take 2 to 5 years to appear, and a suspicious history should lead to computed tomography or magnetic resonance imaging of the sacroiliac joints, if the sacroiliac joints are normal on plain radiographs.

The class I human leukocyte antigen B27 (HLA-B27) can also be helpful when AS is suspected, as up to 90% of patients with AS are positive for the HLA-B27 gene. HLA-B27 is thought to play an important role in disease pathogenesis, although it is not diagnostic of AS, as it occurs in 5% to 8% of the white population.[24] Notably, one third of whites with chronic back pain and a positive B27 gene will have AS. Inflammatory back pain plus a positive B27 is diagnostic of AS. Surprisingly, the erythrocyte sedimentation rate and C-reactive protein can be normal in the presence of active spinal inflammation.

ETIOLOGY AND PATHOGENESIS

Inflammation begins as HLA-B27 class I protein antigens interact with circulating cytotoxic T lymphocytes. This HLA-B27 presentation mechanism is known as the arthritogenic peptide hypothesis.[25] Furthermore, a second stimulatory factor has been hypothesized that includes microtrauma or chronic bacterial deposition in the bowel or joints, leading to an upregulation of cytokine production and subsequent increases in the inflammatory response. One important cytokine produced is tumor necrosis factor α (TNF-α).[1,6,26–29] A possible role of *Pseudomonas aeruginosa* producing an inflammatory response by mimicking the HLA-B27 antigen has been suggested.[1]

Inflammation of the fibrocartilage present in tendon and ligament attachments to bone, also known as enthesitis, is a unique feature of all spondyloarthropathies.[26,27,30] The disease appears to begin with enthesitis in the sacroiliac and lumbar vertebral joints.[24,26,31] Inflammation is followed by fibrosis and ossification of the attached ligaments and intervertebral disc spaces. Erosion of bone at the ligamentous attachment of the intervertebral disc to the vertebral body and calcification along the anterior longitudinal ligament leads to vertebral body squaring, evident on lateral lumbar spine films. In an attempt to repair inflamed and eroded vertebral bodies, bony growth ensues resulting in syndesmophyte formation across the disc space. Eventually, the pattern of ossification progresses to the thoracic and cervical regions of the spine, resulting in kyphotic deformity. This ossified spine, also known as the "bamboo" spine, has secondary osteoporosis due to chronic immobility, leaving the vertebral bodies and ossified discs brittle, fused, and easily susceptible to fracture.[24,26,31]

SPONDYLODISCITIS

Pain and progression of deformity in the globally ankylosed patient raises the suspicion of spondylodiscitis. The most common location is in the lower thoracic and upper lumbar region, but the cervicothoracic junction may also be involved. The exact cause is unknown. A definite history of precipitating trauma or evidence of infection is missing in most cases.[32,33] Many believe that these lesions represent pseudarthrosis resulting from the instability of a chronic nonunion.[34] Histologic studies also suggest pseudarthrosis.[35] Radiographically, these lesions often appear like disc space infection and are referred to as Andersson lesions.[33]

Conservative treatment with a nonsteroidal antiinflammatory drug, rest, and physiotherapy is suggested when symptoms are minimal.[33] For established cases with persistent symptoms, surgical intervention is indicated to treat pseudarthrosis. Posterior surgery alone may be adequate when the sagittal balance can be restored with shift of the plumb line behind the vertebral body and compression applied with the instrumentation.[36] Rarely, these lesion may cause spinal stenosis with neurologic symptoms. An anterior approach with excision of the pseudarthrosis tissue, bone grafting, and instrumentation may be recommended in these cases.[37]

MEDICAL MANAGEMENT

AS treatment focuses on pain management and long-term disease modification, with the goal of preventing disability.

Four treatments are central to patient care: (1) patient education, (2) exercise, (3) nonsteroidal anti-inflammatory drugs, and (4) immune system–modifying agents.[38] Patients should be informed of the long-term prognosis, including disease progression and the risk of fractures related to fusion and the associated osteoporosis. Regular stretching and vigorous aerobic exercise appear to provide immediate gains in flexibility and may help decrease secondary osteoporosis of the spine by reducing immobility.[39,40] Nonsteroidal anti-inflammatory drugs are useful analgesics, with several having randomized trial proof of efficacy including indomethacin, naproxen, and celecoxib.[38] Nonsteroidal anti-inflammatory drugs reduce pain and morning stiffness but do not have a major role in slowing the course of the disease.[38,41] In patients with inflamed peripheral joints, sulfasalazine has been shown to be effective in several randomized trials, whereas the immunosuppressant methotrexate and corticosteroids can also sometimes be helpful. None of these agents control spinal inflammation, however.[38]

True changes in the natural history of AS will occur through novel approaches to immune modulation.[41–44] Several randomized trials published since 2002 have documented that TNF-α inhibition has an important effect on pain, inflammation, and quite possibly disease progression. Infliximab is approved in Europe and etanercept is approved in the United States for the treatment of AS, with trials of adalimumab currently under way. The TNF-α inhibitors are indicated in persons with persistent spinal inflammation despite good trials of at least two nonsteroidal anti-inflammatory drugs and in those with peripheral arthritis who have failed either sulfasalazine or methotrexate. There are some data that antiosteoporotic agent pamidronate has disease-modifying activity, especially for the spine. It appears that the synovium is particularly susceptible to cytokines such as TNF-α.[27,45] Inhibition of TNF-α with etanercept (an immunoglobulin G molecule linked to a TNF-β receptor that blocks receptor action) or antibodies directed at TNF-α antibodies (infliximab) have shown significant and rapid reduction of active axial inflammation in AS.[41,42,45] Preliminary studies with these drugs have suggested that they also have structure-modifying abilities.

CERVICAL SPINE FRACTURES

Published reports suggest that extension fractures of the cervical spine are the most common fractures of the fused spine. However, the exact type of fracture depends on the mechanism of the injury.[46–48] The heightened prevalence of cervical spine extension fracture reflects the common injury mechanism, wherein an individual falls forward striking the forehead.[46,49]

The severity of fractures in AS is disproportionate to the trivial nature of the trauma. This reflects the extremely brittle nature of the cervical and thoracic spine, secondary to osteoporosis.[24,31] The fractures of the osteoporotic spine have been likened to the snapping of a stick or long bone fractures.[50,51] The fracture commonly involves all three columns of the spine,[52] with secondary dislocation and neurologic deficit.[49,50,53]

Transdiscal fractures appear to be common in the cervical as well as the thoracolumbar spine.[31,47,54] A proposed theory suggests that although ossification occurs across the disc space, it remains the least rigid portion of the spine and most likely region to fracture in trauma.[54]

Nonoperative Management of Cervical Fractures

In fractures in which all three columns are not involved and no dislocation or neurologic deficit exists, surgery is not necessary and bracing may be sufficient. In these stable fractures, immobilization in a halo, Miami, or SOMI brace is sufficient. Orthotics are often recommended for as long as 3 months with frequent sequential radiographs and examinations.[48,49] Some accounts suggest that conservative, nonoperative management of fractures in AS produces better outcomes, shorter hospital stays, and lower costs.[48,55] Of the four recent cervical spine fractures treated at our institution with orthotics, only one had minimal deficit on admission. Fractures were located at C5–6 in one, C6–7 in two, and at C7 in the fourth. Immobilization for 3 to 6 months was achieved by a halo in three and a Philadelphia collar in one. All four have remained stable without the need to resort to surgery (Fig. 128-1).

Surgical Management of Cervical Fractures

Spinal instability with disruption of all three columns[52] is often associated with neurologic deficit and requires surgical intervention in the form of anterior and/or posterior instrumentation and fusion.

In cases of fractures with dislocation, deformity, and cord compression, axial traction along the axis of the spine for reduction with weights not in excess of 10 lb is often necessary.[56] Owing to the extent of instability, traction has to be applied with caution, to avoid overdistraction or increased anterior or posterior displacement. Stabilization is generally achieved through a posterior approach by means of posterolateral screws with plates or rods (Fig. 128-2). Screw placement can be difficult in the ankylosed cervical spine due to lack of distinct bony landmarks and fused facets.[57,58] Three of seven subaxial cervical spine fractures were associated with deficit. Fractures were located at C5–6 in three, at C6–7 in three, and C7–T1 in the last. Preoperative traction was applied in four, immobilization with collar in two, and a halo in one. Six underwent posterior fusion alone, and one in the surgeon's opinion required both anterior plating and posterior rodding. Two patients showed neurologic improvement; the third who had a complete lesion was unchanged.

OCCIPITOCERVICAL FRACTURES AND DISLOCATIONS

Fractures of the axis in AS are unusual and only rarely have been reported in the literature.[59,60] The vast majority of cervical spine fractures in AS are subaxial. Occipitocervical dislocations in AS have been reported, and these too are infrequently encountered.[61,62] The hypermobility of the atlantoaxial joint may be compensatory to the rigidity of the rest of the spine, culminating in laxity of the transverse ligament. This chronic C1–2 instability and secondary cranial settling can result in compression of the C1 and

C2 nerve roots and cervicomedullary junction. Patients will present with occipitocervical pain and in advanced cases myelopathy. When symptomatic, treatment for reduction, decompression, and stabilization is necessary. Owing to osteoporosis and ligamentous insufficiency, immobilization with bracing is unlikely to succeed. When the atlantoaxial instability is reducible by preoperative traction, a posterior occipitocervical fusion will suffice. On the other hand, when the dislocation is irreducible, transoral odontoidectomy followed by posterior occipitocervical fusion is necessary. Of the five patients with AS and occipitocervical instability presenting at our institution, symptoms and findings included cervicomedullary compression with pain, numbness, spastic quadriparesis, and dysphagia. All five underwent transoral odontoidectomy followed by contemporaneous or subsequent posterior occipitocervical fusion with titanium loop, wires, and bone grafting (Fig. 128-3). Postoperative immobilization was carried out with Minerva bracing in four and a Philadelphia collar in one for 5 months. All patients showed improvement in strength, pain, numbness, and dysphagia. However, the three patients with spasticity remained mildly hyperreflexic at latest follow-up.

THORACIC AND LUMBAR SPINAL FRACTURES

In the thoracic and lumbar spines, extension fractures occur as a result of falling backward on the kyphotic spine.[63] In the presence of three-column disruption involving the vertebral bodies or discs, and the neural arch, with or without neurologic deficit, stabilization is undertaken. Stabilization is achieved with pedicle screws and/or hooks and rods and bony fusion. Owing to the loss of bony and joint landmarks in AS, placement of screws and hooks can be difficult.[63]

In a retrospective review at the University of Iowa, 266 patients with a diagnosis of AS were identified. Seven thoracic and six lumbar fractures were found in 10 men and three women, who ranged in age from 43 to 79 years.[63] Nine of 13 presented with negative spinal angulation or extension deformity as demonstrated in Figure 128-4. The predominance of extension fractures is a reflection of the kyphosis, brittleness, and osteoporosis that develops in the AS spine. The fragility of the ankylosed spine in our population is highlighted by the fact that 10 patients had only minor trauma, such as falls from their own height, lifting, or transfers.

Nonoperative Management of Thoracic and Lumbar Fractures

Three patients were treated nonoperatively; two were intact, and the third who presented with neurologic deficit had a multitude of medical problems including diabetes, emphysema, obesity, and cirrhosis contraindicating surgery. Nondisplaced fractures were located at T10, L1–2, and L4–5. Bed rest was undertaken for as long as 1 week or until pain subsided followed by gradual mobilization. Irrespective of operative or nonoperative management, thoracolumbar clam shell or Jewett braces were worn for at least 3 months. Sequential radiographs were obtained to confirm healing. Neurologic status improved or remained intact.

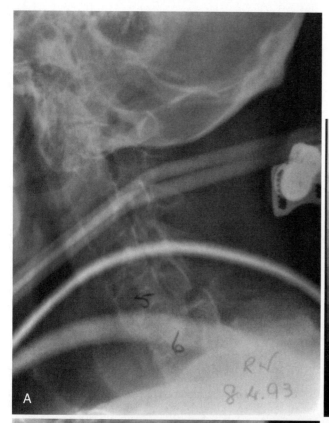

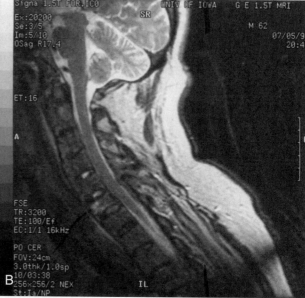

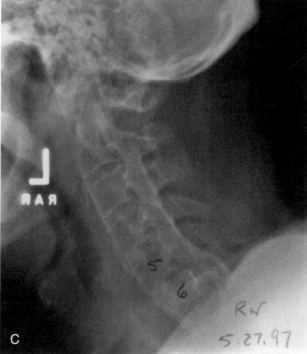

FIGURE 128-1 A 62-year-old man with ankylosing spondylitis was involved in a car accident with secondary C5–6 fracture and minimal subluxation as shown on plain films (*A*) and T2-weighted magnetic resonance imaging (*B*). He was neurologically intact. Treatment consisted of immobilization in a SOMI brace for 6 months. Nearly 4 years later, he remains neurologically intact, and his fracture is healed (*C*).

Surgical Management of Thoracic and Lumbar Fractures

Of the 10 patients who underwent surgery, five presented with neurologic deficit. Six fractures were located in the thoracic spine and the other four in the lumbar spine. Eight of the 10 patients underwent posterior decompression and stabilization with sublaminar hooks in four (see Fig. 128-4) and pedicle screws in six. Instrumentation spanned at least two levels above and two levels below the fracture. Only two patients were thought to require both anterior and posterior instrumentation. Four patients diagnosed with posterior cord compression underwent additional laminectomy.

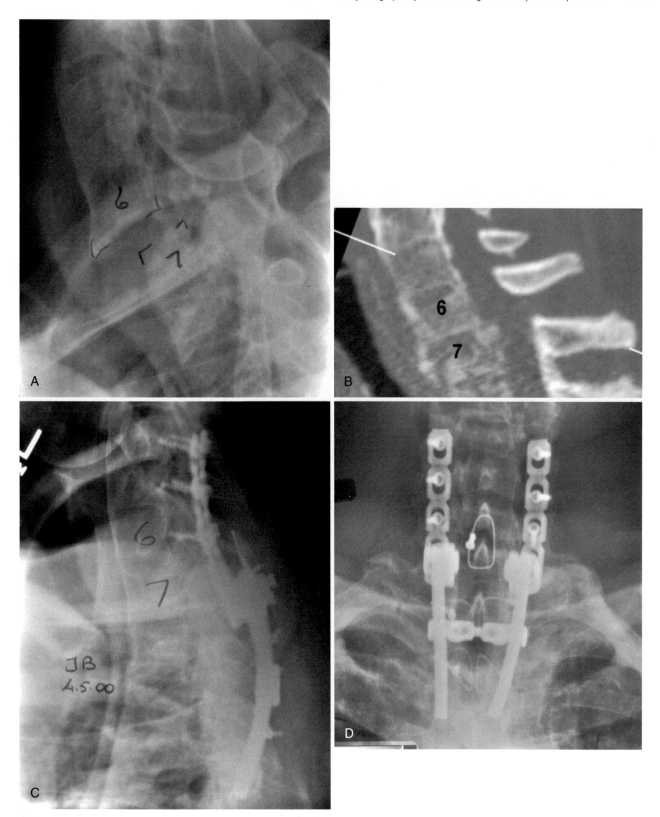

FIGURE 128-2   A 64-year-old man with ankylosing spondylitis fell from ground level, sustaining a C6–7 fracture-dislocation as shown on plain film (*A*) and computed tomographic sagittal reconstructions (*B*). He was neurologically intact and was placed in neutral traction before surgery. Stabilization was accomplished with posterior lateral mass and pedicle screw fixation from C4–T2, as demonstrated on lateral (*C*) and anteroposterior (*D*) plain films taken 2 years after surgery.

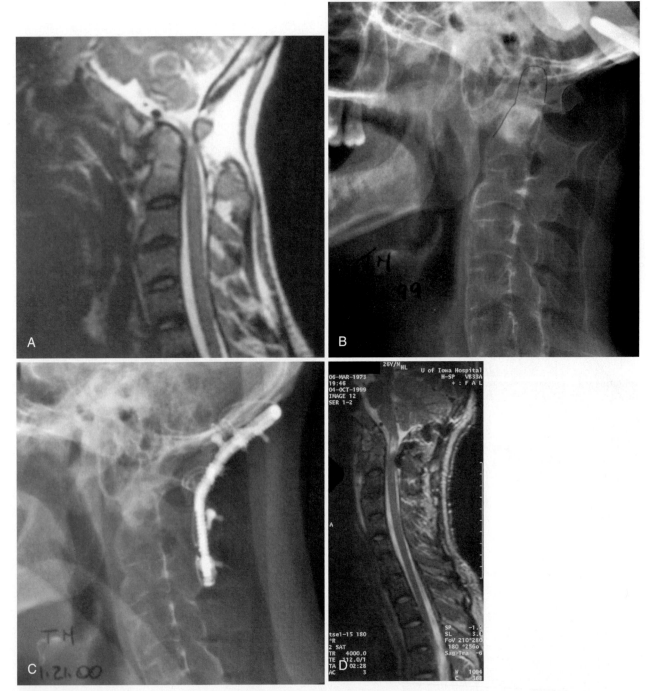

FIGURE 128-3 A 26-year-old man with a C1–2 dislocation and cervicomedullary compression including pain, numbness, weakness, and hyperreflexia. Preoperative magnetic resonance imaging (A), and lateral plain film (B) show the gap between the anterior arch of C1 and dens and ventral cervicomedullary compression. He was placed in halo traction followed by transoral odontoidectomy as well as posterior occiput-C3 fusion using a titanium loop, cables, and rib graft (C). Except for some mild residual spasticity, his symptoms resolved.

Of the five patients who had neurologic deficit, two demonstrated neurologic improvement after treatment, whereas three showed no change. Spinal deformity was corrected as a result of surgery in six of the 10 operated patients by 12 ± 10 degrees (mean $\pm$ SD).[63]

COMPLICATIONS

Common complications after fractures and surgery include epidural hematoma and pulmonary infection. Although spinal epidural hematomas can arise from the fracture itself, pulmonary complications occur secondary to impaired ventilation and prolonged bed rest and immobilization.[47,48,51,64] Increased rates of pneumonia are attributed to decreased lung capacity, kyphotic deformity, and apical fibrosis.[31,19,20]

SPINAL DEFORMITY

A progressive generalized kyphosis is typical of AS. Generalized kyphosis leads to loss of sagittal balance; the

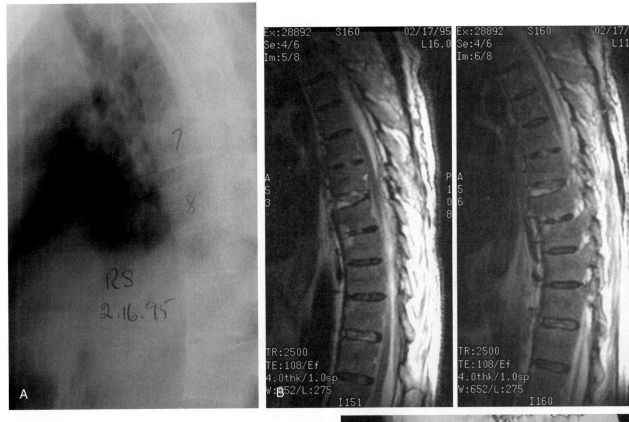

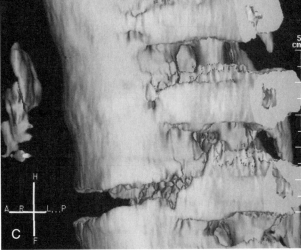

FIGURE 128-4 A 43-year-old man with a T7–8 transdiscal extension fracture due to a car accident as seen on lateral plain film (*A*), magnetic resonance imaging (*B*), and 3-dimensional computed tomographic reconstruction (*C*).

(Continued)

plumb line from C-7 passes in front of the lumbosacral junction. In the initial stages, the patients try to compensate sagittal balance by knee flexion and hyperextension at hips. When the hips are also involved with the disease leading to fixed flexion deformity, the sagittal balance is decompensated. Hyperextension of the cervical spine may help forward gaze. However, in the late stages, the cervical spine is also ankylosed, leading to global ankylosis and kyphosis and a characteristic "chin on chest" posture, which interferes with forward gaze and jaw opening. Patients now try to look forward by rolling the eyeballs cranially. Kyphosis may progress until the lower rib cage rests on the iliac crest, and this may cause compression of the abdominal viscera and reduced vital capacity due to restriction of diaphragmatic excursion.

Indications for Deformity Correction

Surgical intervention is indicated when kyphosis is decompensated. That means that the patient cannot maintain a horizontal gaze when the hips and knees are extended and eyeballs are in the neutral position.[65] In practice, however, the feasibility of surgical intervention considering the general condition of the patient and the morale and earnest desire of the patient to accept the risks are more important deciding factors before considering surgery.

Preoperative Planning

The goals of deformity correction are to restore sagittal balance and correct gaze angle. The degree of gaze angle

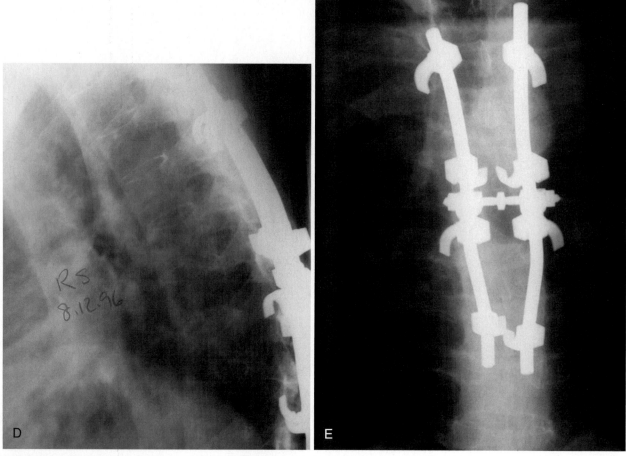

FIGURE 128-4 Cont'd   Surgical correction consisted of a posterior fusion with hooks as seen on lateral (*D*) and anteroposterior (*E*) plain films obtained 18 months later. The patient had no neurologic deficit and has resumed normal activity.

correction needed is determined by the chin-brow to vertical angle.[66] This is an angle between the line drawn from the chin to the brow and a vertical line. The sagittal balance correction is estimated from the degree of posterior shift of the plumb line required to bring it back to the sacrum. A proper estimate of gaze angle and sagittal balance correction should be made from the lateral radiograph taken when the patient stands with relaxed hips and knees, without making an effort to correct the spinal balance or forward gaze to prevent underestimation.

The level of osteotomy to correct a global kyphotic deformity has a disparate effect on gaze angle and sagittal balance. The visual angle (by which the gaze is redirected forward) will always be the same as the osteotomy angle (the angle by which the spine is redirected at the osteotomy) site irrespective of the level of the osteotomy. However, osteotomy at a lower level in the spine will produce greater correction of the sagittal balance (posterior shift of the plumb line) compared with osteotomy at a higher level.[67,68] Figure 128-5 explains the disparate relationship between the osteotomy level and restoration of gaze angle and sagittal balance.

Ideally, kyphotic deformity is best corrected when the osteotomy is placed at the site of maximal deformity. However, the common site for a single-level osteotomy is at

L2–3 level for two reasons: (1) it is safer to do the spinal osteotomy below the level of the cord to prevent catastrophic neurologic damage and (2) osteotomy at a lower level produces greater degree of sagittal balance correction. A single-level lumbar osteotomy usually achieves a correction between 30 and 45 degrees. Most authors estimate the effect of the planned osteotomy at a given level (usually at L2–3), on the posterior shift of the plumb line, from a cutout of a transparent paper tracing over the full-length lateral radiograph (Fig. 128-6). If this angle appears to be smaller than the estimated gaze angle correction, additional smaller osteotomies are planned at a higher level, which have a greater effect on the shift of the gaze angle than the shift of the plumb line. This usually involves a cervicothoracic osteotomy at a later date.

The presence of a hip flexion deformity severely affects both the sagittal balance and the gaze angle, and this must be corrected by total hip replacement before spinal osteotomy is undertaken.

When both lumbar and cervical osteotomy is needed, we perform the lumbar osteotomy in the first stage, achieving maximal correction of the sagittal balance. Cervical osteotomy is performed subsequently for fine-tuning the sagittal balance and gaze angle correction.

FIGURE 128-5 Level of osteotomy has a disparate effect on sagittal balance and gaze angle. Restoration of sagittal balance is achieved by posterior shift of the plumb line (X). The correction of the gaze angle (γ and G) is always the same as the corresponding osteotomy angle (δ and D), respectively. $\delta = \gamma$ and D = G. When osteotomy is performed at a lower level (M), an osteotomy angle δ is needed for restoration of the sagittal balance (X) (*A*). When osteotomy is performed at a higher level (N), a larger osteotomy angle (D) is needed (D > δ) for the same degree of sagittal balance restoration (*B*). Because the osteotomy angle is always same as the gaze angle correction (D = G), the correction of the gaze angle will be larger (G > γ) with a higher level of osteotomy. This may lead to overcorrection of the gaze angle upward. (From Sengupta DK, Khazim R, Grevitt MP, Webb JK: Flexion osteotomy of the cervical spine: A new technique for correction of iatrogenic extension deformity in ankylosing spondylitis. Spine 26:1068–1072, 2001.)

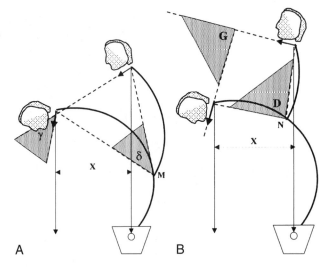

Lumbar Osteotomy: Historical Aspects and Types of Osteotomy

The different techniques of osteotomy described in the lumbar spine may be classified into three basic types.

Smith-Peterson Osteotomy (Monosegmental Anterior Open Wedge Osteotomy)

In this technique, a large wedge of bone is resected from the posterior elements including the lamina and the facet joints and pedicle in the lumbar spine, usually at the L2 level, just below the level of the spinal cord.[65,69–80] The wedge is then closed by hyperextension of the spine with manual pressure. This manipulation causes disruption of the anterior longitudinal ligament and opens up a large gap in the anterior aspect of the vertebral column.

Polysegmental Posterior Closing Wedge Osteotomy

In this technique, multiple small posterior wedge osteotomies are made through the facet joints.[62,81–84] Closing these wedges by osteoclasis gives a more gradual correction and creates only small bony defects anteriorly, thus avoiding the serious vascular and neurologic complications.

Pedicle Subtraction Osteotomy (Lumbar Monosegmental Posterior Closing Wedge Osteotomy)

In this technique, the posterior element of one vertebra including the lamina, facet joints, pedicles, and a posterior wedge of the vertebral body is resected by a transpedicular decancellation procedure (Fig. 128-7).[79,85,86] The wedge is

FIGURE 128-6 Preoperative planning for deformity correction. Chin-brow to vertical angle in this case measures 30 degrees. The sagittal vertical axis drops 13 cm in front of the S-1 (*A*). A silhouette of the spine is drawn on a tracing paper, and the level of the osteotomy is marked at the L3 vertebra (*B*). The tracing paper is now cut at the level of osteotomy and rotated backward, centering the anterior border of the L3 vertebra until the projected plumb line drops over the sacrum (*C*). The angle of rotation gives an estimate of the angle of osteotomy needed to restore the sagittal balance, which is 28 degrees in this case. This osteotomy will also correct the gaze angle by 28 degrees, which is close to full correction of the chin-brow to vertical angle in this case. If larger gaze angle correction would be required in this case, additional cervical osteotomy or polysegmental thoracic osteotomy might be planned instead. The *arrow* indicates the amount of bone to be resected from the posterior elements of the spine, which on closure after osteoclasis at the anterior border of L3 will reproduce the effect of the osteotomy as planned.

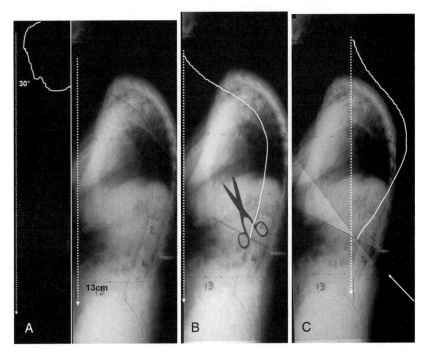

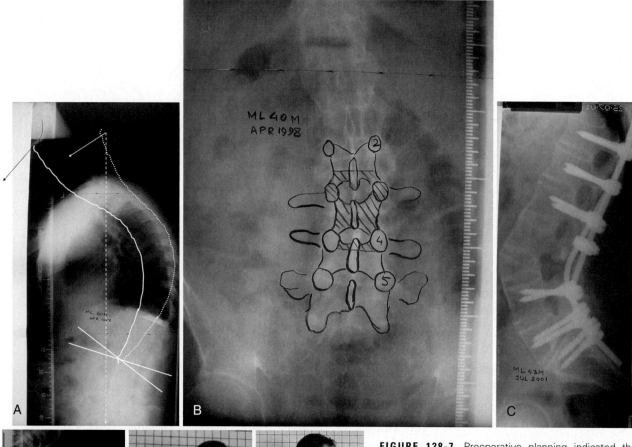

FIGURE 128-7 Preoperative planning indicated that only 30 degrees of corrective osteotomy at the L3 level would adequately restore the sagittal balance but not the gaze angle, which needed approximately 50 degrees of correction (*A*). A 20-degree osteotomy is therefore planned at the L3 level and the amount of bone to be resected is marked out (*B*). Posterior closing wedge osteotomy performed with subtraction of the L3 pedicle (*C*). Three more polysegmental osteotomies were performed in the thoracic spine, with approximately 10 degrees of correction at each level to compensate for the deliberate undercorrection at the lumbar spine (*D*). The net effect was total visual angle correction by 50 degrees and at the same time adequate correction of the sagittal balance. Pre- and postoperative clinical pictures show satisfactory correction of both the sagittal balance and visual angle (*E* and *F*).

closed by hyperextension of the lumbar spine, hinging on the anterior cortex of the vertebral body.

Surgical Technique

The desired angular connection is 40 degrees when restoring sagittal balance and gaze connection. For such a procedure it is preferable to perform a single-level pedicule subtraction osteotomy below the level of conus, usually at L2 or L3. For a larger degree of correction, additional osteotomies are performed at one or two levels in the thoracic spine, averaging 10 to 20 degrees of correction at each level, usually as a staged procedure.

Patient positioning is extremely important. For extreme deformities, a trial of positioning is performed with the awake patient on an appropriate operating table as preoperative planning. The table is broken in the middle like a jackknife before surgery. After osteotomy, the table is gradually flattened to complete the osteoclasis under control. A sudden movement, particularly translation, must be avoided at the osteotomy site to prevent vascular or neurologic catastrophe. A minimum of three levels are instrumented on either side of the osteotomy levels. Once the pedicle screws are inserted, the osteotomy is performed. The apex of the osteotomy is usually placed at the anterior aspect of the vertebral body at the selected level. The minimal amount of bone to be removed from the posterior element is determined from the cutout on the tracing paper at the time of the preoperative planning (see Fig. 128-6). Frequently, the laminectomy is made wider and the remaining laminae must be undercut to prevent impingement on the cauda equina as the osteotomy is closed. The facet joints and the pars above and below the pedicle of the selected level are resected, exposing the exiting nerve roots both above and below the pedicle. This part of the dissection is very similar to that for a standard transforaminal lumbar interbody fusion procedure. The nerve roots are protected, and the pedicles are then removed. The disc and posterior annulus are then excised, and the dorsal part of the vertebral body is removed by transpedicular decancellation.

Once the pedicle subtraction is performed on one side, a short temporary rod is fixed to the pedicle screws at that time. This prevents any accidental translation of the osteotomy site as the pedicle subtraction is completed on the second side. A precontoured definitive rod is then fixed to the distal screws on the second side. The pedicle screws immediately cranial to the osteotomy site should preferably have longer, breakable heads (reduction screws) (Fig. 128-8). The temporary rod is then loosened and osteoclasis is completed, which often feels like the snap of a green tree, by a controlled, gentle effort. The definitive rod on the second side is reduced into the pedicle screws. Finally, the temporary rod on the first side is replaced with a definitive rod. The rods are cross-linked above and below the osteotomy. Before closing, the nerve roots should be checked again to

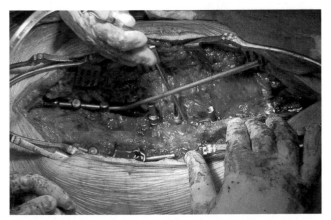

FIGURE 128-8 Operative picture of pedicle subtraction osteotomy. A temporary rod is inserted in the near side. The precontoured definitive rod is fixed to the caudal screws on the far side. The pedicle screws immediately cranial to the osteotomy site are reduction screws (long, breakable extension at the screwhead). The pedicle subtraction is done and the osteoclasis is about to be completed.

make sure they are free from being impinged by closing of the osteotomy gap. The whole procedure is performed under spinal cord monitoring, and a wake-up test is done in case of loss of monitoring signals (Fig. 128-9).

Although a minimum of three levels are instrumented on either side of osteotomy, the proximal instrumentation is often extended above the apex of the kyphosis, to the upper thoracic level, to prevent proximal instrumentation failure. The proximal extension of the instrumentation may be done at a second stage, when additional osteotomies are needed at one or two thoracic levels according to the preoperative planning. Generous chevron osteotomies are done through the facet joints and these are closed by applying compression with the instrumentation. Postoperatively, a molded thoracic lumbar sacral orthosis is used for mobilization out of bed until the osteotomy is consolidated.

Results and Complications

Bridwell and colleagues[87,88] reported 33 patients with a minimum of 2 years of follow-up. Most patients reported improvement in pain and self-image and reported overall satisfaction based on ultimate Scoliosis Research Society questionnaire (SRS-24). There was one pseudarthrosis in the lumbar spine through an area of pedicle subtraction osteotomy (area of previous laminectomy and nonunion), six patients had thoracic pseudarthroses (levels other than the osteotomy level), and one patient had pseudarthrosis at L5–S1. Two patients had acute angular kyphosis at the thoracolumbar junction at the proximal end of the construct. In five patients who experienced transient neurologic deficits, their deficits resolved after central canal enlargement.

Van Royen and De Gast[79] made a structured review of the three methods of lumbar osteotomy. From 856 cases reported in 41 articles published between 1945 and 1998, they selected 523 cases that met the inclusion criteria for analysis of outcome data. They found the average correction ranged between 37 and 40 degrees. Closing wedge osteotomy achieved 3.8 degrees less correction than the other two methods. In contrast, loss of correction was common with open wedge and polysegmental osteotomies but least with closing wedge osteotomy. Rupture of the aorta or its branches was reported only after open wedge osteotomy in 4 of 451 cases. Vascular injuries occurred only when the osteotomy was performed at the L1–2 or L2–3 level but not when it was below the L3 level. Neurological complications were reported in 2.7% after open wedge procedure and 2% after closing wedge procedure. Perioperative mortality was reported in 5.8% with open wedge osteotomy, 2.4% with polysegmental osteotomy, and only 1.3% with closing wedge osteotomy. The data were not suitable for any statistical analysis.

Cervical Osteotomy

Cervicothoracic deformity itself does not produce a significant problem with the sagittal balance but interferes with the forward gaze. A corrective osteotomy therefore should be planned at the cervicothoracic junction, which has less effect on posterior shift of the plumb line, but the gaze angle is corrected by the same magnitude as the osteotomy angle.

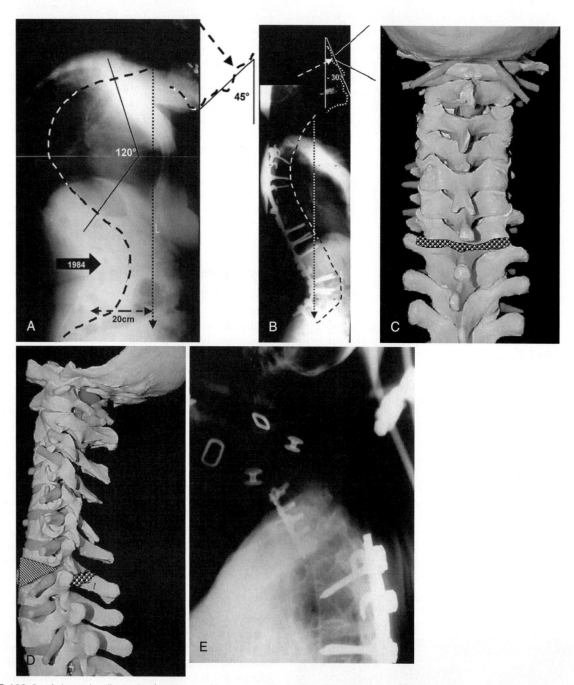

FIGURE 128-9 *A,* Lateral radiograph of a 40-year-old woman with global kyphotic deformity from ankylosing spondylitis who underwent corrective osteotomy of the lumbar spine in 1984. Ten years later, she presented with recurrence of kyphotic deformity measuring 120 degrees, predominantly in the thoracic spine (*A*). The plumb line from odontoid was 20 cm in front of S1. The chin-brow angle measured 45 degrees, limiting the field of vision to within 2.5 m of her feet (*B*). She was treated with multiple osteotomies at T6 and at T8, with posterior stabilization from T2 to L5. The sagittal balance was well corrected, but the gaze angle was deviated upward. The chin-brow angle measured –30 degrees, and the patient could not see anything within 3 m of her feet (*C* and *D*). A flexion osteotomy was performed at the level of C7, as shown in a spine model. A posterior transverse osteotomy was made through the lamina of C7–T1 followed by an anterior closing wedge osteotomy at C7 and plate fixation (*E*). Postoperative lateral radiographs show the corrected position immobilized in a halo.

The preferred site of cervical osteotomy is the C7–T1 level because the vertebral artery and vein, which enters through the transverse foramen at the C6 vertebra, are less likely to be injured when the neck is extended. In addition, the spinal canal is relatively wide at this level. The risk of quadriplegia is the major concern in cervical osteotomy. Urist[89] first described a case of cervical osteotomy under local anesthesia with the patient in sitting position in 1953. The only large series was reported by Simmons[77] of 42 patients, under local anesthesia, using a technique described by Urist, except the deformity was corrected by manipulation at operation, followed by postoperative immobilization in a halo jacket. In 1997, McMaster[90] described internal fixation with a Luque wire in three of his 15 cases to prevent subluxation at the osteotomy site. The only case of a flexion osteotomy to correct iatrogenic extension osteotomy was reported by Sengupta and colleagues[68]

Surgical Technique

Although operating under local anesthesia may be safer, the author (D.K.S.) prefers to operate with the patient under general anesthesia in the prone position, with the head stabilized on Mayfield tongs fixed to the halo. Intubation may be particularly difficult. Awake intubation under local anesthetic with a fiber-optic laryngoscope is recommended. Somatosensory and motor-evoked potentials are monitored.

The caveat in cervical osteotomy is to prevent translation at the site of osteotomy during surgery before the instrumentation stabilizes the spine. Use of transparent drapes for inspection, and application of a preoperative halo to control the head position after osteotomy appear to be helpful. After routine posterior exposure of the spine, lateral mass screws are placed at C4, C5, and C6, and pedicle screws in T2, T3, and T4. A dorsal-based wedge is resected from the whole of the C7 lamina. Parts of the adjacent segment laminae are also resected and undercut to prevent impingement of the C8 nerve roots when the osteotomy is closed. The osteotomy is extended laterally through the fused C7–T1 facet joints, and the C7 and T1 pedicles are removed with the drills to decompress the C8 nerve roots. Before the osteotomy is completed by extension of the neck, a temporary malleable rod is inserted on one side[91] to prevent sudden translation at the osteotomy, similar to that described previously for the pedicle subtraction osteotomy. A 4-mm precontoured definitive rod is inserted into the lateral mass screws cranially. The osteotomy is completed by extending the neck gradually by a gentle, controlled effort, holding the head by the halo and carefully watching the head position through the transparent drapes. Once the osteoclasis through the remaining vertebral body is completed, the precontoured rod lies close to the pedicle screws in the thoracic spine, and the instrumentation is completed. The temporary rod is then replaced with a definitive 4-mm rod.[92] Additional anterior cervical plate fixation at the osteotomy site ensures no postoperative translation. Postoperatively, halo jacket immobilization is used for 6 to 8 weeks followed by a period of molded collar wear until the osteotomy is consolidated.

SUMMARY POINTS

1. AS has a protracted clinical course that is generally managed by medications and lifestyle changes.
2. Owing to osteoporosis and the brittle nature of the spine in AS, cervical and thoracolumbar fractures can result from minimal trauma, with secondary grave neurologic consequences.
3. Due to the instability of fractures in a brittle spine, special consideration of traction and surgery is necessary in AS.
4. Deformity of the spine in AS can constitute a major disability warranting correction.

REFERENCES

1. Keat A: Seronegative spondyloarthropathies: Ankylosing spondylitis. In Klippel JH, Crofford LJ, Stone JH, Weyand CM (eds): Primer on Rheumatic Diseases, 12th ed. Atlanta: The Arthritis Foundation, 2001, pp 250–255.
2. Boumpas DT, Illei GG, Tassiulas IO: Psoriatic arthritis. In Klippel JH, Crofford LJ, Stone JH, Weyand CM (eds): Primer on Rheumatic Diseases, 12th ed. Atlanta: The Arthritis Foundation, 2001, pp 233–237.
3. Arnett FC: Seronegative spondyloarthropathies: Reactive arthritis and enteropathic arthritis. In Klippel JH, Crofford LJ, Stone JH, Weyand CM (eds): Primer on Rheumatic Diseases, 12th ed. Atlanta: The Arthritis Foundation, 2001, pp 245–250.
4. van der Linden S, Valkenburg HA, Cats A: Evaluation of diagnostic criteria for ankylosing spondylitis: A proposal for modification of the New York criteria. Arthritis Rheum 27:361–368, 1984.
5. Dougados M, van der Linden S, Juhlin R, et al: The European Spondylarthropathy Study Group preliminary criteria for the classification of spondylarthropathy. Arthritis Rheum 34:218–227, 1991.
6. Mielants H, Veys EM, Cuvelier C, De Vos M: Course of gut inflammation in spondylarthropathies and therapeutic consequences. Baillieres Clin Rheumatol 10:47–64, 1996.
7. Mielants H, Veys EM, Cuvelier C, de Vos M: Ileocolonoscopic findings in seronegative spondylarthropathies. Br J Rheumatol 27(Suppl 2): 95–105, 1988.
8. Brophy S, Pavy S, Lewis P, et al: Inflammatory eye, skin, and bowel disease in spondyloarthritis: Genetic, phenotypic, and environmental factors. J Rheumatol 28:2667–2673, 2001.
9. Ansell B, Bywaters G, Doniach I: The aortic lesion of ankylosing spondylitis. B Heart J 20:507–515, 1958.
10. Cosh JA: The heart and the rheumatic diseases. Rheumatol Phys Med 11:267–280, 1972.
11. Siede WH, Seiffert UB, Merle S, et al: Alkaline phosphatase isoenzymes in rheumatic diseases. Clin Biochem 22:121–124, 1989.
12. Robinson AC, Teeling M, Casey EB: Hepatic function in ankylosing spondylitis. Ann Rheum Dis 42:550–552, 1983.
13. Sheehan NJ, Slavin BM, Kind PR, Mathews JA: Increased serum alkaline phosphatase activity in ankylosing spondylitis. Ann Rheum Dis 42:563–565, 1983.
14. Kendall MJ, Lawrence DS, Shuttleworth GR, Whitfield AG: Haematology and biochemistry of ankylosing spondylitis. BMJ 2:235–237, 1973.
15. Smith D, Spencer D, Allam B, et al: Serum alkaline phosphatase in ankylosing spondylitis. J Clin Pathol 32:853–854, 1979.
16. Linssen A, Rothova A, Valkenburg HA, et al: The lifetime cumulative incidence of acute anterior uveitis in a normal population and its relation to ankylosing spondylitis and histocompatibility antigen HLA-B27. Invest Ophthalmol Vis Sci 32:2568–2578, 1991.
17. Vilar MJ, Cury SE, Ferraz MB, et al: Renal abnormalities in ankylosing spondylitis. Scand J Rheumatol 26:19–23, 1997.
18. Jones DW, Mansell MA, Samuell CT, Isenberg DA: Renal abnormalities in ankylosing spondylitis. Br J Rheumatol 26:341–345, 1987.
19. Carter R, Riantawan P, Banham SW, Sturrock RD: An investigation of factors limiting aerobic capacity in patients with ankylosing spondylitis. Respir Med 93:700–708, 1999.
20. Boushea DK, Sundstrom WR: The pleuropulmonary manifestations of ankylosing spondylitis. Semin Arthritis Rheum 18:277–281, 1989.
21. Chakera TM, Howarth FH, Kendall MJ, et al: The chest radiograph in ankylosing spondylitis. Clin Radiol 26:455–459, 1975.
22. Lauritzen H, Medina J, Loken MD: Pulmonary disease in patients with ankylosing spondylitis [abstract]. Am Rev Respir Dis 98:126, 1968.
23. Rosenow E, Strimlan CV, Muhm JR, Ferguson RH: Pleuropulmonary manifestations of ankylosing spondylitis. Mayo Clin Proc 52:641–649, 1977.
24. Fox M, Onofrio B: Ankylosing spondylitis. In Menezes AH, Sonntag VH (eds): Principles of Spinal Surgery. New York: McGraw-Hill, 1996, pp 735–750.
25. Lopez de Castro JA: The pathogenetic role of HLA-B27 in chronic arthritis. Curr Opin Immunol 10:59–66, 1998.
26. Benjamin M, McGonagle D: The anatomical basis for disease localisation in seronegative spondyloarthropathy at entheses and related sites. J Anat 199:503–526, 1998.
27. McGonagle D, Gibbon W, Emery P: Classification of inflammatory arthritis by enthesitis. Lancet 352:1137–1140, 1998.
28. McGonagle D, Emery P: Enthesitis, osteitis, microbes, biomechanics, and immune reactivity in ankylosing spondylitis. J Rheumatol 27:2302–2304, 2000.
29. Keller C, Webb A, Davis J: Cytokines in the seronegative spondyloarthropathies and modification by TNF blockage: A brief report and literature review. Ann Rheumatol Dis 62:1128–1132, 2003.
30. Maksymowych WP: Ankylosing spondylitis—at the interface of bone and cartilage [editorial]. J Rheumatol 27:2295–2301, 2000.

31. Weinstein P, Karpman R, Gall E, Pitt M: Spinal cord injury, spinal fracture and spinal stenosis in ankylosing spondylitis. J Neurosurg 67:609–616, 1982.

32. Kabasakal Y, Garrett SL, Calin A: The epidemiology of spondylodiscitis in ankylosing spondylitis—a controlled study. Br J Rheumatol 35:660–663, 1996.

33. Rasker JJ, Prevo RL, Lanting PJ: Spondylodiscitis in ankylosing spondylitis, inflammation or trauma? A description of six cases. Scand J Rheumatol 25:52–57, 1996.

34. Chan FL, Ho EK, Fang D, et al: Spinal pseudarthrosis in ankylosing spondylitis. Acta Radiol 28:383–388, 1987.

35. Fang D, Leong JC, Ho EK, et al: Spinal pseudarthrosis in ankylosing spondylitis: Clinicopathological correlation and the results of anterior spinal fusion. J Bone Joint Surg Br 70:443–447, 1988.

36. Hehne HJ, Becker HJ, Zielke K: Spondylodiscitis in kyphotic deformity of ankylosing spondylitis and its healing affected by dorsal correction osteotomies: Report of 33 patients. Z Orthop Ihre Grenzgeb 128:494–502, 1990.

37. Escosa Bage M, Garcia Navarrete E, Pascual Garvi JM, Sola RG: Surgical treatment of spondylodiscitis in ankylosing spondylitis: Two cases report. Rev Neurol 33:964–966, 2001.

38. Koehler L, Kuipers JG, Zeidler H: Managing seronegative spondarthritides. Rheumatology 39:360–368, 2000.

39. Russel P, Unsworth A, Haslock I: The effect of exercise on ankylosing spondylitis: A preliminary study. Br J Rheumatol 32:498–506, 1993.

40. Inman R: Seronegative spondyloarthropathies: Treatment. In Klippel JH, Crofford LJ, Stone JH, Weyand CM (eds): Primer on Rheumatic Diseases, 12th ed. Atlanta: The Arthritis Foundation, 2001, pp 255–258.

41. Gorman JD, Sack KE, Davis JC Jr: Treatment of ankylosing spondylitis by inhibition of tumor necrosis factor alpha. N Engl J Med 346:1349–1356, 2002.

42. Braun J, Brandt J, Listing J, et al: Treatment of active ankylosing spondylitis with infliximab: A randomized controlled multicenter trial. Lancet 359:1187–1193, 2002.

43. Stone M, Lax M, Payne U, et al: Clinical and imaging correlates of response to treatment with infliximab in patients with ankylosing spondylitis. J Rheumatol 28:1605–1614, 2002.

44. Maksymowich WP, Jhangri GS, Fitzgerald AA, et al: A six month randomized, controlled, double-blind, comparison of intravenous pamidronate (60 mg versus 10 mg) in the treatment of nonsteroidal antiinflammatory drug-refractory ankylosing spondylitis. Arthritis Rheum 46:766–773, 2002.

45. Keffer J, Probert L, Cazlaris H, et al: Transgenic mice expressing human tumour necrosis factor: A predictive genetic model of arthritis. EMBO J 10:4025–4031, 1991.

46. Foo D, Bignami A, Rossier AB: Two spinal cord lesions in a patient with ankylosing spondylitis and cervical spine injury. Neurology 33:245–249, 1983.

47. Hunter T, Dubo HI: Spinal fractures complicating ankylosing spondylitis: A long-term follow-up study. Arthritis Rheum 26:751–759, 1983.

48. Apple DF Jr, Anson C: Spinal cord injury occurring in patients with ankylosing spondylitis: A multicenter study. Orthopedics 18:1005–1011, 1995.

49. Fox MW, Onofrio BM, Kilgore JE: Neurological complications of ankylosing spondylitis. J Neurosurg 78:871–878, 1993.

50. Graham GP, Evans PD: Spinal fractures in patients with ankylosing spondylitis. Injury 22:426–427, 1991.

51. Grisolia A, Bell RL, Peltier LF: Fractures and dislocations of the spine complicating ankylosing spondylitis: A report of six cases. J Bone Joint Surg 49:339–344, 1967.

52. Denis F: The three column spine and its significance in the classification of acute thoracolumbar spinal injuries. Spine 8:817–831, 1983.

53. Osgood CP, Abbasy M, Mathews T: Multiple spine fractures in ankylosing spondylitis. J Trauma Inj Infect Care 15:163–166, 1975.

54. Graham B, Van Peteghem PK: Fractures of the spine in ankylosing spondylitis: Diagnosis, treatment, and complications. Spine 14:803–807, 1989.

55. Rowed DW: Management of cervical spinal cord injury in ankylosing spondylitis: The intervertebral disc as a cause of cord compression. J Neurosurg 77:241–246, 1992.

56. Detwiler KN, Loftus CM, Goderad JC, Menezes AH: Management of cervical spine injuries in patients with ankylosing spondylitis. J Neurosurg 72:210–215, 1990.

57. Taggard DA, Traynelis VC: Management of cervical spinal fractures in ankylosing spondylitis with posterior fixation. Spine 25:2035–2039, 2000.

58. Cooper PR, Cohen A, Rosiello A, Koslow M: Posterior stabilization of cervical spine fractures and subluxations using plates and screws. Neurosurgery 23:300–306, 1988.

59. Miller FH, Rogers LF: Fracture of the dens complicating ankylosing spondylitis with atlantoccipital fusion. J Rheumatol 18:771–774, 1991.

60. Peh WC, Ho EK: Fracture of the odontoid peg in ankylosing spondylitis: Case report. J Trauma Inj Infection Crit Care 38:361–363, 1995.

61. Wilkinson M, Bywaters EGL: Clinical features and course of ankylosing spondylitis. Am Rheum Dis 17:209–228, 1958.

62. Sharp J, Purser DW: Spontaneous atlanto-axial dislocation in ankylosing spondylitis and rheumatoid arthritis. Ann Rheumatol Dis 20:47–77, 1961.

63. Hitchon P, From A, Brenton M, et al: Fractures of the thoracolumbar spine complicating ankylosing spondylitis. J Neurosurg 97:218–222, 2002.

64. Foo D, Rossier AB: Post-traumatic spinal epidural hematoma. Neurosurgery 11:25–32, 1982.

65. Giehl JP, Hehne HJ, Zielke K: Kyphosis correction in ankylosing spondylitis using transpedicular instrumentation. In Bridwell KH, DeWald RL (eds): The Textbook of Spinal Surgery. Philadelphia: Lippincott–Raven, 1997, pp 1159–1167.

66. Simmons EH: Ankylosing spondylitis: Surgical considerations. In Rothman RH, Simeone FA (eds): The Spine, 3rd ed. Philadelphia: WB Saunders, 1992, pp 1447–1511.

67. Lazennec JY, Saillant G, Saidi K, et al: Surgery of the deformities in ankylosing spondylitis: Our experience of lumbar osteotomies in 31 patients. Eur Spine J 6:222–232, 1997.

68. Sengupta DK, Khazim R, Grevitt MP, Webb JK: Flexion osteotomy of the cervical spine: A new technique for correction of iatrogenic extension deformity in ankylosing spondylitis. Spine 26:1068–1072, 2001.

69. Briggs H, Keats S, Schlesinger PT: Wedge osteotomy of spine with bilateral intervertebral foraminotomy: Correction of flexion deformity in five cases of ankylosing arthritis of the spine. J Bone Joint Surg Br 29:1075–1082, 1947.

70. Camargo FP, Cordeiro EN, Napoli MM: Corrective osteotomy of the spine in ankylosing spondylitis: Experience with 66 cases. Clin Orthop 208:157–167, 1986.

71. Goel MK: Vertebral osteotomy for correction of fixed flexion deformity of the spine. J Bone Joint Surg Am 50:287–294, 1968.

72. Herbert JJ: Vertebral osteotomy: Technique, indications and results. J Bone Joint Surg Am 30:680–689, 1948.

73. Herbert JJ: Vertebral osteotomy for kyphosis, especially in Marie-Strumpell Arthritis. J Bone Joint Surg Am 41:291–302, 1959.

74. Law WA: Osteotomy of the spine. Clin Orthop 66:70–76, 1969.

75. Lichtblau PO, Wilson P: Possible mechanism of aorta rupture in orthopaedic correction of rheumatoid spondylitis. J Bone Joint Surg Am 38:123–127, 1956.

76. McMaster MJ, Coventry MB: Spinal osteotomy in ankylosing spondylitis: Technique, complications, and long-term results. Mayo Clin Proc 48:476–486, 1973.

77. Simmons EH: Kyphotic deformity of the spine in ankylosing spondylitis. Clin Orthop 128:65–77, 1977.

78. Smith-Petersen MN, Larson CB, Aufranc OE: Osteotomy of the spine for correction of flexion deformity in rheumatoid arthritis. J Bone Joint Surg Am 27:1–11, 1945.

79. Van Royen BJ, De Gast A: Lumbar osteotomy for correction of thoracolumbar kyphotic deformity in ankylosing spondylitis: A structured review of three methods of treatment. Ann Rheum Dis 58:399–406, 1999.

80. Weatherley C, Jaffray D, Terry A: Vascular complications associated with osteotomy in ankylosing spondylitis: A report of two cases. Spine 13:43–46, 1988.

81. Halm H, Metz-Stavenhagen P, Schmitt A, Zielke K: Surgical treatment of kyphotic spinal deformities in ankylosing spondylitis using the Harrington compression system: Long-term results based on the MOPO scales in the framework of a retrospective questionnaire. Z Orthop Ihre Grenzgeb 133:141–147, 1995.

82. McMaster PE: Osteotomy of the spine for fixed flexion deformity. J Bone Joint Surg Am 44:1207–1216, 1962.

83. Puschel J, Zielke K: Corrective surgery for kyphosis in Bekhterev's disease—indication, technique, results [(author's transl)]. Z Orthop Ihre Grenzgeb 120:338–342, 1982.

84. Wilson MJ, Turkell JH: Multiple spinal wedge osteotomy: Its use in a case of Marie Strumpell spondylitis. Am J Surg 77:777–782, 1949.

85. Scudese VA, Calabro JJ: Vertebral wedge osteotomy: Correction of rheumatoid (ankylosing) spondylitis. JAMA 186:627–631, 1963.
86. Thomasen E: Vertebral osteotomy for correction of kyphosis in ankylosing spondylitis. Clin Orthop 194:142–152, 1985.
87. Bridwell KH, Lewis SJ, Edwards C, et al: Complications and outcomes of pedicle subtraction osteotomies for fixed sagittal imbalance. Spine 28:2093–2101, 2003.
88. Bridwell KH, Lewis SJ, Lenke LG, et al: Pedicle subtraction osteotomy for the treatment of fixed sagittal imbalance. J Bone Joint Surg Am 85:454–463, 2003.
89. Urist MR: Osteotomy of the cervical spine: Report of a case of ankylosing rheumatoid spondylitis. J Bone Joint Surg Am 40:833–843, 1958.
90. McMaster MJ: Osteotomy of the cervical spine in ankylosing spondylitis. J Bone Joint Surg Br 79:197–203, 1997.
91. Mehdian SM, Freeman BJ, Licina P: Cervical osteotomy for ankylosing spondylitis: An innovative variation on an existing technique. Eur Spine J 8:505–509, 1999.
92. Webb JK, Sengupta DK: How do I do it—osteotomy of the cervicothoracic region. In Vaccaro AR, Albert TJ (eds): Tricks of the Trade of Spine Surgery. New York: Thieme, 2002, pp 35–37.

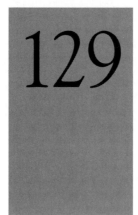

129 Disorders of the Spine Related to Plasma Cell Dyscrasias*

SANFORD KEMPIN and NARAYAN SUNDARESAN

Although all lymphocytic neoplasias may invade the bone, it is the peculiar nature of malignancies of the most mature B cell, the immunoglobulin-secreting cell, that bone destruction dominates the clinical presentation. These disorders are collectively known as the plasma cell dyscrasias and include a broad spectrum of disease presentations (Table 129-1), some of which manifest significant bone destruction[1-10] and others of which exhibit minimal or absent bone destruction.[10-15] This property is not unique to B cells because certain rare T-cell disorders may also manifest this tendency to bone destruction.

The unique clinical presentations of the lymphocytic neoplasias are derived from their phenotypic and ultimately genotypic properties. The B-cell maturational pathway is shown in Figure 129-1. Examples of lymphocytic neoplasias in which bone destruction may occur as a primary phenomenon or with secondary invasion include acute lymphocytic leukemia,[16,17] large cell lymphomas,[18] T-cell leukemia/lymphoma (human T-lymphotropic virus 1 associated),[19] and the plasma cell disorders. These latter disorders can be divided into two major categories: those in which bone involvement is rare or absent, such as benign monoclonal gammopathy and Waldenström's macroglobulinemia,[11-13] IgE myeloma,[14,15] and α, γ heavy chain diseases,[10] and those in which bone lesions are major clinicopathologic manifestations. These latter disorders, the subject of this review, include solitary plasmacytomas without apparent bone marrow involvement (solitary plasmacytoma of bone [SPB]) and those destructive lesions that represent contiguous spread of a primary bone marrow disease, multiple myeloma. Not infrequently extramedullary plasmacytomas may metastasize to bone marrow, and the two disorders then become indistinguishable.[8]

SOLITARY PLASMACYTOMAS OF BONE

Plasmacytomas are tumors composed of malignant plasma cells. When not a part of a systemic bone marrow disease (multiple myeloma), they present either as an SPB or at other sites as extramedullary plasmacytoma, most commonly in the upper airway passages, gastrointestinal tract, lymph nodes, and spleen.[8] Occasionally, more than one bone lesion may be present in the absence of bone marrow involvement. SPBs and extramedullary plasmacytomas may be secretory or nonsecretory and are occasionally associated with light chain urinary excretion (Bence Jones proteinuria). Shaw[23] and Cutler and colleagues[24] were the first to describe solitary plasmacytomas of bone and long survival with surgical resection.

These tumors represent about 3% of plasma cell neoplasms.[25] The disorder is more common in men (3:1) and is seen most frequently in those older than age 50.[8] The frequency of various bone locations as the site of solitary plasmacytomas is shown in Table 129-2.[26-33] The spine is the initial site of presentation in approximately 25% to 50% of cases,[8,27] and the thoracic vertebrae represent nearly one half of the reported cases.[34] Occasionally, the intervertebral disc is the site of occurrence.[35]

Diagnosis

Histologically, these lesions consist of well to poorly differentiated plasma cells, and most lesions contain the entire spectrum of plasma cell maturation (Fig. 129-2; see Color Plate). The cytoplasm is basophilic, and the nucleus is eccentric with pyknotic chromatin ("clock face"). Nucleoli are observed, particularly in plasmablasts. Lesions may be classified as predominantly well differentiated or poorly differentiated.

TABLE 129-1 ■ Plasma Cell Dyscrasias

Disorders	Bone Destruction	References
Benign monoclonal gammopathy	Absent	11
Waldenström's macroglobulinemia	Absent	12,13
Solitary plasmacytoma	Present (localized)	132
Multiple plasmacytomas	Present	132
Multiple myelomas		
IgG	Present	1,2,6
IgA	Present	1,2,6
IgD	Present	5,20
IgE	Rare	14,15,96
Light chain disease	Present	7
Heavy chain disease		
α Heavy chain	Absent	22
γ Heavy chain	Rare	10
δ Heavy chain	Present	3
μ Heavy chain	Rare	9
Nonsecretory	Present	21

*This chapter has been adapted from Sundaresan N, Schmidek HH, Schiller AL, Rosenthal DI (eds): Tumors of the Spine: Diagnosis and Clinical Management. Philadelphia: WB Saunders, 1990.

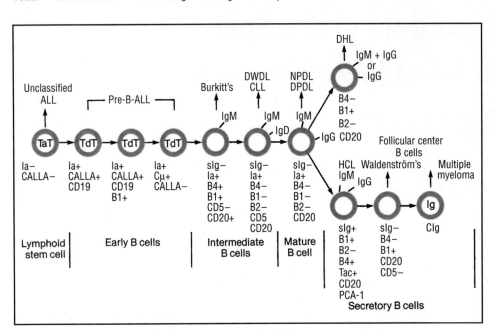

FIGURE 129-1 Phenotypic correlation of B-cell neoplasia. (Adapted from Longo D, Klima P, Korsmyer S: ABCO Educational Booklet, 1966.)

Amyloid has occasionally been observed in blood vessels and interstitium,[8,32] although systemic amyloidosis has only rarely been reported.[32] Immunohistochemical studies of a series of solitary plasmacytomas of bone demonstrated IgG but no other heavy chain in the cytoplasm. Light chain analysis demonstrated a κ-to-λ ratio of approximately 1:1.[32] Woodruff and colleagues[33] reported on a series of 12 patients with SPB, in which one patient was found to have an IgA serum paraprotein and one to have urinary λ chains (two of 12 = 16%). A higher incidence of paraproteinemia was found by Meis and colleagues[32]; 77% of patients with SPB in this series subsequently demonstrated a monoclonal protein, although only eight of 17 were detected at diagnosis (47%). A similar frequency of paraprotein secretion was described by Bataille and Sany,[27] as six of 18 (30%) demonstrated a paraprotein (IgG-κ = 3; IgG-λ = 1; κ light chain = 2). Wiltshaw[8] reported that seven of 11 patients at initial presentation had increases in the immunoglobulin fraction as a single narrow band (immunoelectrophoretic study results not reported). In three patients, a paraprotein developed after dissemination (total, 10 of 11 patients).

Radiographically, the lesions are predominantly osteolytic and have been described as either multicystic (multilobular "soap bubble") lesions, seen predominantly in the long bones, ilium, and mandible, or sharply demarcated destructive lesions.[36] These latter are seen predominantly in the spine[8] (Fig. 129-3A, B). Occasional osteosclerotic lesions have been reported.[27,37–40] Bone scintigraphy findings may be normal or may show reduced uptake[41] in spite of radiographic evidence of destruction.[40] Purely lytic lesions are likely to yield a negative result on radionuclide scanning.[42] Computed tomography and magnetic resonance imaging have been used to diagnose vertebral lesions[43–45] (see Fig. 129-3C to E). Spinal angiography is frequently used to evaluate tumor neovascularity and to identify spinal cord blood supply (see Fig. 129-3F). Plasmacytomas are hypervascular tumors and frequently invade the adventitia of the vertebral artery, especially lesions involving the cervical spine (Fig. 129-4). Thus presurgical embolization may be required to obliterate tumor blood supply before surgery.

The pathogenesis of these neoplasms is not known. They may arise from plasma cells already in bone structures, although lymphatic nodules are not generally found in bone, and thus they are unlikely to arise de novo. Their origin in circulating lymphocytes and clonogenic plasma cells appears possible, although it is difficult to understand the solitary nature of some plasmacytomas by this route. More likely, local spread from bone marrow lymphoid nodules in close proximity to a still undefined localized bone lesion is the origin of the plasmacytoma. The vast majority (83% in Wiltshaw's

TABLE 129-2 ▪ Location of Solitary Plasmacytomas of Bone

Ref.	No. of Patients	S	R	H/F	ST/C/SC	IL/IS/SA	C-V	T-V	L-V
Woodruff et al[133]	12	—	4	1	3	1	—	2	1
Corwin et al[31]	12	—	2	2	1	4	—	3	—
Bataille et al[8]	18	—	2	1	3	1	1	6	4
Bacci et al*[3]	15	—	—	—	—	—	2	8	5
Loftus et al*[79]	6	—	—	—	—	—	—	1	5
Feldman et al*[42]	11	—	—	—	—	1	—	5	5
Meis et al[86]	22	2	4	2	5	3	—	4	2
Chak et al[24]	20	2	2	—	1	6	—	8	1

*Series reporting only spinal plasmacytomas

S, skull; R, ribs; H/F, humerus/femur; ST/C/SC, sternum/clavicle/scapula; IL/IS/SA, ilium/ischium/sacrum; C-V, cervical vertebrae; T-V, thoracic vertebrae; L-V, lumbar vertebrae.

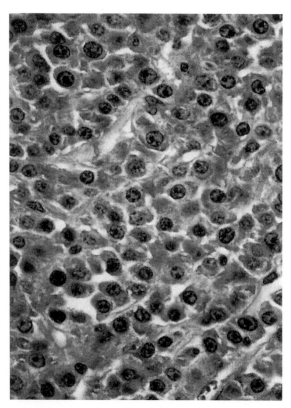

FIGURE 129-2   Plasmacytoma by light microscopy (see also Color Plate.)

series) of primary osseous plasmacytomas occur in bones with active hematopoiesis, suggesting a contiguous spread from the marrow cavity. The high incidence of eventual generalized dissemination gives some credence to this concept. The cause of these neoplasms is not known. Associations of plasmacytomas with previous injury to bone may be the basic underlying cause. There is no known association with previous radiation; however, exposure to asbestos has been linked to the appearance of lymphoid and plasma cell malignancies.[46] Infection, if chronic, could conceivably set up a nidus for lymphocyte and plasma cell proliferation.[47]

The initial presenting symptom in SPB in almost all patients is pain, the distribution of which depends upon the location of the lesion. The mean duration of pain before diagnosis in the series of Bataille and Sany[27] was 6 months. Spinal solitary plasmacytomas may involve the cord or nerve root, with subsequent pain in a radicular distribution,[30] and occasionally paraplegia.[26] In one series, almost 25% of patients with spinal SPB underwent laminectomy because of neurologic involvement. In addition to pain, the secretion of a paraprotein may result in a variety of clinical syndromes, including coagulation abnormalities, hyperviscosity, renal failure, and amyloidosis. In general, the level of paraprotein is considerably lower in SPB (24% to 54%)[48] than in multiple myeloma, and these syndromes are uncommon. An unusual paraneoplastic syndrome has been

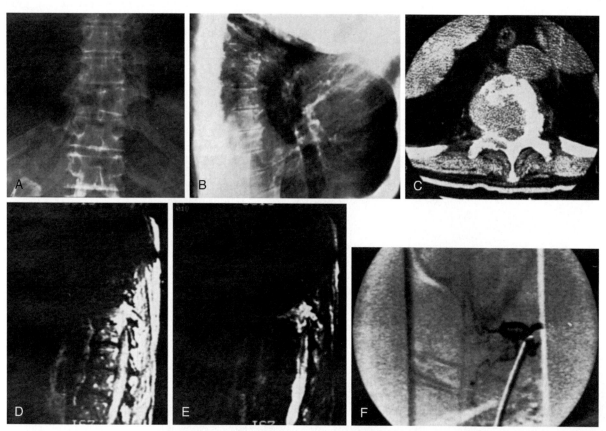

FIGURE 129-3   *A,* Multilobular plasmacytoma demonstrating a lytic defect of T9. *B,* Large lytic defect of the T9 vertebral body demonstrating a wedge compression fracture. *C,* Computed tomography of T9 shows replacement of the vertebral body by plasmacytoma. *D,* Magnetic resonance imaging (MRI) (T1-weighted image) shows an abnormal signal in the T9 body. *E,* MRI (T2-weighted image) in the same patient shows the subarachnoid space and a paraspinal soft-tissue mass. *F,* Spinal arteriography demonstrates the anterior spinal artery arising from the left T9 vascular pedicle.

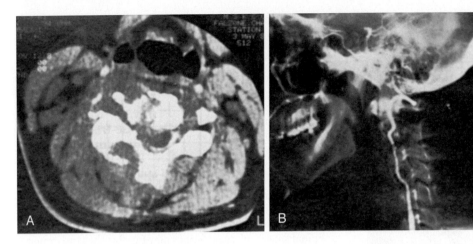

FIGURE 129-4 *A,* Computed tomography of the cervical spine, axial section, shows a soft-tissue tumor with bone destruction extending to the foramen transversarium. *B,* Left vertebral arteriography demonstrates irregularities along the C3–4 segment, indicating tumor invasion of the adventitia.

associated with an osteosclerotic tumor of the thoracic vertebrae consisting of polyneuropathy, skin hyperpigmentation, edema, and hypertrichosis.[49]

The differential diagnosis of osteolytic bone lesions includes prostate cancer[50] and breast cancer.[40] The diagnosis of SPB can be made by needle biopsy.[51] Care must be taken with this procedure in view of a reported episode of massive bleeding related to the biopsy.[52] For spine plasmacytomas, myelography is recommended to determine the extent, if any, of epidural compression. Once the diagnosis of an SPB is made, a search for systemic disease is undertaken. A complete skeletal survey and MRI[53] are necessary to determine the solitary nature of the lesion. A bone marrow aspiration and biopsy are performed. Serum and urinary (24-hour concentrated specimen) paraprotein studies should be performed. The presence of a paraprotein does not necessarily mean that the disease is systemic in nature. The level can be followed to document eradication of the disease as well as recurrence or persistence of a focus of plasma cells.

Treatment

Once staging confirms the presence of a spinal SPB, radiation therapy may be considered the treatment of choice for minimally involved vertebrae. The dose of radiation should be at least 3500 cGy,[54,55] a dose that in one study was found to be associated with no local recurrences for SPB of the spine.[54] Higher doses have been recommended by others (4000–5000 cGy).[1,56] Once enough bone destruction has occurred to result in destabilization (Fig. 129-5), and pain or a neurologic deficit has occurred, resection of tumor and a stabilization procedure should be carried out promptly (Fig. 129-6). This returns the patient promptly to functional status, and further therapy, either radiotherapy or chemotherapy, can then be undertaken.

Several reviews have addressed the role of surgery for these tumors, and numerous techniques, with both anterior and posterior vertebral approaches, have been used.[57–66] If the lesion has not been completely resected,

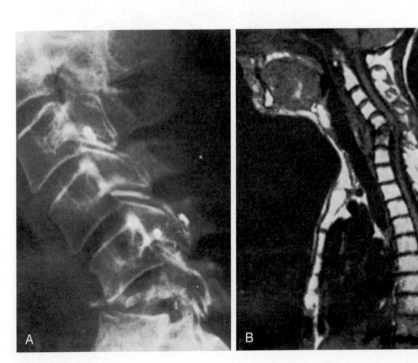

FIGURE 129-5 *A,* Compression fracture with subluxation of the C6 vertebra. This finding should prompt consideration of surgical stabilization in addition to radiation. *B,* T1-weighted image shows an abnormal signal in the C7 body with extension into the posterior elements.

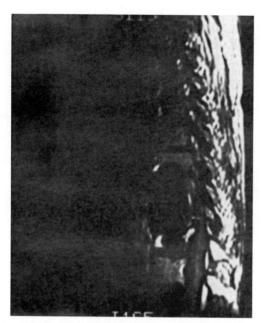

FIGURE 129-6 Postoperative magnetic resonance imaging shows resection of a T9 tumor and replacement of a resected segment with methyl methacrylate. (The same patient is shown in Figure 129-3.)

Prognosis

The evolution of surgically removed and/or radiated solitary plasmacytomas of the spine depends on the completeness of staging for systemic disease at initial presentation, as well as various recognized prognostic factors. Although soft tissue plasmacytomas have an excellent prognosis,[33,56,78] soft-tissue extension from bone disease appears to be a poor prognostic factor; in five of eight patients (60%) in one study multiple myeloma developed. Multiple plasmacytomas are harbingers of systemic disease, although survival rate is better than that for multiple myeloma.[8,25] Both prominence of nucleoli and cellular immaturity (poorly differentiated plasma cells) of SPB are significantly related to the development of multiple myeloma.[32] The presence of either a serum or a urine paraprotein has been documented in 24% to 54% of patients[29,48]; however, its presence does not necessarily suggest dissemination into multiple myeloma because only one fourth of patients (25%) in one series had this complication. Bataille and Sany[27] found older age, spinal involvement, and persistence of a monoclonal protein to be poor prognostic factors for the subsequent development of dissemination. The prognosis for patients presenting with paraplegia may be quite satisfactory after aggressive surgical and radiotherapeutic approaches.[34,75–77] The occurrence of a second isolated plasmacytoma after therapy is occasionally compatible with long-term disease-free survival and cure without dissemination into multiple myeloma.

The results of treatment of plasmacytomas of the spine are outlined in Table 129-3. Bacci and colleagues[26] reported on 15 patients. Therapy included radiation therapy alone (11 patients), surgery and radiation therapy (four patients), and systemic chemotherapy (three patients). One half of the patients had multiple myeloma from 1 to 8 years (mean, 3.5 years) after initial diagnosis. Loftus and colleagues[31] reported on a series of six patients with isolated plasmacytoma of the lower thoracic and lumbar regions. Bone marrow studies and protein electrophoresis were not performed in all patients. All patients underwent laminectomy and spinal fusion (autologous bone and Harrington rods). One half of the patients ultimately experienced systemic disease. Feldman and colleagues[30] reported on 11 cases of solitary plasmacytoma of the spine; in four metastatic plasmacytoma developed and in three medullary disease developed after 1, 4, and 20 years. These patients received radiation therapy and chemotherapy. The degree of initial surgical resection was not stated. Chak and colleagues[28] reported on a series of 20 patients with SPB, of whom nine presented with spinal disease (45%). These lesions were predominantly thoracic (eight of nine). The patients were initially treated with surgical resection (partial) followed by radiotherapy (3000 to 6000 cGy). Multiple myeloma evolved from seven of nine solitary plasmacytomas

postoperative radiation to a total of 3500–5000 cGy must be given. The role of postoperative radiation and adjuvant chemotherapy in the absence of gross residual disease and the role of chemotherapy after radiation therapy have not been rigorously tested. However, for those patients in whom a high risk of dissemination is likely to be present despite apparent complete resection, the use of systemic adjuvant therapy is recommended. Examples of such patients include those with soft-tissue extension or cellular immaturity and older patients. Since Bataille and Sany[27] found spinal disease itself to have a poorer prognosis than other sites of SPB, one might consider all patients with spinal SPB at risk of recurrence and dissemination and apply adjuvant chemotherapy. Alkylating agents (melphelan), steroids, and anthracyclines (doxorubicin) are active agents. However, long-term adjuvant therapy must be shown to be effective before definitive recommendations. For example, chronic alkylating agent therapy is associated with some risk of leukemia,[67,68] and it would be necessary in a randomized study to prove its ultimate benefit. New active agents for the treatment of multiple myeloma such as thalidomide,[69] Revlimid,[70] and bortezomib[72,73] have not been tested for this clinical situation. Disappearance of a paraprotein after therapy should be documented, and its recurrence or appearance after therapy signifies residual disease or dissemination.[34,73,74]

TABLE 129-3 ▪ Results of Therapy of Plasmacytomas of the Spine

Ref.	No. of Patients	Therapy	NED/MM	Time to MM Mean (Range) (yr)
Bacci et al[26]	15	XRT, SURG, CTH	7/8	3.5 (1–8)
Loftus et al[31]	6	SURG	3/3	
Feldman et al[30]	11	XRT, CTH, (SURG)	7/4	8 (1–20)
Chak et al[28]	9	XRT, SURG	2/7	

XRT, radiotherapy alone; SURG, surgery; CTH, chemotherapy; NED, no evidence of disease; MM, multiple myelomas.

and was responsible for death in four patients. In this series, two patients have not had multiple myeloma. Therefore, in most patients described in the literature with solitary plasmacytoma of the spine, the condition ultimately progressed into multiple myeloma,[26,27] as opposed to peripheral lesions, for which the incidence is considerably lower.[26] Therefore, systemic chemotherapy is warranted in this group of patients after local therapy has been applied. The type and duration of this therapy, however, should be determined by clinical trials.

MULTIPLE MYELOMA

Involvement of the spine in multiple myeloma is always present but not always symptomatic. As a systemic disorder beginning initially in the bone marrow and spreading outward to the bone surrounding the marrow cavity and to other bone structures, soft tissues, organs, and blood (leukemia phase), multiple myeloma may be considered the most osteophilic of all lymphoproliferative diseases and the one in which bone involvement and subsequent destruction are the predominant clinical manifestations.

Multiple myeloma is a disease of adult life, with an incidence ranging from 2.0 to 3.1 per 100,000.[79,80] Only rarely have pediatric cases been reported.[81,82] The incidence is somewhat higher in males than females.[1] The median age at presentation is 62 years[6] and increases with age.[83] Multiple myeloma appears to be a more frequent manifestation of lymphoproliferative disease in blacks than in whites, with an incidence in one series of 2.1 per 100,000 whites and of 4.0 per 100,000 blacks.[80,84] The age at which myeloma appears in blacks is younger than that in whites, and a higher frequency of thoracolumbar fractures and solitary plasmacytomas was found in one study.[85]

Diagnosis

The disorder begins as a neoplastic proliferation of plasma cells in association with stromal elements in areas of hematopoietically active bone marrow (vertebrae, ribs, skull, pelvis, sternum). Genetic abnormalities,[86] including abnormalities of oncogenes[87] and suppressor genes, are present[86] particularly when fluorescence in situ hybridization (FISH) is performed.[88] The microenvironment of the bone marrow favors a close interaction of plasma cells and stromal elements. This interaction results from cytokines,[89] proteoglycans,[90] and adhesion molecules on plasma cells,[91] as well as products produced in stromal elements favoring plasma cells proliferation.[92,93] The formed tumors erode adjacent bone structures and osteolytic lesions arise. The bone resorption can be observed microscopically, demonstrating prominent osteoclast activating factor (OAF) activity in areas of resorption but few if any plasma cells in direct contact with bone structures. A number of other molecules have been shown to exert similar effects and include IL-1B,[94] TNF-B,[95,101] IL-6,[96] and osteoprotegerin.[97] The bone marrow stroma/microenvironment also contribute to bone resorption by interaction with myeloma cells and osteoclasts.[98] The extent of skeletal metastases appears to be correlated with production of osteoclast-activating factor by myeloma cells[99] and may be dependent on endogenous prostaglandin E synthesis.[100] Evidence from a 1986 study suggests that tumor necrosis factor and lymphotoxin play

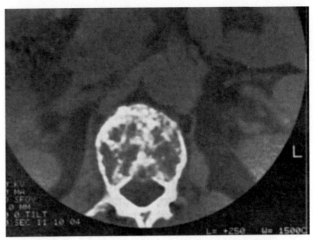

FIGURE 129-7   Axial computed tomography of L2 shows multiple lytic lesions in the body, which can be confused with osteoporosis.

significant roles.[101] Grossly, the marrow is replaced by small grayish pink soft nodules (less than 1 cm), with intervening normal bone marrow. Histologically, the nodules consist of plasma cells of relatively uniform size. The cytoplasm is intensely basophilic; the nucleus has the typical "cartwheel" appearance. Multinucleate large and bizarre-looking plasma cells may occasionally be noted. A more diffuse infiltration may result in generalized bone rarefaction or osteoporosis.[102] Occasionally, multiple myeloma demonstrating numerous lytic lesions in a single vertebral body may mimic osteoporosis and, therefore, should be considered in the differential diagnosis of osteoporotic compression fractures (Fig. 129-7).

The pathophysiologic characteristics of multiple myeloma are directly related to the presence of the myeloma cells in the bone marrow, their direct proximity to bone, as well as their proliferative and secretory capacity. The result of bone marrow replacement by myeloma cells is most often anemia, not an uncommon presenting symptom.[6,103] Most often the anemia is normochromic and normocytic; however, macrocytosis and occasionally megaloblastosis may be present.[104] Red blood cell autoagglutination (rouleau formation) is commonly observed. Patients may present with neutropenia and thrombocytopenia; the incidence of these latter two complications is approximately 16% and 13%, respectively.[6] The expansion of the tumors within the marrow cavity results in pain, a common presenting symptom. As the tumors expand further, bone destruction with hypercalcemia and fractures occur. Hypercalcemia is present in 30% of patients at diagnosis and during the course of the illness may be present in as many as two thirds of the patients.[105] Occasionally, calcium-binding paraproteins may protect against the clinical manifestations of hypercalcemia.[106] The secretion of a monoclonal paraprotein can be documented in almost all patients, with IgG-secreting myelomas the most common[107] (Table 129-4). The presenting clinical features of the disorder and their relationship to the immunochemical class are shown in Table 129-5, taken from a review by Hobbs.[108] Pseudohyponatremia and reduced anion gap,[109] and a hyperviscosity syndrome[110] may all result. Impaired hemostasis due to interference in blood coagulation is commonly observed[111] and is related to

TABLE 129-4 ▪ Types of Monoclonal Proteins Produced by Myeloma Cells

Type of Protein	Patients (%)
IgG	52
IgA	21
IgM	2
IgD	<0.01
IgE	
Light chain secretion (κ or λ) only	11
Heavy chain secretion (γ, α, μ) only	<1
Two or more monoclonal proteins	0.5
No monoclonal protein in serum or urine	1

From Pruzanski W, Ogryzlo MA: Abnormal proteinuria in malignant diseases. Adv Clin Chem 13:355, 1970.

interference in fibrin polymerization,[112,113] inhibitors of clotting factors (particularly factor VIII),[114] accelerated clearance of clotting factors,[115,116] and platelet function abnormalities.[111] Impaired renal function is related to the tubular damage induced by immunoglobulin light chain (particularly λ light chain) metabolism by renal tubular cells with subsequent tubular cast formation[117] as well as to hypercalciuria and nephrocalcinosis, hyperuricosuria, and plasma cell infiltration of the kidneys.[117]

The diagnosis of multiple myeloma is not difficult if symptoms are present. In general, such patients complain of skeletal pain and a decreased performance status related to anemia, renal failure, or infections. Radiographs of painful regions often disclose osteolytic lesions, and a skeletal survey demonstrates multiple osteolytic lesions throughout the skeleton. Other malignant neoplasms may mimic the skeletal findings (breast cancer, prostate cancer, renal cancer, and other malignant lymphomas).[118] A complete blood count demonstrates anemia, and a blood smear examination is likely to demonstrate rouleau formation and occasional plasmacytoid lymphocytes and plasma cells. A biochemical profile demonstrates an elevated globulin fraction and increased blood urea nitrogen and creatinine levels if renal impairment is present, hypercalcemia (30% at diagnosis), and hyperuricemia. The alkaline phosphatase concentration

is frequently normal or only slightly elevated. Metabolic bone disease such as hyperparathyroidism may mimic some of the findings such as bone destruction, hypercalcemia, and renal dysfunction, but the bone marrow findings are normal and the protein studies demonstrate no monoclonal proteins. A bone marrow study demonstrates increased numbers of plasma cells, many of which are large and atypical with binucleate forms. In general, more than 30% of the nucleated marrow elements are plasma cells. Occasionally, a lesser percentage may be present, but their atypia satisfies the criteria for multiple myeloma. Bone marrow samples should be studied for cytogenetic, cytometric abnormalities, and plasma cell labeling index.[1] The differential diagnosis of marrow plasmacytosis includes chronic infections, liver disease, and other neoplasms. Serum protein electrophoresis, immunoelectrophoresis, and immunofixation are necessary to determine the presence of the abnormal protein and to define its class; serum free light chain analysis may also be used. Urine should be concentrated and screened as well for the presence of light chains. A β_2-microglobulin level is obtained as a prognostic factor and followed during therapy.[119] Once the patient is completely evaluated and the diagnosis established, the patient is staged according to the Myeloma Staging System[120] (Table 129-6). The classification is based on the tumor mass as manifested by various clinical parameters, including hemoglobin value, serum calcium level, bone radiographic results, level of M-component, and renal function. Prognostic factors that indicate an aggressive course include certain immunoglobulin classes,[121,122] proteinuria greater than 40 mg/dL,[120,123] a serum albumin concentration less than 3 g/dL,[120,123] poor performance status,[124] and excessive weight loss.[125] The influence of neurologic deficit, particularly related to spinal disease, has not been specifically examined as a prognostic factor, although a large measure of the performance status is related to this problem.

Treatment

The treatment of multiple myeloma must take into account the systemic nature of the disease, its metabolic complications, and the almost universal destruction of the skeleton, with pain as the predominant clinical manifestation and

TABLE 129-5 ▪ Clinical Features at the Time of Diagnosis in 212 Patients with Myelomatosis of Different Classes

Clinical Feature	Class			κ^2 Tests	
	γG	γA	BJ	Classes Compared	Significance
No. of patients	112	54	40		
Mean serum level M-protein (g/100/mL)	4.3	2.8	±	γG : γA	P < .001
Mean doubling time of M-protein (mo)	10.1	6.3	3.4	γG : γA : BJ	P < .02
Lytic bone lesions (%)	55	65	78	γG : BJ	P < .02
Hypercalcemia (%)	33	59	62	γG : γA + BJ	P < .001
Serum urea > 79 mg/100 mL (%)	16	17	33	γG : + γA : BJ	P < .02
Normal immunoglobulins < 20 mean normal (%)	68	30	19	γG : γA + BJ	P < .001
Hospital admissions because of infection* (%)	60	33	20	γG : γA + BJ	P < .005
Detected amyloidosis† (%)	0.5	7	10		

*In 48 γG, 21 γA, 20 BJ myelomata followed up to 3 years.
†In 228 γG, 102 γA, 94 BJ myelomata.
From Hobbs JR: Immunochemical classes of myelomatosis: Including data from a therapeutic trial conducted by a medical research council working party. Br J Haematol 16:599–606, 1969.

TABLE 129-6 ▪ Myeloma Staging System

Stage	Criteria	Measured Myeloma Cell Mass (cells x $10^{12}/m^2$)

I	All of the following:
	1. Hemoglobin value > 10 g/100 mL
	2. Serum calcium value (normal < 12 mg/100 mL)
	3. On roentgenogram, normal bone structure (scale 0) or solitary bone plasmacytoma only
	4. Low M-component production rates
	   a. IgG value < 5 /100 mL
	   b. IgA value < 3 g/100 mL
	   c. Urine light chain M-component on electrophoresis < 4 g/24 hr
		<0.6
		(low)

II	Fitting neither stage I nor stage III	0.6–1.20 (intermediate)

III	One or more of the following:
	1. Hemoglobin value < 8.5 g/100 mL
	2. Serum calcium value > 12 g/100 mL
	3. Advanced lytic bone lesions (scale 3)
	4. High M-component production rates
	   a. IgG value > 7 g/100 mL
	   b. IgA value > 5 g/100 mL
	   c. Urine light chain M-component on electrophoresis > 12 g/24 hr	

Subclassification:
A = Relatively normal renal function (serum creatinine value < 2 mg/100 mL)
B = Abnormal renal function (serum creatinine value > 2 mg/100 mL)

From Durie BJM, Salmon SE: A clinical staging system for multiple myeloma: Correlation of measured cell mass with presenting clinical features, response to treatment, and survival. Cancer 36:842–854, 1975. Copyright © 1975 American Cancer Society. Reprinted with permission of Wiley-Liss, Inc., a subsidiary of John Wiley & Sons, Inc.

neurologic deficit as its major manifestation of morbidity. Treatment of patients with stage I disease in the absence of clinical symptoms is controversial because the time of evolution into symptomatic disease may be quite prolonged. There are no studies that demonstrate an advantage to treating the disease at diagnosis versus waiting until symptoms arise.[126] Unfortunately, the first clinical manifestations may be epidural compression and neurologic compromise. It is not known whether early therapy may prevent these complications. Once symptoms arise and it is clear that the disease is progressing, treatment is instituted with specific antineoplastic agents, radiation therapy, and therapy of complications. Alkylating agents remain the predominant chemotherapy agents used; they include cyclophosphamide,[127] melphalan,[128] and bis-chloroethyl-nitrosourea.[129] Cyclophosphamide and melphalan appear equally effective, with a higher response rate than nitrosoureas.[129,130] Both cyclophosphamide and melphalan do not appear to demonstrate cross-resistance.[131] Pulse prednisone and pulse dexamethasone are highly active agents that cause regression of the myeloma mass, control hypercalcemia and proteinuria, and improve myelosuppression.[132] The combination of melphalan and prednisone appears superior to either alone.[134] Previously used combinations include multiple alkylating agents and vincristine,[135] and alkylating agents and doxorubicin HCl (Adriamycin).[136] Although it would appear from results cited that more aggressive combination programs appear more effective, particularly for patients in an advanced stage (stage III), this assumption is not universally accepted.[137] Until recently the use of infusional vincristine, Adriamycin, and dexamethasone (VAD) represented the initial treatment of choice for many investigators.[138] However, recent studies demonstrating the superiority of thalidomide plus dexamethasone (Thal-Dex) compared to VAD now make this the treatment of choice as

front-line therapy.[139] New active agents include thalidomide,[69] lenalidomide, an analogue of thalidomide,[140] and bortezomib.[141] Such agents are likely to enter into front-line therapy in the future. High-dose melphalan therapy with autologous bone marrow rescue was reported in 1986.[142] Stem cell transplantation has become initial standard therapy for patients without significant comorbiditites and was superior to chemotherapy with respect to survival and response.[143] Interferon is an active agent in myeloma[144] and has been combined with chemotherapy.[145] Although significant progress has been made using chemotherapy, molecular biologic therapy, and stem cell transplantation, the disease is only rarely curable.

Radiation therapy when used judiciously with chemotherapy represents an important therapeutic tool, particularly for the palliative therapy of painful bone lesions and neurologic syndromes related to tumor compression of central and peripheral nervous system structures. Myelosuppression and subsequent decrease in chemotherapy tolerance (the mainstay of therapy) should limit the use of this modality to specific disease-related complications. Painful extremity lesions can be treated over a short period (3 to 5 days) with total doses of 500 to 1500 cGy. More proximal lesions, such as in ribs or vertebrae, may be treated with even a single dose of 800 cGy. Paraspinal lesions generally are more resistant, and doses of 3000 cGy over several weeks need to be administered.[146] Radiation therapy has occasionally been used in the form of total body irradiation, but results have only been palliative.[147] Other wide-field techniques have been used for resistant disease, particularly with intractable pain syndromes; they include half body (both upper and lower)[148] as well as whole bone marrow irradiation.[149] Lack of response to radiotherapy suggests the presence of pathologic fractures needing orthopedic intervention.

Although every bone in the body may be involved in the myelomatous process, it is the spine that tends to dominate the clinical course of this disease, because of both its support function as well as its protective function with respect to the central and peripheral nervous system. The most common symptom of spine involvement is pain, as it is the most common presenting symptom in myeloma. In one study, 87% of patients with myeloma presented with back pain,[150] and in another 75% presented with pain from multiple bone sites.[151] The quality of pain is described as sharp or lancinating and is frequently radiating in type. The pain may be related to bone destruction with subsequent collapse of the vertebrae as well as nerve root compression. Spinal cord compression may be present in as many as 10% of patients during the course of their disease.[152–154] Because pain is often the presenting symptom of a process that may ultimately lead to cord compression and paraparesis, the initial workup of this symptom must include a careful neurologic examination. Radiographic studies should include complete spinal films (generally performed as part of the initial diagnostic evaluation) as well as computed tomography studies. This latter study is particularly useful in determining the degree of myelomatous involvement and destruction of the vertebral body and pedicles, extraosseous spread of the tumor, and cause of spinal cord compression (tumor, collapsed vertebrae, or both).[155,156] A myelogram is obtained if there is any evidence of neurologic deficit. Bisphosphonates are almost universally used to delay skeletal events, prolong survival, and treat hypercalcemia.[158]

Prognosis

Once the appropriate diagnosis of the cause of the pain or neurologic deficit is made, the most appropriate local therapy (either surgery, radiotherapy, or both) is quickly applied in addition to systemic therapy. Surgery plays an important role in the plasma cell disorders with spinal involvement with respect to both diagnosis and therapy. Multiple myeloma rarely presents as an isolated lytic lesion of the vertebral column, and diagnosis is generally made by bone marrow examination. The role, therefore, of surgery, in multiple myeloma is more a therapeutic one. Spine involvement with myeloma represents a particularly difficult surgical problem. The general condition of the patient may be quite poor with infections, renal failure, and hypercalcemia. Hemostatic abnormalities make surgical approaches to the spine particularly hazardous. However, when pain and neurologic deficit are caused by vertebral body destruction and collapse, surgery is necessary to decompress the spinal cord and nerve roots. Vertebral body resection and stabilization by a variety of techniques are often necessary to relieve symptoms and prevent paraplegia. The extent of vertebral resection depends on the radigraphic investigations that determine the extent of involvement, the degree of vertebral destruction, and technical factors related to local anatomic structures. A variety of techniques have been developed with respect to both surgical approaches[62,158–161] and techniques of stabilization after resection.[59,61,63,65,66,159–165]

Figure 129-8 outlines in schematic form the workup of a patient with myeloma and back pain and a therapeutic decision tree. In the absence of a neurologic deficit, an anatomic localization of the cause of the pain is necessary. This can be accomplished by a computed tomography scan. If a paraspinal mass or vertebral destruction without destabilization is present, chemotherapy is begun. An orthopedic or back support is useful because collapse of vertebral tissue may ensue once the myelomatous tissue is destroyed and until new bone forms. If symptoms are not relieved or worsen, repeat computed tomography scan and myelography are performed. If no vertebral destabilization is present or epidural compression is diagnosed, radiotherapy is given and chemotherapy continued. If symptoms continue or worsen,

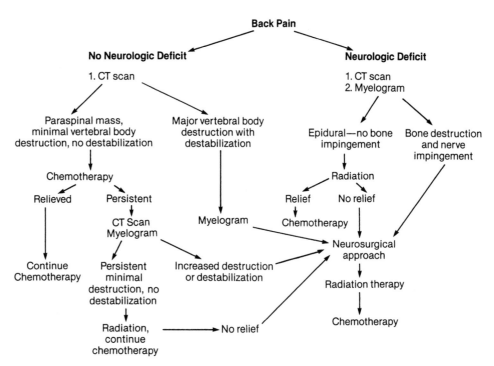

FIGURE 129-8 Therapeutic decision tree for spinal involvement in multiple myeloma and solitary plasmacytoma.

a neurosurgical approach is necessary. The presence of a neurologic deficit at diagnosis demands an aggressive diagnostic and therapeutic approach to prevent further nerve damage or subsequent paraparesis or paraplegia. Once the computed tomography scan and myelogram define the extent of the disease, a number of surgical approaches, resection, and stabilization techniques are available. Radiotherapy is necessary after these surgical techniques because rarely can all tumor be removed and the reported results appear to show a better result with a combined modality approach,[166,167] although this concept has not been rigorously tested in a clinical trial.

REFERENCES

1. Munshi NC, Tricot G, Barlogie B: Plasma cell neoplasms. In DeVita VT, Hellmann S, Rosenberg SA (eds): Cancer: Principles and Practice of Oncology. Philadelphia: JB Lippincott, 2001, pp 2465–2499.
2. Callander NS, Roodman GD: Myeloma bone disease. Semin Hematol 38:276–285, 2001.
3. Vilpo JA, Irjala K, Viljanen MK, et al: Delta heavy chain disease: A study of a case. Clin Immunol Immunopathol 17:584, 1980.
4. Fishkin BG, Orloff N, Scaduto LE, et al: IgE multiple myeloma: A report of the third case. Blood 39:361–367, 1972.
5. Ioachim NJ, McKenna PJ, Halperin I, Chung FJ: IgD myeloma: Immunology and ultrastructure. Ann Clin Lab Sci 8:209–218, 1978.
6. Kyle RA: Multiple myeloma: Review of 869 cases. Mayo Clin Proc 50:29, 1975.
7. Shustik C, Bergsagel DE, Pruzanski W: κ and λ light chain disease: Survival rates and clinical manifestations. Blood 48:41–51, 1976.
8. Wiltshaw E: The natural history of extramedullary plasmacytoma and its relation to solitary myeloma of bone and myelomatosis. Medicine 55:217–238, 1976.
9. Brouet JC, Seligmann M, Danon F, et al: U-chain diseases: Report of two new cases. Arch Int Med 139:672–674, 1979.
10. Buxbaum JN, Alexander A: Heavy-chain diseases. In Beutler E, Lichtman MA, Coller BS, et al (eds): Williams Hematology, 6th ed. New York: McGraw-Hill, 2001, pp 1327–1336.
11. Kyle RA: Monoclonal gammopathy of undetermined significance and solitary plasmacytoma. Implications for progression to overt multiple myeloma. Hematol Oncol Clin North Am 11:71–87, 1997.
12. Kipps TJ: Waldenström macroglobulinemia. In Beutler E, Lichtman MA, Coller BS, et al (eds): Williams Hematology, 6th ed. New York: McGraw-Hill, 2001, pp 1317–1325.
13. Kyle RA, Garton JP: The spectrum of IgM monoclonal gammopathy in 430 cases. Mayo Clin Proc 62:719–731, 1987.
14. Mills RJ, Fahie-Wilson MN, Carter PM, Hobbs JR: IgE myelomatosis. Clin Exp Immunol 23:228–232, 1976.
15. Ogawa M, Kochwa S, Smith C, et al: Clinical aspects of IgE myeloma. N Eng J Med 281:1217–1220, 1969.
16. Nies BA, Kundel DW, Thomas LB, Freireich EJ: Leukopenia, bone pain, and bone necrosis in patients with acute leukemia: A clinicopathologic complex. Ann Intern Med 62:698–705, 1965.
17. Willson JKV: The bone lesions of childhood leukemia: A survey of 140 cases. Radiology 72:672–681, 1959.
18. Rosenberg SA, Diamond HD, Jaslowitz B, Craver LF: Lymphosarcoma: A review of 1269 cases. Medicine 40:31–84, 1961.
19. Wachsman W, Golde DW, Chen IS: HTLV and human leukemia: Perspectives. Semin Hematol 23:245–256, 1986.
20. Kubat R, Svehla F, Horacek J: A case of IgD plasmacytoma with unusual neurological symptoms. Folia Haematol (Leipz) 104:366–375, 1977.
21. Cavo M, Galieri P, Gobbi M, et al: Nonsecretory multiple myeloma: Presenting findings, clinical course and prognosis. Acta Haematol 74(1):27–30, 1985.
22. Martin IG, Aldoori MI: Immunoproliferative small intestinal disease: Mediterranean lymphoma and alpha heavy chain disease. Br J Surg 1:20, 1994.
23. Shaw AFB: A case of plasma cell myeloma. J Pathol Bacteriol 26:125–126, 1923.
24. Cutler M, Buschke F, Cantril ST: The course of single myeloma of bone: A report of 20 cases. Surg Gynecol Obstet 62:918–932, 1936.
25. Knowliag MA, Harwood AR, Bergsagel DE: Comparison of extramedullary plasmacytomas with solitary and multiple plasma cell tumors of bone. J Clin Oncol 1:255–262, 1983.
26. Bacci G, Savini R, Calderoni P, et al: Solitary plasmacytoma of the vertebral column: A report of 15 cases. Tumori 68:271–275, 1982.
27. Bataille R, Sany J: Solitary myeloma: Clinical and prognostic features of a review of 114 cases. Cancer 48:845–851, 1981.
28. Chak LY, Cox RS, Bostwick DG, Hoppe RT: Solitary plasmacytoma of bone: Treatment, progression and survival. J Clin Oncol 5:1811–1815, 1987.
29. Corwin J, Lindberg RD: Solitary plasmacytoma of bone vs. extramedullary plasmacytoma and their relationship to multiple myeloma. Cancer 43:1007–1013, 1979.
30. Feldman JL, Guedri M, Ohana N, et al: Solitary plasmacytoma of the spine. Ann Med Interne (Paris) 135:259–264, 1984.
31. Loftus CM, Michelsen CB, Rapoport F, Antunes JL: Management of plasmacytomas of the spine. Neurosurgery 13:30–36, 1983.
32. Meis JM, Butler JJ, Osborne BM, Ordonez NG: Solitary plasmacytoma of bone and extramedullary plasmacytomas: A clinicopathologic and immunohistochemical study. Cancer 59:1474–1485, 1987.
33. Woodruff RK, Malpas JS, White FE: Solitary plasmacytoma. II Solitary plasmacytoma of bone. Cancer 43:2344–2347, 1979.
34. Delauche-Cavallier MC, Laredo JD, Wybier M, et al: Solitary plasmacytoma of the spine: Long-term clinical course. Cancer 61:1707–1714, 1988.
35. Demirel T: Root compression syndrome S1, simulated by a circumscribed plasmacytoma in the intervertebral disc. Neurosurg Rev 4:37–39, 1981.
36. Paul LW, Pohle EA: Solitary myeloma of bone: A review of the roentgenologic features, with a report of four additional cases. Radiology 35:651–666, 1940.
37. Mustoe TA, Fried MP, Goodman ML, et al: Osteosclerotic plasmacytoma of maxillary bone (orbital floor). J Laryngol Otol 98:929–939, 1984.
38. Roberts M, Rinaudo PA, Vilinskas J, Owens G: Solitary sclerosin plasma cell myeloma of the spine: Case report. J Neurosurg 40:125–129 1974.
39. Sartoris DJ, Pate D, Haghighi P, et al: Plasma cell sclerosis of bone: A spectrum of disease. J Can Assoc Radiol 37:25–34, 1986.
40. Savage D, Garrett TJ: Multiple myeloma masquerading as metastatic breast cancer. Cancer 57:923–924, 1986.
41. Rossleigh MA, Smith J, Yeh SD: Scintigraphic features of primary sacral tumors. J Nucl Med 27:627–630, 1986.
42. Valat JP, Eveleigh MC, Fouquet A, Born P: Bone scintigraphy in multiple myeloma. Rev Rhum Mal Osteoart 52:707–711, 1975.
43. Helms CA, Vogler JB III, Genant HK: Characteristic CT manifestations of uncommon spinal disorders. Orthop Clin North Am 16:445–459, 1985.
44. Lingg G, Miller RP, Fischedick AR, et al: Diagnostic possibilities of computer tomography in spinal and paraspinal space occupying lesions. Rontgenblatter 38:207–212, 1985.
45. Fruehwald FX, Tscholakoff D, Schwaighofer B, et al: Magnetic resonance imaging of the lower vertebral column in patients with multiple myeloma. Invest Radiol 23:193, 1988.
46. Kagan E, Jacobson R: Lymphoid and plasma cell malignancies: Asbestos-related disorders of long latency. Am J Clin Pathol 80:14–20, 1983.
47. Baitz T, Kyle RA: Solitary myeloma in chronic osteomyelitis. Arch Intern Med 113:872, 1964.
48. Dimopoulos MA, Moulopoulos A, Delasalle K, Alexanian R: Solitary plasmacytoma of bone and asymptomatic multiple myeloma. Hematol Oncol Clin North Am 6:359, 1992.
49. Iwashita H, Ohnishi A, Asada M, et al: Polyneuropathy, skin hyperpigmentation, edema, and hypertrichosis in localized osteosclerotic myeloma. Neurology 27:675–681, 1977.
50. Maharaj B, Kalideen JM, Leary WP, Pudifin DJ: Carcinoma of the prostate with multiple osteolytic metastasis simulating multiple myeloma: A case report. S Afr Med J 70:227–228, 1986.
51. Schajowicz F, Hokama J: Aspiration (puncture or needle) biopsy in bone lesions. Recent Results Cancer Res 54:139–144, 1976.
52. Rubins J, Quazi R, Woll JE: Massive bleeding after biopsy of plasmacytoma: Report of two cases. J Bone Joint Surg 62:138–140, 1980.
53. Moulopoulos LA, Dimopoulos MA, Weber D, et al: Magnetic resonance imaging in the staging of solitary plasmacytoma of bone. J Clin Oncol 11:1311, 1993.
54. Mill WB, Griffith R: The role of radiation therapy in the management of plasma cell tumors. Cancer 45:647–652, 1980.
55. Tong D, Griffin TW, Laramore GE, et al: Solitary plasmacytoma of bone and soft tissues. Radiology 135:195–198, 1980.
56. Liebross RH, Ha CS, Cox JD, et al: Solitary bone plasmacytoma: Outcome and prognostic factors following radiotherapy. Int J Radiat Oncol Biol Phys 41:1063, 1998.

57. Colyer RA: Surgical stabilization of pathological neoplastic fractures. Curr Probl Cancer 10:117–168, 1986.

58. Faccioli F, Luna J, Bricolo A: One-stage decompression and stabilization in the treatment of spinal tumors. J Neurosurg Sci 29:199–205, 1985.

59. Jelsma RK, Kirsch PT: The treatment of malignancy of a vertebral body. Surg Neurol 13:189–195, 1980.

60. Lesoin F, Bonneterre J, Lesoin A, Jomin M: Neurologic manifestations of spinal plasmacytomas. Neurochirurgie 28:401–407, 1982.

61. Lobosky JM, Kitchon PW, McDonnell DE: Transthoracic anterolateral decompression for thoracic spinal lesions. Neurosurgery 14:26–30, 1984.

62. Louis R, Casanova J, Baffert M: Surgical techniques in tumors of the spine. Rev Chir Orthop 62:57–70, 1976.

63. Lucantani D, Galzio R, Zenobii M, et al: Spinal cord compression by solitary plasmacytoma. J Neurosurg Sci 27:125–127, 1983.

64. Onimus M, Schraub S, Bertin D, et al: Treatment of secondary cancer of the spine. Rev Clin Orthop 71:473–482, 1985.

65. Panjabi MM, Goel VK, Clark CR, et al: Biomechanical study of cervical spine stabilization with methylmethacrylate. Spine 10:198–203, 1985.

66. Sundaresan N, Galicich JH, Lane JM: Harrington rod stabilization for pathological fractures of the spine. J Neurosurg 60:282–286, 1984.

67. Karchmer RR, Amare M, Larsen WE, et al: Alkylating agents as leukemogens in multiple myeloma. Cancer 33:1103–1107, 1974.

68. Kyle RA, Pierre RV, Bayrd ED: Multiple myeloma and acute myelomonocytic leukemia: Report of four cases possibly related to Melphalan. N Engl J Med 283:1121–1125, 1970.

69. Singhal S, Mehta J, Desikan R, et al: Antitumor activity of thalidomide in refractory multiple myeloma. N Eng J Med 341:1565, 1999.

70. Richardson P, Anderson K: Immunomodulatory analogs of thalidomide: An emerging new therapy in myeloma. J Clin Oncol 22:3269–3276, 2004.

71. Richardson PG, Barlogie B, Berenson B, et al: Clinical factors predictive of outcome with bortezomib in patients with relapsed, refractory multiple myeloma. Blood, 2005 (in press).

72. Krauth MT, Bankier A, Valent P, Kalhs P, Drach J: Sustained remission including marked regression of a paravertebral plasmacytoma in a patient with heavily pretreated, relapsed multiple myeloma after treatment with bortezomib. Leuk Res, 2005 (in press).

73. Carter PM, Rushman RW: Solitary plasmacytoma of the clavicle. Proc R Soc Med 67:1097–1098, 1974.

74. Myer JE, Schulz MD: "Solitary" myeloma of bone: A review of 12 cases. Cancer 34:438–440, 1974.

75. Jameson RM: Prolonged survival in paraplegia due to metastatic spinal tumours. Lancet 1:1209–1211, 1976.

76. Kyle RA, Elveback LR: Management and prognosis in multiple myeloma. Mayo Clin Proc 51:751–760, 1976.

77. Yentis I: The so-called solitary plasmacytoma of bone. J Fac Radiol 8:132–144, 1956.

78. Holland J, Trenkner DA, Wasserman TH, Fineberg B: Plasmacytoma: Treatment results and conversion to myeloma. Cancer 69:1513, 1992.

79. Kyle RA, Nobrega FT, Kurland LT: Multiple myeloma in Ohmsted County, Minnesota. Blood 33:739–745, 1969.

80. McPhedran P, Heath CW, Jr, Garcia J: Multiple myeloma incidence in metropolitan Atlanta, Georgia: Racial and seasonal variations. Blood 39:866–873, 1972.

81. Hewell GM, Alexanian R: Multiple myeloma in young persons. Ann Intern Med 84:441–443, 1976.

82. Porter FS, Jr: Multiple myeloma in a child. J Pediatr 62:602–604, 1963.

83. Devesa SS, Silverman DT, Young JL, Jr, et al: Cancer incidence and mortality trends among whites in the United States, 1947–84. J Natl Cancer Inst 79:701, 1987.

84. Cohen HJ, Crawford J, Rao MK, et al: Racial differences in the prevalence of monoclonal gammopathy in a community-based sample of the elderly. Am J Med 104:439, 1998.

85. Shulman G, Jacobson RJ: Immunocytoma in black and white South Africans. Trop Geogr Med 32:112–117, 1980.

86. Feinman R, Sawyer J, Hardin J, Tricot G: Cytogenetics and molecular genetics in multiple myeloma. Hematol/Oncol Clin North Am 11:1, 1997.

87. Greil R, Fasching B, Loidl P, Huber H: Expression of the c-myc protooncogene in human multiple myeloma and chronic lymphocytic leukemia: An in situ analysis. Blood 78:180–191, 1991.

88. Drach J, Ackermann J, Fritz E, et al: Presence of a P53 gene deletion in patients with multiple myeloma predicts for a short survival after conventional-dose chemotherapy. Blood 92:802, 1998.

89. Hata H, Xiao H, Petrucci MT, et al: Interleukin-6 gene expression in multiple myeloma: A characteristic of immature tumor cells. Blood 81:3357, 1993.

90. Ridley RC, Xiao H, Hata H, et al: Expression of syndecan regulates human myeloma plasma cell adhesion to type I collagen. Blood 81:767, 1993.

91. Huang N, Kawano MM, Harada H, et al: Heterogeneous expression of a novel MPC-1 antigen on myeloma cells: Possible involvement of MPC-1 antigen in the adhesion of mature plasma cells to bone marrow stromal cells. Blood 82:3721, 1993.

92. Podar K, Anderson KC: The pathophysiologic role of VEGF in hematologic malignancies: Therapeutic implications. Blood 105:1383–1395, 2005.

93. Vacca A, Ria R, Samararo F, et al: Endothelial cells in the bone marrow of patients with multiple myeloma. Blood 102:3340–3348, 2003.

94. Cozzolino F, Torcia M, Aldinucci D, et al: Production of interleukin-1 by bone marrow myeloma cells. Blood 74:380, 1989.

95. Garrett IR, Durie BGM, Nedwin GE, et al: Production of lymphotoxin, a bone resorbing cytokine by cultured human myeloma cells. N Eng J Med 291:526, 1989.

96. Bataille R, Klein B: The bone resorbing activity of interleukin-6. J Bone Min Res 9:1144, 1991.

97. Lacey DL, Timms E, Tan HL, et al: Osteoprotegerin ligand is a cytokine that regulates osteoclast differentiation and activation. Cell 93:165, 1998.

98. Roodman GD: Mechanisms of bone lesions in multiple myeloma and lymphoma. Cancer 80:1557, 1997.

99. Durie BGM, Salmon SE, Mundy GR: Multiple myeloma: Clinical staging and role of osteoclast activating factor in localized bone loss. In JE Horton, TM Tarpley, WF Davis (eds): Mechanisms of Localized Bone Loss. Calcif Tissue Abstr (Special Suppl) 1978, pp 319–329.

100. Bockman RS: Lymphokine mediated bone resorption requires prostaglandin synthesis. In Prostaglandin and Cancer: First International Conference. New York: Alan R. Liss, 1982, pp 555–559.

101. Bertolini DR, Nedwin GE, Bringman TS, et al: Stimulation of bone resorption and inhibition of bone formation in vitro by human tumor necrosis factors. Nature 319:516–518, 1986.

102. Schajowicz F: Marrow tumors. In Schajowicz F (ed): Tumors and Tumorlike Lesions of Bone and Joints. New York: Springer-Verlag, 1981, pp 243–302.

103. Kopp WL, Mackinney AA, Jr, Wasson G: Blood volume and hematocrit value in macroglobulinemia and myeloma. Arch Intern Med 123:394–396, 1969.

104. Hoffbrand AV, Hobbs JR, Kremenchuzky S, Mollin DL: Incidence and pathogenesis of megaloblastic erythropoiesis in multiple myeloma. J Clin Pathol 20:699–705, 1967.

105. Bergsagel DE, Griffith KM, Haut A, Stuckey WF, Jr: The treatment of plasma cell myeloma. Adv Cancer Res 10:311–359, 1967.

106. Jaffe JP, Mosher DF: Calcium binding by a myeloma protein. Am J Med 67:343–346, 1979.

107. Pruzanski W, Ogryzlo MA: Abnormal proteinuria in malignant diseases. Adv Clin Chem 13:335–382, 1970.

108. Hobbs JR: Immunochemical classes of myelomatosis: Including data from a therapeutic trial conducted by a medical research council working party. Br J Haematol 16:599–606, 1969.

109. Murray T, Long W, Narins RG: Multiple myeloma and the anion gap. N Engl J Med 292:574–575, 1975.

110. Pruzanski W, Watt JG: Serum viscosity and hyperviscosity and syndrome in IgG multiple myeloma: Report on 10 patients and a review of the literature. Ann Intern Med 77:853–860, 1972.

111. Perkins HA, MacKenzie MR, Fudenberg HH: Hemostatic defects in dyproteinemias. Blood 35:695–707, 1970.

112. Coleman M, Vigliano EM, Weksler ME, Nachman RL: Inhibition of fibrin monomer polymerization by lambda myeloma globulins. Blood 39:210–223, 1972.

113. Davey FR, Gordon GB, Boral LI, Gottlieb AJ: Gammaglobulin inhibition of fibrin clot formation. Ann Clin Lab Sci 6:72–77, 1976.

114. Glueck HE, Hong RA: A circulating anticoagulant in IA-multiple myeloma: Its modification by penicillin. J Clin Invest 44:1866–1881, 1965.

115. Brody JI, Haidar ME, Rossman RE: A hemorrhagic syndrome in Waldenström's macroglobulinemia secondary to immunoadsorption of factor VIII: Recovery after splenectomy. N Engl J Med 300:408–410, 1979.

116. Furie B, Greene E, Furie BC: Syndrome of acquired factor X deficiency and systemic amyloidosis: In vivo studies of the metabolic fate of factor X. N Engl J Med 297:81–85, 1977.

117. Defronzo RA, Cooke CR, Wright JR, Humphrey RL: Renal function in patients with multiple myeloma. Medicine 57:151–166, 1978.

118. Rossi JF, Bataille R, Chappard D, et al: B cell malignancies presenting with unusual bone involvement and mimicking multiple myeloma: Study of nine cases. Am J Med 83:10–16, 1987.

119. Bataille R, Durie BGM, Grenier J: Serum β2 microglobulin and survival duration in multiple myeloma: A simple reliable marker for staging. Br J Haematol 55:439–447, 1983.

120. Durie BGM, Salmon SE: A clinical staging system for multiple myeloma: Correlation of measured cell mass with presenting clinical features, response to treatment, and survival. Cancer 36:842–854, 1975.

121. Hobbs JR: Growth rates and responses to treatment in human myelomatosis. Br J Haematol 16:607–617, 1969.

122. McIntyre OR, Acute Leukemia Group B: Correlation of abnormal immunoglobulin with clinical features of myeloma. Arch Intern Med 135:46–52, 1975.

123. Report of the Medical Research Council's Working Party for Therapeutic Trials in Leukemia: Report on the first myelomatosis trial. I: Analysis of presenting features of prognostic significance. Br J Haematol 24:123–139, 1973.

124. Carbone PP, Kellerhouse LE, Gehan EA: Plasmacytic myeloma: A study of the relationship of survival to various clinical manifestations and anomalous protein type in 112 patients. Am J Med 42:937–948, 1967.

125. Salmon SE, Durie BGM: Cellular kinetics in multiple myeloma. A new approach to staging and treatment. Arch Intern Med 135:131–138, 1975.

126. Kyle RA, Greipp PR: Smoldering multiple myeloma. N Engl J Med 302:1347–1349, 1980.

127. Korst DR, Clifford GO, Fowler WM, et al: Multiple myeloma. II: Analysis of cyclophosphamide therapy in 165 patients. JAMA 189:758–762, 1964.

128. Bergsagel DE, Sprague CC, Austin C, Griffith KM: Evaluation of new chemotherapeutic agents in the treatment of multiple myeloma. IV: L-phenylalanine mustard (NSC-8806). Cancer Chemother Rep 21:87–99, 1962.

129. Cornwell GG III, Pajak TF, Kochwa S, et al: Comparison of oral melphalan, CCNU and BCNU with and without vincristine and prednisone in the treatment of multiple myeloma. Cancer 50:1669–1675, 1982.

130. MRC Working Party for Therapeutic Trials in Leukaemia: Myelomatosis: Comparison of melphalan and cyclophosphamide therapy. BMJ 1:640–641, 1971.

131. Bergsagel DE, Cowan DH, Hasselback R: Plasma cell myeloma: Response of melphalan-resistant patients to high-dose, intermittent cyclophosphamide. CMAJ 107:851–855, 1972.

132. Alexanian R, Yap BS, Bodey GP: Prednisone pulse therapy for refractory myeloma. Blood 62:572–577, 1983.

133. Alexanian R, Barlogie B, Dixon D: High-dose glucocorticoid treatment of resistant multiple myeloma. Ann Int Med 105:8, 1986.

134. Alexanian R, Bonnet J, Gehan E, et al: Combination chemotherapy for multiple myeloma. Cancer 30:382–389, 1972.

135. Lee BJ, Sahakian G, Clarkson BD, Krakoff IH: Combination chemotherapy of multiple myeloma with alkeran, cytoxan, vincristine, prednisone, and BCNU. Cancer 33:533–538, 1974.

136. Salmon SE, Haut A, Bonnet JD, et al: Alternating combination chemotherapy and levamisole improves survival in multiple myeloma: A Southwest Oncology Group Study. J Clin Oncol 1:453–461, 1983.

137. Bergsagel DE: Editorial: Progress in the treatment of plasma cell myeloma? J Clin Oncol 1:510–512, 1983.

138. Barlogie B, Smith L, Alexanian R: Effective treatment of advanced multiple myeloma refractory to alkylating agents. N Engl J Med 310:1353–1356, 1984.

139. Cavo M, Zamagni E, Tosi P, et al: Superiority of thalidomide and dexamethasone over vincristine-doxorubicin-dexamethasone (VAD) as primary therapy in preparation for autologous transplantation for multiple myeloma. Blood 106:35–39, 2005.

140. Richardson PG, Schlossman RL, Weller E, et al: Immunomodulatory drug CC-5013 overcomes drug resistance and is well tolerated in patients with relapsed multiple myeloma. Blood 100:3063–3067, 2002.

141. Richardson PG, Sonneveld P, Shuster MW, et al: Bortezomib or high dose dexamethasone for relapsed multiple myeloma. N Eng J Med 352:2546–3548, 2005.

142. Barlogie B, Hall R, Zander A, et al: High-dose melphalan with autologous bone marrow transplantation for multiple myeloma. Blood 67:1298–1301, 1986.

143. Attal M, Harousseau JL, Stoppa AM, et al: A prospective, randomized trial of autologous bone marrow transplantation and chemotherapy in multiple myeloma: Intergroupe Francais du Myelome. N Eng J Med 335:91, 1996.

144. Constanzi JJ, Cooper MR, Scarffe JH, et al: Phase II study of recombinant alpha-2 interferon in resistant multiple myeloma. J Clin Oncol 3:654–659, 1985.

145. Tribalto M, Mandelli F, Cantonetti M, et al: Recombinant alpha 2-interferon as post maintenance therapy for responding multiple myeloma: Clinical results of a multicentric trial. New Trends Ther Leuk Lymphoma 2:61, 1987.

146. Benson WJ, Scarffe JH, Todd IDH, et al: Spinal-cord compression in myeloma. BMJ 1:1541–1544, 1979.

147. Von Scheefe C: Light chain myeloma with features of adult Fanconi syndrome: Six years remission with one course of melphalan. Acta Med Scand 199:533, 1976.

148. Jaffe JP, Bosch A, Raich PC: Sequential hemi-body radiotherapy in advanced multiple myeloma. Cancer 43:124–128, 1979.

149. Coleman M, Saletan S, Wolf D, et al: Whole bone marrow irradiation for the treatment of multiple myeloma. Cancer 49:1328–1333, 1982.

150. Talerman A: Clinico-pathological study of multiple myeloma in Jamaica. Br J Cancer 23:285–293, 1969.

151. Malpas JS: General management of myeloma. In Delamore IW (ed): Multiple Myeloma and Other Paraproteinemias. Edinburgh: Churchill Livingstone, 1986, p 339.

152. Brenner B, Carter A, Tatarsky I, et al: Incidence, prognostic significance and therapeutic modalities of central nervous system involvement in multiple myeloma. Acta Haematol 68:77–83, 1982.

153. Bruckman JE, Bloomer WD: Management of spinal cord compression. Semin Oncol 5:135–140, 1978.

154. Carmacho J, Arnalich F, Anciones B, et al: The spectrum of neurological manifestations in myeloma. Medicine 16:597–611, 1985.

155. Helms CA, Genant HK: Computed tomography in the early detection of skeletal involvement with multiple myeloma. JAMA 248:2886–2887, 1982.

156. Solomon A, Rahamani R, Seligsohn U, Ben-Artzi F: Multiple myeloma: Early vertebral involvement assessed by computerized tomography. Skeletal Radiol 11:258–261, 1984.

157. Berenson JR, Lichtenstein A, Porter L, et al: Long-term pamidronate treatment of advanced multiple myeloma patients reduces skeletal events: Myeloma Aredia Study Group. J Clin Oncol 16:593, 1998.

158. Carter PM, Rushman RW: Solitary plasmacytoma of the clavicle. Proc R Soc Med 67:1097–1098, 1974.

159. Conley FK, Britt RH, Hanbery JW, Silverberg GD: Anterior fibular strut graft in neoplastic disease of the cervical spine. J Neurosurg 51:677–684, 1979.

160. Lesoin F, Jomin M, Pellerin P, et al: Transclival transcervical approach to the upper cervical spine and clivus. Acta Neurochir (Wien) 80:100–104,1986.

161. Sundaresan N, Galicich JH, Lane JM, Greenberg HS: Treatment of odontoid fractures in cancer patients. J Neurosurg 54:187–192, 1981.

162. Lipson SJ, Hammerschlag SB: Atlantoaxial arthrodesis in the presence of posterior spondyloschisis (bifid arch) of the atlas: A report of three cases and an evaluation of alternative wiring techniques by computerized tomography. Spine 9:65–69, 1984.

163. Sunder-Plassmann M: Dorsal inter and extracorporeal osteosynthesis for tumours of the thoracic vertebral bodies. Neurochirurgia (Stuttg) 23:99–105, 1980.

164. Sunder-Plassmann M: Vertral osteosynthesis for the treatment metastatic tumours of the superior thoracic spine. Neurochirurgia (Stuttg) 23:106–111, 1980.

165. Colyer RA: Surgical stabilization of pathological neoplastic fractures. Curr Probl Cancer 10:117–168, 1986.

166. Dahlstrom U, Jarpe S, Lundstrom FD: Paraplegia in myelomatosis: A study of 20 cases. Acta Med Scand 205:173–178, 1979.

167. Desproges-Gotteron R, Treves R, Loubet R, et al: Spinal cord compression caused by malignant non-Hodgkins lymphoma. Semin Hop Paris 54:704–712,1978.

130 Innovations in Anterior Cervical Spine Surgery

RONAN M. DARDIS, ADRIAN CASEY, JESUS LAFUENTE,
and RICHARD W. GULLAN

BACKGROUND

Over the last few decades the anterior approach to the cervical spine has become well recognized as the optimal route for surgical treatment of ventral cervical cord or root compression.[1-7] Even now, however, there continues a controversy as to which procedure is best at the level of the intervertebral disc. In particular there remains debate on the value of fusion, with autografts or allografts, and nonfusion techniques[2,8,9] including arthroplasty.

The original anterolateral approaches described by Smith and Robinson[10] and Cloward[11] have withstood the test of four decades and there are now many variants of these pioneering operations. Because the predominant changes associated with cervical spondylosis are situated ventral to the spinal cord, and the cord itself tolerates lateral traction poorly, the anterolateral approach allows safe and satisfactory direct decompression. Developing from simple intervertebral space decompression are the present-day two-level, three-level, and four-level discectomies with fusion; vertebrectomy; and newer fusion techniques using allografts, metallic and nonmetallic cages containing bone, and biosynthetic materials.[12-14] The long-term results of these procedures are, as in the past, very satisfactory, but there remain some reservations to the ideal operation.

Recently a "sea change" opportunity has also occurred. The concept of an artificial joint replacing a degenerative symptomatic herniated cervical disc has become a reality.[15-17] There are many conceptual advantages to disc arthroplasty over the conventional and modified anterior cervical discectomy and fusion operations. The premise that interbody fusion of the cervical spine leads to acceleration in the degeneration of adjacent disc levels due to increased stress from the fusion is gaining acceptance.[18-25]

The first nongrafted anterior cervical discectomy review was published by Hirsch in 1960 (reference 26), and the debate has raged since that time about the necessity of an interspacing graft. The proponents of an interspace graft suggest that along with the safer anterior approach, the opportunity to maintain disc space height and the natural lordosis of the cervical spine, the inclusion of a graft arrests spur formation and often leads to resorption of spurs in response to fusion.[4,8,9,27-29] Moreover, proponents propose that there is reduced posterior compression as a result of unbuckling of the ligamentum flavum. The neuroforaminal height may also be maintained with the inclusion of a graft. This aspect may be particularly important if osteophyte removal from the foramen is less than complete. The degree of osteophyte removal is variable and can depend on the surgeon.

Hirsch[26] noted that contralateral arm pain may be due to a neuroforaminal height loss when a graft is not included. The inclusion of a graft is often suggested to be more necessary in spondylotic cervical spine disease than in simple soft disc herniation.

Clinicians opposed to the necessity of graft insertion for every anterior cervical discectomy argue that although grafting should be performed when instability exists or potentially exists (e.g., extensive vertebral body resection, two or more levels operated on, or a previous laminectomy), discectomy without fusion is otherwise an excellent alternative.[1,8,9,30] This procedure has markedly reduced operative time, blood loss, and length of stay along with producing fewer complications. Moreover, as the disc space collapses, fusion occurs spontaneously in approximately 50% to 70% of cases. Although this spontaneous fusion can lead to kyphosis, the preoperative curvature of the spine is often maintained. It is acknowledged that anterior cervical discectomy without grafting is usually associated with longer postoperative neck and interscapular pain, but in long-term follow-up (mean 6 years), low-intensity neck and arm pain occur at the same rate regardless of grafting. Obviously, donor site problems are not associated with simple anterior cervical discectomy. Watters and Levinthal[9] compared simple discectomy and discectomy with grafting and found no significant difference in the average time for return to work (12 vs. 10 weeks), although the neck pain and arm pain lasted significantly longer in the nongrafted group. Long-term graft site pain was not considered to be a problem by all grafted patients contacted, despite some reports suggesting pain in 40% (reference 31). These authors did note that anterior cervical grafting was associated with many more complications, but that all but one of those complications was graft related. Watters and Levinthal[9] concluded that neither simple anterior discectomy nor discectomy with autologous grafting is the ideal procedure.

The ideal fusion procedure for cervical radiculopathy would include a material that could maintain height and lordosis while awaiting and perhaps promoting fusion. We have used carbon fiber cages (Brantigan I/F Cages, DePuy AcroMed, Raynham, MA), which are manufactured from long-fiber Hercules A5-4 carbon fibers in a polymer marix of polyetherketone-etherketone (DePuy AcroMed, Raynham, MA). The cage is fashioned into a trapezoidal shape to match the axial and anteroposterior dimensions appropriate for anterior cervical fusion. The cages are available in a variety of sizes. The hollow inner volume of the cage allows space for either autologous cancellous bone or proprietary porous hydroxyapatite coral bone filler for packing to ensure bone fusion. The cage itself provides support and has toothlike serrations that resist displacement of the prosthesis once placed in final position. The radiolucency of carbon fiber allows good assessment of bone healing. The modulus of elasticity is similar to cortical bone, thereby preventing stress shielding. The wedge shape in the anteroposterior direction aids the promotion of optimal cervical lordosis.

However, the proponents of the cervical arthroplasty believe reconstruction of a failed intervertebral disc with a functional disc prostheses should offer the same benefits as fusion while providing motion, thereby protecting adjacent level discs from the abnormal stresses associated with fusion. Theoretically, such a device would also be beneficial because it would eliminate sources of inflammation and potential instability associated with the abnormal kinematics of a degenerate disc, and restore natural load sharing and kinematic properties.[32] The facets would also be unloaded.

However, there are obvious difficulties in designing an intervertebral arthroplasy implant. Unlike the design of a hip implant, which replaces a relatively simple ball and socket joint, a cervical spine implant must serve the function of mobility, load bearing, and possibly load dampening.

In various series of 28 to 146 patients who had undergone anterior cervical arthrodesis, between 25% and 89% who were followed for a lengthy period developed new degenerative changes at adjacent levels.[25] Biomechanical studies performed in vitro in the lumbar spine have demonstrated increased load, segmented motion, and intradiscal pressure at levels adjacent to simulated arthrodeses.[33-35] Moreover, in a detailed biomechanical evaluation Di Angelo and colleagues found that an artificial cervical joint, in this case the Bristol Cervical Joint (Medtronic Sofamor Danek, Memphis, TN), did not alter the motion patterns at the operated site or at the adjacent segments. Application of a graft and plate, however, significantly reduced motion at the operated site, which was compensated for by increased motion at adjacent segments.[36]

THE BRYAN CERVICAL DISC PROSTHESIS

The Bryan cervical disc prosthesis (Spinal Dynamics Corp., Mercer Island, WA) is designed to permit motion similar to the normal cervical functional spinal unit. The prosthesis is intended to treat stable cervical degenerative disc disease without fusion, thereby providing the patient with the capability for motion at the treated level (Fig. 130-1).

The device consists of a polyurethane-wrapped low-friction, water-resistant elastic nucleus located between, and articulating with, two titanium alloy surfaces (shells). The bone-contacting surface of each shell includes a titanium porous coating to encourage bony ingrowth and long-term stability. A polyurethane sheath surrounds the nucleus and is attached to the shells with titanium wire, forming a closed compartment. Titanium alloy seal plugs provide for retention of a sterile saline lubricant. Anterior stops on each shell help to prevent posterior migration of the device. The design allows for a normal range of motion in flexion/extension, lateral bending, axial rotation, and translation.

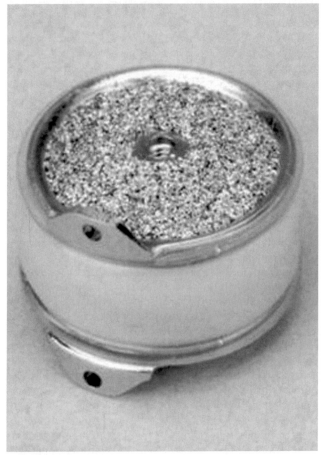

FIGURE 130-1   Bryan cervical disc prosthesis. (Courtesy of Spinal Dynamics Corp., Mercer Island, WA.)

Many biomechanical and surgical considerations were incorporated into the design of the Bryan disc.

- It is semiconstrained over the normal range of motion and is thus able to function synergistically with the remaining anatomic structures (annulus, ligaments, facets, and muscles), which may themselves be degenerate. This allows the coupled vertebral motions typical of the normal cervical spine.
- The prosthesis is part of a system that includes instrumentation and a surgical technique that ensures accurate placement of the prosthesis with minimal resection of supporting bone and soft tissue.
- It utilizes precise bone preparation techniques combined with porous bone ingrowth fixation,[37] allowing it to be mechanically stable both immediately and chronically.
- If necessary, the design permits conversion to a fusion procedure.

NATURAL HISTORY OF CERVICAL SPONDYLOSIS

The degenerative process that occurs as the spine ages can lead to various disease states. Apart from the intervertebral disc space, numerous other structures are influenced by aging and repetitive use. The degenerative process is not a disease in itself, however, and 75% of men and 70% of women in their 60s have at least one level of disc degeneration on a lateral cervical x-ray film without any symptoms.[38] A review by Lee and Turner[39] of 95 patients with cervical spondylosis revealed that of the 51 patients who presented with cervical radiculopathy but no evidence of myelopathy, none progressed to develop myelopathy, 45% resolved spontaneously without recurrence, 30% continued to have mild symptoms or an intermittent pattern, and 25% had persistent or progressive symptoms. Of the 41 patients who had clinical and radiographic evidence of myelopathy, those with mild disability at initial presentation had the best prognosis with no significant progression during the study period of 19 years. Of the 15 patients who presented with severe disability secondary to myelopathy, 14 remained severely disabled after 10 to 20 years of follow-up.

Gore and colleagues[40] retrospectively evaluated 205 patients with neck and arm pain. Almost 80% improved over the 10-year review, with almost all reporting complete loss of pain without recurrence on conservative therapy only. Epstein and Epstein[41] reported on the combined results of four series of patients who were managed conservatively for cervical myelopathy. Of 114 patients, 36% improved, 38% remained unchanged, and 26% deteriorated.

SURGICAL INDICATIONS IN CERVICAL DISC DISEASE

Surgical intervention can improve the outcome results. Ebersold and colleagues[42] reviewed 100 patients with documented cervical myelopathy over 10 years. Of the 33 patients undergoing anterior decompression and grafting, 24 patients showed immediate functional improvement and 9 were unchanged. Surgical decompression was recommended only if progressive, incapacitating neurologic symptoms and confirmatory signs of myelopathy were present. During long-term follow-up, functional outcome was noted to decline. These authors also expressed concern that anterior decompression with fusion may cause accelerated degeneration of spinal segments above and below the graft site, causing recurrent cord compression. As stated previously, the surgical treatment of radiculopathy is associated with an excellent outcome.[1-4,7,10]

The result of surgery is absolutely related to patient selection. The patient must have appropriate clinical complaints for the disease process proposed and must have clinical signs appropriate to the levels of the proposed disc herniation or spondylosis. The radiographic diagnostic studies must confirm what is a virtual clinical certainty. The abnormal finding on imaging must be consistent with the patient's clinical symptoms and physical signs. If the triad of appropriate symptoms, signs, and imaging does not occur, a trial of conservative therapy should be recommended.[2]

CERVICAL RADICULOPATHY

Cervical radiculopathies may exist as isolated mononeuropathies or, more rarely, bilaterally or multisequentially at several sites (mononeuropathy multiplex). Cervical radiculopathy may or may not be associated with a myelopathy. In the instance of myeloradiculopathy, the cause of compression is usually spondylotic disease.[43] Cervical radiculopathy most frequently involved C5–C6, C6–C7, and C4–C5,

in that order of frequency. An acute disc prolapse causes neck pain with radiation into the arm (brachialgia), scapula, or chest. The pain may be associated with sensorimotor and reflex deficits in a specific distribution. The hard disc is a degenerative spur mainly associated with outgrowth from the uncovertebral joint, but it may be accompanied by spur formation in the immediate adjacent posterior portion of the disc. Osteophyte formation results from subperiosteal bone formation resulting from elevation of the periosteum by disc bulging. A spondylotic ridge will then form. As a result of the cervical lordosis, the disc bulge and the resulting osteophyte formation tend to occur toward the spinal canal.[44] The radicular symptoms and signs associated with either hard or soft disc are probably the result of neural compression and perineural inflammation. Surgery is indicated in the following situations[45]:

- Progressive neurologic deficit
- Static neurologic deficit with radicular pain
- Persistent or recurrent arm pain that is not responsive to a trial of conservative therapy

CERVICAL MYELOPATHY

Cervical spondylotic myelopathy occurs only in patients whose cervical spinal canal is narrower than 14 mm in sagittal diameter.[46,47] The severity of the myelopathy tends to correlate with the extent of spinal canal narrowing. When the degenerative changes of osteophyes and ligamentous hypertrophy are superimposed on a primary spinal stenosis, a cervical spondylotic myelopathy results. Compression of the spinal cord by disc material or tractions of the cord against osteophytes is etiologically important, particularly in the case of an acute myelopathy.[48,49] In chronic myelopathy, however, the influences of disc degeneration, spur formation, foraminal encroachment, and a congenitally narrow canal are probably potentiated by motion.

Whether compromise of radicular vessels is important in the pathogenesis remains uncertain. The anterior spinal artery supplies the ventral two thirds of the cord, and this region shows the most pathologic changes.[50] Since the work of Marr and Druckman,[51] efforts have been made to classify the subtypes of cervical spondylotic myelopathy. Ferguson and Caplan[52] categorized spondylosis with nerve involvement into four distinct but overlapping syndromes. Crandall and Batzdorf[53] devised a classification system based on the differential susceptibility of various spinal cord tracts in cervical spondylotic myelopathy. Gregorias and co-workers[54] took Crandall's work further and identified five distinct syndromes, including: (1) a transverse lesion syndrome with corticospinal, spinothalamic, and dorsal column involvement; (2) a motor system syndrome with corticospinal tract and anterior horn cell dysfunctions; (3) a mixed syndrome with root and cord findings presenting with radicular pain and long tract involvement; (4) a partial Brown-Séquard syndrome; and (5) an anterior cord syndrome with distal arm weakness.

The indications for surgery are as stated by Bohlmann[55]:

- Progressive impairment of function without sustained remission
- Failure to demonstrate improvement in myelopathy after cervical immobilization (with a collar)

Anterior approach, using Robinson's technique, should be undertaken for (1) one-level, two-level, or three-level pathology; (2) primarily at the disc level; (3) anterior cord compression; (4) fairly stable cervical alignment.[56] Ebersold and colleagues[42] found that age, severity of disease, number of levels operated, and the preoperative grade were not predictive of outcome. The only variable related to potential deterioration postoperatively was the duration of symptoms preoperatively.

NECK PAIN

Anterior cervical discectomy is rarely indicated for neck pain alone.

DIAGNOSTIC EVALUATION

After careful history taking and demonstration of appropriate signs on examination, confirmatory radiologic imaging is required before surgical intervention. Although simple radiography is an inexpensive, readily accessible starting point, it is severely limited by its inability to visualize neural structures directly or indirectly, and the presence or absence of neural compression is indeterminable.[57] If there is any delay in obtaining true confirmatory imaging, routine cervical radiography should be undertaken to exclude other disease processes, such as malignancy, arthritis, and infection.[58] When Friedenberg and Miller[59] compared 92 asymptomatic patients with those complaining of neck and arm pain, no difference was found between the two groups in radiographic findings, with the exception of a greater incidence of disc degeneration at C5–C6 and at C6–C7 in the symptomatic group.

Currently, published studies support the preferential use of magnetic resonance imaging (MRI) in the confirmatory diagnosis of cervical radiculopathy.[60] In cervical radiculopathy, the data support the use of either computed tomography (CT) myelography or MRI.[57] As an initial test, MRI has an obvious advantage because of its noninvasive nature. Furthermore, the increased MRI signal seen in the cord on T2-weighted images can indicate injury taking place at cord level[61] (Fig. 130-2). To show cord compression by spondylosis, T1-weighted imaging is required because T2-weighted scans exaggerate obstruction of the subarachnoid space and can feign a spinal stenosis. This investigation cannot be used in patients with paramagnetic material in their bodies.

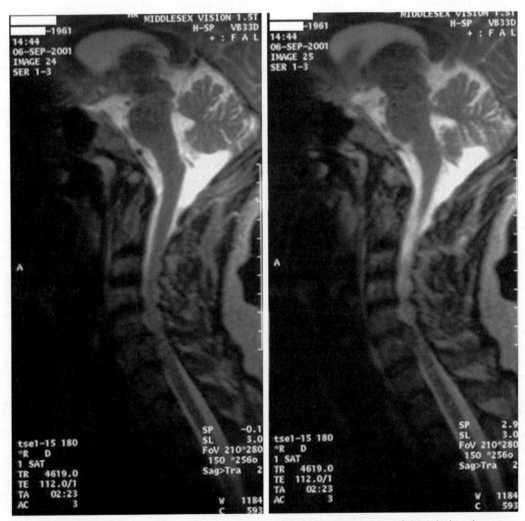

FIGURE 130-2 A sagittal T2-weighted MRI scan displaying compression of the spinal cord.

If titanium material was used for plating in previous cervical fusion, artifacts in postoperative MRI are significantly reduced.

If a Bryan cervical disc prosthesis is to be placed, the MRI axial images are obtained with slices parallel to the vertebral bony end plates. In these cases the stability of the cervical spine is assessed with flexion and extension views.

On occasion we have noted that, particularly in cases involving lateral encroachment of the neural foramen, the excellent cross-sectional imaging of bony prominences by CT myelography or 3-dimensional reconstruction CT can be useful in preoperative planning. It also allows a degree of dynamic imaging with flexion and extension views during myelography. This imaging can be helpful in visualizing posterior indentation by the ligamentum flavum. Moreover, all patients undergoing arthroplasty also had a routine CT scan to assess the disc size preoperatively, along with routine MRI scanning and plain flexion-extension radiographs to ascertain cervical stability.[62]

Electromyography and nerve conduction studies are rarely required, but they can provide additional objective evidence of root compression in patients with relatively minor neurologic findings. Moreover, they are useful in differentiating root, plexus, peripheral nerve, and muscle disorders that may mimic cervical radiculopathy, and they may help to uncover a second problem that coexists with the cervical radiculopathy, such as a carpal tunnel syndrome or ulnar neuropathy.

COMPLICATIONS OF ANTERIOR CERVICAL SURGERY

The complication rate for anterior cervical disc surgery is, in experienced hands, low. The reported series suggest a complication rate of 0% to 13% (references 63 through 65). Hoarseness is the most common reported complication and is usually due to retractor pressure on the larynx. Dysphagia, laryngeal edema, or a sensation of a lump in the throat because of pharyngeal constrictor muscle swelling can also be attributed to retractor blade placement. Careful selection of blade size and meticulous placement reduce these complaints. Recurrent laryngeal injury is another cause of postoperative hoarseness, which may be permanent. Flynn reported its occurrence rate to be 0.14% of all cases.[66] Recurrent laryngeal injury composed 17% of all neurologic complications in his large review. He noted that it frequently resulted in litigation. We do not routinely dissect out the recurrent laryngeal nerve on the right side and in several hundred cases have not found laryngeal nerve palsy to be a particular problem. More serious neurologic deficit occurs approximately once in every 355 cases. Flynn noted that despite the cause of new-onset postoperative myelopathy, reoperation may have little influence on the ultimate status of the neurologic deficit. Moreover, Flynn suggested that most of the surgeons whose patients experienced myelopathic complications were unable to determine the cause. Major bleeding is rare in anterior disc surgery.[66] Any postoperative collection of blood, however, can lead to neurologic compromise or respiratory embarrassment. Drains are only partially useful, and meticulous hemostasis is required. Injury to the carotid artery is rare but reported. The vertebral artery can be damaged if drilling is performed

too far laterally. The resulting hemorrhage can prove difficult to stop. As a last resort, an endovascular technique under radiologic guidance stems the flow.

Esophageal or tracheal perforation occurs in less than 1% of cases; careful placement of retractor blades minimizes the risk. If esophageal perforation is recognized intraoperatively, it should be repaired immediately, and a general surgeon should be notified while the lesion is amenable to optimal surgical correction in the operating room.

Displacement of the bone graft occurs in 5% of cases, although this is rarely posteriorly with the attendant risk of cord compression. Our experience with the carbon fiber cervical cage is that it is secure, having the benefit of toothlike serrations to provide a stable interface when placed in the intervertebral space, along with its slightly greater height anteriorly. An appropriate size must be selected to maximize the security. Similarly, the Bryan disc is very secure because it is placed into optimally milled end plates.

We reviewed 150 consecutive anterior cervical discectomies with insertion of the Brantigan carbon fiber cage at King's College Hospital. There was no surgical mortality. There were no cage related complications. Removal or revision of a cage was never necessary. There was no retropulsion or change in position of any of the cages. Fourteen patients complained of transient dysphagia. Four had transient hoarseness all of whom improved.

We present here a preliminary report of results we obtained at the National Hospital for Neurosurgery, Queen Square, London. Since March 2001, 54 patients have been enrolled in an observational clinical study. Of these patients, 89% complained of radiculopathy and 20% had a myelopathy. All patients underwent preoperative cervical spine radiographs (neutral and flexion-extension views). Four patients had had previous cervical fusion performed at one level.

We noted that the duration of operation ranged from 50 to 270 minutes (mean, 100 minutes; median, 75 minutes). All patients were followed up at 6 weeks, 6 months, and 1 year. The results were very encouraging and are awaiting publication in a peer-reviewed journal.

The complications noted by us included seven cases of mild dysphonia, all of which had resolved by the first postoperative clinic appointment. One patient required an operation to remove the prosthesis following a fall that caused anterior subluxation of the inferior disc plate. The patient had no neurologic deficits and complained of axial neck pain only. An interbody fusion cage was inserted after removal of the Bryan disc prosthesis.

Upon postoperative radiologic review of the series at 12 months, the range of motion was 2 degrees and 17 degrees with a mean of 8 degrees. The outcome measures are due to be published in the near future. The results of the original European consortium have been reported.[15] About 10% developed heterotrophic ossification, which can be prevented by nonsteroidal antiinflammatory drugs.

OPERATIVE PROCEDURES

Brantigan Carbon-Fiber Cage Placement

The procedure is undertaken under general anesthesia with the patient supine and the cervical spine in the neutral or very mimimally extended position. Hyperextension of the neck requires greater forces to retract the pharynx and larynx to expose the anterior cervical spine. We simply place a pillow partly under the shoulders and rolled up under the neck. The endotracheal tube is carefully secured and passes superiorly over the head out of the way of the surgeon and assistant. Rarely, if a graft is to be harvested from the iliac crest, it is beneficial to have a sandbag under the right hip.

Routinely, a collar incision is used, placed in a skin crease or along a Langer line. It is technically easier for a right-handed surgeon using the high-speed air drill under the microscope to operate from the right side. The risk of injury to the recurrent laryngeal nerve is higher on the right, but the risk to the thoracic duct is diminished. The position of the incision is important; the incision should be at the upper level of the cricoid cartilage to expose C5–C6 and just below the level of the cricoid for C6–C7 exposure. In high cervical disc prolapses, we perform lateral screening with a metallic marker after draping to localize the incision.

The skin incision is taken to the platysma, but the platysma is split rather than cut in the line of the incision. Undercutting the subcutaneous tissues facilitates this approach, which gives an excellent postoperative cosmetic result. The investing cervical fascia is divided along the anterior border of the sternocleidomastoid to define the plane between the carotid sheath laterally and larynx, trachea, and esophagus medially. The superior belly of the omphyoid is identified passing from the hyoid bone inferolaterally. Usually, it is possible to divide the fascia around this and gently retract it up or down, but occasionally it is necessary to divide it usually at its midtendinous segment. During the preliminary dissection, it is essential to feel the pulsation of the carotid sheath laterally and to continue dissection in a posteromedial direction toward the spine (Fig. 130-3).

The anterior cervical spine is initially palpated after retraction of the esophagus and trachea using a Langenbeck retractor. Occasionally, a prominent anterior osteophyte at the disc level can aid in identification of the level. The prevertebral fascia is divided in the midline. Although this plane of dissection is usually bloodless, small draining veins

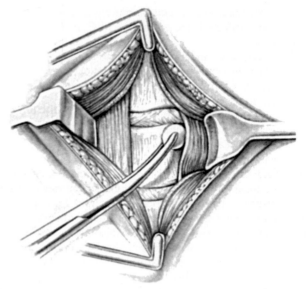

FIGURE 130-4 The longus colli muscles are reflected to each side to expose the anterior cervical spine. (From Brantigan JW: Surgical technique for anterior cervical discectomy and fusion using the cervical I/F cage. Courtesy of DePuy AcroMed, Raynham, MA.)

may require diathermy and division. It is rare that the superior thyroid artery crosses the path of surgery. It is wise to ligature the artery formally if it is to be divided. The authors make no effort to identify the recurrent laryngeal nerve. It readily mobilizes along with the trachea and esophagus away from the midline to the opposite side.

The prevertebral fascia is reflected laterally below the longus colli muscle. We find blunt dissection with a peanut sponge to be helpful or (Fig. 130-4), alternatively, carefully using cutting diathermy. At this stage, the disc level is formally identified with cross-table lateral radiograph screening. The marking needle is placed into the anterior portion of the disc.

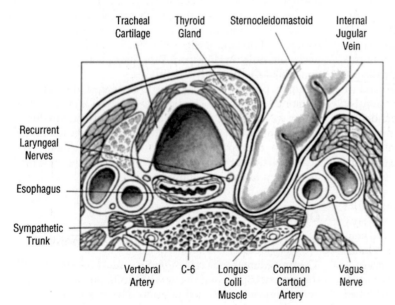

Tracheal Cartilage — Thyroid Gland — Sternocleidomastoid — Internal Jugular Vein

Recurrent Laryngeal Nerves

Esophagus

Sympathetic Trunk

Vertebral Artery — C-6 — Longus Colli Muscle — Common Cartoid Artery — Vagus Nerve

FIGURE 130-3 Cross-sectional view of the neck demonstrating the plane of cleavage between the carotid sheath laterally and the trachea and esophagus medially. (From Brantigan JW: Surgical technique for anterior cervical discectomy and fusion using the cervical I/F cage. Courtesy of DePuy AcroMed, Raynham, MA.)

Once the correct level has been identified, self-retaining Caspar (or similar) retractors are inserted under the medial borders of the longus colli muscle, and while the needle is withdrawn, a small piece of the center of the disc is cut out. This action ensures no later mistakes in recognizing the correct level. We prefer not to use vertebral body distractors, although they are gaining increased popularity. Anterior osteophytes overlying the disc space are removed using a rongeur or the high-speed air drill. The annulus is incised and removed with a pituitary rongeur or curet. The disc is removed with curets. In any technique requiring a graft, good lateral exposure is necessary, no less so using a carbon fiber cage. The dissection is continued until the upslope of the uncovertebral joints on either side is identified. Further dissection or drilling may damage the vertebral arteries.

The operating microscope is introduced once most of the disc space has been cleared. The high-speed drill is used to remove remaining cartilaginous end plate and annulus. For hardened degenerate disc, the drill is used from the early stages. Spherical burrs of appropriate size are used; we feel that it is safer to use a slightly larger burr because this has less potential to penetrate through the back of the disc and damage the cord. Downward pressure is never applied to the drill head; instead the drill is stroked in an axial plane parallel to the end plate. Posterior osteophytes can be thinned down by the drill, then gently cracked off with a small curet or Kerrison upcutting rongeur. The use of bone wax for vertebral bleeding should be kept to a minimum because this interferes with fusion.

During the entire procedure, the risk to three important structures—the spinal cord and the right and left vertebral arteries—must be considered. In severely spondylotic spines, it is possible to be skewed to one side early in the procedure. It is always imperative to stay in the midline.

Once the posterior osteophyte is removed, the annulus is nibbled with a Kerrison punch. This step, however, can be particularly trying when the tissues are grossly thickened and degenerate. The posterior longitudinal ligament is teased open with a blunt hook and a sickle-shaped knife (Karlin knife). It is then removed with a small upcutting punch. Although it is the practice of some clinicians not to remove posterior osteophytes on the grounds that they reabsorb after fusion,[67] we always attempt formal clearance. Exposure of the dura confirms adequate decompression. Careful exploration with a small blunt probe alongside the root foramen allows confirmation that the root is free.

The end plates are prepared with rasps, which ensure parallel roughened end plates consisting of subchondral bone. It is important both in the Smith-Robinson technique and with the carbon fiber cage to preserve as much subchondral bone as possible, so that it can function as a load-bearing surface.

Trial sizes of the cage are selected (Fig. 130-5). Having selected the correct trial cage that fits snugly, the actual cage implant is fitted to the insertion tool. The implant cage is slightly larger than the trial size, which, along with the serrations, allows for a snug fit.

If autologous cancellous bone is used to fill the cage, a small linear incision is made over the anterosuperior iliac crest. The periosteum is incised with cutting diathermy and elevated to allow a small window of about 0.75 cm² to be cut in the outer cortex. A curet is then used to remove

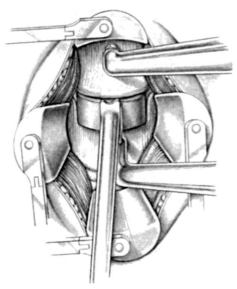

FIGURE 130-5 Trial sizes are placed in the prepared space to ensure that each surface is flat and the space is equally tapered from front to back. (From Brantigan JW: Surgical technique for anterior cervical discectomy and fusion using the cervical I/F cage. Courtesy of DePuy AcroMed, Raynham, MA.)

sufficient cancellous bone to fill the carbon fiber cage, and the cortical window is replaced. The periosteum, subcutaneous layer, and skin layer are sutured. If, alternatively, a substitute material is used, such as porous hydroxyapatite (Pro Osteon, Interpore Cross, Irvine, CA), this material should be preclotted before insertion in the cage. The cage is then inserted into position and gently tapped into place. It is important that the cage should not protrude. Gentle manipulation of the neck confirms that the cage is secure (Fig. 130-6). If meticulous hemostasis is confirmed,

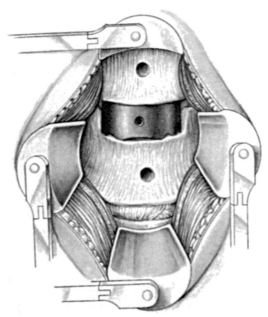

FIGURE 130-6 Final position of the Brantigan cervical I/F cage. (From Brantigan JW: Surgical technique for anterior cervical discectomy and fusion using the cervical I/F cage. Courtesy of DePuy AcroMed, Raynham, MA.)

closure proceeds. If there are any doubts, a small suction drain is placed in the depth of the wound before closure. The split platysma is drawn together with polyglycolic acid suture (Vicryl), and a subcuticular stitch of clear 3-0 Vicryl is inserted. The advantage of sutures over staples is that they can be removed quickly if a life-threatening cervical hematoma develops. A dressing and soft collar, which is for comfort only, is applied before extubation.

Bryan Cervical Disc Prosthesis

At the National Hospital for Neurology and Neurosurgery, Queen Square, London, all patients are considered for surgery and part of the ongoing CEDRIC trial comparing the Bryan cervical disc system with a standard fusion cage.

A multiple-step process is undertaken, ensuring the accurate placement of the prosthesis with minimal resection of the supporting bone. However, it must be remembered that the operation is essentially very similar to a standard anterior cervical discectomy. The notable exception is that the drilling is controlled by a jig. This constrains the drilling apparatus in a similar fashion to the jig in a total knee replacement.

Using customized instrumentation, the following steps are undertaken:

Step 1. Preoperative procedures are as follows. On the smaller of the two vertebral body end plates at the target disc space, a prosthesis template is overlaid to select the prosthesis size. Bryan cervical discs are currently available in diameters of 14 to 18 mm

Step 2. The patient and fluoroscope unit are positioned with an inclinometer attached to the image intensifier of the C arm. The neck is supported on a rolled towel and the head is placed on a firm doughnut. The patient is stabilized with strapping. A lateral view reveals the direction in which the disc space is oriented in relation to the inclinometer pendulum using a goniometer (Figs 130-7 and 130-8).

Step 3. After sterile preparation of skin and patient draping, the specialized retractor frame is attached to the operating table. The frame is aligned so that it is appropriately parallel and perpendicular to the operating table using a spirit level.

Step 4. A routine approach to the anterior cervical spine using a transverse incision centered at the target space is undertaken. Once the anterior spine has been accessed, the longus colli muscles are stripped at the medial edge with the toothed retractor blades, which are attached to the table-mounted retractor system. Rostrocaudal retractors are not required by us (Fig. 130-9).

Step 5. Using a template for the previously determined prosthesis size, the annulus fibrosis is marked for the width of the incision and then excised between these marks. The nucleus pulposus and soft interior portion of the deep anulus are removed with curets and rongeurs. The cartilaginous end plates are curetted away, leaving the bone intact.

Step 6. Any soft tissue and bony protrusions are then drilled away to create a flat surface, but the disc space is not entered with the burr to remove anterior osteophytes. Instead a Kerrison rongeur is used to remove the anterior lip of bone

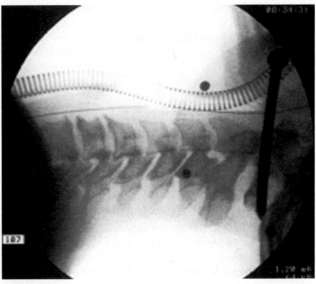

FIGURE 130-7 A multiple-step process is undertaken to ensure accurate placement of the Bryan cervical disc prosthesis with minimal resection of the supporting bone. Figures 130-7 through 130-18 illustrate these steps. See text (Step 2) for details. (From Bryan Cervical Disc System. Single-Level Surgical Technique. As described by Vincent Bryan, MD, Spinal Dynamics, Medtronic Sofamor Danek.)

from the cephalal vertebral body, keeping the shaft of the rongeur parallel to the caudal end plate.

Step 7. Using the two "cam distractors" of increasing widths (6.5–8.5 mm), the disc space is distracted using an alternating clockwise-counterclockwise rotary motion. Care is taken not to damage the end plates. A distraction of 8.5 mm is achieved and held for 30 to 60 seconds to stretch the ligaments and joint capsules. The surgeon then has two choices—either to continue with the decompression and perform the drilling and milling later, or, as is the more common practice, proceed with the specialized drilling and end-plate milling, and once the end plate has been milled for the specific Bryan disc size (14–18 mm), a standard microsurgical decompression is performed. We find this latter technique to be quicker.

Step 8. The transverse centering tool is now inserted into the disc space. The spirit level is placed on the transverse centering tool and adjusted until the bubble is centered in the lateral direction. The sliding pointer of the tool as a guide is used to mark the center point of the cephalal vertebral body (Fig. 130-10).

Step 9. To obtain sagittal centering, the sagittal wedge is placed in the target disc space. The wedge is pressed into the disc space until the stop contacts the anterior surface of the caudal vertebral body (Fig. 130-11A and B).

Step 10. The dual-track milling guide slides onto the sagittal wedge, and the adjustable protractor, set at the angle obtained earlier with the goniometer (as described in Step 2), is placed over the sagittal wedge. The spirit level allows adjusting of the dual-track milling guide to ensure that it is level. The cephalad and caudal pins are then inserted (Fig. 130-12).

Step 11. The anchor posts are placed.

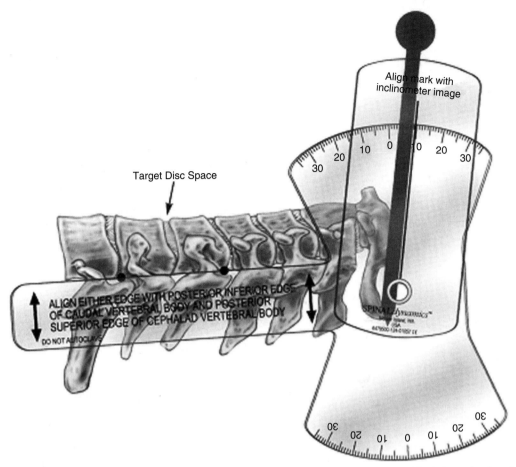

Target Disc Space

Align mark with inclinometer image

ALIGN EITHER EDGE WITH POSTERIOR INFERIOR EDGE OF CAUDAL VERTEBRAL BODY AND POSTERIOR SUPERIOR EDGE OF CEPHALAD VERTEBRAL BODY

DO NOT AUTOCLAVE

30 20 10 0 10 20 30

SPINAL DYNAMICS

30 20 10 0 10 20 30

FIGURE 130-8 See text (Step 2) for details. (From Bryan Cervical Disc System. Single-Level Surgical Technique. As described by Vincent Bryan, MD, Spinal Dynamics, Medtronic Sofamor Danek.)

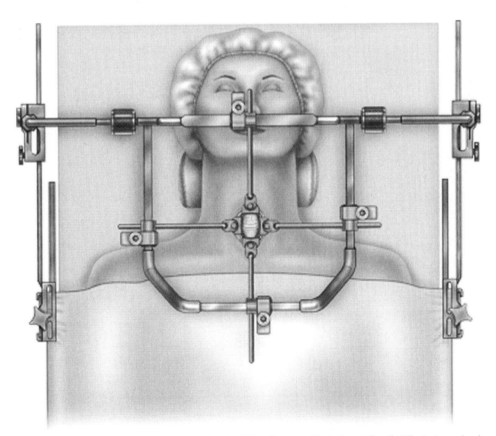

FIGURE 130-9 See text (Step 4) for details. (From Bryan Cervical Disc System. Single-Level Surgical Technique. As described by Vincent Bryan, MD, Spinal Dynamics, Medtronic Sofamor Danek.)

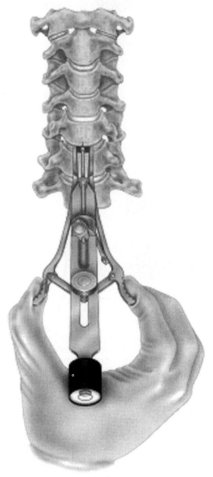

FIGURE 130-10   See text (Step 8) for details. (From Bryan Cervical Disc System. Single-Level Surgical Technique. As described by Vincent Bryan, MD, Spinal Dynamics, Medtronic Sofamor Danek.)

Step 12. The sagittal wedge is removed to allow for insertion of the milling drill.

Step 13. Milling depth is determined using the milling depth gauge (Fig. 130-13).

Step 14. Burring depth is confirmed by selecting the burring ring that corresponds to the previously selected prosthesis size (Step 1; e.g., 14–18 mm). It is screwed onto the burring block. The burring depth gauge is inserted into the burring block.

The gauge set screw is unlocked and the gauge probe lowered to the approximate level of the posterior longitudinal ligament. Then the 4-mm fluted drum burr is inserted in the centered burring handpiece (Fig. 130-14).

Step 15. The centered burring handpiece is attached to the drive system and the disc space cleared using a side-to-side motion (Fig. 130-15).

Step 16. Once the disc space has been cleared, the end plates are milled precisely using the milling disc. Both the superior and inferior end plates are milled (Fig. 130-16).

Step 17. The disc space is distracted and the milling guide brace and anchor posts are removed.

Step 18. The Bryan prosthesis is prepared for insertion. It is filled with sterile saline and then compressed, allowing excess saline to escape. The port of entry is then sealed (Fig. 130-17).

Step 19. The prosthesis is placed into the disc space using an implant inserter (Fig. 130-18).

Step 20. Surgery is completed after confirming hemostasis. A drain is usually inserted. The platysma is closed with 2-0 Vicryl, and a clear 2-0 Vicryl is used on the subcuticular layer covered with sterile strips.

Of course no collar is required.

FIGURE 130-11   *A* and *B,* See text (Step 9) for details. (From Bryan Cervical Disc System. Single-Level Surgical Technique. As described by Vincent Bryan, MD, Spinal Dynamics, Medtronic Sofamor Danek.)

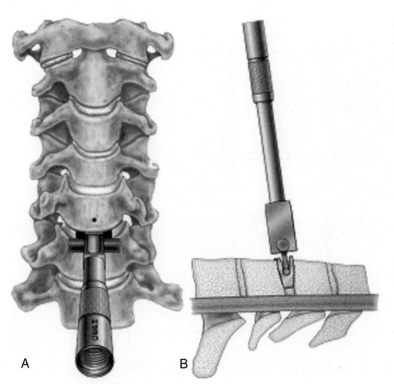

A   B

FIGURE 130-12 See text (Step 10) for details. (From Bryan Cervical Disc System. Single-Level Surgical Technique. As described by Vincent Bryan, MD, Spinal Dynamics, Medtronic Sofamor Danek.)

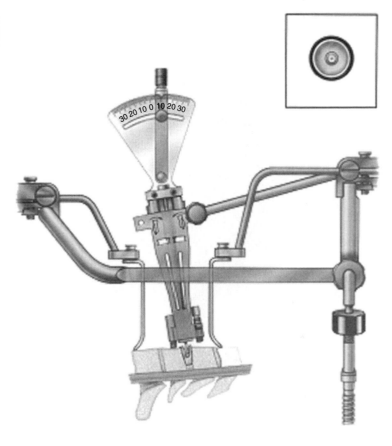

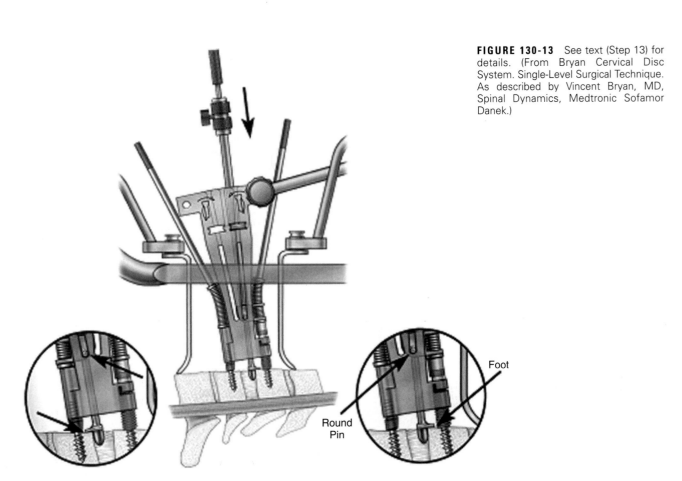

FIGURE 130-13 See text (Step 13) for details. (From Bryan Cervical Disc System. Single-Level Surgical Technique. As described by Vincent Bryan, MD, Spinal Dynamics, Medtronic Sofamor Danek.)

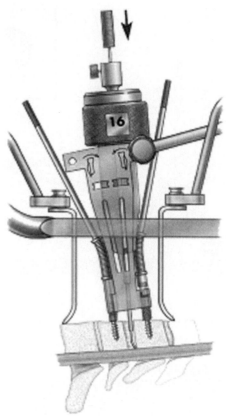

FIGURE 130-14   See text (Step 14) for details. (From Bryan Cervical Disc System. Single-Level Surgical Technique. As described by Vincent Bryan, MD, Spinal Dynamics, Medtronic Sofamor Danek.)

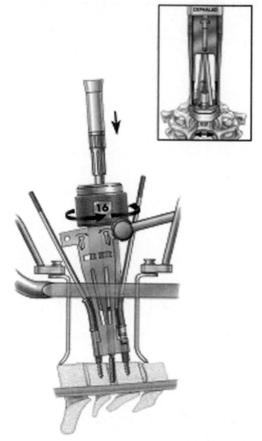

FIGURE 130-15   See text (Step 15) for details. (From Bryan Cervical Disc System. Single-Level Surgical Technique. As described by Vincent Bryan, MD, Spinal Dynamics, Medtronic Sofamor Danek.)

POSTOPERATIVE MANAGEMENT

All Bryan disc patients are commenced on the nonsteroidal anti-inflammatory rofecoxib (Vioxx) 12.5 mg daily for 6 weeks to decrease the possibility of heterotrophic calcification.

These patients undergo immediate mobilization. Physiotherapy is commenced at 6 weeks (core stability with gentle mobilization).

All patients are monitored overnight, to watch for the rare possibility of acute laryngeal swelling or a delayed hematoma causing respiratory embarrassment. If a drain is placed, it is removed the following morning. Postoperative radiography is performed later that day. This timing is preferred because the potential for cage dislodgement is perhaps greatest during extubation. After 6 weeks, flexion-extension

FIGURE 130-16   See text (Step 16) for details. (From Bryan Cervical Disc System. Single-Level Surgical Technique. As described by Vincent Bryan, MD, Spinal Dynamics, Medtronic Sofamor Danek.)

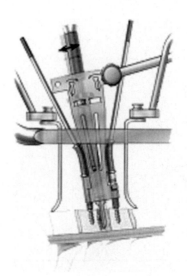
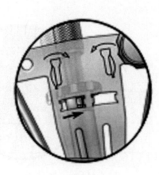

FIGURE 130-17 See text (Step 18) for details. (From Bryan Cervical Disc System. Single-Level Surgical Technique. As described by Vincent Bryan, MD, Spinal Dynamics, Medtronic Sofamor Danek.)

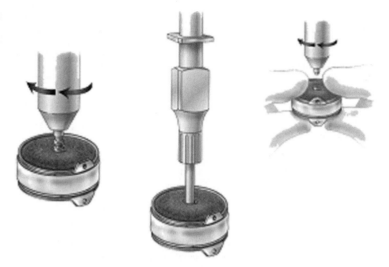

lateral radiography is performed to ensure security of the implant and stability of the level.

CONCLUSIONS

The currently available surgical techniques for treatment of anterior cervical disc pathology produce good clinical results in the majority of patients. Since their introduction in the 1950s, these surgical techniques and modalities have undergone modification over the decades, improving both surgical technique and patient outcome. A few major limitations still remain. There is an increased risk of adjacent level degeneration necessitating further surgery, a risk of pseudarthrosis and resultant immobility of the cervical spine after fusion techniques.

There has been great success with prostheses developed for some of the other joints prone to degenerative changes such as the hip and knee. It is no surprise, therefore, that continuing efforts would be made to develop a successful cervical disc replacement.

The Bryan cervical disc prosthesis promises to usher in a new era in the management of cervical spine disease. The low morbidity and excellent postoperative outcomes to date (Table 130-1) suggest that the procedure will have a greater role in the management of cervical spondylotic disease in the future.

FIGURE 130-18 See text (Step 19) for details. (From Bryan Cervical Disc System. Single-Level Surgical Technique. As described by Vincent Bryan, MD, Spinal Dynamics, Medtronic Sofamor Danek.)

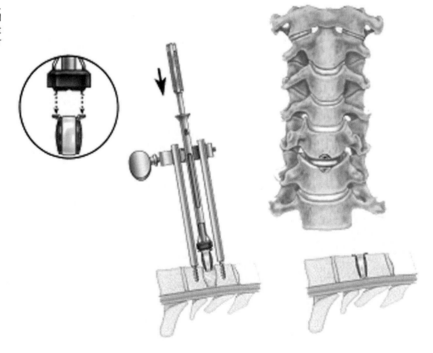

TABLE 130-1 Summary of Clinical Follow-up after Anterior Cervical Spine Surgery

Follow-up	Clinical Success Rate (n)	Sample Size	Excellent (n)	Good (n)	Fair (n)	Poor (n)	No Data* (n)
6 Months	**86% (52)**	**60**	**68% (41)**	**8% (5)**	**10% (6)**	**8% (5)**	**5% (3)**
Radiculopathy	88% (47)	53	71% (38)	8% (4)	9% (5)	8% (4)	4% (2)
Myelopathy	72% (5)	7	44% (3)	14% (1)	14% (1)	14% (1)	14% (1)
1 Year	**90% (27)**	**30**	**80% (24)**	**3% (1)**	**7% (2)**	**10% (3)**	
Radiculopathy	89% (24)	27	78% (21)	4% (1)	7% (2)	11% (2)	
Myelopathy	100% (3)	3	100% (3)				

*Missed follow-up or incomplete patient and/or surgeon forms.

REFERENCES

1. Hadley MN, Sonntag VKH: Cervical disc herniations: The anterior approach to symptomatic interspace pathology. Neurosurg Clin N Am 4:45–52, 1993.
2. Bertalanffy H, Eggert HR: Clinical long-term results of anterior cervical discectomy without fusion for treatment of cervical radiculopathy and myelopathy. Acta Neurochir (Wien) 90:127–125, 1988.
3. Martins AN: Anterior cervical discectomy with and without interbody bone graft. J Neurosurg 44:290–295, 1996.
4. Maurice-Williams RS, Dorward NL: Extended anterior cervical discectomy without fusion: A simple and sufficient operation for most cases of cervical degenerative disease. Br J Neurosurg 10:261–266, 1996.
5. Brodke DS, Zdeblick TA: Modified Smith-Robinson procedure for anterior cervical discectomy and fusion. Spine 17:427–430, 1992.
6. Robertson JT: Anterior operations for herniated cervical disc and for myelopathy. Clin Neurosurg 25:245–250, 1978.
7. Robertson RA, Walker AE, Ferlick DE: The results of anterior interbody fusion of the cervical spine. J Bone Joint Surg Am 44:1569–1587, 1962.
8. Sonntag VK, Klara P: Controversy in spine care: Is fusion necessary after anterior cervical discectomy? Spine 21:1111–1113, 1996.
9. Watters WC, Levinthal R: Anterior cervical discectomy with and without fusion, results, complications and long term follow up. Spine 19:2343–2347, 1994.
10. Smith GW, Robinson RA: The treatment of certain cervical spine disorders by anterior removal of the intervertebral disc and interbody fusion. J Bone Joint Surg Am 40:607–623, 1958.
11. Cloward RB: The anterior approach for removal of ruptured discs. J Neurosurg 15:602–614, 1958.
12. Caspar W, Barbier DD, Klara PM: Anterior cervical fusion and Caspar plate stabilization for cervical trauma. Neurosurgery 25:491–502, 1989.
13. Kaufman HH, Jones E: The principles of bony spinal fusion. Neurosurgery 24:264–270, 1989.
14. Mahnin TI, Brown MD: Bone allografts in spinal surgery. Clin Orthop 154:68–73, 1981.
15. Goffin J, Casey A, Kehr P, et al: Preliminary clinical experience with the Bryan cervical disc prosthesis. Neurosurgery 51:840–847, 2002.
16. Sekhon LH: Cervical arthroplasty in the management of spondylotic myelopathy. J Spinal Disorder Tech 16:307–313, 2003.
17. Cummins B, Robertson J, Gill S: Surgical experience with an implanted artificial cervical joint. J Neurosurg 88:943–948, 1998.
18. Baba H, Furusawa N, Imura S, et al: Late radiographic findings after anterior cervical fusion for spondylotic myeloradiculopathy. Spine 18:2167–2173, 1993.
19. Cherubino P, Benazzo F, Borromeo U, et al: Degenerative arthritis of adjacent spinal joints following anterior cervical spinal fusion: Clinicoradiologic and statistical correlation. Ital J Orthop Traumatol 16:533–543, 1990.
20. Clements DH, O'Leary PF: Anterior cervical discectomy and fusion. Spine 15:1023–1025, 1990.
21. Doehler JR, Kahn MR, Hughes SP: Instability of the cervical spine after interbody fusion: A study on its incidence and clinical significance in 21 patients. Arch Trauma Surg 104:247–250, 1985.
22. Goffin J, van Loon J, Van Calenbergh F, et al: Long-term results after anterior cervical fusion and osteosynthetic stabilisation for fractures and/or dislocations of the cervical spine. J Spinal Disord Tech 8:499–508, 1995.
23. Pospiech J, Stolke D, Wilke JH: Intradiscal pressure recordings in the cervical spine. Neurosurgery 44:379–385, 1999.
24. Matsunaga S, Kababyama S, Yamamoto T, et al: Strain on intervertebral discs after anterior cervical decompression and fusion. Spine 24:670–675, 1999.
25. Hillibrand AS, Carlson GD, Palumbo MA, et al: Radiculopathy and myelopathy at segments adjacent to the site of a previous anterior arthrodesis. J Bone Joint Surg Am 81A:519–528, 1999.
26. Hirsch C: Cervical disk rupture: Diagnosis and therapy. Acta Orthop Scand 30:172–186, 1960.
27. Teramoto T, Ohmori K, Takatsu T, et al: Long term results of the anterior cervical spondylosis. Neurosurgery 35:64–68, 1994.
28. Murphy MA, Trimble MB, Piedmonte MR, Kalfas IH: Changes in the cervical foraminal area after anterior discectomy with and without a graft, Neurosurgery 34:93–96, 1994.
29. Rish BC, McFadden JT, Penix JO: Anterior cervical fusion using homologous bone grafts: A comparative study. Surg Neurol 5:119–121, 1976.
30. Yamamoto I, Ikeda A, Shibaya N, et al: Clinical long-term results of anterior discectomy without interbody fusion for cervical disc disease. Spine 16:272–279, 1991.
31. Savolainen S, Rinne J, Hernesniemi J: A prospective randomised study of anterior single level cervical disc operations with long-term follow-up: Surgical fusion is unnecessary. Neurosurgery 43:51–55, 1998.
32. Theodore N, Sonntag V. Spinal surgery: The past century and the next. Neurosurgery 46:767–777, 2000.
33. Chow D, Luk K, Evans J, et al: Effects of short anterior lumbar interbody fusion on the biomechanics of neighbouring infused segments. Spine 21:549–555, 1996.
34. Dekutoski M, Schandel M, Ogitrie J, et al: Comparison of in vivo and in vitro adjacent segment motion after lumbar fusion. Spine 19:1745–1751, 1994.
35. Lee C, Langrana N: Lumbosacral spinal fusion: A biomechanical study. Spine 9:574–581, 1984.
36. Di Angelo D, Robertson J, Metcalf N, et al: Biomechanical testing of an artificial cervical joint and an anterior cervical plate. J Spinal Disorder Tech 16:314–323, 2003.
37. Rouleau J, Conta R, Bryan V: In vivo stability of a cervical disc prosthesis. IV, Combined Meeting Orthopaedic Research Societies of the USA, Canada, Europe and Japan (Rhodes, Greece), June 3–7, 2001.
38. Fridenberg ZB, Miller WT: Degenerative disk disease of the cervical spine. J Bone Joint Surg Am 45:1171–1178, 1968.
39. Lee F, Turner JWA: Natural history and prognosis of cervical spondylosis. BMJ 2:1607–1610, 1963.
40. Gore DR, Sepic SB, Gardner GM, Murray MP: Neck pain: A long term follow-up of 205 patients. Spine 12:1–5, 1987.
41. Epstein JA, Epstein NE: The surgical management of cervical spinal stenosis, spondylosis and myeloradiculopathy. In Sherk HH, Dunn EJ, Eismont FJ, et al (eds): The Cervical Spine, 2nd ed. Philadelphia: JB Lippincott, 1989, pp 625–643.
42. Ebersold MJ, Parc MC, Quast LM: Surgical treatment for cervical spondylotic myelopathy. J Neurosurg 82:745–751, 1995.
43. Chestnuts RC, Abitbol JS, Farfin S: Surgical management of cervical radiculopathy indications, techniques and results. Orthop Clin North Am 23:461–474, 1992.
44. Benzel E: Biomechanics of Spine Stabilization. Rolling Meadows, IL: American Association of Neurological Surgeons, 2001.
45. Herkowitz HN: Surgical management of cervical radiculopathy: Anterior fusion. In Rothman RH, Simeone FH (eds): The Spine, 3rd ed. Philadelphia: WB Saunders, 1992, pp 597–606.
46. Crandall PH, Batzdorf U: Cervical spondylotic myelopathy. J Neurosurg 25:57–66, 1966.

47. Adams CBT, Longue V: Studies in cervical spondylotic myelopathy. Brain 94:587–594, 1971.
48. Stookey B: Compression of the spinal cord due to vertebral extradural cervical chondromas: Diagnosis and surgical treatment. Arch Neurol Psychol 20:275–291, 1928.
49. Brain WR: Rupture of the intervertebral disc in the cervical region. Proc R Soc Med 41:509–511, 1948.
50. Gooding MR, Wilson CB, Hoff ST: Experimental cervical myelopathy: Effects of ischaemia and compression of the acute cervical spinal cord. J Neurosurg 43:9–17, 1975.
51. Marr WG, Druckman R: The pathology of the spinal cord lesions and their relationship to the cervical features in protrusions of the cervical intervertebral discs. Brain 76:70–91, 1953.
52. Ferguson RJL, Caplan LR: Cervical spondylotic myelopathy. Neurol Clin 3:373–382, 1985.
53. Crandall PH, Batzdorf U: Cervical spondylotic myelopathy. J Neurosurg 25:57–66, 1966.
54. Gregorias FK, Estrim T, Crandall PH: Cervical spondylotic radiculopathy and myelopathy: A long term follow-up study. Arch Neurol 33:618, 1976.
55. Bohlmann H: Cervical spondylosis with moderate to severe myelopathy. Spine 2:151–162, 1977.
56. Abitol JS, Garfin SR: Surgical management of cervical disc disease: Anterior cervical fusion. Semin Spine Surg 4:233–238, 1989.
57. Bell G, Ross J: Diagnosis of nerve root compression, myelography, computed tomography and MRI. Orthop Clin North Am 23:405–419, 1992.
58. Rahim K, Stambough J: Radiographic evaluation of the degenerative cervical spine. Orthop Clin North Am 23:395–403, 1992.
59. Friedenberg ZB, Miller WT: Degenerative disc disease of the cervical spine: A comparative study of asymptomatic and symptomatic patients. J Bone Joint Surg Am 45:1171–1178, 1963.
60. Whitecloud TS: Modern alternatives and techniques for one-level discectomy and fusion. Clin Orthop 359:67–76, 1999.
61. Matsuda Y, Miyazaki K, Kenj T, et al: Increased MR signal intensity due to cervical myelopathy. J Neurosurg 74:887–892, 1991.
62. White AA, Johnson RM, Panjabi MM, et al: Biomechanical analysis of clinical stability in the cervical spine. Clin Orthop 109:85–106, 1975.
63. Hronson N, Bagab M, Filtzer DL: Results of using the Smith-Robinson approach for herniated and extruded cervical discs: Technical note. J Neurosurg 32:721–722, 1970.
64. Tew JM, Mayfield FH: Complications of surgery of the anterior cervical spine. Clin Neurosurg 23:424–434, 1976.
65. Lundsford LD, Bissonnette DJ, Jannetta PJ, et al: Anterior surgery for cervical disc disease. J Neurosurg 53:11, 1980.
66. Flynn TB: Neurological complications of anterior cervical interbody fusion. Spine 7:536–539, 1982.
67. Murphy MG, Gado M: Anterior cervical discectomy without interbody bone graft. J Neurosurg 37:71–74, 1972.

131 Anterior Approaches in Multisegmental Cervical Spondylosis

VOLKER SEIFERT and MICHAEL ZIMMERMANN

Surgical treatment of cervical myelopathy resulting from multisegmental cervical spondylosis (MSCS) is performed by anterior or posterior approaches. The operative procedures that have been employed for MSCS include multisegmental anterior fusion, corpectomy, and graft placement as well as laminectomy and laminoplasty. Considering the complex nature of the underlying disease involving more than one cervical segment as well as the pathobiomechanical features of the spondylotic cervical spine, adequate decompression of the spinal cord, and correction of hypermobility should be achieved by surgery in one stage to have positive immediate and long-term benefits for the patient with progressive myelopathy. Because the offending bony lesions, which are largely responsible for the development of the myelopathic process, are located anteriorly in most patients, neurosurgeons have increasingly used the anterior approach for decompression of the cervical cord. The application of the surgical microscope and microsurgical techniques has been shown to be extremely helpful for the atraumatic and radical performance of the decompressive procedure. Moreover, osteosynthetic techniques are now available and can be used for augmentation of the necessary subsequent bone graft fusion. Based on these prerequisites, vertebral body replacement combined with microsurgical decompression and anterior plating has emerged as an aggressive therapeutic approach for the treatment of MSCS.

PATHOLOGIC CONSIDERATIONS

Although a detailed discussion of the complex pathologic and pathobiomechanical changes responsible for the development of cervical spondylotic myelopathy (CSM) is beyond the scope and intention of this chapter, a brief survey of current concepts is justified. CSM is the result of progression of severe degenerative processes affecting the cervical spinal column and supportive structures, the nerve roots, and the spinal cord itself. The multifactorial cause of CSM involves mechanical, vascular, and dynamic factors, which are of additive importance for the development of the disease.[1-3] The reduced size of the cervical spinal canal, of either congenital or acquired origin, and the development of anterior osteophytes with further compromise of the canal size are considered to be the major mechanical factors in the pathogenesis of CSM (Fig. 131-1). The normal anteroposterior diameter of the cervical spinal canal varies greatly among individuals, ranging from 16 to 18 mm at C3–7, with the spinal cord diameter ranging from 8.5 to 11.5 mm.[4]

It has been established by several authors that in patients with CSM, the average diameter of the lower cervical spine is approximately 3 mm less than in cases with spondylosis without CSM. Wolf and colleagues[5] demonstrated that a canal size of less than 10 mm in anteroposterior diameter was likely to be associated with CSM, whereas the average canal size of patients with CSM evaluated by Adams and Logue[6] was less than 12 mm. These findings have been confirmed by other authors.[7-10]

Although compromise of the cervical spinal canal is probably the most important component in the pathogenesis of CSM, further narrowing of the cervical canal by bony osteophytes, especially when located anteriorly, and ossification of the posterior longitudinal ligament[11,12] and hypertrophy of the ligamentum flavum[13] result in further deformation and compromise of the cord, aggravating the effects of the narrow canal.[14] Especially under flexion and extension, bony osteophytes may act as a fulcrum over which the spinal cord in motion is stretched.

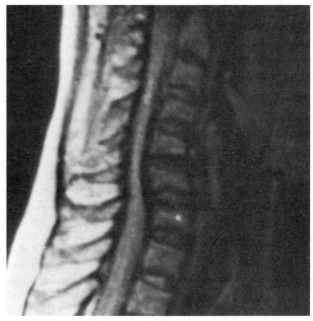

FIGURE 131-1 Magnetic resonance imaging examination (T2 weighted) demonstrates multisegmental cervical canal stenosis from C4 to C6 with anterior compression of the cervical cord.

In regard to the contribution of vascular factors to the pathogenesis of CSM, there is still some controversy.[15] The initial hypothesis, however, put forward by Mair and Druckmann,[16] that ischemic changes in the spinal cord are the result of compression of the anterior spinal artery by anteriorly located osteophytes, does not correspond with comparative studies of experimental occlusion of the anterior spinal artery in animals and the histopathologic patterns of ischemic intramedullary changes detectable in postmortem studies of patients with severe CSM.[17] Several authors have stressed the importance of compression and occlusion of intramedullary vessels rather than anterior spinal artery compression.[18] This compression and occlusion is considered to be the result of tensile stresses and central shear forces acting on the intramedullary arteries in the presence of congenital or acquired cervical canal compromise. As Hukuda and Wilson[19] have pointed out, however, the effects of cervical cord compression and repeated ischemia affecting the cervical cord are likely to be additive for the development of CSM.[20]

Considering that severe cervical spondylosis motion of the cervical cord in flexion and extension leads to aggravation of either spondylotic cord compression or medullary ischemia, increased mobility of the cervical spine represents a significant dynamic factor in the pathogenesis of CSM.[21,22] In this regard, it has been shown that the spinal cord, compromised by spondylotic encroachments, is more vulnerable to adverse tensile stresses, which are likely to occur under the condition of pathologic increase in segmental vertebral column motion,[21] resulting in further aggravation of the preexisting cervical cord injury.

SURGICAL CONSIDERATIONS

Indication for surgery in patients with MSCS is primarily based on the progression of clinical symptoms of advanced cervical myelopathy and on the radiographic detection of multisegmental spondylosis. The clinical diagnosis of CSM is based on the clinical picture, the summary of data derived from a number of radiographic procedures, and the exclusion of other possible nonmechanical causes of long tract alteration.[23] Additional electrophysiologic examinations, such as recording of somatosensory-evoked potential responses, may add helpful information for establishing the diagnosis in selected cases[24] but should not be regarded as an alternative for a thorough neurologic examination. The condition sine qua non for the clinical diagnosis of spondylotic myelopathy is the presence of spastic paraparesis or tetraparesis accompanied by gait abnormality. Severe nuchal, shoulder/arm, or radicular pain and sensory deficits or sensations, although present in a large number of patients with myelopathy, are not reliable in terms of clinical diagnosis.[23] Additionally, the severity of the above-mentioned signs and symptoms varies considerably among patients, which is why different clinical grading systems have been developed in the past (e.g., those of Nurick[25] Harsh and colleagues,[26] and the Japanese Orthopedic Association [JOA]) for the evaluation of pre- and postoperative neurologic status. Although these grading systems are far from satisfactory, they are widely used to classify the degree of myelopathy in patients, while allowing comparison of different forms of conservative or surgical treatment.

Once the suspicion of the clinical diagnosis of cervical myelopathy has been raised, a number of radiographic procedures can be used in combination or alternatively to confirm the existence of relevant bony compression and injury of the cervical cord. Over the years, plain radiographs and cervical myelograms have been used exclusively for the diagnosis of spondylotic myelopathy, and the diagnostic accuracy of myelography still represents the gold standard with which the sophisticated methods of computed tomography (CT) and magnetic resonance imaging (MRI) must be compared.[27,28] Despite the wide and rapid availability of CT and MRI, the authors continue to use myelography in selected cases and for the performance of dynamic studies in flexion and extension of the cervical spine. The virtue of the plain CT scan lies in the fact that it is still the best radiographic method for the demonstration of the presence and amount of bony cord compression by clearly showing the pathologic anatomy in regard to anterior osteophytes and bony narrowing of the cervical canal using the bone-window technique. Moreover, this technique can be used postoperatively to document the amount of surgical bony decompression.[29] The additional question of the degree of bony impingement of the cervical cord can be answered reliably only by CT myelography, which has lost its rank to the superior imaging qualities of MRI. The usefulness of MRI for the imaging of cervical myelopathy has been shown by a number of reports; however, a discussion of the different modes of MRI application is beyond the scope of this chapter, and these modes have been detailed extensively elsewhere.[28,30–33]

Additional clinicoradiographic studies have demonstrated that the severity of compressive alteration of the cervical cord can be evaluated by increased MRI signal intensity within the cord on T2-weighted images.[34] The major advantage of the modern imaging techniques, however, whether CT or MRI, is the ability to clearly demonstrate the pathoanatomic relationship between the extent and especially the location of the offending compressive bone lesions and the amount of cord compromise, which now can be used to tailor the kind and extent of the operative approach. CT and MRI have impressively confirmed earlier suggestions derived from surgical experience or myelography that in CSM the relevant bony compression is located anteriorly in more than 75% of patients.[17] These findings have questioned the routine application of posterior approaches to the cervical spine in CSM, which have been in use for the treatment of this entity for many years. Although there are a vast number of series reporting outcomes from both the anterior and posterior approaches, comparative analyses are rare.[12,17,35–40]

Summarizing those few comparative studies reported in the literature, anterior approaches have a success rate of approximately 75% compared with 60% for posterior approaches. Although in most of these studies, only single-level myelopathic disease has been treated, the question of the appropriate surgical approach becomes even more complicated when more than one cervical segment is affected by the spondylotic process. Posterior approaches, such as multilevel laminectomies, or canal-expanding techniques, such as laminotomy or laminoplasty, have been used primarily for the treatment of MSCS.[41–45] A large amount of data has been accumulated from anterior surgery for the treatment of cervical disc disease as well as for tumor and trauma of the cervical spine, with a high percentage of good or excellent results.[46–49] Considering these experiences, despite technical problems and dissatisfying results from extensive posterior surgery in patients with MSCS, vertebrectomy combined with radical microsurgical removal of anterior osteophytes has emerged as a highly efficient and relatively atraumatic procedure for the treatment of this disease.[37,50] The convincing concept of vertebrectomy, for which the words *corpectomy* and *spondylectomy* are used synonymously in the literature, lies in the ability to treat the two main pathogenetic factors of cervical myelopathy, bony compression of the cervical cord and multisegmental spinal hypermobility, during a single surgical procedure. Single-level or multilevel corpectomy with removal of the posterior longitudinal ligament and microsurgical osteophytectomy eliminates cord compression, whereas hypermobility is treated by bone graft fusion and is, according to the preference of the surgeon, augmented by osteosynthesis.

SURGICAL TECHNIQUE

Patients are given prophylactic antibiotics intravenously before skin incision and thereafter every 8 hours for a total of 36 hours. The patient is placed supine on the operating table under general anesthesia. In cases of severe anterior compression, intubation is performed using a fiberoptic device. The head is slightly extended and secured in a three-point skull fixation device. A standardized approach along the medial border of the sternocleidomastoid muscle to the anterior cervical spine is employed (Fig. 131-2). After a transverse skin incision, the subcutaneous fat is separated generously from the underlying platysma muscle. The platysma is incised, and the incision is extended vertically in the craniad and caudad direction. The anterior rim of the sternocleidomastoid muscle is mobilized by sharply

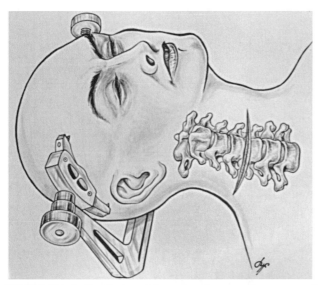

FIGURE 131-2 Positioning of the patient for a vertebrectomy and osteosynthesis. The head is slightly extended and fixed in a Mayfield clamp. A horizontal incision is used, which is appropriate for a vertebrectomy up to three levels. If more levels are to be removed, a vertical-oblique incision along the anterior border of the sternocleidomastoid muscle is more convenient.

dissecting the areolar tissue along its medial border. The cleavage plane between the carotid artery and the esophagus is identified and further dissected by either blunt or sharp preparation. After the spine is exposed, the avascular tissue covering the vertebral bodies and discs is incised vertically along the anterior aspect of the affected vertebra. Using intraoperative fluoroscopic control, the disc spaces above and below the planned level of vertebrectomy are identified and marked by an incision of the anterior longitudinal ligament. The medial border of the longus colli muscle is cauterized bilaterally, stripped from the adjacent vertebra, and retracted with a retractor. The Caspar cervical spine instrumentation system (Aesculap Co., Tuttlingen, Germany) is routinely used for the complete procedure.[47]

The surgical microscope is brought into place, and both cervical discs are removed down to the level of the posterior longitudinal ligament (Fig. 131-3). The ligament is incised and removed until the dura in the depth of the cervical disc space is well exposed. When the removal of more than one vertebra is planned, the appropriate disc spaces between the segments are also removed. The screws of the vertebral body distractor are inserted into the vertebra above and below the planned vertebrectomy site, the vertebral body distractor is slipped over the screw shafts, and gradual distraction is performed, which allows an excellent, unobstructed view along the exposed disc spaces. The vertebrectomy is now performed, starting with rongeurs of different sizes and a high-speed drill, by which the mass of the vertebral body is removed until only the posterior cortical margin is left (Fig. 131-4). The remaining parts of the vertebra and the posterior longitudinal ligament are removed completely under high magnification with a diamond drill and small biting forceps (Fig. 131-5). Because the dural surface has already been exposed after radical disc space evacuation, this delicate part of the spondylectomy can be performed safely under direct vision of the dura and under the prerequisite that the illumination and magnification of the surgical microscope is used. Lateral resection of the vertebral body and posterior longitudinal ligament is performed to the lateral gutter on both sides.

Usually, some bleeding from larger epidural veins located in the lateral gutter occurs but can be controlled easily with hemostatic foam and placement of cottonoids. Radical removal of osteophytes at the posterior margin of the remaining vertebrae craniad and caudad to the spondylectomy site is performed with the diamond drill and microrongeurs, which are used in an undercutting technique. Radical decompression of the exposed dural space from all offending bony lesions is absolutely necessary. This decompression can be judged to be complete when the pulsating dura is bulging into the operative vertebrectomy defect (Fig. 131-6). Not infrequently the pulsatile movements of the cerebrospinal fluid can be observed through the thinned dura. After radical corpectomy is completed, an appropriate bone graft is harvested from the iliac crest and is shaped to a rectangular size and fitted to the vertebrectomy defect using a cutting forceps and a high-speed drill (Fig. 131-7). Apart from the rectangular form of the graft, no special configuration is necessary. Even in multisegmental spondylectomy, iliac bone is preferred to a fibular strut graft because it can be more easily contoured according to the lordotic curvature of the cervical spine, which is important if a plating procedure is planned.

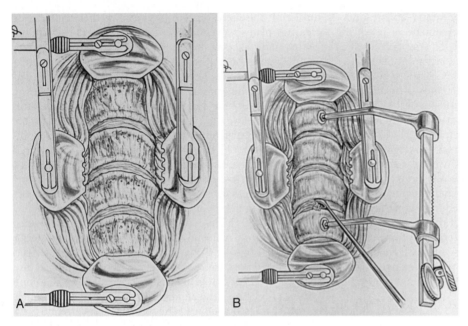

FIGURE 131-3 The cervical spine is exposed using the routine anterior approach. Retractors are placed under the medial border of the longus colli muscle bilaterally and in a cranial and caudal direction (A). After the anterior part of the appropriate discs are partially emptied by rongeurs, the CASPAR vertebral body distractors are slipped over the screw shafts, and gradual distraction is performed. With the aid of the surgical microscope, the disc spaces are completely cleared with rongeurs and sharp spoons of different sizes down to the level of the posterior longitudinal ligament, which is also removed (B).

After vertebral body replacement, the distraction instrumentation is removed, so that the bone graft is locked in place by the self-retracting forces of the adjacent vertebra (Fig. 131-8). Osteosynthesis is performed using a titanium plate of appropriate length. Overlapping of nonfused interspaces should be avoided because this leads to excessive plate motion and possible plate breakage. If the plate length is chosen correctly, it should allow insertion of the screws approximately into the midportion of the vertebral body at both ends of the plate. The plate should be bent before placement, so that it fits tightly to the cervical lordosis and to the graft. Under radiographic control, two drill holes measuring 2 mm each are made in the vertebra above and

below the spondylectomy level. These holes can be made safely using an adjustable drill guide, while hand advancement of the screw within the vertebral body is observed using fluoroscopic control (Fig. 131-9). After the length of the drill canal, which should almost reach the posterior vertebral cortex, has been measured, four 3.5-mm self-tapping spongiosa screws are inserted that are approximately 1 mm longer than the measured length of the drill canal. The screw tip should lie in the posterior vertebral cortex or as close to it as possible. In general, the length of the spongiosa screws is 20 to 22 mm in adults. After all four screws are placed, they are tightened one after another in an opposite fashion under fluoroscopic control to secure the plate safely

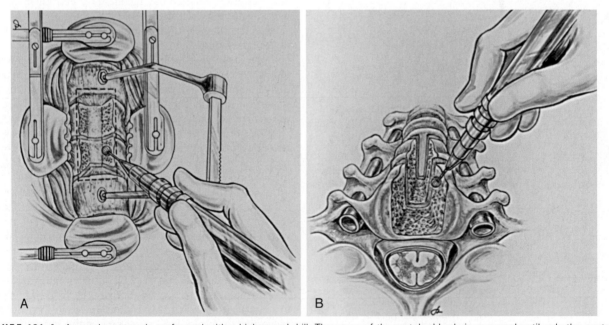

FIGURE 131-4 A vertebrectomy is performed with a high-speed drill. The mass of the vertebral body is removed until only the posterior cortical margin is left. Direct (A) and axial (B) views are shown.

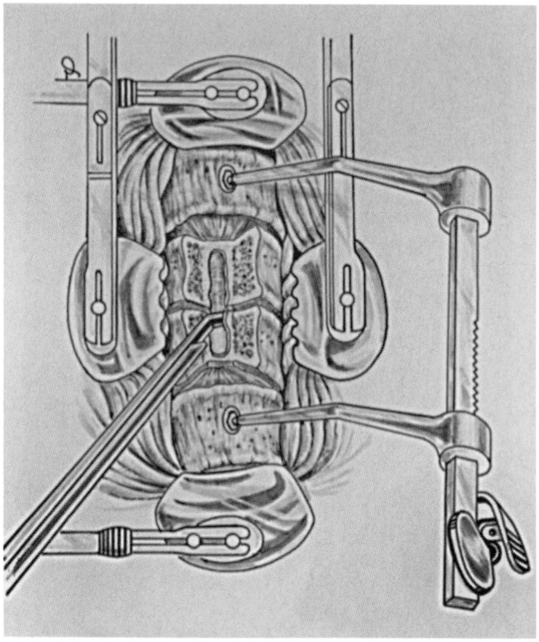

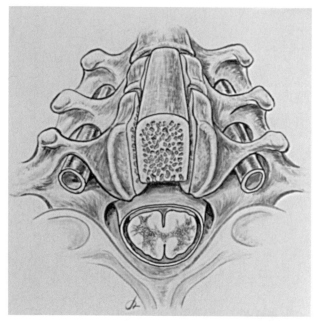

FIGURE 131-5 Using high magnification, the remaining parts of the vertebra and the posterior longitudinal ligament are removed with a diamond drill and microrongeurs. Note that the dura has been well exposed in the depth of the operating field, so that the bone and ligament can be removed safely. Under these conditions, adequate epidural decompression in cranial, caudal, and lateral directions must be performed.

FIGURE 131-7 After a radical vertebrectomy and epidural decompression are completed, an appropriate bone graft is harvested from the iliac crest, shaped to a rectangular size, and placed into the vertebrectomy defect. Apart from the rectangular form of the graft, no special shaping of the bone graft is necessary. The bone graft itself is locked in place by the self-retracting forces of the adjacent vertebrae after the distraction instrumentation has been removed.

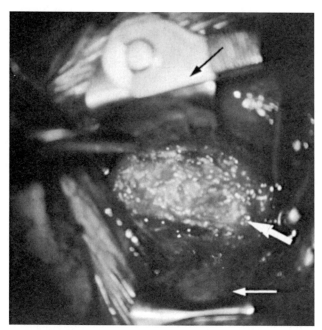

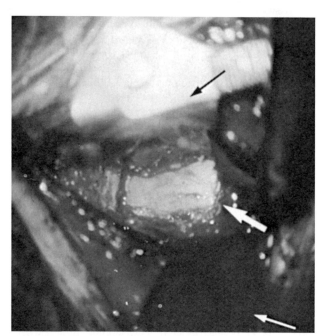

FIGURE 131-6 An intraoperative view after a two-level vertebrectomy, which is seen through the surgical microscope. The dura (*wide arrow*), which is bulging into the operative defect, is visible in the depth of the operating field. Retractor blades are marked by *narrow arrows*.

FIGURE 131-8 The same operative field is shown as in Figure 131-7 after insertion of an iliac bone graft (*wide arrow*). Retractor blades are marked by *narrow arrows*.

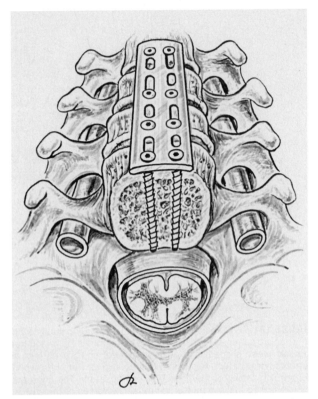

FIGURE 131-9 An intraoperative sketch with a horizontal cut through a vertebral body demonstrates the ideal position of the plate and screw tips.

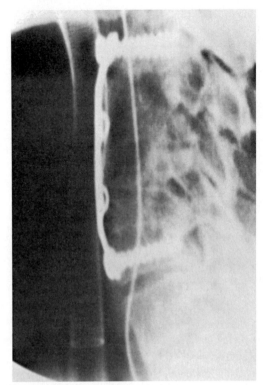

FIGURE 131-10 An example of intraoperative fluoroscopic control demonstrates good positioning of the screws and plate, which adhere tightly to the graft. The screws have been inserted in the midportion of the respective vertebra and have been advanced up to the posterior vertebral cortex.

into position. One or two additional screws of 14 mm length can be used for securing the graft in position (Fig. 131-10). After meticulous hemostasis is achieved, a drain is inserted, and the wound is closed in layers. In the case of a single-level vertebrectomy, only a soft collar is used. When more than one vertebra has been removed, a Philadelphia collar-type orthosis is applied, which should be worn for 12 weeks. Because of the immediate stability provided by the osteosynthesis, the application of a halo device is not considered to be necessary. The day after surgery, the drain is removed, and the patient is mobilized. Seven days after surgery, a control radiograph of the cervical spine is performed, and the patient is discharged.

RESULTS

Compared with the extensive literature that exists regarding the surgical treatment of CSM, larger detailed reports on the use of vertebrectomy and subsequent stabilizing techniques in the treatment of MSCS are scarce and have predominantly appeared in the orthopedic literature. Evaluating the results of 13 large series on corpectomy in MSCS, the percentage of improvement reported ranged from 73% to 100%. Different series on this form of treatment in patients with CSM are difficult to compare. The complex nature of the clinical picture of the myelopathic disease makes evaluation of preoperatively existing signs and symptoms as well as of postoperative results difficult. The authors of these series use either description of myelopathic symptoms or different grading systems of myelopathy such as those of Nurick,[25] Harsh and colleagues,[26] and the JOA for

the evaluation of pre- and postoperative neurologic status, or individual scores, which does not allow adequate comparison of results. Moreover, the differences in the surgical techniques used are considerable, such as the extent of vertebrectomy and decompression, the use of macrosurgical or microsurgical techniques for removal of compressive epidural structures, the type and configuration of the inserted graft, and whether an osteosynthetic procedure is performed.

In the first published description of this technique, Whitecloud and La Rocca[51] in their series of 18 patients with symptomatic MSCS reported an improvement of 100%. The authors stated, however, that clinical outcome is difficult to tabulate and compare. Despite the fact that excellent results with relief of all preoperative symptoms and improvement in abnormal clinical findings could not be achieved, significant relief of pain, functional recovery, and improvement of the overall neurologic status, although not further detailed, were noted in all patients.

Hanai and colleagues[52] in their study of subtotal vertebrectomy for CSM used the more specific evaluating score of the JOA, in which a score of 17 points is considered normal in motor, sensory, and bladder function. The preoperative score in their patients ranged from 5 to 14 points. Marked improvement was noted shortly after the operation in all patients, with long-lasting relief of symptoms in almost all patients. The postoperative JOA score ranged from 9 to 16 points. No patient reported deterioration of the symptoms at the final consultation.

Boni and colleagues,[53] evaluating the results of 29 cases of CSM treated by resection of the central portion of multiple vertebral bodies followed by iliac graft stabilization, reported good results in 53% and moderate improvement in 39%.

Bernard and Whitecloud[54] evaluated their results in 21 patients with CSM treated with aggressive anterior multilevel resection of compressive bony structures and stabilization by autogenous fibular strut graft. Significant improvement was found in 19 of 21 patients.

Doi and colleagues[55] reported their limited experiences in six patients with CSM and ossification of the posterior longitudinal ligament treated by multilevel partial vertebrectomies and stabilization by a vascularized fibular graft. Results were again evaluated by the JOA score and Hirabayashi's improvement score, classifying the clinical results into four grades from excellent to poor outcome. The mean preoperative JOA score was 9.6, and the mean postoperative score was 13.9. Five overall good or excellent results and one fair result were found.

Comparable satisfactory results of larger groups of patients who underwent anterior multilevel decompression and fusion were reported by Senegas and colleagues,[56] with 73% improvement in 45 patients; by Rengachary and Redford,[57] with 86% improved patients in a group of 22 patients with CSM; and by Zdeblick and Bohlman,[58] with 100% improvement in their small series of eight patients with cervical kyphosis and myelopathy. Okada and colleagues[59] reported their results in 37 patients with spondylotic myelopathy treated by partial or subtotal corpectomy followed by strut bone grafting. Patients were graded preoperatively according to the Nurick scale. A satisfactory postoperative result was obtained in 29 patients (78%). All but one of the 37 patients had improved walking ability after surgery. During follow-up, one patient reverted to the preoperative status after initial improvement, and three patients deteriorated, which was the result of new spondylotic changes associated with stenosis of the cervical spinal canal. Yonenobu and colleagues[39] evaluated their results of three different forms of surgical treatment in 90 patients with cervical myelopathy. Extensive laminectomy was performed in 24 patients, anterior fusion in 50 patients, and subtotal vertebrectomy and fusion in 21 patients. Compared with the other two procedures, the results of subtotal vertebrectomy were considered to be significantly better. Kojima and colleagues[60] reported their results with anterior cervical vertebrectomy and interbody fusion in 45 patients with multilevel spondylosis, ossification of the posterior longitudinal ligament, or a combination of both diseases. In their study, the results of the operations were evaluated by the classification of Harsh and colleagues.[26] Although this classification does not include neurologic symptoms and signs of the upper extremities, it was considered by the authors to be convenient and practical for neurologic symptoms and signs in the lower extremities. Improvement of one grade or more in Harsh's myelopathic scale was classified as a good result. In this regard, 16 of the 19 patients with MSCS had good results (84%). Eleven of 12 patients with ossification of the posterior longitudinal ligament had good results (92%), and 12 of 14 patients with both cervical spondylosis and ossification of the posterior longitudinal ligament had good results (86%).

In two studies, Saunders and colleagues[61] and the authors' group[50] evaluated the results of multilevel corpectomy and fusion. In their detailed study, Saunders and colleagues[61] followed 40 cases over a period of 2 to 5 years.

Patients' myelopathic symptoms were graded by the classification of Nurick with additional evaluation of resolution of preoperative central cord syndrome.[62] The outcome was defined as a cure if the patient was satisfied with the operation, with no complaints and no other signs than active reflexes or residual minor hand intrinsic atrophy. Improvement was defined as a change of at least two grades in the Nurick classification or resolution of hyperpathia and dysesthesia (or both). Failure was defined as fewer changes than described or regression of improvement. By these criteria, the long-term cure rate was 57.5%, and the failure rate was 15%. There was no documentation of worsening of myelopathic symptoms. In the initial report of the authors' group, the results in 22 patients with MSCS treated by spondylectomy, microsurgical decompression, and fusion using iliac bone graft were detailed. It is the only study in the series discussed here in which an additional osteosynthetic procedure with metal plates and screws was performed. Additionally, it is the only study in which the postoperative ability to return to work was evaluated. In 19 of 22 patients, the clinical symptoms consisted of typical signs of advanced myelopathy, including gait disturbance, severe impairment of sensory and motor function, and bladder dysfunction. Pain radiating into the upper extremities as well as into the craniocervical region was present in 15 patients. In three patients, incapacitating pain was the most prominent symptom of cervical spondylosis, accompanied by only moderate spastic paresis and hyperreflexia.

In 14 patients, one vertebra was removed; in seven patients, two vertebrae were removed; and in one patient, three vertebrae were removed. The level of single vertebrectomy was at C5 in eight patients, at C4 in two patients, at C6 in two patients, and at C3 and C7 in one patient each. Spondylectomy incorporating two vertebrae was performed four times at the C4–5 level, two times at the C5–6 level, and one time at the C3–4 level. In one patient, C4, C5, and C6 were removed. Of the 19 patients with advanced myelopathic disease, 14 patients were symptom free or had only minor residual symptoms (73.7%). Three patients complained of persistent phases of nuchal or cervicobrachial pain, which could be controlled by the temporary use of analgesics or the application of a soft collar. Symptoms of myelopathy were still present in two patients; however, both patients considered the severity of their disease to be less than before surgery, and neither patient was incapacitated by the myelopathic process. Three patients with excruciating pain secondary to severe cervical spondylosis had significant pain relief. Regarding the socioeconomic results of surgery, of 15 patients who were employed before surgery but not able to perform regular work because of their disease, 13 patients returned to a full-time job. Radiographic follow-up examinations at different intervals showed solid bony fusion in all patients (Fig. 131-11). These data from the authors' initial study on the use of vertebrectomy, microsurgical decompression, and osteosynthesis have been confirmed by more recent experiences, including more than 150 patients with MSCS treated in the described manner, in which an overall percentage of 75% good or satisfactory results have been found.

MacDonald and colleagues[63] performed anterior cervical corporectomy and fibular allograft fusion for cervical myelopathy in 36 patients. Four vertebrae were removed in

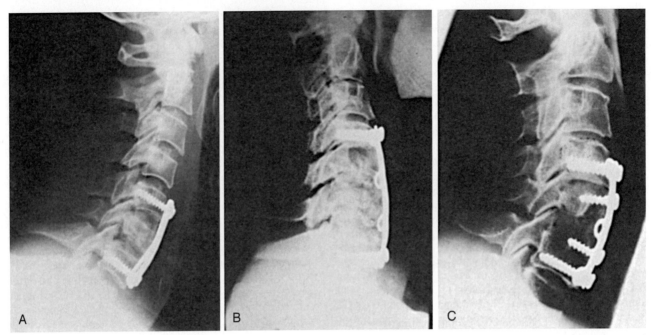

FIGURE 131-11 Typical examples of follow-up radiographs in three different patients. Good positioning of the inserted iliac bone graft and the osteosynthetic material is shown. In the patient in Figure 131-5C, additional screws have been inserted in the graft. However, from a biomechanical point of view, this is not absolutely necessary to achieve a stable and solid bone fusion.

six patients, three in 19, and two in 11 patients. Instrumentation was used in 15 cases. The operative mortality rate was 3% (one patient), and two patients died 2 months postoperatively. Postoperative complications included early graft displacement requiring reoperation (three patients), transient dysphagia (two patients), cerebrospinal fluid leak treated by lumbar drainage (three patients), myocardial infarction (two patients), and late graft fracture (one patient). One patient developed transient worsening of myelopathy and three developed temporary radiculopathies. All patients achieved stable bone union and the mean Nurick grade at an average of 31 ± 20 months (range, 0 to 79) postoperatively was 2.4 ± 1.6 ($p < 0.05$). Cervicobrachial pain improved in 10 (59%) of the 17 patients who had preoperative pain, and myelopathy improved at least one grade in 17 patients (47%, $p < 0.05$). Twenty-six surviving patients (72%) were followed for more than 24 months, and stable, osseous union occurred in 97%.

Fessler and colleagues[64] analyzed the results of 93 patients who underwent multilevel anterior corporectomy for CSM. Symptomatic improvement was achieved for 92% of patients ($p < 0.001$). Nurick scores reflected improvement for 86% of patients, with the conditions of 13% remaining unchanged and only one patient showing worsening. Preoperative myelopathy severity was weakly correlated with age ($p < 0.05$) but was not correlated with gender or number of levels decompressed. Patients treated with anterior corporectomy showed an average improvement of 1.24 points on the Nurick scale, compared with an improvement of 0.07 points for patients treated with laminectomy ($p < 0.001$) and a deterioration of 0.23 points

for patients undergoing conservative treatment ($p < 0.001$). Complications were more likely to occur in older patients ($p < 0.05$). The number of levels decompressed was not significantly correlated with complications.

For the anterior group, good results were reported by Saunders and colleagues[65] in 1998. In their retrospective analysis of 31 cases of four-level corpectomies, they reported that 25 patients improved by at least 1 Nurick grade, which was 89% of surviving patients (80% of entire group). One patient died postoperatively of a pulmonary embolism on day 3. Complications also occurred in other eight cases (total complication rate, 29%).

Wada and colleagues[40] compared subtotal corporectomy ($n = 23$) and laminoplasty ($n = 24$) for multilevel cervical myelopathy. No significant difference in neurologic recovery was found between the two groups 1 and 5 years after surgery. Axial pain was observed in 15% of the corporectomy group and in 40% of the laminoplasty group ($p < 0.05$). The corporectomy group needed longer operative time ($p < 0.001$) and tended to have more blood loss. Six patients in the corporectomy group needed posterior interspinous wiring because of pseudarthrosis.

In 2002, Edwards and colleagues[12] compared the results of corporectomy ($n = 13$) and laminoplasty ($n = 13$) for multilevel cervical myelopathy. Both multilevel corporectomy and laminoplasty arrested progression of cervical myelopathy or led to significant neurologic recovery and pain reduction in the majority of patients. There was a higher incidence of complications in the corporectomy group. The authors concluded that laminoplasty may be the preferred method of treatment for multilevel cervical myelopathy in the absence of preoperative kyphosis.

Illustrative Cases

CASE REPORT 1

The patient was a 50-year-old man from Turkey. Over a period of more than 2 years before presentation to the clinic, the patient had increasing pain in the neck with diffuse distribution into both arms. Chiropractic treatment did not result in any amelioration of symptoms. Within 6 months, the patient's clinical condition deteriorated to Nurick's disability classification grade 4, with gait disturbance, weakness, and paresthesia in both arms. When admitted to the clinic, the patient had severe gait abnormality and needed assistance during walking. During clinical examination, the patient demonstrated tetraspasticity with exaggerated deep tendon reflexes and a positive Babinski sign. Cervical myelography demonstrated almost complete block of the contrast media at the level of C5 (Fig. 131-12). Additional CT myelography showed significant compression and obstruction of the epidural space by extensive cervical spondylosis at the levels C4–5, C5–6, and C6–7 (Fig. 131-13). Because of the multisegmentality of the compression, it was decided to perform a two-level spondylectomy of C5 and C6 with microsurgical decompression at all three cervical segments. Within 6 months after surgery, the severe myelopathy showed significant improvement, with almost complete resolution of the preoperative tetraspastic signs and paresis, to Nurick's grade 2. Postoperative plain radiographs and CT scan demonstrated good position of

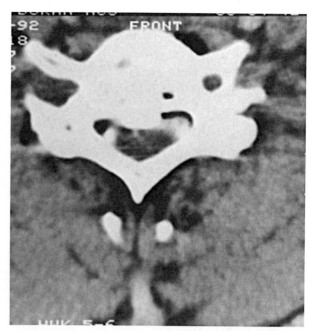

FIGURE 131-13 Case report 1: A preoperative computed tomography myelogram at the C5 vertebra level demonstrates a narrow cervical canal and anterior compression by midline osteophytes.

the bone graft and implanted osteosynthetic material (Fig. 131-14). CT scan of the spondylectomy area demonstrated complete resection of the midline compressive spondylotic bone with wide decompression (Fig. 131-15).

CASE REPORT 2

A 64-year-old woman had long-standing rheumatoid arthritis and had already undergone several operations for joint correction in both hands. Gradually over several years, she developed signs of progressing compromise of the cervical cord and nerve roots. When she was first seen at the authors' institution, the patient reported pain in the neck radiating into the occiput and into both arms. Wearing a soft collar reduced the pain. Plain radiographs in flexion and extension demonstrated only slight widening of the atlantoaxial distance. Additionally, there were radiographic signs of subaxial rheumatoid involvement of the cervical spine most pronounced at the C3–4 and C5–6 levels. No CT scan was performed at that time. Except for exaggerated deep tendon reflexes, there were no signs of cord compression. No indication for corrective or decompressive surgery was seen at that time. Over the next few months, the pain became increasingly worse and the patient was admitted again. Apart from the neck pain, the patient described bilateral excruciating pain sensations radiating in both arms. Additionally, she now exhibited signs of cord involvement and cervical myelopathy with spastic tetraparesis and gait abnormality. CT scan of the cervical spine at the C3–4 and C5–6 segments demonstrated narrowing of the cervical canal by posterior osteophytes at the C4 level and asymmetrical cervical canal stenosis at C5 (Fig. 131-16). MRI examination confirmed partially asymmetrical cervical

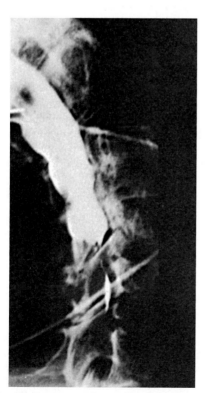

FIGURE 131-12 Case report 1: Preoperative cervical myelogram in a patient with multisegmental cervical spondylosis demonstrates almost complete arrest of the contrast media at the C5 level.

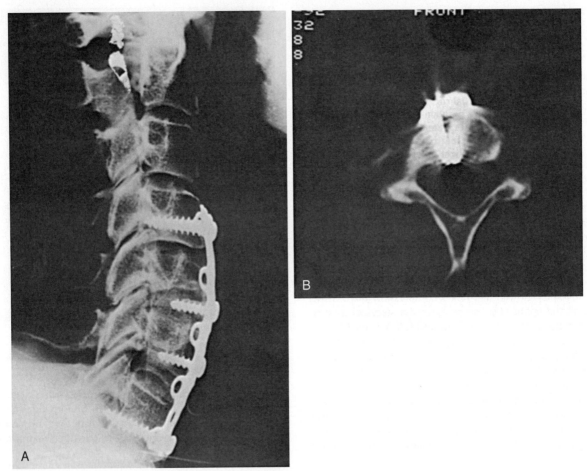

FIGURE 131-14   Case report 1: *A*, Postoperative radiograph 9 months after surgery demonstrates the good position of the inserted graft and osteosynthetic material. The slightly oblique projection gives the impression that screws in C7 have penetrated too far. However, a computed tomography scan (*B*) demonstrates that the screw tips are both placed exactly in the posterior vertebral cortex.

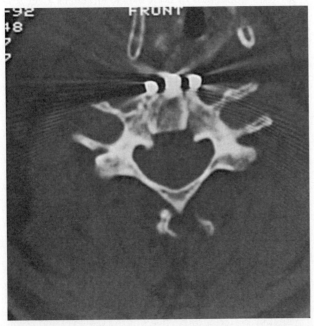

FIGURE 131-15   Case report 1: A postoperative computed tomography scan through the vertebrectomy and graft area demonstrates wide bone decompression and exact placement of grafted iliac bone.

canal stenosis with cervical cord compression (Fig. 131-17). Functional studies of the cervical spine in flexion and extension revealed subaxial hypermobility at the C5–6 level, which contributed to the progressing myelopathy. Because of the multisegmental involvement of cervical canal stenosis at least over two vertebrae and three segments, it was decided to perform a corpectomy of vertebrae C4 and C5 with resection of adjacent osteophytes and fusion. Intraoperatively, it was found that the posterior longitudinal ligament was thickened because of rheumatoid pannus, which compounded the effect of the bony compression of the cervical cord. All compressive bony elements as well as the posterior longitudinal ligament were meticulously removed, followed by bone grafting and osteosynthesis (Fig. 131-18). Postoperatively, the patient developed a temporary weakness of the right arm, which resolved completely within a few weeks. Although the preoperative excruciating pain subsided almost immediately after surgery, the myelopathic symptoms resolved slowly over the subsequent months. At follow-up, the patient was still pain free and ambulatory. Plain CT scan as well as sagittal CT reconstruction confirmed that wide bony decompression had been achieved by surgery (Fig. 131-19).

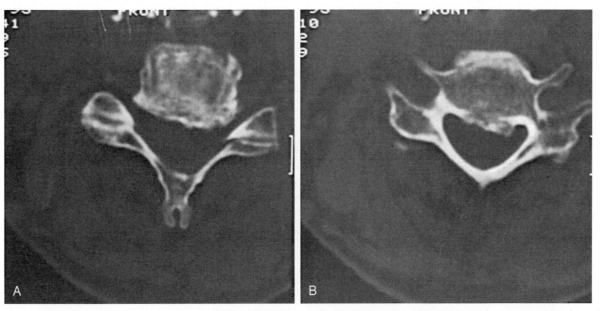

FIGURE 131-16 *A* and *B,* Case report 2: These preoperative computed tomography scans demonstrates the narrow cervical canal and asymmetrical bone encroachment of the cervical cord.

COMPLICATIONS

The complications of the presented procedure, in the experience of the authors and reported in the literature, are usually due to traumatic handling of the prevertebral soft tissue during the approach to the cervical spine, incomplete decompression, and graft-related problems. In the authors' series of more than 50 patients with CSM treated with spondylectomy, microsurgical decompression, and osteosynthesis, no mortality and no worsening of the preoperative neurologic condition occurred. Complications attributable to the surgical procedure were as follows: postoperative loosening of a single screw was detectable on follow-up

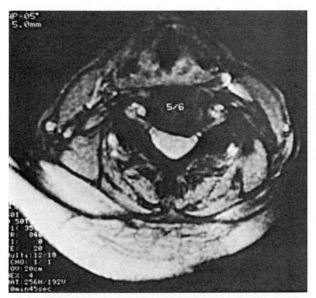

FIGURE 131-17 Case report 2: This preoperative magnetic resonance imaging scan shows asymmetrical bone compression of the cervical cord and nerve root.

radiographs in four patients; however, in none of the patients did this lead to any sort of morbidity or loosening of the affected plate. Breakage of a plate after 12 months of uneventful postoperative follow-up occurred in one patient. Solid bony fusion had occurred at that time, and because the patient refused plate removal, the plate has been left in place, without any adverse effects so far. Transient pain at the graft donor site occurred in 70% of the patients but was controllable with oral analgesics. Despite routine placement of a drain, two large hematomas developed at the graft donor site. One resolved spontaneously, and one hematoma had to be evacuated. Transient recurrent laryngeal nerve palsy occurred in three patients but resolved spontaneously after 4, 10, and 12 weeks. One patient had a superficial wound infection at the cervical incision, and another patient had a minor infection at one of the penetration points of the three-point skull fixation device. Both infections healed without specific therapy.

The most severe complication was a prevertebral abscess in one patient secondary to an infection with *Staphylococcus aureus.* Five days after surgery, the patient reported having severe pain in the cervical area and difficulty swallowing. A plain radiograph of the lateral cervical spine revealed extensive widening of the prevertebral soft tissue. Under general anesthesia, the wound was reopened, drained, and irrigated with an antibiotic solution. The plate and the bone graft were left in place. A drain was placed, and the patient was treated with intravenous antibiotics for 2 weeks followed by oral antibiotic therapy for another 6 weeks. The patient made a complete recovery with resolution of the preoperative myelopathic symptoms. Several radiographic follow-up examinations demonstrated satisfactory bony fusion without signs of screw or plate loosening. The overall complication rate, including minor complications, in this series is 20%. No adverse long-term sequelae attributable to the surgical procedure could be noted.

Complications of vertebrectomy and fusion reported in the literature differ widely not only between different authors

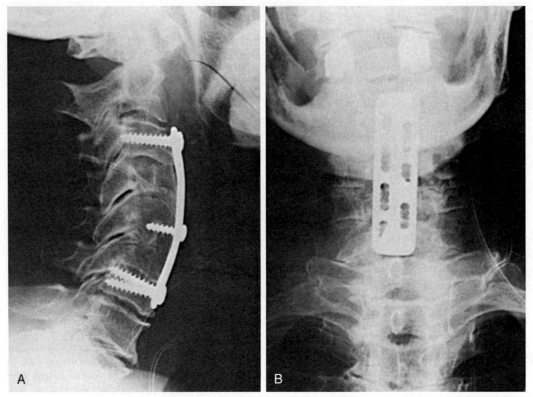

FIGURE 131-18   Case report 2: Early postoperative radiographic examination in lateral (*A*) and anteroposterior (*B*) projection demonstrates good position of the graft and the osteosynthetic material.

but also in regard to the techniques employed. Comparisons of graft-related problems in the literature are difficult because most vertebrectomy studies to date consist of simple graft intrusion without additional osteosynthesis.

Whitecloud and La Rocca,[51] in their early report in 1976 of a series of patients treated with fibular strut graft after spondylectomy and without osteosynthesis, reported graft extrusion in three patients, in one of whom graft dislodgment recurred four times. Splitting of the graft during insertion occurred in one patient. Postoperative abscess after infection with *S. aureus* occurred in another patient. Hoarseness persisted more than 1 month in one patient, and dysphagia for more than 3 days occurred in three patients. Donor site complications were noted in four patients.

In the article by Hanai and colleagues[52] on subtotal vertebrectomy without osteosynthesis, no severe operative complications were reported. In one patient, laryngeal pain occurred 1 day after surgery, continued for 10 days, and finally

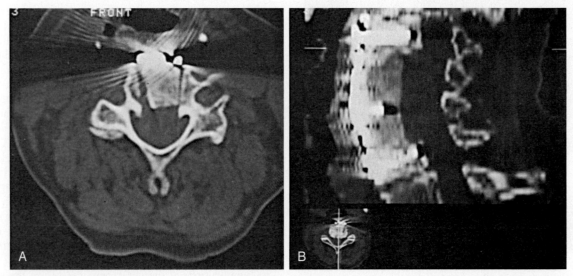

FIGURE 131-19   Case report 2: Postoperative computed tomography (CT) scan (*A*) and CT reconstruction (*B*) show wide bony decompression and adequate position of the bone graft

disappeared 1 month after operation. In three patients, the grafted iliac bone showed minimal displacement within 1 week after surgery, but no further displacement occurred after that.

Kojima and colleagues[60] reported on 45 patients treated with single-level or multilevel vertebrectomy without plating technique. In four patients, the graft extruded anteriorly within 5 days postoperatively; in one patient, the graft extruded 3 weeks after the operation. Dysphagia occurred in one patient, and Horner syndrome and temporary hoarseness developed in two patients. A transient subcutaneous cerebrospinal fluid leak was seen in three patients and was treated with spinal drainage.

The most severe complication after vertebrectomy was reported by Emery and colleagues,[66] who presented seven cases of upper airway obstruction after multilevel corpectomy for myelopathy. All patients had required reintubation, and the early compromise of the upper airway was believed to be due to edema. Five patients had no sequelae, but two died of complications related to the obstruction. Six of the patients had a history of heavy smoking and one of asthma. The authors point out that extra caution should be used in the postoperative management of the airways when multilevel corpectomy is performed in patients who have these preexisting conditions. Saunders and colleagues,[61] in their study on central corpectomy without osteosynthesis, reported an overall complication rate of 47.5%, with a 7.5% incidence of persistent sequelae. These consisted of C5 radiculopathy in one patient, swallowing dysfunction again in one patient, and hypoglossal nerve palsy in one patient. Graft-related problems (extrusion and fracture) without sequelae occurred in two patients. Awasthi and Voorhies,[67] in their technical report on the use of bone-bank fibular strut graft in six patients, reported no surgical morbidity, no mortality, and no graft extrusions, although follow-up in this series was short.

DISCUSSION

In most degenerative diseases involving the cervical spine, the relevant compressive abnormality of discogenic or bony origin is located anterior to the spinal cord. Posterior approaches to the cervical spine, although in use for many years for the treatment of soft disc disease as well as spondylotic processes, have been considered unsatisfactory by many neurosurgeons because of the inability to approach adequately and remove the offending epidural lesions, when they are primarily in an anterior location and because of the inherent possibility of late instability. This possibility is even truer in cases of MSCS. For this entity, an extensive laminectomy and different forms of laminotomy or laminoplasty procedures have been proposed.[12,40–42,44,45,68] In both techniques, however, the anterior compression, resulting from narrowing of the vertebral bodies in the case of significant cervical canal stenosis or bony osteophytes at multiple segments, cannot be alleviated. The anterior compression of the medulla remains unchanged, leaving an additional fulcrum for the spinal cord in motion. Moreover, it has been described that extensive laminectomy procedures in patients with MSCS by the loss of posterior elements significantly aggravate the preoperatively existing increased spinal mobility,[69,70] which is regarded as an important dynamic factor in the pathogenesis of CSM. Additionally,

the possible risk of formation of scar tissue because of exposure of the thecal sac to the dorsal musculature has been mentioned as a potential drawback of this procedure.[44] Although laminotomy or laminoplasty may to some extent prevent or diminish the occurrence of late postoperative instability, these procedures are not easy to perform along the cervical spine and may be fraught with the complication of cervical cord injury.

The anterior approach to the cervical spine developed and popularized by Bailey and Badgley,[71] Cloward,[72] Dereymarker and Muller,[73] and Smith and Robinson[74] has gained wide acceptance among neurosurgeons, especially since the addition of the surgical microscope.[75,76] The surgical technique for the anterior approach to the spine along the anteromedial border of the sternocleidomastoid muscle and through the areolar prevertebral soft tissue is to a large extent a standardized procedure that is performed rapidly and is relatively atraumatic for the patient.[47,72,77] Technical adjuncts, such as the instrumentation developed by Caspar and colleagues,[47] have greatly facilitated the procedure, allowing a wide exposure from C2 to T1. A large amount of data relating to experiences with anterior microsurgical disc excision and removal of osteophytes has been collected for patients with degenerative disease. The combination of these experiences with those gained from vertebrectomy and plating in patients with cervical tumor and trauma has paved the way for the application of these techniques in patients with MSCS. Additionally, since the advent of MRI, the pathoanatomic relationship between the offending multisegmental bony lesion and the extent of spinal cord compression can be precisely demonstrated preoperatively and used for proper planning of the surgical strategy.

In patients with MSCS, generally there are two surgical options when using an anterior approach. One is to resect the discs at all levels involved, remove the appropriate posterior osteophytes, and perform a Cloward or Smith-Robinson procedure, probably followed by an anterior plating technique, spanning the fused segments.[78–80] As has been already stressed, however, in most patients with cervical myelopathy caused by severe MSCS, the bony compression results not only from osteophytic lesions but also, and not infrequently more relevant to the development of the myelopathic process, from additional compression because of anterior narrowing of the spinal canal by the vertebral body itself. In these cases, a multilevel osteophytectomy would lead only to an incomplete decompression of the spinal cord. Additionally, from a biomechanical point of view, a plating procedure crossing several grafted disc spaces is not as stable as when an extensive vertebrectomy and bone graft replacement have been performed.[81–83] Inevitable micromotions along the multiple grafted disc spaces may frequently lead to early screw and plate loosening with consequent instability. Moreover, the pathologic hypermobility along the grafted segments that is still present using this technique consequently leads to new formation and growth of compressive osteophytes.

These drawbacks are avoided in patients with MSCS when the second surgical option, consisting of a single-level or multilevel vertebrectomy followed by graft placement and an appropriate osteosynthesis, is used. The procedure, although complex looking, is relatively straightforward. In the authors' experience, it is also a safe procedure, especially in regard to the pathology and patient age group treated. The most severe complication of corpectomy reported in the literature has been upper airway obstruction,[66] which, in the authors' experience, can be reliably prevented by meticulous dissection and atraumatic handling of the prevertebral tissue during the approach to the cervical spine. Major complications did not arise in the patient group reported here, however, and in none of the patients was worsening of the preoperatively existing myelopathic symptoms noted. Moreover, the success rate in terms of recovery from preoperative myelopathy as well as from incapacitating pain is satisfactory, as is the percentage of patients being able to return to work after surgery.

A few technical details in regard to the decompressive procedure, the choice and configuration of graft material, and the final plating technique are appropriate. It is the authors' contention that the surgical result in patients with MSCS is directly related to the radical extent of epidural decompression, which is related to the consequent use of the surgical microscope. The high rate of unsatisfactory recovery reported after anterior macrosurgical procedures for cervical myelopathy is largely the result of incomplete removal of all bony lesions. Radical resection of the posterior rim of the vertebral bodies involved and the adjacent cranial and caudal osteophytes, using different sized rongeurs down to microrongeurs as well as small-sized diamond drills, is the first and most important step of epidural decompression. Removal of bone should also be performed in the direction of the lateral gutter on both sides. For removal of osteophytes and lateral decompression, the application of an undercutting technique is usually more effective and especially safer than the extensive use of a high-speed drill.

Radical removal of the posterior longitudinal ligament has been performed in all the authors' patients with MSCS as part of the decompression. One might argue that removal of the posterior longitudinal ligament adds a considerable risk to the procedure. Because the authors always remove the posterior longitudinal ligament PLL to expose the dura in the depth of the disc space before vertebrectomy, however, its complete resection after removal of the vertebral bodies has not been considered extremely difficult or even risky. Although true ossification of the posterior longitudinal ligament has not been found in the authors' patient group, not infrequently hardening or some sclerotic change in the posterior longitudinal ligament, adding considerably to the bony compression, was detected. In rheumatoid patients with subaxial MSCS, ingrowth of compressive pannus in the posterior longitudinal ligament could be noted also. Moreover, removal of the posterior longitudinal ligament allows an excellent overview of the spondylectomy region with adequate evaluation of the radical extent and completeness of epidural decompression.

In all the authors' patients, an appropriate bone graft was harvested from the iliac crest and used for vertebral body replacement. The use of fibular strut graft was avoided because of unsatisfactory earlier experiences using this material. The main reason for using exclusively iliac bone graft is that the graft can be obtained in almost any length and size wanted. The possibility to contour the bone graft according to the curvature of the cervical spine allows an almost anatomic remodeling of the cervical lordosis, which is additionally important for the following plating technique. Proper fitting

of the graft into the vertebrectomy defect is much easier and especially more rigid when an individually designed iliac bone graft is used, instead of a usual straight configured fibular strut graft. Stability of the iliac bone graft in comparison with a fibular strut graft, under clinical circumstances, is, in the authors' experience, underestimated. Compression fracture of the iliac bone graft did not occur in any of the authors' patients, including older patients and those with osteoporosis. Because a plating procedure was always performed after graft placement, no additional configuration of the graft was performed apart from contouring it according to the spondylectomy defect and the cervical lordosis. When the graft is inserted in the surgical defect, the Caspar retractor is removed, after which the graft is kept in place by the adjacent vertebrae and their self-retracting forces. Extrusion of the graft is reliably prevented by the subsequent plating technique, which spans the graft and keeps it in place. The necessity for special graft configurations (e.g., the keystone or dovetailed graft) that have been developed and used to avoid graft extrusion[37,67] is avoided.

Apart from prevention of graft extrusion, the additional application of an anterior osteosynthetic technique after vertebrectomy and graft placement using a plate and screws adds to the immediate and long-term stability of the fusion. The applicability and validity of an anterior plating procedure of the cervical spine have been established by a number of studies.[47–49,63,64,84] The authors' experience in degenerative and traumatic and tumorous diseases using the Caspar system or different locking plates has been equally satisfactory.[85] The following points concerning the procedure need to be stressed, however. Correct choice of the plate length is important. The plate should not cover more than two thirds of the adjacent vertebrae, allowing screw insertion almost in the middle of the respective vertebrae. Impingement on the adjacent intact disc spaces or even vertebrae should be avoided. Inevitable motions in these neighboring segments lead to plate movement with the inherent risk of plate breakage, screw loosening, or both. To avoid extensive traction forces on the inserted screws, the plate should be prebent according to the lordosis of the cervical spine and placed tightly against the spine and the graft. Making the drill holes and insertion of the screws into the vertebral bodies is probably the part of the procedure that holds the highest potential for cervical cord injury. Using some precautions, however, it can be performed safely and without additional risk to the patient. First, continuous fluoroscopic control is absolutely mandatory. The consequent use and correct adjustment of a drill guide, which is routinely purchased with the Caspar system, reliably prevent undue penetration of the drill and injury of the dura and cervical cord. Usually in adult patients, a screw length of 20 to 22 mm is sufficient to reach the posterior vertebral cortex. The authors have never used screws longer than that and only rarely shorter ones. One should try to penetrate the posterior cortex or at least put the screw tip as close as possible to it. In the authors' experience with more than 400 anterior plating procedures along the cervical spine, posterior cortex puncture is not absolutely necessary to avoid screw loosening. An experimental study has substantiated this experience by showing that the pull-out strength of Caspar screws is not improved by posterior cortical penetration in an isolated vertebral body model.[86] New plate and screw systems avoiding the necessity of reaching the posterior vertebral body cortex will further increase the safety and applicability of osteosynthetic techniques along the cervical spine.

REFERENCES

1. Bohlman HH, Emery SE: The pathophysiology of cervical spondylosis and myelopathy. Spine 13:843–846, 1988.
2. Panjabi MM, White AA III: Biomechanics of nonacute cervical spine trauma. In Sherk HH (ed): The Cervical Spine, 2nd ed. Philadelphia: JB Lippincott, 2003, pp 91–96.
3. Parke WW: Correlative anatomy of cervical spondylotic myelopathy. Spine 13:831–837, 1988.
4. Burrow HR: The sagittal diameter of the spinal canal in cervical spondylosis. Clin Radiol 14:77–86, 1963.
5. Wolf BS, Khilnani M, Malis L: The sagittal diameter of the bony cervical spinal canal and its significance in cervical spondylosis. J Mt Sinai Hosp 23:283–292, 1956.
6. Adams CB, Logue V: Studies in cervical spondylotic myelopathy. II: The movement and contour of the spine in relation to the neural complications of cervical spondylosis. Brain 94:568–586, 1971.
7. Edwards WC, LaRocca H: The developmental segmental sagittal diameter of the cervical spinal canal in patients with cervical spondylosis. Spine 8:20–27, 1983.
8. Hashimoto I, Tak YK: The true sagittal diameter of the cervical spinal canal and its diagnostic significance in cervical myelopathy. J Neurosurg 47:912–916, 1977.
9. Kessler JT: Congenital narrowing of the cervical spinal canal. J Neurol Neurosurg Psychiatry 38:1218–1224, 1975.
10. Ogino H, Tada K, Okada K, et al: Canal diameter, anteroposterior compression ratio, and spondylotic myelopathy of the cervical spine. Spine 8:1–15, 1983.
11. Murakami N, Muroga T, Sobue I: Cervical myelopathy due to ossification of the posterior longitudinal ligament: A clinicopathologic study. Arch Neurol 35:33–36, 1978.
12. Edwards CC, Heller JG, Murakami H: Corpectomy versus laminoplasty for multilevel cervical myelopathy: An independent matched-cohort analysis. Spine 27:1168–1175, 2002.
13. Stoltmann HF, Blackwood W: The role of the ligamenta flavum the pathogenesis of myelopathy in cervical spondylosis. Brain 87:45–50, 1964.
14. Cusick JF, Myklebust JB: Biomechanics of cervical spondylotic myelopathy. Contemp Neurosurg 9:1–8, 1987.
15. Jellinger K: Spinal cord arteriosclerosis and progressive vascular myelopathy. J Neurol Neurosurg Psychiatry 30:195–206, 1967.
16. Mair WG, Druckman R: The pathology of spinal cord lesions and their relation to the clinical features in protrusion of cervical intervertebral discs: A report of four cases. Brain 76:70–91, 1953.
17. Cusick JF: Pathophysiology and treatment of cervical spondylotic myelopathy. Clin Neurosurg 37:661–681, 1991.
18. Hoff JT, Nishimura M, Pitts L: The role of ischemia in the pathogenesis of cervical spondylotic cervical myelopathy: A review and new microangiographic evidence. Spine 2:100–108, 1977.
19. Hukuda S, Wilson CB: Experimental cervical myelopathy: Effects of compression and ischemia on the canine cervical cord. J Neurosurg 37:631–652, 1972.
20. Hukuda S, Ogata M, Katsuura A: Experimental study on acute aggravating factors of cervical spondylotic myelopathy. Spine 13:15–20, 1988.
21. Barnes MP, Saunders M: The effect of cervical mobility on the natural history of cervical spondylotic myelopathy. J Neurol Neurosurg Psychiatry 47:17–20, 1984.
22. Batzdorf U, Batzdorff A: Analysis of cervical spine curvature in patients with cervical spondylosis. Neurosurgery 22:827–836, 1988.
23. Clark CR: Cervical spondylotic myelopathy: History and physical findings. Spine 13:847–849, 1988.
24. Yiannikas C, Shahani BT, Young RR: Short-latency somatosensory-evoked potentials from radial, median, ulnar, and peroneal nerve stimulation in the assessment of cervical spondylosis: Comparison with conventional electromyography. Arch Neurol 43:1264–1271, 1986.
25. Nurick S: The natural history and the results of surgical treatment of the spinal cord disorder associated with cervical spondylosis. Brain 95:101–108, 1972.
26. Harsh GR, Sypert GW, Weinstein PR, et al: Cervical spine stenosis secondary to ossification of the posterior longitudinal ligament. J Neurosurg 67:349–357, 1987.

27. Badami JP, Norman D, Barbaro NM, et al: Metrizamide CT myelography in cervical myelopathy and radiculopathy: Correlation with conventional myelography and surgical findings. AJR Am J Roentgenol 144:675–680, 1985.
28. Karnaze MG, Gado MH, Sartor KJ, et al: Comparison of MR and CT myelography in imaging the cervical and thoracic spine. AJR Am J Roentgenol 150:397–403, 1988.
29. Clifton AG, Stevens JM, Whitear P, et al: Identifiable causes for poor outcome in surgery for cervical spondylosis: Post-operative computed myelography and MR imaging. Neuroradiology 32:450–455, 1990.
30. Brown BM, Schwartz RH, Frank E, et al: Preoperative evaluation of cervical radiculopathy and myelopathy by surface-coil MR imaging. AJR Am J Roentgenol 151:1205–1212, 1988.
31. Czervionke LF, Daniels DL: Degenerative disease of the spine. In Atlas SW (ed): Magnetic Resonance Imaging of the Brain and Spine. New York: Raven Press, 1991, pp 855–864.
32. Haughton VM: MR imaging of the spine. Radiology 166:297–301, 1988.
33. Mehalic TF, Pezzuti RT, Applebaum BI: Magnetic resonance imaging and cervical spondylotic myelopathy. Neurosurgery 26:217–226, 1990.
34. Matsuda Y, Miyazaki K, Tada K, et al: Increased MR signal intensity due to cervical myelopathy: Analysis of 29 surgical cases. J Neurosurg 74:887–892, 1991.
35. Henderson CM, Hennessy RG, Shuey HM Jr, et al: Posterior-lateral foraminotomy as an exclusive operative technique for cervical radiculopathy: A review of 846 consecutively operated cases. Neurosurgery 13:504–512, 1983.
36. Hukuda S, Mochizuki T, Ogata M, et al: Operations for cervical spondylotic myelopathy: A comparison of the results of anterior and posterior procedures. J Bone Joint Surg Br 67:609–615, 1985.
37. Saunders RL: Anterior reconstructive procedures in cervical spondylotic myelopathy. Clin Neurosurg 37:682–721, 1991.
38. Verbiest H: The management of cervical spondylosis. Clin Neurosurg 20:262–294, 1973.
39. Yonenobu K, Fuji T, Ono K, et al: Choice of surgical treatment for multisegmental cervical spondylotic myelopathy. Spine 10:710–716, 1985.
40. Wada E, Suzuki S, Kanazawa A, et al: Subtotal corpectomy versus laminoplasty for multilevel cervical spondylotic myelopathy: A long-term follow-up study over 10 years. Spine 26:1443–1447, 2001.
41. Casotto A, Buoncristiani P: Posterior approach in cervical spondylotic myeloradiculopathy. Acta Neurochir (Wien) 57:275–285, 1981.
42. Hirabayashi K, Watanabe K, Wakano K, et al: Expansive open-door laminoplasty for cervical spinal stenotic myelopathy. Spine 8:693–699, 1983.
43. Jeffreys RV: The surgical treatment of cervical myelopathy due to spondylosis and disc degeneration. J Neurol Neurosurg Psychiatry 49:353–361, 1986.
44. Kimura I, Oh-Hama M, Shingu H: Cervical myelopathy treated by canal-expansive laminoplasty: Computed tomographic and myelographic findings. J Bone Joint Surg Am 66:914–920, 1984.
45. Tsuji H: Laminoplasty for patients with compressive myelopathy due to so-called spinal canal stenosis in cervical and thoracic regions. Spine 7:28–34, 1982.
46. Camins MB, Rosenblum BR: Osseous lesions of the cervical spine. Clin Neurosurg 37:722–739, 1991.
47. Caspar W, Barbier DD, Klara PM: Anterior cervical fusion and Caspar plate stabilization for cervical trauma. Neurosurgery 25:491–502, 1989.
48. Dickman CA, Sonntag VKH, Marcotte PJ: Techniques of screw fixation of the cervical spine. BNI Q 8:9–26, 1992.
49. Goffin J, Plets C, Van den BR: Anterior cervical fusion and osteosynthetic stabilization according to Caspar: A prospective study of 41 patients with fractures and/or dislocations of the cervical spine. Neurosurgery 25:865–871, 1989.
50. Seifert V, Stolke D: Multisegmental cervical spondylosis: Treatment by spondylectomy, microsurgical decompression, and osteosynthesis. Neurosurgery 29:498–503, 1991.
51. Whitecloud TS, La Rocca H: Fibular strut graft in reconstructive surgery of the cervical spine. Spine 1:33–43, 1976.
52. Hanai K, Fujiyoshi F, Kamei K: Subtotal vertebrectomy and spinal fusion for cervical spondylotic myelopathy. Spine 11:310–315, 1986.
53. Boni M, Cherubino P, Denaro V, et al: Multiple subtotal somatectomy. Technique and evaluation of a series of 39 cases. Spine 9:358–362, 1984.
54. Bernard TN Jr, Whitecloud TS III: Cervical spondylotic myelopathy and myeloradiculopathy: Anterior decompression and stabilization with autogenous fibula strut graft. Clin Orthop 17:149–160, 1987.

55. Doi K, Kawai S, Sumiura S, et al: Anterior cervical fusion using the free vascularized fibular graft. Spine 13:1239–1244, 1988.

56. Senegas J, Guerin J, Vital JM, et al: [Extended spinal decompression using an anterior approach in the treatment of myelopathies caused by cervical arthrosis]. Rev Chir Orthop Reparatrice Appar Mot 71:291–300, 1985.

57. Rengachary S, Redford J: Partial median vertebrectomy and fibular grafting in the management of cervical spondylotic myelopathy [abstract]. J Neurosurg 70:325A, 1989.

58. Zdeblick TA, Bohlman HH: Cervical kyphosis and myelopathy: Treatment by anterior corpectomy and strut-grafting. J Bone Joint Surg Am 71:170–182, 1989.

59. Okada K, Shirasaki N, Hayashi H, et al: Treatment of cervical spondylotic myelopathy by enlargement of the spinal canal anteriorly, followed by arthrodesis. J Bone Joint Surg Am 73:352–364, 1991.

60. Kojima T, Waga S, Kubo Y, et al: Anterior cervical vertebrectomy and interbody fusion for multi-level spondylosis and ossification of the posterior longitudinal ligament. Neurosurgery 24:864–872, 1989.

61. Saunders RL, Bernini PM, Shirreffs TG Jr, et al: Central corpectomy for cervical spondylotic myelopathy: A consecutive series with long-term follow-up evaluation. J Neurosurg 74:163–170, 1991.

62. Maroon JC, Abla AA, Wilberger JI, et al: Central cord syndrome. Clin Neurosurg 37:612–621, 1991.

63. MacDonald RL, Fehlings MG, Tator CH, et al: Multilevel anterior cervical corpectomy and fibular allograft fusion for cervical myelopathy. J Neurosurg 86:990–997, 1997.

64. Fessler RG, Steck JC, Giovanini MA: Anterior cervical corpectomy for cervical spondylotic myelopathy. Neurosurgery 43:257–265, 1998.

65. Saunders RL, Pikus HJ, Ball P: Four-level cervical corpectomy. Spine 23:2455–2461, 1998.

66. Emery SE, Smith MD, Bohlman HH: Upper-airway obstruction after multilevel cervical corpectomy for myelopathy. J Bone Joint Surg Am 73:544–551, 1991.

67. Awasthi D, Voorhies RM: Anterior cervical vertebrectomy and interbody fusion: Technical note. J Neurosurg 76:159–163, 1992.

68. Itoh T, Tsuji H: Technical improvements and results of laminoplasty for compressive myelopathy in the cervical spine. Spine 10:729–736, 1985.

69. Mikawa Y, Shikata J, Yamamuro T: Spinal deformity and instability after multilevel cervical laminectomy. Spine 12:6–11, 1987.

70. Oiwa T: [Experimental study on the post-laminectomy deterioration in cervical spondylotic myelopathy—influences of the meningeal treatment and persistent spinal cord block]. Nippon Seikeigeka Gakkai Zasshi 57:577–592, 1983.

71. Bailey RW, Badgley CE: Stabilization of the cervical spine by anterior fusion. Am J Orthop 42A:565–594, 1960.

72. Cloward RB: Vertebral body fusion for ruptured cervical discs. Am J Surg 98:722–727, 1959.

73. Dereymarker A, Muller J: Nouvelle cure chirurgicale des discopathies cervicales: La meniscotomie par voie ventrale, suivie d'arthrosdese par greffe intercorporale. Neurochirurgie 2:233–234, 1956.

74. Smith GW, Robinson RA: The treatment of certain cervical-spine disorders by anterior removal of the intervertebral disc and interbody fusion. J Bone Joint Surg Am 40:607–624, 1958.

75. Caspar W: A new surgical procedure for lumbar disc herniation causing less tissue damage through a microsurgical approach. Adv Neurosurg 4:74–77, 1977.

76. Dunsker SB: Anterior cervical discectomy with and without fusion. Clin Neurosurg 24:516–521, 1977.

77. Whitecloud TS III: Anterior surgery for cervical spondylotic myelopathy. Smith-Robinson, Cloward, and vertebrectomy. Spine 13:861–863, 1988.

78. Kadoya S, Nakamura T, Kwak R, et al: Anterior osteophytectomy for cervical spondylotic myelopathy in developmentally narrow canal. J Neurosurg 63:845–850, 1985.

79. Yang KC, Lu XS, Cai QL, et al: Cervical spondylotic myelopathy treated by anterior multilevel decompression and fusion: Follow-up report of 214 cases. Clin Orthop 161–164, 1987.

80. Abumi K, Panjabi MM, Duranceau J: Biomechanical evaluation of spinal fixation devices. Part III. Stability provided by six spinal fixation devices and interbody bone graft. Spine 14:1249–1255, 1989.

81. Kaufman HH, Jones E: The principles of bony spinal fusion. Neurosurgery 24:264–270, 1989.

82. White AA III, Panjabi MM: Biomechanical considerations in the surgical management of cervical spondylotic myelopathy. Spine 13:856–860, 1988.

83. Suh PB, Kostuik JP, Esses SI: Anterior cervical plate fixation with the titanium hollow screw plate system: A preliminary report. Spine 15:1079–1081, 1990.

84. Seifert V, Zimmermann M, Stolke D, et al: Spondylectomy, microsurgical decompression and osteosynthesis in the treatment of complex disorders of the cervical spine. Acta Neurochir (Wien) 124:104–113, 1993.

85. Maiman DJ, Pintar FA, Yoganandan N, et al: Pull-out strength of Caspar cervical screws. Neurosurgery 31:1097–1101, 1992.

86. Sonntag VK, Kalfas I: Innovative cervical fusion and instrumentation techniques. Clin Neurosurg 37:636–660, 1991.

132 Surgical Management of Cervical Spondylotic Myelopathy

RICK J. PLACIDE, AJIT A. KRISHNANEY,
MICHAEL P. STEINMETZ, and EDWARD C. BENZEL

INTRODUCTION

Cervical spondylotic myelopathy (CSM) is caused by a reduction of the sagittal diameter of the cervical spinal canal as a result of congenital and degenerative changes in the cervical spine.[1-3] It is the most common type of spinal cord dysfunction in patients over the age of 55 years and it is the most common cause of acquired spastic paraparesis (quadriparesis) in adults.[4,5] Risk factors for spondylosis include cigarette smoking, frequent lifting, and diving.[6]

The degenerative changes of cervical spondylosis occur in the five articulations that comprise the cervical motion segment: the intervertebral disc, the two facet joints, and the two false uncovertebral joints (of Luschka). The normal aging process of the spine results initially in disc desiccation and results in loss of disc height. This change is thought to bring the uncovertebral joints into contact, thereby disrupting the normal biomechanics of the facet joints. Osteophyte formation, ligamentum flavum hypertrophy, and facet and uncovertebral joint eburnation may then occur as a reaction to the abnormal biomechanics.[6,7] These degenerative changes most commonly occur at C5–6 and C6–7.[8] White and Panjabi classify these changes as "static" factors involved in the pathogenesis of cervical spondylotic myelopathy.[9] Also included in this category are congenital spinal canal stenosis (less than 13 mm anterior-posterior diameter) and disc herniation. White and Panjabi also describe "dynamic" factors, which are abnormal forces placed on the spinal column and cord during flexion and extension under normal physiologic loads. For example, repetitive traumatic compression of the spinal cord against an osteophyte during normal flexion and extension of the cervical spine is defined as a dynamic factor.[4,10,11]

In addition to the direct mechanical compression of neural elements, CSM may also be the result of spinal cord ischemia. Ischemia can result from compression of large arterial feeders to the spinal cord such as the anterior spinal artery, reduced flow through the penetrating arteries of the spinal cord or the pial plexuses, or impairment in venous outflow resulting in venous hypertension.[4,12-14]

The natural history of CSM appears to be one of progressive disability.[15,16] In fact, Clarke and Robinson asserted that once the disorder was recognized, neurologic function did not return to normal.[3] In their series, 75% had episodic progression, 20% had slow, steady progression, and 5% had a rapid onset of symptoms followed by a prolonged period of stable disease. Nurick observed that patients with mild disability tended to have a better prognosis while patients over the age of 60 years tended to progress.[17] Moreover, patients who have had symptoms longer than 2 years show no improvement despite treatment.[4,18]

Pathologic Anatomy and Cervical Spondylotic Myelopathy

The patient with cervical spondylosis presents to the physician with complaints of neck pain related to degenerative changes, neurologic symptoms from spinal cord and nerve root compression, or a combination of complaints. CSM is the clinical result of spinal cord compression, and there are many factors with the potential to contribute to decreased space available for the spinal cord within the spinal canal.

There are static, degenerative factors, including intervertebral disc bulging, dorsal vertebral body osteophytes, ossification of the posterior longitudinal ligament, uncovertebral and facet joint hypertrophy, ligamentum flavum, and facet joint capsule laxity and infolding. Collapse of the intervertebral disc space has the potential to lead to a degenerative cascade. As the disc space height decreases, the uncovertebral joints approximate and are loaded abnormally, increasing the likelihood of degenerative spurring. Disc space collapse also causes a rostral-caudal translation, leading to similar degenerative spurring in the facet joints and laxity and buckling of the facet capsules and ligamentum flavum. All of these contribute to static narrowing of the spinal canal (Fig. 132-1).

Dynamic factors include abnormal translation or angulation during flexion and extension of the cervical spine. Flexion can increase spinal cord compression in the presence of disc protrusions or posterior vertebral body osteophytes as the cord is draped over these structures. Extension/hyperextension may narrow the spinal canal and increase compression on the cord as well by infolding or buckling of the ligamentum flavum and facet joint capsules. If there is existing loss of disc space height, this dorsal soft-tissue buckling is usually exaggerated. The morphology of the spinal cord has been shown to change with flexion and extension. Flexion tends to stretch the spinal cord, which can be magnified in the presence of disc protrusions and vertebral

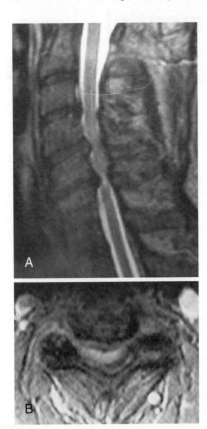

FIGURE 132-1 *A,* Sagittal T2-weighted magnetic resonance image of the cervical spine. Significant circumferential stenosis of the cervical spinal canal is demonstrated. Multiple levels are involved, and there is straightening of the spine. The stenosis results from a combination of osteophyte formation, disc bulging, uncovertebral joint hypertrophy, and buckling of the facet capsule and ligamentum flavum. *B,* Axial image of the same. The spinal cord has assumed a "Napoleon's hat" configuration.

body osteophytes. Cervical spine extension causes the spinal cord to shorten and thicken, making it more susceptible to compression from a buckling ligamentum flavum and other injuries as well.

In addition to these static and dynamic causes for spinal cord compression, congenital narrowing can be associated with myelopathy. Congenital cervical spine stenosis is said to exist if the ventral-dorsal diameter of the spinal canal is less than 13 mm. The normal adult canal diameter in the subaxial cervical spine is approximately 17 to 18 mm. Congenital stenosis, with superimposed degenerative and/or dynamic compressive pathology, increases the likelihood of developing myelopathy. Recognizing the presence of congenital stenosis in the face of significant degenerative changes is crucial, as it may affect surgical decision making.

Patient Presentation and Physical Examination

The patient with CSM can present with any number of subjective complaints and objective findings related to spinal cord compression. Subjective findings can range from subtle paresthesias of the hands to significant problems with upper extremity dexterity and gait/balance difficulties. Often, the patient will attribute early symptoms such as numbness in

the fingers or mild balance disturbance to expected aging changes. The patient may also complain of axial neck pain due to the degenerative changes of spondylosis.

Cervical spondylosis can be divided into three groups based on clinical presentation: (1) myelopathy, (2) radiculopathy, and (3) myeloradiculopathy. Vascular or ischemic pathology is also a known cause of cervical myelopathy; however, this chapter will discuss myelopathy and myeloradiculopathy secondary to spondylosis. Myelopathy in CSM is related to spinal cord compression manifested by vague paresthesias and upper motor neuron signs. The patient with myeloradiculopathy presents with a combination of findings due to myelopathy and radiculopathy (nerve root compression and related lower motor neuron findings).

During the assessment of the patient with suspected CSM, a directed review of systems (ROS) is an important portion of the evaluation, since patients may dismiss or not think to volunteer mild symptoms. Questions are generally directed toward the upper extremity, lower extremity, and bladder function. This is consistent with the myelopathy grading system described by Benzel (modification of the myelopathy scale devised by the Japanese Orthopaedic Association).[19] Upper extremity dysfunction can be ascertained by assessing for handwriting deterioration, increasing frequency of dropping objects, difficulty with fine motor skills such as fastening clasps or buttons, and the feeling of numbness and tingling in the hands. The term *myelopathy hand* had been used to describe nondermatomal paresthesias in the hands, a sense of clumsiness in the hands, and interosseous wasting.[20,21] Myelopathy hand can be confused with peripheral nerve compression syndromes such as carpal tunnel, cubital tunnel, and thoracic outlet syndrome. Questioning regarding lower extremity function is directed toward balance and gait dysfunction, which is related in part to spasticity. Paresthesias and weakness in the lower extremities may also be a prominent complaint. Finally, inquiring about bladder function is important. Bladder dysfunction is not as common a finding as extremity problems but may be present in the form of incontinence or retention.[22]

The physical examination of the patient with suspected CSM includes a generalized neurologic examination, which can then focus more specifically based on the history. A thorough examination can differentiate CSM from those problems stemming rostral and caudal to the cervical spine and from motor neuron disease and peripheral neuropathy. The examination begins with observation of the patient's posture, gait, and general appearance and fluidity of movements. Posture assessment may demonstrate sagittal and/or coronal imbalances. Gait examination may show a wide-based, spastic gait, and subtle changes may manifest only when the patient is asked to increase the pace of walking. Cranial nerve evaluation is included. Extremity function includes a motor and sensory examination from C4 to T1 and L2 to S1 bilaterally. Note that when assessing thoracic sensory levels, patients with cervical myelopathy can have variable sensory levels localizing to the thoracic spine.[23] Deep tendon reflexes (DTRs) are typically hyperactive. This is not always the case because coexisting peripheral neuropathy such as diabetes can alter DTRs. Coexisting lumbar spinal stenosis can present with hyperactive upper extremity reflexes but normal or hypoactive lower extremity reflexes. Additional reflexes include Babinski's reflex and assessment for clonus in the lower extremities, and Hoffman's reflex, the inverted radial reflex, and finger escape sign in the upper extremities. Other reflexes that may help localize the site of compression are the pectoralis reflex, scapulohumeral reflex, and jaw jerk. Finally, cervical spine range of motion may be restricted. Associated findings may include a positive Spurling's sign and Lhermitte's sign.

Radiologic Evaluation

Once an appropriate history and thorough physical examination are completed, a radiographic assessment is needed to complete the evaluation. Imaging studies by themselves do not diagnose myelopathy, because the level of spondylosis and cord compression do not always correlate clinically with patient complaints and physical findings. Imaging studies used in the workup of CSM include plain radiographs, magnetic resonance imaging (MRI), and computed tomography (CT) scan with or without myelography.

Plain radiographs are still an important part for the evaluation of the patient with CSM. The views obtained include anteroposterior (AP), lateral, flexion/extension, and obliques. AP radiographs allow for the evaluation of coronal alignment (scoliosis) and for the presence of anomalies such as cervical ribs or large C7 transverse processes (sometimes associated with fibrous bands). The lateral view provides the most information. It demonstrates the sagittal balance or the amount of lordosis/kyphosis. The lateral view also demonstrates the amount of disc space narrowing, vertebral body osteophytes, the AP diameter of the spinal canal, and sometimes the ossification of the posterior longitudinal ligament. The Pavlov ratio is determined using lateral radiographs.[24] It is the ratio of the sagittal diameter of the spinal canal to the sagittal diameter of the vertebral body. A ratio of less than 0.8 has been associated with an increased risk for developing myelopathy. Lateral flexion/extension views evaluate for translation and angulation abnormalities, which can provide information regarding dynamic cord compression. Flexion/extension views, combined with a static lateral view, demonstrate the ability of the patient to achieve lordosis, either globally or focally, which can be important for deciding between surgical approaches. Lastly, oblique views provide information about foraminal narrowing, particularly due to uncovertebral joint spurring.

MRI is invaluable for evaluation of soft-tissue compressive structures as well as assessing the spinal cord itself. The intervertebral disc and ligamentous and capsular structures are all well visualized in the axial and sagittal planes. Perhaps the greatest advantage of MRI in CSM is its ability to directly visualize the spinal cord. Parenchymal changes such as myelomalacia signal changes and syrinx formation are readily identified (Fig. 132-2). MRI may also have a prognostic role. High-signal-intensity abnormalities on T2-weighted images and low-signal-intensity changes on T1-weighted MRIs are not uncommon findings in patients with CSM. A recent retrospective review correlating MRI findings to operative outcomes suggested that low-signal-intensity changes on the T1-weighted images preoperatively indicated a poor prognosis.[25] The addition of gadolinium is useful in cases of suspected infection or tumor and in patients with prior spine surgery.

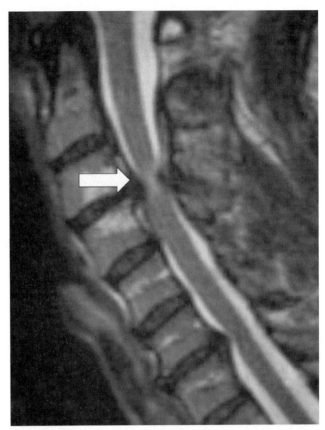

FIGURE 132-2 Sagittal T2-weighted magnetic resonance image of the cervical spine. Significant stenosis is demonstrated at the C3/4 interspace. High signal intensity in the spinal cord in located at that level (*white arrow*). This may indicate spinal cord contusion.

Myelography combined with CT can serve several important roles. The myelogram can be evaluated with the cervical spine in flexed and extended postures, providing details regarding dynamic compression. The CT provides the most detailed information about bony pathology such as osteophytes and ossified posterior longitudinal ligament (OPLL), and in the case of significant OPLL, can influence the decision on surgical approach. It is better at differentiating bony from soft tissue than MRI, and it has been suggested that CT myelography and MRI should be considered complementary, not interchangeable.[26]

Nonsurgical Treatment

Controversy exists regarding the natural history of patients with spondylotic myelopathy. This stems from the lack of randomized prospective studies on the issue and the reflection that the majority of studies that exist in the literature contain a heterogeneous population of patients. The natural history of cervical myelopathy is a slow, stepwise progressive deterioration. Lees and Turner reported episodic, stepwise deterioration in 75% of their patients.[16] Patients with mild symptoms had the best prognosis with regard to lack of progression.

Conservative treatment consists of measures aimed at decreasing symptoms and increasing function. Options include cervical orthoses, physical therapy, medication, and epidural steroids. Medications include anti-inflammatories, analgesics (opioids), muscle relaxants, and steroids. Some or all of these conservative measures may lead to some improvement in 30% to 50% of patients, depending on the grading criteria utilized.[27,28] This is especially true for those with only mild symptoms, that is, mild hand and arm symptoms but without impairment of daily tasks.

Careful conservative management may be considered for those with mild myelopathy, but caution should be taken with those with moderate to severe symptoms. No difference at 2 years was observed between those who received surgical decompression and those who did not in patients with only mild myelopathy.[29] In contrast, those with severe myelopathy rarely improve with conservative measures. Fourteen of fifteen patients with severe disability remained so in one series.[16]

Ultimately, most patients with cervical spondylotic myelopathy undergo surgery. Those with moderate or severe symptoms should undergo early surgical decompression. Many surgical studies have demonstrated that shortening symptom duration prior to decompression results in improved outcome.[30] Those with only mild symptoms may be closely followed and decompression performed when there is deterioration or lack of improvement.

OPERATIVE MANAGEMENT

Ventral Approach

The ventral approach to the cervical spine to address spondylosis has been successfully used for nearly 50 years.[31–33] This approach provides direct access for spinal cord and nerve root decompression secondary to herniated intervertebral discs, dorsal vertebral body osteophytes, ossified posterior longitudinal ligament, and uncovertebral joint hypertrophy. Another important benefit of the ventral approach is the ability to correct kyphotic deformity through discectomy or corpectomy.[34] Although some advocate ventral discectomy without arthrodesis in certain clinical situations, decompression in the setting of CSM is accompanied by a stabilization procedure with the goal of arthrodesis (artificial disc placement would be an exception). Ventral decompression options include discectomy (either single or multiple levels), corpectomy (either single or multiple levels), or a combination of discectomy and corpectomy. Arthrodesis can be accomplished by using autograft or allograft bone, or a combination. A variety of metallic and carbon fiber cages have been used, typically packed with autograft or allograft bone, and all of these options can be performed with or without a ventral cervical plate (Fig. 132-3).

Discectomy versus Corpectomy

There is little debate that when spinal compressive pathology is isolated to the level of the disc space, ventral discectomy and fusion is the treatment of choice. This includes disc herniations, spondylotic, vertebral body spurring, and OPLL. If spinal cord compression is present at multiple levels but still localized to the disc space, multilevel discectomies with bone graft at each disc space is appropriate. In the case of a degenerated, narrowed disc space with posterior osteophytes, consideration should be given to decompressing through the narrowed disc space. These large osteophytes can be associated with OPLL, extending beyond the disc

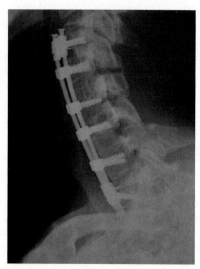

FIGURE 132-3   Lateral cervical radiograph of the cervical spine. The patient underwent multiple cervical discectomies and fusion versus one large contiguous corpectomy. This construct, which uses multiple points of intermediate fixation, has a theoretical mechanical and fusion potential advantage.

space, either rostrally, caudally, or both. Attempting to reach behind the vertebral body through a collapsed disc space may risk neurologic injury. Distraction of the disc space to improve exposure prior to osteophyte removal may compromise the neural structures as well. In this case, corpectomy may provide safer and more complete decompression. When addressing compression due to OPLL, preoperative imaging must define the anatomy of the ligament. The ossification may occur in segments or could be a continuous bony bar, which may necessitate multiple corpectomies or consideration of a posterior decompressive procedure.

Another issue when considering discectomy versus corpectomy is the fusion rate. Certainly, the literature demonstrates successful fusion rates for single-level ventral discectomy as high as 96%.[35] However, as the number of discectomies increases, so does the nonunion rate.[36,37] A corpectomy procedure has the advantage of having fewer sites to fuse (one rostral and one caudal), compared with a multilevel discectomy procedure (rostral, caudal at all intervening sites). In one retrospective review, the corpectomy group had a significantly higher fusion rate when compared with a multilevel discectomy group. However, there were more graft-related complications in the corpectomy group, the clinical outcomes were not significantly different, and these procedures were done without instrumentation.[38] Multiple-strut instrumented fusions have a theoretical mechanical and fusion potential advantage, particularly when utilizing intermediate points of fixation.[34]

Autograft versus Allograft

The use of autograft bone for ventral cervical spine arthrodesis has long been the standard with which to compare other techniques. Structural autograft is typically in the form of tricortical iliac crest or fibula. However, the morbidity associated with these harvest procedures has lead to the use of structural allograft alternatives. Iliac crest bone graft harvest has been associated with a high incidence of local pain, lasting up to a year in one third of patients. Other potential pitfalls include injury to the lateral femoral cutaneous nerve, fracture of the ilium, hematoma formation, and infection. Donor site complications have been reported to be as high as 20%.[39]

The literature provides mixed results when comparing autograft and allograft for ventral discectomy and fusion procedures. Some investigators report equivalent rates of fusion between autograft and allograft recipients while others demonstrate clearly superior results when using autograft.[40-43] A common finding, whether using autograft or allograft, is that increasing the number of discectomies per patient also increases the pseudoarthrosis rate.

The comparison of autograft and allograft for ventral cervical corpectomy is less well studied compared with single-level discectomy. Corpectomy autograft options are tricortical iliac crest and fibula. The predominant corpectomy allograft is the fibular strut graft, although various allograft options exist. Presently, the literature supports the use of both autograft and allograft for cervical corpectomy.[44-46]

Instrumentation versus No Instrumentation

The addition of ventral plating to the cervical spine stemmed from the interest to provide immediate stability, increase arthrodesis rates, and prevent graft dislodgement. Biomechanical testing has demonstrated the ability of ventral cervical plating to enhance construct stability. This increased stability has translated into improved fusion rates clinically, in single as well as multilevel ventral discectomy procedures.[47-49] However, the use of ventral plates for cervical corpectomies has not been as promising, especially for multilevel corpectomies. Graft displacement is reported to be the most common complication following cervical corpectomy (Fig. 132-4). One study failed to show any benefit by the application of a plate to patients with a single-level corpectomy, while others demonstrated satisfactory outcomes with plating in single- and multilevel corpectomies.[46,50]

The specifics of each plate may play a role in outcomes. For example, a static plate (one that does not allow settling) will offload the graft and will be a load-bearing device instead of a load-sharing device. Fusion at the rostral and caudal graft–host interface relies on axial loading. If the implant bears the entire load, this will tend to decrease graft loading and increase implant failure. Newer plate systems allow for some settling, sharing of the load between the implant and graft, and more normal loading characteristics during flexion and extension (Fig. 132-5). Published trials using these implants in corpectomy cases are not yet available. One fact that seems to be agreed upon is if decompression requires three or more contiguous corpectomies, supplemental dorsal stabilization should be seriously considered to help limit ventral graft-related complications.

TECHNIQUE: VENTRAL CERVICAL SPINE APPROACH

Several approaches are used to facilitate access to the ventral cervical spine. They include the transoral approach (with or without splitting of the mandible), the retropharyngeal

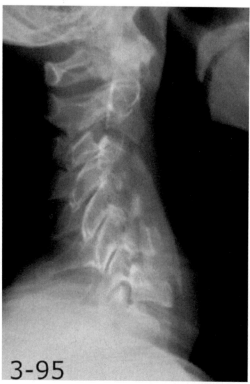

FIGURE 132-4 Lateral radiography of the cervical spine 9 months following a C4, 5, 6 corpectomy. There has been interval collapse of the C3 vertebral body and focal kyphosis of the upper cervical spine.

approaches to the upper cervical spine, and the approach to the subaxial spine described by Robinson and Smith, Cloward, and others. The latter is the most commonly employed approach for discectomy and corpectomy procedures between C2 and T1. This exposure facilitates access to the ventral cervical spine for decompression of the nerve roots and spinal cord, as well as arthrodesis. This approach uses the relatively bloodless plane between the sternocleidomastoid (SCM) muscle and the carotid sheath laterally

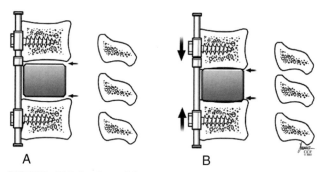

A   B

FIGURE 132-5 An axially dynamic ventral spine implant is pictured. *A,* After the intervertebral bone graft and implant are placed and the patient is supine, there are theoretical areas of no force transmission through the bone graft, or gaps, as depicted by the small arrows. When a rigid implant is placed, the spine is fixed in this position. No load is shared with the bone grafts, and all of the load is borne by the implant. This may result in construct failure. *B,* With an axially dynamic implant, when the patient assumes the upright position, the implant permits the spine to settle, and slides along the rods (*large arrows*). The theoretical gap disappears and the bone grafts share the load with the implant.

and the trachea and esophagus medially. The incision can be performed transversely within or in line with the naturally occurring skin creases or longitudinally along the medial border of the SCM. The longitudinal approach is typically reserved for more extensile, multilevel decompression procedures. The transverse incision approach is described here.

The incision should be placed at the approximate level of pathology by using surface anatomic landmarks. For a transverse incision, these include the hyoid bone (just rostral to the C3–4 level), the thyroid cartilage (at about C4–5), and the cricoid cartilage (approximately C5–6). The approach can be made on the left or right side. The recurrent laryngeal nerve takes a less predictable course on the right side, but there exists no evidence to suggest that this leads to an increased incidence of injury to this nerve following a right-sided exposure. When using a left-sided approach in the low cervical spine and cervicothoracic junction, the surgeon should keep in mind the proximity of the thoracic duct to the lateral confines of the exposure. Unless specific patient-related issues dictate the approach, surgeon comfort and familiarity, as well as surgeon's hand dominance, should be used to determine the side of exposure.

Prior to induction of anesthesia, one should carefully consider the method of intubation. Consideration should be given to awake, fiberoptic intubation in cases of severe stenosis or positional symptoms.

The patient is positioned in the supine position, with the upper extremities tucked at the side. A small towel roll may be placed between the scapulae to provide mild extension of the spine. Another towel roll can be placed to support the natural cervical lordosis. The head can be stabilized with a donut-shaped headrest or with traction using Gardner-Wells tongs or an occipital-mandibular harness. The use of a nasogastric tube or esophageal stethoscope may predispose to esophageal injury from retraction against a firm object within the esophagus.

The incision begins in the midline and is carried laterally to the ventral border of the SCM in a transverse nature, in line with the natural neck creases. The skin incision is carried into the subcutaneous fat, which can be wiped with gauze to expose the platysma. The platysma is then divided in line with the skin incision and undermined. Deep to the platysma lies the superficial layer of the cervical fascia, which is incised in line with the skin incision. Dissection is then carried longitudinally along the medial border of the SCM, exposing the middle layer of the cervical fascia. The omohyoid muscle may become visible at this point in a mid to low cervical spine exposure and can be retracted or divided to satisfy exposure. The natural plane of dissection can be palpated between the SCM and carotid sheath laterally and the trachea and esophagus medially. A combination of blunt and careful sharp dissection can be used to create a small defect in the middle layer of the cervical fascia, at which point the plane deep to this fascial layer is exposed longitudinally along the medial aspect of the SCM. The prevertebral fascia is visualized and the vertebral bodies palpated. Hand-held retractors are held in place with just enough retraction to palpate the vertebral bodies and intervertebral discs. The placement of a spinal needle for an intraoperative lateral radiograph for level confirmation may be performed at this time. Iliac crest bone graft can be harvested while waiting for the developing of the radiograph.

Certainly, there are a variety of subtle and not so subtle differences among surgeons. However, what follows are general approach techniques.

Discectomy

Once the appropriate level is confirmed radiographically, electrocautery is used to elevate the medial aspect of the longus colli muscle to widen the exposure, visualize the uncovertebral joints, and provide a place under which a self-retaining retractor system can be positioned. Placing the blades of the retractors under the medial border of the longus colli muscle serves to protect the trachea and esophagus medially, the carotid sheath contents laterally, and the sympathetic chain bilaterally. Once the retractors are in place, several optional requests can be made of our anesthetic colleagues prior to proceeding with the decompression. Ensure that the temporal pulse can be palpated on the side of the carotid retraction (make sure it is palpable preoperatively). Additionally, ask the anesthesiologist to deflate and reinflate the endotracheal tube cuff, as there is some evidence this may decrease injury to the recurrent laryngeal nerve.[51]

The discectomy is begun by performing an annulotomy with a no. 15 scalpel, taking care not to penetrate too deeply. Anterior and overhanging vertebral body osteophytes are removed with rongeurs and a high-speed burr. The annulus and disc material is removed using various-sized pituitary, Kerrison, and Leksell rongeurs and straight and angled curets. End-plate cartilage must be completely removed. After complete discectomy and cartilaginous end plate removal, a 3- to 4-mm high-speed burr can be used to finalize end plate preparation until punctuate bleeding is noted. Caution must be exercised to avoid overaggressive end plate removal resulting in exposure of cancellous vertebral body bone. This may predispose to unwanted graft settling into the softer bone. If the disc space is significantly narrowed, annulotomy can be followed by intervertebral distraction to enhance visualization. The Caspar distractor is one such device. Care must be taken to avoid overdistraction where several millimeters is usually sufficient. Complete discectomy includes exposure of the posterior longitudinal ligament (PLL) and the uncinate processes bilaterally. The decision to remove the PLL or not is a matter of the pathology at hand and surgeon preference. Certainly, when preoperative imaging demonstrates disc extrusion beyond the PLL, then the ligament needs to be resected to safely complete the decompression. A small nerve hook can be used to gain access between the PLL and the thecal sac, followed by the use of Kerrison rongeurs to remove the ligament. Anterior foraminotomies can be performed if the clinical situation warrants. A nerve hook can be passed behind the uncinate process to assess the foramen and can be used in a gentle sweeping fashion to retrieve any free disc fragments, avoiding injury to the exiting nerve root. If uncovertebral joint osteophyte formation is noted on preoperative imaging, a 1- or 2-mm Kerrison rongeur can be used to remove the hypertrophied bone.

Once decompression is complete, attention is directed to inserting the bone graft. Several autograft and allograft options exist and the choice of graft type will depend on the clinical situation and surgeon preference. The size of the graft will depend on the patient's anatomy and will be measured once the decompression is complete. The height of the graft can be measured using calipers or intervertebral "lollipop" type spacers. The height of the graft is approximately 2 mm greater than the original disc height.[52] The depth should be measured to avoid spinal cord compression and to allow 1 to 2 mm of countersinking beyond the anterior border of the vertebral body. If plate stabilization is to be used, it is applied at this point.

Corpectomy

Corpectomy, or removal of most or all of the vertebral body, can be performed through the same surgical approach as with a discectomy. Perioperative concerns and patient positioning are also the same. One difference is that if fibular autograft is to be used, the leg will need to prepared and draped appropriately. Once the exposure is complete and the correct levels are radiographically confirmed, discectomies are performed as described above on the rostral and caudal ends of the vertebral body to be removed.

The vertebral body can then be removed in several ways. If fibular allograft is to be used as a strut graft, various-sized rongeurs can be used to remove, save, and morselize the vertebral body bone to pack inside of the canal of the strut graft. The other option is to use a high-speed burr to remove the vertebral body. The width of the corpectomy varies depending on individual patient anatomy and can range from 15 to over 20 mm. A corpectomy width of 16 to 18 mm is typically sufficient for decompression. Careful assessment of preoperative imaging (CT, MRI) can help determine appropriate decompression width. Another important factor to consider when evaluating the imaging studies preoperatively is the location of the vertebral arteries on the axial CT or MRI at the level(s) of planned decompression. Anomalous vertebral artery anatomy can place the artery at risk during a corpectomy because the artery can course closer to the midline than would otherwise be expected.[53] Even without aberrant vertebral artery anatomy, excessively wide decompression places the vertebral arteries at risk. This is less of a concern with discectomy due to the uncovertebral joints.

The cancellous bone of the vertebral body is highly vascularized and bleeding can be expected. This can be controlled by application of small amounts of bone wax. Removal of the vertebral body, whether using rongeurs or a high-speed burr, is performed until the posterior cortical wall of the vertebral body is reached. Maintaining visualization of the discectomy sites will help guide the depth of the corpectomy. Once the vertebral body is removed to the level of the posterior cortical bone, a Kerrison rongeur can be used to remove this thin layer of bone. The decompression can be fine-tuned with undercutting of the lateral walls of the corpectomy to widen the decompression at the level of the spinal cord. When decompression is adequate, preparations can be made for graft insertion.

There are several sources of bone graft for corpectomy defects and several ways to secure them in place. Graft options include structural iliac crest and fibular autograft, fibular allograft, allograft bone dowels, and metallic cages. Again, the clinical situation and surgeon preferences and experience help make this determination. As with discectomy, the decompression defect needs to be measured and the appropriate size

graft fashioned. Distraction across the defect can be performed internally by means of an intervertebral distractor or externally through traction using Gardner-Wells tongs or a harness device. The rostral and caudal vertebral body end plates can be gently hollowed out using a high-speed burr to serve as docking sites for the strut graft. The ends of the strut can be rounded in a similar manner to provide optimal graft–host bony contact. There are a variety of creative options to help secure the strut between the vertebral bodies, and one such option is that proposed by Whitecloud and LaRocca.[54] Instrumentation can then be applied if appropriate.

COMPLICATIONS ASSOCIATED WITH VENTRAL APPROACH TO THE CERVICAL SPINE

As with any surgical procedure, the ventral approach to the cervical spine for decompression and fusion is associated with potential complications. These can occur intraoperatively or postoperatively and include neurologic, vascular, and visceral injury. Others include wound infection, pseudoarthrosis, and hardware failure. The ventral approach to the cervical spine is a relatively safe and reliable procedure. Maintaining an awareness of the potential complications can help in avoiding them.

Neurologic Injury

Injury to the spinal cord or nerve roots is an uncommon occurrence with the ventral approach to the cervical spine. Neurologic complications reported by the Cervical Spine Research Society have an incidence of just over 1%, with dorsal approaches having a greater incidence than ventral approaches.[55] When discussing spinal cord injury specifically, the incidence of injury is much lower. Identifiable causes include spinal cord compression, blunt trauma, and ischemia.

Injury of the recurrent laryngeal nerve (RLN) is a known complication of ventral cervical spine surgery. The reported incidence ranges from 1% to 11%.[56] Overzealous retraction and endotracheal tube cuff pressure seem to be several intraoperative factors that can be controlled.[51] Approaching from the right has also been suggested as a factor that increases the risk for injury to the RLN. This is due to the less predictable and often oblique course the nerve takes through the operative field. Although the anatomy of the nerve differs from right to left, there is no evidence that the side of exposure increases or decreases the incidence of injury. On the other hand, previous ventral spine surgery or a procedure such as thyroid surgery may influence the surgeon's approach. If the right side is the preferred side, but the patient has had previous left-sided surgery, a left-sided approach should be considered. If this is not possible, then preoperative otolaryngology assessment of vocal cord function should be sought. If the previous surgery damaged the left RLN, proceeding with a contralateral approach risks complete vocal cord paralysis.

The sympathetic chain courses on the anterolateral surface of the longus colli muscle. It is prone to injury if retractors are not secured below the medial edge of the longus colli on each side. Injury to the sympathetic chain will manifest with Horner's syndrome, classically presenting with ptosis, meiosis, and anhydrosis.

Vascular Injury

The major vascular structures with potential injury during a ventral cervical spine exposure are the carotid and vertebral artery. The carotid artery should be easily palpable during the procedure, and attention to detail on the exposure prevents injury. Using blunt self-retaining retractors and occasional release of the retractors help decrease carotid artery trauma. Additionally, the surgeon can mark the location of the ipsilateral temporal pulse, then ask the anesthesiologist to make sure the pulse is palpable once any retractors are in place. The vertebral artery is at the highest risk for injury during corpectomy. Unlike at the level of the disc, where the uncovertebral joints provide some protection to the vertebral artery by limiting lateral dissection, the same protection is not present at the level of the vertebral body. Accordingly, preoperative imaging in the form of the axial images of a CT scan or MRI should be evaluated to determine a safe width for the corpectomy.[53] These studies also demonstrate anomalous vertebral arteries. If a vertebral artery injury occurs, direct pressure with thrombin-soaked Gelfoam to control the hemorrhage is the first step. A variety of options have been proposed in the literature, including packing and observation, delayed endovascular procedures, artery ligation, and direct repair.[57,58]

Visceral Injury

Injury to the esophagus (or trachea) is rare during ventral exposure to the cervical spine, but it has a potential for significant complications. Esophageal injury can range from contusion with temporary postoperative dysphasia to frank perforation with life-threatening complications. Postoperative dysphasia lasting more than 8 weeks may require additional investigations such as swallowing studies or otolaryngology evaluation.

Perforation of the esophagus can happen during the intraoperative period from sharp or excessive retraction and motorized instruments. Perforation can also occur in the postoperative period due to the esophagus wearing against prominent hardware or bone or from hardware failure.[59] The reported incidence ranges from 0.2% to 0.9%.[56] Early recognition and aggressive treatment, including irrigation and débridement, repair, broad-spectrum antibiotics, and total parenteral nutrition, should be sought to help prevent the devastating effects of mediastinitis and sepsis.

Infection

Ventral cervical spine exposures have a relatively low incidence of wound infections. Preoperative antibiotics such as cephazolin should be administered and continued for 24 hours postoperatively. Copious irrigation throughout the procedure is suggested. Superficial infection (cellulitis) can be managed with a short course of intravenous or oral antibiotics. A deep space infection can be treated with surgical irrigation and débridement and intravenous antibiotics, typically 4 to 6 weeks. Instrumentation and graft should be left in place until arthrodesis occurs and healing can be expected to occur. If the infection persists and hardware must be removed, external immobilization should be considered. This could range from a simple orthosis to halo immobilization, depending on the stability of the spine.

Pseudoarthrosis

Pseudoarthrosis or nonunion is the failure of a bony union to take place. This complication is often related to poor technique and planning. The bone graft–host site preparation is crucial. Maximal surface area contact between the host vertebral end plates and bone graft improves fusion chances. Autograft bone is likely to yield improved fusion rates, and increasing the number of fusion sites decreases fusion rates.[36,37] Patient factors associated with lower fusion rates include smoking, diabetes, and any other immuno-compromised states. The use of a ventral cervical plate has been shown to increase the fusion rates in smokers, improve fusion rates with allograft bone, and increase the fusion rate in multilevel discectomy procedures.[47–49] Note that a pseudoarthrosis does not necessarily mean a poor outcome. Revision of a pseudoarthrosis is indicated if there are neurologic signs or symptoms or if the nonunion has led to deformity and mechanical axial pain that is resistant to nonoperative measures.

Implant Failure

Failure of the instrumentation can occur in several ways. The implant can loosen, causing the screws to back out, for example. The other failure mode is fracture of the implant. Either the plate can break (typically where the cross-sectional area of the plate is the least) or the screw(s) can break (Fig. 132-6). The reason for implant failure should be sought and is typically associated with a pseudoarthrosis. Loose and fractured hardware can be observed closely, but progressive implant migration has the potential for serious complications; therefore, serious consideration should be given to its removal.

Construct Failure

Construct failure with the possibility of deformity may also be seen (see Fig. 132-4). The incidence of such depends on the surgical technique (i.e., discectomy vs. corpectomy) and the number of levels operated on. This complication is usually suspected by increasing cervical pain at a point at which fusion would be expected and/or by new neurologic deficit. Surgical revision may be required.

OPERATIVE MANAGEMENT

Dorsal Approach

As described above, most patients with cervical myelopathy eventually undergo surgical decompression. Options include ventral approaches, such as discectomy and corpectomy, posterior approaches, including laminectomy and laminoplasty, and combined approaches. Analysis of the sites of compression, number of levels involved, and spinal alignment generally dictate the most appropriate surgical approach. In general, dorsal approaches are reserved for patients with multilevel involvement, predominantly dorsal or circumferential compression, and a straight or lordotic cervical alignment.

The aforementioned indications are relative and therefore not absolute. The location of spinal cord compression is intuitive and may be gleaned from review of neuroimaging.

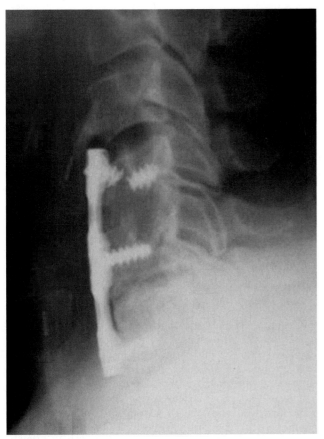

FIGURE 132-6 Lateral radiography of the cervical spine 12 months following a C4/5, C5/6 ventral cervical decompression and fusion with a ventral plate. The rostral screw has fractured and subsidence has occurred. Note the relationship of the rostral portion of the plate to the rostral C4 vertebral body. Despite the fracture, fusion has occurred.

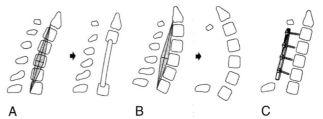

A   **B**   **C**

FIGURE 132-7 The choice of the appropriateness of a ventral or dorsal approach to the cervical spine depends in most part on the orientation of the spine. This may be determined by examination of a lateral cervical radiograph or midline sagittal magnetic resonance image of the cervical spine. A line may be drawn from the dorsocaudal aspect to the C2 to the dorsocaudal aspect of the C7 vertebral bodies. A kite-shaped zone is then added, the width of which depends on the surgeon's own biases and preferences (*A* and *B*). If the kite is completely dorsal to the vertebral bodies (*B*), the spine is in lordosis and a dorsal decompression (i.e., laminectomy) is indicated. If the kite is completely ventral to the dorsal aspects of the vertebral bodies (*A*), the spine is in kyphosis, and a ventral decompression (i.e., corpectomy) is indicated. Often the spine is intermediate or, more appropriately, in a straightened configuration. Essentially, the kite is only partly dorsal to the dorsal aspect of the vertebral bodies. Either a dorsal or ventral decompression may be used in this situation. A laminectomy plus lateral mass fixation may be appropriate (*C*). (From Benzel EC [ed]: Biomechanics of Spine Stabilization, 2nd ed. Rolling Meadows, IL: American Association of Neurological Surgeons, 2001.)

Contraindications

Laminectomy should probably be avoided in patients with kyphosis, in children, and in those with large ventral epidural masses. Laminectomy may be performed safely in children and in those with kyphosis, but a strong consideration for the addition of instrumentation and fusion should be given. Those with ventral epidural masses should undergo a ventral decompressive, with or without concomitant laminectomy.

TECHNIQUE: DORSAL CERVICAL SPINE APPROACH

Laminectomy

The patient is positioned prone on the operating room table with the head fixed in a three-point headholder or on a horseshoe attachment. Hyperextension of the spine should be avoided. All pressure points are carefully padded. After the appropriate skin incision, the dorsal spine is approached with monopolar cautery. The paraspinal muscles are stripped from the spinous processes to the edge of the facets bilaterally. The muscles are easily dissected in the subperiosteal plane using monopolar cautery. Bleeding is controlled with bipolar cautery and Gelfoam as needed. If C2 is not included in the decompression, we do not recommend removal of its muscle attachments. They provide stability at the upper cervical spinal level.

Following exposure and hemostasis, the levels to be decompressed should be fully identified. Many techniques exist to perform the laminectomy. A high-speed drill is used to create a trough on either side of midline at the facet–lamina junction. The trough should be carried down to the thin inner cortical margin of the lamina. A small rongeur is then used to complete the troughs to the level of the dura bilaterally. The laminae may then be removed

If multiple consecutive levels are involved in the stenosis (three or more), some would consider laminectomy over ventral multilevel corpectomy. This indication appears to be more surgeon dependent than borne out of the scientific literature. The most important issue regarding the choice of laminectomy, however, is preoperative spinal alignment. Laminectomy may be considered in cases of cervical lordosis and possibly straightening (see Fig. 132-7) of the spine, but avoided in kyphosis. Benzel has described a useful technique in determining effective cervical alignment.[60] On a sagittal midline MRI of the cervical spine, a line is drawn from the dorsocaudal aspect of C2 to the dorsocaudal aspect of the C7 vertebral body. A perpendicular line is then drawn in the middle of the prior line. The width of this perpendicular line is determined by the surgeon's experience and preferences. The lines are then connected, which creates an area that resembles a kite. If all cervical vertebral bodies lie in front or ventral to the kite, the spine is lordotic, and laminectomy is appropriate (Fig. 132-7). If the kite lies within the vertebral bodies, the spine is kyphotic, and laminectomy alone is not indicated. There are situations is which the dorsal vertebral bodies only line partly within the kite. In this circumstance, the spine is straight, and a ventral or dorsal approach may then be utilized.

en bloc. This technique avoids the need to place an instrument between the laminae and dura. Any remaining ligamentum flavum may then be removed sharply. Lateral decompression (i.e., nerve root) may then be performed, if necessary. Small no. 2 and no. 1 rongeurs may be used to perform the lateral decompression with care not to remove greater than 50% of the facet for fear of instability.[61]

Bleeding may be easily controlled with Gelfoam and/or bone wax. The muscles are next closed in layers and the skin sutured according to the surgeon's preference.

We limit the patient's activity for 6 weeks following surgery (i.e., no lifting greater than 15 pounds or strenuous activity). Patients are encouraged to participate in aerobic type activities as tolerated, such as walking. We do not routinely use cervical collars.

Laminoplasty

The indications for laminoplasty versus laminectomy are surgeon dependent. Theoretically, laminoplasty should provide some aspect of stability and may then be useful in cases where current or future stability is in question. Furthermore, there is a theoretical reduced chance of epidural scar formation following laminoplasty compared with laminectomy.[62] For example, it is useful in children with spinal cord tumors in which a multilevel laminectomy would be required.

As with laminectomy, many techniques exist for performing laminoplasty. Detailing all of them is beyond the scope of this chapter. A high-speed drill is used to create a trough along the lamina–facet junction on one side. This is usually the side contralateral to the side of most significant compression. A trough is also drilled in the opposite side. A Kerrison rongeur is then used to fully remove the bone along the ipsilateral trough. The block of laminae is cracked open like a book, with the contralateral trough serving as the hinge. The block of laminae is then held open by the placement of titanium miniplates at each level. Alternatively, a small block of bone (autograft or allograft) may be placed between the laminae and facet. Suture, wire, or miniplates may then be used to secure the laminoplasty. Bone chips may be placed on the hinged side to aid in stability. The spinous processes may also be split in the midline (rostral to caudal) and the laminae opened similar to French doors. A spacer of bone may be secured between the split spinous processes to maintain them in an "open" position. The closure is then similar to laminectomy.

Patients are maintained in a cervical collar for 6 weeks following the procedure. Patients should be followed after laminoplasty and evaluated for maintenance of an open canal and the state of the fusion if bone graft was placed.

RESULTS

Laminectomy

Laminectomy appears to result in the restoration of neurologic function in some patients or at least halt the progression of the disease following surgery. Overall 68% to 85% of patients can be expected to have a good or excellent outcome.[69–72]

Epstein et al reported on 1355 patients treated for cervical myelopathy.[73] In those patients who were treated with a posterior approach, either extensive or limited laminectomies, 60% to 85% were improved. Age and gender had no

effect on the results, although the investigators noted that no patient older than 70 years had an excellent result.

Of 84 patients reported by Collias and Roberts, improvement was seen in 70% of patients, stable neurologic status was seen in 29%, while 2% were worse following posterior decompression for cervical myelopathy.[74] The patients who were worse following surgery had errors in their preoperative diagnosis. One patient had amyotrophic lateral sclerosis while the other had an astrocytoma of the spinal cord.

Laminectomy appears as effective as ventral procedures for the treatment of cervical spondylotic myelopathy.[75] Some researchers have reported slightly superior results with ventral procedures.[71] Although it is difficult to directly compare the two procedures based on reports in the literature, proper patient selection is probably the most important predictor of outcome following a dorsal procedure compared with ventral strategies.

Laminoplasty

Studies have demonstrated that laminoplasty can increase and maintain spinal canal diameter. In one report, the area of the spinal cord increased 7.4%, while the dural sac area increased 33.8%.[66] Furthermore, clinical improvement has been demonstrated. Lee et al performed laminoplasty on 25 patients with myelopathy.[67] Eighteen months following surgery, 84% of patients demonstrated improvement in gait, 87% improved with regard to upper extremity function (numbness and tingling), while 77% improved in bowel and bladder function. Miyazaki et al reported a 75.5% neurologic improvement following laminoplasty.[68]

Ultimately laminoplasty leads to fusion of the dorsal elements (i.e., those levels included in the laminoplasty). This results in a loss of cervical range of motion by 30% to 70%.[65] This may alleviate axial neck pain following surgery.

COMPLICATIONS ASSOCIATED WITH DORSAL APPROACH TO CERVICAL SPINE

The most dreaded complication following a dorsal approach is kyphosis (Fig. 132-8). The incidence may be as high as 21% following laminectomy.[63] Careful patient selection and meticulous surgical technique should lessen this complication. Theoretically, laminoplasty should have a lower incidence of postoperative kyphosis.

Nerve root injury may also be encountered following a dorsal procedure. It was reported to occur in 13% of cases in one study. It involved C5 and C6 most often with mainly motor symptoms. The researchers reported a mean recovery time of 5.4 months.[64]

Infection and wound breakdown may be higher with dorsal procedures compared with ventral ones (personal experience). Patients should be optimally mobilized and have adequate nutrition to attempt to lessen these complications. The incidence may be greater following laminoplasty because of an elevated block of laminae.[65]

Other potential complications include epidural hematoma. The incidence may be less following laminoplasty because of the retained block of laminae.[65] CSF leak or vertebral injury may be encountered. Careful dissection and bone removal shall lessen these complications.

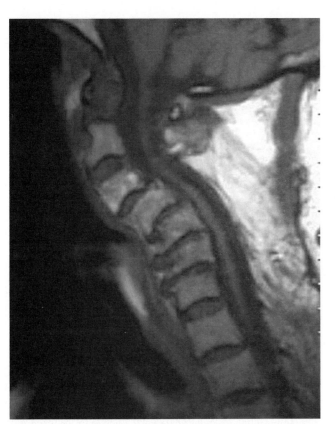

FIGURE 132-8   Sagittal T1-weighted magnetic resonance image of the cervical spine. The patient underwent a multisegment cervical laminectomy 2 years prior. The patient now presents with worsening cervical pain and a kyphotic deformity. (From Benzel EC [ed]: Biomechanics of Spine Stabilization, 2nd ed. Rolling Meadows, IL: American Association of Neurological Surgeons, 2001.)

Combined Approach (Ventral and Dorsal)

Once the decision for surgical intervention is made, three options are possible: ventral, dorsal,[76–80] and combined ventral and dorsal.[76,81–85] While all three options have proponents and detractors, the goals of surgery remain the same: decompress the neural elements and stabilize the spine if necessary. The advantages of the dorsal approach include familiarity, ease of decompression of multiple levels, and the ability to extend the decompression and/or fixation and fusion rostrally to the occiput or caudally to the thoracic spine. The major disadvantage of dorsal decompression is the requisite disruption of the posterior tension band resulting in a high rate of postlaminectomy kyphosis.[60,63] This complication has led a number of researchers to caution against laminectomy or laminoplasty in patients with a preexisting kyphosis, or even the relative kyphosis seen in patients with a "straightened" cervical spine[60,84] (see Fig. 132-7). In some cases, a mild kyphosis can be corrected with a combination of dorsal decompression and posterior fixation, but this requires the presence of a flexible deformity.[76] However, ventral compression of the neural elements cannot be directly addressed with a purely dorsal approach.

The ventral approach allows the surgeon to directly decompress the spinal cord in cases of ventral pathology via discectomy, multiple level discectomies, or corpectomy.

Moreover, it affords the surgeon the ability to perform a ventral release prior to any attempts to correct a cervical deformity. Although this strategy has been shown to be highly effective for patients with short segment stenosis, multisegment constructs have been plagued by historically high rates of pseudoarthrosis, bone graft subsidence, and graft dislocation.[80,84] These complications are the result of the often suboptimal bony fixation sites and the reliance on screw fixation as the only method of bony fixation allowed by the ventral approach.[60] Some of these factors may be mitigated by the use of multiple points of fixation and the use of dynamic implants, but their true effectiveness has yet to be proven.[60] A purely ventral approach, moreover, does not allow access for dorsal decompression of the spinal cord.

The use of a combined dorsal and ventral strategy affords all of the previously mentioned advantages of each and limits the disadvantages of each approach alone. Both dorsal and ventral compression can be addressed directly, resulting in a 360-degree decompression of the spinal cord. Optimal correction of sagittal plane deformities may be achieved by taking advantage of the mechanical advantage of dorsal fixation and osteotomies in conjunction with anterior releases and reconstruction of the ventral load-bearing column via interbody fusion techniques afforded by the ventral approach.[60,82,85] The addition of dorsal fixation to a ventral construct may also serve to reduce the rates of pseudoarthrosis, especially in multisegment constructs. The dorsal fixation loads the ventral interbody graft, creating a compressive moment as well as increasing translational and torsional resistance, thereby increasing fusion rates via Wolff's law.[60] This may be especially useful in patients with poor bone quality, prior failed surgeries, or medical comorbidities that could compromise healing. However, a combined anterior-posterior fusion strategy may obviate the need for external orthoses in many cases.[82,86] Some researchers recommend dorsal fixation when a fibular allograft is employed ventrally because it may take up to 2 years for a long strut to incorporate.[87]

The major disadvantage of a combined approach is the increase in morbidity and perceived increased risk for complications when compared with either dorsal or ventral strategies alone. However, acceptably low rates of morbidity and complications of 5% to 11% have recently been reported in the literature.[82,85]

While the majority of patients with cervical myelopathy can be treated by either a ventral or dorsal approach alone, a subset of patients may only be optimally treated by a circumferential approach. In general, a combined anterior-posterior strategy is indicated for any patient with multilevel spondylosis requiring extensive decompression, multilevel spondylosis with congenital cervical stenosis, multilevel spondylosis with kyphosis, postlaminectomy kyphosis, swan-neck deformity, or posttraumatic kyphosis.[6] Moreover, a circumferential strategy should be considered in patients with poor bone quality, patients with comorbidities that may inhibit bony fusion or wound healing, and any patient that has failed a prior attempt at deformity correction (Fig. 132-9). While no specific contraindications to the combined approach exist, it should be used with discretion due to the relative increase in morbidity and surgical risk when compared with either a dorsal or ventral strategy in isolation.[6]

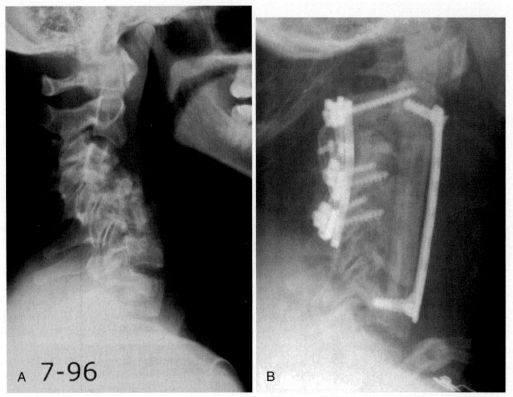

FIGURE 132-9 *A,* Lateral cervical radiograph 20 months following an attempt to correct cervical kyphosis and stenosis by utilizing a ventral corpectomy and strut graft without instrumentation. There has been collapse of the C3 vertebral body, subsidence, graft collapse, and kyphosis. *B,* Revision required a combined ventral/dorsal procedure. The previous strut graft was removed and replaced and a ventral plate was placed. A separate C2–C4 dorsal instrumentation and fusion was performed at the same setting. The kyphosis was corrected with the ventral procedure.

CONCLUSION

CSM is a common spinal disorder caused by a number of congenital and degenerative etiologies. Unfortunately, the natural history of CSM is one of progressive neurologic decline. Although some mild cases may be treated conservatively, most are treated surgically. The primary goal of surgical intervention in CSM is decompression of the neural elements to prevent disease progression. Secondarily, stabilization and fusion may often be indicated to prevent or correct deformity and to prevent further repetitive neural trauma. This goal can be accomplished through a variety of ventral, dorsal, and combined (ventral and dorsal) approaches as described above. The ideal approach for any given patient depends on a number of factors, including extent of disease (single level versus multilevel), the site of spinal cord compression (dorsal, ventral, or both), the extent of cervical kyphosis, the general medical condition of the patient, and the surgeon's experience and comfort with the approach. We generally prefer the ventral approach for patients with single level or limited disease, with mild kyphosis, or with purely ventral pathology. The dorsal approach is advocated for patients with multilevel or dorsal pathology. A combined approach is utilized for patients who require more extensive deformity correction than is possible via a ventral approach alone or for patients who have failed prior surgery. Regardless of the surgical strategy employed, we favor early intervention in most cases

of CSM, given the apparent association between duration of symptoms and neurologic outcome.

REFERENCES

1. Montgomery DM, Brower RS: Cervical spondylotic myelopathy: Clinical syndrome and natural history. Orthop Clin North Am 23:487–493, 1992.
2. Heller JG: The syndromes of degenerative cervical disease. Orthop Clin North Am 23:381–394, 1992.
3. Clarke E, Robinson PK: Cervical myelopathy: A complication of cervical spondylosis. Brain 79:483–510, 1956.
4. Rao R: Neck pan, cervical radiculopathy, and cervical myelopathy: Pathophysiology, natural history and clinical evaluation. Instr Course Lect 52:479–488, 2003.
5. Yonenobu K: Cervical radiculopathy and myelopathy: When and what can surgery contribute to treatment? Eur Spine J 9:1–7, 2000.
6. Truumees E, Herkowiz HN: Cervical spondylotic myelopathy and radiculopathy. Instr Course Lect 49:339–360, 2000.
7. Adams CB, Logue V: Studies in cervical spondylitic myelopathy. Brain 94:557–594, 1971.
8. Brown MD: The pathophysiology of disc disease. Orthop Clin North Am 2:359–370, 1971.
9. White AA, Panjabi MM: Biomechanical considerations in the surgical management of cervical spondylotic myelopathy. Spine 13:856–860, 1988.
10. McCormick WE, Steinmetz MC, Benzel EC: Cervical spondylotic myelopathy: Make the difficult diagnosis then refer for surgery. Cleve Clin J Med 70(10):899–904, 2003.
11. Bernhardt M, Hynes RA, Blume HW, White AA: Current concepts review: Cervical spondylotic myelopathy. J Bone Joint Surg Am 75:119–128, 1993.
12. Shimomura Y, Hukuda S, Mizuno S: Experimental study of ischemic damage to the cervical spinal cord. J Neurosurg 28:565–581, 1954.

13. Ferguson RJL, Caplan LR: Cervical spondylotic myelopathy. Neurol Clin 3:373–382, 1985.
14. Verbiest H: The management of cervical spondylosis. Clin Neurosurg 20:262–294, 1973.
15. Spillane JD, Lloyde GHT: The diagnosis of lesions of the spinal cord in association with "osteoarthritic" disease of the cervical spine. Brain 75:177–186, 1952.
16. Lees F, Turner JWA: Natural history and prognosis of cervical spondylosis. BMJ 2:1607–1610, 1963.
17. Nurick S: The natural history and the results of surgical treatment of the spinal cord disorder associated with cervical spondylosis. Brain 95:101–108, 1972.
18. Phillips DG: Surgical treatment of myelopathy with cervical spondylosis. J Neurol Neurosurg Psychiatry 36:879–884, 1973.
19. Benzel EC, Lancon J, Kesterson L, et al: Cervical laminectomy and dentate ligament section for cervical spondylotic myelopathy. J Spinal Disord 4(3):286–295, 1991.
20. Ono K, Ebara S, Fuji T, et al: Myelopathy hand: New clinical signs of cervical cord damage. J Bone Joint Surg Br 69:215–219, 1987.
21. Voskuhl RR, Hinton RC: Sensory impairment in the hands secondary to spondylotic compression of the cervical spinal cord. Arch Neurol 47(3):309–311, 1990.
22. Sakakibara R, Hattori T, Tojo M, et al: The location of the paths subserving micturition: Studies in patients with cervical myelopathy. J Auton Nerv Syst 55(3):165–168, 1995.
23. Adams KK, Jackson CE, Rauch RA, et al: Cervical myelopathy with false localizing sensory levels. Arch Neurol 53(11): 155–1158, 1996.
24. Pavlov H, Torg JS, Robie B, Jahre C: Cervical spinal stenosis: Determination with vertebral body ratio method. Radiology 164:771–775, 1987.
25. Morio Y, Teshima R, Nagashima H, et al: Correlation between operative outcomes of cervical compression myelopathy and MRI of the spinal cord. Spine 26(11):1238–1245, 2001.
26. Shafaie FF, Wippold FJ, Gado M, et al: Comparison of computed tomography myelography and magnetic resonance imaging in the evaluation of cervical spondylotic myelopathy and radiculopathy. Spine 24:1781–1785, 1999.
27. LaRocca H: Cervical spondylotic myelopathy: Natural history. Spine 13:854–855, 1988.
28. Way YL, Tsau JC, Huang MH: The prognosis of patients with cervical spondylotic myelopathy. Kaohsiung J Med Sci 13:425–431, 1997.
29. Fouyas IP, Statham PF, Sandercock PA: Cochrane review on the role of surgery in cervical spondylotic radiculomyelopathy. Spine 27:736–747, 2002.
30. Yamazaki T, Yanaka K, Sato H, et al: Cervical spondylotic myelopathy: Surgical results and factors affecting outcome with special reference to age differences. Neurosurgery 52:122–126, 2003.
31. Robinson RA, Smith GW: Anterolateral cervical disc removal and interbody fusion for cervical disc syndrome. Bull Johns Hopkins Hosp 96:223–224, 1955.
32. Smith PN, Knaub MA, Kang JD: Anterior cervical approaches for cervical radiculopathy and myelopathy. Instr Course Lect 52:455–463, 2003.
33. Cloward RB: The anterior approach for removal of ruptured cervical disks. J Neurosurg 15:602–617, 1958.
34. Steinmetz MP, Kager C, Benzel EC: Anterior correction of postsurgical cervical kyphosis. J Neurosurg (Spine 2) 97:277–280, 2002.
35. Emery SE, Bolesta MJ, Banks MA, et al: Robinson anterior cervical fusion: Comparison of the standard and modified techniques. Spine 19:660–663, 1994.
36. Emery SA, Fisher JR, Bohlman HH: Three-level anterior cervical discectomy and fusion: Radiographic and clinical results. Spine 22:2622–2625, 1997.
37. Swank ML, Lowery GL, Bhat AL, et al: Anterior cervical allograft arthrodesis and instrumentation: Multilevel interbody grafting or strut graft reconstruction. Eur Spine J 6:138–143, 1997.
38. Hilibrand A, Fye M, Emery S, et al: Improved arthrodesis with strut grafting after multilevel anterior cervical decompression. Spine 27:146–151, 2002.
39. Whitecloud TS III: Complications of anterior cervical fusion. Instr Course Lect 27:223–227, 1978.
40. Young WF, Rosenwasser RH: An early comparative analysis of the use of fibular allograft versus autologous iliac crest graft for interbody fusion after anterior cervical discectomy. Spine 18:1123–1124, 1993.
41. Shapiro S: Banked fibula and the locking anterior cervical plate in anterior cervical fusions following cervical discectomy. J Neurosurg 84:161–165, 1996.
42. Bishop RC, Moore KA, Hadley MN: Anterior cervical interbody fusion using autogeneic and allogeneic bone graft substrate: A prospective comparative analysis. J Neurosurg 85:206–210, 1996.
43. An HS, Simpson JM, Glover JM, et al: Comparison between allograft plus demineralized bone matrix versus autograft in anterior cervical fusion: A prospective multicenter study. Spine 20:2211–2216, 1995.
44. Bernard TN Jr, Whitecloud TS III: Cervical spondylotic myelopathy and myeloradiculopathy: Anterior decompression and stabilization with autogenous fibula strut graft. Clin Orthop 221:149–160, 1987.
45. Eleraky MA, Llanos C, Sonntag VK: Cervical corpectomy: Report of 185 cases and review of the literature. J Neurosurg 90(Suppl 1):35–41, 1999.
46. Mayr MT, Subach BR, Comey CH, et al: Cervical spinal stenosis: Outcome after anterior corpectomy, allograft reconstruction, and instrumentation. J Neurosurg 96:10–16, 2002.
47. Wang JC, McDonough PW, Endow K, et al: The effect of cervical plating on single-level anterior cervical discectomy and fusion. J Spinal Disord 12:467–471, 1999.
48. Wang JC, McDonough PW, Kanim LE, et al: Increased fusion rates with cervical plating for three-level anterior cervical discectomy and fusion. Spine 26:643–647, 2001.
49. Kaiser MG, Haid RW, Subach BR, et al: Anterior cervical plating enhances arthrodesis after discectomy and fusion with cortical allograft. Neurosurgery 50(2):229–236, 2002.
50. Epstein NE: Reoperation rates for acute graft extrusion and pseudoarthrosis after one-level anterior corpectomy and fusion with and without plate instrumentation: Etiology and corrective management. Surg Neurol 56:73–81, 2001.
51. Apfelbaum RI, Kriskovich MD, Haller JR: On the incidence, cause, and prevention of recurrent laryngeal nerve palsies during anterior cervical spine surgery. Spine 25(22):2906–2912, 2000.
52. An HS, Evanish CJ, Nowicki BH, et al: Ideal thickness of Smith-Robinson graft for anterior cervical fusion: A cadaveric study with computed tomographic correlation. Spine 18:2043–2047, 1993.
53. Curylo LJ, Mason HC, Bohlman HH, et al: Tortuous course of the vertebral artery and anterior cervical decompression: A cadaveric and clinical case study. Spine 25(22):2860–2864, 2000.
54. Whitecloud TS III, LaRocca H: Fibular strut graft in reconstructive surgery of the cervical spine. Spine 1:33, 1976.
55. Graham JJ: Complications of cervical spine surgery: A five-year report on a survey of the membership of the Cervical Spine Research Society by the Morbidity and Mortality Committee. Spine 14:1046–1050, 1989.
56. Patel CK, Fischgrund JS: Complications of anterior cervical spine surgery. Instr Course Lect 52:465–469, 2003.
57. Pfeifer BA, Freidberg SR, Jewell ER: Repair of injured vertebral artery in anterior cervical procedures. Spine 19:1471–1474, 1994.
58. Golfinos JG, Dickman CA, Zabramski JM, et al: Repair of vertebral artery injury during anterior cervical decompression. Spine 19:2552–2556, 1994.
59. Newhouse KE, Lindsey RW, Clark CR, et al: Esophageal perforation following anterior cervical spine surgery. Spine 14:1051–1053, 1989.
60. Benzel EC: Biomechanics of Spine Stabilization. American Association of Neurological Surgeons: Illinois, 2001.
61. Zdeblick TA, Abitbol JJ, Kunz DN, et al: Cervical stability after sequential capsule resection. Spine 18(14):2005–2008, 1993.
62. Kawaguchi Y, Kanamori M, Ishihara H, et al: Minimum 10-year follow-up after en bloc cervical laminoplasty. Clin Orthop Rel Res 411:129–139, 2003
63. Kaptain GJ, Simmons N, Replogle RE, et al: Incidence and outcome of kyphotic deformity following laminectomy for cervical spondylotic myelopathy. J Neurosurg (Spine 2) 93:199–204, 2000.
64. Dai L, Ni B, Yuan W, Jia L: Radiculopathy after laminectomy for cervical compression myelopathy. J Bone Joint Surg Br 80:846–849, 1998.
65. Yonenobu K, Yamamoto T, Ono K: Laminoplasty for myelopathy: Indications, results, outcome, and complications. In Clark CR, Ducker TB, Dvorak J, et al (eds): The Cervical Spine, 3rd ed. Philadelphia: Lippincott-Raven, 1998, pp 849–864.
66. Aita I, Hayashi K, Wadano T, Yabuki T: Posterior movement and enlargement of the spinal cord after cervical laminoplasty. J Bone Joint Surg Br 80(1):33–37, 1998.

67. Lee TT, Manzano GR, Green BA: Modified open-door cervical expansile laminoplasty for spondylotic myelopathy: Operative technique, outcome, and predictors for gait improvement. J Neurosurg 86:64–68, 1997.

68. Miyazaki K, Hirohuji E, Ono S, et al: Extensive simultaneous multisegmental laminectomy and posterior decompression with posterolateral fusion. J Jpn Spine Res Soc 5:167, 1994.

69. Fujiwara K, Yonenobu K, Ebara S, et al: The prognosis of surgery for cervical compression myelopathy: An analysis of the factors involved. J Bone Joint Surg Br 71:393–398, 1989.

70. Epstein NE, Epstein JA: Operative management of cervical spondylotic myelopathy: Techniques and results of laminectomy. In Clark CR, Ducker TB, Dvorak J, et al (eds): The Cervical Spine, 3rd ed. Philadelphia: Lippincott-Raven, 1998, pp 839–848.

71. Herkowitz NH: A comparison of anterior cervical fusion, cervical laminectomy, and cervical laminoplasty for the surgical management of multiple level spondylotic radiculopathy. Spine 13:774–780, 1988.

72. Malone DG, Benzel EC: Laminotomy and laminectomy for spinal stenosis causing radiculopathy or myelopathy. In Clark CR, Ducker TB, Dvorak J, et al (eds): The Cervical Spine, 3rd ed. Philadelphia: Lippincott-Raven, 1998, pp 817–823.

73. Epstein JA, Janin Y, Carras R, Lavine LS: A comparative study of the treatment of cervical spondylotic myeloradiculopathy: Experience with 50 cases treated by means of extensive laminectomy, foraminotomy, and excision of osteophytes during the past 10 years. Acta Neurochir (Wien) 61:89, 1982.

74. Collias JC, Roberts MP: Posterior surgical approaches for cervical disc herniation and spondylotic myelopathy. In Schmidek HH (ed): Operative Neurosurgical Techniques: Indications, Methods, and Results, 4th ed. Philadelphia: Harcourt, 2000, pp 2016–2028.

75. Gorter K: The influence of laminectomy on the course of cervical myelopathy. Acta Neurochir (Wien) 33:265, 1976.

76. Abumi K, Shono Y, Taneichi H: Correction of cervical kyphosis using pedicle screw fixation systems. Spine 24:2389–2396, 1999.

77. Butler JC, Whitecloud TS III: Postlaminectomy kyphosis: Causes and surgical management. Clin Orthop North Am 23:505–511, 1992.

78. Cattrell HS, Clark GJ, Jr: Cervical kyphosis and instability following multiple laminectomies in children. J Bone Joint Surg Am 49:713–720, 1967.

79. Herman JM, Sonntag VK: Cervical corpectomy and plate fixation for post-laminectomy kyphosis. J Neurosurg 80:963–970, 1994.

80. Zdeblick TA, Hughes SS, Riew KD, et al: Failed anterior cervical discectomy and arthrodesis: Analysis and treatment of thirty-five patients. J Bone Joint Surg Am 79:523–532, 1997.

81. Heller JG, Silcox DH III, Sutterlin CE III: Complications of posterior cervical plating. Spine 20:2442–2448, 1995.

82. McAfee PC, Bohlman HH, Ducker TB: One stage anterior cervical decompression and posterior stabilization: A study of one hundred patients with a minimum of two years of follow-up. J Bone Joint Surg Am 77:1791–1800, 1995.

83. Savini R, Parisini P, Cervellati S: The surgical treatment of late instability of flexion-rotation injuries in the lower cervical spine. Spine 12:178–182, 1987.

84. Albert TJ, Vacarro A: Postlaminectomy kyphosis. Spine 23:2738–2745, 1998.

85. Schultz KD, McLaughlin MR, Haid RW, et al: Single-stage anterior-posterior decompression and stabilization for complex cervical spine disorders. J Neurosurg (Spine 2) 93:214–221, 2000.

86. Rushton SA, Albert TJ: Cervical degenerative disease: Rationale for selecting the appropriate fusion technique (anterior, posterior and 360 degree). Orthop Clin North Am 29:755–777, 1998.

87. Bohlman HH, Emery SE: The pathophysiology of cervical spondylosis and myelopathy. Spine 13:843–846, 1988.

133 Surgical Management of Ossification of the Posterior Longitudinal Ligament

TAKAO ASANO and SHIGERU HIRABAYASHI

INTRODUCTION

Ossification of the posterior longitudinal ligament (OPLL) was first described by Key in 1838.[1] It then remained unnoticed for a long time until Tsukimoto reported on an autopsy case presenting the syndrome of compression of the spinal cord caused by ossification within the cervical spinal canal.[2] As the occurrence as well as the pathogenetic significance of OPLL was confirmed by succeeding reports in Japan[3–7] and in other countries,[8–12] OPLL gradually became established as a disease entity that is distinguishable from ankylosing spinal hyperostosis,[13] ankylosing spondylitis, and diffuse idiopathic skeletal hyperostosis (DISH).[14] Meanwhile, the Investigation Committee on OPLL of the Japanese Ministry of Public Health and Welfare was organized in 1974, and the annual reports of the committee have served as milestones in every aspect of research on OPLL in Japan.[15]

PREVALENCE

According to the committee report on the 2162 patients registered for clinical analysis,[15] the radiographic prevalence of OPLL in Japanese adults has been estimated to be around 2%. However, the incidence of asymptomatic OPLL increases markedly with advancing age and is as high as 3.2% in people older than 50 years.[16] Nakanishi and associates[17] reported that asymptomatic OPLL was found in 11% of persons in the sixth decade of life when the cervical spine was examined by lateral tomography. Histologic evidence of OPLL was observed in 20% of the 350 autopsied cases without a previous history of OPLL.[18]

Although the incidence of OPLL in East Asian countries was about the same as in Japan (1.4%), it was as low as 0.16% among whites.[15] However, a 1982 review of 1000 consecutive radiographs of the spine in adults older than 20 years in New York City revealed OPLL in 0.7%,[19] and in 1.7% in a similar 1987 study in Italy.[20] In this regard, nearly 50% of patients with DISH had concomitant OPLL on cervical roentgenograms.[14,21] Because the prevalence of DISH is 3% in adults older than 40 years[22] and 12% to 15% in patients older than 65 years,[14,23] OPLL may be a much more common entity among whites than previously believed.

PATHOLOGY

The posterior margin of the vertebral body, where the posterior longitudinal ligament is attached firmly to the spine, is the common site of occurrence of OPLL. From there, ossification proceeds rostrally and caudally along the ligament.

Histopathologically, enchondral ossification has been found in most specimens, and in some cases of massive OPLL, intramembranous ossification has been found as well (Fig. 133-1A, B). Whether or not OPLL is preceded by hypertrophy of the ligament remains controversial, but hypertrophy or ossification of the ligament has been demonstrated in the vicinity of the prolapsed disc material in some cases. Therefore, the prolapsed nucleus pulposus may exert some influence on the nearby ligament, leading to induction of bone formation.[24] Proliferation of small vessels in the ligament was observed at the initial stage of ossification.[18] The origin of bone-forming cells is believed to be the undifferentiated mesenchymal cells in the ligaments. Results of a 1992 histochemical investigation indicate that some bone-inducing substances, such as transforming growth factor-β and bone morphogenetic protein, are involved in the progression of OPLL.[25]

A genetic study of 1030 relatives of probands with cervical OPLL in 347 families revealed OPLL in 26.2% of the parents and 28.9% of the siblings of the probands.[26] Although these prevalences were significantly higher than in the general population, the possibility of polygene inheritance was ruled out. Insomuch as OPLL is likely a disorder controlled by autosomal-dominant inheritance, its genetic aspect has become a target of intensive research using molecular biologic techniques. According to a recent study using multipoint linkage analysis,[27] evidence of linkage to OPLL was detected on chromosomes 1p, 6p, 11q, 14q, 16q, and 21q and subsequent extensive linkage disequilibrium and association studies disclosed that single-nucleotide polymorphisms (SNPs) in the collagen 6A1 gene (COL6A1) were strongly associated with OPLL.

CLINICAL FEATURES

Like that of cervical spondylosis, the clinical manifestation of OPLL is radiculopathy, myelopathy, or both. In the 2162 registered patients discussed earlier, the most common initial symptom of OPLL was pain or dysesthesia in the upper extremities (48%), followed by neck pain (42%), pain or dysesthesia in the lower extremities (19%), motor dysfunction in the lower extremities (15%), motor dysfunction in the upper extremities (10.4%), and bladder disturbance (1%).[15] Those symptoms developed insidiously at approximately age 50 years in both sexes, without any particular cause in 85% of the patients.

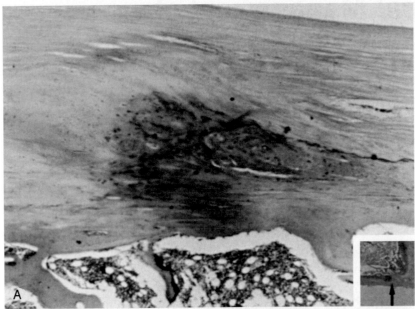

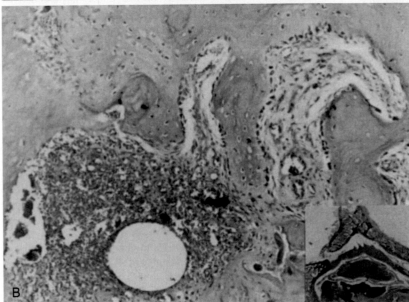

FIGURE 133-1 Types of ossification processes of ossification of the posterior longitudinal ligament (OPLL). *A,* Enlarged view of the area indicated by an arrow in the inset. An enchondral ossification process of the posterior longitudinal ligament in its initial stage was observed at the upper posterior edge of the C6 vertebral body (hematoxylin and eosin stain, ×25). A 46-year-old man with C4 segmental type of OPLL. *B,* Enlarged view of the area indicated by an arrow in the inset. An intramembranous ossification process of the posterior longitudinal ligament was observed at the anterior aspect of a massive OPLL at the C4 level (hematoxylin and eosin stain, ×25). A 65-year-old man with C2–C5 continuous type of OPLL.

However, an acute development or aggravation of tetraparesis after minor trauma was noticed in 21%. The downward development of symptoms from the upper to the lower extremities was more common than the reverse. Acute aggravation of neurologic deficits within a year or two after the onset was particularly common in relatively young patients (30 to 40 years of age).[28] Although the presenting symptoms or signs usually correspond to the cervical level where the cord compression is most pronounced, cervical OPLL is frequently accompanied by lesions in the thoracolumbar region. The possibility of multiple lesions calls for special attention in the neurologic evaluation of patients with cervical OPLL.

PREOPERATIVE EVALUATION

Laboratory Examinations

Routine laboratory results, including blood cell counts; serum protein, serum calcium, phosphorus, and alkaline-phosphatase levels; C-reactive protein; rheumatoid arthritis test; and

erythrocyte sedimentation rate, were shown to be within normal limits.

Human leukocyte antigens (HLAs), such as HLA-BW40 and HLA-SA5, were relatively more common among OPLL patients, but HLA-A27, which frequently produced a positive result in patients with ankylosing spondylitis, yielded a negative finding in those with OPLL.[15] OPLL is common in obese persons, who often have glucose intolerance, indicating a close relation between the ossifying tendency of the ligaments and glucose metabolism. OPLL is a common complication of metabolic or hereditary diseases, such as acromegaly, hypoparathyroidism, vitamin D–resistant rickets, constrictive muscular dystrophy, and spondyloepiphyseal dysplasia tarda.[29]

Diagnostic Procedures

Most OPLL can be easily diagnosed by lateral roentgenography of the cervical spine. Because a small OPLL is likely to be overlooked in the roentgenogram, sagittal tomography or computed tomography (CT) should be performed in

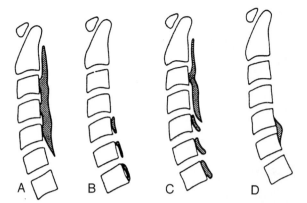

FIGURE 133-2 Classification of the cervical ossification of the posterior longitudinal ligament on a lateral roentgenogram. Continuous (A), segmental (B), mixed (C), and localized (D). (Reprinted with permission from Investigation Committee on OPLL.)

suspected cases. According to its shape indicated by lateral roentgenography, cervical OPLL has been classified into segmental, continuous, mixed, and localized types (Fig. 133-2),[30] which constituted 39%, 27%, 29%, and 8% of the registered cases, respectively.[15] OPLL was most frequently observed at C5, and the number of vertebral bodies involved was an average of 3.1. The narrowing ratio of the spinal canal, which is calculated as the ratio of the maximum anteroposterior (AP) thickness of the ossified ligament to the AP diameter of the spinal canal in the mixed, continuous, segmental, and localized types, was 42%, 41%, 25%, and 30%, respectively. Patients with OPLL frequently show concomitant ossification of the anterior longitudinal ligament (62%), the posterior longitudinal ligament in the thoracolumbar region (37%), and the yellow ligament (37%).[31] The association with ankylosing spinal hyperostosis or DISH was significantly more common in the mixed or continuous type than in the segmental type. Hence, a radiologic survey of the entire spine is mandatory in every patient with cervical OPLL.

Follow-up of the natural course of the disease for more than 10 years[32] revealed that an increase in either length or thickness took place in approximately 76% of patients with cervical OPLL. Marked (>2 mm) growth was observed in 40% of patients. In patients with the segmental type, the growth was less marked than in those with the other types, but transformation to the mixed or the continuous type was observed in about half of the cases. Interestingly, growth of OPLL has been shown to be markedly accelerated by laminectomy,[31] a result that is partly ascribed to increased mobility to the cervical spine. Regrowth of OPLL is much less frequent after laminoplasty or the anterior approach.[33]

Myelography usually reveals that OPLL causes a longitudinal, rodlike filling defect in the anterior aspect of the cervical spinal cord. This defect is easy to find in the AP projection but is often difficult to identify in the lateral view because the contrast material present in the patent subarachnoid space lateral to the compressed cord obscures the filling defect near the midline. More exact information can be obtained by carrying out CT immediately after myelography.

Because OPLL mostly consists of ossified mass, CT is the most reliable method for its identification in the cervical

and thoracolumbar regions. In conjunction with myelography, it clearly demonstrates the sizes and shapes of both the OPLL and the cord, as well as the spatial relationship between them. Commonly, the initial symptom of the OPLL located near the midline is myelopathy, and that of the more laterally located OPLL is radiculopathy with or without some features of lateral cord compression.

Although CT provides better osseous detail, magnetic resonance imaging (MRI) offers superior soft-tissue resolution. Because MRI cannot depict ossification, OPLL is demonstrated as a low-signal intensity band between the bone marrow of the vertebral body and the dural sac on T1- and T2-weighted images (Fig. 133-3).[34] Although detectability of OPLL by MRI is inferior to that afforded by CT, MRI provides invaluable information about the underlying pathologic course of cord damage and of the OPLL. In this regard, a surge of interest has focused on the clinical significance of increased signal intensity on T2-weighted images within the compressed spinal cord.[34–39] Such an increased signal intensity was found in 11.7% of patients with cervical spondylosis and in 16.1% of those with OPLL, and its frequency was proportional to the severity of clinical myelopathy as well as to the degree of spinal canal compression.[34,39] Inasmuch as the pathophysiologic basis of such an abnormality was presumed to be myelomalacia or cord gliosis secondary to a long-standing compressive effect,[36] its correspondence to the various pathologic changes within the spinal cord[40] requires further study. In the MRI images of OPLL, a band of intermediate or high signal intensity surrounded by a thick area of hypointensity was frequently found. This signal was considered to represent bone marrow within areas of ossification.[34] Recently, attention has been directed to detection by MRI of the calcification front (the enthesis) as well as the hypertrophic posterior longitudinal ligament. In the future, such information will greatly contribute to prognostication of the disease.

In the past, electrophysiologic investigation on the compressed cervical spinal cord was undertaken to determine the site of the lesion responsible for the neurologic symptoms, particularly in cases of OPLL with multilevel distribution. Potentials evoked by electrical stimulation, applied either on the peripheral nerve or directly on the spinal cord, were recorded at the spinal level or at the head level. Injury potentials, which indicate the site of cord damage, have been recorded directly from the spinal cord.[41] However, the drawback of the previous electrophysiologic examinations was that they could not detect lesions of the motor pathway in a selective fashion. The advent of magnetic stimulation made direct stimulation of the cortical motor area possible. By the use of this method, the conduction velocity within the motor pathway at the cervical level was shown to be significantly reduced in patients with cervical myelopathy.[42] This technique may be useful in determining the level of cord injury resulting from OPLL.

Correlation between the Neurologic Status and the Findings of Diagnostic Procedures

The advent of various modern diagnostic methods has enabled us to illustrate clearly the size and location of the OPLL together with the status of cord compression. How these findings correlate with the patient's neurologic

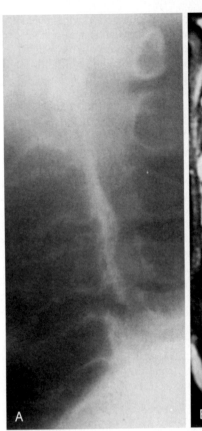
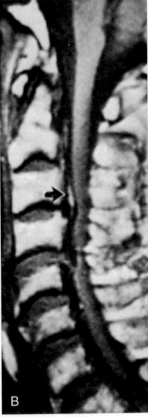
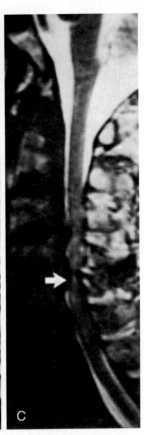

FIGURE 133-3 A lateral tomogram and magnetic resonance images of the mixed type of ossification of the posterior longitudinal ligament (OPLL). *A*, Lateral tomogram. *B*, T1-weighted magnetic resonance imaging (MRI) scan. The OPLL extends from C2 to C7, exerting maximal compression on the spinal cord at the level of the C4–C5 interspace. The arrow indicates the area of high intensity within the OPLL, namely the bone marrow. *C*, T2-weighted MR scan. The arrow indicates the small areas of high intensity at the level of C4–C5.

condition or prognosis has been a matter of great concern. It has been widely admitted that a narrowing ratio of more than 40% as estimated from the plain roentgenogram, CT, or MRI is generally associated with a high incidence of neurologic deficits.[28,30] Frequently, however, a patient with a greater narrowing of the spinal canal remains relatively asymptomatic.[15,17] Furthermore, in patients with a narrowing ratio of greater than 40%, the type of ossification, the extent of OPLL, the narrowest level of the available spinal canal, and the minimal AP diameter had no significant correlation with the severity of clinical symptoms.[43] Although the contour of compressed spinal cord is clearly delineated by CT myelography, no correlation was revealed between the degree of cord transformation (the ratio of the transverse diameter of the cord to its AP diameter) and the severity of preoperative clinical symptoms.[44,45] The only significant correlation revealed is that between the postoperative Japan Orthopedic Association score (discussed later) and the preoperative cross-sectional area of the cervical spinal cord as measured by CT myelography.[44,45] Complete recovery after decompressive surgery cannot be expected when the cross-sectional area of the cervical cord is less than 50% of normal.[45]

PATIENT SELECTION

Conservative Therapy

Because mobility of the cervical spine is a major factor influencing the development of symptoms, strict bed rest with or without skull traction has been the representative mode of conservative therapy for symptomatic OPLL. This therapy is effective, particularly in patients with modest symptoms.[15] As long as the cord is persistently compressed by the OPLL, however, relief of the symptoms is neither complete nor long lasting. Because recurrence or aggravation of symptoms is likely without decompressive measures,[33,46] conservative therapy has only a limited role in the treatment of OPLL. Surgical treatment should not be so delayed that irreversible cord damage occurs.

Indication for Surgical Treatment

The most widely accepted view is that surgical treatment is indicated for patients who have neurologic deficits hindering activities of daily life despite the conservative treatment. However, there is a trend toward a more radical view that patients who have radiologic evidence of severe cord compression should undergo prophylactic decompression regardless of the severity of symptoms. Inasmuch as the issue is still controversial, difficulty in establishing strict criteria of surgical indication stems from the fact that no single diagnostic method that exactly predicts the outcome exists. Therefore, all patients with OPLL are potential candidates for surgical treatment, although indiscriminate surgery should be condemned.

For the sake of decompression, the most reasonable and straightforward method is to remove the OPLL itself. Although the anterior approach can achieve this goal, it not only is more invasive than the posterior approach but also is accompanied by the risk of complications. In the past, pros and cons of these approaches have been debated.[45,47] To maintain balance in this respect, each approach is described by each of the authors according to his personal experience.

SURGICAL TECHNIQUES

Anterior Approach

The anterior approach by the Cloward technique was applied to OPLL for the first time by Onji and colleagues,[4] with reportedly disastrous results. For a considerable period after this report, the anterior approach had been only occasionally employed in the treatment of OPLL and aimed merely at the removal of the concurrent ruptured disc or the stabilization of the mobile portion of the cervical vertebrae. The technique of corpectomy (vertebrectomy) and strut bone graft, which has been employed in cases of trauma, infection,[48] or multiple-level cervical spondylosis,[49] was also employed for the resection of OPLL in Japan. Through the pioneering work at various institutes,[45,50–57] the feasibility of the anterior approach for OPLL has come to be widely recognized. One of the authors (T. A.) has also employed the anterior approach for the treatment of OPLL and multiple-level cervical spondylosis since 1978. Because the general procedure of the anterior approach is described in detail elsewhere,[48,56,58] we discuss only the techniques that are particularly relevant to OPLL.

With the patient in the supine position, the operating table is slightly flexed, and the head and the neck are elevated to lower the intravenous pressure. The head is held in slight extension. Patients with instability of the cervical spine due to trauma or prior laminectomy, with marked cord compression, or with planned postoperative halo-vest immobilization, are equipped with the halo and are subjected to skull traction. The left iliac crest, from which the graft is obtained, is elevated by a pad underneath. Either a longitudinal skin incision along the anterior border of the sternomastoid muscle or a transverse skin incision is used, depending on the number of consecutive interspaces to be operated on. When the lower part of C2 needs to be exposed, a horizontal incision in the submandibular area may be added at the top of the longitudinal incision, especially in a stout, short-necked patient. Special maneuvers[59] are required to develop the surgical plane above C2. After the prevertebral fascia is reached, the cervical level is determined by intra-operative lateral roentgenography. The plane is widened as much as necessary, and the prevertebral fascia is incised in the midline. The medial insertion of the bilateral longus colli muscles is coagulated and separated from the underlying vertebral bodies. The blades of the Cloward retractor should always be placed under the reflected longus colli muscle to prevent inadvertent damage to the esophagus, the carotid artery, and the other surrounding structures. Then, the intervertebral discs are removed together with the cartilaginous plate until the posterior half of the annulus fibrosus is exposed.

The area of corpectomy is determined by the findings of preoperative CT. In principle, the corpectomy should allow enough access to the lateral border of the attachment of the OPLL to the vertebral bodies. The wider the area of corpectomy, the easier the procedure. However, resecting too much of the vertebral body should be prevented because fusion of the bone graft with the remaining lateral surface or surfaces of the vertebral body increases the postoperative stability of the cervical spine. A longitudinal groove of 10- to 15-mm width is first made in, or a little lateral to, the midline, according to the width and the location of the OPLL. Through the emptied interspaces above and below, the vertebral body is resected by use of a Leksell rongeur. At this step, the cortical bone in the posterior aspect of the vertebral body is left unresected. The obtained bone chips are preserved for later use.

Then, the operating microscope is introduced. At each interspace, the remaining disc material, the annulus, and the adjacent fibrous tissue are removed by use of small, angled curets or a miniature bone punch, until the anterior surface of the OPLL is exposed. The lateral margins of the OPLL are confirmed at each interspace, and the groove is enlarged posteriorly by oblique excision of the posterior half of the vertebral bodies by use of an air drill with a diamond burr (Fig. 133-4). The cortical bone in the posterior aspect of the vertebral bodies is usually contiguous with the OPLL. This part of the OPLL is only flattened, and the drilling is advanced toward the epidural space abutting the lateral border of the OPLL. In this procedure, the optical axis must be kept in the right direction.

Both the microscope and the operating table should be frequently manipulated to obtain an adequate visual field.

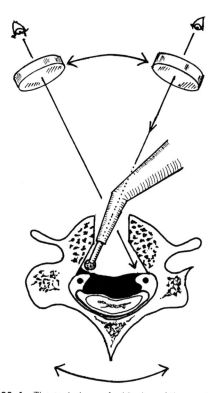

FIGURE 133-4 The technique of widening of the posterior half of the gutter. The drilling is directed toward the epidural space lateral to the ossification of the posterior longitudinal ligament (*black area*), minimizing the danger of cord damage. The *closed circles* indicate the epidural space with the engorged venous plexus. To obtain an adequate visual field, the angle of microscope as well as the position of the operating table must be adjusted frequently.

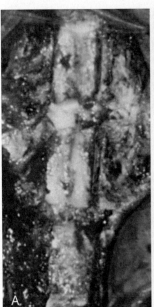 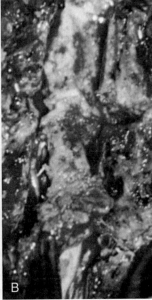 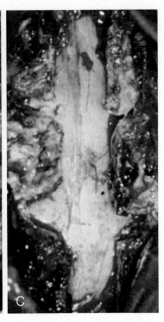

FIGURE 133-5 Intraoperative photographs. *A,* The extent of corpectomy. *B,* Elevation of the isolated ossification of the posterior longitudinal ligament from its lower end. *C,* Complete decompression of the cord and the root sleeves.

Because a narrow visual field tends to lead to incomplete removal of OPLL, further widening of the groove should be performed without hesitation, if it is felt necessary. If the drilling within the vertebral body has proceeded in the right direction, the epidural space is opened. Subsequent bleeding from the venous plexus can be easily controlled by packing with small pieces of thrombin-soaked absorbable gelatin sponge (Gelfoam). If the incision has gone medially, the dura attached to the posterior surface of the OPLL is exposed. When the dura is tightly adherent to the OPLL, it may be torn during the drilling, and the underlying arachnoid space and the cord may be seen. This indicates that the drilling must be directed more laterally.

After the procedure described, the whole OPLL is bilaterally isolated from the vertebral bodies (Fig. 133-5A). Then, attention is directed toward the caudal end of the OPLL. The posterosuperior edge of the vertebral body, which is usually contiguous with the OPLL, is resected by the use of an air drill. Because the thickness of the OPLL is diminished near the rostral and caudal margins, ample space usually exists between the OPLL and the dura to allow the use of small curets and bone punches. The underlying dural sac is exposed between the dural sleeves. The OPLL is completely isolated from the vertebral bodies if a similar maneuver is carried out with the rostral end.

If the OPLL is to be removed, its rostral end is drilled thin so that it can bend like a hinge. Then, the caudal end of the OPLL is gradually elevated by use of a small, curved bone curet as a lever, while the dura is separated from the OPLL (Fig. 133-5B). If the OPLL is completely isolated, either end is firmly grasped by an instrument to prevent its downward movement while the other end is elevated. As the space between the dura and the OPLL is widened, a small bone punch may be used to reduce the size of the OPLL. This step helps to identify the area of dural adhesion, which can be separated by blunt dissection in most cases. The dura that cannot be separated from the OPLL may be excised, thereby leaving the arachnoid membrane intact.

In this way, the OPLL can be lifted up from the dura and removed in toto. A defect of the dura is covered by fascial patch, which is fixed to the dura by a few stitches. Alternatively, the OPLL may be resected by the use of an air drill, leaving a paper-thin layer of bone attached on the dura.[52] In our view, this technique is time consuming and is no less risky than the isolation-elevation technique described earlier because drilling must be carried out all over the posterior surface of the OPLL in close proximity to the underlying dura and the spinal cord.

Although the OPLL can be successfully resected by this procedure in most cases, a large OPLL with a wide area of dural adhesion presents a special problem. The larger the OPLL, the more difficult its removal becomes, particularly when a wide area of dural adhesion is present. In the past, it has been recommended not to remove the part of the OPLL that is tightly adherent to the underlying dura.[45,50,51,53] Going a step further, Yamaura[45] advocated not removing but merely isolating the OPLL (the anterior floating method). If adequate space anterior to the dural sac was created, the OPLL isolated from the vertebral bodies was shown to migrate anteriorly because of cerebrospinal fluid (CSF) pressure, resulting in sufficient decompression of the cord. The long-term result of this operation compared favorably with that of the preceding ones, and further growth of the isolated OPLL was observed in only one of the 33 cases during the follow-up period of over 5 years.[60] Because the risk of OPLL removal is not negligible, this operation certainly appears to deserve a trial.

Regardless of whether the OPLL is removed or merely isolated, decompression of the root sleeves should then be carried out. This procedure can be performed by use of an air drill and other instruments, using the same technique employed in the resection of osteophytes around the joints of Luschka. A generous corpectomy may be added in the lateroposterior part of the vertebral body to ensure complete decompression of the root sleeves at every interspace involved (Fig. 133-5C). During this procedure, attention

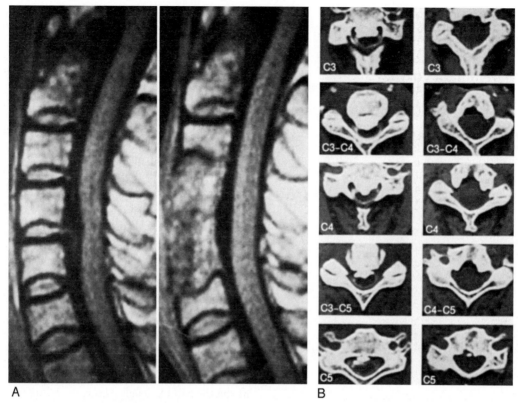

FIGURE 133-6   Preoperative and postoperative magnetic resonance imaging (MRI) and computed tomographic (CT) scans. *A,* the preoperative MRI showing ossification of the posterior longitudinal ligament (OPLL) extending from C3 to C6 (*left*); the postoperative MRI of the same patient (*right*). Note the complete decompression of the cord and the positioning of iliac bone graft. *B,* The preoperative CT myelography of the OPLL extending from C2 to C6 (*left*). The postoperative CT of the same patient (*right*). Note the extent of corpectomy and resection of the OPLL at each level. There is complete, bilateral union between the bone graft and the vertebral bodies.

should also be directed to the residual OPLL, which might be present in the lateral aspect of the dural sac. Together with the residual OPLL, the adjacent ligament is resected as completely as possible to curtail regrowth of OPLL.

After the spinal cord and the root sleeves are completely decompressed (Fig. 133-6), hemostasis is secured, and a bone graft is resected from the iliac crest. A bone graft as long as 8 to 9 cm can be obtained from the iliac crest, and this length usually suffices to fill a groove extending over as many as four consecutive interspaces. A longer bone graft, when necessary, can be obtained from the tibia or fibula. Then, the bone graft is fashioned with keys at either end, and troughs are made in the end plates of the adjacent vertebrae to prevent anterior or posterior extrusion of the graft (see Fig. 133-6A, right).[48] The bone graft is further shaped to fit the groove and is tamped into place while the skull is longitudinally retracted. The interspaces and the slit between the graft and the vertebral bodies are amply filled with the bone chips previously harvested. Then, an intraoperative lateral cervical roentgenogram is obtained to confirm that the graft is correctly positioned.

The operative field is thoroughly irrigated with saline solution that contains antibiotics, and the wound is closed in layers. The author uses the halo vest when more than three interspaces are involved, as is usually the case in patients with OPLL. However, for a few days after the operation, those patients are put on mild skull traction on the bed, using the already equipped halo so that any immediate

postoperative complications can be readily addressed. The halo is furnished with the vest after the patient's condition is stabilized.

Ambulation or a rehabilitation program is started within about a week. The halo vest immobilization is continued for several weeks, and then a cervical collar is used for the next month. In the author's personal experience, however, the use of Halo stabilization does not always prevent the occurrence of deposition or fracture of the bone graft. As Epstein suggests,[56] the addition of the posterior wiring immediately after anterior cervical corpectomy with fusion seems to be recommendable, particularly when the corpectomy involves multiple levels.

Results

In earlier papers reporting favorable results of the anterior approach,[50–55] various scales were employed to evaluate the patient's preoperative and postoperative neurologic status. To compare the surgical results in an unbiased manner, however, the use of a common scale is indispensable. The criteria for evaluation of the operative results of patients with cervical myelopathy formulated by the Japan Orthopedic Association have been widely used for this purpose in Japan (Table 133-1). Postoperative improvement is expressed as the recovery rate:

$$[\text{postoperative condition} - \text{preoperative condition}] \times 100 /$$
$$[17 - \text{preoperative condition}]$$

TABLE 133-1 ▪ The Japanese Orthopedic Association Score for Evaluation of Cervical Myelopathy

I. Motor function
  Upper extremity: feeding oneself with chopsticks or a spoon
  (0) Total disturbance: unable to feed oneself
  (1) Severe disturbance: unable to use chopsticks, but able to use a spoon
  (2) Moderate disturbance in the use of chopsticks
  (3) Mild disturbance in the use of chopsticks
  (4) Normal
II. Motor function
  Lower extremity: gait
  (0) Total disturbance: unable to walk
  (1) Severe disturbance: need aid on flat ground
  (2) Moderate disturbance: need aid on stairs
  (3) Mild disturbance: need no aid on stairs but unstable
  (4) Normal
III. Sensory function
  Upper extremity, lower extremity, and trunk
  (0) Apparent sensory loss or paresthesia
  (1) Mild sensory loss or paresthesia
  (2) Normal
IV. Bladder function
  (0) Total disturbance: complete retention or complete incontinence
  (1) Severe disturbance: incomplete retention, incomplete incontinence, or straining
  (2) Mild disturbance: frequency or hesitation
  (3) Normal

In Satomi and Hirabayashi's series,[33] the average recovery rate after the anterior approach ($n = 16$) was 57.7%, whereas that occurring after the expansive laminoplasty ($n = 54$) was 62.8%. Yamaura reported that 83.3% of a total of 71 patients with OPLL who underwent the anterior approach had a good outcome (recovery rate >25%).[45] Kamikozuru[60] showed that in 33 cases, the percentages of excellent (>80%), effective (50% to 79%), improved (20% to 49%), unchanged (0 to 19%), and worse (<0%) groups were 33.3%, 30%, 24.2%, 12.1%, and 0%, respectively. In the author's consecutive series, ongoing since 1978, 60% (12 of 20) had an excellent outcome; 35% (7 of 20) had an effective outcome; 5% (1 of 20) were unchanged; and 0% were worse according to the same scale. The average preoperative Japan Orthopedic Association score was 9.6, and the postoperative score was 15.0, yielding an average recovery rate of 77.5%. Inasmuch as mere comparison of the presented values may be of little significance because the operative outcome depends on various preoperative factors, such as age, duration of symptoms, and extent of cord atrophy, the generally favorable results of the anterior approach[45,50–57] support its feasibility and effectiveness as a therapy for cervical OPLL.

Complications

Multifarious complications have been reported with the anterior approach for OPLL or other lesions, including extrusion or fatigue fracture of the bone graft, palsy of the recurrent laryngeal or hypoglossal nerve, hematoma, wound infection, esophagocutaneous fistula, CSF fistula, stress ulcer, swallowing dysfunction, pseudoarthrosis, and aggravation of neurologic deficits. Among these, extrusion of the bone graft is common. In the author's (T.A.) series, one patient required repositioning of the graft because of complete extrusion of the inferior end, and another required reoperation because of the fatigue fracture of the graft. Severe C5 radicular pain occurred in one patient, but the pain disappeared a few weeks later. Postoperative aggravation of neurologic deficits occurred in one patient with a large OPLL of continuous type from C2 to C6 who had been bedridden for more than a year because of progressive tetraparesis. After resection of the OPLL from C4 to C6 by the anterior approach, tetraparesis became complete. Because this effect partly resulted from insufficient decompression at the C3 level, emergent expansive laminoplasty from C2 to C6 was carried out. A few months later, tetraparesis was gradually reduced to the level of the preoperative condition. In two other cases, postoperative CT revealed a remaining mass of OPLL behind the vertebral bodies. Although the patient's myelopathy was markedly improved, some radicular symptoms persisted at the corresponding level. Local regrowth of OPLL at the lateral margin of the corpectomized area took place in two patients.

Restrictions on the Indications

For technical reasons, several restrictions should be placed on the indications for the anterior approach. First, because the anterior approach is generally more invasive than the posterior approach, it should be withheld in patients with advanced age or in poor physical condition. Second, OPLL in the C1 and C2 levels cannot be treated by the conventional anterior approach. Because decompression of the cord at this level can be easily achieved by the posterior approach, carrying out an extensive exposure such as the anterior retropharyngeal approach[59] would be unrewarding, unless it is otherwise indicated. Third, the longitudinal extent of OPLL resection is somewhat limited in the anterior approach. Although the anterior floating method involving as many as six interspaces has been safely carried out with the fibular graft,[45,55] complications certainly increase as the range of OPLL resection, namely, the length of the bone graft, becomes greater. Presently, the maximal range of OPLL that can be safely treated by the anterior approach is considered to be four consecutive interspaces. In fact, the anterior approach is sufficient for most patients with OPLL because the average number of vertebral bodies involved is 3.1.[15] Fourth, the anterior approach might increase the danger of cord damage in patients with an extremely narrowed spinal canal. In consideration of the preceding reports of operative results, there is no indication that the anterior approach generally carries more risk than the posterior approach. Nonetheless, an attempt at removal of a very large OPLL carries an undeniably significant risk for cord damage. Either isolation of the OPLL (the anterior floating method) or the posterior approach seems to be the procedure of choice for such cases.

Posterior Approach

Posterior decompression for OPLL can be successfully carried out by laminectomy in the traditional fashion, namely, piecemeal excision of the laminae, if it is performed very carefully.[61] However, partial decompression is always accompanied by bulging of the dural sac, which may lead to angulation and subsequent damage of the cord. To prevent such a complication, Kirita[28] developed an "extensive, simultaneous laminectomy," in which the laminae are drilled paper thin before they are simultaneously excised. Later, facet fusion was added to this technique to stabilize the spine.[62] In 1972, Ohyama and co-workers[63] first introduced "expansive lamina-Z-plasty" to secure the postoperative stability of the cervical spine, afford the osseous protection of the spinal cord, and minimize the invasion of scar tissue into the spinal canal. Since then, various methods of expansive laminoplasty[63–70] have been devised. The long-term surgical results of those posterior decompressive methods were generally favorable,[71–73] and the postoperative stability of the cervical spine as well as the osseous covering of the spinal cord were well maintained. Compared with laminectomy, laminoplasties have shown a lower incidence of regrowth of OPLL, presumably because of postoperative stiffness of the neck.

Tension Band Laminoplasty

Because of contractures of the posterior elements accompanied by ectopic bone formation in laminoplasty, the postoperative stiff neck was so severe that 30% to 50% of the preoperative range of flexion-extension movement was lost. Because this became a major cause of discomfort and poor quality of activities of daily living, Tsuzuki and colleagues[69] developed the tension band laminoplasty, which aimed to minimize postoperative contracture of the neck.

The tension band laminoplasty is based on the mechanistic principle that unilateral reflection of the laminae in the open-door fashion causes stretching of the spinous ligaments and flaval ligaments when these are kept intact. They behave as a tension band, exerting force on the laminae to close the opened space (Fig. 133-7A). This compressing

force stabilizes the spacers inserted into the opened space when the cervical spine is in the neutral position. Furthermore, every neck movement only adds to the compressing force on the spacers as follows: (1) flexion increases the tension band effect of ligaments; (2) extension causes overlapping of the laminae, which then generates force to close the opened space; (3) on lateral bending or rotation, overlapping of both the laminae and facets acts in combination with the tension band effect of the spinous ligament to compress the spacers further; and (4) a circumductory movement of the neck is a combination of these movements. Consequently, the spacers remain stable even before union takes place; hence, early postoperative mobilization of the cervical spine is possible.

SURGICAL TECHNIQUE

After the patient is placed in the prone position, the head is fixed in slight flexion by the use of a three-pin skull fixator. The posterior aspect of the laminae of the cervical spine is exposed through the mid-dorsal approach. While the paravertebral muscles are detached and retracted bilaterally from the laminae, the whole spinoligamentous complex is kept intact. The supraspinous ligament together with the tendinous attachment of trapezius muscle is preserved as a wide band that is 1 to 1.5 cm wide on each side, so that the blood supply to the ligaments is maintained (Fig. 133-8A). In the high cervical region, the funicular and laminar portions of the nuchal ligament are also preserved (Fig. 133-8B). In principle, the spinal canal is enlarged from one above to one below the longitudinal extent of anterior impingement resulting from OPLL. A longitudinal groove of 3 mm in width is made by an air drill along the lamina–facet junction line on each side of the laminae, leaving the cancellous portion and the inner cortical layer. Then, the inner cortical layer of the longitudinal groove of the opening side is drilled thin, and together with the underlying ligamenta flava, it is severed longitudinally by a Kerrison punch with a 1-mm-wide blade.

The laminae are opened while the neck is kept in a neutral position. At first, the spinous process is pushed by a finger that feels its resistance (Fig. 133-8C). If hard resistance is felt, the groove in the hinge side is deepened slightly with an air drill. This procedure is repeated until the lamina is opened wide enough to insert a spacer of required width. In our experience, a spacer up to 10 mm in width can be inserted under good compressive force. The force resulting from the tension band effect of ligaments and that resulting from elasticity of the lamina at the site of greenstick fracture act in combination to hold the spacer in place. As measured on the lateral roentgenogram obtained with a tube film distance of 1 m, the insertion of a spacer of 8-mm width enlarges the AP diameter by 3 to 5 mm, and that of 10-mm width by 6 to 7 mm. A metal spacer is temporarily inserted until hole-making procedures for thread fixation are completed (see Fig. 133-7B). Thereafter, a permanent spacer that may be either an autograft or ceramic is used. When more than two facet joints need to be fixated in a continuous fashion, a spacer of adequate length is used. If necessary, the lamina of C2 can also be enlarged in the same manner described earlier. In this instance, however, the bone at the bottom of the groove in the hinge side must be kept as thick as possible to secure postoperative stability of the lamina. Generally, the AP diameter of the spinal canal at C5 can be enlarged up to 1.5 times in case of C3 to C7 enlargement.

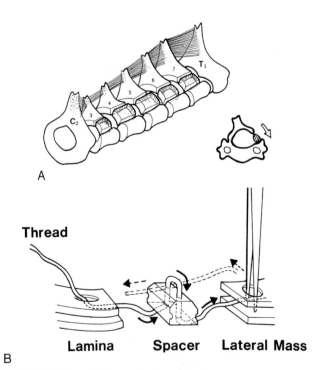

Thread

Lamina   Spacer   Lateral Mass

B

FIGURE 133-7   *A*, The mechanistic principle of the tension band laminoplasty. *B*, The technique of threading a spacer. The tip of a thread is hardened by a surgical skin-adhesive material, which makes it easier to pass a thread through holes in bones and a spacer.

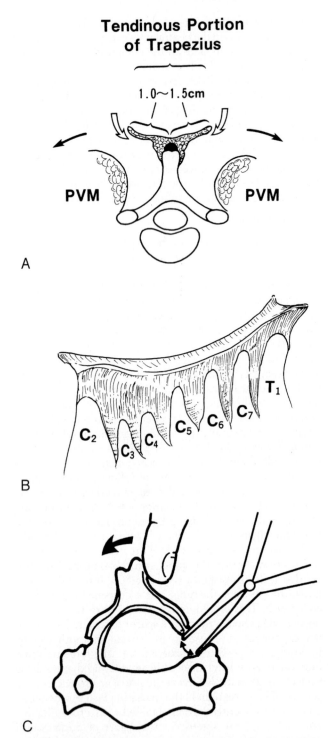

**Tendinous Portion
of Trapezius**

1.0~1.5cm

PVM   PVM

A

B

T_1

C_2 C_3 C_4 C_5 C_6 C_7

C

FIGURE 133-8 *A,* Approaches to preserve the spinoligamentous complex. *B,* An oblique view of the preserved spinoligamentous complex after exposure. *C,* The technique of opening a lamina. PVM, paravertebral muscle.

If more enlargement is required, the canal of C2 should be included (Fig. 133-9). Such an enlargement of the spinal canal is considered to provide ample space for the spinal cord to comply with the future growth of OPLL, which might be accelerated by preservation of mobility of the cervical spine. After the insertion of spacers, the erector

muscles are reattached firmly to the corresponding spinous processes. On the day after the operation, the patient is allowed to sit up in bed wearing a cervical collar, and on the second postoperative day, to walk. Exercise of the neck without the cervical collar is started soon after hemostasis within the wound is confirmed. The cervical collar is discarded by the end of the second postoperative month, or somewhat later if facetectomy was carried out.

RESULTS

Since 1988, a total of 200 patients (145 males, 55 females, 27 to 83 years of age; average 58.7 years) were followed. The follow-up period ranged from 1 year to 10 years. The mean preoperative and postoperative Japan Orthopedic Association scores were 8.2 and 13.0, respectively, which are comparable with results of other types of laminoplasties.

Union of autograft spacers took place within 3 months. With the ceramic spacers, which were of the bioactive type with a porosity of 40% (Apaceram, Pentax Company, Tokyo, Japan), the occurrence of union could not be judged by postoperative roentgenography because no dependable criteria exist. So far, all the ceramic spacers have remained stable.

About 70% of preoperative range of motion of the neck was regained by the end of the fourth postoperative week. During follow-up, the stability of the neck has been preserved without deformity, postoperative ankylosis of laminae at the site of the grooves, or ectopic bone formation around the ligaments. The mean ratio of postoperative to preoperative range of motion of the neck was 75% on flexion and 50% on extension (Fig. 133-10). No aggravation of neurologic symptoms has been noticed except C5 and C6 radiculopathies, which occurred in 3% of patients.

Double-Door Laminoplasty and Intraspinous Process Spacer

Double-door laminoplasty was developed by Kurokawa[64] in 1980 as one of the methods of laminoplasty for cervical myelopathy (Fig. 133-11). The essence of this operation is to obtain decompression of the spinal cord by splitting of the spinous processes and laminae centrally and retracting them symmetrically in a double-door fashion. Compared with other methods such as tension band laminoplasty, the symmetrical posterior skeletal structures of the cervical spine can be reserved after surgery. In the original procedure, a bone from the iliac crest was grafted using a wire to maintain the position of the split spinous processes, thereby providing a wider space for the spinal cord.

However, pain and discomfort at the donor site of the iliac crest were not uncommon, probably due to injury to the superior gluteal nerve. In 1990, Harata and Ito[70] developed an artificial spacer made of hydroxyapatite, which is used to maintain the position of the split spinous processes instead of grafted bone. Since then, several types of artificial spacers have been used. With the use of a spacer, the surgery time is shortened and the blood loss is decreased. However, inadequate contact between these spacers and the spinous processes have often been reported. Inadequate contact rates were about 30%. In some case, displacement of the spacer occurred, resulting in restenosis of the spinal canal and aggravating the neurologic condition.

One of the authors (S.H.) observed that the inadequate contact may be due to a mismatch of the shape of the spacers

FIGURE 133-9 A case of C2 to C7 tension band laminoplasty with autograft in a 57-year-old man with a preoperative Japan Orthopedic Association score of six points. Tension band laminoplasty from C2 to C7 was carried out with posterior fusion from C2 to C6 using a long iliac graft. One year after the operation, the patient had a complete neurologic recovery. *A–D*, Lateral views on the roentgenogram and computed tomography scan (C4 level). *A* and *B*, Before operation. *C* and *D*, Four years after operation.

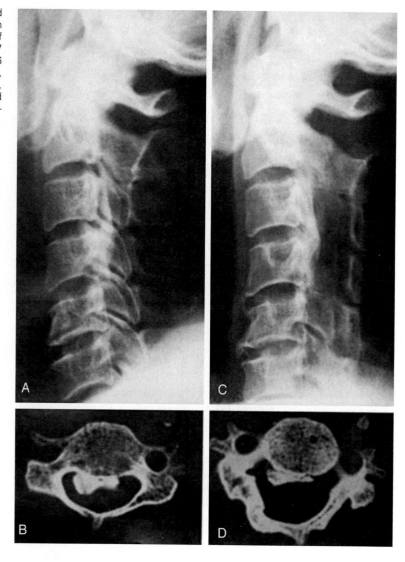

to that of the widened space, and so developed the STSS spacer (Pentax Company, Tokyo, Japan) with an optimal shape in 1994.[74,75] The STSS spacer is made of hydroxyapatite with a 40% porosity. The characteristic shape of the STSS spacer is trapezoidal both on the axial section and on the frontal section. In contrast, the shapes of other spacers are rectangular on the frontal section and trapezoidal on the axial section only. These are the fundamental differences between the STSS spacer and others (Fig. 133-12).

SURGICAL TECHNIQUE

The patient is kept in the prone position. The exposure of the operative field and split of the spinous processes are performed according to Kurokawa's method. A posterior vertical midline incision is made from the base of the skull to the seventh cervical vertebra.

While maintaining the continuity, the nuchal ligament is dissected from one side of the paravertebral muscles. After tracing deeply to the spinous processes along the membranous portion of the nuchal ligament, the muscles that attach to the spinous process of the second cervical vertebra are identified (i.e., semispinalis cervicus, rectus capitus major, obliqueous capitus inferior). They are detached and marked using sutures. The laminae from the second to the seventh cervical vertebrae are exposed to the medial portion of the facet joints laterally.

After that, the spinous processes are split centrally in an order from the second cervical vertebra using an air drill. In splitting the lamina, it is safer to make a triangle-shaped dome first at the base of the spinous process because a good visual field is obtained. Next, the tip of the spinous process and the inner plate of the lamina are split centrally. A complete central split is confirmed by touching yellow ligament using a dissector. Then, gutters are made bilaterally at the medial portion of the facet joint. It is important not to resect too deeply.

Split spinous processes are opened in a double-door fashion. After opening the split spinous processes, the constricting fibrous band above the dura mater and the hypertrophied yellow ligament are resected. In each split spinous process, the transverse length of the widened space can be observed to be longer at the cranial side than at the caudal side.

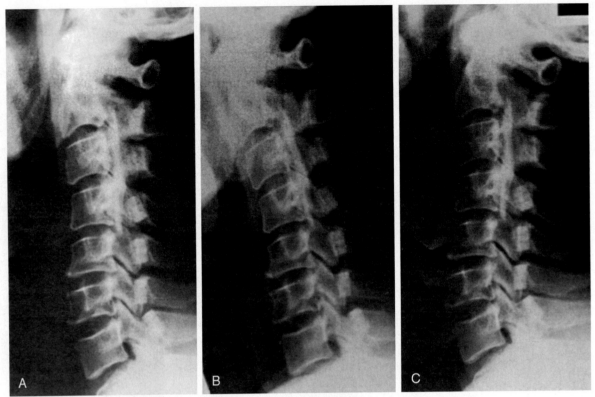

FIGURE 133-10   A case of C2 to C7 tension band laminoplasty with ceramic spacers.

Therefore, the shape of the widened space is trapezoidal both on the axial section and the frontal section. The STSS spacer is well adapted. Good contact is thus obtained at both the cranial side and the caudal side of each spinous process. During the fixation to the spinous process, the STSS spacer rotates slightly in the sagittal plane, and as a result, is more firmly stabilized parallel to each spinous process. A hole to accommodate a suture for fixing the spacer is made at the base of each spinous process. The STSS spacer is fixed using a suture at each spinous process (Fig. 133-13). The appropriate size of the spacer must be selected in accordance with the size of the spinous process.

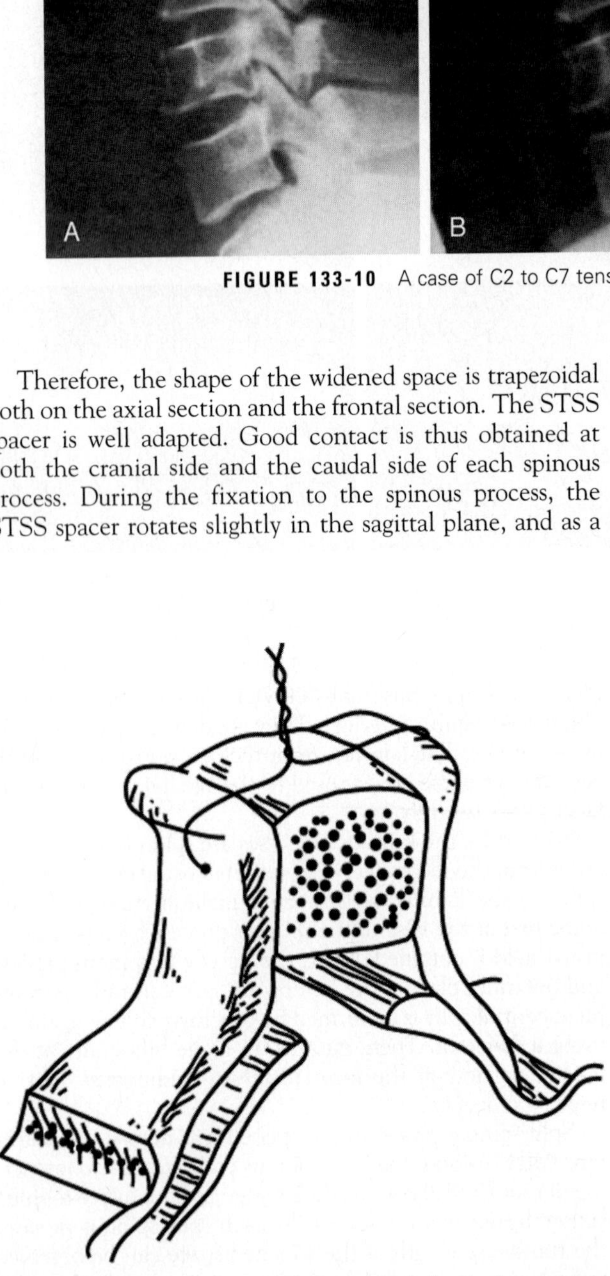

The tension of the muscles, which were detached from the second cervical vertebra, is recovered by suturing each muscle in an X-shaped fashion. After setting a suction drainage, sutures are made in layers. On the day after the operation, the patient is allowed to sit up in bed wearing a cervical collar, and on the second postoperative day, to walk. An outer support of the neck is applied in about 2 months (Fig. 133-14).

RESULTS

In the author's (S.H.'s) consecutive series, ongoing since 1988, 80 patients have undergone double-door laminoplasty. There were 39 patients with cervical spondylotic myelopathy, 31 patients with OPLL, and 10 patients with cervical myelopathy combined with spinal deformity due to rheumatoid arthritis in whom occipitocervicothoracic fusion was additionally performed using spinal instruments of hook and rod system. Of 31 patients with OPLL, 20 patients were male and 11 patients were female.

Their ages at the time of operation ranged from 44 to 81 years, with an average of 61.2 years. The follow-up periods ranged from 6 months to 10 years. From July 1988 to April 1994, 20 patients underwent double-door laminoplasty according to Kurokawa's original method, that is, using the autografted bone from the iliac crest. From May 1994 to April 2003, 11 patients underwent double-door laminoplasty using the STSS spacer.

FIGURE 133-11   A scheme of the original double-door laminoplasty using iliac bone graft with wiring.

FIGURE 133-12 The difference in shape between the STSS and other types of spacers.[66] The upper is the frontal section and the lower is the axial section. The right ones are the STSS spacer on both the above sections. The STSS spacer is trapezoidal both on the frontal and the axial sections, whereas other spacers are rectangular on the frontal section and trapezoidal only on the axial section.

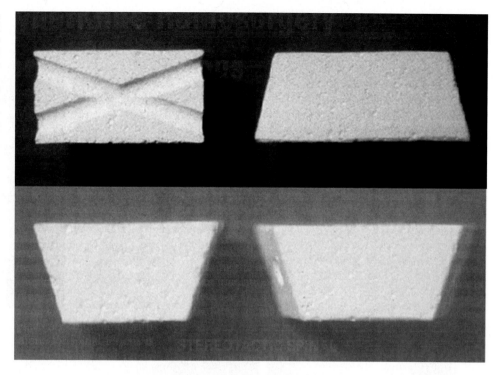

According to the Kurokawa's assessment method[64] in which the neurologic condition is assessed based on the degree of recovery of motor function, over 80% of the patients showed satisfactory recovery after surgery whether the autografted bone or the STSS spacer was used. This is comparable with results of other types of laminoplasties. In patients using the STSS spacer, no displacement or dislocation of the spacer occurred, and good contact between the spacer and the split spinous process was maintained on examination by CT images.

DISCUSSION

It remains unclear what is the minimal extent the spinal canal must be widened to obtain good surgical results. However, it is obvious that a wider spinal canal is preferable to obtain good results, especially in patients with OPLL in whom large-volume lesions occupy the spinal canal anteriorly. One of the authors (S.H.) took notice of the anatomic relationship between the facet joint and the most posterior edge of OPLL, and concluded that in type 2 vertebra in which the most posterior edge of OPLL is dorsal to the horizontal line through the median points of the bilateral facet joint in the anteroposterior direction (Fig. 133-15), the lateral gutters must be particularly made as lateral as possible (i.e., at the medial border of the facet joint) to obtain a wider spinal canal.[74] Therefore, on the preoperative CT film, the relative position between OPLL and the facet joint must be noticed.

Although there is no direct method of confirming the bonding between the spacer and the split spinous process, CT is very useful to estimate it. Kokubun and associates[76] examined histology of spinous processes of the cervical spine implanted by porous hydroxyapatite spacers 1 year after double-door laminoplasty, and confirmed that the bone contact with the spacer on CT images corresponded to bone bonding observed histologically.

In light of their findings, it is reasonable to evaluate the bonding between the spacer and the spinous process from the extent of contact between them based on CT images. Therefore, during operation, the appropriate size of the spacer must be selected in accordance with the size of the

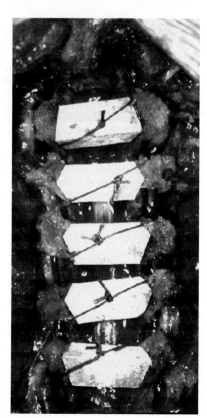

FIGURE 133-13 A photograph during operation using the STSS spacers. The STSS spacer is fixed to split spinous processes by sutures.

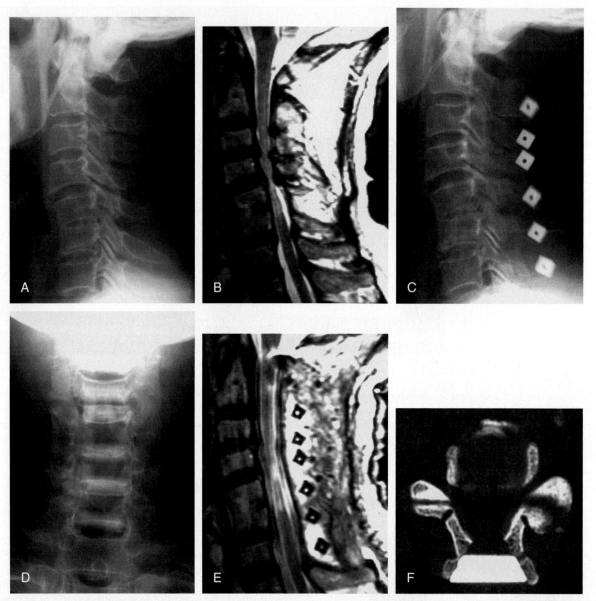

FIGURE 133-14   *A,* Preoperative plain x-ray film of 70-year-old man showing anterior displacement of the C4 vertebral body 20 years after the anterior cervical fusion at C5/C6, which he received after an accident. *B,* Preoperative T2-weighted magnetic resonance image (MRI) of the same patient. The spinal cord is severely compressed between C3/C4 and C4/C5 with the T2-high lesion within the spinal cord at the corresponding levels. *C,* Postoperative plain x-ray film (lateral view) following C1 laminectomy and double-door laminoplasty between C2 and C7. Note that each STSS spacer is fixed parallel to each spinous process. *D,* Postoperative plain x-ray film (anteroposterior view). *E,* Postoperative T2-weighted MRI in the sagittal section. Despite the sufficient widening of the spinal canal, the anteroposterior diameter of the spinal cord did not increase, presumably because of the preexistent cord atrophy. The T2-high lesion within the spinal cord can be clearly seen. The T2-low amorphous lesion at the C2 level is an artifact. *F,* Postoperative CT. The spinal canal is symmetrically opened, and the STSS spacer contacts well with the split spinous processes bilaterally.

spinous process to obtain good contacts, especially at the C3, C4, and C5 levels where the size of the spinous process is relatively smaller than that at the C2, C6, and C7 levels and the spacer tends to protrude from the spinous process. At present, four types of the STSS spacer with several sizes are available.

SUMMARY

For every new patient with symptomatic OPLL, the surgeon must choose between the anterior and posterior approaches.

Here, the relevant issue is not which of the two approaches is generally better or worse, but which can better cope with the particular type of OPLL the patient has. The advantages of the posterior approach over the anterior approach are as follows: (1) it is technically easier and has a lower probability of damaging the spinal cord; (2) the stability of the spine immediately after operation is better, making postoperative management easier; and (3) some degree of spinal movement is maintained, even after an extensive decompression. However, complete decompression of the cord and the root can hardly be achieved by the posterior approach when

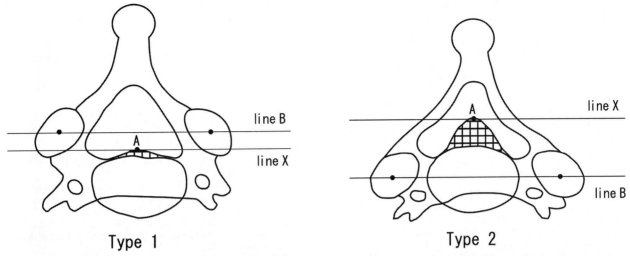

FIGURE 133-15 The difference in shape between type 1 and type 2 vertebrae. The line X is drawn parallel to the posterior wall of the vertebral body, crossing the posterior edge of the space-occupying lesion. Line B connects the midpoints of the joint surfaces of bilateral facets in the anteroposterior direction. In type 1 vertebra, line X is ventral to line B, whereas in type 2 vertebra, line X is dorsal to line B.

there is a severe degree of anterior impingement resulting from the OPLL, particularly of the segmental or localized type. Thus the primary target of the anterior approach is OPLL of the segmental or localized type, and the target of the posterior approach, OPLL of the continuous or mixed type.

However, this categorization by no means poses absolute restrictions on which approach is indicated because the anterior floating method can be safely employed even in the large, continuous OPLL. Furthermore, the influence of regrowth of OPLL on the outcome remains to be determined. Presently, the roles of these two approaches in the therapy of OPLL may better be regarded as complementary rather than mutually exclusive.

If the outcome of the initial approach is unsatisfactory, a second-stage operation by the other approach can be performed. Although the scheme of a two-stage operation is justifiable, selection of the initial approach belongs to the realm of the surgeon's experience and clinical judgment.

REFERENCES

1. Key CA: On paraplegia depending on disease of the ligaments of the spine. Guys Hosp Rep 3:17–34, 1838.
2. Tsukimoto H: On an autopsied case of compression myelopathy with a callus formation in the cervical spinal canal. Arch Jpn Chir 29:1003–1007, 1960.
3. Terayama K, Maruyama S, Miyashita J, et al: Ossification of the posterior longitudinal ligament in the cervical spine. Seikei Geka 15:1083–1095, 1964.
4. Onji Y, Akiyama H, Shimomura Y, et al: Posterior paravertebral ossification causing cervical myelopathy: A report of eighteen cases. J Bone Joint Surg Am 49:1314–1328, 1967.
5. Okamoto Y, Yasuma T: Ossification of the posterior longitudinal ligament of cervical spine with or without myelopathy. J Jpn Orthop Assoc 40:1349–1360, 1967.
6. Yanagi T: Ossification of the posterior longitudinal ligament: A clinical and radiological analysis of 46 cases. Brain Nerve 22:909–921, 1970.
7. Nakanishi T, Mannen T, Toyokura Y, et al: Symptomatic ossification of the posterior longitudinal ligament of the cervical spine. Neurology 24:1139–1143, 1974.
8. Minagi H, Gronner AT: Calcification of the posterior longitudinal ligament: A cause of cervical myelopathy. AJR Am J Roentgenol 105:365–369, 1969.
9. Breidahl P: Ossification of the posterior longitudinal ligament in the cervical spine: "The Japanese disease" occurring in patients of British descent. Australas Radiol 13:311–313, 1969.
10. Bakay L, Cares HL, Smith RJ: Ossification in the region of the posterior longitudinal ligament as a cause of cervical myelopathy. J Neurol Neurosurg Psychiatry 33:263–268, 1970.
11. McAfee PC, Regan JJ, Bohlman HH: Cervical cord compression from ossification of the posterior longitudinal ligament in non-Orientals. J Bone Joint Surg Br 69:569–575, 1987.
12. Trojan DA, Pouchot J, Pokrupa R, et al: Diagnosis and treatment of ossification of the posterior longitudinal ligament of the spine: Report of eight cases and literature review. Am J Med 92:296–306, 1992.
13. Forestier J, Lagier R: Ankylosing hyperostosis of the spine. Clin Orthop 74:65–83, 1971.
14. Resnick D, Guerra J, Robinson CA, et al: Association of diffuse idiopathic skeletal hyperostosis (DISH) and calcification and ossification of the posterior longitudinal ligament. AJR Am J Roentgenol 131:1049–1053, 1978.
15. Tsuyama N: The ossification of the posterior longitudinal ligament of the spine (OPLL): Report of the Investigation Committee on OPLL of the Japanese Ministry of Public Health and Welfare. J Jpn Orthop Assoc 55:425–440, 1981.
16. Ohtsuka K, Terayama K, Yanagihara M: A radiological population study on the ossification of the posterior longitudinal ligament in the spine. Arch Orthop Trauma Surg 106:89–93, 1987.
17. Nakanishi T, Mannen T, Toyokura Y: Asymptomatic ossification of the posterior longitudinal ligament of the cervical spine: Incidence of roentgenographic findings. J Neurol Sci 19:375–391, 1973.
18. Tsuzuki N: Ossification of the posterior longitudinal ligament (OPLL) of the cervical spine: Its incidence and histopathology. Japanisch Dtsch Med Berichte 32:11–22, 1987.
19. Firooznia H, Benjamin VM, Pinto RS, et al: Calcification and ossification of posterior longitudinal ligament of spine: Its role in secondary narrowing of the spinal canal and cord compression. NY State J Med 82:1193–1198, 1982.
20. Terayama K, Ohtsuka K, Berlini L, et al: Ossification of the spinal ligament: A radiographic reevaluation in Bologna, Italy. J Jpn Orthop Assoc 61:1373–1378, 1987.
21. Arlet J, Pujol M, Buc A, et al: Role de l'hyperostose vertérale dans les myélopathies cervicales. Rev Rhum 43:167–175, 1976.
22. Julkunen H, Heinonen OP, Knekt P, et al: The epidemiology of hyperostosis of the spine together with its symptoms and related mortality in a general population. Scand J Rheumatol 4:23–27, 1975.
23. Boachie-Adjei O, Bullough PG: Incidence of ankylosing hyperostosis of the spine (Forestier's disease) at autopsy. Spine 12:403–405, 1987.
24. Tsuzuki N, Imai T, Hotta Y: Histopathological findings of the ossification of the posterior longitudinal ligament of the cervical spine and their significance. J Jpn Orthop Assoc 55:387–397, 1981.

25. Kawaguchi H, Kurokawa T, Hoshino Y, et al: Immunohistochemical demonstration of bone morphogenetic protein-2 and transforming growth factor-β in the ossification of the posterior longitudinal ligament of the cervical spine. Spine 17(Suppl):33–36, 1992.

26. Terayama K: Genetic studies on ossification of the posterior longitudinal ligament of the spine. Spine 14:1184–1191, 1989.

27. Tanaka T, Ikari K, Furushima K, et al: Genomewide linkage and linkage disequilibrium analyses identify COL6A1, on chromosome 21, as the locus for ossification of the posterior longitudinal ligament of the spine. Am J Hum Genet 73:812–822, 2003.

28. Kirita Y, Miyazaki K, Hayashi T, et al: The clinical aspects and the therapeutic results of ossification of the longitudinal ligament of the cervical spine. Rinsho Seikei Geka 10:1077–1085, 1975.

29. Terayama K: Ossification of the posterior longitudinal ligament of the spine. In Suzuta T, Yamauchi Y (ed): Rheumatology-SEAPAL, 1988. Amsterdam: Elsevier Science, 1989, pp 33–37.

30. Seki H, Tsuyama N, Hayashi K, et al: Clinical study on the 185 patients with ossification of the longitudinal ligaments of the cervical spine. Seikei Geka 25:704–710, 1974.

31. The Investigation Committee on OPLL: The follow-up study for more than five years of ossification of the spinal ligament. In The Report of the Investigation Committee on OPLL of the Japanese Ministry of Health and Welfare, Tokyo, 1983, 1984, pp 85–96.

32. The Investigation Committee on OPLL: The follow-up study for more than ten years of ossification of the spinal ligament. In The Report of the Investigation Committee on OPLL of the Japanese Ministry of Health and Welfare, Tokyo, 1985, 1986, pp 71–77.

33. Satomi K, Hirabayashi K: Ossification of the posterior longitudinal ligament. In Rothman RH, Simeone FA (eds): The Spine, 3rd ed. Philadelphia: WB Saunders, 1992, pp 639–654.

34. Yamashita Y, Takahashi M, Matsuno Y, et al: Spinal cord compression due to ossification of ligaments: MR imaging. Radiology 175:843–848, 1990.

35. Hackney DB, Asato R, Joseph PM, et al: Hemorrhage and edema in acute spinal cord compression: Demonstration by MR imaging. Radiology 161:387–390, 1986.

36. Takahashi M, Sakamoto Y, Miyawaki M, Bussaka H: Increased MR signal intensity secondary to chronic cervical cord compression. Neuroradiology 29:550–556, 1987.

37. Koyanagi I, Iwasaki Y, Hida K, et al: Magnetic resonance imaging findings in ossification of the posterior longitudinal ligament of the cervical spine. J Neurosurg 88:247–254, 1998.

38. Ramanauskas WL, Wilner HI, Metes JJ, et al: MR imaging of compressive myelomalacia. J Comput Assist Tomogr 13:399–404, 1989.

39. Takahashi M, Yamashita Y, Sakamoto Y, Kojima R: Chronic cervical cord compression: Clinical significance of increased signal intensity on MR images. Radiology 173:219–224, 1989.

40. Hashizume Y, Iijima S, Kishimoto H, et al: Pathology of spinal cord lesions caused by ossification of the posterior longitudinal ligament. Acta Neuropathol (Berl) 63:123–130, 1984.

41. Shinomiya K, Furuya K, Sato R, et al: Electrophysiologic diagnosis of cervical OPLL myelopathy using evoked spinal cord potentials. Spine 13:1225–1233, 1988.

42. Iizuka T, Azuma H, Tanaka H, et al: Magnetic transcutaneous stimulation of the motor pathway in spinal cord disorders. In Simoji K, Kurokawa T, Tamaki T, Willis WD Jr (eds): Spinal Cord Monitoring and Electrodiagnosis. Berlin: Springer-Verlag, 1991, pp 253–260.

43. Kawaguchi H, Kurokawa T, Machida H, et al: Roentgenological manifestation of ossification of the posterior longitudinal ligament in the cervical spine causing severe spinal canal stenosis: A group comparison with and without marked spinal cord dysfunction. J Jpn Orthop Assoc 65:173–180, 1991.

44. Fujiwara K, Yonenobu S, Ebara S, et al: An analysis of cervical myelopathy due to cervical spondylosis or ossification of posterior longitudinal ligament by CT myelography. Rinsho Seikei Geka 23: 419–424, 1988.

45. Yamaura I: Anterior approach (anterior floating method) and its surgical results for cervical myelopathy caused by ossification of the posterior longitudinal ligament (OPLL). J West Pac Orthop Assoc 27:47–55, 1990.

46. Matsunaga S, Sakou T, Taketomi E, Komiya S: Clinical course of patients with ossification of the posterior longitudinal ligament: A minimum 10-year cohort study. J Neurosurg 100:245–248, 2004.

47. Epstein N: Diagnosis and surgical management of cervical ossification of the posterior longitudinal ligament. Spine J 2:436–449, 2002.

48. Southwick WO, Robinson RA: Surgical approaches to the vertebral bodies in the cervical and lumbar regions. J Bone Joint Surg Am 39:631–644, 1957.

49. Pansini A, Lore F: Une nouvelle technique: La somatotomie méiane longitudinale dans les myélopathies par discarthroses cervicales. Neurochirurgie 1:189–202, 1972.

50. Sakou T, Miyazaki A, Tominura K, et al: Ossification of the posterior longitudinal ligament of the cervical spine: Subtotal vertebrectomy as a treatment. Clin Orthop 140:58–65, 1979.

51. Manabe S, Nomura S: Anterior decompression for ossification of the posterior longitudinal ligament of the cervical spine. Neurol Surg 5:1253–1259, 1977.

52. Abe H, Tsuru M, Ito T, et al: Anterior decompression for ossification of the posterior longitudinal ligament of the cervical spine. J Neurosurg 55:108–116, 1981.

53. Hanai K, Inouye Y, Kawai K, et al: Anterior decompression for myelopathy resulting from ossification of the posterior longitudinal ligament. J Bone Joint Surg Br 64:561–564, 1982.

54. Harsh GR IV, Sypert GW, Weinstein PR, et al: Cervical spine stenosis secondary to ossification of the posterior longitudinal ligament. J Neurosurg 67:349–357, 1987.

55. Kojima T, Waga S, Kubo Y, et al: Anterior cervical ossification of the posterior longitudinal ligament. Neurosurgery 24:864–872, 1989.

56. Epstein N: Anterior approaches to cervical spondylosis and ossification of the posterior longitudinal ligament: Review of operative technique and assessment of 65 multilevel circumferential procedures. Surg Neurol 55:313–324, 2001.

57. Onari K, Akiyama N, Kondo S, et al: Long-term follow-up results of anterior interbody fusion applied for cervical myelopathy due to ossification of the posterior longitudinal ligament. Spine 26:488–493, 2001.

58. Schmidek HH, Smith DA: Anterior cervical disc excision in cervical spondylosis. In Schmidek HH, Sweet WH (eds): Operative Neurosurgical Techniques: Indications, Methods and Results, vol 2, 2nd ed. Orlando, FL: Grune & Stratton, 1988, pp 1327–1342.

59. McAfee PC, Bohlman HH, Riley L, et al: The anterior retropharyngeal approach to the upper part of the cervical spine. J Bone Joint Surg Am 69:1371–1383, 1987.

60. Kamikozuru M: Significance of the anterior floating method for cervical myelopathy due to the ossification of the posterior longitudinal ligament. J Jpn Orthop Assoc 65:431–440, 1991.

61. Nagashima C: Cervical myelopathy due to ossification of the posterior longitudinal ligament. J Neurosurg 37:653–660, 1971.

62. Miyazaki K, Kirita Y: Extensive simultaneous multisegment laminectomy for myelopathy due to the ossification of the posterior longitudinal ligament in the cervical region. Spine 11:531–542, 1986.

63. Oyama M, Hattori S, Moriwaki N: A new method of cervical laminectomy. Cntrl Jpn J Orthop Traumat Surg 16:792–794, 1973.

64. Kurokawa T, Tsuyama N, Tanaka H, et al: Double-door laminoplasty. Bessatsu Seikei Geka (Orthop Surg) 2:234–240, 1982.

65. Hirabayashi K, Watanabe K, Wakano K, et al: Expansive open-door laminoplasty for cervical spinal stenotic myelopathy. Spine 8: 693–699, 1983.

66. Itoh T, Tsuji H: Technical improvements and results of laminoplasty for compressive myelopathy in the cervical spine. Spine 10:729–736, 1985.

67. Iwasaki H: Expansive laminoplasty. Seikei Geka 2(Suppl):228–233, 1987.

68. Tomita K, Nomura S, Umeda S, et al: Cervical laminoplasty to enlarge the spinal canal in multilevel ossification of the posterior longitudinal ligament with myelopathy. Arch Orthop Trauma Surg 107:148–153, 1988.

69. Tsuzuki N, Zhogshi, Abe R, et al: Paralysis of the arm after posterior decompression of the cervical spinal cord. 1. Anatomical investigation of the mechanism of paralysis. Eur Spine J 2:191–196, 1993.

70. Harata S, Ito J: Experimental and clinical studies of the laminoplasty by splitting the spinous process using the hydroxyapatite at the intraspinous spacer. Gekachiryo (Surgical Therapy) 63:583–584, 1990.

71. Kato Y, Iwasaki M, Fuji T, et al: Long-term follow-up results of laminectomy for cervical myelopathy caused by ossification of the posterior longitudinal ligament. J Neurosurg 89:217–223, 1998.

72. Iwasaki M, Kawaguchi Y, Kimura T, Yonenobu K: Long-term results of expansive laminoplasty for ossification of the posterior longitudinal ligament of the cervical spine: More than 10 years follow up. J Neurosurg 96:180–189, 2002.

73. Epstein N: Posterior approaches in the management of cervical spondylosis and ossification of the posterior longitudinal ligament. Surg Neurol 58:194–207, 2002.

74. Hirabayashi S, Koshizuka Y: New method of measuring area of spinal canal after double-door laminoplasty. J Orthop Sci 4:78–82, 1999.

75. Hirabayashi S, Kumano K: Contact of hydroxyapatite spacer with split spinous processes in double-door laminoplasty for cervical myelopathy. J Orthop Sci 4:264–268, 1999.

76. Kokubun S, Kashimoto O, Tanaka Y: Histological verification of bone bonding and ingrowth into porous hydroxyapatite spinous process spacer for cervical laminoplasty. Tohoku J Exp Med 173:337–344, 1994.

134 Circumferential Spinal Fusion (Cervical)

SETH M. ZEIDMAN and THOMAS B. DUCKER

Recently, many surgeons have advanced the concept of circumferential, "front and back," or 360-degree fusion under a single anesthetic as the procedure of choice for a number of conditions affecting the spine.[1-4] Circumferential fusion is a highly demanding, highly specialized technique in spinal surgery with specific indications but substantial associated morbidity.[3,5,6] In the appropriate clinical scenario, this technique is not only useful but may in fact be preferable to a single approach.[3,7,8]

Circumferential and 360-degree fusions are actually misnomers. The approach to the spine is not from all sides but entails simply a combination of anterior and posterior approaches to the spine. Bidirectional is more accurate, but this term does not have the appeal or cachet of circumferential. The convenience of the term circumferential lies in its brevity and present wide acceptance. The ultimate result is a fusion that creates bony consolidation of the motion segment surrounding the spinal canal. Another misnomer is simultaneous combined anterior and posterior fusion, which gives the false impression that two surgical teams are working from opposite sides of the patient at the same time. Though a true simultaneous procedure is occasionally performed, this is the exception rather than the rule. We prefer the use of the term circumferential to indicate a combined anterior and posterior approach. It is brief but descriptive and conveys the fact that the procedure is bidirectional, but it does not suggest the simultaneous performance of a procedure, merely that more than one approach is being used. The critical element is the end result with regard to the spinal segment: the ultimate outcome is a circumferential arthrodesis, at least biomechanically.

The selection of the appropriate surgical approach in the management of an unstable cervical spine is predicated on the biomechanical deficiencies of the bony and ligamentous structures, age of the patient, surgeon's level of experience, and any medical comorbidity. The optimal approach is the least invasive; provides the lowest risk-to-benefit ratio with regard to potential injury of contiguous neural, vascular, and visceral structures; and provides sufficient stabilization to avoid external immobilization, thereby facilitating early mobilization and rehabilitation.[9]

Most conditions of the cervical spine can be effectively treated with either an anterior or a posterior operative technique. Circumferential cervical fusion is a procedure that has traditionally been reserved for those clinical situations in which three-column instability of the spine exists or is surgically created. This is an extrapolation of Denis's three-column model of the thoracic spine to the cervical spine.[10] In the presence of both anterior and posterior ligamentous

and bony disruption, the combined technique provides superior stabilization and thereby prevents acute, chronic, and glacial instability and the consequent late kyphotic deformity.[9,11,12]

Patients with pathologic fractures, multiple levels of vertebral collapse, fixed kyphotic deformities with an incomplete neurologic deficit, and neoplastic conditions with three-column involvement are the most common candidates for the combined technique.[3,6] Traditionally, the two procedures were staged with a separation of several days or even weeks.[6,7] During this time, the patient was maintained either immobile in bed or held in a halo orthosis. The combined procedure decreases the duration of hospitalization and reduces the amount of time that the cervical spine is functionally unstable and at risk for displacement.[5]

In our review of 100 patients who underwent a combined approach, we expanded the initial indications for the procedure to include cervical spondylotic myelopathy, pyogenic vertebral osteomyelitis, rheumatoid arthritis with multiple levels of subaxial subluxation and an incomplete neurologic deficit, and related conditions[3] (Fig. 134-1). Other investigators have published several series reporting additional indications for this highly specialized procedure.[1,2,4,13-19]

There is little disagreement over the advantage of performing both approaches under a single anesthetic in one session of surgery for trauma, failed previous surgery, and a variety of spinal deformities.[5] Not only is correction of deformity improved, but significant savings are made in total anesthetic time, blood loss, incidence of wound infections, hospital stay, and total cost compared with a regimen in which the approaches are performed as staged procedures on separate occasions.[3,5]

INDICATIONS

Acute Cervical Spine Injury

Traditionally, patients with acute cervical injury and an incomplete neurologic deficit were treated first with traction to realign the spine and then with posterior stabilization and arthrodesis. Later, if the neurologic deficit had not resolved or decreased, a second-stage anterior decompression could be performed.[6] These two procedures were subsequently consolidated into a single procedure. A combined, single-stage anterior and posterior approach for acute surgical management of cervical spine injury permits early restoration of anatomic alignment and decompression while optimizing the environment for neurologic recovery[3,7,11] (Figs 134-2 and 134-3).

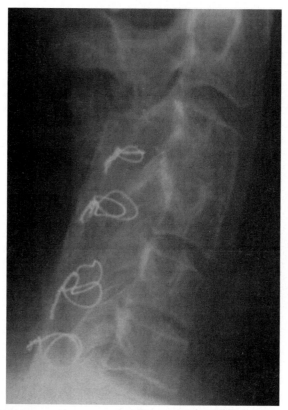

FIGURE 134-1 A myelopathic patient with congenital stenosis and disc herniation of C3–C4 with 1980s anterior decompression and fusion and a posterior laminectomy with lateral mass fusion with wire.

The key to successful management of unstable cervical spinal fractures is the ability to successfully identify those patients in whom a combined anterior-posterior procedure is required. Failure to recognize the presence of three-column instability can result in the failure of either a posterior tension band stabilization or an anterior strut with or without

a plate as a means of gaining cervical spine stability.[8] Failure to identify these patients results in a suboptimal stabilization procedure that may ultimately fail with potentially catastrophic consequences.

Cybulski and associates identified those factors in an acute cervical spine fracture or fracture-dislocation suggestive of three-column cervical spine instability.[8] Three-column cervical spine instability is suspected (1) in the presence of retrolisthesis and angulation of the superior vertebra on the next inferior vertebra, suggesting disruption of the anterior and posterior longitudinal ligaments; (2) in the presence of distraction of the posterior interspinous ligaments sufficient to allow subluxation or dislocation of the facets; or (3) in conjunction with a "shear" dislocation of one vertebra on another.[8] Anterior shearing force through the disc space can disrupt the intervertebral disc, along with disruption of the anterior and posterior longitudinal ligaments, each contributing to the presence of anterior- and middle-column cervical spine instability. Patients in whom three-column instability is identified should be considered for a combined anterior-posterior procedure. The procedure allows for immediate mobilization and should be considered for the management of these particularly unstable cervical spine fractures.

Combined anterior-posterior stabilization procedures also are indicated in patients with posterior ligamentous disruption or facet fractures and simultaneous anterior compression by a herniated intervertebral disc.[12] In this situation, it is mandatory that anterior decompression be achieved first. If posterior stabilization is performed prior to removal of the herniated disc, spinal cord compression may be increased because internal fixation devices increase the cervical lordosis with resultant exacerbation of the neurologic deficit.[9,12]

McNamara and colleagues reported six patients who underwent single-stage anterior decompression and posterior instrumentation and fusion with no late deformity. Five of the patients had incomplete neurologic deficits, and each

FIGURE 134-2 *A,* A 20-year-old athlete with early trauma and fracture dislocation of C4 on C5 had an incomplete cord lesion. A magnetic resonance imaging scan showed disc herniation into the canal. *B,* The disc was removed anteriorly with autograft reconstruction and was followed with posterior triple stabilization of C3 to C5 with single wiring of the destroyed lateral mass on the right.

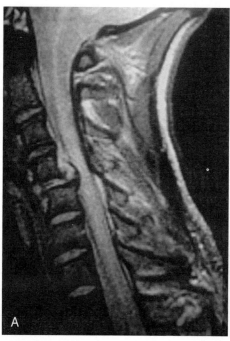

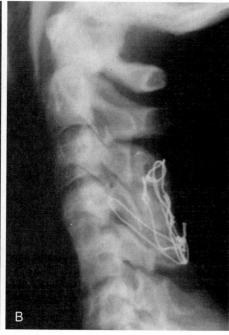

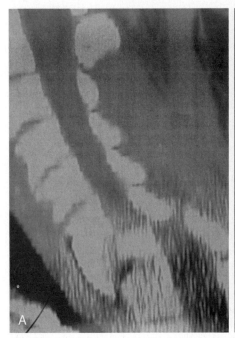
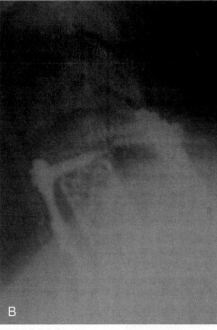

FIGURE 134-3 *A,* A 23-year-old patient with late trauma was rendered quadriplegic with dramatic C7 on T1 fracture dislocation. *B,* Severe pain and arm/hand dysfunction leading to anterior reconstruction with corpectomies, cage reconstruction, and anterior plates. This was followed with posterior limited laminectomy and lateral mass plate fusion.

improved a minimum of one Frankel grade.[11] In patients sustaining multiple-level burst fractures or significant posterior element damage, as is frequently the case after any high-energy or severe fracture, a combined procedure is often necessary.

Kyphotic Deformity

In our series of 100 patients treated with a one-stage anterior cervical decompression and posterior stabilization, cervical instability could be traced to trauma in 31 patients. These patients did not have an acute cervical fracture-dislocation but rather a late kyphotic deformity.[3]

The indications for surgical correction of kyphotic deformity depend on the extent of the deformity, the degree of functional compromise, the age and general condition of the patient (including associated medical comorbidity), the feasibility of correction, and most importantly the desire of a well-informed and educated patient to accept the risks and rehabilitative measures required for correction. In our series, the indication for a combined anterior-posterior procedure was either progression of cervical kyphosis of more than 40 degrees without a neurologic deficit (3 patients) and fixed kyphosis of more than 40 degrees with an incomplete neurologic deficit (28 patients). All the patients had sustained either a flexion compression injury or a burst fracture of a vertebral body combined with posterior ligamentous disruption, resulting in a progressive neurologic deficit with kyphosis of more than 40 degrees due to subluxation, dislocation of the posterior facet joints, or both[3] (Fig. 134-4).

Treatment of the kyphotic deformity consists of an anterior release with or without interbody grafting combined with a posterior instrumentation and arthrodesis procedure. This is a biomechanically robust construct that utilizes the posterior supplementation to assist anterior correction and share the responsibility for stabilizing the spine.[1] Bhojraj and co-workers described a combined anterior-posterior procedure for correction of fixed kyphotic deformity of the cervical spine using a combination of anterior release and posterior osteotomy. The anterior procedure is an open-wedge osteotomy, and the posterior procedure is a closed-wedge osteotomy. This combined procedure permits slow and controlled correction at the preoperatively determined level, rather than rapid, uncontrolled, and often violent correction, which may occur away from the desired level.[1] Both of these techniques have proven to be effective for the successful treatment of kyphotic deformities affecting the cervical spine.

Neoplastic Conditions

Vertebrectomy (corpectomy) and spinal stabilization can improve the quality of life considerably in cancer patients with cervical or cervicothoracic spinal metastases by restoring or preserving ambulation and by controlling intractable spinal pain with acceptable morbidity and mortality.[20] When there is three-column involvement of the spine by metastatic tumor, supplemental posterior instrumentation and arthrodesis are indicated. Supplemental posterior instrumentation prevents severe kyphosis, which is a potential problem in any patient with metastatic disease of the cervical spine, particularly those with involvement of the cervicothoracic junction.[16] A combined anterior-posterior technique should be used for extended tumoral conditions in which anterior fixation does not provide sufficient stability or when more radical surgery is required. Additionally, when the patient is deemed to have a long life expectancy—typically greater than 2 years, such as in breast carcinoma or myeloma—the combined approach should be considered. This provides multiple areas of stabilization that often remain in alignment despite destruction of either the anterior or the posterior elements.[3]

In our series of 100 patients treated with combined anterior cervical decompression and posterior stabilization, 55 patients

FIGURE 134-4 *A,* Fixed kyphosis in a patient with neck and radicular pain primarily at C6 and chin-on-chest deformity. *B,* Corrective surgery with an anterior discectomy and allograft reconstruction and posterior triple-wire fusion stabilization.

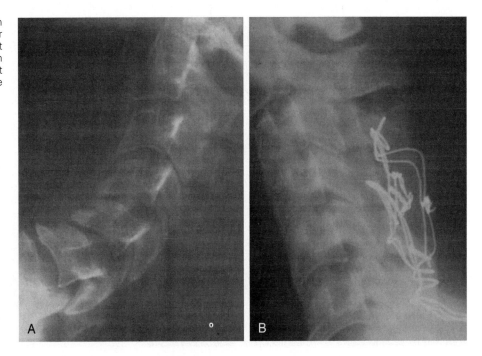

had a neoplasm: 38 had a pathologic fracture, and 17 had an incomplete neurologic deficit. The tumors were characterized as aggressive because they were unresponsive to radiation therapy. The most frequent lesion was carcinoma of the breast that had metastasized to the cervical spine.[3] The first procedure is typically an anterior corpectomy with methylmethacrylate stabilization. The patient is then turned on the operative wedge frame, and the posterior stabilization is performed. Autologous iliac crest bone grafting can be used to provide long-term stabilization. A combined approach decreases the morbidity and the length of hospital stay with no increase in complication rate.

A related problem is the patient with neurofibromatosis and severe dystrophic kyphosis of the cervical spine.[21] These patients can be most successfully treated with a combined anterior-posterior correction. Anterior distractive and posterior compressive corrections are simultaneously applied, keeping the posterior longitudinal ligament intact. Shortening the spinal canal permits dramatic one-stage correction of cervical kyphosis with increased safety and better results.

Cervical Spondylotic Myelopathy

In our series of 100 patients treated with a one-stage anterior cervical decompression and posterior stabilization, seven had cervical spondylotic myelopathy.[3] Additionally, in our series of 300 patients treated with an anterior, posterior, or combined procedure for cervical spondylotic myelopathy, only eight underwent a combined anterior-posterior procedure. Kyphosis associated with a developmentally narrow canal or posterior compression was the most common indication for the combined anterior and posterior approaches[22] (Figs 134-5, 134-6, and 134-7).

Cervical disorders involving three or more levels present a difficult reconstruction problem, especially if the posterior elements are deficient. Segmental fixation with lateral mass plating is an alternative method in situations that would otherwise require a halo. Segmental posterior fixation with

lateral mass plating provides more rigid immobilization than traditional techniques, allows restoration and maintenance of spinal alignment, obviates the need for halo immobilization, and is associated with a low incidence of neurovascular injury.[23]

Ossification of the Posterior Longitudinal Ligament

Ossification of the posterior longitudinal ligament (OPLL) is a challenging clinical condition under any circumstance. These patients have historically been treated with either an expansive laminoplasty or a generous corpectomy and multilevel strut graft fusion.[2] The combined procedure is a reasonable alternative for the management of these complex and difficult situations (Fig. 134-8).

Combined anterior-posterior surgery can be performed in severely myelopathic patients with cervical OPLL. These procedures permit decompression and stabilization with limited blood loss and acceptable risk. Between 1989 and 1996, Epstein performed 22 circumferential procedures in patients with OPLL, including an average 2.5-level anterior corpectomy with 5-level posterior wiring and fusion. Postoperatively, patients improved an average of three grades on the Nurick scale.[2] The use of the combined approach permits total spinal cord decompression and allows improved correction of any kyphotic deformity. Although the surgical procedure is challenging, it yields an excellent clinical outcome and is certainly less difficult than reoperation done from a single approach in a patient who requires subsequent further decompression.

Rheumatoid Arthritis

The treatment of rheumatoid arthritis with combined anterior-posterior fusion is not common but has been reported by a number of investigators with excellent results. Initiation of early treatment, before significant myelopathy has developed, is recommended. Decompression, both via

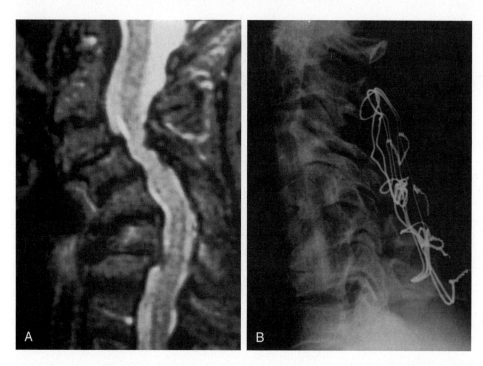

FIGURE 134-5 *A,* Case in 1980 with an S-curved deformity and severe myelopathy. *B,* The patient required anterior fibular strut graft correction (after corpectomies) and posterior laminectomies (1/2 C2, C3, C4), and C2 to C7 standard posterior triple-wire fusion.

realignment and bone resection, followed by fusion of the involved portion of the cervical spine is advocated. The quality of the bone in patients with rheumatoid arthritis is poor. The bone is soft and has a tendency to permit screws to pull out and wires to pull through the bone. Given the characteristics of presently available implant systems,

a circumferential fusion is often preferable to a single approach in these patients. Neck pain can be reliably relieved, although radiculopathy is less positively affected. Myelopathy carries a poor prognosis for relief and it often correlates with near-term death.[24]

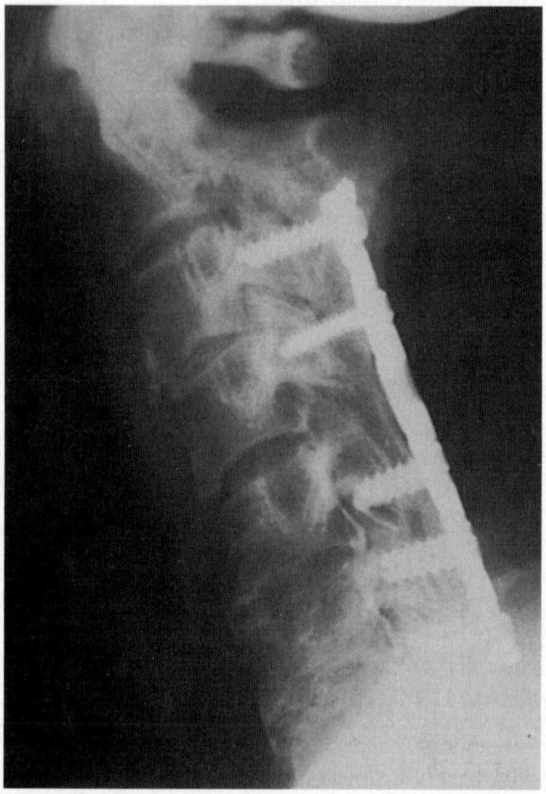

Ankylosing Spondylitis

Severe kyphotic deformities of the cervical spine occur in patients with ankylosing spondylitis. Cervical kyphotic deformity is often severely disabling, with restriction of the field of vision and interference with personal hygiene. The disability can progress to such severity that the patient has a chin-on-chest deformity that prevents opening of the jaw and may interfere with chewing and even swallowing.

The indications for surgical correction of kyphotic deformity in ankylosing spondylitis are the same as those for the correction of any kyphotic deformity.[25] In selecting patients for correction of cervical kyphotic deformity, it is essential to differentiate between long-standing, fixed, relatively painless deformities and recent, painful, progressive deformities. Patients with long-standing deformity who experience the sudden onset of acute painful deformity should be considered to have a fracture until proven otherwise. This can occur even in the face of no history of trauma or possibly trivial trauma.

Patients who present with fixed and frequently painless kyphotic deformity may require a resection/extension osteotomy for correction of their deformity. In considering correction of the kyphotic deformity by cervical osteotomy, the risks should be understood and the basic established principles should be followed to permit maximal correction with a minimal associated risk to the patient.[26]

In the cervical spine, both anterior and posterior approaches have been employed with some success. The risk for late neurologic deterioration is substantial. Because the condition is rare and the treatment is demanding and associated with a high risk for complications, treatment of

FIGURE 134-6 A myelopathic patient with discectomies without fusion at C3–C4 and C6–C7 with posterior lateral mass fusion with plates.

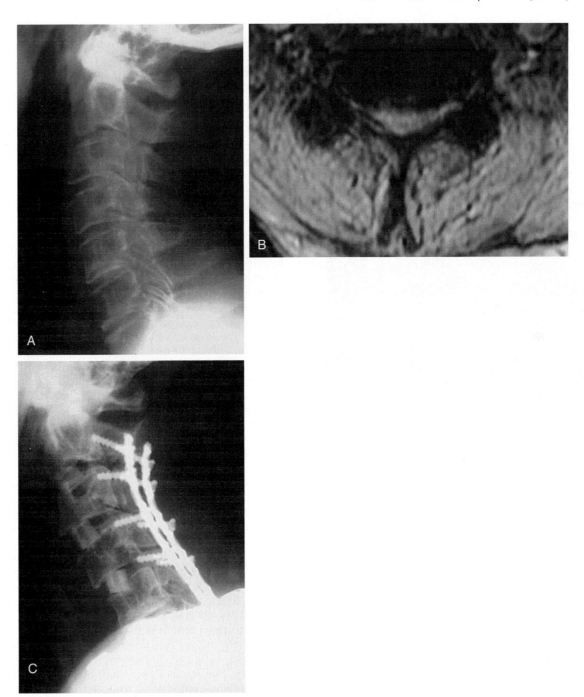

FIGURE 134-7   *A*, A patient with severe myelopathy and congenital stenosis. *B*, The patient had marked focal stenosis at C2–C3, C3–C4, and C4–C5. *C*, Anterior discectomies and extensive decompressions were done at C2–C3, C3–C4, C4–C5 with femoral allograft maintenance of lordosis. Then a posterior laminectomy with lateral mass fusion was done with the patient's own bone. The patient was stout, which made it difficult to do anterior plating at C2. Full decompression was desired at other levels as well.

these patients should be limited to spinal specialists. A combined approach that stabilizes the spine from both sides is preferable.

Pyogenic Vertebral Osteomyelitis

Patients with pyogenic vertebral osteomyelitis often require extensive débridement back to healthy bleeding bone to allow graft incorporation. Anterior débridement and bone grafting are the fundamental principles of surgical treatment. Laminectomy is contraindicated in most cases because it can exacerbate instability and thereby neurologic deterioration. Bone grafting should be performed during the same procedure as the débridement.[15,27]

Several techniques have been employed to optimize the potential for bone growth. These include antibiotic infusions, use of vascularized fibular strut grafts, and use of long mesh cages. Many of these patients benefit from a combined anterior-posterior reconstruction after the extensive anterior débridement required to rid the patient of necrotic or infected bone. In cases with significant kyphotic deformity or extensive anterior involvement, posterior stabilization

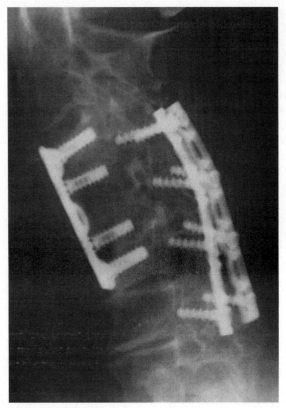

FIGURE 134-8 The patient is myelopathic with ossification of the posterior longitudinal ligament at C2–C3–C4 and fixed kyphosis with canal stenosis. Anterior corpectomies were done with allograft and plate reconstruction, then a posterior laminectomy was done with lateral mass plate stabilization.

and fusion are indicated. Several studies have demonstrated the effectiveness of posterior spinal instrumentation after anterior débridement and arthrodesis.[3,15]

Symptomatic Pseudoarthrosis

One of the primary indications for the combined anterior-posterior arthrodesis is failed anterior cervical fusion. Although not necessarily a simultaneous combined procedure, the net result is a circumferential anterior-posterior arthrodesis.[28]

Symptomatic anterior cervical pseudoarthrosis can be effectively treated by three methods: anterior revision, posterior revision, and circumferential procedures.

Management of cervical pseudoarthrosis by a repeat anterior procedure often requires a difficult dissection in an area that has previously undergone surgery, resection of the nonunion site, and regrafting. The risk for injury to vascular structures, visceral structures (the esophagus), and neurologic structures causes many practitioners to favor a posterior revision technique after a failed anterior cervical arthrodesis with symptomatic nonunion.[28] Because the incidence of failure after reoperation alone is reported to be high, posterior cervical fusion has been proposed as a treatment for anterior pseudoarthrosis. Posterior cervical articular pillar plating and fusion result in a higher probability of fusion than repeat anterior procedures do, even with the addition

of anterior plate stabilization. Posterior fusion and articular pillar plating, whether alone or part of a circumferential procedure, provides the added fixation required to successfully repair failed anterior cervical fusions.[23,28]

TECHNIQUE

All of the procedures are performed on either the operative wedge frame or the Jackson spinal table. One set of somatosensory evoked potentials is recorded prior to placing the patients into traction. The patient is most typically positioned supine at first, with the head held in tong traction. The arms are positioned at the sides, and the shoulders are carefully taped down. We typically place a small gel roll between the shoulder blades to facilitate gentle extension. Patients are instructed to position themselves in a comfortable position. Somatosensory evoked potentials are rechecked after fiberoptic awake intubation. The patient's head and neck are maintained in a neutral position.

The anterior approach is performed to the prevertebral level of the spine. Depending on the underlying pathology, the involved disc or vertebral bodies are rapidly identified and then excised in toto. A discectomy or corpectomy is then performed depending on the diagnosis and the underlying pathology. After this, a strut graft or strut is placed. Many times when there is a fracture-dislocation, anterior instrumentation cannot be placed until the posterior procedure is performed. As a result, many of these cases require an anterior approach to decompress followed by a posterior approach to permit reduction. Some cases even require multiple anterior and posterior approaches to permit optimal configuration of the spine and instrumentation in the ideal sagittal configuration.[12]

Stabilization can be performed in a variety of ways. The most common procedure is to perform either a multilevel corpectomy or multilevel discectomies. Anterior grafting can be performed with either allograft bone or autograft. Each of these techniques has distinct advantages and disadvantages. Certainly the use of autograft iliac crest bone graft is the gold standard, but it comes with very high associated morbidity at the graft site.

When large portions of iliac crest are required to reconstruct the spine, an extensive amount of muscle takedown and sewing of the tendinous attachments back together is necessary. This results in persistent hip and graft site pain, and close questioning of patients often reveals that this is their major complaint after surgery. In contrast, the use of allograft has none of the donor site morbidity associated with autograft, although allografting has its own problems. The incidence of pseudoarthrosis is higher with allograft than with autograft. This can be partially obviated by the use of internal fixation. Anecdotal evidence, however, suggests that the degree of graft incorporation if not quite as good, particularly when a long fibular strut is used.

It was within this context that a move to use mesh cages was introduced. These can be packed with the bone harvested from the site of the procedure (i.e., corpectomy), and bone can be packed around them. Our experience with many of these devices has shown the need to supplement with either anterior plating, combined anterior and posterior internal fixation, or perhaps just posterior instrumentation. Regardless of the instrumentation used, we consider it somewhat unwise to use a large mesh construct as a stand-alone device. Many of these constructs fail with sometimes catastrophic results.

For posterior instrumentation, we use either the standard triple-wire fusion or lateral mass plating.[6,23] Both of these techniques are safe and effective in experienced hands. The triple-wire technique provides excellent fusion results but requires the harvest of a sizable piece of corticocancellous bone graft from the posterior iliac crest. Although morbidity is minimal with this procedure, there is a finite amount of discomfort that can be troubling to the patient.

The alternative is the use of lateral mass plating. Lateral mass plates have enjoyed recent popularity, and they are safe and effective when used well. They do require a firm understanding of the anatomy of the lateral masses as well as the relationship between these structures and the exiting nerve roots and the vertebral arteries. Failure to clearly recognize the potential sources of neural or vascular injury can be devastating for the patient. We tend to use corticocancellous chips from the adjacent spinous processes to pack the facet joints that have been cleared of articular cartilage and decorticated.

It is critical to achieve an excellent substrate to allow fusion to occur both anteriorly and posteriorly. Time spent on carpentry is well worth the expenditure because failure to achieve fusion is dissatisfying for both the clinician and the patient. Procedures designed to correct pseudoarthroses are not as good as the original procedure and do not yield equivalent results.[28]

MORBIDITY

Morbidity is increased with a combined procedure compared with a single operative approach.[3] Given the magnitude of the operative procedure, the severity of the patients' conditions, and the large number of spinal cord injuries, a 10% rate of complications is acceptable.[3] Compared with traditional approaches that have been described in the literature, the single-stage combined anterior-posterior cervical approach is associated with a lower prevalence of postoperative complications involving the airway; a decreased rate of postoperative dislodgment of the graft, failure of the instrumentation, and pseudoarthrosis; and optimal neurologic recovery because of the combined benefits of both anterior and posterior direct decompression of the spinal cord with circumferential arthrodeses. Considering the magnitude of preoperative instability in these patients, we think that one-stage combined anterior-posterior operative reconstruction effectively reduces perioperative complications and optimizes the environment for maximum neurologic recovery.

SUMMARY

Combined anterior-posterior fusion is an extremely demanding technique that can be performed in a variety of ways. Often, the most challenging aspect of these cases is the transition between anterior and posterior surgical approaches. The "turn" often evokes trepidation and concern in the operating room support, anesthesia, and nursing staff. Currently available devices, including the Jackson spinal table and the new Stryker frame (operative wedge frame), have greatly

simplified and minimized the risk inherent in these maneuvers. Still, given the large number of variables involved in any complex case, the morbidity associated with manipulation of the spine about a fixed axis remains significant.

Circumferential arthrodesis is an effective tool to stabilize the spine. In the appropriate clinical scenario, it is perhaps the optimal tool and doing anything less is suboptimal. It requires a certain degree of diligence, meticulousness, and understanding of the overall three-dimensional configuration of the spine and all of the structures required to maintain stability. Although it is associated with greater morbidity than single approaches, it yields results that are far better than with single approaches. In experienced hands, it is a powerful tool and should be used only when clinically and biomechanically indicated.

REFERENCES

1. Bhojraj SY, Dasgupta D, Dewoolkar LV: One-stage "front" and "back" correction for rigid cervical kyphosis: A safer technique of correction for a rare case of adult-onset Still's disease. Spine 18(13):1904–1908, 1993.
2. Epstein NE: Circumferential surgery for the management of cervical ossification of the posterior longitudinal ligament. J Spinal Disord 11(3):200–207, 1998.
3. McAfee PC, Bohlman HH, Ducker TB, et al: One-stage anterior cervical decompression and posterior stabilization: A study of one hundred patients with a minimum of two years of follow-up. J Bone Joint Surg Am 77(12):1791–1800, 1995.
4. Winter RB, Turek-Shay LA: Twenty-eight-year follow-up of anterior and posterior fusion for congenital kyphosis: A case report. Spine 22(18):2183–2187, 1997.
5. Dick J, Boachie-Adjei O, Wilson M: One-stage versus two-stage anterior and posterior spinal reconstruction in adults: Comparison of outcomes including nutritional status, complications rates, hospital costs, and other factors. Spine 17(Suppl 8):310–316, 1992.
6. McAfee PC, Bohlman HH: One-stage anterior cervical decompression and posterior stabilization with circumferential arthrodesis: A study of twenty-four patients who had a traumatic or a neoplastic lesion. J Bone Joint Surg Am 71(1):78–88, 1989.
7. Aebi M, Mohler J, Zach GA, Morscher E: Indication, surgical technique, and results of 100 surgically-treated fractures and fracture-dislocations of the cervical spine. Clin Orthop 203:244–257, 1986.
8. Cybulski GR, Douglas RA, Meyer PR Jr, Rovin RA: Complications in three-column cervical spine injuries requiring anterior-posterior stabilization. Spine 17(3):253–256, 1992.
9. Vaccaro AR, Cook CM, McCullen G, Garfin SR: Cervical trauma: Rationale for selecting the appropriate fusion technique. Orthop Clin North Am 29(4):745–754, 1998.
10. Denis F: Spinal stability as defined by the three column spine concept in acute spinal trauma. Clin Orthop 189:65–76, 1984.
11. McNamara MJ, Devito DP, Spengler DM: Circumferential fusion for the management of acute cervical spine trauma. J Spinal Disord 4(4):467–471, 1991.
12. Zeidman S: Traumatic quadriplegia with dislocation and central disc herniation. J Spinal Disord 4(4):490–497, 1991.
13. Fidler MW: Spinal fusion: A combined anterior and supplementary interspinous technique. Eur Spine J 6(3):214–218, 1997.
14. Law MD Jr, Bernhardt M, White AA III: Cervical spondylotic myelopathy: A review of surgical indications and decision making. Yale J Biol Med 66(3):165–177, 1993.
15. Matsui H, Hirano N, Sakaguchi Y: Vertebral osteomyelitis: An analysis of 38 surgically treated cases. Eur Spine J 7(1):50–54, 1998.
16. Mehdian H, Weatherley C: Combined anterior and posterior resection and spinal stabilization for aneurysmal bone cyst. Eur Spine J 4(2):123–125, 1995.
17. Otsuka NY, Hey L, Hall JE: Postlaminectomy and postirradiation kyphosis in children and adolescents. Clin Orthop 354:189–194, 1988.
18. Safran O, Rand N, Kaplan L, et al: Sequential or simultaneous, same-day anterior decompression and posterior stabilization in the management of vertebral osteomyelitis of the lumbar spine. Spine 23(17):1885–1890, 1998.

19. Viviani GR, Raducan V, Bednar DA, Grandwilewski W: Anterior and posterior spinal fusion: Comparison of one-stage and two-stage procedures. Can J Surg 36(5):468–473, 1993.
20. Weatherley CR, Jaffray D, et al: Radical excision of an osteoblastoma of the cervical spine: A combined anterior and posterior approach. J Bone Joint Surg Br 68(2):325–328, 1986.
21. Craig JB, Govender S: Neurofibromatosis of the cervical spine: A report of eight cases. J Bone Joint Surg Br 74(4):575–578, 1992.
22. Zeidman S, Ducker T: Cervical disc disease. Neurosurg Q 2:116–143, 1992.
23. Wellman BJ, Follett KA, Traynelis VC: Complications of posterior articular mass plate fixation of the subaxial cervical spine in 43 consecutive patients. Spine 23(2):193–200, 1998.
24. Olerud C, Larsson B, Rodriguez M: Subaxial cervical spine subluxation in rheumatoid arthritis: A retrospective analysis of 16 operated patients after 1–5 years. Acta Orthop Scand 68:109–115, 1997.
25. Olerud C, Frost A, Bring J: Spinal fractures in patients with ankylosing spondylitis. Eur Spine J 5(1):51–55, 1996.
26. Simmons E: The surgical correction of flexion deformity of the cervical spine in ankylosing spondylitis. Clin Orthop 86:132, 1972.
27. Gruss P, Friedrich B, Mertens HG, Bockhorn J: Purulent osteomyelitis of the cervical spine with epidural abscess: Operative treatment by means of dorsal and ventral approach. Clin Neurol Neurosurg 79(1):57–61, 1976.
28. Lowery GL, Swank ML, McDonough RF: Surgical revision for failed anterior cervical fusions: Articular pillar plating or anterior revision? Spine 20(22):2436–2441, 1995.

135 Cervical Laminoplasty

DAVID G. MALONE, MITCHELL D. MARTINEAU, and
CHRISTOPHER M. BOXELL

INTRODUCTION

Cervical laminoplasty is a posterior spinal operation where the position of the lamina are altered without intersegmental fusion to augment the volume of the spinal canal. Laminoplasty is primarily used to treat cervical spondylotic myelopathy caused by ossification of the posterior longitudinal ligament, resulting in stenosis of the cervical canal.[1] Laminoplasty is usually performed in cases of multisegmental stenosis of the spinal canal. In the cervical spine, C3 through C7 are most frequently addressed, but C2, T1, and even C1 have been modified by laminoplasty techniques. Many surgeons choose laminoplasty over anterior fusion techniques when more than two levels require decompression. Laminoplasty can be used in other situations where the volume of the cervical spinal canal needs augmentation, but fusion is not desired. All literature to date on laminoplasty is class 3 retrospective data; therefore, at present, laminoplasty is listed as a treatment option for cervical spondylotic myelopathy. Laminoplasty is effective in treating cervical myelopathy caused by stenosis, and long-term studies indicate that laminoplasty can improve symptoms of myelopathy providing many years of improvement in Japanese Orthopedic Association (JOA) scores.[2] No studies demonstrate that laminoplasty is superior to laminectomy alone, laminectomy with posterior fusion, or anterior decompression with fusion for the treatment of cervical spondylotic myelopathy.[3-5] There is no difference in the recovery rates in myelopathic patients treated from a posterior laminoplasty approach versus anterior cervical fusion.

Laminoplasty appears to work by allowing the spinal cord to shift posteriorly into the augmented space.[6] Laminoplasty was first described in 1968, and much of the literature regarding laminoplasty comes from Asia, where cervical myelopathy from ossification of the posterior longitudinal ligament is commonly diagnosed.[7,8]

Theoretical benefits of laminoplasty include preservation of cervical motion, prevention of postlaminectomy kyphosis, lessening of adjacent segment degeneration, and avoidance of development of postlaminectomy membrane formation. Unfortunately, these benefits are not always realized because cervical range of motion diminishes approximately 50% after laminoplasty, and development of kyphotic deformity occurs in 10% to 35% of patients after laminoplasty. Despite the goal of avoiding fusion after laminoplasty, spontaneous intravertebral and intralaminar fusion has been reported frequently after laminoplasty. Additionally, there is a 6% to 60% incidence of chronic neck pain after laminoplasty. This may be more common than in cases of anterior fusion, since one study found a 19% incidence of axial neck pain after anterior fusion versus 60% after laminoplasty.[9,10]

Laminoplasty is thought to decrease the incidence of adjacent level degeneration in the cervical spine. To date, only a few cases of adjacent level degeneration have been reported after laminoplasty. The reported incidence of adjacent level degeneration in patients who had undergone previous anterior cervical fusion, later requiring additional surgery, is estimated to be between 19% and 25% 10 years after the initial surgery. The incidence of adjacent segment degeneration appears to be much less in laminoplasty, but there are no studies presently available to support this claim.[11]

RESULTS OF CERVICAL LAMINOPLASTIES

Because the majority of laminoplasty operations are preformed to treat cervical myelopathy, the preoperative and postoperative conditions are frequently scored using the JOA scoring system for cervical myelopathy (Table 135-1). Several studies comparing cervical corpectomy and several different laminoplasty techniques determined that both techniques are effective in treating cervical myelopathy.

TABLE 135-1 ▪ Japanese Orthopedic Association Score

Motor dysfunction of the upper extremity
  0 = Unable to feed oneself
  1 = Unable to handle chopsticks; able to eat with a spoon
  2 = Handle chopsticks with slight difficulty
  3 = None
Motor dysfunction of the lower extremity
  0 = Unable to walk
  1 = Walk on flat floor with walking aid
  2 = Up and/or down stairs with hand rail
  3 = None
Sensory deficit
  Upper extremity
    0 = Severe sensory loss or pain
    1 = Mild sensory loss
    2 = None
  Lower extremity
    0 = Severe sensory loss or pain
    1 = Mild sensory loss
    2 = None
  Trunk
    0 = Severe sensory loss or pain
    1 = Mild sensory loss
    2 = None
Sphincter dysfunction
  0 = Unable to void
  1 = Marked difficulty in micturition
  2 = Difficulty in micturition
  3 = None

The recovery rates for myelopathy were no different statistically between either procedure.[12–14]

Comparison of the single-door versus double-door laminoplasty techniques show no significant difference in the outcome between these two groups.[15]

Comparison of laminectomy, anterior decompression and fusion, and laminoplasty showed no significant difference in outcome as measured by change in JOA scores.[4,16–19] A comparison of subtotal corpectomy and laminoplasty showed identical results from the two procedures at 1- and 5-year follow-up evaluations. There may be a significant difference in outcome in the special case of massive ossification of the posterior longitudinal ligament, where over 50% of the canal is occupied by ossified posterior longitudinal ligament (OPLL). In this condition, the outcome was much better for the anterior approach patients because none of these patients worsened neurologically, as compared with a 33% neurologic complication rate for the laminoplasty patients.[20]

Laminoplasties can provide rapid improvement of myelopathic symptoms within the first postoperative year as measured on the JOA myelopathy score (Tables 135-1 and 135-2, and Figs. 135-1 and 135-2). Factors predicting recovery have been noted. Urinary bladder function recovers less than other symptoms. Patients older than 60 years improve less than younger patients. Preoperative JOA score, Pavlov ratio, and compression ratio also affect outcomes. Lower JOA scores, lower Pavlov ratios, and lower compression ratios all correlate with less improvement after open-door laminoplasties.[3,21–24] Abnormal spinal cord signal on preoperative magnetic resonance imaging (MRI) scanning has been associated with poor postoperative prognosis.[25] Local kyphosis exceeding 13 degrees is a crucial risk factor for poor recovery after laminoplasty. If kyphosis exceeding 13 degrees is detected, either anterior or posterior fusion should be considered[26] (Fig. 135-3). Transverse area of the spinal cord at the level of maximum compression is also related to outcome, since areas of 42.6 mm² correlated with excellent outcomes and areas of 31 mm² correlated only with good outcomes in postoperative JOA scores.[27] It appears that the ideal enlargement of the canal is 4 mm along an anterior posterior line, and that

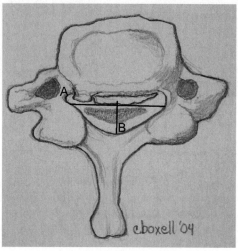

FIGURE 135-1   Compression ratio is the sagittal cord diameter divided by the transverse cord diameter times 100.

a 3-mm posterior cord shift is required for clinical improvement.[6] Reoccurrence of myelopathy postoperatively due to posterior shifting of the cord into the area of split lamina has been reported. This rare event usually occurs in the first few days after laminoplasty and responds to laminectomy of the affected segments.[28]

Risk factors for failure of adequate decompression with laminoplasty have been determined in cases of OPLL (Fig. 135-4). Maximum thickness of the ossification of more than 7 mm, lordosis of less than 10 degrees, or any kyphosis are significantly correlated with continued cord contact in the postlaminoplasty state. If these risk factors are present, then anterior decompression should be considered.[22,29,30] It is recommended that patients be treated surgically as soon as myelopathy is detected. Patients with OPLL usually have improved JOA scores in the postlaminoplasty state, and those last for at least 5 years before myelopathy progresses. Ossification of the posterior longitudinal ligament progresses in 73% of patients after laminoplasty, and younger patients with the mixed or continuous type of OPLL progress most often.[29] Symptomatic progression of OPLL cannot be predicted after laminoplasty, but if symptomatic progression occurs, an anterior approach may be considered. Late neurologic deterioration may be seen in 18% to 60% of cases after cervical laminoplasty, and may be due to instability or development of kyphosis.[31]

Cervical radiculopathy occurs in 7% to 20% of patients after laminoplasty. Radiculopathy most often appears within 2 weeks of surgery, and is evenly split between the hinge and open-door side of the laminoplasty when using the open-door technique. The C5 nerve root appears to be particularly predisposed to postoperative radiculopathy. Performing preoperative electromyogram (EMG) may prevent postoperative C5 palsy. If radiculopathy is found on EMG, selective microforaminotomies should be performed during the laminoplasty procedure.[32,33] There is evidence to suggest that segmental motor paralysis may be due to changes in the central gray matter of the spinal cord, rather than in the nerve root. In those cases, there is a definite delay from the end of surgery to the onset of deficit, and MRI scan may show a high-intensity zone in the spinal cord on T2 images.

TABLE 135-2 ▪ Recovery Rate

$$\text{Recovery rate} = \frac{\text{postoperative score} - \text{preoperative score}}{17 - \text{preoperative score}} \times 100\%$$

Excellent recovery rate: >75%
Good: 50%–75%
Fair: 25%–50%
Poor: <25%

Nurick Scale

0 Signs or symptoms of root involvement, but without evidence of spinal cord disease
1 Signs of spinal cord disease, but no difficulty walking
2 Slight difficulty walking that does not prevent full-time employment
3 Difficulty walking that prevents full-time employment or ability to do all housework, but that is not so severe as to require someone's help to walk
4 Able to walk only with someone's help or with the aid of a frame
5 Chair bound or bedridden

FIGURE 135-2 The Pavlov ratio, also known as the Torg-Pavlov ratio. The ratio is the canal size divided by the vertebral body size. This is determined by using the lateral plain radiograph, and measuring the distance between the posterior vertebral body line and the spinolaminar line, divided by the distance between the anterior vertebral body line and the posterior vertebral body line. The normal value is 1.0 or greater, and stenosis is denoted by a ratio of 0.82 or less.

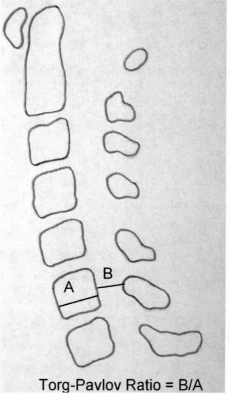

Torg-Pavlov Ratio = B/A

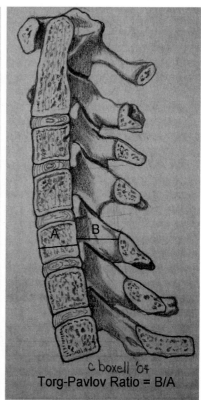

Torg-Pavlov Ratio = B/A

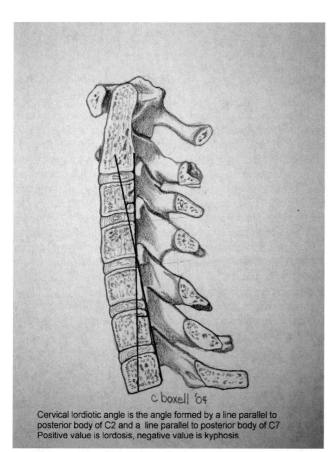

Cervical lordiotic angle is the angle formed by a line parallel to posterior body of C2 and a line parallel to posterior body of C7. Positive value is lordosis, negative value is kyphosis.

FIGURE 135-3 Method of measuring lordosis: the angle formed by a line parallel to the posterior body of C2 and a line parallel to the posterior body of C7. A positive value indicates lordosis, a negative value kyphosis.

The mechanism is unknown, but may be attributable to surgical trauma or possibly due to rapid reperfusion into the ischemic central gray of the cord.[34] Other causes of severe postoperative neck pain or motor paralysis may be due to malposition of osteotomized lamina, surgical trauma, or reclosure of opened lamina.[2] Some patients may develop kyphosis after laminoplasty, and those who develop kyphosis tended to have a poor recovery. Additionally, patients who had preexisting kyphosis had less reversal of myelopathy.[35,36] Some degree of lordosis is lost in 87% of patients after laminoplasty, and this appears to be related to detachment of the semispinalis cervicis muscle on C2, and the nuchal ligament at C6/C7. For this reason, it is recommended that the semispinalis cervicis be left attached whenever possible.[37,38] Laminoplasty techniques have been developed to spare the muscular and ligamentous attachments at the spinous processes. Despite this modification, 26.9% of patients continued to complain of axial neck pain postoperatively, and no good data yet exist to indicate that the extra time spent with this technique is beneficial to patient outcome.[36] One retrospective study of double-door laminoplasty with reconstruction of the extensor musculature found that there was no influence in either the development or resolution of axial pain symptoms. This suggests that muscle reconstruction techniques may have merit in decreasing axial pain postoperatively after laminoplasty. It appears that preventing denervation of the paraspinal muscles by limiting dissection to the lateral border of the facet complex, reconstructing the extensor musculature, avoiding damage to the facet joint when making the lateral gutter hinges, and providing muscular exercise in the postoperative period all contribute to less axial neck pain.[39]

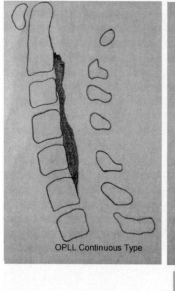

OPLL Continuous Type

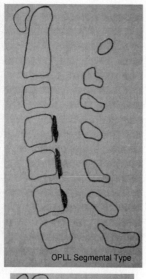

OPLL Segmental Type

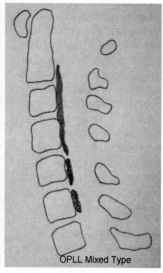
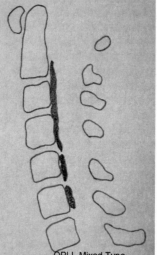

OPLL Mixed Type

FIGURE 135-4 Ossified posterior longitudinal ligament types: continuous, segmental, mixed, and localized.

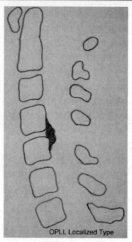

OPLL Localized Type

Fusion spontaneously occurs in patients after laminoplasty and may involve multiple levels. Intervertebral body fusion has been reported in 18% of patients who have undergone laminoplasty, and interlaminar fusion has been seen in 80% of patients who have undergone laminoplasty.[40]

Neck pain exists in up to 80% of patients after cervical laminoplasty, and seems to be greater in those who have more operated levels, and in those who have less range of motion postoperatively.[41] This may be related to damage to the facet capsules, or the paravertebral muscles. The nuchal muscles may be reduced to 80% of their preoperative size in those patients who have undergone laminoplasty.[42] This is likely due to denervation of the musculature from dissecting lateral to the facet joints, and may play a role in persistent postoperative neck pain. Neck pain appears to correlate with an imbalance in the ratio of strength between the flexor and extensor muscles in the postlaminoplasty state.[43] Comparing laminoplasty to anterior fusion for the incidence of postoperative chronic neck and shoulder pain reveals the incidence is 60% in the laminoplasty group as compared with 19% in anterior cervical fusion.[9]

Occupational recovery after cervical laminoplasty for OPLL depends on the severity of preoperative myelopathy, and the degree of postoperative recovery. Return to work rates vary depending on job demands, with 95% of light sedentary laborers, 50% of standing laborers, and 35% of heavy laborers returning to work.[44]

Long-term follow-up of open-door laminoplasty indicates that the canal size increases 48% initially, and decreases slightly to 40% after 5 years. The average loss of motion on flexion is 35%, and the average loss of motion on extension is 57%.[45] Approximately 8% of patients have preserved neck motion after laminoplasty. Ten years after laminoplasty by the double-door technique, 78% of patients maintain their initial improvement in degree of myelopathy.[46] Causes of late deterioration in patients with OPLL who have undergone laminoplasty include thoracic myelopathy from ossification of the yellow ligament, minor trauma, and rarely progression of OPLL at the operative levels.[2,40] Adjacent segment degeneration can occur after laminoplasty, but compared with anterior cervical fusion, laminoplasty may present fewer predispositions for development of adjacent segment degeneration.[47]

TYPES OF CERVICAL LAMINOPLASTY

Four basic types of laminoplasty exist, but only three have gained in popularity. The earliest form of laminoplasty was called the Z-plasty type (Fig. 135-5). In this type of laminoplasty the spinous processes are removed, and the lamina are thinned to the inner cortical region. An opening is made along the long axis of the lamina, and two lateral troughs are made. The canal is augmented by then shifting the lamina and securing them to each other to maintain the

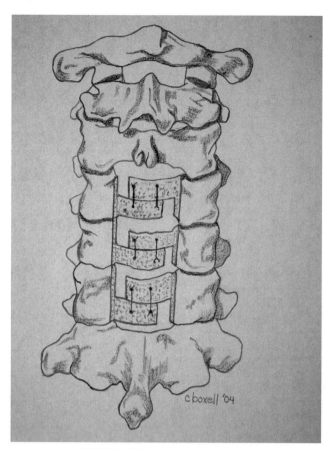

FIGURE 135-5 Z-plasty technique.

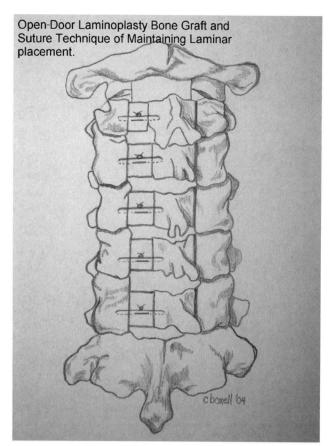

FIGURE 135-6 Open-door technique.

new alignment. This procedure has been largely abandoned as technically demanding without superior results, as compared with the other techniques. The open-door or Hirabayashi-type laminoplasty utilizes a thinned hinge on one side of the lamina, and a complete cut though the lamina on the opposite side (Fig. 135-6). The double-door or Kurokawa-type laminoplasty uses hinges fashioned bilaterally just medial to the junction of the lamina and facet, and a midline bicortical cut (Fig. 135-7). In both the double-door and open-door types of laminoplasty, the bicortical cut area is opened and may be fixed by a variety of techniques to maintain the augmented position. En bloc laminoplasty is utilized in cases where it is desirable to operate inside the spinal canal. This necessitates the removal of the lamina, but in contrast to conventional techniques, the lamina are reconstructed. En bloc laminoplasty offers several advantages because it lessens postoperative scarring and facilitates reoperation. In en bloc laminoplasty, the lamina are removed as a whole by cutting bicortical slots just medial to the junction of the lamina and facet. The entire complex of spinous process, lamina, and intraspinous ligament are removed as a unit and replaced at the conclusion of the procedure. Foraminotomies have been added to each of these techniques to treat radiculopathy as well as myelopathy. A variety of techniques have been utilized to preserve muscle attachments to the spinous processes to aid in reconstruction of the posterior tension band.[48]

TECHNIQUES AND MATERIALS

Patient Positioning

Typically, a general endotracheal anesthetic is used and the patient is given a preoperative dose of antibiotics and steroids. Positioning is accomplished by placing a pin-type headrest, and turning the patient prone. Chest rolls elevate the thoracic cage and decompress the abdomen, thereby lowering venous pressure and diminishing operative blood loss. The head and neck are positioned in a neutral or slightly flexed posture, and the headrest mechanism is locked. The shoulders are taped down to the table with 4-inch adhesive tape to increase lateral x-ray penetration and to improve the view during intraoperative imaging. Closing is facilitated by untaping the shoulders at the end of the procedure. A standard midline approach is utilized, dissecting down to the fascia. At this point in the procedure, a choice exists between standard bilateral subperiosteal dissection, and a posterior element–sparing approach.

Preservation Technique of the Posterior Cervical Elements in Laminoplasty

Along one side only, the lateral attachments to the spinous processes are dissected in a subperiosteal plane, exposing the lamina and facet complex. Next, an oscillating saw is used to cut the spinous processes approximately 5 mm from

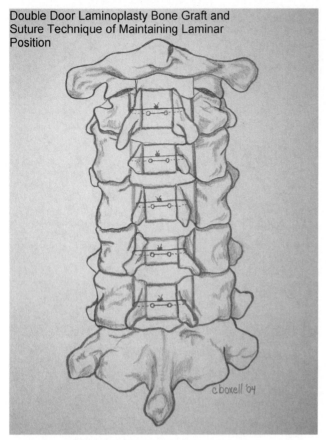

Double Door Laminoplasty Bone Graft and Suture Technique of Maintaining Laminar Position

FIGURE 135-7   Double-door technique.

facet complex. A central bicortical cut is made to split the spinous processes and lamina in the midline. With this technique, bilateral foraminotomies can be performed at each level if required.[49,52,53]

Constructing and Opening the "Hinge"

The hinge is key to overall success in any laminoplasty operation. A high-speed air drill, with either a diamond bit or bone-cutting bit, is utilized. The bit should be around 3 mm in diameter, and an acorn-type bone-cutting bit works well for this task (Fig. 135-8). When making the hinge, care must be taken so that the lamina is not thinned to the point that it fractures, or that it offers no springlike resistance to deformation. This resistance holds the bone graft material in place. The proper resistance of the hinge is found by making the complete laminar cut first, then drilling the hinge side. The resistance is checked once the lamina is thinned from the outer cortex through the cancellous bone. Once the inner cortex of the lamina is identified, the resistance is checked with gentle finger pressure. The inner cortex of the lamina is thinned until gentle finger pressure opens the laminoplasty segment.[10] When performing double-door laminoplasty, an interlaminar spreader may be used to open the hinges. This will probably be required if the spinous process has been resected, as in a posterior element–sparing technique. The ligamentum flavum must be opened, with

the base of the lamina. At this point, subperiosteal dissection is performed along the opposite lamina and facet complex to completely expose the lamina and facet complexes bilaterally. Care must be taken during this part of the dissection to avoid damaging either facet complex. The spinous processes, with their ligamentous attachments, are retracted to one side. Either a double- or single-door laminoplasty is then performed.[49]

Bony Dissection for Open-Door Laminoplasty

To perform an open-door laminoplasty, bone is dissected in two locations. Along one side, a unicortical cut is made to construct one hinge. On the other side, the lamina is cut bicortically to make the "door" that opens. The hinge can be fashioned on either side, which mandates that the bicortical cut is made on the opposite side. The location of the bicortical cut is at the junction of the lamina and facet complex. The hinge is made at the same location on the opposite side.[50,51]

Bony Dissection for Double-Door Laminoplasty

To perform a double-door laminoplasty, bone is dissected in three locations. Two hinges are constructed; they are located bilaterally at the junction of the lamina and

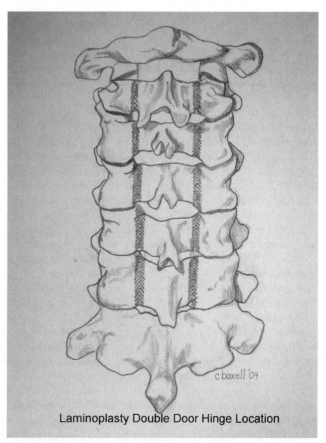

Laminoplasty Double Door Hinge Location

FIGURE 135-8   Cuts for double-door hinge location.

care taken to avoid lacerating the epidural venous plexus, prior to rotating the lamina and opening the segment. This can be done in a variety of ways—with a dural guide, or simply with a scalpel.[54] Bleeding can be lessened by using the bipolar electrocautery to coagulate the epidural veins during section of the ligamentum flavum.

Maintaining the Final Laminar Position

For long-term improvement of myelopathy, the laminae must remain in their altered position. A known complication is a phenomenon called "spring back." This occurs when the canal augmentation is lost when the opened door closes postoperatively. It appears to be related to operative failure in up to 38% of noninstrumented cases.[25] Instrumentation lowers the complication rates in laminoplasty. Historically, there have been a variety of changes in technique and materials to maintain the augmented volume of the spinal canal. Originally, suture and fat graft were used to maintain expansion. Later, placing bone in the area of complete bicortical opening strengthened this region and helped maintain the expansion. Iliac crest, spinous process, and rib from autogenous or allograft sources, as well as custom-designed hydroxyapatite spacers have all been utilized. Titanium miniplates from either standard sources or of custom design are useful for maintaining alignment (Figs. 135-9 and 135-10). Miniplates are extremely useful

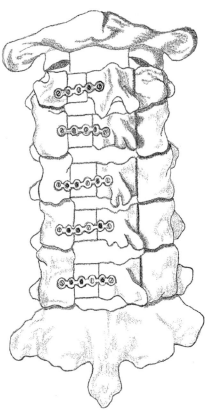

FIGURE 135-10 Open-door laminoplasty with miniplates and intervening bone graft.

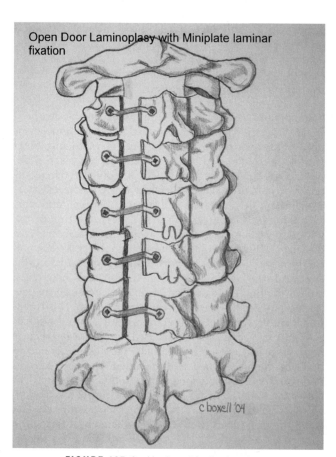

Open Door Laminoplasty with Miniplate laminar fixation

c boxell '04

FIGURE 135-9 Hardware for laminoplasty.

for fixating the bone graft to the opened area of the laminoplasty, thereby preventing the spring back phenomenon. During the opening of the door in the laminoplasty procedure, the bony hinge can fracture. In the event of this complication, miniplates can be used to repair the fracture.[55–57] Artificial titanium laminae have also been utilized for this procedure.[58] In cases of open-door laminoplasty where no instrumentation is desired, commercially available suture anchors placed in the center of the lateral mass of the hinge side have been successful in maintaining canal volume augmentation.[59] A nonabsorbable suture is passed through a hole drilled in the spinous process, and fixated either to a suture anchor, or to the facet capsule to maintain the altered position of the lamina. In double-door laminoplasty, holes are drilled with a right-angle drill through the apex of the spinous process and through the intervening bone graft. A nonabsorbable suture is passed through the holes and tied to maintain the bone graft between the split lamina. Titanium screws have replaced the role of suture in many cases.[60]

T-Laminoplasty

A modification of the double-door technique called the T-laminoplasty was reported in 1995, and is not to be confused with T-saw laminoplasty, although a T-saw may be used in the procedure. The name T-laminoplasty comes from the T shape of the resected spinous process that is used as a bone graft between the split lamina. In T-laminoplasty, a standard midline incision with bilateral subperiosteal dissection is performed over the affected levels, including the level immediately superior and inferior to the pathologic levels. The spinous processes are removed, leaving a 5-mm projection from the lamina. The lamina is cut in the midline using a small drill or craniotome, and the lateral lamina is thinned to the point of plastic deformation when force is placed laterally through the midline cut. Ligamentum flavum in the interlaminar spaces is removed. A 1-mm hole is drilled from medial to lateral in the lamina on each side. The saved, resected spinous processes are sutured into place utilizing the holes in the lamina.[61]

T-Saw Laminoplasty

T-saw laminoplasty was described by Tomita in 1998 and uses a threadwire saw to perform the midline cut as a modification to the double-door type of laminoplasty. This allows less bone loss, less operative time, less blood loss, and less chance of dural injury.[62] The patient is positioned prone with the head neutral or lordotic to prevent kyphosis. The ligamentum flavum is resected and a protective sleeve is passed under the lamina. The wire saw is then passed under the lamina and using a reciprocating motion the lamina is split (Fig. 135-11). If kyphosis is present, cutting multiple levels in one pass is dangerous as the saw may bowstring into the canal, causing catastrophic neurologic injury. The outer cortex is then cut along the junction of the lamina

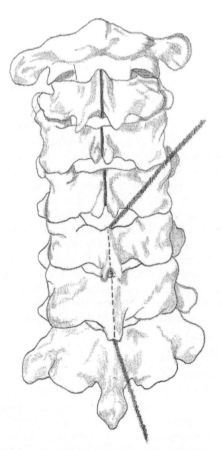

FIGURE 135-11 Midline T-saw cut for double-door laminoplasty.

and facet complex, taking care to preserve the facets. The lamina are then expanded and a spacer of either bone, or porous hydroxyapatite is tied into place with suture. Root injury has been reported with the T-saw technique, and occurred in the thoracic spine when the saw was threaded underneath a nerve root.[63]

Closure and Reconstruction of the Posterior Tension Band

Reconstruction of the posterior muscles and posterior tension band may diminish postoperative complications. Once the canal augmentation portion of the laminoplasty is completed, reconstruction of the posterior tension band begins. In double-door laminoplasty, holes are drilled in the apex of the spinous process, and corresponding holes are drilled in the segment of bone that is used to keep the split lamina apart. A nonabsorbable suture is threaded through the holes and tied to perform the reconstruction. In the open-door laminoplasty, holes are drilled through the apex of the spinous processes and through the base of the corresponding sections on the lamina. Nonabsorbable suture is threaded through these holes and tied to reconstruct the tension band. Additionally, in open-door laminoplasty, sutures are usually placed in a figure-of-eight fashion around the most superior, nonoperated spinous process, and the most superior, operated spinous process. A similar suture is placed around the spinous processes at the inferior end of the construct as well. Any dissection of the muscles from the C2 spinous process should be reattached by suturing them back to their original position. If needed, holes should be drilled with a right-angle drill to provide a point of fixation for the suture.

EN BLOC LAMINOPLASTY

Laminoplasty can be utilized in a nonexpansible method. In this case, the laminae are replaced in their original positions. This approach is especially useful when intradural pathology is addressed through a laminectomy approach, particularly for benign tumor with a propensity for recurrence. The approach will be made easier in the event of reoperation, because there will be much less epidural scarring. This technique also allows for reconstruction of the posterior ligamentous tension band. Bicortical cuts are made at the junction of the lamina and facet processes, and the intraspinous ligament is cut, usually at one end only. A threadwire saw works well for the bilateral bony cuts, and by angling the saw from medial to lateral during the sawing process, a trapezoidal cut can be made. This trapezoidal cut prevents the lamina from sinking into the canal. A high-speed drill can also be used for this task, but it is more difficult to make a trapezoidal cut. The ligamentum flavum is then sectioned, and the laminae are moved from the operative field, allowing access to the spinal canal. To reconstruct the laminae, miniplates or suture are used to fixate the laminae to their original positions. The intraspinous ligament is then reconstructed by suturing the spinous processes to the levels above and below in a figure-of-eight type stitch.[63]

POSTOPERATIVE CARE

Early ambulation is encouraged. Patients should be mobilized on the first day of surgery. They should be placed in a rigid cervical collar and maintained for 8 to 12 weeks. At that point, cervical spine radiographs with flexion extension views are performed to assess stability. MRI or computed tomography scans can be utilized to check canal volume augmentation if surgical outcome does not meet expectations.[64]

REFERENCES

1. Hirabayashi K, Watanabe K, Wakano K, et al: Expansive open-door laminoplasty for cervical spinal stenotic myelopathy. Spine 8:693–699, 1983.
2. Satomi K, Nishu Y, Kohno T, Hirabayashi K: Long-term follow-up studies of open-door expansive laminoplasty for cervical stenotic myelopathy. Spine 19(5):507–510, 1994.
3. Nagata K, Ohashi T, Abe J, et al: Cervical myelopathy in elderly patients: Clinical results and MRI findings before and after decompression surgery. Spinal Cord 34:220–226, 1996.
4. Nakano N, Nakano T, Nakano K: Comparison of the results of laminectomy and open-door laminoplasty for cervical spondylotic myeloradiculopathy and ossification of the posterior longitudinal ligament. Spine 13(7):792–794, 1988.
5. Ratliff JK, Cooper PR: Cervical laminoplasty: A critical review. J Neurosurg (Spine 3) 98:230–238, 2004.
6. Sodeyama T, Gota S, Mochizsuki M, et al: Effect of decompression enlargement laminoplasty for posterior shifting of the spinal cord. Spine 24(15):1527–1532, 1999.
7. Hirabayashi K: Expansive open-door laminoplasty for cervical spondylotic myelopathy. Shujutsu 32:1159–1163, 1978.
8. Morimoto T, Yamada T, Okumora Y, et al: Expanding laminoplasty for cervical myelopathy-spinous process roofing technique. Acta Neurochir (Wien) 138:720–725, 1996.
9. Hosono N, Yonenobu K, Ono K: Neck and shoulder pain after laminoplasty a noticeable complication. Spine 21:1969–1973, 1996.
10. Kuwaguchi Y, Matsui H, Ishihara H, et al: Axial symptoms after en bloc cervical laminoplasty. J Spinal Disord 12:392–365, 1999.
11. Wang MY, Green BA, Vitarbo E, Levi A: Adjacent segment disease: An uncommon complication after cervical expansive laminoplasty: Case report. Neurosurgery 53(3):770–773, 2003.
12. Edwards CC, Heller JG, Murakami H: Corpectomy versus laminoplasty for multilevel cervical myelopathy. Spine 27:1168–1175, 2002.
13. Ieasaki M, Ebara S, Miyamoto S, et al: Expansive laminoplasty for cervical radiculomyelopathy due to soft disc herniation: A comparative study of laminoplasty and anterior arthrodesis. Spine 21:32–38, 1996.
14. Kawakami M, Tamaki T, Iwasaki H, et al: A comparative study of surgical approaches for cervical compressive myelopathy. Clin Orthop Rel Res 381:129–136, 2000.
15. Yue WM, Tan CT, Tan SB, et al: Results of cervical laminoplasty and a comparison between single and double trap-door techniques. J Spinal Disord 13:329–335, 2000.
16. Hasegawa K, Homma T, Chiba Y, et al: Effects of surgical treatment for cervical spondylotic myelopathy in patients greater than or equal to 70 years of age: A retrospective comparative study. J Spinal Disord Techniques 15:458–460, 2002.
17. Wada E, Suzuki S, Kanazwa A, et al: Subtotal corpectomy versus laminoplasty for multilevel cervical spondylotic myelopathy a long term follow-up study over 10 years. Spine 26:1443–1448, 2001.
18. White AA, Panjabi MM: Biomechanical considerations in the surgical management of cervical spondylotic myelopathy. Spine 13:856–860, 1988.
19. Yoshida M, Tamaki T, Kawakami M, et al: Indication and clinical results of laminoplasty for cervical myelopathy caused by disc herniation with developmental canal stenosis. Spine 23:2391–2997, 1998.
20. Tani T, Ushida T, Ishida K, et al: Relative safety of anterior microsurgical decompression versus laminoplasty for cervical myelopathy with a massive ossified posterior longitudinal ligament. Spine 27:2491–2498, 2002.
21. Chung SS, Lee CS, Chung KH: Factors affecting the surgical results of expansive laminoplasty for cervical spondylotic myelopathy. Int Orthop 26:334–338, 2002.
22. Fujimura Y, Nishi Y, Chiba K, et al: Multiple regression analysis of the factors influencing the results of expansive open-door laminoplasty for cervical myelopathy due to ossification of the posterior longitudinal ligament. Arch Orthop Trauma Surg 117:471–474, 1998.
23. Handa Y, Kubota T, Ishii H, et al: Evaluation of prognostic factors and clinical outcome in elderly patients in whom expansive laminoplasty is performed for cervical myelopathy due to multisegmental spondylotic canal stenosis: A retrospective comparison with younger patients. J Neurosurg (Spine 2) 96:173–179, 2002.
24. Lee TT, Manzano GR, Green BA: Modified open door cervical expansive laminoplasty for spondylotic myelopathy: Operative technique, outcome, and predictors for gait improvement. J Neurosurg 86:64–68, 1997.
25. Mochida J, Nomura T, Chiba M, et al: Modified expansive open-door laminoplasty in cervical myelopathy. J Spinal Disord 12:386–391, 1999.
26. Suda K, Abumi K, Ito M, et al: Local kyphosis reduced surgical outcomes of expansive open-door laminoplasty for cervical spondylotic myelopathy. Spine 28:1258–1268, 2003.
27. Yamazaki T, Yanaka K, Sato H, et al: Cervical spondylotic myelopathy: Surgical results and factors affecting outcome with special reference to age differences. Neurosurgery 52:122–126, 2003.
28. Kimura S, Homma T, Uchiyama S, et al: Posterior migration of cervical spinal cord between split lamina as a complication of laminoplasty. Spine 20:1284–1288, 1995.
29. Kawaguchi Y, Kanamori M, Ishihara H, et al: Progression of ossification of the posterior longitudinal ligament following en bloc cervical laminoplasty. J Bone Joint Surg Am 83:1798–1802, 2001.
30. Yamazaki A, Homma T, Uchiyama S, et al: Morphologic limitations of posterior decompression by midsagittal splitting method for myelopathy caused by ossification of the posterior longitudinal ligament in the cervical spine. Spine 24:32–34, 1999.
31. Hoshi K, Kurokawa T, Nakamura K, et al: Expansive cervical laminoplasties—Observations on comparative changes n spinous process lengths following longitudinal lamina divisions using autogenous bone or hydroxyapatite spacers. Spinal Cord 34:725–728, 1996.
32. Sasai K, Saito T, Akagi S, et al: Preventing C5 palsy after laminoplasty. Spine 28:1972–1977, 2003.
33. Uematsu Y, Tokuhashi Y, Matsuzake H: Radiculopathy after laminoplasty of the cervical spine. Spine 23:2057–2062, 1998.
34. Chiba K, Toyama Y, Matsumoto M, et al: Segmental motor paralysis after expansive open-door laminoplasty. Spine 27:2108–2115, 2002.
35. Kawaguchi Y, Kanamori M, Ishihara H, et al: Minimum 10-year follow-up after en bloc cervical laminoplasty. Clin Orthop Rel Res 411:129–139, 2003.
36. Kawakami M, Tamaki T, Ando M, et al: Preoperative instability does not influence the clinical outcome in patients with cervical spondylotic myelopathy treated with expansive laminoplasty. J Spinal Disord Techniques 15:277–283, 2002.
37. Iizuka H, Shimizu T, Tateno K, et al: Extensor musculature of the cervical spine after laminoplasty. Spine 26:2220–2226, 2001.
38. Sasai K, Saito T, Adagi S, et al: Cervical Curvature after laminoplasty for spondylotic myelopathy—Involvement of yellow ligament, semispinalis cervicis muscle, and nuchal ligament. J Spinal Disord 13:26–30, 2000.
39. Yoshida M, Tamaki T, Kawakami M, et al: Does reconstruction of posterior ligamentous complex with extensor musculature decrease axial symptoms after cervical laminoplasty? Spine 27:1414–1418, 2002.
40. Iwasaki M, Kawaguchi Y, Kimura T, Yonenobu K: Long-term results of expansive laminoplasty for ossification of the posterior longitudinal ligament of the cervical spine: More than 10 years follow-up. J Neurosurg (Spine 2) 96:180–189, 2002.
41. Kawaguchi Y, Matsui H, Ishihara H, et al: Axial symptoms after en bloc cervical laminoplasty. J Spinal Dis 12:392–395, 1995.
42. Fujimura Y, Nishi Y: Atrophy of the nuchal muscle and change in cervical curvature after expansive open-door laminoplasty. Arch Orthop Trauma Surg 115:203–205, 1996.
43. Nakama S, Nitanai K, Oohashi Y, et al: Cervical muscle strength after laminoplasty. J Orthop Sci 8:36–40, 2003.
44. Kamizono J, Matsunaga S, Hayashi K, et al: Occupational recovery after open-door type laminoplasty for patients with ossification of the posterior longitudinal ligament. Spine 28:1889–1892, 2003.
45. Baba H, Maezawa Y, Furusawa N, et al: Flexibility and alignment of the cervical spine after laminoplasty for spondylotic myelopathy. Int Orthop 19:116–121, 1995.

46. Seichi A, Takeshita K, Ohishi I, et al: Long-term results of double-door laminoplasty for cervical stenotic myelopathy. Spine 26:479–487, 2001.

47. Iseda T, Goya T, Nakano S, et al: Serial changes in signal intensities of the adjacent discs on T2-weighted sagittal images after surgical treatment of cervical spondylosis: Anterior interbody fusion versus expansive laminoplasty. Acta Neruochir (Wien) 143:710, 2001.

48. Nakano N, Nalano T: Clinical results following enlargement of the cervical spinal canal by means of laminoplasty. Jpn Orthop Assoc 62:1139–1147, 1988.

49. Tani S, Isoshima A, Nagashima Y, et al: Laminoplasty with preservation of posterior cervical elements: Surgical technique. Neurosurgery 50:97–102, 2002.

50. Morimoto T, Uranishi R, Nakase H, et al: Extensive cervical laminoplasty for patients with long segment OPLL in the cervical spine: An alternative to the anterior approach. J Clin Neurosci 3:217–222, 2000.

51. Nakano N, Nakano T: Clinical results following enlargement of the cervical spinal canal by means of laminoplasty. Jpn Orthop Assoc 62:1139–1147, 1988.

52. Kawakami M, Tamaki T, Ando M, et al: Relationships between sagittal alignment of the cervical spine and morphology of the spinal cord and clinical outcomes in patients with cervical spondylotic myelopathy treated with expansive laminoplasty. J Spinal Disord Techniques 15:391–397, 2002.

53. Koshu K, Tominaga T, Yoshimoto T: Spinous process splitting laminoplasty with an extended foraminotomy for cervical myelopathy. Neurosurgery 37:430–435, 1995.

54. Tsuji H: Laminoplasty for patients with compressive myelopathy due to so-called spinal canal stenosis in the cervical and thoracic regions. Spine 7:28–34, 1982.

55. Frank E, Keenan T: A technique for cervical laminoplasty using mini plates. Br J Neurosurg 8:197–199, 1994.

56. O'Brien MF, Peterson D, Casey AT, Crockard HA: A novel technique for laminoplasty augmentation of spinal canal area using titanium miniplate stabilization. Spine 21:474–484, 1996.

57. Shaffrey CI, Wiggins GC, Piccirille CB, et al: Modified open-door laminoplasty for treatment of neurological deficits in younger patients with congenital spinal stenosis: Analysis of clinical and radiographic data. J Neurosurg (Spine 2) 90:170–177, 1999.

58. Fornari M, Luccarelli G, Giombini S, Chiapparini L: Artificial lamina-assisted laminoplasty performed in seven cases. J Neurosurg (Spine 1) 91:43–49, 1999.

59. Wang JM, Roh KJ, Kim DJ, Kim DW: A new method of stabilizing the elevated lamina in open-door laminoplasty using an anchor system. J Bone Joint Surg Br 80:1005–1008, 1998.

60. Takayasu M, Takagi T, Nishizawa T, et al: Bilateral open-door cervical expansive laminoplasty with hydroxyapatite spacers and titanium screws. J Neurosurg (Spine 1) 96:22–28, 2002.

61. Hamburger C: T-laminoplasty—A surgical approach for cervical spondylotic myelopathy: Technical note. Acta Neurochir (Wien) 132:131–135, 1995.

62. Tomita K, Kawahara N, Toribatake Y, et al: Expansive midline T-saw laminoplasty (modified spinous process-splitting) for the management of cervical myelopathy. Spine 23:32–37, 1998.

63. Hara M, Takayasu M, Takagi T, Yoshida J: En Bloc Laminoplasty Performed with a Threadwire Saw: Technical Note. Neurosurgery 48, 2001.

64. Edwards CC, Heller JG, Wilcox DH: T-saw laminoplasty for the management of cervical spondylotic myelopathy. Spine 25:1788–1794, 2000.

136 Surgical Techniques for Stabilization of the Subaxial Cervical Spine (C3–C7)

JONATHAN J. BASKIN, PAUL D. SAWIN, ROGER HARTL, CURTIS A. DICKMAN, and VOLKER K. H. SONNTAG

Many pathologic processes that affect the biomechanical integrity of the subaxial cervical spine (i.e., the cervical spine from C3–C7) ultimately require management with rigid internal fixation of the vertebral column. Over the past few decades, innovations in spinal instrumentation that confer immediate segmental stability along the vertebral column have been developed for posterior and anterior procedures.

The definition of spinal instability is not without controversy. Similarly, the best means of achieving open fixation of the unstable cervical spine is subject to debate. The approach to a patient's pathology must be individualized; consequently, the information presented here should be considered only one facet of a thoughtful approach to managing patients with spinal pathology. An operative approach must consider several basic issues: Is spinal instability present? If so, is nonoperative management reasonable? Does neural compression need to be addressed as a primary concern? Given instability, what is the best means of achieving reconstruction and stabilization from the perspectives of biomechanics, patient morbidity, and cost? This chapter provides a technical overview of some of the more popular methods for stabilizing the subaxial cervical spine from posterior and anterior approaches. Spinal instability substantial enough to warrant internal fixation is presumed, as is a complete evaluation that excludes from surgery patients with inappropriately high comorbidities.

ANATOMIC AND BIOMECHANICAL CONSIDERATIONS

White and Panjabi[1] define spinal stability as the ability of the vertebral column to tolerate physiologic loads with "no initial or additional neurological deficit, no major deformity, and no incapacitating pain." The osseous and ligamentous interrelationships of the vertebral column are complex and not fully explained by a single conceptual model.[2] Rotation and translation can occur simultaneously about three-dimensional axes that are determined by the articular and ligamentous interfaces.[2-5] Ligaments serve as elastic tension bands that facilitate normal motion but limit excessive movement of the vertebrae.[2,4,6] Discs provide shock-absorbing capabilities and rotational and translational interfaces; they also decrease the energy transmitted directly to the bones.[2] The vertebrae provide structural support and scaffolding, protect the neural elements, and interface to limit some and

facilitate other movements.[2] The neural and muscular systems coordinate the integrated movements of the spine. Injury to any of the components of the vertebral column can cause instability. Not all unstable injuries, however, require surgical repair.

Several methods have been developed to identify and quantify cervical instability. White and colleagues[7] proposed a point system predicated on the radiographic appearance of the fracture and the presence or absence of a neurologic deficit (Table 136-1). Denis's[8] three-column classification scheme, initially developed to evaluate acute thoracolumbar fractures, is also often extrapolated to assess cervical spine injuries (Table 136-2). Although these grading strategies are useful for gauging the presence and degree of structural compromise, they should be recognized as merely guidelines that must be used in the context of each patient's specific injury. Neither strategy has been subjected to stringent evaluation in randomized outcome studies comparing surgical and nonsurgical treatments. In practice, the presence of instability can be inferred from static radiographs (e.g., plain film, computed tomography [CT], magnetic resonance imaging [MRI], or myelography). In patients with cervical pain but who have no evidence of myelopathy or radiculopathy, instability can be confirmed safely by dynamic studies (flexion-extension views on plain radiography, MRI, or fluoroscopy).

TABLE 136-1 ■ Criteria for Instability in Subaxial Cervical Spine Injuries

Criterion	Point Value*
Anterior elements nonfunctional	2
Posterior elements nonfunctional	2
Sagittal plane translation > 3.5 mm	2
Sagittal plane angulation > 11 degrees	2
Positive stretch test	2
Spinal cord injury	2
Nerve root injury	1
Abnormal disc-space narrowing	1
Dangerous loading anticipated	1

*Clinical instability if point value > 5.
From White AA, Johnson RM, Panjabi MM, et al: Biomechanical analysis of clinical stability in the cervical spine. Clin Orthop 109:85–96,1975.

TABLE 136-2 ▪ Denis's Three-Column Classification Scheme for Acute Spinal Injuries*

Column	Anatomic Constituents
Anterior	Anterior longitudinal ligament Anterior annulus fibrosus Anterior vertebral body
Middle	Posterior longitudinal ligament Posterior annulus fibrosus Posterior vertebral body
Posterior	Posterior neural arch Articular facets Supraspinous/intraspinal ligaments

*Clinical instability with injury to two or more columns.
From Denis F: The three column spine and its significance in the classification of acute thoracolumbar spinal injuries. Spine 8: 817–831,1983.

In contrast to thoracolumbar fixation devices that can be applied in various modes (distraction, compression, neutral, flexion, extension, or lateral bending), cervical implants are typically applied in a neutral mode. The reductive forces that can be applied by cervical devices are small and usually insufficient to achieve spinal reduction. As a rule, these implants are used to maintain alignment after reduction has been achieved using axial traction. Once surgical stabilization is deemed appropriate for a given patient, the orientation of approach (anterior or posterior) and method of fixation must be decided. The most biomechanically sound construct attempts to match the implant with the site and type of instability. Bone and instrumentation deform and reform as stress is applied.[9] Over time, even the most rigid constructs permit some segmental motion across the sites of fixation. Ultimately, repetitive loading causes the implant to fail unless osseous fusion ensues. Internal fixation does not supplant careful surgical technique directed toward achieving bone fusion.

Posterior cervical constructs provide stability through several load-bearing mechanisms. Mechanically, all of them function to restore the posterior tension band and resist flexion forces. Certain techniques, such as simple interspinous wiring, provide almost no stability in extension, lateral bending, or axial rotation.[10] Conversely, osteosynthetic articular mass plates are the most rigid posterior cervical devices available. In addition to functioning as tension bands, they provide three-point bending and nonfixed moment arm, cantilever beam fixation. These more complex mechanisms of load bearing confer stability in flexion, extension, lateral bending, axial rotation, and axial loading. Selecting an appropriate posterior fixation construct requires understanding these implant characteristics. If the degree of instability is mild, restoring the tension band may be all that is required. More substantial instability necessitates a more aggressive operative strategy.

POSTERIOR SUBAXIAL CERVICAL FUSION

The earliest cervical fusion procedures used autogenous bone grafts that were applied to the posterior elements in an onlay fashion. Because these constructs possessed little inherent stability, extended periods of traction, bed rest, and external orthoses were required to maintain proper alignment while awaiting an osseous union to develop. In 1891, Hadra[11] ushered in the era of internal spinal fixation by using wire to secure adjacent cervical vertebrae that were rendered unstable by trauma or Pott's disease. This technique represented a significant conceptual leap, in that it heralded the use of nonbiologic materials to restore spinal stability. Subsequently, numerous posterior fusion techniques incorporated wire as a means of fixating the spinous processes, laminae, and articular processes of the cervical spine. Given their historical success, many of these methods remain viable options for the treatment of cervical instability in modern neurosurgical practice.

More recently, instrumentation systems, such as osteosynthetic plates and screws and interlaminar clamps, have revolutionized the surgical armamentarium for stabilizing this region of the vertebral column. By imparting intrinsic strength and load-sharing properties to the construct, they facilitate the development and maturation of the fusion response while concomitantly protecting the neural elements from trauma and deformity. These implants minimize or even obviate the need for external orthotic immobilization during the postoperative period and enhance the patient's comfort, ensure compliance, and enable early mobilization and rehabilitation.

An overview of standard posterior subaxial cervical fusion techniques follows. Because the focus of this chapter is technical, the operative indications and rationale for selecting one mode of stabilization over another are addressed only cursorily. Often, different fixation methods offer acceptable alternatives to address a given instability problem. The selection of a stabilization technique should consider the following variables: the nature and extent of the patient's instability; the structural elements that remain available for incorporation within a fixation construct; the patient's general medical condition, underlying disease state, neurologic status, and bone quality; the requirement for postoperative bracing; the patient's comfort or compliance; and the cost of the implant.

Indications

The goals in performing internal fixation and fusion of the subaxial cervical spine can be summarized as follows: (1) to restore stability to the structurally compromised spine, (2) to maintain alignment after correction of a deformity, (3) to prevent progression of a deformity, and (4) to alleviate pain.[1] Instability of the subaxial cervical region can arise from trauma, degenerative disease, infection, inflammatory conditions, or neoplasia or iatrogenically as a consequence of a previous surgical intervention (Table 136-3). Regardless of cause, the surgeon must carefully gauge both the nature and the extent of instability when formulating a treatment plan.[12,13] The nature of instability is established by assessing the integrity of specific anatomic structures that normally confer stability on each cervical motion segment. The extent of instability is a product of the number of affected motion segments and the number of spinal columns involved for each segment. These criteria dictate whether operative stabilization is required and, if so, which techniques would suffice.

TABLE 136-3 ▪ Indications for Posterior Cervical Arthrodesis

Type of Traumatic Cervical Instability	Location
Fractures	Articular facet fractures
	Fractures of the laminae, pedicles
	Vertebral body fractures*
Ligamentous injury	Articular facet dislocation (unilateral, bilateral)
	Posterior ligamentous incompetence
	Anterior ligamentous incompetence*
Degenerative cervical instability	Spondylosis
	Articular facet arthropathy
	Intervertebral disc degeneration
Iatrogenic cervical instability	Postlaminectomy, reversal of lordosis
	Postlaminectomy, established kyphosis*
	Postfacetectomy
Inflammatory/infectious instability	Rheumatoid arthritis
	Ankylosing spondylitis
	Osteomyelitis
Neoplasia	Benign
	Malignant

*Consider anterior stabilization.
    From Sawin PD, Sonntag VKH: Techniques of posterior subaxial cervical fusion. Oper Tech Neurosurg 1(2):72–83, 1998.

Traumatic Instability

Although many patients with cervical spine injuries do not require surgery, instability resulting from trauma is the most frequent indication for posterior fixation of the subaxial cervical spine.[12–14] The initial management of traumatic vertebral column injury consists of spinal realignment (if required), neural decompression (when indicated), and stabilization. Conservative management is most appropriate when the injury is mainly osseous, neural compression is absent, and spinal alignment is acceptable. Primary ligamentous incompetence is often refractory to nonoperative measures.[15,16] Internal fixation is considered when conservative management is inappropriate or ineffectual. As noted, posterior techniques are most effective when used to address dorsal pathology, such as posterior ligamentous instability, facet dislocations, and posterior element fractures. Fractures of the posterior elements typically necessitate incorporation of at least one intact level above and below the injury to achieve a stable construct. Many of the posterior wiring techniques require intact posterior elements to be efficacious. Consequently, fractures of the spinous processes, laminae, or articular facets can preclude the use of some methods and favor others. These nuances are addressed as the individual fixation techniques are described.

Anterior ligamentous incompetence, vertebral body fractures, and intervertebral disc injuries are most appropriately addressed via an anterior approach, particularly in patients with compromise of the ventral spinal canal and incomplete neurologic deficits. In such cases, a ventral approach permits neural decompression and spinal stabilization, optimizing neurologic outcome.[17] If the ventral spinal canal is not compromised or neurologic deficits

are complete, a posterior stabilization construct may be acceptable.[14,18] Posterior stabilization, however, should be attempted only when the articular facets at the involved level are intact because these structures must bear substantial axial loads under these conditions. If a posterior approach is selected, multiple segments above and below the level of injury should be incorporated to minimize the risk of progressive kyphosis.[19–21] Posterior fixation can be used to supplement an anterior arthrodesis when instability is severe or when the anticipated load on a ventral construct alone is deemed excessive. The so-called 360-degree or circumferential fusion procedure is reserved for the management of severe three-column instability for which a single approach would not adequately restore stability.[22–25] If a circumferential fusion is required, we typically prefer to perform the ventral and the dorsal procedures in a single operative setting. Alternatively, each can be performed separately in a staged fashion.

Nontraumatic Instability

Neoplastic processes (primary or metastatic) involving the vertebral column can create instability as a consequence of the local destruction of load-bearing elements. Further iatrogenic destabilization may result from attempts at tumor resection. Malignant tumors, whether primary or metastatic, typically mandate multilevel fixation constructs that must incorporate disease-free segments rostral and caudal to the involved levels. A circumferential arthrodesis is often required to restore cervical stability in this setting.

Segmental instability resulting from degenerative disease can be addressed effectively with a variety of posterior techniques. For patients with cervical stenosis, internal fixation immediately after posterior neural decompression can reduce the incidence of postlaminectomy kyphosis and should be considered in selected cases, particularly when a normal cervical lordosis is absent. Posterior fixation is much less effective as a primary treatment of an established kyphosis; such deformities are best managed with ventral reconstruction.[26]

Occasionally, internal fixation is undertaken to safeguard against anticipated instability that could arise as a consequence of future disease progression (as with spinal neoplasia, infections, inflammatory disease, or degenerative disease) or from potentially destabilizing iatrogenic maneuvers (e.g., decompressive laminectomy). The surgeon must be cognizant of the increased demands placed on the construct by the disease process and the duration of that requirement. In certain settings, the implant must bear 100% of the load for the remainder of the patient's life. Ultimately, these individual considerations influence the selection of an appropriate construct.

Operative Technique

Anesthesia and Spinal Cord Monitoring

In patients with cervical instability, laryngoscopy and endotracheal intubation must be approached cautiously. Awake fiberoptic laryngoscopy may be performed with little or no neck manipulation and affords maximal protection from iatrogenic spinal cord injury while the airway is secured. The awake patient can then be positioned and neurologic function assessed before anesthesia is induced.

This technique should be considered in all patients with known or suspected cervical instability who are able to cooperate.[21,27] Alternatively, direct laryngoscopy under intravenous anesthesia can be undertaken cautiously, provided that the head and neck are adequately stabilized in neutral posture throughout the intubation sequence.

Pharmacologic paralysis with neuromuscular blocking agents should be avoided in patients with cervical instability. The cervical musculature maintains some resting tone even during general anesthesia and continues to function as a physiologic splint that contributes to the overall maintenance of alignment. Neuromuscular blockade can exacerbate instability by abolishing this inherent stabilizing influence.

Intraoperatively, spinal cord function can be assessed by somatosensory or motor (or both) evoked potential responses. Continuous spinal cord monitoring is particularly effective as a surgical adjunct in patients with some neurologic function, in whom an alteration in wave morphology would direct reassessment of the patient's position or the location of the implant. Although often employed, the use of these monitoring tools for cervical pathology other than intrinsic spinal cord tumors or vascular malformations remains controversial.

Positioning

Patients with cervical instability must be positioned carefully to avoid inadvertent neurologic injury. The surgeon should supervise all aspects of rotation to the prone position and, with few exceptions, be responsible for maintaining neutral cervical alignment throughout the positioning process. Although the sitting position is used occasionally, most posterior stabilization procedures are performed with the patient prone. Ideally the neck is maintained either in neutral posture or in slight extension.[13,19,20] If axial cervical traction was employed preoperatively, it is typically continued during the operative procedure.[10,13,14,21,28,29] The awake patient may be positioned before general anesthesia is induced. Neurologic function can then be assessed after the patient is turned. Any change in neurologic status mandates urgent radiographic studies to reappraise cervical alignment.

Once adequate exposure has been achieved, the offending pathology is addressed. Spinal deformity that resisted reduction with preoperative axial traction should be corrected with cautious intraoperative manipulation or partial facetectomy or both. If neural compression persists despite adequate reduction, a decompressive procedure is performed. Resection of key load-bearing elements can exacerbate segmental instability, and the surgeon must be prepared to alter the stabilization strategy accordingly.

Wire and Cable Techniques

During the past 50 years, many wire and cable techniques for posterior subaxial fixation have been described. Although each technique has its own nuances, all can be subclassified into three general categories: (1) spinous process wiring, (2) facet wiring, and (3) sublaminar wiring techniques. Although still a viable option in the atlantoaxial region and frequently used to stabilize the occipitocervical junction, sublaminar wiring has largely been abandoned as a means of securing the subaxial motion segments because

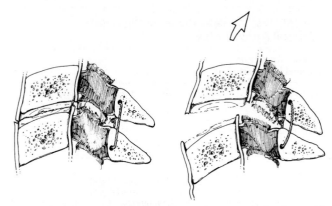

FIGURE 136-1   Three-column injury of the cervical spine stabilized only with posterior cervical wiring. The reconstituted posterior tension band functions to resist flexion deformity, but pathologic hyperextension remains possible. (With permission from Barrow Neurological Institute.)

of the substantial risk for neurologic injury.[14,30,31] Other standard methods (spinous process wiring) provide biomechanical stability that is equivalent or superior to that achieved with sublaminar wiring. Consequently, these risks are rarely justified.[31]

In general, posterior wiring techniques are simple to perform, require no special equipment, and employ inexpensive materials. These methods effectively reconstitute the posterior tension band and consequently resist flexion forces (Fig. 136-1).[10] In most cases, wiring with bone grafting alone does not provide substantial immediate internal stability and must be supplemented with temporary external bracing or, less commonly, with methylmethacrylate.

Wire constructs can be created with monofilament wire, twisted wire, Drummond buttons (Fig. 136-2), or braided cables. Most surgeons prefer to use a larger-gauge wire (16-, 18-, or 20-gauge) for additional strength, although thicker wire is less flexible and more difficult to manipulate. A compromise between strength and malleability is achieved by employing twisted (braided) wires. Two strands of 22-gauge wire braided together are easier to handle and stronger than a single strand of 18-gauge wire.[32] Care must be taken, however, to avoid sawing through bone as the braided wire is passed. Wires should be twisted uniformly and not kinked or bent in an acute angle; bends, notches, and excessive twisting weaken wire and may cause it to break.

Braided multistrand cables have supplanted traditional single-strand or twisted wires for most applications.[33,34] Although more expensive than wire, these devices have the advantages of higher tensile strength, relatively uniform distribution of applied tension, and ease of handling. Braided cables are available in both stainless steel and titanium alloy, and the latter produces less artifact on MRI and CT. Titanium is notch sensitive, however, and more susceptible to fatigue than steel.

Braided cables are tightened using an instrument with a specific, predetermined tension and are fixated with a crimp (Fig. 136-3). The cable's flexibility reduces kinking, makes removing slack easy, and prevents overtightening. Generally, 8 to 12 inch-lb of torque is recommended for normal adult bone.[33] Less torque should be used for osteoporotic or thin bone to prevent the cables from pulling through the bone.

Spinous Process Wiring Techniques

ROGERS WIRING

Interspinous wiring was initially described by Rogers[35,36] in 1942 for the treatment of traumatic cervical instability. Although multiple modifications have been reported, the fundamental technique remains unaltered. In its most basic form, this method is designed to stabilize a single motion segment (two adjacent vertebral levels). Additional segments are incorporated by repeating the maneuver at contiguous levels.

The spinous processes and laminae at the levels to be stabilized are exposed through a standard midline approach. With a right-angle dental drill, a single hole is drilled through the base of the spinous process just dorsal to the spinolaminar junction at each level. A single cerclage wire or cable is looped in opposite directions through the hole in each spinous process, with the superior loop passing above and the inferior loop passing below their respective processes (Fig. 136-4A–C). The free ends of the cable are then pulled to the desired tension (Fig. 136-4D). Provisions are made for bone fusion by thoroughly decorticating the spinous processes and laminae at the instrumented levels and by layering autogenous corticocancellous bone over the site. Graft material can also be insinuated between the cable's parasagittal limbs (as Rogers initially recommended) or within the facet joint space.

In Rogers' original series,[36] all 11 patients achieved solid arthrodesis. This method is technically simple, fast, inexpensive, and biomechanically sound for the treatment of many posterior cervical injuries, provided that the instability is not too complex or severe. A prerequisite for successful Rogers wiring is the presence of intact posterior elements at the levels to be incorporated into the construct. If the posterior elements are pristine, wiring across a single motion segment often suffices. A fracture of a posterior element necessitates incorporation of an additional level above or below the motion segment to be stabilized. Care must be taken to avoid overtightening the wires, which can

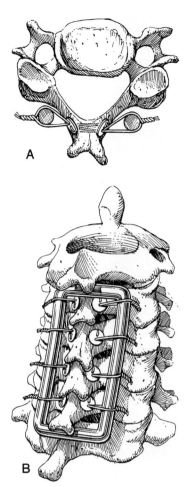

FIGURE 136-2 *A*, Drummond wires are passed through a hole in the base of the spinous process. The wires are threaded through buttons, which are positioned against the spinous process to reinforce the fixation. *B*, Drummond buttons can be used to attach a Luque rectangle for cervical or occipitocervical fixation. (With permission from Barrow Neurological Institute.)

FIGURE 136-3 Songer cable fixation with a tensioner/crimping device. The detachable torque wrench tightens the cable, and the Songer cable is then crimped in final position (*inset*). The excess wire length is then cut. (With permission from Barrow Neurological Institute.)

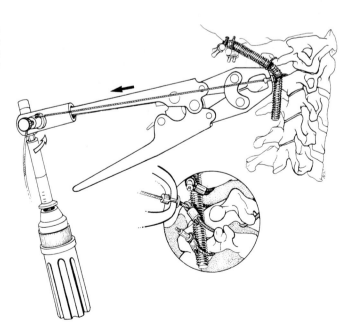

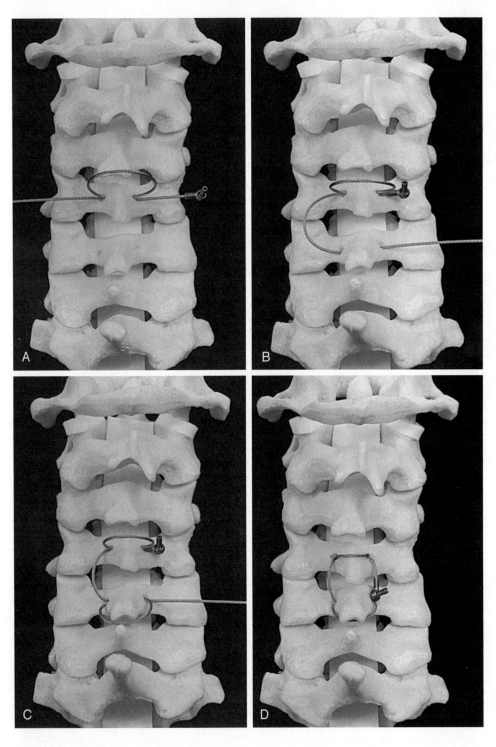

FIGURE 136-4 In the Rogers interspinous wiring technique, a single cable (*A*) is looped through a hole in the base of the superior spinous process, with the loop passing above its respective process. *B*, The free end of the cable is passed through the inferior spinous process. *C*, The inferior loop encircles the inferior spinous process. *D*, The cable is then tightened as desired. (From Sawin PD, Sonntag VKH: Techniques of posterior subaxial cervical fusion. Oper Tech Neurosurg 1[2]:72–83, 1998.)

produce cervical hyperextension with resultant stenosis of the spinal canal or neural foramina.

WHITEHILL MODIFICATION

Whitehill and associates[37] described a variation of the Rogers technique. The fundamental method entails fixation of a single motion segment. A single cerclage wire or cable is passed through a hole in the base of the upper vertebra's spinous process and looped around the inferior edge of the spinous process at the adjacent caudal level, creating a simple interspinous loop (Fig. 136-5A). If additional levels are to

be incorporated into the construct, the wire loops are placed in overlapping fashion (Fig. 136-5B). Decortication and placement of autograft material are performed as previously described to promote fusion. In Whitehill's series, all 22 patients achieved solid arthrodeses.

BENZEL-KESTERSON MODIFICATION

Benzel and Kesterson[38] described another modification of Rogers' basic interspinous wiring technique. This method is also suitable for stabilizing a single motion segment and may be repeated to provide multilevel fixation. A double-stranded

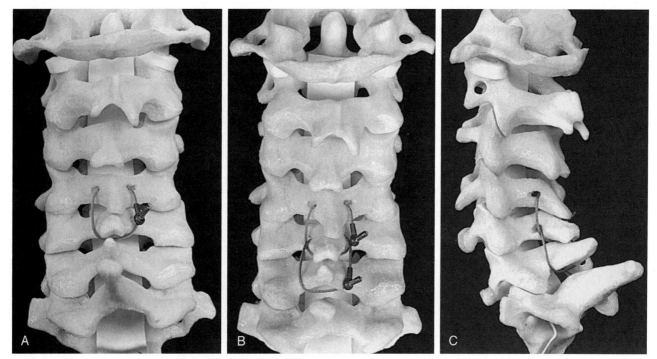

FIGURE 136-5 In the Whitehill interspinous wiring modification, a single cable (*A*) is passed through a hole in the base of the superior spinous process and looped around the inferior margin of the spinous process at the next caudal level. Additional levels can be incorporated in similar fashion, overlapping the wires as shown in posteroanterior (*B*) and lateral (*C*) projections. (From Sawin PD, Sonntag VKH: Techniques of posterior subaxial cervical fusion. Oper Tech Neurosurg 1[2]:72–83, 1998.)

(braided), 22-gauge cerclage wire is passed through a hole in the base of the rostral spinous process and looped around the inferior aspect of the caudad spinous process (Fig. 136-6A) in a manner similar to the Whitehill wiring method. Before the braided wire is tightened, a single strand of 22-gauge wire (the so-called compression wire) is passed through the interspinous space beneath the cerclage wire (Fig. 136-6B). The braided interspinous wire is then tightened but not crimped. A tricortical iliac crest bone graft is split longitudinally, yielding two matched corticocancellous halves. The spinous processes and laminae are decorticated, and the grafts are fashioned to press-fit against the spinous processes (cortical sides out). The compression wire is passed around the outside of both grafts and seated in ventrally placed notches. As the compression wire is tightened, the grafts are secured against the spinous processes and laminae, and the cerclage wire is tightened further and crimped in final position (Fig. 136-6C).

Theoretically, this technique has several advantages. The bone grafts are incorporated as an integral part of the construct, acting as buttresses to provide a measure of torsional stiffness. The second wire compression loads the grafts, enhancing the probability of attaining a successful bone fusion. Furthermore, the interspinous distance is maintained by the grafts as the compression wire is tightened, minimizing the risk for cervical hyperextension.[32] In practice, this method is associated with a high rate of successful fusion (98% in Benzel and Kesterson's series of 50 patients) and long-term stability in individuals with unstable cervical injuries.[38]

BOHLMAN TRIPLE-WIRE TECHNIQUE

The Bohlman[39] triple-wire technique is another common modification of the Rogers interspinous wiring.[40,41]

This method can be used to stabilize a single motion segment (Fig. 136-7), but it is also effective for treating multilevel instability (Fig. 136-8). Holes are created in the spinous processes as previously described. The first (tethering) wire incorporates the two adjacent spinous processes in the manner of Rogers (see Fig. 136-7A). Single wires are then passed separately through the holes in each of the two spinous processes so that the horizontally oriented wires parallel one another (see Fig. 136-7B). Autogenous bone is harvested and split longitudinally into two corticocancellous grafts. The horizontal wires are passed through holes placed midposition in the grafts and tightened. The grafts are thereby secured against the decorticated spinous processes and laminae on each side (see Fig. 136-7C, D).

Similar to the Benzel-Kesterson modification, the Bohlman triple-wire technique integrates the bone graft into the construct, using the corticocancellous struts as buttresses to augment torsional stability and to inhibit flexion and extension. The grafts are placed under compression, optimizing conditions for bony incorporation. The soundness of this construct has been verified by biomechanical testing.[40] Its clinical utility has been confirmed in several studies, most notably in the series of Weiland and McAfee,[41] in which all patients with traumatic cervical instability achieved successful arthrodeses with this technique.

MURPHY-SOUTHWICK MODIFICATION

Murphy and Southwick[42] modified Rogers' interspinous wiring technique to facilitate incorporation of two adjacent motion segments (three vertebral levels) into a single fusion construct. Drill holes are created in the three spinous processes to be incorporated as previously described. The first wire is passed between the upper and middle vertebrae,

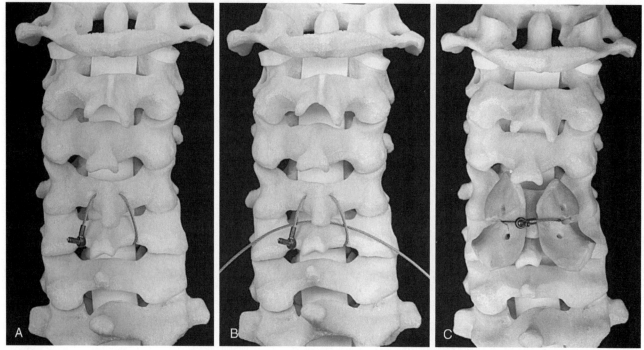

FIGURE 136-6   In the Benzel-Kesterson interspinous wiring modification, a simple interspinous cerclage cable (*A*) is passed in the manner of Whitehill. *B*, A "compression" cable is passed through the interspinous space beneath the cerclage cable, and the interspinous cable is tightened. *C*, The compression cable secures the bone graft against the decorticated spinous processes and laminae and is tightened, augmenting the tension of the interspinous cerclage cable. (From Sawin PD, Sonntag VKH: Techniques of posterior subaxial cervical fusion. Oper Tech Neurosurg 1[2]:72–83, 1998.)

creating a simple interspinous loop (Fig. 136-9A). A second wire secures the middle and lower vertebrae in a similar fashion (Fig. 136-9B). A third wire is passed between the upper and lower vertebrae and tightened (Fig. 136-9C). The laminae are decorticated, and corticocancellous bone grafts are applied in onlay fashion. This technique is effective when two contiguous motion segments require stabilization.

Oblique Facet Wiring

In 1983, Cahill and associates[43] described a technique of oblique facet-to-spinous process wiring for the treatment of segmental cervical instability after trauma. This method was advocated primarily for fixation of subaxial flexion-compression injuries or facet fracture-dislocations because the rotational stability afforded by traditional interspinous wiring techniques may be inadequate to maintain reduction after surgical fixation. This technique is equally useful for stabilization of posterior element fractures that involve the rostral lamina or spinous process of an unstable motion segment, without the need to incorporate an additional vertebral level into the construct.

After routine exposure of the dorsal cervical spine at the level of injury, the inferior articular processes of the rostral vertebra are isolated and the investing facet capsules removed. The facet joint spaces are opened with a small elevator, and articular cartilage is removed with a drill or fine curet. Drill holes are created through the midportion of the inferior articular processes, perforating the bone at right angles to the articular surfaces (Fig. 136-10A). A Penfield dissector protects the

underlying superior articular process, nerve root, and vertebral artery during drilling. A wire or cable is passed through the hole in the articular process and looped beneath an intact spinous process one or two levels below and tightened (Fig. 136-10B). The maneuver is then repeated on the contralateral side (Fig. 136-10C, D). The laminae and spinous process are decorticated, and corticocancellous bone grafts are placed in onlay fashion. The facet joint spaces may be packed with additional graft substrate to stimulate fusion further.

In their series of 18 patients with bilateral facet-to-spinous process wiring, Cahill and associates[43] reported a 100% fusion rate and stable alignment after 3 to 4 months. No additional neurologic morbidity was incurred by the procedure. The investigators recognized the importance of bilateral fixation even in the context of unilateral facet injury: a unilateral facet-to-spinous process wiring construct is not biomechanically sound, and redislocation can occur as a result of persistent rotatory instability.

Facet Wiring

Occasionally the cervical spinous processes and laminae are unavailable as fixation points because of extensive fracture or previous surgical removal. When subaxial instability is present under these conditions, the articular processes can be used as alternative sites for multilevel segmental fixation. In the 1970s, Callahan and colleagues[44] described a method of facet wiring that was initially intended for use after laminectomy to mitigate postlaminectomy kyphosis. Although effective for this indication, facet wiring also can be used when injury to the posterior elements spans multiple

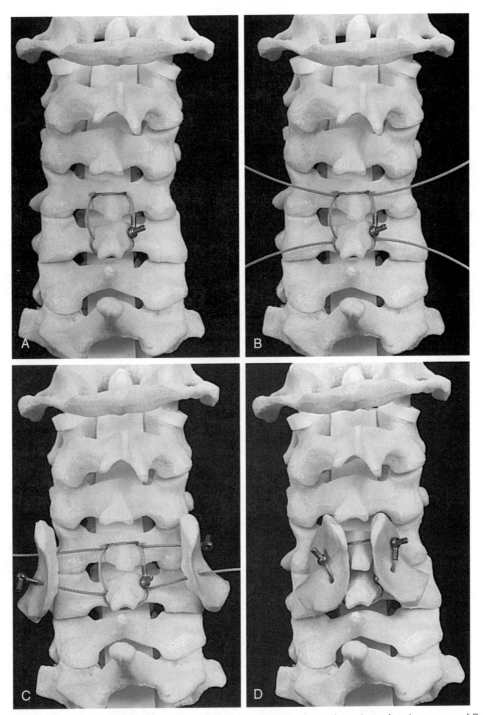

FIGURE 136-7   In the Bohlman triple-wire technique, the first cable (*A*) creates an interspinous loop after the manner of Rogers. *B*, Two separate cables are passed through holes in the superior and inferior spinous processes, respectively. *C*, The ends of these cables are passed through holes in the two autologous bone grafts, and the cables are tightened (*D*), securing the grafts against the decorticated spinous processes and laminae. (From Sawin PD, Sonntag VKH: Techniques of posterior subaxial cervical fusion. Oper Tech Neurosurg 1[2]:72–83, 1998.)

levels, rendering the previously described wire-based fixation methods unfeasible. This technique provides reasonable stability in multiple planes, including axial rotation and translation.

Facet wiring requires dorsal exposure of all levels selected for fusion. The entire lateral mass should be exposed at each level and the facet capsular ligaments removed. The facet joint is opened with a small dissector, and the articular cartilage is removed. A hole is drilled in the inferior articular process at each level to be incorporated, oriented at right angles to the articular surfaces (Fig. 136-11A). A wire or cable is passed through each hole, rostral to caudal, exiting through the joint space (Fig. 136-11B), and the dorsal surfaces of the lateral masses are decorticated.

Two corticocancellous strut grafts of sufficient length to span the entire construct are harvested, either from rib or from the posterior iliac crest. Rib possesses a native curvature that conforms well to the cervical lordosis.

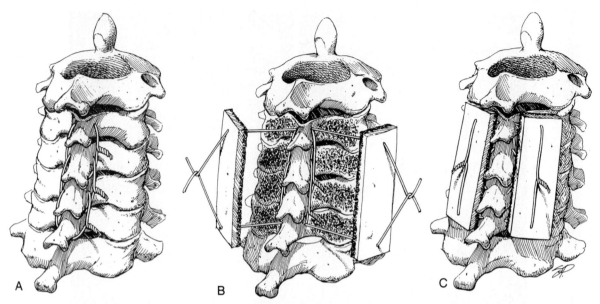

FIGURE 136-8   The Bohlman technique for fixating multiple levels of subaxial instability. *A*, Separate wires are used to create interlocking links at adjacent levels. *B*, Bone struts are wired to the spinous processes. *C*, The grafts are compressed against the bone surfaces, which adds mechanical stability to the spinous process wires. (With permission from Barrow Neurological Institute.)

Its circumferentially intact cortex adds strength, and it can be harvested in long segments for multilevel constructs.[45] The wires should always be passed medial to the graft to prevent displacement of the strut into the spinal canal. The struts are then advanced over the wires and segmentally transfixed against the lateral masses, or they are secured by wrapping the facet wires around (instead of through) the grafts. Additional bone graft can be packed into the facet joints or placed alongside the construct. Typically the facet fusion construct should extend at least one vertebral level above and below the rostral and caudal extent of the laminectomy. The caudal end of the graft can be secured to the first intact spinous process rather than through the articular mass to avoid the chronic pain occasionally associated with violating an unfused facet joint. In lieu of autogenous bone struts, small contoured metal rods or a Luque rectangle can

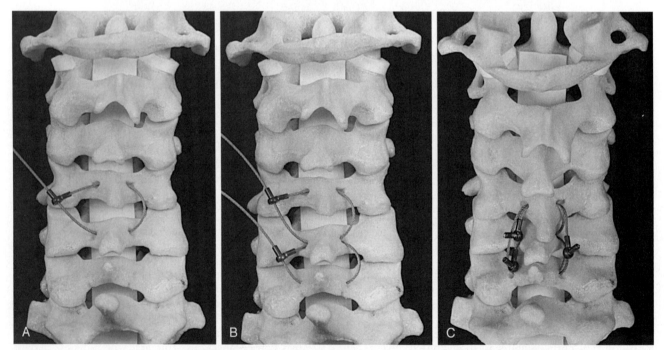

FIGURE 136-9   In the Murphy-Southwick interspinous wiring modification, the first cable (*A*) is passed through holes in the spinous processes of the superior and middle vertebrae, creating a simple interspinous loop. *B*, A second cable incorporates the middle and inferior spinous processes in a similar fashion. *C*, A third cable is passed between the superior and inferior vertebrae and tightened. (From Sawin PD, Sonntag VKH: Techniques of posterior subaxial cervical fusion. Oper Tech Neurosurg 1[2]:72–83, 1998.)

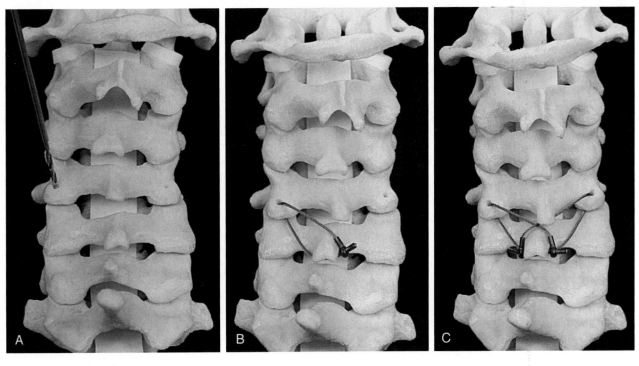

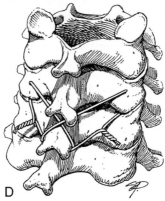

FIGURE 136-10   In the Cahill oblique facet wiring technique, holes (*A*) are drilled through the midportion of the inferior articular facets of the most rostral level to be incorporated, along a trajectory perpendicular to the articular surfaces. *B*, A cable is passed through the hole in the facet and looped beneath an intact spinous process at the level below. *C*, A second cable completes the construct by repeating the facet-to-spinous process wiring maneuver on the contralateral side. *D*, Illustration of a completed construct before placement of onlay grafts. (*A*, *B*, and *C* from Sawin PD, Sonntag VKH: Techniques of posterior subaxial cervical fusion. Oper Tech Neurosurg 1[2]:72–83, 1998. *D*, with permission from Barrow Neurological Institute.)

FIGURE 136-11   In the Callahan facet wiring technique, holes (*A*) are drilled through the inferior articular masses at the levels to be incorporated, at right angles to the articular surfaces. A separate cable is passed through each articular mass in a rostral-to-caudal direction and exits through the joint space. *B*, The cables are passed around autogenous strut grafts and tightened, transfixing the grafts against the articular masses. Note the sparing of the caudal facet joint by securing the graft with a spinous process wire. (With permission from Barrow Neurological Institute.)

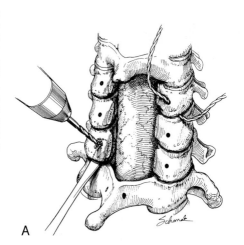

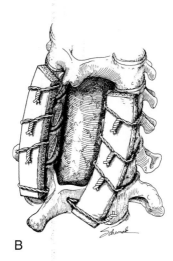

be incorporated into the construct and secured with the segmental facet wires.[46]

Interlaminar Clamps

Subaxial cervical stabilization using interlaminar clamps was first described in 1975.[47] These devices have been used effectively in the treatment of flexion injuries to reestablish the integrity of the posterior tension band. They perform optimally when used to stabilize a single motion segment. Implants are available in a variety of sizes and configurations to conform to the anatomy of individual patients. Initially manufactured of stainless steel, interlaminar clamps are now available in a titanium alloy. The clamp is preassembled with a screw and mounted on clamp applicator forceps.

Interlaminar clamps are relatively quick and easy to apply. After the posterior elements are exposed at the levels to be fused, the leading edge of the lamina above and the trailing edge of the lamina below are thinned bilaterally to augment the interlaminar spaces rostral and caudal to the unstable motion segment (Fig. 136-12A). The appropriate sized clamp is selected and separated into its two major components (fitted laminar hooks). The upper (threaded) half-clamp is hooked over the leading edge of the upper lamina, whereas the lower (unthreaded) half-clamp is hooked under the trailing edge of the lower lamina. A machine screw is placed through the unthreaded lower hook and engages the threads of the hook above. Tightening the screw apposes the two laminae by drawing the hooks together. At subaxial levels, an autologous H graft is used to prevent hyperextension. After the screws are tightened to their final tension, the distal threads of the screws can be stripped or a locking mechanism can be used to prevent screw loosening (Fig. 136-12B). The clamps

have a wide surface area that distributes forces over a broad bone surface. Theoretically the clamps are less likely to pull through osteoporotic bone. Further provisions are made for bone fusion by lightly decorticating the laminae and lateral masses and applying autogenous bone graft.[48,49]

Although good results have been reported for unilateral implants in selected patients,[50] most surgeons advocate bilateral placement of interlaminar clamps to optimize fixation and multiplanar stability.[49,51] Multilevel fixation with these devices should be avoided because the incidence of failure in this setting is excessive.[49,51] With these caveats in mind, interlaminar clamps have demonstrated efficacy in restoring long-term stability to the compromised subaxial cervical spine. The principal disadvantages of this method are the requirement for intact laminae at the level to be instrumented and the risk for increased neurologic deficit caused by metal stenosis from the sublaminar hooks.

Polymethylmethacrylate and Wire Fixation

The basic technique for posterior subaxial fixation with polymethylmethacrylate (PMMA) and wire was described by Branch and associates,[52] although many permutations exist. The posterior elements are exposed in standard fashion; at least one level above and one below the level of injury must be fully visualized. Care should be taken to avoid disruption of the facet capsular ligaments during the dissection. Holes are created in the bases of the spinous processes at all levels to be incorporated, as if preparing for an interspinous wiring. Interspinous wires or cables span the injured segments in a standard configuration and are tightened to achieve adequate reduction (Fig. 136-13A). Stainless-steel pins (Kirschner wires [K wires] are suitable for this

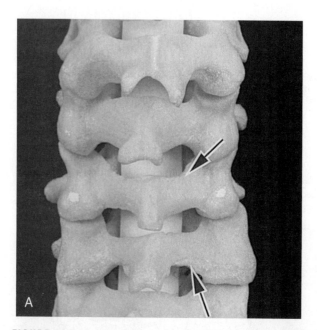

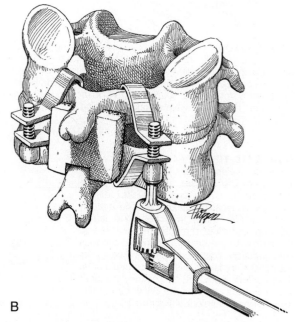

FIGURE 136-12 Interlaminar clamps. *A,* The leading edge of the lamina above and the trailing edge of the lamina below are thinned bilaterally (*arrows*) to increase the interlaminar spaces above and below the segment to be fused. *B,* A bone strut is interposed to add stability, prevent overreduction, and augment chances for fusion. A 90-degree-angled wrench is used to tighten the screws. (*A* from Sawin PD, Sonntag VKH: Techniques of posterior subaxial cervical fusion. Oper Tech Neurosurg 1(2):72–83, 1998. *B,* with permission from Barrow Neurological Institute.)

FIGURE 136-13 Polymethylmethacrylate and wire fixation. *A,* The unstable motion segments are incorporated with a standard interspinous wiring technique. Stainless steel pins are cut about 3 mm long, passed through holes in the spinous processes, and bent slightly to resist backing out. *B,* The entire construct is then encased with polymethy methacrylate. (From Sawin PD, Sonntag VKH: Techniques of posterior subaxial cervical fusion. Oper Tech Neurosurg 1[2]:72–83, 1998.)

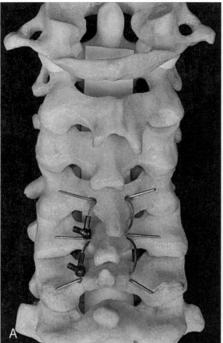
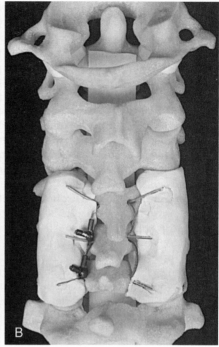

purpose), approximately 1.5 mm in diameter, are cut into 3-cm lengths, passed through the holes in the spinous processes, and bent slightly to prevent them from backing out. These pins provide multiple points of fixation to secure the PMMA to the individual vertebral elements, enhancing interdigitation interface bonding among bone, wire, and cement. The entire construct is then encased in PMMA (Fig. 136-13B).

Wire-reinforced PMMA is an inexpensive, technically simple, and rapid means of restoring the posterior tension band and of providing immediate internal stability in multiple motion planes. In a series of almost 100 patients with traumatic cervical spine injuries, Branch and associates[52] reported long-term stability (mean follow-up, 1.5 years) in 97% of patients treated in this manner. PMMA is not incorporated into the bone-healing process, and we do not use it routinely to bolster fixation constructs.[53,54] As an inert foreign body, it reduces the surface area of bone available for healing and poses an infectious risk. We reserve its use for patients who have life expectancies of less than 1 year (e.g., those with cancer) in whom temporary structural support is needed.

Articular Mass Plates

Posterior stabilization of the subaxial cervical spine has been revolutionized by the advent of articular mass osteosynthetic plates. These devices provide immediate internal stability, are appropriate for single- or multilevel fixation, and do not require intact posterior elements for application. In the United States, three articular mass plate systems are in widespread clinical use (Table 136-4): the AME Haid Universal Bone Plate System (American Medical Electronics, Inc., Richardson, TX, U.S.A.), the Axis Fixation System (Medtronic Sofamor Danek), and the Small Notched Reconstruction Plate (SNRP) System (Synthes Spine, Inc.). All systems are available in titanium alloy. The operative

techniques for placing articular mass plates are similar for all systems and consist of four fundamental steps: (1) sizing and contouring the plate, (2) drilling the articular masses, (3) selecting the appropriate screws, and (4) securing the plate.

SIZING AND CONTOURING PLATES

Plates of identical length are selected to span congruous segments on either side of the spine. When possible, they should be implanted bilaterally and symmetrically. All major plating systems offer plates of different dimensions, affording versatility of application. The shortest plate that allows screw purchase in each articular mass to be instrumented should be selected.[55] Approximating the posterior elements with a clamp or interspinous wiring often enables the application of a plate that initially appeared to be too short.[13] This maneuver can also confer a biomechanical advantage

TABLE 136-4 ■ Selected Features of the Haid, SNRP, and Axis Systems*

Feature	AME Haid	SNRP	Axis
Plate strength	+++	+	++
Plate malleability	+	+++	+++
Screw placement variability	+	++	+++
Screw-plate variety	+	+++	+++
Complexity	+	++	++

*Manufacturers: AME Haid, American Medical Electronics, Inc., Richardson, TX. SNRP, Synthes Spine, Inc., Paoli, PA. Axis, Sofamor-Danek, Inc., Memphis, TN.
  + = Low: ++ = intermediate; +++ = high.
  SNRP, small notched reconstruction plate.
  Modified from Sawin PD, Traynelis VC, Goel VK: Cervical construct design. In Benzel EC (eds): Spine Surgery, Techniques, Complication Avoidance, and Management. New York: Churchill Livingstone, 1998, pp 1129–1140.

because it preloads the construct.[55] Compression loading of the facet joint can also enhance the probability of successful fusion. The facet joints are decorticated with curets, and thin wedges of autologous bone are compressed in the joints to promote fusion.

Ideally, alignment of the instrumented cervical spine should approximate the normal lordotic posture. Articular mass plates are in situ fixators, however, and should not be relied on to alter cervical alignment. The Axis and SNRP plates are readily bent into lordosis; the Haid plate is more stout and does not bend easily. The contact surface of the latter device is contoured to maintain lordosis as the plate is secured. If lordosis cannot be achieved by preoperative traction or intraoperative manipulation, the cervical spine can be instrumented in neutral alignment. It is more appropriate to modify the plate to fit the patient rather than attempting to alter the patient's anatomy to conform to the plate. One exception to this rule is that lateral mass plates should never be bent into kyphosis. If an irreducible kyphotic deformity is encountered, ventral reconstruction should be considered in lieu of, or before, posterior stabilization.

DRILLING ARTICULAR MASSES

Once a plate tandem is selected and custom-contoured, holes are drilled into the articular masses to prepare for screw placement. Various screw trajectories have been described for lateral mass fixation from C3 to C7. Roy-Camille and colleagues and others[10,19] have advocated engaging the drill bit at the center of the lateral mass and proceeding in a direction parallel to the axial plane while angling 10 degrees laterally. The widely used Magerl technique involves drilling from a point 1 to 2 mm medial and rostral to the center of the lateral mass along a trajectory 25 degrees lateral and 40 degrees cephalad.[56] The sagittal angulation is intended to orient the screw parallel to the facet joint. Several variations of the Magerl technique have been described.[13,21,57] In general, a lateral screw trajectory is compulsory to avoid nerve root and vertebral artery injury.[57–59] We advocate the screw placement technique described by Cherny and associates.[20] Drilling is initiated at a point 1 mm medial to the midportion of the lateral mass and proceeds along a course 20 degrees cephalad and 20 to 30 degrees lateral (Fig. 136-14). This trajectory affords reasonable protection from neurovascular injury while attaining sound bicortical screw purchase in the articular masses.[56,57]

Acceptable screw placement can be accomplished in this manner from C3 to C6. The screw trajectory is slightly altered at the transitional C7 vertebral level because of the relatively small size of its articular mass. If lateral mass fixation at C7 is desired, a slightly more lateral and cephalad trajectory accommodates this anatomic constraint. Because the articular mass is small, it is often preferable to obtain pedicular fixation at C7 and T1. The pedicle is entered 1 mm caudal to the C6 to C7 facet joint along a trajectory directed medially 25 to 30 degrees.[13] Each screw hole must be positioned optimally in its articular mass. The holes are oriented with reference to the patient's anatomy, not placed according to the lie of the plate. To minimize this latter tendency, we avoid drilling screw holes through the plate. All articular mass plate designs are sufficiently versatile to accommodate properly positioned screws.

Once the drill bit entry site and trajectory have been determined, the outer cortex of the lateral mass is pierced with an awl or a cutting burr to facilitate initial drilling. The articular masses are drilled with an unprotected drill or a K wire; however, it is preferable to use a drill bit with a depth stop (typically at 15 to 16 mm) to avoid overpenetration. During drilling, toggling must be minimized to avoid creating an irregular or oversized hole. The use of a low-speed drill reduces these concerns.[10] Bicortical screw purchase in the articular mass is desirable, but care must be taken not to penetrate much beyond the anterior cortex.

Screw holes should be placed unilaterally in all articular masses to be instrumented before the contralateral side is addressed. When a three-hole or four-hole plate is implanted, the rostral and caudal holes are usually drilled first. If a three-hole plate is used to bridge a fractured facet or pedicle, no screw should be placed at the site of injury. If the corresponding contralateral elements are intact, the center hole should be drilled and a screw placed on that side.

SCREW SELECTION

Primary screws, 3.5 to 4.5 mm in diameter and 14 to 19 mm long, are usually sufficient to fixate the lateral masses. Typically, safe bicortical fixation is obtained with 3.5 by 15 to 16-mm screws. Bicortical fixation is preferable, although unicortical screw purchase is acceptable. Cancellous screws provide better purchase than those with cortical threads. Articular mass screws may or may not be self-tapping. If the screw is not self-tapping, the posterior cortex of the articular mass should be tapped before the screw is placed.

SECURING THE PLATE

After all articular masses to be instrumented on one side have been drilled, the plate is secured with appropriate screws by tightening them to about 80% of the final torque in a sequential fashion. The contralateral articular masses are then drilled, and the corresponding plate is applied and secured with partially tightened screws. Final screw tightening is then performed on both sides. The screws seat into the plate and become snug with two-finger torque. Overtightening can strip the screw bed and must be avoided. Before the final plate is applied, the facet joints at all instrumented levels are cleared of soft tissue and packed with autogenous corticocancellous graft material to stimulate fusion.

Osteoporosis, irregular or oversized drill holes, or stripping the threads by tapping or overzealous tightening of the screw can result in suboptimal screw purchase. When the purchase is inadequate, a salvage technique must be employed. The primary screw is removed and replaced by a rescue screw of a slightly larger diameter to improve bony purchase. These screws are not placed without peril because the articular mass may fracture. This risk is increased when the articular mass is small or when the entry site is lateral to the facet midline. Alternatively the stripped screw hole can be filled with PMMA and the primary screw reinserted.

Articular mass plates provide unsurpassed immediate stability to the posterior subaxial cervical spine, often obviating the need for postoperative orthotic immobilization. With this technique, successful arthrodesis has been reported in 98% of cases with low operative morbidity.[60] In almost 500 literature-derived cases reviewed by Traynelis,[60] the

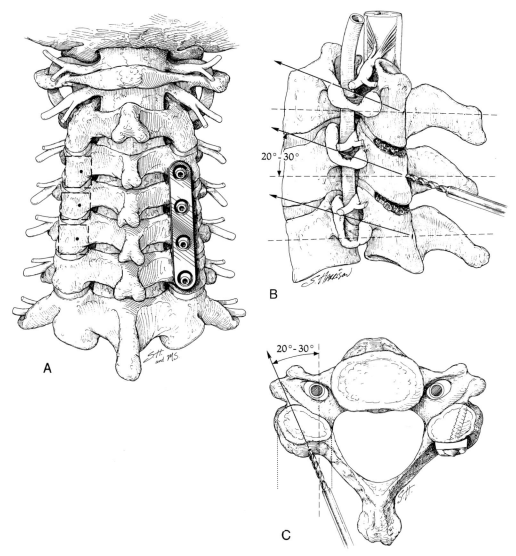

FIGURE 136-14   Articular mass plates (C3–C6). *A*, Holes are drilled in the articular masses at each level to be incorporated (1 mm medial to the center of the lateral mass), along a trajectory 20 degrees cephalad (*B*) and 20 to 30 degrees lateral (*C*). The plate is sized, contoured, and secured against the lateral masses with bicortical screws at each level. The process is then repeated on the contralateral side. (With permission from Barrow Neurological Institute.)

incidence of neurovascular injury was substantially less than 1%. Hardware failure can be anticipated in fewer than 1.5% of cases.[13]

Wound Closure and Postoperative Care

Intraoperative radiographs should always be obtained to confirm acceptable alignment and hardware position before the wound is closed. The wound is then reapproximated in anatomic layers. Absorbable suture is used unless local irradiation is anticipated. In that case, nonabsorbable suture should be considered. New postoperative neurologic deficits must be promptly investigated with imaging studies or surgical exploration or both. Patients manifesting evidence of a new myelopathy receive methylprednisolone in accordance with the North American Spinal Cord Injury Study (NASCIS) III protocol.[61]

The need for postoperative orthotic immobilization is dictated by the extent of preoperative instability, the nature of the underlying disease process, and the quality of the internal fixation. With more rigid implants, such as articular mass plates, orthoses are seldom required. Less rigid constructs must be supplemented by external bracing. Typically, orthotic immobilization is maintained until there is radiographic evidence of fusion on postoperative plain film radiography.

ANTERIOR SUBAXIAL CERVICAL PLATING

Anteriorly based fusion procedures for the subaxial cervical spine can be performed without grafting material (simple discectomy), with grafting material (fusion procedure), and with graft material that is augmented with a screw-plate system (fusion and internal fixation). Even though referred to as a simple discectomy, performing a discectomy without placing a grafting substance generally causes bone fusion between adjacent vertebral bodies. Internal fixation with screw-plate systems is performed solely in conjunction with a grafting procedure.

The use of anterior cervical screw-plate systems for fixation has been associated with improved fusion, greater postoperative comfort, and a more expedient return to work compared with patients who did not receive these implants.[62-67] Several cervical screw-plate systems have been introduced to the commercial market. A decision to use one fixation system over another is based more on an individual surgeon's preference and familiarity rather than on a clearly defined superiority of one system over another. Five cervical screw-plate systems have been used at our institution, and the techniques associated with cervical fusion and fixation procedures are discussed.

Anterior screw-plate systems are an integral part of the armamentarium for facilitating vertebral interbody arthrodesis within the subaxial cervical spine. Early reports that describe the application of bone screws and plates along the anterior cervical spine were directed toward patients who suffered from post-traumatic cervical spine instability. Screw-plate instrumentation has now been incorporated into the management of many pathologic conditions of the vertebral column that require structural stabilization after cervical discectomy or corpectomy. With regard to one-level or two-level cervical discectomies performed for spondylitic disease, it is worth noting that discectomies without fusion or with fusion but without fixation are appropriate procedures that enjoy high rates of clinical efficacy in patients with a normal preoperative lordosis.

Product evolution and advertisement for cervical screw-plate systems have been intense, and several screw-plate systems for internal fixation of the cervical spine are commercially available. In pursuing the practical ideal of versatility, enhanced fusion rates, and ease of application, each new generation of anterior plating system has incorporated subsequent lessons derived from biomechanical research and clinical experience. Most plating systems have had demonstrated success in securing bony unions.

Indications

Because they provide immediate rigid fixation across the span of desired arthrodesis, anterior cervical plates function to optimize the environment for bone fusion. The proximity of this instrumentation to the fusion substrate has multiple benefits: resistance to graft displacement, a reduced incidence of pseudoarthrosis related to micromotion of the graft–vertebral body interface, and, frequently, avoidance of postoperative halo bracing. Degenerative, neoplastic, infectious, inflammatory, traumatic, and iatrogenic (postoperative) causes of vertebral column instability, with or without concomitant neural compression, are well suited for treatment with rigid internal fixation from an anterior (transcervical or retropharyngeal) surgical approach.

At our institution, absolute criteria for performing internal fixation with cervical plate instrumentation include patients who have undergone any extent of formal corpectomy (single or multiple levels) or those with post-traumatic spinal instability. In the latter instance, severe mechanical incompetence might require greater stabilization than an isolated anterior fusion and plate construct can impart.

If so, a second surgical approach to reconstitute the posterior cervical tension band or external bracing with a halo orthosis might be deemed a necessary adjunct for promoting successful fusion. Anterior cervical discectomies accompanied by fusions that involve three or more adjacent levels are now performed routinely in conjunction with anterior instrumentation. Patients treated for degenerative disease limited to one or two motion segments do not routinely require augmentation of the fusion construct with screw plates, assuming that the posterior ligamentous elements are intact. Individual patient characteristics can adversely affect the anticipated success of bone healing. Malnutrition, the active use of tobacco, the presence of significant osteoporosis or other disorders that can result in poor bone quality, the need for exogenous steroids, or a history of previously unsuccessful fusion efforts (at the same or different vertebral levels) often leads to managing patients with an anterior cervical plate. The presence of gross infection at the operative site and sensitivity to metal are the primary contraindications to screw-plate insertion.

Operative Technique

Preoperative Preparation and Positioning

After informed consent for the surgical procedure has been obtained, patients are brought to the operating room wearing antiembolic stockings. Intravenous and intra-arterial access is secured, and a single prophylactic dose of antibiotic is administered about 30 minutes before the skin is incised. Intraoperatively, somatosensory and motor-evoked potential responses are monitored. In patients with evidence of myelopathy or significant compromise of the vertebral canal, baseline evoked potential responses are measured before the patient is intubated or positioned. Muscle relaxants are avoided during anesthesia to provide an immediate indication of neural irritation during the procedure. Patients with post-traumatic cervical instability or preexisting myelopathy related to cervical stenosis undergo fiberoptic or awake intubation. Patients with preexisting myelopathy receive a bolus dose of methylprednisolone followed by drip infusion in accordance with the NASCIS III protocol. The infusion is discontinued postoperatively if the patient's neurologic examination is stable. General endotracheal anesthesia is induced, and a urinary catheter is placed if the procedure is anticipated to exceed 3 hours.

When patients are positioned, bony and soft-tissue prominences are carefully padded to avoid pressure sores or peripheral neuropathies. If an autograft is to be harvested from the iliac crest, the appropriate hip is elevated with a towel roll.[68] An intrascapular towel roll, tape along the lateral aspect of the arms, and soft wrist ties that can be manipulated by the circulating nurse are helpful adjuncts that facilitate intraoperative radiographic visualization of the distal vertebral column.

We prefer the Caspar headholder (Aesculap, San Francisco, CA, U.S.A.) to support the patient's head and cervical spine (Fig. 136-15), even if the patient is already wearing a halo orthosis. The head is maintained in a neutral position, and the neck is maintained neutrally or extended minimally with the assistance of a chin strap. The evoked potentials should be observed carefully for any changes, and

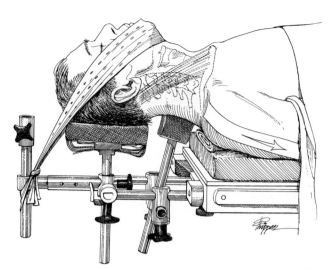

FIGURE 136-15 Patient positioning with the Caspar headholder (Aesculap, San Francisco, CA, U.S.A.). The patient's head is maintained in a neutral position using an elastic chin strap. The cervical spine is carefully maintained in either a neutral or minimally extended posture to recreate the cervical lordosis. Adhesive tape is run along the lateral margin of the shoulder joint and arm and affixed to the foot of the bed to assist with intraoperative fluoroscopic visualization of the distal cervical spine. The tape should not be run directly over the clavicle to avoid a pressure injury to the brachial plexus. An intrascapular roll functions to facilitate operative access by allowing the shoulders to fall below the coronal plane of the cervical spine. Both the scalp leads for evoked potential monitoring and the endotracheal tube (not shown) would be rostral in the operative field. (With permission from Barrow Neurological Institute.)

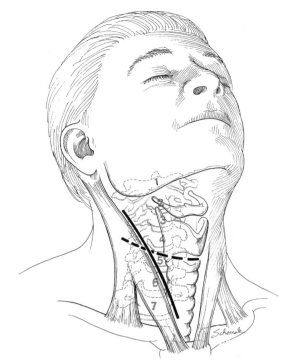

FIGURE 136-16 Orientation to the vertebral column may be estimated by palpating superficial anatomic structures. The hyoid bone sits roughly at the level of the C2 to C3 disc space. The top of the thyroid cartilage can be estimated at the C3 to C4 disc space. The inferior border of the thyroid cartilage can be estimated at the C4 to C5 level. The cricoid ring approximates the level of the C5 to C6 disc space. The C7 to T1 disc space sits approximately one fingerbreadth above the clavicle. We prefer to expose the vertebral column through a transversely oriented skin incision. Adequate extension beyond the midline or across the substance of the sternocleidomastoid muscle allows exposure comparable to that afforded by a longitudinally oriented incision along the medial border of the sternocleidomastoid muscle. Furthermore, the cosmetic result is superior. (With permission from Barrow Neurological Institute.)

intraoperative fluoroscopy should be available to confirm the maintenance of cervical alignment (anatomic or the best attainable) after positioning is completed. At our institution, the convenience and cost effectiveness of using cross-table fluoroscopy from the beginning of the procedure are well established compared with the relative expense and delays associated with obtaining intraoperative plain film radiography. The importance of fluoroscopy for confirming the operative level; for selecting an appropriately sized cervical plate; and for assessing screw trajectories, final screw positions, and alignment of the plate and vertebral column intraoperatively is self-evident.

Skin Incision

The operative approach is directed from the side that is most comfortable for the surgeon and usually corresponds to the patient's right side in a right-handed surgeon. On the right side, the recurrent laryngeal nerve is more susceptible to injury given its relatively anterolateral course outside the tracheoesophageal groove when compared with the left side.[69] Consequently, some surgeons may prefer an approach directed from the patient's left side. If the patient has already undergone a cervical procedure, we pursue operative access from the ipsilateral side. Although this strategy requires contending with scar tissue and altered anatomic planes, it avoids the more daunting possibility of incurring bilateral vagal nerve branch injuries, the unilateral manifestations of which may be subtle and otherwise undetected unless specifically evaluated for after the previous procedures.

A general orientation along the cervical spine can be estimated by external anatomic landmarks (Fig. 136-16),

but intraoperative fluoroscopy ensures more precise placement of the skin incision. Preoperative use of the fluoroscope to define the most rostral and caudal levels of exposure necessary for decompression and stabilization also assists in selection of the optimal orientation for the incision. A transverse incision located within a skin crease is cosmetically superior to a longitudinal incision that follows the medial border of the sternocleidomastoid muscle. When extended adequately (beyond the midline and laterally across the sternocleidomastoid muscle) and accompanied by generous undermining of the platysma muscle, the former incision rarely fails to provide sufficient access and visualization to enable multiple corpectomies to be performed with an accompanying fusion and plating procedure. Particularly long fusion constructs or difficult patient anatomy may make the longitudinal incision more functional, however.

Soft-Tissue Dissection and Exposure of the Vertebral Column

After the patient has been prepared and draped, the skin is sharply incised to the level of the platysma muscle. The platysma layer is traversed. Early attention to broad undermining of this subcutaneous muscle is greatly rewarded by the rostral and caudal extents of surgical exposure that

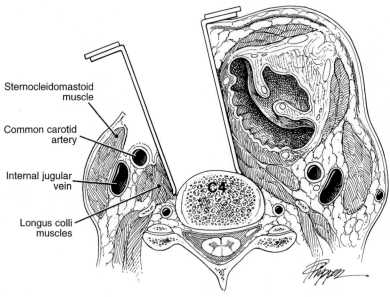

FIGURE 136-17   Illustration showing the relative anatomy and trajectory for an anterior transcervical retropharyngeal approach to the cervical vertebral column. A plane of dissection is maintained lateral to the tracheoesophageal bundle and medial to the carotid sheath. Bilaterally, the longus colli muscles are dissected subperiosteally to provide a submuscular pocket for seating the toothed retractor blades. Failure to seat these blades beneath the longus colli muscles properly places the esophagus and adjacent vascular structures at risk for perforation. When the vertebral column is approached anterolaterally, the tendency is to direct decompression eccentric to the contralateral side. Thus, regardless of whether the operative approach is conducted from the patient's left or right side, it is important to ensure that the ipsilateral neural foramen receives adequate attention and decompression. When anterior cervical plates are applied, the tendency is to place the plates slightly eccentric to the ipsilateral side of dissection. The plates, however, should be applied in as midline of a position as possible to minimize the risk of injuring the vertebral artery and to provide as optimal of a biomechanical construct as possible. (With permission from Barrow Neurological Institute.)

can be attained. The underlying sternocleidomastoid muscle and tracheoesophageal bundle are identified, and the avascular plane between these structures is developed with careful, blunt dissection. A trajectory medial to the carotid sheath is followed, and the underlying vertebral column is palpated (Fig. 136-17). Comparing the osteophytic topography with preoperative or intraoperative radiographs can often help orient the surgeon along the cervical column. Fluoroscopy, however, is helpful to obtain definitive localization along the cervical spine. The prevertebral fascia is opened, and the ventral aspect of the anterior longitudinal ligament is cleaned of overlying soft tissue. The medial insertions of the adjacent longus colli muscles are elevated bilaterally from the vertebral column.

The insertion of self-retaining, serrated (blunt-toothed) Caspar retractor blades (Aesculap) further exposes the anterior vertebral column. Rostral-caudal exposure can be improved by adding a second Caspar retractor (blunt blades) positioned perpendicular to the first (Fig. 136-18). Vertebral body distraction posts can also be added, but at the risk of compromising the structural integrity of the vertebral body and adversely affecting the quality of screw purchase. If ultimately deemed necessary, the distraction posts can be inserted one level rostral and one level caudal to the vertebrae targeted for screw insertion.

Discectomy with or without Corpectomy

Once orientation at the level of pathology has been confirmed, annulotomies are performed, and superficial discectomies are initiated with straight and angled curets (Fig. 136-19A). If an interval corpectomy is necessary, a bone rongeur can be used to resect the anterior half of the

vertebral body, and the Midas Rex drill (Midas Rex Pneumatic Tools, Inc., Fort Worth, TX, U.S.A.) can be used to complete the deeper aspect of bone removal (Fig. 136-19B). If placement of an allograft strut is planned, autologous bone from the vertebrectomy site is saved for packing the

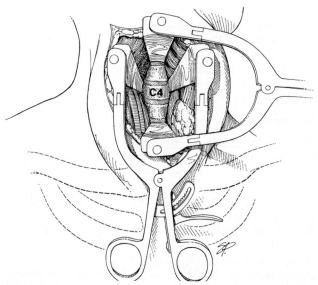

FIGURE 136-18   A second, perpendicularly oriented Caspar retractor system assists with rostral-caudal exposure of the vertebral column. These longitudinally oriented retractor blades are without teeth. Alternatively, the Caspar vertebral body distraction posts can be used to assist with retracting soft tissue in this plane. If the latter system is used, the posts are preferentially placed in the vertebral bodies rostral and caudal to those intended for screw placement. (With permission from Barrow Neurological Institute.)

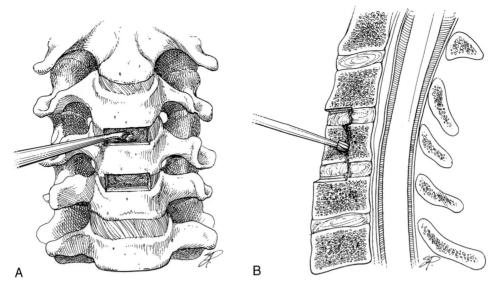

FIGURE 136-19   *A,* Anterior view of partially completed C3 to C4 and C4 to C5 discectomies. Bilaterally, the lateral extent of disc removal is the uncovertebral joints. If a corpectomy is planned, the adjacent disc spaces are similarly first defined, and superficial discectomies are performed before the vertebral body is resected. The superficial aspect of the corpectomy can then be performed easily using either a bone rongeur or a Midas Rex (Midas Rex Pneumatic Tools, Inc., Fort Worth, TX, U.S.A.) drill. Typically, we prefer to use the AM-8 Midas bit to perform the corpectomy. *B,* Sagittal view of a C4 corpectomy. The deeper aspects of the discectomies and corpectomy are performed under the operating microscope to ensure the safe exposure and decompression of the epidural space. Once the epidural space has been identified at the level of the rostral and caudal disc spaces, the remaining posterior cortex of the interval vertebral body is removed with bone punches. (With permission from Barrow Neurological Institute.)

hollow center of the allograft shaft. The operative microscope is routinely used to assist with the removal of deeper bone and soft tissues to facilitate safe exposure of the dura. The epidural space is inspected, and posteriorly based osteophytes are removed from the vertebral bodies and foramen to ensure adequate decompression of the spinal cord and nerve roots.

When completed, the typical lateral extent of tissue removed for discectomies or corpectomies spans 20 mm. Reliable identification of the vertebral midline is crucial to ensure adequate decompression of neural tissue and to avoid vascular complications related to injury of the vertebral artery. Frequently, severe degenerative disease, traumatic disruption, or scarring from previous surgical procedures results in the loss of the otherwise apparent anatomic midline. Typically, however, several anatomic cues remain, and they can be used to provide reference to the midline for decompressive maneuvers and plate positioning (Table 136-5).

TABLE 136-5 ▪ Anatomic Cues for Midline Orientation

Location of longus colli muscles
Location of uncovertebral joints
Curvature of vertebral body (lateral margin/waist)
Location of epidural veins and fat
Curvature of dural tube
Visualization of nerve roots
Palpation of pedicle
Location of sternomanubrial notch (angle of Louis)
Use of anteroposterior fluoroscopy

From Baskin LL, Vishteh AG, Dickman CA, Sonntag VKH: Techniques of anterior cervical plating. Oper Tech Neurosurg 1(2):90–102, 1998.

At this point during the procedure, it is also worthwhile to confirm with the anesthesiologist that the patient's head has not deviated from the midline position established at the beginning of the case.

Grafting and Plate Fixation Techniques

Screw-plate application provides immediate rigid fixation of the cervical spine and functions analogously to an internal halo brace. Only an osseous union can confer long-term stability to the vertebral column, however. Consequently, perhaps the most fundamental principle related to rigid internal fixation is that the presence of instrumentation cannot substitute for a carefully conceived and meticulously prepared fusion site.[70,71] In the absence of an associated bony union, hardware failure is a time-dependent certainty.

We typically use the Robinson-Smith[72] technique for interbody fusion after a cervical discectomy. Techniques to optimize the chances for successful arthrodesis (Table 136-6) at the operative site can be subdivided into those that (1) enhance the natural capacity for bone healing to occur, (2) minimize the extent of iatrogenically induced impediments to bone graft incorporation, and (3) maximize the biomechanical advantage of the hardware construct.

Enhancing the Capacity for Natural Bone Healing

Bone grafts are incorporated with the greatest success when the fusion construct is maintained under a compressive load (Wolff's law).[73] Consequently, the vertical dimension of the graft material is typically sized a few millimeters larger than the measured discectomy or corpectomy defects to ensure mechanical compression of the graft within the recipient bed. At the time of graft placement, the adjacent vertebral bodies are distracted mildly through the use of a disc space

TABLE 136-6 ▪ **Techniques to Optimize Fusion–Hardware Construct**

Maneuver	Benefit
Insert graft under compression	Improves graft incorporation
Maximize surface of implant–bone interface	Improves graft incorporation
Remove soft tissue from fusion interface	Avoids fibrous healing
Maintain integrity of cortical end plate	Prevents telescoping of graft
Irrigate while drilling	Prevents thermal injury with impaired bone healing and resorption
Avoid contouring plate	Avoids fatiguing of implant
Avoid overtightening screws	Prevents stripping screw hole and diminishing bone purchase
Insert angulated screws	Improved pull-out strength
Use longest screws possible	Improved pull-out strength

From Baskin JJ, Vishteh AG, Dickman CA, Sonntag VKH: Techniques of anterior cervical plating. Oper Tech Neurosurg 1(2):90–102, 1998.

spreader, carefully directed axial traction applied by the anesthesiologist, or vertebral body distraction posts.

After the posterior half of the graft has been tamped into place, the vertebral body distraction is released, and the remainder of the graft is advanced. These maneuvers promote seating and avoid excessive impaction of the graft. After final positioning, graft security and an appropriate epidural margin are confirmed by palpation with a nerve hook and with fluoroscopy. All soft tissues are removed from the graft material and interfaces involved with the fusion site (end plate articular cartilage) to prevent the delayed differentiation of fibrous tissue that might hinder bone formation. The creation of smooth, apposing surfaces along the bone graft and vertebral bodies serves to improve fusion by maximizing the area of surface contact at the fusion interfaces.

Iatrogenic Impediments to Fusion Biology

High-speed drills are convenient for denuding articular surfaces within the fusion bed and for shaping the fusion surfaces of the vertebral bodies and graft. During all drilling, consistent irrigation is needed to avoid thermal injury to the osseous tissues that can incite subsequent bone resorption and interfere with fusion. Similarly, the excessive use of monopolar cauterization to expose the vertebral column can impede healing as a result of direct thermal injury and bone devascularization. Using monopolar cauterization for deep tissue dissection also places adjacent soft tissues (e.g., esophagus, recurrent nerve) at greater risk. After discectomy or corpectomy, bone bleeding within the recipient bed can be controlled with a thrombin-soaked Gelfoam sponge, Avitene powder, or bone wax. Applying these substances at the site of the proposed graft–vertebral body interface, particularly bone wax, can potentially hinder fusion and should be minimized.

Optimizing the Fusion and Hardware Construct

Ventral osteophytes should be removed to allow a flush application of the plate to the spinal column. As much of the cortical bone layer as possible needs to be retained, however, because it contributes substantially to an individual

screw's resistance to pulling out. This point is particularly important when screw-plate systems that rely only on unicortical bone purchase are implanted. In contrast to cervical fusion procedures that do not include instrumentation, the graft material is not countersunk away from the ventral margin of the disc space. Instead the anterior border of the bone plug or strut is left in line with the anterior margin of the adjacent vertebral bodies to maximize the contact surface between the plate and the entire fusion construct. For a single-level autograft or allograft, a posteriorly placed trough along the posterior aspect of one of the vertebral bodies protects against graft retropulsion and epidural compression. Autograft struts that span more than one level are secured to the plate with a bicortically anchored bone screw to prevent graft retropulsion. Typically, fibular allograft is too brittle to accept a bone screw, and posterior troughs are created at the upper and lower vertebral levels to protect against its displacement (Fig. 136-20).

Two-finger tightness is the desired final screw torque to avoid stripping the screw hole and diminishing the screw's resistance to pulling out. If the tapped threads are stripped, options for securing the construct include substituting a larger-diameter rescue screw, drilling a new screw hole if variable trajectory placement is possible, moving the entire plate so that a new hole for a fixed trajectory screw can be drilled, or bolstering the initial screw's purchase with methylmethacrylate. Real-time fluoroscopy is used to monitor screw placement, and its use is strongly recommended regardless of the surgeon's experience with screw-plate fixation. If possible, the screw trajectory should capture the denser bone tissue in the subchondral region of the vertebral body, while respecting the vertebral body end plate. Violation of the distal vertebral end plate not only results in a suboptimal screw purchase, but also risks the incorporation of a normal motion segment within the fusion construct. Although the cervical plates can be contoured to maximize contact with the underlying vertebral column, this manipulation fatigues the implant and should be minimized. The longest screws that can be accepted by an individual patient's anatomy are used for plate fixation because they resist pulling out better than their shorter counterparts. When multisegment plating procedures are performed, the plate should be fixated at as many points as possible, particularly at the caudal levels, given the greater failure stresses transmitted to that location. Midsagittal application of the plate fosters optimal load sharing among the fixation points.

When the recipient site is prepared for graft placement, the cortical end plates are thinned sufficiently to expose bleeding bone but are left intact to prevent settling or telescoping of the graft material through the adjacent vertebral bodies. This step is particularly important when implanting allograft material, the rigidity of which makes this complication more common than when autograft is used, especially in patients with soft bone. Settling of the graft adds further mechanical stress to the screw-plate construct, increasing the chances for premature failure of the implant and incomplete fusion of the bone.

Proper attention to graft harvesting (autograft) or preparation (allograft) optimizes the load-bearing capabilities of these materials. We prefer to harvest tricortical iliac crest bone using an oscillating saw to avoid osteotome-related

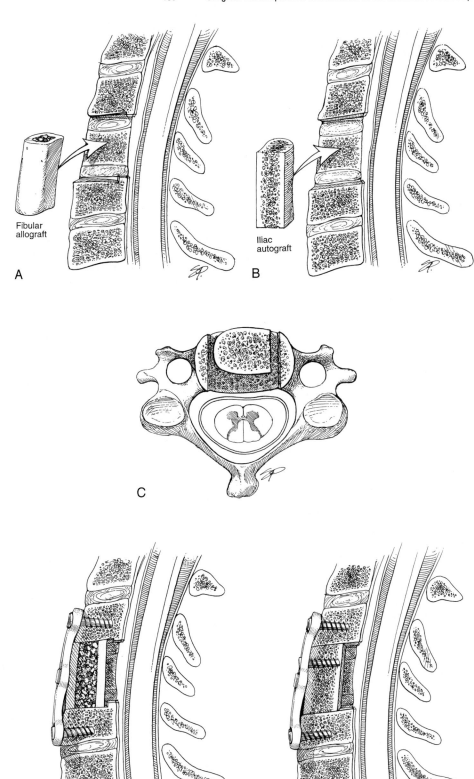

FIGURE 136-20   Sagittal views of corpectomy defects before allograft (*A*) and autograft (*B*) fusion procedures. Because a screw can be used to secure the autograft to the anterior cervical plate, posterior troughs are not necessary to prevent graft retropulsion. Conversely, the allograft material is usually too brittle to accept a screw. Consequently, rostral and caudal troughs are created within the respective vertebral bodies to protect the epidural space. The height of the troughs is 1 to 2 mm, and a concerted effort is made to maintain the integrity of the adjacent vertebral end plates to minimize the risk of the graft construct telescoping through the adjacent vertebral bodies. *C,* Midlevel axial view through a corpectomy defect after insertion of an autologous bone graft illustrates the senior author's preference for orienting autologous graft material. As placed, the cortical margins serve to buttress the anterior and middle column while minimizing the anteroposterior diameter of the graft. This latter point provides an additional margin of safety between the graft material and the epidural space. C4 corpectomy site after allograft (*D*) and autograft (*E*) fusion with plating procedures. In both cases, the graft material is not countersunk; the anterior margin of the graft material is flush with the undersurface of the plate. The allograft material is packed with autologous bone from the corpectomy site to promote fusion. A bicortical screw fixes the autograft to the cervical plates. (With permission from Barrow Neurological Institute.)

microfractures within the graft that would reduce its compressive strength. Failure to reconstitute the freeze-dried allograft in saline for the recommended 30 minutes before shaping or inserting the graft compromises its structural integrity.

Closure

The operative site is finally inspected, under direct visualization and fluoroscopically. Specific attention is directed toward the alignment of the vertebral column after fixation, the position of the graft with respect to the epidural space, and the length of the plate and position of the screws with respect to the rostral and caudal disc spaces. Midline location and vertical orientation of the plate can be assessed fluoroscopically by observing parallel overlap of plate holes and screw trajectories on cross-table views. Bacitracin-containing saline is used to irrigate the wound, and hemostasis is obtained with bipolar cauterization. Self-retaining retractors are removed, and the trachea, esophagus, and carotid sheath are inspected for evidence of injury with a hand-held retractor. If present preoperatively, a persistent carotid pulse above and below the level of self-retaining retractors is confirmed.

The platysma muscle and dermis are closed as separate layers using interrupted polyglycolic acid (Vicryl) sutures, and the skin is further reapproximated with a running subcuticular suture and Steri-Strips. We have found no need to maintain a surgical drain within the operative site, and the routine use of prophylactic postoperative antibiotics in otherwise immunocompetent patients is not supported by the literature.

Orthoses and Postoperative Follow-Up

The nature of the patient's preoperative pathology, the extent of the underlying mechanical instability, and the length of the fusion construct dictate the type of postoperative cervical orthosis prescribed. After screw-plate fixation, most patients are considered to be adequately stabilized if they wear a hard cervical collar when active. They are allowed to wear a soft collar while sleeping. Immediately after surgery, plain film radiographs are obtained. Flexion and extension views are obtained 6 weeks after surgery. If there is evidence of graft incorporation and the instrumentation appears stable on the comparative views, patients are instructed to taper their use of the hard collar and to initiate exercises to strengthen their cervical muscles. In patients who presented with a three-column traumatic disruption of the spinal column or who suffer from an underlying metabolic impediment to healing (i.e., rheumatoid arthritis), use of a halo brace for additional postoperative stabilization should be considered. Multilevel plate constructs are more prone to failure than their shorter counterparts. Postoperatively, patients whose procedures involved three or more corpectomies should be managed in a halo brace.

SCREW-PLATE SYSTEMS

The first reported use of screw-plate fixation of the anterior cervical spine occurred in 1964 and is attributed to Bohler.[74–76] Presently, four varieties of plating systems (Caspar, Aesculap; Synthes Spine; Orion, Medtronic Sofamor Danek; and Codman, Johnson & Johnson Professional Inc.,

Raynham, MA, U.S.A.) constitute most instrumentation used for internal anterior cervical fixation. A fifth system (Atlantis, Medtronic Sofamor Danek) is completing test center trials and is also used at our institution. Concomitantly, several additional systems were introduced to the market, but we have no clinical experience with them.

From biomechanical and biologic perspectives, the ideal plating system would initially provide adequate fixation to promote fusion but would facilitate delayed remodeling at the fusion site by allowing the transmission of physiologic loading (limited stress shielding). Each of the commonly available systems has its own limitations, but clinical success has been achieved with each (Table 136-7). Each system has its own advocates and detractors, and the relative merits of one anterior cervical plate compared with another remain largely subject to the individual surgeon's preferences and familiarity with the different instrumentation.

All of the implants are available in titanium or its alloys, the strength of which is estimated to be 90% that of steel but whose presence causes minimal artifacts on MRI. Later-generation plating systems offer unicortical screw purchase (e.g., Synthes, Orion, Codman, Atlantis), which is technically easier to perform than bicortical screw placement (Caspar). It also poses less potential risk for dural violation and spinal cord injury. Nevertheless, the Caspar system has enjoyed the longest period of clinical use and remains popular with a low incidence of neurologic complications related to screw placement.[62,63] Systems that rely on a unicortical screw purchase require a mechanism for securing the screw head to the plate, and the trend in product development has been for this locking feature to be incorporated within the plate itself (Codman, Atlantis) instead of as a separate component (Synthes, Orion). Fixation at the screw head–plate interface may be described as rigid (constrained system) or nonrigid (nonconstrained). Screws with variable trajectories are, by definition, nonrigidly fixed to the plate by their respective locking mechanisms. In contrast, fixed trajectory screws are rigidly coupled to the plate by locking devices. Selection of a constrained or a nonconstrained fixation construct is determined by the intrinsic instability of the pathology being treated. Patients with traumatic instability are likely better served with a more rigid implant, whereas patients with degenerative instability are more likely to maintain the integrity of a nonrigid construct that permits small amounts of settling over time.

Historically, surgeons have had to choose their plating system, in part based on a preference for placing screws through a fixed (predetermined) or variable trajectory. Although less error is associated with placing fixed trajectory screws, they offer little opportunity for the surgeon to compensate for a patient's abnormal anatomy to achieve an optimal screw purchase or to correct for suboptimal screw tracks or stripped tap holes. Similarly, the ability to contour fixed trajectory plates as desired is limited by the effect that bending would have on the final screw placement. The fixed systems can also be difficult to use at the extremes of cervical placement, where bony structures, such as the mandible or clavicle, can prohibit the necessary placement of instruments for drilling and inserting screws along a predetermined pathway. These issues make variable screws attractive because they offer more diversity in placing the screws; however, they also carry a greater risk for complications related to

TABLE 136-7 ▪ Comparison of Anterior Screw-Plate Systems

Plate	Year Commercially Available	Established Lordotic Cure	Required Screw Purchase	Screw Locking Mechanism	Screw Trajectory	Constrained System	Available Plate Lengths (End-to-End) (mm)	Plate Thickness (mm)	Available Screw Dimensions Diameter (mm) [Length(mm)]	Sample 1997 Catalogue Price ($) Plate Length (mm) ($)	Screw Diameter (mm) ($)
Caspar	1980	No	Bicortical	None	Variable	No	26–90	1.5	3.5 (10–28) 4.5 (17–24)	28 (437.00)	3.5 (9.60)[†] 4.5 (30.00)[†]
Synthes	1991	Yes	Unicortical	Separate 1.85 anchor screw (available at all sites)	Fixed	Yes	22–92	2.0	4.0 or 4.35 (12, 14, or 16)	28 (509.00)	Expansion head 4 (95.50)[†] 4.35 (133.00)[†] Locking (19.50)
Orion	1993	Yes	Unicortical	Separate cover screw (limited to rostral and caudal screw sites)	Fixed	Yes	21.5–110	2.5	4.0 (10–24) 4.35 (11, 13, or 15)	27.5 (529.00)	4.0 (107.00)[†] 4.35 (114.00)[†] Locking (51.00)
Codman	1996	Yes	Unicortical	Integrated cam (all sites)	Variable	No	24–110	2.7	4.5 only (10–26)	28 (458.00)	12 or 15 length (72.00) All other lengths (87.00)
Atlantis	1998	Yes	Unicortical	Integrated locking screw (all sites)	Both	Both	19–110	2.5	4.0 (10–20)* 4.5 (13, 15, or 17)*	27.5 (695.00)	(118.00)[‡]

*Fixed or variable trajectory screw type.
[†]No price difference related to screw length.
[‡]No price difference based on screw length, diameter, or fixed or variable trajectory screw type.
From Baskin JJ, Vishteh AG, Dickman CA, Sonntag VKH: Techniques of anterior cervical plating. Oper Tech Neurosurg 1(2):90–102, 1998.

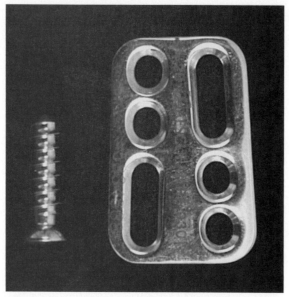

FIGURE 136-21 A Caspar plate and screw. (From Baskin JJ, Vishteh AG, Dickman CA, Sonntag VKH: Techniques of anterior cervical plating. Oper Tech Neurosurg 1[2]:90–102, 1998.)

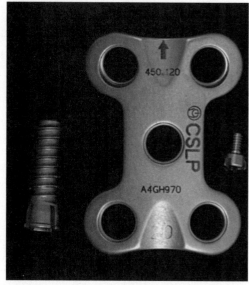

FIGURE 136-22 Synthes plate with fixation and locking screw. (From Baskin JJ, Vishteh AG, Dickman CA, Sonntag VKH: Techniques of anterior cervical plating. Oper Tech Neurosurg 1[2]:90–102, 1998.)

malpositioning the screws than systems with fixed trajectory screws. Of the instrumentation used at our institution, the newly developed Atlantis system is the only one that offers the versatility of fixed, variable, or a combination of these two screw types within a single plate. Depending on the underlying cause of instability, this system can be tailored to offer the properties of a constrained, nonconstrained, or hybrid system as detailed subsequently.

Caspar System

Introduced in 1982, the Caspar osteosynthetic plate (Aesculap) is the only system that requires bicortical screw purchase (Fig. 136-21). The screw trajectory is variable (nonconstrained system), and no locking mechanism secures the screw head to the plate. It is probably the most technically difficult system to use, and the depth of posterior cortical penetration must be determined precisely to avoid compromising the epidural space. The plates are machined without contour in the sagittal plane but can be curved as desired. The slot configuration allows positioning and redirecting the screws as necessary. The recommended screw trajectory is 15 degrees medially and parallel to the adjacent vertebral end plate. The recommended plate length is 2 mm from the rostral and caudal end plates of the vertebral bodies incorporated in the fusion construct.

Synthes

Introduced in 1986, the Synthes (Synthes Spine) is a unicortical system that has historically employed a 14-mm anchor screw with an expansile head that accommodates a separate internal 1.8-mm expansion locking screw (Fig. 136-22). This combination rigidly secures the screw head to the plate. Anchor screws are now available in 12- and 16-mm lengths. Screws are inserted with a predetermined convergent trajectory (constrained system) to resist pulling out. The plate has a fixed rostral and caudal orientation; the upper screws

are angled 12 degrees rostrally to approximate the cervical lordosis, and the lower screws are directed perpendicular to the plate in the sagittal plane. Bending, which further weakens the plate's structure, should be performed away from plate holes to avoid altering the integrity of the locking mechanism. Bending also alters the fixed screw trajectory and can compromise the final trajectory of the screw. The set offers a temporary fixation pin to stabilize the plate while screw sites are drilled.

Orion

The Orion contoured system (Medtronic Sofamor Danek) uses a fixed trajectory screw (constrained system) that is medially convergent (6 degrees) with 15 degrees angulation at the top and bottom (Fig. 136-23). Further plate bending alters

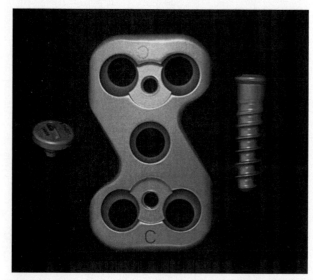

FIGURE 136-23 Orion plate with fixation and locking screw. (From Baskin JJ, Vishteh AG, Dickman CA, Sonntag VKH: Techniques of anterior cervical plating. Oper Tech Neurosurg 1[2]:90–102, 1998.)

the rostral and caudal angulations of screw placement, as with the Synthes system. A separate component locking screw increases the resistance of the bone screw to pulling out. The system also features the option of placing additional screws through a variable interval slot (4.35-mm diameter screws recommended), although screws in this location cannot be formally secured to the plate with a locking screw. Insertion of the locking screw requires an orientation that is truly perpendicular to the plate. Failure to achieve this angle, which may be particularly difficult to attain at the most rostral and caudal levels of the cervical exposure, can result in an inability to insert the locking screws. A self-limiting torque mechanism causes the driver for the locking screw to twist free from the screw head when the locking screw is secured appropriately. Plate sizing must allow for the fixed 15 degrees of angulation. The general recommendation is that the plate length should span just beyond the margins of the graft site to ensure that the screws do not violate the adjacent end plates.

Codman Locking Plate System

The Codman locking plate system (Johnson & Johnson Professional) is a contoured titanium plate (Fig. 136-24) that offers variable trajectories for screw insertion (nonconstrained system) and has no specific rostral or caudal end. A locking cam mechanism integrated into the plate allows unicortical screw fixation. Extremes in screw angulation (>16 degrees) can prevent the cam system from formally engaging the screw head, but the cams can still be positioned to offer some resistance to backout (lock zone between 240 and 270 degrees of rotation). The plate also may be bent, but the curve should be distributed evenly throughout the length of the plate and limited to the thinner, designated bend zones to prevent the locking cam mechanism from failing. The more commonly used 12- and 15-mm drill bits, taps, and screws are color coded (blue and gold) to simplify use of the system. A wide range of screw lengths is available and can be inserted using the variable-depth

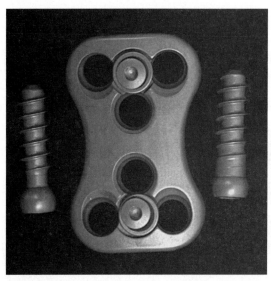

FIGURE 136-25 Atlantis plate with variable (*left*) and fixed (*right*) fixation screws. (From Baskin JJ, Vishteh AG, Dickman CA, Sonntag VKH: Techniques of anterior cervical plating. Oper Tech Neurosurg 1[2]:90–102, 1998.)

drill guide and taps included in the system's kit. With this system, only 4.5-mm diameter screws are available, the size that the other plating systems typically reserve for their rescue screws. The typical recommended screw placement is 10 degrees medially, parallel to the orientation of the adjacent disc space. The recommended plate length is from the rostral subchondral region of the most rostral vertebral body to the caudal subchondral region of the most caudal vertebral body included in the fusion construct.

Atlantis System

With the Atlantis system (Medtronic Sofamor Danek) (Fig. 136-25), fixed and variable screw (Fig. 136-26) trajectories are possible at any plate level. Specific drill guides either lock within the plate in fixed position (12 degrees divergent in sagittal plane, 6 degrees medially convergent) or allow angulation through an arc of approximately 31 degrees relative to the axis of the screw hole (Fig. 136-27). A holding pin, available for hands-off stabilization of the plate during drilling, is small enough in diameter to permit a vertebral body screw to be passed along its path later (Fig. 136-28). The locking screw mechanism is integrated

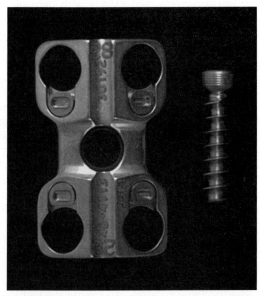

FIGURE 136-24 Codman locking plate with fixation screw. (From Baskin JJ, Vishteh AG, Dickman CA, Sonntag VKH: Techniques of anterior cervical plating. Oper Tech Neurosurg 1[2]:90–102, 1998.)

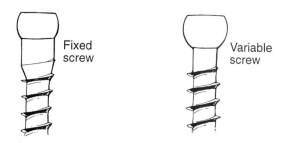

FIGURE 136-26 Illustration showing the fixed and variable trajectory screws (Atlantis system). The configuration of the head and proximal shaft of the fixed screw results in a rigid or constrained interface with the Atlantis plate. (With permission from Barrow Neurological Institute.)

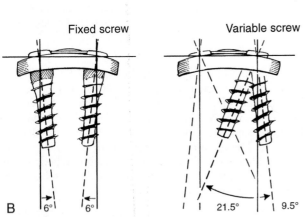

FIGURE 136-27 *A,* Anterior and sagittal views of the Atlantis plate demonstrating the fixed screw trajectory angled 12 degrees rostral to a line perpendicular to the plate at the rostral screw site and a variable screw trajectory at the caudal screw site. Because the screw hole is eccentric on the plate, the arc of rotation possible in the sagittal plane is 6 degrees toward the plate relative to a line perpendicular to the plate or 25 degrees away from this line (4-mm-diameter screw) *B,* Axial view of the Atlantis plate demonstrating the fixed medial (convergent) trajectory of 6 degrees relative to a line drawn perpendicular to the plate and the angulation available with the variable screw (4 mm diameter) relative to the same perpendicular line. The degree of angulation possible in the axial and sagittal planes is less with the larger diameter 4.5-mm screw. (With permission from Barrow Neurological Institute.)

within the plate and is available for all screw sites (vertebral body and autograft strut). The locking screw screwdriver has a torque release feature that indicates sufficient tightening. Similar to any of the other plating systems, extremes of screw angulation can cause the interface of the locking screw with the fixation screw to be incomplete. The plate is manufactured with all of the locking screws present in the open, elevated position. Before the wound is closed, all locking screws should be recessed to minimize the profile of the fixation construct.

Complications

The risks related to screw-plate stabilization of the cervical spine include all of those associated with a routine anterior cervical discectomy with fusion[77,78]: injury to branches of the vagus nerve (recurrent or superior laryngeal nerves); dysphagia; radicular or myelopathic injury; cerebrospinal fluid leakage; infection; anterior or posterior migration of the graft; postoperative hematoma; stroke; and, if autologous graft is used, donor site morbidity. Dislodgment of the screw or plate (with or without fracture of the instrumentation) would typically accompany pseudoarthrosis or a fibrous union at the fusion site and would necessitate revision of the entire graft and instrumentation construct. Morbidity associated with hardware migration also includes tracheoesophageal and neurovascular injuries. It is possible to observe implants that fail in the setting of successful arthrodesis.[79,80] In such a circumstance, the need to remove the hardware is not absolute and would have to be considered in the context of the patient's related symptoms, if any.

DYNAMIC CERVICAL PLATES

One of the main disadvantages of conventional static plating systems is failure of the construct caused by stress shielding of the graft. A rigid construct may eliminate some of the pressure on the strut graft that is actually required for a solid fusion to develop. Recently, interest in dynamic cervical plates for anterior fusion, which address this problem, has grown. The basic difference in design between static and dynamic plates is that dynamic plating systems allow axial screw translation along slots in the plate or along a rod construct. Theoretically, over time this translation should lead to some compression of the plate-graft construct due to axial settling caused by biologic or mechanical shortening of the anterior graft. The ability of the construct to adjust to these changes dynamically may eliminate or reduce stress shielding, improve load sharing, and promote fusion.

Experimental studies have shown that dynamic plates load-share more effectively compared to rigid constructs. Plate stiffness, however, may be less.[81] Three case series with a total of 107 patients undergoing anterior cervical discectomy, vertebrectomy, and plating with dynamic plates showed radiographic fusion in 80% to 96% of patients at a mean follow-up of 1.3 to 3 years.[82–84] One study (case series, class 3 evidence) indicated that the failure rate (i.e., screw pull-out, construct failure, and graft dislodgement) after multiple-level anterior cervical discectomy or corpectomy and fusion may be drastically reduced when dynamic plates are used compared to static plates.[84] Whether dynamic plates improves load-sharing at the cost of compromising stability has not been determined and needs further investigation. It is also unclear whether dynamic plates really offer an advantage over "semiconstrained" plating systems with variable angle screws, which also allow graft subsidence.

At the present time, three types of dynamic plates are available: the DePuy–Acromed DOC system (DePuy-AcroMed, Raynham, MA), the Aesculap ABC plate (Aesculap, Tuttlingen, Germany) and the Medtronic Sofamor Danek Premier plate (Medtronic Sofamor Danek, Memphis, TN). The first system to become available commercially was the DePuy–Acromed DOC system, which is a rod system that can be tailored to an individual patient's anatomy. In the other two systems, the plates have a slot that allows vertical screw translation while the graft settles.

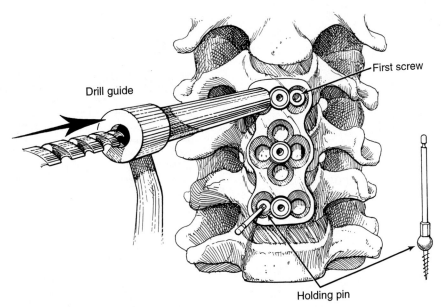

FIGURE 136-28   A holding pin stabilizes the Atlantis plate against the vertebral column while other screw sites are drilled and tapped. The individual plate holes in the Atlantis system can accommodate either a fixed or variable trajectory drill guide or screw, and a locking screw is available for all plate hole sites. (With permission from Barrow Neurological Institute.)

The Aesculap ABC plate is a semirigid construct with variable screw angles and a dual-locking system.

Information about the biomechanical effects of anterior cervical decompression with and without dynamic or static plates is still insufficient. More clinical and biomechanical work is needed to devise the optimal method of treatment that will provide minimal morbidity and maximum stability.

CONCLUSIONS AND SUMMARY

Several anterior cervical plating systems are available for stabilizing and reconstructing a structurally compromised vertebral column. Regardless of what accompanying instrumentation is used, the basis for a successful arthrodesis remains meticulous preparation of the graft and recipient bed. Rigid internal fixation of the cervical spine significantly improves fusion rates, and several available systems have had clinical success in achieving this purpose. The Atlantis plating system provides flexibility by accommodating fixed and variable screw trajectories within any one plate-hole site. Consequently, rigid, nonrigid, or hybrid biomechanical constructs can be created based on the underlying pathology of the vertebral column (Fig. 136-29).

A socioeconomic argument for the use of screw-plate systems is that patients who receive these implants may require shorter hospitalizations and may return to work earlier than those who undergo cervical fusion procedures without plating. For patients in whom cervical immobilization with a halo orthosis would otherwise be considered necessary after a fusion procedure, internal fixation with a screw-plate system provides a more convenient and comfortable alternative. Moreover, when considering the expense of applying a halo brace and maintaining it for a prolonged period under the care of an orthotist and physician, the cost associated with rigid external fixation is significant. As experience with

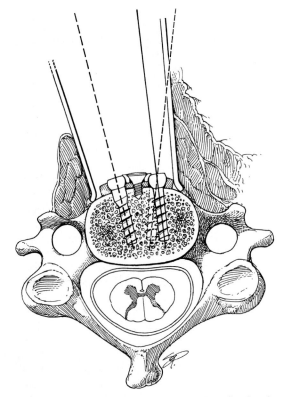

FIGURE 136-29   Atlantis plate system with a fixed trajectory screw used at one position and a variable trajectory screw at the neighboring site. This flexibility allows compensation for a patient's aberrant anatomy or for suboptimal screw positions or purchases. Consequently, the biomechanical stability of the fixation construct can be optimized. (With permission from Barrow Neurological Institute.)

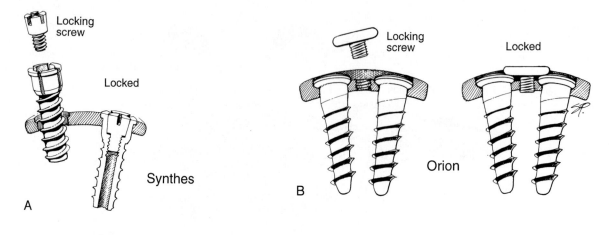

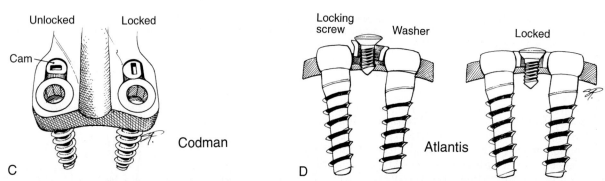

FIGURE 136-30   Comparison of the screw-locking mechanisms offered by the Synthes (*A*), Orion (*B*), Codman (*C*), and Atlantis (*D*) cervical plating systems. (With permission from Barrow Neurological Institute.)

these implants increases, the differences in operative time between procedures that incorporate plating and those that do not continue to narrow. Later generations of screw-plate systems have become progressively easier to insert, offering the convenience of unicortical bone screw purchase and an integrated locking mechanism to prevent retropulsion of the fixation screws (Fig. 136-30).

A fair comparison of the expense of one instrumentation system compared with another must account for the price of the individual bone and locking screws needed to secure the construct, in addition to the actual fixation plate. Individual hospital contracts with manufacturers can dramatically influence the actual cost of inserting one system compared with another. The figures in Table 136-7 reflect current manufacturers' catalogue citations. Additional surgeons' fees for performing internal fixation and the expense and radiation exposure associated with the fluoroscopy necessary to perform this procedure safely are other variables to consider when calculating the cost-to-benefit ratio of screw-plate insertion.

Several mechanically advantageous techniques are available for internal fixation of the subaxial cervical spine. The use of these techniques requires skill, judgment, technical precision, and a thorough knowledge of vertebral anatomy. Wiring techniques are reasonably safe and effective but have mechanical limitations and are not universally applicable. Screw-plate fixation is an excellent alternative to wiring and can be performed from posterior and anterior

approaches. Screw techniques can be used when wiring is impossible, when wiring is inadequate to stabilize the spine, when anterior decompression and stabilization are needed, or when a rigid implant is indicated by the degree of vertebral column instability.

The effective surgical treatment of instability of the cervical spine depends on a thorough knowledge of each patient's pathology. Operative strategies are directed at decompressing neural structures, fixating unstable segments directly, attaining an osseous union, and preserving as much normal cervical mobility as possible.

Stringent criteria must be applied to the selection of the appropriate operative approach to ensure a successful outcome. The method affording the greatest likelihood of attaining internal fixation and fusion, while minimizing the risk to the patient, should be employed. This standard cannot be overemphasized. Techniques should be implemented based on the surgeon's knowledge and technical expertise, the available resources, and the patient's pathology. The financial and biologic costs of surgery should be minimized, and the likelihood of attaining a solid fusion should be maximized.

REFERENCES

1. White AA, Panjabi MM: Biomechanical considerations in the surgical management of the spine. In White AA, Panjabi MM (eds): Clinical Biomechanics of the Spine. Philadelphia: Lippincott-Raven, 1990, pp 511–634.

2. White AA III, Panjabi MM: Clinical Biomechanics of the Spine. Philadelphia: JB Lippincott, 1978.

3. Panjabi MM: The stabilizing system of the spine. I: Function, dysfunction, adaptation, and enhancement. J Spinal Disord 5:383–389, 1992.

4. Frank C, Amiel D, Woo SL, et al: Normal ligament properties and ligament healing. Clin Orthop 196:15–25, 1985.

5. Panjabi MM: The stabilizing system of the spine. II: Neutral zone and instability hypothesis. J Spinal Disord 5:390–397, 1992.

6. Dvorak J, Schneider E, Saldinger P, et al: Biomechanics of the craniocervical region: The alar and transverse ligaments. J Orthop Res 6:452–461, 1988.

7. White AA, Johnson RM, Panjabi MM, et al: Biomechanical analysis of clinical stability in the cervical spine. Clin Orthop 109:85–96, 1975.

8. Denis F: The three column spine and its significance in the classification of acute thoracolumbar spinal injuries. Spine 8:817–831, 1983.

9. Benzel EC: Qualitative attributes of spinal implants. In Benzel EC (ed): Biomechanics of Spine Stabilization: Principles and Clinical Practice. New York: McGraw-Hill, 1995, pp 135–150.

10. Roy-Camille R, Saillant G, Mazel C: Internal fixation of the unstable cervical spine by a posterior osteosynthesis with plates and screws. In Cervical Spine Research Society (eds): The Cervical Spine, 2nd ed. Philadelphia: JB Lippincott, 1989, pp 390–403.

11. Hadra BE: Wiring the vertebrae as a means of immobilization in fractures and Pott's disease. Trans Am Orthop 4:206, 1891.

12. Sawin PD, Traynelis VC, Goel VK: Cervical construct design. In Benzel EC (ed): Spine Surgery, Techniques, Complication Avoidance, and Management. New York: Churchill Livingstone, 1998.

13. Sawin PD, Traynelis VC: Posterior articular mass plate fixation of the subaxial cervical spine. In Menezes AH, Sonntag VKH (eds): Principles of Spinal Surgery. New York: McGraw-Hill, 1996, pp 1081–1104.

14. Cooper PR: Stabilization of fractures and subluxations of the lower cervical spine. In Cooper PR (ed): Management of Posttraumatic Spinal Instability. Park Ridge, IL: American Association of Neurological Surgeons, 1990, pp 111–113.

15. Bucholz RD, Cheung KC: Halo vest versus spinal fusion for cervical injury: Evidence from an outcome study. J Neurosurg 70:884–892, 1989.

16. Sonntag VKH, Hadley MN: Nonoperative management of cervical spine injuries. Clin Neurosurg 34:630–649, 1988.

17. Bohlman HH, Anderson PA: Anterior decompression and arthrodesis of the cervical spine: Long-term motor improvement. I: Improvement in incomplete traumatic quadriparesis. J Bone Joint Surg Am 74:671–682, 1992.

18. Capen DA, Nelson RW, Zigler J, et al: Surgical stabilization of the cervical spine: A comparative analysis of anterior and posterior spine fusions. Paraplegia 25:111–119, 1987.

19. Cooper PR, Cohen A, Rosiello A, et al: Posterior stabilization of cervical spine fractures and subluxations using plates and screws. Neurosurgery 23:300–306, 1988.

20. Cherny WB, Sonntag VKH, Douglas RA: Lateral mass posterior plating and facet fusion for cervical spine instability. BNI Q 7:2–11, 1991.

21. Anderson PA, Henley MB, Gradey MS, et al: Posterior cervical arthrodesis with AO reconstruction plates and bone graft. Spine 16:72–79, 1991.

22. McAfee PC, Bohlman HH: One-stage anterior cervical decompression and posterior stabilization with circumferential arthrodesis: A study of twenty-four patients who had a traumatic or a neoplastic lesion. J Bone Joint Surg Am 71:78–88, 1989.

23. McNamara MJ, Devito DP, Spengler DM: Circumferential fusion for the management of acute cervical spine trauma. J Spinal Disord 4:467–471, 1991.

24. Stauffer ES, Kelly EG: Fracture-dislocations of the cervical spine: Instability and recurrent deformity following treatment by anterior interbody fusion. J Bone Joint Surg Am 59:45–48, 1977.

25. Van Peteghem PK, Schweigel JF: The fractured cervical spine rendered unstable by anterior cervical fusion. J Trauma 19:110–114, 1979.

26. Herman JM, Sonntag VKH: Cervical corpectomy and plate fixation for postlaminectomy kyphosis. J Neurosurg 80:963–970, 1994.

27. Sawin PD, Todd MM, Traynelis VC, et al: Cervical spine motion with direct laryngoscopy and orotracheal intubation: An in vivo cinefluoroscopic study of subjects without cervical pathology. Anesthesiology 85:26–36, 1996.

28. Murphy MJ, Daniaux H, Southwick WO: Posterior cervical fusion with rigid internal fixation. Orthop Clin North Am 17:55–65, 1986.

29. Savini R, Parisini P, Cervellati S: The surgical treatment of late instability of flexion-rotation injuries in the lower cervical spine. Spine 12:178–182, 1987.

30. Geremia GK, Kim KS, Cerullo L, et al: Complications of sublaminar wiring. Surg Neurol 23:629–634, 1985.

31. Sutterlin CE III, McAfee PC, Warden KE, et al: A biomechanical evaluation of cervical spinal stabilization methods in a bovine model: Static and cyclical loading. Spine 13:795–802, 1988.

32. Osenbach RK, Moores LE: Subaxial wire and cable techniques in the cervical spine. Tech Neurosurg 1:128–138, 1995.

33. Songer MN, Spencer DL, Meyer PR, et al: The use of sublaminar cables to replace Luque wires. Spine 16(Suppl):418–421, 1991.

34. Huhn SL, Wolf AL, Ecklund J: Posterior spinal osteosynthesis for cervical fracture/dislocation using a flexible multistrand cable system: Technical note. Neurosurgery 29:943–946, 1991.

35. Rogers WA: Fractures and dislocation of the cervical spine: An end-result study. J Bone Joint Surg Am 39:341–376, 1957.

36. Rogers WA: Treatment of fracture dislocations of the cervical spine. J Bone Joint Surg Am 24:245–258, 1942.

37. Whitehill R, Reger SI, Fox E, et al: The use of methylmethacrylate cement as an instantaneous fusion mass in posterior cervical fusions: A canine in vivo experimental spine. Spine 9:246–252, 1984.

38. Benzel EC, Kesterson L: Posterior cervical interspinous compression wiring and fusion for mid to low cervical spinal injuries. J Neurosurg 70:893–899, 1989.

39. Bohlman HH: Acute fractures and dislocations of the cervical spine: An analysis of three hundred hospitalized patients and review of the literature. J Bone Joint Surg Am 61:1119–1142, 1979.

40. McAfee PC, Bohlman HH: The triple wire fixation technique for stabilization of acute cervical fracture-dislocations. Orthop Trans 9:142, 1985.

41. Weiland DJ, McAfee PC: Posterior cervical fusion with triple-wire strut graft technique: One hundred consecutive patients. J Spinal Disord 4:15–21, 1991.

42. Murphy MJ, Southwick WO: Surgical approaches and techniques: Posterior approaches and fusions. In Cervical Spine Research Society (eds): The Cervical Spine, 2nd ed. Philadelphia: JB Lippincott, 1989, pp 775–791.

43. Cahill DW, Bellegarrigue R, Ducker TB: Bilateral facet to spinous process fusion: A new technique for posterior fusion after trauma. Neurosurgery 13:1–4, 1983.

44. Callahan RA, Johnson RM, Margolis RN, et al: Cervical facet fusion for control of instability following laminectomy. J Bone Joint Surg Am 59:991–1002, 1977.

45. Sawin PD, Traynelis VC, Menezes AH: A comparative analysis of fusion rates and donor-site morbidity for autogeneic rib and iliac crest bone grafts in posterior cervical fusions. J Neurosurg 88:255–265, 1998.

46. Garfin SR, Moore MR, Marshall LF: A modified technique for cervical facet fusions. Clin Neurosurg 230:149–153, 1988.

47. Tucker HH: Technical report: Method of fixation of subluxed or dislocated cervical spine below C1-C2. Can J Neurol Sci 2:381–382, 1975.

48. Aldrich EF, Crow WN, Weber PB, et al: Use of MR imaging-compatible Halifax interlaminar clamps for posterior cervical fusion. J Neurosurg 74:185–189, 1991.

49. Aldrich EF, Weber PB, Crow WN: Halifax interlaminar clamp for posterior cervical fusion: A long-term follow-up review. J Neurosurg 78:702–708, 1993.

50. Holness RO, Huestis WS, Howes WJ, et al: Posterior stabilization with an interlaminar clamp in cervical injuries: Technical note and review of the long-term experience with the method. Neurosurgery 14:318–322, 1984.

51. Schulder M: Interlaminar clamps: Indications, techniques, and results. In Menezes AH, Sonntag VKH (eds): Principles of Spinal Surgery. New York: McGraw-Hill, 1996, pp 1121–1132.

52. Branch CL Jr, Kelly DL Jr, Davis CH Jr, et al: Fixation of fractures of the lower cervical spine using methyl methacrylate and wire: Technique and results in 99 patients. Neurosurgery 25:503–513, 1989.

53. McAfee PC, Bohlman HH, Eismont FJ, et al: Failure of methylmethacrylate stabilization of the spine: A retrospective analysis of 24 cases. In Cervical Spine Research Society (eds): The Cervical Spine, 2nd ed. Philadelphia: JB Lippincott, 1989, pp 838–849.

54. McAfee PC, Bohlman HH, Ducker T, et al: Failure of stabilization of the spine with methylmethacrylate: A retrospective analysis of twenty-four cases. J Bone Joint Surg Am 68:1145–1157, 1968.

55. Gill K, Paschal S, Corin J, et al: Posterior plating of the cervical spine: A biomechanical comparison of different posterior fusion techniques. Spine 13:813–816, 1988.

56. Heller JG, Carlson GD, Abitbol J-J, et al: Anatomic comparison of the Roy-Camille and Magerl techniques for screw placement in the lower cervical spine. Spine 16(Suppl):552–557, 1991.

57. An HS, Gordin R, Renner K: Anatomic considerations for plate-screw fixation of the cervical spine. Spine 16(Suppl):548–551, 1991.

58. Pait TG, McAllister PV, Kaufman HH: Quadrant anatomy of the articular pillars (lateral cervical mass) of the cervical spine. J Neurosurg 82:1011–1014, 1995.

59. Ebraheim NA, Xu R, Yeasting RA: The location of the vertebral artery foramen and its relation to posterior lateral mass screw fixation. Spine 21:1291–1295, 1996.

60. Traynelis VC: Anterior and posterior plate stabilization of the cervical spine. Neurosurg Q 2:59–76, 1992.

61. Bracken MB, Shepard MJ, Holford TR, et al: Administration of methylprednisolone for 24 or 48 hours or tirilazad mesylate for 48 hours in the treatment of acute spinal cord injury: Results of the Third National Acute Spinal Cord Injury Randomized Controlled Trial. National Acute Spinal Cord Injury. JAMA 277:1597–1604, 1997.

62. Caspar W: Anterior stabilization with the trapezial osteosynthetic plate technique in cervical spine injuries. In Kehr P, Weidner A (eds): Cervical Spine I. New York: Springer-Verlag, 1987, pp 198–204.

63. Caspar W, Barbier DD, Klara PM: Anterior cervical fusion and Caspar plate stabilization for cervical trauma. Neurosurgery 25:491–502, 1989.

64. Suh PB, Kostuik JP, Esses SI: Anterior cervical plate fixation with the titanium hollow screw plate system: A preliminary report. Spine 15:1070–1081, 1990.

65. Tippets RH, Apfelbaum RI: Anterior cervical fusion with the Caspar instrumentation system. Neurosurgery 22:1008–1013, 1988.

66. Shapiro S: Banked fibula and the locking anterior cervical plate in anterior cervical fusions following cervical discectomy. J Neurosurg 84:161–165, 1996.

67. Aebi M, Zuber K, Marchesi D: Treatment of cervical spine injuries with anterior plating: Indications, techniques, and results. Spine 16(Suppl):38–45, 1991.

68. Kurz LT, Garfin SR, Booth RE Jr: Harvesting autogenous iliac bone grafts: A review of complications and techniques. Spine 14:1324–1331, 1989.

69. Ebraheim NA, Lu J, Skie M, et al: Vulnerability of the recurrent laryngeal nerve in the anterior approach to the lower cervical spine. Spine 22:2664–2667, 1997.

70. Prolo DJ: Biology of bone fusion. Clin Neurosurg 36:135–146, 1988.

71. Kaufmann HH, Jones E: The principles of bony spinal fusion. Neurosurgery 24:264–270, 1989.

72. Robinson RA, Smith GW: Anterolateral cervical disc removal and interbody fusion for cervical disc syndrome. Bull John Hopkins Hosp 96:223–224, 1955.

73. Wolff J, Maquet P, Furlong R: The Law of Bone Remodeling. Berlin: Springer-Verlag, 1986.

74. Bohler J, Gaudernak T: Anterior plate stabilization for fracture-dislocations of the lower cervical spine. J Trauma 20:203–205, 1980.

75. Cahill DW: Anterior cervical instrumentation. In Menezes AH, Sonntag VKH (eds): Principles of Spinal Surgery. New York: McGraw-Hill, 1996, pp 1105–1120.

76. Klara PM: Anterior cervical plating: A historical perspective and recent advances. In Bunzburg R, Szpalski M (eds): Whiplash Injuries: Current Concepts in Prevention, Diagnosis, and Treatment of the Cervical Whiplash Syndrome. Philadelphia: Lippincott-Raven, 1998, pp 247–257.

77. Bulger RF, Rejowski JE, Beatty RA: Vocal cord paralysis associated with anterior cervical fusion: Considerations for prevention and treatment. J Neurosurg 62:657–661, 1985.

78. Flynn TB: Neurologic complications of anterior cervical interbody fusion. Spine 7:536–539, 1982.

79. Dickman CA, Fessler RG, MacMillan M, et al: Transpedicular screw-rod fixation of the lumbar spine: Operative technique and outcome in 104 cases. J Neurosurg 77:860–867, 1992.

80. McAfee PC, Farey ID, Sutterlin CE, et al: 1989 Volvo Award in basic science: Device-related osteoporosis with spinal instrumentation. Spine 14:919–926, 1989.

81. Brodke DS, Gollogly S, Alexander Mohr R, et al: Dynamic cervical plates: Biomechanical evaluation of load sharing and stiffness. Spine 26:1324–1329, 2001.

82. Bose B: Anterior cervical arthrodesis using DOC dynamic stabilization implant for improvement in sagittal angulation and controlled settling. J Neurosurg 98(Suppl 1):8–13, 2003.

83. Epstein NE: Anterior cervical dynamic ABC plating with single level corpectomy and fusion in forty-two patients. Spinal Cord 41:153–158, 2003.

84. Epstein NE: Fixed vs dynamic plate complications following multilevel anterior cervical corpectomy and fusion with posterior stabilization. Spinal Cord 41:379–384, 2003.

137

Surgical Management of Intramedullary Spinal Cord Tumors in Adults

GEORGES FISCHER, JACQUES BROTCHI,
and KHALID MAHLA

The neurosurgical literature of the intrinsic spinal cord tumors contains many case reports but few series, even for the tumors of glial origin which are the most numerous.[1,2] As a matter of fact these lesions are relatively rare and occur in any age group. Ependymomas are the most common intramedullary spinal cord tumors in adults. Astrocytomas are the most common in children.[3] Hemangioblastomas and cavernomas represent special entities and specific strategies.[4-7] Other tumors of nonglial origin are still more exceptional. It is well known that intramedullary spinal cord tumors have no typical clinical presentation. At present, magnetic resonance imaging (MRI) is the best and, in most cases, the only examination to perform in investigating these cases. Although MRI can be a highly accurate diagnostic tool, it does not always provide accurate differentiation between ependymomas and astrocytomas. Evoked potentials, both sensory and motor, are now standard intraoperative monitoring tools used during the surgery of these lesions.[8] Whenever possible, the neurosurgical goal is the complete removal of spinal cord benign tumors irrespective of the histologic types; however, the surgical treatment of intramedullary spinal cord tumors is not routine surgery. Intramedullary spinal cord tumors remain rare and account for 2% to 4% of central nervous system tumors in adults and 15% of all primary intradural tumors in adults. The surgical approach to try to perform gross total resection is the treatment of choice. The operative duration is often very long and the procedure is always delicate and technically difficult. That is why neurosurgeons specializing in this field of neurosurgery are not numerous.

ANATOMY

The spinal cord is located entirely within the spinal canal. Its rostral end is in continuity with the caudal portion of the medulla, in front of the middle of the atlas anterior arch, to the upper border of the C1 nerve root. The spinal cord has the shape of a roughly cylindrical stem, is ventrally and dorsally slightly flattened, and of whitish color. It is 42 to 45 cm long and 1 cm wide in adults. It has an average weight of 30 g. It presents two enlargements. The cervical enlargement is 10 cm long, extending from the C4 to the T1 vertebral levels. The lumbar enlargement is 8 cm long from T9 to T12 and in continuity with the conus medullaris, which tapers off at the level of the L1–L2 disc space into the filum

terminale, an atrophic remnant of the caudal segment of the embryonic spinal cord.

The ventral surface is marked by a ventral fissure that runs along the entire length of the spinal cord. This 2- to 3-mm deep fissure splits the ventral aspect of the spinal cord into two symmetrical ventral columns 2 to 3 mm wide, the lateral borders of which give rise to the ventral roots. The anterior spinal artery runs along the ventral aspect of the cord but not in the anterior median fissure. The lateral surface of the cord contains a lateral column located between the entrance of the dorsal roots and the exit of the ventral roots. On the dorsal surface there is also a dorsal medial sulcus. Although it is not a fissure, it is also possible to separate its edges, to visualize the sulcocommissural arteries which are clearly identified under the microscope.

The spinal cord consists of gray matter surrounded with white matter. The gray matter has a typical H shape in cross section, and is characterized by a vestigial central or ependymal canal, which runs the entire length of the spinal cord and is a remnant of a larger embryonic central canal, which is nearly always completely obliterated in adults by ependymal cells or neuroglial clusters. Sometimes this vestigial canal may persist over a few millimeters in length, but lies in the central substantia gelatinosa and is lined with ependymal cells. Such an ependymal canal becomes visible on MRI in the shape of a "split central cavity" without pathologic meaning. Otherwise, the vestigial canal may be dilated in hydrosyringomyelic cavities or in the satellite cysts of intramedullary tumors.

The spinal meninges differ from those of the brain due to the presence of a thicker pia mater attached to the inner dural surface by the dentate ligaments. The medial border of each is adherent to the lateral column, all along the spinal cord. The lateral border of each ligament is free, with the exception of the areas adjacent to the roots. These are thick serrations whose apices are attached to the dural between the overlying and underlying root sheaths. The arachnoid consists of a dense impermeable superficial layer adjoining the dura, and of fenestrated dorsal septa which run from the superficial layer of the arachnoid to the pial surface of the spinal cord. That is why the cord is strengthened by the meninges without interference with the free circulation of the cerebrospinal fluid in the subarachnoid space. The spinal dura encloses the spinal cord and the cauda equina from the foramen magnum to the sacrum. The diameter of the dural tube is smaller than that of the spinal canal but much larger than that of the spinal cord. The dura, which forms a cylindrical sheath, is separated from the spinal canal by the epidural space, containing fat and the epidural venous plexuses. That is why the spinal cord is protected by the meninges and the cerebrospinal fluid, and can be slightly mobilized within the spinal canal.

The spinal cord is vascularized by the anterior spinal artery, which arises from the vertebral arteries, in the upper cervical region, and by the pial anastomotic network supplied by the radiculospinal and radiculopial arteries, which run with spinal nerves. Because of their size, two ventral radiculospinal arteries have been distinguished: the artery of the lumbar enlargement (Adamkiewicz's artery), which runs with a spinal nerve on the left side in 75% to 85% of cases, and between T9 and T12 in 75% of cases, and the artery of the cervical enlargement, which follows the course of a nerve root between C4 and C8. The anterior spinal artery has a mean diameter of 200 to 500 μm. The posterior blood supply is provided by discontinuous arteries of smaller size (100 to 200 μm). The pial network and the radially penetrating arteries supply the white matter and the central or sulcocommissural arteries arising from the anterior spinal artery supply the gray matter. Finally, the territory of the anterior spinal artery includes the anterior two thirds of the cord, while the remaining posterior third is supplied by dorsal vessels. The lack of anastomosis between central arteries and the pial network partially justifies the reputation of the midthoracic spinal cord as being "surgically fragile."

Venous drainage takes place first via the intrinsic vessels, which drain in turn into the pial veins. The anterior spinal vein lies dorsal to the artery. The posterior dorsal vein, which is often very large (400 to 1000 μm), has a winding pattern, particularly in the thoracic region and zigzags from one posterior column to the other over the posterior median sulcus.

The surgical approach of the intramedullary tumors depends on the anatomy of the cord and its vessels. The anterior approach to the ventral fissure is blocked by the anterior spinal artery and the branches arising from it. The posterior approach is not blocked by arteries or veins, but there is no open fissure on this side of the spinal cord. It is also possible to open the dorsal medial sulcus, by separating its edges without damaging the dorsal columns and their vessels.

CLINICAL CONSIDERATIONS

Intramedullary spinal cord tumors have no typical clinical presentation, but most adult patients present with complaints of back or radicular pain or paresthesias. Children present with scoliosis or neurologic complaints. The clinical course may be insidious, abrupt in onset, or may progress episodically. The clinical presentation is related to the level of the lesion. However, it is not unusual to see intramedullary spinal cord tumor patients with cervical involvement who have no sensory or motor deficits in the upper extremities. In addition, in patients with intramedullary spinal cord tumors involving the conus, the expected sphincter dysfunction may be absent in 50% of cases. MRI is the diagnostic study of choice in the investigation of spinal cord tumors. However, it is optimal when the images can be correlated with previously obtained clinical data. The therapeutic decision depends on the age, the context, and the state of the patient's clinical functioning at the time of operation, which is graded using the McCormick classification, taking into account both sensory and motor deficits.[1,9]

IMAGING

MRI is the diagnostic modality of choice in the management of intramedullary spinal cord tumors. It is the most effective and sensitive technique for the detection of an intramedullary spinal cord lesion.[1] Any tumoral infiltration produces spinal cord enlargement. Conversely, an enlarged spinal cord may not necessarily be caused by a neoplastic process, particularly when enlargement is limited to one or two vertebral segments. The interpretation of the images allows knowing the location and the extension of the lesion, to distinguish between cystic and solid tumoral components, and to propose a histologic diagnostic formulation. However, apart from hemangioblastomas, lipomas, or pseudotumors like dermoid cysts, epidermoid cysts, and cavernomas, there are no tumor-specific MRIs.

Two thirds of cases of intramedullary spinal cord tumors are glial tumors, and the distinction between ependymoma and astrocytoma is not always possible. Nevertheless, the diagnosis of intramedullary spinal cord ependymoma can be strongly suspected when the tumor is located in the center of the spinal cord, is well delineated, and when the contrast enhancement is intense and homogeneous, especially if the "cap" sign is present (a hypointense signal at the poles of the tumor suggestive of chronic iron deposition in hemosiderin form). Unlike ependymomas, intramedullary spinal cord astrocytomas occur more frequently in children than in adults and can be strongly suspected when the tumoral image is eccentric, when the contrast medium enhancement is heterogeneous, and especially if the tumor image has a poorly defined border. However, as in the case of ependymomas, there is no MRI-pathognomonic appearance in astrocytomas. Insofar as the possibility of cure is gross total resection at the first operation, it appears that all intramedullary spinal lesions with appropriate imaging appearance should be considered to be ependymomas until proven otherwise.

The diagnosis of malignant intramedullary spinal cord tumor can be suspected when the clinical course is short and associated with severe neurologic deficits and when MRI findings are very extensive and poorly delimited with heterogeneous contrast enhancement after the injection of gadolinium.

The surgical strategy is determined by analyzing the MRI data in the three usual planes (sagittal, axial, and coronal) without and after the injection of gadolinium. It is also essential, before a surgical procedure, to localize the lesion within the spinal cord with regard to its lateralization and depth, and to its extension.

INTRAOPERATIVE ELECTROPHYSIOLOGIC MONITORING

Intraoperative monitoring of evoked potentials is a standard monitoring tool for the surgical treatment of the spinal cord lesions. Both sensory and motor evoked potentials

(SEPs and MEPs) monitoring are used to assess the functional integrity of the spinal cord during surgical procedures.[9–11] The perioperative analysis of evoked potentials recording provides invaluable information about the functional status of the spinal cord and shows the abnormalities of the sensory and/or motor pathways, transient or not, which are used to guide the extent of surgical tumor removal. At the end, the monitoring allows to predict the occurrence of postoperative neurologic deficit. Carrying out intraoperative electrophysiologic monitoring is technically difficult but useful during the operative procedure. The use of this technique needs strict collaboration with the neurosurgeon and the electrophysiologic team. A limitation of SEPs monitoring is that the evoked responses may be absent or attenuated preoperatively and cannot be monitored intraoperatively. The evoked potentials may be lost during the procedure, but it is essential to know if the abnormalities are transient or permanent. Dorsal column injury is currently detected during the operation. Irreversible abnormalities are predictive of postoperative sensory deficits. Conversely, the absence of dorsal column conduction changes is a good indicator. However, motor function may be damaged without changes in the SEPs intraoperative recording. That is why monitoring both SEPs and MEPs is useful every time these waveforms are monitorable. The same limitation concerns MEPs monitoring: the patients with severe preoperative motor deficit cannot be monitored. Changes causes by nonsurgical factors are easily recognized by the anesthesiologist. Changes observed during the procedure have to be understood insofar as warning to the surgeon, which allows a change in the surgical approach before the motor pathways are injured. However, in patients with a monitorable preoperative curve of MEPs, a reduction of amplitude that remains until the end of the procedure may predict a postoperative transient motor deficit.

A benefit of monitoring both SEPs and MEPs is the demonstration that surgery of the spinal cord tumors can be followed by complete restoration of spinal cord sensory and motor functions. However, we cannot assert that monitoring is necessary for successful removal of intramedullary tumors. We are conscious that the best chance for good long-term results is a complete surgical resection of the tumor during the first procedure.

OPERATIVE PROCEDURE

General anesthesia is managed taking into account the requirements of intraoperative neurophysiologic monitoring.[1,4,12,13] The surgical procedure is performed while the SEPs and MEPs are recorded. Halogenated volatile anesthetics should be avoided because they modify the SEPs. General anesthesia is established with intravenous opioids and the continuous administration of propofol without bolusing drugs during the operative procedure. MEPs cannot be monitored under complete neuromuscular blockade. Therefore, oral short-acting muscle relaxants are used to facilitate intubation and to avoid the potentially dangerous patient movements. These drugs are not routinely readministered or are kept at a minimum, allowing MEPs monitoring throughout an often lengthy surgical procedure.

When the bladder catheter has been placed, the patient is turned to the prone position on bolster pillows, freeing the abdomen and thorax from pressure. This is the most widely used position for all tumor locations. Head immobilization can be achieved with three-point fixation for procedures above T6, to prevent inadvertent cervical flexion and to prevent pressure sores on the face. The sitting position for cervical intramedullary spinal cord tumors is no longer used by us because of safety issues and for ergonomic reasons, especially for lengthy surgical procedures.

A midline incision is used, centered at the level of the lesion but extending above and below it. It is not necessary to extend the opening over cysts. Bone removal should provide sufficient access to the solid part of the tumor. This step is delicate; either laminectomy or laminotomy can be performed. Hemilaminectomy, proposed for small, mainly extramedullary spinal cord tumors, is inappropriate for surgery of intramedullary spinal cord tumors, since midline exposure is required. Laminectomy, if carried out gently and patiently with removal of small pieces of bone, avoids any damage to the adjacent spinal cord, and preserves the medial facet joints, decreasing the risk for postoperative kyphosis. When an extensive laminectomy or laminotomy is to be performed, we keep one posterior arch intact at every fifth to sixth vertebra. It is possible to work underneath it, and it is of great assistance for the stabilization of the spine. Except for pediatric patients, an osteoplastic laminotomy is unnecessary for two reasons. First, when the tumoral spinal cord is very large, in contact with the laminae, the cord and the roots are more threatened by the surgical instruments during laminotomy than during simple laminectomy. Then, osteoplastic laminotomy may result in a very effective fusion, with a solid block of bone forming the posterior border of the spinal canal. That is to be considered if repeat surgery is contemplated at a later date. For pediatric patients, a laminotomy is performed as a rule, and in infants, unilateral incision of the soft tissues can be performed with surgery through a unilateral laminotomy.

Hemostasis has to be meticulous, and large moistened cottonoids are placed along the symmetrical retracted muscular masses to prevent epidural oozing and to establish a dry and very clean field before opening the dura. Surgical strips are placed in the epidural space, compressing the epidural veins. At this stage, intraoperative ultrasonography may be helpful in locating the solid and cystic areas of the tumor, especially when MRI has not provided enough information.

A midline opening of the dura is performed under magnification from the operating microscope and is extended cranially and caudally to expose the whole tumoral enlargement. Care is taken to not open the arachnoid layer. Dural traction sutures are placed. The arachnoid's membrane is opened separately with microscissors and delicately freed from the posterior or lateral spinal cord. Fine sutures identify the sides of the opened arachnoid's layer and prepare this layer for closure. Careful inspection of the spinal cord may reveal subpial color modification by the tumor. An SEPs electrode is then placed on the dorsal columns and maintained in this position without applying pressure. The tumoral portion of the spinal cord is often enlarged and swollen, smooth and tense, and more or less vascularized. Gentle evaluation of its consistency will confirm the location of solid and cystic areas. The dorsal median sulcus is then identified under high-power magnification. It appears as a distinct median raphe, over which the very tortuous posterior spinal vein runs. Sometimes this sulcus is easily recognized; in other conditions it is identified only by the convergence of vessels toward the midline. The vessels of varying size running vertically over the dorsal columns are dissected and mobilized laterally to expose the posterior sulcus, sacrificing the smallest possible number of vessel branches bridging the two columns, and trying to spare all the thinnest arterial or venous vessels in the sulcocommissural region. However, the problem is not always simple in an eccentrically placed tumor in an enlarged and rotated spinal cord. Such distortion can make midline identification difficult or even impossible when the definition of the posterior median sulcus is lost. Sometimes, the location of the true midline has to be evaluated in relation to the posterior roots on both sides, but this may prove impossible owing to the asymmetrical distortion of the cord or the adherence of the posterior columns. In such cases, the midline is identified above and below this region, and then the two openings may join.

In our view, the midline surgical approach is used except when the lesion is located in one dorsal column and is apparent on the surface without any cortical "mantle," or in the rare case of an exophytic tumor. We do not incise the tissue and we disagree with those authors who recommend laser myelotomy. We prefer to open the spinal cord by spreading the dorsal columns apart with microscissors and microdissectors and to then carefully retract them with warm saline-moistened cottonoids. The surgical field is extended over the entire length of the solid portion of the tumor and continued to expose the rostral and caudal cysts if these are present. The opening of the spinal cord must allow exposure of the poles of the lesion and the cyst walls. Pial sutures improve the surgical exposure and reduce the severity of repeated trauma due to dissection. This can be accomplished using a fine suture without any tension to hold the median pia mater and dura mater close together. One next exposes a sufficient portion of the tumor to obtain a biopsy sample with forceps and scissors but without coagulation. This is immediately followed by histologic examination. Careful hemostasis can now be carried out before proceeding with surgery. This examination sometimes provides a great deal of information when the limits between the tumor and the spinal cord are not clear. Information suggesting an infiltrating or malignant tumor, or both, are crucial in deciding whether further tumor removal should be continued.

Tumor removal begins by reducing the volume of the tumor with an ultrasonic aspirator. The tumor is debulked before looking for a cleavage plane. Intratumoral resection is performed from inside to outside, and this is sometimes facilitated by the presence of a cyst or an intratumoral hematoma. After strict control of hemostasis, dissection can be started laterally, on the side on which resection proves easiest. This dissection is performed by the tip of the microforceps with a gentle traction on the tumor against the countertraction provided by the pial sutures. If the tumor is not too friable, or if there is a capsule, it can be grasped, allowing visualization of a dissectable plane. However, common sense and patience are necessary. If there is any difficulty, we prefer to move the microscope to another area and to come back later; for example, to leave one pole and to go to the other one. The same policy is adopted when SEPs start to alter. Often, the color is helpful in recognizing the

tumor; for example, purple-blue or brown color in recognizing ependymoma and distinguishing it from the normal white spinal cord tissue. In our experience, a clear cleavage plane can usually be found in most ependymomas except in the rare case of a malignant variant. The final objective is total removal of the tumor, which can be performed in most cases. However, the absence of a plane of dissection, particularly in an infiltrating tumor, malignant or not, requires the surgeon to be cautious and avoid continuing tumor removal, which may be dangerous and useless.

Most intramedullary spinal cord tumors have a vascular pedicle arising from the anterior spinal artery. Some large tumors may separate both sides of the spinal cord, resulting in a true diastematomyelia with a high risk for injuring the anterior spinal artery and catastrophic operative results. For the detection of residual tumor, we have observed that bleeding spontaneously stops when tumor removal is macroscopically complete. In case of doubt, ultrasonography may be useful. However, in the absence of a polar cyst, it is not always easy to distinguish between the filiform end of the tumor and the increasingly dense fibrous bend into which it merges. The fibrous gliotic bend should be cut where it enters the center of the cord, but we recommend that the last portion of resected tissue undergo histologic examination.

At the end of the procedure it is necessary to inspect the wall of the cyst or cysts adjacent to the tumor bed. When normal spinal cord tissue can be seen through a transparent cyst wall, surgery can be ended, because the cyst wall adjacent to ependymoma does not contain tumor. After tumor removal, the dorsal columns are released from pial traction and carefully brought together again. We like to approximate the cord with fine interrupted pial sutures whenever possible. The arachnoid may also be partially reconstituted if it was originally preserved. The dura is closed in a watertight fashion always without tension. If the spinal cord remains expanded, because possible residual tumor or edema is present, a duraplasty is performed with fascia, which we prefer to all foreign material. If laminotomy has been performed, the bone is returned to its place, avoiding compression of the spinal cord, with or without internal fixation. After laminectomy, the bone gap can be partly filled with a Surgicel. A nonsuction drain is inserted into the subfascial of subcutaneous space.

OUTCOME

With gross total resection of benign intramedullary spinal cord tumors, radiotherapy or chemotherapy is not required. Complete removal of the lesion is the goal of surgical treatment of intramedullary spinal cord tumors, and this should be performed whenever possible. A tumor cannot be described as "unresectable" if removal has not been attempted. This recommendation concerns all histologic types, astrocytomas included.

Although our results for the surgery of intramedullary tumors have been published previously,[1,4,6,12,13] we reiterate our main conclusions as follows. The evaluation of surgical results with intramedullary spinal cord tumors requires analysis of postoperative functional outcome related to the patient's functional preoperative state. This evaluation must take into account both motor and sensory functions, as proposed by McCormick in a neurologic grading scale, which is useful for evaluating patients before and after surgery.[1]

When early postoperative function was compared with preoperative function at the time of discharge, we have observed that the condition of each patient was at least slightly worse for a few days but improves in a good number of patients. With rare exceptions, patients do not recover from severe preoperative neurologic deficits, and those patients who do not have disabling deficits after surgery are those who exhibited few or no deficits prior to operation. Motor function improves more and over a longer period of time than do sensory disorders when judged in the first postoperative year. That is the reason why surgery is to be performed before the patient experiences neurologic deterioration. The postoperative quality of life depends on the preoperative neurologic status. After the first postoperative year, any increase in motor deficit and any decreases in the patient's functional capacity suggest tumor recurrence usually due to regrowth of a malignant tumor.

When patients wake up in the recovery room, they invariably experience discomfort with diffuse hyperesthesia and paresthesias that can last several days. Due to the separation of posterior columns, they have deep sensory deficits, which can disturb early postoperative reeducation, but in most cases recovery is observed within 6 to 12 weeks. The severity of dysesthesia and pain of various origins is a well-known phenomenon in the early management of intramedullary tumors. Frequently, at some time after surgery, there will be new or worsened dysesthetic complaints of variable severity. Diffuse and permanent paresthesias may reduce the patient's quality of life, and pharmacologic treatment is not very effective. These unpleasant sensations are fortunately often less severe and resolve spontaneously within a few months. However, the paresthesias may not completely disappear and are an annoyance that patients eventually have to adapt to. Generally sensory deficits change little after the third postoperative month, whereas motor function continues to improve at least until the end of the first postoperative year. Finally, even in the best circumstances, the patient's long-term neurologic functional condition will be the same as prior to surgery.

If spinal deformity may be one of the earliest symptoms leading to the discovery of an intramedullary tumor, particularly in children, postoperative spinal deformities present prior to surgery are not exacerbated by surgery.[8,13,14] The sometimes extensive laminectomies required for the surgical treatment of intramedullary tumors may be responsible for severe, but fortunately rather rare, disorders of spinal stability. Four factors are responsible for these severe postoperative deformities: young age, the presence of preoperative spinal deformity, laminectomy involving at least six vertebrae (especially if it includes C2), and malignant neoplasm or adjunctive radiotherapy or both. In the great majority of cases, postoperative spinal deformations such as increased lordosis or scoliosis or, most often, kyphosis or kyphoscoliosis of varying degrees of severity, are spontaneously stabilized within a few months.

Sphincter dysfunction, principally urinary difficulties and sexual difficulties, cannot be dissociated from the paraplegic or tetraplegic picture with which they are associated.

DISCUSSION

The aim of the surgical management of the intramedullary spinal cord tumors is to achieve complete removal of the tumor without causing damage to the spinal cord during the first procedure. No adjunctive radiotherapy is required after removal of a low-grade intramedullary spinal cord tumor. With incomplete removal of a benign intramedullary tumor, low radiation doses are known to be ineffective while higher ratios of radiation are more deleterious to the spinal cord. In such cases we recommend repeat surgery in better hands. It would be better of course to achieve complete resection at the first attempt, even if radical removal is not technically impossible after radiotherapy.

The use of radiotherapy in treating malignant intramedullary tumors is still under debate.[11,15,16] Postoperative radiation therapy is commonly indicated, more often in the pediatric population. However, according to some investigators this treatment has not been validated by a prospective controlled study. The efficacy and harmlessness of radiotherapy have yet to be demonstrated with regard to spinal cord lesions. Although patients respond in the short term, they usually continue to demonstrate a dismal survival rate. There is no convincing evidence in the literature that radiotherapy is of any benefit in preventing recurrence of these kinds of tumors. In the same way, adjuvant chemotherapy has not been shown to change the outcome, except for children, in patients with malignant intramedullary tumors of the spinal cord.[11,17] Despite the poor results in these circumstances, patients who have undergone surgery for malignant intramedullary tumors are often referred to radiotherapists and oncologists in the immediate postoperative period even though there is lack of any proof of efficacy. Recommending radiotherapy without prior biopsy is indefensible.

The surgical management of the intramedullary spinal cord tumors needs a reasonable strategy, which depends on the tumor, the preoperative clinical presentation, and the quality of the first procedure. One needs to consider separately benign or malignant glial tumors and nonglial lesions such as hemangioblastomas and cavernomas.

Intramedullary spinal cord ependymomas (Fig. 137-1) are well-delineated tumors whose total removal is usually possible.[9,12,18,19] Holocord ependymomas can be removed in one or two operative procedures. In these conditions, postoperative radiotherapy is not given to our patients who have a complete or a subtotal removal. When complete tumor removal during the initial operation has not been accomplished due to timidity or caution on the part of the surgeon, we recommend performing a second operation to attempt a total resection. When residual tumor is known to remain and is confirmed on postoperative imaging, we recommend repeating MRI control at more frequent intervals during the first postoperative years. In the rare case of malignant ependymoma, postoperative radiotherapy can be performed because palliation is based more on compassion than proof of efficacy.

Unlike ependymomas, intramedullary spinal cord astrocytomas (Fig. 137-2) occur more frequently in children than in adults.[3,8,11,14,15] The diagnosis is suspected when the tumor is eccentric, shows heterogeneous contrast enhancement, and has a poorly defined border. However, as in the case of ependymomas, there is no pathognomonic appearance. The surgical question is whether complete removal is possible. In one third of cases a spinal cord astrocytoma can be removed as if it were an ependymoma. In low-grade

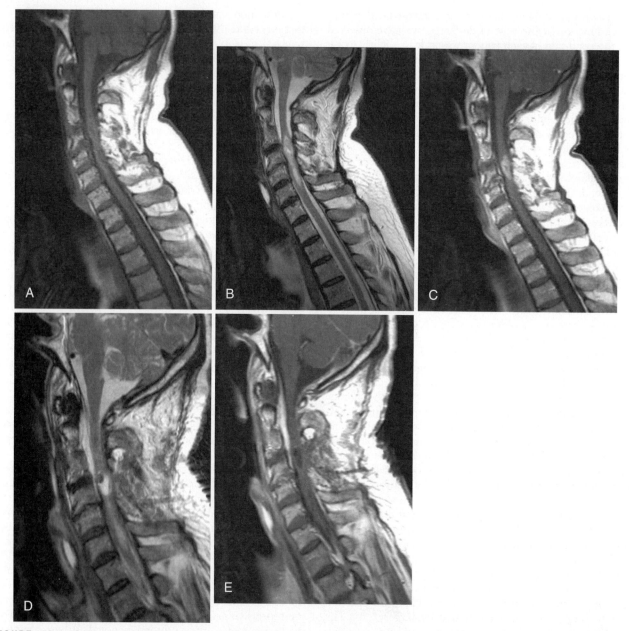

FIGURE 137-1 Grade II cervical ependymoma. *A,* Sagittal T1-weighted image. *B,* Sagittal T2-weighted image. *C,* Sagittal contrast-enhanced T1-weighted image. *D,* Early postoperative magnetic resonance image (MRI): sagittal T2-weighted image. *E,* Early postoperative MRI: sagittal contrast-enhanced T1-weighted image.

astrocytomas we do not prescribe adjunctive radiotherapy, and the recurrence after complete removal of benign astrocytomas is exceptional. The same results are observed after subtotal removal with a long-term follow-up (more than 5 years). After incomplete or partial tumor removal, it is always possible, if clinically required, to repeat surgery. For patients who presented with a malignant astrocytoma, the results remain poor. Irrespective of the treatment, repeat surgery, radiotherapy, or chemotherapy, the disease is usually fatal within 1 to 3 years.

Hemangioblastomas (Fig. 137-3) and cavernomas (Fig. 137-4) are mostly superficial, lying over and into the spinal cord. When they are observed immediately after opening the dura, their complete removal can be performed directly on the posterior or posterolateral aspect of the spinal cord. When they are purely within the spinal cord, surgery is managed through the midline approach, but no debulking is performed. It is now generally agreed that only symptomatic lesions should be treated surgically.

SUMMARY AND CONCLUSIONS

Intramedullary spinal cord tumors are rare. There is no pathognomonic clinical picture for these tumors, although back or neck pain, radicular pain, or diffuse paresthesias are often the first complaints. MRI is the imaging study of choice. Apart from hemangioblastomas, cavernomas, lipomas, and dermoid and epidermoid cysts, there is no tumor-specific MR image for the two thirds of cases that are glial tumors. The imaging diagnosis is sometimes difficult.

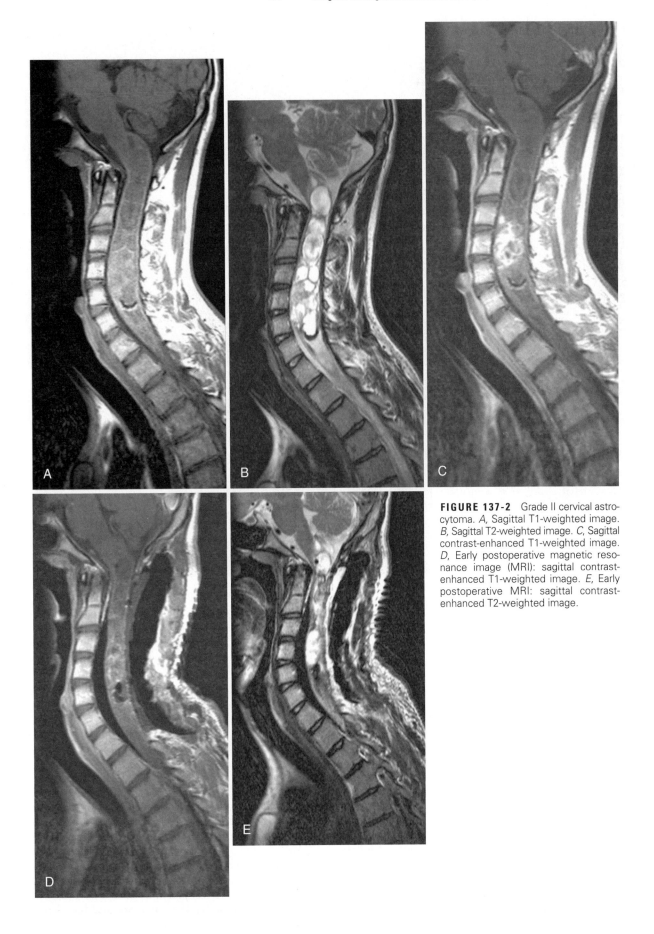

FIGURE 137-2 Grade II cervical astrocytoma. *A,* Sagittal T1-weighted image. *B,* Sagittal T2-weighted image. *C,* Sagittal contrast-enhanced T1-weighted image. *D,* Early postoperative magnetic resonance image (MRI): sagittal contrast-enhanced T1-weighted image. *E,* Early postoperative MRI: sagittal contrast-enhanced T2-weighted image.

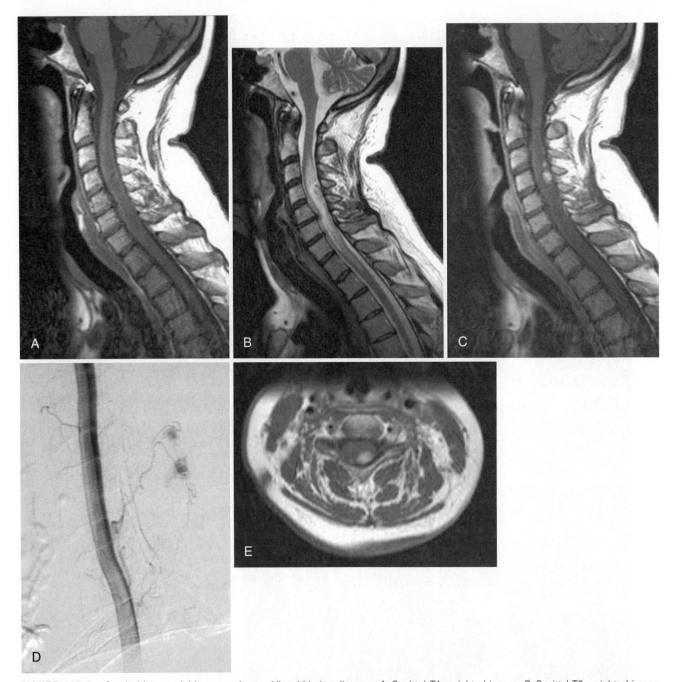

FIGURE 137-3   Cervical hemangioblastomas in von Hippel-Lindau disease. *A,* Sagittal T1-weighted image. *B,* Sagittal T2-weighted image. *C,* Sagittal contrast-enhanced T1-weighted image. *D,* Sagittal vertebral angiogram: two hypervascular nodules can be seen at the C3 level. *E,* Axial contrast-enhanced T1-weighted image at the C3 level.

In addition, the distinction between ependymoma and astrocytoma may require the use of additional histologic staining or immunolabeling techniques. Complete removal of the lesion is the first goal in the treatment of intramedullary spinal tumors. This should be performed whenever possible, that is, when it is possible to visualize a clear and healthy spinal cord. If no such dissectable plane is found, an attempt at complete tumor removal is pointless and hazardous. The presence of an astrocytoma does not necessarily mean that the lesion is an unresectable infiltrating tumor. Complete resection can be macroscopically performed in half of low-grade astrocytoma cases with a long-term follow-up that does not require another operation. Presently we do not believe that there is any place for postoperative radiation therapy apart from the treatment of malignant tumors of the spinal cord, fortunately rare except in children. Even in these circumstances, the efficiency and harmlessness of radiotherapy have not been yet demonstrated.

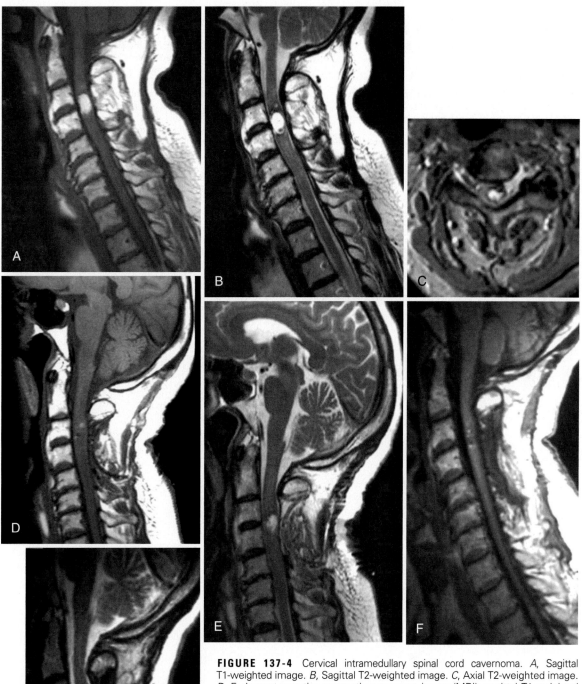

FIGURE 137-4 Cervical intramedullary spinal cord cavernoma. *A,* Sagittal T1-weighted image. *B,* Sagittal T2-weighted image. *C,* Axial T2-weighted image. *D,* Early postoperative magnetic resonance image (MRI): sagittal T1-weighted image. *E,* Early postoperative MRI: sagittal T2-weighted image. *F,* Follow-up MRI, 8 months after surgery: sagittal T1-weighted image. *G,* Follow-up MRI, 8 months after surgery: sagittal T2-weighted image.

Acknowledgments

We are grateful to Professor Danielle Balériaux, Erasme Hospital, Brussels, for providing the medical illustrations.

REFERENCES

1. Fischer G, Brotchi J (eds): Intramedullary spinal cord tumors. New York: Thieme, 1996.
2. Schwartz TH, McCormick PC (eds): Intramedullary spinal cord tumors. Special issue. J Neurooncol 47:187–317, 2000.
3. Constantini S, Epstein F: Pediatric intraspinal tumors. In Choux M, Di Rocco C, Hockley A, Walker M (eds): Pediatric Neurosurgery. London: Churchill Livingstone, 1999, pp 601–613.
4. Brotchi J: Intrinsic spinal cord tumor resection. Neurosurgery 50:1059–1063, 2002.
5. Hsu FPK, Clatterbuck RE, Kim LJ, et al: Intramedullary spinal cord cavernous malformations. Oper Techniques Neurosurg 6:32–40, 2003.
6. Lefranc F, Brotchi J: Surgical strategy in spinal cord hémangioblastomas. Oper Techniques Neurosurg 6:24–31, 2003.
7. Miller DJ, McCutcheon IE: Hemangioblastomas and other uncommon intramedullary tumors. J Neurooncol 47:253–270, 2000.
8. Houten JK, Weiner HL: Pediatric intramedullary spinal cord tumors: Special considerations. J Neurooncol 47:225–230, 2000.
9. Angevine PD, McCormick PC: Spinal cord ependymomas. Oper Techniques Neurosurg 6:9–14, 2003.
10. Kothbauer KF: Intraoperative neurophysiologic monitoring for intramedullary spinal cord surgery. Oper Techniques Neurosurg 6:8, 2003.
11. Sanderson SP, Cooper PR: Intramedullary spinal cord astrocytomas. Oper Techniques Neurosurg 6:1–23, 2003.
12. Brotchi J, Fischer G: Spinal cord ependymomas. Neurosurg Focus 4: Article 2, 1998.
13. Brotchi J, Lefranc F: Current management of spinal cord tumors. Contemp Neurosurg 21:1–8, 1999.
14. Constantini S, Miller DC, Allen JC, et al: Radical excision of intramedullary spinal cord tumors: Surgical morbidity and long-term follow-up in 164 children and young adults. J Neurosurg 93:183–193, 2000.
15. Houten JK, Cooper PR: Spinal cord astrocytomas: Presentation, management and outcome. J Neurooncol 47:219–224, 2000.
16. Isaacson SR: Radiation therapy and the management of intramedullary spinal cord tumors. J Neurooncol 47:231–238, 2000.
17. Lena G, Paredes AP, Scavarda D: Intramedullary spinal cord tumors: Pediatric aspects and adjunct therapies. Oper Techniques Neurosurg 6:41–53, 2003.
18. Hoshimaru M, Koyama T, Hashimoto N, et al: Results of microsurgical treatment for intramedullary spinal cord ependymomas: Analysis of 36 cases. Neurosurgery 44:264–269, 1999.
19. Schwartz TH, McCormick PC: Intramedullary ependymomas: Clinical presentation, surgical treatment strategies and prognosis. J Neurooncol 47:211–218, 2000.

138 CyberKnife Radiosurgery for Spinal Lesions

SAMUEL H. CHESHIER, STEVEN D. CHANG,
STEPHEN I. RYU, and JOHN R. ADLER, JR.

INTRODUCTION

Tumors and vascular malformations of the spine continue to offer unique challenges to the neurosurgeon. A complex anatomy, combined with the delicate and irreplaceable nature of the tightly confined spinal cord, makes the standard open surgical management of many spinal lesions inadvisable. Because of this, treatment strategies employing chemotherapy and irradiation have long been used in conjunction with surgery. However, chemotherapy alone for spinal lesions is associated with significant systemic morbidity and rarely provides a substantial therapeutic benefit. In contrast, conventional radiotherapy as a primary treatment for selected spinal tumors often provides significant palliative benefit and, in rare cases, can even be locally curative.

Standard radiation techniques for treating spinal tumors rely on treatment fields extending up to two vertebral segments above and below the target to compensate for setup errors and patient movement during treatment. Of even greater importance, the close proximity of the spinal cord typically makes it impossible to exclude it from the highest dose regions. These technical limitations result in a significant amount of normal tissue being included in the radiation field, the most important being the spinal cord. In an effort to protect these normal structures, conventional radiation therapy is highly fractionated. Despite such radiobiologic manipulations, the dose tolerance of the spinal cord ultimately precludes the administration of larger and more effective (locally curative) quantities of radiation, thereby limiting the effectiveness of radiation therapy in the definitive management of most spinal tumors.[1] After standard radiotherapy for spinal lesions, relapses within the treatment field are not uncommon.[2–5] Despite the high rate of failure, it is deemed unacceptable to use larger and more therapeutically beneficial doses, given the risk of spinal cord injuries such as radiation-induced myelopathy.

Shaping the irradiation beam to strictly involve the target volume would theoretically maximize the dose to the lesion while minimizing the risk of injury to the spinal cord. The newest radiation therapy technology, intensity-modulated radiation therapy, goes a long way toward achieving this goal.[6,7] This technology enables the shape of the treatment field to more closely match that of the lesion being treated. However, most of the advantages of such dose conformality go unrecognized because the method of targeting radiation remains relatively imprecise. When performing conventional radiotherapy, the radiation beams are aimed at a lesion by manually positioning the patient by means of surface markers attached to the skin. The inherent nature of this process results in limited spatial accuracy and reproducibility. As a consequence, even this most modern of radiation therapy techniques fails to address the unique demands of optimally irradiating the spinal axis. Ultimately, the dilemma with all current irradiation methods is that greater success can only be achieved at the cost of substantially increasing the risk of a devastating complication.

STEREOTACTIC SPINAL RADIOSURGERY

Stereotactic radiosurgery combines the principles of stereotactic localization with multiple radiation beams from a highly collimated radiation source to deliver high-dose irradiation to a target while limiting exposure to normal tissues.[8] Stereotactic radiosurgery has long been used to treat intracranial lesions. Most current radiosurgical methods rely on a rigid frame fixed directly to a patient's skull and presume a fixed relationship between the target and the cranium. In the past 15 years, the results of stereotactic radiosurgery have redefined standards of treatment for a range of intracranial and skull base pathology. Furthermore, the extremely favorable intracranial experience with radiosurgery has inspired the development of new techniques for stereotactically irradiating the spine.

Spinal lesions also often have a more or less fixed spatial relationship to the bony spine. Capitalizing on this, stereotactic methods for targeting within the spine were developed that, not surprisingly, bear a strong resemblance to the many related techniques for intracranial localization that were developed in parallel. Woroschiloff performed the first spinal stereotactic surgery in 1874 when he used a spinal localization device attached directly to the spinous processes to make cord lesions with a knife or electrode in conjunction with electrophysiologic studies.[9] Over the years, modifications of this original design have been employed to perform cervical cordotomies,[10] high cervical tractotomies,[11] and thermocoagulation of lumbosacral centers of the spinal cord.[12] However, it was not until the mid-1990s that Hamilton and colleagues[13–15] developed a spinal stereotactic radiosurgery system using a modified linear accelerator (LINAC) and a skeletal fixation frame.

The spinal radiosurgical system developed by Hamilton and colleagues employed a patient-encircling rigid frame for reference and immobilization. This device could be firmly attached to the spinous processes by means of a series of small incisions made under anesthesia.[16] Although preliminary results were promising, frame fixation was extremely cumbersome and resulted in long procedures.

Moreover, multiple treatments (i.e., treatment fractionation) were impractical.

When treating nonspherical lesions, frame-based stereotactic systems generally use overlapping fixed isocenters to achieve some minimal measure of field shaping. The result of such a scheme is an inhomogeneous dose of radiation within the treatment area that can often be associated with undertreatment of lesions and/or overtreatment of the adjacent spinal cord. Such inhomogeneity is particularly disadvantageous when administering very aggressive doses of radiation immediately adjacent to the spinal cord.

The frameless image-guided radiosurgery system (the CyberKnife) developed by Accuray, Inc. (Sunnyvale, CA) overcomes many of the limitations encountered by Hamilton and colleagues.[13–15] Rather than use an external fixation device, targeting is based on internal radiographic features such as skeletal anatomy or implanted fiducials. Because this design allows real-time images to be acquired during treatment, the system is capable of measuring any change in target location and then precisely retarget the radiation beam to compensate. Finally, in contrast to other radiosurgical techniques, a fixed isocenter is not used by the CyberKnife. As a result, more conformal treatment of irregularly shaped targets is possible, and, if advantageous, greater in-field homogeneity can be achieved.

Since 1994, the CyberKnife has been used at more than 20 sites including Stanford University Medical Center. More than 8000 patients with benign and malignant intracranial lesions have undergone CyberKnife radiosurgery with outcomes similar to those with conventional frame-based techniques.[7,17–27] Because many spinal lesions are histopathologically similar to those in the brain, it is not unreasonable to assume that treatment outcome using the same modality might be comparable. Beginning in 1996, the Stanford CyberKnife has been used to test this hypothesis in a highly selected group of patients. Treatment was initially performed under an investigational device exemption until the U.S. Food and Drug Administration approved the CyberKnife for extracranial applications in 2001. Since that time, the CyberKnife has been successfully used to treat a broad range of lesions throughout the spine, chest, and abdomen.[7,19,25,26,28,29]

INDICATIONS FOR SPINAL RADIOSURGERY

The indications for spinal radiosurgery have evolved rapidly as experience with this relatively new technology has accumulated (Table 138-1). The primary indications include minimal but progressive neurologic deficits, the need for postresection local irradiation, radiographic progression despite previous surgery or irradiation, or treatment of inoperable lesions.[6,7,27] Similar to cranial radiosurgery, spinal lesions appropriate for CyberKnife radiosurgery need to be reasonably well circumscribed and not so large as to negate the benefits of a steep dose gradient. Among the spinal cases selected for CyberKnife treatment, the lesions were usually either unresectable or associated with significant medical comorbidities, thereby precluding surgery. A small subset of patients who have undergone spinal radiosurgery refused open surgical resection. A wide spectrum of spinal pathologies has been treated including primary tumors, metastatic tumors, and vascular malformations (Table 138-2).[7,27]

TABLE 138-1 ▪ Indications and Contraindications of Stereotactic Spinal Radiosurgery

Indications
Progressive but minimal neurologic deficit
Postresection local irradiation
Disease progression despite previous surgery and/or irradiation
Patients with severe medical comorbidities that preclude surgery
Inoperable lesions

Contraindications
Severe neurologic deficit with significant cord compression
Neurologic deficit caused by bony compression
Spinal instability
Lesion not responsive to irradiation
Maximal tolerable doses of irradiation already given to adjacent spinal cord

---

Spinal radiosurgery is contraindicated in patients with significant spinal cord compression causing a substantial neurologic deficit. This contraindication applies particularly to tumors for which the temporal response to treatment is delayed, such as benign lesions. Furthermore, spinal radiosurgery should be avoided when there is evidence of significant spine instability or when a patient's neurologic deficit is caused mainly by bony compression. If the adjacent spinal cord has already received the maximally tolerated dose of radiation, further irradiation can be dangerous. Although it can be a difficult decision to make, this latter group of patients would usually be better treated with surgery and/or chemotherapy, if possible.

TECHNICAL OVERVIEW OF THE CYBERKNIFE SYSTEM FOR SPINAL RADIOSURGERY

The basic components of the CyberKnife are a lightweight 6-MV LINAC mounted on a computer-controlled robotic arm (Fig. 138-1). The robotic arm incorporates an x-ray imaging feedback system consisting of two orthogonally aligned x-ray cameras that acquire radiographs of targeting landmarks during treatment. The components of the imaging system are at fixed positions within the treatment room, providing a stationary frame of reference to locate the patient's spine. Once the spine has been located within the imaging system's coordinate frame, the position of the lesion is known.

TABLE 138-2 ▪ Treated/Treatable Lesions with CyberKnife Radiosurgey

Tumors
Benign
  Neurofibroma, schwannoma, meningioma, hemangioblastoma, chordoma, paraganglioma, ependymomas, epidermoid
Malignant/metastatic
  Breast, renal, non-small cell lung, colon, gastric and prostate metastases; squamous cell (laryngeal, esophageal, and lung) tumors; osteosarcoma; carcinoid; multiple myeloma; clear cell carcinoma; adenoid cystic carcinoma; malignant nerve sheath tumor; endometrial carcinoma; malignant neuroendocrine tumor

Vascular Malformations
Arteriovenous malformation (types 2 and 3), cavernous malformation

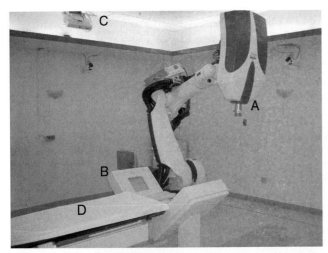

FIGURE 138-1 CyberKnife frameless stereotactic radiosurgery suite. A modified 6-MV X-band LINAC designed specifically for radiosurgery is mounted on a highly maneuverable robotic manipulator (KUKA Roboter GmbH, Augsburg, Germany) (*A*). Two high-resolution x-ray cameras are mounted orthogonally to the headrest (*B*). One of the two x-ray sources is mounted in the ceiling projecting onto the camera (*C*). The treatment couch is mobile, allowing the x-ray sources to image targets at any point along the neuroaxis (*D*).

Targeting is based on the assumption of a fixed relationship between the lesion and the spine. The radiographs acquired by the real-time imaging system are compared by means of computer algorithms to digitally reconstructed radiographs (DRRs) derived from computed tomography scans obtained during treatment planning. The most recent CyberKnife software measures both translation and rotation of the anatomy by iteratively changing the position of the anatomy in the DRR until an exact match of the two radiographs and two DRRs is achieved.[30] This algorithm does not require a database of precomputed DRRs or the array processor used in the previous software, thus eliminating the need to fix the orientation of the patient during treatment. Once the location of the spine is determined, the coordinates are fed to the robotic arm controller, which is involved in targeting the LINAC. This concept enables the system to detect and adjust to changes in spine/patient position in less than 1 second with an accuracy approaching ±0.5 mm.[6,20]

The CyberKnife system is designed so that when a patient is positioned within the treatment area, the target is near the center of an 80-cm³ sphere that is defined with respect to the patient's anatomy. There are 100 equally spaced points on the surface of the sphere called nodes. At each node, the robot defines 12 beams of radiation that intersect various portions of the tumor volume. The robotic arm moves the LINAC to, and stops at, each node, where the beam is precisely aimed and a prescribed dose of irradiation is administered. Treatment plans are formed from a subset of the entire constellation of radiation beams, which maximizes irradiation of the target area and minimizes normal tissue irradiation. In practice, not all nodes are available because objects within the treatment room either interfere with the x-ray beam or prevent the robotic arm from positioning the LINAC at a particular node. During system installation, these obscured nodes are disabled. At least 50 nodes, and as many as 200 beams or more, are used during treatment. Since the robot can aim a beam anywhere within the tumor volume (as opposed to only the center of the

sphere like most radiosurgical systems), highly conformal treatment plans can be created for complex geometries in a nonisocentric manner.[30]

TREATMENT PROCEDURE

Spinal Immobilization

Simple immobilization is used during pretreatment scanning and treatment. It is important to note that the targeting method used by the CyberKnife does not require immobilization. Instead these devices are used for patient comfort, to expedite initial patient alignment, and restrict movement once treatment has commenced. To achieve this goal at Stanford, we employ the Aquaplast mask (WFR Corp., Wyckoff, NJ) in our cervical spine patients (Fig. 138-2A). The mask is made of a thermoplastic mesh and secures the head and neck on a radiolucent headrest. Thoracic and lumbar spine patients are placed in a custom Styrofoam-like body mold called AlphaCradle (Smithers Medical Products, Inc., Akron, OH) (see Fig. 138-2B). To date, all our patients have been treated in the supine position.

Targeting Spinal Lesions with Fiducial Placement

Bony landmarks of the spine can be used to target cervical spine lesions. However, at present, the accuracy of referencing

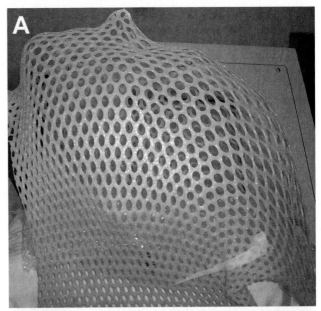

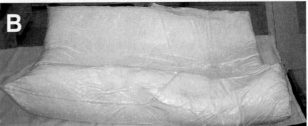

FIGURE 138-2 Simple immobilization devices used during CyberKnife treatment. *A*, Aquaplast mask used in cervical spine patients. *B*, AlphaCradle custom body mold used in lesions below the cervical spine.

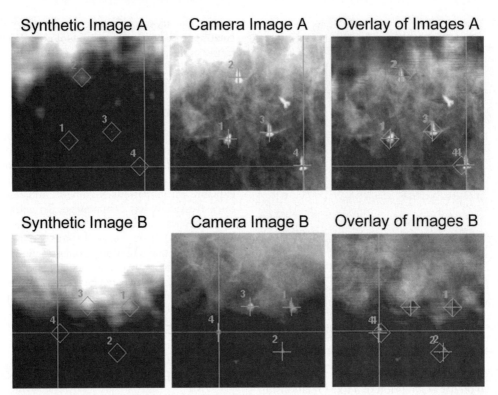

FIGURE 138-3 *Left:* Computed tomography–based, computer-generated images of fiducials within the cervical spine from the perspective of their corresponding orthogonally placed x-ray camera as denoted by A and B. *Middle:* Real-time images of the target area from the same patient in the left column produced by the two orthogonally placed x-ray sources. *Right:* Overlay of synthetic and real-time images that the guidance system uses to aim the robotic arm–mounted LINAC during CyberKnife treatment.

based on these bony landmarks is not completely reliable.[7] The large amount soft tissue surrounding the thoracic and lumbar spine prevents optimal imaging of these regions, also introducing targeting error. To overcome these shortcomings, spatial referencing in these areas is based on tiny metal fiducials placed in bone near the lesion. Fiducials, which are 2 × 6-mm surgical stainless steel self-tapping screws, are placed in a noncoplanar manner on the lamina and/or facets around a spinal target (Fig. 138-3). Under fluoroscopic guidance, the fiducials are inserted into the spinal elements through stab incisions in the skin so as to be at least 25 mm apart. Four to six fiducials are generally employed, although only three are required to define a full spatial transformation in all six degrees of target translation and rotation.[27,30] By virtue of their fixed relationship to the bony spine, any movement in the vertebrae is detected as movement of the fiducials. Such movement is automatically detected and compensated for by the CyberKnife system. Fiducial placement is typically an outpatient procedure that requires less than 30 minutes of operative time. The overall accuracy of CyberKnife spinal radiosurgery guided by fiducials has been calculated to be approximately 1.5 mm.[7]

Treatment Planning

Treatment plans are designed using the Accuray Treatment Planning System that runs on Silicon Graphics workstations (SGI, Mountain View, CA).[17,28,31] Treatment planning begins with a contrast computed tomography scan of the area of interest after the fiducials have been placed. For optimal

imaging, 1.25-mm slices are obtained. This scan is used to generate DRRs that are used for position tracking. The computed tomography scan is downloaded into the Treatment Planning System, and, using the graphics interface, the volume of the target lesion and adjacent radiation-sensitive structures, such as the spinal cord, are defined. An acceptable tolerable dose of irradiation to these areas must be specified (Figs. 138-4 to 138-6). The system uses this contour data to create a 3-dimensional representation of the lesion geometry and define an initial set of beam configurations. The beams are configured so that they are evenly and randomly distributed over the surface of the target with dose weighting to satisfy the specified dose constraints (Fig. 138-7). If the constraints cannot be satisfied, the system uses the previously obtained data and determines a new set of beam configurations with a greater probability of satisfying the constraints. This process continues until a feasible and acceptable set of beams and weights are found. The resulting plan is then presented for review, which can either be accepted or used to redefine new constraint parameters and iterate another solution. At Stanford, each treatment plan is reviewed by a multidisciplinary team consisting of neurosurgeons, radiation oncologists, and radiation physicists before patient treatment.

Treatment Delivery

At the time of CyberKnife radiosurgery, patients are positioned supine on the operating table supported in their customized immobilization devices. Once positioned, images of the relevant spinal anatomy are obtained from the two

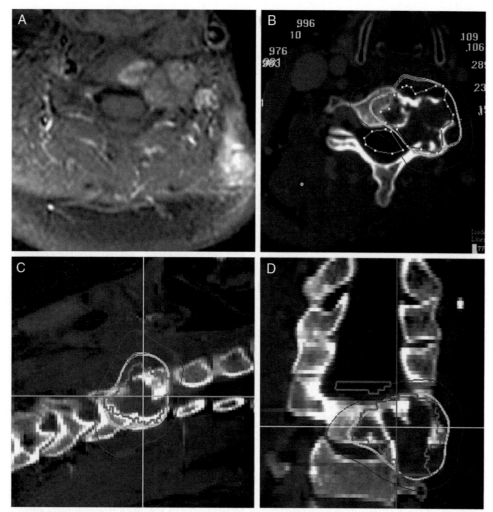

FIGURE 138-4   Treatment plan example in a patient with large malignant neuroendocrine tumor at C5–6 treated with 20 Gy to the 76% isodose line in two stages. (*A*), Pretreatment axial T1 postcontrast magnetic resonance imaging. Axial (*B*), sagittal (*C*), and coronal (*D*) postcontrast computed tomography images used in treatment planning are demonstrated. Red lines (with or without solid squares) demarcate the outline of the lesion, solid green lines demarcate the 76% isodose curve, and the purple lines demarcate the 50% isodose cure. The green line with squares demarcates the critical structure, the spinal cord. (See Color Plate.)

orthogonally placed digital x-ray cameras and compared with the DRRs made from the treatment planning scan. At the start of CyberKnife radiosurgery, the operating table is moved manually to optimally align the real-time x-ray images with the synthetic DRRs. System software searches a defined region of interest within these images for the position of those fiducials and bony landmarks that will be used for targeting (see Fig. 138-3). Once the initial patient position has been manually optimized, the remaining processes are all automatic.[28] The robotic arm moves the LINAC sequentially through the planned beam positions (nodes) delivering the measured dose at each node. At each position, the imaging system reestablishes the location of the target and sends corrective pointing directions to the robotic arm. As a consequence, the aiming of the LINAC beam is repeatedly adapted to position shifts of the patient. Although this can be done at each node, we more typically check position only approximately once per minute when immobilization seems adequate and the patient is cooperative. This process of intermittent retargeting has proven to be reliable and accurate.[32] All treatments are performed on an outpatient basis.

RESULTS: THE STANFORD EXPERIENCE WITH SPINAL RADIOSURGERY

We have treated a wide range of lesions throughout the spinal axis. From March 1999 to December 2003, 73 spinal lesions in 66 patients were treated at Stanford University Medical Center using the above protocol. Ages ranged from 12 to 86 years (mean, 44.5). There were 33 women. Patients were treated in 153 sessions using one to five fractions per lesion (mean, 2.3). The lesions were distributed across the spinal axis in the following manner: 32 cervical, 31 thoracic, 11 lumbar, and 4 sacral (some lesions overlapped the border of spinal regions, i.e., cervicothoracic). The types of lesions treated included benign tumors, metastases, and vascular malformations (Table 138-3). Before treatment, the most common symptoms were myelopathy and pain.

Benign

The most commonly treated lesions were benign tumors (37 patients, 39 lesions). Mean prescription isodose was 20.2 Gy (range, 18.0 to 25.2) with a mean prescription isodose

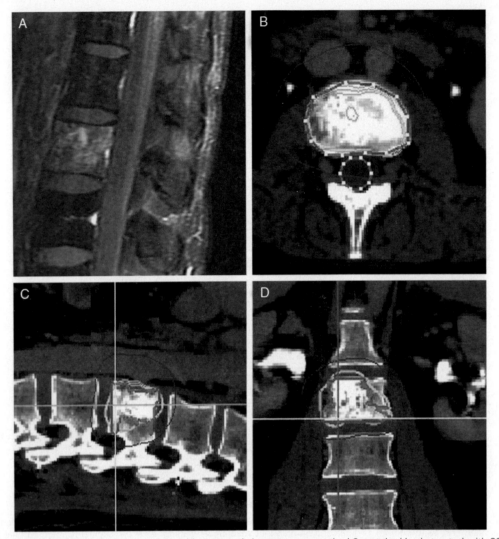

FIGURE 138-5 Treatment plan example in a patient with metastatic breast cancer to the L2 vertebral body treated with 20 Gy to the 83% isodose line in two stages. (*A*), Pretreatment sagittal T1-weighted postcontrast magnetic resonance imaging. Axial (*B*), sagittal (*C*), and coronal (*D*) postcontrast computed tomography images used in treatment planning are demonstrated. Red lines (with or without solid squares) demarcate the outline of the lesion, the solid green lines demarcate the 83% isodose curve, and the purple lines demarcate the 50% isodose cure. The green line with squares demarcates the critical structure, the spinal cord. (See Color Plate.)

line of 79.6% (range, 70% to 90%). The mean maximal dose was 27.6 Gy (range, 20.2 to 34.3). Mean tumor volume was 4.99 mL (range, 0.091 to 33.9). Collimator aperture ranged from 7.5 to 25 mm. Twenty patients had previous surgery, and CyberKnife was used either as a direct adjuvant or to treat recurrent disease. Seventeen patients opted for CyberKnife as primary treatment due to surgically inaccessible lesions, medical comorbidities that precluded surgery, or preference. One 30-year-old woman with neurofibromatosis 2 and a C2 neurofibroma that was causing a significant myelopathy had further progression in her symptoms after CyberKnife treatment. Ten months later, this patient underwent laminectomy and resection of her tumor without incident, after which the myelopathy improved appreciably.

Malignant

Twenty malignant lesions were treated (18 metastatic and 2 primary) in 19 patients. The average prescription isodose was 20.5 Gy (range, 12.0 to 24.0) as defined at a mean isodose

line of 75.5% (range, 64% to 84%). The mean maximal dose was 27.1 Gy (range, 15.0 to 33.8). Malignant tumors were the largest lesions treated with a mean tumor volume of 52.8 mL (range, 3.2 to 168). This reflected the involvement of entire vertebral bodies in many cases. Collimator aperture ranged from 12.5 to 40 mm. Only four patients had previous surgery. Of significance, 11 patients in this group had been treated previously with radiotherapy. Among these patients, it was thought that only CyberKnife radiosurgery could safely administer further irradiation to this location. One patient with a malignant nerve sheath tumor developed a recurrence after CyberKnife radiosurgery and was retreated. One patient died of systemic disease.

Arteriovenous Malformations

Ten arteriovenous malformations (AVMs) were treated with a mean prescription isodose of 21.1 Gy (range, 20.0 to 25.0) and a mean maximal dose was 25.2 Gy (range, 23.4 to 28.9). The mean prescription isodose line was 84% (range, 80%

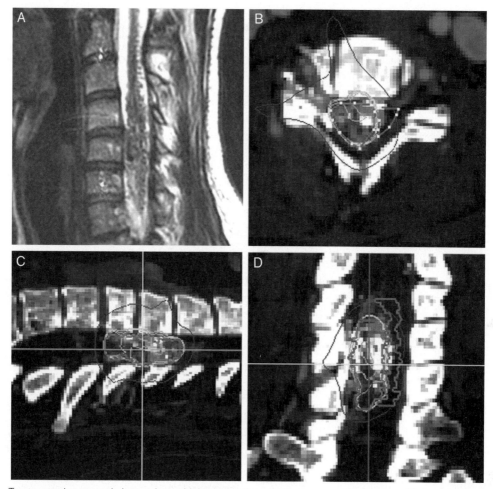

FIGURE 138-6 Treatment plan example in a patient with intramedullary arteriovenous malformation at C5–6 treated with 20 Gy to the 85% isodose line in two stages. (*A*), Pretreatment sagittal T2-weighted magnetic resonance imaging. Axial (*B*), sagittal (*C*), and coronal (*D*) postcontrast computed tomography images used in treatment planning are demonstrated. Red lines (with or without solid squares) demarcate the outline of the lesion, the solid green lines demarcate the 85% isodose curve, and the purple lines demarcate the 50% isodose cure. The green line with squares demarcates the critical structure, the spinal cord. (See Color Plate.)

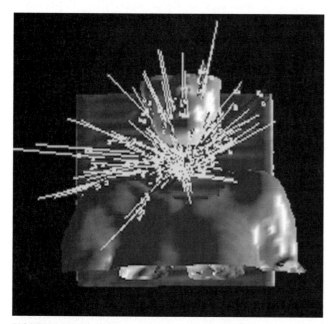

FIGURE 138-7 Three-dimensional reconstruction of actual beam paths used in the treatment of patient in Figure 138-4.

to 90%). The volume of treated AVM averaged 2.33 mL (range, 0.8 to 4.9). Collimators ranged from 7.5 to 15 mm. One patient developed significant myelopathy 3 months after treatment of a cervical AVM. Magnetic resonance imaging demonstrated new hemorrhage within the AVM. After 1 year of follow-up, the patient's symptoms had resolved and the AVM was smaller on magnetic resonance imaging. Two patients have had angiograms 3 years after treatment, and both demonstrate significant reduction in the size of their AVMs.

Intramedullary

Many intramedullary spinal cord lesions have limited treatment options. Some are not surgically resectable, and in others, standard radiation therapy can result in intolerable doses to adjacent cord and/or posttreatment edema. We have treated 15 such intramedullary lesions (10 AVMs and 5 hemangioblastomas). Only one patient in this group developed new weakness posttreatment, which eventually resolved with steroids. Although the CyberKnife may represent a relatively safe treatment option for some patients with intramedullary lesions,

TABLE 138-3 ▪ Treatment Data Summary for 65 Patients Treated with Spinal Radiosurgery

	No. of Patients	Mean Prescribed Isodose (Gy)	Mean Maximal Dose (Gy)	Mean Prescribed Isodose Line (%)
Tumors				
Beingn				
Neurofibroma	7	18.9	29.5	80.9
Meningioma	10	20.3	26.4	78.9
Schwannoma	11	19.0	24.6	79.4
Hemangioblastoma	5	21.3	36.8	78.1
Ependymoma	2	18.0	23.0	79.0
Epidermoid	1*	19.0	22.2	81.0
Chordoma	1	25.0	31.2	80.0
Total	37	20.2	27.6	79.6
Malignant				
Metastatic	18	20.8	25.8	77.6
Primary	1†	20.3	28.4	73.3
Total	19	20.5	27.1	75.5
Vascular Malformations				
Arteriovenous malformation	10	21.1	25.2	84.0

*One patient with two separate lesions.
†One patient with three separate lesions.

longer follow-up will be needed to establish its ultimate effectiveness.

COMPLICATIONS

In the Stanford experience with spinal radiosurgery, no patient reported acute changes in baseline symptoms after treatment. However, as mentioned previously, one patient hemorrhaged within an AVM 3 months after radiosurgery. It is unclear whether this hemorrhage was directly related to the CyberKnife treatment or part of the natural history of the disease. Another patient presented 6 months after CyberKnife radiosurgery of a C3–4 schwannoma with new neck pain and bilateral arm dysesthesias. Although magnetic resonance imaging demonstrated the tumor size to be stable, a new intratumoral cyst had developed and was further compressing the cord. Another patient with a T4 vertebral body metastasis from breast cancer developed a significant myelopathy 4 months after radiosurgery. Spinal magnetic resonance imaging revealed radiation-induced edema in the adjacent thoracic spinal cord. After starting glucocorticoids, she experienced a gradual improvement in her leg weakness. There were two complications with fiducial placement, both occurring with an early generation bone tack as opposed to the more recent self-drilling screw; one such patient required a laminectomy to evacuate a small epidural hematoma and retrieve the fiducial. No complications have occurred with the screw-based fiducials.

SUMMARY

Our preliminary experience with the CyberKnife demonstrates that spinal radiosurgery is feasible and generally safe. To date, the vast majority of patients have derived some clinical benefit from treatment in terms of tumor control and stabilization of symptoms. For the many benign lesions treated to date, much longer follow-up will be needed to determine the ultimate efficacy of spinal radiosurgery.

REFERENCES

1. Kopelson G, Linggood R, Kleinmann G: Management of intramedullary spinal cord tumors. Radiology 135:473–479, 1980.
2. McCuniff AJ, Liang MJ: Radiation tolerance of the cervical spinal cord. Int J Radiat Oncol Biol Phys 16:675–678, 1989.
3. Marcus RB, Millon RR: The incidence of myelitis after irradiation of the cervical spinal cord. Int J Radiat Oncol Biol Phys 17:3–8, 1990.
4. van der Kogel AV: Radiation injury in the central nervous system. In Lunsford D (ed): Stereotactic Radiosurgery. New York: McGraw-Hill, 1993, pp 43–64.
5. Schultheiss TE, Kun LE, Ang KK, Stephens LC: Radiation response of the central nervous system. Int J Radiat Oncol Biol Phys 22:1093–1112, 1995.
6. Ryu S, Fang Yin F, Rock J, et al: Image-guided and intensity-modulated radiosurgery for patients with spinal metastasis. Cancer 97:2013–2018, 2003.
7. Ryu SI, Chang SD, Kim DH, et al: Image-guided hypo-fractionated stereotactic radiosurgery to spinal lesions. Neurosurgery 49:838–846, 2001.
8. Leksell L: The stereotactic method and radiosurgery of the brain. Acta Chir Scand 102:316–319, 1959.
9. Woroschiloff C: Der Verlauf der motorischen und sensililen Bahnen durch das Lendenmark des Kaninchens. Ber Vehr Sachs Ges Wiss Leipzig 26:248–304, 1874.
10. Rand RW, Bauer RO, Smart CR, et al: Experiences with percutaneous stereotaxic cryocordotomy. Bull Los Angeles Neurol Soc 30:705–706, 1965.
11. Hitchock E: An apparatus for stereotactic spinal surgery. Lancet 1:705–706, 1969.
12. Nadvornik P: Woroschiloff's locating device for interventions on the spinal cord and its influence on spinal stereotaxic. Appl Neurophysiol 48:247–251, 1985.
13. Hamilton AJ, Lulu BA, Fosmire H, et al: Preliminary clinical experience with linear accelerator-based spinal stereotactic radiosurgery. Neurosurgery 36:311–319, 1995.

14. Hamilton AJ, Lulu BA: A prototype device for linear accelerator-based extracranial radiosurgery. Acta Neurochir Suppl (Wien) 60: 40–43, 1995.

15. Hamilton AJ, Lulu BA, Fosmire H, Gossett L: LINAC-based spinal stereotactic radiosurgery. Stereotact Funct Neurosurg 66:1–9, 1996.

16. Hamilton AJ: Radiosurgical treatment of spinal metastasis. In Maciunas RJ (ed): Advanced Techniques in Central Nervous System Metastases. Park Ridge, IL: AANS, 1998, pp 255–268.

17. Adler JR, Jr, Chang SD, Murphy MJ, et al: The CyberKnife: A frameless robotic system for radiosurgery. Stereotact Funct Neurosurg 69: 124–128, 1997.

18. Chang SD, Murphy M, Geis P, et al: Clinical experience with image-guided robotic radiosurgery (the CyberKnife) in the treatment of brain and spinal cord tumors. Neurol Med Chir (Tokyo) 38:780–783, 1998.

19. Shaw E, Kline R, Gillin M, et al: Radiation Therapy Oncology Group: Radiosurgery quality assurance guidelines. Int J Radiat Oncol Biol Phys 20:1231–1239, 1993.

20. Murphy MJ, Cox RS: The accuracy of dose localization for an image-guided frameless radiosurgery system. Med Phys 23:2043–2049, 1996.

21. Murphy MJ: An automatic six-degree-of-freedom image restoration algorithm for image-guided frameless stereotaxic radiosurgery. Med Phys 24:857–866, 1997.

22. Chang SD, Meisel JA, Hancock SL, et al: Treatment of hemangioblastomas in von Hippel-Lindau disease with linear accelerator-based radiosurgery. Neurosurgery 43:28–35, 1998.

23. Chang SD, Murphy MJ, Martin DP, et al: Image-guided robotic radiosurgery: clinical and radiographic results with the CyberKnife. In Kondziolka D (ed): Radiosurgery 1999. Basel: Karger, 2000, pp 23–33.

24. Chang SD, Murphy MJ, Martin DP, et al: Frameless stereotactic neurosurgery. In Petrovich Z, Brady IW, Apuzzo ML, et al (eds): Combined Modality Therapy of Central Nervous System Tumors. New York: Springer, 2000, pp 387–396.

25. Murphy MJ, Chang SD, Gibbs IC, et al: Image-guided radiosurgery in the treatment of spinal metastasis. Neurosurg Focus 11:1–7, 2001.

26. Murphy MJ, Martin D, Whyte R, et al: The effectiveness of breath-holding to stabilize lung and pancreas tumors during radiosurgery. Int J Radiat Oncol Biol Phys 29:475–482, 2002.

27. Gerszten PC, Ozhasoglu C, Burton SA, et al: CyberKnife frameless real-time image-guided stereotactic radiosurgery for the treatment of spinal lesions. Int J Radiat Oncol Biol Phys 30:S370–S371, 2003.

28. Murphy MJ, Adler JR, Jr, Bodduluri M, et al: Image-guided radiosurgery for the spine and pancreas. Comput Aided Surg 5:278–288, 2000.

29. Samwel H, Slappendel R, Crul BJ, Voerman VF: Psychological predictors of the effectiveness of radiofrequency lesioning of the cervical spinal dorsal ganglion (RF-DRG). Eur J Pain 4:149–155, 2000.

30. Chang SD, Le QT, Martin DP, et al: The CyberKnife. In Dickman CA, Fehlings MG, Gokaslan ZL (eds): Spinal Cord and Spinal Column Tumors: Principles and Practice. New York: Thieme (in press).

31. Chang SD, Adler JR, Jr, Murphy MJ: Stereotactic radiosurgery of spinal lesions. In Maciunas R (ed): Advanced Techniques in Central Nervous System Metastasis. Park Ridge, IL: AANS, 1998, pp 269–276.

32. Murphy MJ, Chang SD, Gibbs IC, et al: Patterns of patient movement during frameless image-guided radiosurgery. Int J Radiat Oncol Biol Phys 31:1400–1408, 2003.

139 Surgical Approaches to the Cervicothoracic Junction

HOANG N. LE, DANIEL H. KIM, ISSADA THONGTRANGAN, JON PARK, and RICHARD G. FESSLER

Surgical treatment of spinal disorders at the cervicothoracic junction can be a challenging issue because it requires a thorough understanding of the complex anatomy and biomechanical properties of the inherently unstable area. Access to this region is complicated by the presence of major vascular elements as well as important visceral and soft-tissue structures. Precise familiarity with surgical landmarks and associated vital structures around the cervicothoracic junction will guide treatment in terms of both surgical approaches and stabilization techniques. Treatment of this area is complex, as evidenced by a diversity of reported literature from neurosurgeons; orthopedics surgeons; ear, nose, and throat surgeons; and cardiothoracic surgeons. In the treatment of cervicothoracic junction instability, potential pitfalls exist from the initial diagnosis to management to surgical approaches and stabilization techniques.

Pathologic processes in this region are relatively uncommon but can include trauma, degenerative processes, infection, and neoplastic involvement. Neoplastic involvement of the upper thoracic vertebrae accounts for 15% of patients with neoplasms of the spine. Furthermore, 10% of spinal metastases arise from the T1–4 region. Traumatic injuries to the cervicothoracic junction can be as high as 9%.[1] Other pathologic processes that may involve this area include bacterial and tuberculous infections, pathologic fractures secondary to primary bone disease, primary bone tumors, meningeal tumors, vascular malformations, congenital connective tissue and skeletal disorders, trauma, and thoracic disc herniations (Table 139-1). If not carefully investigated, injuries to this area will be often overlooked on routine radiographic studies and may lead to further spinal instability and neurologic compromise. Neurologic involvement is a common sequela to cervicothoracic lesions causing instability and can be as high as 80%.[2,3] Thus treatment for lesions involving the cervicothoracic junction is often surgical, with goals encompassing neural decompression, immediate stabilization, restoration of anatomic spinal alignment, and early rehabilitation.

Posterior approaches, such as laminectomy and pediculectomy, are common approaches that provide poor exposure of the anterior spinal elements and may not be adequate in the management of complex spinal pathology. When performed for disease centered in the vertebral body, laminectomy may be ineffective and have a higher complication rate than anterior or lateral approaches.[4,5] When anterior disease results in unstable anterior and middle columns of the spine, posterior approaches may disrupt spinal stability further.

The limitations imposed by purely posterior exposure have resulted in the development of a variety of anterior and posterolateral surgical approaches to treat lesions in this region of the spine. The first detailed description of a posterolateral approach to the anterior elements of the spine was of the costotransversectomy.[6] Although this technique gave adequate exposure of the middle and low thoracic spine, scapula, levator scapulae, rhomboid, and trapezius musculature, it was less useful in the upper thoracic region. In 1954, Capener[7] described a more extensive posterolateral exposure, the lateral rhachotomy. In 1976, Larson and colleagues[8] reported a modification of the lateral rhachotomy, the lateral extracavitary approach, which provided improved exposure of the middle and lower thoracic spine with somewhat less morbidity. For the cervicothoracic junction, anterior column exposure in both the lateral rhachotomy and lateral extracavitary approaches are limited by the shoulder girdle. The lateral, parascapular, extrapleural operation, a modification of the lateral extracavitary operations, eliminates those obstructions and provides excellent exposure of the thoracic vertebrae up to the inferior end plate of C7.[9]

Purely anterior approaches to the cervicothoracic junction were independently described by Jonnesco[10] and Brunig[11] in 1923. These were supraclavicular approaches and were later used by Royle[12] for spastic paralysis, by Gask[13] for Raynaud's disease, and by Ochsner and DeBakey[14] for thoracic sympathectomy. Because the clavicle was left intact, exposure of the thoracic area was restricted. A modification of this approach, the transmanubrial and transclavicular approach, was described by Sundaresan and colleagues[15] in 1984 and modified by Birch and colleagues[16] in 1990. These modifications call for removal of the medial one third of the clavicle as well as a portion of the manubrium, significantly increasing exposure of the upper thoracic vertebrae.

The third major approach to the anterior vertebral elements of the thoracic spine was first described by Hodgson and colleagues.[17] This approach, the anterolateral thoracotomy, involves resection of the third rib and requires transpleural mobilization of the lung and ligation and division of the intercostal arteries, veins, and hemiazygos vein.

The following sections discuss the clinical presentation of disease at the cervicothoracic junction, preoperative evaluation, anesthetic considerations, relevant regional surgical anatomy of the cervicothoracic junction as it pertains to the surgical approach, biomechanics of the cervicothoracic junction, surgical approaches, and, finally, options for surgical reconstruction and stabilization.

CLINICAL FEATURES

The differential diagnosis of disease processes in this region is listed in Table 139-1. Depending on the exact location of

TABLE 139-1 ▪ Differential Diagnosis of Lesions of the Cervicothoracic Junction

Metastatic tumors
Primary tumors of bone
Primary lymphoma
Intradural, extramedullary tumors
Intradural, intramedullary tumors
Bacterial infections
Tuberculous infections
Vascular malformations
Pathologic fracture (primary metabolic disease of bone)
Connective tissue and skeletal disorders
Traumatic vertebral fractures
Disc herniations

the lesion, disease processes in this region can present as pain without neurologic signs, thoracic myelopathy, C7 or T1 radiculopathy, or a combination of these signs and symptoms. Table 139-2 lists the presenting signs and symptoms in our series of patients with pathologic processes located between C7 and T4. Of these patients, 83% initially presented with generalized upper thoracic back pain. Only 33% presented with radicular pain in the C8 and T1 distributions or in the upper thoracic region. Leg weakness was seen in 58% of the patients, whereas decreased sensation was demonstrated in 92%. Only 35% of the patients demonstrated hand weakness on examination, consistent with the fewer number of patients whose pathology extended as high as C7 and T1. On presentation, 17% of patients had bowel or bladder dysfunction. Ataxia was demonstrated in 25%, and 58% had a positive Babinski sign.

Preoperative Evaluation

Radiographic Evaluation

Radiologic evaluation of this area of the spine begins with anteroposterior and lateral plain radiographs. These radiographs may demonstrate traumatic or pathologic vertebral fractures, infections, evidence of metabolic bone disease, primary or metastatic tumors, and deformities such as kyphosis. Pathologic and traumatic fractures are demonstrated by malalignment, vertebral collapse, and widening of the pedicles on anteroposterior radiograph.

The earliest and most consistent radiographic finding in osteomyelitis or discitis is narrowing of the disc space, which

TABLE 139-2 ▪ Signs and Symptoms at Presentation of Patients with C7–T4 Pathologic Processes (17 Patients)

Signs and Symptoms	Percent of Patients with Signs or Symptoms
Back pain	83
Radicular pain	33
Leg weakness	58
Decreased sensation	92
Hand weakness	35
Bowel or bladder dysfunction	17
Ataxia	25
Babinski sign	58

is present in 74% of patients at presentation.[18] After 3 to 6 weeks, destructive changes in the body can be noted, which usually begin as lytic areas in the anterior aspect of the body adjacent to the disc and end plate. Active bone formation and sclerosis are present in 11% of patients on presentation. Approximately 30% to 70% of the bone must be destroyed before osteomyelitic metastases are visible on plain radiographs.[19] Several classic signs, however, suggest the presence of vertebral metastases, including vertebral collapse, unilateral erosion of a pedicle, *fishmouthing* (cephalad and caudad end plate concavity within the vertebral body), and osteoblastic lesions.

Radionucleotide bone scintigraphy is sensitive, although not specific, in detecting metastatic disease to the spine, infections, and fractures.[20,21] False-negative results have been reported with aggressive lesions, such as lung cancer, renal cell carcinoma, and myeloproliferative diseases, as well as in cases of regional ischemia and in patients with leukopenia.[22–24]

The use of myelography is primarily to evaluate the patency of the subarachnoid space. Myelography can demonstrate the level of a metastatic lesion in the thoracic spine by indentation or complete blockade of the myelographic dye column as it flows through the thoracic spinal canal. In addition, it can demonstrate the presence of intradural extramedullary or intramedullary tumors, thoracic disc herniations, retropulsed vertebral fragments from pathologic or traumatic fractures, and vascular malformations.

After myelography, computed tomography scan aids in the evaluation of metastatic disease to the thoracic spine, the exact location of intradural tumors, thoracic disc herniations, and the presence of vascular malformations. In addition, it defines the extent of paraspinal soft-tissue involvement for the staging of metastatic tumors and surgical planning. Computed tomography also help determine the extent of bone destruction. Finally, computed tomography scans distinguish between osteoporosis and tumor.

Magnetic resonance imaging is the most important diagnostic tool for the evaluation of disease in the thoracic spine. Magnetic resonance imaging permits early diagnosis of infection and recognition of paravertebral or intraspinal abscesses without the risk associated with myelography.[25] Magnetic resonance imaging is also effective in demonstrating the extent of metastatic disease, primary tumors of bone, primary lymphoma, intradural tumors, thoracic disc herniations, and vertebral fractures and may be helpful in spinal vascular malformations. It has been found to be at least as sensitive and accurate as gallium and bone scanning combined.[26] Last, magnetic resonance imaging demonstrates anatomic relationships and surgical corridors.

Metabolic Evaluation

Routine metabolic evaluation of pathology in the cervicothoracic junction should include complete blood count with platelets and differential as well as kidney profile (electrolytes, blood urea nitrogen, and creatinine), liver profile, and erythrocyte sedimentation rate. Other metabolic evaluations that may be helpful include calcium analysis, phosphorus, alkaline phosphatase, serum protein electrophoresis, and serum transferrin analysis. Antinuclear antibody and rheumatoid factor analysis may help in the evaluation for rheumatoid arthritis. Bone marrow aspirate may be helpful in the diagnosis of blood-borne dyscrasias. Specific antigen markers that may contribute to the diagnosis of a specific tumor include carcinoembryonic antigen, serum acid phosphatase, and prostate-specific antigen.

Approach-Related Surgical Anatomy

Lateral, Parascapular, Extrapleural Approach and Anterolateral Thoracotomy Approach

The lateral, parascapular, extrapleural approach to the cervicothoracic junction is an extreme posterolateral approach that allows nearly lateral access to the vertebral bodies. The anterolateral thoracotomy approach is a transthoracic approach through the third rib to the upper thoracic vertebrae that allows access to the anterior and lateral aspects of the vertebrae and control of the mediastinal vasculature. Because of the extensive overlap of anatomy relevant to these two approaches, they are considered together and summarized in three major areas: (1) scapula and parascapular anatomy, (2) posterior thoracic cage, and (3) retromediastinal space and spinal anatomy.

SCAPULAR AND PARASCAPULAR ANATOMY

Posterolateral access to the thoracic cage and vertebral elements is hindered by the scapular and the parascapular shoulder musculature (Fig. 139-1). Mobilization of the scapula anterolaterally is necessary and requires the disruption of the posteromedial shoulder musculature.

The first muscle encountered after skin incision is the trapezius muscle. The trapezius originates along the superior nuchal line and external occipital protuberance and on each spinous process (via the ligamentum nuchae) from C1 through T12. The insertion of the trapezius muscle is divided into upper, intermediate, and lower divisions, which pass to the lateral third of the clavicle, the acromion, and the scapular spine. The lower fibers form an aponeurosis,

which inserts on the tubercle of the lower lip of the scapular spine. These insertions enable the trapezius muscle to function in stabilization and abduction of the shoulder. The trapezius muscle is supplied by the spinal accessory nerve that arises from C1–5 and directly via the ventral rami of C3 and C4. The spinal accessory nerve lies deep to the trapezius muscle but superficial to the levator scapulae. Its arterial supply is from branches of the dorsal scapular artery.

Immediately deep to the trapezius muscle lies the rhomboid major, rhomboid minor, and levator scapulae muscles. The rhomboid major originates on the ligamentum nuchae of the spinous processes T1 through T4, whereas the rhomboid minor originates similarly on the spinous processes of C6 and C7. Both of these muscles insert along the vertebral edge of the scapula: rhomboid minor above and rhomboid major below the scapular spine. The nervous innervation and arterial supply of the rhomboid muscles come from the dorsal scapular nerve and artery. Nervous supply to the levator scapulae muscle is via branches from C3, C4, and C5. Arterial supply to the levator scapulae is also from branches of the dorsal scapular artery. Both of these structures lie deep to the bodies of the muscles and are located somewhat medially under the scapula. In a routine exposure, neither the dorsal scapular nerve nor the dorsal scapular artery or vein is directly exposed.

Immediately deep to the trapezius muscle from C6 through approximately T2 lies the serratus posterior superior muscle. Ventral to this, the splenius arises from the ligamentum nuchae and upper thoracic spine and divides into two parts: the splenius capitis and splenius cervicis. The splenius capitis inserts with the sternocleidomastoid muscle on the superior nuchal line and mastoid process. The splenius cervicis joins the levator scapulae to insert on the transverse processes of C1 through C4. These muscles function in stabilization and rotation of the skull.

In the initial dissection for exposure of the cervicothoracic junction, the spinous process insertions of the trapezius,

FIGURE 139-1 Relationship of the scapula to the incision and surgical approach to the cervicothoracic junction via the lateral parascapular extrapleural approach.

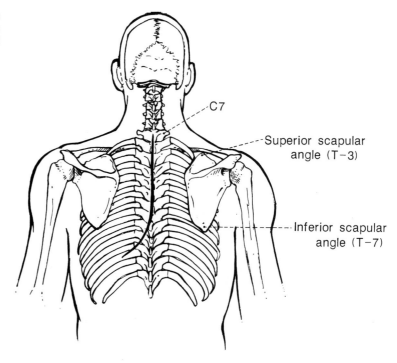

rhomboid, serratus posterior superior, splenius capitis, and splenius cervicis are taken down as a single group for lateral retraction. As these muscles are taken down, the scapula is released from its attachments to the spinous processes and rotates anterolaterally out of the operative field. This maneuver exposes the posterior and posterior lateral rib cage for the remainder of the procedure.

Posterior Thoracic Cage

The next group of muscles encountered is the deep or intrinsic muscles (Fig. 139-2). These include the erector spinae muscles and the transversospinalis muscles. The erector spinae muscles originate as a dense aponeurotic band from the sacrum and divide into three columns below the last rib. The iliocostalis muscle is located most laterally and is inserted into the angles of the ribs and into the cervical transverse processes from C4 through C6. This insertion is achieved through a series of related bundles of muscles that extend over approximately six segments each. Where one muscle is inserted, another arises on its medial side and extends cephalad. The longissimus muscles (thoracis, cervicis, and capitis) are inserted into lumbar and thoracic transverse processes and nearby parts of the ribs between T2 and T12. Muscle bundles arising medial to these, from T1 to T4, are relayed to the cervical transverse processes from C2 through C6. Other bundles arising medially to these insertions extend as broad fleshy bands and attach to the mastoid process deep to the splenius capitis and sternocleidomastoid muscles. These insertions result in the longissimus being the only erector spinae muscle to reach the skull. The spinalis muscle is largely aponeurotic and extends from the upper lumbar to the lower cervical spinous processes.

The transversospinalis group of muscles passes obliquely cephalad from the transverse processes to the spinous processes immediately deep to the erector spinae muscles. These muscles fall into three layers. The most superficial layer, the semispinalis, arises near the tips of the transverse processes and inserts near the tips of the spinous processes approximately five vertebral levels cephalad. In the upper thoracic and lower cervical spine, most of this muscle is composed of the semispinalis capitis. This muscle passes from the upper thoracic transverse processes and lower cervical articular processes (C4 to T4) to the occipital bone between the superior and inferior nuchal lines. Its fibers run nearly vertically, and its medial border is free, separated from its contralateral partner by the ligamentum nuchae. The intermediate layer, the multifidus, arises from the dense aponeurosis of the overlying erector spinae muscle and from all transverse processes up to C4 and inserts into the lower border of each spinous process. This muscle generally spans approximately three levels. The deepest muscles of this group, the rotatores, are small muscles that bridge one interspace. They pass from the root of one transverse process to the root of the spinous process immediately above. The actions of these muscles extend the vertebral column or, when acting individually on one side, bend and rotate the vertebrae. The entire group of erector spinae muscles and transversospinalis muscles can be dissected off the spinous processes, laminae, facets, and transverse processes as a single muscular mass. Control of the musculature in this way exposes all vertebral elements from the tip of the spinous processes to the tip of the transverse processes as well as the costotransverse ligaments, the joints, and the ribs.

Each rib articulates with its own vertebral body, the vertebra above, and the intervertebral disc between them (Fig. 139-3). In the upper thoracic spine, the only exception to this general rule is the first rib, which articulates only with its own vertebral body. The tubercle of each rib also articulates with the transverse process of its own vertebra. Each of these articulations forms separate synovial joints. Those formed with the posterolateral surfaces of each vertebral body are separated by an intra-articular ligament, which is attached to the intervertebral disc. These joints are surrounded by an articular capsule and attached to the vertebral body anteriorly by the radiate ligament. The third synovial joint of this complex, the costotransverse joint, is also surrounded by an articular capsule, which is strengthened laterally by the lateral costotransverse ligament and the costotransverse ligament. In addition, the superior costotransverse ligament joins the neck of the rib to the transverse

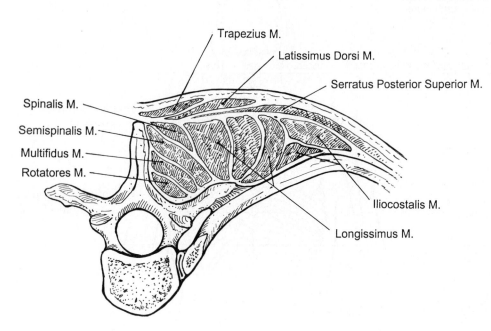

Trapezius M.

Latissimus Dorsi M.

Serratus Posterior Superior M.

Spinalis M.

Semispinalis M.

Multifidus M.

Rotatores M.

Iliocostalis M.

Longissimus M.

FIGURE 139-2 Cross-sectional anatomy of the deep or intrinsic muscle layer of the upper thoracic spine. M., muscle.

FIGURE 139-3 Relationship of each rib and rib head with the transverse process, vertebral bodies, and intervertebral disc. Note that each rib articulates not only with its own transverse process and vertebral body but also with the vertebral body immediately above it. Ant., anterior; Lig., ligament; Sup., superior.

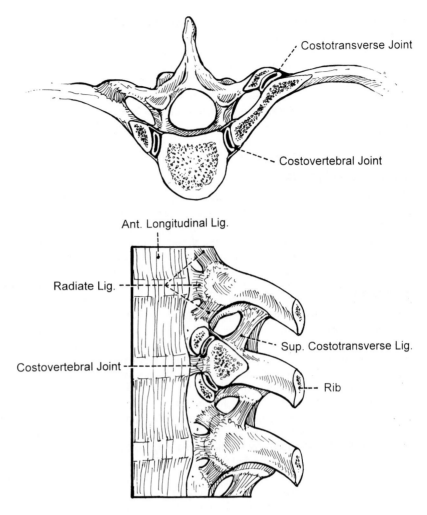

process immediately above. The canal formed between this ligament and the vertebral column transmits the dorsal ramus of the spinal nerve and the dorsal branch of the intercostal artery. The ribs are also attached to one another through the intercostal musculature, which originates medially on each superior rib and inserts laterally on its immediately inferior rib.

After bluntly dissecting the intercostal muscles and costotransverse and radiate ligaments, each rib can be resected. In doing so, a strip of intercostal musculature is isolated between each rib. This strip of musculature contains the intercostal nerve, artery, and vein as they pass laterally between the internal intercostal membrane and the pleura, then between the internal and innermost intercostal muscles. Although there is a great deal of interweaving between nerve, artery, and vein, most frequently the intercostal vein is most cephalad with the intercostal artery close to it but caudad. The intercostal nerve is frequently found separate from these structures and is located most caudad of the three. Immediately ventral to the intercostal bundle and the intercostal muscles lies the pleura.

RETROMEDIASTINAL SPACE AND SPINAL ANATOMY

With blunt dissection, the pleura can be separated from these structures to expose the lateral vertebral elements. The neural foramen can be identified by following the intercostal bundle medially. Within the neural foramen, the dorsal root ganglion can be identified along with the gray and white rami communicantes, which course ventrally to the sympathetic chain and ganglia. The sympathetic chain is contained within a fascial compartment formed by fusion of the mediastinal and prevertebral fascia over the costovertebral articulation.

Because the aortic arch does not extend to the top of the thoracic cavity, the arterial supply to the chest wall in this region has become somewhat specialized. The first two intercostal spaces are supplied by branches of the costocervical trunk through the highest intercostal artery. This artery descends anteriorly to the ventral rami of the eighth cervical and first thoracic nerves on the necks of the first two ribs. The remaining intercostal arteries arise from the posterior surface of the thoracic aorta. Because the aorta is displaced downward and to the left, the upper four aortic, posterior, intercostal arteries ascend to reach the intercostal spaces three through six. Each intercostal artery stretches obliquely across each vertebral body from caudad to cephalad in direct apposition to the periosteum of the vertebral body and is located deep to the azygos or hemiazygos vein, the thoracic duct, and the sympathetic trunk.

The major portion of the ventral ramus of the first thoracic nerve passes cephalad across the neck of the first rib to join the eighth cervical nerve in the brachial plexus. A small intercostal branch runs across the inferior surface of the first rib to enter the first interspace close to the costal cartilage.

The ventral ramus of the second thoracic nerve also usually sends a small branch to the brachial plexus. Occasionally, this branch is large, in which case, the lateral cutaneous branch of the second intercostal nerve is small or absent. Although the intercostal nerves below T1 can usually be sacrificed to facilitate exposure, T1 and C7, which frequently are exposed during this procedure, cannot be sacrificed without causing severe neurologic deficit to hand function. It is occasionally necessary to work around the inferior portion of the brachial plexus in this exposure.

Transmanubrial Approach

The transmanubrial approach is an anterior approach that allows direct access to the vertebral bodies and the pathologic processes contained within them. This approach can be divided into three major steps: (1) the thoracic inlet, (2) the visceral and vascular compartments of the superior mediastinum, and (3) the retromediastinal space.

THORACIC INLET

The superior mediastinum is defined anteriorly by the manubrium, which corresponds to a T2–3 level at the suprasternal notch and a T4–5 level at the sternal angle and lies only 5 cm anterior to these structures. The sternohyoid muscle runs from the ventrocaudal hyoid bone to the dorsal surface of the manubrium, also attaching to the sternoclavicular joint capsule. The sternothyroid muscles attach along the dorsal midline of the manubrium. These muscles are supplied by the ventral rami of C1–3 via the hypoglossal nerve and ansa cervicalis. The sternocleidomastoid muscle arises on the mastoid process and superior nuchal line and attaches to the manubrioclavicular joint. Its nervous supply is from the accessory nerve, and its arterial supply branches from the superior thyroid artery. Careful dissection of the fascial plains enables safe removal of the manubrium and medial third of the clavicle without injury to the brachiocephalic or subclavian veins. This removal reveals the pleural apices, which are covered by an extension of the transthoracic fascia, called Sibson's fascia.

VASCULAR AND VISCERAL COMPARTMENTS OF THE SUPERIOR MEDIASTINUM

The visceral fascia circumscribes the trachea, esophagus, and thyroid gland, defining a visceral compartment, and the carotid sheath circumscribes the carotid arterial system, internal jugular vein, and vagus nerve, defining a neurovascular compartment. These adjacent compartments create a potential space (the viscerocarotid space), which extends from the base of the skull to C7–T4, depending on the location of fusion between the visceral and alar fascia.

In the upper thorax, the visceral compartment continues down to the bronchi, where the fascia fuses with the parietal and visceral pleurae. Between the visceral and parietal pleurae exists a potential intrapleural space. The carotid sheath extends down to the subclavian vessels, where it fuses into the axillary sheath. In the superior mediastinum, the vascular compartment is not circumscribed by its own well-defined fascial sheath but is defined secondarily by independent surrounding fasciae. Ventrally is the transthoracic fascia, the prevertebral fascial extension, caudally is the visceral fascia, laterally are the parietal pleurae, and inferiorly is the pericardium.

The venous structures consist of the brachiocephalic veins with their branches. These veins descend from the neck into the superior mediastinum just posterior to the thymus gland or its remnants. The right brachiocephalic vein is formed just posterior to the medial end of the right clavicle and descends vertically into the superior mediastinum. The left brachiocephalic vein is formed just posterior to the medial end of the left clavicle and descends diagonally to join the right brachiocephalic vein just posterior to the right first costal cartilage to form the superior vena cava. Tributaries draining into the brachiocephalic veins are the vertebral and first, posterior, intercostal veins in the neck and the internal thoracic, thymic, and inferior thyroid veins in the superior mediastinum. On the left, the superior intercostal vein (which drains the second and third intercostal spaces) also drains into the left brachiocephalic vein.

The arterial structures consist of the aortic arch and brachiocephalic, left common carotid, and left subclavian arteries with their branches. The aortic arch initially ascends posteriorly to the superior vena cava but also turns diagonally posterior, then inferior just anterior and to the left of the vertebral column. A second concave turn occurs as the arch curves around the anterolateral visceral compartment to reach the vertebral column. The brachiocephalic artery is the first branch off the aortic arch and ascends vertically and slightly rightward to branch into the right common carotid and subclavian arteries posterior to the right sternoclavicular joint. The left common carotid artery arises next off the arch and ascends essentially vertically into the carotid sheath without branching in the superior mediastinum. The left subclavian artery is the third branch and ascends superiorly and leftward to curve around the thoracic inlet and into the axillary sheath without branches in the superior mediastinum.

The carotid sheath is a circumferential sheath of fused middle and deep fascial layers of deep fascia around the carotid arterial system and internal jugular vein and vagus nerve. At the thoracic inlet, the carotid sheath merges with the subclavian vasculature to form part of the axillary sheath. The esophagus and trachea are encompassed in the visceral fascia, which extends throughout the superior mediastinum. Between these two adjacent compartments lies the viscerocarotid space. Blunt dissection of this space exposes the alar fascia and the retropharyngeal space. In the superior mediastinum, the left brachiocephalic vein runs obliquely from left inferior to right superior. Caudally the field is limited by the aortic arch and its branches, which obstruct access to the T3 and T4 vertebrae. Major structures potentially crossing this retropharyngeal and retromediastinal space are the right recurrent laryngeal nerve and the lymphatics terminating in the thoracic duct. The left recurrent laryngeal nerve branches off the vagus in the superior mediastinum, loops around the ligamentum arteriosum, and ascends within the visceral fascia between the esophagus and trachea. The right recurrent laryngeal nerve can cross the retropharyngeal or retromediastinal space anywhere from C7 to T3.

The thoracic duct runs dorsal and to the left of the esophagus between the visceral and alar fascia in the superior mediastinum and ascends to the C7 level, where it lies laterally in a plane dorsal to the carotid sheath. It then courses caudally and ventrally to the branches of the thyrocervical trunk and phrenic nerve to terminate at the junction of the left internal jugular and subclavian veins. A lymphatic trunk located on the right side follows a similar course to the thoracic duct.

RETROMEDIASTINAL SPACE

By incising the alar and mediastinal fascia, the median compartment of the retromediastinal space is entered. The prevertebral fascia covers the vertebral bodies and envelops the longus colli muscles. Autonomic branches to the cardiopulmonary plexuses may be seen in this region and can be sacrificed if necessary.

CERVICOTHORACIC BIOMECHANICS

The cervicothoracic junction extends from C7 through T4 and includes the lower brachial plexus, the thoracic outlet, and the superior mediastinum. Biomechanically, the cervicothoracic junction is exposed to large forces, particularly in flexion and distraction. Anatomically, this region is characterized by a narrow spinal canal, narrow pedicles, and the transition from lateral masses to transverse processes. As with other areas of the spine, structures affecting spinal stability include the vertebral bodies and intervertebral discs, anterior and posterior longitudinal ligaments, and the interarticulating facet joints and ligamentous complex posteriorly. Anterior elements are the primary structures that transfer compressive forces between the adjacent vertebral bodies. Posterior spinal components have little weight-bearing function but are important for the attachment of supporting ligaments and resisting extremes of motion. The anterior and posterior longitudinal ligaments are important in preventing flexion and extension, whereas intertransverse and capsular ligaments are effective in inhibiting lateral bending and axial rotation. The rib cage and its articulation with the sternum anteriorly also increase the stability of the thoracic spine. Biomechanical studies have also shown a significant role of the costotransverse joints and rib cage in the thoracic spine, especially with lateral bending and axial rotation.[27] Berg[28] describes this sternal rib complex as constituting the fourth spinal column. At the cervicothoracic junction, disruption to any two spinal columns should be view as unstable and should be treated accordingly.

Pathologic processes such as trauma, degenerative processes, infection, and neoplastic involvement in combination with the abrupt change in the biomechanical function of this area can predispose the cervicothoracic segment to instability. This area is unique in being a transition area from a mobile lordotic cervical spine to a rigid kyphotic thoracic spine.[29] Furthermore, the cervicothoracic junction, much like the thoracolumbar junction, represents an area under stress as the transfer of weight occurs between spinal columns.[30] In addition, the vertebral index decreases from the C6 to T1 vertebrae, causing added stress to be applied to a more narrow and slender upper thoracic vertebrae.[31] Previous surgeries at the cervicothoracic junction have been well known to destabilize the region. Several authors have reported increasing spinal deformity caused by a previous cervicothoracic junction laminectomy.[3,32,33] Furthermore, spinal fusions ending at the cervicothoracic junction can also be a contributing factor to iatrogenic cervical instability.[34] Progressive instability of this area ultimately leads to kyphosis and spinal cord compression. This predisposition to neurologic injury may be related to a combination of a smaller spinal canal size at the cervicothoracic junction and a tenous blood supply.[2,3]

Relative to other parts of the spine, very few studies have addressed the biomechanics and fixation stability of the cervicothoracic junction. Only two clinical studies specifically addressed fixation at the cervicothoracic junction.[35,36] The vast majority of biomechanical studies in this region have been about the cervical spine in general. All biomechanical tests on cervical cadaveric spines have shown superior rigidity of the posterior screw fixation techniques as compared with anterior techniques.[37] Under laboratory conditions, none of the wiring techniques were able to achieve the stability of the intact segment and performed poorly with forces other than flexion.[37,38] In extension and torsion, lateral mass screws and plating devices have shown increased stability over posterior wiring alone.[39] Analysis of posterior screw pullout revealed a correlation with the length of screw passage through bone.[40] Biomechanical, transpedicular screw fixation of the lower cervical spine has provided the most stability to the unstable cervical spine.[41] However, a high rate of pedicle violation was noted even when a partial laminectomy was used for screw placement.[42]

Only three studies to date have looked at the biomechanics of spinal fixation specifically at the cervicothoracic junction.[43–45] Bueff and colleagues[43] compared three different fixation devices at the cervicothoracic junction: an anterior plate, a posterior plate, and a posterior hook-rod system. They found that the hook-rod system provided as much as six times the stiffness of the intact spine, whereas the anterior plate provided stiffness similar to that of the intact spine. Clinically, stand-alone anterior fixation at the cervicothoracic junction may lead to a high failure rate.[46] Vaccaro and colleagues[45] examined the use of a novel plate-rod construct for stabilization across the cervicothoracic junction and concluded that the device supported the maximal loading conditions experienced by the native cervical spine. The third biomechanical study examined the mean stiffness of three different posterior fixation systems used for cervicothoracic stabilization after a two- or three-column injury.[44] This included one plate-screw system, and two recently available rod-screw systems. All three systems were able to effectively stabilize the cervicothoracic junction in flexion/extension, lateral bending, and axial rotation for a two-column injury. When a three-column injury was introduced to the already fixated two column–injured cadaveric cervical spine, all systems failed to provide adequate stability, especially in extension. These results suggest that additional anterior stabilization is warranted when a three-column injury occurs at the cervicothoracic junction, but posterior stabilization is sufficient for a two-column injury.

Choice of Surgical Approach

The appropriate choice of surgical approach to the cervicothoracic junction depends on the exact location of the pathologic process. Surgical approaches to the cervicothoracic junction can be divided into four different categories: (1) anterior transcervical approaches (supraclavicular, transclavicular/transmanubrial, transsternal); (2) anterolateral transthoracic approach; (3) posterolateral approaches (costotransversectomy, lateral extracavitary, lateral parascapular extrapleural); and (4) posterior approaches (laminectomy, transpedicular). The latter approach is not recommended because it provides limited exposure of the anterior column and may cause further instabilities.

In patients with long, thin necks, a supraclavicular approach to T2 is sometimes possible. However, the angle of approach and the thoracic kyphosis may not provide the optimal view for decompression and stabilization. The transmanubrial approach exposes the vertebral bodies directly anteriorly and allows excellent exposure of the lower cervical vertebrae as well as T1 and T2. Depending on anatomic variations, T3 may also be accessible. Exposure of T4, however, is rarely possible. To obtain this exposure, dissection of the vascular compartment of the superior mediastinum is required. The exposure is limited by the anatomic positions of the left brachiocephalic vein, subclavian veins, aortic arch, and great vessels and the degree of thoracic kyphosis. Potential anatomic risks are injury to the carotid sheath structures, trachea, esophagus, recurrent laryngeal nerves, aortic arch and its branches, vertebral arteries, brachiocephalic and subclavian veins, sympathetic trunk and stellate ganglion, spinal cord, and pleural apices. The most significant advantage of this approach is the simultaneous excellent exposure of the cervical and the upper thoracic spine. The relative disadvantages are that the corpectomy is performed blindly with regard to the thecal sac and posterior spinal stabilization cannot be performed without repositioning the patient or performing a second procedure. Anterior plates may be applied easily through this approach down to T2 and occasionally T3.

The anterolateral transthoracic approach exposes the vertebral bodies anterolaterally after an extensive mobilization of the scapula. Excellent exposure of T3 and T4 can be achieved, but access to T1 and T2 is limited by the narrowing of the thoracic inlet. The lower cervical vertebrae are not accessible through this approach. To obtain this exposure, the intrapleural space is dissected to reach the paramedian compartment of the retromediastinal space. Potential anatomic risks include injury to the neurovascular supply to the shoulder musculature, lungs, superior mediastinal structures (aorta and its branches, trachea, esophagus, thoracic duct), sympathetic trunk and stellate ganglion, lower trunk and posterior cord of the brachial plexus, and intercostal, long thoracic, and thoracodorsal nerves. Relative advantages of this approach include rapid exposure of the anterior spinal elements and excellent control of intercostal segmental arteries. The relative disadvantages of this approach to the cervicothoracic junction are the transmuscular mobilization of the scapula, the intrapleural dissection, the long depth of field, and the inability to obtain exposure of the lower cervical vertebrae.

The lateral, parascapular, extrapleural approach is an extended posterolateral approach that allows direct lateral exposure of the vertebral bodies. Excellent exposure of T1–4 vertebral bodies can be obtained, and the inferior portion of C7 may be exposed under the T1 nerve root. To obtain this exposure, the thoracoscapular space is dissected after anatomic mobilization of the scapula, and the paraspinal musculature is mobilized to open directly into the paramedian compartment of the retromediastinal space. Potential anatomic risks include injury to the dorsomedial parascapular musculature, pleura and lungs, superior mediastinal structures, sympathetic trunk and stellate ganglion, and spinal cord.

Relative advantages of this approach are decompression of neural tissue under direct visualization, a totally extrapleural dissection, simultaneous exposure of C7 through T4, and simultaneous posterior stabilization through the same incision and patient position. Relative disadvantages of this approach are a more tedious paraspinal muscle dissection, and it does not allow simultaneous exposure of any cervical vertebrae beyond the inferior-most aspect of C7. Aggressive paraspinal muscle dissection may lead to significant muscle atrophy. In selected patients, adequate exposure can be obtained via a traditional costotransversectomy or lateral extracavitary approach.

Anesthetic Considerations

General anesthesia has been used for all patients undergoing any of these three surgical approaches. In general, we prefer a combined protocol of enflurane (Ethrane) inhalant and intravenous sufentanil. Three types of intubation have been used in patients undergoing surgery of the cervicothoracic junction: (1) routine single-lumen endotracheal intubation, (2) double-lumen endotracheal intubation, and (3) single-lumen endotracheal intubation with high-frequency ventilation. Routine, single-lumen endotracheal intubation is the most rapidly performed but requires that the ipsilateral lung expand and contract within the surgical field during anterolateral thoracotomy or lateral parascapular extrapleural surgical procedures. Double-lumen intubation is a much longer procedure but allows unilateral deflation of the lung during the critical periods of corpectomy and spinal cord decompression. Single-lumen intubation with high-frequency ventilation also can be performed rapidly and enables the lung to be retracted out of the surgical field with minimal reinflation during corpectomy and decompression but allows simultaneous ventilation of the remainder of the ipsilateral lung. We have found single-lumen intubation with high-frequency ventilation to be the ideal ventilatory technique for anterolateral or posterolateral procedures of the upper thoracic spine. Single-lumen intubation with standard ventilation is adequate for transmanubrial and transclavicular procedures.

Surgical Techniques

Lateral, Parascapular, Extrapleural Approach

The posterior aspect of the neck and back from the nuchal line to the sacrum is prepared and draped for surgery in a sterile fashion. The incision begins midline three spinous processes above the intended surgical area and is brought to three spinous processes below before curving gently to the surgical side of approach. A myocutaneous flap is then developed by incising the deep fascia at the spinous processes and dissecting them off sharply to expose the trapezius muscle. The trapezius and rhomboid muscles are then dissected off the spinous processes, and the plane of loose areolar tissue located between these muscles and the paraspinal muscles is identified. By developing this plane, the skin and the trapezius and rhomboid muscles can be reflected together toward the medial border of the scapula (Fig. 139-4). The inferior fibers of the trapezius muscle must be transected to reflect this flap, and care must be taken to leave an identifiable cuff of muscle for reapproximation.

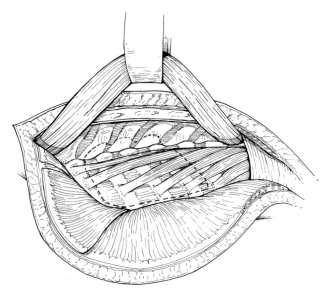

FIGURE 139-4 Reflection of the trapezius and rhomboid muscles laterally and paraspinal muscle mass medially to expose the dorsal and lateral spinal elements and ribs.

Aggressive dissection of the levator scapulae muscles in the cervical region maximizes exposure of the cervicothoracic junction. Mobilization of the myocutaneous flap in this fashion enables the scapula to fall laterally out of the surgical field, which provides wide exposure of the lower cervical region, upper dorsal rib cage region, and dorsal vertebral elements.

The deep cervical fascia and thoracolumbar fascia cover the splenius and erector spinae muscles. Dissection of this paraspinal muscle mass from the spinous processes and dorsal spinal elements enables retraction of this muscle mass medially to the contralateral side. This retraction exposes the entire dorsal rib cage and dorsal vertebral elements from the tip of the spinous process to the transverse process.

Subperiosteal dissection of the appropriate ribs can then be performed to free the neurovascular bundles and intercostal muscles. The costotransverse and costovertebral ligaments are incised, and the rib is removed from its costovertebral tip to the posterior bend of each rib. This can be as much as 3 cm in a standard costotransversectomy approach or as much as 5 cm in the lateral extracavitary approach. The intercostal neurovascular bundles are next dissected free of the intercostal muscles, and the intercostal arteries are ligated and transected. For exposure of the intervertebral disc, the intercostal nerves can be retracted out of the surgical field. To resect a vertebral body, however, one or more intercostal nerves need to be resected to gain adequate exposure. T1 nerve root and above should be preserved whenever possible so that hand function is not affected.

The intercostal nerve can be traced to identify the vertebral foramen. The sympathetic chain can then be identified on the lateral vertebral surface. The rami communicantes are transected, and the intercostal arteries are ligated and transected as well. Displacing the sympathetic chain anterolaterally via subperiosteal dissection reveals the vertebral body, pedicle, and foramen. Removal of the transverse process, lamina, and pedicles, using either a high-speed drill or Kerrison punch (using the intercostal nerve as a guide),

exposes the lateral thecal sac. Direct visualization of the neural elements is available during the remaining decompression. Corpectomy can then be performed using either a high-speed drill or curet, as described previously. The anterior longitudinal ligament and, if possible, the posterior longitudinal ligament are preserved to serve as protective barriers to the thecal sac and superior mediastinal structures (Fig. 139-5). Vertebral reconstruction is performed using a rib graft or fibular allograft strut. If the pathologic process is malignant, Steinmann pins and methyl methacrylate are used. Alternatively, metal cages packed with autologous bone can be introduced for vertebral body reconstruction.

Any sacrificed nerve roots are ligated proximal to the dorsal root ganglion, and the remainder of the nerve is removed. Appropriate posterior spinal fixation is then performed. Before wound closure, the operative field is filled with saline to check for evidence of an air leak. If an air leak is present, a small (French number 22 or 24) chest tube is placed into the wound and brought out through a separate stab wound below the incision. Two Hemovac drains are then placed, and a layered wound closure is performed.

Anterolateral Transthoracic Approach

For the anterolateral transthoracic approach to the cervicothoracic junction, the patient is placed in the lateral decubitus position with the appropriate side up. The skin is incised from the paraspinous area at approximately T1 and taken distally along the medial border of the scapula to the seventh rib. This incision is continued first laterally, then anteriorly, then medially to the costal cartilage of the third rib (Fig. 139-6). The trapezius, latissimus dorsi, rhomboid major, and serratus posterior muscles are divided, after which the third rib is identified. The scapula is then retracted cephalad and medially using a scapular retractor.

In identifying the third rib, it is important to recall that the first rib is located somewhat medially to the second rib. Confirmation of location frequently can be made by identifying the attachment of the scalenus anterior or medius muscles on the second rib. A subperiosteal dissection of the third rib is performed, and the rib is resected from its angle

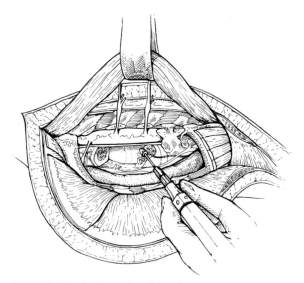

FIGURE 139-5 Operative field after a corpectomy and neural decompression.

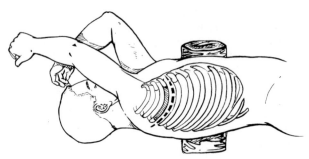

FIGURE 139-6 Patient position and skin incision for right anterolateral transthoracic approach to the upper thoracic spine.

to the costal cartilage. The chest spreader can then be inserted and opened, exposing the pleura and underlying lungs, aorta, and spine.

The parietal pleura can be opened by incising the pleura from the costochondral cartilage to the midvertebral body. After deflating and retracting the lung, the spine is clearly exposed (Fig. 139-7). The pleura can then be incised cephalad and caudad to expose the pathologic vertebrae. This exposure clearly identifies the intervertebral discs and the intercostal arteries and veins that lie in the midvertebral body. Appropriate intercostal arteries and veins are dissected, ligated, and cut. Vertebrectomy can then be performed as described previously.

After resection of the pathologic vertebral elements and vertebral reconstruction, closure is begun by first inserting a chest tube and bringing it to water seal. The pleura is then

sutured closed. Ribs are reapproximated with wire. Each muscle layer is independently reapproximated using 0 polyglycolic acid (Vicryl) sutures. Subcutaneous 2-0 Vicryl sutures and skin staples are used to close the wound.

Transmanubrial and Transclavicular Approach

The patient is positioned supine with the head turned slightly to the side contralateral to the approach. A T-shaped incision is made with the transverse limb of the incision located in a skin crease 2 cm above the clavicle extending from the contralateral sternocleidomastoid to 2 to 3 cm lateral to the ipsilateral sternocleidomastoid (Fig. 139-8). The vertical portion of the incision extends in the midline midway down the sternal body. The platysma muscle is divided in the line of the skin incision, and a wide mobilization of the platysma is performed cephalad and caudad to the incision. The external jugular vein is identified and divided; supraclavicular nerves are identified and protected where possible. Medial branches of these nerves frequently are sacrificed.

The sternocleidomastoid muscle is next identified and dissected free from deeper structures. The medial half of the clavicle and the manubrium are freed from the pectoralis major muscle by subperiosteal dissection. Careful dissection of the superficial and middle layers of the deep cervical fascia allows safe reflection of the sternocleidomastoid, sternohyoid, and sternothyroid muscles from the manubrium and clavicle with preservation of their neurovascular supply. Opening the suprasternal space of Burns (a suprasternal midline space created by a leaflet split in the superficial layer of deep fascia) allows subperiosteal dissection of the manubrium, leaving

FIGURE 139-7 Operative exposure of the upper thoracic spine through a T3 anterolateral transthoracic approach.

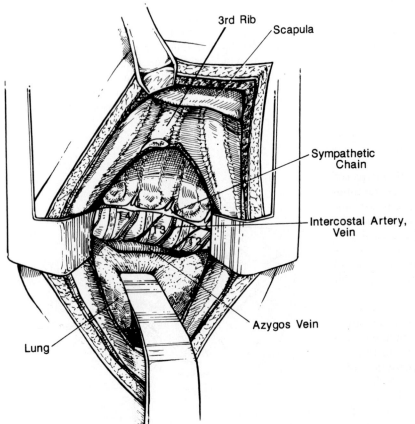

3rd Rib

Scapula

Sympathetic Chain

Intercostal Artery, Vein

Azygos Vein

Lung

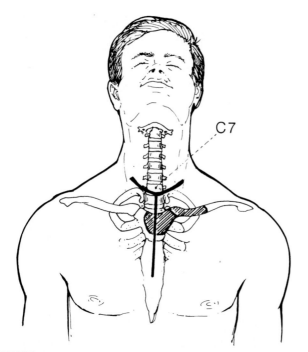

FIGURE 139-8 Patient position and skin incision for a transmanubrial/transclavicular approach to the cervicothoracic junction.

the periosteum along with an anterior extension of the transthoracic fascia for protection of the brachiocephalic veins. Next, the omohyoid muscle is divided between identifying sutures, and the anterior aspect of the internal jugular vein and common carotid artery are identified.

After appropriate protection of the deeper structures, the ipsilateral two thirds of the manubrium are cut using a high-speed drill. Similarly, the first costal cartilage is divided leaving the clavicular manubrial joint intact. After drilling holes

for the eventual application of a fixation plate, the clavicle is divided at its midpoint. The manubrium, sternoclavicular joint, and medial half of the clavicle are then elevated on the pedicle of the sternocleidomastoid muscle. This elevation exposes the infrahyoid muscles, trachea, brachiocephalic veins and tributaries, brachiocephalic artery and branches, subclavian and common carotid arteries, scalenus anterior muscle, phrenic nerve, brachial plexus, and part of the first rib. Blunt dissection can then be performed medial to the carotid sheath to expose the alar and mediastinal fascia. Incision of these fasciae enters the retromediastinal space and exposes the prevertebral fascia covering the vertebral bodies and longus colli muscles (Fig. 139-9).

After placement of appropriate retractors, removal of the pathologic process can be performed by any of several techniques. Soft tumors can be removed through curettage and suction. Bony elements can be removed through use of a high-speed drill and Kerrison punch.

After complete decompression of the spinal cord, reconstruction is begun using either autologous or allograft bone: tricortical iliac crest or fibula is adequate. After bony reconstruction, stabilization can be achieved through placement of an anterior plate screwed to the intact vertebrae above and below the pathologic levels or by placement in a halo brace.

The wound is then closed in layers over vacuum drainage. If the pleura has been opened, a chest tube is inserted through a separate stab wound, threaded into the pleural space, and connected to an underwater seal. The osteomuscular flap is then returned to its appropriate position. The manubrium is reattached using wires, and the clavicle is reattached using plate and screws.

Reconstruction and Stabilization

Many operations at the cervicothoracic junction, whether for tumor, trauma, neural decompression, or deformity,

FIGURE 139-9 Operative exposure of the cervicothoracic junction via transmanubrial/transclavicular approach. M., muscle.

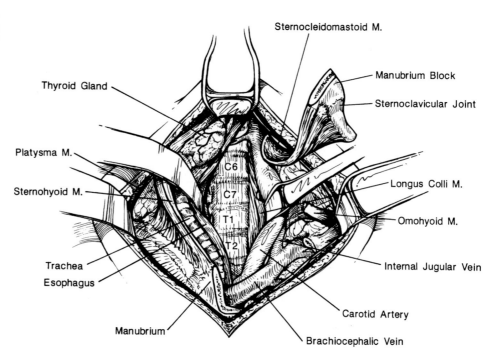

require reconstruction and spinal stabilization. Similar to the thoracolumbar region, the cervicothoracic junction experiences large biomechanical forces because of the large lever arm exerted by the rigid thoracic cage and the normal transition from lordosis to kyphosis that it encompasses. Although anterior reconstruction and stabilization from C7–T4 closely resemble those of the midcervical spine in principle and practice, this region poses special anatomic problems for posterior instrumented fusion. A wide variety of options for instrumented fusion exist at present, and this field is constantly evolving (Table 139-3).

Anterior Reconstruction

After any of the anterior approaches for corpectomy and fusion described previously, a substantial construct is required to bear the axial loads normally exerted on the anterior and middle columns. Several options exist. In tumor cases, it is frequently unnecessary to achieve a solid bone fusion given that patients with metastatic cancer to the spine generally have a short life expectancy. Further, many of these patients undergo radiation therapy and chemotherapy, which inhibit bone growth. A methyl methacrylate cast held in place with vertically embedded Steinmann pins is a commonly used alternative. This construct may be created rapidly in the operating room and provides immediate stability.

In patients with lesions that are the result of trauma, infection, degenerative disease, and benign tumors, stabilization with instrumentation that results in bone fusion is generally desirable. Most neurosurgeons have considerable experience with anterior cervical fusions and stabilization. The difficulties of exposure notwithstanding, anterior cervicothoracic fusions are not substantially different. In many cases, fibular strut grafts or iliac crest autografts supplemented with an anterior cervical plate and screws provide excellent structural results (Fig. 139-10). Application of an anterior cervical plate does, however, require a straight anterior approach. A Harms cage packed with autograft is another option for structural anterior support and eventual fusion. Recent additions of expandable cages and metal spacers may help to facilitate placement and reconstruction. Last, the use of free vascularized fibular

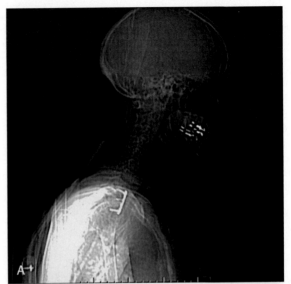

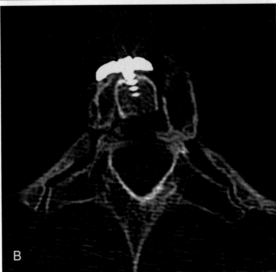

FIGURE 139-10 *A,* Sagittal view of anterior plate and screw fixation after a T2 corpectomy with an iliac crest bone graft. *B,* An axial computed tomography view of the iliac crest bone graft stabilized by an anterior screw.

strut grafts has been increasingly reported, particularly in deformity correction.[47]

Posterior Stabilization

A growing number of options for posterior cervicothoracic instrumentation now exist. They range from the application of a simple tension band to complex hook, rod, and screw constructs. The application of tension bands effectively resists flexion and distraction. In cases of pure ligamentous disruption, a tension band may be the only intervention required. Tension bands usually take the form of interspinous wiring, which, when given the long lever arm from the instantaneous axis of rotation, can exert tremendous resistive forces. This simple technique is safe, fast, and a useful adjunct to other techniques.

The Luque rectangle in combination with sublaminar wires or Songer cables has been a mainstay of internal fixation at the cervicothoracic junction. It forms a relatively rigid construct, which combines segmental fixation with resistance

TABLE 139-3 ▪ **Options for Reconstruction and Stabilization**	
Anterior	**Posterior**
Structural Graft	
Iliac crest autograft	Iliac crest autograft
Rib	Laminectomy bone
Fibular allograft	
Vascularized fibular autograft	
Methyl methacrylate	
Instrumentation	
Anterior cervical plate	Interspinous wires
Harms cage	Luque rectangle/sublaminar wires
Steinmann methyl	Pediatric CD hooks and rods
methacrylate pins	AO plates/lateral mass or
	pedicle screws

to flexion, torsion, and, to some extent, translation. Passage of sublaminar wires carries some risk of spinal cord injury but has been generally safe in practice. This technique requires the posterior elements to be intact and of good-quality bone. The construct should cover at least two levels above and two below the region of instability.

Pediatric Cotrel-Dubousset systems employing laminar hooks and rods have been applied at the cervicothoracic junction (Fig. 139-11). Although biomechanically this construct is extremely stable, it requires intact posterior elements at the points of fixation. More importantly, the narrowness of the cervicothoracic spinal canal may prohibit placement of laminar hooks.

In cases in which the posterior elements have been disrupted by trauma or removed surgically, posterior internal fixation becomes more difficult. A number of good options now exist, however. Since the pioneering work of Roy-Camille and colleagues[48] with lateral mass plates in the cervical spine, plate and rod–based methods of fixation for the cervicothoracic junction have been progressively developed, particularly in the placement of cervical and thoracic pedicle screws.[49] Current additions of minipolyaxial screws, dual-diameter rods, cervical cross-links, and interconnectors have facilitated posterior instrumentation greatly. Because the cervicothoracic junction is under significant biomechanical stress, surgical fixation should incorporate several segments above and below the injured site. For the most part, current stabilization techniques of the cervicothoracic junction will require experience with cervical lateral mass or pedicle screw placement, upper and lower thoracic pedicle screw placement, and the use of thoracic transverse, pedicle, and laminar hooks. Sublaminar wiring techniques can add to construct stability when cross-links are used and the lamina is intact. This will be especially useful in the cervical area because there will be

a tendency for cervical screw pullout. By using two cross-links as part of a screw-rod construct, quadrilateral stability can also be achieved.

Anatomic understanding of the cervicothoracic junction is required for accurate screw placement and choosing the appropriate fixation technique. Because the cervicothoracic junction represents a transition zone, significant anatomic variations are common. The lower cervical laminae are thinner and weaker compared with those of the upper thoracic vertebrae. This, together with a narrow spinal canal, often limits the use of hook-rod stabilization at the cervicothoracic junction. Use of lateral mass screws should take into consideration the location of the vertebral artery and the spinal nerves. Compared with T1, the C7 vertebrae have a closer anatomic relationship with the vertebral artery. Based on cadaveric studies, at C7, the vertebral artery is on average 18 mm from midline and 17 mm from the posterior cortex of the lateral mass.[50] At T1, it is 22 mm from the midline of the vertebral body and 22 mm from the posterior cortex of the transverse process. The vertebral artery will be at risk of injury if a lateral mass screw is too long or directed less than 14 degrees laterally from the midpoint of the lateral mass of C7. These neurovascular relationships may change with significant kyphotic/scoliotic deformity of the spine and can subject them to greater risk of injury with posterior screw fixation. Aiming too caudal with the lateral mass screws may lead to spinal nerve injury. Furthermore, the C6 and C7 lateral masses are the thinnest in the cervical spine because they are in transition to becoming transverse processes. A gentle touch will be needed to obtain adequate screw purchase of the lateral masses at C6 and C7.

Although in the midcervical spine, the facet/lateral mass forms a substantial complex into which a screw may be

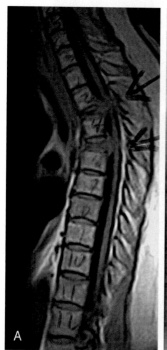 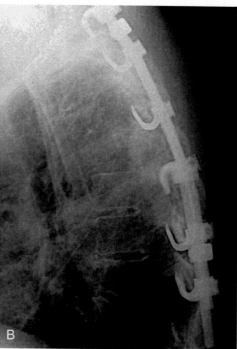 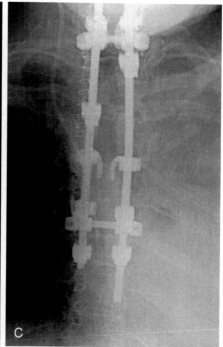

FIGURE 139-11   *A,* T2 and T4 pathologic fractures from metastatic carcinoma on a T1-weighted sagittal view (*B*). *C,* Laminar-hook and dual-rod construct after decompression of compromised spinal canal through lateral parascapular extrapleural approach.

securely anchored, this complex frequently provides inadequate screw purchase at C7 and below. Traditional techniques of lateral mass plating may not produce a biomechanically stable construct at the cervicothoracic junction. Pedicle screw constructs, however, have shown excellent biomechanical stability in this region (Fig. 139-12).

A number of careful anatomic studies of the cervicothoracic pedicles have been conducted to assess the feasibility and safety of placing cervicothoracic pedicle screws. An and colleagues[51] found it difficult to determine pedicle alignment in a cadaveric study. Stanescu and colleagues[52] and Panjabi and colleagues[53] both found highly variable pedicle dimensions and angles. The mean pedicle width increases on average from 5 mm at C5 to 8 mm at T1 and then decreases to 4.5 mm at T5. Although the pedicles at C7, T1, and T2 are frequently large enough to permit placement of a 3.5-mm screw, those above and below were usually significantly smaller. Karaikovic and colleagues[54] studied 53 Euro-American cervical spines finding outer pedicle widths equal to or smaller than 4 mm in 13.2% at C5 and C6 and 6.6% of C7 pedicles. Miller and colleagues[55] placed 3-mm pedicle screws in cadaveric cervical spines blindly according to the technique of Jeanneret and colleagues[56] and via a small laminotomy. They found potentially dangerous violations of the pedicle in 10 of 38 blind placements and one of 40 placements after laminotomy.

In the thoracic spine, this group compared the Roy-Camille technique with the open lamina technique. They found grade II and III pedicle violations in 48 of 95 screws and 10 of 94 screws. T3 to T5 will often have small narrow pedicles that prevent their screw placement. Incorporating this area will often require the use of thoracic hooks. The pedicle angle also decreases from 50 degrees medially at C5 to 11 degrees medially at T5. However, the pedicle length increases gradually from C5 to T5 without any significant differences between adjacent vertebral levels. The mean distance of the spinal nerve to the superior and inferior pedicles ranged between 0.8 and 2.3 mm with greater separation between the nerve and the superior pedicle. Thus pedicle screw violation of the superior cortex may place the nerve at higher risk of injury than inferior cortex violation.

Despite the foregoing anatomic concerns, cervicothoracic pedicle screws have been successfully employed in clinical practice. Abumi and colleagues[57] used pedicle screws in 13 patients with fracture/dislocations of the lower cervical spine with uniformly good results and a lack of complications. In another series,[58] they placed 191 cervical pedicle screws (most by landmarks) linked to plates or rods, reporting only one transient screw thread–related radiculopathy. Chapman and colleagues[36] analyzed 23 patients instrumented posteriorly using AO plates with cervical lateral mass screws

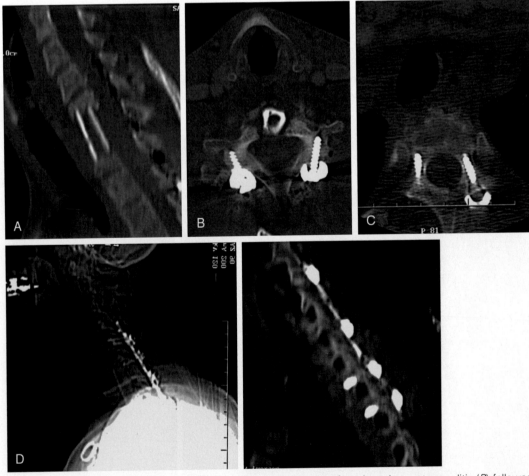

FIGURE 139-12   *A,* T1 to T3 iliac crest autograft placement after T2 corpectomy for tuberculous osteomyelitis (*B*) followed by posterior stabilization with lateral mass screw placement at C7 and transpedicular screw fixation (*C*) at T2 and T3. *D,* Sagittal view of a lower cervical lateral mass and upper thoracic transpedicular screw fixation.

and thoracic pedicle screws. They reported a 100% fusion rate, no neurovascular complications, and no hardware complications requiring reoperation. Albert and colleagues[35] reviewed 21 patients who were treated with pedicle screws at C7 placed by an open lamina technique. They found no neurovascular complications and no instrument failures at the 1-year follow-up examinations. Given their greater biomechanical stiffness, higher resistance to pullout, and broader applicability of pedicle screw constructs, they have provided versatility for cervicothoracic stabilization.

DISCUSSION

The anatomic relationships of the upper thoracic spine have made surgical access to this region challenging. Attempts to approach this area have frequently used procedures designed for approaching the vertebral elements of the lower thoracic region and thoracolumbar junction (e.g., costotransversectomy, lateral rachiotomy, and lateral extracavitary procedure). The scapula, trapezius, rhomboid, and levator scapulae muscles limit the exposure provided by these procedures. Approaches designed specifically for this region include the transmanubrial and transclavicular, anterolateral thoracotomy, and lateral parascapular extrapleural approaches.

Among these approaches, the transmanubrial and transclavicular approach of Sundaresan and colleagues[15] provides the best approach for pathologic processes that include both the lower cervical and the upper thoracic region. It gives excellent access from the lower cervical region to T2 and occasionally to T3. To obtain this exposure, dissection of the vascular compartment of the superior mediastinum is required to reach the median compartment of the retromediastinal space. The exposure is limited by the anatomic positions of the left brachial cephalic vein, subclavian veins, aortic arch, and great vessels as well as the degree of thoracic kyphosis. Potential risks include injury to the carotid sheath structures, trachea, esophagus, recurrent laryngeal nerves, aortic arch, vertebral arteries, sympathetic trunk and stellate ganglion, spinal cord, and pleural apices. The distinct advantage of this approach is the simultaneous exposure of the cervical and thoracic spine. The disadvantages are that the corpectomy is performed blindly until the thecal sac can be identified and posterior stabilization cannot be performed without a second procedure.

The transthoracic approach through the third rib exposes the vertebral bodies from an anterolateral approach but requires extensive mobilization of the scapula and a relatively long surgical depth of field. Exposure of T3 and T4 vertebral bodies is generally adequate, but access to T1 and T2 is limited by the narrowing of the thoracic inlet. The intrapleural cavity is opened to reach the paramedian compartment of the retromediastinal space. Potential risks include injury to the neurovascular supply of the shoulder musculature, lungs, superior mediastinal structures, sympathetic trunk and stellate ganglion, lower trunk and posterior cord of the brachial plexus, and intercostal, long thoracic, and thoracodorsal nerves. Advantages of this approach include excellent access to superior mediastinal vasculature if necessary for control. Relative disadvantages of this approach are the extensive mobilization of the scapula,

TABLE 139-4 ■ Recommended Surgical Approaches

Transmanubrial/transclavicular
  Pathology extends from C6 or C7 to T1 or T2 but not below T2
Lateral parascapular extrapleural or anterolateral thoracotomy
  Pathology limited to T3 and/or T4
Lateral parascapular extrapleural
  Pathology extends up to but not beyond C7/T1 disc

intrapleural dissection, long depth of field, inability to reach T1 and T2, and inability to perform posterior stabilization in the same procedure.

The lateral, parascapular, extrapleural approach is an extended posterolateral approach that allows excellent exposure of T1–4 vertebral bodies but limited exposure of C7. To obtain this exposure, the thoracoscapular space is dissected to mobilize the scapula partially, and the paraspinal musculature is mobilized to open directly into the paramedian compartment of the retromediastinal space. Potential anatomic risks include the dorsal medial parascapular musculature, pleura and lungs, superior mediastinal structures, sympathetic trunk and stellate ganglion, and spinal cord. The advantage of this approach is that decompression of neural tissue is performed under direct visualization at all times, with minimal manipulation of the thecal sac. Simultaneous exposure of C7–T4 is easily achieved. In addition, posterior stabilization can be performed simultaneously through the same incision. The relative disadvantage is that only the inferior aspect of C7 is available through this approach and it is partially obstructed by the T1 nerve root and rami communicantes to the stellate ganglion.

SUMMARY

Surgical approaches to the cervicothoracic junction can be divided into three main groups. Depending on the location and extent of pathology, one or another may be more appropriate. Considerations for selection of the most appropriate surgical approach are listed in Table 139-4. Pathology that extends from the lower cervical to the upper thoracic region but that does not extend below T2 is most easily approached through a transmanubrial and transclavicular approach. Pathology limited to T3 and T4 can be easily accessed through either the lateral parascapular extrapleural or the anterolateral thoracotomy approaches. Pathology that includes T3 or T4 and extends cephalad to (but no further than) the C7–T1 disc space is more easily approached through the lateral, parascapular, extrapleural approach.

REFERENCES

1. Nichols CG, Young DH, Schiller WR: Evaluation of cervicothoracic junction injury. Ann Emerg Med 16:640–642, 1987.
2. Sapkas G, Papadakis S, Katonis P, et al: Operative treatment of unstable injuries of the cervicothoracic junction. Eur Spine J 8:279–283, 1999.
3. An HS, Vaccaro A, Cotler JM, Lin S: Spinal disorders at the cervicothoracic junction. Spine 19:2557–2564, 1994.
4. Sundaresan N, DiGiacinto GV, Hughes JEO, Krol G: Spondylectomy for malignant tumors of the spine. J Clin Oncol 7:1485–1491, 1989.
5. Siegal T: Surgical decompression of anterior and posterior malignant epidural tumors compressing the spinal cord: A prospective study. Neurosurgery 17:424–432, 1985.
6. Menard V: Etude Pratique sur le Mal de Pott. Paris: Masson, 1900.

7. Capener N: The evolution of lateral rachotomy. J Bone Joint Surg 36:173–179, 1954.

8. Larson SJ, Holst RA, Hemmy DC, Sances A: Lateral extracavitary approach to traumatic lesions of the thoracic and lumbar spine. J Neurosurg 45:628–637, 1976.

9. Fessler RG, Dietze DD Jr, MacMillan M, Peace D: Lateral parascapular extrapleural approach to the upper thoracic spine. J Neurosurg 75:349–355, 1991.

10. Jonnesco T: Le sympathique cervico-thoracico. Paris: Masson, 1923.

11. Brunig F: Technik der kombinierten Resektionsmethode samtlicher sympathischen Nervenbaum am Halse. Zentralbl Chir 50:1056–1059, 1923.

12. Royle ND: Observations on the alteration of the circulation of the brain by surgical means in diseases of the central nervous system. BMJ 1:1063–1068, 1932.

13. Gask GE: The surgery of the sympathetic nervous system. Br J Surg 21:113–130, 1933.

14. Ochsner A, DeBakey M: Peripheral vascular disease. Surg Gynecol Obstet 70:1058–1072, 1940.

15. Sundaresan N, Shah J, Foley KM, Rosen G: An anterior surgical approach to the upper thoracic vertebrae. J Neurosurg 61:686–690, 1984.

16. Birch R, Bonney G, Marshall RW: A surgical approach to the cervicothoracic spine. J Bone Joint Surg Br 72:904–907, 1990.

17. Hodgson AR, Stock FE, Fang HSY, Ong GB: Anterior spinal fusion: The operative approach and pathological findings in 412 patients with Pott's disease of the spine. Br J Surg 48:172–178, 1960.

18. Sapico BL, Montgomerie JZ: Vertebral osteomyelitis in intravenous drug abusers: Report of three cases and review of the literature. Rev Infect Dis 2:196–206, 1980.

19. Edelstyn GA, Gillespie PJ, Grebbell FS: The radiological demonstration of osseous metastases. Clin Radiol 18:158–162, 1967.

20. O'Mara RE: Bone scanning in osseous metastatic disease. JAMA 229:1915, 1974.

21. Butler EG, Dohrmann PJ, Stark RJ: Spinal subdural abscess. Clin Exp Neurol 25:67–70, 1988.

22. Galasko CS: Skeletal metastases. Clin Orthop 210:18–30, 1986.

23. Schlaeffer F, Mikolich DJ, Mates SM: Technetium Tc 99m diphosphonate bone scan: False normal findings in elderly patients with hematogenous vertebral osteomyelitis. Arch Intern Med 147:2024–2026, 1987.

24. Staab EV, McCartney WH: Role of gallium 67 in inflammatory disease. Semin Nucl Med 8:219–234, 1978.

25. Bruns J, Maas R: Advantages of diagnosing bacterial spondylitis with magnetic resonance imaging. Arch Orthop Trauma Surg 108:30–35, 1989.

26. Paushter DM, Modic MT, Masaryk TJ: Magnetic resonance imaging of the spine: Applications and limitations. Radiol Clin North Am 23:551–562, 1985.

27. Oda I, Abumi K, Lu D, et al: Biomechanical role of the posterior elements, costovertebral joints, and rib cage in the stability of the thoracic spine. Spine 21:1423–1429, 1996.

28. Berg EE: The sternal-rib complex: A possible fourth column in thoracic spine fractures. Spine 18:1916–1919, 1993.

29. An HS, Wise JJ, Xu R: Anatomy of the cervicothoracic junction: A study of cadaveric dissection, cryomicrotomy, and magnetic resonance imaging. J Spinal Disord 12:519–525, 1999.

30. Pal GP, Routal RV: A study of weight transmission through the cervical and upper thoracic regions of the vertebral column in man. J Anat 148:245–261, 1986.

31. Boyle JJ, Singer KP, Milne N: Morphological survey of the cervicothoracic junctional region. Spine 21:544–548, 1996.

32. Yasuoka S, Peterson HA, MacCarty CS: Incidence of spinal column deformity after multilevel laminectomy in children and adults. J Neurosurg 57:441–445, 1982.

33. Inoue A, Ikata T, Katoh S: Spinal deformity following surgery for spinal cord tumors and tumorous lesions: Analysis based on an assessment of the spinal functional curve. Spinal Cord 34:536–542, 1996.

34. Drennan JC, King EW: Cervical dislocation following fusion of the upper thoracic spine for scoliosis: A case report. J Bone Joint Surg Am 60:1003–1005, 1978.

35. Albert TJ, Klein GR, Joffe D, Vaccaro AR: Use of cervicothoracic junction pedicle screws for reconstruction of complex cervical spine pathology. Spine 23:1596–1599, 1998.

36. Chapman JR, Anderson PA, Pepin C, et al: Posterior instrumentation of the unstable cervicothoracic spine. J Neurosurg 84:552–558, 1996.

37. Ulrich C, Arand M, Nothwang J: Internal fixation on the lower cervical spine—biomechanics and clinical practice of procedures and implants. Eur Spine J 10:88–100, 2001.

38. Wellman BJ, Follett KA, Traynelis VC: Complications of posterior articular mass plate fixation of the subaxial cervical spine in 43 consecutive patients. Spine 23:193–200, 1998.

39. Ulrich C, Woersdoerfer O, Kalff R, et al: Biomechanics of fixation systems to the cervical spine. Spine 16(3 Suppl):S4–S9, 1991.

40. Heller JG, Estes BT, Zaouali M, Diop A: Biomechanical study of screws in the lateral masses: Variables affecting pull-out resistance. J Bone Joint Surg Am 78:1315–1321, 1996.

41. Kotani Y, Cunningham BW, Abumi K, McAfee PC: Biomechanical analysis of cervical stabilization systems: An assessment of transpedicular screw fixation in the cervical spine. Spine 19:2529–2539, 1994

42. Miller RM, Ebraheim NA, Xu R, Yeasting RA: Anatomic consideration of transpedicular screw placement in the cervical spine: An analysis of two approaches. Spine 21:2317–2322, 1996.

43. Bueff HU, Lotz JC, Colliou OK, et al: Instrumentation of the cervicothoracic junction after destabilization. Spine 20:1789–1792, 1995.

44. Kreshak JL, Kim DH, Lindsey DP, et al: Posterior stabilization at the cervicothoracic junction: A biomechanical study. Spine 27: 2763– 2770, 2002.

45. Vaccaro R, Conant RF, Hilibrand AS, Albert TJ: A plate-rod device for treatment of cervicothoracic disorders: Comparison of mechanical testing with established cervical spine in vitro load testing data. J Spinal Disord 13:350–355, 2000.

46. Boockvar JA, Philips MF, Telfeian AE, et al: Results and risk factors for anterior cervicothoracic junction surgery. J Neurosurg 94(1 Suppl): 12–17, 2001.

47. Kaneda K, Kurakami C, Minami A: Free vascularized fibular strut graft in the treatment of kyphosis. Spine 13:1273–1277, 1988.

48. Roy-Camille R, SG, Mazel C: Internal fixation of the unstable cervical spine by a posterior osteosynthesis with plates and screws. In Sherk HH, Dunn EJ, Eismont FJ, et al (eds): The Cervical Spine, 2nd ed. Philadelphia: JB Lippincott, 1989, pp 390–403.

49. Xu R, Ebraheim NA, Ou Y, Yeasting RA: Anatomic considerations of pedicle screw placement in the thoracic spine: Roy-Camille technique versus open-lamina technique. Spine 23:1065–1068, 1998.

50. Xu R, Ebraheim NA, Tang G, Stanescu S: Location of the vertebral artery in the cervicothoracic junction. Am J Orthop 29:453–456, 2000.

51. An HS, Gordin R, Renner K: Anatomic considerations in plate-screw fixation of the cervical spine. Spine 16(Suppl):548–551, 1981.

52. Stanescu S, Ebraheim NA, Yeasting R, et al: Morphometric evaluation of the cervico-thoracic junction. Spine 19:2082–2088, 1994.

53. Panjabi MM, Duranceau J, Goel V, et al: Cervical human vertebrae: Quantitative three-dimensional anatomy of the middle and lower regions. Spine 16:861–869, 1991.

54. Karaikovic EE, Daubs MD, Gaines RW, Jr: Morphologic characteristics of human cervical pedicles. Spine 22:493–500, 1997.

55. Miller RC, Bonner JA, Wenger DE, et al: Spinal cord localization in the treatment of lung cancer: Use of radiographic landmarks. Int J Radiat Oncol Biol Phys 40:347–351, 1998.

56. Jeanneret B, Gebhard JS, Magerl F: Transpedicular screw fixation of articular mass fracture-separation: Result of an anatomical study and operative technique. J Spinal Disord 7:222–229, 1994.

57. Abumi K, Itoh H, Taneichi H, Kaneda K: Transpedicular screw fixation for traumatic lesions of the middle and lower cervical spine: Description of the techniques and preliminary report. J Spinal Disord 7:19–28, 1994.

58. Abumi K, Kaneda K: Pedicle screw fixation for nontraumatic lesions of the cervical spine. Spine 22:1853–1863, 1997.

140 Video-Assisted Thoracoscopic Discectomy

JOSHUA M. AMMERMAN and ANTHONY J. CAPUTY

INTRODUCTION

History of Thoracic Disc Disease

The surgical management of disorders of the thoracic spine began in 1814 when H. J. Cline attempted to treat a fracture of the thoracic spine by laminectomy.[1] In 1911, Middleton and Teacher undertook the first surgical procedure for a thoracic disc herniation, which was later described by Benjamin.[2] In this case, the patient was paraplegic and subsequently died.

Historically, the diagnosis of a thoracic disc herniation was a challenge. Given the lack of imaging, the diagnosis was required to be made solely on clinical history and physical findings. In addition, early surgical results were largely dismal. The evolution of diagnostic imaging and surgical techniques in the last half of the 20th century has resulted in a significant improvement in the diagnosis and outcome of patients with thoracic disc herniation.

Thoracic disc herniation is a relatively infrequent clinical diagnosis, accounting for 0.25% to 0.75% of all disc herniations and approximately 4% of the operative cases.[3,4] The symptoms of thoracic disc herniation are variable and often nonspecific; as such, many patients experience a protracted clinical course with a delay in diagnosis. A current series focused on computed tomography myelography and magnetic resonance imaging has shown that there is an 11% to 14.5% incidence of thoracic disc herniations.[5,6] Woods and colleagues[7] found disc herniations in 37% of the 60 asymptomatic patients evaluated by magnetic resonance imaging.

There has been a significant evolution of the surgical management of thoracic disc herniation. Early surgical therapy consisted of laminectomy, which often resulted in paraplegia, and carried a combined operative mortality as high as 10%.[8] In 1969, Perot and Munro reviewed 91 laminectomies for thoracic disc herniations and found no neurologic improvement in 40 of the patients and progressive paraplegia in 16 of these patients.[9] Others have also reported similarly poor outcomes with laminectomies for thoracic disc herniation.[10–12] Variations on the surgical technique were employed with laminectomies, including the use of decompression alone, decompression and transdural removal of disc material, and decompression with transdural rhizotomy and sectioning of the dentate ligaments, but all these successive approaches had similarly poor outcomes. The only exception to this pattern of poor surgical outcomes was the series reported by Horwitz and colleagues[13] in 1955 in which five consecutive cases of thoracic disc herniation treated with laminectomy resulted in a good outcome. In 1998, Fessler and Sturgel[14] reviewed and reported on 60 years of the literature in which

they compared the mortality and morbidity rates with the various surgical approaches to the thoracic spine. They concluded that laminectomy does not provide adequate access to safely treat thoracic disc herniations.

In response to the uniformly poor outcome after midline dorsal approaches to thoracic disc disease, surgical alternatives were developed using the anterior or extended posterolateral approaches with the costotransversectomy, transpedicular, and the lateral extracavitary approach.[9,15–17] Maiman and colleagues[18] in their report on the lateral extracavitary approach for thoracic disc herniation reviewed 23 cases. None of the patients in the review experienced any new deficits postoperatively. This surgical technique, however, required significantly more soft-tissue dissection and manipulation, with the paraspinous muscles being mobilized medially, resulting in devascularization and denervation. This was found to contribute to poor wound healing and increase in perioperative kyphosis. In addition, the lateral parascapular extrapleural approach, as developed by Fessler, provided exposure to the upper thoracic spine, which was comparable with the lateral extracavitary approach. However, it presents the risk of significant shoulder girdle dysfunction due to lateral scapular mobilization.[19] These approaches, despite their complexity, yielded significantly improved surgical and neurologic outcomes when compared with laminectomy for thoracic disc herniations.

The use of a transpleural approach to the thoracic spine dates to 1958 when Crafoord and colleagues[20] reported the use of this technique for herniated thoracic discs. In 1969, Perot and Munro[9] reported the use of this approach in two patients, and in the same year Ranasohoff and Spencer[15] reported the results of a similar approach for three patients. Since that time, the benefits of the anterior transthoracic approach have been supported by other published series.[21–23]

In 1988, Bohlmann and Zedeblick[24] recommended the anterior transthoracic approach over the costotransversectomy to treat herniated thoracic discs. This anterior transthoracic approach required a thoracotomy with rib resection and frequently resulted in significant perioperative morbidity including pulmonary dysfunction, and intercostal neuralgia, and shoulder girdle ... dysfunction.[25–27]

History of Spinal Endoscopy

The beginnings of endoscopic surgery date to 1807 when Philip Bozzini developed an endoscopic device that he called the *Lichtleiter*.[28] This, like other earlier endoscopic devices, was primarily used to explore body orifices using reflected light. Later, optical lenses were incorporated, and in 1910, Jacobeus[29,30] reported the first use of an endoscope to explore the thoracic cavity. He used a cystoscope to examine the pleural cavity in the treatment of tuberculosis and eventually expanded its use to the diagnosis of malignant and benign pulmonary diseases.[31,32] Since that time, thoracoscopes have been adapted to treat a variety of pulmonary disorders including penetrating chest injuries.[33–35]

Spinal endoscopy began in 1931 when Burman[36] published a report on a technique he called "myeloscopy." He described the use of an arthroscope to examine cadaveric spines and explore the lumbar thecal sac. In 1938, Pool[37,38] expanded on Burman's work and used a hot lamp system with improved visualization of the thecal space to examine more than 400 patients between 1938 and 1942. Despite the initial success of Barman and Pool, spinal endoscopy did not immediately gain widespread acceptance. Optical resolution and the light intensity were poor, and the instruments were far too large to easily explore and work in the confines of this small surgical space. Advances in fiber optics and the development of modern video technology have led to resurgence in interest in endoscopic approaches to the spine. Small cold light sources and video display monitors have replaced the older hot reflected light and lens tube systems.

In 1983, Hausmann and Forst[39] used a nucleoscope to inspect the disc space for loose fragments after an open discectomy, and in 1992, Shreiber and Leu[40] successfully performed a percutaneous discoscopy. The procedure was rapidly applied to surgery for thoracic disc herniations.[41,42]

The anterior approaches provide an unsurpassed exposure of the ventral aspect of the spinal column. It not only provides a large working area in which the adjacent anatomic structures became clearly identified but also provides the optimal angle for removal of intervertebral discs and allows easy inspection of the spinal cord. If necessary, repair of the dura in cases of intradural disc herniations can be performed via this approach. The anterior approach has become the preferred approach of many spinal surgeries for most thoracic spinal pathology other than far lateral lesions.[2,9,15]

The risk associated with the anterior transpleural approach is that of injury to the adjacent vascular and visceral structures. There is additional associated morbidity with prolonged pulmonary dysfunction, incisional pain, and pain associated with thoracostomy tube drainage that contributes to the potential adverse consequences. Comparative studies have shown a lower rate of pulmonary morbidity with thoracoscopic procedures when compared with open thoracotomy. Thoracoscopy minimizes the incidence of intercostal neuralgia and avoids shoulder girdle dysfunction. In addition, there are reduced blood loss and a proven reduction in hospital length of stay.[43–45]

The dramatically improved optics and lighting of rigid glass endoscopes as developed by physicist Harold Hopkins in 1970 nurtured the rapid growth of endoscopic surgical techniques.[46] Landreneau and colleagues[45] reported 106 such cases in 1993 in which they compared video-assisted thoracoscopic surgery (VATS) with thoracotomy. The patients who underwent VATS had less pain and improved pulmonary function and superior shoulder girdle function when compared with thoracotomy patients. That same year, Mack and colleagues published a report demonstrating the potential of VATS to provide reliable access to the ventral surface of the thoracic spine.[47] In 1995, Caputy and colleagues[48] demonstrated the successful use of VATS

in performing thoracic discectomy on both cadaveric and porcine models. In that same study, the clinical use of thoracoscopic dissection was also reported.

Although the benefit of VATS is usually compared only with the alternative thoracotomy, data also suggest that it is a less morbid procedure than a costotransversectomy. Rosenthal and Dickman[49] reported a series of 55 patients who underwent thoracoscopic discectomy and compared the rate of complications of the thoracoscopic procedures with both the patients undergoing open thoracotomy and the patients undergoing costotransversectomy for thoracic disc herniations. There were no instances of postoperative neurologic deterioration in either the thoracoscopic or thoracotomy group, but of those patients undergoing costotransversectomies, 7% experienced new neurologic deficits after surgery. Intercostal neuralgia, both temporary and permanent, has been a significant problem associated with thoracotomy. The use of VATS has significantly reduced the incidence of this painful disorder. In that same series, there was a 16% rate of intercostal neuralgia in the VATS group compared with 50% in patients who had a thoracotomy. In all patients in the thoracoscopic group with intercostal neuralgia, the condition was temporary and resolved completely within 1 to 2 weeks. In those patients undergoing costotransversectomy, there was a 20% rate of intercostal neuralgia.[49]

SURGICAL ANATOMY

Thoracic Cavity Anatomy

The surgical anatomy includes the external anatomy of the chest, the intrathoracic visceral and vascular anatomy, the contents of the posterior mediastinum, the ribs, vertebrae, and neural elements.

A thorough knowledge of the anatomy of the thoracic cavity is critical for a successful procedure as well as complication avoidance. The muscles of the chest wall, primarily the serratus anterior, pectoralis major, and latissimus dorsi, form important landmarks for thoracoscopic portal placement. The serratus anterior forms the medial wall of the axilla. The pectoralis major demarcates the anterior axillary line and serves as the anterior boarder for trocar insertion, whereas the latissimus dorsi denotes the posterior axillary line and the posterior boarder for trocar placement. Attention should also be paid to the mammary gland overlying the anterior and lateral thoracic wall. Its origin just anterior to the midaxillary line, from the second to the sixth rib, is at risk during trocar introduction.[50]

Once inside the thoracic cavity, transparent parietal pleura covers the anterior, posterior, and superior aspects of the chest cavity. It reflects over the great vessels, trachea, esophagus, and spinal column and is easily separated from these structures. Commonly, the parietal pleura is studded with anthracotic pigment, indicating exposure to smoke or other inhaled pollution over the patient's lifetime. Chronic inflammation of the pleura can render it opaque and prevent visualization of the underlying structures.

The normal lung is pink, soft, and covered by visceral pleura. The right lung is composed of three lobes, whereas the left has two lobes. Each is divided by one or two fissures. Deflation and retraction of the lung permit visualization of the majority of the intrathoracic structures.

In the center of the chest cavity lies the mediastinum, containing the heart and great vessels. The heart is enclosed within the glistening pericardial sac with the phrenic nerve overlying the lateral surface. Accessing the right side of the thoracic cavity permits visualization of the right subclavian and brachiocephalic vessels. The right pulmonary artery, right main stem bronchus, and distal trachea can also be seen with retraction of the lung. Inspection of the left side of the chest cavity displays the left subclavian artery, descending aorta, and internal mammary vessels. The left carotid artery is difficult to visualize in its position deep to the brachiocephalic venous trunk.

An inferior view of the chest cavity is defined by the diaphragm. Divided into two halves, it originates from the xiphoid process, upper lumbar vertebrae, and lower six ribs. During full expiration, the right hemidiaphragm ascends to the level of the fourth intercostal space and the left to the level of the fifth rib. This fact must be considered at the time of trocar placement to avoid diaphragmatic perforation and violation of the peritoneal cavity.

The complex vascular anatomy of the paravertebral area as demarcated from the intrathoracic perspective requires a detailed understanding before embarking on thoracoscopic procedures. The posterior intercostal arteries of the first two vertebral segments arise from the superior intercostal artery branch of the costocervical trunk of the subclavian artery. The lower posterior intercostal arteries arise segmentally directly from the aorta. The segmental branches on the right are longer and transverse a greater distance than segmental branches on the left. These arteries leave the aorta and travel on the side of the vertebral body between the intravertebral discs. These arteries are crossed, immediately anterior to the rib head articulation, by the sympathetic chain. The arteries then course superiorly under the tip of the transverse process merging with the vein and nerve in the costal groove. At this point, the artery gives off a branch that continues in a posterior course over the transverse process to supply the muscles of the back. Before passing over the transverse process, however, it sends a spinal branch through the intravertebral foramen, which supplies the spinal cord (Fig. 140-1). The primary blood supply to the lower thoracic spinal cord is via the great radicular anastomotic artery of Adamkiewicz. This vessel most often enters from the left side between T8 and L3. Disruption of this radicular artery may lead to spinal cord infarction and paraplegia. Consideration should be given to spinal angiography for location of this vessel before exposure of the lower thoracic spine.[51] However, this is generally unnecessary when a thoracoscopic technique is used.

The posterior intercostal vein courses in the intercostal space adjacent to and in a rostral position with the posterior intercostal artery. Blood from the spinal cord, spine, and posterior muscles converge at the level of the rib head. The segmental vein courses over the lateral aspect of the vertebral body merging, dependent on the location, with the azygos, hemiazygos, or superior intercostal vein.

The first intercostal vein ascends over the first rib and arches above the pleura to terminate in the corresponding brachycephalic or vertebral vein. The second and third intercostal veins unite to form a superior intercostal vein. On the right, this vein drains into the terminal part of the azygos vein, and on the left, it branches into the brachycephalic vein. At all levels below the third intercostal region,

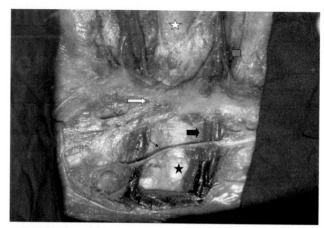

FIGURE 140-1 Anatomic dissection displaying the relevant surgical anatomy of the retropleural space with the vertebral column oriented in the horizontal plane. Highlighted are the rib (*open star*), intervertebral disc (*black star*), segmental vessels (*black arrow*), intercostal neurovascular bundle (*gray arrow*), splanchnic nerve (*thin arrow*), and sympathetic chain (*open arrow*). Note the relationship of the intervertebral disc to the segmental vessels and sympathetic chain.

the veins empty into the azygos vein on the right and into the accessory hemiazygos vein on the left. The hemiazygos and accessory hemiazygos veins cross to the right side of the thoracic cavity emptying into the azygos vein. The azygos vein then ascends and empties into the superior vena cava just before it passing through the pericardium.

To avoid injury to the phrenic nerve and subsequent diaphragm paralysis, a more thorough discussion of its course is warranted. Once it leaves the cervical plexus, the phrenic nerve accesses the thoracic cavity via the thoracic inlet and runs along the lateral border of the brachiocephalic trunk. On the right, the nerve continues along the superior vena cava, over the right side of the heart, and into the diaphragm. On the left, the nerve runs between the left common carotid and subclavian vessels until it meets the diaphragm.

The sympathetic chain and ganglia lie in the retropleural space over the rib heads in the upper chest cavity, across the segmental vessels, and move medially to lie over the vertebral bodies in the caudal portion. It is made up of ganglia linked by interganglionic cords. This chain is located anterior to the rib head of the thoracic vertebrae and crosses the segmental vessels. The medial branches of the upper five ganglia supply the thoracic aorta via the thoracic aortic plexus. The medial branches of the lower ganglia coalesce to form the splanchnic nerves. The anterior rami of the thoracic nerves form an intercostal nerve. Each nerve is connected to the ganglion of the adjacent sympathetic trunk by a gray and a white communicating ramus. They pass forward in the intercostal space below the intercostal vessels. The sympathetic preganglionic nerve fibers are conveyed through white rami to the sympathetic trunk. They in turn synapse with the cells of the sympathetic ganglia. These ganglion cells of the sympathetic chain send out postganglionic fibers through the gray rami, which return to join the spinal nerves.

The vagus nerves and their recurrent branches also lie within the thoracic cavity. The left vagus nerve runs between the left common carotid artery and subclavian artery, then passes between the left pulmonary artery and the aortic arch.

It continues in close proximity to the esophagus where it forms the anterior vagal trunk. The left recurrent laryngeal nerve arises below the aortic arch and ascends into the neck in the tracheoesophageal groove. The right vagus nerve runs anterior to the right subclavian artery and deep to the brachiocephalic vein. It then gives off its recurrent branch and continues along the trachea and ends as the posterior vagal trunk along the esophagus.[52]

Thoracic Spinal Anatomy

The thoracic vertebrae are distinguished from their lumbar and cervical counterparts by their articulation with the ribs. There are two points of connection of the ribs with the thoracic vertebral column. One is at the vertebrae, and the second is at the transverse process. On the second through ninth thoracic vertebrae, these articulations are shared by adjacent vertebrae by a demifacet. The rib head articulation thereby covers the intervening intravertebral disc. The 1st, 10th, 11th, and 12th rib heads articulate with a single vertebra. The articular capsule surrounds the joint and becomes continuous with the intervertebral fibrocartilage of the annulus. A radiate ligament connects the rib head with the side of the vertebral bodies spanning the adjacent vertebrae and the annulus. Anterior to this ligament are the ganglia of the thoracic sympathetic trunk and the pleura. Contained by the radiate ligaments are the synovial membranes of the demifacets and the intra-articular ligament connecting the rib head to the annular fibers belonging to the demifacets. The second point of attachment of the rib to the vertebrae is by the costotransverse articulation. This is a synovial articulation connecting the tubercle of the rib with the transverse process of that vertebral segment.

The thoracic vertebrae increase in size as one moves caudal in the spine and form a nearly circular vertebral canal with the anteroposterior dimensions being equal to the transverse dimensions. The demifacets articulate with the vertebral bodies. At the vertebrae above the articulation, this articulation is lateral and at the root of the pedicle. The articulation with the vertebrae below is near the inferior vertebral notch covering the pedicle and is in close proximity to the transverse process and the superior facet. The facet joints of the vertebrae are oriented in a coronal plane with the inferior facet of the superior vertebrae overlapping the superior facet of the inferior vertebrae as do shingles on a roof. The 1st cervical as well as the 9th, 10th, 11th, and 12th vertebrae have no demifacets. The synovial joints with the rib are contained over the vertebrae and lateral pedicle of that single vertebra. The ribs of the 11th and 12th vertebrae have no articulations with transverse processes.

PREOPERATIVE EVALUATION

The preoperative evaluation involves both an anatomic and functional evaluation of the patient's pathology. An anatomic evaluation is used to define the structural spinal pathology and to correlate the physical findings with that pathology. An initial radiographic evaluation is done using magnetic resonance imaging, which will delineate the degree of compromise of the spinal cord and exiting nerve roots. Bright signal on T2-weighted sequences, indicating myelomalacia, may be appreciated within the spinal cord. Sagittal views permit the vertebrae to be counted, localizing the pathologic level.

The axial images aid in planning which side is optimal in approaching the pathology and may provide information on the adjacent vascular structures. Myelography with postmyelogram computed tomography scanning has been invaluable in defining the bony anatomy of the thoracic spine and in localizing the pathologic changes within the context of the broader anatomy of the thoracic cavity. It allows a determination as to whether the disc pathology is soft or calcified, and it may provide a preoperative indication of the involvement of the dura with an adherent calcified disc (Fig. 140-2).

Plain radiographs of the thoracic and lumbar spine are essential in the preoperative evaluation for VATS procedures. An accurate rib count can be obtained and any calcified pathology may also be noted to aid at the time of surgery in determining the correct operative level. As previously mentioned, location of the artery of Adamkiewicz, via angiography, is of paramount importance if there is an anticipated left-sided surgical approach involving disc herniations between T8 and L2.

Preoperative functional evaluations in a patient include an estimate of both anesthetic and pulmonary risks. Patients who are elderly or smokers or those patients with preexisting pulmonary or cardiac disease are at greater risk of complications. The anesthetic evaluation is similar to the evaluation that is routinely performed before any thoracotomy. In general, however, the patients undergoing VATS for spinal pathology have less pulmonary dysfunction when compared with patients undergoing VATS for primary pulmonary or cardiac pathology.

The greatest pulmonary and anesthetic risks are seen in those patients engaged in heavy smoking. Smoking cessation should be encouraged before surgery. Cessation of smoking for as short of a period as 1 week before surgery will reduce pulmonary secretions and may improve ciliary function. Refraining from smoking for 24 hours will increase the available oxygen by reducing the levels of carboxyhemoglobin. Preoperative pulse oxymetry and/or blood gas measurements are useful in predicting postoperative pulmonary complications. Patients with a preoperative PO_2 of less than 60 mm Hg and a resting PCO_2 of greater than 50 mm Hg are at increased risk of pulmonary complications. These preoperative levels will also serve as a baseline for the operative procedure.

In at-risk patients, further screening may be obtained by the use of pulmonary function tests. A forced vital capacity that is 50% of predicted and a maximal ventilatory ventilation of 50% of predicted may also be associated with postoperative pulmonary complications.

Patients with a history of cardiac disease are also at an increased risk of perioperative complications. A history of a myocardial infarction increases the risk of a perioperative myocardial infarction to 17%. A screening preoperative electrocardiogram may aid in determining the risk by highlighting arrhythmias and signs of ischemic change or infarction. A thallium stress test or coronary angiogram may be indicated in older patients or in patients with a known history of coronary artery disease.

SURGICAL INDICATIONS

Indications for VATS include disc herniation, sympathectomy, vertebral biopsy to evaluate for tumor or infection, vertebrectomy, bone graft or instrumentation, anterior

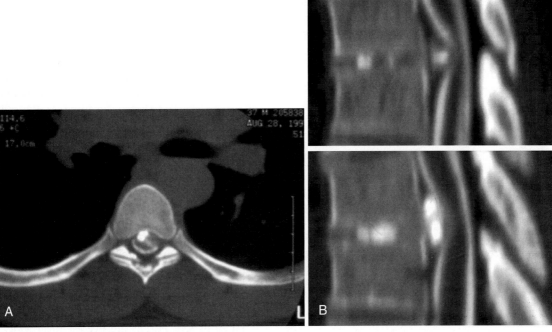

FIGURE 140-2 Axial (*A*) and sagittal (*B*) postmyelography computed tomography scans demonstrate ventral compression of the thecal sac by a large, calcified disc fragment.

release for spinal deformity correction, or other ventral thoracic spine pathology. The thoracoscopic approach provides access to the entire thoracic spine from T1–2 to T11–12. There is a steep learning curve required to master the technique. Practice with cadaveric specimens in the laboratory before the actual operating room application has been strongly advocated.

Degenerative discs may be excised at a single or multiple levels through the VATS approach. Access to the upper and lower extremes of the thoracic spine may be difficult in some individual cases. Approaches to the lower thoracic discs may require retraction of the diaphragm, and adequate exposure of the levels below T9–10 on the right may not be possible due to the elevated diaphragm on that side. Surgical approaches are most frequently from the right because of the eccentric placement of the aorta, but the lateralization of the disc pathology is the predominant reason for selecting a side for the approach.

Absolute contraindications to VATS include a fused pleural space, inability to tolerate single-lung ventilation, severe acute respiratory insufficiency, and positive pressure ventilation with high airway pressures. Relative contraindications include previous thoracotomy, a history of empyema, or previous traumatic chest injury or chest tube placement that could contribute to extensive pleural adhesions.

ANESTHESIA

Patients undergoing a thoracoscopic procedure require single-lung ventilation to facilitate the surgical exposure. Single-lung ventilation is routinely achieved by the use of either a double-lumen endotracheal tube or the bronchial blocker technique. The preferred method of single-lung ventilation is with the use of a double-lumen endotracheal tube; however, this endotracheal tube may be too large for patients weighing less than 50 kg, and, in that instance, bronchial blockers are used. Double-lumen endotracheal tubes are formed by two catheters attached to each other side by side (Fig. 140-3). Each catheter will independently ventilate one of the lungs. Bronchial blockers are catheters that are placed within the lumen of a single endotracheal tube. The blocker is placed fiberoptically to block one of the main stem bronchi while the endotracheal tube is positioned in the

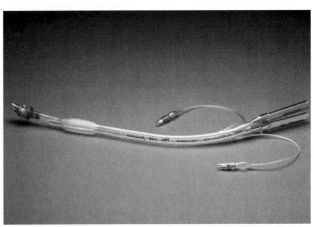

FIGURE 140-3 A double-lumen endotracheal tube used for single-lung ventilation.

trachea and will ventilate the nonblocked lung. This blocking technique has many disadvantages including the tendency of the balloon blocker to back out of the bronchus and partially obstruct the trachea. Bronchoscopy should be used to confirm proper positioning of the endotracheal tube and reconfirm once positioning is complete. Invasive blood pressure monitoring and somatosensory evoked potentials are other techniques employed in this procedure.

SURGICAL TECHNIQUE

Positioning

The lateral decubitus position is used for most VATS procedures. In most cases, the lesion is approached from the right unless the pathology is distinctly lateralized to the left. The approach from the right is preferred because there is more working space between the azygos vein and the rib head and there is less risk of injury to the aorta and heart. An axillary roll is placed between the axilla and the operating table on the patient's down side, while the upward, nondependent upper extremity is supported at right angles to the body. The dependent lower extremity is slightly flexed and all bony prominences are padded. The patient is secured to the operating table with 3-inch tape, and the stability of this position is tested by rolling the table from side to side before the patient is prepped and draped.

Operating Room Setup

After positioning, the anesthesiologist is placed at the patient's head to control the endotracheal tube and facilitate lung collapse and single-lung ventilation. The surgeon and first assistant stand on the abdominal side of the patient, and a second assistant is positioned on the patient's dorsal side. Two video monitors are positioned one on each side of the patient's head. The nurse is positioned at the foot of the table opposite the principal surgeon. A thoracotomy set is to be immediately available for use should proper exposure

not be attained via the VATS exposure or should excessive bleeding occur. A thoracic surgeon should also be available.

Endoscopic Instruments

Open radiolucent portals are used because they do not obstruct the fluoroscopy or radiographic localization during surgery. The portals most commonly used are 10 mm in diameter but can range from 3 to 18 mm. Smaller portals cause less pressure on the neurovascular bundle. Rigid portals are used for the initial thoracoscopy but may be substituted for flexible models during the actual surgical decompression to minimize the tissue pressure in the intercostal area.

After initial portal placement, the pleural cavity is inspected. The lung is further deflated by suctioning through the endotracheal tube to the isolated lung. The table is tilted in the patient's ventral direction, 30 degrees toward the principal surgeon. This allows displacement of the lung and the mediastinal contents in a more anterior direction away from the spinal column, improving the exposure of the operative area. The use of the Trendelenburg or reverse Trendelenburg position will improve the exposure of the lower and upper spine, respectively.

Three to four portals are needed to provide a surgical working area for a VATS discectomy. These ports are arranged in a reverse L pattern (Fig. 140-4). The first portal is placed in the anterior axillary line at the sixth or seventh intercostal space to avoid injury to the diaphragm. After the initial lung inspection, two or three more portals are inserted under direct inspection. These portals are centered on the area of interest. Two additional ports are placed, one rostral and the other caudal to this initial port. A fourth port may be placed at the caudal corner of the reverse L pattern if further lung or diaphragm retraction is required in the case of lower thoracic lesions. One of the ports will be used for the endoscope. It is usually the more posterior port, along the posterior axillary line. The remaining ports along the anterior axillary line serve as the working channels. Proper placement

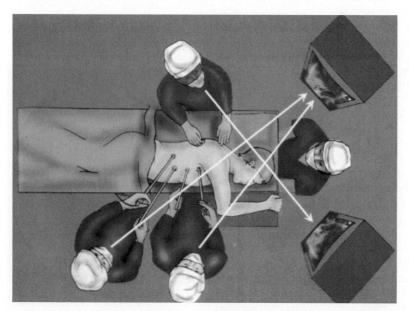

FIGURE 140-4 Standard operating room setup for thoracoscopic discectomy. The patient has been placed in the left lateral position, and thoracoscopic portals have been inserted in the reverse L pattern. Monitors are displayed on either side of the patient to permit viewing of the operative field by both the primary surgeon and the assistant(s).

of the ports is critical to ensure that the surgical instruments inserted through any given port are not inhibiting the use of a second instrument inserted through a second port. Ports that are placed too close together may cause "fencing" when the instruments crowd the operative area and make contact with the shaft of the other instruments, thereby inhibiting the free movement of the primary surgical instrument.

The imaging equipment consists of the endoscope, light source, camera, video monitors, and video recorders. The endoscopes may be either rigid or flexible, but the most frequently used scope is a rigid rod-lens system in which the image is transmitted through a series of quartz rods to a camera mounted at the end. The field of view through the lens can vary from 0 to 70 degrees, but the 30-degree lens is preferred because it affords the greatest visualization of the operative field. In addition, better angles of inspection of the surgical area and the thoracic cavity are afforded by the use of a 30-degree scope.

The illumination is provided by a remote halogen or xenon light source transmitted through fiber-optic cables. The video camera sensor is attached directly to the end of the endoscope, and the camera sends its output directly to the monitor where the image is displayed. The cameras are now of high resolution, which produces intense, accurate color images.

Instruments that are used by the thoracic surgeons for VATS procedures have become the mainstay for VATS discectomy. These instruments are longer and have been adapted with pistol grips. They include scissors and dissectors with articulating heads that allow the tip to be repositioned for greater visualization during the surgical dissection (Fig. 140-5). Other instruments have been developed to aid in the specific needs unique to the thoracic cavity, such as fan retractors and suction irrigation devices.

The existing instruments common to spinal surgery have been modified by lengthening and by providing a greater variety of tip angles. These include a variety of periosteal elevators, and curets, rongeurs, and dissectors. Modified long drill bits with coarse diamond bits are now available (Midas Rex, Fort Worth, TX) (Fig. 140-6).

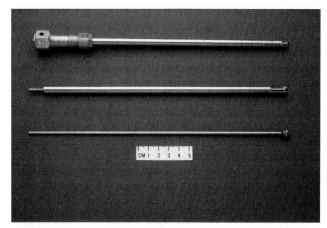

FIGURE 140-6   Extended diamond drill bits for removal of vertebral elements and calcified disc herniations. Long protective collars accompany these bits to shield the intrathoracic viscera, nerves, and vascular structures.

Description of Procedure

Once the ports have been placed and the exposure of the spinal column complete, the level must be determined. The ribs are counted from the apex of the thoracic cavity. The first rib is usually not visualized because it is covered by the subclavian fat pad. It can, however, be palpated and the ribs counted to determine the level of operative interest. This is confirmed by the use of an image intensifier or intraoperative radiograph. Once the level has been confirmed, the rib head is palpated and the pleura over the proximal rib and disc space is incised. The segmental vessels are dissected, mobilized, and isolated. For single-level disc pathology, ligation is usually not required. However, if necessary, they are then ligated with endoscopic hemoclips and cut with the endoscopic cautery scissors. The pleura is then further mobilized by the use of a Cobb elevator to expose a 3-cm segment of the rib head. The rib head is removed by using a high-speed pneumatic drill with a rough-cut diamond burr (Midas Rex). The diamond burr provides tactile feedback and significantly aids in controlling bone bleeding and thereby increases the visibility at the operative site. An alternate method of removing the rib involves sectioning a 2- to 3-cm segment of rib head en bloc to be used for an arthrodesis.

Once the rib head has been removed and the lateral disc space clearly identified, the spinal canal must be defined. To accomplish this, the pedicle immediately posterior to the costovertebral articulation is exposed. The upper one third of the pedicle is typically removed using the diamond burr and a Kerrison rongeur. An extended rostral removal of the pedicle may be necessary if the disc herniation is large or calcified. Removing this portion of the pedicle exposes the anterior portion of the vertebral canal and the posterior longitudinal ligament. The normal dura and the epidural space are identified. Epidural venous bleeding may be encountered, and it is generally controlled by the use of the bipolar cautery or Avitene (CR Bard, Murray Hill, NJ). The decompression of the spinal canal and the removal of the disc material may now take place under direct visualization. A portion of the vertebral body on either side of the disc is

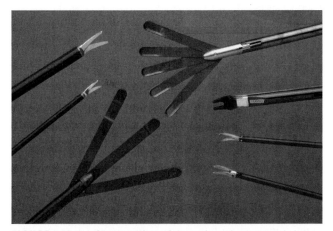

FIGURE 140-5   Close-up view of the various thoracoscopic instruments including fan retractors for displacing the lung and graspers/scissors for performing soft-tissue dissection and disc removal.

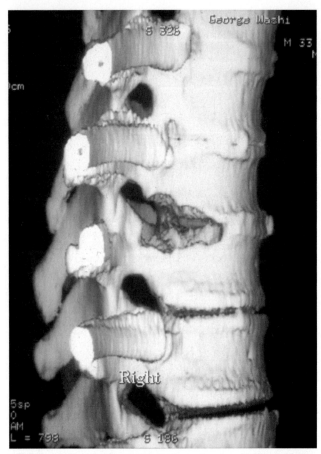

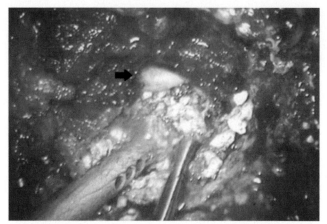

FIGURE 140-8   Intraoperative thoracoscopic view of herniated disc material being removed with a thoracoscopic pituitary rongeur. The dural margin is visible (*arrow*), allowing direct visualization of the thecal sac during completion of the decompression.

FIGURE 140-7   Postoperative 3-dimensional computed tomography reconstruction of the thoracic spine shows the area of disc and vertebra removal needed to perform the discectomy. It should be noted that the cephalad portion of the lower pedicle has been removed to expose the lateral thecal sac and define the anterior margin of the vertebral canal. The cavity created provides a working space into which disc material can be pulled to decompress the spinal cord.

removed to create a working channel (Fig. 140-7). This is accomplished using a shielded diamond burr to fashion a pyramid-shaped space. The disc material is pulled away from the thecal sac into this cavity (Fig. 140-8).

The amount of bone removed to create this space is determined by the size of the disc herniation and the amount of associated canal compromise. The working channel must be large enough to afford visualization of the normal dura rostral and caudal to the disc herniation. For large calcified discs or when an intradural fragment is identified, an extended vertebral body resection may be necessary. After the spinal canal has been exposed through this working channel, the disc material may be pulled away from the spinal cord into this created working space. If the disc material is soft, then it may be removed with a pituitary forceps or a curet. In the case of a calcified disc, however, care must be taken to sequentially dissect it away from the dura. The decompressed spinal canal is inspected and palpated to the level of the contralateral pedicle. If an intradural fragment is encountered, then it should be carefully dissected from the adjacent pia-arachnoid. A dural repair is accomplished with a tissue patch and fibrin glue. A lumbar drain is placed postoperatively.

Although a generous vertebral body resection may be required to adequately decompress the spinal cord in some cases of disc herniation, it is usually not necessary to perform an arthrodesis, and alone, it does not produce instability of the thoracic spine. If the patient has had a previous laminectomy or posterolateral procedure, then an arthrodesis may be indicated.

The surgical bed and thoracic cavity is irrigated copiously to remove blood and bone debris. The chest cavity and lungs are inspected, and a chest tube is inserted under direct visualization using one of the existing portal sites. The chest tube is set to water seal rather than to suction. The remaining ports are removed, and the wounds are closed in sequential layers. The chest tube is removed when there is no air leak, drainage is less than 15 mL/24 hour, and lung reexpansion is documented on a chest radiograph.

OUTCOMES AND COMPLICATIONS

Outcome results for patients undergoing thoracoscopic discectomy have been widely available since the late 1990s. In 1999, Rosenthal and Dickman[45] reported on their experience with 55 patients undergoing thoracoscopic discectomy and compared their patients with a smaller subset undergoing thoracotomy. They reported a 1-hour reduction in operative time and a 50% reduction in blood loss, narcotic use, and hospital length of stay. They also noted a 16% incidence of intercostal neuralgia in the thoracoscopy group as compared with the thoracotomy group, which carried a 50% incidence. Regarding neurologic outcome, of the 36 patients with preoperative myelopathy, 27 had neurologic improvement and all patients' neurologic examinations stabilized. Nineteen patients were treated for radiculopathy with improvement in all patients.[49]

In 2000, Johnson and colleagues[53] reported their prospective series of 36 patients undergoing thoracoscopic discectomy compared with 8 patients undergoing thoracotomy. Their results matched those reported earlier, demonstrating a statistically significant reduction in hospital length of stay and narcotic use in the thoracoscopy group. They also reported a 30% complication rate in the thoracoscopy group versus a greater than 100% (i.e., more than one complication per patient) complication rate in the thoracotomy group. However, they were not able to show a statistically significant difference in ultimate neurologic outcome between the two groups.

Anand and Regan[54] recently evaluated the long-term outcome after thoracoscopic discectomy for thoracic disc disease. They examined 100 consecutive patients who underwent thoracoscopic discectomy with an average of 4 years of follow-up. Five percent of patients required a reoperation during the follow-up interval, including one nonunion. Seventy percent of those treated had achieved a 20% improvement on their Oswestry score (their definition of a clinical success) at their last visit, and 84% of the patients were satisfied with their results.

In 1995, McAffe and colleagues[55] addressed the issue of complications related to the thoracoscopic approach. They reported on 78 patients undergoing thoracoscopic discectomy. They found an 8% incidence of intercostal neuralgia and a 6% incidence of postoperative atelectasis, both figures are significantly less that those reported for thoracotomy. Only one case required conversion to thoracotomy for significant plural adhesions.

CONCLUSIONS

The surgical treatment of thoracic disc herniations has undergone a rapid and dramatic evolution in the past century. The surgical technique for the treatment of thoracic disc herniation has progressed from an era when the laminectomy was the sole surgical approach and the outcome was often defined by dramatic mortality and morbidity rates to the present when the field now has a variety of effective surgical approaches, with the routine expectation of satisfactory surgical outcomes. VATS is a new modality that provides an excellent surgical alternative to treat anterior thoracic spine pathology in a minimally invasive manner. VATS discectomy permits safe, effective visualization and ventral decompression of the thoracic spinal cord and nerve roots, with less risk of neurologic injury as compared with standard posterior spinal approaches. The VATS discectomy has several advantages over the alternative anterior approaches to the thoracic spine. The risks of pulmonary dysfunction, postoperative pain, and extended hospital stay are reduced with this minimally invasive technique. Despite its advantages, thoracoscopic discectomy caries a steep learning curve that requires specific specialized training to develop a familiarity with the instruments and techniques.

REFERENCES

1. Hayward G: An account of a case of fracture and dislocation of the spine. J Med Sci 4:1–3, 1815.
2. Benjamin V: Diagnosis and management of thoracic disc disease. Clin Neurosurg 38:577–605, 1983.
3. Arce CA, Dohrmann GJ: Herniated thoracic disks. Neurol Clin 3: 383–392, 1985.
4. Ridenore TR, Haddad PW, Hichson PW, et al: Herniated thoracic disks: Treatment and outcome. J Spinal Disord 3:218–224, 1993.
5. Awwad EE, Martin DS, Smith KR, et al: Asymptomatic versus symptomatic herniated thoracic discs: Their frequency and characteristics as detected by computed tomography after myelography. Neurosurgery 28:180–186, 1991.
6. Williams MP, Cherryman GR, Husband JE: Significance of thoracic disc herniation demonstrated by MR imaging. J Comput Assist Tomogr 13:211–214, 1989.
7. Woods KB, Schellhas KP, Garvey TA, et al: Thoracic discography in healthy individuals: A controlled prospective study of magnetic resonance imaging and discography in asymptomatic and symptomatic individuals. Spine 24:1548–1555, 1999.
8. Horowitz NH, Rizzoli NV: Postoperative Complications of Extracranial Neurological Surgery. Baltimore: Williams & Wilkins, 1987.
9. Perot PL, Munro DD: Transthoracic removal of midline thoracic protrusions causing spinal cord compression. J Neurosurg 31:452–458, 1969.
10. Benson MD, Byrnes DP: The clinical syndromes and surgical treatment of thoracic intervertebral disc prolapse. J Bone Joint Surg Am 70:1038–1047, 1988.
11. Logue V: Thoracic intervertebral disc prolapse with spinal cord compression. J Neurol Neurosurg Psychiatry 15:221–247, 1952.
12. Mixter WJ, Barr JS: Rupture of the intervertebral disc with involvement of the spinal canal. N Engl J Med 221:210–215, 1934.
13. Horwitz NH, Whitcomb BB, Reilly FG: Ruptured thoracic discs. Yale J Biol Med 28:322–330, 1955.
14. Fessler RG, Sturgill M: Review: Complications of surgery for thoracic disc disease. Surg Neurol 49:609–618, 1998.
15. Ranasohoff J, Spencer F, Siew F, Gade L, Jr: Transthoracic removal of thoracic disks: Report of three cases. J Neurosurg 31:459–461, 1969.
16. Huhme A: The surgical approach to intervertebral disk protrusions. J Neurol Neurosurg Psychiatry 23:133–137, 1960.
17. Patterson RH, Arbit E: A surgical approach through the pedicle to protruded thoracic disks. J Neurosurg 48:768–772, 1978.
18. Maiman DJ, Larson SJ, Luck E, Elghatit A: Lateral extracavitary approach to the spine for thoracic disk herniation: Report of 23 cases. Neurosurgery 41:178–182, 1984.
19. Fessler RG, Dietze DD, Jr, MacMillan M: Lateral parascapular extrapleural approach to the upper thoracic spine. J Neurosurg 75: 349–355, 1991.
20. Crafford C, Hiertonn T, Lindblom K, Olsson SE: Spinal cord compression caused by a protruded thoracic disc: Report of a case treated with anterolateral fenestration of the disc. Acta Orthop Scand 28:103–107, 1958.
21. Bohlmann HH, Zdeblick: Anterior excision of herniated thoracic discs. J Bone Joint Surg Am 70:1038–1047, 1988.
22. Otani K, Yoshida M, Fujii E, Nakai S, Shibasaki K: Thoracic disc herniation: Surgical treatment in 23 patients. Spine 13:1262–1267, 1998.
23. Otani K, Nakai S, Fujimura Y, Manzoku S, Shibasaki K: Surgical treatment of thoracic disc herniation using the anterior approach. J Bone Joint Surg Br 64:340–343, 1982.
24. Bohlman HH, Zdeblick TA: Anterior excision of herniated thoracic discs. J Bone Joint Surg Am 78:1038–1047, 1988.
25. Faciszewski T, Winter RB, Lonstein JE, et al: The surgical and medical perioperative complications of anterior spinal fusion surgery in the thoracic and lumbar spine in adults: A review of 1223 procedures. Spine 20:1592–1599, 1995.
26. Naunheim KS, Barnett MG, Crandall DG, et al: Anterior exposure of the thoracic spine. Ann Thorac Surg 57:1436–1439, 1994.
27. Sundaresan N, Shah J, Foley KM, et al: An anterior surgical approach to the upper thoracic vertebrae. J Neurosurg 61:686–690, 1984.
28. Bozzini PH: Lichtleiter, eine Erfindung Zur Anschauung innerer Teile und Krankheiten. J Prak Heilk 24:107, 1806.
29. Nitze M: Beobachtungs and untersuchungsmethode fur Harnrohre Harnblase und rectum. Wien Med Wochenschr 24:649–652, 1879.
30. Jacobeus HC: Uber die Moglichkeit die Zystoskopie bei Untersoachangen seroser Hohlmongen asznwenken. Munch Med Wochenschr 57:2090–2092, 1910.
31. Jacobeus HC: The cauterization of adhesions in pneumothorax treatment of tuberculosis. Surg Gynecol Obstet 32:493–500, 1921.
32. Jacobeus HC: The practical importance of thoroscopy in surgery of the chest. Surg Gynecol Obstet 34:289–296, 1922.
33. Branco JMC: Thoracopy as a method of exploration in penetrating injuries of the chest. Dis Chest 12:330, 1946.
34. Kux M: Thoracic endoscopic sympathectomy in palmar and axillary hyperhydrosis. Arch Surg 113:264–266, 1978.
35. Hatch HB, DeCamp PT: Diagnostic thoracopy. Surg Clin North Am 46:1405–1410, 1966.
36. Burman MS: Myeloscopy or the direct visualization of the spinal canal and its contents. J Bone Joint Surg 13:695–696, 1931.
37. Pool JL: Direct visualization of the dorsal nerve roots of the cauda equine by means of the myeloscope. Arch Neurol Psychol 39: 1308–1312, 1938.

38. Pool JL: Myeloscopy, intrathecal endoscopy. Surgery 11:169–182, 1942.

39. Hausmann B, Forst R: Nucleoscope instrumentarium for endoscopy of the intervertebral disc space. Arch Orthop Trauma Surg 102:37–59, 1983.

40. Schreiber A, Leu HJ: Percutaneous nucleotomy: Technique with discoscopy. Orthopedics 14:439–444, 1991.

41. Horowitz MB, Moosey JJ, Julian T, et al: Thoracic diskectomy using video-assisted thorascopy. Spine 9:1082–1086, 1994.

42. Rosenthal D, Rosenthal S, Somone A: Removal of a protruded thoracic disc using microsurgical endoscopy: A new technique. Spine 19:1087–1091, 1994.

43. Ferson PF, Landreneau RJ, Dowling RD, et al: Comparison of open versus thorascopic lung biopsy for diffuse infiltrating pulmonary disease. J Thoracic Cardiovasc Surg 106:194–199, 1993.

44. Kaiser LR: Video assisted thoracic surgery current state of the art. Ann Surg 220:720–734, 1994.

45. Landreneau RJ, Hazelrigg SR, Mack MJ, et al: Post operative pain related morbidity: Video-assisted thoracic surgery versus thoracotomy. Ann Thorac Surg 56:1285–1289, 1993.

46. Gow JG: Harold Hopkins and optical systems for urology—an appreciation. Urology 52:152–157, 1998.

47. Mack MJ, Regan JJ, Bobechko WP, Acuff TE: Application of thoracoscopy for diseases of the Spine. Ann Thorac Surg 56:736–738, 1993.

48. Caputy A, Starr J, Riedel C: Video-assisted endoscopic spinal surgery: Thorascopic diskectomy. Acta Neurochir (Wien) 134:196–199, 1995.

49. Rosenthal D, Dickman CA: Thorascopic microsurgical excision of herniated thoracic discs. Neurosurg Focus 6:4, 1999.

50. Liljenqvist U: Anatomic principles of thoracoscopic spine surgery. In Mayer HM (ed): Minimally Invasive Spine Surgery. New York: Springer, 2000.

51. Benaventre OR, Barnett HM: Spinal cord infarction. In Carter LP, Spetzler RF, Hamilton MG (eds): Neurovascular Surgery. New York: McGraw-Hill, 1995.

52. Jasuja ML: Intrathoracic anatomy: An endoscopic perspective. In Dieter RA (ed): Thoracoscopy for Surgeons: Diagnostic and Therapeutic. New York: Igaku-Shoin, 1995.

53. Johnson JP, Filler AG, McBride DQ: Endoscopic thoracic diskectomy. Neurosurg Focus. 9, 2000.

54. Anand N, Regan JJ: Video assisted thoracoscopic surgery for thoracic disk disease: Classification and outcome study of 100 consecutive cases with a 2-year minimum follow-up period. Spine 27:871–879, 2002.

55. McAffe PC, Regan JR, Zdeblick T, et al: The incidence of complications in endoscopic anterior thoracolumbar spinal reconstructive surgery: A prospective multicenter study comprising the first 100 consecutive cases. Spine 20:1624–1632, 1995.

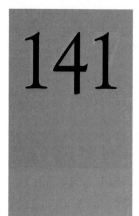

141 Endoscopically Assisted Surgical Management of Thoracic and Lumbar Fractures

RUDOLF BEISSE

Within the past 30 years, the management of thoracic and thoracolumbar spinal fractures has evolved from conservative management with external orthoses and bed rest to operative intervention with decompression, reconstruction, and internal fixation with metallic instrumentation. As a result of the relative central location of the vertebral column within the cylinder of the human torso, posterior approaches are attractive because they avoid the ventrally located visceral cavities. However, because traumatic injuries typically disrupt the anterior load-bearing integrity of the vertebral column, reconstruction that uses only posterior surgical techniques can often result in suboptimal long-term outcomes.

When comparing stand-alone posterolateral fusion with pedicle screws for cases of spinal injury with significant destruction of the anterior column with the use of supplemental anterior reconstruction, numerous clinicians have observed a significantly higher degree of correction loss for posterior-only reduction and fixation.[1-5] By comparison, anterior and anterolateral reconstruction with bone grafting or insertion of a cage in combination with plate stabilization offers the biomechanical advantage of immediate anterior load-bearing column restoration as well as a superior biologic milieu for later healing and arthrodesis. As such, ventral operative treatment of the spine has been used with great success to treat spinal deformity, infection, and fracture.[6-8] The wide exposure and extensive soft-tissue disruption of these approaches often causes much postoperative morbidity.[9,10] For thoracotomy, the most common of these complications includes intercostal neuralgia, post-thoracotomy syndromes, paresis of the abdominal muscles, and hemiparesis of the diaphragm after extensive detachment and mobilization for cases of thoracolumbar fracture.[11-13] During an open transthoracic exposure, the majority of injury to the chest wall is inflicted simply by obtaining access to an area of focal abnormality that is often far smaller than the exposure itself.

As such, surgeons have sought to minimize this degree of exposure-related injury by minimizing the size of the approach through the ribcage by the use of thoracoscopically assisted surgical techniques. The development of sophisticated endoscopic dissection tools and video imaging led to the birth of video-assisted thoracoscopic surgery (VATS) by cardiothoracic surgeons in the late 1980s.[13-15]

The first reports on the use of thoracoscopy on the spinal column date from 1993. Here Mack and colleagues[15]

describe using the procedure for the diagnosis and treatment of various diseases of the thoracic spine. As early as 1994, there are accounts of possible applications in degenerative and metastatic diseases.[15] The first edition of an atlas of endoscopic spinal surgery by Regan and colleagues[16] appeared in 1995.

In parallel, and partly based on these reports, the first endoscopic operations were carried out at the Trauma Center Murnau, Germany in 1996, to treat fractures in the thoracic and lumbar spine, after a preparation period of a year, and subsequently described the current standard techniques of bone and intervertebral disc resection, decompression of the spinal canal, and reconstruction of the anterior spinal column through vertebral body replacement and a plate implant as an overall concept for the endoscopic treatment of fractures in the spinal column.[17-19]

The operative technique developed and described here is now based on the experiences of more than 500 endoscopically performed spinal procedures.[20]

TREATMENT CONCEPT

The anatomic configuration of the fracture type is classified by use of the Magerl classification (Arbeitsgemeinschaft für Osteosynthesefragen–Association for the Study of Internal Fixation [AO] classification) schemata.[21] All patients with type B and C injury patterns (distraction and/or rotation) as well as patients with type A lesions with a higher degree of preoperative instability, dislocation, or neurologic deficit undergo mandatory posterior reduction and fixation first. Patients with only anterior column pathology type A1.2, A1.3, A2, and A3.1 and higher can be treated with a single anterior reconstruction including partial corpectomy and discectomy, vertebral body replacement, and anterior instrumentation providing angular stability.

Overall, the range of indications for the technique described here can be defined as follows:

1. Unstable fractures of the thoracic and lumbar spine in the region between T3 and L3.
2. Post-traumatic, degenerative, and tumor-related narrowing of the spinal canal.
3. Discoligamentary instability.
4. Malposition of healed fractures with or without instability.
5. Revision surgery, implant removal.

6. Tumor and metastasis surgery with intervertebral body replacement, possibly after previous embolization of the supplying vessels.

PREOPERATIVE CONSIDERATIONS AND ANESTHESIA

The investigation covers all the general surgical risks as well as the particular risks of endoscopic surgery. These include, among other things, injury to large vessels, injury to central and peripheral nerve structures, sympathetic deafferentation symptoms and sympathectomy syndromes, and injury to the organs in the thoracic and upper abdominal cavity. The possibility of switching from an endoscopic to an open procedure should also be investigated.

The operations are performed under general anaesthesia. Double-lumen endotracheal single-lung ventilation is preferred to facilitate intrathoracic visualization. Proper placement of the double-lumen endotracheal tube is routinely confirmed under direct bronchoscopic inspection. For postoperative pain relief, a peridural analgesic catheter is inserted in the thoracic region. In standardized fashion, a Foley catheter, a central venous line, and an arterial line for continuous blood pressure assessment are placed. Routine bowel preparation is commonly used to decrease intra-abdominal pressure, thereby facilitating mobilization and retraction of the diaphragm dome.

SURGICAL TECHNIQUE

Technical Prerequisites

Compared with standard open thoracotomy, thoracoscopic procedures require the use of specialized video equipment as well as modified surgical instrumentation.

Image Transmission

A video endoscopy system is used that includes a high-resolution video system with a three-chip camera, 30-degree angled rigid scope, powerful xenon light source, and at least two monitors placed on each side of the patient, ideally with the second monitor's image reversed to facilitate the assistant's orientation. Image recording systems can be added to the video tower if desired. Obscuring of the optic in the warm, moist environment of the thoracic cavity can be prevented by moistening the tip of the optic with a sterile antimisting cloth or fluid.

Instruments

The instruments used are as follows:

1. Long instruments for thoracoscopic dissection of the prevertebral soft-tissue and segmental vessels, as for resection of the bone, ligaments, and discs; osteotomes; hook for dissection; blunt probe; hook probe; rongeurs and curets; graft holder; and reamer. Today there are sets of instruments available to use with the endoscopic technique. In choosing instruments, one should look for a scale marked on both sides of the instruments for bone and intervertebral disc resection and an antiglare, nonreflective surface finish. A suitable length and large handles make it possible to guide the instruments with both hands and to work safely and securely with them.

2. Instruments to use for implantation (e.g., cannulated awl, screwdriver, sleeves and Kirschner [K] wires). Instruments and implants primarily designed for endoscopic instrumentation are recommended.

3. Disposable instruments such as lung and diaphragm retractor, clip applicator, and ultrasonic knife.

Patient Preparation (Positioning, Trocar Placement)

As in open surgery access, the central and upper thoracic spine is approached from the right and the thoracolumbar transition usually from the left. We have moved away from dictating fixed reference vertebrae for approaching from right or left. If the CT scan shows us the aorta localized on the left side of the spine, we will choose the access from the right, and vice versa.

The patient is moved into a lateral recumbent position and stabilized with supports above the sacrum, the pubic symphysis, and the shoulder blades. Special attention must be paid to the ergonomic flow of the operative area. As such, the upper arm of the patient is abducted and elevated parallel to the floor to facilitate endoscope placement and manipulation. Similarly, the fluoroscopic C arm should be brought into the field to ensure that the arc and the tilt paths are free of obstruction to allow spinal image acquisition in both planes (Fig. 141-1).

The primary surgeon and the assistant holding the camera stand immediately posterior to the patient and face the main flat screen monitor. The C arm is located on the same side behind the patient. The second assistant is located on the opposite side of the surgeon. The video monitors are placed at the lower end of the operating table on opposite sides to allow for easy viewing by the surgeons. Sterile draping is extended from the middle of the sternum anteriorly to the spinous processes posteriorly as well as from the axilla down to the iliac crest.

Portal Placement and General Approach Technique

The position of the portals in relation to one another and to the operating site on the spine influences the entire course of the operation. The injured spinal section is therefore first projected exactly orthograde onto the lateral chest or abdominal wall using the radiographic image amplifier and then drawn on the skin with a marker pen indicating the line of the anterior and posterior edges as well as the end plates of the affected segments. The operating portal is the first position to be marked exactly over the target area and then, corresponding with this, the portal for the optic is drawn in over the spine, two or three intercostal spaces above the mark for the operating portal for thoracolumbar access or underneath it for access to the central or upper thoracic spine (Fig. 141-2).

The portal for the suction and rinsing instrument is approximately four fingerbreadths from the operating portal in a ventral and cranial direction. If the distance from the operating portal is too great, the unfavorable angle makes it impossible to suck and rinse right to the bottom of the

FIGURE 141-1 Patient positioning and intraoperative setup. Primary surgeon (*A*), first assistant (*B*), second assistant holding the camera (*C*).

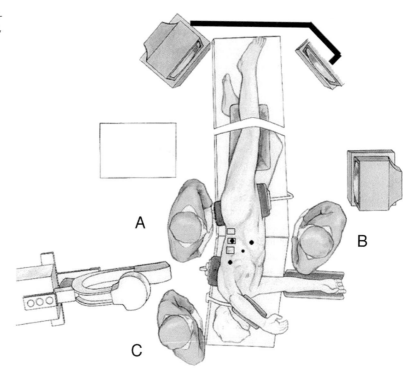

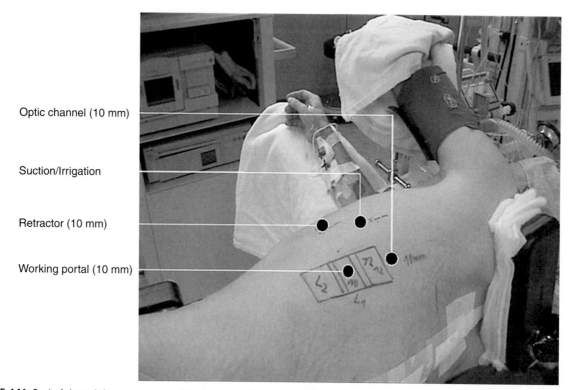

Optic channel (10 mm)

Suction/Irrigation

Retractor (10 mm)

Working portal (10 mm)

FIGURE 141-2 Left lateral thoracoscopy position is prepared with a typical portal arrangement after having confirmed the portal placement directly under lateral fluoroscopic control.

operating site. By contrast, the portal for the diaphragm and lung retractor should be placed as far as possible ventrally to avoid this instrument, which protrudes from the thorax, conflicting with the working instrumentation in the operating portal.

To keep the risk of injury to the diaphragm and the organs beneath it to a minimum, we always start by opening the portal lying in the farthest cranial position. In doing this, we prefer to make the access in the form of a minithoracotomy so that we can recognize, visually or by palpation, adhesions that occasionally occur between the lung and the thoracic wall. After an incision approximately 1.5 cm in length has been made in the skin, the muscle layers of the thoracic wall are cut through with a zigzag incision following the direction of the fibers, and the opening is gradually widened by the insertion of Langenbeck hooks. After collapsing the lung to commence single-lung ventilation, we perforate the pleura and introduce the first trocar. The 30-degree angled optic is introduced, and the other trocars and instruments are inserted in the positions described previously (Fig. 141-3).

Access to the Thoracolumbar Junction (T11–L2)

Lesions located above the T12–L1 disc can be approached thoracoscopically from above without dividing the diaphragm because both crura and arcuate ligaments, which form the lumbar part of the diaphragm, are located below

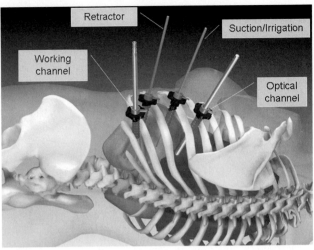

FIGURE 141-4 Thoracoscopic approach to the thoracolumbar junction: typical portal arrangement.

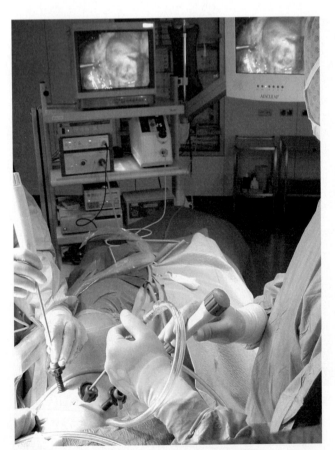

FIGURE 141-3 Typical ergonomic setup of the thoracoscopic operative procedure.

the T12–L1 disc space. However, in lesions located below the T12–L1 disc space, the spine is surrounded by the diaphragmatic crura, psoas muscles, and arcuate ligaments, thus requiring diaphragmatic detachment for adequate exposure. To open up the entire thoracolumbar transition of the spine for endoscopic surgery, we have been able to reduce to a minimum the previous total detachment of the diaphragmatic insertion performed in the open procedure.[22–23]

This is made possible by an anatomic peculiarity of the pleural cavity and the diaphragmatic insertion, the lowest point of which, the costodiaphragmatic recess, is projected onto the spine with a perpendicular projection just about on the base plate of the second lumbar vertebra (Fig. 141-4).

The actual incision can be made with a monopolar hook electrode or an ultrasonic knife. A 2- to 3-cm-long incision is usually sufficient for the instrumentation of the first lumbar vertebra and must be lengthened to 4 to 5 cm for the instrumentation of L2. Although radial incision of the diaphragm is associated with an increased risk of hernia from bowel incursion, we preferentially use a semicircular incision following the diaphragm's contour, thereby leaving a 1-cm rim of the attachment to facilitate closure at the end of the procedure (Fig. 141-5).

After the diaphragm has been split, the retroperitoneal fat and the peritoneal sac are pushed away from the fascia of the psoas muscle. A fan-shaped retractor with blunt tips will be inserted and serves double duty by also exposing the diaphragmatic crus on the spine and holding the dome of the diaphragm away. To expose the thoracolumbar junction, the psoas muscle with its tendinous insertions is dissected carefully from the vertebral bodies to avoid damaging the segmental vessels hidden underneath.

After having performed the procedure at the spine, the gap in the diaphragm can be closed with a hernia stapler. We prefer endoscopic suturing, also from a cost perspective. Small incisions as long as 2 to 3 cm close by themselves without needing sutures. Having made a semicircular incision, the domelike shape of the diaphragm naturally makes the edge of the diaphragm come up against and adhere to the lateral thoracic wall under the pressure in the abdomen,

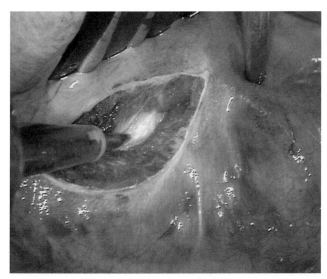

FIGURE 141-5 Thoracoscopic approach to the thoracolumbar junction: incision of the diaphragm at its crural attachments to the spine and the ribs.

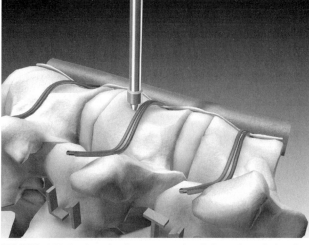

FIGURE 141-6 Anterior instrumentation I: insertion of the first Kirschner wire using a radiolucent Kirschner-wire introducer for percutaneous fluoroscopic placement through the working portal.

so that only a few adaptive sutures are needed to bring about a secure closure of the incision in the diaphragm.

Thus the entire thoracic spine and the upper region of the lumbar spine from T3 to L2 is accessible endoscopically using the thoracoscopic technique.

ENDOSCOPIC RECONSTRUCTION OF THE ANTERIOR SPINAL COLUMN

In principle, the treatment of spinal injuries consists of four stages: (1) correcting the malposition; (2) decompression of the spinal canal, if necessary; (3) replacement or partial replacement of the vertebral body and the disc(s); and (4) retention to ensure stable healing.

Operative Technique Step by Step

The operative procedure described here uses the MACS TL implant.[24,25] This system uses a cannulated polyaxial titanium screw connected to a clamping element that serves as an independent staple and foot plate for the final construct.

As a first step, K wires are placed in the vertebral bodies caudal and cranial to the injured segment(s). The ideal entry point for the K wires in the dorsoventral diameter is at the transition from the rear to the central third of the vertebra and is chosen to be the same as that for the vertebral body screws that are inserted immediately thereafter (Fig. 141-6).

After inserting K wires with a targeting instrument under radiographic image amplification, the screw, clamp, and a connecting "centralizer" are assembled and introduced through the working channel. Therefore, the working channel is dilated by removing the thoracoscopic portal and enlarging it with a small hand-held speculum. Once inside, the cannulated screws are then endoscopically guided onto the target over the K wires. Before completely advancing the screws, the K wires are removed through the cannulated screws and holder to avoid inadvertent advancement of the wires and perforation of the contralateral cortex. The screw

direction to be aimed at is one running parallel to the posterior edge and close to the end plate. After the two clamping elements have been placed in position, the site of the screws is checked with the image amplifier and captured for the surgeon on the monitor (Fig. 141-7).

Partial Corporectomy and Discectomy

The doorlike opening of the pleura can be made with the monopolar dissection hook or an ultrasonic knife following a virtual connecting line between the two screws acting as important landmarks and defining a "safety zone." We then expose the segment vessels, which are not infrequently included in the vertebral body fracture zone. They are mobilized using a rasp and a right-angled Overholt clamp, drawn down and ligated with titanium vascular clips.

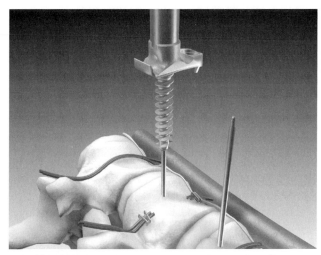

FIGURE 141-7 Anterior instrumentation II: insertion of a cannulated polyaxial titanium screw connected to a clamping element that serves as an independent staple and foot plate for the final construct.

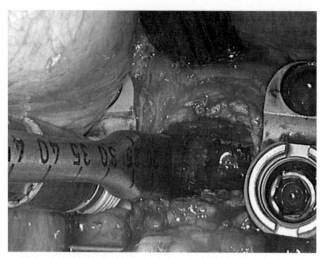

FIGURE 141-8 Anterior instrumentation III: performing partial corpectomy and discectomy with the clamping elements in place serving as landmarks.

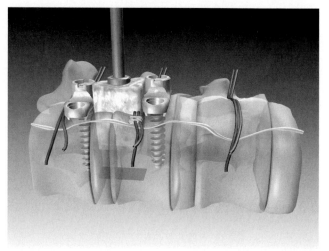

FIGURE 141-9 Anterior instrumentation IV: the interpositional bone graft is inserted and press-fit into the graft bed.

After the vessels have been separated, the rasp is used to expose the vertebral body.

The extent of the partial corporectomy is marked in a ventrodorsal direction with a sharp endoscopic osteotome, and the adjacent intervertebral disc spaces are opened with an intervertebral disc knife. The (partial) corpectomy is performed using rongeurs, sharp scoops, and curets (Fig. 141-8).

Repositioning

For repositioning and distracting the injured segments, we use the distraction module belonging to the MACS TL implant, which is placed via sleeves onto the bone screws. A hydraulic distraction device restores the distance between the posterior edges while lordosis of the spinal section is achieved through manual pressure from behind. The distraction module load bearer on the rear of the spine secures the result of the repositioning maneuver so that both measuring the necessary length of the bone graft or basket implant and the interposition of the vertebral body replacement can be done under reposition conditions.

Vertebral Body Replacement

If an iliac crest graft is being used, this is tapped in the area of the iliac crest cortex with a 2.5-mm drill, and the threaded graft holder is screwed in. To protect the soft tissue as the bone graft passes through the thoracic wall, the graft is cloaked in an antifriction plastic cover. After replacing the operating trocar with the retracting forceps, narrow Langenbeck hooks are introduced into the portal and the bone graft is pushed through between the ribs. Grafts longer than 2 cm are introduced lengthwise and only connected to the graft holder inside the thorax (Fig. 141-9).

The bone graft should be tamped in with press-fit far enough to lie centrally in the vertebra.

A distractible titanium cage can also be used,[26] especially in patients with poor bone quality or whose iliac crest was considered to be inadequate. Using distractible cages, additional reduction can be achieved by further increasing the

height of the cage within the graft side and then filling and surrounding the cage with morselized autologous cancellous bone harvested from the corpectomy. The side is covered with a collagen fleece to prevent the dislocation of the cancellous bone.

Fitting the Plate

At this time, an endoscopic caliper is used to measure the size of the plate to be used. The plate is introduced lengthwise into the chest cavity, laid onto the clamping elements, and definitively fixed in place with swivel nuts and a starting torque of 15 Nm. A special feature of the MACS TL system makes it possible to screw the bone screws in further and thus bring the implant into direct contact with the side wall of the vertebra, thereby increasing the stability of the implant fixation. Guide sleeves are used to insert the ventral screws, which complete the stable angle fitting procedure (Fig. 141-10).

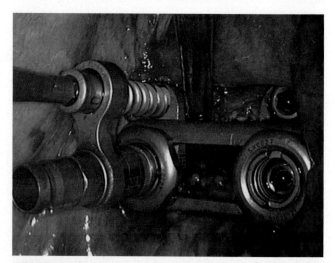

FIGURE 141-10 Anterior instrumentation V: a guiding centralizer sleeve is attached on the clamping element to allow placement of the angled ventral body screw.

Alternate tightening of the four bone screws permits optimization of the frictional connection between the screws, plate, and vertebral body. As a final step, the polyaxial mechanism of the dorsal screws is locked using a locking screw.

ANTERIOR ENDOSCOPIC DECOMPRESSION OF THE SPINAL CANAL

The surgical technique presented here, with an endoscopically performed anterior decompression of the spinal canal, has been developed based on an analysis of typical fracture patterns and taking into account the particular features of the endoscopic procedure.[27] Vertebral fractures with stenosis of the spinal canal almost always exhibit several typical changes. The posterior vertebral body wall (middle column) is fragmented and dorsally displaced (retropulsed) into the spinal canal causing compression of the spinal cord and cauda equina. The retropulsed fragment is frequently trapped pincer-like between the two relatively intact pedicles[28] (Fig. 141-11).

In burst fractures, the retropulsed fragment frequently remains attached to the annular fibers of the cranial intervertebral disc space.

The important step is the identification and resection of the ipsilateral pedicle. This allows movement of the trapped, retropulsed fragment compressing the spinal canal

and provides an anterior direct endoscopic view of the dural sac. The image detail of the high-resolution 30-degree angled optic provides an excellent view of the posterior longitudinal ligament and the dural sac.

The working channel is located directly over the affected vertebral body. After access has been gained and all portals are in place, we recommend placing the screws into the vertebral bodies above and below the level selected for corpectomy. This maneuver will provide the surgeon with intraoperative landmarks, which can be of great value as changing the camera position during endoscopic surgery is necessary, and without clear intraoperative landmarks, the surgeon can become disoriented. After this, the adjacent intervertebral discs are incised and removed, and the central part of the vertebral body is resected with osteotomes and rongeurs. Initially, the posterior vertebral body wall is preserved to avoid further canal compromise during the partial corpectomy.

At this point, the pedicle of the vertebral body at the level of spinal canal compression must be identified. In a traumatic burst fracture, the pedicles are nearly always preserved and the retropulsed fragment is usually located medial to the pedicles and trapped in between, like in a pincer. Therefore, we recommend resecting the ipsilateral pedicle before attempting to remove the retropulsed fragment. The base of the pedicle and the neural foramen can be localized with a small nerve hook. Once identified, the resection of the base

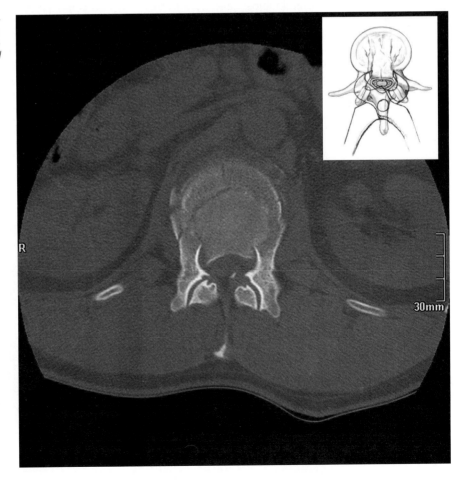

FIGURE 141-11 Anterior decompression I: typical vertebral body fracture with an associated retropulsed fragment. The mostly intact pedicles trap the *retropulsed* fragment like a pincer.

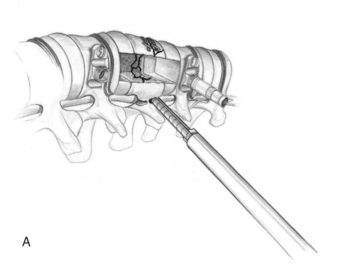

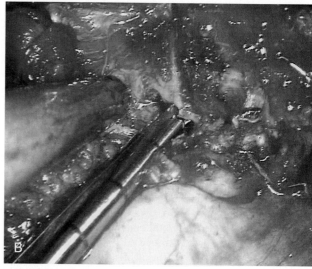

FIGURE 141-12 Anterior decompression II: resection of the pedicle to expose the lateral dural sac (*A* and *B*).

of the pedicle will open the spinal canal and it is possible to visualize the retropulsed fragment (Fig. 141-12).

After the ipsilateral pedicle is completely resected, the retropulsed fragment is cautiously moved away from the dural sac and toward the corpectomy defect under direct endoscopic visualization (Fig. 141-13).

Complete decompression of the dural sac is confirmed in the direct endoscopic view and radiographically with fluoroscopy (Fig. 141-14).

After completion of the decompression, the dura is covered with Gelfoam. The corpectomy defect can be reconstructed with an interbody bone graft or a cage. We routinely perform an endoscopic anterior fixation with a constrained screw-plate system.

POSTOPERATIVE TREATMENT

The First 24 Hours after the Operation

A radiographic check with the image amplifier is carried out in both planes in the operating room before the sterile drapes are removed. The patient is normally extubated while still in the operating room. Artificial respiration for 24 hours postoperatively is recommended for patients with a higher level of surgical risk (age, chronic pulmonary disease, cardiovascular primary illness, post-traumatic thoracic or pulmonary contusion).

We carry out medicinal thrombosis prophylaxis with low molecular heparin because, despite the use of a minimally invasive technique, the operation must be regarded as

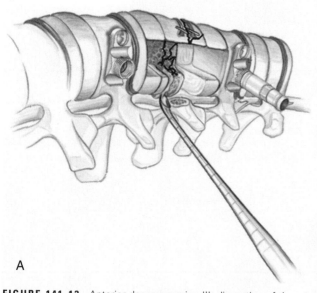

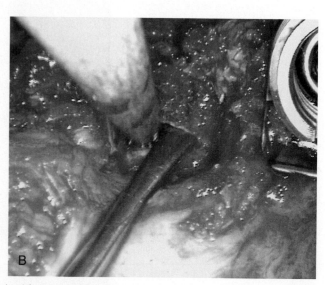

FIGURE 141-13 Anterior decompression III: dissection of the retropulsed fragment under direct visualization of the dura. Removal of the fragment (*A* and *B*).

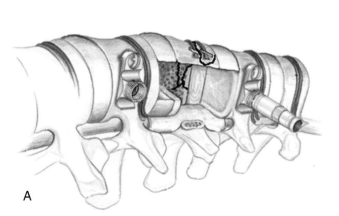

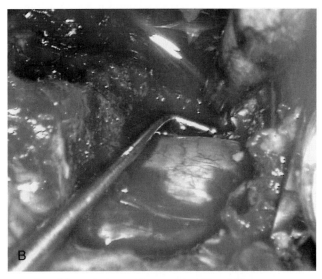

FIGURE 141-14   Anterior decompression IV: the decompression of the spinal canal is completed (*A* and *B*).

entailing risks with regard to the development of a thrombosis and a pulmonary embolism. This is especially true for patients with neurologic deficits (paraplegics). Immediately postoperatively, the patient is placed in the intensive care unit overnight. On the morning of the first postoperative day, the thoracic drainage is clamped and a radiograph is obtained to monitor the thorax. If the lung has expanded fully and pneumothorax has been excluded, the thoracic drainage is removed and the patient is transferred to the normal ward.

The First Weeks after the Operation

From the first postoperative day, the patient is mobilized without a corset, avoiding torsion and kyphosis. Lung function is improved through intensive breathing exercises with instruction.

Active and passive physiotherapy is employed in the first week with standing upright, walking exercises, and back training for approximately 1 hour per day. From the second week, substantial intensification takes place, with water therapy after the sutures have been removed on the 10th day. The patient is discharged from the hospital after 8 to 12 days. The therapy is continued in a rehabilitation center.

Radiographic Monitoring of the Healing Process

On the second postoperative day, conventional radiography in both planes and computed tomography of the section of the spine operated on are performed to check its position and the position of the implant. Further radiographic checks are performed in the ninth postoperative week and after 6 and 12 months to make certain that the fusion is successful. The ventral implant is not removed if healing proceeds normally.

RESULTS

In a 5-year period from May 1996 to May 2001, 371 patients underwent endoscopic spinal surgery.[17,29] The surgery comprised anterior reconstruction and fusion using a vertebral body replacement and an anterior titanium fixation system. In 84% of cases, a tricortical iliac crest graft was used to replace the vertebra, and in 16% of cases, a titanium basket implant was used. The average age of the patients was 36 years, the youngest patient being 16 and the oldest 75. The majority of the injuries (72%) were located in the area of the thoracolumbar transition. The injuries were split according to the AO-ASIF classification into 65% type A injuries, 22% type B, and 17% type C.

TREATMENT CONCEPT

The type of surgery was chosen according to the nature of the injury. Sixty-five percent of the cases involved injuries with type B and C distraction and rotation elements or patients with a neurologic defect associated with higher grade structural damage to the vertebral body, and these patients were primarily repositioned and stabilized dorsally using an internal fixator. In 35% of the cases, it was exclusively the anterior spine that was affected by type A compression injuries, and these were reconstructed and stabilized in an exclusively ventral endoscopic procedure.

Fifteen percent of our patients with significant narrowing of the spinal canal and simultaneous neurologic deficit were treated by anterior decompression of the spinal canal. Corresponding with the high rate of injuries to the thoracolumbar transition, 51% of our patients underwent endoscopic diaphragm splitting, which was subsequently closed using the method described previously. Despite using merely adaptation suturing, no case of diaphragmatic hernia was observed.

The concept of the least extensive fusion possible resulted in an almost equal rate of mono- and bisegmental fusions (46%/49%). In 5% of cases, the pattern of injury necessitated multisegmental fusion.

As far as the rate of fusion is concerned, an investigation of the first 30 patients operated on endoscopically showed a fusion rate of 86% within a 6-month period using the Z-Plate. Initial results using the stable angle MACS TL system indicate an increase in the rate of fusion.

The average duration of surgery when we introduced the endoscopic procedure was 6 hours, with a maximal duration of as long as 9 hours. We have gradually been able to reduce these extremely long operating times to an average of 2 to 3 hours. The shortest operating time was 70 minutes for a monosegmental fusion on the thoracolumbar transition.

We recently reported our results of procedures with endoscopically performed anterior decompression (Beisse, unpublished). Corresponding with a canal clearance of 110%, neurologic improvement was found in 25% of our patients with initial complete paraplegia and 65% of the patients with an incomplete neurologic deficit. The rate of more than 100% is explained by the fact that the resection of the posterior vertebral wall and the intervertebral disc results in some expansion of the spinal canal cross-sectional area compared with an intact vertebral segment. These results correspond with the data in the literature.[30–34]

PAIN REDUCTION AND REHABILITATION

The benefit of thoracoscopy in comparison with open thoracotomy has been reported in several publications.[35–38] The reduction of postoperative pain was also demonstrated in one of our previous studies, in which 30 patients operated on endoscopically in the first year were compared with a group of 30 patients who had undergone open surgery. We observed in the group treated endoscopically an average reduction in both the duration of administration of pain relief (31%) and the overall dose (42%) in comparison with the patients who had open surgery treatment. The injury to the spine was the only relevant injury in both groups. Eighty percent of the patients treated endoscopically returned to their previous employment.

Illustrative Cases

PATIENT 1 (FIG. 141-15)

An 18-year-old female patient sustained a type C1.3.2 compression/rotation fissured fracture of the 12th thoracic vertebra in a car accident.

Because of the unstable fracture type with displacement of a large fragment of the posterior margin, we performed dorsal redressment and stabilization with an internal fixator on the day of the accident. Four days after the first operation, the ventral endoscopic operation was performed with partial corporectomy of T12, graft interposition and monosegmental anterior stabilization with a 60-mm-long MACS TL plate and screw system (Twin Screw). This case impressively demonstrates the potential of the implant with the possibility of:

1. Angle-stable anterior reconstruction
2. The shortest possible monosegmental fusion with preservation of the caudal section of the fractured vertebra
3. True osteosynthesis of the fissured fracture in T12 through the use of bicortical screws
4. The possibility of implanting under endoscopic conditions with the corresponding functional and cosmetic advantages for the young patient (see Fig. 141-15E)

PATIENT 2 (FIG. 141-16)

A 44-year-old man was involved in a high-speed motor vehicle accident and experienced a Pincer fracture type A2.3 of the first lumbar vertebra according to the AO-ASIF classification without any neurologic deficit. Primary dorsal reduction and fixation was performed on the day of accident. Six days after the primary dorsal stabilization, anterior endoscopic reconstruction was performed via endoscopic detachment of the diaphragm. Bisegmental anterolateral instrumentation was performed from T12 to L2 using the MACS TL system and a Synex cage filled with autologous cancellous bone.

PATIENT 3 (FIG. 141-17)

A 54-year-old man sustained a burst fracture of the first lumbar vertebra in a skiing accident with a rotational component type C1.3.3 and severe canal compromise secondary to a retropulsed fragment. The patient had a Frankel grade D injury. After primary dorsal reduction (ligamentotaxis) and stabilization using an internal fixator, endoscopic anterior decompression followed by anterior reconstruction and instrumentation was performed 4 days after the first operation.

OPEN CONVERSION AND COMPLICATIONS

Our overall operative conversion rate from a thoracoscopic procedure to an open thoracotomy was 1.2% (4 patients) in the series of 371 patients. We had to convert in two of the first four operations alone, in one case because of bleeding from spongy bone that at that time could not be stopped endoscopically and in the other case because of a technical difficulty with the implant. The third conversion was made necessary by a small leak in the aorta during a revision operation to correct a loosened implant. The source of the bleeding was sewn up after thoracotomy and clamping of the aorta. In the fourth case involving injury to the upper thoracic spine, we did not succeed in positioning the trocars in the narrow space between the ribs. We therefore performed a thoracotomy and resection of one rib.

As far as injuries to organs are concerned, we must report a perforated spleen in a 52-year-old female patient. In the closing phase of the operation, a so-called pleura-cath was introduced in addition to thoracic drainage to facilitate the removal of residual effusion after the withdrawal of the thoracic drainage after 2 to 3 days. Under gradual relaxation of the patient, a coughing response occurred with a consequent leaping up of the diaphragm and perforation of the spleen through the diaphragm with a hollow needle. The spleen was removed by subsequent laparotomy. After this incident, we did not introduce any more pleura catheters.

We identified seven patients (2.1%) with partial implant loosening; a revision operation was performed on five of them because of the accompanying loss of correction. In five of these seven cases, the former partially stable angle Z-Plate system was used, and the MACS TL system in the other two. The two latter patients had advanced osteoporosis and were treated exclusively ventrally.

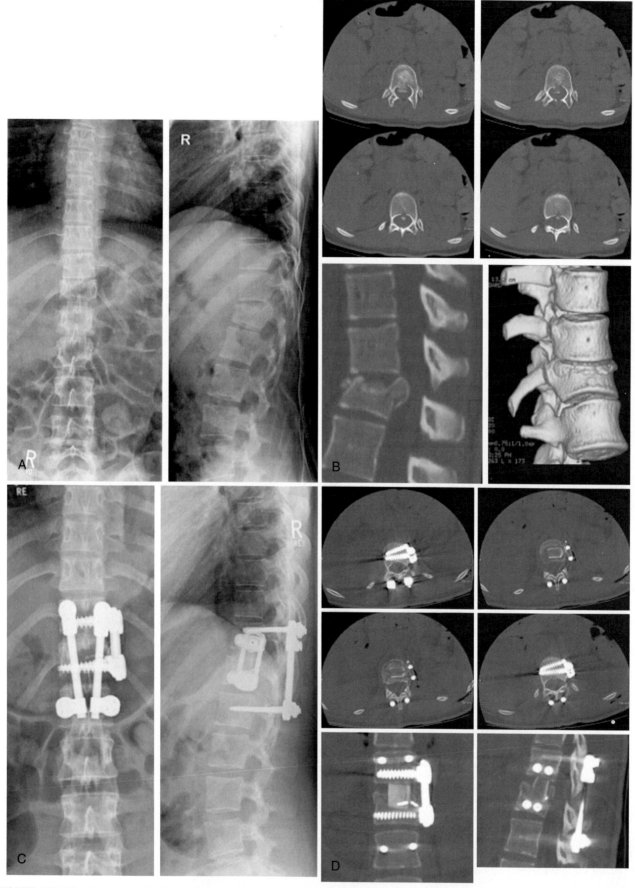

FIGURE 141-15 Case example of a compression/rotation fissured fracture type C1.3.2 (Arbeitsgemeinschaft für Osteosynthesefragen–Association for the Study of Internal Fixation [AO] classification). Preoperative radiographs (*A*). Transversal computed tomography layer and 2- and 3-dimensional reconstruction of the injury (*B*). Postoperative radiographic check after initial dorsal bisegmental stabilization and subsequent thoracoscopic monosegmental ventral fusion with the MACS TL system of T11–12 (*C*). Transversal computed tomography layers show the bicortical screw fixation of the caudal section of T12, position check of tricortical iliac crest graft, and 2-dimensional reconstruction to check position after monosegmental stabilization of T11–12 (*D*).

(Continued)

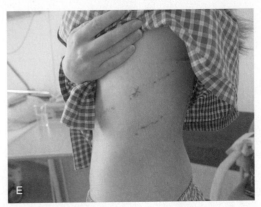

FIGURE 141-15   Cont'd Clinical and cosmetics result after suture removal 10 days postoperatively (*E*).

In terms of postoperative complications, we observed one (0.3%) profound and five (1.5%) superficial infections in the area of the operating portal, which we originally used as a channel for thoracic drainage. After we had transferred the draining tube to one of the ventrally lying portals under less stress from the surgery itself, these complications did not recur. Among the neurologic complications, we observed the lesion of the L1 root through the use of monopolar current in an extensive diaphragm-splitting procedure as well as damage to the thoracolumbar nerve on the side of the body being lain on due to the patient position. Both healed completely. Access-related complications requiring surgery, such as ventricular pleural effusions, pneumothorax, and intercostal neuralgia, occurred with a frequency of 5.4%. In treating ventricular pleural effusion,

FIGURE 141-16   Case example of a type A2.3 pincer fracture. Preoperative radiographs in both planes (*A*), 2-dimensional computed tomography reconstruction (*B*), postoperative radiographs after primary dorsal reduction and fixation with an internal fixator and secondary ventral reconstruction using the Synex Cage and MACS TL System for anterior instrumentation (*C*), 2-dimensional computed tomography reconstructions (*D*). Clinical and cosmetic results after partial suture removal 8 days postoperatively (*E*).

(Continued)

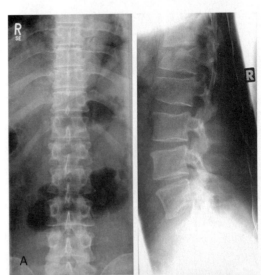

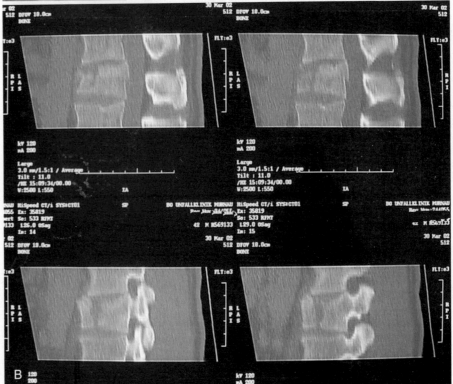

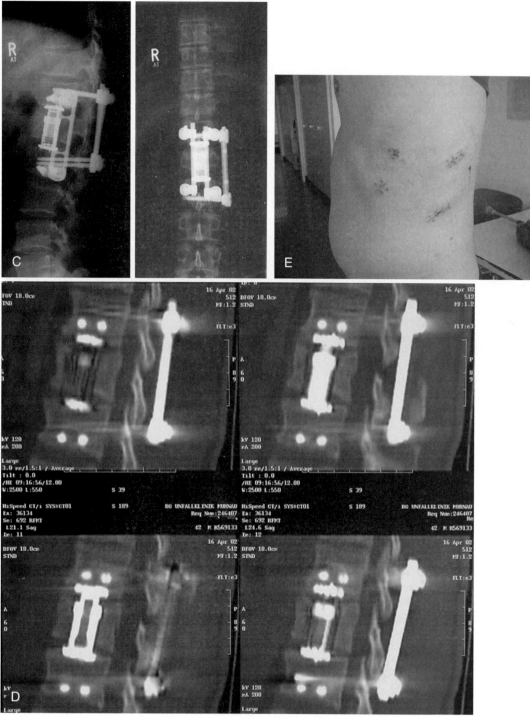

FIGURE 141-16 Cont'd

early thoracoscopic revision with adhesiolysis and suction has proved effective.

Performing endoscopic anterior decompression, we recently reported 11 complications in 30 procedures; 5 alone were associated with the harvesting of the bone graft taken from the iliac crest used as vertebral body replacement and should not be considered strictly related to the endoscopic procedure. However, in the past 2 years, we have made increasing use of expandable titanium cages that can be placed endoscopically. Compared with iliac crest grafts, the cages are biomechanically more stable and have a lower risk of graft dislodgment. Other complications that were associated with endoscopic surgery were pleural effusions and an intercostal neuralgia. These complications are observed with much higher frequency for open thoracotomy.[10]

CONCLUSION

The initial period of endoscopic spinal surgery was characterized by the lack of coordinating instrumentation and

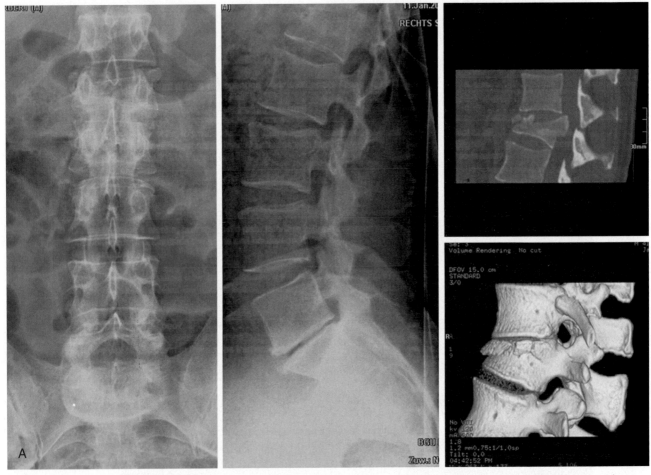

FIGURE 141-17 Case example of a burst fracture with a rotational component type C1.3.3 and severe canal compromise secondary to a retropulsed fragment. Preoperative radiographs and computed tomography with reconstructions (*A*), postoperative radiographs and computed tomography reconstructions (*B*); postoperative fine cut axial computed tomography slices for the assessment of spinal canal reconstruction (*C*).
(*Continued*)

implants suitable for endoscopic use, which, together with the still small amount of experience, resulted in longer operation times. In the past 8 years, endoscopic procedures in the treatment of spinal trauma have developed in importance from optional additional operations to a standard concept of spinal trauma therapy. They are based on the classic spinal surgery principles of repositioning, reconstruction, and retention of the anterior section of the spine. This development was helped by a continuous improvement in instruments that make it possible to perform even subtle operations such as anterior decompression of the spinal cord with optical conditions that can only be compared with those of a surgical microscope. The advantages of endoscopic treatment of thoracic and thoracolumbar fractures and instabilities include the following:

1. Small intercostal incisions without the need for rib resection or rib retractors
2. Excellent direct intraoperative visualization of the abnormality with a magnified 30-degree optical lens
3. Treatment of multisegmental lesions without the need for rib osteotomy or resection
4. Potential for effective anterior decompression of the spinal canal

5. Significantly reduced injury and destabilization of the chest wall

The disadvantages of endoscopic spinal procedures include a slightly increased anesthesiologic complexity with the need for double-lumen intubation and a steep learning curve for the surgeon and surgical team, which can be eased by attending labs and workshops as well as performing surgery with an experienced thoracoscopic spine surgeon at the beginning. The results demonstrate the benefit of thoracoscopic over open spinal fracture treatment, which justifies the steep learning curve of the minimally invasive procedure.

Given a suitable injury pattern, the high primary and angle stability of modern implants make it appear possible to carry out an exclusively ventral treatment, avoiding the dorsal procedure with its traumatizing effect on soft tissue.

Limitations can be imposed by the extent of the malposition to be corrected, injury to dorsal structures, and poor bone quality, which in each case requires additional dorsal reconstructive and stabilizing measures. The level of safety of endoscopic surgery is reflected in the lower complication rate and operating time, which is shorter or at least comparable with that of the open procedure. The basic intention

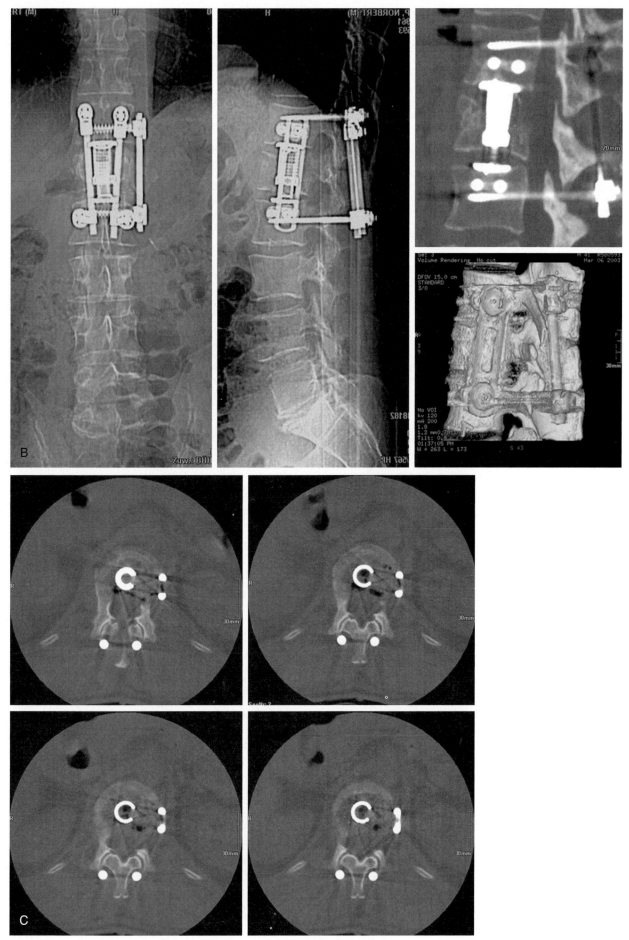

FIGURE 141-17 Cont'd

in introducing endoscopic techniques—to reduce access morbidity—can be fully realized.

Acknowledgment

The author thanks Axel Stahlhut-Klipp (www.framdivision.de) for his cooperation in the 3-dimensional drafting of this work.

REFERENCES

1. Aebi M, Etter C, Kehl T, et al: Stabilization of the lower thoracic and lumbar spine with the internal spinal skeletal fixation system. Indications, techniques, and first results of treatment. Spine 12:544–551, 1987.
2. Daniaux H: [Transpedicular repositioning and spongioplasty in fractures of the vertebral bodies of the lower thoracic and lumbar spine]. Unfallchirurg 89:197–213, 1986.
3. Knop C, Blauth M, Bastian L, et al: Fractures of the thoracolumbar spine: Late results of dorsal instrumentation and its consequences. Unfallchirurg 100:630–639, 1997.
4. Liljenqvist U, Mommsen U: [Surgical treatment of thoracolumbar spinal fractures with internal fixator and transpedicular spongiosaplasty]. Unfallchirurgie 21:30–39, 1995.
5. Olerud S, Karlstrom G, Sjostrom L: Transpedicular fixation of thoracolumbar vertebral structures. Clin Orthop 227:44–51, 1988.
6. Hodgson AR, Stock FE: Anterior spinal fusion a preliminary communication on the radical treatment of Pott's disease and Pott's paraplegia. Br J Surg 44:266–275, 1956.
7. Hodgson AR, Stock FE, Fang HS, et al: Anterior spinal fusion: The operative approach and pathological findings in 412 patients with Pott's disease of the spine. Br J Surg 48:172–178, 1960.
8. Kirkaldy-Willis WH, Thomas TG: Anterior approaches in the diagnosis and treatment of infections of the vertebral bodies. J Bone Joint Surg Am 47:87–110, 1965.
9. Dajczman E, Gorden A, Kreisman H, et al: Longterm postthoracotomy pain. Chest 7:270–273, 1991.
10. Faciszewski T, Winter RB, Lonstein JE, et al: The surgical and medical perioperative complications of anterior spinal fusion: Surgery in the thoracic and lumbar spine in adults. Spine 20:1592–1599, 1995.
11. Anetzberger IL, Friedl HP: Wirbelsäule. Stuttgart/New York: Thieme-Verlag, 1997.
12. Blauth M, Knop C, Bastian L: Brust- und Lendenwirbelsäule: Springer-Verlag, 1997.
13. Coltharp WH, Arnold JH, Alford WC, Jr, et al: Videothoracoscopy: Improved technique and expanded indications. Ann Thorac Surg 53:776–779, 1992.
14. Mack MJ, Aronoff RJ, Acuff TE, et al: Present role of thoracoscopy in the diagnosis and treatment of diseases of the chest. Ann Thorac Surg 54:403–409, 1992.
15. Mack MJ, Regan J, Bobechko WP, et al: Applications of thoracoscopy for diseases of spine. Ann Thorac Surg 56:736–738, 1993.
16. Regan JJ, McAfee P, Mack M: Atlas of endoscopic spine surgery. St. Louis: Quality Medical Publishing, 1995.
17. Beisse R, Potulski M, Bühren V: Endoscopic techniques for the management of spinal trauma. Eur J Trauma 27:275–291, 2001.
18. Beisse R, Potulski M, Bühren V: Thoracoscopic assisted anterior fusion in fractures of the thoracic and lumbar spine. Orthop Traumatol 7:54–66, 1999.
19. Potulski M, Beisse R, Buhren V: [Thoracoscopy-guided management of the "anterior column." Methods and results]. Orthopade 28:723–730, 1999.
20. Beisse R, Potulski M, Buhren V: Endoscopic surgery of the thoracic and lumbar spine—A report on 500 treatments. Osteosynthesis and Trauma Care 4:196–205, 2003.
21. Magerl F, Aebi S, Gertzbein SD, et al: A comprehensive classification of thoracic and lumbar injuries. Eur Spine J 3:184–201, 1994.
22. Beisse R, Potulski M, Bühren V: Thoracoscopic-assisted approach to thoracolumbar fractures. In Mayer HM (ed): Minimally Invasive Spine Surgery. Berlin/Heidelberg/New York: Springer-Verlag, 2000, pp 175–186.
23. Beisse R, Potulski M, Temme C, et al: [Endoscopically controlled division of the diaphragm: A minimally invasive approach to ventral management of thoracolumbar fractures of the spine]. Unfallchirurg 101:619–627, 1998.
24. Beisse R, Potulski M, Beger J, et al: Development and clinical application of a thoracoscopic implantable frame plate for the treatment of thoracolumbar fractures and instabilities. Orthopade 31:413–422, 2002.
25. Schultheiss M, Hartwig E, Wilke H-J, et al: A new endoscopically-implantable stabilization system for the treatment of thoracolumbar fractures–design and comparative biomechanical study. Eur Spine J 8:53–57, 1999.
26. Knop C, Lange U, Bastian L, et al: Biomechanical compression tests with a new implant for thoracolumbar vertebral body replacement. Eur Spine J 10:30–37, 2001.
27. Beisse R, Muckley T, Schmidt MH, Hauschild M, Buhren V: Surgical technique and results of endoscopic anterior spinal canal decompression. J Neurosurg Spine 2:128–136, 2005.
28. Lemons VR, Wagner FC, Montesano PX: Management of thoracolumbar fractures with accompanying neurological injury. Neurosurgery 30:667–671, 1992.
29. Khoo LT, Beisse R, Potulski M: Thoracoscopic-assisted treatment of thoracic and lumbar fractures: A series of 371 consecutive cases. Neurosurgery 51:104–117, 2002.
30. Esses SI, Botsford DJ, Kostuik JP: Evaluation of surgical treatment for burst fractures. Spine 15:667–673, 1990.
31. Esses SI, Botsford DJ, Wright T, et al: Operative treatment of spinal fractures with the AO internal fixator. Spine 16:146–150, 1991.
32. Frankel HL, Hancock DO, Hyslop G, et al: The value of postural reduction in the initial management of closed injuries of the spine with paraplegia and tetraplegia. I. Paraplegia 7:179–192, 1969.
33. Kaneda K, Taneichi H, Abumi K, et al: Anterior decompression and stabilization with the Kaneda device for thoracolumbar burst fractures associated with neurological deficits. J Bone Joint Surg Am 79:69–83, 1997.
34. Okuyama K, Abe E, Chiba M, et al: Outcome of anterior decompression and stabilization for thoracolumbar unstable burst fractures in the absence of neurologic deficits. Spine 21:620–625, 1996.
35. Hazelrigg SR, Landreneau RJ, Boley TM, et al: The effect of muscle-sparing versus standard posterolateral thoracotomy on pulmonary function, muscle strength, and postoperative pain. J Thorac Cardiovasc Surg 101:394–400, 1991.
36. Landreneau RJ, Hazelrigg SR, Mack MJ, et al: Postoperative pain-related morbidity: Video-assisted thoracic surgery versus thoracotomy. Ann Thorac Surg 56:1285, 1993.
37. Landreneau RJ, Wiechmann RJ, Hazelrigg SR, et al: Effect of minimally invasive thoracic surgical approaches on acute and chronic postoperative pain. Chest Surg Clin N Am 8:891, 1998.
38. Passlick B, Born C, Mandelkow H, et al: [Long-term complaints after minimal invasive thoracic surgery operations and thoracotomy]. Chirurg 72:934–939, 2001.

142 Surgical Techniques in the Management of Thoracic Disc Herniations

NATHAN E. SIMMONS

INTRODUCTION

The management of thoracic disc herniations presents a paradox to the casual observer. One of the most accepted features of thoracic disc disease is its infrequency in comparison with the more common cervical and lumbar disc herniations. Given such a low incidence, one might assume that only a limited number of operative procedures are available to treat the condition. Yet for such a "rare" entity, a remarkably wide array of effective surgical techniques has been developed. The surgeon therefore needs to understand the indications and limitations of these procedures to apply them in the clinical setting.

The initial use of laminectomy for the treatment of thoracic discs was met with uniformly unacceptable results.[1,2] As a result, numerous methods have been developed to treat thoracic disc herniations. Unfortunately, no standard algorithm exists to aid the surgeon in selecting the best procedure for a given patient. Each technique offers a combination of advantages and compromises that needs to be evaluated for each patient. Despite the relatively low prevalence of symptomatic thoracic herniated discs, any surgeon managing a moderate proportion of spinal disease in his or her practice will invariably become confronted with this condition. Therefore, a basic understanding of the available surgical options and the indications and limitations of each procedure is vital.

This chapter discusses the major open surgical approaches to the herniated thoracic disc and offers guidance in the selection of one procedure over another. Thoracoscopic indications and procedures are discussed elsewhere in this text.

IMPORTANT CONCEPTS

1. Thoracic disc herniations, although uncommon, will be encountered by spine surgeons.
2. Laminectomy is an unacceptable alternative for thoracic disc herniations.
3. Posterior techniques include the transpedicular, Stillerman's transfacet pedicle sparing, transcostovertebral, costotransversectomy, and lateral extracavitary.
4. Posterior approaches are generally favored in cases of more lateral, noncalcified, extradural disc herniations.
5. Anterior approaches include the transthoracic, retropleural, and transsternal.
6. Anterior techniques offer better ventral exposure for discs that are centrally located, calcified, and/or intradural.
7. Complication rates for the common posterior and anterior procedures are similar.

Thoracic disc herniations comprise a minority of the disc herniations evaluated by a spine surgeon. This reflects the relative immobility of the thoracic spine as compared with the cervical and lumbar regions and thus the low incidence of degenerative changes. Contemporary series suggest that thoracic herniated discs represent less than 1% of all symptomatic discs and, accordingly, represent less than 1% of all disc operations.[1] This establishes an incidence of 1 symptomatic patient per 1 million individuals per year.[2-4]

The majority of thoracic herniated discs are asymptomatic. As many as 37% of patients harbor an asymptomatic herniated thoracic disc as defined on randomly sampled magnetic resonance imaging scans.[5] More conservative estimates propose this number lies in the range of 10% to 15%.[1,6,7]

The majority of symptomatic discs are found in the lower third of the thoracic region, with most being found between the T8 and T11 levels.[1,7] Discs in the upper third of the thoracic spine are rare. Herniated discs in the thoracic spine commonly present centrally within the canal (77% to 94%) and are often calcified (22% to 65%).[1,8] A small but very important 6% to 7% of discs prove to be intradural.[9]

Symptomatic thoracic herniated discs present with a wide array of findings. Stillerman and colleagues[8] presented an exhaustive review of their personal findings in 71 patients with thoracic disc disease as well as a meta-analysis of 13 series encompassing 247 patients (Table 142-1). Both of these surveys demonstrated that sensory changes were seen in more than 60% of cases. Pain was a finding in greater than half of the patients but was actually more likely to be axial than the typically presumed radicular pattern. Motor weakness and spasticity/hyperreflexia were present in 55% to 58% of patients. As with many cervicothoracic lesions, bowel and bladder dysfunction was one of the least common symptoms, appearing in only 24% to 35% of patients.[8]

The radiographic identification of these lesions is obviously most commonly performed with magnetic resonance imaging. Magnetic resonance imaging allows visualization of the disc herniation and the surrounding neural elements (Fig. 142-1). However, computed tomography/myelography remains a viable imaging technique with excellent resolution of the affected region, despite the inconvenience and invasiveness of the procedure. Plain computed tomography scanning also serves a supportive role as it often assists magnetic resonance imaging in evaluating whether a given disc

TABLE 142-1 ▪ Comparison of the Present Study and Earlier Thoracic Disc Series

Factor	13 Contemporary Series (1986–1997)	Present Study
Demographics and Disc Characteristics		
No. of patients/no. of discs	247/263	71/82
Sex (F/M)	112/95 (1.18/1)	37/34 (1.09/1)
Age, yr	18–79	19–75
Trauma	37% (59/161)	37% (26/71)
Levels (total)	T1–L1 (244)	T4–L1 (82)
Level/frequency (no.)	T8–9: 17% (41)	T9–10: 26% (21)
	T11–12: 16% (39)	T8–9: 23% (19)
	T10–11: 11% (26)	T10–11: 17% (14)
Calcified	22% (33/151)	65% (53/82)
Intradural	6% (5/90)	7% (6/82)
Canal location		
Central/centrolateral	77% (113/146)	94% (77/82)
Lateral	23% (33/146)	6% (5/82)
Multiple discs	8% (20/242)	14% (10/71)
Presenting Signs and Symptoms		
Localized/axial pain	56% (111/199)	61% (43/71)
Radicular pain	51% (94/185)	16% (11/71)
Sensory deficit	64% (145/226)	61% (43/71)
Bowel/bladder deficit	35% (72/208)	24% (17/71)
Motor impairment	55% (114/208)	61% (43/71)
Results*		
Pain/total	76% (106/140)	87% (47/54)
Localized/axial	80% (39/49)	86% (37/43)
Radicular	74% (29/39)	91% (10/11)
Sensory deficit	NR	84% (36/43)
Bowel/bladder deficit	80% (47/59)	77% (13/17)
Motor impairment	69% (65/94)	58% (25/43)

*Number resolved or improved/total number of patients in groups reporting this result.
NR, not reported.
From Stillerman CB, Chen TC, Couldwell WT, et al: Experience in the surgical management of 82 symptomatic herniated thoracic discs and review of the literature. J Neurosurg 88:623–633, 1998.

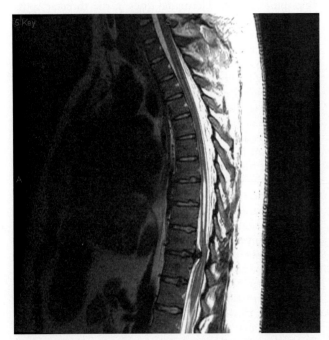

FIGURE 142-1 Sagittal T2-weighted magnetic resonance imaging demonstrates a thoracic herniated disc and associated syrinx.

is calcified and offers a better analysis of the bony anatomy (Fig. 142-2).

Surgical selection of patients is much like that for degenerative processes afflicting the remainder of the spine. That is, the indications for surgery are by no means objectified and established but rather are physician defined. As with most cervical lesions, myelopathy with or without bowel/bladder involvement is a nearly absolute operative indication. Surgical treatment of thoracic herniated discs for radiculopathy, back pain, or sensory changes is much more difficult to uniformly define. The natural history of thoracic disc herniations is not completely understood. Brown and colleagues[10] followed 40 patients with symptomatic thoracic disc herniations and determined that 77% returned to work symptom free without surgical intervention. Therefore, an argument can be made to manage patients without significant neurologic insult (weakness, spasticity) in a fashion similar to those with degenerative cervical and lumbar conditions. These nonoperative measures can include a combination of rest, physical therapy, oral antiinflammatory medication (steroidal and/or nonsteroidal), and/or steroid injections.

If a patient has myelopathy or nonmyelopathic symptoms not amenable to conservative measures, surgical intervention may be necessary. At this point, a surgeon must decide on an operative approach. Again, a wide variety of techniques

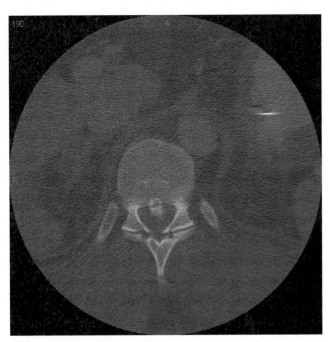

FIGURE 142-2 Axial computed tomography scan of same patient demonstrates calcification of the herniated disc.

can be used for thoracic disc herniations, each method possessing its own advantages and compromises.

One of the reasons for the development of this variety of procedures is the surgical constraint of the thoracic spine anatomy. In this region, the spinal cord lies within the relatively narrow thoracic spinal canal and the thecal sac cannot be manipulated as freely as within the lumbar region. Therefore, the operative approach needs to minimize manipulation of the dura and spinal cord. Although this feature is similar to the cervical region, the anterior approaches to the thoracic region (excluding the very superior thoracic spine) are more involved than standard anterior cervical procedures. Thus the ideal procedure would afford the surgeon a ventral view of the region while maintaining the more straightforward technical aspect of a posterior approach. As a result of these requirements, more aggressive posterior procedures have been developed in attempts to gain greater "anterior" perspectives and circumvent the need for more involved anterior thoracic exposures.

Considerations for an operative approach for herniated thoracic discs include the following:

1. Level of the herniation
2. Mediolateral localization of the herniation (location with respect to canal/cord and foramen/root and the resultant symptoms)
3. Complicating factors of the disc itself (intradural, calcification)
4. Presence of multiple disc herniations
5. Health of the patient
6. Experience of the surgeon

Although not inclusive, the following guidelines can be made in terms of operative approaches.

Posterior approaches can be employed at any level. Their utility depends largely on the laterality of the disc; that is, the more lateral the disc, the more accessible and successful

a posterior approach might prove. The one caveat is that a standard posterior laminectomy is not an adequate approach for any thoracic disc herniation. Laminectomies for thoracic disc herniations have been repeatedly shown to carry unacceptable rates of morbidity. Excepting a truly foraminal herniated disc or a case of isolated stenosis from thoracic spondylosis (and not a disc herniation), the laminectomy should not be used. Rather, standard posterior approaches include the transpedicular, Stillerman's transfacet pedicle sparing, transcostovertebral, costotransversectomy, and lateral extracavitary. In that order, these procedures offer gradually increasing exposures toward the midline of the canal despite the incursion of increasingly larger and more destructive incisions/dissections. Unfortunately, no posterior approach allows a true ventral view of the spinal canal and dura. Therefore, features favoring a posterior approach include more laterally located discs, soft discs without evidence of calcification, and extradural lesions. Often these approaches are better tolerated by the patient than anterior approaches, making them more attractive in individuals with comorbidities, especially in regards to pulmonary disease. Last, the anatomy encountered by the surgeon with these procedures is very familiar and mastering even the more aggressive posterior procedures is usually quickly attained by most surgeons.

Anterior approaches (transsternal/transmanubrial, transthoracic, anterolateral/retropleural) can be used selectively at varying levels. The transmanubrial/transsternal approach is best suited for superior thoracic lesions above T4 (below this level, the aortic arch and associated veins become an obstacle). Below T4, anterior approaches are either transthoracic or retropleural. All the anterior approaches afford the surgeon a more direct view of the ventral dura and disc herniation. This allows for greater ease in the management of calcified or intradural herniations. Central discs are also more directly accessed through these approaches. The downside of these operations is usually a more substantial operative event for the patient, requiring a greater period of recovery and the contraindication in patients with significant comorbidities. Multiple disc herniations need to be within one to two levels of one another to be accessed ventrally. The surgical approach and anatomy are somewhat foreign to most neurosurgeons and require focused training and repetitive procedures to maintain proficiency. This can be somewhat overcome by cardiothoracic surgeons aiding in the exposure of these regions, but the neurosurgeon must still manage the bony dissection, which is not as familiar to many surgeons as the anatomy encountered in typical posterior spinal procedures.

INTRAOPERATIVE LOCALIZATION

Although radiographic localization is often taken for granted in the cervical and lumbar regions, it poses a significant hurdle in the thoracic spine. Lower thoracic levels can often be imaged with standard lateral radiographs. However, in some larger patients and certainly in mid- to upper thoracic regions, lateral radiographs are very difficult to interpret and have no reference with which to localize appropriate levels.

First and foremost, a surgeon needs to identify the level of a herniated disc using the same method by which the preoperative level is diagnosed. That is, if the preoperative investigations identify the affected thoracic level counting

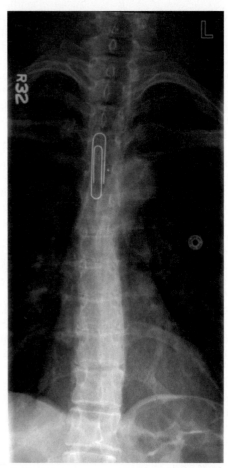

FIGURE 142-3 Preoperative anteroposterior radiograph for incision localization.

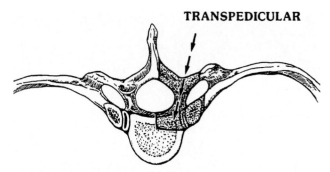

FIGURE 142-4 Schematic demonstrates the region of bony removal in transpedicular approach. (From Fessler RG, Sturgill M: Review: Complications of surgery for thoracic disc disease. Surg Neurol 49:609–618, 1998.)

down from C1, then the surgeon should not necessarily use the sacrum as a reference point intraoperatively, as a lumbarized sacral segment could obviously cause an error in localization. Rather, the surgeon can employ an intraoperative anteroposterior (AP) radiograph and count down from the first thoracic ribs, or the sacrum can be used to count upward, if this has been confirmed as an accurate means of reference. A preoperative localization can be easily performed by taping a radiopaque marker to the patient and obtaining a standard AP radiograph (Fig. 142-3).

Lateral radiographs are of limited utility in the thoracic spine, and AP radiographs must often be used to adequately visualize spinal elements and levels. The surgeon has the option to prepare the operating table for the insertion of AP radiograph cassettes or to use a radiolucent operating table with intraoperative fluoroscopy. Either option is effective, but reliance on exclusively lateral thoracic radiographs can prove to be very difficult to interpret.

DESCRIPTION OF INDIVIDUAL PROCEDURES

Posterior Procedures

Transpedicular

The transpedicular approach is perhaps the most commonly considered procedure when confronted with a thoracic disc herniation. Its origins date to the initial description of

Patterson and Arbit[11] in 1978, which represent a modification of Carson's[12] 1971 technique. The transpedicular approach allows the surgeon relatively straightforward access into the most lateral region of the spinal canal ventral to the spinal cord (Fig. 142-4). The patient is placed in a prone position on gel rolls or a Wilson frame and a vertical midline incision is centered over the level of interest. Sharp dissection is carried deeply to the thoracodorsal fascia. A unilateral exposure can be performed to minimize trauma to the contralateral paravertebral musculature. Once through the thoracodorsal fascia, a subperiosteal dissection is performed with Cobb elevators until the lateral facets are exposed on the affected side.

Viewing the facet joints, the surgeon needs to then develop an idea as to the location of the pedicle and the associated nerve root. The thoracic pedicle to be drilled is centered 1 to 2 mm beneath the edge of the inferior facet of the superior vertebra (Fig. 142-5). For example, a T7–8 disc herniation will aim to drill the T8 pedicle, which is centered just below the inferior edge of the T7 inferior facet.

By using a combination of the pneumatic drill and Kerrison rongeurs (generally no larger than 2 mm), a lateral laminotomy is performed to visualize the lateral edge of the thecal sac. This visualization allows the surgeon to safely proceed with further bone resection. The removal of bone is then extended laterally to the medial facet joint and ventral pedicle. Once the dorsal aspect of the facet is drilled adequately to visualize the exiting nerve root, the axis of the pedicle can be discerned. At this point, the interior of the pedicle is drilled, allowing the superior and medial cortex to act as a protective barrier against the nerve root and thecal sac, respectively. Often this drilling is undertaken with the aid of the operating microscope. Once the drilling has been performed to the depth of the disc space/vertebral body, a curet can be used to fracture and remove the remaining cortical shell of the pedicle, being careful to fracture the remnant pedicle away from the dura.

The increased lateral exposure obtained by removing the superomedial pedicle allows the surgeon to view a portion of the lateral disc space/spinal canal tangentially under the nerve root and thecal sac. The lateral aspect of the herniated disc is then incised and disc material removed from centrally within the disc space. This allows the surgeon to displace more medial herniated tissue into the disc space (the force being directed away from the spinal cord) using

FIGURE 142-5 Transpedicular approach after drilling of facet and superior pedicle. (From Kumar R, Dunsker SB: Surgical management of thoracic disc herniations. In Schmidek HH, Sweet WH (eds): Operative Neurosurgical Techniques, 4th ed. New York: WB Saunders, 2000, pp 2122–2131)

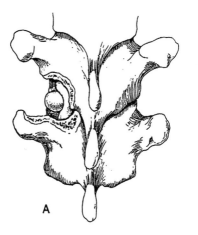
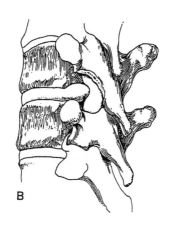

A

B

down-biting curet. Once this is completed, the disc fragments can be removed safely without disturbing the dura.

Closure resembles that of posterior lumbar and cervical procedures.

Transfacet Pedicle Sparing

This technique shares many similarities with the transpedicular approach but avoids the resection of the pedicle. Devised by Stillerman and colleagues,[13] the technique employs a setup similar to that used in the transpedicular technique. The patient is positioned prone. Stillerman and colleagues recommend the use of AP fluoroscopy for verification of the proper level during the exposure. A linear midline incision is used, and the standard dissection and subperiosteal exposure is performed so as to expose the ipsilateral facet joint.

At this point, the proper disc level and overlying facet joint are verified with fluoroscopy. As with the transpedicular procedure, a pneumatic drill is used to penetrate the medial aspect of the facet joint. Unlike the previous procedure, the inferiorly lying pedicle is not entered with the drill. Once in the neural foramen, blunt dissection can be performed to visualize the disc space lying at the inferior

aspect of the foramen (Fig. 142-6). The exiting nerve root is usually found in the extreme superior aspect of the foramen and therefore is often not encountered (except in the higher thoracic spine). Once the annulus is identified, the disc removal proceeds in a fashion similar to that of any of the other posterior procedures.

Transcostovertebral Approach

Another more recent posterolateral approach has been described by Dinh and colleagues[3] in which only the posterior cortex of the rib head is removed, thus allowing for an increased lateral exposure while not incurring the potential disadvantages of complete rib resection. In this procedure, the patient is once again positioned on the operating table in a prone position. A midline incision is used, typically spanning the adjacent superior and inferior disc spaces. A standard subperiosteal dissection is performed, but the exposure is extended laterally to visualize the transverse process. At this point, the transverse process is removed to reveal the underlying rib head. Using a diamond-tipped drill, the lateral one half of the facet joint and the upper one third to one half of the pedicle are removed (Fig. 142-7).

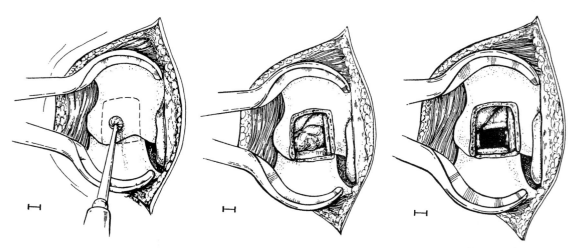

FIGURE 142-6 Sequential views of the transfacet pedicle-sparing procedure illustrate facet drilling, identification of nerve root and disc material, and removal of disc herniation. (From Stillerman CB, Chen TC, Diaz Day J, et al: The transfacet pedicle-sparing approach for thoracic disc removal: Cadaveric morphometric analysis and preliminary clinical experience. J Neurosurg 83:971–976, 1995.)

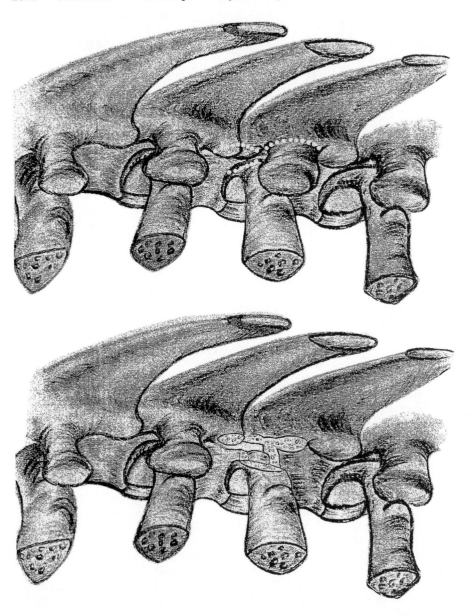

FIGURE 142-7 Transcostovertebral approach demonstrates intended region of bony removal (*white dots*) and resultant exposure of the lateral annulus. (From Dinh DH, Tompkins J, Clark SB: Transcostovertebral approach for thoracic disc herniations. J Neurosurg 94:38–44, 2001)

This allows visualization of the spinal cord and exiting nerve root. Further ventral drilling is performed through the posterior cortex of the rib head until the annulus is identified medially. The authors emphasize that the key to this procedure is "staying within the costovertebral joint and drilling outward circumferentially to include immediate adjacent structures such as the posterior cortex of the rib head and the lateral endplates above and below the annulus."[3] Once the annulus is exposed, the disc can be removed in the standard fashion by central decompression of the disc and removal of the herniation via the newly formed central cavity.

The advantages of this procedure are the increased lateral exposure to the disc space while leaving the ventral portion of the rib and, consequently, the pleura. Inspection for violation into the thoracic cavity is performed before closure, but generally no chest tube is required.

Early during their experience, the authors noted a postoperative radiculopathy that appeared in several patients when the nerve root was maintained. Their recommendation is now to transect the nerve root proximal to the ganglion to prevent this occurrence. In doing so, the authors have not noted any adverse complications.

Costotransversectomy

The next progression in terms of a greater lateral exposure through a posterior incision is the costotransversectomy. Recognition has been awarded to both Hulme and Menard for the development of this procedure.[9,14]

This technique offers a more lateral working corridor than the transpedicular route and hence affords a better view of the anterior spinal canal (Fig. 142-8). To do so, the costotransversectomy incurs a more extensive muscular and bony dissection, often leading to more postoperative discomfort.

The patient can be positioned in a variety of ways, ranging from prone to a partial lateral position. Skin incisions for this approach have also varied, ranging from curvilinear (convexity toward midline) to straight paramedian. Generally, these incisions are much longer than the transpedicular

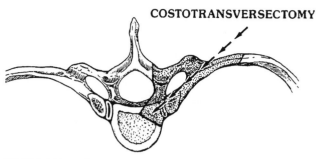

FIGURE 142-8 Bony removal in costotransversectomy procedure. (From Fessler RG, Sturgill M: Review: Complications of surgery for thoracic disc disease. Surg Neurol 49:609–618, 1998.)

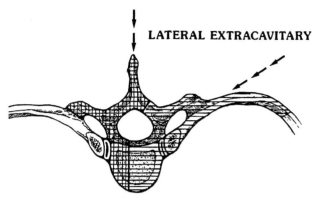

FIGURE 142-9 Bony removal in the lateral extracavitary approach. Note the larger amount of rib to be resected as compared with the costotransversectomy. (From Fessler RG, Sturgill M: Review: Complications of surgery for thoracic disc disease. Surg Neurol 49:609–618, 1998.)

counterparts, spanning anywhere from two to three segments above and below the affected region.

The skin and muscle (trapezius, erector spinae) layers are reflected medially to allow visualization of the ribs and transverse processes. The bony resection begins by identifying the adjoining rib to the lower vertebral body (e.g., rib 8 for a T7–8 disc). The rib is then dissected free of investing fascia and pleura. A Cobb or periosteal elevator can be used to initiate this procedure, but Doyen dissectors are generally used to complete the bulk of the dissection. The rib is then disarticulated and removed with rongeurs from the costotransverse and costovertebral joints. Additionally, the corresponding transverse process should be resected.

Anatomic landmarks at this point include the corresponding pedicle, the neurovascular bundles of the resected rib and superior rib, and the underlying pleura. The pleura can be retracted ventrally under a malleable retractor. Attention is next turned to drilling the pedicle just inferior to the affected disc space. This allows identification of the lateral thecal sac and the exiting nerve root. The herniated disc is then visualized from its inferior aspect, where it is incised laterally for disc removal. As in the transpedicular approach, the lateral herniated disc is initially removed, followed by removal of the central nucleus pulposus. Once a cavity has been created within the disc, careful mobilization of the more medial herniated material from the canal into the center of the disc space is performed. The herniated disc can then be removed safely with pituitary rongeurs.

Closure requires inspection of the pleura for violations into the thoracic cavity. The operative site is flooded with irrigation under positive pressure ventilation. Small tears can be closed with sutures. Larger tears will require closure and the placement of a chest tube.

Lateral Extracavitary

The term lateral extracavitary approach was first coined by Larson and colleagues[15] in 1976 for a technique for treating traumatic thoracic spine injuries. However, this was a modification of Capener's[16] 1954 technique for treating tuberculous spondylitis.[17]

The lateral extracavitary approach represents the most aggressive posterior approach. It therefore offers the greatest visualization of the anterior canal via a posterior incision but requires a much more significant dissection than a transpedicular approach. The "lateral" nomenclature should not fool one into believing that the entirety of the anterior dura is as well visualized as in anterolateral procedures.

This procedure is still a posterior approach, despite its lateral viewing corridor.

This procedure typically uses one of two incisions: a hockey stick incision with the vertical segment centered over the affected level or a curvilinear incision with the convexity facing medially. The major difference between the lateral extracavitary approach and the costotransversectomy is that a larger lateral resection of the inferior rib is performed (Fig. 142-9). This allows a lower viewing angle toward the canal. If a hemilaminectomy is performed, the nerve root overlying the disc space can be ligated, incised, and then used to rotate the thecal sac dorsally. Removal of the disc material is performed in the same manner as the preceding techniques. If necessary, portions of the vertebral body can be drilled to facilitate disc manipulation. If this is performed, then portions of resected rib can be placed as strut grafts between the vertebral bodies.

Closure is performed in a manner similar to the costotransversectomy.

Anterior Procedures

Unlike the posterior procedures, the lung will substantially obscure visualization of the disc space in transthoracic procedures. In the lower thoracic spine, the lung can be mobilized superiorly and held out of the operative site with table-mounted retractors. In the mid- and upper thoracic spine, adequate visualization is best obtained by placing a dual-lumen endotracheal tube, which allows the lung to be collapsed during the discectomy.

For this procedure, the patient is placed in a lateral position on a bean bag. The patient can be positioned so that the break of the operating table is directly beneath the intended operative level. This allows the surgeon to "flex" the operating table, thus causing affected disc space to "open" during the operation. The lower leg is left straight while the upper leg is flexed somewhat to allow relaxation of the psoas muscle (if a more inferior level is being addressed). Appropriate padding is placed, being sure to protect the peroneal nerves and brachial plexus.

Either the right or left side can be used for a transthoracic procedure, but several criteria need to be considered. The side of greater herniation is used if any asymmetry exists. Left-sided approaches are generally recommended for all central lesions except those in the upper (T4 or higher) thoracic spine. In doing so, one avoids the dome of the liver, vena cava/azygous system, and thoracic duct. Severe scoliosis may require the surgeon to approach from the side of the convexity rather than work within the narrow confines of the concavity. Last, previous surgery or notable pulmonary disease may make one thoracic cavity preferable to another.

Transthoracic Procedure (Adapted from Vollmer and Simmons[18])

A curvilinear incision is made from the posterior angle of the rib to several centimeters beyond the anterior axillary line. The decision as to which rib to dissect can be clarified by obtaining a preoperative AP chest radiograph and drawing a line directly lateral to the affected disc space. This line will intersect the rib directly lateral to this region, offering the most direct exposure. Typically, this tends to be the lower associated rib in the upper and midthoracic spine, whereas in the lower thoracic spine, often the 10th rib is adequate for discectomies. Muscles are divided with electrocautery. Once the subscapular space has been entered, the surgeon can verify the appropriate level by reaching superiorly, palpating the first rib, and then counting downward. Additionally, a second AP radiograph will provide added confirmation of the level. Cobb and Doyen elevators are used to perform a subperiosteal dissection of the rib, which can then be removed and used later for bone grafting, if necessary. The neurovascular bundle is identified and traced to the neural foramen. After the rib is removed, the pleural cavity is sharply entered. A rib spreader is then inserted to provide additional exposure within the thoracic cavity.

Once the appropriate level is identified by the above methods, the lung is retracted/deflated. The parietal pleura is incised longitudinally, extending over adjacent vertebral bodies, and a subperiosteal dissection performed until the disc space and vertebral bodies are well visualized. Care is taken to preserve the intersegmental vessels running at the midportions of the vertebral bodies. The sympathetic chain is then mobilized away from the vertebral bodies in a dorsal direction. The intercostal nerve is dissected from the pleura and used to identify the location of the neural foramen and pedicle.

The rib head is removed with rongeurs, drills, or both. Resection of the rib allows access to the posterolateral aspect of the disc and the intervertebral foramen. At this point, the surgeon needs to identify the disc margins, the intervertebral foramen, and the pedicles above each foramen. The pedicle inferior to the desired disc space can be drilled away with a diamond-tipped drill to allow greater visualization of the exiting nerve root and thecal sac. Due to the typically narrow thoracic disc spaces, the posterolateral portions of the vertebral bodies may need to be drilled away to adequately access the disc space itself. Larger and more centrally located disc herniations will often require more aggressive drilling, in some cases even extending beyond the midpoint of the ventral spinal canal (Fig. 142-10). Exposure of this portion of the disc allows an incision to be made in the lateral annulus. Using curets, the dorsal herniation can then be manipulated into the cavity created by the initial disc removal.

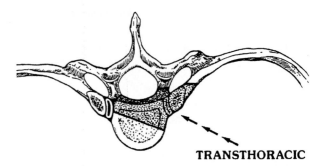

TRANSTHORACIC

FIGURE 142-10 Bone removal employed in the transthoracic procedure. (From Fessler RG, Sturgill M: Review: Complications of surgery for thoracic disc disease. Surg Neurol 49:609–618, 1998.)

This portion of the procedure can be performed under loupe magnification, although the operating microscope allows superior magnification and illumination.

Often after decompression, notable bleeding from epidural veins is encountered. This is usually easily dealt with by using a combination of gentle tamponade with hemostatic agents (Gelfoam or the equivalent) and/or bipolar electrocautery at lower settings. In most instances, no graft is required unless the bony removal of the vertebral bodies is significant.

Closure

The initial step of the closure involves rinsing the thoracic cavity with warm saline. This maneuver accomplishes two goals: (1) the removal of bone fragments and dust generated during the exposure and (2) inspection for air leaks as the lung is ventilated. If necessary, the lung can again be deflated for closure. A chest tube should be placed along the posterior thoracic wall and passed through a separate incision adjacent to the surgical incision. The ribs are reapproximated using heavy suture (no. 5 Ticron or similar), tied in an interrupted fashion over at least three points. Overlying muscular layers are closed with a running suture, being careful to adhere to corresponding muscular planes. Subcutaneous tissues and skin may be closed in standard fashion. The chest tube should be placed to water-suction and monitored for air leak and postoperative drainage. Generally, the tube can be removed after drainage decreases to less than 200 mL/8 hours and no air leak or pneumothorax is noted after 8 to 12 hours of water seal.

If cerebrospinal fluid leakage is noted during the operation, attempts can be made to primarily repair the tear, although this may often prove very difficult to perform. If direct repair is not an option, a patch graft of autologous tissue (muscle, fascia) or processed allograft or xenograft (e.g., Duragen) can be placed over the leak site. Recombinant fibrin glue can also be used. Additionally, a lumbar drain should be placed before recovery from anesthesia to aid in the avoidance of a cerebrospinal fluid fistula. The chest tube needs to be removed as early as possible and before discontinuation of the lumbar drain.

Retropleural Thoracotomy

Although the transthoracic approach offers a clear visualization of the thoracic spinal canal, it carries the inherent

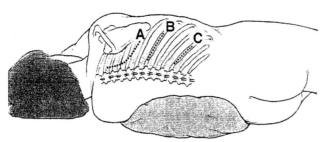

FIGURE 142-11 Incisions for the retropleural thoracotomy in the upper (*A*), mid- (*B*), and lower (*C*) thoracic regions. (From McCormick PC: Retropleural approach to the thoracic and thoracolumbar spine. Neurosurgery 37:908–914, 1995.)

complications of entering the thoracic cavity. McCormick[19] introduced the retropleural approach as an alternate means of ventrolateral access to the spine.

Positioning is similar to that of the transthoracic procedure. The patient is placed in a lateral position on a beanbag, preferably with the lesion lying directly over a break in the operating table. The incision is slightly smaller than in the transthoracic procedure. In the midthoracic spine, the incision is placed over the rib of interest, extending from several centimeters off midline to the posterior axillary line. Higher thoracic lesions necessitate a "hockey stick" incision, while lower thoracic lesions are best approached by making an incision over the 10th rib (Fig. 142-11).

Again, the muscular dissection remains similar to the transthoracic procedure. The inferior rib of the affected level is dissected free from investing fascia. An 8- to 10-cm segment of rib is removed, leaving the proximal portion still attached to the transverse process and vertebral body.

Once this portion of the rib is removed, the endothoracic fascia is identified. This layer of tissue encompasses the entire thoracic cavity and the parietal pleura. By incising this fascia along the longitudinal axis of the recently removed rib, the parietal pleura is exposed (Fig. 142-12).

Using blunt dissection, the parietal pleura can be gently dissected free from the inner aspect of the fascia toward the spine. When necessary, the remaining portion of rib can be disarticulated and removed to allow additional exposure. A malleable retractor is placed over the parietal pleura to prevent entrance into the thoracic cavity and to facilitate the exposure of the disc space.

The periosteum and investing tissues are then dissected off the vertebral body. The neural foramen is identified, along with the pedicle and the superiorly lying disc space. At this point, disc space manipulation remains the same as in the transthoracic procedure. The end plates and pedicle are removed via a pneumatic drill (Fig. 142-13). Closure is also the same, being sure to check for tears in the parietal pleura and closing these with sutures as needed. A chest tube is generally not needed unless a large tear in the pleura is encountered.

TRANSSTERNAL APPROACH TO THORACIC SPINE (T1–5)

The transsternal approach affords access to the upper thoracic spine, from T1 to T4/5. The lower limit of this approach depends on individual anatomic variability as defined by the level of the aortic arch, which allows only minimal manipulation.

An orogastric tube can be placed in the esophagus to improve intraoperative identification of this structure. Several incisions can be used to perform this procedure including a midline T-shaped incision or a vertical incision over the sternal region, which curves to one side or another as it extends superiorly into the lower cervical region. The upper portion of the dissection is similar to that of an anterior

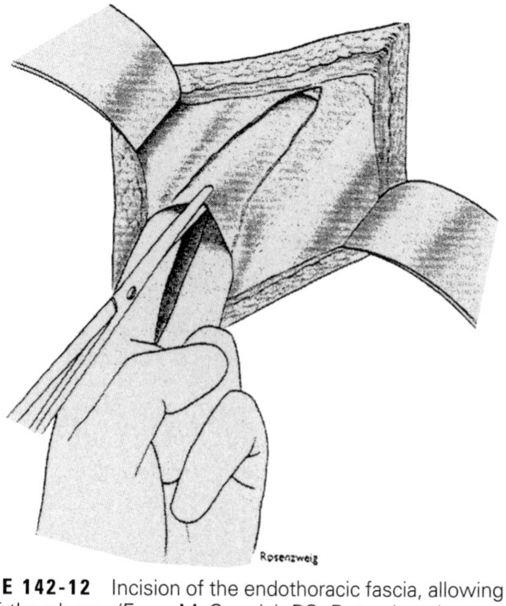

FIGURE 142-12 Incision of the endothoracic fascia, allowing exposure of the pleura. (From McCormick PC: Retropleural approach to the thoracic and thoracolumbar spine. Neurosurgery 37:908–914, 1995.)

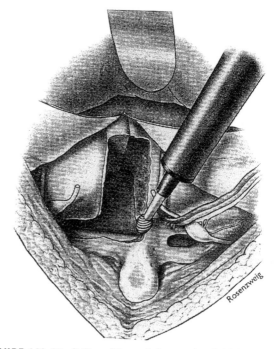

FIGURE 142-13 Drilling of the end plates and pedicles in a transthoracic or retropleural thoracotomy. (From McCormick PC: Retropleural approach to the thoracic and thoracolumbar spine. Neurosurgery 37:908–914, 1995.)

cervical procedure. Fascial attachments to the sternum are removed, and the surgeon can insert a finger to bluntly dissect along the underside of the sternum. The sternum is then opened with a sagittal saw, whereupon a sternal retractor is placed. At this point, the major vessels are identified, along with the pericardium and thymus. The inferior thyroid artery and vein can be ligated for additional exposure.[20] The thymus is reflected to the patient's right side, affording a window of operative exposure just medial to the left common carotid artery.[9] Disc manipulation is then carried out in the fashion similar to that of anterior cervical surgery. In addition to the vascular and neurologic structures, care must be taken to avoid injury to the thoracic duct, which ascends along the esophagus and eventually runs behind the left subclavian artery to enter the internal jugular vein.

Fortunately, the demand for transsternal surgery is low, owing to the infrequency of upper thoracic herniated discs and the posterior procedures generally offering access with less morbidity. In the few cases requiring a transsternal approach, assistance by cardiothoracic surgeons is often invaluable.

COMPLICATIONS

Since the abandonment of laminectomy for thoracic disc herniations, morbidity and mortality rates have dropped significantly.[2] Obviously, the type of complication differs with the specific procedure, as pneumonia and hemo-/chylothorax is more commonly seen after a transthoracic procedure than after a transpedicular procedure. Again, complications of some procedures may be accepted outcomes in others. For example, a pleural tear is an undesirable outcome during a costotransversectomy, but a pleural incision is intentionally performed in a transthoracic procedure.

Despite these difficulties in comparing the complication rates, the morbidity and mortality associated with currently accepted procedures appear similar.[2,21] Fessler and Sturgill[2] demonstrated that, since 1986, reported complication rates for all thoracic disc surgeries ranged from 8% to 16%. When analyzed with respect to procedure, morbidity rates were 9% for transpedicular, 12% for costotransversectomy, 12% for lateral extracavitary, and 11% for transthoracic procedures. No mortality was noted.

Infection rates ranged from 1% to 3%, which compare favorably with those of other spinal surgeries.[2] Neurologic worsening was seen in approximately 1% of cases.[2,9]

In regards to the newer procedures mentioned in this chapter, reports of the transfacet-pedicle sparing procedure of Stillerman and colleagues[13] and the transcostovertebral approach of Dinh and colleagues[3] mentioned no complications in the their analyses of 6 and 22 patients, respectively.

CONCLUSION

Most neurosurgeons will encounter symptomatic thoracic disc herniations from time to time in their practices. Successful management of these lesions requires a thorough understanding of the spectrum of available procedures.

REFERENCES

1. Debnath UK, McConnell JR, Sengupta DK, et al: Results of hemivertebrectomy and fusion for symptomatic thoracic disc herniation. Eur Spine J 12:292–299, 2003.
2. Fessler RG, Sturgill M: Review: Complications of surgery for thoracic disc disease. Surg Neurol 49:609–618, 1998.
3. Dinh DH, Tompkins J, Clark SB: Transcostovertebral approach for thoracic disc herniations. J Neurosurg 94:38–44, 2001.
4. Wood KB, Blair JM, Aepple DM, et al: The natural history of asymptomatic thoracic disc herniations. Spine 22:525–529, 1997.
5. Wood KB, Garvey TA, Gundry C, et al: Magnetic resonance imaging of the thoracic spine: Evaluation of asymptomatic individuals. J Bone Joint Surg Am 77:1631–1638, 1995.
6. Awaad EE, Martin DS, Smith KR, Jr, et al: Asymptomatic versus symptomatic herniated thoracic discs: Their frequency and characteristics as detected by computed tomography after myelography. Neurosurgery 28:180–186, 1991.
7. Kumar R, Dunsker SB: Surgical management of thoracic disc herniations. In Schmidek HH, Sweet WH (eds): Operative Neurosurgical Techniques, 4th ed. New York: WB Saunders, 2000, pp 2122–2131.
8. Stillerman CB, Chen TC, Couldwell WT, et al: Experience in the surgical management of 82 symptomatic herniated thoracic discs and review of the literature. J Neurosurg 88:623–633, 1998.
9. Stillerman CB, McCormick PC, Benzel EC: Thoracic discectomy. In Benzel EC (ed): Spine Surgery. New York: Churchill Livingstone, 1999, pp 369–387.
10. Brown CW, Deffer PA, Akmakjian J, et al: The natural history of thoracic disc herniation. Spine 17:S97–S102, 1992.
11. Patterson RH, Arbit E: A surgical approach through the pedicle to protruded thoracic discs. J Neurosurg 48:768–772, 1978.
12. Carson J, Gumpert J, Jefferson A: Diagnosis and treatment of thoracic intervertebral disc protrusions. J Neurol Neurosurg Psychiatry 34:68–77, 1971.
13. Stillerman CB, Chen TC, Diaz Day J, et al: The transfacet pedicle-sparing approach for thoracic disc removal: Cadaveric morphometric analysis and preliminary clinical experience. J Neurosurg 83:971–976, 1995.
14. Hulme A: The surgical approach to thoracic intervertebral disc protrusions. J Neurol Neurosurg Psychiatry 23:133–137, 1960.
15. Larson SJ, Holst RA, Hemmy DC, et al: Lateral extracavitary approach to traumatic lesions of the thoracic and lumbar spine. J Neurosurg 45:628–637, 1976.
16. Capener N: The evolution of lateral rhachotomy. J Bone Joint Surg Br 36:173–179, 1954.
17. Delfinia R, Lorenzo ND, Ciappetta P, et al: Surgical treatment of thoracic disc herniation: A reappraisal of Larson's lateral extracavitary approach. Surg Neurol 45:517–523, 1996.
18. Vollmer DG, Simmons NE: Transthoracic approaches to thoracic disc herniations. Neurosurg Focus 9:1–6, 2000.
19. McCormick PC: Retropleural approach to the thoracic and thoracolumbar spine. Neurosurgery 37:908–914, 1995.
20. Knoller SM, Brethner L: Surgical treatment of the spine at the cervicothoracic junction: An illustrated review of a modified sternotomy approach with the description of tricks and pitfalls. Arch Orthop Trauma Surg 122:365–368, 2002.
21. Mulier S, Debois V: Thoracic disc herniations: Transthoracic, lateral, or posterolateral approach? A review. Surg Neurol 49:599–608, 1998.

143 Management Options in Thoracolumbar Fractures

PATRICK W. HITCHON, KURT M. EICHHOLZ,
AARON M. FROM, and JAMES C. TORNER

Both surgery and recumbency have been adopted successfully in the treatment of spinal fractures. The selection of operative versus nonoperative treatment in thoracic and lumbar fractures should be not random but based on clinical as well as radiologic criteria. In the absence of neurologic deficit, instability with three-column injury,[1-3] or intractable pain, recumbency is favored. Treatment in these cases consists of bed rest generally for 3 to 7 days, with gradual monitored mobilization thereafter.[4-6] The resolution of pain is generally a good index of when mobilization can commence.

Surgical intervention is generally indicated in patients with partial or complete neurologic deficit, persistent pain, or spinal instability with three-column injuries.[5,6] Such fractures include fracture dislocations, burst fractures with angulation greater than 20 degrees, a canal smaller than 50% of normal, and 50% or more loss in vertebral body height. The increased use of spinal implants has resulted partly from improvements in imaging techniques, a better understanding of spinal stability, and refinements in spinal implants and their ease of use. The application of customized or off-the-shelf thoracolumbar clamshell or similar braces is individualized and recommended after either recumbency or surgery.

RECUMBENCY

Recumbency treatment for up to 3 months in spinal fractures was advocated in the work of Ludwig Guttmann[7] and Frankel[8] at the Stoke Mandeville Hospital. Surgical management for fractures was reserved for open fractures, secondary to missile injuries or to fractures with progressive neurologic deficit. In 1949, Nicoll[9] reported on his analysis of 166 thoracic and lumbar fractures in 152 miners in England, the majority of whom were treated with immobilization and bed rest. A good anatomic result did not always equate with a good functional outcome. Postural nonsurgical reduction of thoracic and lumbar fractures was adopted by Bedbrook[10,11] and by Davies and colleagues in Australia,[12] and immobilization for 6 to 10 weeks followed by bracing was recommended. Surgery was indicated in the few cases of irreducible fractures, locked facets, gunshot wounds, and neurologic deterioration. In his analysis of 143 thoracic and lumbar fractures, Bedbrook noted that an angulation of 40 degrees was often well tolerated without functional impairment.

Subsequent reports[13-27] rekindled interest in recumbency in the management of thoracic and lumbar fractures. This approach was associated with a stable or improved neurologic status, despite progression in spinal angulation. In addition, computed tomography (CT) scans revealed remodeling of

the spine with partial resolution of the compromised canal.[14,16,18,27] At our center, 32 patients with thoracolumbar burst fractures (T12–L2) were treated with recumbency and followed prospectively for a mean of over 1 year.[4-6] Among these 32 patients, 26 had a Frankel score of E (intact) and 6 a score of D (minimal motor deficit). Angular deformity measured (means ± standard deviation) 5.6 ± 7 degrees (range = 1.4–16 degrees), and residual spinal canal on CT compared with the average of the normal rostral and caudal canal measured 65% ± 18% . Patients were kept on bed rest generally for 1 week or less, or until their pain resolved. They were mobilized thereafter in thoracolumbar orthosis for 3 to 5 months with sequential radiographs.

In this recumbency group, total charges including hospital and physician charges were calculated at $27,000 ± $19,600 per patient, versus $62,900 ± $38,900 ($p = 0.0001$) in a comparable group of 36 patients treated with surgery. Neurologic improvement occurred irrespective of recumbency or surgical treatment. Whereas on admission the incidences of deficit in the recumbency and surgical groups were 19% and 86%, respectively, these numbers decreased to 3% and 72%, respectively, at follow-up. At final follow-up, angulation progressed in the recumbency group to 13.5 ± 8.5 (Fig. 143-1). Where sequential CT scans were obtained, remodeling of the spinal canal with time in the recumbency group was seen (Fig. 143-2). It is therefore difficult to justify surgery in the treatment of thoracic and lumbar fractures in patients who are intact, without three-column injuries,

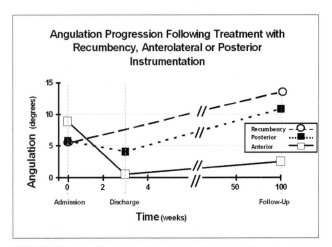

FIGURE 143-1 Progress of spinal angulation with time in patients with thoracolumbar burst fractures treated with recumbency, and with anterolateral or posterolateral surgery.

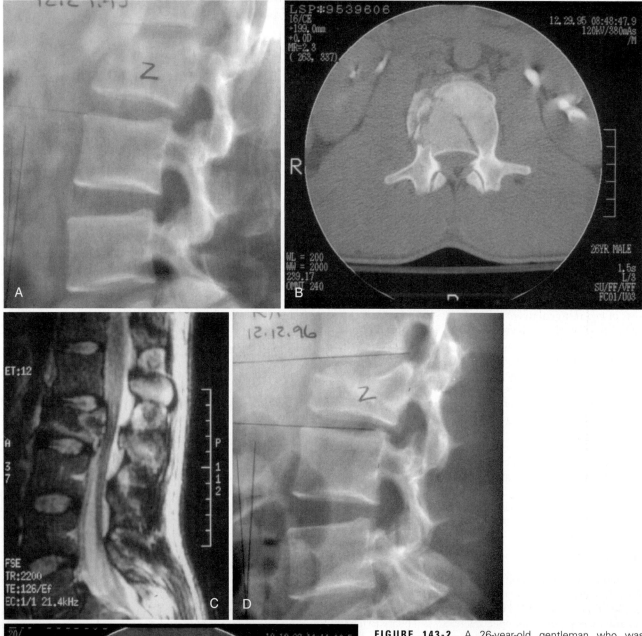

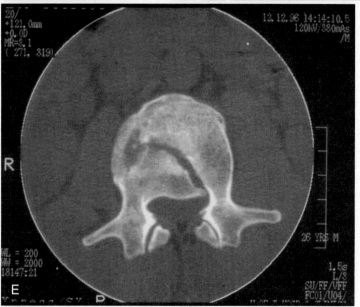

FIGURE 143-2 A 26-year-old gentleman who was involved in a single-car accident was intact but had multiple injuries including head, bladder laceration, and extremity fractures. *A,* Lateral radiographs of the spine show a burst fracture of L2 with loss in height. *B,* CT scan shows the burst fracture of L2 with at least 50% compromise of the AP diameter of the canal. *C,* T2-weighted MRI scan reveals the burst fracture, with posterior displacement of bone and compression of the cauda equina. For his spinal and right ankle fracture, he was treated with recumbency for 17 days, and was discharged 2 days later. He wore his customized thoracolumbar orthosis for 3 months and has since returned to his previous employment. *D,* Radiographs obtained 1 year later show an angular deformity at L2 measuring 8 degrees compared with 5 degrees on admission. *E,* A follow-up CT scan shows remodeling of the spinal canal.

angulation less than 20 degrees, and residual canal greater than 50% of normal.[13–27]

SURGICAL TREATMENT

All patients now undergo plain anteroposterior (AP) and lateral supine radiographs and CT scans in the emergency room. Magnetic resonance imaging (MRI) is usually done shortly thereafter. In accordance with published randomized studies,[28,29] patients with spinal cord injury are treated with methylprednisolone for 1 day if started within 3 hours of injury, or 2 days if started between 3 and 8 hours after injury. Patients are usually kept on bed rest before surgery because of pain and/or neurologic deficit. Surgery for cord or cauda equina compression is undertaken when the patient is deemed stable from his other injuries, and rarely is undertaken emergently in the face of worsening neurologic status. Surgery may have to be delayed because of hemodynamic instability or infection that may compromise a 4- to 6-hour operation. In the face of clinical worsening, however, surgery may be undertaken urgently (within 24 hours) without an increase in morbidity when compared to delayed surgery (24–72 hours[30]).

Thoracic Spine

Where ventral cord compression is present in the thoracic spine, as in the case of pathologic fractures from metastatic disease or infection, anterolateral transthoracic or transsternal decompression and stabilization might be necessary. On the other hand, the midline posterior approach is preferred for thoracic spine fractures where anterior decompression is unnecessary, as in dislocations or flexion compression fractures. The surgeon is striving to achieve reduction of angular deformity or dislocation, and establish stability (Figs. 143-3 to 143-5). Due to the stability of the thoracic spine afforded by the rib cage, the majority of thoracic spinal fractures are of the flexion compression type. In cases of severe trauma, however, fracture dislocations are encountered, though less frequently. Thus the majority of thoracic spinal fractures are treated by the posterior approach.

This operation is performed with the patient prone on gel or foam rolls, with the legs wrapped in pneumatic pulsatile stockings. If a frame is to be used to position the patient prone, it should be radiolucent and should not elevate the patient excessively for the surgeon's comfort. The table is positioned flat, such that the instrumentation will align the spine anatomically. The skin incision is linear, midline, and located over the area of interest as confirmed by intraoperative fluoroscopy. The incision is extended to expose at least two levels above and below the site of instability. In case of dislocation, the facets are partially resected by rongeur or air drill to facilitate reduction. Generally excessive distraction or the use of an outrigger is not necessary. Furthermore, distraction in the presence of neurologic function is dangerous and if not monitored can lead to stretching of the cord and aggravation of a partial deficit. An adequate laminotomy is made to allow inspection of the canal directly or by ultrasound for displaced bone or disc fragments. When small fragments of bone are retropulsed into the canal, decompression can be achieved using small impactors or reversed curets through unilateral or bilateral transpedicular or transfacetal approach.

Burst fractures with significant bone in the canal are best treated through thoracotomy or a posterolateral extracavitary approach.[31,32]

Once reduction has been achieved, it is maintained using rods with anchors—be they screws, hooks, or sublaminar wires.[33,34] Correction is achieved using the principle of three-point fixation.[35] The rostral and caudal ends of the rods constitute two points of fixation, and the third is the apex of the deformity that is ventrally displaced by tightening of the anchors. At least two instrumented levels are needed caudal and rostral to the level of fracture. Pedicle screw fixation, by engaging the pedicles and posterior and anterior halves of the body, secures all three columns and provides the best option for stabilization.[33] Pedicle screws usually come in sizes of 5, 6, and 7 mm, and in the thoracic spine, 5- or 5.5-mm screws are generally used. The upper third of the thoracic spine might be difficult but not impossible to engage with pedicle screws. Thus in the upper thoracic spine the surgeon may resort to hooks. The entry point for pedicle screws is easily identified in the lumbar spine and is located at the intersection of the horizontal axis of the transverse process and superior facets. In the thoracic spine, the transverse process is more posterior, and the entry point to the pedicle is located at the base of the superior facet. A skeleton in the operating room is helpful to correlate bony landmarks. Where the anatomy has been distorted by fracture, an angled curet may be used to identify the medial margin of the pedicle through a laminotomy, and its lateral margin underneath the transverse process. Pedicle screw insertion is generally though not necessarily performed under fluoroscopic monitoring in the lateral (the authors' choice) or AP projections. The AP projection helps identify the bull's eye or pedicle on end, whereas the lateral projection helps identify the appropriate trajectory and avoidance of the disc space with the screw. Once anchors are in place, the set screws are tightened to the rods in compression to maintain reduction.

The transverse processes are eburnated with an air drill, or preferably bone rongeur preserving the bone chips. Posterolateral bone fusion is accomplished using autogenous bone harvested from the spinous processes and laminae supplemented with demineralized bone matrix or iliac crest bone if necessary. More recently, where autogenous bone has been deemed insufficient, hydroxyapatite-impregnated strips supplemented with bone marrow aspirate have proven effective (Helos, DePuy Spine, Raynham, MA). Grafts are packed lateral to the hardware over the eburnated transverse processes. The principle of rodding long and fusing short is adopted here. Although the hardware may extend five or six levels, the bony fusion extends over three levels only. Thus if the hardware can be removed at a future time, not sooner than 18 months, the patient may regain some spinal mobility. Crosslinks are placed between the rods to provide further rigidity, particularly against axial rotation. Usually one crosslink is used for every three spinal levels (see Figs. 143-3 to 143-5).

The authors prefer to use pedicle screws whenever possible. Sublaminar hooks engaging at least two levels above and below the level of instability are an acceptable alternative and can be applied without the need for fluoroscopy. However, unlike pedicle screws that engage all three columns,[33] hooks engage the posterior column or neural arch only. In our experience the failure rate with sublaminar wires and hooks is higher than that encountered with pedicle screws.

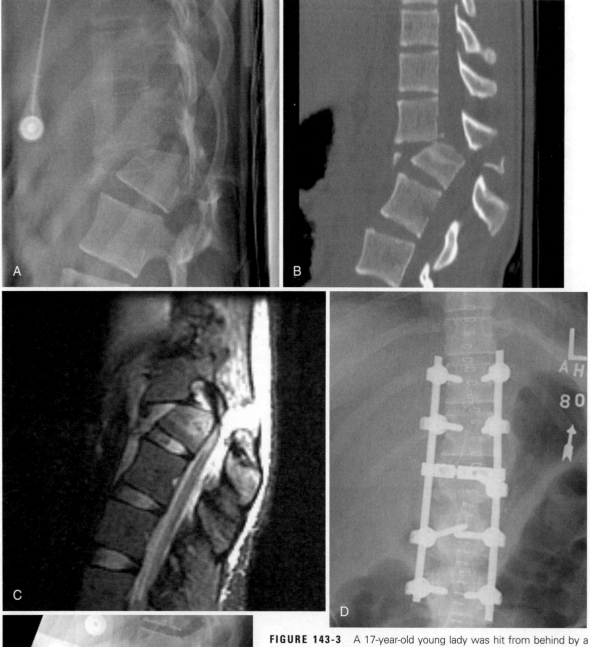

FIGURE 143-3   A 17-year-old young lady was hit from behind by a friend who was immediately behind her on a haunted house slide. The patient experienced immediate lower extremity paralysis. A fracture dislocation at T12–L1 was revealed on plain lateral radiograph (*A*), reformatted sagittal CT (*B*), and MRI (*C*). The patient was treated with pedicle screw fixation as seen on AP (*D*) and lateral (*E*) radiographs. Angular correction was corrected, and she remains paraplegic.

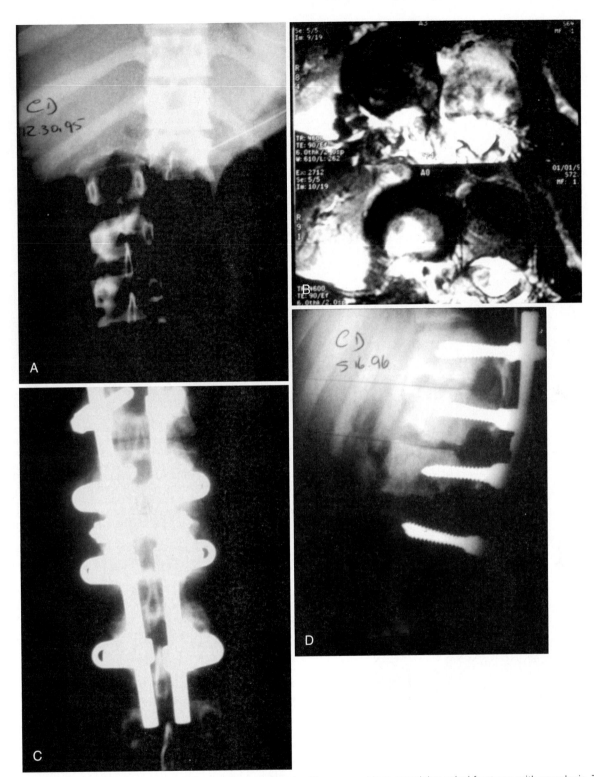

FIGURE 143-4   An 18-year-old unrestrained young man was involved in a car accident, sustaining spinal fractures with paraplegia. The AP radiograph (*A*) demonstrates a fracture dislocation of the lumbar spine with right lateral displacement of L1 relative to L2. T2-weighted axial MRI scan through the fracture site (*B*) demonstrates both vertebral bodies L1 and L2 on the same slice. AP radiograph (*C*) and lateral radiograph (*D*) obtained 5 months postoperatively demonstrate pedicle screw and rod fixation from T12 to L2 inclusive. Normal alignment has been restored without change in neurologic status.

When hooks are applied, a claw configuration applied to the same lamina rostrally and caudally at the ends of the construct is recommended (see Fig. 143-5). An additional pair of sublaminar hooks directed rostrally and a pair directed caudally are also applied, for a total of at least six hooks above and six hooks below the fracture. To avoid failure, three basic principles of posterior instrumentation have to be emphasized: (1) multiple points of fixation, (2) screw triangulation, and (3) transverse connectors to maintain triangulation, prevent rod twisting, or screw withdrawal.

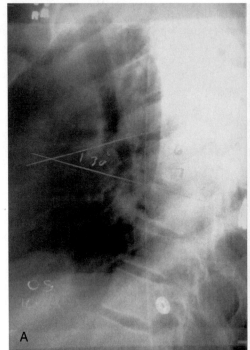

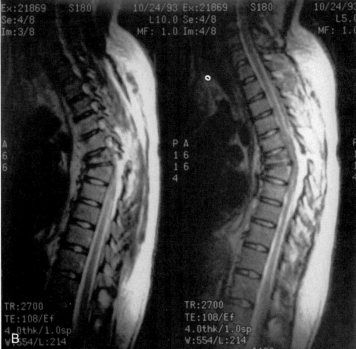

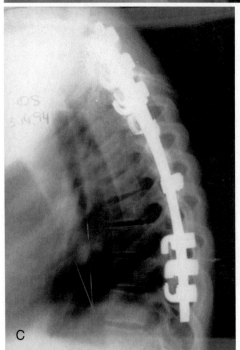

FIGURE 143-5 A 17-year-old young lady lost control of her car, driving it into a ditch while reaching for a can of soda. She was able to walk and seek help from a nearby home. She complained of severe back pain and leg numbness. On examination she had a T6 sensory level, and 4/5 bilateral motor weakness of the iliopsoas and quadriceps muscles. *A,* Plain radiographs revealed flexion compression fractures of T6–T7. *B,* MRI shows the spinal cord compressed and tethered anteriorly by the wedging of T6–T7. At surgery the patient had laminar fractures of T4 and T5, bilateral pars fractures of T6, as well as multiple transverse process fractures. Claw hooks were therefore applied on T2 and T9, with rostral hooks on T3 and caudal hooks on T8. *C,* Additional sublaminar wires were applied on T4. Six months postoperatively the patient was intact, though complaining of interscapular discomfort from the hardware.

Thoracolumbar Spine (T11–L4)

The anterior or anterolateral approach is undertaken where the spinal cord or cauda equina are under ventral compression from bone fragments. Under such circumstances it is difficult or impossible to decompress the canal and proceed with anterior grafting or stabilization through a midline posterior approach. In the case of the thoracolumbar, or lumbar spine (T11–L4), reconstruction of the anterior two columns[1] is achieved through a transthoracic, or flank retroperitoneal approach.[36-39] Although the posterolateral extracavitary, or costotransversectomy approach is also

viable,[31,32] the authors prefer the anterolateral approach described herein.

Due to the left-sided location of the aorta at the thoracolumbar junction, and to avoid injury to the more fragile vena cava, the approach is from the left side. The decubitus patient is maintained with a bean bag (Fig. 143-6). Particular care is taken to stabilize the head and neck, and a well-padded sling supports the left arm. A soft pad is placed in the dependent axilla to prevent compression injury to the long thoracic nerve. The upper knee is slightly bent, and the knees, heels, and ankles are also padded. Wide adhesive tape across the greater trochanter and shoulder straps the patient to the

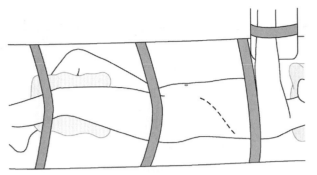

FIGURE 143-6 For the anterolateral approach to the thoracolumbar spine, the patient is laid in the decubitus position with the left side up. Position is maintained by means of a bean bag as well as wide adhesive tape across the hip and left shoulder.

operating table and allows tilting such that the spinous processes are perfectly aligned between the pedicles on cross-table lateral fluoroscopy. Thigh-high pneumatic compression stockings or the equivalent are placed to reduce the incidence of postoperative deep venous thrombosis. A warming blanket or convection air heat apparatus may be placed over the lower extremities to maintain body temperature.

Fluoroscopy allows the identification of the fracture site, and an oblique incision of 8 to 9 inches (20.5–23 cm) length is outlined centered over the involved vertebra (Fig. 143-7). The exposure to the spine is performed with the active participation of a general surgeon familiar with this approach. The incision extends from a point lateral to the edge of the rectus muscle posteriorly to the edge of the paraspinal muscles. The appropriate interspace to be entered is chosen allowing access to the fracture and adjacent vertebral bodies. The interspace selected is generally two levels above the fracture level (e.g., for decompression at T12, the 10th interspace may be the most appropriate). The rostral rib is generally the larger, and an appropriate length is harvested for use in the bone fusion. The periosteum and intercostal muscles are then reflected off the rib circumferentially without injuring the pleura. In areas where the diaphragm must be incised as in the

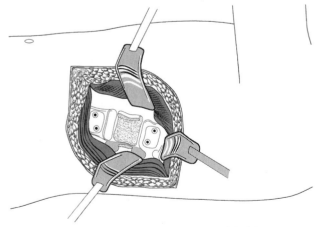

FIGURE 143-7 Through an 8-inch (~20.5 cm) incision, exposure of the spine is achieved with a table-mounted vascular retractor, with blades retracting the peritoneal contents anteriorly, the diaphragm or parietal pleura rostrally, and the psoas muscle posteriorly. The corpectomy, and rostral and caudal disc excision are complete, and the canal is decompressed.

case of fractures of T11 or T12, a rim of muscle is tagged and left on the rib to facilitate reattachment at the time of closure.

Lower incisions that do not overlie the rib cage are carried through the layers of the abdominal wall down to the transversalis fascia. The latter is retracted anteriorly, and through it the surgeon can visualize the kidney and ureter. The spleen is located above the kidney and may be seen or palpated. Blunt dissection is used to define the space behind the transversalis fascia, and is carried down (posteriorly) to the psoas muscle (see Fig. 143-7). A table-mounted self-retaining retractor, preferably with radiolucent blades, can then be used to displace the psoas muscle posteriorly, and the diaphragm or lung and ribs superiorly, and the kidney and abdominal contents anteriorly. The most appropriate position for the retractor post is anteriorly just below the patient's right arm. Using electrocautery, the psoas muscle is incised at its attachment to the vertebral bodies and further retracted posteriorly, exposing the pedicles and neural foramina of the fractured and adjacent vertebrae. The psoas muscle is a variable in exposure, and can prove a major hindrance if large. Intraoperative fluoroscopy is a must during these procedures for level identification as well as applying the instrumentation. The segmental artery at the fracture level is ligated and the corpectomy undertaken. To avoid spinal cord ischemia or infarction, ligation of these intercostal vessels should be undertaken sparingly and only when absolutely necessary. The discs adjacent to the fractured body are excised, preserving the integrity of the end plates that will appose the graft. Corpectomy of the fractured vertebra is accomplished with rongeurs and not an air drill, and the bone morsels saved for the fusion. The corpectomy and decompression are easily accomplished with fresh fractures but may be quite tedious with older fractures necessitating careful use of osteotomes, or, if necessary, power drills. Overzealous use of sharp or power tools can lead to dural lacerations, and thus caution is warranted. The ipsilateral pedicle of the involved vertebra is also removed and the canal visualized from the side. The decompression is accomplished to the contralateral pedicle and between the end plates of the adjacent vertebrae.

The dura can be felt with a Penfield dissector and inspected with a small laryngeal mirror. Bleeding from decompressed and torn epidural veins can be excessive and is best controlled with beef collagen or thrombin-soaked Gelfoam. Small dural tears can be difficult to suture, especially when the dura is attenuated. Thus closure is accomplished with commercially available fibrin glue and Gelfoam. The corpectomy does not have to include the anterior longitudinal ligament but must be large enough to accommodate the largest feasible iliac crest autograft, femoral allograft, or prosthesis. The adjacent end plates are kept intact to provide rigid apposition to the graft. Most suitable anterior constructs consist of titanium dual 5.5-mm rods, and bicortical bone screws 6 or 7 mm in diameter driven through plates that come in small, medium, or large sizes (DePuy Spine, Raynham, MA, and Medtronic Sofamor Danek, Memphis, TN).[40] Application of the plates in the lower thoracic spine may necessitate excision of the head of the rib with a bone rongeur through the open wound. The largest plate or staple is used provided the prongs on it are all embedded in the lateral aspect of the rostral and caudal bodies. The entry point for the screws is usually 5 to 10 mm from the floor of the canal and the adjacent end plate, with a trajectory 10 degrees

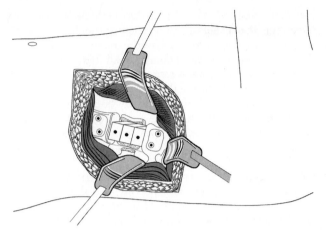

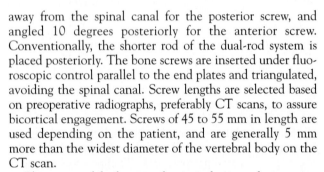

FIGURE 143-8 Plates and bicortical screws are inserted into the bodies rostrally and caudally. After distraction is applied to the anterior screws, the carbon fiber hollow prosthesis packed with the patient's own vertebral and rib graft is pressed into place.

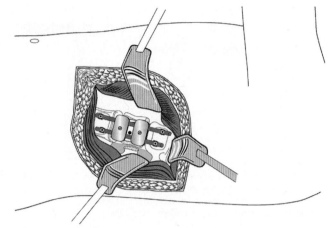

FIGURE 143-9 The spinal construct complete with the vertebral body prosthesis, and dual-rod and screw fixation applied in compression. Two transverse connectors bridge the rods.

away from the spinal canal for the posterior screw, and angled 10 degrees posteriorly for the anterior screw. Conventionally, the shorter rod of the dual-rod system is placed posteriorly. The bone screws are inserted under fluoroscopic control parallel to the end plates and triangulated, avoiding the spinal canal. Screw lengths are selected based on preoperative radiographs, preferably CT scans, to assure bicortical engagement. Screws of 45 to 55 mm in length are used depending on the patient, and are generally 5 mm more than the widest diameter of the vertebral body on the CT scan.

Placement of the bone graft or prosthesis, and correction of angular deformity is achieved by applying distraction between the anterior screws. Since the anterior screws are farther away from the end plates, distraction can be applied to these screws while allowing room for the insertion of the graft or prosthesis. Correction of angular deformity can be further augmented by gentle manual pressure on the spine. The prosthesis can be a titanium mesh cage[41] or stackable carbon fiber cages, packed with the patient's own bone from the corpectomy or rib, augmented if necessary with allograft (Fig. 143-8). The length of the prosthesis or graft selected is obtained using a compass or micrometer to measure the distance between the distracted end plates. The largest dimension of the prosthesis is selected to share the anterior load and avoid telescoping into the adjacent bodies. Impaction of the prosthesis into the corpectomy defect is facilitated by using fluted blades or sleds. Graft insertion is monitored with fluoroscopy to assure it is flush or countersunk in the corpectomy defect so as not to obstruct the placement of the dual rods and cross connectors. At this point it is important to rotate the image intensifier to examine the position of the graft in the lateral projection. Before fixation of the construct, one must make certain that the prosthesis is not infringing on the canal. The rods are then placed within the bone screws, and the set screws are maximally tightened at one end. One or two crosslinks between the rods are then applied and fixed. Using the crosslink for counterpressure, the screws at the other end are compressed and those set screws are then tightened (Fig. 143-9). Additional autologous graft is placed in and around the implant and the construct covered with Gelfoam. The wound is closed

in layers with vacuum drainage of the wound, or chest tube if the chest has been entered. Postoperative pain requirements are significantly reduced by the infiltration of the wound with 0.25% Marcaine (bupivacaine).

Due to the small size of S1 and the obstruction by the iliac crest, it is impossible to place a lateral implant spanning L4 to S1. Thus L4 and L5 burst fractures are often treated nonsurgically[22] or through a posterior approach. If anterior decompression involves two levels of the thoracolumbar spine, or in cases of additional posterior column involvement with dislocation, supplementary posterior instrumentation may be necessary. Only 2 of our 53 patients have needed both anterior and posterior instrumentation, and in each case the posterior approach had not been anticipated and was performed in a separate setting. Anterior and posterior instrumentation can be staged or, more conveniently, performed during the same session if assured of its necessity.

Mobilization in a thoracolumbar orthosis is started on the first postoperative day, or after removal of the chest tube with sequential radiographs at 45 degrees in the patient's room and at 90 degrees in the radiology department. Incentive spirometry, as well as physical and occupational therapy commence as soon as the patient is able. The vacuum drain is generally removed on day 2 or 3 or when the output is less than 100 mL per shift. Patient-controlled analgesia is usually turned off after the third day, unless the patient had been on large doses of narcotics preoperatively. The brace is worn for 3 to 5 months. Radiographs and clinic visits are scheduled at 6 weeks and 3, 6, and 12 months postoperatively (Fig. 143-10).

DISCUSSION

Our results and those of others show that several parameters must be examined before resorting to selection of treatment options. This selection should be not random but based on clinical as well as radiologic criteria including neurologic deficit, angulation, residual canal, and possibly vertebral body height.[5,6,42,43] Surgery was undertaken in the presence of neurologic deficits either total or partial, and persistent pain. The intent of surgery was to provide neural decompression, fracture reduction, and stabilization. In flexion compression

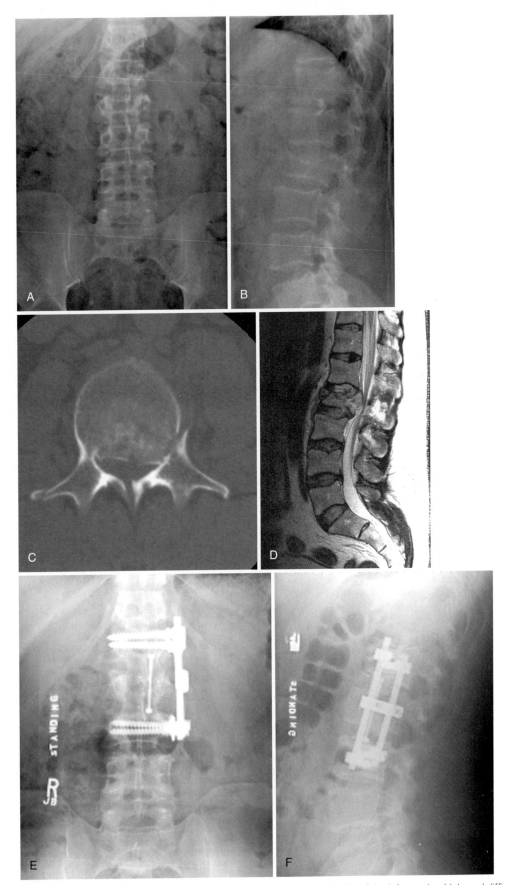

FIGURE 143-10 A 45-year-old man fell off a horse, incurring severe back pain, dysesthesias of the left anterior thigh, and difficulty in urination. On examination he had no leg or sphincter weakness. Plain AP (*A*) and lateral (*B*) radiographs showed a fracture of L2, with loss in height and increased angulation. CT scan shows the burst fracture of L2 (*C*), with retropulsion of bone and a residual AP diameter of the canal of 50%. Sagittal MRI scan shows the fracture of L2, loss in height, angulation, and canal compromise (*D*). Six weeks postoperatively, AP (*E*) and lateral (*F*) radiographs show the dual-rod and screw instrumentation with a stackable carbon fiber vertebral prosthesis packed with the patient's own bone. Other than mild pain, the patient is neurologically intact.

fractures where the anterior column alone is affected with loss of height but no compromise of the canal,[1,2] surgery is generally not needed. Also, patients with burst fractures who are intact with angular deformity less than 20 degrees and a residual spinal canal greater than 50% of normal, nonoperative treatment is sufficient.[5,6,15,20,23,27] It is important to note that surgical intervention is associated with operative risk, high cost, and the possibility of hardware removal at a future time. It was only the occasional patient with total paralysis who showed neurologic improvement with any treatment in any of the aforementioned reports. Nevertheless, neurologic recovery has been described with decompression, even though delayed in incomplete lesions.[32,35,44,45] Such reports and others would favor surgical intervention in patients with neurologic deficit, intractable pain, or instability.

Anterior devices for the treatment of compressive lesions of the spine have been shown to be safe, providing for decompression of neural elements, correction of angular deformity, and stabilization.[35,37–39] The anterior approach is better suited than a posterior route in the removal of retropulsed bone, and reestablishing a solid anterior column without sacrificing the integrity of the posterior column. In addition, the anterior approach to vertebral body fractures generally requires fixation of only one level rostral and caudal to the fractured body. To optimize fusion, bone grafts are better maintained under compression, and this is provided through an anterior, but not posterior approach. Posterior approaches for burst fractures not only sacrifice the facets on at least one side for decompression, but generally entail fixation to at least two levels rostral and caudal to the site of pathology. Also, the complication rate of posterior instrumentation has not been negligible. In one series of 70 patients with thoracic and lumbar fractures,[46] 25% of screws adjacent to the fracture bent or broke, 4 patients had their hardware removed for pain or prominence, in 2 patients hardware was removed for infection, and 3 underwent revision surgery. Nevertheless, in small series,[47] posterior instrumentation in thoracolumbar burst fractures have been shown to be safe, simple, and cost effective.

To identify the advantages of one approach over the other, the following retrospective study was conducted. A total of 112 burst fractures of the thoracolumbar spine from T11 to L5 have been managed operatively. Fifty-three patients (38 males and 15 females) underwent anterolateral corpectomy, followed by grafting and instrumentation with dual rods and screws in 34, and by plates and screws in 19. In 59 patients (44 males and 15 females) decompression was achieved through a posterior approach by either transpedicular or costotransversectomy routes followed by instrumentation and posterolateral fusion. A variety of posterior devices were used, including pedicle screws, hooks, and sublaminar wires. Patients were followed for an average of 142.2 weeks (range, 0–752 weeks).

For ease of statistical analysis, the Frankel score was converted to a numerical scale, with A equivalent to 1 with complete neurologic deficit below the level of the lesion, and E equivalent to 5 with normal motor and sensory function. Mean preoperative Frankel scores in the anterior and posterior groups were (mean ± SD) 3.9 ± 1.0 and 3.5 ± 1.4, respectively. Preoperative angular deformity in the anterior and posterior groups measured 8.8 ± 11.9 degrees and

5.8 ± 12.4 degrees, respectively (see Fig. 143-1). On preoperative CT scan the residual canal at the fracture site averaged $43.3\% \pm 17.1\%$ in the anterior group and $41.2\% \pm 21.5\%$ in the posterior group. Follow-up Frankel scores had improved to 4.3 ± 0.8 and 3.9 ± 1.4, for a mean change of 0.4 in both anterior and posterior groups. At latest follow-up angular deformity corrected to 2.5 ± 9.2 degrees in the anterior group but progressed to 10.9 ± 13 degrees in the posterior group, with a significant difference between the two ($p < 0.01$, two-tailed Student's t-test). Neurologic improvement seems to occur in thoracolumbar fractures irrespective of approach. Randomized and evidence-based guidelines for the treatment of these fractures are lacking.[48] Angular deformity is more successfully corrected and maintained with the anterior approach. In burst fractures where neurologic deficit, and angular deformity occur, the anterior approach with anterior column reconstruction seems to have the advantage.[49–53]

Not only does an implant correct and maintain proper alignment, but its stiffness enhances fusion. Fusion rates in the spine have been shown to be enhanced with instrumentation whether anterior or posterior.[54–59] Thus the more rigid implant is less likely to fail and is able to maintain correction and enhance fusion rates. In vitro biomechanical testing in cadaveric spines[40] showed that the stiffness of the construct (spine + implant) was attributable to many variables, including the constraint of the screws to the plate or rods, the bicortical engagement of the screws, and the ability of these devices to compress the graft between the vertebral end plates. Devices that consist of dual-rod and bicortical screw fixation generally provide the same attributes, with the greatest ease of application.

Acknowledgments

This research was funded by the Injury Prevention Research Center Pilot Project (IPRCPP) Research Fund at The University of Iowa.

REFERENCES

1. Denis F: The three column spine and its significance in the classification of acute thoracolumbar spinal injuries. Spine 8:817–831, 1983.
2. Gertzbein SD: Spine update: Classification of thoracic and lumbar fractures. Spine 19:626–628, 1994.
3. McCormack T, Karaikovic E, Gaines RW: The load sharing classification of spine fractures. Spine 19:1741–1744, 1994.
4. Hitchon PW, Torner JC: Recumbency in thoracolumbar fractures. Neurosurg Clin N Am 8:509–517, 1997.
5. Hitchon PW, Torner JC, Haddad SF, Follett KA: Thoracic and lumbar fractures: Management analysis. In Hitchon PW, Traynelis VC, Rengachery S (eds): Techniques in Spinal Fusion and Stabilization. New York, Stuttgart: Thieme Medical Publishers, 1995, pp 338–344.
6. Hitchon PW, Torner JC, Haddad SF, Follett KA: Management options in thoracolumbar burst fractures. Surg Neurol 49:619–627, 1998.
7. Guttmann L: Surgical aspects of the treatment of traumatic paraplegia. J Bone Joint Surg Br 31:399–403, 1949.
8. Frankel HL, Hancock DO, Hyslop G, et al: The value of postural reduction in the initial management of closed injuries of the spine with paraplegia and tetraplegia. Part I. Paraplegia. 7:179–192, 1969.
9. Nicoll EA: Fractures of the dorso-lumbar spine. J Bone Joint Surg Br 31:376–394, 1949.
10. Bedbrook GM: Spinal injuries with tetraplegia and paraplegia. J Bone Joint Surg Br 61:267–284, 1979.
11. Bedbrook GM: Treatment of thoracolumbar dislocation and fractures with paraplegia. Clin Orthop Relat Res 112:27–43, 1975.
12. Davies WE, Morris JH, Hill V: An analysis of conservative (non-surgical) management of thoracolumbar fractures and fracture-dislocations with neural damage. J Bone Joint Surg Am 62:1324–1328, 1980.

13. Cantor JB, Lebwohl NH, Garvey T, Eismont FJ: Nonoperative management of stable thoracolumbar burst fractures with early ambulation and bracing. Spine 18:971–976, 1993.
14. Chakera TMH, Bedbrook G, Bradley CM: Spontaneous resolution of spinal canal deformity after burst-dispersion fracture. AJNR Am J Neuroradiol 9:779–785, 1988.
15. Domenicucci M, Preite R, Ramieri A, et al: Thoracolumbar fractures without neurosurgical involvement: Surgical or conservative treatment. J Neurosurg Sci 40:1–10, 1996.
16. Johnson R, Herrlin K, Hagglund G, Stromqvist B: Spinal canal remodeling after thoracolumbar fractures with intraspinal bone fragments. Acta Orthop Scand 62:125–127, 1991.
17. Knight RQ, Stornelli DP, Chan DPK, et al: Comparison of operative versus nonoperative treatment of lumbar burst fractures. Clin Orthop Relat Res 293:112–121, 1993
18. Krompinger WJ, Fredrickson BE, Mino DE, Yuan HA: Conservative treatment of fractures of the thoracic and lumbar spine. Orthop Clin North Am 17:161–170, 1986.
19. Mumford J, Weinstein JN, Spratt KF, Goel VK: Thoracolumbar burst fractures. Spine 18:955–970, 1993.
20. Rechtine GR, Cahill D, Chrin AM: Treatment of thoracolumbar trauma: Comparison of complications of operative versus nonoperative treatment. J Spinal Disord 12:406–409, 1999.
21. Reid DC, Hu R, Davis LA, Saboe LA: The nonoperative treatment of burst fractures of the thoracolumbar junction. J Trauma 28:1188–1194, 1988.
22. Seybold EA, Sweeney CA, Fredrickson BE, et al: Functional outcome of low lumbar burst fractures: A multicenter review of ooperative and nonoperative treatment of L3–L5. Spine 24:2154–2161, 1999.
23. Shen WJ, Liu TJ, Shen YS: Nonoperative treatment versus posterior fixation for thoracolumbar junction burst fractures without neurologic deficits. Spine 26:1038–1045, 2001.
24. Tator CH, Duncan EG, Edmonds VE, et al: Comparison of surgical and conservative management in 208 patients with acute spinal cord injury. Can J Neurol Sci 14:60–69, 1987.
25. Weinstein JN, Collalto P, Lehmann TR: Thoracolumbar "burst" fractures treated conservatively: A long-term follow-up. Spine 13:33–38, 1988.
26. Willen J, Anderson J, Toomoka K, Singer K: The natural history of burst fractures at the thoracolumbar junction. J Spinal Disord 3:39–46, 1990.
27. Wood K, Butterman G, Mehbod A, et al: Operative compared to nonoperative treatment of a thoracolumbar burst fracture without neurological deficit: A prospective, randomized study. J Bone Joint Surg Am 85:773–781, 2003.
28. Bracken MB, Shepard MJ, Collins WF, et al: Methylprednisolone or naloxone treatment after acute spinal cord injury: 1 year follow-up data. J Neurosurg 76:23–31, 1992.
29. Bracken MB, Shepard MJ, Holford, TR, et al: Administration of methylprednisolone for 24 or 48 hours or tirilazad mesylate for 48 hours in the treatment of acute spinal cord injury. JAMA 277:1597–1604, 1997.
30. McLain RF, Benson DR: Urgent surgical stabilization of spinal fractures in polytrauma patients. Spine 24:1646–1654, 1999.
31. Larson SJ, Holst RA, Hemmy DC, Sances A: Lateral extracavitary approach to traumatic lesions of the thoracic and lumbar spine. J Neurosurg 45:628–637, 1976.
32. Maiman DJ, Larson SJ, Benzel EC: Neurological improvement associated with late decompression of the thoracolumbar spinal cord. Neurosurgery 14:302–307, 1984.
33. Hitchon PW, Brenton MD, Black AG, et al: In vitro biomechanical comparison of pedicle screws, sublaminar hooks, and sublaminar cables. J Neurosurg Spine 99:104–109, 2003.
34. Hitchon PW, Follett KA: Transpedicular screw fixation of the thoracic and lumbar spine. In Hitchon PW, Traynelis VC, Rengachery S (eds): Techniques in Spinal Fusion and Stabilization. New York, Stuttgart: Thieme Medical Publishers, 1995, pp 240–247.
35. Transfeldt EE, White D, Bradford DS, Roche B: Delayed anterior decompression in patients with spinal cord and cauda equina injuries of the thoracolumbar spine. Spine 15:953–957, 1990.
36. Cohen M, McAfee P: Kaneda anterior spinal instrumentation. In Hitchon PW, Traynelis VC, Rengachary S (eds): Techniques in Spinal Fusion and Stabilization. New York, Thieme, 1995, pp 264–278.
37. Kaneda K, Taneichi H, Abumi K, et al: Anterior decompression and stabilization with the Kaneda device for thoracolumbar burst fractures associated with neurological deficits. J Bone Joint Surg Am 79:69–83, 1997.
38. McAfee PC: Complications of anterior approaches to the thoracolumbar spine: Emphasis on Kaneda instrumentation. Clin Orthop Relat Res 306:110–119, 1994.
39. McAfee PC, Bohlman HH, Yuan HA: Anterior decompression of traumatic thoracolumbar fractures with incomplete neurological deficit using a retroperitoneal approach. J Bone Joint Surg Am 67:89–104, 1985.
40. Dvorak MF, Kwon BK, Fisher CG, et al: Effectiveness of titanium mesh cylindrical cages in anterior column reconstruction after thoracic and lumbar vertebral body resection. Spine 28:902–908, 2003.
41. Hitchon PW, Goel VK, Rogge TN, et al: In vitro biomechanical analysis of 3 anterior thoracolumbar implants. J Neurosurg Spine 93:252–258, 2000.
42. Bohlman HH: Current concepts: Review treatment of fractures and dislocations of the thoracic and lumbar spine. J Bone Joint Surg Am 67:165–169, 1985.
43. White AA, Panjabi MM: Clinical Biomechanics of the Spine, 2nd edition. Philadelphia: Lippincott, 1990, Chapter 5, pp 278–378.
44. Benzel EC, Larson SJ: Functional recovery after decompressive operation for thoracic and lumbar spine fractures. Neurosurgery 19:772–778, 1986.
45. Bohlman HH: Late anterior decompression for spinal cord injury: Review of 100 cases with long term results. Orthop Trans 4:42–43, 1980.
46. McLain RF: Functional outcomes after surgery for spinal fractures: Return to work and activity. Spine 29:470–477, 2004.
47. Danisa OA, Shaffrey CI, Jane JA, et al: Surgical approaches for the correction of unstable thoracolumbar burst fractures: A retrospective analysis of treatment outcomes. J Neurosurg 83:977–983, 1995.
48. Verlaan JJ, Diekerhof CH, Buskens E, et al: Surgical treatment of traumatic fractures of the thoracic and lumbar spine: A systematic review of the literature on techniques, complications, and outcome [Review]. Spine 29:803–814, 2004.
49. Esses SI, Botsford DJ, Kostuik JP: Evaluation of surgical treatment for burst fractures. Spine 15:667–673, 1990.
50. Gertzbein ST: Scoliosis Research Society, Multicenter Spine Fracture Study. Spine 17:528–540, 1992.
51. McLain RF, Burkus JK, Benson DR: Segmental instrumentation for thoracic and thoracolumbar fractures: Prospective analysis of construct survival and five-year follow-up. Spine J 1:310–323, 2001.
52. Parker JW, Lane JR, Karaikovic EE, Gaines RW: Successful short segment instrumentation and fusion for thoracolumbar spine fractures, a consecutive 4 1/2 year series. Spine 25:1157–1169, 2000.
53. Schnee CL, Ansell LV: Selection criteria and outcome of operative approaches for thoracolumbar burst fractures with and without neurological deficit. J Neurosurg 86:48–55, 1997.
54. Dickman CA, Yahiro MA, Lu HTC, Melkerson MN: Surgical treatment alternatives for fixation of unstable fractures of the thoracic and lumbar spine. A meta-analysis. Spine 19(20 Suppl):2266S–2273S, 1994.
55. Garfin S: Summation. Spine 19(20 Suppl):2300S–2305S, 1994.
56. Johnston CE, III, Ashman RB, Baird AM, Allard RN: Effect of spinal construct stiffness on early fusion mass incorporation experimental study. Spine 15:908–912, 1990.
57. Steffee AD, Brantigan JW: The variable screw placement spinal fixation system report of a prospective study of 250 patients enrolled in Food and Drug Administration clinical trials. Spine 18:1150–1172, 1993.
58. Yuan HA, Garfin SR, Dickman CA, Mardjetko SM: A historical cohort study of pedicle screw fixation in thoracic, lumbar, and sacral spinal fusions. Spine 19(20 Suppl):2279S–2296S, 1994.
59. Zdeblick TA: A prospective, randomized study of lumbar fusion preliminary results. Spine 18:983–991, 1993.

144 Vertebroplasty and Kyphoplasty

CLIFFORD J. ESKEY

Vertebroplasty and kyphoplasty are minimally invasive, percutaneous procedures in which a fast-setting polymer is injected into a pathologic vertebral body with the goal of relieving pain or disability. These treatments have been applied to painful osteoporotic compression fractures, painful neoplasms, and structurally compromised vertebrae. They represent a young and evolving technology for treating a common and important problem that had resisted medical and open surgical treatments. The remarkable anecdotal success of the procedures has spurred rapidly increasing clinical usage and scientific investigation.

Before the introduction of vertebroplasty and kyphoplasty, treatment of compression fractures consisted of bed rest, pain control (with nonsteroidal antiinflammatory medications, calcitonin, and narcotics), and back bracing.[1] This regimen is often effective, and most people will eventually find relief from their pain as the fracture heals. However, a substantial number will fail to heal within 3 to 6 weeks. These people will often suffer persistent back pain and a risk of gradually worsening kyphotic deformity. Even in those whose compression fractures do heal over time, the recovery period is time consuming, requiring at least several weeks. The experience is often profoundly unpleasant and can be marked by periods of insufficient pain control, delirium, and constipation. Such patients are sometimes bedridden, with the attendant risks of deep venous thrombosis, pulmonary embolism, and pneumonia. The prolonged immobility accelerates bone resorption and predisposes one to additional injury. Finally, the long-term effects of even a healed fracture may be substantial: kyphotic deformity, decreased lung capacity, and altered forces on intervertebral discs and facet joints.

The vertebroplasty procedure was introduced in France in 1984 by a group who used the technique to treat symptomatic vertebral hemangiomas.[2] They found that the "internal casting" provided by polymethylmethacrylate (PMMA) injected into the pathologic vertebral body provided substantial pain relief. This success led to expansion of the procedure to the treatment of pain from myeloma and metastatic neoplasms of the vertebrae[3]; these indications remain the most common ones for the use of vertebroplasty in Europe. In 1993 the technique was introduced in the United States,[4] where its chief use has been to treat the pain from osteoporotic compression fractures. Kyphoplasty was introduced in 1999 as the proprietary technology of Kyphon Inc. Kyphoplasty differs from vertebroplasty by adding the insertion and inflation of a balloon before cement delivery. It has the added goal of restoring vertebral body height and spine alignment.[5] Both procedures are now practiced throughout the world, with the number of procedures and practitioners (including radiologists, orthopedic surgeons, neurosurgeons, and anesthesiologists) growing rapidly.

INDICATIONS

The primary indication for vertebroplasty and kyphoplasty is a painful, unhealed compression fracture. These fractures may be the result of osteoporosis, hematopoietic or lymphoid neoplasm (e.g., leukemia, multiple myeloma), or hematogenous metastasis. People with no fracture but pain resulting from lytic metastatic neoplasm or the rare symptomatic hemangioma are also candidates for vertebroplasty. People with chronically nonhealing traumatic fractures (e.g., osteonecrosis) may be candidates. In all these circumstances, there should be congruent historical, physical, and imaging findings. Vertebroplasty can also be performed prophylactically to stabilize a weakened vertebra before planned surgery.

CONTRAINDICATIONS

There are few absolute contraindications to vertebroplasty and kyphoplasty. These contraindications are: (1) recent systemic or spinal infection, (2) uncorrected bleeding diathesis, (3) insufficient cardiopulmonary health to tolerate sedation or general anesthesia, and (4) fracture-related compromise of the spinal canal sufficient to result in myelopathy or radiculopathy. In addition, these procedures are generally not performed for fractures that are painless or have already healed.

There are also specific fracture features that do not represent absolute contraindications but substantially increase the risk or technical difficulty of the procedure. Disruption of the posterior cortex increases the risk of posterior cement leakage and, therefore, the risk of spinal cord or nerve root compression; this feature is rare in osteoporotic compression fractures but frequent in burst fractures and metastatic neoplasm. Substantial canal narrowing (without clinical evidence of myelopathy or radiculopathy) increases the risk that even a small amount of cement leakage will produce neurologic compromise. Marked loss of vertebral body height makes the procedure more difficult since there may be little space for needle placement. Poor visualization of osseous structures on fluoroscopy increases the risk of improper needle placement and cement leakage but can be overcome with the use of computed tomography (CT). Treatment of patients whose fractures have these features should only be performed by the most experienced practitioners.

PREPROCEDURE EVALUATION

The primary goal of the preprocedure evaluation of patients for vertebroplasty and kyphoplasty is to confirm that the cause of the person's pain is an unhealed vertebral compression. The pain of an acute fracture can be difficult to distinguish from the many other sources of pain in the back. Many people with osteoporotic vertebral compression fractures are elderly, and they often suffer from more than one pathologic process that may produce back pain. Furthermore, vertebroplasty and kyphoplasty are relatively new procedures, and many physicians have little knowledge of these procedures and their indications. Thus the practitioner of these procedures will often be asked to consult on people who ultimately probably will not benefit from either procedure. The excellent outcomes reported to date with these procedures are grounded in the careful selection of appropriate candidates.

History

The classic symptoms from an acute vertebral compression fracture include deep pain with sudden onset, midline location, and exacerbation by motion and standing. These fractures may occur with little or no trauma. The pain often diminishes little in the first week, then fades gradually over the next several weeks to 3 months.[1] Lateral radiation may be present, but persistent radiation of the pain in a radiculopathic pattern is rare. When there is substantial kyphosis, patients may also suffer from difficulty breathing, anterior chest wall pain, and gastrointestinal discomfort.

In addition to evaluating the nature of the pain, the interview should include assessment of the effect of the pain on activities of daily living and sense of well-being. Such measures are at least as important as an index of the pain itself. One can quantify these factors using such questionnaires as the Owestry Disability Questionnaire, Roland-Morris Disability Questionnaire, and Medical Outcomes Study 36-Item Short-Form Health Survey (SF-36). Such indices can be used in conjunction with a visual analogue pain scale to follow the success of treatment.

The physician should inquire about treatment of the underlying disease process. For osteoporotic patients the interview is an opportunity to make sure that appropriate treatment of the osteoporosis is under way. The severity of osteoporosis and the use of antiosteoporosis medications will substantially alter the risk of additional fractures. For patients with neoplasm, timing of the treatment may be affected by ongoing chemotherapy and radiation. Finally, the physician should search for possible contraindications to the procedure such as use of warfarin (see above).

Physical Examination

The practitioner should perform a directed physical examination. This examination includes inspection of the back, palpation for focal areas of tenderness, and correlation of the site of pain with anatomic landmarks. In difficult cases, examination of the sites of pain and tenderness can be performed with fluoroscopic assistance to localize the pain to specific anatomic structures. Although point tenderness at the spinous process is the typical finding in unhealed compression fractures, the absence of typical focal tenderness does not preclude the presence of such a fracture. Imaging is a more reliable test than this portion of the physical examination.[6] Assessment of lower extremity neurologic function is especially important in patients with symptoms suggestive of myelopathy, radiculopathy, or spinal stenosis.

Evaluation of the heart and lungs is necessary for the safe use of sedation for the procedure.

Imaging

Imaging of the spine is undertaken in all cases to confirm the clinical diagnosis and to plan the procedure. Radiographs are the imaging study of choice for the initial imaging evaluation (Fig. 144-1). Anteroposterior (AP) and lateral views should be obtained. This study allows one to confirm the presence of fracture, determine the location of fractures, assess the degree of height loss and kyphosis, and identify anatomic variants. Whenever possible, comparison to prior studies is particularly valuable. A single radiograph almost never allows one to distinguish a new or unhealed fracture from a chronic, healed fracture. With prior radiographs ("old gold") for comparison, new compression fractures can be identified. If serial radiographs taken several weeks apart show a new compression fracture in a patient with classic history and symptoms, no further imaging may be necessary. However, since back pain is a difficult diagnostic problem and since recent prior studies are rarely available, most patients benefit from additional imaging.

Magnetic resonance imaging (MRI) is the test of choice for this additional evaluation. The main goals of this imaging are to: (1) distinguish new or unhealed fractures from healed fractures, (2) evaluate the risk of worsening central canal or neural foramen compromise during the procedure, and (3) identify other causes of pain. For these purposes, the single most useful sequence is a T2-weighted sequence with fat saturation. We prefer using inversion recovery (i.e., a STIR sequence) to achieve the fat suppression, since it is less sensitive to magnetic field inhomogeneity than the frequency-selective fat saturation techniques. On any of these MR sequences, recent or unhealed fractures show hyperintense signal within the bone marrow (Fig. 144-2). This signal

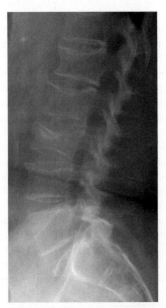

FIGURE 144-1 Lateral radiograph of the lumbar spine. The loss of height and wedge deformity signal compression fractures at L1–L4. It is not possible to determine the age of these fractures from a single radiograph.

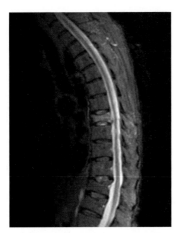

FIGURE 144-2 MR imaging with a sagittal STIR sequence. The hyperintense signal in the T7 vertebral body is consistent with an unhealed compression fracture. While there is also wedge deformity at T11 and T12, the absence of signal abnormality identifies these compression fractures as old and healed.

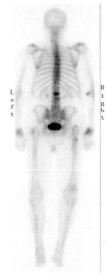

FIGURE 144-3 Bone scan. Areas of increased uptake in the L1 and L2 vertebra represent bone turnover in recent or unhealed fractures.

may be present as amorphous areas filling much of the vertebral body or as discrete curvilinear fracture clefts. In contrast, healed fractures have marrow signal similar to that of unfractured vertebra. These sequences also provide an adequate evaluation of the spinal canal and will show most alternative causes of pain that might mimic fracture. Additional imaging using a sagittal T1-weighted sequence and axial T1- and T2-weighted images does provide additional information but is rarely necessary in the vertebroplasty evaluation. In most patients with a typical clinical history and physical examination for osteoporotic compression fracture, the STIR sequence alone is adequate, and one can reserve the full set of MR sequences for patients whose pain is atypical. Postcontrast imaging is best reserved for cases of suspected neoplasm. In patients who cannot tolerate MRI (e.g., those with a pacemaker), bone scan is the test of choice. Bone scan does not provide any evaluation of the soft tissues or spinal canal, but it does allow the differentiation of healed and recent fractures. The recent fractures will take up the injected ^{99m}Tc-medronate tracer in much higher concentrations (Fig. 144-3). The relative sensitivity and specificity of bone scan and MRI for this purpose have not been established.

CT is not necessary for most osteoporotic compression fractures but is very useful for preprocedure evaluation of burst fractures and metastases. In these circumstances, there may be substantial loss of integrity of the posterior vertebral body cortex (Fig. 144-4). This loss increases the risk of the procedure, specifically the risk of posterior leakage of cement or posterior displacement of bone or tumor.[7] CT provides the best means for assessing this cortex. CT is also the test of choice for postprocedure evaluation of unexpected symptoms (see later section on Risks).

PROCEDURE—VERTEBROPLASTY

Sedation

Analgesia for vertebroplasty and kyphoplasty can be achieved with moderate sedation, but in some cases intubation and general anesthesia are needed. This process begins with the informed consent. Fully informing the patient of what to expect in the operating room or procedure suite facilitates patient comfort, cooperation, and satisfaction. Vertebroplasty has generally been performed with moderate sedation. At our

FIGURE 144-4 Loss of posterior vertebral body integrity. *A,* MRI shows metastasis with pathologic compression fracture at T1. *B,* CT scan demonstrates more clearly the extensive destruction of the posterior cortex.

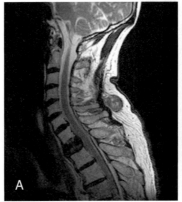
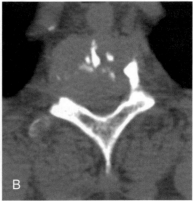

institution and many others, intravenous midazolam and fentanyl are the drugs of choice. Continuous monitoring is performed with electrocardiogram, blood pressure measurements, and pulse oximetry. The drug delivery and monitoring are performed by certified nursing personnel. In patients with substantial preexisting respiratory or cardiac disease, an anesthesiologist is asked to evaluate the patient and determine if monitored anesthesia care is warranted.

Patient Positioning

The ideal patient position for thoracic and lumbar procedures is prone. This position allows one to place the needle from either side and simplifies positioning of the biplane fluoroscopy unit or C arm. Furthermore, this position and proper cushion support maximizes extension of the fractured segments, promoting kyphosis reduction.[8] Although the patient can be rotated slightly, substantial patient angulation can make this a more difficult procedure. A special table and cushions may be used to support the head and body, but good results can also be achieved with a flat fluoroscopy table and careful placement of simple cushions. The patient's arms should be placed sufficiently toward the head to keep them out of the path of the fluoroscope. Patients can usually be placed in the prone position despite their painful compression fracture. If necessary, moderate sedation can be induced before the patient is moved. Care must be taken when transferring these patients, since many of them are of advanced age and have fragile bones.

Antibiotic Prophylaxis and Skin Preparation

Antibiotic prophylaxis can provided for vertebroplasty in one of two forms. Intravenous antibiotics such as 1.0 g cefazolin can be administered during the procedure. Alternatively, the PMMA can be mixed with an antibiotic, such as 1.2 g tobramycin, as the cement is being prepared. There are no hard data to support or oppose these practices, but there are case reports of periprocedure spine infections after these procedures (see later section on Risks). The risk of infection is minimized with the use of standard operating room procedures for sterile preparation of the skin, draping, operator scrub, and sterile gowns, masks, and gloves.

Image Guidance

Imaging guidance is necessary to ensure the success and safety of vertebroplasty. Generally the needle placement and cement placement are performed with fluoroscopy, but, in rare cases, CT may be necessary. Fluoroscopy has inherently lower contrast resolution and makes greater demands on imaging technique, on the operator's knowledge of radiographic anatomy, and on the operator's ability to integrate planar data into a 3-dimensional picture. However, the compelling reasons for using fluoroscopy whenever possible are the lower radiation dose and the ability to monitor the cement distribution continuously as the injection proceeds.

There are no established minimum standards for the fluoroscopic equipment used in vertebroplasty. However, the key to avoiding complications in this procedure is the ability to see the needles, bone landmarks, and opacified cement at all times. Visualization of the opacified cement puts the greatest demand on imaging equipment. At least one C-arm unit is necessary. A dedicated biplane fluoroscopy suite is optimal. The quality of these fluoroscopic systems varies widely, and many of the older C-arm systems used for general orthopedic work put the operator at a disadvantage. The newer image intensifiers and digital fluoroscopy systems available from numerous vendors provide the best image quality and lowest radiation exposure. Shielding to minimize operator exposure to scatter radiation is strongly recommended if one performs this procedure routinely.

Needle Placement

Once the patient is properly positioned in the fluoroscopy unit, the needle trajectory can be planned. Once an approach has been selected (see later), the skin is anesthetized with a small amount of subcutaneous lidocaine or bupivicaine. Following the planned needle trajectory, the periosteum is anesthetized in a similar fashion. The planned trajectory can be assessed and adjusted from flouroscopic views of this smaller needle at the bone surface. A small nick is made in the skin, and an 11- or 13-gauge needle is placed.

There are two principal approaches for needle placement: transpedicular and parapedicular. The transpedicular approach has the advantage of a long intraosseous path protecting the postganglionic nerve roots, and protecting the soft tissues from cement leakage along the tract. However, in pedicles that have a long axis parallel to the sagittal plane, this approach limits one's ability to achieve a final needle tip position near the midline. The parapedicular approach may then be the technique of choice. For either approach, there are two image guidance strategies.

The first strategy uses an ipsilateral oblique view to place the fluoroscopy beam and needle tract perfectly parallel to each other (Fig. 144-5). The image intensifier is first rotated to a true AP position, aligning the spinous process midway between the pedicles. The craniocaudad angulation is changed to bring the pedicles to the midportion of the vertebral body. The image intensifier is then rotated to bring the ipsilateral pedicle so that its medial cortex is at the middle third of the vertebral body. This rotation can only be continued so long as the medial cortex of the pedicle remains clearly visible. The needle will be placed so that it is "end on" to the image intensifier and appears as a small circle. Once the needle has been advanced to the bone surface, small corrections in the craniocaudad angulation can be made using a true lateral view (care is needed to angle this view so that the pedicles project over each other). The needle is then advanced through the pedicle, maintaining the "end-on" appearance of the needle. Once the needle has traversed the pedicle, it is advanced using the lateral view to the junction of the anterior and middle thirds of the vertebral body.

The second strategy replaces the AP ipsilateral oblique view with the straight AP view. This strategy may be preferred if manipulation of the C arm is difficult. Here the craniocaudad angulation is adjusted to bring the vertebral body end plates perpendicular to the image (Fig. 144-6). The skin entry site is placed about 1 cm superior and lateral to the center of the pedicle but must be adjusted for thickness of the posterior paraspinal soft tissues. The needle is advanced

FIGURE 144-5 Needle placement with "end-on" approach. *A,* Initial AP view. *B,* Craniocaudad angulation to place pedicle at the vertical middle of vertebral body. *C,* Ipsilateral oblique view to place pedicle over medial aspect of vertebral body. *D,* Ipsilateral oblique view with needle (*black circle*) in proper alignment. This view is maintained as the needle is advanced through the pedicle. Care is taken to avoid the medial cortex of the pedicle. *E* and *F,* Lateral and AP views with final needle location.

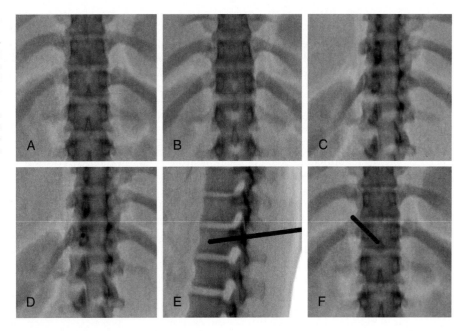

anteriorly, medially, and caudally. By the time it reaches the bone surface, the tip should project over the upper outer cortex of the pedicle. Again, small corrections in the craniocaudad angulation can be made using a true lateral view. The needle is advanced so that its tip projects over the center of the pedicle on both AP and lateral views. The tip should project over the medial pedicle cortex as the needle traverses the posterior third of the vertebral body. The final position is again adjusted on the lateral view.

The image guidance for a parapedicular approach is quite similar. The needle is placed lateral and superior to the lateral cortex of the pedicle and enters the vertebral body at its junction with the pedicle. The position at which bone is encountered (i.e., at the junction of the pedicle and vertebral body) is more anterior on the lateral view.

The advance of the large needles is achieved with either a drilling motion or tapping with a small hammer. The needle position should be checked frequently in the oblique view for two reasons. First, it is important to ensure that the needle does not violate the medial cortex of the pedicle. Second, needle trajectory cannot be markedly altered once the needle has passed even a small distance into the pedicle. Accurate placement is also aided by positioning the needle centrally in the field of view to avoid inaccuracies from parallax.

The planning for the lateral position of the tip should be adjusted depending on the shape of the vertebral body and on whether a unipedicular or bipedicular approach is used. Vertebroplasty for osteoporotic vertebral compression fractures was initially performed using two needles and a bipedicular approach. This technique allows reliable filling of both halves of the vertebral body, independent of the precise lateral position of the needle tip within its half of the vertebral body. More recently, many practitioners have adopted a unipedicular approach. With this technique, a near-midline position of the needle tip provides more reliable filling of the vertebral body. In our experience both techniques work well, and we base our approach on the number of levels to be treated and configuration of the fractured vertebra. For example, in a severely collapsed vertebra, there is often substantially more marrow space at the lateral aspects of the vertebral body. In this circumstance, a bipedicular approach with lateral positioning of the needle tip provides reliable bilateral filling with little risk of symptomatic cement leakage[9] With more lateral tip positions, it is important to remember that the vertebral body is round and that the anterior cortex of the vertebra along the needle trajectory is posterior to the radiopaque line of anterior cortex on the fluoroscopic image.

FIGURE 144-6 Needle placement with AP approach. *A,* AP view with site of skin entry (*black dot*). *B,* Needle appearance as it enters the posterior pedicle surface. *C,* Needle appearance when it has been advanced to the midpoint of pedicle on the lateral view. If the needle tip is more medial at this point, there is risk for traversing the medial pedicle cortex.

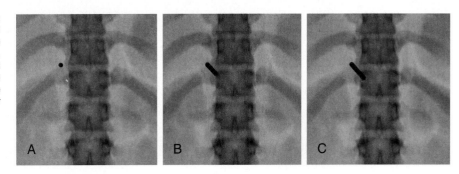

Cement Placement

Both vertebroplasty and kyphoplasty currently employ polymethylmethacrylate (PMMA) cements. These PMMA cements include Codman Cranioplastic (DePuy CMW), Secour (Parallax), Spineplex (Stryker), KyphX (Kyphon), and Osteobond (Zimmer). These cements either contain or must be modified with sterile barium sulfate powder to provide sufficient radioopacity. The barium sulfate is necessary to improve the visibility of the cement on fluoroscopy, making the procedure safer. Further alteration of the cement may be introduced by adjusting proportions of the PMMA powder and liquid monomer. The desired consistency of the cement, when ready for injection, is roughly similar to toothpaste. Working time varies from 10 to 20 minutes. There are a variety of delivery systems available for the cement. These systems vary from a few 1-mL syringes, a spatula, and a mixing bowl, to self-contained, integrated, mixing and delivery devices. The syringe or delivery system is connected to the needle cannula and the cement is slowly injected.

As the cement flows from the needle cannula, careful fluoroscopic monitoring helps ensure that the cement remains within the vertebra. The critical view for this portion of the procedure is the lateral, since posterior leakage should be assiduously avoided. This view also shows venous or intradiscal leakage to good advantage. Some practitioners have advocated the fluoroscopic monitoring of an injection of iodinated contrast before the cement instillation,[4] but this practice is not necessary for the safe placement of cement.[10]

The endpoints for cement injection are: (1) leakage of cement beyond the marrow space, (2) cement reaching the posterior quarter of the vertebral body, and (3) cement filling the vertical expanse of the vertebra and extending across the midline. Injection stops when any of these criteria is met (Fig. 144-7). Since the cement will tend to follow any pathway of least resistance, it is rare to achieve a complete vertebral body cast. It is tempting to inject until a "pretty" fluoroscopic picture is achieved. However, filling until one has achieved a complete cast of the vertebra is not necessary to provide pain relief or stability[11] and, when taken to extremes, will lead to higher rates of cement leakage and clinical complications.[12] Even with these guidelines, however, there is substantial variation in philosophy and practice between practitioners regarding the optimum amount and pattern of cement deposition.[13]

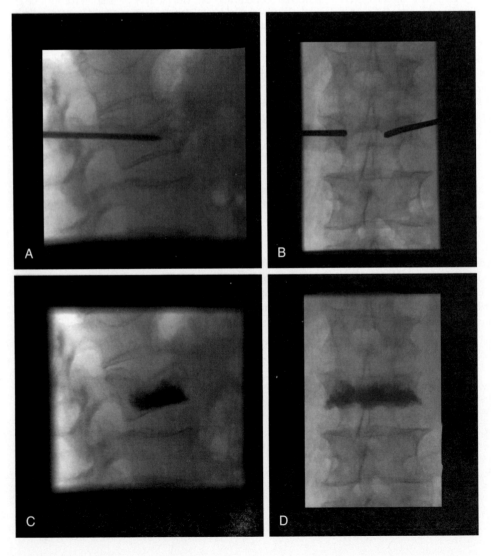

FIGURE 144-7 Vertebroplasty. *A* and *B*, Final needle positions for a bipedicular technique shown on lateral and AP radiographs, respectively. *C* and *D*, Cement filling at end of procedure on lateral and AP radiographs, respectively. Installation was stopped when cement reached the posterior quarter of the vertebral body.

Postprocedure Monitoring

Manual compression is applied to the puncture sites, and sterile bandages are placed. Postprocedure radiographs are obtained. The patient is gently returned to the supine position. The patient is monitored for 2 hours with standard postanesthesia monitoring and neurologic assessment. The patient is then allowed to attempt supervised ambulation. As long as there is no increased pain or disability the patient is allowed to return home with postprocedure instructions that include 3 days of limited activity and monitoring of the puncture sites. If there is no postprocedure improvement in pain or if there are new symptoms, the patient is assessed by a physician and usually undergoes CT of the treated area.

PROCEDURE—KYPHOPLASTY

Much of the kyphoplasty procedure follows steps and guidelines similar to those described for vertebroplasty. The patient preparation, sedation, positioning, and image guidance are largely the same. Kyphoplasty has traditionally been performed with general anesthesia. There is justification for this difference: The procedure time is longer, larger cannulas are used, and there is greater manipulation of osseous structures. However, some institutions have been able to overcome these obstacles for most patients and the procedure is performed with moderate to deep sedation with success.[5,14]

The key differences between kyphoplasty and vertebroplasty are the cannula introducer system, the balloon tamp and pressurization system, and the details of cement delivery. These features add to the time and complexity of the procedure but increase the likelihood of height restoration and kyphosis reduction.

The initial needle placement is similar to that of vertebroplasty, but the needle is only advanced to the posterior aspect of the vertebral body. The needle is exchanged for a cannula and introducer system over a guide pin. The introducer fits within and protrudes beyond the cannula; it has a beveled tip that allows the system to be advanced into the vertebral body when it is tapped with a small hammer. The system is advanced to the posterior aspect of the vertebral body. The introducer is then exchanged for a hand-operated drill bit. This drill is carefully advanced to the anterior aspect of the vertebral body, 3 to 4 mm posterior to the anterior cortical margin (Fig. 144-8). In general, a near-midline position of the needle tip on the AP view is desired. The drill or introducer is removed, and the space thus created is smoothed with gentle tamping. The deflated balloon is advanced into this small cavity so that the posterior balloon marker is sufficiently anterior to the cannula tip. A second system is then placed from the other side in a similar manner. Once both balloons are in place, each balloon tamp, attached to a locking syringe with digital manometer, is slowly inflated with iodinated contrast.

FIGURE 144-8 Kyphoplasty. *A,* Lateral view with cannula at the posterior aspect of the vertebral body and drill advanced to the anterior aspect of the vertebral body. *B,* Balloons in place before inflation. *C,* Balloons inflated. *D,* Final view after cement deposition.

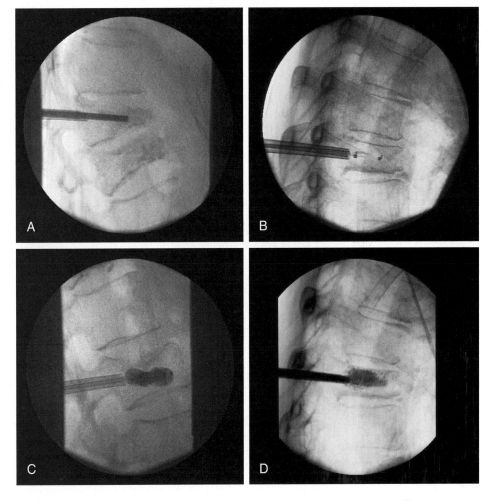

The inflation is performed synchronously and is monitored with both the pressure transducer and intermittent fluoroscopy. Inflation continues slowly until (1) the kyphotic deformity is corrected, (2) the balloon tamp reaches one of the cortical margins, or (3) the system reaches maximum pressure of 300 psi or maximum balloon volume. The balloon is then deflated. Cement is prepared and placed into tubular bone fillers. Sufficient time is allowed for the cement to reach a doughy consistency, with loss of the "sheen" of the initially mixed cement. The cement used in kyphoplasty generally has a greater viscosity than that which many practitioners use for vertebroplasty. The loaded bone filler is placed through the cannula into the cavity, and cement is slowly hand-injected under fluoroscopic guidance. The cement fills the cavity, matching or slightly exceeding the volume of the inflated balloon tamp.

Kyphoplasty has traditionally been performed with bilateral needle and balloon placements, but unilateral balloon placement has also been used with success.[5] For either approach, the needle placement is slightly more demanding than that for vertebroplasty, since the introducer system is larger, and the cement placement depends more directly on the needle position.

The equipment for kyphoplasty continues to evolve. There are several balloon sizes and configurations that improve the ability of the system to achieve vertical expansion of the vertebral body before inflation must end. There is now a curet available that allows the operator to focally disrupt the integrity of the osseous matrix before full balloon inflation, improving chances for height gain and kyphosis reduction. A simplified version of the needle-introducer-cannula system is now available that may reduce the time of the procedure.

RISKS

Vertebroplasty and kyphoplasty are minimally invasive procedures with only small risk of morbidity and mortality. However, careful attention to technique and first-rate imaging equipment are necessary, since one is working near the spinal cord and aorta with large needles and a fluid material. With such care the overwhelming majority of complications should be minor.

The single most common complication reported for vertebroplasty and kyphoplasty is rib fracture. In the largest case series the reported incidence is 3%.[15,16] These fractures presumably result from even minor trauma to the osteoporotic skeleton during transfer of the patient or needle placement. Since such fractures can occur in these patients with even normal movement, they may be difficult to prevent entirely.

Leakage of cement beyond the confines of the vertebra is a complication unique to these procedures. The cement is injected, and, therefore, filling of the vertebra is dependent on a pressure gradient between the needle tip and the cement's destination. The cement will flow along pathways of least resistance. These pathways include fracture clefts and venous channels. Even with careful fluoroscopic monitoring, small amounts of cement leakage are very common, occurring in more than two thirds of treated vertebrae.[15] The incidence of such leakage varies substantially in reported series and is probably a function of such factors as operator experience and approach to cement

filling (see earlier section on Cement Placement). In most circumstances, a small amount of extraosseous cement produces no symptoms or long-term morbidity. These leaks include those that occur along the anterior and lateral surfaces of the vertebral body and those into the intervertebral disc. However, even small amounts of cement adjacent to a nerve root can produce radicular pain. Early small case series describe rare cases of such symptomatic leaks. One study that is a significant outlier contains many cases of epidural leakage with a high symptomatic complication rate and relatively poor efficacy[12]; the approach to cement injection used in this study is more aggressive than those used elsewhere, highlighting the dangers of such an approach. The large case series published by experienced operators report a risk of symptomatic cement leakage about the vertebral body that varies from 0% to 1% for the treatment of osteoporotic fractures[10,15,16] and is up to 4% to 8% for the treatment of metastases.[7,17] For kyphoplasty, the overall risk of leakage is less. Kyphoplasty permits greater control of cement instillation through the creation of a cavity into which a predetermined volume of cement is placed and the use of more viscous cement. The per-patient rates of leakage reported in the small series published to date are 0% to 20%.[14,18–21] Symptomatic leakage about the vertebral body has occurred but seems to be quite rare.[22]

When radiculopathy is produced by cement leakage, the pain usually can be treated with a short course of intravenous or oral steroids or nerve root block. In some cases, there is sufficient foraminal cement to cause frank root compression; in these cases surgical decompression may be the treatment of choice.[17] In rare cases, sufficient cement has been placed in the spinal canal to cause cord compression or cauda equina syndrome; surgical decompression is then warranted.[23]

If cement passes into perivertebral veins, it can be carried to the lungs and produce symptomatic pulmonary embolism. The reported incidence of this phenomenon is quite low, and it has occurred during both vertebroplasty and kyphoplasty. Although the morbidity is usually mild,[15,24] substantial cement embolization has occurred necessitating endovascular or surgical intervention. Since even these cases of large embolism were unrecognized during cement placement, they highlight the need for good cement opacification, high-quality equipment, and vigilant fluoroscopic monitoring.

Other rare complications reported in the larger case series for these procedures include transient fever, transient hypotension, unexplained pain exacerbation, hematoma, pedicle fracture, noninfectious discitis, and spinal infection. Death has occurred in a few patients in the periprocedure period, generally from cardiovascular complications of uncertain etiology.[25]

BENEFITS

Pain Relief and Activity

The first goal of vertebroplasty and kyphoplasty is pain relief. This pain relief is often immediate (as soon as the patient has reached the recovery room) and complete. Most practitioners have had bedridden patients in severe pain leave the same day smiling and pain free. Most patients are able to stop or reduce their use of analgesic medications and resume activities of daily living. This anecdotal evidence was borne out in small case series that testified to the marked pain relief and improved function in about 90% of patients.[26]

The more rigorous data on the efficacy of these procedures chiefly consist of large case series. For vertebroplasty, large case series published in peer-reviewed journals have examined the results in hundreds of patients with osteoporosis. Evans and co-workers[16] reported results in 245 patients retrospectively interviewed for pain, ambulation, and activities of daily living at a mean of 7.2 months after the procedure. Mean pain score (1 = none, 10 = most severe) decreased from 8.9 ± 1.7 to 3.4 ± 2.7. A pain level of only 1 or 2 was reported by 49% of patients. Ambulation and activities of daily living were markedly improved and analgesic use decreased. Hodler and colleagues[15] studied 152 patients, assessing pain with the visual analogue scale immediately after the procedure and in a cross-sectional study at a mean of 8.8 months after the procedure. Immediately after vertebroplasty, pain was absent in 58% of patients and improved in another 28%. At later follow-up, the postprocedure pain level was stable in 67%, worsened in 22%, and improved in 8%. One prospective but nonrandomized study has compared vertebroplasty with medical management.[27] Patients with acute pain ascribed to compression fracture were given the choice of immediate treatment with vertebroplasty. Patients choosing vertebroplasty had substantially better pain control and physical function at 24 hours than those choosing narcotic analgesia and prolonged bed rest. Average length of hospital stay was reduced from 15 to 9 days. Consistent with the known natural history of patients with compression fractures (i.e., those not subjected to a trial of conservative management), follow-up at 6 weeks and at 6 to 12 months showed only minor average benefit. Longer term studies have been performed but include only small numbers of patients; the pain relief afforded by vertebroplasty seems largely stable at 4 to 5 years.[28,29] The pain resulting from neoplasm and hemangioma frequently responds to vertebroplasty. Studies dedicated to such patients show improvement rates similar to or slightly lower than those for osteoporotic fractures.[3]

Kyphoplasty has shown similar ability to reduce pain in the published case series. Coumans and co-workers[18,21] reported results from 78 patients with compression fractures from osteoporosis and multiple myeloma. There was marked improvement in many of the SF-36 indices and the Owestry disability index. The average score on a visual analogue pain scale decreased from 7.0 to 3.2 and was stable at 12 to 14 months. Dudeney and colleagues[19] reported similar results in 18 patients with multiple myeloma. Ledlie and Renfro[20] studied results from 96 patients using visual analogue scale and ambulation indices. Pain decreased from 8.6 to 2.7 at 1 week and 1.4 at 1 year; ambulation was markedly improved. Phillips and co-workers[30] reported results from 36 patients with osteoporotic compression fractures. There was a decrease in average visual analogue pain score from 8.6 to 2.6 at 1 week, with a further decrease to 0.6 at 1 year. Sixty-two percent of patients reported a return to prefracture function.

Fracture Stabilization

Stabilization of the vertebral body is usually a secondary goal of vertebroplasty and kyphoplasty. Many vertebrae that have compression fractures will continue to lose height over time as they undergo additional fractures. Vertebroplasty and kyphoplasty prevent this additional pain and additional deformity in almost all cases. Case series with long-term follow-up have generally not reported any recurrent fractures at treated levels.[17,28] However, a small incidence of repeat fracture in treated vertebrae has been reported in the setting of osteoporosis.[31] In patients with metastatic neoplasm, vertebroplasty has been performed for stabilization of pathologic but unfractured vertebrae. In this setting, no fracture has been reported in short-term follow-up.[3]

Height Restoration and Kyphosis Correction

Kyphoplasty has the added goal of restoring or improving vertebral body height and mechanical alignment at the fracture. The height loss and kyphosis associated with compression fractures can lead to decreased pulmonary capacity and quality of life. Furthermore, it has been proposed that the kyphotic deformity alone may predispose patients to chronic pain and the risk of additional injury. There are clearly cases in which marked height restoration and kyphosis reduction can be achieved with kyphoplasty (Fig. 144-9). There is anecdotal evidence of patients for whom kyphoplasty provides substantial relief of not only pain but also breathing difficulty and deformity.

Several case series have quantified the apparent height gain achieved with kyphoplasty. Lieberman and colleagues[21] were able to reduce fractures of varying age by 36% on average. While many fractures proved irreducible, 16% of the treated vertebrae had greater than 70% height restoration. Ledlie and Renfro,[20] treating patients with more recent fractures, produced on average a 68% restoration of anterior vertebral body height that was stable at 1 year. In patients with myeloma, Dudeney and co-workers[19] produced complete height restoration in 10% of treated levels, no change in 31% of treated vertebrae, and an average of 56% restoration in the remaining treated levels. Some apparent height restoration has been seen in vertebroplasty as well,[8] but there are only rare cases in which more than 50% of the height loss was restored.

The data available for this height restoration must be approached with some caution. The measurements of height restoration for both kyphoplasty and vertebroplasty have been based on questionable methods. First, none of the studies seem to have employed skilled, unbiased, and blinded readers in the evaluation of the radiographs. Second, investigators have attempted to measure height gain in the treated vertebrae themselves, using only lateral radiographs or using different imaging modalities before and after the procedure. The complex shape of fractured vertebrae can lead to measurement error when less compressed aspects of the vertebrae (usually the lateral margins) become more conspicuous as they fill with cement. It is possible to have substantial apparent gains in height without any true change. Given the distribution of cement, this problem is more likely to arise in the evaluation of vertebroplasty. A more appropriate measure would be the distance between the inferior end plate of the vertebra above and superior end plate of the vertebra below the fracture.

The restoration of alignment following kyphoplasty has been studied in only a few reports. Phillips and colleagues[30]

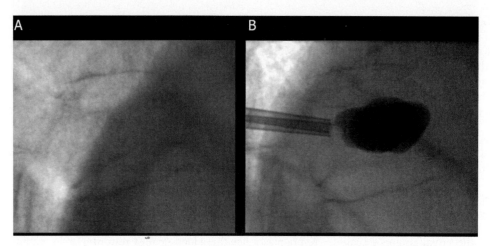

FIGURE 144-9 Restoration of vertebral body height and reduction of kyphosis after kyphoplasty. *A,* Preprocedure. *B,* Balloon inflation.

found 58% of fractures treated with kyphoplasty to be partially reducible; in the reducible fractures, mean Cobb angle correction was 14 degrees. The mean for all levels was 9 degrees. Theodorou and co-workers[14] reported substantially improved kyphosis with a mean angle correction for all fractures of about 10 degrees, representing a 62% reduction of the deformity. Mild kyphosis correction has also been seen with vertebroplasty, with a mean angle correction of 4 degrees, representing a 17% reduction of deformity.[8]

FUTURE DIRECTIONS

Cement Choices and Fracture Risk

Vertebroplasty and kyphoplasty both employ similar polymethylmethacrylate cements. There are several PMMA formulations available, and they have different setting and mechanical properties.[32] These cements are formulated to have sufficiently low viscosity and long working time to allow for percutaneous injection through large needles. The cured cement reliably increases the strength and stability of the vertebra. Thus far, the cements appear to have no adverse effects when placed into the vertebral body. However, there are concerns with the durability and long-term effects of these cements.

It has been proposed that the presence of the intravertebral PMMA creates stresses that can lead to fractures in adjacent vertebrae. The substantiation for this comes from retrospective analyses showing a substantially greater risk of fracture at levels adjacent to treated vertebra.[29,33] In the larger of these two studies, two thirds of the new fractures occurred in vertebrae adjacent to treated levels. However, regional variation in stresses and in bone integrity at baseline could explain the results obtained in the published studies. It is clear that fractures are much more common in the lower thoracic and upper lumbar spine. Even without cement augmentation, a new fracture is more likely to occur near a previously fractured vertebra. Convincing assessment of any risk induced by cement augmentation awaits a prospective trial with an untreated control group.

Newer bioactive cement materials may replace PMMA. The materials developed and tested to date consist of various formulations of either bisphenol-α-glycidol resin mixed with ceramic filler or calcium phosphates.[34] The advantage of these materials is that they more closely match the physical properties of native bone and will remodel over time. However, the physical properties of these cements (e.g., viscosity, compressive strength, heat release) are different from the PMMA cements, and it is not clear if they will provide the same pain relief and long-term stabilization seen with PMMA. Nevertheless, early clinical results in vertebroplasty are promising.[35]

Surgery versus Medical Management

Although both practitioners and patients have provided strong anecdotal support for the efficacy of vertebroplasty and kyphoplasty, these procedures have yet to undergo the rigors of a randomized controlled trial. A recent study in which patients receiving "sham" treatment for osteoarthritis of the knee had better outcomes than a widely practiced arthroscopic procedure highlights the need for such trials. Since a placebo effect can be strong when pain and disability are the outcome variables, there is a need for such a trial that includes a "best medical management" group. Such trials are difficult and expensive, but one such trial, including a "sham" treatment group, is currently under way for vertebroplasty.

Even the role of a short period of medical management is controversial. Although many practitioners follow the initially published guideline of a 3- to 6-week trial of conservative management (so long as patients tolerate the narcotics, immobility, and braces), some advocate immediate treatment. This approach seeks to minimize the period of pain and disability, minimize the risks of relative immobility, and prevent further vertebral collapse. However, since many fractures heal with conservative management alone, further study is needed to justify routine use of such early treatment.

Vertebroplasty versus Kyphoplasty

One of the chief controversies in the treatment of compression fractures revolves about the relative merits of vertebroplasty and kyphoplasty. The competition between these alternatives has been fostered by the procedures' academic and corporate proponents, with most practitioners exclusively performing only one of the alternatives. The partisan nature of the debate is evident in the many review articles that discuss both procedures. Despite the strong feelings on both sides and plenty of anecdotal evidence, there is no truly evidence-based means of selecting one procedure over the other.

Vertebroplasty has the advantages of simplicity and lower cost. The procedure requires about half the time of kyphoplasty.[5] The materials are less expensive by a factor of 5 to 10. Both procedures can be performed with moderate sedation, but the procedure time, larger cannulas, and balloon inflation of kyphoplasty make greater demands on the analgesia; many kyphoplasty practitioners perform the procedure with general anesthesia. Vertebroplasty is also backed by more years of published experience.

Kyphoplasty does offer the chance to reduce malalignment associated with many compression fractures. For some patients, reduced pulmonary capacity and altered posture are an important part of the disability resulting from the fracture. Even subclinical loss of pulmonary capacity and altered balance may contribute to morbidity or mortality. There may be long-term pain benefits to mechanical realignment. However, the argument that kyphoplasty can produce substantial clinical benefits above those of vertebroplasty remains unproven. Although there is potential for greater safety in kyphoplasty, the published experience shows similar clinically relevant complication rates. Kyphoplasty certainly seems to provide pain control at least as effectively as vertebroplasty. It does produce more correction of height loss and deformity. However, we do not know if this achievement translates into the substantial clinical benefit necessary to offset its greater cost.

A randomized prospective study would best address whether kyphoplasty or vertebroplasty provides better safety, short-term efficacy, and long-term efficacy for the treatment of painful vertebral body fractures. Furthermore, the simple proposal that one procedure is superior to the other may be overly simplistic. In fact, these may be complementary procedures whose use can be based rationally on patient and fracture characteristics. For example, patients with recent fractures may see substantial additional benefit from kyphoplasty, whereas those with older fractures may not. Even though the technology, particularly that of kyphoplasty, continues to evolve, the time for a randomized, prospective study is near. This study will probably be time consuming and expensive but, given the large number of patients involved and cost of the procedures, is more than merited.

REFERENCES

1. Silverman SL: The clinical consequences of vertebral compression fracture. Bone 13:S27–S31, 1992.
2. Galibert P, Deramond H, Rosat P, et al: Preliminary note on the treatment of vertebral angioma by percutaneous acrylic vertebroplasty. Neurochirurgie 33:166–168, 1987.
3. Jensen ME, Kallmes DE: Percutaneous vertebroplasty in the treatment of malignant spine disease. Cancer J 8:194–206, 2002.
4. Jensen ME, Evans AJ, Mathis JM, et al: Percutaneous polymethyl-methacrylate vertebroplasty in the treatment of osteoporotic vertebral body compression fractures: Technical aspects. AJNR Am J Neuroradiol 18:1897–1904, 1997.
5. Ortiz AO, Zoarski GH, Beckerman M: Kyphoplasty. Tech Vasc Interv Radiol 5:239–249, 2002.
6. Gaughen JR, Jensen ME, Schweickert PA, et al: Lack of preoperative spinous process tenderness does not affect clinical success of percutaneous vertebroplasty. J Vasc Interv Radiol 13:1135–1138, 2002.
7. Weill A, Chiras J, Simon JM, et al: Spinal metastases: Indications for and results of percutaneous injection of acrylic surgical cement. Radiology 199:241–247, 1996.
8. Teng MM, Wei CJ, Wei LC, et al: Kyphosis correction and height restoration effects of percutaneous vertebroplasty. AJNR Am J Neuroradiol 24:1893–1900, 2003.
9. Peh WCG, Gilula LA, Peck DD: Percutaneous vertebroplasty for severe osteoporotic vertebral body compression fractures. Radiology 223:121–126, 2002.
10. Vasconcelos C, Gailloud P, Beauchamp NJ, et al: Is percutaneous vertebroplasty without pretreatment venography safe? Evaluation of 205 consecutive procedures. AJNR Am J Neuroradiol 23:913–917, 2002.
11. Cotten A, Dewatre F, Cortet B, et al: Percutaneous vertebroplasty for osteolytic metastases and myeloma: Effects of the percentage of lesion filling and the leakage of methyl methacrylate at clinical follow-up. Radiology 200:525–530, 1996.
12. Ryu KS, Park CK, Kim MC, et al: Dose-dependent epidural leakage of polymethylmethacrylate after percutaneous vertebroplasty in patients with osteoporotic vertebral compression fractures. J Neurosurg 96:56–61, 2002.
13. Gilula L: Is insufficient use of polymethylmethacrylate a cause for vertebroplasty failure necessitating repeat vertebroplasty? AJNR Am J Neuroradiol 24:2120–2121, 2003.
14. Theodorou DJ, Theodorou SJ, Duncan TD, et al: Percutaneous balloon kyphoplasty for the correction of spinal deformity in painful vertebral body compression fractures. J Clin Imaging 26:1–5, 2002.
15. Hodler J, Peck D, Gilula LA: Midterm outcome after vertebroplasty: Predictive value of technical and patient related fractures. Radiology 227:662–668, 2003.
16. Evans AJ, Jensen ME, Kip KE, et al: Vertebral compression fractures: Pain reduction and improvement in functional mobility after percutaneous polymethylmethacrylate vertebroplasty—retrospective report of 245 cases. Radiology 226:366–372, 2003.
17. Deramond H, Depriester C, Galibert P, et al: Percutaneous vertebroplasty with polymethylmethacrylate: Technique, indications, and results. Radiol Clin North Am 36:533–546, 1998.
18. Coumans JV, Reinhardt MK, Lieberman IH: Kyphoplasty for vertebral compression fractures: 1-year clinical outcomes from a prospective study. J Neurosurg 99(1 Suppl):44–50, 2003.
19. Dudeney S, Lieberman IH, Reinhardt MK, et al: Kyphoplasty in the treatment of osteolytic vertebral compression fractures as a result of multiple myeloma. J Clin Oncol 20:2382–2387, 2002.
20. Ledlie JT, Renfro M: Balloon kyphoplasty: One-year outcomes in vertebral body height restoration, chronic pain, and activity levels. J Neurosurg 98:36–42, 2003.
21. Lieberman IH, Dudeney S, Reinhardt MK, et al: Initial outcome and efficacy of "kyphoplasty" in the treatment of painful osteoporotic vertebral compression fractures. Spine 26:1631–1638, 2001.
22. Garfin SR, Reilley MA: Minimally invasive treatment of osteoporotic vertebral body compression fractures. Spine J 2:76–80, 2002.
23. Shapiro S, Abel T, Purvines S: Surgical removal of epidural and intradural polymethylmethacrylate extravasation complicating percutaneous vertebroplasty for an osteoporotic lumbar compression fracture: Case report. J Neurosurg 98:90–92, 2003.
24. Padovani B, Kasriel O, Brunner P, et al: Pulmonary embolism caused by acrylic cement: A rare complication of percutaneous vertebroplasty. AJNR Am J Neuroradiol 20:375–377, 1999.
25. Jensen ME, Evans AJ: Cardiovascular collapse and death during vertebroplasty. Radiology 228:902–903, 2003.
26. Zoarski GH, Snow P, Olan WJ, et al: Percutaneous vertebroplasty of osteoporotic compression fractures: Quantitative prospective evaluation of long-term outcomes. J Vasc Interv Radiol 13:139–148, 2002.
27. Diamond TH, Champion B, Clark WA: Management of acute osteoporotic vertebral fractures: A nonrandomized trial comparing percutaneous vertebroplasty with conservative therapy. Am J Med 114:257–265, 2003.
28. Perez-Higueras A, Alvarez L, Rossi RE, et al: Percutaneous vertebroplasty: Long-term clinical and radiological outcome. Neuroradiology 44:950–954, 2002.

29. Grados F, Depriester C, Cayrolle G, et al: Long-term observations of vertebral osteoporotic fractures treated by percutaneous vertebroplasty. Rheumatology 39:1410–1414, 2000.

30. Phillips FM, Ho E, Campbell-Hupp M, et al: Early radiographic and clinical results of balloon kyphoplasty for the treatment of osteoporotic vertebral compression fractures. Spine 28:2260–2267, 2003.

31. Gaughen JR, Jr., Jensen ME, Schweickert PA, et al: The therapeutic benefit of repeat percutaneous vertebroplasty at previously treated vertebral levels. AJNR Am J Neuroradiol 23:1657–1661, 2002.

32. Jasper LE, Deramond H, Mathis JM, et al: Material properties of various cements for use with vertebroplasty. J Mat Sci Mat Med 13:1–5, 2002.

33. Uppin AA, Hirsch JA, Centenera LV, et al: Occurrence of new vertebral body fracture after percutaneous vertebroplasty in patients with osteoporosis. Radiology 226:119–124, 2003.

34. Larsson S, Bauer TW: Use of injectable calcium phosphate cement for fracture fixation: A review. Clin Orthop 395:23–32, 2002.

35. Nakano M, Hirano N, Matsuura K, et al: Percutaneous transpedicular vertebroplasty with calcium phosphate cement in the treatment of osteoporotic vertebral compression and burst fractures. J Neurosurg Spine 97:287–293, 2002.

145 Technique of Complete Spondylectomy in the Thoracic and Lumbar Spine

BERTIL STENER[†]

The term complete spondylectomy (or vertebrectomy) is used to describe the removal of all parts of one or more vertebrae. Above the sacrum, the author has performed complete spondylectomy for extirpation of tumors in eight patients; the first operation was carried out in May 1968 (see reference 1) and the second in February 1969 (see reference 2). The following description of the technique of complete spondylectomy in three different regions of the spine is based on this experience.

REMOVAL OF MIDDLE THORACIC VERTEBRAE INCLUDING CONSIDERABLE PARTS OF ADJACENT VERTEBRAE

If a malignant tumor, originating in the body of a middle thoracic vertebra, protrudes anteriorly into the mediastinum so that it extends over the adjacent bodies, it may be suitable to include in the surgical specimen the anteroinferior half of the vertebral body above and the anterosuperior half of the vertebral body below the originally affected vertebra. With such oblique transvertebral osteotomies, it is possible to avoid entering the tumor. A technique is described for the removal of the whole of T7 and about half of T6 and T8 (Fig. 145-1).

The whole operation can be performed from behind with the patient in the prone position. Using the incision illustrated in Figure 145-1B, a flap is raised bilaterally, consisting of skin; subcutaneous tissue; and the underlying trapezius, rhomboids, and latissimus dorsi muscles. The erector spinae muscles are detached from the spinous processes, the laminae, and the medial part of the transverse processes of T3–T10 on both sides; they are then severed transversely, level with T7. The dural sac is exposed by removal of the spinous process and the inferior articular processes of T6; by removal of the lamina, the superior and inferior articular processes,

and the transverse processes of T7; and by removal of the superior articular processes of T8 (see Fig. 145-1A). Both pleural cavities are then opened by resecting the seventh rib bilaterally from the costotransverse joint to the midaxillary line. To gain adequate exposure within the thorax, the fifth, sixth, and eighth ribs are transected just lateral to the costotransverse joint, with care taken not to damage unnecessarily the intercostal nerves and vessels. After dissecting adjacent mediastinal organs free from the tumor, the intervertebral discs between T5 and T6 and between T8 and T9 are exposed. Then starting at the anterior edge of these discs, oblique osteotomies are done through the bodies of T6 and T8; using a Gigli saw, the osteotomy is directed posteroinferiorly through the body of T6 and posterosuperiorly through the body of T8 (see Fig. 145-1A). The last part of the osteotomy is performed with a chisel directed transversely from one side to the other. The specimen (see Fig. 145-1C) becomes loose and can be pushed forward enough to allow one of the pedicles of the vertebra to pass anterior to the spinal cord, whereas the entire specimen is taken out through one of the thoracotomy openings.

Reconstruction of the spine is performed according to Figure 145-1A. ASIF plates with 12 holes, having been bent to fit the thoracic curve, are fastened, one on each side of the spinous processes, with double 1-mm-thick stainless-steel wires to the transverse processes of T3–T6 and T8–T10. At the upper and lower ends, the plates are secured to each other by wires. Thereafter, one corticocancellous block of bone is taken from the posterior part of each ilium using separate incisions. The blocks are given the form illustrated in Figure 145-1A (*bottom right*), and they are inserted side by side between T6 and T8. By pressing them posteriorly, a good contact is obtained between the obliquely cut ends and the obliquely cut vertebral bodies. A transverse bore hole is made through the superior and inferior ends of the blocks and through the bodies of

[†]Bertil Stener passed away on November 30, 1999, at the age of 79 years. A graduate of Uppsala University, Sweden, he embarked on a very successful career, first as a general surgeon and then as an orthopedic surgeon. He was Professor and Chairman of the Department of Orthopedic Surgery, Sahlgren University Hospital, Gothenburg, Sweden, from 1970 to 1986. Dr. Stener made several important scientific contributions to orthopedic surgery involving the neurophysiology of ligamentomuscular protective reflexes and the analysis of hand ligament injuries. His most prominent contribution was in the field of musculoskeletal tumor surgery. His report on total spondylectomy for primary skeletal sarcoma in 1971 (J Bone Joint Surg Br 53:288–295) was the first of its kind and was followed by several others on tumor surgery of the spine. He wrote 61 scientific articles on tumors of soft tissue and bone. Dr. Stener was an honorary member of several prestigious societies, among them the American Academy of Orthopedic Surgeons. He was an esteemed teacher and renowned guest lecturer all over the world.

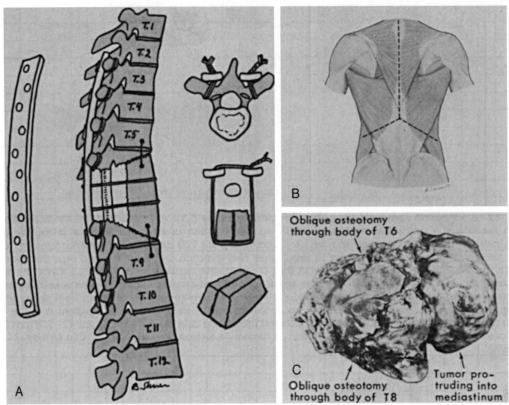

FIGURE 145-1 Complete spondylectomy for chondrosarcoma. *A,* Reconstruction of the spine after removal of the anteroinferior half of the body, the inferior articular processes, and the spinous process of T6, all of T7, and the anterosuperior half of the body and the superior articular processes of T8. Two ASIF plates have been fastened with double steel wires to the transverse processes of T3–T6 and of T8–T10. Two iliac bone blocks with obliquely cut ends have been put together and inserted between the obliquely cut bodies of T6 and T8. The blocks have been fastened to the spine with silk threads passed through holes in the blocks and the vertebrae. Further fixation has been provided by two steel wires fastened to the plates and gripping the bone blocks. *B, Interrupted lines* indicate incisions by which a flap could be raised on either side, consisting of not only the skin and subcutaneous tissue but also the underlying trapezius, rhomboids, and latissimus dorsi muscles. *C,* Right aspect of the surgical specimen. The tumor protruded from the body of T7 not only anteriorly and to either side but also posteriorly into the spinal canal (not visible here). The patient, a 49-year-old man, could walk with sticks after a block vertebra had been created by the inserted iliac grafts and the remaining parts of T6 and T8. He was still free from evidence of tumor when he died of an unrelated disease 23 years after the operation. This is the first case in which a patient with a primary malignant tumor of the spine has been permanently cured by a complete spondylectomy. (*A,* From Stener B: Total spondylectomy in chondrosarcoma arising from the seventh thoracic vertebra. J Bone Joint Surg Br 53:288–295, 1971.)

T5 and T9. Via these bore holes, the blocks are fastened to the spine with sutures of nonabsorbable material. Further fixation is provided by two steel wires gripping around the anterior cortical surface of the blocks and fastened to the steel plates. The wires are tightened so that the cancellous surfaces meeting at the superior and inferior ends of the blocks are pressed firmly together.

After reconstruction of the spine, two suction tubes are inserted into each pleural cavity, one anteriorly and one posteriorly. The thoracotomy wounds are closed, and the trapezius, rhomboids, and latissimus dorsi muscles are reattached to the spine. After completion of the operation, it is advisable to put the patient in a bed allowing convenient changing of position, prone to supine and vice versa.

REMOVAL OF LOW THORACIC VERTEBRAE AND THE FIRST, SECOND, AND THIRD LUMBAR VERTEBRAE

At T11, T12, L1, L2, and L3 levels, the whole operation can be performed from behind in one stage with the patient in the prone position. The author has removed T11, T12, L1, L2, and L3 in six patients.[1,3–7] It is important that the patient is positioned to avoid compression of the inferior vena cava.

A suitable incision for removal of L3 is illustrated in Figure 145-2A; a similar incision is used for other levels. The erector spinae muscles are exposed by raising, on each side, a flap consisting of skin, subcutaneous tissue, and the aponeurotic part of the thoracolumbar fascia. The erector spinae muscles are completely detached from the spine so that they can be retracted laterally while working on the posterior elements of the vertebrae (*central arrows* in Fig. 145-2B) and medially while exposing bilaterally the vertebral bodies, the aorta, and the vena cava (*lateral arrows* in Fig. 145-2B). It is advisable to ligate and divide, at a safe distance from their origin, the segmental arteries and veins at the affected level and the two adjacent levels.

The continued technique is illustrated in Figure 145-3, which shows a complete spondylectomy of L1. The dural sac is exposed by removing those posterior elements of the affected vertebra that are free from tumor (see Fig. 145-3C).

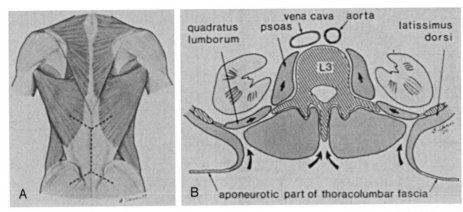

FIGURE 145-2   Posterior approach for a complete spondylectomy (L3). *A, Interrupted lines* indicate incisions through the skin, the subcutaneous tissue, and the aponeurotic part of the thoracolumbar fascia. The angles formed between the midline incision and the lateral extensions are 120 degrees. The superior lateral extensions divide the latissimus dorsi muscles more or less in their fiber direction. By raising the two flaps, the underlying erector spinae muscles are exposed as shown in *B*. *B*, Diagrammatic transection level with L3. Once the erector spinae muscles have been detached from the spine, they can be retracted laterally to expose the posterior elements of the spine (*middle arrows*) and medially to expose the vertebral bodies from both sides, which is done by transecting the quadratus lumborum and psoas muscles (*lateral arrows*). The patient is in the prone position during the whole operation. This approach was used in the case illustrated in Figure 145-5. (From Stener B: Complete removal of vertebrae for extirpation of tumors: A 20-year experience. Clin Orthop 245:72–82, 1989.)

For better exposure, it is usually necessary also to remove parts of the posterior elements of the adjacent vertebrae (see Fig. 145-3*D* and *E*). If the nature of the tumor indicates performing the spondylectomy with wide margins, it is advisable to ligate and divide the spinal nerve roots at the tumor level close to their exit from the dural sac. An osteotomy is then performed through the vertebral bodies above (see Fig. 145-3*C*) and below the affected vertebra so that the discs confining the lesion are included in the specimen. Once the two transvertebral osteotomies have been performed, the specimen is gently removed (*arrow* in Fig. 145-3*C*), with care taken not to damage the contents of the dural sac.

After removal of the specimen, the spine is reconstructed using the method illustrated in Figures 145-3*D* and *E*, and 145-4. Approaching from the right and using a handsaw, a groove is made inferiorly in the vertebral body above the gap and superiorly in the vertebral body below the gap. After diminishing the gap somewhat, three corticocancellous blocks of bone from the posterior ilium (see Fig. 145-4*A*) are inserted and fixed with three screws. With the patient in the prone position, the large, matchbox-like graft is inserted into the grooves obliquely from the right, and the screws are inserted obliquely from the left (see Figs. 145-3*D* and *E* and 145-4*B*). Strips of cancellous bone (omitted in the drawings) are placed outside the reconstructed part of the spine (see Fig. 145-3*F* and *G*). Posteriorly, metallic fixation is used above and below the inserted grafts. Meurig-Williams plates, fastened to spinous processes as shown in Figures 145-3 and 145-4, have been used successfully in two cases (T11 and L1), but in a third case (L3) ASIF plates were used to obtain good immediate stability. Plates with 12 holes were placed in the sagittal plane, one on each side of several spinous processes above and below the resected part of the spine. The plates were wired to the spinous processes in such an oblique way that the tightening of the wires resulted in axial compression of the inserted grafts (Fig. 145-5).

The described use of corticocancellous iliac grafts for reconstruction of the spine has consistently resulted in the formation of a block vertebra, allowing vertical loading after about 4 months.

REMOVAL OF THE FOURTH LUMBAR VERTEBRA

For complete removal of the fourth lumbar vertebra, it is advisable to use an anterior and a posterior approach. There are two reasons for this: one is the close relation of the lower lumbar spine to the large vessels (aorta, vena cava, common iliac arteries, and veins); the other is the hindrance caused by the iliac wings in exposing the body of L5 from behind.

Figure 145-6 illustrates a technique for complete spondylectomy of L4 that was successful for total removal of a giant cell tumor. The biologic behavior of these tumors allows such intralesional surgery. The operation was performed in two stages: first through an anterior approach, then, 4 weeks later, through a posterior approach. For the anterior approach, a large V-shaped incision (see Fig. 145-6*B*) was made through the abdominal wall down to the parietal peritoneum, which was pushed away for exposure of the aorta, the vena cava, and the common iliac arteries and veins. The large myocutaneous flap, with the underlying viscera enclosed in the peritoneal sac, was retracted to the left while working on the right side and to the right while working on the left side. After ligation and division of the third, fourth, and fifth lumbar arteries and veins on both sides, a space was dissected free between the large vessels and the lower lumbar spine. Thus released, the aorta and the vena cava could be retracted to either side as required for suitable exposure. The diseased body of L4 was then removed along with the adjacent intervertebral discs. Corticocancellous blocks of iliac bone, easily available through the anterior approach from the inside of the pelvic wings, were inserted between the bodies of L3 and L5

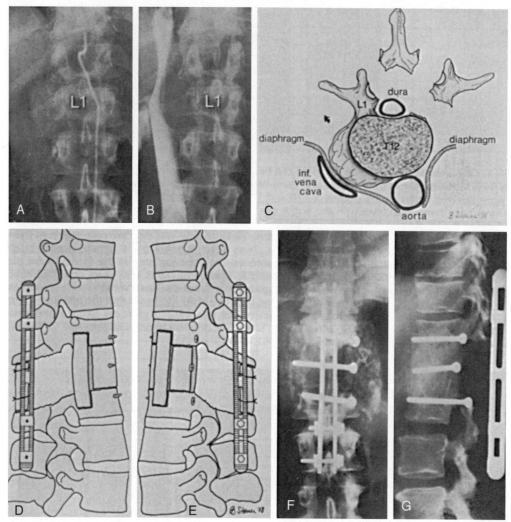

FIGURE 145-3 Complete spondylectomy for metastasis of renal cancer. As revealed by the late phase of aortography (*A*), the tumor has expanded outside the affected vertebra (L1) on the right side, making an impression in the inferior vena cava (*B*). The right crus of the diaphragm, located between the tumor and the vena cava (*C*), facilitated removal of the whole L1, including the adjacent discs and parts of T12 and L2, without damaging the vein. The spinous process, lamina, and left pedicle were free from tumor and could be removed separately to allow extraction of the specimen (*arrow*) without damaging the dural sac with its contents. *D* and *E*, The spine was reconstructed using three corticocancellous blocks of iliac bone. The largest graft, formed as a matchbox, was placed obliquely in grooves made inferiorly in the body of T12 and superiorly in the body of L2; it was inserted posteriorly on the right side (*D*) and came out anteriorly on the left side (*E*). The three grafts were fixed with three screws inserted posteriorly on the left side (*E*). Meurig-Williams plates were used for posterior fixation; pieces of rib were placed between them for creating a bony bridge between the spinous processes of T12 and L2. *F* and *G*, Pieces of cancellous iliac bone were placed outside the inserted grafts as visible on radiographs taken 4 weeks after operation. After 4 months, when a block vertebra had been created, the patient, a 56-year-old man, was allowed to start walking. Eventually, he regained function good enough for playing tennis. Unfortunately, he died from pulmonary metastases after 15 months. (From Stener B, Henriksson C, Johansson S, et al: Surgical removal of bone and muscle metastases of renal cancer. Acta Orthop Scand 55:491–500, 1984.)

(see Fig. 145-6C). The largest bone block, formed as a matchbox, was inserted in the coronal plane in grooves made inferiorly in the body of L3 and superiorly in the body of L5. For fixation of the blocks, axial compression was achieved using a Dwyer tension wire (see Fig. 145-6C). During the posterior approach, all remaining parts of L4 and some posterior parts of L3 and L5 were removed along with all residual tumor. Strips of cancellous iliac bone were placed on each side along a Harrington compression rod joining L2 to L5 (see Fig. 145-6C). After the anterior and the posterior operations, the patient was placed in a bed allowing convenient turning without jeopardizing the reconstruction of the spine.

The author has used this technique only for the removal of a giant cell tumor. If L4 is affected by a tumor, a chordoma for instance, which must be removed without being exposed in any place, let alone being entered, the described technique must be modified as required for achieving a suitable margin. It is advisable in this case to start with the posterior approach for removal of the posterior elements of L4 that are free from tumor, as illustrated in Figure 145-3C.

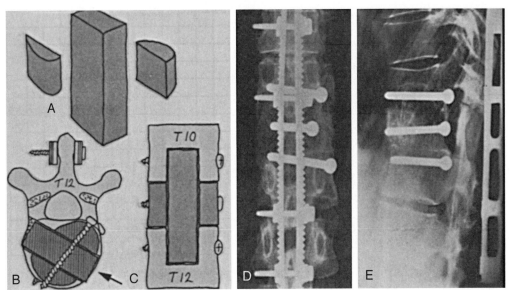

FIGURE 145-4 Complete spondylectomy for a giant cell tumor. *A* to *C,* Reconstruction of the spine after complete removal of T11, including the adjacent discs and parts of T10 and T12. Three corticocancellous blocks of iliac bone (*A*) were inserted between the bodies of T10 and T12 and were fixed by three screws (*B*) and (*C*). In *B,* the grafts have been transected level with the screw used to hold them together. The aspect of the vertebral bodies and grafts in *C* is indicated by an *arrow.* (For the sake of simplicity, the posterior parts of the vertebrae have been omitted.) With the patient in the prone position, the large graft was inserted obliquely from the right and the screws obliquely from the left. Meurig-Williams plates were fastened to two spinous processes above and two below the resected part of the spine. Strips of cancellous iliac bone (omitted in the figures) were placed outside the inserted grafts, laterally and anteriorly. *D* and *E,* Roentgenograms 2 years after operation. *D,* Anteroposterior view (see *B*); *E,* lateral view. The bone grafts have formed a block vertebra with the remaining parts of the bodies of T10 and T12. The patient, a 33-year-old woman, gave birth to a child 3½ years after the operation. She remains well after 23 years. (*A* to *C,* from Stener B: Total spondylectomy for removal of a giant-cell tumor in the eleventh thoracic vertebra. Spine 2:197–201, 1977; *D* and *E,* from Stener B: Complete removal of vertebrae for extirpation of tumors: A 20-year experience. Clin Orthop 245:72–82, 1989.)

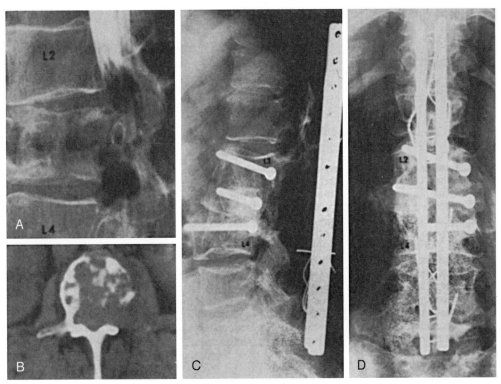

FIGURE 145-5 Complete spondylectomy for chordoma. The tumor has grown outside the body of L3 as revealed by myelography (*A*) and computed tomography (*B*). After removal of the whole of L3 and parts of L2 and L4, the spine was reconstructed by inserting iliac bone grafts anteriorly, using the method illustrated in Figure 145-4*A* to *C,* and by wiring ASIF plates to spinous processes posteriorly in such an oblique way that the tightening of the wires resulted in axial compression. *C* and *D,* Roentgenograms 15 months after operation. A block vertebra has been created by the grafts and the remaining parts of L2 and L4. The patient, a 51-year-old woman, who was unable to walk and suffered severe pain before the operation, regained walking ability and became free from pain. After about 7 years, having developed a severe osteoporosis, she sustained a stress fracture through the reconstructed part of the spine. Needle biopsy did not show any signs of recurrent tumor. She died of an unrelated disease 10 years after the operation. (From Stener B: Surgical treatment of giant cell tumors, chondrosarcomas, and chordomas of the spine. In Uhthoff HK [ed]: Current Concepts of Diagnosis and Treatment of Bone and Soft Tissue Tumors. Berlin: Springer-Verlag, 1984, p 240.)

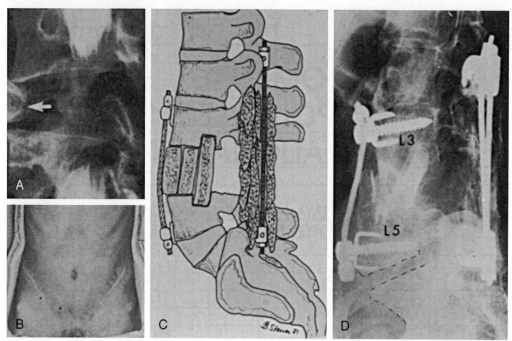

FIGURE 145-6   Complete spondylectomy for a giant cell tumor. *A,* The lumen of the dural sac has been obliterated by the tumor, which has destroyed the body of L4 almost completely; a small remaining part (*arrow*) is displaced anteriorly. *B,* A postoperative scar indicates the anterior extraperitoneal approach. *C,* After removal of the whole of L4 and parts of L3 and L5, the spine was reconstructed using corticocancellous bone blocks and a Dwyer tension wire anteriorly, and strips of cancellous iliac bone and a Harrington compression rod on both sides posteriorly. *D,* Roentgenogram 2 years after operation. Fusion has occurred between the bone grafts and the remaining parts of L3 and L5. The patient, a 23-year-old woman, remains well after 18 years. She has borne three children after the operation and works as an occupational therapist. (From Stener B: Surgical treatment of giant cell tumors, chondrosarcomas, and chordomas of the spine. In Uhthoff HK [ed]: Current Concepts of Diagnosis and Treatment of Bone and Soft Tissue Tumors. Berlin: Springer-Verlag, 1984, p 234.)

REFERENCES

1. Stener B, Johnsen OE: Complete removal of three vertebrae for giant cell tumour. J Bone Joint Surg Br 53:278–287, 1971.
2. Stener B: Total spondylectomy in chondrosarcoma arising from the seventh thoracic vertebra. J Bone Joint Surg Br 53:288–295, 1971.
3. Stener B: Resección de columna en el tratamiento de los tumores vertebrales. Acta Orthop Latinoam 1:189–199, 1974.
4. Stener B: Total spondylectomy for removal of a giant-cell tumor in the eleventh thoracic vertebra. Spine 2:197–201, 1977.
5. Stener B: Surgical treatment of giant cell tumors, chondrosarcomas, and chordomas of the spine. In Uhthoff HK (ed): Current Concepts of Diagnosis and Treatment of Bone and Soft Tissue Tumors. Berlin: Springer-Verlag, 1984, pp 233–242.
6. Stener B, Henriksson C, Johansson S, et al: Surgical removal of bone and muscle metastases of renal cancer. Acta Orthop Scand 55:491–500, 1984.
7. Stener B: Complete removal of vertebrae for extirpation of tumors: A 20-year experience. Clin Orthop 245:72–82, 1989.

146 Endoscopic and Minimally Invasive Surgery of the Spine

HAREL DEUTSCH and JOHN RATLIFF

INTRODUCTION

Minimally invasive approaches and techniques have been incorporated in all fields of surgery including spinal surgery. Benefits include improved patient outcomes, quicker recovery, and decreased health care costs. Minimally invasive spinal surgery has a long history. Introduction of the operative microscope is an example of the early incorporation of less invasive techniques to spinal surgery.[1] Chemonucleolysis, percutaneous discectomy via cannula, percutaneous laser discectomy, intradiscal electrotherapy, and percutaneous vertebral polymethylmethacrylate augmentation vertebroplasty are all minimally invasive spine procedures.

Introduction of the endoscope to perform a laparoscopic cholecystectomy in 1987 revolutionized general surgery. Endoscopic techniques have been expanded to many other general surgical procedures and also to spinal procedures.[2] The endoscope was adopted in spinal surgery and was initially used in thoracoscopic discectomies, thoracic sympathectomies, and other thoracic procedures.[3,4] Substantial benefits were realized over open thoracotomy techniques.

The most common spinal surgery is lumbar spine surgery. Minimally invasive approaches to standard lumbar surgeries were contemplated. Laparoscopic transperitoneal anterior lumbar interbody fusions developed. Laparoscopic lumbar techniques failed to disseminate widely due to difficulties with the technique and significantly longer operative times.[5,6] Patients' hospital stays were shorter by 1 to 2 days, but overall the advantages were moderate. Long-term outcomes were not different, and the incidence of complications was higher with laparoscopic surgery than with the open technique.[7] More recently, posterior lumbar minimally invasive procedures based on a muscle-splitting approach were developed. Data are still being collected prospectively to determine whether a minimally invasive muscle-splitting approach offers significant benefit over standard procedures. Early indications are promising.

MUSCLE-SPLITTING APPROACH

The development of a tubular retractor system in 1994 allowed a posterior muscle-splitting approach to the spine.[8] Sequential graduated dilators allow the introduction of a tubular retractor (Fig. 146-1). The muscle-splitting approach avoids traumatizing muscle tissue, a routine feature of standard, open spinal exposures. Tubular retractors were initially used to perform a microendoscopic discectomy.[9,10] Potential advantages include less postoperative pain, quicker recovery, and preservation of normal paravertebral muscle function.

An endoscope was used initially for visualization through the tubular retractor. The microendoscopic discectomy procedure has a high learning curve. Endoscopic procedures require a different skill set and visualization lacks depth perception because of the absence of stereoscopic vision. Initial nonrandomized comparisons indicated minimal to moderate benefit of the microendoscopic discectomy procedure.[11] The procedure was not adopted widely.

Subsequent instrumentation advancements (METRx; Medtronic Sofamor Danek, Minneapolis, MN) allowed a larger working channel and the introduction of the operative microscope or even loupe magnification. The combination of better instrumentation and more standard visualization techniques allowed the tubular retractor muscle-splitting approach to gain more popularity for microendoscopic discectomies.

Palmer and colleagues[12] effectively applied a muscle-splitting approach to lumbar stenosis decompression.

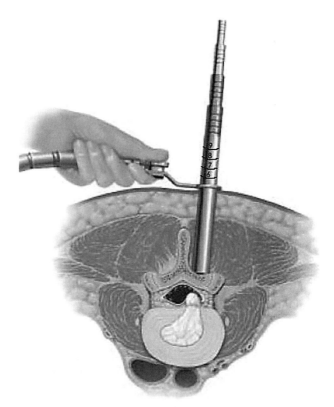

FIGURE 146-1 Tubular sequential dilators allow less traumatic dissection. A final tubular retractor maintains exposure of spinal elements. (Medtronic Sofamor Danek, Minneapolis, MN.)

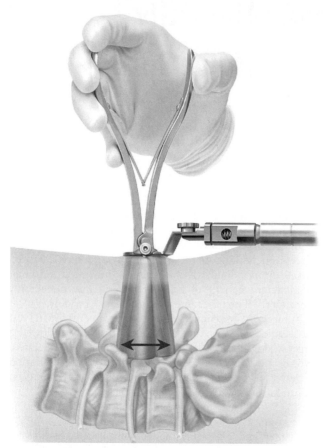

FIGURE 146-2 An expandable inverted-cone tubular retractor (X-Tube, Medtronic Sofamor Danek, Minneapolis, MN) provides a wider exposure of spinal elements through a small skin incision and via a muscle-splitting approach. (Medtronic Sofamer Danek, Minneapolis, MN.)

Further instrumentation developments have eased the transition to minimally invasive spinal fusion. The X-tube (Medtronic Sofamor Danek), an expandable tubular retractor with an inverted cone design, provides wider visualization of thoracic and lumbar spinal anatomy through a minimally invasive approach, likely easing the learning curve for these techniques (Fig. 146-2).

MINIMALLY INVASIVE POSTERIOR LUMBAR INTERBODY FUSION

Cloward[13] described a posterior lumbar interbody fusion (PLIF) technique in the 1950s. He reported excellent results, although the procedure was not widely adopted. The introduction of rigid pedicle screw systems and other instrumentation advancements caused spine surgeons to revisit the PLIF procedure.[14] Recent authors have reported excellent result with PLIFs. Freeman and colleagues[15] reported an 83% success rate with a PLIF done with posterior pedicle screws with a 5-year follow-up in 60 patients. Similar results have been described with transforaminal lumbar interbody fusion (TLIF) procedures.[16–18] Minimally invasive techniques were developed to achieve a PLIF.[19] Foley and colleagues[20] described initial excellent results in 12 patients undergoing a minimally invasive TLIF procedure.

General operative procedure follows the classic PLIF technique, with modification for the minimally invasive approach.[21] The learning curve for any minimally invasive spinal procedure is significant. Use of a larger working channel may ease the transition.

We use a Jackson table for positioning. Anteroposterior and lateral fluoroscopy is used to visualize the pedicles, facets, and spinous processes for the involved level. A "bull's-eye" view of the pedicles is obtained. Angles for percutaneous pedicle screw placement are obtained and noted. Skin incisions are planned to overlie the facet joints of the involved level. The angle of entry of the working channel determines the angle of attack for the interbody procedure. A more lateral approach is chosen for a TLIF to ease placement of the interbody cage across midline, whereas entry points closer to midline are used for a PLIF procedure (Fig. 146-3).

The skin is sharply incised approximately 4 cm lateral to midline, followed by sharp incision of the lumbar fascia and blunt finger dissection of the facet joint complexes bilaterally. Use of finger dissection limits the risk of inadvertent neural injury during dissection through misplacement of small muscle dilators. Sequential dilators are then passed percutaneously and docked on the appropriate facet joint. Finally, bilateral working channels are docked on the facet complex (Figs. 146-4 and 146-5).

Appreciation of surface anatomy through a working channel is one of the more difficult aspects of the minimally invasive learning curve. The angle of approach is different from that of an open procedure. The spinous process and lamina, usually the first bony vertebral landmarks identified, are obscured by muscle. The surgeon must recognize and

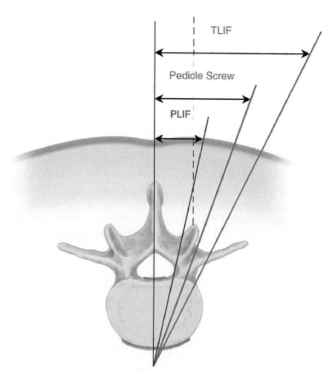

FIGURE 146-3 The initial angle of entry determines the final orientation at the disc space level. By choosing a more lateral entry point, the canal may be avoided and appropriate angulation of interbody instruments facilitated for a transforaminal lumbar interbody fusion (TLIF) procedure. PLIF, posterior lumbar interbody fusion. (Medtronic Sofamer Danek, Minneapolis, MN.)

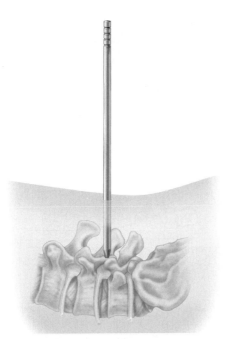

FIGURE 146-4 Dilators are passed and docked on the relevant facet joint complex (Medtronic Sofamor Danek, Minneapolis, MN). Sequential dilators or tissue trocars are used to divide muscle fibers and expose the facet joints and lamina. An up-and-down sweeping motion with the smaller dilators completes the majority of the dissection. (Medtronic Sofamer Danek, Minneapolis, MN.)

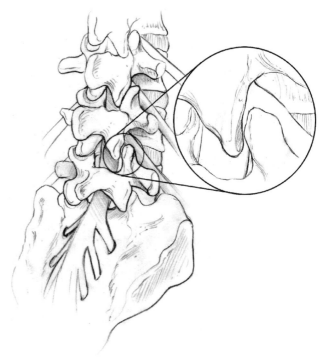

FIGURE 146-6 The view through the tubular retractor. The facet and the pars are usually visualized and provide anatomic markers to indicate that the tube is properly placed.

orient his or her approach based on the facet joint complex and pars interarticularis. Lateral dissection to expose the transverse processes may be of aid. The surgeon must allow adequate time to obtain orientation (Fig. 146-6).

Decompression begins with bilateral laminectomies and medial facetectomies. Extensive facet resections are completed to minimize nerve retraction during the interbody portion of the procedure. The ligamentum is removed, and

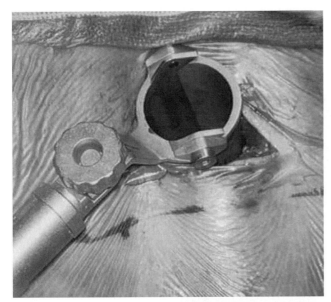

FIGURE 146-5 After completing the soft-tissue dissection, the working channel is positioned, proper placement is checked with fluoroscopy, and the retractor is secured to the operating room bed.

foraminotomies completed following standard technique. The thecal sac and traversing nerve roots are identified.

A thorough discectomy is performed using appropriate curets and disc space shavers. The end plates are decorticated to provide a fusion bed. Autograft or a biologic agent is obtained to fill the interbody space. Sequential dilators are used to restore disc space height. Interbody cages may be used to maintain disc space distraction during bony arthrodesis. We routinely augment our interbody construct with posterior pedicle screws (Fig. 146-7). Posterolateral arthrodesis is also possible by exposing the transverse process and appropriate decortication and placement of autograft.[22]

TRANSFORAMINAL LUMBAR INTERBODY FUSION

Operative Procedure

The minimally invasive TLIF procedure is similar to the PLIF procedure. In the TLIF procedure, the entire facet complex is removed and the disc is encountered further laterally. The minimally invasive approach is particularly well suited for the TLIF approach because the dilators allow a more lateral-to-medial orientation than possible with open exposure. TLIF only requires a one-sided approach, whereas a PLIF requires bilateral dilation and introduction of two retractors.

The patient is positioned prone on a Jackson table. A 3-cm incision is made overlying the affected level and carried down through the posterior lumbar fascia. Sequential dilators are introduced until a 26-mm wide X-tube retractor (Medtronic Sofmor-Danek) is placed centered on the appropriate disc space. The X-tube is secured to the bed

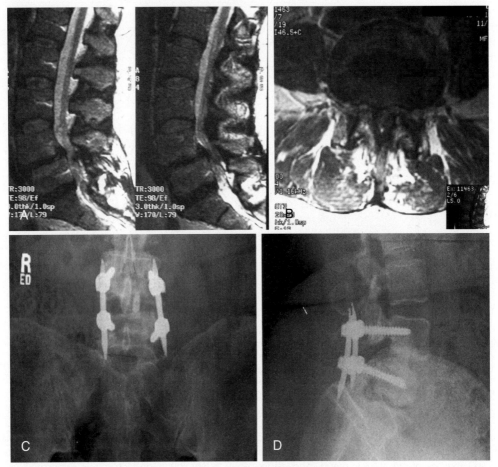

FIGURE 146-7 *A,* Sagittal T2-weighted magnetic resonance imaging (MRI) demonstrates L4–5 lumbar spondylolisthesis. *B,* Axial MRI shows severe lumbar stenosis. *C,* Postoperative anteroposterior radiograph shows bilateral screws placed percutaneously. *D,* Lateral postoperative radiograph shows an interbody fusion across the L4–5 space at 6 months.

using an articulated arm device. Smaller ports with only an 18-mm diameter are used by others. We use headlight and loop magnification alone in our minimally invasive PLIF and TLIF procedures. A complete facetectomy is performed using a high-speed air drill.

The disc space is identified and epidural veins coagulated. An aggressive discectomy is performed under direct visualization. The angle allowed with a minimally invasive approach allows the surgeon to reach across to the other side of the disc space. Osteotomes are used to remove the posterior vertebral body osteophyte. The disc space is distracted using paddle interbody distracters (Fig. 146-8). Autograft is placed anteriorly within the disc space. Options for an interbody graft include machined allograft,

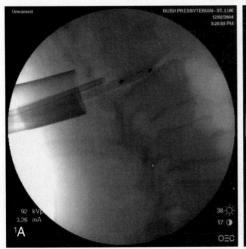
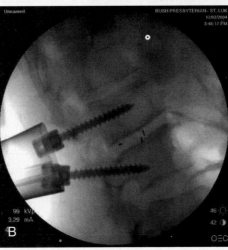

FIGURE 146-8 Transforaminal lumbar interbody fusion interbody distraction. *A,* Paddle distractors are used to dilate the interspace initially. *B,* A bullet-shaped implant helps to further distract the interspace and hold distraction. Pedicle screws are then placed.

PEEK interbody graft (Capstone, Sofmor-Danek, Memphis, TN), carbon fiber (DePuy-Acromed, Rayman, MA), or titanium interbody implant (Geo, Interpore-Cross, Irvine, CA). Local bone derived from the facetectomy is collected and placed within the disc space. Harvested iliac crest bone graft is also placed in the interbody graft.

Percutaneous Pedicle Screw Placement

The interbody arthrodesis is augmented with posterior pedicle screws. Percutaneous pedicle screws are also used to augment an anterior lumbar interbody fusions or in conjunction with a posterolateral arthrodesis. All percutaneous pedicle screw systems feature the same basic steps: localization and cannulation of the pedicle percutaneously, muscle splitting via dilator, tapping of the pedicle screw course, screw insertion, and rod delivery. The most difficult portion in learning percutaneous pedicle screw fixation is pedicle identification and cannulation with fluoroscopy.[23]

The angle of the fluoroscope may be used to guide pedicle screw insertion. Preoperative films are studied in the axial plain to ascertain pedicle angulation. Sagittal alignment is obtained via intraoperative imaging. The fluoroscope is sighted down the long axis of the pedicle, and a Jamshedi needle is used to "bull's-eye" the target pedicle (Fig. 146-9). A Kirschner wire is inserted via the Jamshedi needle in the

pedicle, and the transpedicular course is verified by lateral fluoroscopy and anteroposterior fluoroscopy. Muscle dilation is used to introduce a cutting tap to tap the pedicle and then a screw is advanced over the Kirschner wire into the pedicle.

Another routinely used option for pedicle screw fixation in our practice is mini-open pedicle screw placement via the tubular retractor. After completing an interbody fixation, pedicle screw entry points are visualized through the tubular retractor and confirmed via lateral fluoroscopy. The cortical bone over the pedicle is scored by high-speed drill, and a blunt-tipped pedicle probe is advanced into the vertebral body. The remainder of the fixation follows standard open technique. A single level rod can easily be inserted via tubular retractor (Fig. 146-10). Another option, especially useful in multilevel cases, is placement of Jamshedi needles and Kirschner wires via the tubular retractor followed by removal of the retractor, tapping, and screw insertion following a minimally invasive percutaneous screw technique.

POSTEROLATERAL ENDOSCOPIC THORACIC DISCECTOMY

Patterson and Arbit[24] described the transpedicular approach to thoracic disc herniations in 1978. Mulier and colleagues[25] reviewed 331 thoracic discectomy cases and

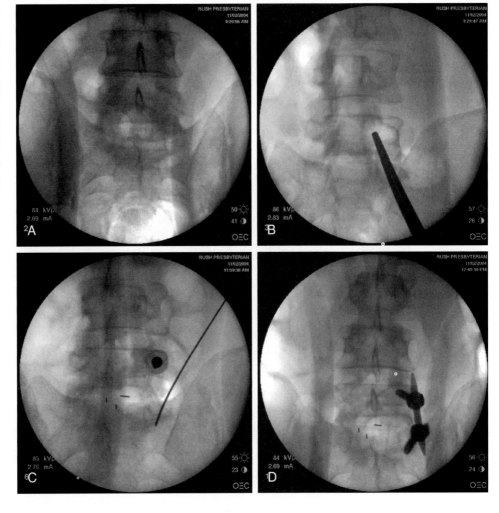

FIGURE 146-9 *A,* An anteroposterior radiographic view is initially obtained. *B,* The fluoroscope angle is modified to allow direct on-end visualization of the relevant pedicle, here the left L5 pedicle. *C,* A Jamshedi needle is inserted percutaneously in the pedicle, followed by a Kirschner wire. Here, a Kirschner wire is inserted in S1, and a Jamshedi needle is "bull's-eyeing" the L5 pedicle. *D,* The pedicle screw course is tapped and a screw inserted. A rod may be placed via a percutaneous delivery system or via the tubular retractor.

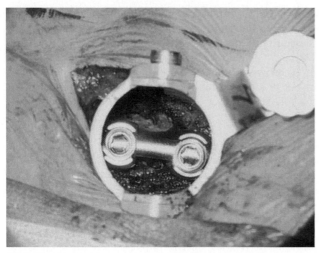

FIGURE 146-10 Intraoperative view through a tubular retractor shows the exposed dura and pedicle screws and rod in place.

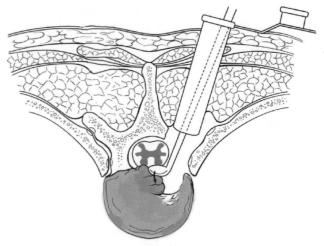

FIGURE 146-11 Placement of the tubular retractor and bone removal necessary to access the disc space for a thoracic discectomy.

reported partial or total neurologic recovery in 93% after a transthoracic procedure versus 87% after a posterolateral technique and 80% after a lateral approach. Pulmonary complications occurred in 7% of transthoracic techniques versus 5% in lateral and 0% in posterolateral techniques. Anterior approaches have the advantages of minimal spinal cord manipulation and direct access to relevant pathology. Disadvantages include the morbidity associated with transthoracic surgery, long instrument reach, and unfamiliar surgical approach.

Video-assisted thoracoscopic surgery for thoracic disc herniation has been demonstrated to be effective and substantially reduce the morbidity and overall recovery.[26,27] Video-assisted thoracoscopic surgery is technically difficult and requires careful collaboration with a thoracic surgeon.

Jho[28] first described a transpedicular minimally invasive posterior thoracic discectomy using an endoscope. Perez-Cruet and colleagues[29] reported a minimally invasive posterior approach using a tubular METRx retractor for thoracic discs in seven patients. Five of seven patients demonstrated excellent results. An endoscope was used in conjunction with a tubular retractor. The retractor allows a muscle-splitting approach and a better lateromedial angle than the open procedure. The angle allows better ventral decompression without spinal cord manipulation (Fig. 146-11). Additionally, the angled endoscope allows inspection of the ventral spinal cord. Thoracic discs lateralized to one side are appropriate for the minimally invasive transpedicular discectomy. Central discs are more appropriate for an anterior approach (Fig. 146-12).

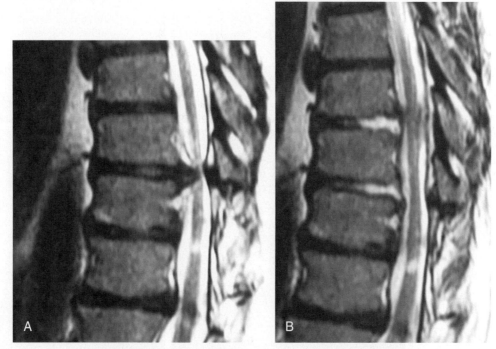

FIGURE 146-12 Thoracic discectomy. *A,* Preoperative magnetic resonance imaging (MRI) shows a large thoracic disc with spinal cord compression. *B,* Postoperative MRI shows no further spinal cord compression.

CERVICAL MINIMALLY INVASIVE PROCEDURES

Fessler and colleagues[30] described the use of a tubular retractor to perform a cervical foraminotomy. The authors found that the average hospital stay decreased from 68 hours to 20 hours. The overall clinical outcome was comparable with that of patients undergoing an open cervical foraminotomy. The retractor allows a muscle-splitting approach, and otherwise the procedure is performed in a standard fashion. Special care is taken to ensure that the dilators dock on the lateral mass complex rather than the central lamina where the spinal cord is located. Before placing the dilators, the posterior fascia is divided widely to ensure easy retractor placement. The procedure is performed either with a microscope or endoscopic visualization.

Wang and colleagues[31] described the placement of lateral mass screws in the cervical spine using a tubular retractor in a small number of patients. Other minimally invasive techniques in the cervical spine have been explored, but so far posterior minimally invasive techniques have not been widely adopted.

CONCLUSION

The tenants of minimally invasive surgery are not new to spinal surgery. Spinal surgery's history represents a gradual evolution to more effective and more minimally invasive methods. Reducing the direct and indirect cost of spinal care is very important because of the high prevalence of spinal pathology in the population and the increasing use of surgery to address degenerative pathology. The muscle-splitting approach and minimally invasive PLIF and TLIF applications are promising to significantly speed recovery from lumbar surgery. Percutaneous pedicle screw placement has significant advantages in some situations such as the posterior augmentation of an anterior lumbar interbody fusion. Further data demonstrating the effectiveness of minimally invasive techniques and instrumentation refinement will speed the embracement of the technology by practitioners.

REFERENCES

1. Malis J: Technical contributions of Leonard I. Malis. Mt Sinai J Med 172–181, 1997.
2. Fuchs K: Minimally invasive surgery. Endoscopy 34:154–159, 2002.
3. Han P, Kenny K, Dickman CA: Thoracoscopic approaches to the thoracic spine: Experience with 241 surgical procedures. Neurosurgery 51(5 Suppl):S88–S95, 2002.
4. Oskouian RJ, Johnson JP, Regan JJ: Thoracoscopic microdiscectomy. Neurosurgery 50:103–109, 2002.
5. Chung SK, Lee SH, Lim SR, et al: Comparative study of laparoscopic L5-S1 fusion versus open mini-ALIF, with a minimum 2-year follow-up. Eur Spine J 12:613–617, 2003.
6. Zdeblick TA, David SM: A prospective comparison of surgical approach for anterior L4-L5 fusion: Laparoscopic versus mini anterior lumbar interbody fusion. Spine 25:2682–2687, 2000.
7. Liu J, Ondra SL, Angelos P, et al: Is laparoscopic anterior lumbar interbody fusion a useful minimally invasive procedure? Neurosurgery 51:155–158, 2002.
8. Thongtrangan I, Le H, Park J, Kim DH: Minimally invasive spinal surgery: A historical perspective. Neurosurg Focus 2004;16:E1.
9. Foley KT, Smith MM: Microendoscopic discectomy. Tech Neurosurg 3:301–307, 1997.
10. Kawaguchi Y, Matsui H, Tsuji H: Back muscle injury after posterior lumbar spine surgery: A histologic and enzymatic analysis. Spine 21:941–944, 1996.
11. Muramatsu K, Hachiya Y, Morita C: Postoperative magnetic resonance imaging of lumbar disc herniation: Comparison of microendoscopic discectomy and Love's method. Spine 26:1599–1605, 2001.
12. Palmer S, Turner R, Palmer R: Bilateral decompression of lumbar spinal stenosis involving a unilateral approach with microscope and tubular retractor system. J Neurosurg 97:213–217, 2002.
13. Cloward R: The treatment of ruptured lumbar intervertebral discs by vertebral body fusion: Indications, operative technique, after care. J Neurosurg 10:154–168, 1953.
14. Steffee AD, Sitkowski DJ: Posterior lumbar interbody fusion and plates. Clin Orthop 227:99–102, 1988.
15. Freeman B, Licina P, Mehdian SH: Posterior lumbar interbody fusion combined with instrumented postero-lateral fusion: 5-year results in 60 patients. Eur Spine J 9:42–46, 2000.
16. Lowe T, Tahernia AD, O'Brien MF, Smith DA: Unilateral transforaminal posterior lumbar interbody fusion (TLIF): Indications, technique, and 2-year results. J Spinal Disord Tech 15:31–38, 2002.
17. Rosenberg W, Mummaneni PV: Transforaminal lumbar interbody fusion: Technique, complications, and early results. Neurosurgery 48:569–574, 2001.
18. Salehi S, Tawk R, Ganju A, et al: Transforaminal lumbar interbody fusion: Surgical technique and results in 24 patients. Neurosurgery 54:368–374, 2004.
19. Leu HF, Hauser RK: Percutaneous endoscopic lumbar spine fusion. Neurosurg Clin N Am 7:107–117, 1996.
20. Foley K, Holly LT, Schwender JD: Minimally invasive lumbar fusion. Spine 28:S26–S35, 2003.
21. Khoo L, Palmer S, Laich DT, Fessler RG: Minimally invasive percutaneous posterior lumbar interbody fusion. Neurosurgery 51:166–181, 2002.
22. Boden SD, Moskovitz PA, Morone MA, Toribitake Y: Video-assisted lateral intertransverse process arthrodesis: Validation of a new minimally invasive lumbar spinal fusion technique in the rabbit and nonhuman primate (rhesus) models. Spine 21:2689–2697, 1996.
23. Foley KT, Gupta SK: Percutaneous pedicle screw fixation of the lumbar spine: Preliminary clinical results. J Neurosurg 97(Suppl 1):7–12, 2002.
24. Patterson RJ, Arbit E: A surgical approach through the pedicle to protruded thoracic discs. J Neurosurg 48:768–772, 1978.
25. Mulier S, Debois V: Thoracic disc herniations: transthoracic, lateral, or posterolateral approach? A review. Surg Neurol 49:599–608, 1998.
26. Han PP, Kenny K, Dickman CA: Thoracoscopic approaches to the thoracic spine: Experience with 241 surgical procedures. Neurosurgery 51(5 Suppl):S88–S95, 2002.
27. Regan JJ, Mack MJ, Picetti GD 3rd: A technical report on video-assisted thoracoscopy in thoracic spinal surgery: Preliminary description. Spine 20:831–837, 1995.
28. Jho H: Endoscopic transpedicular thoracic discectomy. J Neurosurg 91:151–156, 1999.
29. Perez-Cruet M, Kim BS, Sandhu F, et al: Thoracic microendoscopic discectomy. J Neurosurg 1:58–63, 2004.
30. Fessler RG, Khoo LT: Minimally invasive cervical microendoscopic foraminotomy: An initial clinical experience. Neurosurgery 51(5 Suppl):S37–S45, 2002.
31. Wang M, Prusmack CJ, Green BA, et al: Minimally invasive lateral mass screws in the treatment of cervical facet dislocations: Technical note. Neurosurgery 52:444–448, 2003.

147 Microsurgery of Ruptured Lumbar Intervertebral Disc

EDWARD C. TARLOV and SUBU N. MAGGE

Lumbar and sciatic pains are among the symptoms for which patients most commonly seek medical advice.[1] Because these symptoms are so widespread in the general population and are increasing, the diagnosis and care of patients with lumbar and sciatic pain forms and will continue to form the majority of most neurosurgical practice. Only a small proportion of symptomatic patients we see benefit from disc surgery. In the referral practice at the Lahey Clinic, about 10% of the patients we see require discectomy. The remainder are best treated by conservative programs of exercise, courses of physiotherapy, encouragement to pursue their normal activities, and the tincture of time.

In recent years, improvements in the techniques of fusion procedures have led to wider applications of these surgeries to patients with back pain. This large subject is not in the scope of this chapter.[2] In addition, the alternative now exists to fusion with use of the newly approved artificial disc, theoretically to preserve the motion segment and lessen the stresses on the adjacent disc levels. The motion segment comprises the facet joints and disc, and thus far, experiences in Europe have indicated that disc arthroplasty can disrupt the normal function of the facets. The complexities of the motion segment, including axial shock absorption, flexion, and translocation, have not yet been reproduced by any prosthesis, and it is our belief that the practical value of disc replacement remains unclear.

The title of this chapter emphasizes the importance of confining surgical treatment to those instances in which a lumbar disc is found clinically and on imaging studies to have ruptured.[3-9] The outcome of surgery for a degenerative slightly bulging disc is likely to be disappointing to the doctor and patient. Magnetic resonance imaging (MRI) is the mainstay of diagnosis. Approximately 10% of the population, because of claustrophobia, is unable to undergo standard MRI. In these patients, so-called open MRI can be carried out, but the quality of the images is severely degraded. Patients who have undergone previous surgery require gadolinium enhancement to identify postoperative changes and to distinguish these from disc herniations. In patients strongly suspected of disc herniation and when MRI is unsatisfactory or impossible, computed tomographic (CT) myelography remains a valuable imaging modality.

Radiologists who interpret these studies, because they usually do not have an opportunity to correlate the patients' symptoms, have a tendency to overinterpret the images. A report of "normal for this patient's age" almost never appears. In spite of advanced imaging technology, the onus of correct diagnosis rests more than ever on clinical judgment, correlating the patient, symptoms, and imaging studies.

Better imaging has done little to improve the outcome of surgery. Many asymptomatic patients have abnormal imaging study findings.[10]

The natural history of degenerative and spondylitic changes in the lumbar spine is one of gradual progression over years. Facet arthropathy is ubiquitous in the population and is seen on CT scans of most adult spines. CT, with its bone detail, shows these changes more clearly than MRI. Disc degeneration, also ubiquitous, is best demonstrated in its earliest stages by changes seen on MRI. Most degenerated discs remain confined to the intervertebral space with slight to moderate bulging. As part of the degenerative process in discs, the annulus can degenerate relatively more than the nucleus, resulting in herniation of a part of the nucleus, compressing the adjacent nerve root or roots. This process is described later. It is not commonly recognized that disc and facet degeneration can cause referred pain in the buttock and down the thigh. All too often, it is assumed that if there is leg pain there must be nerve root compression. This is not the case. This important point cannot be overemphasized. True sciatica radiating down the back of the thigh, below the knee, and involving the calf may indicate nerve root compression by herniated disc. Less well-defined pains, particularly those predominantly involving the buttock or thigh without radiation in a full sciatic distribution, bilateral pain in buttocks of thighs, and pains that vary from side to side are most likely to be referred pain from facet arthropathy or disc degeneration. Nonspinal pathology, including osteoarthritis about the hip and trochanteric bursitis, may also be involved. In general, patients with these pains will not be helped by surgery, regardless of what myelograms or scans are believed to demonstrate. In other words, patients with back pain alone are unlikely to be helped by microdiscectomy surgery, even if scans, as they often do, demonstrate disc protrusions. Also, there are patients with typical sciatica and intense disabling pain in whom high-quality imaging studies demonstrate no nerve root compression. In these patients, no surgery is advisable. In time, the symptoms usually subside.[11]

MECHANISM OF DISC HERNIATION AND NATURAL HISTORY

A better understanding of the forces that lead to disc herniation may help in advising patients about activity, including work. There has been a tendency for physicians to be overly cautious in this regard, often advising limitation of activity or work and thus promoting an outlook that is detrimental to a patient's feeling of health and economic well-being.

In fact, the back is beautifully engineered and quite strong. The forces leading to disc herniation result from the relative proportion of degeneration and loss of vertical height of the annulus and nucleus. From observation of the distortion of neural elements resulting from a disc herniation, there is considerable force involved. The extruded disc fragment most commonly is forced to pass to one side of the posterior longitudinal ligament by the confining effect of the posterior longitudinal ligament itself. From clinical observations, it seems likely that the sequence leading to disc herniations is that shown in Table 147-1 and Fig. 147-1.

During the normal course of life, dehydration and degenerative changes lead to a loss of height of the lumbar intervertebral discs. This loss usually occurs at the expense of both annulus and nucleus. In some patients, a disproportionate loss of nuclear material occurs with relatively less degenerated annulus. Ordinarily, the degenerative changes of nucleus and annulus lead only to a loss of height of the interspace. If there is a preferentially greater loss of annulus, however, the axial pressures on the nucleus from the weight of the body and the pull of the paraspinous muscles leads to excessive pressure on the remaining portion of the nucleus, which is unsupported by the degenerated narrowed annulus. This is transferred to centrifugal pressure, which together with shearing forces may produce tearing of the fibers of the annulus, allowing extrusion of nuclear material. After the excess nucleus has herniated, the disc is structurally stable. The forces on the degenerated nucleus and annulus are in balance, and there is no vector force driving further nuclear material out, unless the annulus further degenerates. Mixed situations may occur in which there is loss of substance in one part of the nucleus, resulting in gas formation, and excessive pressure in another part of the nucleus. In such an instance, a herniation with intradiscal gas may occur (Fig. 147-2).

It is not widely appreciated that disc herniation usually does not result from trauma but rather is the result of degenerative changes in the annulus as outlined above. Truly herniated discs rarely result from automobile accidents or work-related injuries. Patients with truly herniated discs rarely arrive at the hospital by ambulance. Truly herniated discs rarely cause long periods of inability to work. A lack of appreciation of these facts has led to the widespread abuse of workers' compensation laws and litigation.

CLINICAL EVALUATION: INDICATIONS FOR IMAGING AND SURGERY

The most common indication for lumbar surgery to excise the herniated portion of a lumbar intervertebral disc is persistent severe pain in a sciatic distribution together with imaging findings clearly indicating a disc herniation in a patient who is likely to be helped by the operation. Patients with severe sciatic pain in whom a bona fide disc herniation has clearly been demonstrated usually have good results from surgery. Disc herniation ordinarily occurs as an isolated event at one level. It is extremely unusual to have more than one bona fide disc herniation at the same time. A diagnosis of multiple disc herniations is usually incorrect. Judging the severity of a patient's pain can be difficult. There is obviously no quantitative method of doing so. A very severe pain for a short period may be tolerable, whereas a less severe pain persisting for a long period may be intolerable. Patients' tolerances of pain vary widely. Often it requires all of the physician's cognitive skills and intuition to make a wise judgment in this area.

Workers' compensation laws are a severe deterrent to health. True disc herniation rarely occurs in the work place, but muscular and ligamentous strain is common. All too often, the patient injured in the workplace is subjected to excessive testing, overdiagnosis, and overtreatment, all of which can lead to loss of confidence and disability. Patients with workers' compensation issues must be judged especially carefully and a very clear diagnosis established before any surgery is contemplated. Acute or post-traumatic symptoms are occasionally attributed to spinal stenosis or spondylitic changes. Both are chronic conditions, and the attributing of acute symptoms to them is frequently an error.

The usual lateral disc herniation at L4–L5 compresses the L5 root. The usual lateral disc herniation at L5–S1 compresses the S1 root. Occasionally, a more medial disc herniation at L4–L5 may compress the L5 root. The same principles apply at higher levels of the lumbar spine. A deficit may not

---

TABLE 147-1 ▪ Degenerative Changes Leading to Disc Space Narrowing, Vacuum Phenomenon, Disc Bulging, and Disc Herniation

Status of Disc	Status of Nucleus and Annulus	Stresses	Comment
Normal disc	Normal annulus, normal nucleus	Stresses proportionately borne by nucleus and annulus	
Degenerated narrowed disc	Loss of substance in both annulus and nucleus	Stresses proportionately borne by nucleus and annulus	
Vacuum disc phenomenon	Disproportionate loss of substance, greater in nucleus	Stresses disproportionately borne by annulus	Gas in interspace
Preherniation of disc	Disproportionate loss of substance	Stresses disproportionately borne by nucleus	Axial forces translated in nucleus to centrifugal forces leading to herniation
Herniated disc		Once herniation has occurred, stresses borne proportionately by remaining nucleus and annulus herniated fragment of nucleus exerts pressure on adjacent root, causing sciatica	
Postoperative disc			May have gas in interspace

FIGURE 147-1 Exploded views of vertebrae and disc in axial section. Theoretical diagrams of changes in the lumbar discs leading to disc herniation and extrusion. *A,* Normal annulus and nucleus. Axial forces (*arrows*) balanced by elastic properties of nucleus and annulus. *B,* Degenerated disc. Annulus and nucleus have proportionately narrowed. Axial forces still balanced by elastic properties of the disc. Some flexibility may be lost due to loss of height of disc. *C,* Degenerated disc with vacuum disc phenomenon. Annulus relatively preserved. Relatively more degenerative change has occurred in the nucleus, leading to loss of substance in the nucleus. Axial forces are mainly borne by the annulus. There is no pressure on the nucleus. Gas is seen in the nucleus due to loss of substance of involuted nucleus. *D,* Preherniated disc. Annulus has degenerated more than nucleus. Bulk remaining nucleus, unsupported by degenerated axially narrowed annulus, is now under increased pressure. Axial forces are now translated to centrifugal forces within the nucleus (*small arrows*), which can lead to disc herniation. *E,* Bulging disc. Some fibers of annulus on the right in the diagram of disc are stretched or incompetent, allowing elevated intranuclear pressure to displace disc material from the interspace into the epidural space. *F,* Frank disc extrusion. Incompetent fibers of the annulus have ruptured. Shearing forces can be the final event leading to this problem, either in the midportion of the annulus or at the margin of annulus. Axial pressure translated to centrifugal forces (*small arrows*) seen in *D* lead to extrusion of disc material into the epidural space.

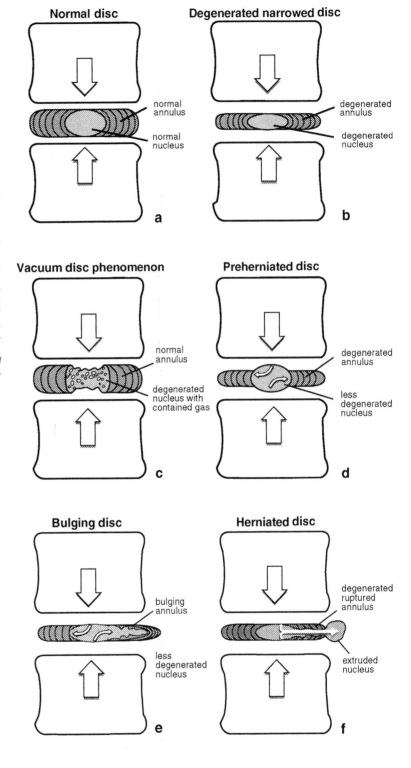

be present. Although there may be a weakness of the tibialis anterior and extensor hallucis longus with involvement of the L5 nerve root, it is quite common, even with a very large disc rupture at L4–L5, to have no obvious neurologic deficit because of the overlapping distribution of adjacent roots. This, too, is a limitation of neurologic examination. If pain is improving, a residual deficit may improve along with it over a slightly longer time. Therefore, if pain is diminishing, a weakness of dorsiflexion of the foot is not in

itself necessarily an indication for surgery. A severe foot drop with sciatic pain is an indication for surgery. Even with prompt surgery, recovery from severe foot drop does not always occur.

Cauda equina syndrome is a neurosurgical emergency. However, it can sometimes be difficult to diagnose. The event may occur acutely. Experienced neurologic consultation may not be available. Sometimes the deficit is more pronounced than the pain. Widespread sensorimotor loss and impairment

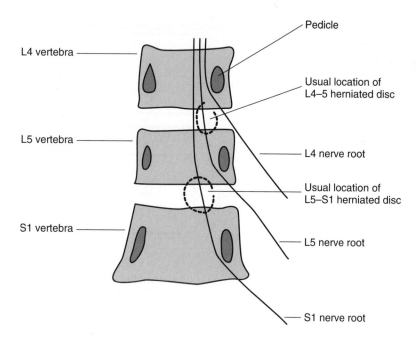

FIGURE 147-2 Diagrammatic representation of the relationships of the lumbar intervertebral spaces, pedicles, and nerve roots at L4, L5, and S1. The L4 root is seen passing caudal to the pedicle of L4 and laterally. A disc herniation at L4–L5 commonly compresses the L5 root. It can be appreciated that a further lateral disc herniation will compress the L4 root and a larger or more medial disc herniation at L4–L5 can compress the S1 root.

of bladder function may be present. The condition is unusual. It can result from massive disc herniation. In this situation, the preponderance of evidence supports urgent surgery. However, recovery does not always occur even with prompt surgery, and the dysfunction of bowel and bladder may become long-term disabling problems.

The early diagnosis of cauda equine syndrome may not be possible, and even in the best of circumstances the diagnosis is sometimes delayed. Medical history taking has elements of art.

IMAGING

Once a clinical diagnosis of lumbar disc herniation has been made in a patient whose severity of pain is sufficient to warrant surgery, preoperative imaging studies are in order. When no surgery is being contemplated, imaging is probably not warranted. Sometimes, imaging studies are carried out in response to patients' requests that an MRI be done. Scanning is theoretically harmless, but the danger of overdiagnoses is great, particularly because the radiologist's report may be given to the patient, triggering a cycle of events often leading to unwarranted surgery. Then, too, there is a tendency to carry out excessive studies even when a diagnosis is clear on one study. To a large extent, these problems of imaging are reduced when patients and doctors have an incentive to reduce the costs of care by avoiding unnecessary tests.

High-quality CT scanning can demonstrate disc herniation in patients who are not obese and who have not undergone previous surgery, but MRI is superior to CT scanning in terms of accuracy for diagnosis of disc herniation. Both studies tend to be overinterpreted by radiologists, because they do not have the opportunity to see the patient and correlate signs and symptoms.

In patients strongly suspected on clinical grounds of having disc herniation and whose CT or MRI scans are unrevealing, it is justifiable to carry out CT myelography with water-soluble intrathecal contrast, followed by CT scanning. This is still our most accurate diagnostic test. Even when scar tissue is present from previous surgery, an accurate diagnosis of nerve root displacement should be possible in almost all cases. The use of CT scanning permits using smaller quantities of intrathecal contrast agent and a diminution of side effects. In its present form, MRI scanning requires the patient to lie still for a prolonged period. Some patients in severe pain cannot do so even with medication. For some, even CT scanning, which requires less time, is intolerable. For these patients, too, CT myelography, when skillfully carried out, can offer more flexibility of positioning. CT myelography may also be more acceptable to patients who are claustrophobic.

It is important to emphasize the pathology of lumbar disc rupture. The strong posterior longitudinal ligaments in the midline cause most disc herniations to occur paracentrally in the spinal canal. Disc herniations rarely affect both legs; the pain syndrome is unilateral in the majority of patients. Midline bulging of discs occurs so commonly that it should hardly be considered pathologic. Lateral views on myelography, as well as on CT and MRI, scans that demonstrate disc bulging usually do not indicate a situation likely to benefit from surgery.

A system of grading disc ruptures to distinguish among free fragments, major disc ruptures, and normal discs with minimal bulging is used. Disc grade 0 or grade I indicates there is little or no bulge; grade II if there is a marked herniation with a few fibers of annulus intact; and grade III if there is an extruded free fragment. Grade II and grade III are the pathologic conditions most likely to be helped by surgery (Fig. 147-3).

The importance of true sciatic pain, radiating down the back of one leg or below the knee, for the diagnosis of true disc herniation and prediction of favorable result from surgery cannot be overemphasized. Atypical variations that are not

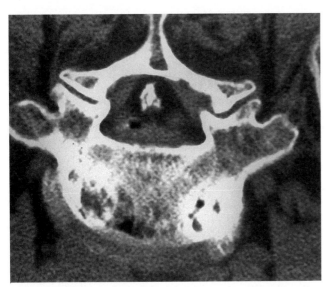

FIGURE 147-3 Computed tomography scan showing extruded disc fragment with gas in the fragment. Prior degenerative changes in the nucleus apparently led to gas formation. Subsequent degenerative changes in the annulus, as outlined in Figure 147-1, may lead to herniation of the degenerated nucleus.

true sciatica, however, namely pain confined to the buttock or back of the thigh and variable sciatic pain involving both legs, are negative factors and tend to be correlated with poor outcome from surgery. Occasionally a large disc herniation or extrusion is seen in a patient with back pain only. Variations in nature do occur, and if other predictive factors are favorable, good results of disc surgery can occur.

Progressively worsening neurologic deficit is often included among indications for surgery. It is extremely unusual for a disc rupture to cause a progressive neurologic deficit. This condition should be removed from the standard list of surgical indications. Intractable pain is also listed as an indication for disc surgery and should also be removed. The pain from disc rupture typically fluctuates, and most motivated patients often do not stop work because of it. In general, injuries that occur in the workplace do not cause disc rupture; even twisting and shearing forces that are necessary to rupture the annulus usually do not occur after lifting and after falls in the workplace. The failure of conservative treatment is not an indication for surgery in the absence of a bona fide disc rupture. Among the contraindications to surgery is a first episode of sciatic pain without an adequate trial of conservative management. There are, however, occasional instances in which pain is so severe that it may be worse with bed rest, and early surgery is advisable.

With widespread use of MRI and CT scanning, the combination of negative CT and MRI results makes it extremely unlikely that a surgically remediable disc rupture will be found. For this reason, exploratory lumbar surgery is almost never advisable.

TIMING OF SURGERY

Judging the severity of a patient's pain can be difficult. Severe pain is the usual indication for surgery. For this reason an operation for removal of a herniated disc is usually carried out fairly promptly, because the patient who needs surgery is usually in fairly intense pain and the operation is not totally elective. If the patient has a profound foot drop or quadriceps weakness, the chances of good motor recovery are enhanced if the operation is carried out promptly. Sometimes, even with immediate surgery, a profound deficit does not recover, but if the deficit is not quite complete, there is a reasonable chance for recovery if the pressure on the nerve root is promptly relieved.

The healing of a lumbar disc herniation has been documented, in which the herniated disc material absorbs over a long period of time. We have seen a number of instances in which bona fide disc extrusion has been imaged and, over a period of months or longer, has been shown to resolve. However, well-documented cases are unusual. The radiologic findings have not always correlated with the clinical findings. There are instances in which the herniation appears better but the patient's symptoms are worse or vice versa. The remarkable healing process of the spine can lead to reduction in symptoms in most patients. It is only with unremitting sciatic pain and significant disc herniation that surgery is clearly of value.

Risk factors negatively influencing the results of surgery include an unclear diagnosis; atypical symptoms; equivocal imaging studies; very long duration of symptoms; workers' compensation claims; litigation; drug, cigarette, or alcohol dependence; obesity; and concurrent medical problems. Once all factors have been considered and it has been determined that surgery is likely to be very helpful, the patient should be preoperatively informed of the possibility of infection, bleeding, cerebrospinal fluid (CSF) leak, incontinence, persistent neurologic deficit, root injury, paralysis, recurrent herniation, rupture of the abdominal vessels or viscera, and death. The physician needs to be reassuring in manner and should, if his or her experience warrants, indicate that such problems are unlikely to occur.

OPERATIVE TECHNIQUES

Magnification and improved illumination have unquestionably increased the accuracy of surgery and reduced tissue trauma (Figs 147-4 to 147-15).[12–20] Microsurgical disc surgery can be carried out with powerful loupes and fiberoptic headlight illumination or with the operating microscope. In our practice at the Lahey Clinic with a large volume of intervertebral disc surgery, we have not been able to detect a significant difference in clinical outcome between these two techniques. Patient selection and high-quality imaging studies remain major determinants of surgical outcome.

A variety of patient positions have been used for lumbar disc surgery. The prone position, with rolls placed under the chest and iliac crests and the table flexed, is commonly used. The preference of one of us (E.T.) is for the knee-chest position, in which the laminae are spread apart, the depth of the wound is reduced to a minimum, the epidural veins are decompressed, and the great vessels in the abdomen hang away from the spine to some extent. It is important to avoid neck extension during any prone operation, in order to prevent cervical spinal cord injury (Fig. 147-5A). The preference of the other of us (S.M.) is for the use of the Jackson table with the Wilson frame (Fig. 147-5B).

Posterolateral Disc Herniation

Most herniated discs occur in a posterolateral position within the spinal canal (Fig. 147-4). We estimate that 70% of ruptured lumbar discs are in this location. We therefore employ a paramedian incision on the side of the herniation. Regarding surface landmarks, a surgeon's relaxed hand with the thumb and little finger spread apart corresponds to the size of the sacrum in almost all patients. If the surgeon's little finger is placed on the tip of the coccyx, the thumb in this relaxed position will lie on the lumbosacral interspace. This has been of greater help to me in localizing this level than any other method.

Intraoperative radiographs should be used to confirm the level of pathology. In most instances, the presence of a large disc herniation is the confirmation that the correct level is being exposed. It is important to emphasize that if only patients with major disc ruptures are undergoing surgery, the correct level is the level with the obvious disc rupture. This is often a free fragment or at least an obvious major prolapse (grade II or grade III) if the patients are well selected.

Several errors must be made for the surgeon to operate on the wrong level. If the patient has no disc rupture, there is no correct level for surgery. This is an error made more often than one might like to think. The same is true for minimally herniated discs. The taking of radiographs in such instances can confirm the appropriate anatomic level being operated on, but there is usually a more fundamental

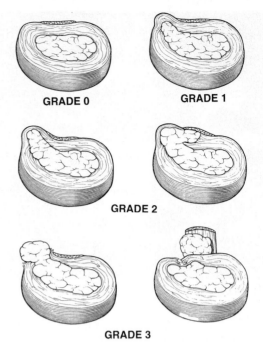

FIGURE 147-4   Gradations of disc bulging and herniation. Normal disc: grade 0. Slightly bulging disc: grade 1. Moderate disc herniation: grade 2. Extruded disc: grade 3.

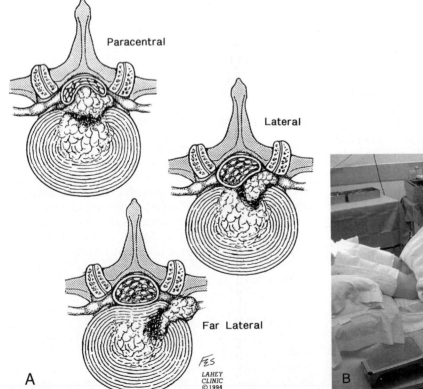

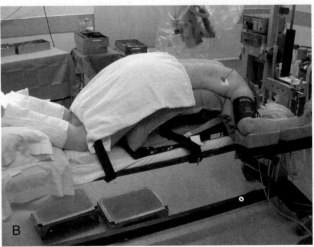

FIGURE 147-5   *A,* Position of disc herniation. Most herniations (estimated at 80%) occur in the posterolateral quadrant, compromising the spinal canal and medial foramen. Posterior longitudinal ligament forces herniation to one side of midline. An estimated 10% of herniations occur laterally in the lateral foramen or lateral to the foramen, where the root existing above may be compromised. Preoperative recognition of location of herniation helps in operative planning. (From Fager CA: Atlas of Spinal Surgery. Philadelphia: Lea & Febiger, 1989.) *B,* Patient positioned prone on a Wilson frame on the Jackson table. The abdomen is free and all pressure points are well padded.

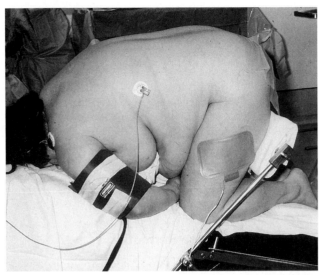

FIGURE 147-6 Knee-chest position. Note that the abdomen is dependent. This lowers the pressure in the epidural veins. Laminae are separated and brought more superficial by the flexed position. The patient's buttocks are supported on a seat. In obese patient such as this, surgery can be relatively bloodless. (From Fager CA: Atlas of Spinal Surgery. Philadelphia: Lea & Febiger, 1989.)

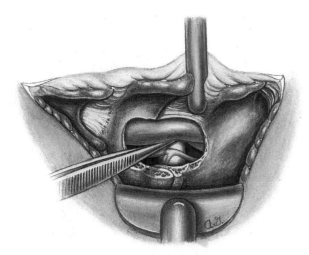

FIGURE 147-8 Extruded fragment is visible beneath the epidural vein at the level of the interspace. (From Fager CA: Atlas of Spinal Surgery. Philadelphia: Lea & Febiger, 1989.)

problem: No matter what level is operated on, the outcome will likely be poor. If a large disc rupture is expected and no disc rupture is found, then one is at the wrong level. If no disc rupture is expected, the operation should probably not have been carried out to begin with.

Regarding the technique of dissection, the muscles can be placed on slight tension using a periosteal elevator to retract them laterally, and then using the cutting cautery at low setting, the attachments of the paraspinous muscles to the spine are divided. Two Markham or Williams retractors

are used to maintain the exposure. The Leksell rongeur is used to start the hemilaminectomy. This rongeur has a special feature incorporated into its design; it can be held to cut in a nearly vertical position. Its lower cutting jaw should never be inserted beneath the lamina because of the danger of injury to the underlying nerve root. Alternatively, a high-speed drill can be used to perform the hemilaminectomy. The initial exposure is then widened with a thin foot plate Kerrison rongeur. The yellow ligament is carefully excised, being drawn dorsally with toothed forceps as it is cut to avoid dural injury. The Kerrison punch, which may pick up a fold of dura, also must be used with great care to avoid dural or root injury. A dural tear, if recognized and repaired, is usually of no consequence. Bony removal is carried out laterally above and below the level of herniation.

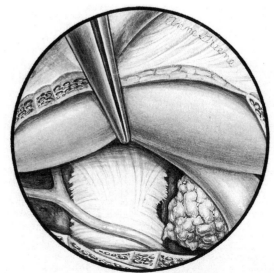

FIGURE 147-7 Left-sided exposure. Dural sac retracted medially. Nerve root seen at right. Extruded fragment of a disc can be seen to have extruded caudally from a marginal tear in the annulus. (From Fager CA: Atlas of Spinal Surgery. Philadelphia: Lea & Febiger, 1989.)

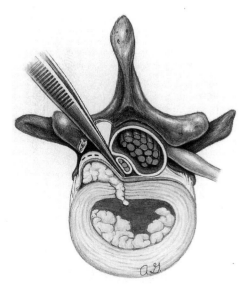

FIGURE 147-9 Extruded fragment seen in the foramen, displacing the root and dural sac medially. (From Fager CA: Atlas of Spinal Surgery. Philadelphia: Lea & Febiger, 1989.)

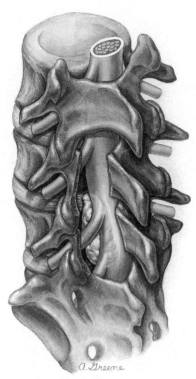

FIGURE 147-10   Large extruded fragment straddling the L5 nerve root. Wider bony exposure is required for safe removal of an extensive lesion. (From Fager CA: Atlas of Spinal Surgery. Philadelphia: Lea & Febiger, 1989.)

The yellow ligament is excised and the root exposed. Bipolar coagulation of the epidural veins is carried out.

The nerve root is gently retracted medially over the dome of the herniation. A conjoined root may be apparent on preoperative studies but may sometimes be recognized only at this stage. Medial retraction of a conjoined root may be difficult, and it may be necessary to work in the limited space beneath the axilla of the root rather than in the safer zone lateral to the shoulder of the retracted root. If a free fragment is present, it is removed from the epidural space at this point. If a herniated fragment is contained within a portion of the annulus, an incision in these thinner annular fibers is made. The therapeutic portion of the operation is removal of the epidural mass. It is safest to limit the operation to this maneuver. It is not clear to what extent curettage of the interspace is helpful, and it raises the level of risk of the operation slightly. Removal of the herniated portion of the disc is likely to be sufficient to provide relief (Fig. 147-16). It has not been shown that recurrence is any less likely if curettage of the interspace is carried out.

Paracentral Disc Herniation

Slight central disc bulging of lumbar discs is common and ordinarily of no clinical significance. The posterior longitudinal ligament forces most disc herniations to a posterolateral position. Occasionally (we estimate in 15% of instances), significant disc herniation may occur just to one side of the midline. Such a disc herniation can obstruct a major portion of the spinal canal. In these cases a larger bony exposure is performed rostrocaudally and sometimes across the midline

to include a portion of the contralateral lamina. It need not be extended all the way laterally on the other side, and one should preserve the facet joint on the other side. The disc can be removed from the side of the patient's symptoms or, if symptoms are bilateral, from the side of the more severe symptoms. We almost never carry out fusion in these instances and have not encountered postoperative instability in relation to this condition. A wide exposure both rostrocaudally and laterally is helpful in reducing the possibility of neural injury in large central disc herniations. This is particularly important because instances of postoperative cauda equina syndrome have occurred when the operative exposure is not wide enough owing to excessive retraction of already compromised nerve roots.

Extraforaminal Disc Herniation

Far lateral or extraforaminal lumbar disc herniation occurs in about 15% of instances. These lesions are ordinarily evident on CT scan or MRI scan as a mass lateral to the foramen on the axial views. Parasagittal images on MRI are particularly helpful in showing the relationship of the disc, nerve root, and pars interarticularis laterally in the foramen.

There are two general approaches to deal with these far lateral disc herniations. A purely lateral approach has been devised through a muscle-splitting incision.[21–23] Paraspinal muscles are split parallel to their fibers to expose the facets and transverse processes. The intertransverse membrane is divided and careful dissection carried out to expose the pedicle, serving as the superior boundary of the foramen, and the pars interarticularis, which establishes the roof of the foramen. The exiting nerve root can be seen under the pars. The root is then mobilized, usually caudally, to remove the herniated disc fragment. If the disc fragment is in the medial aspect of the foramen, we find it safer to begin dissection medially in the familiar territory of the interlaminar space, widening the standard hemilaminectomy approach laterally so as to have the nerve root well in view. The more lateral approaches do not afford an early exposure of the nerve root, and careful dissection is required. However, they offer a direct route to truly lateral pathology that preserves the facet complex and decreases the risk for any instability. At L5–S1, a lateral exposure can be difficult because of the overriding iliac crest. Here it may be necessary to perform a complete facetectomy and work from within the interspace itself to draw the herniated portion medially.

Minimally Invasive Approaches

Recent improvements in surgical access devices have allowed exposure of the interlaminar space with minimal disruption of the soft tissues. The basic principles involve sequential dilation of the muscle and fascia about the interlaminar space leading to the placement of a tubular retractor mounted to the operating table (Fig. 147-17). For selected patients, we have used the MetRx system (Medtronic), although a variety of systems are available. An initial 2-cm long incision is made 2 to 3 cm off midline. A guidewire is then placed under fluoroscopic guidance to engage the inferior edge of the lamina at the base of the spinous process. Sequentially larger tubes are then placed to dilate the soft tissues and expose the interlaminar space. An operating

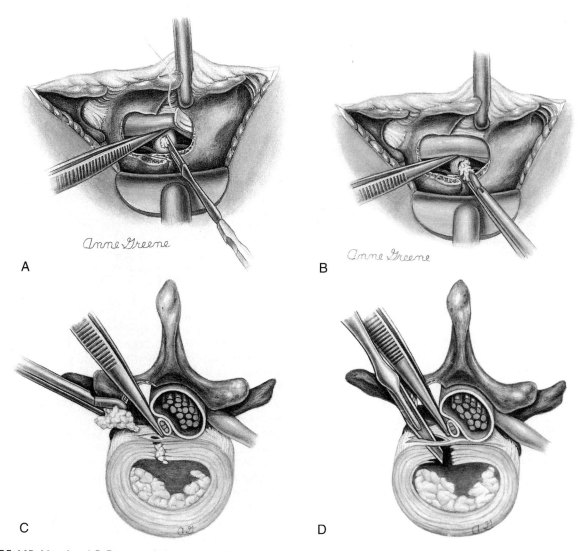

FIGURE 147-11 *A* and *B,* Fragment being grasped. Dissection from a medial to lateral direction avoids increasing pressure on nerve root. *C,* Fragment being brought out of epidural space. *D,* The annulus is being incised so that interspace can be explored for loose fragments of nucleus. (From Fager CA: Atlas of Spinal Surgery. Philadelphia: Lea & Febiger, 1989.)

FIGURE 147-12 Proximity of common iliac arteries, iliac veins, and ureters to anterior surface of the L4–L5 annulus. Curettage within the interspace increases the risks of surgery and likely has no effect on the incidence of recurrence. The incidence of recurrence is suspected to relate more to degenerative changes in the annulus (see Fig. 147-1 and Table 147-1). (From Fager CA: Atlas of Spinal Surgery. Philadelphia: Lea & Febiger, 1989.)

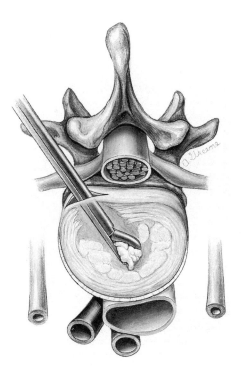

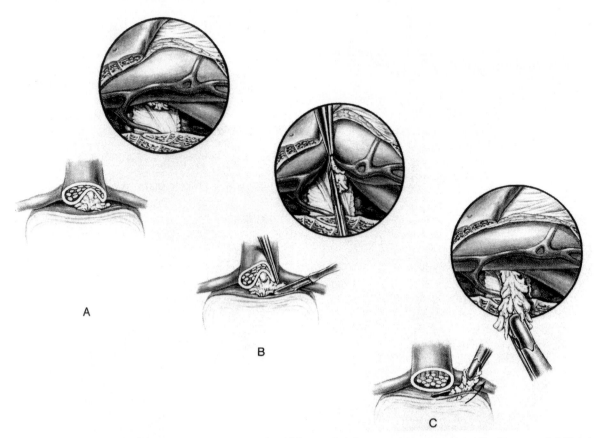

FIGURE 147-13   Steps in gentle retraction of the dural sac, in which extruded disc material is drawn laterally. At surgeon's initial view (*A*), extruded fragment may not be obvious. As dissection proceeds, the extruded fragment comes into view (*B* and *C*). (From Fager CA: Atlas of Spinal Surgery. Philadelphia: Lea & Febiger, 1989.)

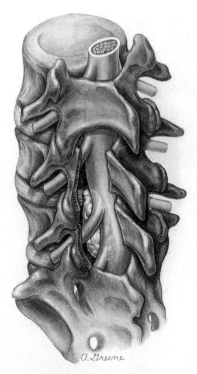

FIGURE 147-14   Wider exposure is necessary for safest removal of paracentral disc herniation. (From Fager CA: Atlas of Spinal Surgery. Philadelphia: Lea & Febiger, 1989.)

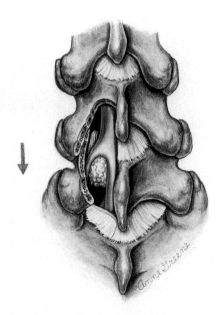

FIGURE 147-15   Caudal migration of fragment requires its removal via the axilla of the nerve root. Similar exposure is necessary for a conjoined nerve root. (From Fager CA: Atlas of Spinal Surgery. Philadelphia: Lea & Febiger, 1989.)

microscope or endoscope is used to visualize the interspace and the operation proceeds using specialized bayoneted rongeurs and dissecting instruments. This technique is useful for all but far lateral disc herniations. We must stress, however, that while minimal access may minimize the "invasiveness" of surgery, only correct diagnosis and successful neural decompression can lead to a successful outcome for the patient.

Reoperative Surgery for Lumbar Disc Herniations

Disc herniation recurs in 5% to 10% of patients followed for 10 years. Obesity may be a risk factor. Although hard physical work can cause back symptoms, it is not clear that recurrent disc herniation is any more common in the physically stressed population than in the general population. The caveats that apply to primary disc surgery are equally important with recurrent symptoms.[24,25]

Imaging studies can be difficult to interpret in patients who have previously undergone surgery. If the findings on enhanced MRI or CT scanning are clear and correlate with the patient's symptoms, no further studies are required. If the CT and MRI studies are unclear, CT myelography provides definitive results in most cases. Formation of scar tissue is the natural result of surgery. All too often scar tissue is implicated as a cause of recurrent symptoms in patients who have previously undergone disc surgery when, in fact, failure of original diagnosis, degenerative spondylosis, or nerve root injury at prior surgery is the cause of continued pain. Arachnoiditis has similarly been inappropriately invoked as a cause of symptoms in many instances. In reoperative surgery, the extensive dissection of scar tissue can be traumatic. If a

bona fide recurrent disc herniation has been diagnosed, it is safest to enter the scar tissue at the site where disc herniation is suspected and to remove the herniated portion of the disc, leaving most of the scar undisturbed. This is important in speeding postoperative recovery and avoiding additional trauma.

INTRADISCAL PROCEDURES

With the advent of endoscopic surgery and the associated publicity, the public has come to expect that less invasive operations will provide better results. In actual fact, good results of a procedure depend mainly on proper patient selection, the correct diagnosis, and gentle manipulation of the tissues. A large body of literature has been accumulating on theoretically less invasive intradiscal techniques. Percutaneous techniques for disc aspiration also have been introduced. These procedures have mainly been applied to the "contained" disc (i.e., the disc that has not herniated) and are directed at the contents of the interspace. The rationale is to remove normal disc tissue, trusting that herniation will reduce itself into the space created within the normal disc. The percutaneous technique does not address the extruded fragment directly, and it has not been shown that procedures on the interior of the disc itself provide any better outcome than the natural course of healing.

COMPLICATIONS ASSOCIATED WITH LUMBAR DISCECTOMY

Complications have been extensively treated.[26-29] One of the most catastrophic complications associated with lumbar

FIGURE 147-16 Facet has been excised to access foraminal extrusion.

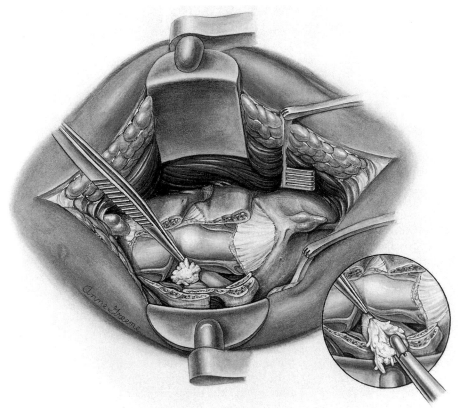

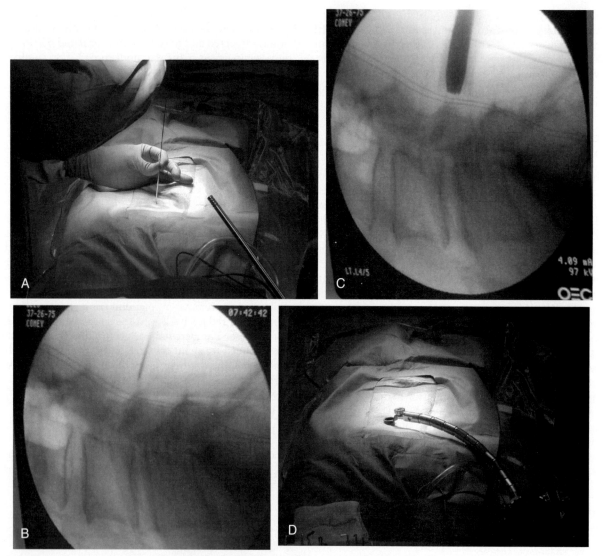

FIGURE 147-17   *A* and *B,* Guidewire placed under fluoroscopic guidance to engage the inferior aspect of the L4 lamina. *C* and *D,* Sequential dilation under fluoroscopic guidance leads to placement of table-mounted 16-mm MetRx retractor (Medtronic).

disc surgery is arterial injury to the iliac arteries or veins if a curet or rongeur is inserted through the interspace and through the anterior annulus damaging these vessels. Occasionally, the anterior annulus itself is not patent, and an instrument may pass through it without evident change in resistance. Marking the instruments in such a way as to warn of a deep penetration has not always been helpful. Ventral perforation has occurred even in the hands of the most experienced neurosurgeons. A sudden drop in blood pressure should alert the surgical team to this possibility. Visible bleeding in the interspace is evident in fewer than 10% of cases. With major hypotension, it is important to terminate the operation, place the patient supine on the operating table, and call for the help of a vascular surgeon. If a vascular surgeon is not available, an incision can be made and a hand placed through a midline abdominal incision onto the spine to compress the aorta until help arrives. The rupture ordinarily involves the common iliac artery and/or the iliac vein. Both the artery and the vein can be injured, in which case an arteriovenous fistula may

subsequently form. Occasionally, injuries to the bowel or ureter, or both, have been reported; these, too, require early recognition and corrective surgery.

CSF leak in the course of a lumbar discectomy is a problem. Occasionally, the site of the CSF leak is ventrally placed and not accessible. If the area of the leak is reinforced with Surgicel and the deep layers of fascia and skin are well repaired, the leak can heal itself. If a dural tear is amenable to repair, this procedure is best carried out immediately. Ordinarily, there are no consequences of dural repair, provided that the nerve root has not been injured.

There are occasional instances in which a dural defect allows a root to herniate through it, trapping the root and resulting in postoperative radicular pain. Evidence of CSF leak in connection with persistent radicular pain after surgery should alert the surgeon to this possibility. Imaging studies may be unrevealing, and surgery to replace the herniated portion of the root in the dural sac and repair the dura may be helpful.

SF-36™ HEALTH STATUS SURVEY

INSTRUCTIONS: This survey asks for your views about your health. This information will help keep track of how you feel and how well you are able to do your usual activities.

Answer every question by marking the appropriate oval. If you are unsure about how to answer a question, please give the best answer you can.

Before beginning this questionnaire. . .
Please pencil in your ID number in the squares to the right and then darken in the appropriate oval below each number.

If you don't know what ID number to use, ask the person who gave you this questionnaire.

Now begin with the questions below.

SIDE 1

MARKING INSTRUCTIONS
- Use a No. 2 Pencil ONLY.
- Make dark heavy marks that fill the oval completely.
- Erase unwanted marks cleanly.
- Make no stray marks on this answer sheet.

PROPER MARK   IMPROPER MARKS

START HERE - Leave out spaces, dashes, etc.

ID NUMBER

1. In general, would you say your health is:
   1. ① Excellent
      ② Very good
      ③ Good
      ④ Fair
      ⑤ Poor

2. **Compared to one year ago,** how would you rate your health in general now?
   2. ① Much better now than 1 year ago
      ② Somewhat better now than 1 year ago
      ③ About the same as 1 year ago
      ④ Somewhat worse now than 1 year ago
      ⑤ Much worse now than 1 year ago

3. The following items are about activities you might do during a typical day. Does **your health now limit you** in these activities? If so, how much? (Mark one oval on each line.)

	Yes, Limited A Lot	Yes, Limited A Little	No, Not Limited At All
a. Vigorous activities, such as running, lifting heavy objects, participating in strenuous sports	①	②	③
b. Moderate activities, such as moving a table, pushing a vacuum cleaner, bowling, or playing golf	①	②	③
c. Lifting or carrying groceries	①	②	③
d. Climbing several flights of stairs	①	②	③
e. Climbing one flight of stairs	①	②	③
f. Bending, kneeling, or stooping	①	②	③
g. Walking more than a mile	①	②	③
h. Walking several blocks	①	②	③
i. Walking one block	①	②	③
j. Bathing or dressing yourself	①	②	③

4. During the **past 4 weeks,** have you had any of the following problems with your work or other regular daily activities **as a result of your physical health?** (Mark one oval on each line.)

	Yes	No
a. Cut down the amount of time you spent on work or other activities	①	②
b. Accomplished less than you would like	①	②
c. Were limited in the kind of work or other activities	①	②
d. Had difficulty performing the work or other activities (for example, it took extra effort)	①	②

PLEASE TURN CARD OVER TO COMPLETE QUESTIONNAIRE

A

FIGURE 147-18 *A* and *B,* Medical Outcomes Study short form, a 36-item multiple choice questionnaire. This form has been validated worldwide for over a decade in 7.5 million patients in many disease categories. (SF-36 Health Survey, Copyright 1992 Medical Outcome Trust. All Rights Reserved. Reproduced with permission of the Medical Outcome Trust.)

(Continued)

This is Side 2 of this Questionnaire.
Make sure you complete the OTHER side first.   SIDE 2

5. During the **past 4 weeks,** have you had any of the following problems with your work or other regular daily activities **as a result of any emotional problems** (such as feeling depressed or anxious)? (Mark one oval on each line.)

5.

	Yes	No
a. Cut down the <u>amount of time</u> you spent on work or other activities	a.①	②
b. <u>Accomplished less</u> than you would like	b.①	②
c. Didn't do work or other activities as <u>carefully</u> as usual	c.①	②

6. During the **past 4 weeks,** to what extent has your physical health or emotional problems interfered with your normal social activities with family, friends, neighbors, or groups? (Mark one oval.)

6. ① Not at all   ④ Quite a bit
    ② Slightly   ⑤ Extremely
    ③ Moderately

7. How much **bodily** pain have you had during the **past 4 weeks?** (Mark one oval.)

7. ① None   ④ Moderate
    ② Very mild   ⑤ Severe
    ③ Mild   ⑥ Very severe

8. During the **past 4 weeks,** how much did **pain** interfere with your normal work (including both work outside the home and housework)? (Mark one oval.)

8. ① Not at all   ④ Quite a bit
    ② A little bit   ⑤ Extremely
    ③ Moderately

9. These questions are about how you feel and how things have been with you **during the past 4 weeks.** For each question, please give the one answer that comes closest to the way you have been feeling. How much of the time during the **past 4 weeks . . .** (Mark one oval on each line.)

9.

	All of the Time	Most of the Time	A Good Bit of the Time	Some of the Time	A Little of the Time	None of the Time
a. Did you feel full of pep?	a.①	②	③	④	⑤	⑥
b. Have you been a very nervous person?	b.①	②	③	④	⑤	⑥
c. Have you felt so down in the dumps that nothing could cheer you up? ...	c.①	②	③	④	⑤	⑥
d. Have you felt calm and peaceful?	d.①	②	③	④	⑤	⑥
e. Did you have a lot of energy?	e.①	②	③	④	⑤	⑥
f. Have you felt downhearted and blue?	f.①	②	③	④	⑤	⑥
g. Did you feel worn out?	g.①	②	③	④	⑤	⑥
h. Have you been a happy person?	h.①	②	③	④	⑤	⑥
i. Did you feel tired?	i.①	②	③	④	⑤	⑥

10. During the **past 4 weeks,** how much of the time has your **physical health or emotional problems** interfered with your social activities (like visiting with friends, relatives, etc.)? (Mark one oval.)

10. ① All of the time   ④ A little of the time
    ② Most of the time   ⑤ None of the time
    ③ Some of the time

11. How **true** or **false** is **each** of the following statements for you? (Mark one oval on each line.)

11.

	Definitely True	Mostly True	Don't Know	Mostly False	Definitely False
a. I seem to get sick a little easier than other people.	a.①	②	③	④	⑤
b. I am as healthy as anybody I know.	b.①	②	③	④	⑤
c. I expect my health to get worse.	c.①	②	③	④	⑤
d. My health is excellent.	d.①	②	③	④	⑤

12.

12a. Which are you? ....   a. ○ Male .... ○ Female

b. How old were you on your last birthday? ....   b. ○ Less than 35   ○ 65-74
                                                            ○ 35-44   ○ 75-84
                                                            ○ 45-54   ○ 85 and older
                                                            ○ 55-64

13. Have you ever filled out this form before? ....   13. ○ Yes
                                                                       ○ No
                                                                       ○ Don't remember

Thank you for your time.   14. **DO NOT MARK HERE**   ⒶⒷⒸⒹⒺ
                                    NOT LAST CARD   ○

B

This printed form of the SF-36 Health Status Survey is for use on the RT-2000 Response Terminal made by Response Technologies, Inc. - East Greenwich, RI 02818

FIGURE 147-18   Cont'd

Failure to relieve symptoms is probably the most common complication of lumbar disc surgery,[30–32] and it often results from improper initial diagnosis or it may relate to surgical trauma. Its incidence can be minimized by careful attention to the preoperative assessment and to the gentlest possible surgical technique. This complication cannot be avoided completely.

POSTOPERATIVE CARE

Our routine is to place few limitations on the patient's activity following surgery, relying on the patient's level of pain to regulate it. No normal activity is likely to cause injury to the disc, muscle, or incision. The disc itself is as structurally strong after surgery as it was before. The annulus and the

MOS SF-36™ HEALTH SURVEY

SITE: 1

DATE: 07-23-1994

ID:　00000000101　　　　SEX: Male　　　AGE: 35-44

HEALTH SCORES

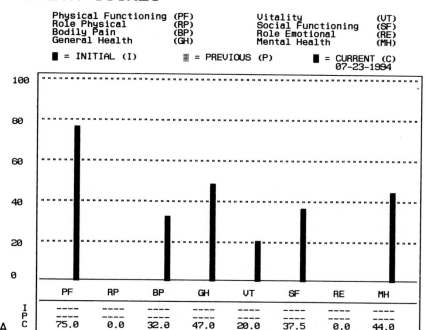

PF	RP	BP	GH	VT	SF	RE	MH
I ----	----	----	----	----	----	----	----
P ----	----	----	----	----	----	----	----
C 75.0	0.0	32.0	47.0	20.0	37.5	0.0	44.0

A

MOS SF-36™ HEALTH SURVEY

SITE: 1

DATE: 08-07-1994

ID:　00200000101　　　　SEX: Male　　　AGE: 45-54

HEALTH SCORES

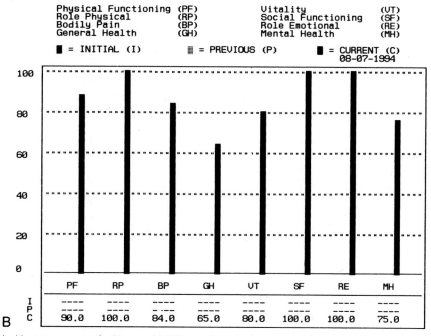

PF	RP	BP	GH	VT	SF	RE	MH
I ----	----	----	----	----	----	----	----
P ----	----	- .---	----	----	----	----	----
C 90.0	100.0	84.0	65.0	80.0	100.0	100.0	75.0

B

FIGURE 147-19　*A*, Health status survey of a 23-year-old, 330-pound nursing home aide who developed sciatica while lifting a patient at work. Studies showed an extruded disc at L4–L5. The health survey here shows impairment in spheres of physical role functioning, bodily pain, vitality, and mental health areas. In summary, the Medical Outcomes Study short form (SF-36) shows marked impairment. *B*, Health status survey in a 54-year-old laborer who underwent surgery for L4–L5 disc herniation 4 years previously. He is working fully in a stressful job without apparent limitations. SF-36 shows essentially normal levels of function for his age. Serial measurements before and after surgery would show the effect of intervention. Patient-generated information such as this is no more subjective than a surgeon's view that a patient is doing well.

remaining portion of the nucleus support the axial and shearing forces as well after the surgery as before. Patients are kept in the hospital overnight. They ordinarily can return to work within a short time. There is no medical contraindication to allowing sedentary workers to return to work in a few days. Because of muscular pain, a laborer may prefer to stay out of work a little longer, but most patients should be back to work within 1 month of surgery and many within days or weeks. The mechanism of disc herniation (Fig. 147-1 and Table 147-1) render it unlikely that any particular activity will raise the risk for recurrent disc herniation. Even competitive athletes are usually able to return to their sports within months.

OUTCOME ANALYSIS

An important development in the measurement of health status is the use of sophisticated patient-based questionnaires to evaluate a patient's functional status, level of pain, and general health.[32-36] Heretofore, health status has been judged on the basis of pathologic findings and the physician's subjective opinion. As new procedures are developed, their proponents have a bias. We are in need of methods to evaluate neurosurgical treatment and to allow it to be compared with the general range of medical and surgical treatments available today.

The Medical Outcomes Study short form, a 36-question survey (MOS-SF-36) (Fig. 147-18), has been tested for over a decade in very large populations and in many disease states; the method is just coming into use in neurosurgery. The health status of a patient is assessed by having the patient answer a set of 36 questions. The questionnaire must be filled out by the patient, without the help of others. A computerized scoring instrument is used to determine the results. Its use is very simple and does not consume the physician's time. The carefully designed set of questions is weighted and scored to reflect physical functioning, bodily pain, general health, vitality, social functioning, emotional role, and mental health. The resulting scores can be plotted as a curve and can give an assessment of the patient's status without the bias of the physician.

The MOS-SF-36 is a generic health survey not specific to lumbar surgery but it lends itself well to evaluating patients with sciatica before and after treatment. Our preliminary studies show that the MOS-SF-36 can be used to assess the impairments of patients with sciatica before and after surgery (Figs 147-18 and 147-19). The patients are shown to be worse immediately after lumbar surgery, even if preoperative pain is diminished. Longer-term postoperative pain is diminished. Longer postoperative follow-ups will measure the efficacy of the procedures we carry out.

SUMMARY

We believe that the future of lumbar disc surgery will depend on better and more widespread understanding of the natural history of the degenerative process and on tailoring of surgery to the specific instances in which significant nerve root compression is truly present. The simplest methods to effectively release nerve root compression will no doubt be the ones widely used in the future. At present, the safest, simplest, and most reliable technique is still open surgery

as described here using magnified vision and the gentlest possible neurosurgical techniques.

REFERENCES

1. Tarlov E, D'Costa D: Back Attack. Boston: Little, Brown, 1985.
2. Nachemson RA, Mirza AS: Spinal fusion surgery—The case for restraint. N Engl J Med 350(7):722–726, 2004.
3. Apostolides PJ, Jacobowitz R, Sonntag VK: Lumbar discectomy microdiscectomy: "The gold standard." Clin Neurosurg 43:228–238, 1996.
4. Fager CA: Atlas of Spinal Surgery. Philadelphia: Lea & Febiger, 1989.
5. Haglund MM, Moore AJ, Marsh H, Uttley D: Outcome after repeat lumbar microdiscectomy. Br J Neurosurg 9(4):487–495, 1995.
6. Heifertz MD: Lumbar disc herniation: Microsurgical approach. Neurosurgery 52(1):160–164, 2003.
7. Javedan S, Sonntag VK: Lumbar disc herniation: Microsurgical approach. Neurosurgery 52(1):160–164, 2003; & Neurosurgery 53(1):248, 2003.
8. Moore AJ, Chilton JD, Uttley D: Long term results of microlumbar discectomy. Br J Neurosurg 8(3):319–326, 1994.
9. Roberts MP: Lumbar disk herniation: Standard approach. Neurosurg Clin N Am 4:91–99, 1993.
10. Boden SD, Auris DO, Dina TS, et al: Abnormal; magnetic resonance scans of lumbar spine in asymptomatic patients. J Bone Joint Surg Am 72:430–408, 1990.
11. Robertson T: The rape of the spine. Surg Neurol 39:5–12, 1993.
12. Bavinski G, Schoeggl A, Trattnig S, et al: Microsurgical management of postoperative disc space infection. Neurosurg Rev 26(2):102–107, 2003.
13. Henriksen L, Schmidt K, Eskesen V, Jantzen E: A controlled study of microsurgical versus standard lumbar discectomy. Br J Neurosurg 10(3):289–293, 1996.
14. Khoo LT, Fessler RG: Microendoscopic decompressive laminotomy for the treatment of lumbar stenosis. Neurosurgery 51(Suppl):146–154, 2002.
15. O'Brien MF, Peterson D, Crockard HA: A posterolateral microsurgical approach to extreme-lateral lumbar disc herniation. J Neurosurg 84(6):1077, 1996.
16. Park YK, Kim JH, Chung HS, Suh JK: Microsurgical midline approach for decompression of extraforaminal stenosis in L5-S1. J Neurosurg 98(3 Suppl):264–270, 2003.
17. Perez-Cruet MJ, Foley KT, Isaacs RE, et al: Microendoscopic lumbar discectomy: technical note. Neurosurgery 515(5 Suppl):129–136, 2002.
18. Schoeggl A, Maier H, Saringer W, et al: Outcome after chronic sciatica as the only reason for lumbar microdiscectomy. J Spinal Disord Tech 15(5):414–419, 2002.
19. Tureyen K: One level, one-sided lumbar disc surgery with and without microscopic assistance—One year outcome in 114 consecutive patients. J Neurosurg 99(3 Suppl):247–250, 2003.
20. Watkins RG, Williams LA, Watkins RG III: Microscopic lumbar discectomy results for 60 cases in professional and olympic athletes. Spine J 3(2):100–105, 2003.
21. Hood RS: Far lateral lumbar disc herniation: Standard approach. Neurosurg Clin N Am 4:117–124, 1993.
22. Viswanathan R, Swamy NK, Tobler WD, et al: Extraforaminal lumbar disc herniations: Microsurgical anatomy and surgical approach. J Neurosurg 96(2 Suppl):206–211, 2003.
23. Schlesinger SM, Fannhauser H, de Tribolet N: Microsurgical anatomy and operative techniques for extreme lateral lumbar disc herniation. Acta Neurochir 118:117–129, 1992.
24. Silvers HR, Lewis PJ, Asch HL, et al: Lumvar diskectomy for recurrent disk herniation. J Spinal Disord 7(5):408–419, 1994.
25. Schoeggl A, Reddy M, Matula F: Functional and economic outcome following microdiscectomy for lumbar disc herniation in 672 patients. J Spinal Disord Tech 16(2):105, 2003.
26. Tarlov E (ed.): Complications of Spinal Surgery. Chicago: American Association of Neurological Surgeons, 1991.
27. Kothbauer KF, Seiler RW: Transdural cauda equina incarceration after microsurgical lumbar discectomy: Case report. Neurosurgery 47(6):1449–1451, 2000.
28. Geh R, Zanetti M, Boos N: Subacute subdural haematoma complicating lumbar microdiscectomy. J Bone Joint Surg Br 82(7):1042–1045, 2000.

29. Shaikh S, Chung F, Imarengiaey C, et al: Pain, nausea, vomiting and ocular complications delay discharge following ambulatory microdiscectomy. Can J Anaesth 50(5):514–518, 2003.

30. Lundin A, Magnuson A, Axelsson K, et al: The effect of perioperative corticosteroids on the outcome of microscopic lumbar disc surgery. Eur Spine J 12(6):625–630, 2003.

31. Mack PF, Hass D, Lavyne MH, et al: Postoperative narcotic requirement after microscopic lumbar discectomy is not affected by intraoperative ketorolac or bupivacaine. Spine 26(6):658–661, 2001.

32. Turner JA, Ersek M, Herron L, et al: Patients outcome after lumbar spinal fusions. JAMA 268:907–911, 1992.

33. Ware JE: SF-36 Health Survey Manual and Interpretation Guide. Boston: The Health Institute, New England Medical Center, 1993.

34. Tarlov AR: Shattuck Lecture: The increasing supply of physicians, the changing structure of the health services system and the future practice of medicine. N Engl J Med 308:1235–1244, 1983.

35. Tarlov AR, Ware JE, Greenfield S, et al: The Medical Outcome Study: An application of methods for monitoring the results of medical care. JAMA 262:925–930, 1989.

36. Stewart AR: Measuring Function and Well Being: The Medical Outcome Study Approach. Durham, NC: Duke University Press, 1992.

148

Far Lateral Lumbar Disc Herniations: Diagnosis and Surgical Management

NANCY E. EPSTEIN and JOSEPH A. EPSTEIN

Far lateral disc herniations (FLDs) comprise between 6.5% and 12% of lumbar disc herniations.[1–6] The resection of FLDs can be accomplished using laminotomy, hemilaminectomy, laminectomy, or endoscopic discectomy techniques (Figs 148-1 to 148-9). The extent of facet resection is quantitated by the extent of accompanying stenosis and the location of the disc herniation. Either medial facetectomy with foraminotomy or the intertransverse approach may be used primarily in younger patients without significant attendant stenosis. Minimally invasive endoscopic techniques typically involve significant disruption of the ipsilateral facet joint and are often performed with posterior lumbar interbody fusion and pedicle-screw instrumentation placed either openly or percutaneously. Where patients have significant stenosis in conjunction with an FLD, a full facetectomy with laminectomy may be accompanied by an instrumented lumbar fusion. Additionally, older individuals may also be managed with simultaneous in situ fusions. The extreme lateral approach performed either "open" or endoscopically can be used without removing a significant amount of bone, avoiding the need for simultaneous fusion.

Compromising pathology can include far lateral stenosis associated with degenerative spondylolisthesis, degenerative scoliosis, or limbus vertebral fractures. The extent and type of facet resection required for decompression should be measured by the individual patient's pathology, and no single technique is universally appropriate.[3] Clinical, neurodiagnostic, surgical alternatives, and outcomes (Medical Outcomes Trust Short Form 36 [SF-36] questionnaire) in patients undergoing FLD surgery are reviewed.

MATERIALS AND METHODS

Anatomy

Microdissection of more than 200 spines in cadavers by Schlesinger and colleagues revealed that with caudal movement in the lumbar spine, the bony structures increasingly overlay the intervertebral foramen, resulting in less available space in the lateral and subarticular recesses (see Fig. 148-9).[7] Hence, progressively more bone removal is required from the medial pars interarticularis and portions of the superior facet joint inferiorly at lower lumbar levels to adequately expose the nerve root and ganglion. Typically, at the L5 and S1 level, where the interpedicular diameter is widest, almost no facet removal is required to expose the superiorly exiting nerve root as it extends into the foramen.

Cadaveric studies of the lumbar spine, using sagittal sections as well as biomechanical assessment, document that the foramen contains four distinct ligaments.[8] These four "bands" extend radially from the nerve root sleeve. The first attaches posteriorly to the overlying facet capsule, while two attach respectively to the superior and inferior pedicles, and the fourth is tethered to the disc annulus anteriorly.

Definition of the Far Lateral Compartment

The superior and inferior pedicles constitute the cephalad and caudad borders of the "far lateral" compartment. The annulus defines the ventral floor, while the superior articular

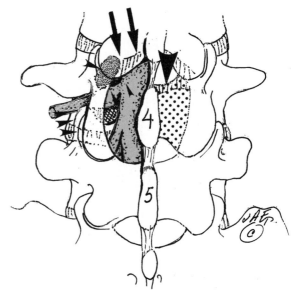

FIGURE 148-1 The intertransverse approach to a far lateral disc is illustrated here on the left at the L4–L5 level. A left-sided hemilaminectomy with a medial facetectomy and foraminotomy are performed both at the cephalad L3–L4 and caudad L4–L5 levels. This affords simultaneous exposure of the exiting L4 and L5 nerve roots, respectively. Note that the midportion of the facet joint is preserved. Extreme lateral exposure is then afforded by removing the lateral-most aspect of the superior articular facet. Once the intertransverse ligament and fascia have been excised, direct visualization of the L4 nerve root far laterally is provided. This exposure is optimal for lateral, foraminal, and FLDs without attendant foraminal stenosis or degenerative olisthy.

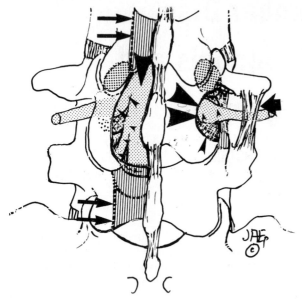

FIGURE 148-2   The intertransverse approach illustrated includes a left-sided L4 hemilaminectomy with L3–L4 and L4–L5 medial facetectomies and foraminotomies providing medial exposure of the intertransverse process (*large arrowhead, large and small double arrows, triple arrows*). A right-sided extreme lateral exposure of the far laterally exiting L4 nerve root at the L4–L5 level (*small double arrows*) is illustrated. Note that resection of the lateral aspect of the inferior and superior L5 articular facets (*large double arrowheads, small single arrowhead*), along with removal of the intertransverse ligament and fascia (*large single arrow*) provide optimal exposure.

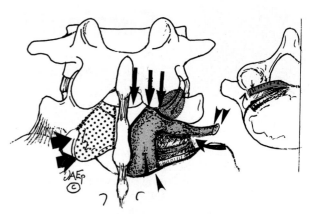

FIGURE 148-4   Full facetectomy for excision of lateral, foraminal, and far lateral type III-B calcified limbus vertebral fracture is illustrated. A right-sided hemilaminectomy with medial facetectomy at the L4–L5 level (*triple arrows*) combined with a full facetectomy at the L5–S1 level provides adequate visualization of the superior, foraminal, and far lateral exiting L5 nerve root (*small double arrows*) as it is tethered over a lateral, foraminal, and far lateral Type III-B calcified limbus vertebral fracture (*curved arrow*). A transaxial view on the right demonstrates the crucial foraminal location of the limbus fracture (*single small arrow*). Also observe the extent of L5 laminar resection illustrated to the far left (*large double arrows*).

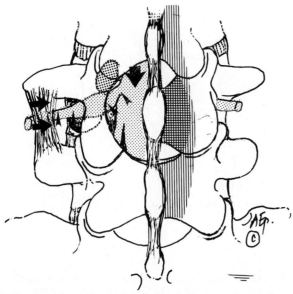

FIGURE 148-3   This illustration of the medial exposure for a far lateral disc excision includes a left-sided hemilaminectomy of L4 followed by medial facetectomy and foraminotomy, exposing the superiorly exiting L4 and inferiorly exiting L5 nerve roots (*large arrow*). Note that the L4 nerve root is also visualized far laterally with partial removal of the intertransverse ligament and fascia and lateral-most aspect of the superior articular facet. On the right side, should significant lateral recess stenosis be present at both the L3–L4 and L4–L5 levels, hemilaminectomies involving the L3, L4, and L5 hemilamina may simultaneously be accomplished.

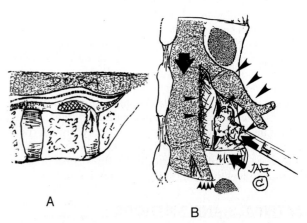

A   B

FIGURE 148-5   Bone removal required for excision of foraminal and far lateral sequestrated disc herniation on the right at the L5–S1 level is illustrated. *A,* On a paramedian sagittal drawing, the sequestrated disc arising from the L5–S1 level has migrated cephalad (*single arrow*) and foraminally into the L5–S1 foraminal and far lateral compartment. *B,* A dorsal view illustrates the thecal sac from the L4–L5 to the L5–S1 level (*large arrow*) following right-sided L4 and L5 hemilaminectomy. Full right-sided facetectomy provides exposure of the L5 nerve root (*large triple arrows*), particularly foraminally as it exits underneath the L5 pedicle. Note how the sequestrated disc fragment (*small triple arrows*) has moved laterally beyond the lateral aspect of the posterior longitudinal ligament (*small double arrows*). A small pituitary rongeur is then introduced to gently excise the free fragment of disc while the attendant limbus vertebral fracture arising from the superior aspect of the sacrum may be excised with a down-biting curet, tamp, and mallet technique (*large double arrows*).

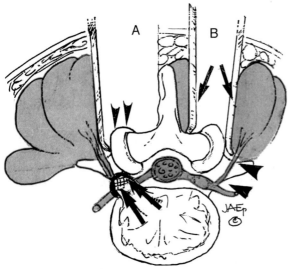

FIGURE 148-6 Median and paramedian muscle-splitting approaches to FLD excision. *A,* The medial exposure for FLD excision. Dissection is carried down the midline, exposing the spinous processes and lamina medially, and the facet joint (*small double arrows*) and transverse processes laterally and far laterally. If a purely far lateral disc is present, the lateral portion of the exposure provides visualization of the nerve root once the intertransverse ligament and fascia are removed, while medial exposure through a laminotomy or hemilaminectomy allows for medial disc excision. *B,* The paramedian muscle-splitting approach (*large long double arrows*) allows more direct exposure of the facet joint and far lateral compartment over the transverse processes for FLD excision (*large double arrowheads*).

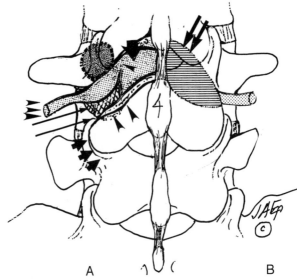

FIGURE 148-8 The transpars technique for the excision of FLDs. *A,* The initial dissection occurs at the disc level superior to the FLD. For example, shown here is a laminotomy that was completed superiorly at the L3 (*large arrow*) and L4 levels (*double small arrows*). This is then succeeded by excision of the pars interarticularis, overlying the L4–L5 neural foramen. This exposure affords direct visualization of the lateral (*small single arrow*), foraminal, and far lateral exiting L4 nerve root (*triple small arrows*). Observe the sequestrated disc selectively underlying the foraminal segment of the nerve root (*long double arrows*). Note that the left-sided L4–L5 facet and its ligamentous attachments are left intact (*large triple arrows*). *B,* On the right side of the diagram, the extent of laminar bone resection required to provide this exposure (*long double arrows*) is demonstrated.

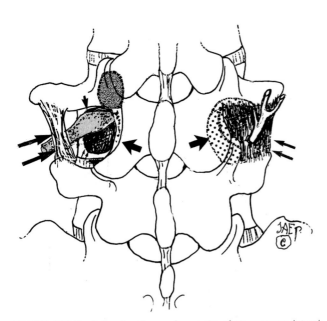

FIGURE 148-7 Following the performance of an extreme lateral exposure (*large arrow*), the left L4 nerve root (*small single arrow*) is seen exiting into the far lateral compartment at the L4–L5 level. Note the continuation of the L4 root beyond residual fibers of the intertransverse ligament and fascia (*double arrows*). On the right, the extent of lateral resection of the superior and inferior L5 articular facets and pars are illustrated (*single arrow*), combined with visualization of the arterial investment of the intertransverse ligament (*double arrows*).

facet with the combined facet joint are found dorsally. Narrowing of the far lateral compartment occurs when underlying degenerative changes related to spondyloarthrosis, degenerative spondylolisthesis, spondylolisthesis with lysis, scoliosis, and limbus vertebral fractures limit available space.

Viswanathan and colleagues further assessed the vasculature of the extraforaminal (EF) compartment in three cadavers.[9] They defined the superolateral location of an arterial arcade supplying the exiting nerve root and, therefore, recommended that dissection be confined to its inferomedial aspect.

Frequency and Location of Far Lateral Discs

Far lateral discs reportedly constitute between 6.5% and 12% of all lumbar herniations and typically include free fragments located superolateral to the disc space of origin.[1,3,10–16] Sequestrated discs located foraminally comprise 3%, while those extending both intra- and extraforaminally include 4% of all FLDs.[17] FLDs compress the superiorly exiting nerve root and its dorsal root ganglion, producing deficits referable to the involved nerve roots. A far lateral lesion at L3–L4 contributes to L3 root compromise, while far lateral pathology at the L4–L5 and L5–S1 levels contribute to L4 and L5 root signs.

The majority of FLDs occur at the L3–L4 or L4–L5 levels, typically followed by L5–S1 (see references 2–4, 11, 14). More cephalad involvement at L1–L2 and L2–L3 is usually

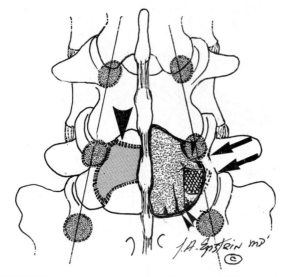

FIGURE 148-9 Progressive caudal divergence of the pedicles in the lumbar spinal canal results in increasingly greater dorsal compromise of the far lateral compartment by overlying facet joints. Anatomically, this results in the need for increasing lateral excision of the superior and inferior articular facets, plus progressive shaving of the lateral portion of the pars interarticularis. On the left of the figure illustrated here, a left L5 hemilaminectomy is shown (*large arrow*). On the right, laminar removal combined with medial facetectomy and foraminotomy at both the L4–L5 and L5–S1 levels has afforded adequate visualization of the laterally and foraminally exiting L5 (*large double arrows*) and S1 roots, respectively (*small double arrows*). Because the interpedicular distance at L5–S1 is wide, often medial facetectomy alone suffices for lateral and foraminal disc exposure. However, if there is a truly far laterally extruded disc and/or ossified component of a limbus vertebral fracture, greater excision of the lateral aspect of the facet joint and pars may be warranted because the facet overlies a greater extent of the far lateral compartment at this level.

rare, except where reported by An and co-workers with a 28% frequency.[10] In Porchet and colleagues' series of 202 patients undergoing microsurgical resection of foraminal and far lateral disc herniations, frequency was reported as: L1–L2 (1 patient), L2–L3 (9 patients), L3–L4 (48 patients), L4–L5 (86 patients), and L5–S1 (58 patients).[1]

Clinical and Neurologic Parameters

Patients presenting with FLDs are often in their mid-fifties, with a range from 19 to 78 years of age, with the ratio of males to females varying from 1:1 to 2:1 (see references 1–3, 10). Severe radicular pain usually results when the dorsal nerve root ganglion becomes compressed and inflamed in the far lateral compartment. This pain is often excruciating and unremitting, while the degree of back pain is minimal. Those compromising the femoral nerve L2–L4 roots complain of pain radiating into the hip, thigh, and medial aspect of the calf. Signs include a positive reverse Laségue maneuver (femoral stretch test), iliopsoas and/or quadriceps weakness, a diminished or absent patellar response, and appropriate dermatomal sensory loss. The more proximal location of complaints requires differentiation from intrinsic hip and/or knee pathology. Radiologic and magnetic resonance imaging (MRI) studies may identify intrinsic hip or knee disease, while arterial Doppler tests may help define whether claudication is present.

As an example, an FLD at the L4–L5 interspace compressing the L4 nerve root will typically result in a positive femoral stretch test, weakness involving the tibial anticus and the extensor hallicus longus, a diminished Achilles response, and decreased pin appreciation in the L4 distribution.

OTHER PATHOLOGY CONTRIBUTING TO FAR LATERAL ROOT COMPROMISE

Limbus Vertebral Fractures

Fractures of the vertebral limbus with or without lateral, foraminal or far lateral stenosis and/or disc herniation may contribute to nerve root compression.[18,19] Limbus vertebral fractures occur in four types (I–IV): Type I consists of a cortical rim separation that extends across the full width of the disc space resulting in central and foraminal stenosis; type II includes both cortical and cancellous elements with predominant midline intrusion on the thecal sac; type III fractures are often found foraminally or far laterally, may be noncalcified-cartilaginous (III-A) or ossified elements (III-B); type IV fractures involve the full sagittal length of the vertebral body, from one disc space to the next, and are often located centrally resulting in significant thecal sac as well as nerve root compromise. Any of these fractures may arise from the cephalad or caudad vertebral end plate.

Removal of limbus vertebral fractures located foraminally or far laterally often necessitates a full facetectomy to adequately expose the nerve root over its entire course.[18] Resection warrants removal of the annulus from within the interspace, and subsequent delivery of the ossified limbus fracture into the previously created cavity with a down-biting curet, tamp, and mallet fragmenting technique. Exposure for this type of decompression and resection may also be accomplished using microscopic endoscopic approaches with simultaneous fusion combining posterior lumbar interbody fusion and percutaneous pedicle screw instrumentation techniques.

Stenosis and Spondylosis

Lumbar spinal stenosis and FLDs may coexist.[8,12,19] Significant simultaneous stenosis, demonstrated in 72% of older patients using myelogram–computed tomography (myelo-CT) studies, requires more extensive surgical decompression.[2] An and colleagues similarly noted that 50 patients with FLDs and stenosis also required more extended decompressions.[10] Epstein reported on 857 patients undergoing surgery for lumbar stenosis; 40 patients demonstrated FLDs and 5 far lateral stenosis.[12,13,19]

The surgical resection of FLDs is complicated by spondylostenosis with foreshortened, vertically oriented pedicles, thickened lamina, massive facet arthrosis, and varying degrees of olisthy accompanying other degenerative changes. Whereas a laminotomy or hemilaminectomy with medial facetectomy may suffice for decompression where stenosis is minimal, particularly at the L5–S1 level, multilevel laminectomy with the intertransverse approach or full facetectomy may be warranted to address more complex pathology. Intraoperative localization of the appropriate level, before endangering the facet joint, is critical and often requires an initial x-ray film locating the correct interspinous ligament and a second radiogram with a Penfield elevator placed at the involved interspace. Where more extensive facet resection is necessary, simultaneous fusion may be required.

Degenerative Spondylolisthesis

Grade I degenerative spondylolisthesis or olisthy is most often encountered at L4–L5, followed in descending order of frequency at the L3–L4, L2–L3, and L5–S1 levels.[15,16,20] Grade I olisthy is defined as a slip representing 25% of the vertebral body width and is usually limited by locking of sagittally oriented, hypertrophied posterior facet joints.[20] Disc herniations are encountered 4.3% to 20% of the time in conjunction with degenerative spondylolisthesis.

FLDs occurring at the level of a slip require a full unilateral facetectomy with instrumented fusion to avoid progressive instability in patients younger than 65 years of age, while those over the age of 65 may be managed successfully with in situ posterolateral intertransverse fusion.[3,15] Good-to-excellent results are cited in up to 80% of patients.

Spondylolisthesis with Spondylolysis

When spondylolysis accompanies spondylolisthesis, the exiting nerve root is already maximally compressed beneath the mobile and interrupted pars interarticularis. Here, safe removal of an extruded or sequestrated disc fragment requires exposure of the nerve root along its entire intracanalicular, foraminal, and extreme lateral course. Many of these patients require simultaneous instrumented fusions, by either open pedicle screw-rod constructs or endoscopic posterior lumbar interbody fusions with percutaneous application of instrumentation. Good-to-excellent outcomes are typically reported in 80% to 85% of cases.[16]

Degenerative Scoliosis

Geriatric patients (>65 years of age) may exhibit far lateral compressive root syndromes attributed to degenerative scoliosis confirmed on both MRI and CT studies. In these patients, accompanying rotational and conformational deformities exaggerate the extent of foraminal root compression usually in the concavity of the curve. Whereas far lateral lesions may respond to unilateral decompression alone, unless spontaneous intervertebral fusion is demonstrated, an accompanying bilateral fusion should be performed.

NEURODIAGNOSTIC EVALUATIONS

Magnetic Resonance Imaging

On MRI studies, far lateral soft disc herniations are located lateral to the pedicles and appear isointense or hypointense. Obliteration of the normally hypointense fat pad surrounding the dorsal root ganglion may signal the presence of an FLD. Transaxial and parasagittal MRI studies provide transverse and longitudinal evidence of foraminal and far lateral nerve root compression (Figs 148-10 to 148-12). CT will more readily document bony or ossified pathology, providing a direct hyperdense image, rather than the hypointense signal seen on MRI.

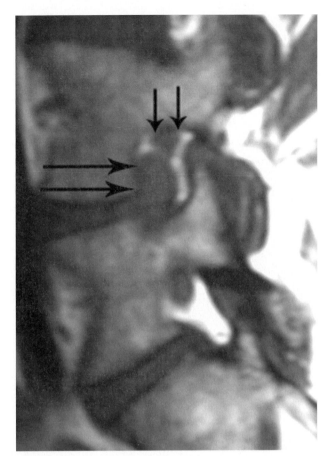

FIGURE 148-10 The paramedian sagittal right-sided T1-weighted MRI scan at the L4–L5 level demonstrates a foraminal and far lateral disc herniation at the L4–L5 level (*single long arrows*). Marked compression of the exiting L4 root can readily be visualized in the foramen (*double short arrows*).

Gadolinium DTPA (diethylenetriamine-pentaacetic acid)-enhanced MRI helps to differentiate FLDs from other enhancing neoplasms.[21] Postoperative enhanced MRI scans may distinguish between scar formation (enhancing) and recurrent disc herniations (nonenhancing).[22]

Computed Tomography and Myelogram–Computed Tomography Scans

Computed tomography studies, with multiplanar reformations (2-dimensional–3-dimensional) or enhanced with iodine-based dyes, help establish the diagnosis of FLDs with attendant far lateral pathology (Figs 148-13 to 148-16).[5,21] FLDs appear isodense. Anatomic abnormalities secondary to limbus vertebral fractures, facet arthropathy, olisthy, and scoliosis appear hyperdense on CT-based studies. Additional intrathecal contrast better defines central, lateral, and proximal foraminal stenosis, since beyond the foramen, the root is no longer invested with a subarachnoid space. Myelo-CT studies, providing better definition of the extent of the stenosis, may significantly influence operative procedures performed in the elderly.[2] CT discography may facilitate the demonstration of a far lateral lesion by revealing extravasation of dye far laterally.

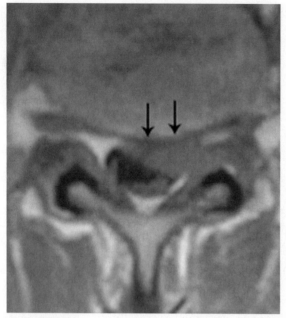

FIGURE 148-11 On this transaxial T1-weighted left-sided MRI study obtained at the L4–L5 level, a lateral and foraminal disc herniation (*double arrows*) is readily visualized. Note, on the right side the foraminal L4 nerve root is clearly visualized, surrounded by hypointense fat, while on the left side the foraminal nerve root appears swollen and compromised by disc material extending to and through the neural foramen.

CONSERVATIVE MANAGEMENT

The efficacy of conservative management in patients with FLDs, utilizing steroidal and nonsteroidal medications, epidural steroid injections, and physiotherapy, remains controversial. In Rust and Olivero's series of 17 patients, symptoms resolved in 12 (71%) patients without surgery.[23] Transforaminal injections of local anesthesia and depo-steroids provided immediate relief in 27 of 30 of Weiner and Fraser's patients, and long-term relief in 22 of 28 patients; only 3 subsequently required surgery.[24] In contrast, other studies reveal that only 10% of patients with FLDs can be successfully managed without surgery.[3,4] The greater the pain syndrome and the more severe the neurologic signs, the more likely patients will be offered and accept surgery as a course of management.

CRITICAL ADJUNCTS TO FAR LATERAL DISC SURGERY

Utility of Corticosteroids and Bupivacaine Hydrochloride

Performing a randomized, controlled trial, Mirzai and colleagues documented the efficacy of administering both corticosteroids preoperatively and bupivacaine intraoperatively during lumbar disc surgery.[25] The antiinflammatory mechanism of the steroids includes the inhibition of phospholipase A2, which plays an important role in alleviating pain production. Before the incision, the skin was infiltrated with 10 mL of 1% lidocaine with 1:200,000 epinephrine. At the time of wound closure, an additional 20 mL of 0.9% saline was given to the patients in group I (22 patients) and 20 mL of 0.25% bupivacaine to those in group II (22 patients). Postoperative pain medications were markedly reduced for the first 12 hours for those receiving the bupivacaine, while no significant differences were observed in heart rate or blood pressure.

DIFFERENT FACET RESECTION TECHNIQUES

Medial Facetectomy

Excision of the medial 25% of the facet joint in conjunction with a laminotomy or hemilaminectomy may allow for

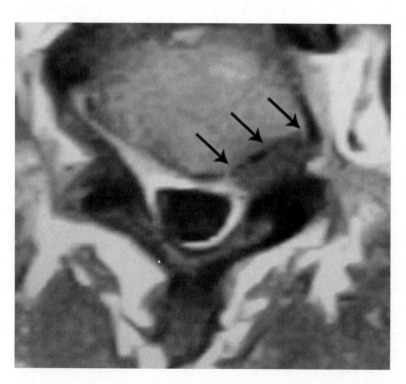

FIGURE 148-12 On this transaxial T1-weighted MRI study obtained at the L5–S1 level, a left-sided foraminal disc herniation (*triple arrows*) is seen focally compressing the L5 nerve root. Note the anomalous configuration of this transitional L5–S1 level.

FIGURE 148-13 This parasagittal 3-dimensional CT study reveals marked foraminal compromise and grade I olisthy at the L4–L5 level (*single arrows*). Note how narrowed this foramen is compared with the cephalad L3–L4 and L2–L3 foramina (*double arrows*).

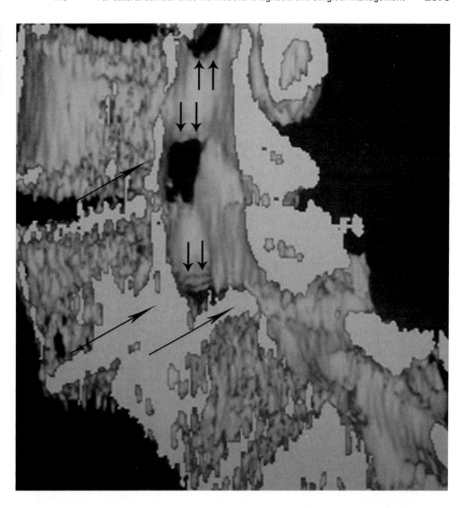

resection of a proximal foraminal FLD at the L5–S1 level (see Fig. 148-3). However, only limited foraminal exposure would be provided by this degree of facet removal, particularly where coexistent degenerative changes are present. Furthermore, the blind passage of angulated down-biting curets or Woodson dissectors into the foramen and far lateral compartment with limited facet removal may inadvertently damage the foraminal nerve root.

Full Facetectomy

Any type of far lateral stenosis, whether attributable to spondylosis, degenerative spondylolisthesis, spondylolisthesis with lysis, scoliosis, or limbus fractures, may require a complete facetectomy to achieve sufficient exposure of the far lateral compartment (see Figs 148-4 and 148-5). The full facetectomy, the procedure most familiar to surgeons, and the one offering the most complete visualization of the nerve root along its entire course, is associated with the lowest incidence of inadvertent root injury and of retained disc fragments. Even radiographically documented instability is relatively rare. In only 1 of 41 of Garrido and Connaughton's patients undergoing FLD surgery including full facetectomy was fusion necessary.[5] In Epstein's initial series, only 1 of 60 patients with FLDs required a fusion.[2] Only 4 of 170 subsequent patients with FLDs required fusions, and all 4 demonstrated grade I olisthy at the L4–L5

level, the level of their far lateral herniations.[3] This rarely occurs at the L5–S1 level, where the iliotransverse ligament provides excellent support if the L5 vertebra is located below the intercrestal line.

Transpars Technique

The transpars approach to FLDs is fraught with numerous deterrents (see Fig. 148-8). First, it requires that the far laterally exiting nerve root be isolated utilizing a laminotomy at the superior interspace. Second, it has to be followed laterally extending below the superior pedicle, thus requiring sacrifice of the pars interarticularis. Third, it is followed foraminally and far laterally by removing the entire inferior articular facet. Major disadvantages of this approach include the lack of access to the disc medially, increasing the chances of recurrent or residual disc herniation, while disrupting the pars and facet joint, and increasing instability. Of the 170 patients undergoing FLD surgery in the author's series, this approach was employed only once.[3]

Isolated Extraforaminal (Extreme Lateral) Approach

The extreme lateral or EF exposure, utilizing midline or paramedian muscle-splitting approaches, directly exposes the far lateral compartment (see Figs 148-6 and 148-7).[5,17,26]

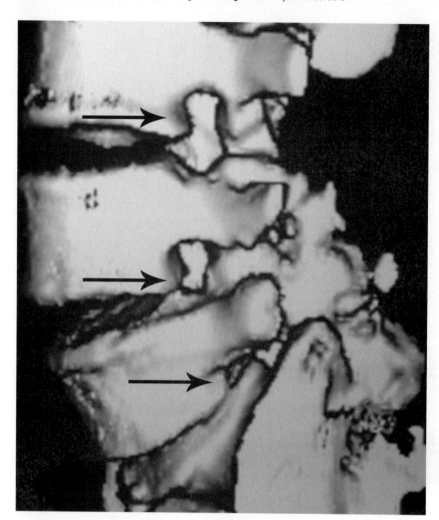

FIGURE 148-14 This oblique left-sided 3-dimensional CT study shows the neural foramina (*arrows*) and far lateral compartments at multiple lumbar levels from L3–L4 through L5–S1. Note that the foramen boundaries include the superior and inferior pedicles, the ventral disc annulus, and dorsal superior articular facet.

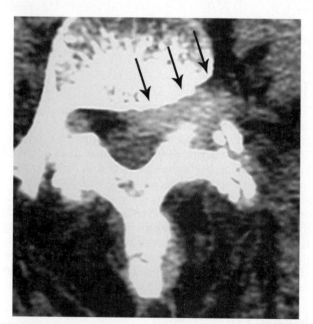

FIGURE 148-15 This noncontrast transaxial CT study at the L4–L5 level reveals marked left-sided lateral, foraminal, and far lateral compromise of the exiting L4 nerve root attributed to the combination of disc herniation, degenerative grade I olisthy, and significant rotational deformity (scoliosis) (*triple arrows*). A full unilateral facetectomy with instrumented L4–L5 fusion was required.

Excising the intertransverse ligament and fascia exposes the cephalad nerve root exiting along a diagonal superomedial to inferolateral course. One risk of the EF exposure is potential injury to the iliolumbar artery, which may be identified on preoperative MRI studies, particularly if enlarged and located near the disc space.[27]

The EF technique is chosen where pathology is confined to the far lateral compartment.[17] Darden and co-workers excised 25 FLDs using the muscle-splitting approach.[28] Two years postoperatively, 48% of patients exhibited excellent, 32% good, and 20% fair or poor results. Notably, low back pain and persistent dysesthesias remained the major complaints, conditions that could not be radiographically correlated with evidence of instability. Pain relief was achieved in 85% of Siebner and Faulhauer's 40 patients undergoing EF resection of far lateral lesions.[17] Their success was attributed to the preservation of stability offered by the limited bony decompression and facet excision. Performing a microsurgical far lateral approach to foraminal and EF lesions, Porchet and colleagues determined that in 202 cases, outcomes using the MacNab classification were excellent (31%), good (42%), fair (20%), and poor (7%).[1] In Hodges and colleagues' study of 25 patients using extreme lateral approaches to FLDs without any medial bone resection, postoperative neuropathic pain typically resolved over a 4- to 6-week period, while Visual Analog

FIGURE 148-16 Marked central, lateral, and foraminal stenosis is present at the L4–L5 level secondary to ossification of the yellow ligament (OYL) (*triple arrows*). OYL typically begins foraminally at the margin of the capsular ligament, extends medially through the neural foramen into the lateral recess, and finally approximates the midline. This noncontrast transaxial CT study demonstrates OYL compromise at the L4–L5 level.

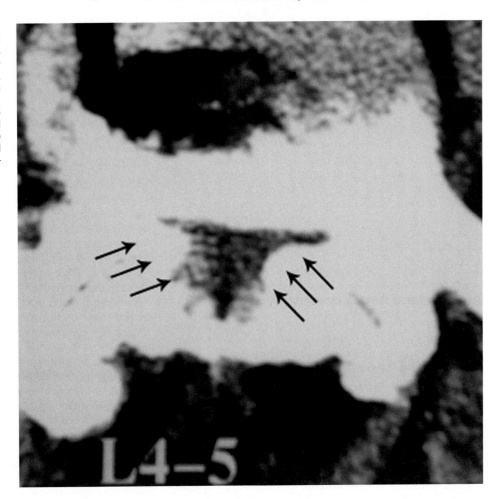

Pain Scale scores were 7.7 and 4.2, respectively, the mean postoperative Oswestry scores being 50.7% and 34.7% (see reference 29).

For patients who have had previous surgery, the isolated EF exposure provides access to the far lateral lesion while avoiding epidural scarring. However, limitations of this technique include a higher recurrent disc herniation rate, since the disc space is not evacuated medially, and the lack of access to foraminal and intracanalicular changes including spondyloarthrotic pathology. In the study of Porchet and colleagues, 11 of 202 FLDs excised extraforaminally recurred, 4 in the same extreme lateral location, 5 paramedially, and 2 contralaterally.[1]

Intertransverse Technique: Medial Facetectomy–Extraforaminal Exposure

The intertransverse (ITT) exposure combines the medial facetectomy with the extreme lateral approach (see Figs 148-1 and 148-2).[30] Medially, the thecal sac and proximally exiting nerve root are exposed, allowing for evacuation of disc and decompression of lateral recess stenosis. The pars interarticularis and the midportion of the facet joint are preserved. The EF exposure includes removal of the lateral-most aspect of the superior articular facet.

Advantages of the ITT procedure include simultaneous medial and far lateral exposure, limiting the risk of disc recurrence or an exacerbation of postoperative symptoms attributable to lateral recess compromise.[30,31] The extent of facet resection required to perform the ITT procedure raises concerns regarding the concurrent need for stabilization; some studies have demonstrated that the risk of instability was not significantly altered by the varying degrees of facet resection—under 50% (group I), 50% to 75% (group II), and 76% to 100% (group III).[31]

Endoscopic Techniques

Transforaminal arthroscopic and endoscopic techniques are employed for foraminal and far lateral disc excision. Kambin and co-workers observed an 82% success rate with limited causalgias in 40 patients with lateral recess stenosis and sequestrated foraminal disc herniations undergoing posterolateral arthroscopic procedures.[32] Ditsworth utilized a transforaminal endoscopic approach in 100 of 533 patients with FLDs and found that 91% of these procedures were successful.[33] Guidable endoscopes extended transforaminally allowed for excision of sequestrated fragments.

Lew and colleagues utilized a transforaminal percutaneous endoscopic discectomy technique for the resection of foraminal and far lateral disc herniations.[6] Excellent to good outcomes were attained in 85% of these 47 patients an average of 18 months postoperatively, and 90% returned to work. However, 11% of patients required second open procedures to address residual pathology at the same levels.

Ditsworth additionally performed 110 transforaminal endoscopic procedures over a 6-year period.[33] With a 2-year minimum follow-up, MacNab's criteria showed an excellent-to-good postoperative outcome in 95%.

Employing a posterolateral endoscopic technique, Yeung and Tsou evaluated 307 patients undergoing routine lumbar disc excision, with or without far lateral disc excisions.[34] Notably, utilizing MacNab's criteria, good-to-excellent results were obtained in 89.3% of patients, while poor outcomes were noted in only 10.7%. Major and minor complications were observed in 3.5% of individuals; results were comparable to open procedures.

Anterolateral Retroperitoneal Approach

Anterolateral retroperitoneal approaches to far lateral lumbar disc herniations commence with a left-sided incision above the 12th rib, followed by retroperitoneal dissection, retraction of soft tissues and the psoas muscle, and exposure at the appropriate level. Accompanying anterior lumbar interbody fusion may be completed with titanium cages or allograft bone dowels. If the procedure is performed laparoscopically, less perineural and peridural scar formation occurs, while offering the advantage of undisturbed posterior elements. Disadvantages include the morbidity of the transabdominal, retroperitoneal, or laparoscopic approaches, the risk of an anterior meningocele, and poor visualization of the medial portion of the nerve root thereby risking root damage, and/or a retained or recurrent disc fragment.

Utilizing the lateral retroperitoneal approach, 171 patients had modified anterior interbody fusions while 26 had total disc replacement in Weinhert and Wiechert's study.[35] The average intraoperative blood loss was 100 mL, and pseudoarthrosis occurred in only 5% of patients. Dezawa and co-workers similarly performed retroperitoneal laparoscopic lateral approaches to 22 FLDs in the lumbar region, avoiding damage to the facet joints and posterior elements.[36] They used a powered mechanical lift and flat inflatable retractor to separate the psoas major and quadratus lumborum. This exposure was optimal for L5–S1 lesions or around the conus at L1–L2.

FUSION

Fusion Requirements

The greater the extent of facet resection, the higher the risk of instability. Whereas the EF exposure does not compromise the facet joint, the medial facetectomy excises 25% of the medial facet joint, the ITT approach sacrifices 25% or more of the superolateral facet joint (the amount varies according to level involvement), while the full facetectomy sacrifices the entire inferior articular facet and the medial portion of the superior articular facet. Nevertheless, several studies have shown that full facet resection only rarely results in the need for secondary stabilization.[2,3,5]

Pedicle Fixation

Pedicle screw-rod fixation techniques, particularly for stabilization following full facetectomy for FLD excision carries limited morbidity and should be considered in patients under 65 years of age. Posterior lumbar interbody fusion and percutaneous fusion techniques may also be considered.

Percutaneous Pedicle Screw Fixation Techniques

Khoo and colleagues combined microendoscopic posterior lumbar discectomy, interbody fusion, and percutaneous pedicle screw-rod instrumentation including METRx, Tangent, and Sextant (Sofamor Danek, Memphis, TN) techniques for performing lumbar disc excision whether routine or far lateral in location.[37] Decompressions and constructs were validated in three cadavers at six motion segments and in three living patients.

Foley and Gupta noted that standardized techniques for pedicle screw instrumentation in the lumbar region involved extensive exposures and muscle dissection.[38] The clinical alternative proposed was a new device for percutaneous placement of pedicle screw instrumentation. This was accomplished by developing an extension sleeve that allowed for remote manipulation of a polyaxial screw head and engagement of the screw/locking mechanism. The Sextant device also allowed for a precut contoured rod to be placed between two screw heads percutaneously. Twelve patients (six males and six females, ranging in age from 23 to 68 years) were included in the original study. Ten of these patients had attendant spondylolisthesis, while two had nonunions associated with prior fusions. Single-level fusions were performed in 10 patients (6 at L5–S1, 3 at L4–L5, and 1 at L2–L3), whereas 2 patients had two-level fusions (from L3 to L5 and from L4 to S1). They were followed from 10 to 19 months (mean of 13.8 months). All patients had successful fusions utilizing this technique. The device successfully allowed for pedicle screws and rods to be introduced without disrupting paraspinal tissues.

Resorbable Posterior Interbody Fusion Devices

Lowe and Coe performed 60 instrumentation-assisted posterior transforaminal lumbar interbody fusions employing a resorbable polymer cage combined with autogenous bone graft in patients with degenerative lumbar disease.[39] Outcome studies are still pending. This procedure may prove particularly useful for the excision of FLDs where unilateral facetectomy and fusion are required.

Interbody Fusion Cages

Lumbar fusion can also be attained utilizing interbody fusion cages, placed either anteriorly (laparoscopically for anterior lumbar interbody fusion) or posteriorly (endoscopically for posterior lumbar interbody fusion). However, close evaluation of the results of these procedures reveals significant attendant morbidities. McAfee and colleagues reviewed 20 patients who required reoperations secondary to the placement of interbody fusion cages. They utilized the Bagby and Kuslich

(BAK: Sulzer-Spine Technologies, Minneapolis, MN) and 2-Ray threaded fusion cages (Surgical Dynamics, Norwalk, CT).[40] Of the 20 cages that failed, 8 were anteriorly placed and 12 posteriorly. The average interval between first and second procedures was 32 weeks (range, 1–156 weeks). Failure correlated with inadequate initial annular distraction, utilization of a cage that was too small, cerebrospinal fluid fistula, pseudomeningocele, use of local bone graft rather than iliac crest, anterior insertion too far laterally resulting in symptoms of a far lateral disc, and failure to define the midline during anterior surgery. All 20 patients were re-explored posteriorly at the level of presumed nerve root compression. In four instances, cages had migrated into the spinal canal. Five patients deemed fused on preoperative studies demonstrated pseudarthrosis intraoperatively. Of these, nine patients required posterior fusion with pedicle screw instrumentation.

Further investigation regarding simultaneous implantation of 13-mm, 15-mm, and 17-mm cylindrical interbody fusion cages was evaluated by Wong and colleagues in an Asian population.[41] The feasibility of implanting paired fusion cages into 150 Asian males was based on preoperative MRI assessments. Their analysis included whether paired cages could be implanted from the L3–L4 through the L5–S1 levels without full facetectomy. They determined that without sacrificing the facets, no lumbar segment could accommodate dual cages. With a unilateral facetectomy, only a few select individuals could receive dual cages at any of these levels; most required full bilateral facetectomy for paired-cage placement, significantly affecting stability at each of the involved levels.

Differing morbidities associated with the placement of interbody fusion cages must also be considered. Elias and colleagues evaluated complications in 67 posterior lumbar interbody fusions performed using titanium-threaded cages.[42] Of these patients, 15% (10 patients) developed cerebrospinal fluid fistulas, 25% of patients required transfusions (average blood loss 670 mL), 4.5% experienced minor wound problems, and one patient expired. Patients were hospitalized for an average of 4.25 days. Three months postoperatively, 42% exhibited significant low back pain; in 15% pain persisted over the first postoperative year. One patient sustained a permanent motor deficit accompanied by sexual dysfunction, while 15% exhibited postoperative pseudoarthrosis. Seven additional patients demonstrated lucency around an implant, whereas two showed posterior cage migration. Fourteen patients required additional pedicle screw instrumentation for persistent back pain and instability.

Resorbable Anterior Interbody Fusion Devices

Di Angelo and co-workers performed in vitro biomechanical studies to evaluate the efficacy of anterior stabilization on cage-assisted lumbar interbody fusions in a multilevel human cadaveric spine model.[43] Three spinal procedures were analyzed utilizing harvested bone, bilateral multilevel cages, and cages with bioabsorbable anterior plates. Testing included flexion/extension, lateral bending, and axial rotation movements. Anterior resorbable plating decreased local motion and increased stiffness at the level of stabilization, in theory promoting fusion.

PREOPERATIVE PSYCHOMETRIC TESTING UTILIZED FOR PATIENT SELECTION

Recognizing and establishing the diagnosis of depression should be an integral part of preoperative patient selection for routine and FLD surgery, since it seems to significantly influence postoperative outcome. Kjellby-Wendt and colleagues studied the predictive value of psychometric testing in 50 patients before undergoing routine lumbar disc surgery—14 females and 36 males, averaging 40 years of age.[44] The Back Depression Inventory, the Stat-Trait Anxiety Inventory, and the Visual Analog Pain Scale were used preoperatively, and at 3 and 12 months postoperatively. Two years following surgery, 37 patients were pleased with their outcomes, while 10 were not and 3 could not be located. Those with histories of prior surgery exhibited more depression and were less satisfied with secondary surgical results; they also experienced greater anxiety and postoperative pain. Utilizing a combination of three questionnaires may successfully predict those patients who would be dissatisfied with postoperative results (78%) and those who would be content with postoperative results (76%). The combined three instruments may function as useful prognosticators in selecting optimal surgical candidates.

OUTCOMES OF FAR LATERAL DISC SURGERY

Different success rates have been reported following FLD surgery. An and colleagues observed a combined 92% incidence of good-to-excellent outcomes.[10] Siebner and Deckler, and Darden and colleagues observed an overall 85% rate of good-to-excellent results following EF surgery for FLDs.[17,28] Utilizing the ITT, full facetectomy, and medial facetectomy approaches for FLD excision, the author encountered 79%, 70%, and 68% good-to-excellent outcomes, respectively.[3,4] Porchet and co-workers observed excellent and good scores in 73% of patients undergoing microsurgical foraminal and far lateral disc resections.[1] Utilizing transforaminal percutaneous endoscopic discectomy techniques, Lew and colleagues noted excellent and good responses in 85%, with Ditsworth reporting a 95% success rate.[1,6,33] Hodges and co-workers found mean preoperative and postoperative Oswestry scores were 50.7% and 34.5% (see reference 29).

FAR LATERAL DISC PROCEDURES IN 170 PATIENTS

Clinical Data

Between 1984 and 1994, 170 of the authors' patients had FLD surgery.[3] Patients were followed a mean of 5 years, averaged 55 years of age, and included 112 males and 58 females. The majority had subclinical symptoms for over 2 years, but almost all experienced a subacute or acute exacerbation within 6 months of neurosurgical evaluation.

On preoperative physical examination, patients exhibited atrophy (31 patients) and positive mechanical findings: ipsilateral knee contractures (143 patients), positive femoral stretch tests (reverse Lasegue maneuvers) (145 patients), and positive Laségue maneuvers (159 patients). Motor deficits

(126 patients), reflex abnormalities (167 patients), and radicular sensory abnormalities (135 individuals) were frequently observed. However, evidence of massive central canal compromise and cauda equina syndromes were rarely seen (7 patients).

Preoperative Magnetic Resonance Imaging and Computed Tomography Studies

Both MRI- and CT-based studies were performed before surgery. MRI demonstrated the soft tissue elements and disc material, while CT more clearly identified accompanying spondyloarthrosis, stenosis, scoliosis, and/or limbus vertebral fractures. The L4–L5 level was most frequently involved (68 patients), followed in descending order by L3–L4 (63 patients), L5–S1 (33 patients), L2–L3 (4 patients), and L1–L2 (2 patients). Far lateral stenosis was identified in 30 patients, with 23 showing grade I degenerative spondylolisthesis.

Flexion-Extension Radiographs, Definition of Instability, and Secondary Fusions

Baseline and 3-month postoperative dynamic films were utilized to assess spinal instability. Where greater than 4 mm of active motion was demonstrated or where there was "fish-mouthing" at the involved level, patients were deemed radiographically unstable. In four patients with preoperative grade I olisthy at the L4–L5 level who additionally had full facetectomy performed at L4–L5 for the excision of lateral discs, fusions were secondarily required because instability was confirmed on both 3- and 6-month postoperative dynamic radiographs. The first patient in 1986 was managed with a Hibbs fusion, while the three subsequent patients underwent pedicle screw-rod instrumentation. Currently, patients with olisthy at the level of FLDs have fusions performed primarily utilizing either open or percutaneous techniques.

Surgical Procedures

Lumbar spondyloarthrosis, stenosis, degenerative spondylolisthesis, and scoliosis accompanied FLDs in 36 of 170 patients.[3] Laminectomies and more extensive facet resections were required to address the greater pathology; full facetectomy (58%), the ITT approach (medial facetectomy combined with extreme lateral approach, 25%), and medial facetectomy alone (17%). In 134 patients, less severe stenosis was managed with more restricted facet resections: full facetectomy (38%), medial facetectomy (24%), and intertransversectomy (37%).

Notably, 25 of 170 patients required second procedures, and 6 required third operations, following initial FLD surgery. These additional operations included the removal of recurrent lateral and far lateral discs (15 patients), decompression of recurrent far lateral stenosis (15 patients), and in one instance, resection of a previously undiagnosed neurofibroma.[3] The average interval between first and second operations was 49 months (range of 40 months to 7.5 years).

Outcomes

Surgeon-based outcome assessment utilized Odom's criteria: excellent (no deficit), good (mild residual radiculopathy requiring minimal analgesia), fair (moderate residual radiculopathy or unchanged requiring moderate analgesia), and poor (increased radiculopathy requiring increased analgesia). Excellent outcomes were achieved in 73 patients, good outcomes in 51 patients, fair outcomes in 26 patients, and poor outcomes in 20 patients. The incidence of combined good-to-excellent outcomes was comparable across all three facet resection techniques: 79% for the ITT approach, 70% for the full facetectomy, and 68% for the medial facetectomy.

COMMON ERRORS IN FAR LATERAL DISC SURGERY

Frequent mistakes in FLD surgery include: operating at the wrong level, making an incorrect diagnosis (e.g., diabetic amyotrophy), operating on the wrong side, and improper patient selection (prohibitive comorbidities). Converting to a full facetectomy exposure should be employed in any instance where the anatomy becomes too confusing, and the extent of arthrosis, spondylosis, and olisthy too severe.

OUTCOME STUDY OF FAR LATERAL DISC SURGERY USING SHORT FORM-36

Patient-based outcome measures are increasingly employed to assess surgical outcomes and set standards for operative policy.[13] The Medical Outcomes Trust Short Form (SF-36) is a well-tested, patient-based outcome instrument, which has been successfully employed for over 2 decades in more than 260 medical and surgical settings. It is easily administered in 15 minutes over the telephone or in the office.

The SF-36 measures eight Health Scales reflecting different dimensions of outcome: Physical Function, Role Physical, Bodily Pain, General Health, Vitality, Social Function, Role Emotional, and Mental Health. Thirty-six generic questions are rated on graded scales. From these data, raw scores are calculated for each of the eight Health Scales and are then converted to a transformed scale (0% to 100%) (raw score – lowest possible raw score for that health scale, divided by the raw score range multiplied by 100). Difference scores also take into account patients' normative data based on age and sex obtained from 2474 individuals in the general U.S. population.

The SF-36 was completed by 76 (45%) of 170 patients in our far lateral disc series from 1984 to 1994 (see references 3, 4, 14). One individual performed telephone interviews, and 100% of those contacted successfully completed the questionnaire. The average period between the last visit to the surgeon (the time of the surgeon-based assessment) and the administration of the questionnaire was 2.8 years (standard deviation of 2.3) with a range of 0.6 to 10.2 years. Those completing the outcome questionnaires averaged 60 years of age and included 43 males and 33 females.

Along with the SF-36 patient-based outcome measure, the surgeon's assessment of outcome, employing Odom's critiera, was also obtained. The surgeon, an average of 9.1 months following surgery, last examined 76 patients, and their outcomes were categorized as excellent (32 patients = 42%), good (24 = 31.5%), fair (12 = 16%), and poor (8 = 11%). The median time between the operation and the surgeon's outcome analysis was 4.5 months (average 9.1 months): 75% less than 9 months and 90% less than 22 months). The longest interval between surgery and final clinical assessment was 75 months. There was a statistically nonsignificant correlation (Spearman rank-order of 0.13) between the surgeon's evaluation and the time since surgery, the trend tending toward better outcome ratings for increased time since surgery.

Modest correlation was established between the surgeon's assessment and SF-36 scores. A positive trend indicated a correlation between the patient's and the surgeon's measures except regarding the General Health scale. A significant positive correlation was established between six of the eight SF-36 Health Scales and the surgeon-based assessment. Correlation coefficients using the Spearman rank-order correlation r varied from 0.329 to 0.205 for these six scales; correlation coefficients for General Health and Mental Health were lower (0.088 and 0.160). A difference score was obtained by subtracting the specific age- and sex-matched norm from the patient's SF-36 transformed score. The mean difference score was then obtained by averaging these data across the eight categories.

There was a discrepancy between the patient's self-analysis and the surgeon's evaluation over longer postoperative intervals. A 4.5-year cutoff point was chosen maintaining 75% (56 patients) of patients in the cohort, while providing a reasonable postoperative time frame. Correlations for this shorter period were greater than those established for all 76 patients followed for up to 10 years, varying from 0.187 to 0.378 with all but General Health and Social Function passing statistical significance.

Correlations between the surgeon's assessment and SF-36 responses were modestly positive. For patients seen within the last 4.5 years, the surgeon's assessment was a relatively good predictor of mean SF-36 outcome scores. Physical Function, Role Physical, and Bodily Pain best correlated on a descending scale with the surgeon's assessment of physical function.

Future outcome studies should prospectively require that the surgeon-based outcome measure and SF-36 be administered at each postoperative visit. Critical data assessment should be performed, particularly at 6 months and 2 years postoperatively.

Acknowledgments

I would like to thank the Joseph A. Epstein Neurosurgical Education Foundation for their support of this research and the editorial assistance of Ms. Sherry Grimm.

REFERENCES

1. Porchet F, Chollet-Bornand A, de Tribolet N: Long-term follow up of patients surgically treated by the far-lateral approach for foraminal and extraforaminal lumbar disc herniations. J Neurosurg 90(1 Suppl):59–66, 1999.
2. Epstein NE, Epstein JA, Carras R, Hyman R: Far lateral lumbar disc herniations and associated structural abnormalities. An evaluation in 60 patients of the comparative value of CT, MRI, and myelo-CT in diagnosis and management. Spine 15:534–539, 1990.
3. Epstein NE: Evaluation of varied surgical approaches used in the management of 170 far-lateral lumbar disc herniations: Indications and results. J Neurosurg 83:648–656, 1995.
4. Epstein NE: Review article: Different surgical approaches to far lateral lumbar disc herniations. J Spinal Disord 8:383–394, 1995.
5. Garrido E, Connaughton PN: Unilateral facetectomy approach for lateral lumbar disc herniation. J Neurosurg 76:342–343, 1992.
6. Lew SM, Mehalic TF, Fagone KL: Transforaminal percutaneous endoscopic discectomy in the treatment of far-lateral and foraminal lumbar disc herniations. J Neurosurg 94(2 Suppl):216–220, 2001.
7. Schlesinger SM, Frankhauser H, de Tribolet N: Microsurgical anatomy and operative technique for extreme lateral lumbar disc herniations. Acta Neurochir (Wien) 118:117–129, 1992.
8. Grimes PF, Massie JB, Garfin SH: Anatomic and biomechanical analysis of the lower lumbar foraminal ligaments. Spine 25:2009–2014, 2000.
9. Viswanathan R, Swamy NK, Tobler WE, et al: Extraforaminal lumbar disc herniations: Microsurgical anatomy and surgical approaches. J Neurosurg 96:206–211, 2002.
10. An HS, Vaccaro A, Simeone FA, et al: Herniated lumbar disc in patients over the age of fifty. J Spinal Disord 3:143–146, 1990.
11. Ebeling U, Reulen HJ: Are there typical localizations of lumbar disc herniations? A prospective study. Acta Neurochir (Wien) 117:143–148, 1992.
12. Epstein JA, Epstein NE: Lumbar spondylosis and spinal stenosis. In Wilkins RH, Rengachary SS (eds): Neurosurgery, 2nd edition. New York: McGraw-Hill, 1996, pp 3831–3840.
13. Epstein NE, Epstein JA: Surgery for spinal stenosis. In Wiesel SW, Weinstein JN, Herkowitz H, et al (eds): The Lumbar Spine, 2nd edition. Philadelphia: WB Saunders, 1996: pp 737–757.
14. Epstein NE, Hood DC: A comparison of surgeon's assessment to patient's self-analysis (Short Form 36) after far lateral lumbar disc surgery: An outcome study. Spine 22:2422–2428, 1997.
15. Epstein NE: Decompression in the surgical management of degenerative spondylolisthesis: Advantages of a conservative approach in 290 patients. J Spinal Disord 11:116–122, 1998.
16. Epstein NE: Primary fusion for the management of "unstable" degenerative spondylolisthesis. NeuroOrthopaedics 23:45–52, 1998.
17. Siebner HR, Faulhauer K: Frequency and specific surgical management of far lateral lumbar disc herniations. Acta Neurochir (Wien) 105:124–131, 1990.
18. Epstein NE: Lumbar surgery for 56 limbus fractures, emphasizing non calcified type II lesions. Spine 17:1489–1496, 1992.
19. Epstein NE, Epstein JA: Lumbar decompression for spinal stenosis: Surgical indications and techniques with and without fusion. In Frymoyer JW, Ducker TB, Kostuik JP, Whitecloud TS (eds): The Adult Spine, 2nd edition. Philadelphia–New York: Lippincott-Raven, 1997, pp 2055–2088.
20. Epstein BS, Epstein JA, Jones MD: Degenerative spondylolisthesis with an intact neural arch. Radiol Clin North Am 15:227–239, 1977.
21. Winter DD, Munk PL, Helms CA: CT and MR of lateral disc herniation: Typical appearance and pitfalls of interpretation. Can Assoc Radiol J 40:256–269, 1989.
22. Glickstein MF, Sussman SK: Time-dependent scar enhancement in magnetic resonance imaging of the postoperative lumbar spine. Skeletal Radiol 20:333–337, 1991.
23. Rust MS, Olivero WC: Far lateral disc herniations: The results of conservative management. J Spinal Disord 12:138–140, 1999.
24. Weiner BK, Fraser RD: Foraminal injection for lateral lumbar disc herniation. J Bone Joint Surg Br 79:804–807, 1997.
25. Mirzai H, Tekin I, Alincak H: Perioperative use of corticosteroid and bupivacaine combination in lumbar disc surgery: A randomized controlled trial. Spine 27:343–346, 2002.
26. Wiltse LL, Bateman JG, Hutchinson RH: The paraspinal sacrospinalis-splitting approach to the lumbar spine. J Bone Joint Surg 50A: 919–921, 1960.
27. Harrington JF: Far lateral disc excision at L5–S1 complicated by iliolumbar artery incursion: Case report. Neurosurgery 48:1377–1379, 2001.
28. Darden BV, Wade JF, Alexander R, et al: Far lateral disc herniations treated by microscopic fragment excision. Techniques and results. Spine 20:1500–1505, 1996.
29. Hodges SD, Humphreys SC, Eck JC, et al: The surgical treatment of far lateral L3–L4 and L4–L5 disc herniations. A modified technique and outcomes analysis of 25 patients. Spine 24:1243–1246, 1999.
30. Jane JA, Haworth CS, Broaddus WC: A neurosurgical approach to far-lateral disc herniation. Technical note. J Neurosurg 72: 143–144, 1990.
31. Postacchini F, Cinotti G, Guimna S: Microsurgical excision of lateral lumbar disc herniation through an interlaminar approach. J Bone Joint Surg (Br) 80:201–207, 1998.

32. Kambin P, Casey K, Obrien E, Zhou I: Transforaminal arthroscopic decompression of lateral recess stenosis. J Neurosurg 84:462–471, 1996.

33. Ditsworth DA: Endoscopic transforaminal lumbar discectomy and reconfiguration: A postero-lateral approach into the spinal canal. Surg Neurol 49:588–597, 1998.

34. Yeung AT, Tsou PM: Posterolateral endoscopic excision of lumbar disc herniations. Surgical technique, outcome, and complications in 307 consecutive cases. Spine 27:722–731, 2002.

35. Weinhert K, Wiechert K: Microsugical anterior approaches to the lumbar spine for interbody fusion and total disc replacement. Neurosurgery 51(5 Suppl):159–165, 2002.

36. Dezawa A, Yamane T, Mikami H, et al: Retroperitoneal laparoscopic lateral approach to the lumbar spine: A new approach, technique, and clinical trial. J Spinal Disord 13:138–143, 2000.

37. Khoo LT, Palmer S, Laich DT, et al: Minimally invasive percutaneous lumbar interbody fusion. Neurosurgery 51(5 Suppl):166–171, 2002.

38. Foley KT, Gupta SK: Percutaneous pedicle screw fixation of the lumbar spine: Preliminary clinical results. J Neurosurg 97(1 Suppl): 7–12, 2002.

39. Lowe TG, Coe JD: Resorbable polymer implants in unilateral transforaminal interbody fusion. J Neurosurg 97(4 Suppl):464–467, 2002.

40. McAfee PC, Cunningham BW, Lee GA, et al: Revision strategies for salvaging or improving failed cylindrical cages. Spine 24:2147–2153, 1999.

41. Wong HK, Goh JC, Goh PS: Paired cylindrical interbody cage fit and facetectomy in posterior lumbar interbody fusion in an Asian population. Spine 26:572–577, 2001.

42. Elias WJ, Simmons NE, Kaptain GJ, et al: Complications of posterior lumbar interbody fusion when using a titanium threaded cage device. J Neurosurg 93(1 Suppl):42–45, 2000.

43. Di Angelo DJ, Scifert JL, Kitchel S, et al: Bioabsorbable anterior lumbar plate fixation in conjunction with cage-assisted anterior interbody fusion. J Neurosurg 97(4 Suppl):447–455, 2002.

44. Kjellby-Wendt G, Styf JR, Carlsson SG: The predictive value of psychometric analysis in patients treated by extirpation of lumbar intervertebral disc herniations. J Spinal Disord 12:375–379, 1999.

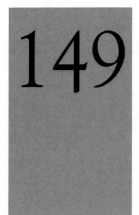

149 Anterior Lumbar Interbody Fusion: Mini-Open Laparotomy Approach

PETER F. ULLRICH, JR.

Anterior lumbar interbody fusion (ALIF) of the lower lumbar segments has become an increasingly popular technique over the last 20 to 25 years.[1–8] The many advances in surgical technique allow the procedure to be done through a small anterior incision with a minimum of postsurgical morbidity.[9,10] Approaching the lumbar spine anteriorly allows for excellent visualization of the entire disc space and, compared with the posterior approach, it allows for a much more complete disc removal and fusion bed preparation. It requires very little soft tissue disruption and little to no disruption of the neural elements.

Other advantages to an ALIF include the following:

- Bone graft and instrumentation is placed at the center of rotation, increasing the rigidity of the construct.[11]
- Lumbar lordosis and sagittal alignment are restored.
- There is a vascular bed for the fusion.
- Bone graft is placed in a favorable healing environment (in compression with little soft tissue competition).[9]
- A large surface area is provided for bone-to-bone contact.
- Foraminal height is restored, leading to indirect nerve root decompression.[12]
- Deformities can be reduced by releasing the anterior column (e.g., reduction of an isthmic spondylolisthesis).[1,4]

The two main disadvantages of the procedure are: (1) In cases requiring posterior decompression and/or fixation a second incision is necessary, and (2) there is a fairly steep learning curve to the approach and the instrumentation. Most spinal surgeons are more comfortable approaching the lumbar disc space posteriorly, and many spine surgeons do not have ready access to an experienced general surgeon (vascular surgeon) to help provide anterior access to the lumbar disc space.

INDICATIONS

Anterior lumbar interbody fusions are effective for:

- Stabilizing painful motion segments (degenerative disc disease).[1,4]
- Providing anterior column support in patients with instability.[1,13]

- Foraminal distraction and indirect decompression of a nerve root.[12]
- Patients who have had multiple disc herniations at the same level.
- Treatment of a posterior lumbar pseudoarthrosis.[1,3,4]

Degenerative Disc Disease

"Stand-alone" ALIFs became popular in the late 1990s after the Food and Drug Administration (FDA) approved the use of threaded titanium cages for the procedure.[6,7] Unfortunately, many of these procedures failed, and although some of the failures were technical, most were due to improper patient selection.[14] The initial FDA-approved criteria for patients receiving a stand-alone ALIF with threaded titanium cages were for disc space desiccation ("black disc") with discogram-confirmed discogenic pain at one or two levels, or for patients with grade I or less spondylolisthesis. The initial indications for ALIF surgery were overly broad and did not account for the failure of anterior cages to adequately stabilize "tall" disc spaces or to provide fixation in patients with posterior instability (e.g., isthmic spondylolisthesis). Many surgeons have now refined the broader indications for a stand-alone ALIF to include only patients with discogenic pain from a collapsed disc space.

In Kuslich's original prospective multicenter study on the use of BAK cages for chronic low back pain, 84% were found to have pain relief at 2-year follow-up.[6] A later study found that these results were maintained at 4-year follow-up.[7] In a retrospective review of 130 of our patients who had had threaded titanium cages used for L5–S1 degenerative disc disease, 86% of commercial insurance patients and 75% of workman's compensation patients had substantial relief of their pain (unpublished data). There was a 3% revision rate (posterior fusion) in this series of patients with between 1 and 7 years of follow-up. These results indicate that at least in patients with L5–S1 degenerative disc disease, stand-alone cages are efficacious and do not necessarily require a posterior stabilization procedure.

Using narrower indications for surgery can improve the clinical outcomes of ALIF for degenerative disc disease. If the disc space is collapsed, the annulus will be stiffer. A lumbar disc that still has a lot of disc height is inherently more mobile, making anterior fixation alone less capable of adequately stabilizing the spine. The cages were designed to act as an interference device and do not provide direct fixation of the disc space. Much of the stabilizing force of an anterior cage is provided by placing tension on the annulus, and in those patients who do not have a collapsed space it is difficult to obtain adequate tension of the annulus. Without preloading the construct with tension on the annulus, there is less rigidity in flexion/extension.[15] Subsidence of the implant can be a problem in tall discs, and if subsidence does occur, the tension effect of the annulus is further compromised, leading to inadequate fixation of the lumbar spine segment.

The ideal candidate for a stand-alone ALIF is a patient with one-level degenerative disc disease, preferably at L5–S1, with a lot of disc space collapse (Figs. 149-1 and 149-2). As a spinal segment, L5–S1 has the least motion of the lumbar segments because it is deep within the pelvis and has the large sacroiliac ligaments running from the transverse process of L5 to the sacral ala. This limits the amount of flexion/extension moment arm across the facet joints posteriorly. L4–L5 is the first segment outside of the pelvis, and the facet joints are more sagittally oriented, allowing for more flexion/extension motion. This increased motion makes it more difficult to fuse this level. Posterior fixation provides a tension bond to limit flexion/extension.

Two levels (e.g., L4–L5 and L5–S1) can be fused but only in patients with a lot of disc space collapse. Likewise, L4–L5 can be fused as a stand-alone ALIF if there is a lot of disc space collapse and no opening of the posterior elements on flexion/extension radiographs.

Determining whether a degenerated disc space is a pain generator or whether it is undergoing a natural degenerative

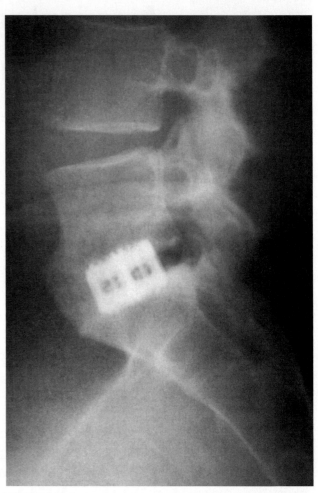

FIGURE 149-2   Lateral radiograph 2 years after an anterior lumbar interbody fusion with a BAK cage (Zimmer). A solid anterior sentinel fusion can be seen anterior to the cage.

(e.g., aging) process is truly an art. There is no universally agreed-upon definition of what actually constitutes degenerative disc disease, and exhaustive review of this topic is beyond the scope of this chapter. However, the patient with only one collapsed disc space and normal segments at all the other levels is likely to have this finding as a result of damage to the disc space. Patients who have multiple levels of collapse can have either degeneration due to a normal aging process or a variant of juvenile disc disorder (formerly known as Scheuermann's disease), where all of the disc spaces are weak. In general, a one-level fusion in an otherwise healthy lumbar spine is much more likely to be successful than a multilevel fusion in a patient with multilevel changes on the magnetic resonance imaging (MRI) scan. A computed tomography (CT) discogram can be useful to determine if a patient's pain is discogenic, although its usefulness is still controversial.[16–20]

Anterior Column Support for Spinal Instability

Anterior column support when treating conditions that are grossly unstable (e.g., isthmic spondylolisthesis) is often desirable[1,4] (Fig. 149-3). It can help as an adjunct to posterior fusion, enhance reduction of the segment, and greatly

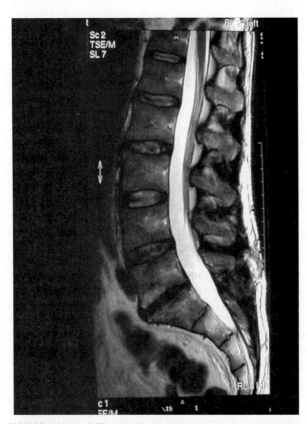

FIGURE 149-1   MRI showing characteristic degenerative changes on T2-weighted sagittal image. Note that the other discs are well preserved.

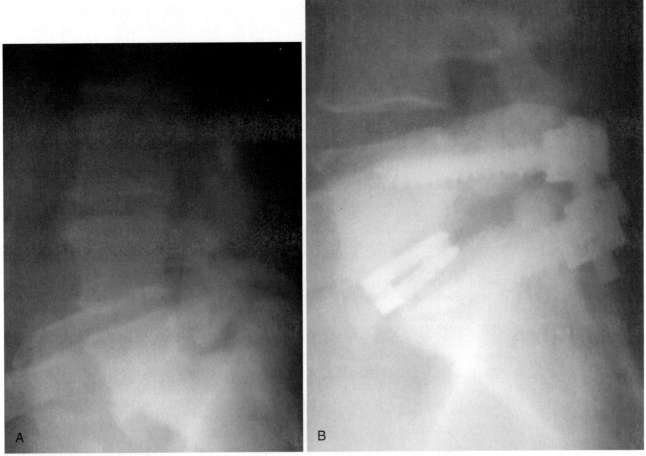

FIGURE 149-3 *A,* Lateral radiograph shows severe disc space collapse and a grade II isthmic spondylolisthesis. *B,* Postoperative radiograph shows excellent reduction of the spondylolisthesis, along with restoration of the disc height and lordosis at the L5–S1 level.

increase the surface area for a bony fusion. Posterior lumbar interbody fusions and transforaminal lumbar interbody fusions can also provide anterior column support, but the ALIF procedure provides for much better preparation of the disc space, a larger implant, and the ability to restore the normal sagittal alignment of the lumbar spine through distraction.

Foraminal Stenosis

Anterior lumbar interbody fusion can also provide needed disc space distraction to open up a foramen.[12] Much as an anterior cervical discectomy and fusion can open up a cervical foramen, the ALIF can provide for the same sort of indirect decompression of an existing nerve root (Fig. 149-4). In patients who have either gross instability (e.g., isthmic spondylolisthesis) or a tall disc space, supplemental posterior fixation should be considered. Stand-alone ALIF can be considered in patients with either a significant amount of disc space collapse and/ or at L5–S1. Any anterior fusion construct relies on putting tension on the annulus to help hold the implant/graft in place. In patients who have a tall disc space and a relatively compliant annulus, this tension cannot be established and there is a tendency for the annulus to loosen with time. In a collapsed disc space with a very stiff annulus, adequate tension can often be obtained and the implant will be stable without added posterior fixation.

Recurrent Lumbar Disc Herniations

Anterior lumbar interbody fusions can be useful to prevent recurrent lumbar disc herniations, since the majority of the nucleus pulposus is removed during the procedure. At the time of surgery an attempt can be made to remove a recurrent disc herniation through the anterior approach, although unfortunately a posterior approach for a revision may be necessary if the fragment cannot be reached anteriorly.

Pseudoarthrosis

In cases with posterior fusion complicated by a pseudoarthrosis, anterior fusion provides an anterior column support and a large well-vascularized fusion area. It has been shown to be effective as a salvage procedure,[1,4,5] and carries the benefit of not having to approach the spine through a scarred and fibrosed environment.

CONTRAINDICATIONS

Anterior lumbar interbody fusion procedures are not recommended for those individuals who have osteoporosis. The stability is compromised if the anterior intervertebral subchondral bone is not strong enough to withstand axial loads. Generally, patients older than 60 are not good candidates,

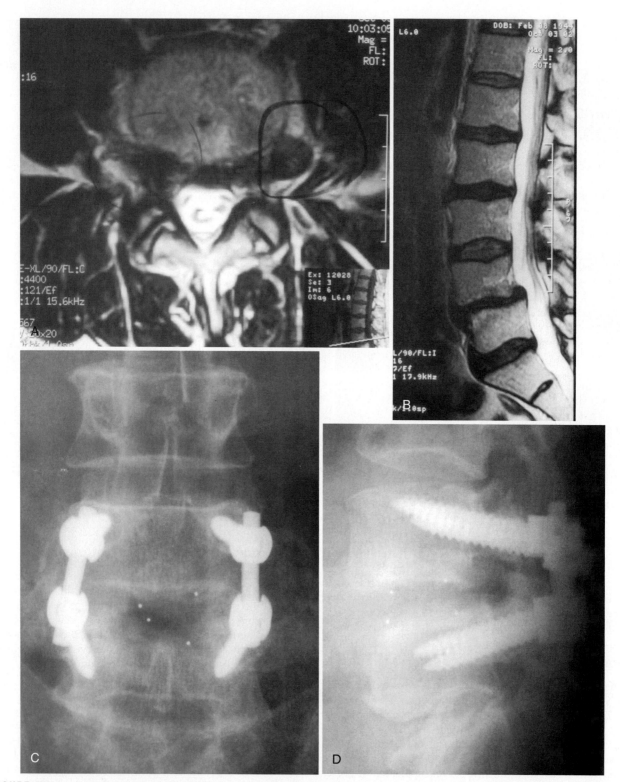

FIGURE 149-4 *A* and *B,* Axial and sagittal MRI scans show L4–L5 isthmic spondylolisthesis showing bilateral foraminal stenosis. *C* and *D,* Postoperative radiographs show excellent foraminal distraction and restoration of the normal lordosis.

and if there is any question about the strength of the bone, a preoperative dual-energy x-ray absorptiometry scan can help quantify the amount of preoperative osteoporosis.

Other relative contraindications include patients with active discitis or osteomyelitis, significant atherosclerosis or abdominal aneurysms, prior radiation treatment to abdomen/pelvis, or morbid obesity.[5] Patients who have had

prior abdominal or pelvic surgery can usually still undergo approach through a mini-open laparotomy exposure. Revision lumbar surgery after a previous retroperitoneal exposure can be difficult, especially within the first several months after the procedure, because the retroperitoneal plane fibroses down, eliminating a clear dissection plane. Eventually, the fibrosis remodels and loosens, and patients with a remote history of an anterior exposure are generally easier to approach than those who have had a recent retroperitoneal dissection. Fibrosis is not a problem within the first 2 to 3 weeks after surgery, so if a revision is likely to be needed, it is much easier to do it immediately.

TECHNIQUE

The mini-open technique for retroperitoneal exposure of the lower lumbar disc segments has been well described in the past by David Selby[9] and Robert Henderson.[10] This chapter provides some practical revisions to the technique, but this is a technique that has stood the test of time. There have been reports of laparoscopic approaches, but they are generally technically more challenging and do not significantly lessen the morbidity of the procedure. They also carry a potentially higher risk of intraoperative complications.[21–26]

In my personal experience, after performing approximately 750 anterior cases, all with the same general surgeon, this is a very reproducible technique that carries a minimum of morbidity. In general, these procedures take between 30 and 60 minutes, and it has been years since we have had a major vessel injury. We had two cases with major vessel injuries early on in the series that were repaired at the time of surgery with no postoperative sequelae, but have not had any subsequent major vessel injuries. For a one-level ALIF, blood loss is typically 50 mL or less, and the patient can normally be discharged the same day or the next morning.

Room Setup

Patient is placed on the operating table in the supine position with either a kidney rest or a rolled-up towel placed under the lumbar spine to recreate lordosis. The legs should be partially flexed and the knees spread apart ("frog-legged") to reduce tension on the iliopsoas. The arms are folded across the chest on a pillow and taped in place. The operating table should be set up such that the C arm can be easily rotated underneath (Fig. 149-5).

Generally, a general vascular surgeon is used to provide the access portion of the surgery and to mobilize the vessels. It is best if this surgeon stands on the patient's left side, and his or her responsibility will be to protect the left common iliac vein during the fusion portion of the procedure. Standing on the patient's left allows for better visualization of the left common iliac vein. The operating spine surgeon stands on the right side, and an assistant stands cephalad to the surgeon on the same side. The surgical technologist stands caudal on the right side (Fig. 149-6). It is then best to bring the C arm in from the left side, where it can be rotated under the table and come in the lateral position between the spine surgeon and the assistant.

Exposure of Disc Space

For the vast majority of ALIF procedures, the lower lumbar disc spaces will need to be approached. A lower abdominal incision in a horizontal fashion can provide access to two disc spaces, but a vertical incision is needed for three or more spaces. A horizontal incision lies within Langer's lines and allows for faster healing and a much more cosmetic scar. The ideal starting position for L5–S1 is midway between the umbilicus and the pubic symphysis, and for L4–L5 it is midway between the umbilicus and the L5–S1 level. L3–L4 is just below the umbilicus (Fig. 149-7).

After the incision, dissection is carried through the subcutaneous fat and down onto the rectus abduminus fascia, which can be split vertically in the outer one third with cautery. Usually it is best to carry a horizontal arm laterally on the cephalad portion of the fascial incision. Blunt dissection is then best carried out lateral to the rectus abduminus, which is mobilized medially. This provides excellent access to the midline, because the rectus is very mobile. It is much easier to find a retroperitoneal plane laterally (especially in the inferior portion of the wound). The retroperitoneum is much more attached to the undersurface

FIGURE 149-5 Photo of room setup. Spine surgeon is in the middle on patient's left. Surgical technologist is to right and assistant to the left of the surgeon. Exposing surgeon is on opposite side of table. C-arm fluoroscopy is brought in between the spine surgeon and the assistant.

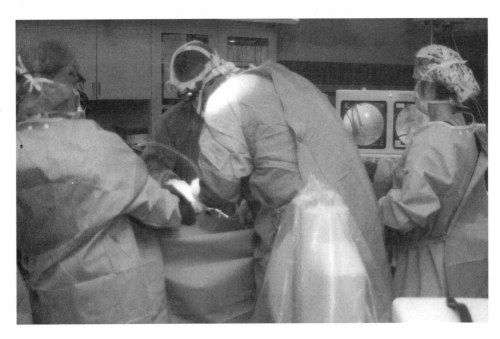

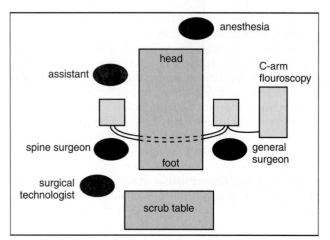

FIGURE 149-6 Diagram of operating room setup. (Copyright © 2004 NeuroSpine Center of Wisconsin.)

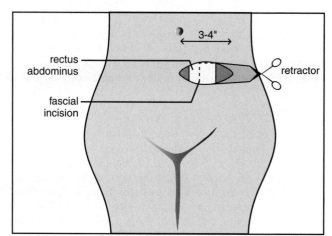

FIGURE 149-8 Horizontal incision has been made and the rectus abdominus is exposed. The anterior sheath is horizontally incised and a vertical arm is carried cephalad. (Copyright © 2004 NeuroSpine Center of Wisconsin.)

of the rectus abdominus in the midline, which makes mobilizing the rectus from medial to lateral much more difficult. It also leads to a higher incidence of breaching the peritoneum (Fig. 149-8).

The exposing surgeon can bluntly dissect with his or her finger inferiorly and laterally along the rectus. In this region the peritoneum easily sweeps away from the remainder of the transversalis and the posterior sheath, and these structures can be released cephalad with electrocautery. Going lateral to the rectus does sometimes require transection of the neurovascular bundle that enters the rectus from the lateral side. One or two levels can be transected, but if three levels need to be exposed, this can unilaterally paralyze the rectus muscle. In those cases where three levels need to be exposed, a medial approach to the rectus is advisable.

The peritoneum is then swept off the psoas, over the left great vessels, and finally over the disc space (Fig. 149-9). Care should be taken to carry the ureter with the peritoneum. At the L5–S1 level, exposure of the disc space is started on the side of the left common iliac vein (Fig. 149-10). The prevertebral fascia is bluntly dissected up off the space, and the middle sacral vessels generally must be cauterized with a

bipolar electrocautery or ligated. Care should be taken not to use unipolar cauterization, because the current can travel and damage the presacral plexus. This leads to an increased risk of postoperative retrograde ejaculation in males.

We have found that the handheld Wiley vein retractors work best to gently retract the blood vessels (Fig. 149-11). Generally, we place one on the superior aspect toward the right and then one on the right-side vessels. The exposing surgeon then uses a "peanut" pusher (Kitner) to hold the left common iliac vein out of the way. By standing on the left side of the patient, the general surgeon will have a clear view to the vein. A cerebellar self-retaining retractor is used to hold the skin edges apart. It is advisable that both surgeons wear a headlight and loupes to allow adequate visualization through a small incision.

Exposure at the L4–L5 level is somewhat more difficult. At this level, the exposure is on the left side of the aorta. To mobilize it across the midline, it is often necessary to ligate the left iliolumbar (first ascending lumbar) vein. This vein comes off the left common iliac vein and can act as a tether.

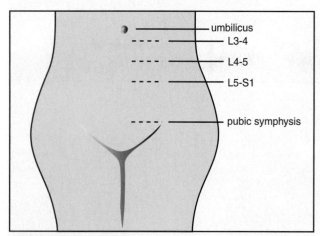

FIGURE 149-7 The L5–S1 level is midway between the umbilicus and pubic symphysis. The L4–L5 incision is midway between the L5–S1 incisional level and the umbilicus. (Copyright © 2004 NeuroSpine Center of Wisconsin.)

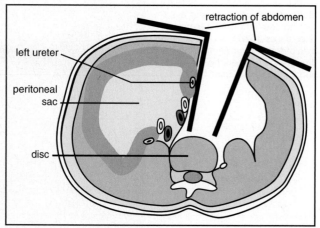

FIGURE 149-9 Peritoneum is reflected from the left to the right side by blunt dissection. Care should be taken that the ureter stays with the peritoneum as it is reflected up off the iliopsoas. (Copyright © 2004 NeuroSpine Center of Wisconsin.)

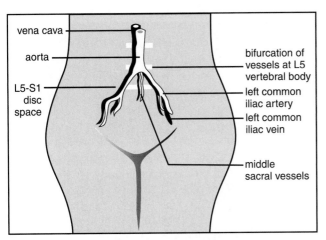

FIGURE 149-10 L5–S1 disc is at the level of the bifurcation of the great vessels. The L4–L5 level is just cephalad to the bifurcation. (Copyright © 2004 NeuroSpine Center of Wisconsin.)

If it is avulsed with retraction, the vein itself will retract into the psoas, and one can be left with a very difficult sidewall repair of the left common iliac vein. It is best for the exposing surgeon to look at and decide if the iliolumbar vein is tethering the aorta at all and, if there is any question, it should be ligated before attempting to expose the L4–L5 disc interspace.

Discectomy

After the disc interspace has been cleared of the prevertebral fascia, the center of the disc space is marked by making a small cut in the annulus and inserting a small screw (or other metal marker) (Fig. 149-12). The C-arm fluoroscopy machine is then brought in to confirm that this is marking the center of the disc space, and before removing the screw the center is marked with a marking pen. It is vital to find the center of the disc before removing the disc itself, especially for those discs that are more oval. It is easy to mistakenly dissect on one side of the disc space or the other, and this may result in

placement of the anterior hardware and/or bone graft into the foramen instead of the center of the disc space.

Care should be taken when marking the center of the disc space that a true anteroposterior film is obtained. If the pedicles are not equidistant from the spinous process on the AP view with the C arm fluoroscopy, the table should be turned until the spinous process is centered. One must also be certain that the technologist operating the C arm has rotated it to 90 degrees to the horizontal plane. To visualize L5–S1, the gantry of the C arm should be rotated 30 to 45 degrees cephalad (Ferguson view) to account for the lordosis at this level (Fig. 149-13). After the center of the disc space has been accurately marked, the C arm is turned into the lateral position. The rest of the case can be done in this position. While the assistant holds the upper Wiley vein retractor, the general surgeon can hold the right common iliac vessels with another Wiley vein retractor and the left common iliac vein with a "peanut" (or Kitner) pusher. At L4–L5, the aorta and left common iliac artery can be held by the assistant and the iliopsoas by the exposing surgeon.

A No. 15 blade on a long handle is used to cut the annulus. It is advisable to cut away from the vein, and once the blade is placed into the annulus, care should be taken to use the blade only within the disc space until the cut has been completed. Slipping is more likely if the blade comes out of the disc space with each cut. After the annulus has been cut from the vertebral end plates, an angled chisel or Cobb elevator is used to dissect the remainder of the disc from the end plates. Curets and pituitary rongeurs are used to remove the disc material back to the posterior longitudinal ligament. After starting the discectomy, the vessels are often more mobile. Therefore, if it is difficult to mobilize the vessels, start the discectomy and mobilize the vessels afterward. It is best to do a complete discectomy, because this will allow for a much better fusion bed and allow more bone graft to be placed in the interspace. It is often difficult to see in the posterior disc space, so great care should be taken to remove the posterior disc down to the posterior longitudinal disc space. Disc material left in this location can compromise the fixation of an intervertebral device and impede the fusion process.

FIGURE 149-11 Wiley vein retractors are held by the assistant above the incision and the general surgeon. The skin is retracted with a self-retaining retractor (e.g., cerebellar).

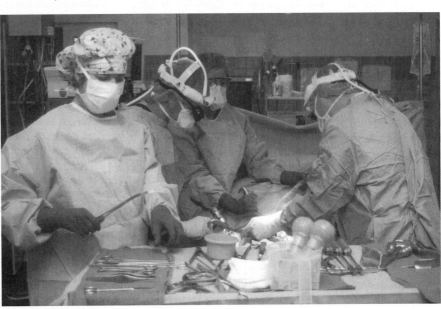

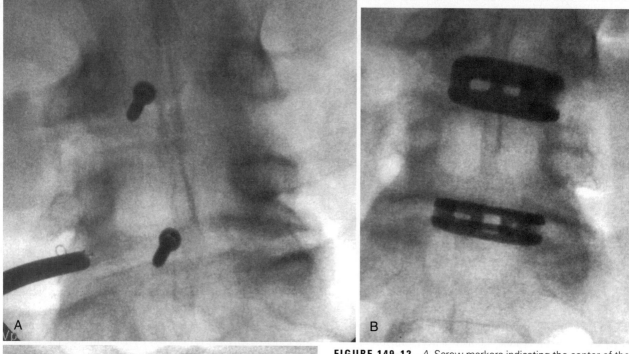

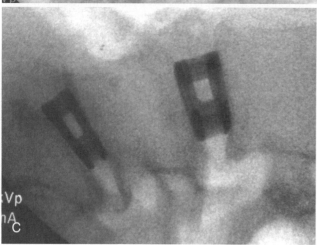

FIGURE 149-12 *A,* Screw markers indicating the center of the disc space. The metallic marker is to the patient's right, and the markers are therefore slightly offset to the right. Appropriate adjustments can then be made when marking the disc space. Note that the spinous process is in the center between the pedicles. If it is not, the table can be rotated until the spinous process lies directly in between the pedicles. *B* and *C,* Anteroposterior and lateral C arm fluoroscopy views of Endoskeleton cages (Orthovita) that have been placed in the center of the disc space during the anterior portion of an antero-posterior fusion.

COMPLICATIONS

Vascular Injuries

The most dreaded complication of an ALIF is a major vascular injury. The most at risk vessel is the left common iliac vein, and great care should be taken to protect it throughout the case. The combined skill of the spine surgeon and a vascular surgeon can help reduce the risk of major vascular injuries, and it is invaluable to have a surgeon who is experienced in the repair of vascular injuries. There is a fairly steep learning curve to exposing the spine through a minimally invasive approach, but the reality is that this is a procedure that can be done with very little morbidity. The reported incidence of major vascular injuries with an anterior approach has been placed at 1.0% to 1.8%.[6,27,28]

It is highly unusual to have an arterial injury, because the major arteries have a very strong exterior lining. It is the thin-walled veins that are at risk. Fortunately, venous blood is under very low pressure, and if a venous injury is encountered, the bleeding can be controlled with direct pressure. If bleeding is encountered, cross clamping the vein is not necessary and can potentially lead to further vein damage. Caudal and cephalad control of the bleeding around the injury should be gained with a sponge stick, and the tear should be directly repaired with 4-0 polypropylene (Prolene) or similar suture.

There have been isolated reports of atherosclerotic arterial plaque being dislodged because of traction to the common iliac arteries and/or aorta. This can result in loss of blood flow to the lower limbs and necessitate immediate embolectomy.[29]

Retrograde Ejaculation

The very small presacral plexus lies over the L5–S1 disc interspace. It is responsible in males for coordinating ejaculation, and if it is injured, the ejaculate will no longer be ejected from the body but follow the path of least resistance

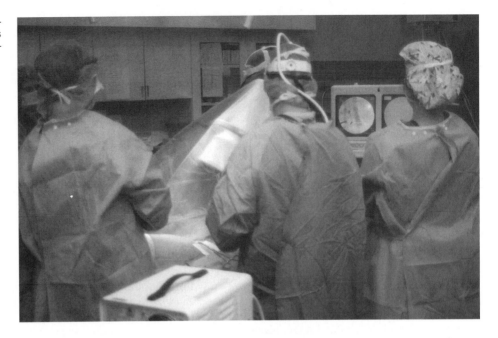

FIGURE 149-13 C-arm fluoroscopy is angled at 30 degrees (Ferguson view) to get a true anteroposterior view of the L5–S1 level.

into the bladder. The major problem with this is that it makes impregnation much more difficult (though still possible); the feeling of orgasm and sexual function are largely the same, however. Fortunately, many cases will resolve spontaneously within a year. Refraining from the use of electrocautery around the disc space reduces considerably the postoperative incidence of this complication. Flynn and Price listed the rate of this complication at 0.42% after interviewing 20 surgeons with 15 to 20 years of experience.[30] Carl and colleagues put the rate at 1.2% after 655 surgeons responded to a questionnaire.[31] In the Kuslich and colleagues study with the initial experience of the BAK cages, the rate was 4.0% in males.[6] Although this is probably an underreported complication because patients are embarrassed to bring it up and many surgeons do not ask postoperatively, the true incidence is probably between 1% and 2%.

Impotence

Impotence should be an uncommon complication and can be largely eliminated by not dissecting into the pelvis. The most caudal dissection should be at the top of the sacrum, since there is no advantage to dissecting into the pelvis. Flynn's review placed the postoperative impotence rate at 0.44%,[31] but there are a lot of psychologic issues and other known anatomic variables that make it difficult to assess the rate as a true postoperative complication.

Sympathetic Chain Injuries

The sympathetic chain runs on the lateral side spine at the L4–L5 level and under the common iliac veins at L5–S1. Injury to these nerves can result in loss of regulation of the blood flow to the lower limbs. The common result is an increase of blood flow to the left leg, which can create a noticeable difference in skin temperature when compared with the right. Interestingly, patients do not complain of the warmth in the left leg; instead, they complain that their right leg feels cold. This complication is usually temporary, although it may take up to a year to resolve.

It is more common after exposing the L4–L5 level than the L5–S1 level.

Reflex Sympathetic Dystrophy

A more serious form of the injury is the development of a reflex sympathetic dystrophy (or chronic regional pain syndrome). The cause of this is unknown, but early recognition and treatment is crucial. If recognized early, it can be treated with a sympathetic injection followed by physical therapy. Alpha blocker antihypertensive medication can also be useful to block sympathetic discharge. If missed, the sympathetically mediated pain cycles become more entrenched and it can be increasingly difficult to effectively treat this condition if not recognized early.

The usual clinical course of reflex sympathetic dystrophy is that patients do well directly after surgery, but within a week they develop pain in one leg or the other that is difficult to describe. It is not made worse with activity, and most patients will actually feel better while active. On exam, they are generally neurologically intact and have a negative tension sign (straight leg raising test). The hallmark of this complication is that the pain quickly resolves after injecting the sympathetic chain at the L2–L3 level on the affected side with lidocaine. The only pain that should be relieved by a sympathetic block is sympathetically mediated pain, and relief can be quite dramatic. It can be performed as many times as necessary until the pain fully resolves. If the injection confirms the diagnosis of a reflex sympathetic dystrophy, physical therapy should be started in the immediate postoperative course.

ANTERIOR LUMBAR CAGES

Originally, all interbody fusions were done with either a structural autograft or a structural allograft. Harvesting a structural autograft from the iliac crest is associated with fairly significant morbidity, and eventually femoral allografts filled with morselized autograft became more popular.

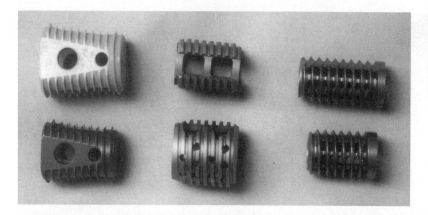

FIGURE 149-14 Representative sample of threaded titanium cages. *Bottom left,* LT titanium cage (Medtonic Sofamor Danek); *top left,* LT PEEK cage (Medtronic Sofamor Danek); *middle top,* Proximity cage (Zimmer); *middle bottom,* BAK titanium cage (Zimmer); *top right,* Unite titanium cage (Stryker); *bottom right,* Ray cage (Stryker).

In September 1996, the FDA approved the first threaded anterior interbody device (BAK-Zimmer Spine). Threaded cages provided much better stability, but there is only limited surface area for bony fusion. Most of the contact area is metal to bone. Since that time, there have been literally dozens of different designs and materials used as cages for interbody fixation.

There are basically three types of available implants.[32] Here is a representative sample of the different implants, although there are many types of each group.

- Threaded titanium cages: Ray cage (Stryker), BAK (Zimmer), LT (Medtronic Sofamor Danek) (Fig. 149-14)
- Vertical rings: Implex (Zimmer), Femoral Ring Allograft (Synthes), Syncage (Synthes), Endoskeleton cage (Orthovita), In Fix (Spinal Concepts), Pyramesh (Medtronic Sofamor Danek) (Fig. 149-15)
- Open boxes: Brantigan carbon fiber cage (Depuy Spine), Vertigraft allograft (Depuy Spine), Vertical cage (Synthes) (Fig. 149-16)

The devices can be constructed of different materials:[32,33]

- Allograft bone
- Metal
- Carbon fiber
- PEEK (polyetheretherketone)

Basically, all interbody devices, whether they are bone or of a manufactured material, are interference devices. They fit between two bones and do not fix the bones together. No matter which device is chosen by the surgeon, care should be taken to insert it in between the vertebral end plates. Disc space preparation and device insertion should be closely followed by C-arm fluoroscopy in a lateral position to ensure that the implant is not driven into one vertebral body or the other. Especially with threaded cages, the S1 vertebral end plate is denser than the inferior end plate of L5, and the tendency is to skive off the S1 end plate and place the device into the L5 vertebral body.

When preparing the disc space to insert an interbody device, as much of the vertebral end plate subchondral bone as possible should be left intact. Subsidence is a potentially major postoperative problem, and the more bone that is removed, the more likely the bone will not be strong enough to withstand the axial load placed upon it. Cage extrusion is not nearly as common a problem as subsidence. Initially, it was felt that as large a threaded cage as possible should be inserted to put tension on the annulus and prevent extrusion. Unfortunately, the larger the cage, the more subchondral bone is reamed out to insert the device. A vertical ring allograft or metal device, or an open-box PEEK or carbon fiber cage will require less destruction of the end plate, although many of these devices may need to be supported with posterior fixation.

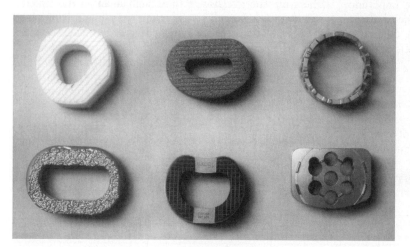

FIGURE 149-15 Representative sample of vertical ring cages. *Clockwise from upper left,* Femoral ring allograft (Synthes); Implex (Zimmer); Pyramesh (Medtronic Sofamor Danek); In Fix (Spinal Concepts); Syncage (Synthes); Endoskeleton (Orthovita).

FIGURE 149-16 Representative sample of impactable cages. *Top left,* titanium vertical cage (Synthes); *bottom left,* PEEK vertical cage (Synthes); *top middle,* Brantigan carbon fiber cage (Depuy Spine); *bottom middle,* Vertigraft allograft (Depuy Spine); *right,* plastic model of the stackable carbon fiber cage (Depuy Spine).

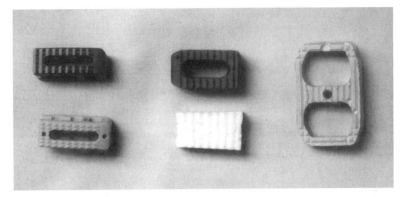

There are pros and cons to each of the dozens of different designs and materials available for fusing the interspace. There is interplay between stability, surface area for fusion, biologic reaction, and radiolucency. Threaded titanium cages are very stable but do not allow a lot of surface area for fusion. Only 8% to 10% of the surface area is bone-to-bone contact. With a ring implant, adequate stability is achieved with peripheral fixation on the outer apophysis and provides equivalent stability as implants with more metal-to-bone contact. Leaving the inner ring open allows for much more fusion area (e.g., bone-to-bone contact).[34-36]

Other implantable cages including allograft, PEEK, and carbon fiber are strong in compression and generally have a lot of surface area for fusion, but may not be as stable in shear, rotation, lateral bending, or flexion/extension. They are, however, radiolucent and allow for better assessment of fusion mass postoperatively.[36]

In general, most of the implants will provide for adequate stability if posterior stabilization is used. In cases that will require posterior stabilization (e.g., isthmic spondylolisthesis), an implant that allows for greater surface area and, therefore, more bone-to-bone contact for the fusion, is more important than overall stability. In stand-alone cases, a more stable implant should be chosen (e.g., threaded or ring titanium implants).

BONE GRAFT

The gold standard for obtaining a solid fusion is still autograft bone from the patients' iliac crest.[37-39] Unfortunately, this requires a second incision over the iliac crest and carries the risk of postoperative complications such as infection, chronic pain, or meralgia paresthetica. The environment of the disc interspace lends itself well to obtaining a solid fusion. There is a lot of clinical research currently being done to investigate the use of manufactured products to use as a bone graft substitute, obviating the need to harvest the patients' own bone. The lumbar disc space is to an extent a privileged environment, since many of the biologic factors that are necessary for a fusion (e.g., bone morphogenic protein and osteoprogenitor cells) are readily available within the large bone surface areas of vertebral bodies.[37] As opposed to a posterior lumbar fusion, there is little fibrous ingrowth competition, since the surface area is not covered in muscle. Finally, the bone is placed in compression, and this is a much more favorable environment for bone healing than is tension (Wolff's Law).

At the time of this publication, the only FDA-approved product for a bone graft substitute for a lumbar interbody fusion is Infuse (Medtronic Sofamor Danek), which is human recombinant bone morphogenic protein-2 (BMP-2).[40] Its approval is for use in threaded titanium cages in the lumbar disc interspace, inserted through an anterior exposure. Research shows that it grows bone at least as well as autograft.[40,41] However, it is very expensive, and there are some contraindications to using BMP-2, because it is a growth factor (particularly in children, women who are trying to become pregnant, and patients with a known carcinoma).

Many other bone graft substitutes are available that are FDA approved, but their approval for use in the spine is as a bone void filler.[37,42] These are osteoconductive products that are primarily composed of calcium sulfate, calcium triphosphate, or hydroxyapatite. In the privileged environment of the lumbar disc space, osteoconductive products may suffice for bone growth, especially in an immobilized segment.[37] However, more research is necessary to determine clinically if osteoconductive products can make the claim that they can be used as a bone graft substitute for ALIFs.

CONCLUSIONS

Anterior lumbar interbody fusion, when done through a mini-open laparotomy approach, allows for excellent stabilization of the intervertebral disc space with a minimum of morbidity. Although there is a steep learning curve, it is a very anatomic approach to the spine. It does not require any mobilization of the nerve roots and no muscle dissection. Fusing the anterior disc space through an anterior approach provides for an excellent fusion bed, complete removal of the disc space, restoration of the normal disc height, and foraminal distraction. Bone placed in compression tends to fuse better, and bone graft substitutes may eliminate the need to harvest autologous bone. There are currently a multitude of products that provide for stabilization of the intervertebral disc space, although in many cases posterior stabilization should be considered to augment the anterior construct. In certain cases, a stand-alone ALIF is adequate (e.g., in an L5–S1 collapsed disc space).

In the near future, it will become even more important for spine surgeons to become facile with a mini-open laparotomy approach to the lumbar spine. Artificial disc technology requires an anterior approach for each of the four designs of total disc replacements currently in investigational device exemption studies. Besides the earlier listed indication for

ALIFs, more of these newer technologies will require spine surgeons to be able to approach the spine anteriorly, and a mini-open laparotomy approach lends itself particularly well to approaching the lower lumbar disc spaces.

REFERENCES

1. Crock HV: Anterior lumbar interbody fusion: Indications for its use and notes on surgical technique. Clin Orthop Relat Res 165:157–163, 1982.
2. Kozak JA, Heiken AE, O'Brien JP: Anterior lumbar fusion options: Technique and graft materials. Clin Orthop Relat Res 300:45–51, 1994.
3. Raney FL, Adams JE: Anterior lumbar disc excision and interbody fusion used as a salvage procedure. J Bone Joint Surg 47B:211–220, 1965.
4. Duggal N, Mendiondo I, Pares HR, et al: Anterior lumbar interbody fusion for treatment of failed back surgery syndrome: An outcome analysis. Neurosurgery 54:636–643, 2004.
5. Penta M, Fraser R: Anterior lumbar interbody fusion: A minimum 10-year follow-up. Spine 22:2429–2434, 1997.
6. Kuslich SD, Ulstrom CL, Griffith SL, et al: The Bagby and Kuslich method of lumbar interbody fusion, history, techniques, and 2-year follow-up results of a United States prospective, multicenter trial. Spine 23:1267–1278, 1998.
7. Kuslich SD, Danielson G, Dowdle JD, et al: Four-year follow-up results of lumbar spine arthrodesis using the Bagby and Kuslich lumbar fusion cage. Spine 25:2656–2662, 2000.
8. McAfee PC: Interbody fusion cages in reconstructive operations on the spine. J Bone Joint Surg Am 81:859–880, 1999.
9. Selby DK, Henderson RJ: Anterior lumbar fusion. In White AH, Rothmann RH, Ray CD (eds.): Lumbar Spine Surgery: Techniques and Complications. St Louis: CV Mosby, 1987, p 383–395.
10. Henderson RK: Anterior approach for lumbar fusions and associated morbidity. In White AH, Schofferman JA (eds.): Spine Care: Diagnosis and Treatment. St Louis: CV Mosby, 1995, pp 1112–1125.
11. Lee CK, Noshir LA: Lumbosacral spinal fusion: A biomechanical study. Spine 9:574–581, 1984.
12. Chen D, Fay LA, Lok J, et al: Increasing neuroforaminal volume by anterior distraction in degenerative lumbar spine. Spine 20:74–79, 1995.
13. Oda I, Abumi K, Yu BS: Types of spinal instability that require interbody support in posterior lumbar reconstruction: An in vitro biomechanical investigation. Spine 28:1573–1580, 2003.
14. McAfee PC, Cunningham BW, Lee GA, et al: Revision strategies for salvaging or improving failed cylindrical cages. Spine 24:2147–2153, 1999.
15. Patwardhan AG, Carandang G, Ghanayen AJ: Compressive preload improves the stability of the anterior lumbar interbody fusion cage constructs. J Bone Joint Surg Am 85:1749–1756, 2003.
16. Derby R, Howard MW, Grant JM, et al: The ability of pressure-controlled discography to predict surgical and nonsurgical outcomes. Spine 24:364–372, 1999.
17. Carragee EJ, Vittum D, Tanner C: The deceptive discogram: Positive provocative discography as a misleading finding in the evaluation of back pain. Proceedings of the 12th annual meeting of the North American Spine Society, October 1997, New York.
18. Wetzel TF, LaRocca SH, Lowery GL, et al: The treatment of lumbar spinal pain by discography: Lumbar arthrodesis. Spine 19:792–800, 1994.
19. Gill K, Blumenthal SL: Functional results after anterior lumbar interbody fusion at L5–S1 in patients with normal and abnormal MRI scans. Spine 17:940–942, 1992.
20. Kokkonen SM, Kurunlahti M, Tervonen O: Endplate degeneration observed on magnetic resonance imaging of the lumbar spine: Correlation with pain provocation and disc changes observed on computed tomography discography. Spine 27:2274–2278, 2002.
21. Zdeblick A, David SM: A prospective comparison of surgical approach for anterior lumbar fusion: Laparoscopic versus mini anterior lumbar interbody fusion. Spine 25:2682–2687, 2000.
22. Lieberman IH, Willsher MB, Litwin MD, et al: Transperitoneal laparoscopic exposure for lumbar interbody fusion. Spine 25:509–574, 2000.
23. Regan JJ, Yuan H, McAfee PC: Laparoscopic fusion of the lumbar spine: Minimally invasive spine surgery: A prospective multicenter study evaluating open and laparoscopic fusion. Spine 24:204–211, 1999.
24. Mathews HH, Evans MT, Mulligan HJ, et al: Laparoscopic discectomy with anterior lumbar interbody fusion: A preliminary review. Spine 20:1797–1802, 1995.
25. Escober E, Transfeldt E, Garvey T, et al: Video-assisted versus open anterior lumbar spine fusion surgery: A comparison of four techniques and complications in 135 patients. Spine 28:729–732, 2003.
26. Kaiser MG, Haid RN, Subah BR, et al: Comparison of the mini-open versus laparoscopic approach for anterior lumbar interbody fusion: A retrospective review. Neurosurgery 51:97–103, 2002.
27. Rajaraman V, Vingan R, Roth P: Visceral and vascular complications resulting from anterior lumbar interbody fusion. J Neurosurg Spine 91:60–64, 1999.
28. Baker JK, Reardon PR, Reardon MJ, et al: Vascular injury in anterior lumbar surgery. Spine 22:691–699, 1997.
29. Hackenberg L, Liljenquist U, Halm H: Occlusion of the left common iliac artery and consecutive thromboembolism of the left popliteal artery following anterior lumbar interbody fusion. J Spinal Disord 14:365–368, 2001.
30. Flynn JC, Price CT: Several complications of anterior fusion of the lumbar spine. Spine 9:489–492, 1984.
31. Carl AL, Kostuick JP, Abitol JJ, et al: Interdiscal cage complications: A general consensus. Presented at the annual meeting of the North American Spine Society, Chicago, 1999.
32. Weiner BK, Fraser R: Spine update: Lumbar interbody cages. Spine 23:634–640, 1998.
33. Wimmer C, Krisner M, Gluch H, et al: Autogenic versus allogenic bone graft in anterior lumbar interbody fusions. Clin Orthop Relat Res 360:122–126, 1999.
34. Steffen T, Tsantrizos A, Irmgard F, et al: Cages: Designs and concepts. Eur Spine J 9(Suppl 1):589–594, 2000.
35. Steffen T, Tsantrizos A, Aebi M: Effect of implant design and endplate preparation on the compressive strength of interbody fusion constructs. Spine 24:1077–1084, 2000.
36. Tsantrizos A, Andreou A, Aebi M, et al: Biomechanical stability of five stand-alone anterior lumbar interbody fusion constructs. Eur Spine J 9:14–22, 2000.
37. Boden SD: Overview of the biology of lumbar spine fusion and principles for selecting a bone graft substitute. Spine 27:526–531, 2002.
38. Finkemeier CG: Current concepts review: Bone-grafting and bone-graft substitutes. J Bone Joint Surg Am 84:454–464, 2002.
39. Vaccaro AR, Chiba K, Heller JG, et al: Contemporary concepts in spine care: Bone grafting alternatives. Spine J 2:206–215, 2002.
40. Burkus KJ, Transfeldt E, Kitchel SH, et al: Clinical and radiographic outcomes of anterior lumbar interbody fusion using recombined human bone morphogenic protein-2. Spine 27:2396–2408, 2003.
41. McKay B, Sandhu HS: Use of recombinant human bone morphogenic protein-2 in spinal fusion applications. Spine 27:566–585, 2002.
42. Ohyama T, Kibo Y, Iwata H: Beta-tricalcium phosphate as a substitute in interbody fusion cages in the canine lumbar spine. J Neurosurg Spine 97:350–354, 2002.

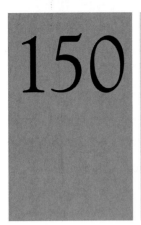

150 Surgical Management of Degenerative Lumbar Stenosis and Spondylolisthesis

HARGOVIND DEWAL, AFSHIN E. RAZI, and THOMAS J. ERRICO

LUMBAR SPINAL STENOSIS

The surgical management of lumbar spinal stenosis and degenerative spondylolisthesis is critically shaped by whether a spinal arthrodesis (instrumented or noninstrumented) is performed along with the decompressive procedure. Although the conditions under which these choices are made have not been fully and absolutely defined, the literature provides positive guidelines once the disorders are definitively diagnosed. Differentiation of these conditions is therefore a first step toward optimal management. Complaints from patients with lumbar stenosis and degenerative spondylolisthesis include back and leg pain; neurologic symptoms such as numbness, tingling, and dysesthesia; and subjective weakness often exacerbated by either prolonged standing or walking. Fixed neurologic deficits may be absent or subtle in the form of reflex changes and/or mild bowel or bladder difficulties. Significant fixed motor paralysis and/or significant bowel or bladder symptoms are less common, and may be seen in neglected cases or, even less commonly, in acute presentations. However, patient symptomatology does not definitively differentiate pure lumbar stenosis from degenerative spondylolisthesis.

Common nonoperative measures to treat a diagnosis of either stenosis or spondylolisthesis include active physical therapy, pharmacologic management, and injection techniques for steroid medications. Failure of an adequate and coordinated program of conservative care is an indication for consideration of operative treatment. Since rapid neurologic deterioration is relatively rare, the vast majority of surgery for lumbar stenosis/degenerative spondylolisthesis is elective.

RADIOLOGIC IMAGING

The differentiation of pure lumbar stenosis from degenerative spondylolisthesis begins with plain radiographs and dynamic lateral flexion and extension x-rays. The patient's symptoms should correlate with the pathologic anatomy noted on all preoperative imaging studies. Greater than 4 mm of anterior translation of the superior vertebral body on the inferior body constitutes degenerative spondylolisthesis.[1] Standing lateral flexion and extension x-rays may provide additional evidence of dynamic instability to supine lateral flexion and extension views.

Neural compression is documented well by magnetic resonance imaging (MRI). Increased sophistication in the technology and interpretation of MRI scans, with or without supplemental computed tomography (CT) images, has decreased the "mandatory" usage of CT-myelography for all surgical patients. Some radiologic facilities will supplement MRIs with select CT cuts through the spine areas where maximal compression has occurred. A CT image better defines the bony architecture of the spinal column, while an MRI scan better depicts the soft neural structures. The CT scan also provides information on the extent of the neural compression due to bone involvement. Neural compression is usually due to a reduction of the spinal canal from posterior protrusion of the disc material, hypertrophy of both the facets and ligamentum flavum, and from the listhesis.

SURGICAL INTERVENTION

The purpose of any surgical intervention is to decrease pain, improve function, and prevent neurologic deterioration. The goal of surgical decompression is to decompress all of the neural elements that are producing the patient's symptoms. Degenerative changes may span multiple vertebral levels on imaging studies, but not all levels may be involved in the production of the patient's symptoms at the time of examination.

Simple laminectomy alone is the standard surgical treatment for lumbar spinal stenosis that is not associated with spondylolisthesis or degenerative scoliosis. The goal of decompression is to relieve the thecal sac and nerve root from any local impingements causing pressure or irritation: centrally from the spinal canal, through the lateral recess, and into the neural foramen. When fusion is to be performed, there is less concern about the precise amount of facet removal. However, care must be taken to avoid destroying the pars interarticularis, which will unnecessarily destabilize the spine, potentially diminishing the fusion rate.

The lamina, hypertrophic ligamentum flavum, and osteophytic areas of facet joints may all contribute to the stenosis and therefore require removal. The excess ligamentum flavum should be removed prior to the facetectomy. Part of the facet joint may be removed by means of an undercutting of the medial aspects of both facets. Fusion must be considered if greater than 50% of either facet is removed. Decompression should be performed in a caudal to cranial direction, usually to the level of the pedicle of the vertebra below the involved level. This is accomplished in three steps: First, the central canal is decompressed using a high-speed burr or an osteotome. Second, both lateral recesses are decompressed by partially removing the medial aspect of each inferior facet, with subsequent undercutting of the respective superior facets. Third and last, a fine instrument, such as a blunt dental tool or a Frazer dural angled elevator, is used to assess the degree of foraminal stenosis as well as the adequacy of foraminal decompression. The actual decompression is performed using a fine Kerrison rongeur placed just dorsal to the nerve root. The neural foramen is adequately decompressed when the nerve root can be gently retracted about 1 cm medially. Visualization of the pars interarticularis must be maintained to avoid excessive bone removal (Fig. 150-1).

A limited laminectomy, or hemilaminectomy, has also been described for the treatment of spinal stenosis.[2] In this procedure, the central portion of the neural arch is preserved. Thus, the interspinous and supraspinous ligaments remain intact, minimizing spinal instability. Hemilaminectomy is indicated for patients with unilateral stenosis and unilateral symptoms. However, this procedure potentially makes it difficult to decompress the contralateral side or to perform adequate decompression of the ipsilateral foramen. This is due, in part, to the difficulty in angling instruments laterally to enter the foramen in the presence of an intact spinous process and midline ligaments.

The procedure is started in identical fashion to a laminectomy; however, care must be taken not to violate the spinous process and interspinous and supraspinous ligaments. Laminotomy of the inferior lamina is performed laterally from the midline to the base of the inferior facet. In order to gain access to the medial aspect of the superior facet, a partial facetectomy of the inferior facet is performed medially. This can be done using a high-speed burr. Undercutting of the superior facet is then performed with the aid of a Kerrison rongeur. The neural foramen is subsequently checked for whether the nerve root has been adequately decompressed. Some researchers advocate performing a contralateral nerve root decompression through a unilateral hemilaminotomy, facilitated by tilting the table toward the surgeon and using a microscope. However, there is an increased risk for creating a dural tear with this approach due to working through a small access portal. If a dural tear does occur in this situation, a full bilateral laminectomy is needed for further exposure and subsequent repair of the dural tear.

An alternative to hemilaminectomy is a hemilaminotomy procedure where two hemilaminotomies are performed on the adjacent hemilaminae. Partial facet excision is then performed for greater lateral decompression, as described for hemilaminectomy. Another published method is a lumbar laminoplasty, a treatment used in active manual workers.[3] It is a procedure similar to cervical laminoplasty. Affected spinous processes are removed at the base, and bilateral unicortical grooves are made at the junction of the lamina and facets. The laminae are then split in the midline and the canal is opened. Spinous processes or bone allograft is placed between the open laminae and held secure with suture or steel wire through previously made holes in the laminae and grafts. A body cast is mandatory postoperatively for a minimum of 2 weeks in order to avoid stress on the construct during ambulation.[3]

Discectomy is generally not required in the treatment of lumbar spinal stenosis. True herniations are uncommon.

However, the surgeon should assess each case for the possibility of a concomitant disc herniation or hard ridge that might compress the root. In the presence of a markedly bulging disc or in the case of a true soft disc herniation that is contributing to significant nerve root compression, a discectomy may be needed. This being said, a discectomy may also cause subsequent spinal instability, since both anterior and posterior elements are sacrificed. In this circumstance, some surgeons recommend arthrodesis at the time of surgery. Spinal stability should be maintained during decompression by preserving both the pars interarticularis and the facet joints. However, in many cases, much of the facet joint may need to be removed for adequate decompression of the involved nerve root. If more than 50% of the facet joint is removed, postoperative instability may occur. In addition, excessive removal or thinning of the pars interarticularis may lead to postoperative fracture and/or instability. If postoperative instability is suspected based on the degree of decompression performed, then arthrodesis is recommended in addition to decompression.

Surgeons are often faced with the question of whether to decompress stenotic levels that are not symptomatic. In general, if a given stenotic area is not believed to be contributing to a patient's symptoms, decompression of that particular level is not considered mandatory. Certain patients may present with a clear monoradiculopathy with multilevel stenosis. An isolated, single unilateral decompression can sometimes be performed. Some patients present with more complex symptomatology. A preoperative selective nerve root block may assist in confirming the symptomatic level or side.

DECISION MAKING IN SURGICAL INTERVENTION

First and foremost, decision making in the treatment of lumbar stenosis involves differentiating between the two entities: stenosis on spondylolisthesis as the cause of the patient's symptomatology. Pure lumbar stenosis is frequently found in combination with significant osteoarthritic changes, often with large osteophyte formations. Pure degenerative spondylolisthesis is frequently manifested as a grade I spondylolisthesis of L4 on L5, and is more frequent in females than males. There is an overlap of radiologic findings between these two entities that requires further categorization. Each level of the lumbar spine can be assessed preoperatively for individual stability based on disc height, angular motion of the end plates, translation as measured on plain radiographs, or fixed or mobile translation as evaluated on dynamic radiographs. Unfortunately, the preoperative assessment of stability loses significance after destabilizing decompressive procedures are performed.

Increasingly, the lumbar spine is iatrogenically destabilized by hemilaminectomy, central laminectomy, concomitant discectomy, partial facetectomy, total facetectomy, and violation and destruction of the pars interarticularis. Guidelines based on biomechanical studies have suggested that it is safe to remove unilaterally or bilaterally up to 50% of either the medial or lateral facets without destabilizing the motion segment. This guideline may not apply in the clinical setting of a motion segment with greater than 4 mm of fixed translation, even if the disc space is bone on bone

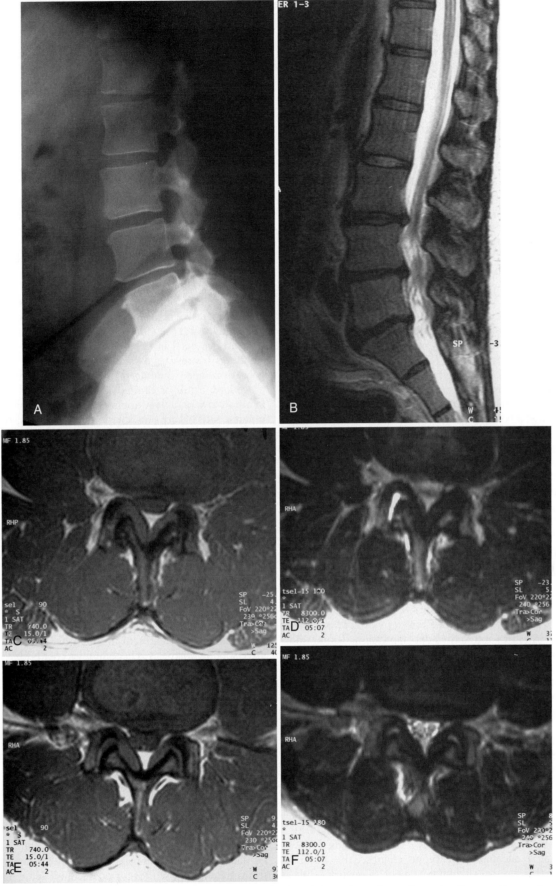

FIGURE 150-1 A 54-year-old man with bilateral neurogenic claudication. *A*, Lateral standing radiograph with no evidence of spondylolisthesis. *B*, T2 sagittal magnetic resonance imaging scan. *C* and *D*, T1 and T2 axial images at the L3–L4 level indicating central and lateral recess stenosis. *E* and *F*, T1 and T2 axial images at the L4–L5 level indicating central and lateral recess stenosis. Treatment included L3–L4 and L4–L5 posterior laminectomies.

with no angular or translational movement demonstrated on preoperative dynamic radiographs. Similarly, postoperative stability cannot be guaranteed in lumbar stenosis without translational instability even if, unilaterally, 100% of the medial facet is resected while 100% of the lateral facet is left intact (equal to a 50% facet joint resection). It is important to understand that the 50% rule means leaving 50% of a facet with functional medial and lateral components.

Clearly, violation of the pars interarticularis during a decompressive procedure creates an immediate predilection for a painful postoperative instability. Iatrogenic violation of the pars not only produces increased instability but also decreases the probability of a successful fusion, even with the addition of instrumentation.

SURGICAL OUTCOME FOR SPINAL STENOSIS

Surgical outcome for lumbar spinal stenosis is quite varied. In a prospective, nonrandomized observational cohort study of patients with spinal stenosis followed for 1 year, 55% of surgical patients reported definite improvement. This was in contrast to the nonsurgical patients, of whom only 28% reported a satisfactory outcome.[4] In a prospective study of 105 consecutive patients undergoing decompressive laminectomy, a 63% to 67% rate of satisfactory results was reported at 2 years. This result deteriorated to 52% at 5-year follow-up.[5] Sixteen percent of these patients underwent reoperation for severe back pain and/or recurrence of their stenosis during the 5-year period. Risk factor for poor outcome was correlated to a preoperative duration of symptoms of more than 4 years, significant comorbidity, and preoperative back pain. In another series of 140 patients treated surgically, at an average follow-up of 3 years, 71% reported an improvement in back pain and 82% improvement in leg pain.[6] In a longer follow-up of 2.8 to 6.8 years of 88 patients with decompression laminectomy, Katz concluded that 11% of patients had poor results at 1 year.[7] This poor satisfactory result later increased to 43% with a reoperation rate of 17% at final follow-up. Again, poor outcome was correlated to preoperative comorbidities and limited decompression. Turner and colleagues performed a meta-analysis of the lumbar stenosis literature and noted a 64% mean proportion of good to excellent results over the long term.[8]

Most studies indicate that decompression alone is adequate in pure lumbar stenosis without significant spondylolisthesis or other deformity. In a prospective randomized study, by Grob and colleagues, 45 patients underwent decompression or decompression with arthrodesis for pure stenosis. There was no significant difference in clinical outcome among patients.[9] Overall satisfactory results were 78% for patient-related outcome data in all groups, including decompression without arthrodesis, decompression plus fusion of the most significant stenotic segment, and decompression with arthrodesis of all stenotic levels. They concluded that lumbar spine decompression alone changed the natural history of this disease with improvement in quality of life. They also determined that arthrodesis is indicated when stenosis is associated with degenerative spondylolisthesis, scoliosis or kyphosis, recurrent stenosis at the same level, stenosis adjacent to a prior fusion, aggressive facetectomy,

or need for a disc excision. Other prospective randomized studies have concurred on the role of fusion for stenosis associated with degenerative spondylolisthesis.[10,11]

Complications associated with surgical intervention for lumbar stenosis are more common in cases of increased preoperative morbidities, advancing age, and complex surgical procedures. Two studies have demonstrated a relationship between mortality rate and age. One study showed a higher mortality rate of 0.6% in patients older than 75 years (about ninefold compared with patients younger than 75 years) with a complication rate of 17.7% (compared with 9.1%).[12] The second study showed similarly increased rates for patients older than 80 years.[13] The most commonly cited comorbidities in the literature are osteoarthritis, cardiac disease, rheumatoid arthritis, and chronic pulmonary disease. However, the risk factors most closely correlated with a poor outcome are preoperative complaints of predominantly low back pain, followed by preoperative comorbidities. Complications of decompression procedures are postoperative neurologic deficit, dural tear, cerebrospinal fluid fistulas and pseudomeningoceles, facet fractures, infection, and vascular injury.

When conservative measures have failed, stenosis is a condition aptly managed by a surgical decompressive procedure: a full or limited laminectomy, a double hemilaminotomy, or a laminoplasty. The majority of patients report a satisfactory outcome following surgery, though the absolute duration of long-term benefits has not been established. If stenosis is associated with an uncommonly found disc herniation, significant degenerative spondylolisthesis, degenerative scoliosis, or aggressive decompression, arthrodesis is recommended.

SPINAL STENOSIS WITH DEGENERATIVE SPONDYLOLISTHESIS

Degenerative spondylolisthesis is described as the anterior translation of one vertebral body over another adjacent vertebra in the absence of a defect of the pars interarticularis. The listhesis may cause lower back pain, radicular pain, and/or symptoms of neurogenic claudication (Fig. 150-2). The main goal of treatment in spinal stenosis with degenerative spondylolisthesis is decompression of both the exiting and traversing nerve root. The role of arthrodesis, with or without instrumentation, in the treatment of spinal stenosis with degenerative spondylolisthesis is controversial. In a retrospective review of 290 patients who underwent decompression laminectomy with 10-year follow-up, the reported outcome was excellent in 69%, good in 13%, fair in 12%, and poor in 6%. Reoperation rate for pseudoarthrosis was only 2.7%.[14] A prospective randomized study conducted by Herkowitz and Kurz compared the results at 3-years' follow-up of decompression alone versus decompression and intertransverse arthrodesis in patients with one level of spinal stenosis and degenerative spondylolisthesis.[10] Only 44% of patients with decompression without fusion reported a satisfactory outcome compared with 96% of patients reporting the same outcome who received decompression plus fusion. Patients who underwent concomitant arthrodesis had significantly better results. Moreover, despite the pseudoarthrosis rate of 36% in patients who underwent decompression and in situ fusion, all had good to excellent results.

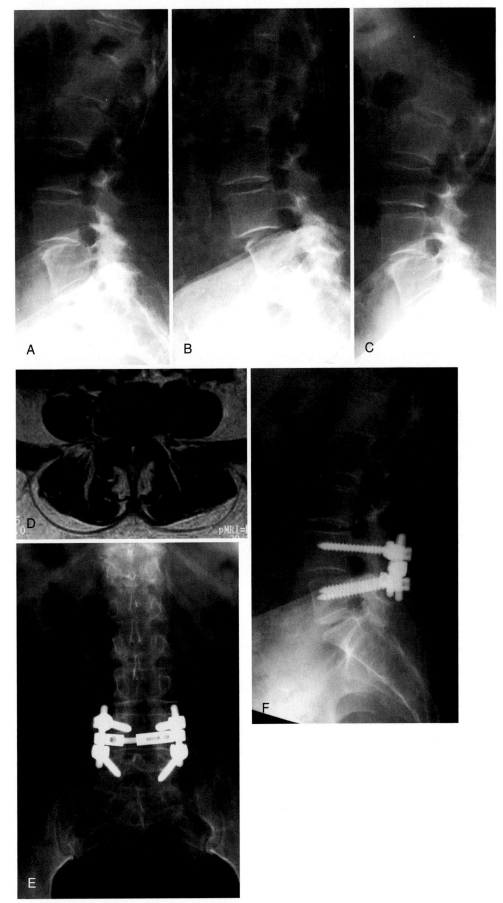

FIGURE 150-2 A 71-year-old woman with a history of low back pain and bilateral neurogenic claudication with degenerative spondylolisthesis of L4–L5. *A,* Lateral standing preoperative radiograph with evidence of spondylolisthesis at L4–L5. *B,* Lateral flexion radiograph demonstrating increased anterior translation relative to that shown in the neutral radiograph. *C,* Lateral extension radiograph with reduction of anterior translation. *D,* Axial magnetic resonance imaging scan at L4–L5 indicating central and lateral recess stenosis. *E* and *F,* Anteroposterior (*E*) and lateral (*F*) images at 2-year follow-up for posterior L4–L5 laminectomy, pedicle screw fixation, and posterolateral bone grafting using autogenous iliac crest graft.

Significant progression of the slip did not occur in either group. The investigators concluded that those patients with degenerative spondylolisthesis and stenosis should undergo concomitant arthrodesis at the time of decompression.

An attempted meta-analysis of the literature on degenerative spondylolisthesis was performed by Mardjetko and colleagues.[15] This analysis demonstrated that patient outcome was significantly better when concomitant arthrodesis was performed ($p < 0.0001$). A satisfactory clinical result was found in 69% of the 260 patients who received decompression without spinal arthrodesis; progression of the spondylolisthesis occurred in 31% of these patients. Ninety percent of those who had a surgical decompression with posterolateral arthrodesis achieved a satisfactory clinical outcome, with progressive listhesis in only 17%.

An instrumented arthrodesis has been shown to produce higher fusion rates; however, the clinical outcome of decompression with instrumented spinal fusion for this entity is not completely known.[16] Although a pseudoarthrosis occurred in 36% of those with an in situ arthrodesis in the investigation above, in the study of Herkowitz and colleagues,[10] the clinical results ranged from excellent to good in all patients. The investigators concluded that, at a mean follow-up of 3 years, a radiographic finding of pseudoarthrosis did not preclude a successful result. Fischgrund and colleagues examined 67 patients undergoing decompression and arthrodesis with or without instrumentation.[17] Patients undergoing the instrumented arthrodesis demonstrated an 87% fusion rate, while those patients undergoing a noninstrumented arthrodesis had a 45% fusion rate. However, the higher fusion rate of the instrumented group did not improve their clinical outcome. A landmark follow-up study of longer duration by Kornblum and colleagues reviewed 47 of the original patients who were diagnosed with single-level symptomatic spinal stenosis and spondylolisthesis and treated by decompression and in situ arthrodesis.[11] These patients were observed over 5 to 14 years, with an average follow-up of 7 years and 8 months. They found that long-term clinical outcome was excellent or good in 86% of patients with solid arthrodesis, but only 56% in those patients who developed a pseudoarthrosis. Significant differences in residual back and lower limb pain was discovered between the two groups, with the solid fusion group performing significantly better in the symptom, severity, and physical function categories on self-administered questionnaires. Those patients who achieved a solid fusion had improved clinical results, which demonstrated the benefit of a successful arthrodesis over pseudoarthrosis with respect to back and lower limb symptomatology compared with their prior short-term studies.

Reviewing the current literature, one may conclude that in the short-term, those patients who at least have an arthrodesis attempted, even if it results in pseudoarthrosis, will do better than those patients who have no attempt at arthrodesis. Although this "fibrous union" may benefit patients in the short term, long-term results deteriorate in patients who do not have a solid fusion. Based on the literature, one can conclude that those patients who receive instrumentation at the same time as arthrodesis will have a higher fusion rate. Combining a higher fusion rate using instrumentation with the desirable long-term clinical effect of achieving a solid fusion makes the case for using

instrumentation in the treatment of degenerative spondylolisthesis.[10,11,15,16,18,19] Because fusion performed with instruments will improve the likelihood of a solid fusion, this would suggest that an instrumented arthrodesis in the treatment of degenerative spondylolisthesis is preferred over noninstrumented fusion.

CONCLUSIONS

For patients who are indicated for surgery for either degenerative lumbar stenosis or spondylolisthesis, the choice and combination of procedures planned is critically tied to a careful diagnosis supported by a thorough correlation of symptoms and radiographic evaluation. In the perioperative planning, there must be a consideration of the extent of disease, adequacy of decompression, and instability that may be surgically produced. Pure lumbar stenosis may be managed by simpler surgical procedures with risk for fewer complications, but if the stenosis is already complicated by degenerative or iatrogenic instability, arthrodesis should at least be considered. If stenosis is accompanied by degenerative spondylolisthesis, arthrodesis is strongly indicated. For the primary condition of degenerative spondylolisthesis, the choice of fusion is unambiguous, with instrumentation being weighed in the balance. Most recently, however, research appears to indicate that an instrumented arthrodesis, as opposed to a noninstrumented procedure, may provide the patient's best opportunity for long-term clinical benefit.

REFERENCES

1. Wiltse LL, Newman PH, Macnab I: Classification of spondylolisis and spondylolisthesis. Clin Orthop 117:23–29, 1976.
2. Postacchini F, Cinotti G, Perugia D, et al: The surgical treatment of central lumbar stenosis. Multiple laminotomy compared with total laminectomy. J Bone Joint Surg Br 75:386–392, 1993.
3. Matsui H, Tsuji H, Sekido H, et al: Results of expansive laminoplasty for lumbar spinal stenosis in active manual workers. Spine 17(Suppl): 37–40, 1992.
4. Atlas SJ, Deyo RA, Keller RB, et al: The Maine Lumbar Spine Study, Part III. 1-year outcomes of surgical and nonsurgical management of lumbar spinal stenosis. Spine 21(15):1787–1794, 1996.
5. Jonsson B, Annertz M, Sjoberg C, et al: A prospective and consecutive study of surgically treated lumbar spinal stenosis. Part II. Five year follow-up by an independent observer. Spine 22:2938–2944, 1997.
6. Herron LD, Mangelsdorf C: Lumbar spinal stenosis. J Spinal Disord 4:26–33, 1991.
7. Katz JN, Lipson SJ, Larson MG, et al: The outcome of decompressive laminectomy for degenerative lumbar spinal stenosis. J Bone Joint Surg Am 73:809–813, 1991.
8. Turner JA, Ersek M, Herron L, et al: Surgery for lumbar spinal stenosis: Attempted meta-analysis of the literature. Spine 17:1–8, 1992.
9. Grob D, Humke T, Dvorak J: Degenerative lumbar spinal stenosis. Decompression with and without arthrodesis. J Bone Joint Surg Am 77(7):1036–1041, 1995.
10. Herkowitz HN, Kurz LT: Degenerative lumbar spondylolisthesis with spinal stenosis. A prospective study comparing decompression with decompression and intertransverse process arthrodesis. J Bone Joint Surg Am 73:802–807, 1991.
11. Kornblum MB, Fischgrund JS, Herkowitz HN, et al: Degenerative lumbar spondylolisthesis with spinal stenosis: A prospective long-term study comparing fusion and pseudarthrosis. Spine 29(7):726–733, 2004.
12. Deyo RA, Cherkin DC, Loeser JD, et al: Morbidity and mortality in association with operations on the lumbar spine. The influence of age, diagnosis, and procedure. J Bone Joint Surg Am 74(4):536–543, 1992.
13. Deyo RA, Ciol MA, Cherkin DC, et al: Lumbar spinal fusion. A cohort study of complications, reoperations, and resource use in the Medicare population. Spine 18(11):1463–1470, 1993.

14. Epstein NE: Decompression in the surgical management of degenerative spondylolisthesis: Advantages of a conservative approach in 290 patients. J Spinal Disord 11(2):116–122, 1998.
15. Mardjetko SM, Connolly PJ, Shott S: Degenerative lumbar spondylolisthesis. A meta-analysis of literature 1970–1993. Spine 19(Suppl):2257–2265, 1994.
16. Gibson JN, Grant IC, Waddell G: The Cochrane review of surgery for lumbar disc prolapse and degenerative lumbar spondylosis. Spine 24:1820–1832, 1999.
17. Fischgrund JS, Mackay M, Herkowitz HN, et al: 1997 Volvo Award winner in clinical studies. Degenerative lumbar spondylolisthesis with spinal stenosis: A prospective randomized study comparing decompressive laminectomy and arthrodesis with and without spinal instrumentation. Spine 22:2807–2812, 1997.
18. Thomsen K, Christensen FB, Eiskjaer SP, et al: 1997 Volvo Award winner in clinical studies. The effect of pedicle screw instrumentation on functional outcome and fusion rates in posterolateral lumbar spinal fusion: A prospective, randomized clinical study. Spine 22(24):2813–2822, 1997.
19. Zdeblick TA: A prospective, randomized study of lumbar fusion. Preliminary results. Spine 18(8):983–991, 1993.

151

Image-Guided Spine Surgery

LANGSTON T. HOLLY and KEVIN T. FOLEY

INTRODUCTION

The development of novel intraoperative navigational techniques has been an important advancement in the field of spine surgery. Current intraoperative spinal navigational techniques have evolved from the previous standards of direct visualization, serial radiography, and C-arm fluoroscopy. These techniques, commonly referred to as image guidance or image-guided surgery (IGS), provide simultaneous, multiplanar visualization of spinal anatomy. IGS allows virtually any surgical instrument to be tracked in reference to the displayed anatomy in real time. This can be particularly helpful when a spine surgeon places an instrument or implant into unexposed or partially exposed spinal structures that may not be directly visible, such as the pedicle or vertebral body.

A thorough knowledge of surgical anatomy and technique remains the most essential aspect of a spinal surgeon's navigational expertise, yet the information acquired from image guidance can assist even the most experienced surgeon. The beneficial effects of IGS on the safety and accuracy of a variety of spinal instrumentation procedures have been well documented in the medical literature. As a result, image guidance has become an increasingly accepted and practiced form of spinal intraoperative navigation.

However, there are some significant limitations to IGS. These include the fact that current image guidance techniques have a learning curve that can result in surgeon frustration and longer operating room times, especially early in the surgeon's IGS experience. Also, although image guidance is more accurate than conventional navigational techniques, it is not perfect. Failure to appreciate these limitations can result in a surgical misadventure. IGS technology is best thought of as a supplement to, not a replacement for, the spine surgeon's experience and judgment.

CONVENTIONAL INTRAOPERATIVE SPINAL NAVIGATION

Prior to the advent of image guidance, intraoperative spinal navigation was based on the surgeon's knowledge, experience, and judgment combined with information gathered from serial radiography or fluoroscopy. Monitoring of nerve and/or spinal cord status can provide data regarding the function of these structures (and, indirectly, whether or not a spinal instrument or implant may be placing this function at risk), but is only an indirect indicator of instrument position.

Plain radiography is still frequently used by many surgeons to assist in localizing the skin incision and/or the proper anatomic level for procedures such as microdiscectomy. One of the drawbacks of plain radiography is that a significant amount of time can elapse while the films are being obtained and processed. This time factor is multiplied when

unsuitable images are obtained, as they must be repeated. The other disadvantage of radiography is that only static images can be acquired; thus, information regarding instrument position within the surgical field cannot be immediately updated.

C-arm fluoroscopy addresses many of these concerns, and therefore many surgeons use fluoroscopy as their principle modality of intraoperative spinal navigation. Fluoroscopy can be used to acquire multiple images in succession, or it can be used continuously to obtain immediate updates of an instrument's position. A variety of spinal instrumentation procedures can be performed using fluoroscopy. The major disadvantage is the potential for significant occupational radiation exposure, particularly when continuous fluoroscopy is used.[1,2] Moreover, when using a single fluoroscope, images can only be obtained in a single plane at a time. If another plane of view is desired, the C arm must be repositioned. Two separate fluoroscopes are needed for intraoperative navigation during procedures that require simultaneous biplanar fluoroscopy, such as odontoid screw placement. Lastly, a C arm itself is quite cumbersome and can create ergonomic limitations that hinder access to the surgical field.

Factors such as anatomic variability, poor imaging, and complex anatomy can increase the difficulty of intraoperative spinal navigation. Clearly, conventional methods of intraoperative spinal navigation have some significant limitations. For instance, several laboratory and clinical studies have shown that lumbar pedicle screw insertion using standard techniques yields misplacement rates that range from 20% to 30%.[3-5] In contrast, pedicle screw misplacement rates using image guidance range from 0% to 4%.[6-8] Spinal image guidance was developed to address the shortcomings of conventional intraoperative navigation and to optimize the accuracy and safety of spinal instrumentation procedures. This manuscript details the spinal applications of contemporary IGS as well as image-guided technology of the near future.

EVOLUTION OF SPINAL IMAGE GUIDANCE

Spinal image guidance was adapted from intracranial frameless stereotaxy, which used skin surface markers for registration (matching of the image anatomy to the surgical anatomy). These superficial markers were initially used for spinal applications as well. Unfortunately, significant registration inaccuracy due to relative movement between the mobile skin surface and the underlying bony anatomy occurred. Several clinical studies determined that spinal image guidance was not clinically feasible due to these concerns.[9,10]

Despite this initial difficulty, interest in spinal image guidance continued and an effective method of registration soon emerged. Foley and Smith[6,11] described the use of anatomic landmarks on the dorsal aspect of the spine as fiducial (registration) markers in association with a dynamic reference array (DRA). These anatomic fiducials replaced the skin surface markers and provided reliable registration accuracy. The markers also augmented the flexibility of the system, as the registration points could be added or changed intra-operatively. The DRA attached directly to the spine and further enhanced accuracy by alerting the computer work-station to any changes in spine position that occurred during the procedure. Kalfas and colleagues[12] and Nolte and colleagues[13] also performed some of the early investiga-tional research using similar image-guided techniques to improve the safety of lumbar pedicle screw placement.

Once the issues regarding registration inaccuracy were solved, the popularity of spinal image guidance began to increase. As technology improved, second-generation computed tomography (CT) and fluoroscopy-based systems were soon developed. Surgeons expanded the use of image guidance to more complex procedures throughout the entire spine such as C1–2 transarticular screw placement[14,15] and thoracic pedicle screw insertion.[12,16]

PREOPERATIVE COMPUTED TOMOGRAPHY–BASED IMAGE GUIDANCE

Description of the System

A number of different manufacturers offer spinal image guid-ance systems that utilize preoperatively-obtained CT scans. There systems generally share the same basic components and functions, yet there are some differences in the exact hardware and software capabilities. A typical system is com-posed of multiple parts, including an electro-optical camera array, a DRA, and various customized surgical instruments (screwdrivers, awls, probes, etc.). A computer workstation functions as the primary system interface and runs the system software. Light emitting diodes (LEDs) or reflective spheres are attached to the DRA and surgical instruments so that they can be tracked by the electro-optical camera array. The LEDs are known as active arrays, whereas the reflective spheres are termed passive arrays. An optical tracking digi-tizer controls the camera firing and tracking of the LEDs or spheres, and measures the 3-dimensional (3D) location of the arrays in the operating room. This information is then relayed to the computer workstation, and the spatial location of the instruments is displayed in reference to the patient anatomy on the computer monitor. The use of both active and passive arrays on different instruments allows for simultaneous tracking of multiple instruments. Nonoptical localization technologies (mechanical, sonic, electromagnetic) have also been used in the past but are presently not routinely used.

Description of the Technique

A CT scan of the relevant spinal levels is obtained preop-eratively using a specific scan protocol. The majority of image guidance systems require thin (1 to 3 mm), contiguous axial slices and a scan field of view between 12 and 14 cm. The scan data are then transferred to the computer workstation either via a network connection, digital audio tape, compact disc, or optical disc. The data are reformatted by the computer workstation into coronal, axial, sagittal, and 3D views of

the spinal anatomy. These reconstructed images provide the opportunity for surgical preplanning since the size of structures such as the pedicles and lateral masses can be accurately measured. A virtual implant of any dimension can be directed along any desired trajectory. At this stage the surgeon can confidently determine the feasibility of complex surgical procedures, determining both proper implant size and location prior to entering the operating room. This is particularly helpful in technically challenging procedures such as thoracic pedicle screw and C1–2 transarticular screw place-ment, which can be made even more difficult by anatomic variation between patients.

Patient registration begins by choosing a minimum of three to four distinct anatomic points (fiducials) on the refor-matted CT images of each level involved in the procedure. This step is critical because it provides the means to pre-cisely match the operative anatomy to the image anatomy displayed on the computer workstation monitor. Once the surgical exposure has been completed, discrete anatomic landmarks such as the tips of the transverse processes and apex of the spinous process are identified and usually serve as satisfactory registration points. A DRA is firmly attached to the spine and positioned such that it does not hinder the operation. A registration probe fitted with LEDs or passive spheres is then used to touch the anatomic points in the surgical field that match those selected on the work-station monitor. This method of registration is called paired-point matching. Paired-point matching can be sup-plemented by surface matching, a process in which a large number of random points are selected on the exposed surface of the vertebral level of interest. This provides the computer with a contour map of the vertebra and serves to reduce the registration error. The electro-optical camera tracks the position of the vertebra via the DRA. This allows the regis-tration accuracy to be maintained despite patient or camera movement as long as the DRA remains fixed to the spine.

The computer workstation calculates a registration error, a relative index of the accuracy of the match between the computer display and the surgical anatomy. Procedure-specific limitations of acceptable registration error exist,[1] but in general, mean fiducial errors of less than 1.5 mm are con-sidered adequate for most spinal procedures. It is important to keep in mind that different manufacturers calculate registration errors in different fashions. Also, registration errors are only one component of system localization accu-racy. This accuracy must be confirmed before any surgical navigation is attempted. Verification of system accuracy occurs when the probe tip is placed on several different anatomic points on the exposed spine and the computer monitor displays the virtual probe touching the correspond-ing points on the CT images. If the locations of the virtual and real probes do not correlate, then the registration process must be repeated.

Once the verification process has been completed, spinal anatomy previously hidden from direct surgical view (such as the pedicles or underlying vertebral body) is now easily visualized on the workstation monitor. The trajectory and tip location of image-guided surgical instruments are dis-played in relationship to the anatomy in multiple planes. Navigation can be carried out by emulating the entry points and trajectories that were previously selected during the sur-gical planning stage. Alternatively, a new implant path may be selected intraoperatively. Every step of the procedure, including drilling, tapping, and screw placement, can be performed under image guidance. Any necessary changes in instrument trajectory can be made simply by observing the workstation monitor. This allows the surgeon to avoid critical neurovascular structures and improve the accuracy and safety of implant placement.

Disadvantages of Preoperative Computed Tomography–Based Image Guidance

Although preoperative CT-based image guidance is a highly effective method of intraoperative navigation, there are some notable disadvantages to the technology. The systems require a preoperative scan to be performed using a specific protocol. This can add cost and time to the preoperative workup, particularly if the patient has already had a diagnostically adequate but non-image-guided-compatible scan performed. The registration process appears relatively straightforward in experienced hands, but there is a significant learning curve involved with properly selecting the anatomic landmarks and matching them to the image anatomy. Complex anatomy can accentuate the learning curve and can add significant time to registration and ultimately to the operative procedure. Lastly, since the CT images are obtained preoperatively with the patient in one position and the surgery is commonly performed in a different position, intersegmental relationships between adjacent vertebral levels can differ. This is particularly true in cases of spinal instability such as those resulting from trauma or inflammatory processes of the atlantoaxial junction. Isthmic spondylolisthesis can result in a position-dependent change in the anatomic relationship between the lamina and vertebral body. In these instances the preoperative data set may not accurately reflect the intraoperative anatomy, potentially leading to navigational inaccuracy. At the very least, potential changes in intersegmental vertebral relationships mandate the use of a separate registration process for each vertebral level to be navigated. In addition, the surgeon should strongly consider that a grossly unstable segment should only be navigated with an attached DRA. Otherwise, motion of that segment induced by the force of a probe or drill might lead to a lack of correlation of the image and surgical anatomy and a resultant navigational misadventure.

INTRAOPERATIVE COMPUTED TOMOGRAPHY–BASED IMAGE GUIDANCE

Instead of using a preoperatively obtained CT data set, spinal image guidance can be carried out with a CT scanner based in the operating room combined with the same IGS equipment mentioned above.[17] The scan can be obtained after the spine has been exposed and discrete fiducials (such as 2 mm diameter marker screws) have been implanted. This greatly simplifies registration and increases registration accuracy as compared with the use of anatomic fiducials. The use of a CT scanner in the operating room also obviates the problem of intersegmental motion between scan acquisition and operative positioning. Disadvantages include the cost of purchasing a dedicated intraoperative CT system (in addition to an IGS system), the need to use a specially

designed OR table, the cost of implanted fiducials, and certain ergonomic issues and sterility (e.g., draping issues).

FLUOROSCOPY-BASED IMAGE GUIDANCE

Fluoroscopy-based image guidance, termed "virtual fluoroscopy," is a method of intraoperative navigation that combines computer-aided surgical technology with C-arm fluoroscopy.[18] Most spine surgeons are comfortable using standard fluoroscopy during instrumentation procedures, as it provides real-time intraoperative visualization of spinal anatomy. The major limitation of fluoroscopy is the amount of occupational radiation exposure.[2,19] The other significant disadvantage is that images can only be obtained in one plane at a time. The union of computer technology and fluoroscopy enhances the advantages of fluoroscopy and minimizes its disadvantages. Once the system is calibrated with spatial and fluoroscopic information from at least one projection (an automated process), the computer then generates a model of the saved fluoroscopic images that permits the superimposition of a tracked surgical instrument. No surgeon-derived registration step is necessary. The real-time, multiplanar position of the instrument is displayed on the workstation monitor in reference to the previously acquired fluoroscopic images. Since the saved fluoroscopic images used for navigation are obtained while the surgical team stands away from the operative field, occupational radiation exposure is significantly reduced. Furthermore, the need for tedious C-arm repositioning is eliminated because the system can use multiple saved projections and effectively performs as a multiplanar imaging unit. During navigation the fluoroscope can be removed from the operative field altogether, thereby optimizing the surgical team's comfort and ergonomics.

Description of Technique

As with CT-based image guidance, there are several different manufacturers that provide commercially available virtual fluoroscopy systems. A standard virtual fluoroscopy system consists of an image-guided computer system, a C-arm fluoroscope, a calibration target that attaches to the C arm, and customized surgical instruments that can be tracked by the system. The DRA is attached to the patient, and then intraoperative fluoroscopic images of the patient are obtained and automatically relayed to the computer workstation for processing. In the next step the relative position of the C arm and the patient is measured by an electro-optical camera that can track the location of the calibration target and the DRA. The computer then calibrates the previously obtained images by referencing the spatial measurements acquired in the last step. Finally, the computer determines the position of the surgical instrument and generates an overlay of the instrument onto the calibrated fluoroscopic images. The actual position of the instrument in reference to the saved images can be simultaneously displayed in multiple planes.

Disadvantages of Fluoroscopy-Based Image Guidance

The system allows for simultaneous 2-dimensional (2D) guidance in multiple planes, yet fluoroscopy-based image guidance does not provide the axial images that CT-based IGS provides. The quality of the images is totally dependent on the resolution of the acquired fluoroscopic projections. Consequently, in osteopenic, obese, or spinal deformity patients, image interpretation may be difficult and navigation adversely affected. Lastly, although occupational radiation exposure is significantly reduced compared with conventional fluoroscopy, there is still some exposure that does not occur with CT-based systems.

IMAGE-GUIDED SPINAL APPLICATIONS

Lumbar Spine

The initial laboratory and clinical studies into the efficacy of spinal image guidance were limited to the lumbar spine. This was in part stimulated by research that revealed that the actual lumbar pedicle screw misplacement rates using conventional techniques were higher than previously thought. Weinstein and colleagues[20] placed T11–S1 pedicle screws in eight cadaver specimens using anatomic landmarks and fluoroscopy. They determined that 21% of the pedicles manifested evidence of cortical violation. Schulze and colleagues[5] reviewed postoperative CT scans in a large series of patients who underwent lumbar fusion procedures by experienced surgeons and determined that 20% of the screws perforated the pedicle wall. In comparison, Foley and Smith[6] performed a cadaver study patterned after the work of Weinstein and colleagues using image guidance instead of fluoroscopy for navigation. T11–S1 pedicle screws were placed in six cadavers, and postoperative CT scans and visual inspection revealed no evidence of pedicle wall violation. Kalfas and colleagues[12] placed 150 lumbar pedicle screws in 30 patients using image guidance and determined that 149 of the screws were placed satisfactorily.

Thoracic Spine

Until recently, hook and claw constructs have been traditionally used for dorsal thoracic instrumentation procedures. Thoracic pedicle screws are now preferred by many surgeons because of their biomechanical superiority, increased tolerance of corrective force application, and sparing of additional motion segments. However, thoracic pedicle screw placement, particularly in the midthoracic region, can be technically difficult. The thoracic pedicles are smaller in size than their lumbar counterparts and have quite a variable and complex 3D morphology. This is compounded by the fact that high-quality intraoperative anteroposterior and lateral fluoroscopic views of the thoracic spine are frequently difficult to acquire.

Consequently, clinical and laboratory investigations of thoracic pedicle screw placement using conventional techniques have shown significant screw misplacement rates. Liljenqvist and colleagues[21] placed 120 thoracic pedicle screws in 32 patients with scoliosis and found that 25% of the screws were misplaced. Vaccaro and colleagues[22] placed 90 screws in T4–T12 pedicles and determined that 41% violated the pedicle wall. In contrast, Youkilis and colleagues[16] reported a series of 266 thoracic pedicle screws placed in 65 patients over a 4-year period using image guidance. They determined that the pedicle perforation rate was 8.5%,

significantly lower than that reported with conventional techniques.

Cervical Spine

Intraoperative navigation in the cervical spine presents a unique set of challenges that are ideally suited for image-guided applications. The cervical region is prone to pathologic entities that can distort familiar anatomy such as traumatic, inflammatory, and neoplastic, conditions that can make traditional spinal navigation more difficult and risky. The small bony anatomy and intimate relationship with the vertebral artery and spinal cord increase the need for precise screw placement during cervical instrumentation procedures. Although a standard entry point and trajectory have been described for some of these procedures, recent data suggest that screw placement should instead be tailored to the individual patient anatomy. Foley and colleagues[23] performed cervical spine CT scans on a number of patients and then determined the entry points and trajectories for C1–2 transarticular screw placement using an image guidance system. They found wide variations of optimal screw entry points between patients and concluded that following a preset path, rather than one dictated by the individual anatomy, may result in screw misplacement and patient injury.

Several anatomic investigations have analyzed the suitability of the atlantoaxial complex for C1–2 transarticular screw placement. Cadaver studies by Madawi and colleagues[24] and CT evaluations by Paramore and colleagues[25] similarly determined that approximately 20% of patients have anomalous vertebral artery anatomy on at least one side that precludes safe screw placement using conventional techniques. Mandel and colleagues[26] evaluated 205 sets of C1 and C2 vertebrae with both CT and anatomic measurements to establish which patients would be at risk for vertebral artery injury during C1–2 transarticular screw placement. They found that the screws could not be safely placed in patients with C2 pars interarticularis widths and heights less than 5.0 mm.

Bloch and colleagues[14] studied the effect of image guidance on C1–2 transarticular screw placement in 17 cadaver specimens. In this study, screws were placed in any specimen whose C2 pars interarticularis height or width was greater than 4.0 mm. Bilateral screws were placed in 16 specimens; the remaining specimen had significant narrowing of the pars interarticularis by the vertebral artery that precluded screw placement bilaterally. Based on conventional criteria using fluoroscopy and landmarks alone, 23% of the specimens would have been unable to accept a transarticular screw on at least one side. In contrast, image guidance reduced this incidence to 6% because of the precision provided by this technology.

Image guidance can also be used to improve the safety and accuracy of lateral mass screw placement. Although lateral mass screws are frequently placed using a standard entry point and trajectory, anatomic variation can lead to screw misplacement when a uniform methodology is employed. Clinical studies have shown lateral mass screw misplacement rates to be as high as 14%.[27] Heller and colleagues[28] reviewed 78 cases of lateral mass screw placement and determined that 5% suffered a clinically significant nerve root injury. Foley and colleagues[29] reported the use of image guidance to place 100 lateral mass screws in 10 cadaver specimens. The specimens were evaluated visually and radiographically; all screws were safely placed without evidence of nerve root, facet joint, or vertebral artery injury.

2-Dimensional–3-Dimensional Registration

The ideal spinal navigation system would combine the convenience of virtual fluoroscopy (C arm based, no need for anatomic registration) with the anatomic visualization provided by CT-based systems. One means of doing this is to correlate intraoperatively acquired 2D fluoroscopic images with preoperatively-acquired 3D CT images. This process, termed 2D-3D registration, exists. Several manufacturers provide software packages that perform this function. However, there are disadvantages to this approach. First of all, the process is not automated (surgeon input is required). Second, there is still a need to obtain a properly formatted preoperative CT. Lastly, the accuracy of current 2D-3D registration techniques is questionable. Future IGS development will likely include enhancements of the 2D-3D registration process.

3-Dimensional C-arm Fluoroscopy

Three-dimensional C-arm fluoroscopy (3D fluoroscopy) is a significant advancement in the rapidly developing field of image guidance and potentially represents the future of intraoperative spinal navigation. Unlike a standard fluoroscope, an isocentric C arm can automatically rotate around the patient while maintaining the relevant spinal anatomy in its center. With the addition of specialized software, such a C arm can effectively function as a CT scanner. The automated image acquisition takes approximately 2 minutes. The images are then reconstructed to provide axial, coronal, and sagittal views of the anatomy. The multiplanar constructions are of high quality and with regard to anatomic detail are comparable with images produced by an actual CT scanner.

The isocentric C arm can be used in conjunction with IGS technology to create a novel method of spinal image guidance. This requires that the C arm be fitted with a calibration target and that a DRA be attached to the patient. An electro-optical camera can then track the position of the DRA in reference to the C arm while image acquisition takes place. The reconstructed images are transferred to the computer workstation and automatically uploaded into the IGS software in a process that takes 1 minute. Since the images are obtained with reference markers on both the C arm (the target) and patient (the DRA), anatomic registration is not necessary for navigation. This process is similar to virtual fluoroscopy, except that the images are identical to those provided by CT-based systems.

There are many advantages of this innovative technology. The isocentric C arm provides 3D reconstructed images of the patient on the operating table. Therefore, the risk for navigation inaccuracy due to intervertebral alignment differences between the preoperative CT data set and the intraoperative position is eliminated. Since the system can display three adjacent lumbar vertebrae, separate registration solutions are unnecessary. The need for a preoperative CT scan with a specific image-guided protocol is eliminated. The surgeon-driven registration process is completely obviated, as navigation can commence immediately after the images have been transferred to the workstation. Since spinal exposure is unnecessary, this provides an ideal opportunity for the integration of IGS with minimally invasive techniques such as percutaneous pedicle screw placement, minimally invasive decompression, and thoracoscopy. The isocentric C arm can serve as a standard C-arm fluoroscope, maximizing its use in the operating room when image-guided cases are not being performed (no "down time") and allowing a single device to serve as both C arm and CT during image-guided cases. Lastly, a postoperative scan can be performed in the operating room to ensure accurate implant placement and/or to evaluate the thoroughness of a decompressive procedure.

Laboratory Experience

Laboratory testing was carried out to measure the application accuracy of 3D fluoroscopy. A Siemens Iso-C 3D fluoroscope (Siemens Medical Solutions, Erlangen, Germany) was fitted with a calibration target and tracked with the StealthStation Treon image-guided surgery system (Medtronic Navigation, Louisville, CO). A phantom with multiple spherical targets and an attached DRA was imaged with the Iso-C 3D fluoroscope. The images were imported into the Treon through an Ethernet cable connecting the two devices. The spherical targets were then touched with a customized probe with a concave tip that matched the sphere surface and localized the centers of the spheres. The distance between the tip of the image-guided probe and the center of each sphere was measured on the IGS display. The mean localization error was 1.1 mm with a standard deviation of 0.4 mm.

In order to test the efficacy of 3D fluoroscopy for intraoperative navigation, we performed a cadaver study placing image-guided percutaneous pedicle screws.[30] Three intact cadavers were used as specimens. A small skin incision was made to allow access to the spinous process immediately rostral to the most cephalad level to be instrumented. A percutaneous DRA was firmly attached to this spinous process. The Iso-C 3D fluoroscope was fitted with a calibration target and used to obtain images of the levels of interest (three adjacent vertebrae). These images were transferred to the Treon computer workstation. A drill guide fitted with LEDs was then used to determine the proper trajectory for percutaneous screw placement. A small skin incision was made (15 mm) and the drill guide was advanced to the appropriate pedicle entry point as displayed on the workstation monitor. A hand drill was advanced through the guide and through the appropriate pedicle, using image-guided feedback. The drill was removed and a K wire was inserted through the drill guide and into the pedicle pilot hole. Sequential tubular dilators were inserted over the K wire, with the last dilator being left in place to serve as a protective sheath for an image-guided tap. The tap was removed and a percutaneous screw was inserted, followed by removal of the K wire. In this fashion, bilateral pedicle screws were inserted from T1 to L5 in the three cadavers. All pedicles that were at least 4.0 mm in diameter were instrumented. Thirty lumbar pedicle screws and 64 thoracic pedicle screws were placed (eight thoracic pedicles were less than 4.0 mm in diameter). The largest possible screw, ranging from 4.0 to 6.5 mm diameter, was inserted. Postprocedure, CT scans with 1 mm slice thickness were obtained using a GE High Speed Advantage scanner (GE Healthcare Technologies, Waukesha, WI). The scans were reconstructed so as to allow evaluation of screw placement accuracy. Eighty-nine of 94 screws (95%) were placed completely within the cortical pedicle margins. This included all 30 lumbar screws (100%) and 59 of 64 thoracic screws (92%). The mean diameter of all thoracic pedicles was 6.0 mm (range 2.9 to 11.0 mm); the mean diameter of the five pedicles that suffered wall violations was 4.6 mm (range 4.1 to 6.3 mm). Two of the violations were less than 2 mm outside of the cortex and the three others were between 2 and 3 mm.

Clinical Experience

Three-dimensional fluoroscopy has been used at the University of Tennessee to place pedicle screws in several clinical cases, all of which involve percutaneous fixation of the lumbar spine. The following case is illustrative.

A 36-year-old man with a long history of severe mechanical low back pain and bilateral leg pain presented for treatment. Plain films and magnetic resonance imaging showed evidence of a grade I L5–S1 spondylolisthesis with degenerative disc disease and retrolisthesis at L4–5. He had previously undergone a thorough trial of nonoperative therapy including nonsteroidal anti-inflammatory drugs, physical therapy, and chiropractic manipulation. His neurologic examination was completely normal. He underwent a two-level anterior lumbar interbody fusion procedure at L4–5 and L5–S1 using threaded cortical bone dowels and bone morphogenetic protein. Posterior percutaneous pedicle screws and rods were then placed from L4 to S1 using the Sextant system.[31] The Iso-C 3D fluoroscope, in conjunction with the StealthStation Treon, was used to determine the proper skin entry site and navigate through the pedicles. With the same device, fluoroscopy was used to make certain that inadvertent K-wire advancement did not occur. All steps of pedicle cannulation were performed under 3D image guidance. A postprocedure scan was performed in the operating room prior to closure and confirmed accurate screw placement. A formal thin-cut postoperative CT scan was also performed and revealed that all four screws were safely placed within the cortical margins of the pedicles. The patient's preoperative leg pain resolved, and he was discharged home in improved condition.

CONCLUSION

Intraoperative spinal navigation technology has advanced rapidly in recent years. Although traditional methods of intraoperative spinal localization still have an important role to play in the field of spine surgery, it is clear that short-comings with these modalities exist. Image guidance addresses many of these concerns and provides detailed views of "hidden" spinal anatomy that can be used for surgical planning and navigation. As a result, image guidance has repeatedly been shown to increase the accuracy of many spinal instrumentation procedures and enhance patient safety. Certainly, there are drawbacks to and limitations of image-guided spinal surgery. Ongoing advances in this field address these limitations and appear quite promising.

REFERENCES

1. Rampersaud YR, Simon DA, Foley KT: Accuracy requirements for image-guided spinal pedicle screw placement. Spine 26(4):352–359, 2001.
2. Sanders R, Koval KJ, Dipasquale T, et al: Exposure of the orthopaedic surgeon to radiation. J Bone Joint Surg 75:326–330, 1993.
3. Castro WH, Halm H, Jerosch J, et al: Accuracy of pedicle screw placement in lumbar vertebrae. Spine 21(11):1320–1324, 1996.
4. Laine T, Lund T, Ylikoski M, et al: Accuracy of pedicle screw insertion with and without computer assistance: A randomized controlled clinical study in 100 consecutive patients. Eur Spine J 9(3):235–240, 2000.
5. Schulze CJ, Munzinger E, Weber U, et al: Clinical relevance of accuracy of pedicle screw placement. A computed tomographic-supported analysis. Spine 23(20):2215–2220, 1998.
6. Foley KT, Smith MM: Image-guided spine surgery. Neurosurg Clin North Am 7:171–186, 1996.
7. Merloz P, Tonetti J, Pillet L: Pedicle screw placement using image-guided techniques. Clin Orthop 354:39–48, 1998.
8. Schwarzenbach O, Berlemann U, Jost B, et al: Accuracy of computer-assisted pedicle screw placement. An in vivo computed tomography analysis. Spine 22(4):452–458, 1997.
9. Brodwater BK, Roberts DW, Nakajima T, et al: Extracranial application of the frameless stereotactic operating microscope: Experience with lumbar spine. Neurosurgery 32:209–213, 1993.
10. Roessler K, Ungersboeck K, Dietrich W, et al: Frameless stereotactic guided neurosurgery: Clinical experience with an infrared based pointer device navigation system. Acta Neurochir 139:551–559, 1997.
11. Foley KT, Smith KR, Bucholz RD: Stereotactic applications in spine surgery. Contemporary Update on Disorders of the Spine, Snowbird, Utah, January 1994.
12. Kalfas IH, Kormos DW, Murphy MA, et al: Application of frameless stereotaxy to pedicle screw fixation of the spine. J Neurosurg 83:641–647, 1995.
13. Nolte LP, Zamorano LJ, Jiang Z, et al: Image-guided insertion of transpedicular screws. A laboratory set-up. Spine 20(4):497–500, 1995.
14. Bloch O, Holly LT, Park J, et al: Effect of frameless stereotaxy on the accuracy of C1–2 transarticular screw placement. J Neurosurg 95(1 Suppl):74–79, 2001.
15. Foley KT, Smith MM: Frameless stereotactic guidance of C1-2 transarticular screw placement: Clinical experience. J Neurosurg 86(2):360A, 1997.
16. Youkilis AS, Quint DJ, McGillicuddy JE, et al: Stereotactic navigation for placement of pedicle screws in the thoracic spine. Neurosurgery 48(4):771–781, 2001.
17. Haberland N, Ebmeier K, Hliscs R, et al: Intraoperative CT in image-guided surgery of the spine. Med Mundi 43(4):24–31, 1999.
18. Foley KT, Simon DA, Rampersaud YA: Virtual fluoroscopy: Computer-assisted fluoroscopic navigation. Spine 26(4):347–351, 2001.
19. Rampersaud YR, Foley KT, Shen AC, et al: Radiation exposure to the spine surgeon during fluoroscopically assisted pedicle screw insertion. Spine 25:2637–2645, 2000.
20. Weinstein JN, Spratt KF, Spengeler D, et al: Spinal pedicle fixation: Reliability and validity of roentgenogram based assessment and surgical factors on successful screw placement. Spine 13:1013–1018, 1988.
21. Liljenqvist UR, Halm HF, Link TM: Pedicle screw instrumentation of the thoracic spine in idiopathic scoliosis. Spine 22(19):2239–2245, 1997.
22. Vaccaro AR, Rizzolo SJ, Balderson RA, et al: Placement of pedicle screws in the thoracic spine II: An anatomical and radiographic assessment. J Bone Joint Surg 77(8):1200–1206, 1995.
23. Foley KT, Silveri CP, Vaccaro AR, et al: Atlantoaxial transarticular screw fixation: Risk assessment and bone morphology using an image guidance system. J Bone Joint Surg Br 80(Suppl):245, 1998.
24. Madawi AA, Casey AT, Solanki GK, et al: Radiological and anatomical evaluation of the atlantoaxial transarticular fixation technique. J Neurosurg 86:961–968, 1997.
25. Paramore CG, Dickman CA, Sonntag VKH: The anatomical suitability of the C1-2 complex for transarticular screw fixation. J Neurosurg 85:221–224, 1996.
26. Mandel IM, Kambach BJ, Petersilge CA, et al: Morphologic considerations of C2 isthmus dimensions for the placement of transarticular screws. Spine 25:1542–1547, 2000.
27. Graham AW, Swank ML, Kinard RE, et al: Posterior cervical arthrodesis and stabilization with a lateral mass plate: Clinical and computed tomographic evaluation of lateral mass screw placement and associated complications. Spine 21(3):323–329, 1996.
28. Heller JG, Carlson GD, Abitol JJ, Garfin SR: Anatomic comparison of the Roy-Camille and Magerl techniques for screw placement in the lower cervical spine. Spine 20(22):2442–2448, 1995.

29. Foley KT, Smith KR, Smith MM: Frameless stereotactic guidance of cervical spine lateral mass screw placement. In Nolte LP, Ganz R (eds): Computer Assisted Orthopaedic Surgery (CAOS). Bern, Switzerland: Hogrefe & Huber Publications, 1999, pp 89–98.

30. Holly LT, Foley KT: The placement of percutaneous thoracolumbar pedicle screws using three-dimensional fluoroscopy. J Neurosurg (Spine 3) 99:324–329, 2003.

31. Foley KT, Gupta S: Percutaneous pedicle screw fixation of the lumbar spine: Preliminary clinical results. J Neurosurg 97(1 Suppl):7–12, 2002.

152 Surgical Management of Segmental Spinal Instability

MICHAEL C. PARK, J. FREDERICK HARRINGTON, JR.,
LOUIS G. JENIS, and GERHARD M. FRIEHS

White and Panjabi[1] have described instability as the loss of the spine's ability under physiologic loads to maintain a pattern of displacement so as to avoid neurologic deficit, deformity, and pain. Spondylolisthesis, trauma, and congenital abnormalities in the lumbar spine can easily fulfill these criteria. However, a significantly larger proportion of patients without gross deformity of the spine but significant pain may not necessarily fulfill these instability criteria. Such patients may be labeled with a "failed back syndrome" when chronic, unremitting back pain follows one or more surgical procedures, or may be described as having "mechanical back pain" if similar pain is not associated with previous surgery or deformity. Other descriptors include "degenerative disc disease" or "internal disc disruption" when chronic pain is associated with radiographic or magnetic resonance imaging (MRI) abnormalities at the disc space. These patients have in common pain without gross deformity in the motion segment (the disc space and facet joints). The condition was termed segmental spinal instability by Frymoyer and Selby.[2] The precise pathophysiologic dynamic of this kind of back pain is not completely understood. However, through basic research, imaging, and procedures such as facet injections and discography, we have developed a greater understanding.

SEGMENTAL SPINAL INSTABILITY

Frymoyer[3] has classified degenerative segmental instabilities into primary instabilities related to the degenerative process alone, and secondary instabilities, those related in part to previous lumbar spine surgeries or procedures (Table 152-1). All relate to degenerative change within the facets or discs or to facets and discs degenerated or weakened by surgical intervention. Kirkaldy-Willis and Hill[4] postulated that until the degenerative process has stiffened an injured motion segment adequately, pain will persist. It is well appreciated that chronic back pain occurs more often in middle age,[5] and that low back pain is much less common in the seventh decade of life and beyond, although degenerative changes are most advanced in these decades. For a variety of reasons, the arthritic process of stiffening and strengthening is inadequate compensation for the demands placed on the lumbar spine in many middle-aged patients.

Kinematics studies of range of motion under conditions of physiologic loading suggest that what is most likely to cause pain is not degeneration per se, but variations in velocity within the neutral zone, that is, that part of usual and normal range of motion requiring little or no loading force.[6] These variations in velocity probably arise from degeneration and irregularity of disc and facet joint surfaces. Biomechanical studies have shown that complex and continuous load sharing occurs between the two components of the motion segment.[7] Because of load sharing, pain may often emanate from more than one source in a single motion segment.[8–10]

Degeneration in the disc space appears to begin with the breakdown of the proteoglycan, link, and core proteins that provide the hydrostatic and shock-absorbing qualities of disc material.[11–13] Some factors that exacerbate this process are surgical disc removal, end-plate trauma, tears in the disc annulus,[14,15] end-plate thickening leading to decreased nutrients to disc material,[16,17] and cigarette smoking.[18,19] As the volume and elasticity of the disc material decrease, the supporting ligaments of the disc space become lax, and the kinematic relationships between disc and facets change.[20] Disc shrinkage further concentrates stresses in the margins of the end plates, which precipitates arthritic spurring in an attempt to stiffen this lax region.[21] Although these arthritic changes serve eventually to stiffen and strengthen this region, the process may be slow and pain may manifest when kinematic changes first develop, especially when combined with disc space abnormalities.[22,23]

Unfortunately, there is no clinical test that can directly measure and quantify these physiologic abnormalities

---

TABLE 152–1 ■ **Degenerative Segmental Instabilities**

Primary Instabilities

Axial rotational instability
Translational instability
Retrolisthetic instability
Progressing degenerative scoliosis
Disc disruption syndrome

Secondary Instabilities

After disc excision, subclassified according to the pattern of instability as described under primary instabilities
After decompressive laminectomy
Accentuation of preexisting deformity
New deformity (i.e., no deformity existed at the time of original decompression); further subclassified as for primary instabilities
After spinal fusion
Above or below a spinal fusion, subclassified as for primary instabilities
Pseudoarthrosis
After chymopapain injection

Adapted from Frymoyer JW: The role of spine fusion. In Loeser JD (ed): Neurosurgery Clinics of North America. Philadelphia: WB Saunders, 1991, p 931.

associated with painful degeneration. Reliance is placed on the clinical history and examination, flexion-extension radiographs, MRI, facet injections, and discography.

PATIENT SELECTION

An important concern is the chronicity of the pain. Chronic back pain is usually defined as that lasting 3 months or longer, because most musculoskeletal pain abates in that time.[24-26] Only patients who have pain at least this long should be considered for surgical evaluation. It is important to take a careful history of the duration, location, and quality of the pain to differentiate segmental instability pain from radicular pain, spinal stenosis pain, sacroiliac pain, or degenerative disease of the hip. Although the degree of pain can be variable, patients to be considered for invasive treatment should have significant pain on a daily basis that makes work or routine activities difficult or impossible.

Segmental instability pain is usually centered in the midline and is not associated with paresthesias in the foot unless the patient has had previous or coincident radiculopathy. Segmental instability pain can radiate into the buttocks but usually goes no lower than the knees, and is coincident with worsening midline pain or frank muscle spasm. When the facet joint is a prominent component of the pain, a more unilateral buttock pain may be experienced, but without the shooting quality and paresthesias associated with radicular pain. Recumbency usually provides relief, and pain usually is not worse at night.

On physical examination, the degree of tenderness or muscle spasm in the back to palpation can be quite variable. The patient's spine should be palpated in the flexed position to observe for thoracic or lumbar scoliosis. Muscle tenderness, if present, is not necessarily over the dysfunctional motion segment. Decreased range of motion is the most consistent physical examination finding, and is limited by pain. Frequently, there is a specific pain in moving from flexion to a fully upright position that results in a "catch" that causes patients to brace themselves with their hands on the anterior thigh. Nerve root tension signs are absent, although hip flexion may often precipitate back pain. Tenderness over the sacroiliac joint strongly suggests sacroiliitis, but the diagnosis is not made unless there is pain with gapping, compression, and pressure maneuvers of the sacroiliac joint. Injecting the sacroiliac joint with lidocaine and steroids can be diagnostic or theraputic.[27] It is important to observe nondirected patient movements to see if these behaviors are consistent with those elicited by the physician; if inconsistent, the patient may be exaggerating.

Plain radiographs should be observed for traction spurs, indicative of incomplete or unsuccessful ankylosis of the motion segment associated with low back pain,[28] for scoliosis, or for lytic defects of the pars interarticularis. Computed tomography (CT) can be used to confirm suspected bony abnormalities seen on plain radiography, particularly pars interarticularis fractures or degenerative changes of the facet joints.[29] However, MRI is the most important imaging modality because of its sensitivity for degenerative changes in the disc space region. On T2-weighted images, a good approximation of the degree of disc material degeneration can be inferred from the loss of signal related to proteoglycan and water loss in the disc.[30] Berns and colleagues[31] described three types of degenerative change in bony end plates. Type 1 is the least advanced, with decreased signal on T1-weighted images and increased signal on T2-weighted images, indicating early fibrovascular tissue invasion; type 2 shows increased signal on T1-weighted images, indicating increased fat and perhaps more advanced degenerative change; and type 3 changes demonstrate low signal on both T1- and T2-weighted images consistent with cortical bone signal. Patients with degenerative segmental instability should have at least one of these MRI abnormalities (Fig. 152-1).

Although imaging modalities, particularly MRI, have facilitated the diagnosis of segmental spinal instability, we believe that MRI supplemented with a conservative care program that includes a psychological profile of the patient plus discography is the most complete way to screen patients for treatment. This type of evaluation, and time invested with the patient, may lead to optimum patient selection and, therefore, the best long-term outcomes.

ROLE OF DISCOGRAPHY

A trial of external bracing has been felt to be of benefit in patient selection for surgery,[32] but we believe that the more anatomic and physiologic specific data obtained from a combination of MRI and provocative discography are far more informative. We believe that water-soluble contrast discography (Omnipaque 300, Amersham Health, Princeton, NJ) is particularly helpful to confirm adequate sensitivity of MRI for painful internal disc disruption. Holt[33] was the first to demonstrate a relationship between the development of a concordant pain response to injection in a lumbar disc space and a positive response to fusion surgery, and many reviews since have confirmed this.[34-36] It appears that pain on injection of the disc is relatively specific for patients with back pain, because only 17% of discs injected in healthy volunteers are painful.[37] Complication rates in general are low, but include discitis and nerve root injury. Infection rates are low with the use of intravenous or intradiscal antibiotics.[38] Whether surgical results are improved when discography is used together with available imaging studies is controversial.[39-41] The radiographic integrity of posterolateral or titanium alloy cage and allograft bone interbody fusion are difficult to determine. Because of this uncertainty, and continuously evolving surgical methods, the question is still not definitively answered. We often find concordant pain elicited even at normal levels by MRI. This information is useful in our surgical planning.

The goal of any discography session is to identify any number of concordant pain responses and one nonpainful "control" level. A control level usually is signaled when a disc injection is experienced as a slightly uncomfortable pressure sensation clearly unlike the patient's usual back pain. Disc degeneration can be graded on a 5-point scale[42] (Fig. 152-2), but the patient's subjective experience is more important than the morphology of the disc. However, the radiographic appearance of the disc can help explain a concordant pain response because annular tears are more frequently appreciated by discography than by MRI, and are highly associated with concordant pain[43] (Fig. 152-3). Discography should be performed with a minimal amount of sedation. If the patient is awake and alert, or at most minimally sedated, both the physician and patient understand

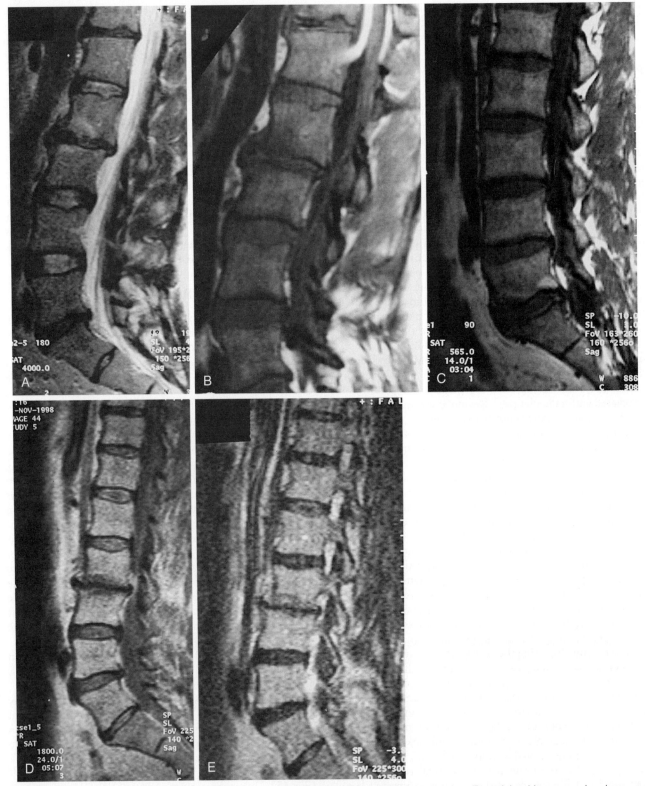

FIGURE 152-1   *A* and *B,* Modic type 1 end-plate degenerative change with a decreased signal on T1-weighted images and an increased signal on T2-weighted images, which is indicative of fibrovascular change. *C,* Type 2 change is considered to be more advanced with fatty invasion of the end-plate region and an increased signal on T1-weighted images. *D* and *E,* Type 3 change is most advanced and demonstrates a decreased signal on both T1- and T2-weighted images, which is indicative of cortical bone formation.

FIGURE 152-2 Classification of discograms. (From Adams MA, Dolan P, Hutton WC: The stages of disc degeneration as revealed by discograms. J Bone Joint Surg Br 68:36–42, 1986.)

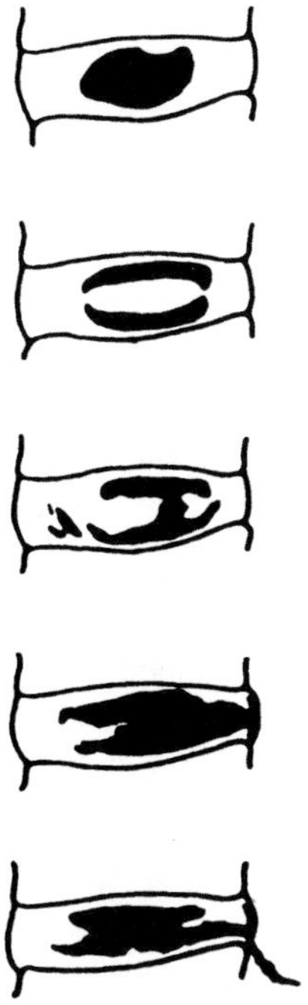

Discogram type		Stage of disc degeneration
1. Cottonball		No signs of degeneration. Soft white amorphous nucleus
2. Lobular		Mature disc with nucleus starting to coalesce into fibrous lumps
3. Irregular		Degenerated disc with fissures and clefts in the nucleus and inner annulus
4. Fissured		Degenerated disc with a radial fissure leading to the outer edge of the annulus
5. Ruptured		Disc has a complete radial fissure that allows injected fluid to escape. Can be in any state of degeneration

what particular pain is being sought in the procedure, and false-positive responses are minimized.

Concordant pain responses are usually obtained with the first milliliter of contrast injection. Sometimes, in patients with annular tears and contrast extravasation, more contrast is needed. If concordant pain has not developed after injection of 2 mL, the level is considered asymptomatic. If contrast extravasation is seen, we inject up to 3 mL before making a final determination. If the patient has pain, and once a determination has been made about the disc, we inject 1 mL of 1% lidocaine into the disc to give relief and make evaluations at subsequent levels clearer during the session. For equivocal responses, we bring the patient back later for

a lidocaine discogram instead of a provocative injection. If relief is significant, this information can be helpful.

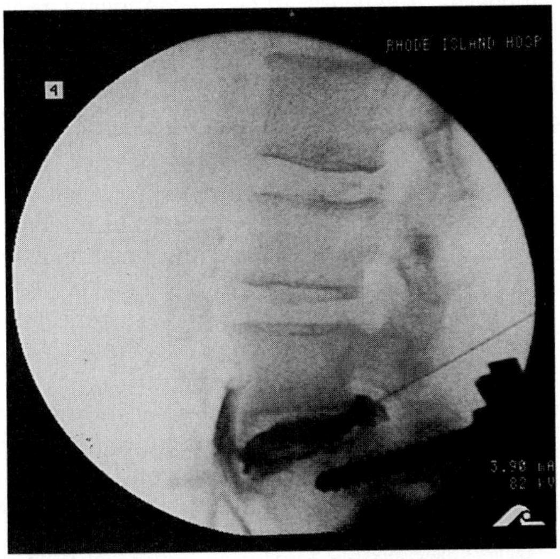

When concordant pain is present at three levels in a patient without previous back surgery at a painful level, we are unlikely to recommend fusion surgery, although joint-preserving procedures such as intradiscal electrothermal therapy (IDET) or disc prostheses may be considered. A somatoform disorder that inhibits a favorable response to surgery is a consideration in patients with concordant pain for whom a nonpainful level cannot be obtained.

OTHER PREOPERATIVE CONSIDERATIONS

Complicating matters even further are Workers' Compensation or disability claims. Remaining ill can be financially rewarding under some circumstances, and financial considerations may either consciously or unconsciously promote the unwell state.[44,45] Psychological testing has not been able to screen those patients for whom the "compensation neurosis" is a major factor, and so it can be difficult to discern how secondary gain is affecting the patient's health status.[46-48] We believe that time spent in a goal-oriented conservative care program emphasizing fitness, aerobic exercise, and a healthy lifestyle can clarify these situations. Fitness, weight, and strength should be tracked and quantified, and hopefully improved before any intervention is considered. Because of its deleterious effects on joints and on bone fusion, smoking cessation is demanded in our clinic before any surgical fusion is considered. We demand participation in a vigorous program of conservative care where these parameters are monitored before surgery is performed. Patients with secondary gain issues often eliminate themselves from surgical consideration by their inability to

FIGURE 152-3 Discogram demonstrating contrast extravasation through an annular tear.

concentrate on goal-directed behaviors. Whether biological fusion enhancers like bone morphogenic protein (BMP-2) (INFUSE, Medtronic Sofamor Danek, Memphis, TN, U.S.A.) can overcome the deleterious effects of smoking on fusion is not yet known, but these substances should be considered for use if for some reason surgery is performed on smokers, or in patients with abnormalities of bone metabolism.

TREATMENT

Treatments beyond the routine use of oral pain relievers can be divided into six categories: (1) surgical fusion, (2) facet rhizotomy, (3) epidural electrical spinal cord stimulation (SCS), (4) intrathecal opiates, (5) IDET, and (6) prosthetic disc replacement. These treatments have not been compared with each other in a randomized, retrospective fashion, so their true relative efficacies remain uncertain. The newest treatments, IDET and prosthetic disc replacement, are exciting from a conceptual standpoint because they treat microinstability pain without sacrificing the motion segment. If these techniques prove to be effective long-term treatments of microinstability pain and avoid later adjacent segment pain syndromes seen over time with fusion, a significant advance in treatment will have occurred. However, at this point in time fusion remains the standard of surgical treatment of focal microinstability in the lumbar spine that has exhausted conservative measures. For patients with multilevel disease, for those whose pain generator appears to be in the facet, and for patients who fail to make attainable lifestyle changes necessary to reduce long-term strain on the low back, pharmacologic treatment, facet rhizotomy, spinal epidural stimulation, or intrathecal opiates may be preferable strategies.

Fusion

As stated by Nachemson,[49] there are still no prospective studies that have a strictly defined patient population or a complete, long-term follow-up to determine accurately the efficacy of fusion procedures. Surgical fusion makes sense because it hastens the apparent end result of the osteoarthritic process, a stiffer but stronger spine.[50] Fusing more than two levels decreases range of motion and leads to high levels of stress on remaining motion segments that may cause segmental instability and pain at the next functioning motion segment.[51,52] Unless surgery has been performed previously at more than two levels, we do not recommend fusion of more than two levels in this patient group.

Prospective cohort studies and retrospective studies of the use of posterolateral fusion with or without instrumentation for patients with segmental spinal instability demonstrated good or excellent outcomes in 39% to 82% of patients.[53–57] Newer interbody methods use implants that are simultaneously osteoconductive and stabilizing, which may lead to higher fusion rates.[58–61] The approach may be anterior with temporary displacement of major arteries and veins, anterior lumbar interbody fusion (ALIF), or posterior between nerve roots, posterior lumbar interbody fusion (PLIF). In reality, the decision of which fusion process to employ in a particular patient can be complex and difficult in the absence of literature-based standards or recommendations. Existing literature is mostly retrospective, providing only evidence-based

options of treatment modality. Therefore, in addition to the complex and difficult process of patient selection, the process of choosing a fusion procedure is also complex and difficult, and without certainty.

The choice of procedure may simply rest on the resources at hand. For example, if an experienced vascular or general surgeon is not available to help access the spine in the region of the great vessels, many ALIF procedures are contraindicated unless the spine surgeon has an exceptional background. However, in most cases, the decision rests on knowledge of sometimes subtle advantages of one approach over another for specific situations. In our clinic, we have tried to take advantage of this knowledge to get the best outcomes and avoid complications.

There are two main strengths of the anterior approach to the lower lumbar spine. The first is that manipulation of nerve roots can be completely avoided, a worthwhile goal since when nerve root injury or irritation occurs, pain may last indefinitely.[62] The second advantage of the anterior approach is that a relatively large percentage of the vertebral end plate can be accessed and a large interbody implant can be used to cover a relatively large amount of the surface area of the end plate.[63,64]

The most obvious disadvantage of the anterior approaches is damage to the large arteries and veins overlying the spine.[62] Damage to the aorta, iliac arteries, or lumbar segmental vessels during surgery are generally well tolerated in most patients.[62,64,65] However, in patients with calcified or otherwise atherosclerotic vessels, there is a risk for further embolism or occlusion, which could threaten blood flow to the lower extremities, and even to the spinal cord. Calcification of the aorta or iliac arteries represents a contraindication to the anterior approach. Damage to the large venous structures during surgery can actually be life threatening since control of hemorrhage and surgical repair are more difficult. The potential for retrograde ejaculation related to disruption of the spinal sympathetic plexus is 2% to 40% and can make men desiring to have children essentially sterile.[66,67] Any man planning a family should be aware of this possibility preoperatively.

The advantage of a posterior approach is that decompression of the spinal canal and neural foramen can be treated simultaneously.[63] Obviously, the bony confines of a stenotic lumbar spinal canal cannot be changed from the anterior approach. Distraction of the disc space from the anterior approach can lessen foraminal stenosis by increasing the height of the foramen.[63] However, in many cases, the neural foramen is narrow in an anterior to posterior direction. Under these circumstances, a posterior approach is the best way to increase the width of the foramen in the dorsal to ventral direction while also increasing foraminal height. From the posterior approach, the surgeon can also directly inspect the position of pedicle screws vis-à-vis the neighboring nerve roots. This may be an advantage if placing pedicle screws in the presence of deformity.

Posterior lumbar interbody fusion with instrumentation appears to be an effective method of arthrodesis, particularly since a new generation of allograft, metallic and reabsorbable polymer-based implants, and implantation preparation instrumentation have been developed over the past few years.[63,68–70] During PLIF, symptomatic disc herniations are removed and foraminal stenosis is improved during the process of implant insertion into the disc space. Following implant insertion, further foraminotomy is facilitated because the nerve root has been partially decompressed by distraction afforded by the interbody spacer. We find PLIF the procedure of choice for levels with associated foraminal stenosis. The drawback of the method is that the process is performed in close proximity to the exiting nerve roots above and below the disc space.[62,71] An incidence of nerve root irritation has been described, and this complication can greatly affect outcome.

Transverse lumbar interbody fusion (TLIF) refers to posterior placement of interbody spacers as in PLIF, but from a unilateral and somewhat more oblique orientation to the dorsal ventral axis. This method has similar advantages to the PLIF approach. However, because insertion of interbody spacers is unilateral, fewer nerve roots are exposed to the risk for irritation, and generally, the time of surgery is reduced.[62] This is an ideal approach at L4–L5 and rostrally where both the end plates and the lateral epidural space is smaller than at L5–S1. Relatively more facet is removed unilaterally than in PLIF to establish a working space. Disadvantages are that at times it can be difficult to insert equivalent size or number of implants as in the standard PLIF approach, and this difference could affect overall fusion rates.

Intertransverse or posterolateral fusion has the advantage that it can be performed without direct exposure of nerve roots that are vulnerable to injury, and has been the standard method of fusion in the lumbar spine for decades. Iliac crest bone harvest and bone harvested during laminectomy have been used. Problems with this method include pseudoarthrosis at a rate of 5% to 10% per level fused and persistent discomfort from the bone harvest site at the posterior iliac crest. The disadvantages of the posterior approach are that open exposure techniques are quite painful in the perioperative period and that the nerve roots are relatively susceptible to injury from surgical manipulation.

If posterolateral fusion to the transverse process is performed, most patients will require at least 3 days of intravenous narcotics. While performing an interbody fusion, the rostral nerve root in the area of disc space exposure is particularly susceptible to injury, especially when there has been a previous posterior surgery and when there is a spondylolisthesis. Under these two conditions, the rostral nerve root may be poorly visualized in a scar, or it may actually overlie the disc space. Thus scraping, tapping, and chiseling maneuvers may inadvertently injure the nerve root despite the efforts to control for this. Finally, metallic implants, dead space, and avascular tissue planes during closure set conditions whereby infection can develop more often than in anterior procedures.

Thus we use the anterior approach in younger patients without signs of atherosclerosis by clinical examination and without significant calcification of the great vessels, with adequate foraminal size in the dorsal ventral direction, with adequate bony dimensions to the spinal canal, and with pain related to the L4–L5 and/or L5–S1 joint space levels, with two-level fusions always having supplemental posterior instrumentation fixation. Posterior approaches are used under other circumstances, and always include supplemental instrumentation. These include intertransverse or posterolateral fusion, as well as PLIF and TLIF.

Stand-alone intertransverse fusion is a reasonable choice after laminectomy with degenerative spondylolisthesis and without significant loss of height of the neural foramen at that level. However, for a variety of reasons, intertransverse fusion is often used to supplement an interbody fusion to create a "360-degree" fusion. With an associated interbody construct, we have avoided iliac crest harvest and have instead used a combination of allograft bone chips, laminectomy bone, and biological bone fusion enhancers with good results.

Facet Rhizotomy

Facet rhizotomy is an alternative for patients with relatively normal-looking disc spaces on MRI who have responded with more than 75% pain relief to a facet injection. Studies have shown that results are best in patients who have not had previous surgery, and we do not usually recommend this procedure at levels previously subjected to surgery.[72] Even in the patients who have not previously undergone surgery, successful results are seen only in 30% to 50% of patients 2 years after the procedure.[72–75] The main reason for its lack of effectiveness is probably that most of the ventral innervations of the facet joint is unaffected by the procedure. However, because significant complications are rare in this minimally invasive outpatient procedure, it may be worthwhile in certain patients with buttock and back pain without severe disc disease on MRI.

Epidural Spinal Cord Stimulation

The concept of SCS therapy for the suppression of pain is based on the gate control theory developed in 1965.[76] Low-threshold, large-diameter nerve fiber collaterals in the spinal cord are believed to inhibit transmission of pain signals to the brain. The sensation of electrical stimulation of the dorsal spinal cord is usually perceived as paresthesia in the respective dermatomal distributions; the constant, nagging pain is traded for a warm, tingling sensation in the affected area. The epidural electrode arrays implanted today most likely provide electrical stimulation to the posterior columns, the dorsal horn, dorsal root entry zone, and dorsal roots.[77] Therefore, the previously used term dorsal column stimulation may be somewhat misleading.

For a patient to be eligible for SCS therapy, there must be no identifiable neurocompressive lesion on diagnostic studies. In other words, patients who do not have frank instability, disc herniations, or spinal, neuroforaminal, or lateral recess stenosis that would require surgical repair are in general considered candidates for SCS. The pain has to be refractory to nonsurgical means, including physical therapy, chiropractic treatment, nerve blocks, and behavioral or psychological approaches to pain treatment. It is advisable to exercise a multimodality approach to SCS treatment and include a psychologist or psychiatrist in the decision-making process for SCS therapy, especially to identify potential depression or other mood disorders, although there is still debate over whether certain psychological profiles can be used as predictors of good outcome for SCS treatment.[78–80] Patients with leg pain usually respond better to SCS therapy than patients with back pain.[81] However, newer hardware designs with up to 16 electrodes per array and the use of multiple implanted arrays arranged parallel to each other have shown promising results for pain relief in the lower back and both legs.[82]

A good response to SCS therapy is achieved when patients report pain relief of at least 50%. Prospective studies show that this pain relief is achieved in 50% to 70% of patients in the first 2 years after implantation.[83–88] Five years and more after implantation, the positive response rate drops slightly to around 50%.[83,89–92] Compared with alternative therapies, SCS was found to be cost effective, especially when compared with expensive surgical alternatives or drug therapies with lower efficacy.[93,94]

Intrathecal Morphine

Morphine or morphine-like medications are available as oral, intramuscular, intravenous, subcutaneous, sublingual, nasal, and intrathecal preparations. However, the intrathecal route of administration allows for application of the medication directly to the site of action in the spinal cord and brain without having to cross the blood-brain barrier. This results in a dramatic increase in effectiveness, decrease in the required dose (0.3% to 1% of the oral or intravenous route), and decrease in side effects such as lethargy, somnolence, or constipation. When considering intrathecal opioid therapy, it is especially important to bear in mind the difference between drug tolerance, physical drug dependence, and drug addiction.[95] Unfortunately, misinterpretation of these terms has often led to undertreatment of pain. With the increased use of intrathecal opioid therapy in nonmalignant diseases, the often irrational fear of long-term opioid administration is being questioned.

Because of the potential lifelong commitment to a medication pump, intrathecal morphine therapy is usually reserved for patients who are poor candidates for fusion or SCS, or have insufficient pain relief with SCS therapy. The importance of patient selection applies to intrathecal drug therapy even more than with other therapies.[96] In addition to the general contraindications to surgery, there are also specific contraindications to intrathecal morphine therapy, which include active untreated depression and other psychopathologies,[97] so we recommend a thorough psychological evaluation before implantation.

Selected patients become potential intrathecal opioid pump recipients when a test trial of intrathecal opioid produces at least 50% reduction in pain with no intolerable side effects.[96] Studies have shown that patients report, on the average, 40% to 60% reduction in pain in the first 2 years after implantation.[98–101] Three years or more after implantation, approximately 65% to 75% of patients report continued good to excellent pain relief and satisfaction with the procedure.[102–104] Although there is development of tolerance to opioids in 35% of patients with intrathecal therapy, it is much slower than with other delivery forms. In one study, the average intrathecal morphine requirement was found to be less than 5 mg/24 hours after more than 3 years of intrathecal therapy.[100] It is estimated that intrathecal opioid therapy is less expensive than comparable alternative treatment if the duration of therapy exceeds 22 months.[105–107]

Intradiscal Electrothermal Therapy

As previously stated in this chapter, microinstability pain is felt to originate from laxity and unpredictability in lumbar motion segments in the neutral zone. Theoretically, treatment that changes these parameters could be helpful in reducing

back pain. In 1998, Saal and Saal introduced IDET.[108] In this percutaneous procedure, a copper coil is introduced into the disc space for the purpose of heating the disc annulus. As a result of a 17-minute burn at 90°C, cross-linking bonds between collagen fibers stiffen annular collagen.[109] In addition, some loss of annular denervation may also occur.[110] The combined effect of the stiffening of collagen fibers and potential loss of nerve receptors can provide relief from microinstability pain.

This is a particularly attractive strategy in treating patients who have not previously undergone surgery and younger patients with relatively normal amounts of disc cartilage left in the disc space. The motion segment is preserved, albeit in an altered state.[111] Discography is recommended prior to the procedure to confirm which discs are pain producing. Two-year follow-up in a controlled trial showed that 54% had achieved at least 50% pain relief, no longer used opioids, and were at work.[112,113] These are degrees of effectiveness well above the placebo effect. Beyond 2 years, efficacy has not been determined. As for almost all treatments for microinstability, there have been no prospective comparisons of this treatment with other older or more established treatments such as fusion. At this point in time, insurance coverage is not universally available for this procedure.

Prosthetic Disc Replacement

The concept of pain relief with fusion for degenerative disc disease likely relates to elimination of causative factors. Load redistribution, load sharing, and eradication of inflammatory components are possible mechanisms involved with pain relief. The clinical outcomes of fusion are reasonable given the appropriate diagnostic determination of the pain generator and a technically sound procedure. However, lumbar fusion is not without potential drawbacks, including pseudoarthrosis, persistent pain, instrumentation failure, persistent donor graft site pain, and adjacent segment degeneration. The lumbar artificial disc is a motion preservation device that may become an alternative to arthrodesis. Replacement of a degenerated joint by a prosthetic device has been successfully performed for painful and degenerated knees and hips for several years.[114] Therefore, a disc prosthesis could offer relief from degenerative spine pain related to microinstability in the disc space.

Lumbar disc prosthesis has several obvious advantages over other forms of treatment for microinstability pain. First, normal range of motion of the lumbar spine can be maintained. Second, preservation of the motion segment should lessen or eliminate the problem of adjacent disc level irritation seen with fusion, which is a prominent reason why fusion operations may not give permanent relief. The indications for the disc replacement include symptomatic degenerative disc disease with minimal facet joint sclerosis or narrowing at L5–S1 and mechanical back pain in patients that have failed a conservative treatment program. Postlaminectomy syndrome with mechanical back pain is also a reasonable indication. However, the complexity of the entire lumbar motion segment may make diagnosis of the most appropriate patients for the procedure more difficult. In cases where there is microinstability related to the facet joint, a disc prosthesis may not relieve pain and/or prosthesis insertion could change conditions enough to initiate microinstability pain in the facet joint at the same motion segment or in other motion segments. Therefore, the device is contraindicated in situations involving posterior element insufficiency, including spondylolysis and spondylolisthesis. Thus patient selection will remain an important component to achieve successful outcomes. Both discography and diagnostic facet injections will be necessary to ensure proper patient selection.

The ideal disc motion preservation device is one that alleviates pain, preserves flexibility and stability, and can withstand normal biomechanical forces while limiting stress transference to adjacent levels. The key design factors that differentiate disc spacer devices relate to the replacement of the nucleus versus total disc and the degree of constraint of the implant. Numerous devices and implants have been developed and designed over the past three decades, and several companies have expended significant financial resources in attempts to bring to market a suitable implant.

The LINK SB-Charité III device (Johnson & Johnson, Raynham, MA) is a total disc replacement device that has been well described. The device has a sliding, nonconstrained

intermediate "mobile" core made of ultra-high-density polyethylene between two cobalt chrome end plates (Fig. 152-4A). A radiopaque marker wire is embedded around the circumference of the core for identification of the position on radiographs. The end-plate design allows for restoration of lordosis based on thickening of the anterior aspect of the device of up to 0 to 10 degrees. The importance of the nonconstrained sliding core relates to the translation that occurs during segmental motion. In a normal intervertebral segment during flexion, the cranial vertebral body translates anteriorly while the center of rotation within the nucleus of the disc shifts posteriorly. The Charité device mimics this mechanical range of motion and attempts to restore normal mechanics of motion (Fig. 152-4B). Similar translation of the sliding core occurs with extension, coronal plane bending, and axial rotation. Restoration of translation of the vertebral body and core will reestablish facet motion and, at least theoretically, prevent high stresses in the posterior articulation. The ProDisc design (Synthes, West Chester, PA) differs by having a single polyethylene core,

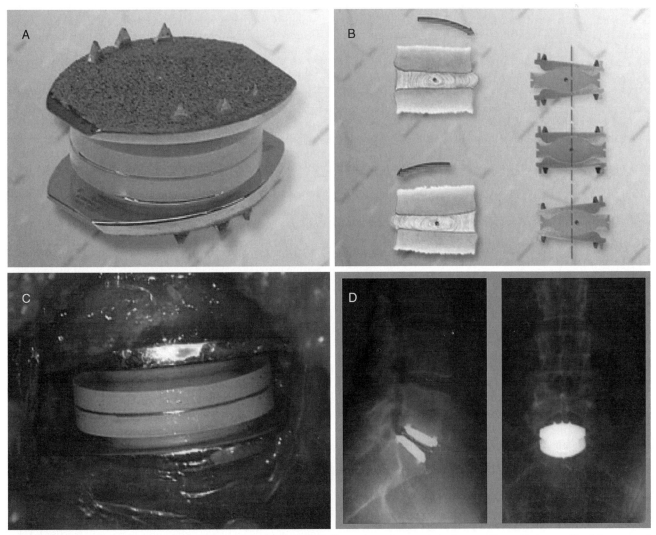

FIGURE 152-4 Lumbar disc prosthetic device. *A,* LINK SB-Charité III consists of two cobalt-chrome alloy end plates with sliding core of ultra-high-molecular-weight polyethylene. *B,* The implant allows physiologic motion of intervertebral segments in every direction, mimicking mechanical range of motion. *C,* Intraoperative image of the implanted device. *D,* Postoperative lateral and anteroposterior view plain radiographs of the properly implanted device. (Courtesy of Johnson & Johnson.)

which is relatively more constrained to its base plate during voluntary movements. Several-year follow-up after insertion of both devices at a single level suggests that patient satisfaction is at least equal to patients undergoing single-level fusion.[115-119]

Many of the prostheses in trials contain polyethylene weight-bearing surfaces used previously in hip and knee prostheses. This material is known to fragment with time and causes a chronic inflammatory reaction that contributes to fibrosis in the artificial joint and deterioration of the bone implant interface, although the degree of fragmentation appears less than with hip and knee prostheses due to less extensive forces that are conferred on a lumbar spine implant. Although the concern for the device failure exists, no laboratory data or clinical cases have demonstrated such failure, despite more than 10 years in existence and use of these devices.[114] Whether due to wear or some other factor, it is likely that prostheses will require revision over the lifetime of a young or middle-aged recipient. Scar around the great vessels in the region of the lumbar spine makes a second access relatively complicated with attendant risks. Despite these concerns, the development of disc prostheses could revolutionize the care of chronic low back pain.[120]

Over the past decade, lumbar prosthetic discs have been developed and inserted in patients outside of the United States (Fig. 152-4C and D).[114,120] Significant follow-up over several years has been obtained with both the LINK SB-Charité and ProDisc designs in Europe, with promising results.[115-119] Presently, the Food and Drug Administration (FDA) is monitoring prospective studies of these different implants.[121-123] The first Charité was implanted in the United States in March 2000 during an FDA-approved Investigational Device Exemption (IDE) study involving 15 sites. Commercial release of the device is expected by 2005. It is probable that lumbar prosthetic discs will be generally available in the United States within the next 2 years.

SURGICAL TECHNIQUE

Standard Versus Minimally Invasive Methods

From the patient's standpoint, the most onerous aspects of fusion surgery can be the significant and often severe perioperative pain created by the surgical dissection required to obtain exposure for fusion. Recently, less invasive and less painful forms of spinal exposure have been developed for most spinal fusion operations. These promise a future of less pain and shorter hospital stays, and these are worthwhile goals. However, in general these new methods increase technical difficulty. These technical challenges may increase the chances for complications, including nerve root injury, or may lead to less optimal conditions for fusion, particularly if the surgeon does not already have extensive experience with an open technique. It should be kept in mind that obtaining a complete decompression and solid arthrodesis will always be more important than the degree of perioperative discomfort.

Anterior Lumbar Interbody Fusion

Anterior lumbar interbody fusion is generally performed open using an anterior retroperitoneal approach or laparoscopically through the peritoneal cavity. Allograft threaded cylindrical bone dowels and machined and nonmachined femoral ring allografts are available (Fig. 152-5). One difference between dowels and femoral rings is that the dowels are designed to cut through the end plate while techniques or femoral allografts are more end-plate sparing. Titanium alloy interbody cages packed with autograft or bone growth enhancers have shown good to excellent results in manufacturer-sponsored and subsequent studies. It is obvious that titanium alloy will never be integrated with bone, but this handicap does not seem to prevent fusion if the surface area of the implant is more porous than metal and if the patient's bone healing is good. Fusion with biological bone enhancers such as BMP-2 (INFUSE) may increase rates of fusion, speed the time to fusion, and may make up for native deficiencies in bone metabolism that may retard successful fusion. In our clinic, most patients undergoing ALIF also undergo some form of minimally invasive supplemental instrumentation posteriorly or anteriorly to obtain the highest fusion yield.

Despite the availability of several different products, the methods of insertion are remarkably similar. It is important to adhere to the following principles during insertion to optimize outcome: (1) ascertain with fluoroscopy the midline in the axial plane before insertion, (2) secure and mobilize overlying vascular structures, (3) obtain maximal distraction of the disc space, and (5) make sure the implant position is clear of the thecal sac and nerve roots.

Open Technique

Implant size is estimated from the width of the next rostral disc space, which is assumed to be near in width to the maximally distracted disc space at surgery, and the interpedicular distance and the anteroposterior (AP) diameter of the vertebral body. Although final decisions are made at surgery, this analysis may help the surgeon anticipate potential problems at surgery created by extensive osteophytes and nonparallel end plates, which might make distraction complicated, or a narrow interpedicular distance, which might cause implant erosion into the neural foramen.

Unless the neurosurgeon has special experience and appropriate privileges, this procedure requires collaboration with a general or vascular surgeon. The patient undergoes a bowel preparation protocol beginning the night before surgery. The patient is placed in the supine position on an imaging-compatible operating room table such that both AP and lateral images can be obtained through the lumbar spine (Fig. 152-6). A Foley catheter is inserted along with an arterial line and large-bore venous access in case of rapid blood loss. Pneumatic stockings are placed to decrease venous stasis. If cages are being used and more than one level is being fused, fusion bone is obtained from the posterior iliac crest with the patient in a lateral decubitus position before making the abdominal incision. For allograft dowels and cage insertion, adequate bone can be obtained from a unilateral anterior iliac harvest with the patient supine. A less invasive alternative is replacement of autograft with BMP-2 (INFUSE).

A left-sided paramedian incision is used to expose the spine. The length of the incision depends on which levels are being fused. At L5–S1, the inferior extent of the incision ends just above the pubis bone, and for the L3–L4 level, the skin incision can extend rostrally just above the umbilicus. With experience, the incision can be as small

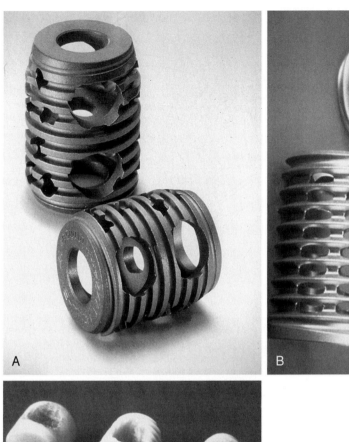

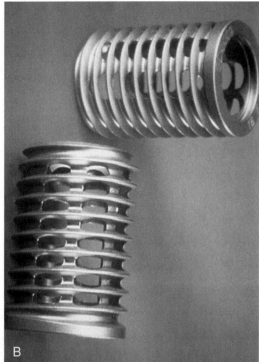

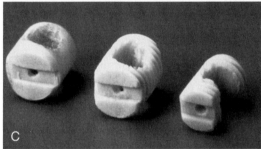

FIGURE 152-5 Common interbody devices: *A*, BAK cage. (Courtesy of Sulzer Spine Tech.) *B*, Ray cage. (Courtesy of Surgical Dynamics.) *C*, Danek machine threaded allograft bone dowels. (Courtesy of Medtronic Sofamor Danek.)

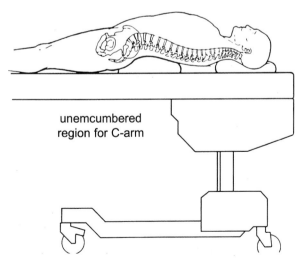

FIGURE 152-6 Intraoperative setup for open anterior lumbar interbody fusion. (Courtesy of Surgical Dynamics.)

as 5 cm in length in the nonobese patient. The posterior rectus muscle sheath is then separated from the peritoneum by sharp and blunt dissection beginning at its lateral margin. The rectus is then separated from the midline to allow its lateral retraction. The peritoneum and abdominal contents are retracted to the patient's right as the rectus is retracted to the patient's left. Dissection continues in the retroperitoneal plane. The ureter is visualized and retracted to the right with the abdominal contents, exposing the great vessels in the area (Fig. 152-7A). Retraction is maintained with a Buchwalder or modified Thompson-Farley retractor.

Of the various disc space exposures, that of L5–S1 is the most straightforward. The surgeon can easily palpate the acute angle with the sacrum between the left and right iliac arteries, and the proper level is confirmed fluoroscopically. Between the internal iliac arteries and over the disc space, a variable number of middle sacral vessels and sympathetic nerves are encountered; these are dissected, doubly tied with 3-0 silk, and cut, exposing the plane of the disc space (see Fig. 152-7B). Because of the possibility of indiscriminate damage to the sacral plexus, monopolar cautery is avoided. At L4–L5, dissection is usually complicated by the presence

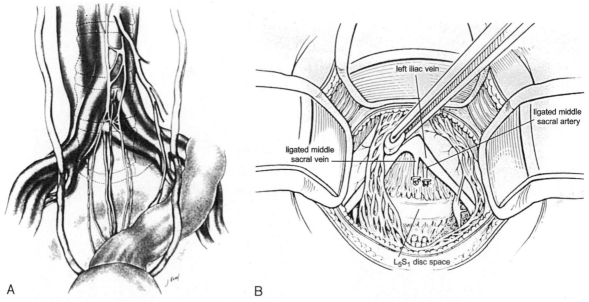

A

B

FIGURE 152-7 *A,* Exposure of the retroperitoneum after retraction of the peritoneal contents. (Courtesy of Surgical Dynamics.) *B,* Blunt dissection of the sacral plexus and tying or clipping of middle sacral vessels to gain access to the disc space at L5–S1. (Courtesy of Surgical Dynamics.)

of the left iliac vein and its tributary, the left gluteal vein, which tethers it in position near or over the L4–L5 disc space. Exposure at L4–L5 usually requires double-suture ligation of the left gluteal vein, which allows mobilization of the left iliac vein to the patient's right and away from the disc space. Occasionally, with a high iliac vein and artery bifurcation, dissection of L4–L5 can be achieved continuing in the midline. Ligation of segmental arteries at one level above and one level below may be necessary to mobilize the left iliac artery to the right (Fig. 152-8). Exposure above,

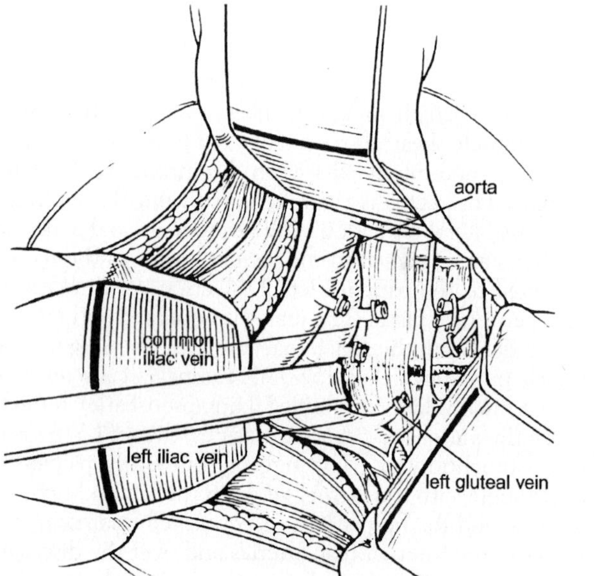

at L3–L4, is similar to that at L4–L5, but exposure is not recommended above the L3–L4 disc space because of the presence of nearby large aortic branch vessels.

Once exposure is obtained, a spinal needle is placed specifically in the ventral midline of the disc space (Fig. 152-9). AP fluoroscopy is used to guide the needle to the midline, and the needle is removed and the insertion point marked with ink or cautery. The anterior disc annulus is incised at the margin of the vertebral body above and below, and symmetrically in extent to the midline, and large enough to accommodate the implant or implants being used. Using a mallet, sequentially larger distractors are inserted into the disc space until withdrawal of the distraction plug is difficult, the disc space is distracted, and the distractor is flush with bone on fluoroscopic images (Fig. 152-10). It may be advisable to drill away very large osteophytes. If distractors seem to "bounce" out of the disc space, removing more disc material with a pituitary rongeur may eliminate this problem.

Occasionally, and particularly at L4–L5 or rostrally, it becomes clear at this stage that exposure or size of the vertebral body is inadequate to insert paired implants. In this situation, one large midline implant with good disc space distraction is preferred over two implants impinging the neural foramen laterally. If it is necessary to remove disc fragments in the spinal canal, the operating microscope can be used to perform a discectomy through one of the access holes created by the distractors while the other is left in place to maintain separation of the vertebral bodies.

For cylindrical titanium cages and cylindrical bone dowels, tapping and implant insertion are similar (Fig. 152-11). A single- or double-barreled drill tube is then slid over the shaft of the distractor and impacted into the ventral surface of the vertebral body above and below by teeth that extend 3 to 4 mm beyond the face of the drill tube, or by "tangs," which are metal flanges the width of the distracted disc space (Fig. 152-11B and C). Care is taken to ensure that

FIGURE 152-8 Ligation of lumbar intersegmental arteries and tributaries of the iliac vein to gain access to the L4–L5 disc space. (Courtesy of Surgical Dynamics.)

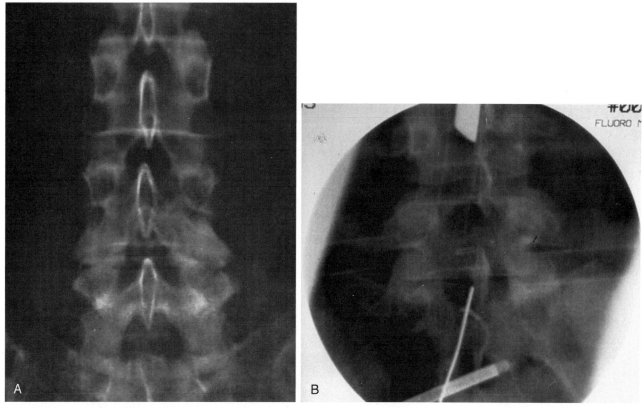

FIGURE 152-9 *A* and *B,* Midline determination on an anteroposterior fluoroscopic image with a spinal needle. The needle tip is only 1 to 3 mm below the surface to reduce parallax. Note that the tip is in line with the spinous processes and midway between the pedicles at this level.

these teeth or tangs are clear of any vessels in the region while sliding the tube into position. Lateral fluoroscopy is used to ensure that the teeth or tangs are sunk fully to bring the face of the tube flush with the ventral surface, and that the rostral and caudal aspects of the tube are equidistant from and parallel to the nearest end plate. The tangs maintain distraction of the disc space as the distraction plugs are removed.

A reaming device of appropriate width for the drill tube with a preset depth of penetration is inserted into the

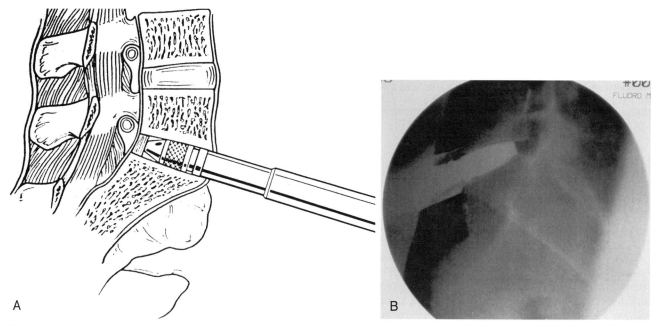

FIGURE 152-10 *A,* Diagrammatic view of disc space maximally dilated. Tight purchase is related to tight contact between the distractor and the end plate. *B,* Fluoroscopic image showing maximal contact between the distractor and the end plate. (Courtesy of Sulzer Spine Tech.)

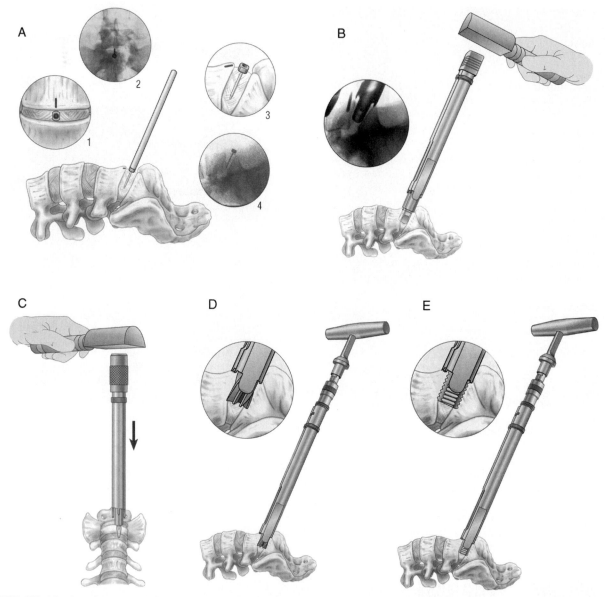

FIGURE 152-11 Anterior approach for placing threaded cylindrical constructs. *A,* For block discectomy, centering pin is used to fluoroscopically confirm the midline of the disc. *Insets 1 to 4,* Anteroposterior and lateral views, including fluoroscope images, demonstrating optimal centering pin placement. *B,* After discectomy and vertebral distraction, double-barrel drill tube is firmly seated into the disc space with proper orientation confirmed using fluoroscopy (*inset*). *C,* Single-barrel tube can be used as an option for placement of either single-threaded construct or bilateral constructs without using the double-barrel technique. *D,* Reamer is advanced in a clockwise direction, ideally with multiple passes to remove debris, until it reaches a predetermined depth. Inset shows detailed lateral view. *E,* Tap prepares the reamed space with clockwise movement, taking care to make only one pass and to remove the tap by counterclockwise rotation. (Courtesy of Medtronic Sofamor Danek.)

drill tube while the assistant holds the shaft of the tube (Fig. 152-11*D*). The surgeon checks sagittal orientation fluoroscopically and coronal orientation visually before beginning. Reaming should stop approximately 5 mm from the dorsal surface on lateral fluoroscopy to avoid contact with the spinal canal or neural foramen and should have even and equal penetration into the end plates above and below the disc space (Fig. 152-12). The reaming device is rotated clockwise as it is removed to avoid dropping bone and disc fragments into the canal just created. Under fluoroscopy to verify that the instrument does not enter the spinal canal, large pituitary rongeurs are used to remove loose disc and bone, and then the process is repeated. The lumbar

tapered (LT) cage (Medtronic Sofamor Danek) is an end-plate-sparing implant for nonparallel end plates that does not have an end-plate reaming step (Fig. 152-13).

A tap of appropriate width for the opening is set to a preset depth 2 mm short of the reaming depth. Under fluoroscopy and guided by the drill tube, threads are created with steady pressure (Fig. 152-14). It is important not to tap beyond the reaming depth because this can cause slippage and destroy the threads just created. The tap is removed with counterclockwise rotation to preserve the threads. The titanium implant or bone dowel is then attached to a specialized implant driver for insertion to a preset depth not to exceed the depth of the tapped surfaces (Fig. 152-11*E*).

Harvested bone chips or BMP-2 in a sponge are securely packed into specified portions of the cylindrical cage or bone dowel.

Threaded devices should have obvious purchase on insertion. The correct orientation of the insertion device for proper implant position should be known before insertion begins. Insertion is performed with steady, moderate pressure under fluoroscopic control. If purchase has been inadequate, and if the implant is obviously loose, the drill tube and the implant are removed. The hole is tapped with a larger tap without reaming, and a larger implant is screwed into place. A tight central implant is preferred over two loose implants, so if all else fails, the entire process can be restarted in the midline with a larger implant. If vascular structures are immovable, a single oblique implant centered in the disc midline at its midpoint is also an acceptable strategy. In addition, paired implants with recess, as well as the LT fusion device, are also available, which allow closer approximation of the implants, taking up less space in the disc space for patients with narrowed vertebral body in the coronal plane (Figs. 152-13 and 152-15). If possible, and especially if only one cylindrical implant is used, the disc and end plate between implants are removed, and the space is gently packed with bone.

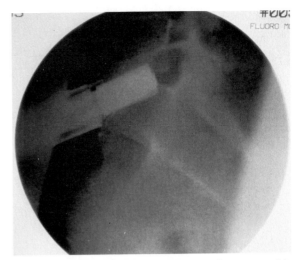

FIGURE 152-12 Reaming incorporating equal amounts of bone above and below the disc space and extending to approximately 5 mm from the posterior margin of the vertebral body on a lateral fluoroscopic view. (Courtesy of Sulzer Spine Tech.)

FIGURE 152-13 *A,* Lumbar tapered fusion device allows symmetric distraction of the vertebral bodies with significantly less reaming of the vertebral end plates. *B,* After a standard en bloc discectomy is performed via an anterior approach, double-barrel tubing and distractors are placed and the cylindrical distractor is removed to create a working cylindrical space while the C-style distractor remains in place. *C,* Top view of the double-barrel tubing showing working space and the C-style distractor. (Courtesy of Medtronic Sofamor Danek.)

A

B

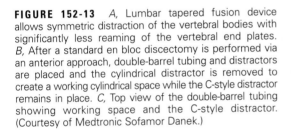

C

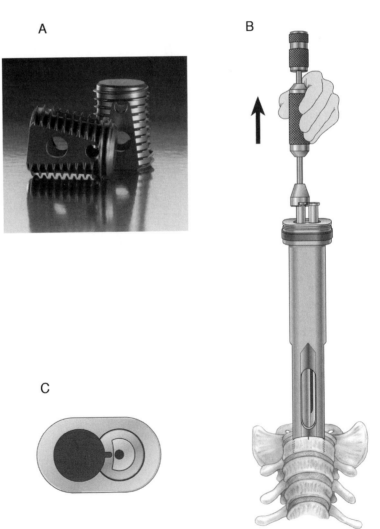

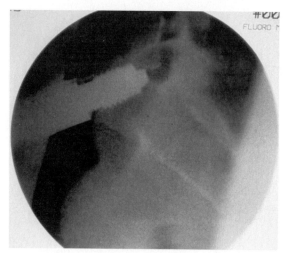

FIGURE 152-14 Tapping from a lateral fluoroscopic view. (Courtesy of Sulzer Spine Tech.)

preparation device that controls the width, depth, and sagittal angle of the end-plate preparation (Fig. 152-16A to C). The femoral ring is then malleted into place under fluoroscopic control, placing the ring as symmetrically as possible into the disc space on fluoroscopic or neuronavigation-derived images (see Fig. 152-16E). This is important to prevent bone extrusion.

The wound is irrigated and the anterior and posterior rectus sheaths are sewn to midline with interrupted 0 Vicryl, followed by subcutaneous and skin closure. A nasogastric tube is inserted. After surgery, patients demonstrate varying levels of bowel dysfunction. Patients are mobilized the day after surgery, extubated when appropriate, and advanced to liquids when nausea subsides and they are passing gas. We use a lumbosacral external orthosis to lessen strain on the fusion site, and patients avoid strenuous activity over the following 3 to 6 months.

Adequate healing is most clearly determined by clinical improvement at least 3 months after surgery. One advantage of allograft bone dowels is that incorporation and remodeling of bone with the adjacent vertebral bodies, with preservation of disc space distraction and a lack of motion on flexion-extension lateral radiographs, can accurately confirm fusion. For titanium implants, the radiographic criteria are more uncertain, but adequate healing and fusion can be assessed by a lack of radiolucency around the implants and

Allograft or autograft femoral ring and titanium ring insertion requires a rather complete removal of disc material prior to implant since there is no reaming step (Fig. 152-16). Depending on the system being used, the end plate is prepared by flattening the convexity of the surface with a hand chisel and or hand drill, or by inserting an end-plate

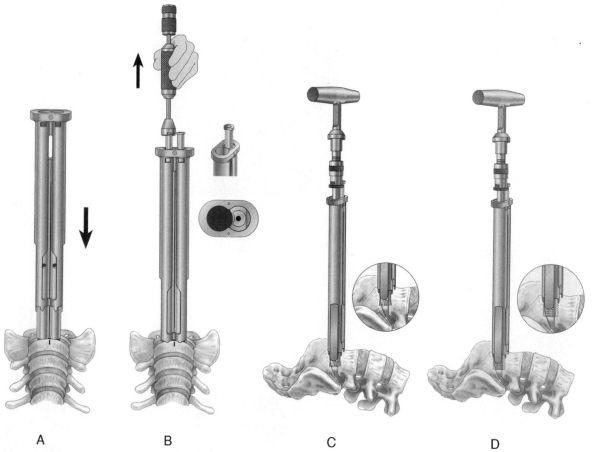

A   B   C   D

FIGURE 152-15 Reduced-profile instruments reduce the lateral dimension requirements, thus allowing insertion of two anterior interbody constructs in a limited disc space. *A,* Once disc space is properly prepared and distracted; double-barrel tubing is seated into the space. *B,* One distractor is removed, thus creating a cylindrical working channel as seen in the top view. *C,* The disc space is reamed via the working channel. *D,* The reamed space is then tapped, in preparation for the construct. (Courtesy of Medtronic Sofamor Danek.)

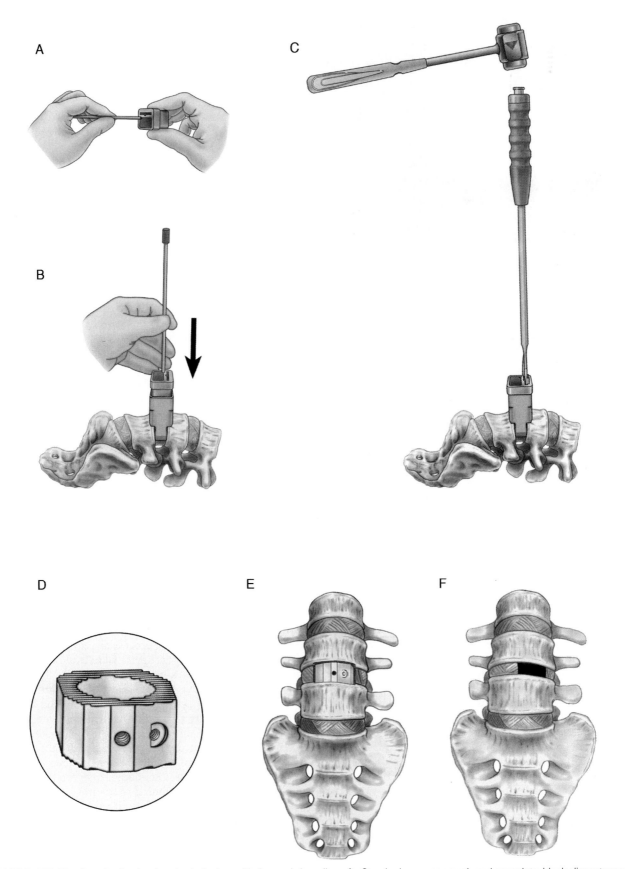

FIGURE 152-16 Anterior lumbar interbody fusion with femoral ring allograft. Standard open approach and complete block discectomy is performed. *A,* Appropriate straight chisel guide is selected and handling rod is inserted for easy handling of the guide. *B,* The chisel is then inserted into a previously seated straight housing. *C,* Top end plate is prepared with the chisel, which is driven into the guide to a predetermined depth. Steps B and C are repeated for the preparation of the bottom end plate. *D,* The femoral graft has a central opening for the autogenous bone and a threaded interface for the inserter. *E,* Final position of the implant after proper placement demonstrating slight countersink from the anterior surface of the vertebral body. *F,* The femoral ring implant can be implanted via an oblique approach as shown by the block discectomy performed obliquely. (Courtesy of Medtronic Sofamor Danek.)

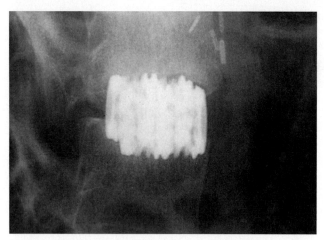

FIGURE 152-17 Radiographic evidence for pseudoarthrosis. Note the lucencies around the cage 9 months after insertion.

an absence of motion on flexion-extension radiographs (Fig. 152-17), and by high-definition CT scans with sagittal and coronal reformatted images. If patients do not improve clinically, and there is no frank motion on flexion-extension radiographs, they should be followed for up to 1 year before a level is considered a nonunion.

Percutaneous Pedicle Screws

Less invasive techniques have evolved for insertion of pedicle screws. For those patients at risk for nonunion, a percutaneous pedicle screw insertion technique may provide additional stability in the postoperative period that may increase the likelihood of successful arthrodesis. We use this technique when BMP-2 is unavailable or contraindicated in a single-level procedure and in all two- or three-level anterior fusions.

The Sextant system (Medtronic Sofamor Danek) is a novel method of percutaneous screw insertion that utilizes the principle that any two points in proximity can be considered as part of a circle (Fig. 152-18). A Jam-Sheedie needle is inserted into the more rostral pedicle, avoiding the rostral lateral mass by working the tip medially from the transverse process under fluoroscopic control (Fig. 152-18A). The Jam-Sheedie needle begins at the lateral margin of the pedicle and is inserted to the middle of the pedicle at its junction with the vertebral body. The needle is inserted into posterior portions of the vertebral body before the stylet is removed and a K wire is inserted to the midpoint of the body on the lateral view. A similar K-wire insertion then occurs at the more caudal level.

Pedicle screw insertion is most conveniently performed at the caudal level first. A series of dilators are placed from the skin to the junction with the posterior pedicle origin (see Fig. 152-18B). A cannulated tap is placed through this dilated pathway, and through the pedicle to the tip of the K wire (Fig. 152-18C). The tap is removed, and a cannulated screw of appropriate depth measured from the relationship of the depth of tap penetration to the end of the dilator is chosen. A screw with a polyaxial screw cap and tightening nut are attached to a housing that fits over the screw cap, and this assembly is inserted and screwed into place over the K wire. The K wire is removed, leaving the screw, screw head, and screw head housing construct in place and sticking out posteriorly (Fig. 152-18D). The same procedure is then performed at the more caudal level. Screws may be placed at adjacent levels and in tandem on the left and right sides for a two-level fusion, or, alternatively, one level may be skipped without screw placement or a third screw may be placed with a housing with an open side to persuade a connecting rod to engage the screw head of the intermediate screw.

The housings have male/female connections that connect while they are rotated 90 degrees in a counterclockwise direction. This allows connection of the sextant to the combined housing (Fig. 152-18E). A small stab wound is made and the sextant is pushed to contact with the rostral screw head. The positioning is checked fluoroscopically. Templates are then placed in slots in the individual screw housings, which determine the proper length of connecting rod. The sextant is removed from the back, and the proper length rod is attached to the sextant by lining up a slot in the distal end of the rod with a holder device that grabs the slotted rod through tightening of a spring-loaded knob at the base of the sextant. The sextant–rod complex is then passed with moderate force through the open heads of the top tightening screws (Fig. 152-18F). The break-off nuts are tightened from distally first to ensure a proper engagement, and a confirmatory fluoroscopic image is a good idea at this time. The nuts are tightened to the break-off point and the housing elements are now easily removed. Staples are used to close all stab wounds.

Facet Screws

This represents another viable form of supplemental instrumentation after anterior fusion procedures. Biomechanical studies have shown that translaminar facet screws have comparable strength to pedicle screw fixation, and have the advantage over pedicle screws of avoiding proximity and damage to the rostral facet complex. This technique is essentially a noninvasive percutaneous technique, requiring only a superficial midline exposure of a spinous process. It is appropriate to use at all lumbar levels.

At L5–S1, the L5 spinous process is exposed to the junction with the lamina. Under fluoroscopy and beginning contralaterally and just superficial to the margin of the lamina, a threaded K wire and power drill are used to drill within the cancellous bone of the lamina, aiming for the pedicle/superior articulating process margin contralaterally. The lamina is observed for superficial extrusion, and resistance is monitored as a measure of potentially harmful passage into the epidural space. If resistance is lost, drilling is stopped and the tract is revised. A cannulated drill and tap are used to create a passageway for a cannulated screw, which is also screwed into place over the K wire. Ideally, the screw tip rests within the pedicle. One must take care not to pass the screw tip into the neural foramen rostrally. The second screw is passed similarly. However, the origin of the contralateral screw will need to be either more rostral or caudal on the lamina to avoid contact with the first screw in the midline. Therefore, at the onset of the procedure, insertion points in the lamina should be determined for both screws to avoid collision.

Ventral Plate at L5–S1

An alternative exists to pedicle screw supplementation of ALIF at L5–S1 only. A chevron-shaped, low-profile plate has been developed that confers additional stability to an

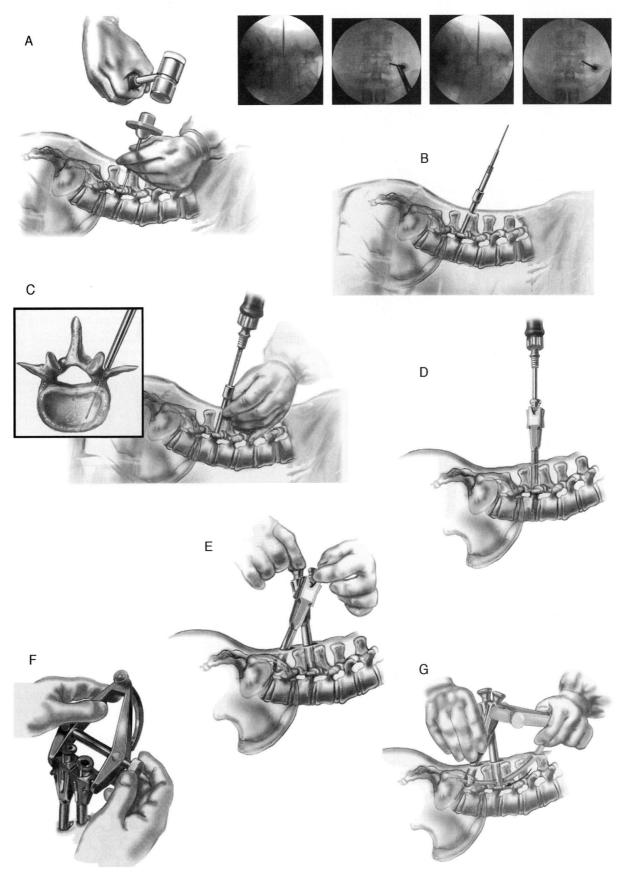

FIGURE 152-18 Percutaneous pedicle screw insertion method using the Sextant system. *A,* After proper location for skin incision and starting point is determined under fluoroscopy, an 11-gauge biopsy needle, or Jam-Sheedie needle, is used for accessing the pedicle. The needle is advanced through the pedicle with the tip starting at the lateral margin of the pedicle, approaching the base of the pedicle on the lateral view and the pedicle center on the anteroposterior view (radiographs, right to left.) *B,* With the guide wire in place, dilators are utilized to make a path through the fascia and muscle. *C,* The tap is placed over the guide wire to prepare the pedicle. Inset shows the axial placement of the guide wire and tap. *D,* The screw assembly with extender is driven into the pedicle while removing the guide wire. *E,* After steps A through D are repeated for placing a second screw on the same side, the extenders are connected. *F,* The rod inserter is attached to the two-screw assembly. *G,* The rod trocar prepares the path, and an appropriate rod is placed through the screw heads. (Courtesy of Medtronic Sofamor Danek.)

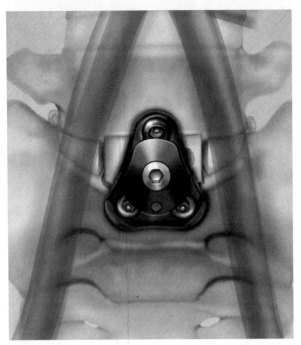

FIGURE 152-19 Anterior lumbar plate, a supplemental fixation for interbody construct for L5–S1. (Courtesy of Medtronic Sofamor Danek.)

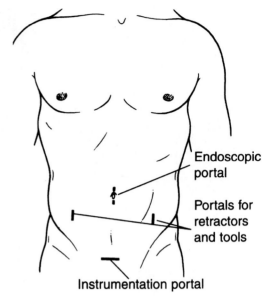

FIGURE 152-20 Portals for laparoscopic anterior lumbar interbody fusion. The working portal is horizontal 3 to 4 cm above the pubis in most patients. (Courtesy of Barrow Neurological Institute.)

L5–S1 ALIF close to that achieved with pedicle screws, while avoiding the additional time required to reposition the patient (Fig. 152-19). A single screw is placed in the midline through a hole in the plate near its rostral point, and two screws enter paired at the sacral promontory after use of an awl and tap at each hole. Screw heads are secured with a covering plate, which is held by a midpoint screw accepted by the base plate.

Laparoscopic Anterior Lumbar Interbody Fusion

The laparoscopic method has the advantage of reducing morbidity related to movement of the abdominal contents and the trauma to the abdominal wall associated with open approaches. Therefore, postoperative pain and recovery time may be lessened. This approach carries a significant learning curve, and it is necessary to collaborate with an experienced laparoscopic surgeon during this period, or beyond. It is most easily performed at the L5–S1 level, where mobilization of the middle sacral vessels and portions of the sacral nerve plexus is required. At L4–L5, the iliac and gluteal veins present a more formidable challenge. Laparoscopic approaches to this level should be performed by experienced laparoscopic surgeons, and in patients in whom preoperative MRI does not show large vessels over the disc space. Preparations should be made to convert to an open technique if necessary.[39] Above L4–L5, the transperitoneal approach is obstructed by the viscera and their feeding vessels. A retroperitoneal lateral approach is available for levels above L4–L5.

The patient is treated with cathartic agents the evening before surgery to empty stool from the large intestine, which facilitates bowel mobilization at surgery. General anesthesia is induced, a Foley catheter is inserted, arterial and central venous access is obtained, and pneumatic compression stockings are placed to decrease venous stasis. Although we

presently prefer to use BMP-2 as a fusion promoter from within the implant, mid–iliac crest harvest in a supine patient usually yields adequate bone graft for most single or two-level implants.

The supine patient's feet and legs are wrapped by Kerlix, which is then secured to the operating room table so that the patient does not slide when placed in the Trendelenburg position. Either CO_2 or gasless methods may be used. Four portals usually are required (Fig. 152-20). Initially, a 1- to 2-mm incision is made at the umbilicus if an insufflation technique is used for a Veress insufflating needle, which is used to insufflate to 10 to 15 mm Hg. A 10-mm portal for a 30-degree endoscope is inserted, which allows the other three portals to be inserted under direct vision. Smaller, 5-mm portals are placed lateral to the rectus sheath for retractors below the umbilicus but 1 to 2 cm rostral to the level of the lesion. The working incision is horizontal and approximately 20 cm wide in the midline, caudal, and in line with the axial plane of the disc space. This position is confirmed by fluoroscopy, and penetration of the abdominal wall is also under laparoscopic visualization to prevent damage to abdominal contents.

Placing the patient in the Trendelenburg position may help mobilize the small intestines. The sigmoid colon may provide more resistance, and an additional right-sided portal may be needed for mobilization and retraction, or the mesentery may be stitched rostrally to the ventral wall of the abdomen to maintain retraction during the procedure. To reach the L5–S1 disc space, the posterior peritoneum is incised at the base of the sigmoid mesocolon with endoscopic scissors, exposing the middle sacral arteries and veins and branches of the sacral plexus over the disc space (Fig. 152-21A). Using endoscopic hemoclips or endoscopic suture ligatures, the middle sacral vessels are mobilized, clipped, or tied and cut to gain access to the disc space, as in the open procedure. The sacral plexus over the disc space is preserved by mobilization whenever possible; monopolar

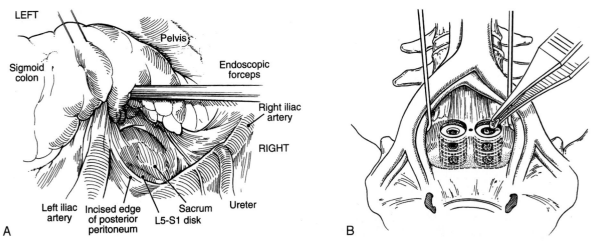

FIGURE 152-21 *A*, Diagrammatic representation ventral to the L5–S1 region after retraction of the sigmoid colon to expose the mesentery above the L5–S1 disc space. (Courtesy of the Barrow Neurological Institute.) *B*, View after the insertion is completed. Note that the implants must be parallel. (Courtesy of Sulzer Spine Tech.)

cautery is never used, and bipolar cautery only when necessary because of concern for the development of retrograde ejaculation in men. Both iliac vessels are retracted laterally.

To expose the L4–L5 disc space, the sigmoid mesocolon mesentery is incised 3 to 5 cm further rostrally. Any ascending lumbar vessels and left-sided segmental vessels at L4 and L5 must be ligated and cut, as in the open procedure. The iliac vein is often over the L4–L5 disc space and may be tethered by the left gluteal vein, which may require double ligation for adequate mobilization of the left iliac vein from the disc space. This may be a formidable task. A sponge stick can temporarily tamponade bleeding if conversion to an open technique is required. In general, all vascular structures are mobilized to the right at this level, which may require a second right-sided retractor portal.

From this point, the process of implant insertion is similar to that in the open procedure, except that paired implants are placed individually with uniportal instruments, and longer tubes that extend from the ventral surface of the spine well through the instrument portal are required. Through holes in the annulus created by the alignment guide, distraction plugs of sequentially larger size are inserted until a snug fit is obtained, the disc space is distracted, and the plug is flush with bone on lateral fluoroscopy, while checking visually for correct AP orientation. As with the open technique, implant size may be changed from preoperative template determinations if disc space distraction determines a larger implant is needed. If an implant one size larger than expected is used, manufacturers have developed a second implant with a concave margin medially that allows the implants to accommodate the height of the disc space without impinging so far laterally as to extend into the foramen.

At this point, one distraction plug may be removed and insufflation preserved by a large, valved trocar placed over the remaining distraction plug and into the instrumentation portal. A drill tube with teeth or tangs that enter the disc space is then inserted over the distraction plug and the teeth are tamped into the bone, leaving the face of the tube flush with the ventral vertebral body. While an assistant holds the drill tube, the distraction plug is removed. A pilot hole is then reamed to the same depth as in the open technique. Just as with the open technique, reaming must extend at

least 3 mm into the vertebral bodies above and below. Under fluoroscopic control, free disc fragments may be removed with large pituitary forceps. The hole is tapped, and the implant or bone dowel is filled with autograft bone or BMP-2. After insertion, any residual space in an implant is filled with bone, and bone chips are also placed between implants in the disc space. Postoperative bone bridging in this region may be indicative of successful fusion through an implant.

The second implant is inserted identically (Fig. 152-21B). On completion of the insertions, the posterior peritoneum is closed with endoscopic suture or clips. Insufflation, if used, is reduced, during which the region is carefully inspected for venous bleeding that might manifest as pressure is lowered. Peritoneum is sutured at removal of the 10-mm or larger portals to prevent an incisional hernia, the fascia is closed at the instrumentation portal, and the subcutaneous layer is closed, followed by a subcuticular stitch. After recovery room observation, intensive care usually is not required. Pain is managed in the first 24 hours by a patient-controlled analgesic pump. Patients are mobilized the following day in a lumbar corset, and discharged when pain is manageable with oral analgesics.

Retroperitoneal Lateral Approach

In the more unusual patient for whom it has been determined that fusion is necessary from the L4–L5 to the L1–L2 disc spaces, cages or bone dowels, or end-plate-preserving allograft spacers or cages, may be used from a lateral retroperitoneal approach. Depending on the size of the patient and the configuration of the disc space, one implant, or occasionally two different-sized implants that more correctly match a more fish-mouthed disc space, may be used. The patient is placed in the right lateral decubitus position with an axillary roll because it is preferable to avoid the inferior vena cava. It is important for the patient to be in an exact lateral position with the coronal plane of the spine perpendicular to the plane of the operating table to simplify fluoroscopy during surgery. Bone is harvested from the mid–iliac crest if necessary.

Fluoroscopy is used to identify the level of the lesion. A 4-cm incision is made parallel to the external oblique muscle centered on the midaxillary line (Fig. 152-22).

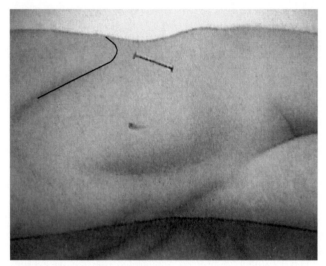

FIGURE 152-22 An oblique incision over the site of pathology in the midaxillary line for the retroperitoneal approach with the patient in a lateral decubitus position. The dark line marks the inferior margin of the rib cage. (Courtesy of H. Yuan, M.D.)

The external oblique, internal oblique, and transversalis layers are sequentially split. The peritoneum and ureter are identified, dissected from the region of the psoas muscle, and retracted anteriorly. Any tear in the peritoneum should be repaired. The genitofemoral nerve can be seen lying obliquely on the ventral surface of the psoas muscle. Retraction is maintained with a Buchwalder or modified Thompson-Farley retractor. The medial aspect of the psoas muscle overlies the disc space. It is mobilized posteriorly and, if necessary, incised longitudinally to get exposure. Extensive cross-sectional division of the psoas muscle is associated with hip flexor weakness and should be avoided.

Segmental vessels are then tied or clipped above and below the disc space. Under fluoroscopy, a spinal needle determines the midpoint of the lateral aspect of the vertebral body, and the drill guide is used to determine if one or two end-plate cutting implants will be inserted. If the decision is for two, distraction begins first at the more posterior site. It is acceptable to place cages or dowels of different sizes at the

two sites from a lateral approach when the disc space end plates are not parallel. Adequacy of distraction is determined by snugness of fit and appearance on AP fluoroscopy. Reaming, tapping, and insertion depths are determined by a preoperative analysis of the width of the end plate, and by AP and lateral fluoroscopy at surgery. The implant should extend to within 5 mm of the contralateral side of the vertebral body to maximize bone-implant contact. Elongated cages up to 40 cm in length are available for this purpose (Fig. 152-23).

When end-plate-sparing allograft bone or similarly shaped cages are to be used, the first step is a large lateral annulotomy with a no. 15 blade followed by subtotal curettage of disc material from the disc space. Then disc cutters, scrapers, and chisels can be used sequentially to prepare the disc space and determine the height and number of implants to be placed. We prefer to place two implants in parallel that fit snugly against the end plates beginning first with the most anterior so that the second implant does not force the first implant back toward the spinal canal. One should consider BMP-2 placement anteriorly within the disc space before implant placement in patients at high risk for nonunion (i.e., in smokers and osteoporotic patients or patients with bone disease). Supplemental instrumentation fixation is used and provided by percutaneous pedicle screws or with use of a lateral plate.

Laparoscopic Retroperitoneal Approach

The patient is placed in the right lateral decubitus position and care is taken to maintain the patient in a straight lateral position with a beanbag or other radiolucent device. A 10- to 12-mm incision is made in the posterior axillary line midway between the 12th rib and the iliac crest. Slowly, the trocar is advanced through the external oblique, internal oblique, and transversalis muscles to ascertain when the peritoneum has been encountered. The peritoneum should be dissected forward bluntly to allow placement of a special balloon trocar (Preperitoneal Distention Balloon System, Spherical Shaped; Origin Medical Systems, Inc., Menlo Park, CA, U.S.A.) (Fig. 152-24). The balloon is then inflated with approximately 1000 mL of air or saline. A laparoscope can be placed inside the balloon during

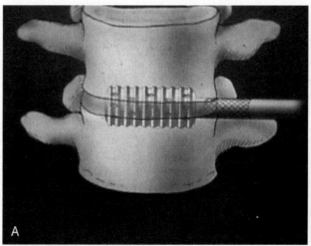
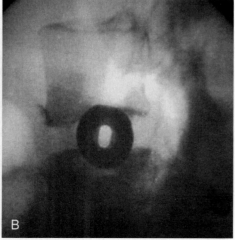

FIGURE 152-23 Anteroposterior (A) and lateral (B) views of a BAK implant after lateral retroperitoneal insertion. (Courtesy of H. Yuan, M.D.)

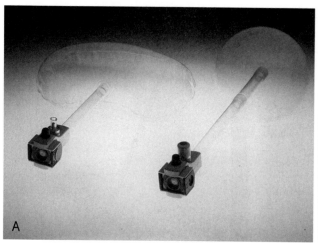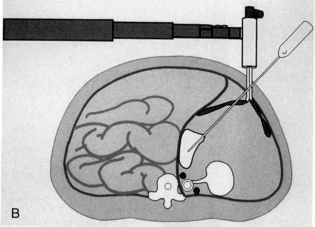

FIGURE 152-24 *A,* One- and two-liter balloons for dilatation of the retroperitoneal space. *B,* Maintenance of the retroperitoneal space with table-mounted paddles during balloon deflation. (Courtesy of Origin Medical Systems.)

inflation so that the psoas muscle, genitofemoral nerve, and ureter can be seen to confirm proper location. Fluoroscopy is used to confirm that the potential space is over the proper level. CO_2 insufflation may be necessary to maintain this potential space, or paddles may be used to tent open the space after balloon deflation.

At least two working portals are then made under direct laparoscopic observation in the midaxillary line. Insufflation also may be necessary through at least one portal. The aorta and iliopsoas muscle are identified. Dissection longitudinally through the psoas muscle posteriorly reveals the disc space and segmental vessels under a layer of fibrofatty tissue. The proper level is determined fluoroscopically. Enough dissection is performed for the drill tubes to be unencumbered by fat, muscle, or blood vessels. Cage or bone insertion then proceeds as with the open approach.

Posterior Fusion Approaches

Pedicle Screws

Although subject to some controversy, an analysis of the literature to date would suggest that pedicle screw instrumentation leads to higher fusion rates with all forms of posterior lumbar fusion techniques. Therefore, pedicle screw fixation is recommended in the treatment of segmental instability, when pseudoarthrosis development is tantamount to failure. The process of insertion of pedicle screws in the middle and lower lumbar spine can be accomplished with a variety of techniques. However, the most important aspect of successful insertion is an understanding of pedicular anatomy as it relates to the anatomical cues available at surgery.

From L3 to S1, the pedicle can be determined to originate dorsally at the confluence of the transverse process or the ala of the sacrum and the origin of the superior articulating facet (Fig. 152-25A). At the rostral end of a fusion construct, it is important that the pedicle screw not impinge in any way on the more rostral inferior articulating facet. If this occurs, it is likely that within a short period of time, that facet may become dysfunctional and painful. Depending on the level of experience of the surgeon, fluoroscopy or neuronavigation and electrophysiologic probes or no real-time

guidance at all may be used to guide insertion and avoid contact with nerve roots. We routinely use some form of guidance.

Initially, a diamond burr marks a shallow pathway in the pedicle that is confirmed as appropriate by AP and lateral views. We then deepen this path to the posterior margin of the vertebral body. From L3/4 to L5–S1, a degree of lateral to medial slant in the screws varies from 10 to 20 degrees. We probe this path to make sure it has not penetrated the cortical margins ventrally, medially, and caudally. Alternately, a handheld probe can dissect into the vertebral body (Fig. 152-25B). If a nice base and sides are palpated, a tap 1 mm smaller than the anticipated size of the final screw is used to tap into the posterior third of the vertebral body. The length of the pedicle screw is estimated, so that it will sit flush to the pars interarticularis region and penetrate into two thirds of the vertebral body (Fig. 152-25C). It should have good purchase and line up as well as possible with adjacent level screws to make rod connection easy.

Posterolateral Fusion

The posterolateral fusion occurs through a decorticated facet articulation and a space bordered ventrally by the transverse processes and intertransverse muscle, laterally by the quadratus lumborum muscle, and medially by the pars interarticularis and the lateral aspect of the lateral mass. More often than not, for patients with segmental instability, this type of fusion is now used as a supplement at the time of a posterior interbody fusion. However, in patients for whom there is determined to be increased risk for nerve or vascular injury with interbody techniques, this remains an adequate operation with a well-known track record of success when performed optimally to lessen rates of pseudoarthrosis. The use of BMP-2 may also hasten the development of fusion and lower the percentages of pseudoarthrosis using this technique, and should be considered in every patient with segmental instability because pseudoarthrosis is tantamount to clinical failure in this patient population.

Exposure requires extension of a traditional laminectomy exposure to include exposure of the entire facet and the dorsal aspect of the spinous processes. This is most easily

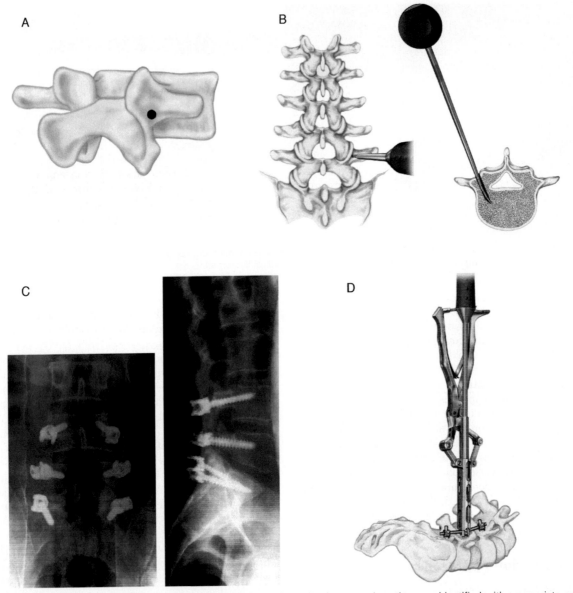

FIGURE 152-25   Pedicle screw placement. *A,* Entry points of the pilot holes for screw insertions are identified with appropriate anatomic landmarks. *B,* Pilot holes are created with a sharp awl or burr, followed by a probe, palpating for any perforation in the pedicle wall. *C,* Intraoperative posteroanterior and lateral plain radiograph demonstrates proper placement of the pedicle screws. *D,* If necessary, the Beale Rod Reducer can be used to fully seat the rod, simplifying the plug insertion process. (Courtesy of Medtronic Sofamor Danek.)

accomplished by first using moderate electrocautery to define a subperiosteal plane over the lateral aspect of the facet mass. Retractor deepening then pulls paraspinous muscles further laterally. Cautery dissection over the smooth and densely opaque pars interarticularis while avoiding cauterizing within the foramen brings the surgeon over the region of the transverse process. The transverse process can usually be palpated with a sucker or Penfield probe. Visualization of the transverse process occurs by cauterizing fibrous attachments from the paraspinous muscle to the inferior aspect of the proximate lateral mass. Almost always, a region of fatty tissue is entered that overlies the transverse process. This fatty tissue may be cauterized or retracted to reveal the transverse process, which is further exposed subperiosteally while avoiding penetration further ventrally where nerve roots are passing obliquely. At this point, the space created laterally is maintained with strip sponges.

Preparation of the fusion bed is very important and occurs after preparation or harvest of autograft or allograft and BMP-2 fusion substrate. When the lateral mass contains both a superior and an inferior articulating process, it is important to decorticate the actual joint space with a cutting burr or an osteotome. Fusion through the facet joint itself is very desirable. With or without an intact facet, decortication of the dorsal surface of the transverse process and pars interarticularis rostrally and the lateral aspect of the superior articulating facet distally with a burr also assures ankylosis between adjacent level structures.

At this point some combination of iliac crest autograft, allograft, and bone fusion enhancers are placed in the decorticated regions to fill in gaps between adjacent level structures and to promote a larger fusion mass. At first, emphasis should be placed on making sure that the bone products contact both transverse processes ventrally.

Then the gap lateral to the lateral mass is also packed with bone chips. Pressure is now applied medially to assure bone contact with the lateral mass more than the quadratus muscle laterally. However, penetration of bone through the intertransverse muscle ventrally between the transverse process is not desirable because bone can contact nerve root that far ventrally. Enough material should be packed dorsally to be level with the pars interarticularis. The bone mass developed should have a solidity to it through compaction medially against the lateral aspect of the lateral mass. The wound is closed meticulously in layers, with great care taken to avoid any gaps in the fascial and skin layers. Sloppy technique at this point may predispose to infection. Drain placement in the fusion bed is optional, depending on the degree of intraoperative bleeding or if there is a significant dead space at closure.

Posterior Lumbar Interbody Fusion

When the plan is for coincident posterolateral fusion, exposure is the same as with posterolateral fusion. If it is felt that coincident posterolateral fusion is unnecessary, exposure may be limited laterally to the joint space junction between the superior and inferior articulating facet masses. The ligamentum flavum is initially retained if present to act as a barrier against dural penetration. The rostral two thirds of the facet complex and two thirds of the pars interarticularis from medially is cut with an osteotome or drilled away. While drilling the lateral mass, the inferior articulating facet over the disc space gives way to the joint surface. At this point, a blunt angled dissector is used to determine the rostral margin of the pedicle. This marks the caudal aspect of the bony resection. The superior articulating facet over the disc space is drilled or cut away with Kerrison punches. The disc space is palpated for, and bipolar cautery and scissors are used to remove veins and fat over the disc space. It may be desirable to remove ligamentum flavum at this point if orientation to the thecal sac is considered helpful (Fig. 152-26A).

Dissection laterally beyond the lateral margin of the pedicle is avoided because this marks the region where the disc space comes in close approximation to the rostral nerve root in its foramen. Instrumentation this far laterally risks injury to this nerve root. The best point for PLIF is in the center of the axilla rather than this far laterally. At this point in the operation, there is no point in exposing rostral to the disc space unless a significant spondylolisthesis exists or the rostral pedicle is very large and compromises the size of the axilla. Under these circumstances, the proximal nerve root may actually be in or very close to the disc penetration site, and so visualizing the nerve root under these circumstances may actually lessen the likelihood of injuring it during disc space preparation. The very same bony dissection is prepared on the contralateral side.

Preparation of the disc space is similar over the range of implants available. The first step is to enter the disc space with a 6-mm osteotome under fluoroscopy or navigation to disrupt the annulus (Fig. 152-26B). A nerve root retractor is used while careful ongoing inspection confirms that neither the proximal nor the distal nerve roots nor the main thecal sac is caught up in the instrumentation process. It may be helpful to make sure that contact with the disc space occurs first medially away from contact with neural structures.

Dilators and scrapers are placed in the disc space until the disc space becomes moderately resistant (Fig. 152-26C). Fusion is less likely if distraction is not adequate, but if distraction is too great, the integrity of the end plate may be compromised, especially if osteoporosis is present, which may also hinder fusion. A variety of cutters and scrapers are available to strip the end plates of all cartilage (Fig. 152-26D through F). The final preparation step is to use a broach or chisel to define parallel margins of the end plates and an adequate opening dorsally for the end plate (Fig. 152-26G).

Implant width is based on the size of the distracted disc space. While continuously retracting and visualizing the nerve roots, the implant is tamped from dorsally to ventrally within the disc space (Fig. 152-26H). Generally, countersinking 5 mm beyond the spinal canal is the best final position (Fig. 152-26I). When spondylolisthesis exists, both the length of the disc space available, the length of the implant, and the posterior wall of the proximal body have to be taken into consideration.

At any point in time during the preparation for and insertion of the implants, epidural bleeding can be troublesome. If it does not respond to direct cautery, then packing with Gelfoam and a patty will usually stop the bleeding. The usual site is under the proximal nerve root or medially. A deep lumbar but not epidural HemoVac drain is an option when persistent bleeding occurs at time of closure. Protection of the nerve roots during PLIF is a high priority. However, if a dural tear occurs, we attempt closure with 4-0 Neurolon. When the tear is either too ventral or distal on the nerve root sheath for access, we will place a fat graft dipped in antibiotic solution over the defect to create a barrier to cerebrospinal fluid (CSF) extravasation and to create a less oxidizing environment around the nerve root. The fat graft is covered with Tisseal tissue adhesive. The wound is closed meticulously in layers. Unless the remaining dural defect is quite large, CSF diversion has not been necessary. However, patients with significant dural tears are kept supine for the first 48 hours after surgery.

Lateral Transforaminal Lumbar Interbody Fusion

To perform a lateral TLIF, a more extensive removal of the lateral mass is necessary to allow for insertion of an implant at a more oblique angle. At L5–S1, and especially in men, the posterior iliac crest may also inhibit the development of the insertional angle. Under these circumstances, a bilateral PLIF approach is required. The difference in exposure between a PLIF and a TLIF is that a complete removal of the superior articulating facet over the disc space is required along with a transection of the pars interarticularis.

Generally, both the proximal and distal nerve roots are visualized. The nerve roots are retracted medially if necessary with a nerve root retractor, although the degree of retraction may be less than with a PLIF. Preparation of the disc space is performed very similarly to the PLIF, except that angled rasps and up-biting pituitary rongeurs are required to get a thorough disc removal across the midline. Both bony and cage implants with longer lengths and appropriate curvatures have been developed to be long enough to cover more disc space area and to extend across the midline. Another option is to pair standard bony or cage implants in a horizontal position. This can be managed by first inserting the implant obliquely and then pivoting the implant with specialized

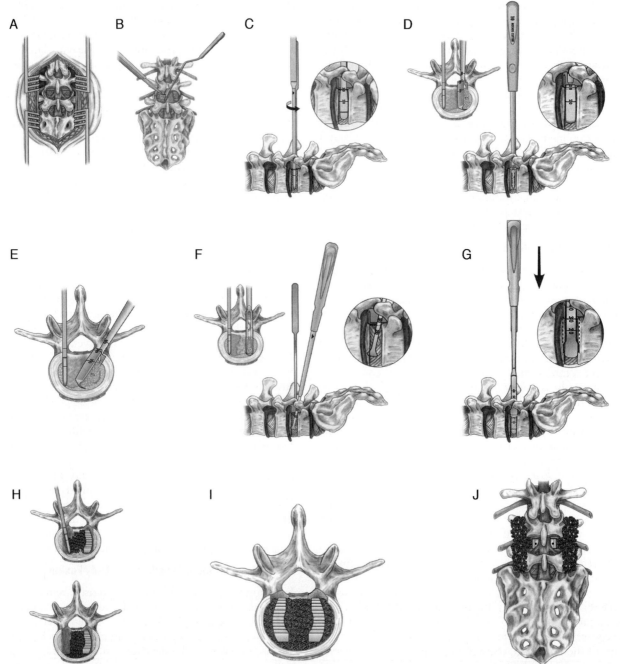

FIGURE 152-26   Posterior lumbar interbody fusion using Tangent System. *A,* Midline incision is made for approach and exposure of the interlaminar space and facet joints at the affected level, with routine exposure of the dura and annulus lateral to the dura via bilateral hemi-laminectomy and partial medial facetectomy. *B,* Conventional discectomy is performed by incising the annulus bilaterally to remove extruded fragments, to decompress neural elements, and to provide entry to the space for distraction with minimal to no nerve root retraction. *C,* Disc space is distracted until original disc space height is achieved and normal foraminal opening is restored, as sequentially larger distractors are placed in alternating fashion from the right to left side of the disc space. Inset shows largest distractor, which is left in place while the oppo-site side disc space is being prepared. *D,* A rotational cutting instrument is inserted into the side opposite the distractor and rotated to remove residual intradiscal material. The instrument can be inserted up to a depth of 30 mm with flat surface parallel to the dura. Inset shows detailed close-up view. *E,* The rotational cutting instrument is rotated and lifted out. *F,* A round scraper is utilized to remove remaining soft tissue or cartilaginous end-plate coverings, as illustrated by the axial and detailed lateral views. *G,* A cutting chisel is seated and impacted into the disc space, thereby removing the residual osteophytes and completing the débridement of the end plate. While a distractor is placed into the above prepared side of the disc space, the opposite side is prepared by repeating steps D to G. *H,* A Tangent Wedge is placed into the previously prepared disc space along with packing of the morselized autograft which is swept against the wedge. The disc distractor is removed in preparation for a second Tangent Wedge placement. *I,* Residual disc space is fitted with autograft cancellous bone. *J,* Extradural space and foramina are probed to ensure adequate decompression. Segmental internal fixation is applied using a standard technique to facilitate satisfactory immobilization. Autograft bone may be placed posterolaterally over the facets and medial transverse processes. (Courtesy of Medtronic Sofamor Danek.)

tamps to a horizontal position. A second similar implant is then passed into the disc space posterior to the first, confined anteriorly by the first implant and posteriorly by the posterior longitudinal ligament.

Facet Rhizotomy

Patient selection begins with a successful facet injection on the side with most pain at either the L4–L5 or L5–S1 level, depending on which motion segment is associated with the greater lordotic angle because stresses on the facet may be greatest there. The patient is placed in the prone position with a roll under the lower abdomen, placing the hips in moderate flexion to open up the facet joint. At a point above the facet joint and 6 mm from midline, the skin and subcutaneous tissue are infiltrated with 1.5% lidocaine. Under lateral and oblique fluoroscopy, a 22-gauge needle is inserted into the midpoint of the facet in both the oblique and axial planes (Fig. 152-27). The facet joint is infiltrated with 1 to 2 mL of a solution containing 40 to 80 mg triamcinolone and 0.5% bupivacaine. A 24-hour pain log is maintained after the procedure, and at least 75% pain relief must be at least transiently obtained to move on to facet rhizotomy. If pain should return after the injection procedure, the patient may proceed to facet rhizotomy. We prefer to inject only one level bilaterally because most patients can tolerate only a single-level rhizotomy at a time, and this allows us to compare results of rhizotomy directly with the facet block.

Rhizotomy is performed at least several days after the facet block. The patient is placed prone as for the injection procedure. The skin is infiltrated in a somewhat wider swath to accommodate varying needle trajectories. Three specific targets are used for L4–L5, and four at L5–S1. At L4–L5, the first target is the descending ramus of L4, which is characteristically at the shoulder of the L4 transverse process. The second target is near the origin of the pars

interarticularis, where there is frequently a branch point of the descending ramus. The third target is found at the shoulder of the L5 transverse process, at the origin of the descending branch of L5. At L5–S1, target points are the shoulder of the L5 transverse process, the origin of the pars interarticularis, the margin of the sacral ala with the superior articulating process, and just above the S1 foramen at the origin of an additional ascending branch (Fig. 152-28).

As demonstrated by Bogduk and colleagues,[124] the narrowest width of a radiofrequency lesion is directly forward from the tip. Therefore, both stimulation and lesioning are performed with the tip of the electrode at as oblique an angle to the bony surface as possible (Radionics RFG-3B; Radionics, Inc., Burlington, MA, U.S.A.). If stimulation (<3 V, 1 msec, 25 to 50 Hz) elicits concordant pain, radiofrequency lesioning is performed at 80°C for 90 seconds. Leg pain or paresthesias during stimulation indicate the electrode is too near the ventral nerve roots. The immediate area is stimulated and lesioned again until the stimulation threshold triples, while ensuring the needle has an oblique trajectory to the bone surface. A repeat procedure is indicated if there is recurrence of pain after at least 75% pain relief for 3 months.

Epidural Spinal Cord Stimulation: Technique

SCS is usually performed in two distinct stages. The first part involves exact placement of the SCS electrode into the epidural space for temporary testing, and the second step is formal implantation of the receiver and electrode arrays. For initial electrode placement, the patient is positioned prone on the operating table with proper padding to allow for a somewhat comfortable position under conscious sedation. The C-arm image intensifier is used to identify the point of entry into the epidural space from T11 to L1, just superior to the conus medullaris. After generous infiltration of local anesthetic, a vertical skin incision is made above the identified spinous processes.

There are two accepted techniques for placement of SCS electrode arrays. The percutaneous approach uses a 14- to 15-gauge Tuohy needle inserted at an angle of approximately 45 degrees and advanced into the interlaminar space under fluoroscopic guidance. The epidural space is identified using the "hanging drop technique" (a small drop of saline on the needle is suddenly sucked into the needle when it reaches the epidural space) or the "loss of resistance technique" (after penetration of the ligamentum flavum, resistance to the needle's further advance is clearly decreased; injection of saline or air becomes very easy). The percutaneous electrode array is then fed into the needle and advanced epidurally to the desired level around T8–T9 under fluoroscopic guidance. An open surgical approach, either a laminotomy or laminectomy, may be required for stenotic spinal canals, for the obese, or for patients with previous surgery in the region of insertion. Deep sedation and generous infiltration of local anesthetic is mandatory if an open technique is chosen. After a small midline laminotomy and ligamentum flavum resection, the electrode is initially inserted under direct vision into the epidural space, but the location of the electrode tip is monitored fluoroscopically.

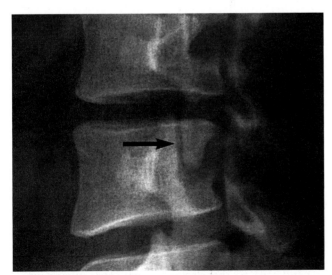

FIGURE 152-27 *A,* Site of needle insertion from the midline for facet injection. *B,* Oblique fluoroscopic view at the midpoint of the facet joint margin serving as the best point for needle insertion during facet joint injection.

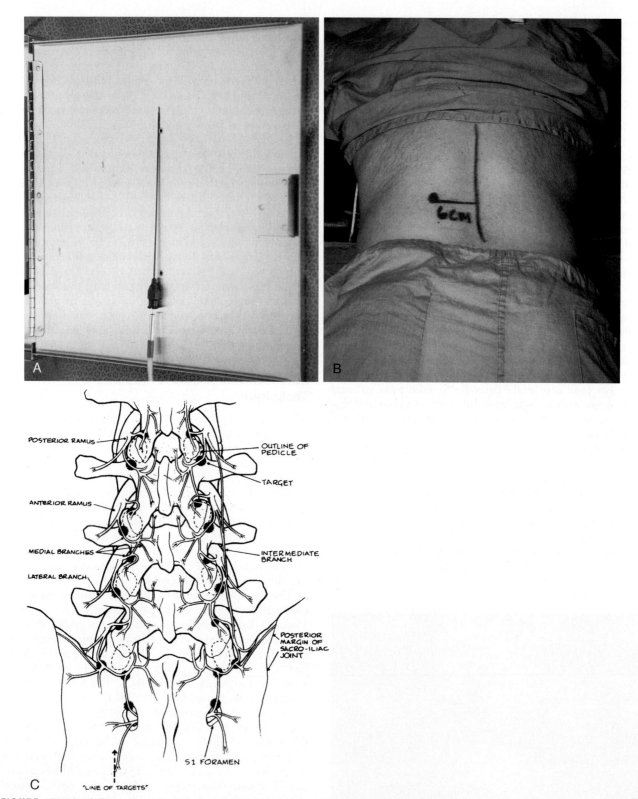

FIGURE 152-28   *A,* Electrode and needle for facet rhizotomy. *B,* Needle insertion begins 6 cm from the midline. *C,* Sites for rhizotomy with a needle electrode. Three sites surround the L4–L5 facet and four at L5–S1.

Depending on the location and distribution of pain, the electrode array is either positioned strictly midline for bilateral and truncal stimulation coverage, or slightly off midline ipsilateral to the pain area. Crude electrode position can be estimated using fluoroscopy. At this point, the patient is awakened from sedation while the intraoperative stimulator is connected to the electrode array. Test stimulation is performed at increasing stimulation amplitudes until the patient reports a moderately strong sensation of paresthesia. The stimulation cannot be effective until the areas of paresthesia are mapped over the areas of pain, which may require multiple adjustments of the electrode array or introduction of multiple electrode arrays for better coverage. As soon as the patient reports coverage of all painful areas with a tingling sensation, the electrode array is sutured to the paravertebral fascia with nonabsorbable sutures. A temporary extension wire is tunneled subcutaneously and secured externally for 3 days to several weeks of test stimulation. The patient is discharged home the same day or on the first postoperative day after instructions on use of the temporary stimulator.

At readmission, the electrode arrays are removed or repositioned if the test stimulation did not give the expected relief of pain. Permanent implantation of the implantable pulse generator is undertaken if the patient is highly satisfied with the pain-suppressing effect and documented at least a 50% reduction of pain. The procedure (phase 2) can be performed in general intubation anesthesia or monitored anesthesia care. The patient is positioned in a lateral position and the area where the electrode implantation was undertaken is exposed again. In addition, a small subcutaneous pocket is created in the flank or buttock according to the patient's preference to allow for placement of the pulse generator. The electrode array is connected to the pulse generator device with an extension wire that is tunneled subcutaneously. The patient can be discharged the same day after instruction on how to adjust the implanted stimulator.

The possible complications associated with SCS include general surgical complications and the specific risk of spinal cord or nerve damage, but neurologic complications have been rare. The infection rate is comparable with the expected rate after implantation of devices in other regions of the body and is generally quoted as 3% to 5%. Electrode migration or dislodgment, which could result in ineffective stimulation patterns, is also possible and best avoided if the patient is instructed to abstain from twisting or bending until the scarring process is completed, approximately 6 weeks after implantation.

Trial and Implantation of Intrathecal Medication Therapy (Morphine Pump)

After patients are selected as potential candidates for intrathecal therapy, a test challenge of intrathecal opioids is performed to assess efficacy and potential side effects. This test can be performed as a single-bolus injection with a spinal tap (usually 1 mg morphine sulfate in preservative-free saline), or an epidural or intrathecal catheter can be temporarily implanted to test longer-term continuous infusion of epidural or intrathecal test medication. In both cases, patients are admitted to the hospital with continuous pulse oximetry and an opioid antidote (naloxone) at the bedside. The pain-relieving effect can be expected to start as soon as 30 minutes after bolus injection and can last up to 24 hours with a single bolus application.

If good pain relief is reported and no or minimal side effects observed, patients are taken to the operating room the following day. The pump implantation procedure is performed with the patient in the lateral decubitus position under regional or general anesthesia. The area of the lumbar spine and flank is prepared and draped. A midline skin incision is made in the lower back around L4–L5, and dissection

is carried down to the level of the paravertebral fascia. A Tuohy needle is inserted at a 45-degree angle into the interlaminar space and advanced into the intrathecal space, which is confirmed by positive CSF return. Under fluoroscopic guidance, the intrathecal catheter is then introduced and advanced intrathecally to the thoracic spinal area. Positive CSF return through the catheter is observed before the Tuohy needle is removed. At this point, the catheter end should be occluded to avoid extra CSF loss, which could collapse the subarachnoid space and lead to placement of the catheter in a subdural or epidural position.

The implantable pump is then prepared for implantation, which, for programmable pumps, requires a purging routine that takes approximately 15 to 20 minutes. An 8-cm skin incision is then made in the flank between the rib cage and the iliac crest, and a subcutaneous pouch is created large enough to hold the pump. The catheter is then tunneled subcutaneously and connected to the pump, which has been filled with the desired medication. The margins of the pump are sutured to Scarpa's fascia to prevent rotation of the device and kinking of the tubing. Patients can usually be discharged home the same day. Immediately after surgery, programmable pumps are set to provide the adequate daily amount of medication. The amount of intrathecal morphine needed per day can be estimated based on a conversion formula.[86]

Possible side effects from intrathecal test injections include post–spinal tap headaches and potential injury to nerve roots (especially in patients with arachnoiditis). Side effects from intrathecal morphine include changes in mental status, respiratory depression, pruritus, gastrointestinal side effects such as constipation, cardiovascular side effects such as hypotension, and other rarely observed phenomena. In our experience, greater than 90% of well-selected patients experience pain relief from the test injections. The surgical pump implantation procedure carries general surgical risks (infection, hemorrhage) as well as the risk for complications with the catheter (kinking, holes in the catheter, catheter breaks) or pump itself (mechanical or electrical failure).

Intradiscal Electrothermal Therapy

IDET is a percutaneous fluoroscopically mediated outpatient procedure performed under light and intermittently heavy sedation (Fig. 152-29). The goal of the procedure is to navigate a precontoured copper wire around the inner margin of the disc annulus posteriorly at the margin with the more central nucleus pulposus. Once in position, the distal end of the copper wire is designed to be heated to 90°C for 16 minutes. This thermal lesion creates chemical reactions that stiffen the annular fibers and causes some proliferation of fibrous cells that stiffen the motion segment and/or denervate the pain fibers within the annulus (Fig. 152-29A). Therefore, it is important to obtain an adequate burn over the entire posterior margin of the disc annulus. This is often inhibited by radial tears in the annulus, which can block circumferential progression of the coil. When complete passage is not passable from a unilateral approach, a bilateral approach is recommended to get complete coverage of the posterior annular margin.

The patient is placed in the prone position with a horizontal lower abdominal roll to initiate a moderate degree of

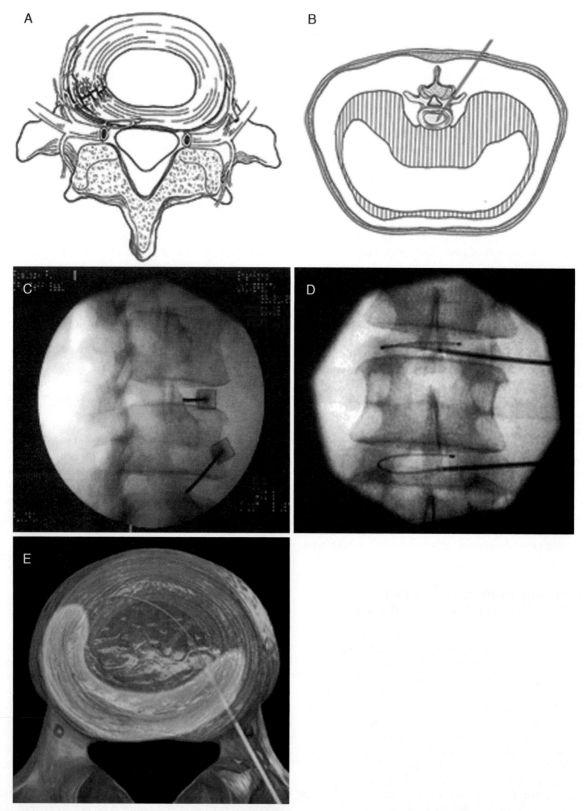

FIGURE 152-29 Intradiscal electrothermal therapy. *A,* Axial view illustration of a fissured disc and pain fibers within the annulus. *B,* With the patient in the prone position, an 8-inch needle and trocar are inserted as shown, targeting the disc space just anterior to the most anterior portion of the pedicle, guided by fluoroscopy. *C,* Proper placement of the needle and trocar as seen by fluoroscopy. *D,* With the trocar removed, an intradiscal electrothermal therapy coil is inserted through the needle shaft under fluoroscopy, passing the coil circumferentially around the annulus past the midline until the tip rests back on the ipsilateral side of insertion but not making a complete circle. *E,* The catheter is then connected to the power source and the catheter is heated, ramping up to the temperature of 90°C over 12 minutes and maintaining it for the next 4 minutes. (Courtesy of Smith & Nephew.)

lumbar flexion. After sterile preparation, the skin and retroperitoneal region are infiltrated with lidocaine solution. An 8-inch needle and trocar are inserted with a similar trajectory to discography, beginning approximately 14 cm from the midline on average (Fig. 152-29B). Should the patient complain of buttock and leg pain, the needle is removed and the trajectory in the sagittal plane is adjusted to avoid the extraforaminal nerve root. The target point at the disc space is just anterior to the most anterior portion of the pedicle at the disc space level as seen on a lateral fluoroscopic image (Fig. 152-29C). Once impacted at the annular margin, the needle is inserted another 10 mm to the inner margin of the disc annulus.

The trocar of the needle is removed, and an IDET coil that has been checked for normal impedance characteristics is then inserted through the needle shaft. A line on the proximal adaptor orients the surgeon to the native two-dimensional plane of the coil outside the disc space. This will let the surgeon know whether twisting the coil will direct the coil rostrally or caudally as it is passing circumferentially in the disc space. The surgeon changes from lateral to an AP projection frequently to assure that the coil is passing anteriorly, then horizontally to the contralateral side, and then posteriorly toward the posterior annular margin. If circumferential passage does not occur, then the coil can be retracted out of the disc space and reinserted. If after three passes the coil does not develop a circumferential trajectory, the needle should be removed and reinserted at a different angle until a circumferential trajectory is achieved. In some patients, particularly men, IDET at L5–S1 is impossible due to relatively rostrally situated tops of the iliac crests that block any potential needle trajectory.

Once the IDET cable has begun a circumferential trajectory, the coil is passed beyond the midline on the AP fluoroscopic image until the tip rests back on the ipsilateral side of insertion, but in less than a 360-degree arc to prevent touching the coil near its insertion point (Fig. 152-29D). The surgeon confirms that the proximal end of the heating element, which is marked by a radiopaque stripe, is inside the disc on an AP view. Due to annular tears and laxity of the annular fibers, it sometimes appears that the coil is inside the spinal canal. As long as the coil passes posteriorly around the convexity of the posterior margin, it should be in a safe position for heating. If the catheter does not continue to follow the convexity and goes into the spinal canal, it should be removed and insertion should be restarted.

If the catheter will not pass further and begins to kink, it should be retracted a centimeter or so and passed again. The catheter should not be forced at this point. This indicates a radial annular tear. The best strategy is to perform a full 16-minute burn in this position. The catheter adaptor is connected to the power source, which then ramps up the temperature to 90°C over 12 minutes, with the next 4 minutes at 90°C (Fig. 152-29E). The patient should be conscious at the onset of the lesioning. However, during the heating process, the patient should be awake enough to say if he or she is having any leg pain. If leg pain develops, the heating is stopped. If no leg pain occurs after 4 minutes and the patient is in pain, then heavier sedation is given. When the catheter has not passed completely, the procedure is repeated from the contralateral side. This usually affords coverage of the entire posterior annulus. At the conclusion

of the heating procedure, the coil and then the needle are removed. Patients wear a lumbar corset and follow limited physical activities for 3 months. The timing of pain relief varies from immediate to gradual over a period of several weeks.

REFERENCES

1. White AA, Panjabi MM: The problem of clinical instability in the human spine: A systematic approach. In White AA, Panjabi MM (eds): Clinical Biomechanics of the Spine, 2nd ed. Philadelphia: Lippincott Williams & Wilkins, 1990, p 278.
2. Frymoyer JW, Selby DK: Segmental instability. Rationale for treatment. Spine 10:280–286, 1985.
3. Frymoyer JW: Low back pain. The role of spine fusion. Neurosurg Clin North Am 2:933–954, 1991.
4. Kirkaldy-Willis WH, Hill RJ: A more precise diagnosis for low-back pain. Spine 4:102–109, 1979.
5. Kelsey JL, White AA: Epidemiology and impact of low-back pain. Spine 5:133–142, 1980.
6. Ogon M, Bender BR, Hooper DM, et al: A dynamic approach to spinal instability. Part I: Sensitization of intersegmental motion profiles to motion direction and load condition by instability. Spine 22:2841–2858, 1997.
7. Gardner-Morse MG, Stokes IA: Structural behavior of human lumbar spinal motion segments. J Biomech 37:205–212, 2004.
8. Pelz DM, Haddad RG: Radiologic investigation of low back pain. CMAJ 140:289–295, 1989.
9. Janevic J, Ashton-Miller JA, Schultz AB: Large compressive preloads decrease lumbar motion segment flexibility. J Orthop Res 9:228–236, 1991.
10. Schwarzer AC, Aprill CN, Derby R, et al: The relative contributions of the disc and zygapophyseal joint in chronic low back pain. Spine 19:801–806, 1994.
11. Lohmander LS, Neame PJ, Sandy JD: The structure of aggrecan fragments in human synovial fluid. Evidence that aggrecanase mediates cartilage degradation in inflammatory joint disease, joint injury, and osteoarthritis. Arthritis Rheum 36:1214–1222, 1993.
12. Neame PJ, Barry FP: The link proteins. Experientia 49:393–402, 1993.
13. Benoist M: Natural history of the aging spine. Eur Spine J 12 (Suppl): 86–89, 2003.
14. Goel VK, Winterbottom JM, Weinstein JN, et al: Load sharing among spinal elements of a motion segment in extension and lateral bending. J Biomech Eng 109:291–297, 1987.
15. Schellhas KP, Pollei SR, Gundry CR, et al: Lumbar disc high-intensity zone. Correlation of magnetic resonance imaging and discography. Spine 21:79–86, 1996.
16. Antoniou J, Goudsouzian NM, Heathfield TF, et al: The human lumbar end plate. Evidence of changes in biosynthesis and denaturation of the extracellular matrix with growth, maturation, aging, and degeneration. Spine 21:1153–1161, 1996.
17. Kauppila LI, McAlindon T, Evans S, et al: Disc degeneration/back pain and calcification of the abdominal aorta. A 25-year follow-up study in Framingham. Spine 22:1642–1647, 1997.
18. Ernst E: Smoking: A cause of back trouble? Br J Rheumatol 32:239–242, 1993.
19. Fogelholm RR, Alho AV: Smoking and intervertebral disc degeneration. Med Hypoth 56:537–539, 2001.
20. Kaigle AM, Holm SH, Hansson TH: Kinematic behavior of the porcine lumbar spine: A chronic lesion model. Spine 22:2796–2806, 1997.
21. Panjabi MM, White AA: Physical properties and functional biomechanics of the spine. In White AA, Panjabi MM (eds): Clinical Biomechanics of the Spine, 2nd ed. Philadelphia: Lippincott Williams & Wilkins, 1990, pp 14–15.
22. Yang KH, King AI: Mechanism of facet load transmission as a hypothesis for low-back pain. Spine 9:557–565, 1984.
23. Indahl A, Kaigle AM, Reikeras O, et al: Interaction between porcine lumbar intervertebral disc, zygapophyseal joints, and paraspinal muscles. Spine 22:2834–2840, 1997.
24. Horal J: The clinical appearance of low back pain disorders in the city of Gothenburg, Sweden. Comparisons of incapacitated probands with matched controls. Acta Orthop Scand Suppl 118:1–109, 1969.
25. Haylor A: Lumbar disc disease. In Dickson RA (ed): Spinal Surgery: Science and Practice. London: Butterworth-Heinemann, 1990, pp 123–126.

26. Bigos S (ed): Report of the Low Back Pain Guidelines. Panel to the Office of Forum of the Agency for Health Care Policy and Research, Department of Health and Human Services. Washington, DC: Department of Health and Human Services, 1993.

27. Maigne JY, Aivaliklis A, Pfefer F: Results of sacroiliac joint double block and value of sacroiliac pain provocation tests in 54 patients with low back pain. Spine 21:1889–1892, 1996.

28. Pate D, Goobar J, Resnick D, et al: Traction osteophytes of the lumbar spine: Radiographic-pathologic correlation. Radiology 166:843–846, 1988.

29. Vallee C, Chevrot A, Benhamouda M, et al: X-ray computed tomographic aspects of lumbar articular synovial cysts with intraspinal development. J Radiol 68:519–526, 1987.

30. Tertti M, Paajanen H, Laato M, et al: Disc degeneration in magnetic resonance imaging. A comparative biochemical, histologic, and radiologic study in cadaver spines. Spine 16:629–634, 1991.

31. Berns DH, Blaser SI, Modic MT: Magnetic resonance imaging of the spine. Clin Orthop 244:78–100, 1989.

32. Olerud S, Sjostrom L, Karlstrom G, et al: Spontaneous effect of increased stability of the lower lumbar spine in cases of severe chronic back pain. The answer of an external transpeduncular fixation test. Clin Orthop 203:67–74, 1986.

33. Holt EP Jr: The question of lumbar discography. J Bone Joint Surg Am 50:720–726, 1968.

34. Colhoun E, McCall IW, Williams L, et al: Provocation discography as a guide to planning operations on the spine. J Bone Joint Surg Br 70:267–271, 1988.

35. Newman MH, Grinstead GL: Anterior lumbar interbody fusion for internal disc disruption. Spine 17:831–833, 1992.

36. Wetzel FT, LaRocca SH, Lowery GL, et al: The treatment of lumbar spinal pain syndromes diagnosed by discography. Lumbar arthrodesis. Spine 19:792–800, 1994.

37. Walsh TR, Weinstein JN, Spratt KF, et al: Lumbar discography in normal subjects. A controlled, prospective study. J Bone Joint Surg Am 72:1081–1088, 1990.

38. Osti OL, Fraser RD, Vernon-Roberts B: Discitis after discography: The role of prophylactic antibiotics. J Bone Joint Surg Br 72:271–274, 1990.

39. Adams MA, Dolan P, Hutton WC: The stages of disc degeneration as revealed by discograms. J Bone Joint Surg Br 68:36–41, 1986.

40. Executive Committee of the North American Spine Society: Position statement on discography. Spine 13:1343, 1988.

41. Nachemson A: Lumbar discography—Where are we today? [Editorial]. Spine 14:555–557, 1989.

42. Simmons JW, McMillin JN, Emery SF, et al: Intradiscal steroids. A prospective double-blind clinical trial. Spine 17 (Suppl):172–175, 1992.

43. Saifuddin A, Braithwaite I, White J, et al: The value of lumbar spine magnetic resonance imaging in the demonstration of anular tears. Spine 23:453–457, 1998.

44. Greenough CG, Fraser RD: The effects of compensation on recovery from low-back injury. Spine 14:947–955, 1989.

45. Taylor VM, Deyo RA, Ciol M, et al: Surgical treatment of patients with back problems covered by workers compensation versus those with other sources of payment. Spine 21:2255–2259, 1996.

46. Frymoyer JW: Predicting disability from low back pain. Clin Orthop 279:101–109, 1992.

47. Gallagher RM, Williams RA, Skelly J, et al: Workers' compensation and return-to-work in low back pain. Pain 61:299–307, 1995.

48. Riley JL 3rd, Robinson ME, Geisser ME, et al: Relationship between MMPI-2 cluster profiles and surgical outcome in low-back pain patients. J Spinal Disord 8:213–219, 1995.

49. Nachemson AL: Lumbar spine instability: Outcome and randomized controlled trials. Bull Hosp Joint Dis 55:166, 1996.

50. Kirkaldy-Willis W, Farfan HF: Instability of the lumbar spine. Clin Orthop 165:110–123, 1982.

51. Lee CK: Accelerated degeneration of the segment adjacent to a lumbar fusion. Spine 13:375–377, 1988.

52. Rahm MD, Hall BB: Adjacent-segment degeneration after lumbar fusion with instrumentation: A retrospective study. J Spinal Disord 9:392–400, 1996.

53. Rompe JD, Eysel P, Hopf C: Clinical efficacy of pedicle instrumentation and posterolateral fusion in the symptomatic degenerative lumbar spine. Eur Spine J 4:231–237, 1995.

54. Lee TC: Transpedicular reduction and stabilization for postlaminectomy lumbar instability. Acta Neurochir (Wien) 138:139–145, 1996.

55. Parker LM, Murrell SE, Boden SD, et al: The outcome of posterolateral fusion in highly selected patients with discogenic low back pain. Spine 21:1909–1917, 1996.

56. Beguiristain JL, Villas C, Preite R, et al: Lumbosacral arthrodesis using pedicular screws and ringed rods. Eur Spine J 6:233–238, 1997.

57. Thomsen K, Christensen FB, Eiskjaer SP, et al: The effect of pedicle screw instrumentation on functional outcome and fusion rates in posterolateral lumbar spinal fusion: A prospective, randomized clinical study. Spine 22:2813–2822, 1997.

58. Martz EO, Goel VK, Pope MH, et al: Materials and design of spinal implants—A review. J Biomed Mater Res 38:267–288, 1997.

59. Hashimoto T, Shigenobu K, Kanayama M, et al: Clinical results of single-level posterior lumbar interbody fusion using the Brantigan I/F carbon cage filled with a mixture of local morselized bone and bioactive ceramic granules. Spine 27:258–262, 2002.

60. Thalgott JS, Klezl Z, Timlin M, et al: Anterior lumber interbody fusion with processed sea coral (coralline hydroxyapatite) as part of a circumferential fusion. Spine 27:E518–E527, 2002.

61. Kim DH, Jenis L, Berta SC, et al: Bone graft alternatives in spinal fusion surgery. Curr Opin Orthop 14:127–137, 2003.

62. Resnick DK: Spinal fusion for discogenic back pain: Patient selection, operative techniques, and outcomes. Tech Neurosurg 8:176–190, 2003.

63. Brodke DS, Dick JC, Kunz DN, et al: Posterior lumbar interbody fusion: A biomechanical comparison, including a new threaded cage. Spine 22:26–31, 1997.

64. Duggal N, Mendiondo I, Pares HR, et al: Anterior lumbar interbody fusion for treatment of failed back surgery syndrome: An outcome analysis. Neurosurgery 54:636–644, 2004.

65. Rajaraman V, Vingan R, Roth P, et al: Visceral and vascular complications resulting from anterior lumbar interbody fusion. J Neurosurg 91:60–64, 1999.

66. Tiusanen H, Seitsalo S, Osterman K, et al: Retrograde ejaculation after anterior interbody lumbar fusion. Eur Spine J 4:339–342, 1995.

67. Sasso RC, Kenneth Burkus J, LeHuec JC: Retrograde ejaculation after anterior lumbar interbody fusion: Transperitoneal versus retroperitoneal exposure. Spine 28:1023–1026, 2003.

68. Ray CD: Threaded titanium cages for lumbar interbody fusions. Spine 22:667–680, 1997.

69. Ray CD: Threaded fusion cages for lumbar interbody fusions. An economic comparison with 360 degrees fusions. Spine 22:681–685, 1997.

70. Kuslich SD, Danielson G, Dowdle JD, et al: Four-year follow-up results of lumbar spine arthrodesis using the Bagby and Kuslich lumbar fusion cage. Spine 25:2656–2662, 2000.

71. Hacker RJ: Comparison of interbody fusion approaches for disabling low back pain. Spine 22:660–666, 1997.

72. Andersen KH, Mosdal C, Vaernet K: Percutaneous radiofrequency facet denervation in low-back and extremity pain. Acta Neurochir (Wien) 87:48–51, 1987.

73. Savitz M: Percutaneous radiofrequency rhizotomy of the lumbar facets: Ten years' experience. Mt Sinai J Med 58:177–178, 1991.

74. Gocer AI, Cetinalp E, Tuna M, et al: Percutaneous radiofrequency rhizotomy of lumbar spinal facets: The results of 46 cases. Neurosurg Rev 20:114–116, 1997.

75. Tzaan WC, Tasker RR: Percutaneous radiofrequency facet rhizotomy—Experience with 118 procedures and reappraisal of its value. Can J Neurol Sci 27:125–130, 2000.

76. Melzack R, Wall PD: Pain mechanisms: A new theory. Science 150:971–979, 1965.

77. Barolat G, Massaro F, He J, et al: Mapping of sensory responses to epidural stimulation of the intraspinal neural structures in man. J Neurosurg 78:233–239, 1993.

78. Burchiel KJ, Anderson VC, Wilson BJ, et al: Prognostic factors of spinal cord stimulation for chronic back and leg pain. Neurosurgery 36:1101–1111, 1995.

79. North RB, Kidd DH, Wimberly RL, et al: Prognostic value of psychological testing in patients undergoing spinal cord stimulation: A prospective study. Neurosurgery 39:301–311, 1996.

80. Kumar K, Toth C, Nath RK, et al: Epidural spinal cord stimulation for treatment of chronic pain—Some predictors of success: A 15-year experience. Surg Neurol 50:110–120, 1998.

81. Turner JA, Loeser JD, Bell KG: Spinal cord stimulation for chronic low back pain: A systematic literature synthesis. Neurosurgery 37:1088–1096, 1995.

82. North RB, Kidd DH, Olin JC, et al: Spinal cord stimulation electrode design: Prospective, randomized, controlled trial comparing percutaneous and laminectomy electrodes. Part I: Technical outcomes. Neurosurgery 51:381–389, 2002.

83. North RB, Ewend MG, Lawton MT, et al: Failed back surgery syndrome: 5-year follow-up after spinal cord stimulator implantation. Neurosurgery 28:692–699, 1991.

84. LeDoux MS, Langford KH: Spinal cord stimulation for the failed back syndrome. Spine 18:191–194, 1993.

85. Broggi G, Servello D, Dones I, et al: Italian multicentric study on pain treatment with epidural spinal cord stimulation. Stereotact Funct Neurosurg 62:273–278, 1994.

86. Ohnmeiss DD, Rashbaum RF, Bogdanffy GM: Prospective outcome evaluation of spinal cord stimulation in patients with intractable leg pain. Spine 21:1344–1351, 1996.

87. Ohnmeiss DD, Rashbaum RF: Patient satisfaction with spinal cord stimulation for predominant complaints of chronic, intractable low back pain. Spine J 1:358–363, 2001.

88. Allegri M, Arachi G, Barbieri M, et al: Prospective study of the success and efficacy of spinal cord stimulation. Minerva Anestesiol 70:117–124, 2004.

89. Kumar K, Nath R, Wyant GM: Treatment of chronic pain by epidural spinal cord stimulation: A 10-year experience. J Neurosurg 75:402–407, 1991.

90. Fiume D, Sherkat S, Callovini GM, et al: Treatment of the failed back surgery syndrome due to lumbo-sacral epidural fibrosis. Acta Neurochir Suppl (Wien) 64:116–118, 1995.

91. Devulder J, De Laat M, Van Bastelaere M, et al: Spinal cord stimulation: A valuable treatment for chronic failed back surgery patients. J Pain Symptom Manage 13:296–301, 1997.

92. Lang P: The treatment of chronic pain by epidural spinal cord stimulation—A 15 year follow up; present status. Axone 18:71–73, 1997.

93. Bell GK, Kidd D, North RB: Cost-effectiveness analysis of spinal cord stimulation in treatment of failed back surgery syndrome. J Pain Symptom Manage 13:286–295, 1997.

94. Krames E: Spinal cord stimulation: Indications, mechanism of action, and efficacy. Curr Rev Pain 3:419–426, 1999.

95. Portenoy RK, Savage SR: Clinical realities and economic considerations: Special therapeutic issues in intrathecal therapy—Tolerance and addiction. J Pain Symptom Manage 14 (Suppl):27–35, 1997.

96. Krames ES, Olson K: Clinical realities and economic considerations: Patient selection in intrathecal therapy. J Pain Symptom Manage 14 (Suppl):3–13, 1997.

97. Krames ES: Intraspinal opioid therapy for chronic nonmalignant pain: Current practice and clinical guidelines. J Pain Symptom Manage 11:333–352, 1996.

98. Paice JA, Penn RD, Shott S: Intraspinal morphine for chronic pain: A retrospective, multicenter study. J Pain Symptom Manage 11:71–80, 1996.

99. Tutak U, Doleys DM: Intrathecal infusion systems for treatment of chronic low back and leg pain of noncancer origin. South Med J 89:295–300, 1996.

100. Winkelmuller M, Winkelmuller W: Long-term effects of continuous intrathecal opioid treatment in chronic pain of nonmalignant etiology. J Neurosurg 85(3):458–467, 1996.

101. Valentino L, Pillay KV, Walker J: Managing chronic nonmalignant pain with continuous intrathecal morphine. J Neurosci Nurs 30:233–239, 243–244, 1998.

102. Levy RM: Quantitative, crossover, double-blind trial paradigm for patient screening for chronic intraspinal narcotic administration. Neurosurg Focus 2:e2, 1997.

103. Angel IF, Gould HJ Jr, Carey ME: Intrathecal morphine pump as a treatment option in chronic pain of nonmalignant origin. Surg Neurol 49:92–98, 1998.

104. Rainov NG, Heidecke V, Burkert W: Long-term intrathecal infusion of drug combinations for chronic back and leg pain. J Pain Symptom Manage 22:862–871, 2001.

105. Hassenbusch SJ, Paice JA, Patt RB, et al: Clinical realities and economic considerations: Economics of intrathecal therapy. J Pain Symptom Manage 14 (Suppl):36–48, 1997.

106. de Lissovoy G, Brown RE, Halpern M, et al: Cost-effectiveness of long-term intrathecal morphine therapy for pain associated with failed back surgery syndrome: Clin Ther 19:96–112, 1997.

107. Kumar K, Hunter G, Demeria DD: Treatment of chronic pain by using intrathecal drug therapy compared with conventional pain therapies: a cost-effectiveness analysis. J Neurosurg 97:803–810, 2002.

108. Saal JA, Saal JS: Thermal characteristics of lumbar disc: Evaluation of a novel approach to targeted intradiscal thermal therapy. Presented at the 13th annual meeting of the North American Spine Society. San Francisco, California, October 28–31, 1998.

109. Shah RV, Lutz GE, Lee J, et al: Intradiskal electrothermal therapy: A preliminary histologic study. Arch Phys Med Rehabil 82:1230–1237, 2001.

110. Saal JS, Saal JA: Management of chronic discogenic low back pain with a thermal intradiscal catheter. A preliminary report. Spine 25:382–388, 2000.

111. Lee J, Lutz GE, Campbell D, et al: Stability of the lumbar spine after intradiscal electrothermal therapy. Arch Phys Med Rehabil 82:120–122, 2001.

112. Bogduk N, Karasek M: Two-year follow-up of a controlled trial of intradiscal electrothermal anuloplasty for chronic low back pain resulting from internal disc disruption. Spine J 2:343–350, 2002.

113. Saal JA, Saal JS: Intradiscal electrothermal treatment for chronic discogenic low back pain: Prospective outcome study with a minimum 2-year follow-up. Spine 27:966–974, 2002.

114. Guyer RD, Ohnmeiss DD: Intervertebral disc prostheses. Spine 28 (Suppl):15–23, 2003.

115. Cinotti G, David T, Postacchini F: Results of disc prosthesis after a minimum follow-up period of 2 years. Spine 15:995–1000, 1996.

116. Lemaire JP, Skalli W, Lavaste F, et al: Intervertebral disc prosthesis: Results and prospects for the year 2000. Clin Orthop 337:64–76, 1997.

117. Ross ERS, Tandon V: A prospective cohort study of the Charite intervertebral disc replacement. J Bone Joint Surg Br 80 (Suppl):46, 1998.

118. Ross ERS, Williamson JB: Intervertebral disc replacement—Six years experience using the Link Charite prosthesis. J Bone Joint Surg Br 82 (Suppl):36, 2000.

119. Tropiano P, Huang RC, Girardi FP, et al: Lumbar disc replacement: Preliminary results with ProDisc II after a minimum follow-up period of 1 year. J Spinal Disord Tech 16:362–368, 2003.

120. Bao QB, Yuan HA: Prosthetic disc replacement: The future? Clin Orthop 394:139–145, 2002.

121. Hochschuler SH, Ohnmeiss DD, Guyer RD, et al: Artificial disc: Preliminary results of a prospective study in the United States. Eur Spine J 11 (Suppl):106–110, 2002.

122. Delamarter RB, Fribourg DM, Kanim LE, et al: ProDisc artificial total lumbar disc replacement: Introduction and early results from the United States clinical trial. Spine 28 (Suppl):167–175, 2003.

123. Zigler JE: Clinical results with ProDisc: European experience and U.S. investigation device exemption study. Spine 28 (Suppl):163–166, 2003.

124. Bogduk N, Macintosh J, Marsland A: Technical limitations to the efficacy of radiofrequency neurotomy for spinal pain. Neurosurgery 20:529–535, 1987.

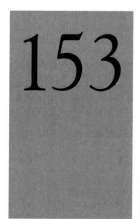

153 Surgical Management of Cerebrospinal Fluid Leakage after Spinal Surgery

STEPHEN R. FREIDBERG

Jason Mixter noted that "after the operative work is finished comes the question of closing the wound . . . the dura is closed tightly with a continuous fine silk stitch. If there is a dural defect, it is patched with a fascial graft carefully applied. This careful closure is to prevent any cerebrospinal fluid leak which is always fraught with danger."[1] Most, although not all, researchers[2-5] agree with Mixter's observation. In this chapter, methods of prevention, diagnosis, and treatment of patients with leakage of spinal cerebrospinal fluid (CSF) are discussed.

CAUSES AND PREVENTION

The presence of spinal dural CSF leakage can change a well-performed operation into one with a serious complication: A dural cutaneous fistula can lead to meningitis, a meningocele can disrupt the muscle as well as the skin closure and may cause spinal cord or nerve root compression, and CSF leakage increases morbidity and the length of hospital stay. Leakage and the formation of a collection of CSF can be noted after the purposeful opening or resection of dura or with the tearing of dura during laminectomy or dural puncture or after spinal trauma. Each of these situations presents specific technical problems that are addressed in this chapter.

Cerebrospinal Fluid Leakage after Laminectomy

Repair of a midline or paramedian dural opening fashioned in the course of intradural exploration should involve a straightforward repair. The dural incision separates dural fibers that, when retraction on them is released, have a natural tendency to fall together. Assuming that the spinal cord need not be decompressed, the incision can be sutured easily in a watertight fashion. The difficulty in elective dural opening arises, for example, when it is necessary to resect dura in the course of removing a tumor, such as a meningioma. When the dural resection is dorsally situated, the defect can be repaired with a patch of fascia. However, in certain situations a sutured dural repair may not be possible. This occurs when the defect in the dura is ventrally situated, is in the axilla of the nerve root, or when the dura is cut perpendicular to the fibers of the dura when removing a dumbbell schwannoma. Other measures, described later, may be necessary to prevent CSF leakage.

Inadvertent CSF leakage during an elective extradural operation can frequently be avoided if the surgeon adheres to careful technique. In my experience, dural laceration occurs most commonly with the use of a Kerrison punch when the dura has not been separated adequately from the overlying bone or ligament in the presence of severe lumbar spinal stenosis or during a reoperation associated with scar tissue. Laceration of the dura may also occur in the course of routine lumbar disc excisions.

When the patient's spine is being operated on for the first time, the dura must be separated from the overlying tissue with a fine dissector before the footplate of a rongeur is placed in the epidural space. Heavy bone should be removed with a Leksell rongeur or a high-speed drill so that the more delicate Kerrison instrument is not required to perform this task. If a drill is used to thin the bone, the motion of the drill must be medial to lateral so that if any slippage occurs, it is away from the dura. When possible, the surgeon should operate superficial to the ligamentum flavum because this structure protects the dura. After bone removal is completed, the ligament should be cut sharply and not torn with a rongeur.

Another source of dural tear and CSF leakage is the sharp bone spicule,[6] which may cause a dural laceration and CSF leakage days after the operation. A similar situation can occur with a medially placed pedicle screw, which tears the dura.[7] In both situations, CSF leakage can develop in a delayed fashion. Bone edges must be smooth, and screws and other hardware must be well placed before final closure.

In a patient who has had previous surgery at the site of reoperation, one should identify normal dura by extending removal of bone rostrally and caudally from the margins of the previous laminectomy. The plane of the normal dura must then be identified so that dissection can proceed safely through the scar to free the dura and the nerve root or roots. When the scar readily separates from the dura, dissection with a blunt dissector is satisfactory. When the scar is firmly adherent to the dura, however, sharp dissection is necessary to prevent a dural tear. When the repeated operation is for a lateral lesion, such as recurrent lumbar disc herniation, bone and scar lateral to the nerve root must be removed. The plane lateral and ventral to the nerve root and dura can then be dissected with minimal retraction and with less chance of dural injury.

Cerebrospinal Fluid Leakage after Anterior Spinal Surgery

Prevention of dural injury during anterior spinal surgery requires the same attention to surgical principles as does laminectomy. The plane of the dura must be identified and the dura separated from the overlying tissue before further bone, ligament, or tumor is removed.

In the cervical spine, cervical corpectomy in patients with ossification of the posterior longitudinal ligament (OPLL) deserves special mention. At times, the lesion from OPLL invades dura, making resection of dura inevitable. Smith and colleagues[8] recommend the use of autogenous fascial or muscle graft and lumbar subarachnoid shunting in this situation. They stress the need to prevent sudden increases in CSF pressure with its resultant vomiting and coughing. At other times, the posterior longitudinal ligament can be dissected from the dura. The dissection should be performed with the knife parallel to the fibers of the dura. Should a laceration occur, suture repair may be possible. When the laceration is perpendicular to the dural fibers, a gap occurs in the defect, and the sutures will pull out.

Anterior vertebral resection at thoracic or lumbar levels of the spine for tumor, degenerative disease, or herniated disc should follow the same principles described previously. Should a dural tear occur and CSF be seen during operation at these levels, sufficient room exists to drill bone to expose the leak adequately and deal with it by direct suture or a patch. A CSF drain may be necessary.

With nonsurgically managed spinal trauma, a CSF leakage under the skin or into a body cavity is unlikely unless the patient has sustained a penetrating injury. If surgery is required for the injury, severe disruption of the dura may be found that requires repair with a fascial graft using a suture technique, if possible, and fibrin glue. Lumbar drainage of CSF to reduce the pressure on the repair is then necessary.[9]

The use of spinal instrumentation at any level of the spine can be a cause of dural laceration. Leakage of CSF has been reported[10] with sublaminar wires and with pedicle screws, especially when they are placed more medially than is appropriate. Great care must be taken with the use of these instruments and devices. Dura must be stripped from the overlying bone and ligament before sublaminar wires are passed. The surgeon who uses any spinal instrumentation must be well trained and careful so that the screws are of appropriate length and are placed at the correct angles.

A CSF fistula in an operative field in which radiotherapy had previously been delivered usually is an extremely difficult problem to manage. The tissues are firm and, when brought together, do not conform to the cavity created by the operation. Sutures hold poorly and they must be tied with excess force to bring the rigid tissues together. Most importantly, the irradiated tissue has a poor blood supply caused by the characteristic vascular changes of radiation, which include hyaline thickening of blood vessel walls. Dealing with this problem is discussed later in this chapter.

DIAGNOSIS

Intraoperative Cerebrospinal Fluid Leakage

Leakage of CSF during surgery is usually obvious. When the dura has been opened on purpose, it should be repaired. When the tear is accidental, CSF usually appears in the operative field. The source of the leakage must be found and, if possible, repaired. Untreated CSF leakage during the operation invites postoperative complications.

Postoperative Cerebrospinal Fluid Leakage

Leakage of CSF during the postoperative period presents in two clinical patterns. The first is that of the low-pressure, posture-related headache that is similar to the common post–lumbar puncture headache. The patient experiences headache and often nausea, lightheadedness, and sweating when he or she assumes a vertical posture. These symptoms are somewhat relieved by lying down. The second clinical problem relates to the wound. A laminectomy wound bulges, and CSF leakage occurs at the suture line. Continual leakage of CSF prevents the incision from healing and increases the possibility of infection. When the nature of wound drainage is in doubt, glucose-oxidase paper is a reliable test for glucose. Although other body fluids may contain some glucose, a strongly positive result is diagnostic of CSF, and no further diagnostic tests are necessary to establish that CSF is passing from the incision.

A collection of CSF after anterior spinal surgery can present as a fluid-filled mass in the anterior neck. Thoracic leakage can result in CSF coming out of a chest tube or a significant collection of pleural fluid, and lumbar CSF leakage can result in a pelvic collection.

After it has been established that CSF leakage exists, the site of leakage must be localized. Various techniques have been used to accomplish this: fluorescein 0.5% and intrathecally injected methylene blue have been used to demonstrate the site of such leakage. Both of these agents are neurotoxic and should not be used.[11,12] The radioisotope technetium 99m diethylenetriamine-penta-acetic acid (^{99m}Tc-DTPA) can be used to demonstrate CSF leakage either by routine scanning or by single-photon emission computed tomography (SPECT).[13] With its ability to perform 3-dimensional reconstruction, SPECT provides better localization than does biplanar scanning. Magnetic resonance imaging (MRI) demonstrates the CSF collection, which has low signal characteristics on T1-weighted imaging, low signal intensity on proton density–weighted imaging, and increased signal on T2-weighted pulse sequences. The best method of demonstrating the exact anatomic location of the leakage, however, is the use of water-soluble, positive-contrast myelography followed by 3-dimensional computed tomography (CT) (Fig. 153-1).[14] The exact site of the fistula tract in relation to the adjacent bony anatomy can be clearly shown, as can the leakage of the contrast agent into the soft tissues or into a pseudomeningocele.

TREATMENT

Most investigators,[2,3] including myself, believe that with confirmation of the diagnosis of persistent spinal CSF leakage, the appropriate treatment is prompt re-exploration of the wound and repair of the dural defect. Not all researchers agree. One should not be dogmatic about this problem. Clearly, some minor leakage heals with nonoperative treatment. Should a soft subcutaneous bulge occur in a well-healed incision in a patient with no symptoms of postural headache, a waiting period is justified. Conversely, early operation must be considered in a patient with a tense or enlarging subcutaneous mass, especially when the incision appears to be breaking down. The morbidity and uncertainty associated

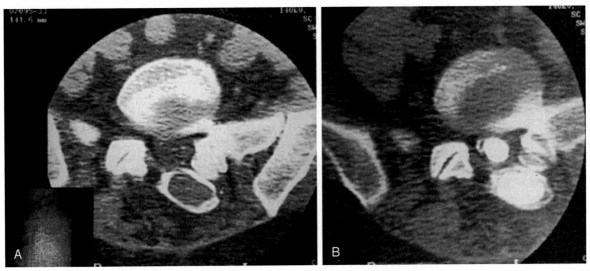

FIGURE 153-1   Computed tomographic view through the lumbar spine at L5–S1. *A,* Status after laminectomy with fusion. An ovoid mass with rim calcification is present in the laminectomy defect to the left of the midline. *B,* Myelogram after administration of iopamidol shows contrast material in the thecal sac and filling into the previously demonstrated ovoid mass, the pseudomeningocele.

with a prolonged nonoperative course of treatment of CSF leakage is not justified.

With a small series of patients, Waisman and Schweppe[5] advocated nonoperative treatment of postoperative leakage. They reported good results with watertight skin closure, the Trendelenburg position, daily subcutaneous taps, and administration of antibiotics. In their series, all wounds cleared within 10 to 28 days. Rosenthal and co-workers[4] described the use of multilayered watertight soft tissue closure in situations in which the dura cannot be closed. They advocated the use of mannitol, 20 g every 4 hours, and nursing supervision to ensure that the patient's head is not raised for 7 days. Our feeling is that treatment with prolonged bed rest is rarely indicated, subjects patients to complications such as phlebitis, pneumonia, and urinary infection, and incurs further hospital expenses. Hodges and colleagues[15] agree with this approach and feel that with a good dural repair, bed rest is not indicated.

The ideal method of dural repair, either as prevention during the primary operation or as treatment of the complication, is watertight suture of the dural defect. The choice of suture material and method of suture closure are important. Because the suture line is rarely exposed to stress, fine suture material, such as a 5-0 or 6-0 braided, coated synthetic, or monofilament suture, can be used. The needle should be swedged to minimize the size of the suture hole. Leakage of CSF can occur from needle holes in the dura. I prefer to suture dura with closely spaced interrupted sutures. This repair is slower and more tedious than a running stitch, but it avoids the unraveling of the entire suture line if the tension is not perfect or if the suture breaks. Cain and associates[16] have shown little difference in the resistance to pressure with interrupted or running locked sutures. Reinforcement with fibrin glue, however, added to the strength of the repair.

The surgical techniques are shown in Figures 153-2 through 153-5. The ability to perform these techniques depends, to some extent, on the character of the dura itself. When the dura is thin and friable, as sometimes occurs in

ossification of the posterior longitudinal ligament or severe lumbar stenosis or when the defect is ventrolateral, a creative, individualized solution is necessary. When the dural defect is at the margin of bone, the laminectomy must be enlarged to gain access to the entire dural defect. Magnification and bright lighting improve the surgical technique.

When the dural defect is linear, a simple suture repair is possible (Fig. 153-2). When the dura is thin or slightly irregular or when CSF is leaking from the suture holes, the sutures should be tied over a thin pledget of muscle. All of the sutures are placed, the muscle is placed over the defect and is held by an assistant, and the sutures are tied (Fig. 153-3).

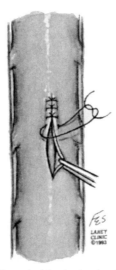

FIGURE 153-2   A linear incision in the dura is repaired with interrupted closely placed 5-0 sutures. (Courtesy of the Lahey Clinic, Burlington, MA.)

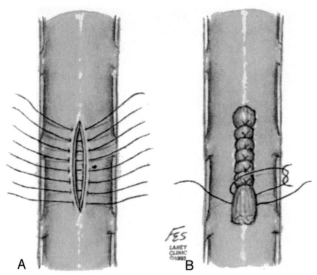

FIGURE 153-3 The sutures are placed, the muscle is placed in the defect, and all sutures are tied. (Courtesy of the Lahey Clinic, Burlington, MA.)

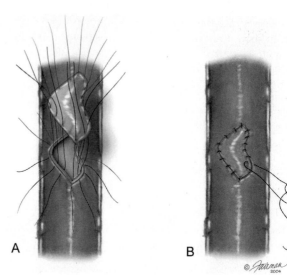

FIGURE 153-5 Parachute technique. The sutures are placed at the dural edge and then through the patch outside of the operative field. The graft is then slid into the defect and tied in place.

When a large dural defect is present, the dura must be patched (Fig. 153-4). The graft is anchored at the corners, then sutured with closely spaced interrupted sutures. The graft is then trimmed to fit with minimal redundancy. A minimal overlap of approximately 1 mm at the suture edge provides adequate tissue to plug the leakage. Excess tissue interferes with the suture line. Heavy fascia is readily available for use in grafting from the tissues superficial to the paraspinal muscles, which can be harvested easily on an as-needed basis and trimmed to fit the dural defect. When such paraspinal fascia is not readily available, fascia lata may be used. A commercial preparation, AlloDerm (Lifecell, Branchburg, NJ, U.S.A.), has been an excellent preparation to use as a patch graft. For difficult to suture wounds a "parachute" technique may

be useful (Fig. 153-5). Sutures are placed at the dural edge and then into the graft which is outside of the field. The graft is then slid into position and tied firmly into place.

Mayfield and Kurokawa[17] described a method of plugging small dural holes that are difficult to suture. This repair is performed through a midline durotomy. A suture is tied to a piece of fat or muscle, and the suture is passed from the durotomy through the dural defect. This suture can then be tied firmly. The graft located on the inside of the dura seals the leakage (Fig. 153-6).

It is not always possible to suture a dural defect directly. Most commonly, this situation occurs with anteriorly situated or anterolaterally situated defects, defects involving nerve root sleeves, or thin friable dura. This is a special

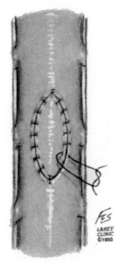

FIGURE 153-4 The patch is held in place with sutures at either end. It is then sutured with interrupted sutures. (Courtesy of the Lahey Clinic, Burlington, MA.)

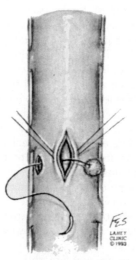

FIGURE 153-6 A pledget of muscle is tied to a suture, which is drawn intradurally and is fastened to plug the hole. (Modified from Mayfield FH, Kurokawa K: Watertight closure of spinal dura mater. J Neurosurg 43:639, 1975.)

problem during corpectomy when placing sutures is not possible. In such situations, tissue adhesives have been used in conjunction with fascial or muscle patches and sometimes as an adjunct to partial suturing. CSF drainage may be required to reduce the hydrostatic pressure on the dural defect until healing takes place.[18] This process needs to be combined with meticulous multilayered soft tissue closure if the repair is to succeed. We have used drains freely in the presence of dural tear and removed them when no further bleeding is observed. CSF fistula has not been a problem.

Fibrin glue is a very useful preparation to seal the edges of a patch, hold it to the dura, and prevent leakage of CSF from suture holes.[19] The preparation that we now use is Tisseel (Baxter Healthcare Corporation, Glendale, CA, U.S.A.). The glue must be used in a dry surgical field for the muscle or fascial graft to adhere to the dura. The graft can then be covered by a layer of absorbable fabric and again anchored with the fibrin adhesive (Fig. 153-7). Hadley and colleagues[20] have demonstrated the clear benefit of a fibrin glue repair compared with direct suture or laser welding of patches in a clivus dural model. Patel and co-workers[21] have closed postoperative CSF leaks in the lumbar spine by percutaneously injecting fibrin glue.

In the patient with a difficult suture line or with an adhesive repair or a persistent CSF leakage, the CSF pressure may be elevated, a condition that does not permit the defect to seal. Reduction of the CSF pressure with lumbar CSF drainage for 4 or 5 days is frequently sufficient to permit the leakage to seal. A few days without leakage from the dural repair will usually allow it to seal completely. The external lumbar drainage is to a closed collection system. There must be a warning here regarding overdrainage of lumbar CSF. Excess CSF drainage can cause downward traction on the cerebellum and brain stem with herniation.[22] CSF drainage should be limited to 10 mL/hour. Should signs of herniation occur, the drainage should be stopped and the patient laid flat or even in a head-down position.

The use of myocutaneous flaps to cover dura in operative fields in which tissue has been irradiated has been invaluable. Irradiated tissue has poor blood supply and poor healing potential.[23] A free flap or a pedicle flap of muscle or muscle and skin with its vascular supply can be moved from a healthy area to the poorly vascularized defect, then sutured to well-vascularized surrounding tissue. This technique has the benefit of not only permitting the skin to heal, but also providing healthy soft tissue that fills in and molds itself to a cavity and seals a hole in the dura. The well-vascularized flap is resistant to bacteria and can be used in the presence of infection.[24,25]

Post–lumbar puncture CSF leakage has been the most common cause of procedure-related symptoms associated with low CSF pressure after diagnostic lumbar puncture, spinal anesthesia, or myelography. Classically a headache develops when the patient assumes the vertical position, and this symptom is relieved when the patient is supine. The cause is the persistent leakage of CSF through a dural rent. This symptom usually clears with nonoperative treatment, rest, and hydration. Before the 1980s, when myelography was performed with iophendylate and a 19-gauge needle, CSF was commonly encountered in the wound during laminectomy performed within a few days of myelography. When the site of the needle puncture was unroofed, a nerve rootlet was seen herniating through, preventing the hole from closing and allowing the leakage to persist. It was necessary to reduce the nerve root hernia and to suture the dura (Fig. 153-8). At times, it was necessary to enlarge the dural defect to reduce the root.

Excellent relief of low-pressure symptoms has been reported with an autologous blood patch injected in the epidural space near the site of the puncture.[26] Szeinfeld and associates[27] demonstrated that 12 to 15 mL of blood spreads over 8 to 10 spinal segments. The spread is easier in a cephalad direction. The injection should be caudad to the lowest interspace in cases of multiple punctures. Although most

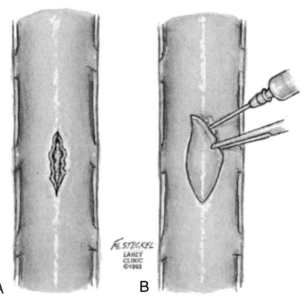

FIGURE 153-7 The patch is held in place with fibrin glue. (Courtesy of the Lahey Clinic, Burlington, MA.)

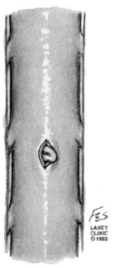

FIGURE 153-8 A nerve rootlet is herniated through a small hole in the dura. (Courtesy of the Lahey Clinic, Burlington, MA.)

blood patches have been placed in the lumbar area, Waldman and associates[28] used this technique successfully in the cervical spine with the injection of 8 mL of blood.

SUMMARY

Postoperative CSF leakage should be treated aggressively. Failure to stop the leakage can lead to infection of the wound and meningitis, inability to heal the wound, and prolonged hospitalization and morbidity. It is reasonable to attempt nonoperative treatment for a short while, but when the response is not prompt, the wound should be re-explored and the dura repaired.

REFERENCES

1. Mixter WJ: Spinal column and spinal cord: Laminectomy. In Lewis D (ed): Practice of Surgery, Vol XII. Hagerstown, MD: WF Prior Company, 1954, p 29.
2. Agrillo U, Simonetti G, Martino V: Postoperative CSF problems after spinal and lumbar surgery: A general review. J Neurosurg Sci 35:93–95, 1991.
3. Eismont FJ, Wiesel SW, Rothman RH: Treatment of dural tears associated with spinal surgery. J Bone Joint Surg Am 63:1132–1136, 1981.
4. Rosenthal JD, Hahn JF, Martinez GJ: A technique for closure of leak of spinal fluid. Surg Gynecol Obstet 140:948–950, 1975.
5. Waisman M, Schweppe Y: Postoperative cerebrospinal fluid leakage after lumbar spine operations: Conservative treatment. Spine 16:52–53, 1991.
6. Horwitz NH, Rizzoli HV: Laminectomy: General complications. In Horwitz NH, Rizzoli HV (eds): Postoperative Complications of Extracranial Neurological Surgery. Baltimore: Williams & Wilkins, 1987, pp 2–29.
7. Faraj AA, Webb JK: Early complications of spinal pedicle screw. Eur Spine J 6:324–326, 1997.
8. Smith MD, Bolesta MJ, Leventhal M, Bohlman HH: Postoperative cerebrospinal-fluid fistula associated with erosion of the dura: Findings after anterior resection of ossification of the posterior longitudinal ligament in the cervical spine. J Bone Joint Surg Am 74:270–277, 1992.
9. Robertson DP, Simpson RK: Penetrating injuries restricted to the cauda equina: A retrospective review. Neurosurgery 31:265–269, 1992.
10. Esses SI, Sachs BL, Dreyzin V: Complications associated with the technique of pedicle screw fixation: A selected survey of ABS members. Spine 18:2231–2238, 1993.
11. Wallace JD, Weintraub MI, Mattson RH, Rosnagle R: Status epilepticus as a complication of intrathecal fluorescein: Case report. J Neurosurg 36:659–660, 1972.
12. Evans JP, Keegan HR: Danger in the use of intrathecal methylene blue. JAMA 174:856–859, 1960.
13. Lewis DH, Graham MM: Benefit of tomography in the scintigraphic localization of cerebrospinal fluid leak. J Nucl Med 32:2149–2151, 1991.
14. Fujimaki H, Saito N, Tosaka M, et al: Cerebrospinal fluid leak demonstrated by three-dimensional computed tomographic myelography in patients with spontaneous intracranial hypotension. Surg Neurol 58:280–285, 2002.
15. Hodges SD, Humphreys C, Eck JC, Covington LA: Management of incidental durotomy without mandatory bed rest. Spine 24:2062–2064, 1999.
16. Cain JE, Randall FD, Barton BR: Evaluation of dural closure methods. Spine 13:720–725, 1988.
17. Mayfield FH, Kurokawa K: Watertight closure of spinal dura mater: Technical note. J Neurosurg 43:639–640, 1975.
18. Macdonald RL, Fehlings MG, Tator CH, et al: Multilevel anterior cervical corpectomy and fibular allograft fusion for cervical myelopathy. J Neurosurg 86:990–997, 1997.
19. Kassam A, Horowitz M, Carrau R, et al: Use of Tisseel fibrin sealant in neurosurgical procedures: Incidence of cerebrospinal fluid leaks and cost-benefit analysis in a retrospective study. Neurosurgery 52:1102–1105, 2003.
20. Hadley MN, Martin NA, Spetzler RF, et al: Comparative transoral dural closure techniques: A canine model. Neurosurgery 22:392–397, 1988.
21. Patel MR, Louie W, Rachlin J: Postoperative cerebrospinal fluid leaks of the lumbosacral spine: Management with percutaneous fibrin glue. AJNR Am J Neuroradiol 17:495–500, 1996.
22. Bloch J, Regli L: Brain stem and cerebellar dysfunction after lumbar spinal fluid drainage: Case report. J Neurol Neurosurg Psychiatry 74:992–994, 2003.
23. Azizkhan RG, Roberson JB Jr, Powers SK: Successful use of a vascularized intercostal muscle flap to seal a persistent intrapleural cerebrospinal fluid leak in a child. J Pediatr Surg 26:744–746, 1991.
24. Chang N, Mathes SJ: Comparison of the effect of bacterial inoculation in musculocutaneous and random-pattern flaps. Plast Reconstr Surg 70:1–10, 1982.
25. Hussussian CJ, Reece GP: Microsurgical scalp reconstruction in the patient with cancer. Plast Reconstr Surg 109:1828–1834, 2002.
26. Weakland HJ: The epidural blood patch—Current practices and concerns. CRNA 5:156–163, 1994.
27. Szeinfeld M, Ihmeidan IH, Moser MM, et al: Epidural blood patch: Evaluation of the volume and spread of blood injected into the epidural space. Anesthesiology 64:820–822, 1986.
28. Waldman SD, Feldstein GS, Allen ML: Cervical epidural blood patch: A safe effective treatment for cervical postdural puncture headache. Anesthesiol Rev 14:23–24, 1987.

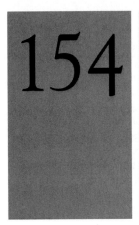

154 Management of Persistent Symptoms after Lumbar Disc Surgery

DONLIN M. LONG

The management of symptoms that persist after lumbar disc surgery varies according to the intensity of the complaints and the temporal relationship to the original procedures. It is not unusual for a patient who has undergone lumbar disc surgery to have some retained symptoms for a while after surgery. The fact that the symptoms persist does not mean they need evaluation. However, if symptoms remain completely unchanged for more than a few days, if they are worsened in any significant way, or if new neurologic deficits, not easily explicable on the basis of the surgical procedure, are present, then prompt diagnosis is required. No matter what the findings, management depends on the severity of symptoms. Most patients with recurrent symptoms after lumbar disc surgery improve spontaneously, and reoperation should be undertaken only when the recurrent symptoms are significant and a defined, reparable cause is present.[1] When symptoms recur more than 1 month after a previous surgical procedure, especially when they develop months to years later, they must be reevaluated according to standard clinical guidelines without direct concern for the previous operative procedure.[2] In my personal series of over 7,000 patients with failed back syndrome, only 30% had a definable problem that might be corrected by reoperation. This 30% could be divided into three approximately equal groups. These groups were those who had developed a new problem, those in whom the original surgery had failed to correct the original problem, and those with a significant complication of the original problem. In approximately two thirds of patients with recurrent complaints, no correctable underlying mechanical cause could be found.[3]

CLINICAL PROBLEM

The first group of patients are those who awaken from surgery with the same or worse pain than they had before. This is an unusual situation, but one that requires relatively urgent evaluation. The speed with which the evaluation proceeds depends on the severity of the complaints and whether there are new neurologic deficits. If there are any new significant deficits, or if the pain is extremely severe, then immediate (not emergent) reimaging is indicated. Magnetic resonance imaging (MRI), even in the early phase, may exaggerate postoperative findings because of changes secondary to edema and inflammation. Nevertheless, MRI is the simplest first step, but computed

tomography (CT) and CT myelography are reasonable alternatives. CT provides a great deal of information concerning bony structures and the presence or absence of blood, but is less useful for recurrent disc herniation. MRI, if available, can be the next choice, but many postoperative patients find MRI difficult to tolerate. CT myelography is often simpler to do and is usually well tolerated by patients, although additional analgesia is often required for postoperative patients to undergo the manipulations required.[4] Considerations include exploration at the wrong space, retained disc fragment, or nerve root injury. It is incumbent on the surgeon to be certain that the goals of surgery have been met appropriately. Only when this is proven can the patient be managed symptomatically.[5] Remember that in some patients, particularly those with existing preoperative deficits, these abnormalities may be exaggerated by the anesthesia. A period of observation before reimaging is warranted if patients are not fully awake and the effect of anesthesia cannot be easily assessed.

The second group of patients is those in whom the initial result appears to be satisfactory but pain recurs after a few days to a few weeks. If the problem is associated with excruciating pain or a profound neurologic deficit, then reevaluation is urgent. If the pain recurrence is less extreme, then waiting expectantly is probably the best course, while the patient is afforded pain relief by analgesia and local therapy measures. However, assuming that the patient's recurrent complaints are severe, evaluation is required.[6] Plain films with flexion and extension demonstrate instability and may show evidence of infection, even at this early phase. White blood cell count with differential and the erythrocyte sedimentation rate provide the best clues to an early infection. MRI is somewhat unreliable during the first 3 months and exaggerates postoperative abnormalities because of inflammation and edema. In my experience, this imaging problem persists for at least 3 months after surgery. Nevertheless, an MRI is the first choice for evaluating the problem. CT may be useful but is much less specific for soft tissue; CT myelography may be required if the problem cannot be resolved adequately by MRI. MRI is more likely to overemphasize an abnormality than to miss something important. The major diagnostic possibilities are infection, retained disc fragment, recurrent disc fragment, residual foraminal compression, usually secondary to progressive disc space collapse, or a missed lateral disc protrusion.[3,7] Postoperative scarring with tethering of the nerve root may be an important issue but should not be used as an excuse, and it is necessary for the surgeon to review all these other possibilities before ascribing the recurrence of pain to epidural scar.[8]

The third category of patients is those who present with recurrent symptoms long after apparently successful disc surgery. Here the diagnostic possibilities are considerably fewer. The most likely is recurrent disc at the same or another space; the development of foraminal stenosis because of progressive disc collapse is the next most likely cause. Progressive spondylolisthesis at the level of prior surgery is a third possibility to explain late recurrence of symptoms. Epidural scarring is often invoked as a cause of these symptoms while epidural scar is undoubtedly ubiquitous. The relationship of scarring to radicular pain is associative at best. The purpose of the imaging studies is to determine if nerve root compression at the same or a different level is present or if there is any evidence of instability. Pars fracture is a relatively common event following disc surgery and may explain the problem. For all of these possibilities, reevaluation is required. The evaluation should include plain films with flexion and extension, MRI, and possibly CT if the lesion is thought to be bony.[3]

Spinal fluid leak with or without an external fistula is another significant problem, but fortunately is rare. It is estimated that durotomy occurs in up to 5% of primary surgeries, including all types of operations. The reincidence is certainly lower following simple discectomy. Our own data indicate that simple uncomplicated durotomy has no influence on eventual outcome of surgery. However, two important situations occur. Leak of cerebrospinal fluid through an incision or from a drain site is important because of the risk for infection. The first step is usually to oversew the wound with a continuous suture of a material that can be left in place. Hermetic closure is usually adequate to solve the problem. If the leak recurs, the surgeon has two options. One is to place an intrathecal lumbar drain well away from the surgical site for a few days of drainage while the wound seals. The other is to open the wound and seal the leak.

The second related problem occurs when fluid simply accumulates in the operative site and compresses the spinal sac and its contents. Symptoms vary from cauda equina syndrome with complete laminectomy to individual root compression. Sometimes only severe back pain is present. There are two options for management. One is image-guided aspiration of the collection followed by separate placement of a lumbar drain if needed. The injection can be supplemented by an epidural blood patch if the surgical exposure allows. The second option is reoperation with closure of the fistula and obliteration of the cyst.

Review of my own data indicates that durotomy occurs in 5% to 7% of patients and is most common in the course of reoperation. As a complication of the primary disc surgery or first laminectomy, durotomy occurs in less than 1% of operations. Closure is by primary suture repair whenever possible. Reinforcement of the repair with an artificial substance such as DuraGen (Synovis Surgical Innovations, St. Paul, MN) or one of the commercially available tissue adhesives such as Tisseel (Baxter Healthcare Corporation, Glendale, CA) is commonplace, but there are no data to indicate that these additives are valuable. When primary closure is not possible due to the location or nature of the

durotomy, then filling the defect with fat and muscle supplemented by a dural substitute or tissue adhesive is typical. Sometimes with very friable dura, including a small patch of fat over the suture line beneath the knots of the dural closure will improve the seal. In my experience, a cerebrospinal fluid fistula through a wound in primary lumbar surgery is an extreme rarity and occurs in less than 1% of reoperations. Return to the operating room for dural closure or obliteration of a fistula occurs on the Johns Hopkins Spine Service once or twice yearly, which means it is required in perhaps 1 in 1,000 operations.

DIAGNOSTIC POSSIBILITIES

Surgical management depends on the problem diagnosed, but the typical procedure relates to recurrent disc fragment, retained disc fragment, foraminal compression, or compression by a focal scar. The treatment of the latter lesion is still controversial; however, it is my belief that a scar that is a focal mass is no different than a recurrent disc herniation. In my experience, excision of the compressive mass, whether it is disc, bony spur, ligament overgrowth, synovium, or scar, is successful for relief of pain.[3]

When the patient has been operated on by another surgeon, it is always well to evaluate the preoperative studies, if possible, to be certain that the abnormality operated on was present and that the surgery chosen was the appropriate operation. All patients still require reevaluation, but when indications for operation initially were lacking, it should not be surprising that the surgery was unsuccessful in the relief of symptoms. Only if an obvious abnormality is found subsequently should reoperation be undertaken.[5] Decompressive surgery corrects only nerve root compression syndrome.[9] Fusion is currently utilized only for demonstrated instability. Unfortunately the definition of stability is much debated, so indications for fusion remain soft. However, recurrent pain alone is inadequate to justify fusion as a part of reoperation.

The use of diagnostic blocks to supplement clinical impressions is increasingly common. It is my view that diagnostic blockades of spinal structures can be used to strengthen clinical judgment but in themselves do not constitute indications for surgery. The relationship of diagnostic blocks with successful outcome of reparative surgeries has not yet been verified in any significant series. Blocks in common use include those that anesthetize the zygapophyseal joints, nerve roots, and intervertebral discs.[10,11] Successful relief of pain by a diagnostic block suggests but does not prove that the structure blocked is a pain generator or at least in the same segment as the pain generator. Successful relief of back pain by zygapophyseal joint blockade may lead to percutaneous neurotomy of the innervation of the blocked joints and strengthen the case for posterior fusion. Relief of pain by individual root block strengthens the supposition that decompression of the root may be useful if anatomic proof of compression is present. Blockade of discs is most controversial.[10] Current data certainly suggest that so-called provocative discography can identify painful discs. What is missing is data that allow verification of outcome of surgery based at least partially on the results of discography. Positive discography has been used to justify both interbody and posterior fusion. This makes intuitive sense but is not yet verified by studies of selectivity and specificity. The hypothesis with all these blocks is that carrying out the block itself will aggravate the patient's typical pain as step 1 and the injection of a local anesthetic into the area will relieve the patient's pain as step 2. When this occurs, the block is called concordant. Blocks may add clinical information in questionable situations but by themselves do not constitute an indication for surgery in my opinion.

A major difficulty in assessing what to do about persistent symptoms is that it is so hard to differentiate the injured nerve root from the compressed nerve root.[11] The history is probably the most useful tool. Patients with nerve root injury typically have burning pain along the distribution of the injured root. It is persistent and not alleviated by rest; in fact, it is improved by virtually nothing, although emotional stress and movement may worsen the pain. There may or may not be an associated neurologic deficit, but the presence of a deficit does not help in diagnosis. Electromyography is not useful because it usually cannot differentiate between the compressed and injured root. It is necessary to obtain imaging studies that exclude the possibility of root compression before suggesting that nerve root injury is the likely probability. Another differentiating point is that nerve root injury pain rarely is relieved by narcotic administration; it requires medical therapy with a group of novel drugs used for neuropathic pain. This treatment regimen is beyond the scope of the current chapter, but is mentioned because the differentiation of nerve root injury pain from compression pain by response to medication is often an important diagnostic point with these patients. MRI and CT are both satisfactory to diagnose cerebrospinal fluid collection when no external leak has occurred. Treatment can be expectant because most will reabsorb spontaneously; when they do not, surgical percutaneous or surgical obliteration may be required.

Once a cause of nerve root compression is identified and physical rehabilitation measures, analgesia, and adequate recovery time have been ineffective for the relief of pain, surgical decompression is indicated. When the pain is extremely severe, or the apparent root compression is associated with a significant neurologic deficit, more urgent surgery is required and the conservative measures are not indicated.[4]

The key to successful surgery is to define the abnormalities exactly so that all appropriate corrections are carried out. If there is significant canal stenosis, the procedure should be planned to correct the stenosis. If there is a recurrent disc mass, scar, or bone spur, then the surgeon has to decompress the root and remove the mass if possible. If the foramen is involved, then foraminotomy is required. When instability is present, fusion should be planned as a part of the operation, but this also is beyond the scope of my discussion.[6,12] However, it is important to recognize that the time-honored practice of recommending fusion because a patient is to have a second operation is unwarranted. Fusions are carried out for demonstrated instability, progressive glacial change, and rarely for prophylactic reasons with specific disease states. Adding a fusion just because a patient is thought to need additional surgery for some reason is inappropriate.[13]

The best candidates for reoperation should have symptoms that are refractory to time and standard conservative measures employed for long enough to be certain they will not be

effective, usually a few weeks to a few months. Moving directly to surgery is indicated when neurologic deficits and/or pain are severe. Imaging studies should demonstrate clear-cut compression from something. Occasionally it may be useful to identify specifically involved nerve roots by diagnostic blockade. Surgery should be planned to correct whatever anatomic abnormality is imaged. Stereotypical operations with or without fusion are unlikely to be successful.[3]

SURGICAL MANAGEMENT

Perioperative Care and Anesthesia

These operations are carried out under general anesthesia. I prefer to perform them with the patient in the prone position, but the lateral position is satisfactory when unilateral decompression is required. I think these operations are too complex to be done under local anesthesia, and I do not use a spinal anesthetic because I think it is, in general, more uncomfortable for the patient. The patient is intubated and turned into the prone position on any frame or support the surgeon prefers. I use prophylactic antibiotics for 24 hours, beginning at the approximate time of surgery, although the evidence that this is an extremely important measure is sparse. Infection is so uncommon in these patients that the use of antibiotics is not a major issue and should be left to the surgeon's choice.[6] Although I do not use monitoring for simple lumbar disc surgery, I usually use electromyographic monitoring when reoperation is required. I find it helpful to know when the nerve root is being manipulated enough to cause electromyographic firing. Preemptive local anesthesia in the skin may in theory reduce postoperative pain, and infiltration of the muscle certainly does. After infiltration, the skin incision is made. The skin incision required for reoperation is somewhat larger than that needed for first-time disc surgery. I like to expose at least the spinous process above and below if unilateral exploration is to be undertaken. If laminectomy is contemplated, then obviously both sides are exposed, again one level above and one level below. Muscles are taken down from spines and laminae with electrocautery, knife, or sharp osteotomes, as the surgeon prefers. The lamina above the area to be explored and the lamina below should be well seen. The dissection is carried far enough laterally to expose the zygapophyseal joints, but it is not necessary to go to the level of the transverse processes. Reoperation can take two forms. The most common is simple re-exploration of an individual nerve root where surgery has previously been carried out (Fig. 154-1). However, if there is significant spinal stenosis, a complete laminectomy is required. The laminectomy has no considerations different from those of laminectomy for any purpose, and is not described in detail here. The techniques for dissecting the previously operated site are the same whether partial hemilaminectomy, hemilaminectomy, or laminectomy is used.

With the previous operative area exposed, the next step is to identify the current operative site with certainty by radiography. If anatomic landmarks are sufficient, radiography is not required, but often they have been distorted by surgery and it is important to be certain that the exploration is at the appropriate level. I personally like a film taken after the procedure is complete which verifies the location of surgery. I do not consider this mandatory, but such

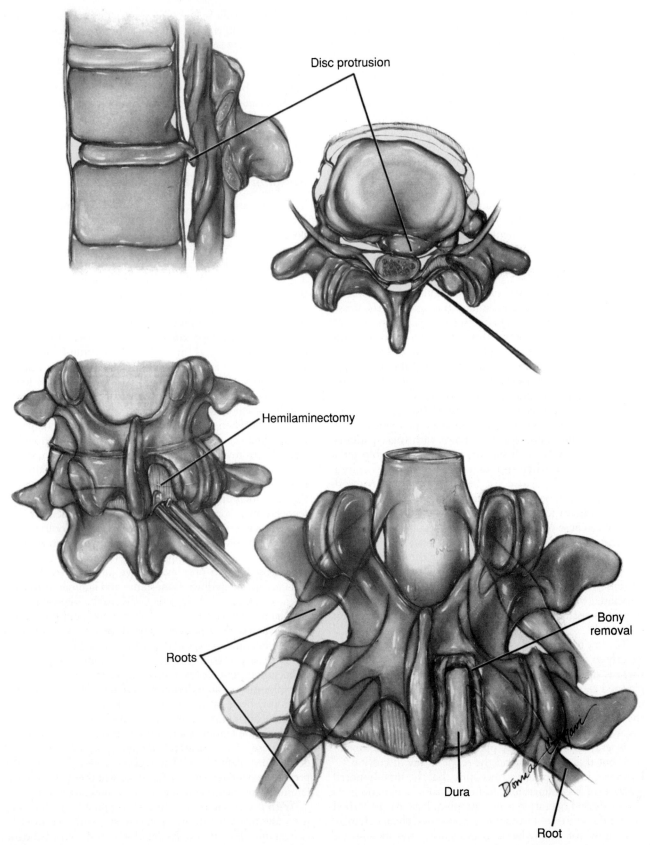

FIGURE 154-1   A simple disc protrusion is demonstrated to illustrate principles of open disc surgery. *Upper panel,* Disc herniation. *Lower panel,* Hemilaminectomy and exposure of dura and nerve root. (From Long DM, McAfee PC: Atlas of Spinal Surgery. Philadelphia: Lippincott Williams & Wilkins, 1992.)

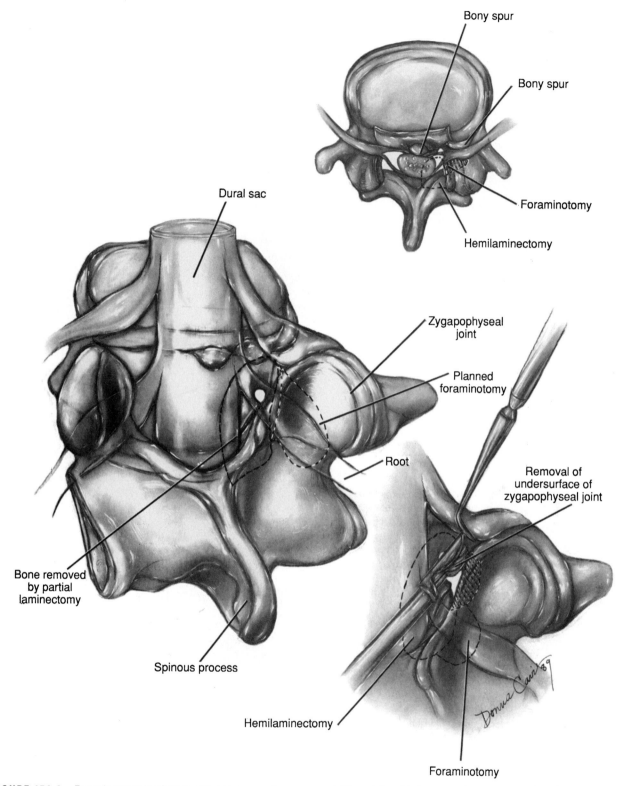

FIGURE 154-2   Foraminotomy is often required to expose the nerve root. The relationship between the nerve root, dorsal root ganglion to laminar pedicle, and zygapophyseal joints is depicted here. (From Long DM, McAfee PC: Atlas of Spinal Surgery. Philadelphia: Lippincott Williams & Wilkins, 1992.)

verification eliminates one of the risks of lumbar surgery. The scar is then freed from the lamina above and the lamina below. An extension of the previous bony removal is carried both up and down until normal ligament or dura is exposed. If the ligament is intact, it can be opened and the epidural space found well away from the operative site. If the ligament is not intact, laminectomy often demonstrates the dura. When unilateral exploration is required, partial or complete laminectomy is done (Figs. 154-2 and 154-3). The spinous process and opposite side are

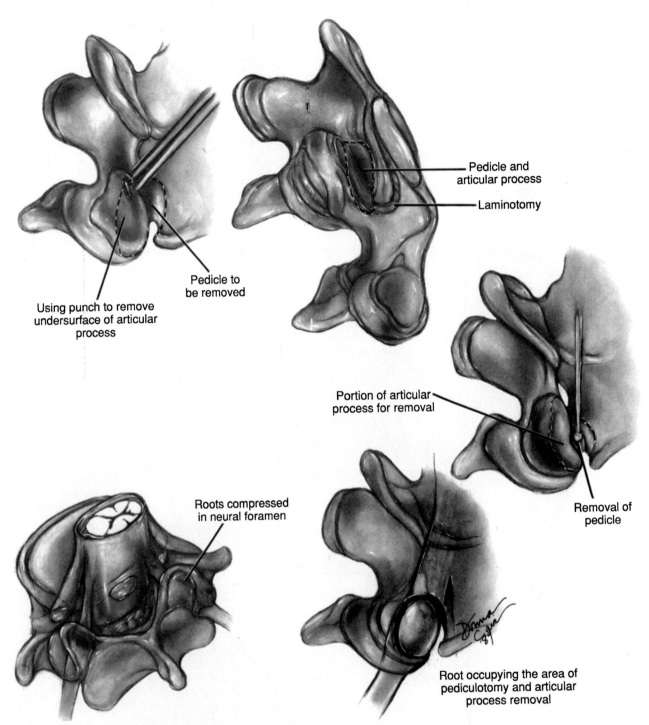

FIGURE 154-3   Details of foraminotomy, which are often very important in reoperation on the lumbar disc. The area of pedicle and articular process to be removed and the extent of the laminotomy are illustrated. The bone may be removed by using a high-speed drill or punch rongeurs. (From Long DM, McAfee PC: Atlas of Spinal Surgery. Philadelphia: Lippincott Williams & Wilkins, 1992.)

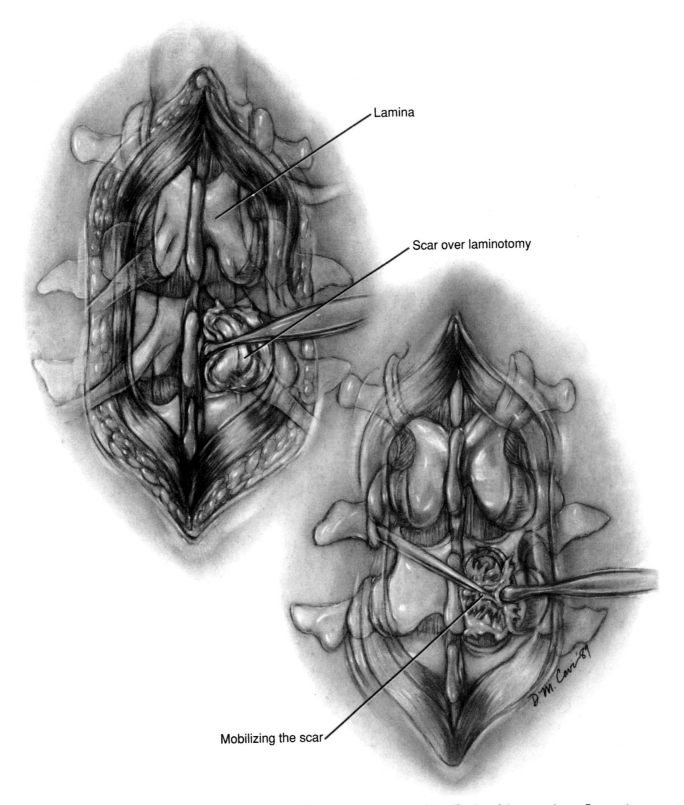

Lamina

Scar over laminotomy

Mobilizing the scar

FIGURE 154-4   Reoperation on the lumbar spine begins with generous exposure and identification of the scarred area. Reoperation may be done by unilateral or bilateral laminectomy. The procedure is easier with bilateral laminectomy because the normal dura is seen. (From Long DM, McAfee PC: Atlas of Spinal Surgery. Philadelphia: Lippincott Williams & Wilkins, 1992.)

left intact. If the patient has an associated spinal stenosis, I believe that complete laminectomy should be done. This makes the additional dissection quite easy because normal dura is exposed above, below, and medial to the original scar. Once the dura is seen above or below the operative site, the dissection begins to remove the previous scar from the dura. I prefer to remove all scar from the dura and do so first with sharp dissectors. Some scars are extremely adherent, and even sharp dissectors, such as the Adson curved periosteal elevator or the Rosen knife, do not lift the scar off the dura easily. In this case, the plane is identified and careful dissection with a small knife blade such as a no. 15 is used to separate scar from dura (Fig. 154-4). If the dura is entered and a cerebrospinal fluid leak occurs, the leak should be repaired immediately so that the spinal sac is not decompressed. The scar is removed completely to the margins of the original exposure. I then free the adhesions from dura and lateral nerve root sheath from bone. The next step is foraminotomy, which is usually done with small punches or a fine chisel or osteotome. The inferior surface of the articular process is undercut so the joint is not entered; care should be taken not to go across the pars interarticularis in the course of the foraminotomy. Sometimes it is impossible not to cross the pars if a complete foraminotomy is to be carried out, in which case the surgeon must decide whether stabilization will be required.

Once the posterior and lateral surfaces of dura and nerve root are exposed, the dura above the lateral margin of the nerve root and the dura below must all be dissected free from the lateral recess, and the nerve root gradually retracted medially or laterally depending on where the offending mass is compressing (Fig. 154-5). The recurrent

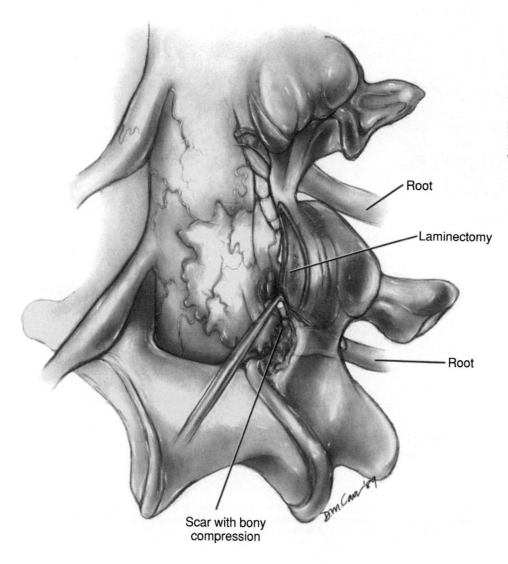

Root

Laminectomy

Root

Scar with bony compression

FIGURE 154-5 Complete laminectomy has been performed, exposing the area of the compressed nerve root, and the dissection of the scar has begun. Care must be taken not to go through the pars or thin it so much that a fracture might occur postoperatively. (From Long DM, McAfee PC: Atlas of Spinal Surgery. Philadelphia: Lippincott Williams & Wilkins, 1992.)

disc or mass can be approached through the axilla of the nerve root or the nerve root may be retracted medially off the mass. Once the nerve root is retracted and the offending mass can be visualized, removal technique depends on the nature of the mass. If it is a recurrent disc, it can usually be handled like any other disc. The fragment is either removed or the mass incised and the fragment removed from beneath ligament and scar (Fig. 154-6). If the problem is simply ligamentous and bony, piecemeal removal is done with small rongeurs or curets. When the problem is a scar, piecemeal removal is also required, but the scar is frequently too firm for the small rongeurs that can be used in this space, and simply excising it with a knife is worthwhile.

It is important to free the entire root, which should be explored circumferentially to ensure that all offending mass has been removed. If the interspace can be entered,

it is wise to remove any additional degenerative disc material that can be obtained without undue tension on the root.

Once I am certain that the root is decompressed and there is no potential compression in the bony foramen if additional disc collapse occurs, a thin, 2- to 3-mm fat graft is harvested from a fresh area of fat, not from the scarred material in the reopened incision (Fig. 154-7). Usually the scarring is thinned to no more than 1 cm, so that it is easy to obtain fat from the immediate vicinity of the wound. I carefully fashion a graft that covers all exposed dura and place it in the epidural space posterior and lateral, but not anterior, to the root and dura. The wound can then be closed in anatomic layers, reapproximating muscle loosely. The strength layer is the lumbar fascia, and this has to be carefully closed. There are no other special considerations in closure.

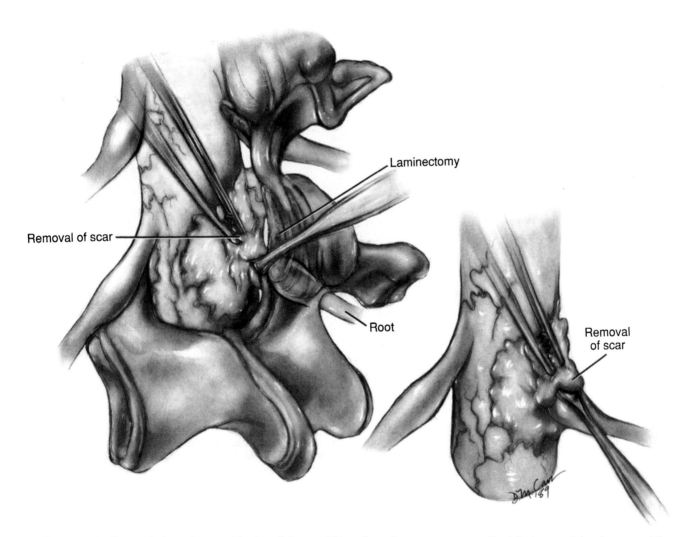

FIGURE 154-6 Removal of scar by a combination of sharp and blunt dissection, as necessary, until relatively normal dura is seen and the nerve root is exposed. (From Long DM, McAfee PC: Atlas of Spinal Surgery. Philadelphia: Lippincott Williams & Wilkins, 1992.)

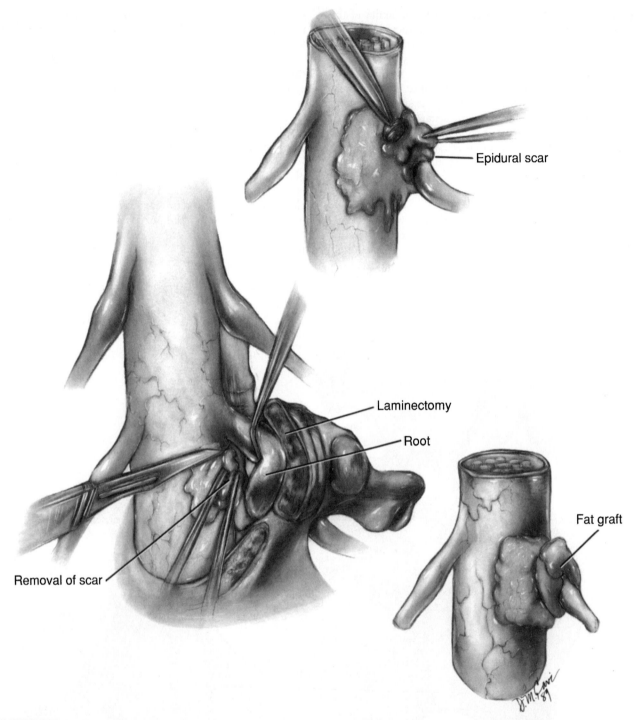

Epidural scar

Laminectomy

Root

Fat graft

Removal of scar

FIGURE 154-7   Further removal of scar, until the nerve root has been well demonstrated. A fat graft may be placed posteriorly or circumferentially, depending on the circumstances after scar removal. (From Long DM, McAfee PC: Atlas of Spinal Surgery. Philadelphia: Lippincott Williams & Wilkins, 1992.)

REFERENCES

1. Long DM: Decision making in lumbar disc disease [Review]. Clin Neurosurg 39:36–51, 1992.
2. Connolly ES, Long DM: Spinal Reoperations. Spine Surgery: Techniques, Complication Avoidance, and Management, Vol 2. New York: Churchill Livingstone, 1999, pp 843–847.
3. Long DM: Reoperation for the failed back syndrome. Summary of a thirty year experience. In Brock M, Schwarz W, Wille-Monduzzi C (eds): First Interdisciplinary World Congress on Spinal Surgery and Related Disciplines. Bologna, Italy: Monduzzi Editore, 2000, pp 9–15.
4. Zeidman SM, Long DM: Failed back surgery syndrome. In Menezes AH, Sonntag VKH (eds): Principles of Spinal Surgery, Vol 1. New York: McGraw-Hill, 1996, pp 657–679.
5. North RB, Campbell JN, James CS, et al: Failed back surgery syndrome: 5-year follow-up in 102 patients undergoing repeated operation. Neurosurgery 28:685–690, 1991.
6. Long D, Watts C: Lessons from recent national back pain projects. In Salcman M (ed): Current Techniques in Neurosurgery, 2nd ed. Philadelphia: Current Medicine, 1996, pp 171–182.
7. Waddell G: Failures of disc surgery and repeat surgery. Acta Orthop Belg 53:300–302, 1987.

8. Bundschuh CV, Modic MT, Ross JS, et al: Epidural fibrosis and recurrent disk herniation in the lumbar spine: MR imaging assessment. AJR Am J Roentgenol 150:923–932, 1988 .
9. Long DM: A review of psychological considerations in the neurosurgical management of chronic pain: A neurosurgeon's perspective. Neurosurg Q 1:185–195, 1991.
10. Bogduk N: Diskography. Am Pain Soc J 3:149–154, 1994.
11. Bogduk N, Aprill C, Derby R: Selective nerve root blocks. In Wilson DJ (ed): Interventional Radiology of the Musculoskeletal System. London: Edward Arnold, 1995, pp 121–132.
12. Long DM, Zeidman SM: Outcome of low back pain therapy. Perspect Neurol Surg 5:41–51, 1994.
13. Deyo RA, Nachemson A, Mirza SK: Spinal-fusion surgery—The case for restraint. N Engl J Med 350(7):722–726, 2004.

155 Spinal Cord Stimulation for Chronic Pain*

RICHARD B. NORTH and BENGT LINDEROTH

A theory of pain transmission published in 1965 inspired researchers to develop a reversible, nondestructive pain therapy that relied on equipment adapted from cardiac pacemakers to deliver electrical stimulation to the spinal cord. The initial results of this therapy, now known as spinal cord stimulation (SCS), were inconsistent, but some patients benefited dramatically. During the past half century, refinements in SCS techniques, equipment, and patient selection criteria (Table 155-1) have led to significantly improved and continually improving clinical results.

BACKGROUND

Melzack and Wall's "gate control theory," which offers a hypothesis to explain the segmental suppression of nociceptive transmission in the spinal cord, provided a theoretical rationale for the use of electrical stimulation in the management of pain.[130] The theory proposes that a "gate" controls the central transmission of pain signals from the dorsal horn of the spinal cord to the brain, with an excess of small fiber afferent input opening the gate and an excess of large fiber afferent input closing it.

TABLE 155-1 ■ Chronic Pain Patient Selection Criteria

1. An objective basis for the patient's pain (with a specific diagnosis). The results of physical examinations and diagnostic imaging studies in patients with failed back surgery syndrome, for example, should be consistent with the reported distribution of the irradiating pain; furthermore, these findings should predominate over functional, nonphysiologic signs.[199]
2. In most patients, spinal cord stimulation (SCS) is more effective in treating the radicular component of neuropathic pain than in alleviating nociceptive components of axial or midline pain.
3. SCS should be a late resort. Reasonable alternative treatments should be exhausted or be comparatively unacceptable (see section on Failed Back Surgery Syndrome under Clinical Results).
4. A multidisciplinary evaluation, with specific attention to psychological issues, must rule out any unresolved major psychiatric problems or personality disorders, significant issues of secondary gains, or major drug habituation problems. Some investigators find formal psychological testing of value in screening patients for SCS.[37,103]
5. The technical feasibility of overlapping pain with paresthesia should be demonstrated through a temporary trial.
6. No on-demand pacemaker or need for a magnetic resonance imaging test.
7. No coagulopathy or sepsis.
8. The patient must be able to control the device.

---

*See also Chapter 110, "Spinal Cord Stimulation and Intraspinal Infusions for Pain."

Because large fibers are more susceptible than small fibers to electrical depolarization, investigators believed they could close the gate (stop pain transmission) if they used low-amplitude stimulation to selectively recruit large fiber activity from a mixed population of nerve fibers. Electrical stimulation of a mixed peripheral nerve can achieve this effect,[179] but stimulation of peripheral nerves at amplitudes close to those required for a therapeutic effect can cause unwanted motor effects. Also, most pain problems involve multiple peripheral nerves. Thus, investigators decided to apply electrical stimulation to the spinal cord where they could "recruit" the primary, large fiber afferents from multiple segments that are conveniently isolated in the posterior columns. As expected, antidromic activation of these primary afferents, whose collateral processes extend into the dorsal horn, allowed clinicians to obtain a wide area of pain relief.

MECHANISM OF ACTION

Figure 155-1 provides a schematic illustration of the mechanisms outlined in the text.

Spinal Cord Stimulation Mechanisms in Neuropathic Pain

Although the electrical stimulation techniques that grew out of the gate control theory have succeeded, the theory remains controversial because, in some pathologic circumstances, large fibers themselves signal hyperalgesia.[26] In such cases, peripheral nerve stimulation or SCS might relieve pain by blocking the conduction of primary afferents into the branch points of dorsal column fibers and collaterals.[25] The mechanism of action of SCS, however, cannot depend solely on blocking conduction (e.g., by impulse collision), because electrical stimulation does not inhibit all types of pain,[118] and therapeutic SCS normally does not evoke pain, which would occur if SCS activated thin high-threshold fibers in the spinothalamic tracts. Furthermore, dorsal column activation has always been more successful than ventral stimulation (i.e., close to the spinothalamic tracts).[116]

In neuropathic pain states, neuronal elements in the involved dorsal horns, especially wide dynamic range neurons in the superficial laminae, become hypersensitive/hyperactive, and SCS suppresses several aspects of this hyperactivity. Furthermore, in rat models of neuropathy using parameters of current similar to those used in humans, SCS effectively relieved allodynia, a common symptom in neuropathic pain syndromes.[203]

In a study that sought to determine if SCS suppresses long-term potentiation of wide dynamic range dorsal horn

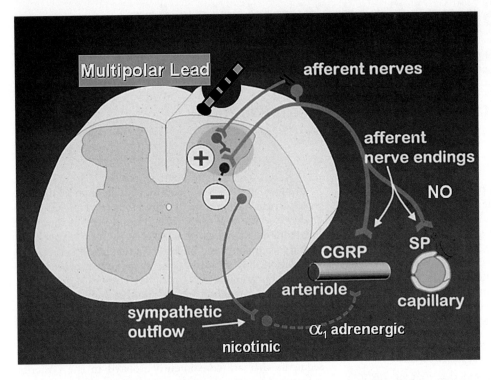

FIGURE 155-1 The extradurally placed, multipolar lead excites fibers in the dorsal columns, resulting in orthodromic activity, giving rise to the paresthesia experienced by the patients, and in antidromic activation channeled into the underlying dorsal horns via the large diameter collaterals. In the dorsal horns, this evokes a complex pattern of transmitter changes, which results in an increase of inhibitory activity and a decrease of pathologic hyperexcitability. (Redrawn after Cui JG, Meyerson B, Linderoth B: Opposite effects of spinal cord stimulation in different phases of carrageenan-induced hyperalgesia. Eur J Pain 3:365–374, 1999.)

neurons, SCS gradually reduced the C-fiber response to the baseline level. A-fibers, on the other hand, were not potentiated by the conditioning stimulus or affected by SCS.[201] This indication that SCS affects C-fibers is noteworthy because previous studies supported the view that SCS primarily influences A-fibers.

Investigators have used finite element computer techniques to model the electrical fields SCS produces in the spinal cord.[30,74,75] These models reveal distributions of current and voltage that agree with measurements from cadaver and primate spinal cords.[170] The models and measurements predict that (1) an electrode's longitudinal position is the most important factor in achieving the desired segmental effect (fibers decrease in diameter as they ascend the fasciculus gracilis)[155]; (2) bipolar stimulation with contacts 6 to 8 mm apart will provide the greatest selectivity for midline, longitudinally oriented fibers; and (3) the electrical field between two cathodes, one on either side of the midline, does not sum constructively in the midline. Clinical experience confirms that the correct position and spacing of SCS electrodes is essential and that, instead of expanding the area of paresthesia, positioning electrodes more cephalad commonly elicits unwanted, excessive local segmental effects.[107]

Psychophysical studies have found that stimulation induces a subtle loss of normal sensation in SCS patients but does not affect acute pain sensibility to an extent that could lead to undesirable side effects, such as Charcot joints.[115,127] Side effects increase with increases in stimulation amplitude and in nerve fiber recruitment; thus, psychophysical studies should include quantitative measures of stimulation adjusted for the range of amplitudes from perception to motor threshold.[109]

In order to explain the sustained pain relief (often lasting from 1 to 3 hours) that patients experience following a 30-minute period of SCS, investigators have hypothesized that SCS affects the release of neurotransmitters in the dorsal horn and brain.[119] Several lines of investigation have shed light on the neurochemical mechanisms that possibly underlie the beneficial effects of SCS: (1) analysis of cerebrospinal fluid revealed that SCS changes the concentration of neurotransmitters and their metabolites[116,134]; (2) administration of opioid antagonists, such as naloxone, does not affect the relief of pain achieved by SCS[60,133]; and (3) administration of γ-aminobutyric acid (GABA) agonists to neuropathic animals suppresses the hyperactivity associated with neuropathic pain, as does SCS.[34,36]

Additional investigations found that SCS induces GABA release in the dorsal horn[184] and that the pain-relieving effect of SCS depends on activation of the GABA-B receptor.[34,36] In fact, SCS inhibits for a period of time the pathologic response properties of dorsal horn neurons often observed in allodynic rats after peripheral nerve injury (elevated firing frequency of wide dynamic range neurons, presence of after-discharge, etc.),[203] conceivably because of an electrically induced increase in GABAergic activity.[135]

In fact, SCS likely prompts the release of a multitude of as-yet-unidentified transmitters and neuromodulators in the dorsal horn as well as supraspinally.[116,120,121,184] In addition to GABA, animal and human studies indicate that SCS releases substance P, serotonin, glycine, adenosine, and noradrenaline in the dorsal horn.[36,119,134] The resultant beneficial effect might depend on a complicated interaction among several of these known substances and several that remain unrecognized.[35]

This emerging knowledge may be used to tailor adjunct pharmacologic therapy to SCS in SCS-nonresponsive patients.[173,200] In fact, the first published report of a clinical trial of adjunct pharmacologic therapy in patients with neuropathic pain who had not responded well to SCS noted that an intrathecal infusion of the GABA-B agonist baclofen via an implanted pump in addition to SCS was beneficial in a subgroup of the 48 patients included in the trial.[114]

Spinal Cord Stimulation Mechanisms in Ischemic Pain

Peripheral Vascular Disease and Peripheral Arterial Occlusive Disease

Ischemic pain is the only type of nociceptive pain that responds to SCS, and the mechanisms involved in the stimulation-induced alleviation of ischemic pain differ fundamentally from those involved in the relief of neuropathic pain.[116,117,135]

SCS appears to exert its beneficial effect in the treatment of ischemic extremity pain primarily by reducing tissue ischemia (through increased or redistributed perfusion to the ischemic area) or by decreasing tissue oxygen demand. In peripheral arterial occlusive disease, experimental studies favor the notion that SCS suppresses efferent sympathetic activity (particularly the activity maintained via nicotinic ganglionic receptors and mainly α_1-adrenoreceptors in the periphery), which results in diminished peripheral vasoconstriction and secondary relief of pain.[117] Furthermore, experimental studies indicate that antidromic mechanisms might also be activated by SCS at intensities far below the motor threshold[32,33,186–188] and that this might result in peripheral calcitonin gene-related peptide (CGRP) release with subsequent peripheral vasodilatation. The balance between the two mechanisms seems to depend on the activity level of the sympathetic system and SCS intensity and probably also on individual factors (genetic differences, diet, etc.).

Investigations of the putative mechanisms underlying the powerful effects of SCS in vasospastic disorders show that pre-emptive SCS might block or reduce vasospasm in ischemic skin flaps in experimental animals[63] and in patients with Raynaud's syndrome.[118] This is consistent with theories that Raynaud's syndrome is caused by a heightened sensitivity or increased density of α-adrenergic receptors[59] in possible combination with dysfunction in the CGRP system.[21] Consequently, a stimulation-induced "normalization" of function in each system could underlie the efficacy of SCS in treating this condition. Figure 155-2 provides a schematic illustration of the possible mechanisms of action of SCS in peripheral ischemia.

Putative Spinal Cord Stimulation Mechanisms in Complex Regional Pain Syndrome

SCS therapy is often effective in complex regional pain syndrome (CRPS) with signs of dysautonomia. In principle, SCS could affect pain syndromes related to sympathetic hyperactivity in at least three ways. The first is by direct action on central hyperexcitability, as discussed above. Second, the direct-coupling hypothesis[15] implies that de novo abnormal contacts develop between peripheral sympathetic and damaged somatosensory fibers. This implies that central inhibition of sympathetic efferent activity, as indicated above, could exert a beneficial net effect on the pain condition. Third, the indirect-coupling concept proposes that damaged sensory neurons might become so hypersensitive to mild degrees of hypoxia that even moderate increases in sympathetic activity with peripheral vasoconstriction could excite the damaged afferent fibers.[15,67] Both types of coupling seem plausible, but the indirect-coupling hypothesis did not get support in a study where SCS therapy in cases of

reflex sympathetic dystrophy (CRPS type I) did not result in peripheral vasodilatation.[87]

In conclusion, the mechanisms underlying the effects of SCS on pain due to ischemia in the extremities, whether from occlusive vascular disease or vasospasm, are different from those active in neurogenic pain. For such ischemic pain, a rebalancing of oxygen supply and demand (i.e., the relief of net ischemia) seems to be the underlying action. SCS-induced vasodilation in a situation with low sympathetic vasoconstrictor tone might also occur as a result of antidromic activation, whereas with a high level of sympathetic activity, stimulation-induced sympathetic inhibition could also contribute to the effect.

Mechanism in Angina Pectoris

The mode of action of SCS in otherwise therapy-refractory angina pectoris appears to be even more complex, and investigators have derived conflicting data from a number of studies in humans and in experimental animals.

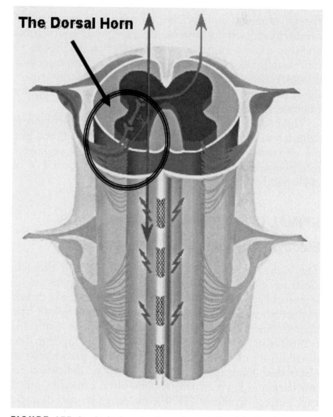

The Dorsal Horn

FIGURE 155-2 In ischemia, the relevant physiologic changes in the central nervous system and nerve roots seem to occur when stimulation of the posterior cord (via some as yet unidentified circuitry) inhibits efference from central sympathetic neurons. Of special relevance in this context is the sympathetic activity relayed via nicotinic receptors in the ganglia and mainly α_1 receptors at the neuroeffector junction. Another route for the influence of spinal cord stimulation on peripheral vessels is antidromic and is activated when excitation of primary afferents releases vasodilatory substances (e.g., calcitonin gene-related peptide) in the periphery. Both of the two mechanisms might be active, and the balance between them seems to depend on the general activity level of the sympathetic system (enhanced, for example, by a cold milieu). (Redrawn after Linderoth B, Foreman RD: Physiology of spinal cord stimulation. Review and update. Neuromodulation 2:150–164, 1999.)

Although the first studies in animals demonstrated direct inhibitory effects of experimental SCS on cardiac nociception,[28] the clinical studies that followed clearly demonstrated that a partial resolution of cardiac ischemia seems to be a pivotal factor in the antianginal SCS effect.[125] On the basis of their findings, some researchers favor a stimulation-induced flow increase or redistribution of blood supply from well-perfused to ischemic regions in the heart as the cardinal underlying factor,[69] while others interpret the reduction of coronary ischemia, manifested in decreased ST changes on the electrocardiogram as well as a reversal of lactate production to extraction, as mainly due to decreased cardiomyocyte oxygen demand.[51] Experimental studies have hitherto been unable to demonstrate a local flow increase in the myocardium[93]; instead, preemptive SCS seems to induce protective changes in the myocardium that increase its resistance to critical ischemia.[27]

Another observation of possible importance is that local coronary ischemia excites the intrinsic cardiac nervous system. This system consists of mixed somatosensory and autonomic ganglia housed in fat pads on the exterior surface of the heart and constitutes the "final common integrator system" of neural activity directed to or from the heart. If this increased activity persists, it might spread dysrhythmia and thus cause a more generalized ischemia. SCS seems to inhibit and stabilize the activity of these neurons, especially during an ischemic challenge, and might in this way protect the heart from more severe ischemic threats resulting, for example, from generalized arrhythmia.[27,55,56]

The last word for the use of SCS in cardiac ischemia is definitely not written yet, and the effects of stimulation might prove to extend far beyond relief of angina (e.g., to cardioprotection against elusive events preceding the appearance of chest pain).

SPINAL CORD STIMULATION DEVICES

Electrode Designs and Placement

The earliest applications of SCS involved high thoracic electrode placement in an attempt to treat pain in all segments caudal to the electrode.[178] This commonly caused excessive, uncomfortable, radicular effects before the desired caudal segments were recruited. When clinicians realized that stimulation paresthesia should overlap the distribution of pain, they adjusted the placement of electrodes accordingly. For the common indication of low back and lower extremity pain, often caused by failed back surgery syndrome (FBSS), for example, low thoracic electrode placement (T9 to T12) is most effective.[12]

In the late 1960s and early 1970s, SCS electrodes were two-dimensional and required a laminectomy or laminotomy for introduction into the epidural, endodural, or subarachnoid space.[23,139,185] Use of these electrodes was problematic because clinicians had no way of determining the ideal spinal level for electrode placement in any given patient and because laminotomy under local anesthesia limits longitudinal access. Furthermore, even when electrodes are placed so that paresthesia overlaps the area of pain, not all patients report pain relief. Thus test stimulation with a temporary electrode became desirable.

Accordingly, in the 1970s, investigators developed percutaneous techniques that involved a Tuohy needle to place temporary catheter-type electrodes,[24,52,76,79] which could be used during screening trials to establish (1) analgesic effect before permanent implantation of a device and (2) the best level for electrode placement. Clinicians soon applied these percutaneous techniques to the implantation of permanent electrodes, thus avoiding the need for laminectomy.[146,205] Use of a percutaneous technique to place multiple, individual electrodes and achieve bipolar stimulation, however, increased the likelihood of electrode migration, a problem that can eliminate bipolar stimulation, can reduce or eliminate pain relief, and often requires surgical revision.

In the early 1980s, to mitigate this complication, electrode manufacturers introduced electrodes with arrays of contacts that can be inserted percutaneously. If such an electrode migrates, its implanted pulse generator can be reprogrammed with a different selection of stimulating anodes and cathodes to recapture paresthesia. This noninvasive, postoperative adjustment can be made with the patient in the erect or supine position in which the device is ordinarily used (as opposed to the prone position in which it is usually implanted). Multicontact, programmable systems rarely require surgical revision and have significantly improved long-term clinical results.[110,145,154]

New electrode designs based on computer models of SCS[74] are being tested clinically.[73] These configurations should make it even easier to steer paresthesia to cover the painful area. Clinicians are also improving results by refining the method of anchoring percutaneously placed electrodes.[165]

Despite these improvements in the use of percutaneous electrodes, properly placed laminectomy electrodes continue to offer advantages. For example, a prospective, randomized, controlled technical comparison involving 24 patients—half of whom received a four-contact percutaneous electrode and half a four-contact insulated laminectomy electrode[153]— yielded significantly superior results with the laminectomy electrode for paresthesia coverage of pain and amplitude (sufficient to double battery life).

Figure 155-3 shows a sample of percutaneous and laminectomy electrodes. The percutaneous electrode is always inserted with local anesthesia, which does not interfere with the ability to monitor paresthesia during test stimulation. The laminectomy electrode can be implanted with local anesthesia or spinal anesthesia (with paresthesia at an only slightly higher than normal threshold to guide positioning).[113]

Implanted Pulse Generators

The prototype SCS device, used exclusively during the first decade of experience, was a passive implant powered by an external radiofrequency transmitter. In these systems, the implanted part of the system delivers the stimulation pulses.

Another type of implanted pulse generator, powered by an internal battery and capable of autonomous operation, was subsequently developed from pacemaker technology. The term *implanted pulse generator* (IPG) has been inaccurately assigned only to this type of system. A more accurate description, which properly distinguishes the two systems, would have IPG mean "internally powered generators." Patients turn these systems on and off and control the amplitude within

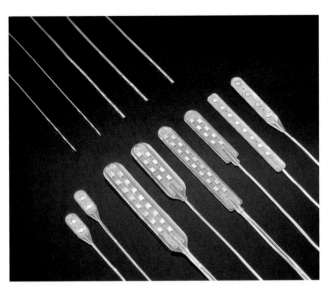

FIGURE 155-3 Contemporary spinal cord stimulation electrodes are arrays with multiple contacts. Some require laminectomy; others may be inserted percutaneously, through a modified Tuohy needle.

preset limits with an external magnet or a handheld "remote control." (Thus even this system is not "totally implanted.") Use of these hand-held devices reduces the necessity for postoperative outpatient consultations and thus saves time and money.

Pulse generators, like cardiac pacemakers, are powered by lithium cells. The power required for SCS, however, commonly exceeds that required for cardiac pacing by one or two orders of magnitude. In order to avoid frequent surgical replacement of the battery, therefore, the physician's decision to offer the patient an IPG must take into account the needed pulse amplitude, pulse width, pulse repetition rate (frequency), electrode impedance or load (determined by size and number of active contacts), and duty cycle (hours of use per day). Thus, for some patients, individual requirements might preclude use of these devices; other patients might be too concerned about battery depletion to use the device as often as necessary to meet its intended purpose. The alternative, external, radiofrequency-coupled power source contains no life-limiting components and thus avoids the expense and potential morbidity of eventual replacement. The obvious cosmetic advantages and convenience of a "totally implanted" power source should be considered in this context.

Figure 155-4 shows representative pulse generators.

SCREENING PROTOCOLS

Neuroaugmentative techniques, such as SCS, have inherent advantages over anatomic procedures (which are intended to correct the structural abnormality causing pain) and ablative procedures (which destroy portions of the nervous system in an attempt to block pain transmission). Not only are neuroaugmentative techniques reversible, they can be tested by a preoperative, therapeutic trial that reproduces the effect of chronic treatment.

Percutaneous placement of a temporary, epidural electrode for a therapeutic trial of SCS is a straightforward procedure and makes it possible to test electrode positions for optimal therapeutic effect and determine if the response warrants permanent implantation. Indeed, most third-party payers in the United States and in some European countries require that patients complete a successful trial before undergoing permanent implantation. Although a brief

FIGURE 155-4 Contemporary implanted pulse generators used for spinal cord stimulation support multiple contacts, which may be programmed noninvasively as anodes and cathodes. Some are powered by implanted batteries (visible here); some accept or require power from an externally worn device.

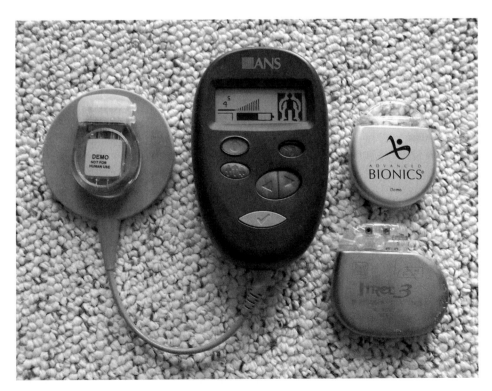

period of intraoperative stimulation immediately before permanent implantation technically meets this requirement, an extended trial provides the following advantages:

1. The physician can place a temporary electrode in a fluoroscopy suite instead of an operating room, which minimizes expense while allowing assessment of a number of anode and cathode positions and stimulation parameters.
2. The patient can provide a realistic assessment of stimulation effects while engaging in everyday activities.
3. Using the temporary electrode to measure current requirements helps the physician decide if a patient with a successful trial should receive a "totally implanted" or external power generator.

A temporary electrode can be secured with a simple skin suture where the lead emerges from the Tuohy needle tract or with a subcutaneous anchor through an incision around the needle. Although anchored electrodes can be converted to a permanent system, it is better not to anchor the electrode but to incur the expense of replacing the electrode for the following reasons:

1. Anchoring and removing an anchored electrode (if the trial fails) must take place in the operating room instead of the fluoroscopy suite. This increases the cost.
2. Anchoring temporary electrodes implies a commitment on the part of the patient and the physician to proceed to internalization, which partially defeats the purpose of the trial.
3. The physician cannot adjust the position of an anchored electrode at the bedside as the patient gains experience with the system. In contrast, if the physician places a temporary percutaneous array at the most cephalad position that shows promise during preliminary testing of the naive patient, the electrode can be incrementally withdrawn at the bedside (instead of in the operating room or fluoroscopy suite) for testing at more caudal positions. Plain radiographs can document successful repositioning.
4. Pain from the anchoring incision might confound the results of the therapeutic trial.
5. Anchoring increases the risk for infection.[95,106]

The criteria for proceeding from a temporary to a permanent device vary considerably. Some clinicians have extended the percutaneous test for as long as 2 months,[128] whereas others implant in a single procedure, relying solely on intraoperative stimulation trials.[54] A retrospective comparison of 15-minute intraoperative versus 5-day screening in 54 patients (33 percutaneous; 21 laminectomy), for example, found that the positive predictive value of each screening test was equivalent for predicting SCS outcome.[202] In this trial, however, the screening success rate was an extraordinarily high 47 of 52 at 5 days. If all clinicians obtained such a high success rate in trials for patients such as these (with chronic low back and/or lower extremity pain), it would not be necessary to conduct an SCS trial. (Indeed, some clinicians forgo trials for angina patients, considering the benefits of SCS to extend beyond pain control in those patients.) Also, the number of patients who failed the prolonged trial (five) was significantly greater than the number who failed the acute trial (one); thus, despite the equivalent predictive

value of each trial, the prolonged trial identified more patients who would fail long-term therapy. In fact, a lower trial success rate is likely to result in a higher long-term success rate.

Some have defined a successful trial as 70% to 75% reported pain relief[40,111,129]; others have required as little as 30%.[16] Some reports note that as few as 40% of patients undergoing temporary electrode placement proceeded to permanent implantation.[39] We conduct 3- to 5-day trials, extending them as necessary, and our patients proceed to permanent implantation after achieving at least 50% relief of pain for 45 to 60 minutes after stimulation as well as demonstrably stable or improved levels of activity and of analgesic use.

The potential morbidity of infection and epidural scarring (which can compromise permanent device implantation), however, and the expense of prolonged, intensive follow-up for screening purposes must be balanced against the potential long-term yield of a prolonged trial.

INDICATIONS FOR SPINAL CORD STIMULATION FOR PAIN

Neuropathic Pain

Failed Back Surgery Syndrome

FBSS has been the most common indication for SCS in the United States, especially when patients' symptoms have not been alleviated by a repeat operation (of course, an operation is required if a patient has a severe neurologic deficit caused by neural compression that can be seen via diagnostic imaging studies or if a patient has gross instability).

When FBSS causes a chief complaint of axial low back pain, achieving pain overlap by paresthesia is technically difficult and might require the use of complex electrode arrays and detailed psychophysical testing.[108,152] In addition, mechanical or nociceptive axial low back pain will not respond as well to SCS as does neuropathic pain.[120,132,171]

Initial case reports indicate that SCS therapy is safe for FBSS patients with cardiac pacemakers or cardioverter defibrillators.[136]

Peripheral Nerve Injury

SCS is used to treat pain from peripheral nerve injury (postherpetic neuralgia, causalgia, and/or CRPS. In the first author's (R.B.N.'s) first 20 years of experience with SCS, however, the 68% rate of successful percutaneous trials in peripheral nerve injury patients was significantly lower than the 87% success rate in patients with FBSS and the 90% success rate in patients with spinal cord injury.[154] Nevertheless, this observation is of limited clinical significance given the availability of percutaneous trials. The other author (B.L.) considers pain due to peripheral nerve injury (with or without signs of disturbed sympathetic function) to be one of the best indications for SCS. For CRPS, SCS placement in the cervical or lumbar regions yields statistically equivalent results.[57]

Stump neuroma pain can be classified as a peripheral nerve injury syndrome and often coexists with and can be difficult to distinguish from postamputation phantom limb pain. SCS is used to treat both stump neuroma pain and phantom limb pain. Pain from pressure applied directly onto a stump neuroma (e.g., from a prosthesis), however, does not respond adequately to SCS. This might be due to the technical difficulty of covering an entire phantom limb with paresthesia or to the degeneration of dorsal column fibers as a consequence of severe nerve damage.

Ischemic Pain

Peripheral Vascular Disease

Clinicians have used SCS to treat pain arising from peripheral vascular disease (PVD) since Cook and associates published their report in 1976.[31] When several investigators presented very encouraging results from confirmatory studies,[8,11,61,65,80,81] the use of SCS for ischemic pain spread rapidly in Europe among neurosurgeons, vascular surgeons, and anesthetists.

Despite fairly wide acceptance of the therapy during the late 1980s and early 1990s, however, ill-defined principles of patient selection resulted in poor long-term outcomes. This situation, combined with a lack of knowledge about the mechanism underlying the beneficial effect of SCS, likely hindered the use and further development of SCS for PVD. During the same period, a technical development in vascular surgery enabled physicians to perform increasingly complicated bypass grafting procedures, endovascular interventions, and so forth. This meant that only extremely fragile patients were deemed unable to benefit from surgery. These patients, often elderly and suffering from advanced arteriosclerosis with concurrent disease (e.g., coronary ischemia, diabetes), generally progressed rapidly toward critical, limb-threatening ischemia.

Thus, in many countries, the use of SCS for PVD decreased considerably. During 1994, for example, Swedish neurosurgeons implanted only 13 SCS systems for PVD.[117] The fact that most of these patients, however, had a satisfactory outcome and more than half achieved very good pain control helped the application of SCS for PVD to survive in a few centers that adopted strict patient selection criteria (Table 155-2).

Typical ischemia (e.g., of the foot) might involve several pain components, including deep, aching ischemic pain; nociceptive pain, which might respond to opioid treatment, arising from ischemic ulcers and from the border of gangrenous zones; and neuropathic pain that might be opioid resistant.[19,176] Usually, SCS alleviates just the ischemic pain component (and this effect is immediate only for vasospastic conditions and angina pectoris).

Clinicians who used SCS to treat ischemic pain wanted to know if SCS has a positive impact on tissue salvation. Initial investigation of this possibility with prospective, randomized studies,[82] however, demonstrated no statistically significant limb-saving effects of SCS in fairly unselected PVD cases. In specific subgroups, however, positive effects emerged (see later section on Ischemic Pain under Clinical Results).

The general recommendation that clinicians should not offer SCS therapy to patients with major tissue loss is, of course, relative. In fact, patients who reach stage IV on the Fontaine Classification System for Peripheral Artery Disease (tissue loss or ulceration)[190] might demonstrate a clear benefit from SCS therapy, and patients with diabetes can do as well as those without this condition.[78]

From initial case reports, it seems likely that a patient undergoing SCS for PVD can later receive a cardiac pacemaker or a dual-chamber cardioverter defibrillator capable

---

TABLE 155-2 ▪ Additional Peripheral Vascular Disease Patient Selection Criteria

1. Severe pain at rest, with or without defined tissue loss.
2. Reconstructive vascular surgery is impossible or contraindicated. Conservative therapies are exhausted.
3. Life expectancy is more than 3 months.
4. Any ulcer is less than 3 cm in diameter (larger ulcers do not heal completely and place patients at risk for infection).
5. If arrest of tissue loss is the primary goal, it should be evaluated objectively.
6. Any gangrene should be dry, and, when patients have gangrene, spinal cord stimulation (SCS) should be regarded as a means of obtaining a more distal amputation.
7. The preoperative transcutaneous oxygen pressure ($TcPO_2$) measured apically on the diseased extremity (usually at the dorsum of the foot) should be 10 to 30 mm Hg.[101] (A comparison of $TcPO_2$ measurements in the supine and seated positions revealed that a gradient exceeding 15 mm Hg predicts a successful outcome in 88% of cases.[62] Another technique is to assess the change in $TcPO_2$ while the patient breathes pure oxygen.[53])
8. During a percutaneous test, the patient should report a significant decrease in the ischemic component of the pain or demonstrate a clear increase in $TcPO_2$ or in some other objective indicator of microflow.
9. The patient should be cooperative and have at least a minimum understanding of the procedure and of the fact that the SCS can alleviate ischemic pain but not nociceptive pain from ulcers and gangrene.

---

of delivering tiered therapies in both the atrium and ventricle with no adverse effect on either therapy.[174]

Angina Pectoris

In the United States, angina is a major reason for hospitalization and is often refractory to standard treatment (administration of appropriate pharmaceuticals and revascularization). As more and more patients live longer with coronary artery disease, the number with intractable angina will increase. Many patients suffering from disabling angina (New York Heart Association [NYHA] Class III to IV) are elderly or have a concurrent disease that makes them unsuitable candidates for invasive, front-line treatment. Some patients with typical symptoms of angina but no signs of obstruction in cardiac circulation suffer from "syndrome X," which has its physiological basis in small vessel disease, vasospasm, or some other disturbance hard to demonstrate and treat with standard techniques.[83]

In the 1980s, transcutaneous electrical nerve stimulation became the first stimulation technique used to treat otherwise intractable angina pectoris,[123,124] and the outcome was remarkably promising. During this period, clinicians were using SCS to treat ischemic pain in the lower extremities, and it was a natural next step for them to position the electrode higher (at the T1 to T2 level) to induce paresthesia to mitigate the pain of otherwise intractable angina.[122,137]

The initial use of SCS for angina was met with skepticism and with fear that paresthesia would conceal important warning signs of a potentially fatal myocardial infarction. Several studies, however, demonstrated that paresthesia does not mask the pain of myocardial infarction or have an adverse impact on arrhythmia.[5,49]

An additional safety question considered the impact of SCS in patients with implanted cardiac pacemakers. A study

TABLE 155-3 ▪ Additional Angina Patient Selection Criteria

1. Severe angina pectoris (New York Heart Association Class III–IV)
2. Significant coronary artery disease refractory to conventional treatment
3. Demonstrated reversible myocardial ischemia
4. Pain alleviation with transcutaneous electrical nerve stimulation
5. No history of acute myocardial infarction
6. No concurrent heart disease (e.g., peri/myocarditis)
7. Ability to cooperate and no severe, untreated mental problems
8. No on-demand pacemaker (relative contraindication)
9. No cardioverter defibrillator
10. No body coil magnetic resonance imaging planned for the near future (relative contraindication)
11. No previous failure of a percutaneous spinal cord stimulation trial
12. Pharmacologic therapy possibilities depleted

to assess this impact involved 18 angina patients being treated concurrently with a pacemaker and thoracic SCS. Under electrocardiographic monitoring, the researchers increased the pacemaker setting and SCS intensity (to the maximum tolerated). They also asked patients for information on any possible interference during long-term treatment. Nothing indicated an adverse reaction to this combination treatment, but the investigators recommend individual patient assessment and have proposed a safety testing procedure.[46]

No one has reported use of SCS for angina in a patient with a cardioverter defibrillator, however, and, given the cervical placement of the SCS electrode, the likely overlap of the electrical fields could result in interference that would necessitate removal of the electrode.[174]

To date, thousands of SCS systems have been implanted for angina, and, with a success rate above 80%, angina has become one of the best indications for SCS.[9] Table 155-3 lists the additional patient selection criteria that must be met for patients with angina who are being considered for SCS therapy.

CLINICAL RESULTS

Neuropathic Pain

The clinical results of SCS for neuropathic pain vary considerably (Table 155-4), and investigators often express results in terms of the number of permanent systems implanted instead of the number of temporary electrodes placed for screening purposes. When the rate of permanent implantation is as low as 40%, adjustment for this factor is more important than when the implantation rate exceeds 75%.

Patient-rated pain relief is the most common outcome criterion, and the standard for "success" is a minimum 50% reported relief. This definition, however, arbitrarily and unduly emphasizes only one of many outcome measures for successful pain management, which include utilization of health care resources, ongoing medication requirements, ability to engage in productive activity or work, and change in neurologic function.

The source of this information is another important consideration; for example, data collected by a disinterested third-party interviewer can differ from those gleaned from a review of physicians' office records and hospital charts. Because this difference likely means that use of the disinterested interviewer reduces bias, many investigators have adopted this technique.

Table 155-4 summarizes the results of reports of SCS trials published since 1995. Although this list of reports might not be exhaustive, it is extensive. As the table indicates, most of these studies are prospective or retrospective trials; a conclusion about the absolute merit of SCS must await the results of more randomized studies—admittedly a difficult undertaking in the case of an interventional pain procedure.

Failed Back Surgery Syndrome

In FBSS patients, retrospective studies indicated that SCS can produce better results with fewer risks than those associated with reoperation.[144,149] Then, in 1994, the first author's (R.B.N.'s) research group published the results of the first prospective, randomized study that compared SCS with reoperation in FBSS patients with and without low back pain. All patients were eligible for and randomized to SCS or reoperation. Patients with unsatisfactory results could "cross over" to the other treatment, and the frequency of this crossover was a primary outcome measure. Of the first 27 patients to reach this point, 10 of 15 reoperation patients versus only 2 of 12 SCS patients crossed over, which indicated that patients were significantly ($p = 0.018$) more likely to be satisfied with SCS treatment than with reoperation.[151] The final results of this study confirmed the initial statistically significant findings, with 14/26 patients randomized to reoperation choosing to cross to SCS for secondary treatment versus only 5 of 24 patients randomized to SCS choosing to also undergo reoperation.[150]

Peripheral Nerve Injury

The other important SCS prospective, randomized trial for neuropathic pain did not offer cross-over.[89,90] Instead, the investigators randomized a group of patients with reflex sympathetic dystrophy (CRPS) to either SCS plus physical therapy ($n = 36$) or to physical therapy alone ($n = 18$), despite the fact that the study subjects had failed 6 months of physical therapy and other pain treatment, including transcutaneous electrical nerve stimulation. Only 24 SCS patients passed the screening trial and received implants. Even though only two thirds of the SCS group received SCS treatment, and the investigators only considered 20 of these patients SCS successes, the intent-to-treat analysis showed significant improvements in pain intensity and global perceived effect in the SCS group versus the physical therapy–only group.

Another neuropathic pain syndrome that often resists therapy is postherpetic neuralgia. In this case, we have only a prospective study to indicate that otherwise intractable pain from herpes zoster and postherpetic neuralgia responds so well to SCS that some patients were able to discontinue the therapy. In this study, the only patients who failed SCS treatment had serious comorbidities.[68]

As mentioned above, SCS can often relieve both phantom limb pain and stump neuroma pain.[96] An analysis in 19 patients with phantom limb pain, for example, found that SCS relieved the pain in 6 (32%), sometimes producing a "dramatic effect" with stimulation needed only infrequently. When SCS failed, deep brain stimulation was successful in 6 of 10 patients.[84]

TABLE 155-4 ▪ Clinical Results of Spinal Cord Stimulation for Neuropathic Pain—A Comprehensive Selection from Reports Published Since 1995

Reference	Study Design (Date)	Number Screened	Number Implanted	Number Followed	Indication (n)	Mean Months of Follow-up (Range)	Results	Complications	Note
Allegri et al[1]	Prospective (4/98–3/01)	170	103		Neuro, 113 FBBS, 29 Vasc, 28	12	Effective 68.4%; Pt sat 71%	Not noted; 10 removals for "inefficacy"	Concluded not necessary to obtain complete paresthesia
Aló et al[2]	Prospective (2/95–10/96)		80	62	FBSS, 32 CRPS, 17 Radicular, 11 Other, 2	48	"Favorable" Only 23 still use	Difficult to determine from tables	Third-party follow-up
Barolat et al[14]	Prospective (5/97–11/99)		54	41	FBSS (>50% low back pain)	6, 12, 24	"Most" had significant relief at 6 and 12 months Pt sat 88%–92%	2 revisions, 3 infections, 2 removals	24-month data not reported (see Sharan et al[117])
Bennett et al[18]	Multicenter (4) Retrospective (1995–1998)	134	134	30 (group 1 = Pisces Quad with Xtrel or Itrel)	CRPS	18.7 (11–33)	VAS reduced significantly (most in group 2) Dissatisfaction: 30% in group 1; 8.5% in group 2	Loss of paresthesia: 16.7% in group 1, 15.5% in group 2, 4 migrations, 1 infection, 4 other	
				71 (group 2 = Dual-Octrode)		23.5 (8–44)			
Budd[20]	Retrospective		20	20	FBSS	60	Improved in pain, functioning, drug use, work status, Q of L	60% (includes 25% battery failure before converted to Xtrel)	Primarily a cost study
Burchiel et al[22]	Prospective	219	182	70	FBBS 64%	12	55% successful pain management No significant change in medication use or work status	Surgical revision required in 12 (17%)	
Dario et al[38]	Prospective (1992–1997)	24	23		FBSS (14 leg pain only; 10 predominant leg pain "some" back pain)	43	21 "good results" Mean VAS decreased from 85–22 for leg pain and 45–40 for back pain		
Devulder et al[42]	Retrospective (13 years)		102	69 (of these 3 lost, 3 died)	FBSS, 69	"Long-term"	43 (62%) continued use with good pain relief 11 returned to work	"Multiple electrode reinterventions"	Third-party follow-up
Forouzanfar et al[57]	Prospective (began 1997)	36	36 (19 cervical; 17 lumbar)	36	CRPS	6, 12, 24	"Much improvement" in 42% of cervical and 47% of lumbar	64% had complications or adverse effects, mainly "technical defects"	
Harke et al[68]	Prospective (1994–2000)	32	32	32	PHN, 28 Acute herpes zoster, 4	29 median (9–38.5)	5 short-term success then unable to comply 23 (82%) long-term pain relief 15 continued use 8 could discontinue		

(Continued)

2173

TABLE 155-4 ▪ Clinical Results of Spinal Cord Stimulation for Neuropathic Pain—A Comprehensive Selection from Reports Published Since 1995—cont'd

Reference	Study Design (Date)	Number Screened	Number Implanted	Number Followed	Indication (n)	Mean Months of Follow-up (Range)	Results	Complications	Note
Heidecke et al[72]	Retrospective	42	42	42	FBSS	46 median (6–74)		8 fractures or disrupted insulation, 4 cable failures	Time to hardware failure = median 24 months (range 5–37)
Hord et al[77]	Retrospective	23	15	15	CRPS	1, 9	15 had "good" pain relief at 1 month 11 at 9 months		Assessed predictive value of sympathetic block response for SCS success
Kavar et al[85]	Prospective (9/94–7/96)	17/23	19	19	FBSS, 21 Spinal pain, 2	18.5 (7–38)	Statistically significant improvement in pain scores (56% benefited)	2 migrations, 2 repositioned pulse generators	
		4/6	2	6	Other, 6		Only one patient obtained pain relief		
Kay et al[86]	Retrospective (1984–1997)		70	70			60% "substantial" pain relief	72 revisions, 6 infections	
Kemler et al[88]	Retrospective (1991–1997)	Yes n=?	23	23	CRPS	32	18 (78%) improved 15 still use SCS	9 patients	
Kemler et al[89]	RCT (3/97–7/98)	36	24	24	RSD (CRPS)	6	Compared with physical therapy alone, significant pain relief and improved HRQOL	2 dural punctures 6 (25%) patients had 11 other complications (4 had long-term complications)	Not clear if 4 with long-term complications are included in the 6 with complications
Kemler et al[90]				21		24	"Intent-to-treat" had pain relief As-treated also improved HRQOL	9/24 had 22 surgical revisions 2/24 removed 22/24 had unpleasant side effects	Claims first report of "impossible to solve" side effects
Kim et al[92]	Retrospective (1/90–12/98)	122	74	60.7%	Neuropathic pain	~48 (~16–98)	34 (45.9%) still used SCS 7 excellent, 17 good, and 10 fair pain relief	36.5% surgically revised: 10.0% infection, 59.2% migration, 16.3% fracture, 12.2% receiver failure, 24 removed	Third-party follow-up
Kumar et al[100]	Retrospective	12	12	12	CRPS	41	Pain relief 50%–75% in 4 >75% in 8	1 fracture, 1 repositioned, 2 replaced	Third-party follow-up
Kumar et al[102]	Retrospective ("past" 15 years)	235	189		FBSS, 114 PVD, 39 Peripheral neuropathy, 30 MS, 13 CRPS, 13 Other, 26	66	111 (59%) satisfactory pain relief 25 rejoined workforce	35 repositioned: 11 infections, 8 malfunctions, 8 fractures, 3 electrical leaks, 3 CSF leaks, 1 hematoma	

Study	Design	N	Patients	Diagnosis	Follow-up (mo)	Results	Complications	Notes
Kumar et al[99]	Prospective	104	60 (44 others considered controls)	FBSS	60	Q of L improved in 27% versus 12% in controls; 88% pt sat; 15% returned to work; Drug intake reduced	Average per patient electrode change = 1/5 years; Pulse generator replaced = 1/4 years; 4 infections	Cost study
Kumar et al[98]	Retrospective	75	67 (unilateral limb pain)	FBSS, 58; Upper limb pain, 10; Other, 7	24 (most 132)	>50% pain relief in 87% initially, 79% at 6 months, 84% at 2 years	40% IPG replacements; 27% revisions (2.7% infection; 13.3% surgical complications)	
Leveque et al[112]	Retrospective (12/92–1/98)	30	16	FBSS	Minimum 6	75% success	24 electrode migrations or failures in 12 patients; 1 infection	Third-party follow-up; More pain decrease with laminectomy
North et al[153]	Prospective RCT comparing percutaneous with laminectomy electrodes	26	24 (12 percutaneous; 12 laminectomy)	FBSS	Soon after implantation	Laminectomy better coverage of pain and amplitudes (double battery life)		Comparison of technical results
Ohnmeiss[156]	Prospective (2-year period)	No	40	All FBSS and "some" CRPS	12, 24	70% improved; Significant relief of leg pain in 26%	4 power source adjustments; 4 migrations; 7 other removals; 3 reimplanted; 1 infection	Third-party follow-up
Ohnmeiss and Rashbaum[157]	Retrospective	41	36	Predominant low back pain (38/41 and 33/36 FBSS)	36	60% improved; 33.3% no change; 6.1% worse	16 revisions in 11 patients (4 removed for loss of pain relief, 6 repositioned, 1 replaced twisted extension wire)	
Quigley et al[162]	Retrospective (1989–2000)	168	102	CRPS, 21; FBSS, 20; Brachial plexus injury, 9; Amputation, 8; PVD, 7; Neuropathy, 25; Other, 12	~49	"Substantial" pain relief in 69	64 revisions in 35 patients; 5 infections	Questionnaires mailed
Rainov et al[163]	Prospective	32	29	FBSS	24–42	Good in 25; Failure in 4	"No major complications"	
Rutten et al[169]	Prospective (1998–2000)	34	34	FBSS	24	Pain and medication reduced; Q of L improved		
Segal et al[175]	Prospective (1992–1995)	27	19	FBSS, 12; CRPS, 6; PVD, 2; Other, 7	19 (6–49)	78% self-rated very good results (vs. 83.3% neurosurgeon rated)	No infections; 1 battery replaced early; 2 lead replacement; 1 connector repositioning; 1 revision of flipped generator (after a roller-coaster ride)	Data from neurosurgeon and from impartial third party

(Continued)

TABLE 155-4 ■ Clinical Results of Spinal Cord Stimulation for Neuropathic Pain—A Comprehensive Selection from Reports Published Since 1995—cont'd

Reference	Study Design (Date)	Number Screened	Number Implanted	Number Followed	Indication (*n*)	Mean Months of Follow-up (Range)	Results	Complications	Note
Sharan et al[177]	Prospective (additional data from Barolat et al[14])		26	Postop, 16; 6-month, 21; 12-month, 20; 24-month, 10	FBSS, 15 Arachnoiditis, 5 Radiculitis, 6 (at least 50% low back pain)	24	6 months 83% 12 months 94% 24 months 75%		Promotes use of complex electrodes and pulse generators
Simpson et al[180]	Prospective	No	41	"Most"	"Damage," 9 FBSS, 4 CRPS, 15 Other neuropathic, 1 Amputation, 5 Raynaud's, 3 Other, 4	59 median (5–135)	68% pain relief (facial pain did not respond)	Surgical revisions to correct 6 fractures, 3 migrations, 5 postural problems, 2 infections, 1 unknown	
Sindou et al[181]	Prospective (1984–2000)	No	95	95	Peripheral, 28 Radicular, 27 Root, 8 Cord lesions, 32	18.8	At least 50% pain relief in 54.7% (52/95) No success in patients with "significantly abnormal" SSEPs 75.4% in pts with normal SSEPs		Patient selection using SSEPs
Slavin et al[182]	Prospective	11	10	1 month in 10; "longer" in 7	FBSS, 5 Other neuropathic, 5 (all significant low back pain)		Insignificant decrease in pain and disability; at last follow-up only 33% continued use	1 infection 1 delayed healing 1 receiver pocket hematoma 1 malfunction 4 problems with positional stimulation	Transverse Tripolar

Study	Design	n	n	n	Diagnosis	Follow-up (mo)	Outcome	Complications	Comments
Tseng[191]	Retrospective	3	4		Cord injury, 2 PHN, 1 FBSS, 1	21 (19–15)	"Satisfactory" pain relief	1 migration	
van Buyten et al[196]	Retrospective (8/95–2/97)	Yes n=?	20	17	FBSS (all low back and leg pain)	28 (20–38)	Leg and back pain significantly decreased globally, In 8 with comparable low back and bilateral leg pain, reduction not significant; 65% would repeat	No serious complications but "external hardware problems occurred"	
van Buyten et al[195]	Retrospective (10 year)	254	217 (screening electrode used for permanent system)	123 (plus 22 died and 22 had explantations)	FBSS 78.4% Radiculopathy 5.6% Other 16%	~48	68% excellent-good 31% resumed work	47 technical problems 13 migrations 37 inappropriate pain or paresthesia 9 CSF leaks 17 infections	Third-party follow-up
van Buyten et al[197]	Prospective	Yes n=?	84 (one got 2 systems; considered 85)	1 (77 pts), 3, 6, 12 months, yearly to 5 years (28 pts)	Low back and/or leg pain, 32 PVD, 37	37.6 (0–68)	55% (45/82) pain relief >50% at 1 month 68% (19/28) at 5 years	24 removed 43 device-related anticipated adverse events required 19 revisions	Assess Itrel 3 System
Villavicencio et al[198]	Prospective (12/92–1/98)	41	27	27 (15 percutaneous; 12 laminectomy)	FBSS, 15 CRPS, 5 Neuropathic, 4 Stroke, 1 Other, 2	31 median (6–66)	89% overall had >50% pain relief (53% of percutaneous and 100% of laminectomy)	16 patients had total of 36 revisions	Third-party follow-up

CRPS, complex regional pain syndrome; CSF, cerebrospinal fluid; FBSS, failed back sugery syndrome; HRQOL, health-related quality of life; IPG, implanted pulse generator; Neuro, neurologic; PHN, postherpetic neuralgia; pt sat, patient satisfaction; PVD, peripheral vascular disease; Q of L, quality of life; RSD, reflex sympathetic dystrophy; SCS, spinal cord stimulation; SSEP, somatosensory evoked potential; VAS, visual analog scale; Vasc, vascular.

SCS is also used to treat myelopathy after spinal cord injury, such as gunshot wounds, and is reportedly effective when patients have only partial spinal cord lesions.[167]

Ischemic Pain

Peripheral Vascular Disease

Investigators use various outcome criteria to determine the impact of SCS on PVD, including relief from pain, limb salvage, and various measures of peripheral microcirculation. In general, SCS exerts a positive effect on most of the measured parameters, but this difference is not always statistically significant. The results of stratified series, however, indicate that careful patient selection is key to a successful outcome.

Two studies compared results in PVD patients randomized to SCS or to conservative treatment. One included 51 patients and found a clear, though not significant, trend for a limb-saving effect of SCS.[82] This study protocol, however, had technical problems: no percutaneous trial was performed, and 12% of the patients randomized to SCS did not receive implants for various reasons. The investigators also observed a tendency for a less satisfactory result in patients with arterial hypertension (excluding the hypertensive patients from analysis significantly reduced the amputation rate among the remaining group). Other researchers consider arterial hypertension to have no impact on outcome.[66]

In the other prospective study—a Dutch multicenter, randomized, controlled trial—120 patients with nonreconstructable PVD were randomized to SCS versus conservative treatment. The first data analysis considered only mortality and limb survival at 2 years' follow-up and found no benefit to limb survival of SCS treatment.[94] Additional analysis of data from baseline capillary microscopy, laser Doppler perfusion, and transcutaneous oxygen pressure ($TcPO_2$) measurements allowed investigators to classify the pretreatment microcirculatory status of their patients as poor, intermediate, or good.[193] By 18 months' follow-up, in each treatment group, those with poor baseline microcirculatory status had a high rate of amputation and those with good baseline microcirculatory status had a low rate of amputation. The only significant difference between the treatment groups was found in the patients with an intermediate baseline microcirculatory status: among patients with a preoperative $TcPO_2$ between 10 and 30 mm Hg, only 24% of those who received SCS underwent amputation versus 48% of those who received standard treatment. By 24 months, the amputation rate had climbed to 48% for SCS and 54% for standard treatment.[183] Each treatment reduced pain, but SCS patients needed fewer analgesics. No other significant treatment differences were found in pain or quality of life.

A 2003 report from the European Peripheral Vascular Disease Outcome Study considered the effect of SCS treatment on limb survival in patients with critical leg ischemia and the effect of using $TcPO_2$ as a screening tool for patient selection.[3] In three comparison groups, the baseline forefoot $TcPO_2$ was less than 30 mm Hg. One group ($n = 41$) obtained pain relief and more than 75% paresthesia coverage after an SCS trial lasting a minimum of 72 hours; the second group ($n = 32$) failed the trial; and the third group ($n = 39$) received no SCS treatment. The SCS treatment group obtained significantly improved pain relief and

$TcPO_2$ scores as well as significantly better limb survival at 12 months.

These results led this investigative group to revisit all of the baseline and treatment (conservative or SCS) $TcPO_2$ data reported on patients with inoperable PVD.[192] They found that 1-year limb salvage was 83% in SCS patients whose baseline supine parameter was greater than 10 mm Hg, baseline sitting-supine was greater than 17 mm Hg, and treatment difference was greater than 4 mm Hg. The general SCS treatment salvage rate regardless of $TcPO_2$ was 68%. The investigators proposed that these parameters would help guide patient selection when the goal of SCS is limb salvage.

A group of Italian investigators, on the other hand, believes that a 50% improved $TcPO_2$ score during a 2-week screening period with a temporary electrode predicts that SCS treatment will lead to limb salvage,[161] regardless of baseline score or disease stage.[159] In the case of diabetes, however, further study by the same investigators found that the stage of neuropathy was inversely related to SCS treatment success[160] independent of the stage of the disease.[158]

These clinical analyses are helping investigators shed light on the optimum patient selection criteria for SCS treatment of PVD. Much remains to be determined, however. A meta-analysis, for example, that included six controlled studies of SCS versus conventional therapy for inoperable critical leg ischemia found positive results for the SCS patients in terms of limb salvage, pain relief, and Fontaine stage attained after treatment but no overall difference in ulcer healing.[194] The only trial included in the meta-analysis that used presence of ischemic ulcers as an inclusion criterion randomized 86 Fontaine stage IV patients with end-stage PVD who were undergoing a 21-day regimen of intravenous prostaglandin E_1 therapy for nonhealing ulcers into a group of 45 who received SCS and a group of 41 who did not, and the SCS group showed significantly better total healing of foot ulcers (69% versus 17%; $p < 0.0001$) but no difference in the frequency of amputations at 1-year follow-up.[29] In each group, healing of ulcers or amputation wounds was best among patients whose $TcPO_2$ rose to an average of 26.0 ± 8.6 mm Hg. This favorable impact of SCS on ulcer healing is echoed in a report of a patient with severe Raynaud's syndrome of long duration in whom, by improving microcirculation, SCS treatment led to complete resolution of all fingertip ulcers as well as of pain.[140]

Every published trial on the use of SCS to treat vasospastic conditions, such as Raynaud's syndrome, demonstrates a positive effect of the therapy.[10,13,58,97,166] This is not surprising because, compared with PVD patients, patients with vasospastic conditions are relatively young, present with relatively few obliterative vessel wall processes, and have symptoms that are often temporarily relieved by destroying or blocking the corresponding sympathetic ganglia. The few published studies, however, involve only small numbers of patients.

Because the long-term results of SCS seem to be superior to those of many other therapies, clinicians should attempt to identify candidates whose ischemic pain has major vasospastic components. A comparison of the outcome of different interventions in a case of vasospasm, for example, revealed that sympathetic blockade and sympathectomy provided only temporary effects, whereas SCS produced a long-lasting increase in blood flow index.[111a] SCS has also been used successfully to treat pain in frostbite.[7]

Angina Pectoris

In general, 80% to 90% of angina patients treated with SCS report marked pain relief with a diminished frequency of anginal attacks, a diminished need for short-acting nitrates (but other medication use is often unchanged), fewer visits to the emergency room, and enhanced quality of life.[9,41,51]

Many investigators report SCS-induced changes in various indices of coronary ischemia during workload, such as reduction in ST segment depression, reversal of cardiac lactate production to extraction, and an increase in working capacity.[70,125,172] In these studies, the multipolar electrode was often placed with its center near T1 to T2. Gonzalez-Darder and associates, however, reported positive effects of SCS with the electrode tip at C2 in 23 angina patients followed at least 3 months.[64] In these patients, SCS decreased the number of angina attacks from an average of 124 per month to 8 per month and led to reclassification of most patients as NYHA class I from a pre-SCS class of III to IV.

A meta-analysis of results of treating angina patients with SCS from 114 centers with a total of 517 patients and a median follow-up of 23 months[50] found that the cardiovascular mortality rate of approximately 5% per year was related to several factors, including sex, cardiovascular history, age older than 71 years, and the use of medications prescribed for severe disease. Nothing indicated that SCS alters long-term mortality in this patient group.

The ESBY Study (electrical stimulation versus bypass surgery) randomized 104 patients with angina to SCS or to coronary artery bypass surgery and found no significant difference in symptom relief.[126] In the bypass group, however, the patients' exercise capacity increased significantly and various indices of ischemia changed positively. This contradiction of previous findings might have resulted from the fact that the investigators discontinued stimulation during the 24 hours before the exercise test because they believed the "antiischemic effect during ongoing stimulation" required no further documentation, and they wanted to determine if the antiischemic effect of SCS would continue despite discontinuation. These investigators concluded that because of the complications sometimes encountered during bypass surgery, SCS should be a therapeutic alternative for patients with increased risk.

Indeed, the impact of discontinuation of stimulation in angina patients remains controversial. Additional data from the ESBY study indicate that the number of anginal attacks decreased significantly in patients who underwent coronary artery bypass surgery and in those with temporarily disconnected SCS but that temporarily discontinuing SCS temporarily stops the antiischemic effects of the therapy.[141] These ischemic results are supported by findings in a study involving 15 angina patients who had been treated with SCS for a mean of 39 ± 27 months and were randomized to 48-hour ambulatory electrocardiograph monitoring with SCS stimulation on or off for 24 hours.[44] During the off periods, the number and duration of ischemic events increased, as did the total ischemic burden (heart rate variability parameters were similar during both periods).

Another study, however, contradicts part of the ESBY conclusion by indicating that temporary SCS dysfunction increases anginal symptoms. In this study, 32 patients had been treated with SCS for an average of 65 months before battery depletion or electrode failure ($n = 7$) led to complete cessation of stimulation. In all patients, the number of anginal attacks, consumption of nitrates, and physical dysfunction (assessed with the Seattle Angina Questionnaire) increased during the time without stimulation and decreased when stimulation was restored.[48] These results permit us to draw two conclusions: at least some of the effects of SCS on angina do not continue without stimulation, and patients do not become tolerant to, and thus do not cease to benefit from, this therapy.

A long-term (4.8 years) follow-up report on the 104 patients in the ESBY Study found no significant difference between the patients treated with coronary artery bypass surgery and those treated with SCS in quality of life and survival.[47] It is clear, then, that SCS is a reasonable therapeutic choice for patients whose disease will not benefit from a surgical procedure or whose overall condition makes such a procedure an unacceptable risk. The SCS versus bypass selection procedure for other patients is less apparent.

Another situation where bypass surgery is not indicated is if the angina patient has syndrome X (see earlier section on Angina under Indications). In this case, SCS can improve the disabling anginal symptoms that have such an adverse impact on quality of life. The first prospective study dealing solely with syndrome X patients treated by SCS followed seven patients for a mean of 11 months.[104] All seven passed a trial stimulation, and, at last follow-up, SCS significantly reduced anginal symptoms and improved physical activity and quality of life. Only four of the patients, however, sustained their improvement throughout the follow-up period (for two this was 14 to 15 months). The three who lost benefit after several months of pain control reported that the distribution of their paresthesia suddenly changed, despite no radiographic evidence of a displaced electrode.

In general, very few complications are reported with SCS therapy for angina.[4] For example, investigators conducting a retrospective, multicenter review of 130 patients with a mean follow-up of 31.4 ± 25.9 months reported only 6.8% minor complications and no major complications.[168] In a subsequent prospective report, members of this investigative team found that the most frequent complication was infection at the site of implantation of the electrode or of the abdominal pocket, and this only occurred in 6 of 104 patients enrolled in a registry and followed for an average 13.2 ± 8 months.[43]

COMPUTERIZED METHODS

The development of programmable, multicontact, SCS electrodes has improved the technical (overlap of pain by paresthesia) and clinical results of SCS. The range of possible anode and cathode assignments for a multicontact array, however, becomes quite large as the number of contacts increases. Furthermore, achieving the best results might require testing each electrode combination over a range of pulse parameters (particularly amplitude).

By noting the amplitude at which the painful target area is first stimulated on a scale that encompasses the range of first perception to discomfort threshold, however, we can compare electrode configurations and stimulus parameters at identical subjective stimulus intensities.[105]

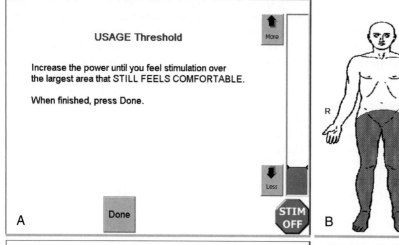

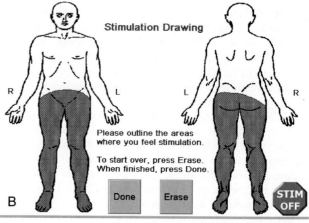

FIGURE 155-5   A computer graphics interface used by patients to control standard, commercially available, radiofrequency-coupled spinal cord stimulation systems. The controls of the device allow greater ease of operation than do the controls of standard radiofrequency transmitters or programming units. *A,* For each new setting, the patient adjusts amplitude with a "thermometer." *B,* The patient uses the graphics tablet to enter "pain drawings," distribution of paresthesia drawings, and ratings on a standard 100-mm visual analog scale; to control amplitude; and to answer "yes-no" questions for psychophysical studies. The computer fills in the area of paresthesia outlined by the patient. *C,* Overlap of pain by stimulation paresthesia is readily calculated from these graphic data, and settings are easily ranked for everyday use by the patient. (Reprinted with permission from North RB, Brigham DD, Khalessi A, et al: Spinal cord stimulator adjustment to maximize implanted battery longevity: A randomized, controlled trial using a computerized, patient-interactive programmer. Neuromodulation 7:13–25, 2004.)

Systematic, quantitative assessment of these effects generates a large volume of data, which would be prohibitively expensive to analyze without a computer.[147,148] Data can be entered by a skilled operator working with the patient or, given a suitable means of control, by the patient working alone. Figure 155-5 illustrates a computer system that presents the patient with a series of contact combination and pulse parameters that the practitioner previously specified. The patient adjusts the stimulation amplitude and draws the area of paresthesia for comparison with drawings of the painful area. Optimal settings are derived from analysis of these results. In a randomized, controlled trial involving 44 patients from two centers, the computerized system produced significantly better technical results at a significantly faster rate than did the manual adjustment method. This occurred regardless of practitioner experience, but results improved with patient experience. The computer results also indicated ways to maximize battery life in implanted power generators (and thus to reduce costs and procedural risk by reducing the frequency of battery replacements).[143]

Additional analysis of data from the same 44 patients to examine this possibility revealed that the use of the computerized system allowed identification of new settings that improved expected battery life for 41 of the patients (95%).[142] With an assumed battery use of 24 hours per day, the average battery life linked to manual settings was 25.4 + 49.5 months versus 55.0 + 71.7 months for the computerized settings. For 72% of the patients, the settings that extended battery life also equaled or improved technical results.

The investigators estimate the attendant savings in batteries to be greater than $300,000 over the life of an average patient, which is 600 times the presumed cost of the computerized method.

Computerized systems that directly control the implanted stimulator also facilitate the investigation of novel modulation schemes and pulse sequences that might be more advantageous than the monotonic pulse sequences used for SCS in the past.

COST EFFECTIVENESS

The high cost of SCS equipment has prompted much debate about the cost effectiveness of the procedure for various indications. It is noteworthy that, other than conducting a few return-to-work analyses, no study has taken into account the economic impact of the patient's suffering and related disability on the patients and on any caregiver families. Finally, the overall cost of SCS treatment will decrease due to improvements in equipment, implantation technique, parameter adjustment technique (including use of computers), and patient selection.

A literature review identified 14 studies that met the broad criteria of providing SCS cost information. Analysis of these reports led the investigators to conclude that the reduction in post-SCS use of health care resources offsets the initial high cost of SCS implantation.[189] The following sections briefly review the findings of 10 of these studies and of two additional reports.

Neuropathic Pain

Failed Back Surgery Syndrome

SCS is a valid alternative to reoperation in FBSS patients,[150,151] and a comparison of 5-year costs for 100 patients with FBSS with those for 100 patients receiving other therapies found that SCS was more cost effective than repeat operation when the repeat operation efficacy rate was less than 80%.[71] In addition, rehabilitation after SCS is much less expensive than rehabilitation after reoperation.

SCS is also less expensive than conventional, medical pain therapy for FBSS. The first report supporting this finding was a 2-year analysis of a series of 14 FBSS patients in whom the decrease in the cost of medication and the ability to return to work more than compensated for the initial high cost of the SCS system.[16] Another group of investigators conducted a 5-year trial in a consecutive series of 104 FBSS patients to compare the cost of SCS treatment (n = 60) with that of the best available conventional pain therapy in those who failed the SCS trial (n = 44 who did not obtain 50% pain relief with a temporary electrode).[99] Each group had the same follow-up protocol in a controlled environment. The cumulative cost per patient in Canadian dollars of SCS treatment was $29,123 versus $38,029 for conventional pain therapy. SCS treatment was more expensive only during the initial half of the study period. SCS also improved productivity: 15% of the SCS patients and none of the conventionally treated patients returned to work.

To compare the cost of SCS treatment for FBSS with the mix of therapies commonly in use (chronic maintenance), including reoperation and medical management, a group of investigators[17] applied the technique of cost-minimization analysis[45] and found that SCS with an efficacy of 56% pays for itself within 2.3 years.

The choice of SCS equipment, the implantation technique, and clinician experience, obviously have a large impact on cost. Battery failure, for example, can result from a less than optimum choice of stimulating parameters. Even when such issues lengthen cost recovery, however, it can still occur within 5 years. In a retrospective study of 20 patients who received SCS for FBSS conducted in the United Kingdom, for example, the mean cost of care in the year prior to SCS was £1,954.18.[20] Extrapolated over 5 years, this would be £9,770.90 compared with £9,782 for SCS. These investigators noted that the SCS cost included a high incidence of battery failure and reflected their change to external generators as well as their decision to modify the receiver site. Even with these factors driving up the total cost of SCS, they achieved cost neutrality in 5 years. They estimated that, without these changes in procedure, they would have achieved cost neutrality in 3.4 years.

Peripheral Nerve Injury

An evaluation of the cost of SCS in a randomized, controlled trial (see earlier section on Clinical Results) in 54 patients

with reflex sympathetic dystrophy (CRPS) compared costs before and after treatment.[91] The investigators presented cost data in 1998 euros for three sets of patients: the SCS plus physical therapy as-randomized group (n = 36; 24 underwent SCS and 12 failed SCS and underwent physical therapy); the physical therapy group (n = 18); and the SCS plus physical therapy as-treated group (n = 24). The data on the as-randomized group (two thirds SCS, one third physical therapy) revealed a mean per patient first year cost of 9,805 euros. The mean as-treated first year cost per patient for SCS plus physical therapy, however, at 12,721 euros was more than twice the 5,741 euro cost of physical therapy alone. The initial year disadvantage for SCS was eliminated by analysis to expected time of death, which yielded a mean as-randomized cost per patient of 171,153 euros in the SCS plus physical therapy group versus 229,624 euros in the physical therapy alone group. These investigators concluded that, in addition to being a more effective therapy for CRPS, SCS becomes cost effective after 3 years.

Ischemic Pain

Angina

Several studies have demonstrated that SCS is a cost-effective treatment for angina. The first was a 1992 cost-benefit analysis that found SCS[164] reduced angina-associated hospitalization costs by US$5,700 per year per patient and reduced home care costs by approximately $2,300 US per year per patient.

Another study compared hospitalization rates from most recent revascularization until SCS implantation, and from implantation until the study date in 19 consecutive NYHA Class III/IV patients with three-vessel disease.[138] Revascularization led to an annual admission rate of 0.97 per patient, whereas the rate following SCS implantation was 0.27. The annual duration of hospitalization was longer during the postrevascularization period (8.3 days) than in the SCS period (2.5 days). This result was underscored when the ESBY investigators (see earlier section on Clinical Results) conducted a 2-year follow-up of their 104 patients in which they considered hospital costs[6] and found that the SCS patients spent significantly fewer days in the hospital, which made SCS significantly less expensive than bypass surgery.

Two reports attempted to determine the cost recovery period of SCS for angina, which apparently is shorter than for FBSS. One relied on data from eight patients treated before April 1999 at a single hospital.[131] The investigators compared costs associated with hospitalization duration and consumption of health care resources for the 12 months preceding and following attempted implantation in the six patients with successful implants with those in the two patients in whom implantation was "technically impossible." The successful SCS patients had significantly fewer days of hospitalization and consumed significantly fewer resources in the period following implantation. The opposite was true for the two unsuccessful SCS patients. The investigators concluded that the cost of SCS implantation for angina is recovered in approximately 15 months.

The other study came to a nearly identical conclusion after conducting a retrospective comparison of hospitalization data before and after SCS implantation in 24 angina patients.[204]

The median annual per patient duration of hospitalization increased during the 3 years prior to SCS implantation from 3 days to 10 and decreased significantly to a median of 0 days in the year after implantation. Thus, in this group, the cost of SCS was recovered within 16 months of implantation.

CONCLUSION

SCS has evolved into a relatively easily implemented, reversible technique with low morbidity for the management of chronic, intractable pain in selected patients. Percutaneous placement of electrode arrays, supported by programmable, implanted electronics, allows noninvasive adjustment of anode and cathode positions and has been a major technical advance. With contemporary devices, the need for surgical revision is significantly less, and clinical results have improved substantially. The cost of an SCS system has often been considered so high that many doctors hesitated to use this treatment modality. Several cost/benefit analyses, however, have demonstrated that beyond the relief of pain and increase in activities of daily life for these patients, the total cost of health care declines for SCS patients as a whole. Improvements in the design, implantation technique, and use (with computer guidance) of SCS systems will only improve this cost-benefit ratio. Thus SCS is a minimally invasive, effective, and economical therapy, given appropriate patient selection. We believe that, at present, SCS is an underused therapeutic modality.

REFERENCES

1. Allegri M, Arachi G, Barbieri M, et al: Prospective study of the success and efficacy of spinal cord stimulation. Minerva Anestesiol 70(3):117–124, 2004.
2. Aló KM, Redko V, Charnov J: Four year follow-up of dual electrode spinal cord stimulation for chronic pain. Neuromodulation 5(2):79–88, 2002.
3. Amann W, Berg P, Gersbach P, et al: European Peripheral Vascular Disease Outcome Study SCS-EPOS. Spinal cord stimulation in the treatment of non-reconstructable stable critical leg ischaemia: Results of the European Peripheral Vascular Disease Outcome Study (SCS-EPOS). Eur J Vasc Endovasc Surg 26(3):280–286, 2003.
4. Andersen C: Complications in spinal cord stimulation for treatment of angina pectoris. Differences in unipolar and multipolar percutaneous inserted electrodes. Acta Cardiol 52(4):325–333, 1997.
5. Andersen C, Hole P, Oxhoj H: Does pain relief with spinal cord stimulation for angina conceal myocardial infarction? Br Heart J 71:419–421, 1994.
6. Andrell P, Ekre O, Eliasson T, et al: Cost-effectiveness of spinal cord stimulation versus coronary artery bypass grafting in patients with severe angina pectoris—long-term results from the ESBY study. Cardiology 99(1):20–24, 2003.
7. Arregui R, Morandeira JR, Martinez G, et al: Epidural neurostimulation in the treatment of frostbite. PACE 12:713–717, 1989.
8. Augustinsson LE, Carlsson CA, Holm J, Jivegard L: Epidural electrical stimulation in severe limb ischemia. Ann Surg 202:104-110, 1986.
9. Augustinsson LE, Linderoth B, Eliasson T, Mannheimer C: Spinal cord stimulation in peripheral vascular disease and angina pectoris. In Gildenberg PH, Tasker R (eds): Textbook of Stereotactic and Functional Neurosurgery. New York: McGraw-Hill, 1997, pp 1973–1978.
10. Augustinsson LE, Linderoth B, Mannheimer C: Spinal cord stimulation in various ischaemic conditions. In Illis L (ed): Spinal Cord Dysfunction. III: Functional Stimulation. Oxford, UK: Oxford Medical Publications, 1992, pp 272–295.
11. Augustinsson LE, Linderoth B, Mannheimer C, Eliasson T: Spinal cord stimulation in cardiovascular disease. Neurosurg Clin N Am 6:157–165, 1995.
12. Barolat G, Massaro F, He J, et al: Mapping of sensory responses to epidural stimulation of the intraspinal neural structures spin man. J Neurosurg 78:233–239, 1993.
13. Barolat G, Myklebust JR, Wenninger W: Effects of spinal cord stimulation on spasticity and spasms secondary to myelopathy. App Neurophys 51:29–44, 1988.
14. Barolat G, Oakley JC, Law JD, et al: Epidural spinal cord stimulation with a multiple electrode paddle lead is effective in treating intractable low back pain. Neuromodulation 4(2):59–66, 2001.
15. Baron R, Binder A, Schattschneider J, Wasner G: Pathophysiology and treatment of complex regional pain syndromes. In Dostrovsky JO, Carr DB, Koltzenburg M (eds): Proceeding of the 10th World Congress on Pain. Seattle, WA: IASP Press, 2003, pp 683–704.
16. Bel S, Bauer BL: Dorsal column stimulation: Cost to benefit analysis. Acta Neurochir 52(Suppl):121–123, 1991.
17. Bell GK, Kidd D, North RB: Cost-effectiveness of spinal cord stimulation in treatment of failed-back surgery syndrome. J Pain Symptom Manage 13:286–295, 1997.
18. Bennett DS, Aló KM, Oakley J, Feler CA: Spinal cord stimulation for complex regional pain syndrome I (RSD): A retrospective multicenter experience from 1995–1998 of 101 patients. Neuromodulation 2(3):202–210, 1999.
19. Bonica J: Pain due to vascular disease. In Bonica JJ (ed): The Management of Pain, 2nd ed. Philadelphia: Lea & Febiger, 1990, pp 502–537.
20. Budd K: Spinal cord stimulation: Cost-benefit study. Neuromodulation 5(2):75–78, 2002.
21. Bunker CB, Terenghi G, Springall DR, et al: Deficiency of calcitonin gene-related peptide in Raynaud's phenomenon. Lancet 336:1530–1533, 1990.
22. Burchiel KJ, Anderson VC, Brown FD, et al: Prospective, multicenter study of spinal cord stimulation for relief of chronic back and extremity pain. Spine 21(23):2786–2794, 1996.
23. Burton CV: Dorsal column stimulation: Optimization of application. Surg Neurol 4:171–176, 1975.
24. Burton CV: Session on spinal cord stimulation: Safety and clinical efficacy. Neurosurgery 1:164–165, 1977.
25. Campbell JN, Davis KD, Meyer RA, North RB: The mechanism by which dorsal column stimulation affects pain: Evidence for a new hypothesis. Pain 5(Suppl):228, 1990.
26. Campbell JN, Meyer RA: Primary afferents and hyperalgesia. In Yaksh TL (ed): Spinal Afferent Processing. New York: Plenum, 1986, pp 59–81.
27. Cardinal R, Ardell J, Linderoth B, et al: Spinal cord activation differentially modulates ischemic electrical responses to different stressors in canine ventricles. Autonom Neurosci 111(1):34–47, 2004.
28. Chandler MJ, Brennan TJ, Garrison DW, et al: A mechanism of cardiac pain suppression by spinal cord stimulation: Implications for patients with angina pectoris. Eur Heart J 14:96–105, 1993.
29. Claeys LG, Horsch S: Transcutaneous oxygen pressure as predictive parameter for ulcer healing in endstage vascular patients treated with spinal cord stimulation. Int Angiol 15(4):344–349, 1996.
30. Coburn B, Sin W: A theoretical study of epidural electrical stimulation of the spinal cord. I: Finite element analysis of stimulus fields. IIEEE Trans Biomed Eng 32:971–977, 1985.
31. Cook AW, Oygar A., Baggenstos P, et al: Vascular disease of extremities: Electrical stimulation of spinal cord and posterior roots. NY State J Med 76:366–368, 1976.
32. Croom JE, Foreman RD, Chandler MJ, Barron KW: Cutaneous vasodilation during dorsal column stimulation is mediated by dorsal roots and CGRP. Am J Physiol 272:H950–H957, 1997.
33. Croom JE, Foreman RD, Chandler MJ, Barron KW: Reevaluation of the role of the sympathetic nervous system in cutaneous vasodilatation during dorsal spinal cord stimulation: Are multiple mechanisms active? Neuromodulation 1:91–101, 1998.
34. Cui JG, Linderoth B, Meyerson BA: Effects of spinal cord stimulation on touch-evoked allodynia involve GABAergic mechanisms: An experimental study in the mononeuropathic rat. Pain 66:287–295, 1996.
35. Cui JG, Meyerson BA, Sollevi A, Linderoth B: Effects of spinal cord stimulation on tactile hypersensitivity in mononeuropathic rats is potentiated by GABA B and adenosine receptor activation. Neurosci Lett 247:183–186, 1998.
36. Cui JG, O'Connor WT, Ungerstedt U, et al: Spinal cord stimulation attenuates augmented dorsal horn release of excitatory amino acids in mononeuropathy via a GABAergic mechanism. Pain 73:87–95, 1997.
37. Daniel M, Long C, Hutcherson M, Hunter S: Psychological factors and outcome of electrode implantation for chronic pain. Neurosurgery 17:773–777, 1985.

38. Dario A, Fortini G, Bertollo D, et al: Treatment of failed back surgery syndrome. Neuromodulation 4(3):105–110, 2001.
39. de la Porte C, Siegfried J: Lumbosacral spinal fibrosis (spinal arachnoiditis): Its diagnosis and treatment by spinal cord stimulation. Spine 8:593–603, 1983.
40. de la Porte C, Van de Kelft E: Spinal cord stimulation in failed back surgery syndrome. Pain 52:55–61, 1993.
41. deJongste MJL, Hautvast RVM, Hillege HL, Lie KI: Efficacy of spinal cord stimulation as adjuvant therapy for intractable angina pectoris: A prospective, randomized clinical study. J Am Coll Cardiol 23:1592–1597, 1994.
42. Devulder J, de Laat M, van Bastelaere M, Rolly G: Spinal cord stimulation: A valuable treatment for chronic failed back patients. J Pain Symptom Manage 13(5):296–301, 1997.
43. Di Pede F, Lanza GA, Zuin G, et al: Immediate and long-term clinical outcome after spinal cord stimulation for refractory stable angina pectoris. Am J Cardiol 91(8):951–955, 2003.
44. Di Pede F, Zuin G, Giada F, et al: A. Long-term effects of spinal cord stimulation on myocardial ischemia and heart rate variability: results of a 48-hour ambulatory electrocardiographic monitoring. Ital Heart J 2(9):690–695, 2001.
45. Eisenberg JM: Clinical economics. JAMA 262:2879–2886, 1989.
46. Ekre O, Borjesson M, Edvardsson N, et al: Feasibility of spinal cord stimulation in angina pectoris in patients with chronic pacemaker treatment for cardiac arrhythmias. Pacing Clin Electrophysiol 26(11):2134–2141, 2003.
47. Ekre O, Eliasson T, Norrsell H, et al: Electrical stimulation versus coronary artery bypass surgery in severe angina pectoris. Long-term effects of spinal cord stimulation and coronary artery bypass grafting on quality of life and survival in the ESBY study. Eur Heart J 23(24):1938–1945, 2002.
48. Ekre O, Norrsell H, Wahrborg P, et al: Temporary cessation of spinal cord stimulation in angina pectoris-effects on symptoms and evaluation of long-term effect determinants. Coron Artery Dis 14(4):323–327, 2003.
49. Eliasson T: Spinal cord stimulation in angina pectoris [Thesis]. Göteborg, Sweden: Stra Hospital, 1994.
50. Eliasson T, Andersen C, deJongste MJL, et al: Long-term mortality and morbidity with treatment of severe angina pectoris with spinal cord stimulation. Hygiea 106:364, 1997.
51. Eliasson T, Augustinsson LE, Mannheimer C: Spinal cord stimulation in severe angina pectoris: Presentation of current studies, indications and practical experience. Pain 65:169–179, 1996.
52. Erickson DL: Percutaneous trial of stimulation for patient selection for implantable stimulating devices. J Neurosurg 43:440–444, 1975.
53. Favre JP, Richard A, Gournier JP, Barral X: Value of spinal cord stimulation for limb salvage in patients with graft failure. In Horsch S, Claeys L (eds): Spinal Cord Stimulation. II: An Innovative Method in the Treatment of PBD and Angina. Darmstadt, Germany: Steinkopff Verlag, 1995, pp 137–145.
54. Feler C, Kaufman S: Spinal cord stimulation: One stage? Acta Neurochir 117:91, 1992.
55. Foreman RD, DeJongste MJL, Linderoth B: Integrative control of cardiac function by cervical and thoracic spinal neurons. In Armour JA, Ardell JL (eds): Basic and Clinical Neurocardiology. London: Oxford University Press, 2004, pp 153–186.
56. Foreman RD, Linderoth B, Ardell JL, et al: Modulation of intrinsic cardiac neuronal activity by spinal cord stimulation: Implications for its therapeutic in angina pectoris. Cardiovasc Res 47(2):367–375, 2000.
57. Forouzanfar T, Kemler MA, Weber WE, et al: Spinal cord stimulation in complex regional pain syndrome: Cervical and lumbar devices are comparably effective. Br J Anaesth 92(3):348–353, 2004.
58. Francaviglia N, Silvestro C, Maiello M, et al: Spinal cord stimulation for the treatment of progressive systemic sclerosis and Raynaud's syndrome. Br J Neurosurg 8:567–571, 1994.
59. Freedman RR, Sabharwal SC, Desai N, et al: Increased α-adrenergic responsiveness in idiopathic Raynaud's disease. Arthritis Rheum 32:61–65, 1989.
60. Freeman TB, Campbell JN, Long DM: Naloxone does not affect pain relief induced by electrical stimulation in man. Pain 17:189–195, 1983.
61. Galley D, Elharrar C, Scheffer J, et al: Intérêt de la neurostimulation épidurale dans les artériopathies des members intétients. Arteres Veines 7:61–71, 1988.
62. Gersbach P, Hasdemir MG, Stevens RD, et al: Discriminative microcirculatory screening of patients with refractory limb ischemia for dorsal column stimulation. Eur J Endovasc Surg 13:464–471, 1997.
63. Gherardini G, Lundeberg T, Cui JG, et al: Spinal cord stimulation improves survival in ischemic skin flaps: An experimental study of the

64. possible mediation via the calcitonin gene-related peptide. Plast Reconstr Surg 103(4):1221–1228, 1999.
64. Gonzalez-Darder JM, Canela P, Gonzalez-Martinez V: High cervical spinal cord stimulation for unstable angina pectoris. Stereotact Funct Neurosurg 56:20–27, 1991.
65. Groth KE: Spinal cord stimulation for the treatment of peripheral vascular disease. In Fields HL, Dubner R, Cervera F (eds): Advances in Pain Research and Therapy, Vol 9. New York: Raven, 1985, pp 861–870.
66. Guarnera G, Mascellari L, Bianchini G, et al: [The role of spinal cord electric stimulation in critical ischemia of the extremity.] Minerva Cardioangiol 44(12):663–667, 1996.
67. Häbler H-J, Eschenfelder S, Brinker H, et al: Neurogenic vasoconstriction in the dorsal root ganglion may play a crucial role in sympathetic-afferent coupling after spinal nerve injury. In Devor M, Rowbotham MC, Wiesemfeld-Hallin Z (eds): Progress in Pain Research and Management. Seattle: IASP Press, 2000, pp 661–667.
68. Harke H, Gretenkort P, Ladleif HU, et al: Spinal cord stimulation in postherpetic neuralgia and in acute herpes zoster pain. Anesth Analg 94(3):694–700, 2002.
69. Hautvast R: Spinal cord stimulation for chronic refractory angina pectoris [Thesis]. Groningen, the Netherlands: Rijksuniversiteit, 1997.
70. Hautvast R, deJongste MJL, Blanksma PK, et al: Effect of spinal cord stimulation on myocardial blood flow assessed by positron emission tomography in patients with refractory angina pectoris. Am J Cardiol 77:462–467, 1996.
71. Health Technology Assessment Information Service: Spinal cord (dorsal column) stimulation for chronic intractable pain. Plymouth Meeting, PA: ECRI, 1993.
72. Heidecke V, Rainov NG, Burkert W: Hardware failures in spinal cord stimulation for failed back surgery syndrome. Neuromodulation 3(1):27–30, 2000.
73. Holsheimer J, Nuttin B, King GW, et al: Clinical evaluation of paresthesia steering with a new system for spinal cord stimulation. Neurosurgery 42:541–549, 1998.
74. Holsheimer J, Strujik JJ, Rijkhoff NJM: Contact combinations in epidural spinal cord stimulation: A comparison by computer modeling. Stereotact Funct Neurosurg 56:220–233, 1991.
75. Holsheimer J, Wesselink WA: Effect of anode-cathode configuration on paresthesia coverage in spinal cord stimulation. Neurosurgery 41:654–660, 1997.
76. Hoppenstein R: Electrical stimulation of the ventral and dorsal columns of the spinal cord for relief of chronic intractable pain. Surg Neurol 4:187–194, 1975.
77. Hord ED, Cohen SP, Cosgrove GR, et al: The predictive value of sympathetic block for the success of spinal cord stimulation. Neurosurgery 53(3):626–632, 2003.
78. Horsch S, Schulte S, Hess S: Spinal cord stimulation in the treatment of peripheral vascular disease: results of a single-center study of 258 patients. Angiology 55(2):111–118, 2004.
79. Hosobuchi Y, Adams JE, Weinstein PR: Preliminary percutaneous dorsal column stimulation prior to permanent implantation. J Neurosurg 17:242–245, 1972.
80. Jacobs MJ, Jorning PJ, Beckers RC, et al: Foot salvage and improvement of microvascular blood flow as a result of epidural spinal cord electrical stimulation. J Vasc Surg 13:354–360, 1990.
81. Jivegard L, Augustinsson LE, Carlsson CA, Holm J: Long-term results of epidural spinal electrical stimulation (ESES) in patients with inoperable severe lower limb ischaemia. Eur J Vasc Surg 1:345–349, 1987.
82. Jivegard LEH, Augustinsson LE, Holm J, et al: Effects of spinal cord stimulation (SCS) in patients with inoperable severe lower limb ischemia: A prospective randomized controlled study. Eur J Endovasc Surg 9:421–425, 1995.
83. Kaski JC, Russo G: Microvascular angina in patients with syndrome X. Z Kardiol 89(Suppl 9):121–125, 2000.
84. Katayama Y, Yamamoto T, Kobayashi K, et al: Motor cortex stimulation for phantom limb pain: Comprehensive therapy with spinal cord and thalamic stimulation. Stereotact Funct Neurosurg 77(1–4):159–162, 2001.
85. Kavar B, Rosenfeld JV, Hutchinson A: The efficacy of spinal cord stimulation for chronic pain. J Clin Neurosci 7(5):409–413, 2000.
86. Kay AD, McIntyre MD, Macrae WA, Varma TR: Spinal cord stimulation—A long-term evaluation in patients with chronic pain. Br J Neurosurg 15(4):335–341, 2001.

87. Kemler MA, Barendse GA, van Kleef M, Egbrink MG: Pain relief in complex regional pain syndrome due to spinal cord stimulation does not depend on vasodilation. Anesthesiology 92(6):1653–1660, 2000.

88. Kemler MA, Barendse GA, van Kleef M, et al: Electrical spinal cord stimulation in reflex sympathetic dystrophy: Retrospective analysis of 23 patients. J Neurosurg 90(1 Suppl):79–83, 1999.

89. Kemler MA, Barendse GA, van Kleef M, et al: Spinal cord stimulation in patients with chronic reflex sympathetic dystrophy. N Engl J Med 343(9):618–624, 2000.

90. Kemler MA, de Vet HC, Barendse GA, et al: The effect of spinal cord stimulation in patients with chronic reflex sympathetic dystrophy: Two years' follow-up of the randomized controlled trial. Ann Neurol 55(1):13–18, 2004.

91. Kemler MA, Furnee CA: Economic evaluation of spinal cord stimulation for chronic reflex sympathetic dystrophy. Neurology 59(8):1203–1209, 2002.

92. Kim SH, Tasker RR, Oh MY: Spinal cord stimulation for nonspecific limb pain versus neuropathic pain and spontaneous versus evoked pain. Neurosurgery 48(5):1056–1064, 2001.

93. Kingma JG Jr, Linderoth B, Ardell JL, et al: Neuromodulation therapy does not influence blood flow distribution or left-ventricular dynamics during acute myocardial ischemia. Auton Neurosci 91(1–2):47–54, 2001.

94. Klomp HM, Spincemaille GH, Steyerberg EW, et al: Spinal-cord stimulation in critical limb ischaemia: A randomised trial. ESES Study Group. Lancet 353(9158):1040–1044, 1999.

95. Koeze TH, Williams AC, Reiman S: Spinal cord stimulation and the relief of chronic pain. J Neurol Neurosurg Psychiatry 50:1424–1429, 1987.

96. Krainick JU, Thoden U, Riechert T: Pain reduction in amputees by long-term spinal cord stimulation: Long-term follow-up study over 5 years. J Neurosurg 52:346–350, 1980.

97. Ktenidis K, Claeys L, Bartels C, Horsch S: Spinal cord stimulation in the treatment of Buerger's disease. In Horsch S, Claeys L (eds): Spinal Cord Stimulation: An Innovative Method in the Treatment of PVD and Angina. Darmstadt, Germany: Steinkopff Verlag, 1995, pp 207–214.

98. Kumar A, Felderhof C, Eljamel MS: Spinal cord stimulation for the treatment of refractory unilateral limb pain syndromes. Stereotact Funct Neurosurg 81(1–4):70–74, 2003.

99. Kumar K, Malik S, Demeria D: Treatment of chronic pain with spinal cord stimulation versus alternative therapies: Cost-effectiveness analysis. Neurosurgery 51(1):106–115, 2002.

100. Kumar K, Nath RK, Toth C: Spinal cord stimulation is effective in the management of reflex sympathetic dystrophy. Neurosurgery 40(3):503–508, 1997

101. Kumar K, Toth C, Nath RK, et al: Improvement of limb circulation in peripheral vascular disease using epidural spinal cord stimulation. A prospective study. J Neurosurg 86:662–669, 1997.

102. Kumar K, Toth C, Nath RK, Laing P: Epidural spinal cord stimulation for treatment of chronic pain—some predictors of success. A 15-year experience. Surg Neurol 50(2):110–120, 1998.

103. Kupers RC, van den Oever R, van Houdenhove B, et al: Spinal cord stimulation in Belgium: A nation-wide survey on the incidence, indications and therapeutic efficacy by the health insurer. Pain 56:211–216, 1994.

104. Lanza GA, Sestito A, Sandric S, et al: A. Spinal cord stimulation in patients with refractory anginal pain and normal coronary arteries. Ital Heart J 2(1):25–30, 2001.

105. Law JD: A new method for targeting a spinal stimulator: Quantitatively paired comparisons. Appl Neurophysiol 50:436, 1987.

106. Law J: Results of treatment for pain by percutaneous multicontact stimulation of the spinal cord. Presented at the American Pain Society meeting, Chicago, November 11–13, 1983.

107. Law J: Spinal stimulation: Statistical superiority of monophasic stimulation of narrowly separated bipoles having rostral cathodes. Appl Neurophysiol 46:129–137, 1983.

108. Law JD: Targeting a spinal stimulator to treat the "failed back surgery syndrome." Appl Neurophysiol 50:437–438, 1987.

109. Law JD, Kirkpatrick AF: Pain management update: Spinal cord stimulation. Am J Pain Manage 2:34–42, 1991.

110. Leclercq TA: Electrode migration in epidural stimulation: Comparison between singles electrode and four electrode programmable leads. Pain 20(Suppl 2):78, 1984.

111. Leibrock L, Meilman P, Cuka D, Green C: Spinal cord stimulation in the treatment of chronic low back and lower extremity pain syndromes. Nebraska Med J 69:180–183, 1984.

111a. Lepantalo M, Rosenberg P, Pohjola J, et al: Epidural spinal cord stimulation in the treatment of limb threatening vasospasm—Report of a case with a five year follow-up. Eur J Endovasc Surg 11:368–370, 1996.

112. Leveque JC, Villavicencio AT, Bulsara KR, et al: Spinal cord stimulation for failed back surgery syndrome. Neuromodulation 4(1):1–9, 2001.

113. Lind G, Meyerson BA, Winter J, Linderoth B: Implantation of laminotomy electrodes for spinal cord stimulation in spinal anesthesia with intraoperative dorsal column activation. Neurosurgery 53(5):1150–1153, 2003.

114. Lind G, Meyerson BA, Winter J, Linderoth B: Intrathecal baclofen as an adjuvant therapy to enhance effect of spinal cord stimulation. Eur J Pain 8:377–383, 2004.

115. Lindblom U, Meyerson BA: Influence on touch, vibration and cutaneous pain of dorsal column stimulation in man. Pain 1:257–270, 1975.

116. Linderoth B: Dorsal column stimulation and pain: Experimental studies of putative neurochemical and neurophysiological mechanisms [Thesis]. Stockholm, Sweden: Karolinska Institute, 1992.

117. Linderoth B: Spinal cord stimulation in ischemia and ischemic pain. In Horsch S, Claeys L (eds): Spinal Cord Stimulation III: An Innovative Method in the Treatment of PVD and Angina. Darmstadt, Germany: Steinkopff Verlag, 1995, pp 19–35.

118. Linderoth B, Foreman RD: Physiology of spinal cord stimulation. Review and update. Neuromodulation 2:150–164, 1999.

119. Linderoth B, Gazelius B, Franck J, Brodin E: Dorsal column stimulation induces release of serotonin and substance P in the cat dorsal horn. Neurosurgery 31:289–297, 1992.

120. Linderoth B, Meyerson BA: Spinal cord stimulation. I: Mechanisms of action. In Burchiel K (ed): Pain Surgery. New York: Thieme, 1999.

121. Linderoth B, Stiller CO, Gunasekera L, et al: Release of neurotransmitters in the CNS by spinal cord stimulation: Survey of the present state of knowledge and recent experimental studies. Sterotact Funct Neurosurg 61:157–170, 1993.

122. Mannheimer C, Augustinsson LE, Carlsson CA, et al: Epidural spinal electrical stimulation in severe angina pectoris. Br Heart J 59:56–61, 1988.

123. Mannheimer C, Carlsson CA, Emanuelsson H, et al: The effects of transcutaneous electrical nerve stimulation in patients with severe angina pectoris. Circulation 71:308–316, 1985.

124. Mannheimer C, Carlsson CA, Eriksson K, et al: Transcutaneous electrical nerve stimulation in severe angina pectoris. Eur Heart J 3:297–302, 1982.

125. Mannheimer C, Eliasson T, Andersson B, et al: Effects of spinal cord stimulation in angina pectoris induced by pacing and possible mechanisms of action. BMJ 307:477–480, 1993.

126. Manneheimer C, Eliasson T, Augustinsson LE, et al: Electrical stimulation versus coronary artery bypass surgery in severe angina pectoris: The ESBY Study. Circulation 97:1157–1163, 1998.

127. Marchand S, Bushnell MC, Molina-Negro P, et al: The effects of dorsal column stimulation on measures of clinical and experimental pain in man. Pain 45:249–257, 1991.

128. Meglio M, Cioni B, Rossi GF: Spinal cord stimulation in management of chronic pain: A 9-year experience. J Neurosurg 70: 519–524, 1989.

129. Meilman PW, Leibrock LG, Leong FTL: Outcome of implanted spinal cord stimulation in the treatment of chronic pain: Arachnoiditis versus single nerve root injury and mononeuropathy. Clin J Pain 5:189–193, 1989.

130. Melzack P, Wall PD: Pain mechanisms: A new theory. Science 150(3699):971–978, 1965.

131. Merry AF, Smith WM, Anderson DJ, et al: Cost-effectiveness of spinal cord stimulation in patients with intractable angina. N Z Med J 114(1130):179–181, 2001.

132. Meyerson BA: Electric stimulation of the spinal cord and brain. In Bonica JJ, Loeser JD, Chapman RC, Fordyce WE (eds). The Management of Pain, 2nd ed. Philadelphia: Lea & Febiger, 1990, pp 1862–1877.

133. Meyerson BA, Boethius J, Terenius L, Wahlström A: Endorphine mechanisms in pain relief with intracerebral and dorsal column stimulation. Presented at the 3rd Meeting of the European Society for Stereotactic and Functional Neurosurgery, Freiburg, Germany, 1977.

134. Meyerson BA, Brodin E, Linderoth B: Possible neurohumoral mechanisms in CNS stimulation for pain suppression. Appl Neurophysiol 48:175–180, 1985.

135. Meyerson BA, Linderoth B: Spinal cord stimulation: Mechanisms of action in neuropathic and ischemic pain. In Simpson BA (ed): Electrical Stimulation and the Relief of Pain. New York: Elsevier, 2003, pp 161–182.

136. Monahan K, Casavant D, Rasmussen C, Hallet N: Combined use of a true-bipolar sensing implantable cardioverter defibrillator in a patient having a prior implantable spinal cord stimulator for intractable pain. Pacing Clin Electrophysiol 21:2669–2672, 1998.

137. Murphy DF, Giles KE: Dorsal column stimulation for pain relief from intractable angina pectoris. Pain 28:365–368, 1987.

138. Murray S, Carson KG, Ewings PD, et al: Spinal cord stimulation significantly decreases the need for acute hospital admission for chest pain in patients with refractory angina pectoris. Heart 82(1):89–92, 1999.

139. Nashold B, Somjen G, Friedman H: Paresthesias and EEG potentials evoked by stimulation of the dorsal funiculi in man. Exp Neurol 36:273–287, 1972.

140. Neuhauser B, Perkmann R, Klingler PJ, et al: Clinical and objective data on spinal cord stimulation for the treatment of severe Raynaud's phenomenon. Am Surg 67(11):1096–1097, 2001.

141. Norrsell H, Pilhall M, Eliasson T, Mannheimer C: Effects of spinal cord stimulation and coronary artery bypass grafting on myocardial ischemia and heart rate variability: Further results from the ESBY study. Cardiology 94(1):12–18, 2000.

142. North RB, Brigham DD, Khalessi A, et al: Spinal cord stimulator adjustment to maximize implanted battery longevity: A randomized controlled trial using a computerized, patient-interactive programmer. Neuromodulation 7(1):13–25, 2004.

143. North RB, Calkins SK, Campbell DS, et al: Automated, patient-interactive, spinal cord stimulator adjustment: A randomized controlled trial. Neurosurgery 52(3):572–580, 2003.

144. North RB, Ewend MG, Lawton MT, et al: Failed back surgery syndrome: Five-year follow-up after spinal cord stimulation implantation. Neurosurgery 28:692–699, 1991.

145. North RB, Ewend MG, Lawton MT, Piantadosi S: Spinal cord stimulation for chronic, intractable pain: Superiority of "multichannel" devices. Pain 44:119–130, 1991.

146. North RB, Fischell TA, Long DM: Chronic stimulation via percutaneously inserted epidural electrodes. Neurosurgery 1:215–218, 1977.

147. North RB, Fowler KR, Nigrin DA, et al: Automated "pain drawing" analysis by computer-controlled, patient-interactive neurological stimulation system. Pain 50:51–58, 1992.

148. North RB, Fowler KR, Nigrin DA, Szymanski RE: Patient-interactive, computer-controlled neurological stimulation system: Clinical efficacy in spinal cord stimulation. J Neurosurg 76:689–695, 1992.

149. North RB, Kidd DH, Campbell JN, Long DM: Dorsal root ganglionectomy for failed back surgery syndrome: A five-year follow-up study. J Neurosurg 74(2):236–242, 1991.

150. North RB, Kidd DH, Farrokhi F, Piantadosi SA: Spinal cord stimulation versus repeated lumbosacral spine surgery for chronic pain: A randomized, controlled trial. Neurosurgery 56:98–107, 2005.

151. North RB, Kidd DH, Lee MS, Piantadosi S: A prospective, randomized study of spinal cord stimulation versus reoperation for failed back surgery syndrome: Initial results. Stereotact Funct Neurosurg 62(1–4):267–272, 1994.

152. North RB, Kidd DH, Olin J, et al: Spinal cord stimulation for axial low back pain: A prospective, controlled trial comparing dual with single percutaneous electrodes. Spine 30:1412–1418, 2005.

153. North RB, Kidd DH, Olin JC, Sieracki JM: Spinal cord stimulation electrode design: Prospective, randomized, controlled trial comparing percutaneous and laminectomy electrodes. Part I: Technical outcomes. Neurosurgery 51(2):381–389, 2002.

154. North RB, Kidd DH, Zahurak M, et al: Spinal cord stimulation for chronic, intractable pain: Two decades' experience. Neurosurgery 32:384–395, 1993.

155. Ohnishi A, O'Brien PC, Okazaki H, Dyck PJ: Morphometry of myelinated fibers of fasciculus gracilis of man. J Neurol Sci 27:163–172, 1976.

156. Ohnmeiss DD, Rashbaum RF, Bogdanffy GM: Prospective outcome evaluation of spinal cord stimulation in patients with intractable leg pain. Spine 21(11):1344–1350, 1996.

157. Ohnmeiss DD, Rashbaum RF: Patient satisfaction with spinal cord stimulation for predominant complaints of chronic, intractable low back pain. Spine J 1(5):358–363, 2001.

158. Petrakis IE, Sciacca V: Does autonomic neuropathy influence spinal cord stimulation therapy success in diabetic patients with critical lower limb ischemia? Surg Neurol 53(2):182–188, 2000.

159. Petrakis IE, Sciacca V: Spinal cord stimulation in critical limb ischemia of the lower extremities: Our experience. J Neurosurg Sci 43(4):285–293, 1999.

160. Petrakis IE, Sciacca V: Spinal cord stimulation in diabetic lower limb critical ischaemia: Transcutaneous oxygen measurement as predictor for treatment success. Eur J Vasc Endovasc Surg 19(6):587–592, 2000.

161. Petrakis IE, Sciacca V: Transcutaneous oxygen tension (TcPO$_2$) in the testing period of spinal cord stimulation (SCS) in critical limb ischemia of the lower extremities. Int Surg 84(2):122–128, 1999.

162. Quigley DG, Arnold J, Eldridge PR, et al: Long-term outcome of spinal cord stimulation and hardware complications. Stereotact Funct Neurosurg 81(1–4):50–56, 2003.

163. Rainov NG, Heidecke V, Burkert W: Short test-period spinal cord stimulation for failed back surgery syndrome. Minim Invasive Neurosurg 39(2):41–44, 1996.

164. Rasmussen MB, Andersen C, Andersen P, Frandsen F: Cost-utility analysis of electric spinal cord stimulation for treatment of angina pectoris. Ugeskr Laeger 154:1180–1184, 1992.

165. Renard VM, North RB: Percutaneous electrode migration in spinal cord stimulation: Problem and solution (in preparation).

166. Robaina FJ, Dominguez M, Diaz M, et al: Spinal cord stimulation for relief of chronic pain in vasospastic disorders of the upper limbs. Neurosurgery 24:63–67, 1989.

167. Rogano L, Teixeira MJ, Lepski G: Chronic pain after spinal cord injury: Clinical characteristics. Stereotact Funct Neurosurg 81(1–4):65–69, 2003.

168. Romano M, Auriti A, Cazzin R, et al: [Epidural spinal stimulation in the treatment of refractory angina pectoris. Its clinical efficacy, complications and long-term mortality. An Italian multicenter retrospective study]. Ital Heart J 1(1 Suppl):97–102, 2000.

169. Rutten S, Komp M, Godolias G: [Spinal cord stimulation (SCS) using an 8-pole electrode and double-electrode system as minimally invasive therapy of the post-discotomy and post-fusion syndrome—Prospective study results in 34 patients] Z Orthop Ihre Grenzgeb 140(6):626–631, 2002.

170. Sances A, Swinotek TJ, Larson SJ, et al: Innovations in neurologic implant systems. Med Instrum 9:213–216, 1975.

171. Sanchez-Ledesma MJ, Garcia-March G, Diaz-Cascajo P, et al: Spinal cord stimulation in deafferentation pain. Stereotact Funct Neurosurg 53:40–55, 1992.

172. Sanderson JE, Brooksby P, Waterhouse D, et al: Epidural spinal electrical stimulation for severe angina: A study of its effects on symptoms, exercise tolerance and degree of ischaemia. Eur Heart J 13:628–633, 1992.

173. Schechtmann G, Wallin J, Meyerson BA, Linderoth B: Intrathecal clonidine potentiates suppression of tactile hypersensitivity by spinal cord stimulation in a model of neuropathy. Anesth Analg 99(1):135–139, 2004.

174. Schimpf R, Wolpert C, Herwig S, et al: Potential device interaction of a dual chamber implantable cardioverter defibrillator in a patient with continuous spinal cord stimulation. Europace 5(4):397–402, 2003.

175. Segal R, Stacey BR, Rudy TE, et al: Spinal cord stimulation revisited. Neurol Res 20(5):391–396, 1998.

176. Seijo F: Ischemic pain: Nociceptive pain or deafferentation pain. In Herreros J, et al (eds): Spinal Cord Stimulation for Peripheral Vascular Disease: Advances and Controversies. Madrid: Editorial Libro del Año, SL, 1994, pp 25–29.

177. Sharan A, Cameron T, Barolat G: Evolving patterns of spinal cord stimulation in patients implanted for intractable low back and leg pain. Neuromodulation 5(3):167–179, 2002.

178. Shealy C, Mortimer J, Reswick J: Electrical inhibition of pain by stimulation of the dorsal columns: A preliminary report. Anesth Analg 46:489–491, 1967.

179. Shetter AG, Racz GC, Lewis R, Heavner JE: Peripheral nerve stimulation. In North RB, Levy RM (eds): Neurosurgical Management of Pain. New York: Springer-Verlag, 1997, pp 261–270.

180. Simpson BA, Bassett G, Davies K, et al: Cervical spinal cord stimulation for pain: A report on 41 patients. Neuromodulation 6(1):20–26, 2003.

181. Sindou MP, Mertens P, Bendavid U, et al: Predictive value of somatosensory evoked potentials for long-lasting pain relief after spinal cord stimulation: Practical use for patient selection. Neurosurgery 52(6):1374–1383, 2003.

182. Slavin KV, Burchiel KJ, Anderson VC, Cooke B: Efficacy of transverse tripolar stimulation for relief of chronic low back pain: Results of a single center. Stereotact Funct Neurosurg 73(1–4):126–130, 1999.

183. Spincemaille GH, Klomp HM, Steyerberg EW, Habbema JD: Pain and quality of life in patients with critical limb ischaemia: Results of a randomized controlled multicentre study on the effect of spinal cord stimulation. ESES study group. Eur J Pain 4(2):173–184, 2000.

184. Stiller CO, Cui JG, O'Connor WT, et al: Release of GABA in the dorsal horn and suppression of tactile allodynia by spinal cord stimulation in mononeuropathic rats. Neurosurgery 39:367–375, 1996.

185. Sweet W, Wepsic J: Stimulation of the posterior columns of the spinal cord for pain control. Clin Neurosurg 21:278–310, 1974.

186. Tanaka S, Barron KW, Chandler MJ, et al: Local cooling alters neural mechanisms producing changes in peripheral blood flow by spinal cord stimulation. Auton Neurosci 104(2):117–127, 2003.

187. Tanaka S, Barron KW, Chandler MJ, et al: Low intensity spinal cord stimulation may induce cutaneous vasodilatation via CGRP release. Brain Res 896:183–187, 2001.

188. Tanaka S, Barron KW, Chandler MJ, et al: Role of primary afferent in spinal cord stimulation-induced vasodilatation: Characterization of fiber types. Brain Res 959(2):191–198, 2003.

189. Taylor RS, Taylor RJ, Van Buyten JP, et al: The cost effectiveness of spinal cord stimulation in the treatment of pain: A systematic review of the literature. J Pain Symptom Manage 27(4):370–278, 2004.

190. TransAtlantic InterSociety Consensus Working Group: Management of peripheral arterial disease (PAD): TransAtlantic InterSociety Consensus. J Vasc Surg 31(1 Part 2; Suppl):39, 2000.

191. Tseng SH: Treatment of chronic pain by spinal cord stimulation. J Formos Med Assoc 99(3):267–271, 2000.

192. Ubbink DT, Gersbach PA, Berg P, et al: The best TcPO$_2$ parameters to predict the efficacy of spinal cord stimulation to improve limb salvage in patients with inoperable critical leg ischemia. Int Angiol 22(4):356–363, 2003.

193. Ubbink DT, Spincemaille GH, Prins MH, et al: Microcirculatory investigations to determine the effect of spinal cord stimulation for critical leg ischemia: The Dutch Multicenter Randomized Controlled Trial. J Vasc Surg 30(2):236–244, 1999.

194. Ubbink DT, Vermeulen H: Spinal cord stimulation for non-reconstructable chronic critical leg ischaemia (Cochrane Review) In: The Cochrane Library, Issue 3. Chichester, UK: Wiley, 2004.

195. van Buyten JP, van Zundert J, Vueghs P, Vanduffel L: Efficacy of spinal cord stimulation: 10 years of experience in a pain centre in Belgium. Eur J Pain 5(3):299–307, 2001.

196. van Buyten JP, van Zundert JV, Milbouw G: Treatment of failed back surgery syndrome patients with low back and leg pain: A pilot study of a new dual lead spinal cord stimulation system. Neuromodulation 2(3):258–265, 1999.

197. van Buyten JP: The performance and safety of an implantable spinal cord stimulation system in patients with chronic pain: A 5-year study. Neuromodulation 6(2):79–87, 2003.

198. Villavicencio AT, Leveque JC, Rubin L, et al: Laminectomy versus percutaneous electrode placement for spinal cord stimulation. Neurosurgery 46(2):399–405, 2000.

199. Waddell G, McCulloch JA, Jummel EG, Venner RM: Non-organic physical signs in low back pain. Spine 5:117–125, 1980.

200. Wallin J, Cui J-G, Yakhnitsa V, Meyerson BA, Linderoth B: Gabapentin and pregabalin suppress tactile allodynia and potentiate spinal cord stimulation in a model of neuropathy. Eur J Pain 6:261–272, 2002.

201. Wallin J, Fiska A, Tjolsen A, et al: Spinal cord stimulation inhibits long-term potentiation of spinal wide dynamic range neurons. Brain Res 973(1):39–43, 2003.

202. Weinard M, Madhusudan H, Davis B, Melgar M: Acute vs. prolonged screening for spinal cord stimulation in chronic pain. Neuromodulation 6:15–19, 2003.

203. Yakhnitsa V, Linderoth B, Meyerson BA: Spinal cord stimulation attenuates dorsal horn neuronal hyperexcitability in a rat model of mononeuropathy. Pain 79(2–3):223–233, 1999.

204. Yu W, Maru F, Edner M, et al: Spinal cord stimulation for refractory angina pectoris: A retrospective analysis of efficacy and cost-benefit. Coron Artery Dis 15(1):31–37, 2004.

205. Zumpano BJ, Saunders RL: Percutaneous epidural dorsal column stimulation. J Neurosurg 45:459–460, 1976.

156 Management of Cauda Equina Tumors

FRANÇOISE LAPIERRE, MICHEL P. WAGER,
and NGUYEN VAN TUAN

Cauda equina tumors (CETs) are seldom reported and their specificity is seldom emphasized, yet they should be considered a distinct entity because of their anatomic localization, their surgical management, and their clinical course. Neurosurgeons should be aware of this surgical anatomoclinic entity, and CETs should be referred to well-trained teams. Some pathologies are virtually specific to the pediatric population and are described in a special paragraph in this chapter.

Most CET tumors involve adolescents or young adults and are slow-growing, benign tumors arising from the nerve sheaths. Some may be the expression of a congenital disease such as neurofibromatosis or von Hippel-Lindau disease. The diagnosis is established following a long time lapse if the initial symptoms are considered, leading to tumors of large or even giant size. This large size is also due, like the previous feature, to the wide free space surrounding the cauda equina. Postoperative functional status is correlated to the preoperative status of patients at the time of the operation.

That most of these tumors are benign justifies an aggressive surgical approach, using magnification techniques and microsurgical instrumentation, and adjuvant therapy is unnecessary, at least after the first procedure. In 1996 the authors performed a retrospective review of the French cases with 231 patients.[1,2] Our personal series comprises 31 patients. It is not always easy to make a distinction between a true CET and a tumor arising from the neighboring structures, even with the magnetic resonance imaging (MRI) data, and it is sometimes necessary to obtain the operative and anatomopathologic findings to correctly classify the tumor. In the literature, many isolated cases are reported, but large series and practical advice for management are seldom encountered.

DEFINITION OF CAUDA EQUINA TUMORS

Primary tumors of the cauda equina arise from the different intrinsic structures of the region, such as the filum, the nerve sheaths, intrinsic vessels of the nerves, conjunctive tissue, and embryologic remnants.[3] Some authors include tumors sprouting from the surrounding tissues (i.e., meningeal envelopes, epidural structures, bone), but this does not seem to be the proper nosologic approach in description of this pathology, even if their clinical features present some similarities. It is in fact relatively difficult to classify metastatic tumors that, though not infrequent, do not constitute a surgical problem.

In infants and children, CETs are often associated with occult dysraphism and are treated with their special features taken into account.

The most common tumors are benign schwannomas, neurofibromas (nerve sheath tumors), ependymomas in their myxopapillary type (filum tumor), hemangioblastomas, lipomas, epidermoid cysts and teratomas, and paragangliomas. Some others may develop on the nerve roots; they include lymphomas, metastasis, and capillary hamartomas. Some chordomas may develop inside the dura in the absence of any patent connection with the sacrum or the spine. Astrocytomas have also been reported; these develop inside the conus medullaris, involving the proximal part of the roots, and are not true tumors of the cauda equina.

CLINICAL PRESENTATION

The involved population is constituted by both sexes, with a slight masculine predominance, which is more marked for ependymomas (nearly 61%).[1,2] Mean age for all CETs is 47 years, but there is a strong correlation between age and tumor type (34.6 years ± 16 for ependymomas, 51 years ± 17 for benign neurinomas).

Symptomatology at the time of diagnosis common to all tumors involves low back pain (60%), radiculopathies (81%), and sphincter dysfunctions (25%). There exists a general rule, which is to pay special attention to bilateral radicular pain. There are some differences linked to the pathologic type: 70% of ependymomas suffer low back pain but only 55% of neurinomas; 75% of ependymomas have radiculopathy, and 93% of neurinomas; 3% of neurinomas present functional sphincter or genital disturbance, and 24% of ependymomas. Other symptoms that seldom reveal the tumor but are never isolated are focal deficit (33%) and amyotrophy (8.5%).

Physical examination discloses a limited range of spinal motion in 50% of patients, a paravertebral spasm in 28%, abolition of one or several reflexes in half, and of this half, 25% have a bilateral abolition of ankle tendon jerk and 13.5% of knee jerk. A motor deficit exists in 42% of cases, often bilateral at L5 and S1 levels (15%) and less frequently at L2, L3, and L4 levels. A sensory deficit exists in 50% of cases at the same levels. Amyotrophy was found in 15%. Saddle hypesthesia or anesthesia exists in 20% of cases bilaterally and in 3.5% unilaterally, most often in ependymomas. The bilaterality of symptoms mainly involves those with ependymoma. Associated genital and sphincter dysfunctions affect 34.2% of patients and should be precisely sought and explored: urinary emergency, episodic incontinence, overflow with retention, and loss of anal and bulbocavernosus reflexes. All patients can walk, some (11%) requiring a stick or a crutch.

The time interval between the first symptom and the diagnosis ranges from 1 month to 264 months. In our series the mean delay was about 2 years, 10 months for 50% of the patients. There is no influence of age but rather a strong correlation with the type of tumor: long-lasting time lapse, 50 months for neurofibromas and paragangliomas; medium, 20 months for neurinomas and ependymomas; short for malignant tumors, especially metastasis. In a few cases intratumoral bleeding caused by a trauma may result in an acute cauda equina syndrome.[4]

Among our cases one patient presented with papilledema and progressive visual loss. He had a long-lasting history of low back pain and sciatica, and MRI revealed a giant cauda equina ependymoma, the removal of which did not improve his visual function. Optic atrophy resulted in blindness. The mechanism of papilledema remains a matter of controversy and in the majority of cases is correlated with large-scale hyperproteinorachy, arachnoiditis, and disturbances of cerebrospinal fluid (CSF) circulation.

DIAGNOSTIC EVALUATION

Electromyography and evoked potentials are of limited value in the investigation of CET.

Plain Radiography

Although performed in almost all patients, plain radiograms are unremarkable in two out of every three cases. They may reveal scoliosis, increased interpedicular distance, or scalloping in large lesions. This last sign is nonspecific and is only the mark of large chronic or slow-growing lesions; it is also encountered in large arachnoid cysts. Erosion of the posterior wall of a vertebral body can be observed in 21% of ependymomas and neurinomas.

Enhanced Computed Tomography Scan

Enhanced computed tomography (CT) scan has been performed in 53.5% of our cases and was not contributive in half; this result is attributable to incomplete examination leading to a CT scan focused on the last three levels, below the level of the tumors. Sometimes misinterpretation arises from a spinal canal completely filled by the hypodense tumor and a radiologist drawing the conclusion that there is no compression. Contrast administration showed intraspinal enhancement in one case out of two, and osseous abnormalities in one out of four. Water-soluble intrathecal injection allows for enhanced visualization of lesions, their size, and shape.

Computed Tomography–Myelography

Myelo-CT scan is used in cases of contraindication or impossibility of obtaining an MRI. The whole lumbar spinal canal must be examined: misdiagnosis was found in two cases of giant tumors with a CT scan limited to the three lowest vertebrae.

Magnetic Resonance Imaging

Magnetic resonance imaging, the gold standard for diagnosis, must include T1- and T2-weighted sequences, with and without gadolinium administration, sagittal and axial views. It demonstrates the existence and the size of the tumor, cystic components, and intratumoral bleeding; it appreciates the vascularity and the relation of the tumor to the conus; finally, it contributes in 100% of the cases. It also rules out other pathologies and leads to a presumptive histopathologic diagnosis.[5]

Myelography, with or without postmyelographic CT scan, is always helpful but is more invasive than MRI, yields less information, and is done only if MRI is contraindicated. In our series spinal cord angiography was performed only once: the tumor was very vascular, and the angiography was followed by embolization of the feeding vessels.

MANAGEMENT DECISIONS

The diagnosis of a CET necessarily mandates operative removal following an exhaustive general and neurologic evaluation of the patient.

In young patients, if the diagnosis of neurinoma or neurofibroma is suspected, signs of neurofibromatosis must be sought. If several criteria of the disease are found, an extensive exploration of the central and peripheral nervous systems is required.

The functional problems and prognosis have to be precisely described to the patient and his or her relatives, and the expectations must be realistic. Patients harboring minor neurologic impairment must be aware that neurologic deterioration may result from the operation, and in all cases a hospitalization in a rehabilitation center will probably be necessary. Sphincter dysfunction is the least likely symptom to improve after surgery if it has existed for several weeks, and may be amplified or appear postoperatively. As in intramedullary spinal tumors, the final outcome depends on the preoperative neurologic status of the patient. Since those tumors are nearly always benign, there is no alternative treatment to surgery; the goals of the operation are tumor removal and preservation or improvement of neurologic function.

Technical Adjuncts to Tumor Removal

The ultrasonic aspirator is less useful than in spinal cord tumors and may be dangerous especially between S2 and S5, where the nerve roots are tightly applied to the tumor.

Laser can be used with low intensity, but classical microsurgery tools and optic magnification are usually sufficient.

Intraoperative stimulation of motor roots may be used for their identification when they are surrounded by tumor tissue,[6] and evoked potential recordings are sometimes used, but they also are far less effective than in spinal cord tumors, and there is no evidence that they improve patient outcome.

SURGICAL TECHNIQUE

Surgery of CET requires 3 to 8 hours, and the patient is positioned prone on soft cushions, avoiding compression of the belly. A bladder catheter is always inserted, and large venous infusion takes place. The head must be kept in flexion to avoid massive loss of CSF.

The incision is median and must be 5 cm above and below the tumor limits.

Laminotomy must be performed systematically in infants and young adults, with reconstruction of a normal anatomy by reinserting the posterior processes; this procedure prevents growth deformation in the young but also decreases the postoperative pain and the frequency of CSF leaks (Fig. 156-1).

The dura mater may be absent in large ependymomas, and caution must be exercised not to injure the roots during the laminotomy. In the event of reoperation, laminectomy is unavoidable. Dura opening must allow for control of the tumor extremities (Fig. 156-2), and the dura is fixed with stitches to the muscles. Dividing of the tumor under optic magnification can begin. The best way to proceed is to start at the upper limit of the tumor (Fig. 156-3) and proceed inferiorly to the lower (Fig. 156-4) and to finish at the central part of the tumor (Fig. 156-5). This strategy allows optimal root control. Most of the roots are pushed against the dura by the tumor. Tumors of the filum terminale displace the roots on the right and left sides of the spinal canal but may develop between the roots, covering and hiding them. It is important to identify the filum, and stimulation can help in doing this.

Since the surgical objective is complete tumor removal, operative biopsy is of little value. Small-size tissue specimens

FIGURE 156-1 Schematic drawings illustrating surgical approach via laminotomy. *A,* Lines of bone incision during laminotomy. Area of removal includes the spinous process and the laminae. *B, C,* Two stages in surgical approach. 1, Spinous process; 2, projection of the tumor on the dura mater (dotted line); 3, the rostral and caudal flaps of the spinous process and laminae, which are lifted and will be replaced and fixed; 4, laminae; 5, cutting line of the laminae; 6, incision of the dura mater.

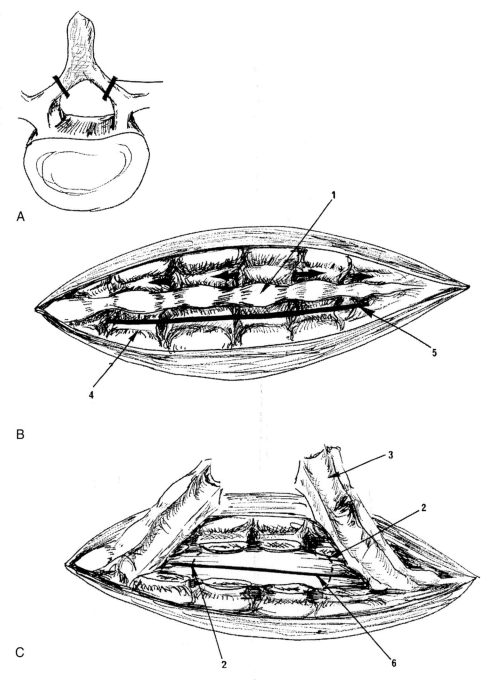

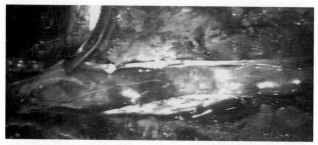

FIGURE 156-2   Operative view showing exposure of a cauda equina ependymoma after opening of the dura mater.

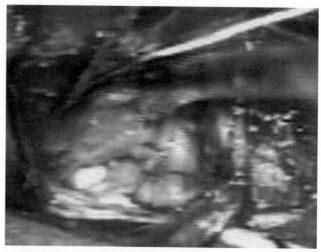

FIGURE 156-4   Operative view of the same case as Figures 156-2 and 156-3 showing debulking of the superior pole of the tumor.

only complicate the situation, and in hemorrhagic lesions it is difficult to distinguish between vascular tumors.

The upper part of the tumor sometimes grows into the lower conus, which has to be divided: the tumor does not usually invade the conus and can be separated from it. With large tumors, debulking is necessary; in such cases (mostly ependymomas), the tumor wall no longer exists and the tumor is always modified by intratumoral hemorrhage of different ages. The adjacent roots must be followed and preserved; bipolar coagulation must be used at a distance from them, and irrigation must be permanent. Of the sacral roots, the thinnest are the most exposed, and one or more is often injured during dissection. After complete tumor removal and careful hemostasis the dura is closed. A dural graft is often necessary.[7] The spine is reconstructed and the lumbar aponeurosis attached to the spinous processes. It is recommended that one leave some aponeurosis attachment during the opening to facilitate this type of closure (Fig. 156-6). The subcutaneous fat and skin are closed as usual. The use of tissue glue is left to the preference of the surgeon. All the removed material is sent for histopathologic examination.

After surgery the bladder catheter is left in situ for at least 3 days, and once the pain has grown less intense, the patient will be trained in self-catheterization until restoration of normal bladder function has been confirmed by urodynamic evaluation.

Pain is controlled with morphine at the early postoperative period. Specific treatment of deafferentation pain (antiepileptic, benzodiazepines, etc.) is instituted according to the type of discomfort described by the patient. Healing must be perfect by the time the patient is discharged to the rehabilitation facility.

An MRI evaluation must be scheduled 3 months after surgery and serves as the reference in long-term follow-up of the patient.

HISTOLOGIC FINDINGS AND THEIR CONSEQUENCES

Adult Pathology

Neurinomas (Schwannomas)

Schwannomas are the most common CET, composing nearly 50% of our series (mean age 51 ± 17 years). The time lapse between the first signs and the diagnosis is 2 years, and radiculopathy exists in nearly all cases, sometimes especially frequently during the night. Sphincter disturbance was present in 9% of patients, sexual dysfunction in 4.4%.

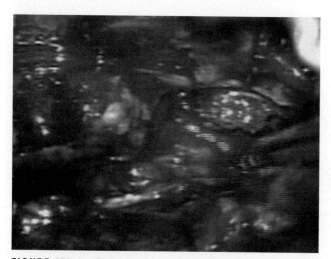

FIGURE 156-3   Operative view of the same case as Figure 156-2 showing debulking of the inferior pole of the tumor.

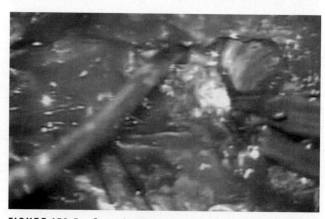

FIGURE 156-5   Operative view demonstrating lateral debulking of the tumor following a nerve root laterally.

FIGURE 156-6 Fixation of the opened lamina with wires. 1, Spinous process; 6, supraspinous ligaments; 7, the opened lamina is fixed with wires.

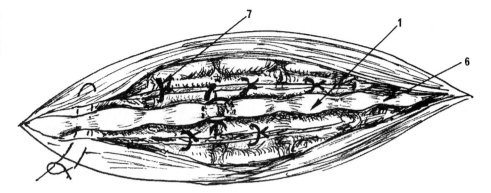

Paravertebral spasm was found in 50% of patients and some degree of motor or sensory deficit in one third of cases.

Neurinomas may develop purely inside the spinal canal or simultaneously in the foramen (hourglass type), which may cause an enlargement of the neural foramen seen on neuroimaging. On CT scan and MRI there is homogeneous enhancement (Figs. 156-7 and 156-8). The tumor is well encapsulated, and complete removal can be achieved in most cases. Magnification allows for identification of the rootlet bearing the tumor and preservation of the other roots (Fig. 156-9). The bearing rootlet is cut 1 cm above and 1 cm below the tumor, some very small satellite tumors or tumor extensions are at times in close proximity to the tumor. At 1 year postoperatively only 3.5% of patients still need a cane to walk and/or have sphincter dysfunction. Sexual disturbance is found in fewer than 1%. Of our 114 cases, 59% had a long-term follow-up (5–10 years), and recurrence occurred in only 1% after 1 year. If there is no recurrence after 2 years, the patient can be considered cured. No malignant transformation of a benign schwannoma has been established. The recurrence found in our series involved

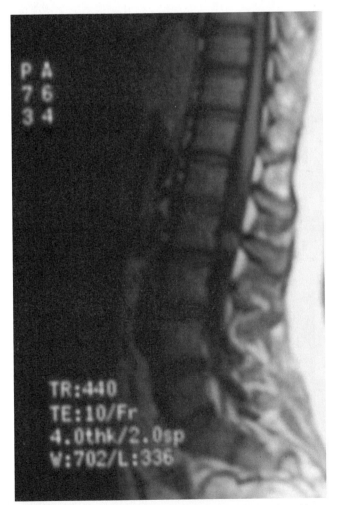

FIGURE 156-7 Sagittal T1-weighted MRI sequence without gadolinium of a benign neurinoma at the L2 level. The lesion is slightly hypointense to conus medullaris.

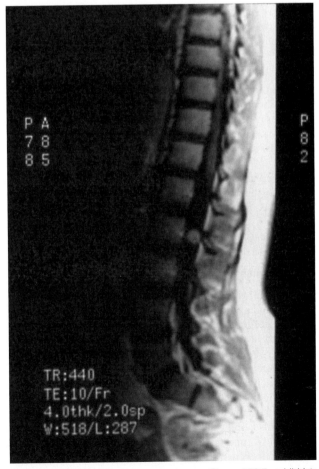

FIGURE 156-8 MRI of the same case as Figure 156-7, exhibiting strong homogeneous enhancement after contrast medium injection.

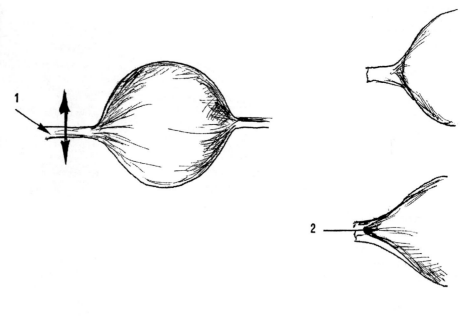

FIGURE 156-9 Diagram demonstrating the relation between the involved nerve root and the tumor. 1, The involved nerve root is cut proximal to the tumor; 2, tumor expansion inside the fascicle; 3, satellite tumor inside of the fascicle.

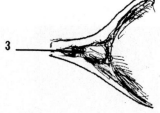

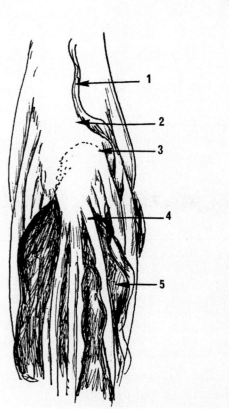

a patient with neurofibromatosis, and in such a special circumstance follow-up must last for years, mainly to detect new sites of the disease. Malignant neurinomas were found only in association with this disease and carry a very poor prognosis, since they are not responsive to any adjuvant therapy.

Neurofibromas are present only in association with neurofibromatosis[8] and are often found in several locations. Surgery requires the removal of several roots and gives poor results. It is the only form of CET requiring pure symptomatic medical management. Malignant evolution is possible and leads to death in a few months.

Ependymomas

The myxopapillary type of ependymoma is characteristic of the cauda equina and arises from the filum terminale below the conus, but in a few cases may develop from the distal part of the filum inside the sacrum[9,10] (Fig. 156-10).

It involves younger patients than those harboring neurinomas (34.6 ± 16 years), with a slight masculine predominance (61%), with the same time interval before diagnostic and for the same reasons: It is slow-growing and may reach giant proportions, filling the lumbar and sacral canal. This benign tumor is often hemorrhagic, with rupture of its walls, tumoral implants in other parts of the spinal canal, and even spread inside the skull: A complete MRI exploration of the central nervous system (CNS) is strongly recommended.[11,12]

FIGURE 156-10 Exposure of a cauda equina ependymoma. 1, Vessel; 2, conus terminalis; 3, projection of the rostral pole of the lipoma (dotted line); 4, dorsal root; 5, ependymoma.

Ependymomas represent 35% of the CET. They constitute a surgical challenge, and even with magnification it is often difficult to ensure that the removal is complete. This soft, brownish tumor follows the root's course, penetrating every cavity it may meet during its growth. Though of a benign histology, ependymomas are more likely to recur.

Clinically, the patient's bothersome symptoms are more severe than in schwannomas, with low back pain in 70%, radiculopathy in 75% bilaterally, sphincter disturbances in 14%, and sexual disturbances in 23%. Bilateral saddle anesthesia is found in 25%.

Scalloping is found on radiography in 22% of the cases. Many patients have had a CT scan performed one or several years before the diagnosis with normal results. This is because the level of the spine examined was below the level of the tumor, or is established because hypodense tumor had completely filled the dura and was not identified. MRI demonstrates a generally hypointense signal on T1-weighted sequences (Fig. 156-11) and a hyperintense one on T2-weighted sequences (Fig. 156-12), often with heterogeneity due to hemorrhage and cystic changes inside

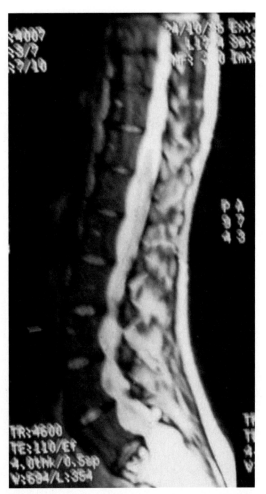

FIGURE 156-12 Sagittal T2-weighted MRI sequence of the same case as Figure 156-10. The tumor appears as hyperintense and slightly unhomogeneous. Scalloping at the L4, L5, and S1 levels is marked.

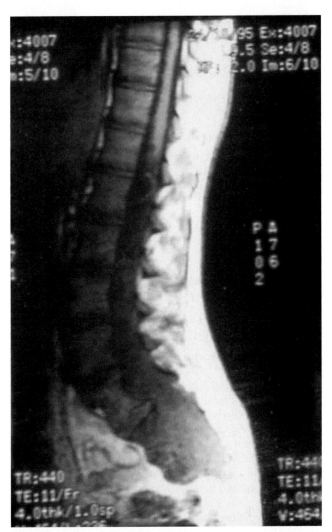

FIGURE 156-11 Sagittal T1-weighted MRI sequence without contrast sequence of a giant ependymoma, demonstrating a signal that is hypointense to conus medullaris.

the tumor. Those hemorrhages will appear as hyperintense on T1 sequences (Fig. 156-13). After gadolinium injection, enhancement is often homogeneous, except in hemorrhagic zones (Fig. 156-14). Large drainage veins exist and contribute to the identification of these hypervascularized lesions.

Total removal was achieved in 85% of the cases in our series. The clinical outcome is often problematic: 23% still have sphincter disturbance and 9% need help for walking after 1 year. Recurrences occurred in 14 cases (17%) 3 months to 25 years after the first surgical treatment. These cases always require reoperation because of neurologic deterioration, especially with respect to urinary and genital functions. Postoperative radiotherapy is no longer prescribed when total removal has been achieved, given the potential for late postradiotherapy complications in a young population. In case of recurrence, patients require reoperation and will often undergo radiation therapy. Irradiation is indicated in aggressive forms with early and multifocal recurrence.[13] No chemotherapy has been shown to be of value in these cases. Recurrences are not particularly more difficult to remove, but most of the time the clinical postoperative outcome will be worse than after the first operation, especially with reference to the sphincter and genital functions.

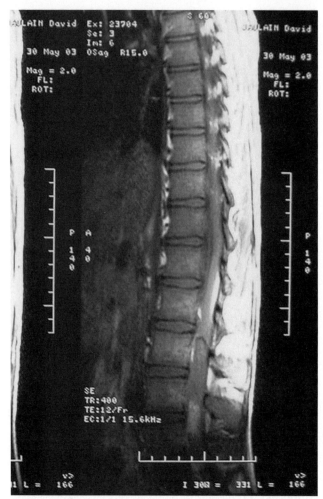

FIGURE 156-13 Sagittal T1-weighted MRI sequence without contrast medium. Ependymoma revealed by intratumoral bleeding.

Paragangliomas

Paragangliomas are benign tumors representing 3.8% of the tumors in our series.[1,2] In only one case did the tumor undergo malignant transformation.[14] They occur most commonly in the head and neck region and originate in the jugular glomus, deriving from the APUD system. They can be found nearly everywhere in the body. In the CNS, they can develop in the pineal or pituitary glands, in the cerebellopontine angle, and in the cauda equina and the filum terminale. There is a male predominance: 62% versus 38% (see reference 15). About 100 cases have been reported in the literature in the last 30 years. They involve adults and young people (mean age 49 years, spanning ages 13–70 years). There are no specific features, and these patients usually present with low back pain or sciatica or both. Functional hormonal activity has been described in only one case despite the neuroendocrine origin. On MRI the lesion is hypo- or isointense to the conus medullaris on T1-weighted sequences (Fig. 156-15) and hyperintense on T2, sometimes inhomogeneous, with cysts. There is a marked enhancement after injection of gadolinium (Fig. 156-16), and sometimes large vessels are seen around the tumor. Hemosiderin may be present, indicating previous hemorrhage. If performed, selective angiography demonstrates a highly vascular mass

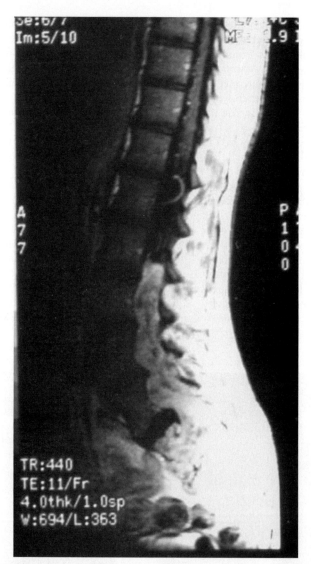

FIGURE 156-14 Sagittal T1-weighted MRI sequence of the same case as Figures 156-10 and 156-11, after gadolinium injection, demonstrating strong enhancement.

in the early arterial series, and selective embolization may simplify surgery. At surgery the tumor is a soft, red, well-circumscribed lesion originating from the filum (85%). Complete removal can generally be achieved, but in a few cases adherence to the conus or the root may leave some small remnants of tumor.

Distinguishing this tumor from an ependymoma may be difficult even in histopathology (pseudorosettes) and performed only after immunohistochemical and electron microscopy methods. The outcome is generally good, and recurrences are exceptional after complete resection. No adjuvant therapy is advised.

Hemangioblastomas compose less than 1% of our series of CETs. The clinical and radiologic presentation is like that of a paraganglioma.[16,17] Hypervascularity of the tumor may cause troublesome intraoperative bleeding. In one of our cases the procedure was stopped, the lesion embolized, and resection performed at a second stage (Figs. 156-17 through 156-19). This patient had a recurrence 3 years later, underwent reoperation, and is free of recurrence at 7 years, with

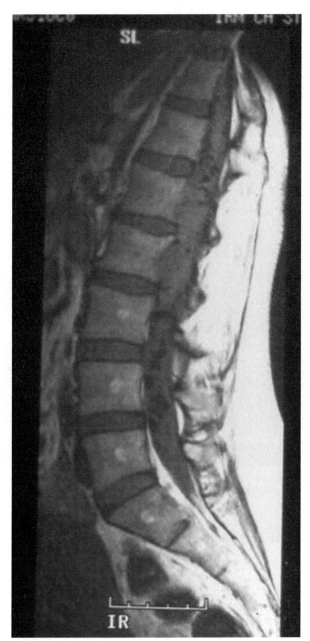

FIGURE 156-15 Sagittal T1-weighted MRI sequence, without gadolinium, of a paraganglioma at the L3 level, illustrating difficulties of differential diagnosis with neurinomas and ependymomas.

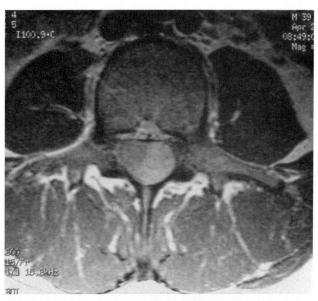

FIGURE 156-16 Axial T1-weighted MRI sequence of the same case as in Figure 156-15, after contrast injection.

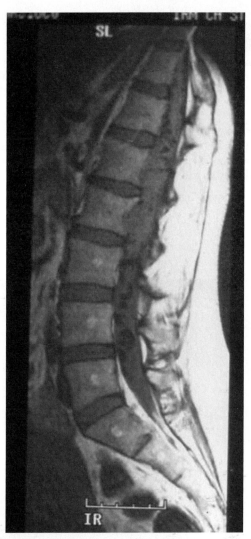

FIGURE 156-17 Sagittal T1-weighted MRI sequence without gadolinium of a hemangioblastoma exhibiting heterogeneity and particularly hyposignals due to drainage veins.

a good functional result. The origin of hemangioblastomas is not clearly established and may not be associated with von Hippel-Lindau disease.[18]

Malignant neurinomas and neurofibromas are always seen in association with neurofibromatosis and carry a very poor functional prognosis.

Metastasis to the Cauda Equina

These are not true cauda equina tumors.[19,20] Multiple localizations taking the form of a "bunch of grapes" are the rule, with dissemination along the roots, and strong gadolinium enhancement on MRI (Fig. 156-20). Sometimes these tumors arise during the evolution of another tumor of the CNS that spreads inside the CSF (ependymoma, pineal

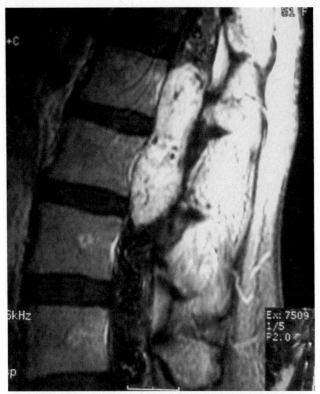

FIGURE 156-18 Sagittal T1-weighted MRI sequence of the same case as Figure 156-17, exhibiting strong enhancement after gadolinium injection.

tumor, medulloblastoma). Surgery is seldom indicated, and its main purpose is to establish a histopathologic diagnosis. Radiotherapy is nearly always indicated, and chemotherapies are adapted to the histology.

Miscellaneous Tumors

An isolated case of chordoma of the filum was reported in 2002.[21]

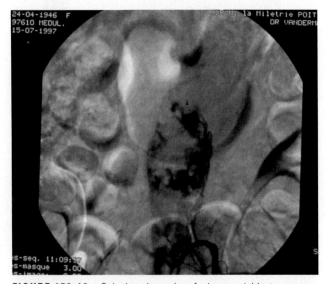

FIGURE 156-19 Spinal angiography of a hemangioblastoma case, showing a hypervascular lesion.

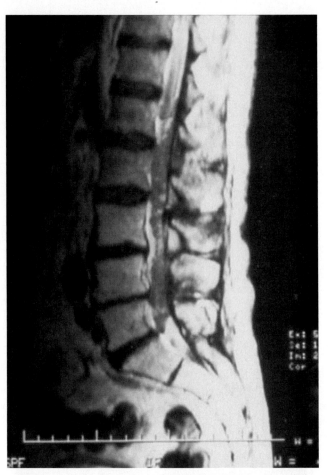

FIGURE 156-20 Sagittal T2-weighted MRI sequence of a multiple leptomeningeal metastasis case, demonstrating dissemination on the roots.

Infant and Child Pathology

Some tumors involve young patients and are often associated with a dysraphic state, either apparent or occult. It is often difficult to interpret pain and neurologic signs in this population, secondary disturbance of the walk being too often correlated with shoe problems rather than to their exact cause. Pes cavus foot deformities and scoliosis are attributed to hereditary or obscure congenital origin; mild amyotrophies and cramps are often misinterpreted. The occurrence of bilateral sciatica in a child without trauma should lead to a neuroradiologic examination. In very young children, sphincter disturbances are often ignored.

Very often the existence of a subcutaneous lipoma, dermal sinus or sinus tract, deviation of the gluteal cleft, flame nevus, hyperpigmentation, or hypertrichosis on the middle line of the back will lead to MRI and the diagnosis of the dysraphism, tethered cord, and/or tumor.

Lipomas are often associated with a large subcutaneous lumbar mass in infants and newborns. On MRI the lipomatous structure is hyperintense on T1-weighted sequences (Fig. 156-21) and hypointense on T2 (Fig. 156-22). Lipomas[22] evolve slowly, and one of the primary aims of surgery is to untether the cord. There is no consensus about the ideal age for surgery, but it has also been established that fully constituted sphincter disturbances occurring during the child's growth are not likely to disappear, and so, for many

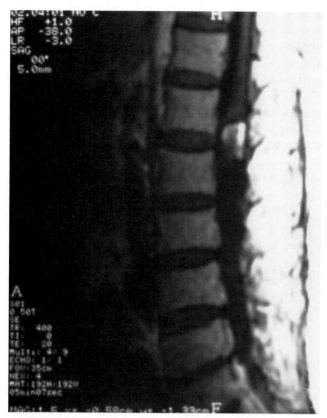

FIGURE 156-21 Lipoma associated with an epidermoid cyst. This lipoma demonstrates a hyperintense signal on this sagittal T1-weighted MRI sequence without contrast medium.

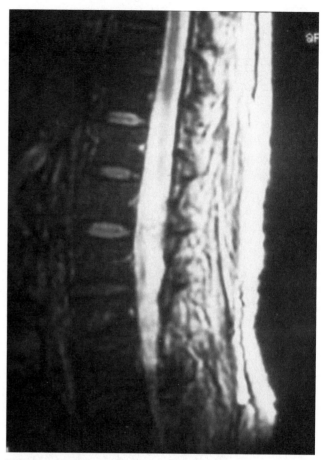

FIGURE 156-22 In the same case as Figure 156-21, the lipoma disappears on this sagittal T2-weighted MRI sequence. Behaving like CSF, the epidermoid cyst is difficult to detect on both MRIs.

surgeons, the earlier the surgery the better. Others prefer to operate only when there is clinical deterioration.

The surgeon must be aware that these tumors always involve the conus medullaris and that the interface between the conus and tumor is intimate and extensive (Fig. 156-23). There always exists a dura defect the location of which may indicate that of cauda equina roots. The lipoma is attached to the distal extremity of the conus, to its dorsal aspect, or else to both.

Nerve roots emerge laterally ventral to the lipoma-conus interface.

Dividing the lipoma from the conus often results in injury and lesions of the conus. On account of the same problems of interface of the lipomas with the roots, dissection must be cautious. The lipoma must be detached from the dura, but the lipoma removal must be limited to avoid root or conus damage. The goal of surgery is to release the cord and debulk the lipoma. A dura graft is then inserted, and laminoplasty takes place. CSF leaks are the most common complication of this procedure and may require external lumbar drainage. Long-term follow-up for more than 20 years does not show evolution of the remnants of the lipoma. Late surgical failures are usually caused by retethering, requiring reoperation.

Dermoid Cysts

Usually dermoid and epidermoid tumors arise from the expansion of a dermal sinus but may be isolated when developing from congenital vestigium or occurring as the iatrogenic complication of implantation of viable dermal or epidermal structures through spinal needles, trocars, or when closing a myelomeningocele.[23]

Clinical presentation is unremarkable, but when a dermal sinus has been neglected, diagnosis is sometimes made at the time of infection of the tumor, which has become an abscess coexisting with bacterial meningitis (two cases in our series).[24] These children are often in poor condition, are operated on emergently, and often have severe sphincteric disturbances.

On MRI, the tumor appears as hypointense on T1-weighted sequences and hyperintense on T2-weighted ones as compared with the conus medullaris, behaving like CSF. CT scan will help in documenting the fatty composition of the tumor.

At surgery these tumors are fatty and include hair and sometimes nails. Total removal can usually be achieved, and the prognosis is good. Dissemination to the CNS may exist, but most of the time this dissemination comprises fatty droplets, with no evolution.

Teratomas

Teratomas are found in the same circumstances as dermoid cysts and can be removed. In all cases, dysraphy has to be treated during the same procedure.

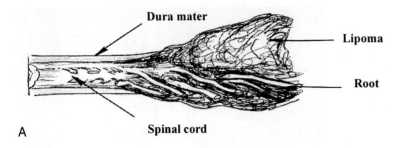

FIGURE 156-23 Schematic drawings of the three types of cauda equina lipomas. *A,* Caudal type. *B,* Dorsal type. *C,* Mixed type.

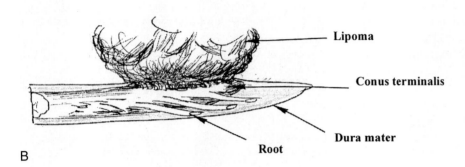

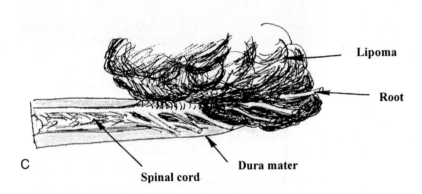

LONG-TERM EVOLUTION AND FOLLOW-UP

In our series of CETs no operative or early mortality occurred. The intermediate mortality (1–5 years) and long-term mortality (>5 years) involved three patients: One malignant schwannoma presented after 2 years, one patient committed suicide, and one patient died of an intercurrent disease.

Functional results have already been reported with each type of tumor but, mainly in ependymomas, recurrence will increase the percentage of sphincter or genital disturbances and during the follow-up 11% of the patients acquired those disturbances.

Postoperative spinal deformity is prevented by laminotomy. In two cases, however, we observed lumbar kyphosis with no functional consequence. Laminotomy cannot be repeated at reoperation, and extensive laminectomy may be responsible for disorders of spinal stability and lumbar pain in the long-term follow-up. No severe spinal deformities occurred in our series, probably because laminotomy was performed on young patients. After laminectomy, kyphosis and kyphoscoliosis are the most common deformations.

Pain is uncommon after 1 year, with complaints related to the low back region in half of cases and radicular pain in the other half, with deafferentation and paresthesias pain.

Neuroradiologic Follow-up

Magnetic resonance imaging is the examination of choice for follow-up. It must include T1- and T2-weighted sequences after contrast T1-weighted sequences, and at least two perpendicular planes (sagittal and axial), and involve the whole CNS except in solitary schwannomas. Early MRI is contributive only if carried out in the 2 days following surgery. Postoperative changes often consist in linear or more extensive contrast enhancement "nontumoral fibrosis," which can mimic or suggest tumor recurrence: Comparison of serial MRI scans, carried out twice a year, enables one to make the right diagnosis. For ependymomas there is no consensus about the duration of the follow-up, since very late recurrences do exist. In all cases, patients and their relatives must be aware of this eventuality and contact their neurosurgeon if functional signs reappear.

CONCLUSIONS

Cauda equina tumors generally carry a favorable prognosis: Most of these tumors are benign, and the aim of treatment is to restore function and prevent recurrences. In our series, no postoperative or short-term deaths could be found. The one death during the 3 postoperative years was that of a patient with a malignant neurinoma. Five years after surgery, 92% of the patients were alive, while 3.8% of patients with ependymomas had died (two). The one suicide was in connection with a neurologic handicap. Very few patients needed adjuvant therapy.

REFERENCES

1. Lapierre F, Bataille B, Vandermarcq P, et al: Tumeurs de la queue de cheval chez l'adulte. Neurochirurgie. 45:29–38, 1999.
2. Wager M, Lapierre F, Blanc JL, et al: Cauda equina tumors: A French multicenter retrospective review of 231 adult cases and review of the literature. Neurosurg Rev 23:119–129, 2000.
3. Russell DS, Rubinstein LJ: Pathology of the Tumors of the Nervous System, first edition London: Edward Arnold, 1990.
4. Cordan T, Bekar A, Yaman O, et al: Spinal subarachnoid hemorrhage attributable to schwannoma of the cauda equina. Surg Neurol 51:373–375, 1999.
5. Hahn M, Hirschfeld A, Sander H: Hypertrophied cauda equina presenting as an intradural mass: Case report and review of literature. Surg Neurol 49:514–519, 1998.
6. Sala F, Krzan MJ, Deletis V: Intra-operative neurophysiological monitoring in pediatric neurosurgery: Why, when, how? Childs Nerv Syst 18:264–287, 2000.
7. Tindall GT, Cooper PR, Barrow DL: The Practice in Neurosurgery, 1st ed. Baltimore: Williams & Wilkins, 1996.
8. Nadkarni TD, Rekate HL, Coons SW: Plexiform neurofibroma of the cauda equina. J Neurosurg (Spine). 91:112–115, 1999.
9. Ricket CH, Kedziora O, Gullotta F: Ependymoma of the cauda equina. Acta Neurochir (Wien) 141:781–782, 1999.
10. Fourney DR, Fuller GN, Gokaslan ZL: Intraspinal extradural myxopapillary ependymoma of the sacrum arising from the filum terminale externa. J Neurosurg (Spine) 93:322–326, 2000.
11. Gelabert-Gonzales M, Prieto-Gonzales A, Abdulkader-Nallib I, et al: Double ependymoma of the filum terminale. Childs Nerv Syst 17:106–108, 2001.
12. Hallacq P, Labrousse F, Streichenberg N, et al: Bifocal mixopapillary ependymoma of the terminal filum: The end of a spectrum? J Neurosurg 9(Suppl 3):288–289, 2003.
13. Lonjon M, Von Langsdorf D, Lefloch S, et al: Analyse des facteurs de récidive et rôle de la radiothérapie dans les épendymomes du filum terminale. Neurochirurgie 47:423–429, 2001.
14. Kulkarni AV, Bilbao JM, Cusimano MC, et al: Malignant transformation of ganglioneuroma into a spinal neuroblastoma in an adult. J Neurosurg 88:324–327, 1998.
15. Aghani N, George B, Parker F: Paraganglioma of the cauda equina region—Report of 2 cases and review of the literature. Acta Neurochir (Wien) 141:81–87, 1999.
16. Tibbs RE, Harkey HL, Raila FA: Hemangioblastoma of the filum terminale: Case report. Neurosurgery 14:221–223, 1999.
17. Nowak DA, Gumprecht H, Blumenta C: Intraneural growth of a capillary haemangioma of the cauda equina. Acta Neurochir (Wien) 142:463–468, 2000.
18. Brisman JL, Borges LF, Ogilvy CS: Extramedullary hemangioblastoma of the conus medullaris. Acta Neurochir (Wien) 142:1059–1062, 2000.
19. Locke J, True LD: Isolated carcinoid tumor of the terminal filum. J Neurosurg (Spine) 94:313–315, 2001.
20. Maxwell M, Borges LF, et al: Renal cell carcinoma: A rare source of cauda equina metastasis. J Neurosurg (Spine) 90:129–132, 1999.
21. Bayar MA, Erdem Y, Tanyel O, et al: Spinal chordoma of the filum terminale. J Neurosurg (Spine) 96:236–238, 2000.
22. Chapman P, Stieg PE, Magge S: Case problems in neurosurgical surgery: Spinal lipoma controversy. Neurosurgery 44:186–193, 1999.
23. Kanev PM, Park TS: Dermoids and dermal sinus of the spine. Neurosurg Clin N Am 6:359–365, 1995.
24. Calvit MF, Guzman A: Timing of surgery in patients with infected spinal dermal sinuses: Report of two cases. Childs Nerv Syst 11:129–132, 1995.

157 Tethered Cord Syndrome in the Adult

R. SHANE TUBBS and W. JERRY OAKES

INTRODUCTION

The tethered cord syndrome (TCS) is essentially fixation of the spinal cord from multiple pathologic entities, thus not allowing normal physiologic motion of this component of the central nervous system. Most of the conditions resulting in TCS are congenital. Those that occur after surgery or injury are not discussed here. The two issues addressed here can be divided into primary tethered cord (i.e., occult spinal dysraphism [OSD]) and secondary tethered cord (i.e., fixation of the spinal cord at the site of previous myelomeningocele repair). This chapter focuses on the tethered cord related to OSD. The primary problem with this condition is not the technical aspects of detethering the spinal cord but in recognizing which patients are at risk of having these problems and what are the earliest possible symptoms and signs that would allow their discovery. Primary TCS, if detected in early infancy and operated on, is likely to yield a neurologically intact child who will have the potential for a normal life. However, most adults who are discovered to have OSD will present with neurologic deficits that are generally not reversible and/or life-altering pain that may be slow to resolve postoperatively.

EMBRYOLOGIC CONSIDERATIONS

Differentiating the extremes of normal from minimal pathologic states is one of the most difficult aspects for the clinician. When the TCS was first described, clinically devastated patients with extreme caudal displacement of the conus medullaris into the sacrum from a thickened and unyielding filum terminale were easily differentiated from normal.[1,2] One important issue regarding a normally positioned conus is where should the "normal" conus reside? To some clinicians, below the L1–2 disc space is abnormally low, whereas to others, below the inferior border of L2 is abnormally displaced. This is confounded by the fact that the conus, which normally has an anteroposterior diameter ranging from 5.0 to 8.0 mm, at times has no definite tip but gradually tapers to a very thick filum.

The human embryo has a distinct tail bud that gradually regresses, and by 30 to 35 mm (9 weeks), it is no longer present externally.[3] The tip of the vertebral coccygeal segments contains an epidermal cell rest, the coccygeal medullary vestige (caudal cell mass). Secondary neurulation involving this inferiorly placed epidermal cell rest seemingly only gives rise to the filum terminale and ventriculus terminalis, which may be identified at stages 18 to 20 (days 43 to 48), at which time it lies adjacent to the coccyx. This ependymal-lined dilatation of the central canal contains neuronal degenerative tissue. The filum terminale is created when the caudal neural tube regresses (retrogressive differentiation) between the ventriculus terminalis and the coccygeal medullary vestige and is first seen at stage 23 (day 52). The distal conus may also arise from the process of secondary neurulation.

Distally, the filum (internal filum terminale) travels to fuse with the dorsal dura mater, usually in the midline, and then continues with this dural sheath as the coccygeal ligament (external filum terminale) to the dorsal coccyx. Historically, in the term infant, the inferior tip of the conus medullaris was described as being located at the L2–3 interspace in 98% of cases and at the L3 level in 1.2% of cases. Presumably, by 3 months of age, the tip of the conus achieved its adult position by "ascending" to the L1–2 interspace. Wilson and Prince[4] have concluded that a conus positioned at L2–3 should be considered normal at any age. Reimann and Anson[5] have compiled both their data and those from three other large series (a total of 801 adult spinal cords) to find that the conus medullaris is found above the L2–3 disc level in approximately 94% of cases, whereas the mean conus lies at the lower third of the L1 vertebrae. Saifuddin and colleagues[6] have also found that the mean termination of the conus is at the lower third of the L1 vertebrae.

It would be logical then to assume that tight fixation of the cord by the filum during in utero development would result in the most caudal position of the conus but that lesser degrees of tension would allow some cephalad migration. It might even be possible that mild tension on a relatively elastic cord could result in a relatively normal position of the conus but with enough microtrauma, over time, that the patient might not become overtly symptomatic until adult life. The degree of caudal descent of the conus might be less impressive in this case and yet the patient becomes symptomatic from intermittent traction and injury, especially spinal flexion, during normal daily activities.

PRESENTATION

The common clinical presentations of OSD include the presence of a cutaneous signature (59%), neurogenic bladder with the development of primary or secondary incontinence or urinary tract infection (18%), leg or foot weakness (12%), leg or foot length discrepancy (6%) (Fig. 157-1), foot deformity (pes cavus, claw toes), and nondermatomal back and leg pain (6%).[7-12] Nonradicular pain is by far the most common chief complaint in adults with OSD and is often seen with physical exertion.

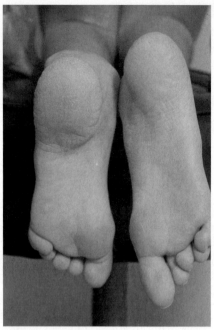

FIGURE 157-1 Foot length discrepancy in a 55-year-old adult with tethered cord syndrome.

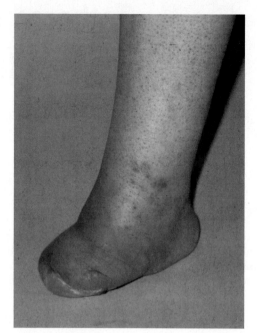

FIGURE 157-3 An additional case of foot amputation in an adult with tethered cord syndrome who had a chronic history of insensation of the left lower extremity distal to the knee.

The weakness seen from distal spinal cord fixation usually has a combination of both upper and low motor neuron signs. Typically, the patient might have decreased muscle bulk (Fig. 157-2) and increased or pathologic reflexes. The combination of both upper and lower motor neuron weakness in the legs should alert the examiner to the possibility of this clinical entity. Much later in the clinical course, rectal incontinence and the occurrence of insensitive foot ulceration may occur (Fig. 157-3). Scoliosis in isolation is an unusual presentation for TCS (Fig. 157-4). Further, Yamada and colleagues[11] examined 40 adult patients with TCS and found 53% with an accentuation of their lumbosacral lordosis.

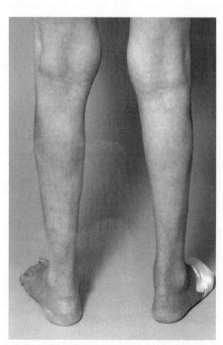

FIGURE 157-2 Atrophy of the leg musculature in a 75-year-old woman with tethered cord syndrome. Note the forefoot amputation on the right side.

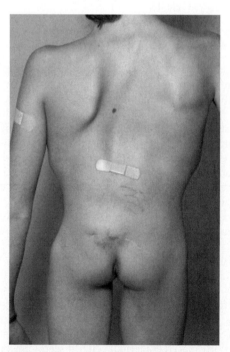

FIGURE 157-4 Severe atrophy of the lower extremities notably in the gluteal musculature. This patient presented with a history of scoliosis and at operation was found to have a fatty infiltrated filum terminale.

ASSESSMENT

Ideally, spinal cord tension and elasticity could be measured and assessed in an objective manner. Currently, that is not technically possible in a noninvasive clinical manner. Therefore, we must rely on more indirect measures such as cord position with magnetic resonance imaging (MRI). If the position of the conus is indeterminate (L3) or even above the L2–3 disc space, one can still look for other associated findings to help explain clinical symptoms. Small accumulations of fat within the filum may be seen in 6% of the normal population but in more than 90% of patients symptomatic from TCS.[13] This finding alone should alert the clinician. Almost all patients with TCS will have bony spina bifida occulta in the low lumbar and/or sacrum. This finding is also seen in a small percentage of the normal population, but when present in a symptomatic patient, TCS must again be entertained. Less clear is the genetic predisposition for the occurrence of open neural tube defects with siblings who have one of the more occult forms of spinal dysraphism. It has also been reported that multiple siblings with TCS have occurred together with parents who both were shown to have bony spina bifida occulta in the lumbosacral area.[14] Bony spina bifida occulta is seen in approximately 4% of the population.

PHYSICAL EXAMINATION

Cutaneous signatures of OSD (midline capillary hemangioma, subcutaneous lipoma, dermal sinus tract, epithelial appendage, focal hirsutism, and an atretic meningocele) (Figs. 157-5 through 157-10) are strong evidence of an underlying problem. Unfortunately, these are present in only about half of patients with isolated TCS from a tight filum terminale.[12] Of particular interest are the capillary hemangioma and epithelial appendage, which are more likely

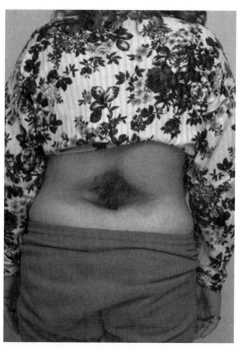

FIGURE 157-6 Adult female patient with a history of severe back pain. Note the area of focal hirsutism, which was found to be associated with a split cord malformation.

to have TCS from a tight filum terminale when seen in isolation. Cutaneous angiomas ordinarily found in other parts of the body are unusual for the lumbosacral region (see Fig. 157-5). In this area, they have been associated with OSD and are often found in conjunction with other skin findings, such as focal hirsutism and subcutaneous lipomas. Capillary hemangiomas are thought to be the least sensitive indicator of intradural pathology with an approximately 10% incidence of associated intradural anomalies when seen in the

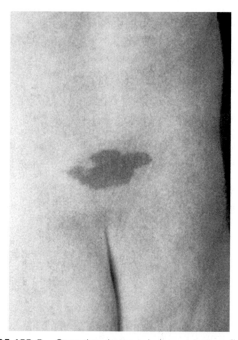

FIGURE 157-5 Operative photograph demonstrates a flat capillary hemangioma of the midline lumbar spine. This patient was found to harbor a conus medullaris at the S1 vertebral level and a thickened fatty filum terminale.

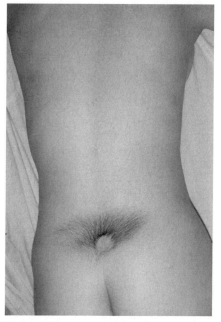

FIGURE 157-7 A female patient with two cutaneous signatures. Note the area of hypertrichosis and a centered atretic meningocele.

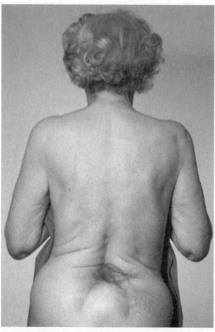

FIGURE 157-8   An elderly patient with a history of leg length discrepancy, urinary dysfunction, and back pain. Note the subcutaneous mass and area of focal hirsutism. This patient was found to have a lipomyelomeningocele with dorsally tethering bands (meningocele manqué).

lumbar region.[10] Some authors admonish the use of capillary and cavernous to describe hemangiomas because they both arise from the same cell type. Dorsal or ventral bands (meningocele manqué) have more of a predilection to be seen with focal hirsutism (see Fig. 157-6) in association with the split cord

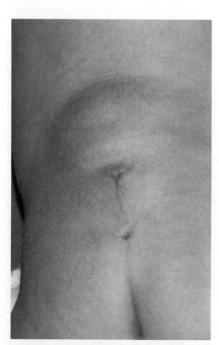

FIGURE 157-9   A patient found to have a subcutaneous mass and dermal sinus. At operation, both a dermal sinus tract and dorsal lipoma of the cord were found.

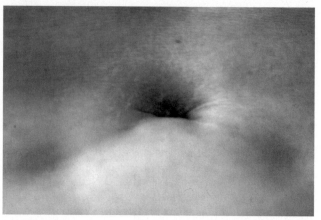

FIGURE 157-10   A large dermal sinus on the midline lumbar back of a 50-year-old man with back pain and increased sensory deficit of the lower extremities.

syndrome or with an atretic meningocele (see Fig. 157-7) without the split cord.

Examination of the paravertebral muscles in patients with TCS will not be observed to spasm as in patients with disc herniation unless these entities coexist. Progressive arching of the feet is often seen in the adult with TCS and should be evaluated as should lower extremity size discrepancies (see Fig. 157-1). The clinician should evaluate for hypalgesia of the lower extremities in patients with potential TCS. This sensory disturbance is often found to be in a patchy distribution. Muscle weakness must be evaluated. On digital rectal examination, the external anal sphincter is often found to be weak in these patients. Straight leg raises are often normal in patients with TCS.[11]

SURGICAL DECISION MAKING

The natural history of a low-lying conus from a fatty infiltrated and thickened filum terminale is now accepted to be progressive loss of neurologic function, usually over years. This knowledge, together with the low risk of surgical intervention and high likelihood of cure with a single procedure, justify operation. Since the inception of the term *tethered spinal cord*, most have intuitively accepted that a spinal cord that is placed under caudal stresses must be located distal to its normal anatomic termination (i.e., L1–2 vertebral levels). As discussed previously, most authorities have declared radiographic coni located inferior to the L2 vertebral level and in patients with symptoms of lower spinal cord dysfunction as abnormally low and thus tethered. This inevitably leads to operative intervention via a detethering procedure. However, we have previously described a series of 13 patients in whom symptoms of a tethered spinal cord were evident clinically, yet radiologically the conus medullaris was found to lie at a widely acceptable normal anatomic site.[15,16] In fact, after a review of the extant literature before our publication in 1993, several authors had operated on patients for symptoms of a distally tethered spinal cord in whom a conus was either retrospectively or prospectively found to terminate at a "normal" vertebral level. This entity is discussed in more detail later. Justifying or entertaining surgical treatment for bona fide symptoms of a tethered cord seems appropriate considering that some authors advocate operative intervention for patients who are asymptomatic and are merely found to have fat within the filum terminale.

Fatty Filum Terminale

The filum terminale is a structure usually less than 2 mm wide. If it is insufficiently elastic (e.g., abnormally thick, fat laden), this supposedly reduces the ability of the cord to move cephalad and thus places undue stress on the distal conus (Figs. 157-11 through 157-13). Incidental fat within the filum is seen in approximately 3.7% to 17% of the normal adult population.[12] In one series, fat was found in 91% of patients with a tethered spinal cord.[13] The lack of denticulate ligaments along the caudal cord (inferior to T12 spinal nerve) allows for less stability and thus more mobility if caudal forces are placed on it. Moreover, we have found that the denticulate ligaments, even cephalically, do little to abort either cranial or caudal traction on the spinal cord.[17] Supposed failure of involution of the terminal spinal cord and/or failure of the lengthening process of the filum terminale results in the syndrome of the "tight filum." This entity, first described by Garceau[1] in 1953, is extremely speculative and is diagnosed on a clinician's ability to interpret the filum terminale on sagittal MRI as being taut. Occasionally, this diagnosis is made at operation. This classification has unfortunately been used for both cases in which the tip of the conus medullaris is at normal and abnormal vertebral levels. In one series of tight filum terminale, the tip of the conus resided inferior to the L2 vertebral level in 86% of the cases (i.e., 14% had a conus at L2 or above).[3] The question to pose is whether a symptomatic patient (tethered spinal cord) can have a normally positioned conus medullaris and a "tight" filum terminale so that with various ranges of motion, an abnormal torque is placed on this thin connection to the conus, thereby stressing this caudal portion of the spinal cord containing sacral and coccygeal spinal segments without malpositioning it. The distal spinal cord becomes attenuated with flexion of the pelvis, and this biomechanical feature causes insult to the spinal cord during motion and increase

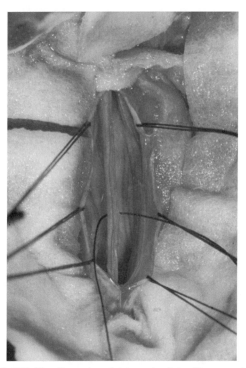

FIGURE 157-12 Operative photograph of the filum terminale in the patient described in Figure 157-11.

in stature. Flexion of the cervical spine has also been shown to increase the tension of the spinal dura mater.

Lipomatous involvement of the distal cord runs the gamut from small accumulations of fat in an otherwise normal filum to extensive involvement of the distal spinal cord. Terminal syrinx, neurenteric cyst, dermal sinus tract and intramedullary dermoid, and split cord malformation (SCM)

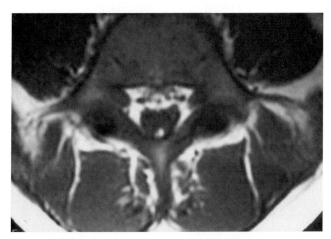

FIGURE 157-11 T1-weighted axial magnetic resonance image of the lumbosacral spine. Note the fatty infiltrated filum terminale. The conus medullaris in this patient was at the L4 vertebral level.

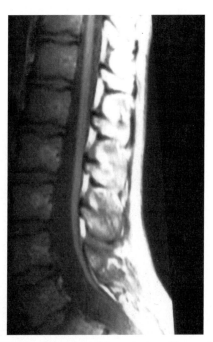

FIGURE 157-13 Elongation of the spinal cord in a patient with a fatty infiltrated filum terminale.

may all have an associated tight filum terminale, which must be sought at the time of surgical exploration.[1,2,7,14]

SPLIT CORD MALFORMATION

The two dominant radiographic characteristics of a type I lesion are the double dural tubes and the osseous or osseocartilaginous midline septa. The type I septa always reach from the posterior surface of the vertebral body to the corresponding neural arches. Rostrally, the hemicords stretch a variable distance (sometimes as much as seven vertebral levels) before rejoining. Here the two hemicords are rostral to the median dural sleeve and therefore reside in a single thecal sac.

Lateral ventral and dorsal nerve roots are frequently seen on the axial computed tomographic myelography and less so on the axial MRI. Occasionally, paramedian dorsal roots are also discernible on computed tomographic myelography or MRI as fine lines stretching between the medial aspect of the hemicords and the median dural sleeve.

The two dominant radiographic characteristics of a type II SCM are the single thecal sac housing the full length of the split segments and the nonrigid (nonosseous and noncartilaginous) nature of the median septum (Figs. 157-14 and 157-15). Because there is crossover regarding these two features between type I and II lesions, the SCM cannot always be classified radiographically before surgery.

When discernible, the type II septum is always at the caudal extreme of the split cord where the hemicords appeared to be closely opposed with the septum and with each other before rejoining into a single structure. In general, the hemicords in a type II lesion are much closer together and the split segment is much shorter than in a type I lesion. This correlation between hypertrichosis and SCM is probably higher than any other combination of cutaneous abnormality and underlying spinal cord lesion.

At least one unrelated tethering lesion (i.e., fatty filum) is found in all lumbosacral and lower thoracic SCMs and in a much smaller number of cervical SCMs. The entire neuraxis should be studied radiographically and if a second tethering

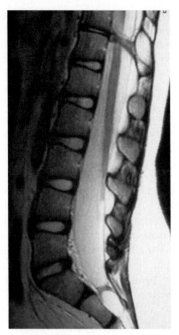

FIGURE 157-15 T2-weighted sagittal magnetic resonance imaging of the lumbosacral spine of the patient described in Figure 157-14. Note the bony septation dividing the spinal canal into two compartments.

lesion is found, it should be treated.[8] The surgical outcome is generally excellent for SCM. The overall surgical morbidity is low but slightly higher with type I lesions (Fig. 157-16).

The radiographic data on the split lengths when correlated with age, lesion type, and level of the septum are compatible with the hypothesis of an endomesenchymal tract transfixing the neural plate during early development of the neural tube.

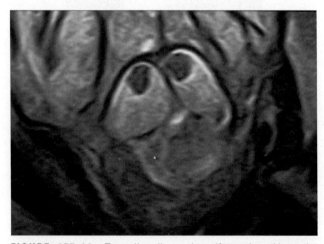

FIGURE 157-14 Type II split cord malformation. Note the hemicords separated by a bony septation.

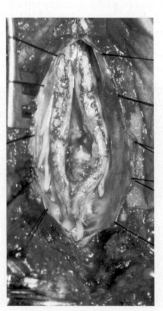

FIGURE 157-16 Operative photograph of the patient described in Figures 157-14 and 157-15. Note the two hemicords and the remains of the bony spicule.

LIPOMYELOMENINGOCELE

Lipomyelomeningocele emphasizes the two most important components of this lesion, which are fat within a dysmorphic conus medullaris. These patients will almost always have a cutaneous abnormality present at birth and tend to come to clinical attention within the first few months to years of life (see Fig. 157-9). There is a clear female-to-male predominance of approximately 1.5:1. The lesion itself is generally composed of a caudally descended conus medullaris infiltrated by fat that continues out of a dural, bony, and fascial defect to emerge as a skin-covered subcutaneous mass that is found in the lumbosacral region (Fig. 157-17). These lesions are frequently accompanied by other forms of occult dysraphism (distal syringomyelia, tethered spinal cord from a thickened filum terminale, dermal sinus tract, dermoid tumor, meningocele manqué, split cord anomaly, and neurenteric cyst).[8,10–12]

Lipomyelomeningoceles present little diagnostic difficulty in most patients. More than 90% will have an obvious soft-tissue swelling over the spine in the lumbosacral region. Associated cutaneous anomalies (dermal sinus tract [see Fig. 157-9], atretic meningocele, hemangioma, and focal hirsutism) are present in more than half of the patients. The typical lesion is fully skin covered with a nontender lumbosacral mass gently rising off the plane of the back. Patients may present with progressive asymmetrical foot deformities (commonly cavovarus but occasionally valgus deformities), foot length discrepancies, and atrophic ulcerations of the skin of the feet. Leg length discrepancy, scoliosis, and lower extremity weakness can all be seen as well. Lipomyelomeningocele is one of the few clinical problems that can have signs of both upper and lower motor neuron disturbances in the same lower extremity. The patient may have muscle wasting with increased tone and exaggerated deep tendon reflexes. If the muscle weakness is confined to the small muscles of the foot, the toes may be splayed. Asymmetrical weakness of the feet and legs is a hallmark of this condition.

Outside of childhood, patients are seen primarily for symptoms of neurogenic bladder. This may take the form of incontinence or repeated bouts of urinary infection. Rectal incontinence does not occur without accompanying urinary incontinence.

In the adult, pain may be the driving force to have the patient evaluated. The pain may be difficult to describe and may be radiating in nature but is rarely in a specific dermatome. There may be limitation of back mobility, especially during flexion. The symptoms related to lipomyelomeningoceles cover many medical specialties and vary with the age of the patient. The majority of patients have insidious problems that can be seen to progress for years. However, a smaller group presents with acute and sudden symptoms, usually weakness or urinary incontinence, which may not be reversible after intervention. Previously minimally symptomatic adult women seem to be at particular risk of the development of symptoms during pregnancy or when placed in the lithotomy position.

Radiographic Diagnosis

Plain spinal radiographs are almost always abnormal. The radiographic hallmark of the lipomyelomeningocele is the presence of a dorsal fusion defect in the lamina, or bony spina bifida. MRI is the imaging procedure of choice for lipomyelomeningoceles, and positioning the patient both prone and supine can detect movement of the spinal cord within the spinal canal and thus provides useful information concerning dorsal fixation of the cord, especially in the postoperative state.

Hydrocephalus is rarely associated with lipomyelomeningoceles, and the Chiari I malformation is seen in approximately 3% of patients.[7] Despite this lack of absolute proof, it is the belief of many neurosurgeons that patients with lipomyelomeningoceles have such a clear likelihood of worsening that prophylactic surgery is justified and recommended. One of the lines of persuasion that the natural history is a progressive loss of function is that older patients rarely present neurologically intact. If one looks at age groups and relates that to the degree of symptomatology, generally, the older the patient is, the more serious are the symptoms. Most neonates have normal neurologic function including urodynamic testing. Adolescents and adults are almost always neurologically disadvantaged. In the past, because of the reluctance of neurosurgeons to explore lipomyelomeningoceles deeply, the superficial aspect of a bulky lipoma might have been excised by a general surgeon. These superficial debulking procedures were the standard of practice through the mid-1970s. They were thought to be justified at the time because of the high risk of manipulating the intradural contents associated with resecting the lipoma and a lack of information on the natural history of the lesion. After a superficial operation, re-exploration is made much more difficult because of the inflammatory response from the previous procedure. Secondary resection of the intradural aspect of lipomyelomeningoceles is associated with an increased risk of iatrogenic injury to the neural elements. Today, there is no

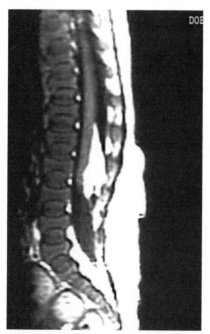

FIGURE 157-17 Intradural component of a lipomyelomeningocele as seen on T1-weighted sagittal magnetic resonance imaging of the lumbosacral spine.

justification for superficial excision of a lipomyelomeningocele alone.

NEURENTERIC CYST

Spinal neurenteric cysts are infrequently reported congenital abnormalities believed to be derived from an abnormal connection between the primitive endoderm and ectoderm during the third week of life. Neurenteric cysts are not confined to the spinal column (Figs. 157-18 and 157-19) but may be found within the brain, mediastinum, abdomen, pelvis, or even in a subcutaneous location. Intraspinal neurenteric cysts represent 0.3% to 0.5% of all spinal "tumors."[9] They are, in fact, not tumors, which differentiates them from teratomas; instead, they are more similar to hamartomas, i.e., displaced nests of endodermally derived tissue. The terminology for these lesions is problematic, as they have been reported as a neurenteric cysts, enterogenous cysts, enteric cysts, gastrocytomas, dorsal enteric fistulae, split notochord syndrome, and teratoid cysts (Fig. 157-20). Part of the confusion in naming these cysts is that they are not uniform; likely they exist as a spectrum of lesions. A consistent association between neurenteric cysts and other forms of OSD has not been reported. A neurenteric cyst is classically reported as a solitary lesion in the cervical region, located anterior or anterolateral to the cord. Bone abnormalities, if present, are likely to involve the anterior column. The most commonly reported location is cervical, followed by thoracic and lumbosacral positions. There is a slight male predominance of approximately 2:1, with the most common locations of the cyst being intradural, extramedullary, and anterior or anterolateral to the cord. The most challenging technical problem for this pathologic entity is that the surgeon is obligated to remove the entire wall of the cyst to avoid its reaccumulation.[9]

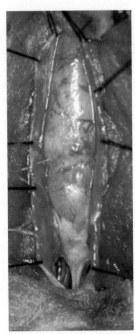

FIGURE 157-19 Operative photograph of a lumbosacral neurenteric cyst.

DERMAL SINUS TRACT

Chronic bouts of meningitis and meningitis involving unusual organisms should alert the clinician to the possibility of a portal connecting the skin to the craniospinal neuraxis. Dermal sinus tracts are seen primarily from the vertex of the skull to the coccyx. These entities are seen most commonly in the occipital region, although many are appreciated in the lumbosacral area (see Fig. 157-10). Cranial dermal sinus tracts normally travel inferiorly toward the deeper neural structures, whereas lumbosacral tracts ascend from their origin to destination. Coccygeal tracts "pits" normally end before the thecal sac and are therefore regarded as innocent. An approximate incidence of this form of OSD is one in 2500 births. Although seemingly benign structures, these small communications between the superficial and deep derivatives of the ectoderm can result in tragic insult to the central nervous system if not adequately addressed.

Perhaps reflecting a common ontogenic disorder, dermal sinus tracts are seen in 15% to 40% of split cord malformations. Approximately 60% of these tracts will

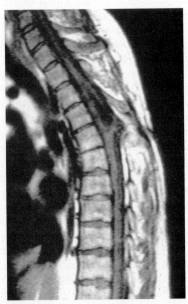

FIGURE 157-18 Magnetic resonance imaging of a patient with an operatively confirmed neurenteric cyst.

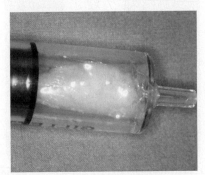

FIGURE 157-20 A syringe filled with the mucin-laden material removed from the patient shown in Figure 157-19.

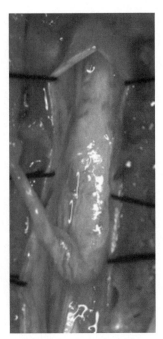

FIGURE 157-21 Operative image of a patient with a dermal sinus tract and intradural dermoid.

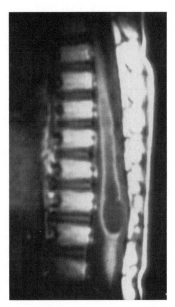

FIGURE 157-22 T1-weighted sagittal magnetic resonance imaging illustrates a terminal syrinx.

violate the spinal subarachnoid space, and of these, approximately one half will attach to the conus medullaris, cauda equina, or filum terminale (Fig. 157-21). The literature supports a small male preponderance. These connections between the skin and underlying structures usually occur in the midline but may be found in a paravertebral location. Common cutaneous findings seen in conjunction with dermal sinus tracts include flat capillary hemangiomas, focal hirsutism, subcutaneous lipomas, signs of local infection, and drainage of debris or fluid from the surface of a tract.[8,10] Many suggest prophylactic removal of all such defects.

Clinicians should have a high index of suspicion and perform a detailed physical examination of the skin of the craniospinal axis when antibiotic therapy is ineffective in treating patients with meningitis.

TERMINAL SYRINX

The term syringomyelia was introduced in 1827 by Ollivier d'Angers to describe a tubular collection of fluid within the spinal cord (Fig. 157-22). The term hydromyelia was introduced later. Hydromyelia refers to a fluid accumulation within the spinal cord that is partially lined with ependyma. A cavity that either does not communicate with, or is outside of, the central canal of the spinal cord is referred to as syringomyelia or more commonly a syrinx. These names were combined to form the term syringohydromyelia, which denotes the uncertainty that practitioners face in evaluating the location of these lesions on imaging. In reality, whether the fluid compartment does or does not have a partial lining of ependymal has little practical significance. The term terminal syrinx denotes a cavity found within the distal third of the spinal cord. A terminal syrinx is seen in 10% to 30% of patients with TCS. The terminal syrinx is usually a secondary result of other pathologic processes causing TCS.

Clinical Features

Symptoms of syringomyelia are easily grouped by the age of the patient at presentation. Because of the likelihood of multiple neurologic findings due to the complexity of the situation, the diagnosis of syringomyelia is often difficult. MRI has dramatically reduced the age at which patients are diagnosed and decreased the severity of their symptoms at presentation.

A common symptom complex of a syrinx consists of dissociated and suspended sensory loss, particularly with diminished pain and temperature appreciation and preservation of position sense and light touch. Lower motor neuron weakness of the hands and arms may also be seen. These patients may develop painless injury in the feet or legs depending on the level of the syrinx. In adults with syringomyelia, symptoms frequently progress. In the past, due to the chronic progressive nature of syringomyelia, earlier authors have categorized this as a chronic degenerative disease. This categorization is inappropriate because the process is often reversible if treated early and can usually be stabilized even when presenting with serious neurologic deficits.

Patients will often complain of numbness as their presenting symptom. It may appear to be radicular but is more commonly nondermatomal in nature. Symptoms tend to be asymmetrical, beginning distally and moving proximally. This is due to interruption or stretching of the crossing spinothalamic fibers in the anterior commissure of the spinal cord. This helps to explain the early involvement of pain and temperature appreciation and preservation of the noncrossing light touch and proprioception fibers. The patient may incur multiple injuries to the toes or feet with painless chronic ulceration. The patient may not appreciate the loss of pain and/or temperature sensation. Pain and temperature loss with the preservation of light touch and proprioception may occur with any intramedullary spinal cord lesion but is classically associated with a syrinx. As the syringomyelia progresses, the patient may develop dysesthetic pain that is often deep and occurs in a nonradicular distribution. It has variously been described as "itching," "burning," or "deep and boring."

The symptomatology, especially pain, may be worsened by Valsalva maneuvers. Patients may also complain of weakness of the lower extremities. As the disease progresses, atrophy of the lower extremities may develop. Late in the disease, the deep tendon reflexes may disappear and fasciculations may develop in the affected muscles. Signs of upper motor neuron disease such as spasticity and hyperreflexia may affect the lower extremities. The Babinski response is usually positive. Bowel or bladder control is usually not affected. The lack of bladder disturbance is such a standard feature that if present one should question the primary diagnosis. Primary spinal cord tumors invading the conus may affect sacral root function and secondarily produce a syrinx. This possibility should be considered if urinary incontinence is a prominent early feature of the patient's problem. Periodic limb movements may occur due to hyperexcitability of the spinal cord.

The progression of syringomyelia occurs in an unpredictable fashion, generally occurring over many years. Neurologic worsening may either be gradual or stepwise but rarely is precipitous. Using MRI in the acute postoperative period is of limited utility to evaluate the collapse of the syrinx, as it may take months for the syrinx to resolve.

Shunting of the syrinx alone has produced a poor long-term outcome. In the presence of a tethered cord, releasing the area of fixation and stenting the syrinx to the subarachnoid space appears to produce a better outcome than stent placement alone. Perhaps the most significant problem seen with the stent or shunt is the reaccumulation of fluid within the syrinx and a return of neurologic difficulty.

Outcomes vary significantly, depending on the time of intervention, nature of the TCS creating the syringomyelia, and location of the lesion. Asymptomatic patients may be followed, but outcome from treatment is directly related to preoperative disability. In adults especially, the collapse of the syrinx does not tightly correlate with the relief from the discomfort. Radiographic resolution of the syrinx does not mean the patient's symptoms are reversed. Patients with tethered spinal cords who undergo tethered cord release with or without syringosubarachnoid shunting will often have collapse of their syrinx.

MENINGOCELE MANQUÉ

Tethering bands from the spinal cord to the surrounding tissue are a rare anomaly. These bands known as meningocele manqué (*manqué*, "that which might have been but is not"; French for "missing") are found in association with multiple other elements of spinal dysraphism. These entities may be seen with MRI (Fig. 157-23) (linear and isointense with the spinal cord on T1-weighted images) but are frequently not appreciated owing to both their small size and loss between imaging slices. However, they are easily demonstrable at operation. These bands are generally composed of aberrant neural tissue with dorsal root ganglion cells, or fibrous tissue with even hamartomatous elements. They frequently penetrate the dura of an associated bony median septum or may simply exit dorsally or rarely ventrally. They need not

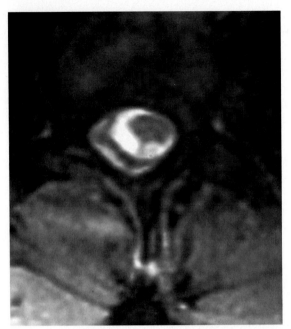

FIGURE 157-23   T2-weighted axial magnetic resonance imaging MRI demonstrates a dorsal tethering band (meningocele manqué).

be associated with a split cord anomaly and may occur distal to the site of spinal dysraphism. On occasion, they pierce the dura and terminate on the undersurface of the laminae. The surgeon should be aware of this condition when removing lamina during an operation on a patient with OSD so as to not inadvertently put tension on the underlying cord or cauda equina. Rarely, dorsal tethering bands are the only reversible pathologic processes seen. In the appropriate clinical setting, exploration of the intradural contents to search for these points of fixation is justified. Often though, retrospectively, it is difficult to determine whether a patient with other findings consistent with OSD and signs of a tethered spinal cord are symptomatic from meningocele manqué or other findings such as fatty filum terminale.[8,12]

Conus in "Normal" Position with Symptoms of a Tethered Cord

The term tethered to most clinicians implies abnormally positioned. Most definitions of normal level of cord termination, as already discussed, are based on the anatomic measurements of Barson,[18] who quite intuitively concluded that his findings in embryos were minimally inaccurate due to the hyperextension of the specimens during dissection. Many series have now shown that incontinence in children who essentially have normal MRI scans of the lumbosacral region and usually have cystometrographic findings indicative of a neurogenic bladder (hyperreflexic detrusor muscle) can be successfully treated by simple sectioning of the filum terminale.[19-24] Transection of the spinal cord superior to the conus medullaris results in an upper motor neuron bladder where the bladder acts automatically, independent of higher cortical centers. It empties when it is sufficiently distended to excite the reflex arc between the conus and the bladder wall.

When the injury is at the conus medullaris or inferior, this arc is interrupted and a flaccid, lower motor neuron bladder results.

Postulation of a tethered cord in the face of a normally positioned conus is thought to be the culprit of neurogenic hyperreflexic bladder by many. These series have had patients with both normal and minimally fat-infiltrated fila.[13,23,24] Improvement of bladder function in these series, in which the number patients ranged from 15 to 31, showed improvements of 58%, 44%, 59%, and 67% at 1, 26, 13, and 20 months, respectively. Most patients in these series demonstrated few if any elements of OSD. However, one should be clear that this is a diagnosis of exclusion and should be carefully considered.

In patients who present with symptoms indicative of a tethered cord yet with imaging demonstrating a "normally" positioned conus medullaris, the approximately same frequency of the following is observed: cutaneous signatures of OSD (46% versus 52%), abnormalities of the extremities (39% versus 32%), bony abnormalities (100% versus 95%), dysraphic abnormalities (62% versus 78%), and neurologic abnormalities (77% versus 87%).[16] In our series, none of the patients with symptoms of a tethered spinal cord and a conus in normal position presented solely with urologic dysfunction.[15,16] One criticism of the normally positioned conus in a patient with symptoms of a tethered spinal cord is that these individuals may have additional vertebrae in the lumbar region, thereby distorting this diagnosis if one does not number vertebrae from a cephalad to caudal direction. Often only imaging of the lumbosacral region is obtained in evaluation of these patients. However, Wilson and Prince[4] found that the degree of potential error introduced into this study by the possible occurrence of undetected transitional vertebrae or six lumbar vertebrae is negligible.

In support of biomechanical stress on the conus medullaris without alteration of its termination site at a normal level is the simple concept that static midsagittal MRI of the lumbosacral region is all revealing in the absence of flexion or extension of the spine. Indeed, even with Barson's historic publication, he states, "Our data represents the vertebral segments as thought they were of constantly equal length both in respect of position and time. This is obviously not so, although no adequate physical measurements exist of the precise size of the various vertebral segments at varying gestational ages and the normal ranges to be expected." Barson also makes an important query with regard to conus position by asking whether the conus level is a result of an unusually short vertebral column or an abnormally long spinal cord or whether both factors play a part.[18]

In our original report of patients with TCS and the conus in a normal position, we reviewed our experience over 12 years with 73 patients with TCS. Of these, 13 (18%, six male and seven female) had a cord termination at or above the L1–2 vertebral disc space. These patients otherwise displayed characteristics usually associated with the patient with an abnormally low conus medullaris. The most common neurologic complaints were lower extremity weakness, spasticity/hyperreflexia, and bladder dysfunction, each occurring in four of 10 (40%) patients. Bowel dysfunction occurred in three of 10 patients (30%). Six of these patients

had cutaneous signatures indicative of OSD, four of 13 (31%) had lumbosacral hemangiomas, one had a lumbosacral subcutaneous lipoma (8%), and one had a midline lumbar skin tag (8%). Five of these patients (39%) presented with extremity abnormalities, including three (23%) with leg length discrepancy and two (15%) with foot deformities. Adipose tissue was found in 92% of patients either radiographically or histologically.[15]

Radiographically, several bony anomalies were identified in this population of patients. Ten of the 13 had bony abnormalities. These abnormalities included scoliosis (three patients), bifid vertebrae (seen in all 10 patients), hemivertebrae, and segmentation errors. Other nonbony dysraphic anomalies included meningocele manqué in two patients, intradural lipoma in four patients, split cord anomaly (without median septa) in two patients, and terminal syringomyelia in two patients. Twelve of the 13 patients underwent surgery. The average follow-up at that time was 2.2 years. Three patients presented as neurologically normal. Seventy-five percent of patients with lower extremity weakness improved with surgery. For urinary complaints, at follow-up, two patients had normal urinary control, one patient had improved control, and one patient in whom there was a neurogenic bladder had no postoperative change. Of patients presenting with bowel complaints, all three had cessation of complaints at follow-up. Two patients presented with back pain that had resolved after their operation. The one patient who did not undergo surgery, presented with low back pain and radicular leg pain that had improved at 6 months follow-up.

Our follow-up publication on TCS and the normally positioned conus compared this subgroup with 60 patients with TCS and a low-lying conus medullaris. Comparison of the parameters of these two groups was not significant at the 5% level in statistical analysis.[16]

Moufarrij and colleagues[25] reported a series of patients with findings of a tethered spinal cord in which three patients had a cord termination at L2 vertebral level. Only one of these patients had a fatty filum terminale. Presenting symptoms in these three patients were gait disturbance with lower extremity weakness, leg cramps with foot inversion, and progressive kyphoscoliosis. The ages of the patients in this group were 4, 6, and 7 years. Interestingly, these patients were noted at operation to have the cut ends of their fila retract 1 to 3 cm. Raghavan and colleagues[26] reported 25 patients with a tethered spinal cord in which four (16%) had coni superior to the middle segment of the L2 vertebrae. Two of the four presented with urinary incontinence, and fatty fila were found in three of the four, one of whom did not present with urinary difficulties.

Urinary Dysfunction and Conus in the Normal Position

Although our description of the tethered cord with a conus in the normal position did include patients who had urinary incontinence, this was only in four patients. In our report, three of the four patients had improved bladder function at postoperative follow-up. Many other reports in the literature have shown that urinary complaints, especially incontinence, are effectively dealt with by sectioning the filum terminale in the face of a conus that is in a "normal" position.[23,27]

Selçuki and Coskun[23] showed in 13 patients aged 5 to 17 years with a proven hyperreflexic neurogenic bladder and who had failed to respond to anticholinergic therapy that on the first postsurgical day 93% were continent. Disappointingly, almost half lost continence within the first month after surgery. Their conclusion was that sectioning of the filum could be used as a supplementary measure in the treatment of incontinence. In a more recent publication from this group, four additional patients were added to the first publication with the results after sectioning of the filum revealing 58.8% with a good outcome, 17.6% with a fair outcome, and 23.5% with a poor outcome. Kondo and colleagues,[21,22] also in two publications, discuss this topic. In their first publication, 15 adults were operated on for bladder dysfunction. Three of these 15 patients were classified as grade I TCS with a "tense" filum of normal diameter and a conus positioned at the L1–2 disc space. These three were deemed normal or improved postoperatively. In their second publication, 27 children (mean age, 9.3 years) were operated on for persistent enuresis. In this study, the conus was basically in the normal position for all patients and the filum was confirmed to be taut in all 27 cases, although it was not discernible whether this was at imaging or at operation. They concluded from this study that they could find no parameters that would predict a favorable outcome in this patient subset with only seven patients benefiting from surgery. Khoury and colleagues,[19,20] also in two publications, discussed sectioning of the filum in the same scenario. In their first publication, 23 patients were operated on, all with normally positioned coni according to myelography. Approximately 72% had resolution of their preoperative incontinence. However, many functionally unstable bladders may do so spontaneously. Subsequently, four patients were added to this series in a more recent publication. Similar results were also observed in this second group.

We believe that there is indeed a subset of the patient population with TCS in whom the tip of the conus lies at even liberally accepted normal levels. We would encourage clinicians treating patients with symptoms of TCS not to treat the patient based simply on imaging but imaging coupled with clinical symptoms and physical examination. It is important to point out that, in lieu of the many publications of conus termination, one accepts that there is no one single "normal" position of the terminal cord but rather a normal range.[28] In addition, one may consider a patient with a supposedly "normally" positioned conus to actually have caudal descent of his or her cord that, if not placed under stress, would have terminated superior to its current location. This would imply that earlier intervention might address an abnormally taut cord before its displacement. Perhaps a superior way of interpreting a "tethered" cord is to view this as tautness of the cord and not necessarily elongation of the distal cord in every case.

SURGICAL MANAGEMENT OF OCCULT SPINAL DYSRAPHISM

The likelihood of significant reversal of lost neurologic function is not entirely predictable, but, in general, the longer and more complete the deficit is, the less likely it is to resolve after surgical intervention. Foot and leg length discrepancy and other bony deformities of the foot from long-standing neural injury will not improve and may even worsen despite full relief of intradural tension.[8] Leg weakness that is not profound is likely to improve as is any sensory disturbance. Lost muscle mass implies a more severe neurologic impairment and will not improve.

Patient and family expectation in regard to return of lost bladder function almost always runs high, but the surgeon's ability to restore the complex integration of detrusor and sphincter motor function is quite limited, making surgery primarily a prophylactic procedure. The likelihood of some improvement in neurologic function and the elimination of pain is high. In the patient with the position of the conus over the L3 vertebral body or below, the rationale of therapeutic or prophylactic surgery is clear.

One of the lines of persuasion that the natural history is a progressive loss of function is that older patients rarely present neurologically intact. If one looks at age groups and relates that to the degree of symptomatology, generally, the older the patient is, the more serious the symptoms. Adults almost always present as neurologically disadvantaged. The likelihood of losing function during surgery in contemporary published series is well below 10%. For example, infants born with a lipomyelomeningocele have a high (88%) likelihood of demonstrating progressive loss of neurologic function, whereas operative worsening is well less than 10%. Late deterioration in the operated group occurs in 13% to 26% followed for at least 5 years. Once the patient has demonstrated clinical worsening, little argument can be made for further conservative therapy.

Preoperative Evaluation

Preoperative evaluation includes appropriate imaging, for example, radiographs of the spine for localization of spina bifida or median septa. Urodynamics is important in establishing preoperative urinary function and its baseline. MRI is the gold standard when visualizing the neuraxis. However, in patients with complex OSD, computed tomographic myelography may still have some use.

Operative Technique

The purpose of surgery for OSD is to release the neural tissue from all points of fixation without damaging any functional neural tissue. Discussion of the surgical nuances of each form of OSD is beyond the scope of this presentation. For illustration, we now describe the operative technique used for the exploration of a lipomyelomeningocele. A laminectomy is performed over the length of the lesion. The ultrasonic aspirator adds significantly to operative efficiency by permitting the relatively atraumatic removal of the fat so that better visualization can be accomplished of the points of fixation. The goal of the procedure is important and is not the total ablation of the subpial fat but rather the substantial debulking of the lipoma and the release of points of fixation. The cleavage plane between the lipoma and cord does not lend itself to total removal of the fat, and, barring some extraordinary circumstance, this should not be attempted.

Surgical treatment of a lipomyelomeningocele presents a technical challenge. A linear midline incision is used to extend above and below the subcutaneous lesion. The skin is separated off the lipoma, and a lateral circumferential plane of dissection is established. The cleavage between the subcutaneous lipoma and the lumbodorsal fascia is distinct and clear. Distally, the lesion may merge with the muscular fibers of the gluteus maximus, confusing the situation. An approach superficial to the muscle fibers is best at this point. As the operator dissects in the plane between lipoma and fascia, the neck of the lipoma as it emerges through the fascial defect will be appreciated. With care, lateral and superficial aspects of the lipoma can be removed at this point to lessen the bulk of the tumor.

A laminectomy of one or two segments immediately cephalad to the lesion is then accomplished. With the exposure of the normal dura under the laminectomy, this layer is then opened. The caudally descended cord is appreciated, and some subpial fat infiltration may be seen. The dural opening is continued caudally in the midline until the lipoma-cord complex is seen rising out of the plane of the spinal canal. Circumferential dissection of the dura to free the lipoma-cord complex is critical in releasing the cord from its restrained movement (Fig. 157-24). The dura at this point may also be infiltrated by fat. The filum terminale is sought and sectioned.

Closure is especially important because constriction of the dorsal or caudal cerebrospinal fluid space will defeat the goal of a free-floating and mobile conus and cauda equina. If there is significant fatty infiltration of the dura mater and its inner surface is irregular, it can be sacrificed at this point. Frequently, sufficient dura is available to allow a redundant primary closure. If inadequate dura is present, lumbosacral fascia can be used as well as an assortment of relatively inert synthetic products. Tight reapproximation of the fascia over the dura should be avoided if this is thought to compromise the redundancy of the dural closure. There is almost always sufficient full-thickness skin to allow adequate cosmetic skin coverage. Patients are maintained in a prone position with a waterproof dressing for several days before assuming the erect position. Neurologically, intact patients operated on prophylactically in infancy are unlikely to demonstrate neurologic loss as a result of the procedure, the incidence being less than 5%. Intradural adhesions of the unoperated patient seem to increase with age.

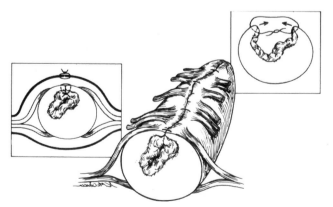

FIGURE 157-24 Operative drawing of a lipomyelomeningocele of the lumbosacral spinal cord. After debulking of the fatty mass, the pial edges are reapproximated with inverted stitches in an attempt to minimize retethering of the cord.

Postoperative Management

Following TCS surgery, patients are observed for pain control and their ability to void. Once these issues are resolved, discharge can be considered. Over the next several days, occupational and physical therapy may be obtained. Acute follow-up imaging is generally not obtained other than in cases of terminal syringomyelia or continued symptoms.

REFERENCES

1. Garceau GJ: The filum terminale syndrome. J Bone Joint Surg Am 35:711–716, 1953.
2. Jones PH, Love JG: Tight filum terminale. Arch Surg 73:556–566, 1956.
3. Fitz CR, Harwood-Nash DC: The tethered conus. AJR Am J Roentgenol 125:515–523, 1975.
4. Wilson DA, Prince JR: MR imaging determination of the location of the normal conus medullaris throughout childhood. AJR Am J Roentgenol 152:1029–1032, 1989.
5. Reimann AF, Anson BJ: Vertebral level of termination of the spinal cord with report of a case of sacral cord. Anat Rec 88:127–138, 1944.
6. Saifuddin A, Burnett SJD, White J: The variation of position of the conus medullaris in an adult population: A magnetic resonance imaging study. Spine 23:1452–1456, 1998.
7. McLone DG: Occult dysraphism and the tethered spinal cord. In Choix M, De Rocco C, Hockley A, et al (eds): Pediatric Neurosurgery. Philadelphia: Churchill Livingstone, 1999, pp 61–78.
8. Iskandar BJ, Fulmer BB, Hadley MN, Oakes WJ: Congenital tethered spinal cord syndrome in adults. Neurosurg Focus 10:1–5, 2001.
9. Rauzzino MJ, Tubbs RS, Alexander E, Grabb PA, Oakes WJ: Spinal neurenteric cysts and their relation to more common aspects of occult spinal dysraphism. Neurosurg Focus 10:1–10, 2001.
10. Chapman PH: Surgical management of occult spinal dysraphism. In Schmidek HH (ed): Schmidek & Sweet Operative Neurosurgical Techniques, vol 2, 4th ed. Philadelphia: WB Saunders, 2000, pp 1897–1907.
11. Yamada S, Iacono RP, Douglas CC, et al: Tethered cord syndrome in the adult. In Yamada S (ed): Tethered Cord Syndrome. Park Ridge, IL: American Association of Neurologic Surgeons, 1996, pp 149–165.
12. Warder DE: Tethered cord syndrome and OSD. Neurosurg Focus 10:1–9, 2001.
13. McLendon RE, Oakes WJ, Heinz ER, et al: Adipose tissue in the filum terminale: A computed tomographic finding that may indicate tethering of the spinal cord. Neurosurgery 22:873–876, 1988.
14. Love JG, Daly DD, Harris LE: Tight filum terminale: Report of condition in three siblings. JAMA 176:31–33, 1961.
15. Warder DE, Oakes WJ: Tethered cord syndrome and the conus in a normal position. Neurosurgery 33:374–378, 1993.
16. Warder DE, Oakes WJ: Tethered cord syndrome: The low-lying and normally positioned conus. Neurosurgery 34:597–600, 1994.
17. Tubbs RS, Salter G, Grabb PA, Oakes WJ: The denticulate ligament: Anatomy and functional significance. J Neurosurg 94:271–275, 2001.
18. Barson AJ: The vertebral level of termination of the spinal cord during normal and abnormal development. J Anat 106:489–497, 1970.
19. Khoury AE, Hendrick EB, McLorie GA, et al: OSD: Clinical and urodynamic outcome after division of the filum terminale. J Urol 144:426–429, 1990.
20. Khoury AE, Balcom A, McLorie GA, Churchill BM: Clinical experience in urological involvement with tethered cord syndrome. In Yamada S (ed): Tethered Cord Syndrome. Park Ridge, IL: American Association of Neurologic Surgeons, 1996, pp 89–98.
21. Kondo A, Kato K, Kanai S, Sakakibara T: Bladder dysfunction secondary to tethered cord syndrome in adults: Is it curable? J Urol 135:313–316, 1986.
22. Kondo A, Gotoh M, Kato K, et al: Treatment of persistent enuresis: Results of severing a tight filum terminale. Br J Urol 62:42–45, 1988.
23. Selçuki M, Coskun K: Management of the tight filum terminale syndrome with special emphasis on normal level conus medullaris (NLCM). Surg Neurol 50:318–322, 1998.

24. Selçuki M, Ünlü A, Ugur H, et al: Patients with urinary incontinence often benefit from surgical detethering of tight filum terminale. Childs Nerv Syst 16:150–155, 2000.

25. Moufarrij NA, Palmer JM, Hahn JF, Weinstein MA: Correlation between magnetic resonance imaging and surgical findings in the tethered spinal cord. Neurosurgery 25:341–346, 1989.

26. Raghavan N, Barkovich AJ, Edwards M, Norman D: MR imaging in the tethered spinal cord syndrome. AJR Am J Roentgenol 152:843–852, 1989.

27. Nazar GB, Casale AJ, Roberts JG, Linden RD: Occult filum terminale syndrome. Pediatr Neurosurg 23:228–235, 1995.

28. Vettivel S: Vertebral level of the termination of the spinal cord in human fetuses. J Anat 179:149–161, 1991.

158 Sacral Resection and Stabilization

DARYL R. FOURNEY and ZIYA L. GOKASLAN

INTRODUCTION

Tumors of the sacrum and related neural, retroperitoneal, and pelvic structures are rare, accounting for 1% to 7% of all spinal tumors that come to clinical attention.[1] The diagnosis of sacral lesions is frequently delayed, and tumors may be far advanced at the time of presentation. The types of tumors encountered in this region are diverse, and treatment options depend on the medical status of the patient, the location and extent of the lesion, and the biological aggressiveness of the tumor type.

Most primary neoplasms affecting the sacrococcygeal region, including chordomas, chondrosarcomas, and giant cell tumors, are resistant to radiation therapy and chemotherapy. Even when these treatments are successful in the short term, rates of recurrent disease are high. Sacral resection is often the only effective alternative for possible cure in these patients.[2-8] In patients with sacral invasion from advanced colorectal carcinoma or other tumors of the pelvic viscera, sacrectomy combined with rectosigmoid resection or pelvic exenteration may result in long-term disease-free survival.[9]

Due to the complex anatomy of the sacral region, aggressive resections are technically demanding procedures that require the expertise of a multidisciplinary surgical team. En bloc sacral resection often involves the purposeful sacrifice of sacral nerve roots. High sacral amputations may even disrupt spinopelvic stability, requiring advanced techniques to reconstruct the continuity of the pelvic ring and spinal column.[10] The technical challenges of such operations and the functional costs for the patient (with respect to anorectal and urogenital dysfunction) are significantly increased when the tumor involves high sacral levels.

This chapter outlines the evaluation of patients with sacral tumors and discusses the relevant clinical, radiologic, and pathologic characteristics of the major tumor types. We will discuss the important anatomic and functional considerations in planning a sacral resection. A step-by-step description of various operative approaches will be discussed. Finally, we will review current methods of spinopelvic reconstruction and stabilization.

ANATOMY

Osseous and Ligamentous Structures

The adult sacrum consists of five fused sacral vertebrae. At birth, each vertebral body is separated by an intervertebral disc. The caudal two bodies undergo fusion at approximately the 18th year of life, and the process of fusion continues rostrally until the S1–S2 interspace finally fuses by 25 to 30 years of age. The development of fused adult sacral vertebrae is dependent on normal weight bearing.

The sacrum is wedge shaped. Its broad base at S1 forms the posterior segment of the pelvic ring. The upper two or three sacral vertebrae articulate with the ilium on either side. Rostrally, the sacrum articulates with the lowest lumbar vertebra. At its apex, the sacrum articulates with the coccyx.

The ventral or pelvic surface is concave. The ventral rami of the first four sacral nerves and their associated vascular elements pass into the pelvis via four pairs of ventral sacral foramina. The transverse ridges between each pair of foramina represent the area where the intervertebral disc was once located. The promontory is the anterior enlargement of the upper portion of the body of S1.

The pars lateralis (lateral mass) is the area lateral to the ventral foramina. The lateral surfaces of the upper two or three sacral vertebrae form an ear-shaped "auricular" surface, which articulates with the ilium on each side. Ventrally, the lateral masses are marked by neural grooves that run laterally from each of the foramina. The large lateral masses of S1 are known as the alae. On the anterior aspect of each ala is a rounded bony groove formed by the lumbosacral trunk.

The dorsal surface of the sacrum is convex in shape and has an irregular surface that includes median, intermediate, and lateral sacral crests representing the fused spinous, articular, and transverse processes, respectively. The shallow grooves between the median and intermediate crests are formed by fused laminae. The dorsal rami of the upper four sacral nerves and associated vascular structures pass through the four pairs of dorsal sacral foramina, located between the intermediate and lateral sacral crests. The dorsal sacral foramina are much smaller than the corresponding ventral sacral foramina. The laminae of the fifth (and on occasion the fourth) vertebra fail to fuse in the midline and form the sacral hiatus, which is the caudal opening of the sacral canal. The sacral cornu, a remnant of the inferior articular process, lie on each side of the sacral hiatus.

Since the lumbosacral and sacroiliac joints transmit the entire weight of the body to the hip bones and lower limbs, these joints and their supporting ligaments must be very strong. The strong dorsal ligamentous complex includes the interosseous ligaments and the dorsal sacroiliac ligaments. The very stout interosseous ligaments connect the sacral tuberosities to the overhanging bone of the iliac tuberosities and represent the single strongest ligaments binding the sacrum to the ilium. The dorsal sacroiliac ligaments are divided into deep (short) and superficial (long) parts.

The deeper ligaments connect the sacral and ilial tuberosities and are composed of horizontally oriented fibers; the more superficial ligaments are oriented vertically and stretch from the posterior superior iliac spine to the tubercles of the lateral sacral crest. The caudal portions of the superficial dorsal sacroiliac ligaments blend with the sacrotuberous ligaments.

The ventral ligamentous complex includes the ventral sacroiliac ligaments and the lumbosacral ligaments. The ventral sacroiliac ligament is a weak fibrous band that attaches to the base and lateral part of the sacrum and to the medial margin of the auricular surface of the ilium.

Three sets of accessory ligaments—the sacrospinous, sacrotuberous, and iliolumbar ligaments—also function to strengthen the pelvic girdle. The iliolumbar ligament originates on the transverse process of L5 and courses caudally and laterally to insert on the ilium. Some fibers stretch ventrally to merge with the ventral sacroiliac ligament as the lumbosacral ligament. The sacrospinous ligament connects the lateral and anterolateral surfaces of the sacrum and coccyx with the ischial spine. This ligament divides the sciatic notch into greater and lesser sciatic foramina. Finally, the sacrotuberous ligament, an extensive structure, originates broadly from the posterior superior iliac spine and the dorsal and lateral aspects of the sacrum and coccyx to form a dense narrow fibrous band that inserts on the ischial tuberosity.

Vascular Anatomy

The abdominal aorta bifurcates at the L4 level. The small median or middle sacral artery arises from the posterior surface of the abdominal aorta close to the bifurcation and descends vertically along the pelvic surface of the sacrum. It gives rise to several small parietal branches that anastomose with the lateral sacral arteries and to small visceral branches that anastomose with the superior and middle rectal arteries. The median sacral artery ends in the coccygeal body, a small cellular and vascular mass located at the tip of the coccyx, the function of which remains unclear.

The aorta divides into the common iliac arteries that travel laterally and inferiorly to divide into the external and internal iliac arteries. The internal iliac artery begins at approximately the level of the L5–S1 disc space where it is crossed by the ureter. It is separated from the sacroiliac joint by the internal iliac vein and the lumbosacral trunk.

The iliolumbar artery may arise form the common iliac artery, although it more commonly is the first branch of the internal iliac artery. This vessel runs superomedially, in close relation to the lumbosacral trunk, passing anterior to the sacroiliac joint and posterior to the psoas muscle. It later turns laterally and upward to divide in the region of the iliac fossa.

The lateral sacral artery is usually the second branch of the internal iliac, although it may also originate from the superior gluteal artery. These vessels, usually a superior one and an inferior one, sometimes arise from a common trunk. They pass medially and descend downward anterior to the sacral ventral rami, giving branches that enter the ventral sacral foramina to supply the spinal meninges and the roots of the sacral nerves. Some branches may pass from the sacral canal through the dorsal foramina to supply the muscles and skin overlying the sacrum. Most tumors arising from the sacrum or presacral space, as well as some intraspinal masses, derive at least a part of their blood supply from the medial and lateral sacral arteries. Enlargement, displacement, or encasement of these vessels may be seen on angiography.

The next two branches of the internal iliac artery are the superior and inferior gluteal arteries. The superior gluteal is a large artery that passes anteriorly across the lumbosacral trunk as the trunk passes over the ala. It then turns posteriorly between the lumbosacral trunk and the ventral ramus of the first sacral nerve to leave the pelvis through the superior part of the greater sciatic foramen, superior to the piriformis muscle. The inferior gluteal artery passes posteriorly to pierce the sacral plexus more inferiorly (most often between S2 and S3) and exits the pelvis through the inferior part of the greater sciatic foramen, inferior to the piriformis muscle.

The venous anatomy of the region generally parallels that of the arterial, but it is more variable. It is important to note some features. First, the vena cava lies to the right of the aorta at the bifurcation of the common iliac vessels. The right common iliac vein passes posterior to the artery, and is therefore much shorter than the left common iliac vein. Second, the middle sacral vein, which is occasionally doubled, drains into the left common iliac vein rather than into the inferior vena cava. Finally, the iliolumbar veins drain into the common iliac veins rather than into the internal iliac veins.

Neural Anatomy

The thecal sac ends blindly at the S2 level. The lower sacral and coccygeal nerves emerge from the sac, as does the extradural portion of the filum terminale. The upper four roots exit the sacrum through the paired ventral and dorsal sacral foramina. The fifth sacral roots, the coccygeal roots, and the filum exit the sacrum caudally through the sacral hiatus. The filum terminale extends to its point of fusion with the periosteum of the first coccygeal segment.

The sacral plexus is formed by the ventral rami of six roots: L4 through S3 and the upper part of S4. The lumbosacral trunk (the conjoined L4–5 roots) crosses the anterior aspect of the ala of the sacrum, descends obliquely in front of the sacroiliac joint, and enters the pelvis deep to the parietal pelvic fascia. It crosses the superior gluteal vessels and joins the first sacral root. The sacral plexus is located on the anterior surface of the piriformis muscle, deep to the parietal (Waldeyer's) fascia. Except for the nerves to the piriformis muscle, the perforating cutaneous nerves, and the nerves to the pelvic diaphragm, essentially all branches of the sacral plexus leave the pelvis through the greater sciatic foramen.

The most important derivatives of the sacral plexus are the sciatic and pudendal nerves. The latter is unique in exiting the greater sciatic foramen only to reenter the lesser sciatic foramen by hooking around the sacrospinous ligament. It supplies the muscles of the perineum, including the external anal sphincter, and provides sensory information to the external genitalia.

The coccygeal plexus is derived from the ventral rami of S4 and S5 as well as the coccygeal roots. It lies on the pelvic surface of the coccygeus muscle. It innervates the coccygeus muscle and provides some perianal sensation.

Both the sympathetic and parasympathetic components of the autonomic nervous system have an intimate relationship with the sacrum. The sacral sympathetic trunk, continuous with the lumbar sympathetic trunk, descends against the ventral surface of the sacrum, converging in front of the coccyx to form the unpaired ganglion impar. Three to four sacral trunk ganglionic enlargements are found on each side of the midline, just medial to the ventral sacral foramina. No white rami communicantes are present in this region; however, the postsynaptic gray rami communicantes from each ganglion join the corresponding sacral or coccygeal nerves for distribution to sweat glands, blood vessels, and erector pilori muscles. In addition, the sacral sympathetic trunks provide fine branches to the superior hypogastric plexus. The superior hypogastric plexus is the caudal continuation of the periaortic sympathetic plexus; it lies on the anterior surface of the fifth lumbar vertebra and upper sacrum in the retroperitoneal tissue. Fibers of the superior hypogastric plexus diverge into right and left hypogastric nerves opposite the first sacral vertebra. The term *hypogastric nerve* may be a misnomer, since the structure is really a narrow plexus of fibers. The hypogastric nerves represent the principal sympathetic inputs to the inferior hypogastric plexus.

The parasympathetic contributions to the pelvic plexi arise from the ventral S2 to S4 nerve roots. These preganglionic fibers form the pelvic splanchnic nerves (nervi erigentes). The parasympathetic system provides motor innervation to the detrusor muscle of the bladder and is primarily responsible for the vascular reflexes that sustain erectile function. The sympathetic system plays less of a role in normal voiding reflexes, but is important for male fertility by promoting timely transport of spermatozoa from the testes to the seminal vesicles and by coordinating reflexes responsible for ejaculation.

DIAGNOSIS

Clinical Presentation

Sacral tumors are rare and difficult to diagnose at an early stage.[1] The major reasons for this delay include (1) the unique capacity of the sacral canal to allow neoplastic expansion without causing symptoms, (2) the often nonspecific nature of complaints when they arise, and (3) the difficulty in obtaining and interpreting adequate imaging studies.

As tumor expands within the sacral canal, it may erode or invade the walls of the sacrum, expand cephalad within the spinal canal, or enter the pelvis via the ventral sacral foramina. A slow-growing regionally expansive neoplasm may attain a large size without causing symptoms early in the course of the illness. Aggressive or malignant tumors tend to present earlier.

The earliest presenting symptom in patients with sacral tumors is pain located in the lower back or sacrococcygeal region.[1,7,11] Referred pain to the leg or buttock may occur secondary to irritation of the first sacral root or iliolumbar trunk.[11] The early presentation of sacral lesions is therefore very similar to that of lumbar spondylosis. By the time a sacral lesion is diagnosed, some patients have been treated and occasionally even operated on for suspected lumbar intervertebral disc pathology.

Abnormalities on plain sacral radiographs may be missed, and routine lumbar myelography, computed tomography (CT), and magnetic resonance imaging (MRI) studies frequently fail to visualize the sacrum below the S2 level. Unfortunately, the true diagnosis is frequently realized late in the course of illness, when bladder or bowel function have been compromised, or when a large presacral mass is noted on rectal or gynecologic examination.

Radiologic Evaluation

A sacral tumor can be easily overlooked on standard radiographs. The curved shape of the sacrum, its position within the pelvic girdle, and overlying bowel gas are frequent sources of obscuration. Destructive changes must be advanced before they become evident on plain x-ray films.[12] Adequate radiographs should display the entire sacrum and coccyx on lateral views, and the sacrum should be visualized en face on anteroposterior views. A malignant process is suggested when lytic lesions without sharply defined borders are seen. Well-defined sclerotic margins, reflecting reactive changes in the surrounding bone, imply the presence of a benign or chronic process.

CT and MRI more readily allow the detection, characterization, and staging of sacral tumors.[12,13] CT has the advantage of providing excellent bony detail and showing tumor matrix calcification. CT is also useful to image the abdomen for evidence of visceral involvement. Major advantages of MRI studies include the detailed depiction of associated soft tissue masses and the ability to assess the anatomy in multiple planes. The rostral extent of sacral involvement, which is particularly critical to surgical planning, is best appreciated on a midsagittal view.

The radionucleotide bone scan is a sensitive but nonspecific indicator of bone destruction that is most useful as part of a systemic workup to rule out widespread bony metastases during the preoperative staging of these patients. Purely osteolytic lesions, such as myeloma, may not be well defined on bone scan. Obscuration of sacral lesions by the accumulation of radioactive material in the bladder may result in falsely negative study results.

In addition to the bone scan, chest radiography and CT of the abdomen are also warranted to rule out metastatic pathology. Intravenous pyelography and/or barium enema may be indicated in evaluating sacral tumors with significant pelvic invasion.[14]

Angiography is useful in defining the vascularity of sacral tumors and for preoperative tumor embolization, especially in the case of highly vascular lesions such as giant cell tumor or aneurysmal bone cyst.[15,16]

Biopsy

The differential diagnosis of sacral tumors is extensive, and although clinical and imaging factors may suggest a more abbreviated differential diagnosis, a biopsy should be performed in virtually all cases. In patients with significant comorbid illness who are not considered candidates for major surgical resections, a biopsy may still be warranted in order to plan radiotherapy or chemotherapy.

The percutaneous CT-guided biopsy involves minimal risk and is currently the method of choice. The site of entry and the trajectory of the needle should be carefully selected such that they can easily be included within the margins of any subsequent resection. If possible, the puncture site should be located in the midline posteriorly. It may be worthwhile to introduce a small droplet of sterile permanent ink into the needle tract to "tattoo" the skin for later identification.

A transrectal biopsy should never be considered, since the otherwise uninvolved rectum may become seeded with tumor cells necessitating later resection.[8] Further, infection of the tumor bed following transrectal biopsy has been documented.

PATHOLOGY

Sacral tumors are categorized as those that originate from the neural elements or their supporting tissues, those arising from bone, and those tumors that are metastatic from distal sites or the result of direct invasion from adjacent pelvic structures. The most common sacral tumors are metastatic, while the most common primary sacral tumor is chordoma.[7,8] Some non-neoplastic entities, including developmental cysts and inflammatory conditions, may mimic sacral tumors on imaging studies. A broad differential diagnosis of the various lesions encountered in this area is provided in Table 158-1.

Congenital Tumors

Sacrococcygeal Teratoma

A teratoma is a lesion containing tissue from all three germ layers, represented by either well-differentiated or immature elements. Skin, teeth, central nervous system tissue, and respiratory and alimentary mucosa may be found within these tumors. Sacrococcygeal teratomas are the most common sacral tumor in neonates, although it is rare in adults.[17,18] They develop during intrauterine growth and may grow large enough to cause dystocia.[19] The diagnosis is often made on prenatal ultrasonography.[20] Postpartum they present as an exophytic mass located between the anus and coccyx, covered by normal skin. Presacral and sometimes combined pre- and postsacral (dumbbell-shaped) lesions also occur.

Chordoma

Chordoma is the most common primary bone tumor of the sacrum.[8,21] Sacral chordomas occur almost twice as frequently in men compared with women and are uncommon in individuals less than 40 years of age.[8] The most common presenting symptom is pain in the lower back or sciatic region.[11] Chordomas may reach a very large size before constipation (from rectal compression) or lower extremity paresis (due to sacral plexus involvement) occurs.

Chordomas are considered congenital in origin because the microscopic appearance of vacuolated "physaliferous" cells resembles that seen in notochordal remnants. The midline location of these tumors also relates to this proposed etiology.[22]

Chordomas are typically slow growing but locally aggressive. Significant extracompartmental growth is often seen by the time of diagnosis. Most sacral chordomas present as surgical stage IB[23] with anterior extension into the pelvis. The tumor often displaces but does not invade the rectum,

TABLE 158-1 ■ Differential Diagnosis of Sacral and Presacral Lesions

Congenital Lesions

Posterior sacral meningocele, meningomyelocele, and lipomyelomeningocele
Developmental cysts
    Dermoid and epidermoid cysts
    Retrorectal tailgut cysts
    Enteric duplication cysts
    Anterior sacral meningocele
    Lateral meningocele
    Occult intrasacral meningocele
    Perineural (Tarlov's) cysts
Tumors
    Primitive neuroectodermal tumors
    Teratoma
    Hamartoma
    Chordoma

Inflammatory Lesions

Osteomyelitis
Abscess (pelvic abscess, perirectal abscess)

Neurogenic Lesions

Schwannoma and neurofibroma
Ependymoma
Ganglioneuroma
Neuroblastoma

Osseous Lesions

Bone island
Osteoid osteoma and osteoblastoma
Osteochondroma
Hemangioma
Aneurysmal bone cyst
Giant cell tumor
Chondrosarcoma
Osteosarcoma
Ewing's sarcoma
Paget's disease (monostotic)

Metastatic Lesions

Hematogenous spread (lung, breast, prostate, kidney, lymphoma)
Locally invasive lesions (colorectal and gynecologic malignancies, sarcoma)

Miscellaneous Lesions

Carcinoid tumor
Lymphoma
Solitary plasmacytoma, multiple myeloma
Meningioma
Hemangiopericytoma

as the tough periosteum and presacral fascia resist the transgression of disease. Metastasis is usually a late event.[7,22]

The usual CT appearance consists of lytic bone destruction in addition to a disproportionately large soft tissue mass. Calcification is present in 30% to 70% of cases.[13] Unlike most bone tumors, chordomas may show reduced uptake or normal distribution of isotope on bone scan.

En bloc excision, whenever possible, is the treatment of choice for sacral chordomas.[7,8,21,22] The extent of surgical resection has been found to play a major role in determining the length of disease-free survival.[22] Although a distinct capsule is often seen within the soft tissues, a radical wide posterior margin of the gluteal muscles should be employed to reduce the risk for local recurrence.[24] The margins of chordoma within bone are often indistinct. Surgical resection should extend at least one whole sacral segment beyond the area of gross disease.[7]

The value of radiotherapy as primary or adjuvant treatment for chordoma has been debated.[8] Supplementary radiotherapy may be a useful adjunct to surgical care, but is not sufficient as stand-alone therapy. In a clinical series spanning 40 years, York and colleagues[7] reported that the addition of radiation therapy significantly prolonged the disease-free interval for patients undergoing subtotal resection (2.12 years versus 8 months). Others have suggested that radiotherapy is of limited value in most cases.[22] Chemotherapy has been of little value in the management of these tumors.

Neurogenic Tumors

Schwannoma and Neurofibroma

Sacral schwannomas are much more common than neurofibromas. They grow within the sacral canal and only rarely expand through the anterior sacral foramina into the presacral space.[25,26] A complete resection of these benign tumors is potentially curative because, with the exception of plexiform neurofibromas, they do not infiltrate beyond their capsular envelope. The surgical approach depends on the size and location of the tumor, especially the degree of intraspinal and presacral extension. The majority of lesions coming to neurosurgical attention will be largely confined to the sacral canal and can be resected completely using a posterior approach. This approach allows direct visualization of the relationship between the sacral nerve roots and the tumor. If there is a small presacral component, limited access to this region may be obtained by transforaminal resection. Tumors with a large presacral component should be removed through an anterior transabdominal approach. Giant intrasacral schwannomas have been described for which radical sacral resection was performed.[25,26]

Ependymoma

Sacral ependymomas are most commonly the benign myxopapillary type. They arise from ependymal cell clusters within the terminal filum and expand the sacral canal.[27] Rare extradural sacrococcygeal ependymomas have been reported, including subcutaneous, presacral, and intrasacral varieties.[28]

Patients with sacral region ependymomas typically present with pain in either a lower back or sciatic distribution. By the time of diagnosis, which averages 2 to 3 years after the onset of symptoms, many patients exhibit some form of cauda equina syndrome.[11] As with other slow-growing sacral tumors that tend to be diagnosed at an advanced stage, ependymomas may be associated with extensive bony destruction and a large soft tissue mass.[27]

A complete en bloc resection is advisable in order to prevent local recurrence or cerebrospinal fluid dissemination. Intradural lesions can be resected completely via a posterior approach.[28] Intraoperative somatosensory-evoked potentials are useful, since dissection of tumor from the roots of the cauda equina may be difficult. The approach to extradural lesions depends on tumor location. Radiotherapy may be useful in cases of subtotal removal or recurrence.

Ganglioneuroma

Ganglioneuromas are rare, slow-growing tumors composed of sympathetic ganglion cells.[29] They are thought to represent the benign counterpart of malignant neuroblastomas. Ganglioneuromas may arise anywhere from the base of the skull to the pelvis. Like neuroblastoma, most ganglioneuromas arise in the abdomen, predominantly from the adrenal gland. The small percentages of pelvic tumors likely arise from sacral extensions of the sympathetic chain. As tumor expands within the pelvis, it may extend through a sacral foramen into the epidural space, causing sacral nerve root compression. The treatment is complete surgical removal.

Osseous Tumors

Less than 10% of all primary bone tumors occur in the spine, with the exception of osteoblastoma, which has a 40% incidence of vertebral involvement.[30] The incidence of sacral involvement among osseous tumors varies considerably. Bone tumors are a histologically diverse group of neoplasms. Some lesions are of low biologic activity, such as osteoid osteoma, osteoblastoma,[30,31] and aneurysmal bone cyst.[32] High-grade lesions include chondrosarcoma and osteosarcoma. Although giant cell tumors are histologically benign, they are locally invasive and have a high risk for recurrence.[33]

Sacral Bone Island

Sacral bone islands are probably much more common than reported. They are developmental variants that consist of compact bone in locations where trabecular bone is expected. These lesions are generally asymptomatic. Radiographically, they appear as well-circumscribed areas of increased density with spiculated edges.[12] They are clinically important in that they occasionally present as a large or growing lesion that may require differentiation from osteosarcoma or blastic metastasis.

Osteoid Osteoma and Osteoblastoma

Osteoid osteoma and osteoblastoma are histologically similar tumors that are distinguished from each other primarily on the basis of size.[31] The lytic defect in osteoid osteoma is less than 1.5 cm in diameter; osteoblastomas are larger than 1.5 cm. Both tumors are most common in young adults. The sacrum and coccyx are considered rare sites.

Osteoid osteomas and osteoblastomas most commonly present with localizing pain.[31] These tumors most often involve the posterior elements of the nonsacral spine,[30] and they tend to involve the body of the sacrum.[31] Intense radionucleotide uptake on bone scan is typically seen. Plain radiography and CT scans show a radiolucent defect with a thick rim of reactive sclerotic bone. Calcification may be present. In osteoblastoma, the margins of the lesion are more frequently ill defined and an epidural soft tissue may be found.[13]

In a review of 21 patients with osteoid osteoma or osteoblastoma of the sacrum treated with curettage, prognosis was generally good with a low incidence of recurrence (less than 10%).[31] Radiotherapy as well as embolization of feeding arteries may be used for the most aggressive lesions.

Aneurysmal Bone Cyst

Aneurysmal bone cysts are non-neoplastic multiloculated sacs of blood thought to result from localized disturbances in osseous blood flow. Sacral lesions are usually aggressive and associated with substantial bone destruction, pathologic fractures, and local recurrence.[32] The most common presenting symptom is low back pain. The radiographic appearance is that of an osteolytic expansile lesion surrounded by a thin shell of sclerotic bone, most often arising in the posterior osseous elements. Both CT and MRI may reveal multiple fluid-fluid levels within the cyst, reflecting hemorrhage with sedimentation, a characteristic feature of this tumor. Neoplasms such as giant cell tumor and osteoblastoma can simulate an aneurysmal bone cyst because of their occasional presentation with fluid-fluid levels.[12] Current management recommendations include preoperative selective arterial embolization and excision-curettage.[32]

Giant Cell Tumor

Giant cell tumor is the second most frequent primary bony tumor of the sacrum after chordoma.[33] Although histologically benign, these osteolytic, expansive bone tumors are locally aggressive and have a high risk for recurrence after curettage alone.[33,34] Sarcomatous degeneration and metastases are not uncommon. The peak incidence is approximately 30 years of age, and the prevalence is slightly higher in women. The most common presenting symptom is pain, although many patients also present with neurologic symptoms, including bladder dysfunction and sphincter weakness.[33]

Most sacral giant cell tumors are located eccentrically in the proximal sacrum. On plain x-ray films, a purely lytic lesion without marginal sclerosis or matrix calcification is typical.[12] On CT scans and MRI, giant cell tumors are frequently heterogeneous lesions due to the presence of necrosis, hemorrhage, and cystic spaces.[13] They are hypervascular on angiography.[16]

Selective arterial embolization is efficacious, with most patients demonstrating an objective early radiographic response to treatment. Long-term follow-up studies have show that the response is durable in approximately one half of the patients.[16]

The treatment of choice is en bloc excision if possible. Complete resection is challenging, since many giant cell tumors involve the upper sacral segments, often crossing the midline. Furthermore, these tumors frequently abut or extend across the sacroiliac joint. Total sacrectomy has been advocated in some cases.[6]

Chondrosarcoma

Chondrosarcomas are a heterogeneous family of malignant tumors in which cells tend to differentiate into cartilage.[35] The majority of sacral chondrosarcomas are low-grade, slow-growing, locally aggressive tumors. Because they commonly involve the upper portion of the sacrum and are eccentrically located, they may destroy the sacroiliac joint. Radiographs and CT images reveal a large destructive lesion with characteristic chondroid matrix mineralization. Calcification may also be visible within the soft tissue component of the tumor.[13]

The treatment of choice is en bloc excision.[35] Significant factors associated with a worse prognosis with respect to local control and/or survival include high histologic tumor grade, increasing patient age, primary surgery outside of a tumor center, incisional biopsy versus a noninvasive diagnostic procedure, and inadequate surgical margins.[35]

Radiation therapy may offer some benefit to patients who are not surgical candidates, but these tumors are considered radio-resistant. Chemotherapy has been applied to high-grade lesions, but appears to be of little benefit.

Osteosarcoma

Osteosarcoma is composed of malignant osteoblasts that form woven bone. Spinal osteosarcoma is rare, but occurs most commonly with the lumbar and sacral regions.[36] Many cases, especially among older patients, are associated with Paget's disease or with previously irradiated lesions. Distant metastases are often present at the time of diagnosis.

Osteosarcoma usually involves the anterior elements of the sacrum or spine. The CT and radiographic appearance varies depending on the amount of ossification of the tumor; however, many lesions are purely lytic.

In a recent study of osteosarcoma, including 15 patients with sacral lesions,[36] a poorer prognosis was reported in patients with large tumors, metastases, and incomplete tumor resection. Patients with sacral osteosarcoma should be treated with a combination of chemotherapy and at least marginal excision for those with surgically accessible tumors.[37] Postoperative radiotherapy may be beneficial.[36]

Ewing's Sarcoma

Ewing's sarcoma of the spine most commonly arises as a metastasis from an extraspinal primary lesion. The spine is the primary site of involvement in only 3.5% to 10% of cases, and the lumbosacral spine is the most frequent site.[38] Sacral lesions are associated with poorer survival rates than nonsacral spinal lesions.[39] Males have a higher incidence than females, and most patients present before the age of 20.[40] Pain is the most common symptom, followed by neurologic deficits.

Radiographs and CT images may reveal lytic, mixed, or sclerotic lesions. There is typically an extensive soft tissue mass spreading into the gluteal and pelvic regions that is best depicted on CT or MRI.[13] Despite these dramatic findings, radionucleotide scanning may show only a slightly increased uptake or even a "cold spot" in the region. Since Ewing's sarcoma of the sacrum is often a secondary lesion, and because primary sacral Ewing's sarcoma tends to metastasize early, a complete evaluation for disseminated disease should be performed in all patients, including CT of the chest and radionucleotide bone scanning.

Histologically, Ewing's sarcoma is a highly cellular tumor. The histologic differential diagnosis includes other round cell tumors such as neuroblastoma, lymphoma, and rhabdomyosarcoma. Ewing's sarcoma is thought to represent the most undifferentiated form of primitive neuroectodermal tumor.[41]

Ewing's sarcoma has one of the highest mortality rates of all bone tumors; however, it is highly responsive to both chemotherapy and irradiation. The role of surgery is controversial.[40,42,43] Multidisciplinary adjuvant therapy may reduce tumor bulk and improve the possibility of resection. Despite the advances of multimodality therapy, the prognosis for patients with Ewing's sarcoma of the spine remains poor.[40]

Metastatic Tumors

Metastatic tumors are by far the most common malignant neoplasms affecting the sacrum.[44] Most result from hematogenous spread. Although the diagnosis of primary sacral neoplasms is frequently delayed, metastatic involvement of the sacrum is usually suspected relatively early because the rapidly progressive and locally invasive nature of these tumors often causes significant low back pain or radicular symptoms affecting the lower extremities.[11]

Radiographically, metastatic tumors usually produce multiple irregular osteolytic, osteoblastic, or mixed lesions. CT and MRI best demonstrate the extent of sacral disease.[12] Radionucleotide bone scan is very sensitive in detecting small osteoblastic lesions, as seen in breast or prostate cancers. Purely osteolytic lesions, such as multiple myeloma, are often undetected on routine bone scanning.

Metastatic involvement of the sacrum usually signifies advanced disease. The goal of treatment in these patients is palliation, which is most often accomplished with local radiotherapy and sometimes chemotherapy. Such tumors are considered for operation only under certain circumstances.[44,45] For example, palliative surgical decompression of neural or pelvic structures may occasionally be indicated. Spinal-pelvic stabilization may be considered in carefully selected patients with severe pain or loss of the ability to ambulate due to a pathologic fracture or instability.[10,45]

In addition to hematogenous metastases from distal sites, the sacrum is often involved by local spread of tumors arising within the pelvic viscera. Locally advanced adenocarcinoma of the rectum is a condition for which the techniques of sacral resection may be a worthwhile consideration, both at primary presentation and in patients with recurrent disease.[9,46,47] Midline posterior tumors adherent to or invading the distal sacrum may be resectable for cure with an extended abdominoperineal resection, including the sacrum.[9] Occasionally, total pelvic exenteration (including a portion of the sacrum) is necessary.[46] Careful patient selection is paramount in ensuring a favorable outcome from these aggressive procedures.[47]

SURGICAL TREATMENT

Indications

The overall status of the patient, the anatomic extent of the tumor, and an appraisal of the biological behavior of the tumor are major factors in determining the goals of surgery. Sacral tumors may be classified as benign tumors, low-grade locally aggressive tumors, and high-grade malignancies. Benign encapsulated tumors can be treated with lesional resection. Primary bony tumors such as chordoma or chondrosarcoma require en bloc excision, including a circumferential margin of uninvolved tissue, to effect cure.[7,8] The surgical goals are similar for some primary localized high-grade malignancies such as osteosarcoma[36] and advanced rectal cancer with sacral invasion.[9] Palliative surgical debulking to preserve or restore neurologic function and reconstruction of spinopelvic junction for painful instability is a consideration for selected patients with metastatic sacral tumors.[10,45]

The need for careful patient selection can never be understated. Sacral resection is associated with a high risk for morbidity, may jeopardize lumbopelvic stability, and may involve inherent functional consequences with regard to motor, bladder, bowel, and sexual functions.

Functional and Biomechanical Considerations

There are several detailed studies that address the functional aspects of sacral amputations.[21,22,48–51] Patients with amputations distal to S3 generally have limited deficits, with preservation of sphincter function in the majority and some reduced perineal sensation. Sexual ability may also be decreased. The highest variability in functional results is seen for transverse resections of S2–3 (including removal of one to all four roots of S2–3).[49] There is seldom any relevant motor deficit; however, many patients have saddle anesthesia and a significant reduction in sphincter control. Section of the S1 roots may result in clinically relevant motor deficits (walking with external support), and almost uniformly results in total loss of sphincter control and sexual ability. Unilateral resection of sacral roots leads to unilateral deficits in strength and sensitivity; however, sphincter control may be either preserved or only partially compromised.[48,51] No matter the level of resection, damage to the lumbosacral trunks or sciatic nerves may cause serious postoperative motor and sensory deficits.[6] Damage to the parasympathetic and sympathetic plexi alone can result in problems with sexual ability and fertility in the male.

Another important consideration is lumbopelvic stability. The lumbosacral junction is a unique region of the spinal column because it is a transition zone where the mobile lower lumbar segments meet the highly immobile sacrum and pelvis.[10] The lumbosacral junction is exposed to the largest loads of any area of the spine. Although it has a greater range of motion than any thoracic or lumbar level in the sagittal (flexion-extension) plane, the lumbosacral junction has a very limited range of motion in the axial plane, as well as during rotation and lateral bending.

Because of the normal lordotic curvature of the lumbar spine, the lumbosacral intervertebral disc possesses a steep angle with respect to the horizontal. The lumbar spine therefore has a tendency to slip forward on the sacrum. The facet joints at L5–S1 are oriented very close to the coronal plane, a configuration that offers the most resistance to spondylolisthesis. The forward tilt of the sacrum causes the body load to be transmitted to the ventral surface of the sacrum as a potential rotatory force, with the axis centered at S2. The dorsal ligamentous complex, including the interosseous and dorsal sacroiliac ligaments, resists forward rotation at the upper end of the sacrum. The sacrospinous and sacrotuberous ligaments are primarily responsible for resisting the tendency of the lower end of the sacrum and coccyx to rotate dorsally. Bony constraints offered by the wedgelike shape of the sacrum within the pelvis, and the interdigitating surfaces of the sacral alae with respect to the iliac bones, provide additional resistance to sacral tipping.

In the resection of sacral tumors, sacroiliac stability is not greatly affected if the sacroiliac joints are left intact.[2,52] Although the sacrospinous and sacrotuberous ligaments are often transected in lower sacral amputations, the strong dorsal ligamentous complex is preserved.

Gunterberg and colleagues[52] studied cadaveric pelvises to evaluate pelvic strength after major amputations of the sacrum. If one third of the sacroiliac joint and the associated ligamentous structures were resected, weakening of the pelvic ring amounted to approximately 30%. Resections between S1 and S2 caused loss of stability of about 50%. In all of these experiments, the load to failure far exceeded physiologic loads. These authors concluded that weightbearing was safe for patients after sacral resection, as long as 50% or more of the sacroiliac joint (corresponding to at least the upper half of the S1 segment) remained intact.

Some partial sacrectomies may involve sacroiliac joint resection on only one side. Without reconstruction, the patient may experience postoperative pain associated with proximal migration of the pelvis. It is generally recommended that lumbopelvic fixation be performed in such cases, unless the contralateral joint is completely intact and there is no anterior pelvic deficiency.[53]

The problem of fatigue fractures as a complication of high sacral amputation appears to be limited. Bergh and colleagues[22] found that only 6 of 18 patients with high sacral amputations (through or above the S1–2 disc) developed fractures, and only 1 of them had permanently disabling pain.

Total sacrectomy results in complete dissociation of the spine and pelvis, and requires specialized surgical stabilization techniques to preserve mechanical support and allow satisfactory walking ability.[6,10]

Preoperative Planning

Appropriate preoperative planning requires a keen appreciation of the anatomic relationships of the sacral region, familiarity with the advantages and limitations of the different exposures, and a clear sense of the surgical objective.

Preoperative CT and MRI studies should be performed above and below the tumor site to define its margins and determine the relationship of the tumor with its surrounding structures. Preoperative angiography and embolization are a worthwhile consideration for many lesions, most notably for giant cell tumor.[16,34] If the tumor mass extends well beyond the osseous confines and invades surrounding visceral structures, then preoperative intravenous pyelography or use of a barium enema may be helpful. In cases in which resection of the bladder wall or rectum is planned, diverting colostomies or diverting urinary procedures may be necessary. These must be planned and considered in advance of the surgical procedure.[14]

Surgical Approaches

When the decision to operate has been made, the particular approach is determined by the extent of sacral destruction, the amount of intrapelvic disease, the presence of sacroiliac joint involvement, and the surgical goal of palliation versus cure.

Exposure of the sacrum is complicated by many factors, including its location deep within the pelvis, its intimate relationships with neurovascular structures and pelvic organs, its lateral iliac articulations, and the dorsal overhang of the iliac crests. In addition, due to the capacity of the sacral canal and pelvis to accommodate regional expansion, tumors of the sacral region may attain enormous dimensions by the time of clinical detection. Because of tumor size and the constraints posed by regional anatomy,

the standard unidirectional approaches (anterior, posterior, perineal, lateral) are frequently combined in order to achieve an adequate exposure. Combined approaches may be performed simultaneously, performed consecutively under the same anesthetic, or staged.

Posterior Transsacral Approach

The major advantages of the posterior transsacral approach are its familiarity and technical ease, wide access to the intraspinal and intradural compartments, and clear identification of neural tissue. It is the procedure of choice for the resection of intraspinal tumors and cysts with little or no presacral extension. The patient is placed in the prone position. Due to the proximity of the incision to the anal orifice, extra care in skin preparation and the use of plastic adhesive barrier drapes is advisable.

The principles of this dorsal approach are familiar to most neurosurgeons. The incision may be midline or transverse, depending on the preference of the surgeon and exposure requirements. During the subperiosteal dissection, blood vessels are frequently encountered penetrating the dorsal sacral foramina. Sacrifice of the dorsal rami is unavoidable, but does not cause serious functional sequelae. As long as the sacroiliac joints are left intact laterally, disruption of the dorsal sacroiliac ligaments to achieve a wider exposure of the canal should not lead to mechanical instability. Laminectomies are performed using standard techniques. Limited access to the caudal presacral space may be achieved by resection of the coccyx and division of the anococcygeal muscles. Following tumor resection, any dural defects should be closed in a watertight fashion, and lumbar spinal drainage is advisable.

The neurosurgical microscope is particularly important in the resection of intradural tumors such as schwannomas and ependymomas, which need to be clearly distinguished from surrounding neural tissue.

Transperineal Approach

The transperineal approach allows easy access to the caudal presacral space with minimal morbidity. It can be used alone for cyst drainage or tumor biopsy, but most frequently it is combined with a posterior midline exposure for low sacral amputations. The transperineal approach is not recommended for tumors higher than the S3 level, since it is difficult to accurately dissect the soft tissues of the upper presacrum using this exposure, thereby increasing the risk for major vascular injury, damage to the rectum and lumbosacral trunk, and violation of the tumor capsule.

The patient is placed in the Kraske position (flexed prone) and a midline incision extending rostrally from the coccygeal region is carried out. Access to the presacral space is afforded by division of the anococcygeal ligament. The caudal sacrum may be osteotomized after transection of several soft tissue attachments, including the gluteus maximus, the sacrotuberous and sacrospinous ligaments, and the piriformis muscle. The transperineal approach is discussed in detail in the section entitled Low Sacral Resection on the next page.

Anterior Approach

Wide access to the ventral sacrum is best obtained by a transabdominal route.[54] This exposure facilitates dissection of the rectum and other pelvic contents from the tumor surface while providing access to the vascular supply of the tumor.

Although an anterior sacral approach may be used for the resection of presacral masses, it is often combined with a staged or simultaneous posterior approach to achieve a high sacral amputation or total sacrectomy. In these circumstances, the ventral exposure is used to gain vascular control, dissect the rectum and other pelvic contents from the tumor, and complete the anterior osteotomy; the posterior approach is used to dissect and transect the dural contents and to complete the sacral amputation.

Synchronous Abdominosacral Approach

Localio and colleagues[3] popularized a one-stage abdominosacral approach with the patient in the lateral decubitus position. Although they utilized a retroperitoneal exposure ventrally, others[4] have employed a transabdominal route. The sacrum is exposed through a separate posterior incision, and division of the anococcygeal ligament allows access to the presacral space. By developing the plane behind the rectum, an effort is made to meet with the abdominal incision. The internal iliac artery and vein can be temporarily occluded while the lateral muscular and ligamentous attachments onto the sacrum and sacroiliac joint are transected at the level of intended amputation. The gluteus maximus, piriformis and coccygeus muscles, as well as the sacrotuberous, sacrospinous and posterior sacroiliac ligaments, are divided bilaterally. The sacroiliac joint and sacrum can then be osteotomized under direct vision both dorsally and ventrally.

Localio and colleagues[3] suggested that the combined synchronous approach not only decreases operative time, but also results in less blood loss than either sequential or staged procedures. Although this technique can be used to simultaneously expose the sacrum anteriorly and posteriorly, it is more difficult to expose both of them well. In addition, it is difficult to carry out complex soft-tissue reconstruction and spinopelvic fixation techniques with the patient positioned laterally. We reserve this type of exposure to cases requiring hemisacrectomy.

Lateral Approach to the Sacroiliac Joint

A combined anteroposterior approach to the sacroiliac joint is useful for the en bloc excision of malignant tumors that involve not only the sacroiliac joint itself, but also the lateral sacral ala and medial iliac wing.[55] Chondrosarcoma is notorious for its often eccentric location within the upper sacrum and typically involves the sacroiliac joint.[35] The technique of en bloc resection for tumor localized to the sacroiliac joint is discussed below.

Sacral Resection

The techniques of sacrectomy were popularized by Stener.[2] Sacral resections may be categorized into two groups: those used for midline tumors (typically chordoma, giant cell tumor, and locally invasive rectal carcinoma) and those used for eccentric lesions (e.g., chondrosarcoma of the sacroiliac joint).

The midline group includes low, middle, and high sacral amputations, total sacrectomy, and hemicorporectomy.

Because of the significant functional consequences of nerve root sacrifice, we define the type of sacral amputation not by the level of the osteotomy, but by the level of nerve root sacrifice. Low sacral amputation involves sacrifice of at least one S4 nerve root (or any level below S4). Midsacral amputation involves the sacrifice of at least one S3 nerve root. High sacral amputation requires sacrifice of at least one S2 nerve root. All of the sacrococcygeal nerve roots are lost during total sacrectomy, but the L5 nerve roots and the lumbosacral trunks should be preserved. Progressively higher sacrectomy is technically more challenging and involves greater blood loss, potential for instability, risk for complications, and loss of sphincter control and sexual ability. In hemicorporectomy, or translumbar amputation, the bony pelvis, pelvic contents, lower extremities, and external genitalia are removed following disarticulation of the lumbar spine and transection of the thecal sac.[56]

The lateral group of sacral resections includes hemisacrectomy and en bloc excision of the sacroiliac joint.

Low Sacral Resection

Low sacral amputation via a combined posterior and transperineal exposure was described by McCarty and colleagues[57] in 1952. This approach provides access to the low presacral/retrorectal space and allows complete resection of small tumors of the middle and distal sacrum. More complicated cases, such as for patients with recurrent tumor or rectal involvement, require staged anterior and posterior procedures. Because the low sacral amputation osteotomy is performed below the level of the sacroiliac joint, it is not inherently destabilizing.

The patient is placed in a Kraske (flexed prone) position over padded bolsters to allow the abdomen to hang free and minimize compression of the inferior vena cava. After careful skin preparation and draping, a midline incision is made extending from the region of the lumbosacral junction to the coccyx. The dorsal exposure should be tailored to incorporate any biopsy incision as well as the underlying tract. The erector spinae muscles are usually dissected subperiosteally and retracted laterally. However, if preoperative imaging studies reveal tumor extending dorsally out of the sacrum, a layer of sacrospinalis musculature and fat should be left to cover the involved regions. Depending on the extent of soft tissue involvement, it may also be advantageous to transect the gluteal maximus several centimeters from its origin, leaving a cuff of gluteal musculature attached to the sacrum laterally. The lateral sacrococcygeal attachments including the sacrotuberous and sacrospinous ligaments and the coccygeus and piriformis muscles are then identified and transected close to their insertions. The pudendal and sciatic nerves as well as the gluteal arteries are carefully identified and preserved. The inferior edge of the sacroiliac joint is cleared of soft tissue using a Cobb elevator.

Division of the anococcygeal ligament allows entry into the presacral space. The rectum is gently mobilized away from the tumor surface by blunt finger dissection. A limited sacral laminectomy, immediately rostral to the level of intended amputation, allows direct visualization of the nerve roots. For example, if the intent is to amputate the sacrum at the bony S3 level with preservation of the third sacral

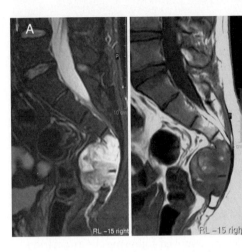
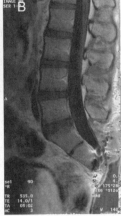
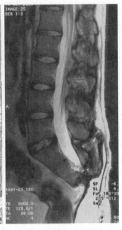

FIGURE 158-1 Preoperative and postoperative magnetic resonance images of a patient with sacral chordoma involving the S4-coccygeal region. The patient underwent dorsal approach S3 and partial S4 laminectomy and high S3 sacral amputation. Transperineal dissection of the rectum was performed to free up the tumor from ventral viscera.

nerve roots, a laminectomy from S1 to S3 is performed. The filum terminale externa is transected and the nerve roots below S3 are doubly ligated and transected within the sacral canal. An osteotomy of the sacral body is then performed using a high-speed drill with a diamond burr. The pelvic structures are protected during the osteotomy by maintaining a finger in the presacral space. This maneuver also provides tactile sensation to help guide the osteotomy (Fig. 158-1).

A large cavity results from this resection; therefore, excellent hemostasis is essential. Suction drains are placed within the cavity and the wound is reapproximated in a layered fashion. Local soft tissue flaps may be necessary to fill the large defect and to facilitate a tensionless closure (Fig. 158-2).

Middle and High Sacral Resection

Sacral amputation above S3 utilizing a staged anterior and posterior approach was initially reported by Bowers.[54] The use of a transpelvic vertical rectus abdominis myocutaneous (VRAM) flap for the reconstruction of large sacral defects has significantly reduced problems with wound breakdown following these aggressive resections.[58]

The first stage is the transabdominal exposure, for which the patient is positioned supine. A midline celiotomy is performed. An initial inspection of the abdominal contents is done both to confirm the resectability of the tumor and to ensure that there are no other intra-abdominal masses that would preclude curative resection. The bowel is packed off, and both ureters and internal iliac vessels are identified.

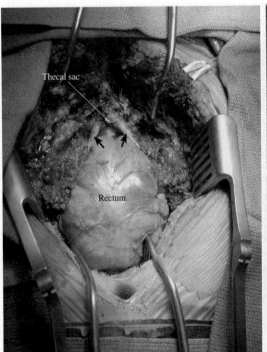
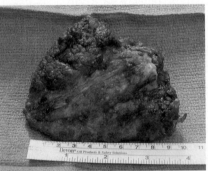
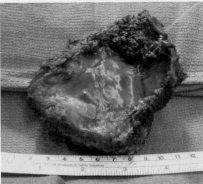

FIGURE 158-2 Postoperative dorsal view of the same patient following en bloc removal of the tumor. Seen are bilaterally preserved S3 roots (*arrows*), posterior rectal wall, and ligated end of the thecal sac. The last two images show a postoperative surgical specimen that was excised en bloc.

Moistened umbilical tapes are loosely applied to secure the common iliac arteries and veins. The internal iliac vessels are doubly ligated and transected, and the anterior and lateral sacral vessels are identified, ligated, and transected. If the rectum is to be spared, the retrorectal peritoneal reflection is incised and the rectosigmoid colon is dissected away from the tumor capsule. Although the sacrum is somewhat devascularized by transection of the hypogastric and tumor vessels, hemostasis of the robust presacral venous plexus is often difficult. Exposure of the tumor proceeds carefully to leave as much normal fatty tissue as possible with the specimen.

Rostral dissection with mobilization of the common iliac vessels is often required for high sacral amputations. The ventral sacral foramina serve as the best landmarks to guide the ventral sacral osteotomy, although the level may also be confirmed using intraoperative radiographs or fluoroscopy. Selecting an area approximately one sacral level above the region of the planned osteotomy, the periosteum is incised in a transverse fashion and reflected downward. The sympathetic trunks are unavoidably cut, along with the hypogastric plexus in the case of very high sacral amputations. If the planned osteotomy incorporates any of the ventral sacral foramina, the sacral nerves exiting at that level are first dissected out and preserved. It is not possible to spare any sacral nerves if the osteotomy must cross the body of S1 above the foramina. The sacral alae are dissected laterally and the lumbosacral nerve trunks are exposed and freed. The nerve trunks are mobilized laterally during the osteotomy.

The anterior osteotomy only incises the anterior cortical bone and should not proceed deep enough to damage the dural contents. Our preference is to use a high-speed drill with a diamond burr rather than an osteotome. The osteotomy proceeds inferolaterally to incorporate a small portion of the sacroiliac joints and anterior ilium. It is important to be able to feel the lateral extent of the anterior osteotomy through the sciatic notch as a guide during the posterior osteotomy.

If the rectum is to be included with the specimen, the superior rectal vessels are identified and ligated and the rectosigmoid junction is mobilized in preparation for division with a mechanical stapler. The bowel is transected and the middle rectal vessels are ligated and divided. The stapled stumps of bowel may be oversewn to decrease the risk for wound soilage. Tumor involvement of other pelvic organs or the endopelvic fascia may require pelvic exenteration if the surgery is to have curative intent.[46]

A Silastic sheet is placed into the plane of dissection between the dorsally situated sacrectomy specimen with its associated presacral mass and the ventral structures including the iliac vessels, ureters, and sacral plexi. The VRAM flap, which is based on the inferior epigastric vessels, is harvested and secured within the pelvis until it is needed for the posterior closure. The anterior abdominal wall is closed in the standard fashion.

We previously preferred to stage these complex procedures on separate days. However, performing both stages sequentially under the same anesthetic has several advantages. During the anterior procedure the distal gastrointestinal tract is denervated, resulting in an expected postoperative ileus. As a result, the second stage may be delayed for 10 to 14 days. Due to the effects of this prolonged interval with regard to flap viability, we did not harvest the VRAM flap

until the beginning of the second stage. Thus, the celiotomy incision had to be reopened with the patient in the supine position before being able to proceed with the posterior approach. With more experience, we can now complete both the anterior and posterior stages within 12 to 14 hours.

The second stage begins with the patient in a Kraske (flexed prone) position on padded bolsters. The abdomen should be allowed to hang free. A midline incision is created from the tip of the coccyx to the lower lumbar level. If the rectum is to be included with the resection, the caudal end of the incision also involves a circumferential incision about the anus. Another alternative is to perform the perineal dissection during the anterior approach, with the patient in the lithotomy rather than the supine position. Any skin and underlying soft tissue that is involved with tumor or may be seeded with tumor cells as a consequence of a previous percutaneous biopsy should be incorporated with the specimen en bloc.

Lateral flaps are elevated to expose the iliac crest. The gluteal maximus is transected laterally, leaving a cuff of tissue attached to the sacrum. The underlying piriformis muscles are also divided bilaterally. The superior and inferior gluteal vessels and the sciatic, pudendal, and posterior cutaneous femoral nerves should be identified and protected. If the resection is to spare the rectum, the anococcygeal ligament is divided and the sacrotuberous and sacrospinous ligaments as well as the coccygeus muscles are divided. If the rectum is to be included, the levator musculature is divided and the anus is freed circumferentially.

A subperiosteal exposure of the posterior elements of the lower lumbar and upper sacral levels is performed and the sacrospinalis muscles are sectioned transversely. A wide L5 and upper sacral laminectomy is completed in order to expose the dural sac. The dural sac is doubly ligated and transected just below the exit of the last nerve root to be preserved. The floor of the sacral canal can thus be exposed for the dorsoventral osteotomy.

The ventral osteotomy cuts are palpated by introducing a finger presacrally via the perineal exposure. The tactile sense provided guides the dorsal osteotomy. The osteotomy is performed in two stages, each beginning in the midline and extending through the lateral sacroiliac joint to exit at the greater sacroiliac notch. Once the specimen is freed, the sacral roots, which have already been sacrificed within the spinal canal, are divided just proximal to their connections with the sciatic nerve.

The gluteal muscles may be reapproximated to each other or to bone. Suction drains are placed deep in the wound and tunneled to remote exit sites. The large sacral defect is closed using the VRAM flap, which is retrieved from the pelvis and sutured into place in a layered fashion. As an alternative, a microvascular free flap reconstruction may be performed. Free flap reconstruction is challenging in the sacral area because of difficult access to adequate recipient vessels.[59] Gluteal rotation flaps are not a reliable option.[58]

Patients with rectal resections are again turned to the supine position, the celiotomy is reopened, and a colostomy is completed.

Total Sacrectomy

Few cases of total sacrectomy have been reported in the literature.[5,6,60–64] Although it is not possible to spare any of

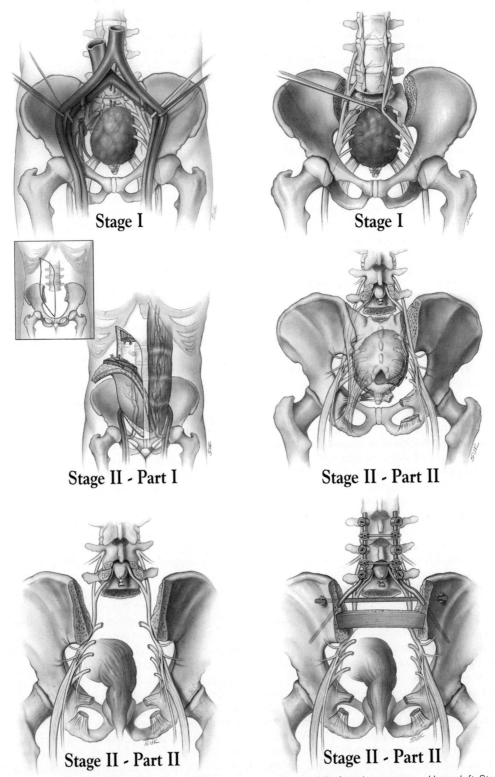

FIGURE 158-3 Artist's renderings depicting the operative fields during stages I and II of total sacrectomy. *Upper left,* Stage I. Ventral view of the lumbosacral region after median celiotomy. The inferior vena cava and aorta (and their main branches) are mobilized, allowing a clear view of the L5–S1 disc space and permitting retraction of these vessels for lumbar trunk (L4–5 nerve roots) identification. Median and lateral sacral vessels along with internal hypogastric vessels are ligated. The S1 foramina and nerve roots are also visualized bilaterally; the tumor usually obscures the lower sacral nerve roots (S2–5). Visualized sacral roots are then transected ventrally while preserving the lumbar trunk. *Upper right,* Stage I. Ventral view of the lumbosacral region with the vessels removed. Nerve roots at S1–3 are transected ventrally. Using a diamond burr, partial (ventral) sacroiliac osteotomy is performed lateral to the lumbar trunk. *Center left,* Stage II, part I. Ventral view of the abdominal wall while the patient is supine. A vascularized rectus abdominus muscle with an island of skin and subcutaneous adipose tissue is harvested from the location outlined in the *inset.* Taking care to preserve the inferior epigastric vessels, this flap is placed in the abdominal cavity and the incision is closed. *Center right,* Stage II, part II. Dorsal view of the lumbosacral region while the patient is in the jackknife position after completion of L5 laminectomy and bilateral L5–S1 foraminotomy. The completed L5–S1 discectomy and dorsal sacroiliac osteotomy are also shown. The thecal sac is ligated distal to the takeoff of the L5 nerve roots bilaterally.

(Continued)

the sacral roots during this procedure, careful preservation of the L4 and L5 nerve roots allows patients to ambulate postoperatively.

The technique is essentially the same as that discussed for high sacral amputation, with some exceptions (Fig. 158-3). During the anterior approach, bilateral ventral osteotomies along the entire length of the sacroiliac joints are performed with the lumbar nerve roots and lumbosacral trunks protected medially. Instead of a transverse osteotomy through the upper sacrum, an L5–S1 discectomy is performed. Finally, the S1–S3 ventral nerve roots are transected at their foramina, if they can be visualized. During the second stage of the procedure, an L5 laminectomy and bilateral L5–S1 foraminotomies expose the L5 nerve roots, which are preserved. The posterior iliac crests are removed with Leksell rongeurs and a high-speed drill is used to complete the sacroiliac osteotomies from the posterior approach. The thecal sac is then ligated below the level of the L5 nerve roots and the L5–S1 discectomy is completed. The sciatic notches are exposed bilaterally and the S1–S5 roots are transected. Following division of the posterior ligamentous attachments, the sacrum can be removed in toto. Lumboilial fixation is required. As described for high sacral amputation, resection of the rectum may be incorporated and the VRAM flap is routinely used to close the sacral defect.[58]

En Bloc Resection of Tumors of the Sacroiliac Joint

The patient is placed in the lateral decubitus position. A curved incision is made just above the margin of the iliac crest, beginning a few centimeters behind the anterior superior iliac spine. The incision extends to the lumbosacral junction where it is joined by a posterior midline lumbosacral incision. The fascia of the abdominal muscles is incised near the iliac crest, leaving a 1-cm cuff attached to the crest to later facilitate closure. The iliacus muscle is stripped from the inner aspect of the iliac wing using a Cobb elevator. As the sacroiliac joint and greater sciatic notch is approached, blunt dissection using a sponge-covered elevator is recommended. Damage to the femoral nerve and major vessels is prevented by remaining deep to the iliacus muscle. The nearby lumbosacral trunk, which passes over the pelvic inlet medial to the ventral surface of the sacroiliac joint, is also at risk during these maneuvers. Medial retraction of the iliacus and psoas muscles as well as the overlying viscera completes the ventral exposure of the sacroiliac joint.

Posteriorly, the attachments of the lumbodorsal fascia and gluteus maximus are detached from the iliac crest. The gluteus maximus is raised with a Cobb elevator in a subperiosteal fashion. It is important to proceed with care in the region of the greater sciatic notch to avoid damage to the sciatic nerve and the superior gluteal vessels. The ipsilateral erector spinae muscles are divided in a transverse fashion below the

level of the sacroiliac joint and raised subperiosteally as a lumbosacral flap, which is retracted laterally and rostrally. Depending on the extent of tumor, additional posterior exposure may be gained by transection of the sacrospinous and sacrotuberous ligaments and the piriformis muscle.

With the superior gluteal vessels mobilized and the neural structures protected, a Gigli saw is passed through the greater sciatic notch and the iliac osteotomy is performed. The anterior structures are retracted medially, and the sacrum is osteotomized in a posteroanterior direction, beginning just lateral to the upper three dorsal foramina. We prefer to use a high-speed drill to perform the osteotomies rather than an osteotome, because of improved hemostasis and finer control. A diamond burr does not tend to entrain adjacent soft tissues. After completing the osteotomies, the entire specimen can be removed en bloc.

Osseous bleeding is controlled with bone wax, and soft tissue hemostasis is obtained. Suction drains are placed within the resection cavity. The gluteus maximus can sometimes be reapproximated to the midline fascia. Anteriorly, the closure is performed in layers. The aponeurosis of the abdominal muscles is reattached to the soft tissue cuff left on the iliac crest during the exposure.

Hemisacrectomy

This surgical procedure generally involves the unilateral removal of the sacroiliac joint and a portion of the ilium along with the hemisacrum. It may be performed as part of a more extensive internal or external hemipelvectomy procedure.[65] The approach is essentially an extension of the lateral approach to the sacroiliac joint: it involves combined simultaneous retroperitoneal and posterior exposures with the patient placed in the lateral decubitus position. Dorsal and ventral osteotomies can thus be performed under direct vision. Resection of all the sacral nerves on one side results in expected deficits in sensitivity and strength; however, sphincter function may be normal or only partially compromised.[2]

SPINOPELVIC STABILIZATION

Partial sacrectomy involving more than 50% of the sacroiliac joint on each side is an indication for spinopelvic stabilization.[52] Pedicle screws provide rigid stabilization and can be used for short segment fixation across the lumbosacral junction.[66] The S1 pedicle is larger than the lumbar pedicles and often can be fitted with 7- to 8-mm screws. Additional bony purchase can be obtained if the screw penetrates the anterior S1 cortex or the superior end plate of S1. Medially directed S1 pedicle screws that are cross-linked and attached to rods create a triangulation effect, which greatly increases torsional stability and resists pullout.[67-71] Triangulation with an oblique orientation also

---

FIGURE 158-3 Cont'd *Lower left,* Stage II, part II. Dorsal view of the lumboiliac region after en bloc removal of the sacrum. The cut ends of nerve roots S1–4 are shown bilaterally, as are the bilaterally preserved lumbar trunk and remaining sciatic nerve. Sacrotuberous and sacrospinous ligament cut ends are also depicted. The dorsal rectal wall is viewed ventrally. *Lower right,* Stage II, part II. Dorsal view of the lumbosacral region after reconstruction. Pedicle screws are seen bilaterally at L3–5 along with rods that are attached to the screws and bent (L-shaped) and embedded between the cortices of the remaining ilia as reported in the Galveston technique. A threaded rod (transiliac bar) is placed ventral to the Galveston rods but dorsal to the lumbar trunk, and the ends outside the iliac cortical surface are secured with C-shaped clamps. The tibial allograft is seen bridging the defect between the remaining ilia. (From Gokaslan ZL, Romsdahl MM, Kroll SS, et al: Total sacrectomy and Galveston L-rod reconstruction for malignant neoplasms. Technical note. J Neurosurg 87:781–787, 1997.)

interferes less with the superjacent facet joint and allows more purchase with a longer screw.[70]

A method to enhance sacral fixation with screws is to place an additional pair of laterally directed bone screws into the sacral alae below the S1 level. This has a biomechanical advantage over a single pair of S1 pedicle screws[68]; however, the bone of the ala is usually of low density, and purchase may be tenuous. Moreover, the risk for neurovascular injury from laterally directed screws in this region must be kept in mind.

S2 (or lower level) pedicle screws are often of little use because the pedicles are very short. Biomechanical testing has shown that pedicle screws placed below the S1 level do not significantly enhance stability.[68] In addition, the thin sagittal dimension of the sacrum at lower levels increases the risk for penetration of its ventral surface, with a potential for injury to the adjacent vascular and visceral structures. Screws at lower sacral levels are often prominent dorsally and may even tent the overlying skin.

Sacral screw fixation may be sufficient for cases in which the fixation length is short (one or two levels) and there is minimal instability. If a long construct is placed, the sacral attachment is subjected to large cantilevered forces that may lead to screw pullout. Finally, the use of sacral screws may be precluded in certain cases, such as when the pedicles, body, or ala of the sacrum is involved with tumor.

A simple method of sacropelvic fixation involves the placement of long, variable-angle bone screws obliquely across the sacroiliac joint into the iliac bones. A tripod effect may be gained by combining the sacroiliac fixation with additional sacral fixation points.[72]

Salehi and colleagues[45] recently described a novel reconstructive technique for spinopelvic stabilization after resection of metastatic sacral tumors involving a modification of the transiliac bar. They used a cage and ilial bolt system for fixation of the spine to the ilium and connected rods that had been affixed to the pedicle screws with satisfactory results.

Reconstruction after Total Sacrectomy

In the case of total sacrectomy, there is no bone for sacral fixation. Iliac fixation is the only procedure to stabilize the spinopelvic junction. A number of different constructs for reconstruction following total sacrectomy have been described in the literature.[5,6,10,14,60-64,73] Some of the early methods involved the placement of transverse sacral bars[5,60] or Steinmann pins[61] to connect the posterior iliac wings. In one report,[60] the bar was placed through the L5 vertebral body. These devices were then connected to the spinal instrumentation, which consisted of Harrington rods[60] or Cotrel-Dubousset rods.[5,61] The major disadvantage of these constructs relates to the soft bone of the posterior ilium, which does not provide firm fixation. Additionally, these methods provide poor rotational stability. Hook-and-rod systems may accidentally disengage from the transverse sacral bars or Steinmann pins.

An alternative form of reconstruction for large sacral defects is the implantation of a custom-made prosthesis[73] designed to fit the individual shape of the pelvis and accommodate for the amount of resection performed. The major disadvantage is that it is impossible to make adjustments during surgery.

The Modified Galveston Technique

Allen and Ferguson from Galveston, Texas, were the first to describe a technique involving the insertion of an angled distal limb of a spinal fixation rod into the posterior iliac bones, just above the sciatic notch.[74] The Galveston technique has since become the benchmark for other spinopelvic fixation systems.[6,68]

In the biomechanical testing of 10 different lumbosacral instrumentation techniques in a bovine model, McCord and colleagues[68] found that the most effective construct entailed medially directed S1 pedicle screws and an iliac purchase in the Galveston-type fashion. The key to the strength of the Galveston construct is explained by the concept of the lumbosacral "pivot point."[68] This point is located at the intersection of the osteoligamentous column in the sagittal plane and the lumbosacral intervertebral disc in the transverse plane. It represents the axis of rotation at the lumbosacral junction. The iliac rod in the Galveston technique extends anterior to the lumbosacral pivot point, providing a long lever arm within the ilium to counteract flexion moments exerted by the lumbar spine.

In cases requiring total sacrectomy, we supplement the Galveston technique by placing a threaded transiliac rod to resist axial rotation of the lumboiliac union[6,10] (Fig. 158-4). This threaded rod helps reconstruct the pelvic ring, thereby preventing the open-book phenomenon. The rod is placed more anteriorly on the ilium, which avoids the slippage associated with anchorage into the softer posterior ilium. Locking collars are placed to prevent lateral migration of the rod. An alternative to the threaded rod (although we have not used this) is to place a large pelvic reconstruction plate, with pedicle screws at the fifth lumbar vertebra going through the plate and bicortical screws securing the plate to each iliac wing.[37]

Custom bending and insertion of the Galveston rod requires some technical skill to achieve the correct position with the rod remaining intracortical. Tube benders are used to create an initial sacroiliac bend of approximately 60 degrees, and then a table vice is used to stabilize the distal ilial segment of the rod while an approximately 110-degree lumbosacral bend is created.[10]

A technically simpler alternative to the Galveston rod are iliac screws (ISOLA iliac screws; AcroMed, Cleveland, OH, U.S.A.), which can be placed independently of the spinal rod, with the two subsequently linked together. Double iliac screw fixation[14] involves the placement of long 7- to 8-mm-diameter threaded screws into the iliac wings and linked to the spinal rods independently. The rods may be connected with a cross-linked bar to better counteract rotational force (Fig. 158-5).

Extensive bone grafting is essential to obtain a fusion. In addition to placing autogenous and allogenic corticocancellous bone extending from the transverse processes to the ilium bilaterally, we place a tibial allogenic strut graft to close the space between the two ilia and help facilitate fusion of the entire defect.[6]

After surgery, the patient remains in bed for 6 to 8 weeks in order to allow at least a fibrous union of the reconstruction before the patient is mobilized. Although bone fusion takes a minimum of 6 months, this fibrous union may be quite effective at providing enough structural support for ambulation.

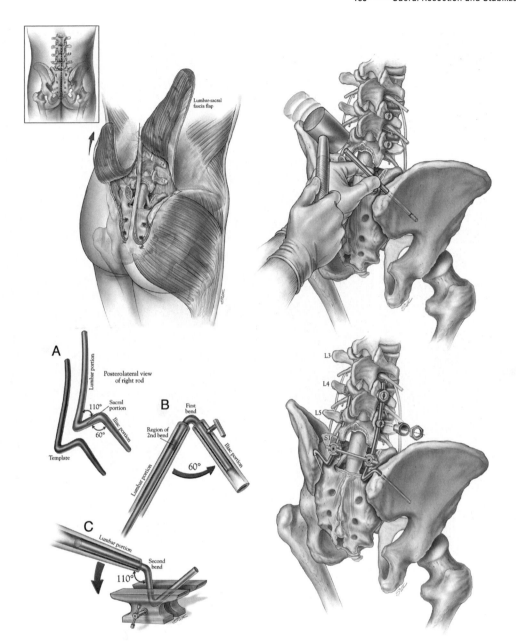

FIGURE 158-4 *Upper left,* Illustration depicting the posterior exposure of the sacrum, medial ilium, and lumbar spine. The lumbosacral fascia/muscular flap is lifted off of the sacrum and retracted cephalad and laterally. *Inset,* The *dashed line* represents the posterior incision. *Upper right,* A 6-mm titanium pilot rod is tapped into the cancellous portion of the ileum to create a path for the contoured rod. This temporary rod is directed 1.5 cm above the sciatic notch and between the two cortices of the ilium. It is tapped into place with a mallet to a depth of 6 to 9 cm. *Lower left,* A 6-mm titanium rod is then contoured to match the template rod (wire) by using tube benders and a table vice. The final shape of the spinal-pelvic rod matches the template rod (A); tube benders are used to create the sacroiliac bend of approximately 60 degrees (B); and the table vice is used to stabilize the sacral and iliac segments of the rod while an approximately 110-degree bend is created between the lumbar and sacral segments (C). *Lower right,* Illustration of the spinal-pelvic fixation. (From Davis KD, Taub E, Duffner F, et al: Activation of the anterior cingulate cortex by thalamic stimulation in patients with chronic pain: A positron emission tomography study. J Neurosurg 92:64–69, 2000.)

We no longer routinely recommend the use of a thoracolumbosacral orthosis after total sacrectomy.

In a series of 13 patients who underwent Galveston fixation following the resection of metastatic or locally aggressive neoplasms of the lumbosacral region, including five patients who required total sacrectomy, solid bone fusion was achieved in four (31%) and partial or unilateral fusion in three (23%).[10] Five patients (38%) had no convincing evidence of fusion on radiographic studies. Since three of these five patients improved clinically, a satisfactory

fibrous union may have occurred. Radiation therapy, chemotherapy, and neoplastic disease processes may have contributed to the lack of bony fusion in some patients. Only one hardware-related complication occurred: the rods fractured bilaterally at the transition point between the lumbar and sacral segments in one patient. This was corrected with double iliolumbar rod fixation. Ambulatory status improved in 62% (eight patients), and spine-related pain, as reflected by visual analogue pain scores and medication consumption, was significantly reduced in 85% of our patients.

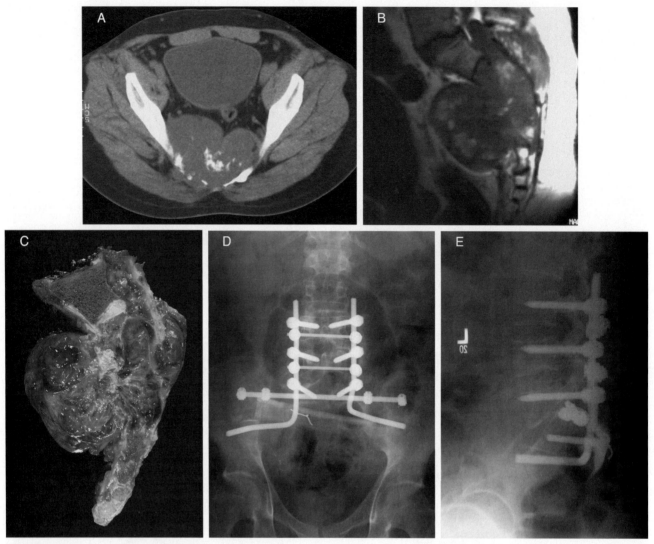

FIGURE 158-5 Preoperative axial computerized tomography scan (*A*) magnetic resonance image (*B*) revealing a sacral chordoma. *C*, Hemisection of gross pathologic specimen demonstrating complete en bloc resection of the sacrum. *D* and *E*, Postoperative anteroposterior and lateral radiographs.

POSTOPERATIVE CARE AND COMPLICATION AVOIDANCE

Patients undergoing major sacral resections are managed in an intensive care unit postoperatively. Since a significant amount of blood may be lost during these procedures, ongoing assessment of fluid and blood product requirements is essential. It is advisable to keep patients intubated for a few days after surgery to ensure that laryngeal edema has subsided and that all fluids given during the operation have been mobilized. Nursing the patient on an air bed helps prevent wound breakdown and decubitus ulcers. The wound should be observed closely for infection, hematoma, or seroma formation. Antibiotics are continued until all suction drains have been removed from the wound. Pneumatic compression devices applied to the lower extremities and small intermittent doses of subcutaneous heparin are important for the prevention of deep vein thrombosis. Denervation of the distal gastrointestinal tract during high sacral resections almost uniformly results in a significant postoperative ileus, with some patients requiring intravenous nutrition for a prolonged period.

Patients are mobilized as soon as possible, depending on functional reserve and the perceived stability of the dorsal pelvic ring. The input of rehabilitation physicians is essential following aggressive sacral resections. Progressive independence with walking, competence with intermittent catheterization, and management of fecal incontinence are some of the goals of rehabilitative therapy. The input of psychosexual counselors and reproductive health specialists may be valuable with regard to sexual function issues.

The highest incidence of wound infection occurs in patients who have received preoperative radiation therapy.[66] We routinely use soft tissue reconstructive techniques such as the transpelvic VRAM flap or a microvascular free flap to help reduce the risk for wound complications in patients who require high sacral resection or total sacrectomy.[58]

Early failure of the lumbosacral instrumentation (i.e., within 6 to 12 weeks) is usually due to screw pullout. This is most commonly caused by repetitive stress at the bone–metal interface. Early failure of the construct may be prevented by the use of multiple sites of fixation in order to best distribute the forces at the bone–implant junction. In some cases, early loosening of the instrumentation may not prevent solid bony fusion; however, close radiologic follow-up is required. Delaying revision surgery is reasonable until it is certain that it is required to achieve an acceptable result.

Since the Galveston rods lie within cancellous bone, any change in the orientation of the rods after the iliac limb has been implanted creates a small void in the bone with the potential for loosening. A 2- to 3-mm lucency around the iliac portion of the rod is often visible on x-ray studies; however, in our experience, this finding alone does not indicate construct failure or pseudoarthrosis.

Reoperation is recommended if evidence of progressive deformity or painful pseudoarthrosis is observed. Revision surgery should address the cause for failure. For example, metal fatigue fracture suggests poor load sharing in the original construct, and new fixation points may need to be added. Screw pullout suggests the need for larger-diameter or longer bone screws to obtain a solid bony purchase on additional cortices. The application of methylmethacrylate may enhance screw fixation in the setting of poor-quality bone.[10]

Surgery for failed spinal fixation should always involve additional bone grafting, preferably with autologous bone. No rigid ventral stabilizing device can be easily applied to the sacrum, although interbody grafts (allogenic or autogenic), cages, and techniques using methylmethacrylate may be applied at the lumbosacral junction.[10]

CONCLUSIONS

All patients with sacral tumors should be evaluated in a multidisciplinary environment. The choices of treatment, including surgery, radiotherapy, chemotherapy, or a combination thereof, must be made on an individual basis with an understanding of the biological nature of the disease. The technical challenges of high sacral amputation and total sacrectomy should not be underestimated. The functional consequences of the procedure should be clearly discussed with the patient preoperatively. The surgeon must be intricately familiar with sacral anatomy and methods to reestablish spinopelvic stability. The collaborative input of oncologic and plastic surgeons is invaluable. The VRAM flap has been of major benefit in obliterating surgical dead space with viable nonirradiated tissues and affecting a tensionless wound closure.

REFERENCES

1. Feldenzer JA, McGauley JL, McGillicuddy JE: Sacral and presacral tumors: Problems in diagnosis and management. Neurosurgery 25:884–891, 1989.
2. Stener B, Gunterberg B: High amputation of the sacrum for extirpation of tumors. Principles and technique. Spine 3:351–366, 1978.
3. Localio SA, Eng K, Ranson JH: Abdominosacral approach for retrorectal tumors. Ann Surg 191:555–560, 1980.
4. Huth JF, Dawson EG, Eilber FR: Abdominosacral resection for malignant tumors of the sacrum. Am J Surg 148:157–161, 1984.
5. Tomita K, Tsuchiya H: Total sacrectomy and reconstruction for huge sacral tumors. Spine 15:1223–1227, 1990.
6. Gokaslan ZL, Romsdahl MM, Kroll SS, et al: Total sacrectomy and Galveston L-rod reconstruction for malignant neoplasms. J Neurosurg 87:781–787, 1997.
7. York JE, Kaczaraj A, Abi-Said D, et al: Sacral chordoma: 40-year experience at a major cancer center. Neurosurgery 44:74–80, 1999.
8. Fourney DR, Gokaslan ZL: Current management of sacral chordoma. Neurosurg Focus 15(2): Article 9, 2003.
9. Weber KL, Nelson H, Gunderson LL, et al: Sacropelvic resection for recurrent anorectal cancer. A multidisciplinary approach. Clin Orthop 372:231–240, 2000.
10. Jackson RJ, Gokaslan ZL: Spinal-pelvic fixation in patients with lumbosacral neoplasms. J Neurosurg 92(1 Suppl):61–70, 2000.
11. Payer M: Neurological manifestations of sacral tumors. Neurosurg Focus 15(2): Article 1, 2003.
12. Disler DG, Miklic D: Imaging findings in tumors of the sacrum. AJR Am J Roentgenol 173:1699–1706, 1999.
13. Llauger J, Palmer J, Amores S, et al: Primary tumors of the sacrum: Diagnostic imaging. AJR Am J Roentgenol 174:417–424, 2000.
14. Zhang HY, Thongtrangan I, Balabhadra RS, et al: Surgical techniques for total sacrectomy and spinopelvic reconstruction. Neurosurg Focus 15(2): Article 5, 2003.
15. Broaddus WC, Grady MS, Delashaw JB Jr, et al: Preoperative superselective arteriolar embolization: A new approach to enhance resectability of spinal tumors. Neurosurgery 27:755–759, 1990.
16. Lin PP, Guzel VB, Moura MF, et al: Long-term follow-up of patients with giant cell tumor of the sacrum treated with selective arterial embolization. Cancer 95:1317–1325, 2002.
17. Rescorla FJ, Sawin RS, Coran AG, et al: Long-term outcome for infants and children with sacrococcygeal teratoma: A report from the Children's Cancer Group. J Pediatr Surg 33:171–176, 1998.
18. Audet IM, Goldhahn RT Jr, Dent TL: Adult sacrococcygeal teratomas. Am Surg 66:61–65, 2000.
19. De Backer A, Erpicum P, Philippe P, et al: Sacrococcygeal teratoma: Results of a retrospective multicentric study in Belgium and Luxembourg. Eur J Pediatr Surg 11:182–185, 2001.
20. Chisholm CA, Heider AL, Kuller JA, et al: Prenatal diagnosis and perinatal management of fetal sacrococcygeal teratoma. Am J Perinatol 16:47–50, 1999.
21. Cheng EY, Ozerdemoglu RA, Transfeldt EE, et al: Lumbosacral chordoma. Prognostic factors and treatment. Spine 24(16):1639–1645, 1999.
22. Bergh P, Kindblom LG, Gunterberg B, et al: Prognostic factors in chordoma of the sacrum and mobile spine: A study of 39 patients. Cancer 88:2122–2134, 2000.
23. Enneking WF: A system of staging musculoskeletal neoplasms. Clin Orthop 204:9–24, 1986.
24. Ishii K, Chiba K, Watanabe M, et al: Local recurrence after S2–3 sacrectomy in sacral chordoma. Report of four cases. J Neurosurg 97(1 Suppl):98–101, 2002.
25. Dominguez J, Lobato RD, Ramos A, et al: Giant intrasacral schwannomas: Report of six cases. Acta Neurochir (Wien) 139:954–959, 1997.
26. Takeyama M, Koshino T, Nakazawa A, et al: Giant intrasacral cellular schwannoma treated with high sacral amputation. Spine 26: E216–E219, 2001.
27. Ginsberg LE, Williams DW, Stanton C: Intrasacral myxopapillary ependymoma. Neuroradiology 36:56–58, 1994.
28. Fourney DR, Fuller GN, Gokaslan ZL: Intraspinal extradural myxopapillary ependymoma of the sacrum arising from the filum terminale externa. Case report. J Neurosurg 93(2 Suppl):322–326, 2000.
29. Marmor E, Fourney DR, Rhines LD, et al: Sacrococcygeal ganglioneuroma. J Spinal Disord Tech 15:265–268, 2002.
30. Boriani S, Capanna R, Donati D, et al: Osteoblastoma of the spine. Clin Orthop 278:37–45, 1992.
31. Biagini R, Orsini U, Demitri S, et al: Osteoid osteoma and osteoblastoma of the sacrum. Orthopedics 24:1061–1064, 2001.
32. Papagelopoulos PJ, Choudhury SN, Frassica FJ, et al: Treatment of aneurysmal bone cysts of the pelvis and sacrum. J Bone Joint Surg Am 83:1674–1681, 2001.
33. Turcotte RE, Sim FH, Unni KK: Giant cell tumor of the sacrum. Clin Orthop 291:215–221, 1993.
34. Althausen PL, Schneider PD, Bold RJ, et al: Multimodality management of a giant cell tumor arising in the proximal sacrum: Case report. Spine 27:E361–365, 2002.

35. Bergh P, Gunterberg B, Meis-Kindblom JM, et al: Prognostic factors and outcome of pelvic, sacral, and spinal chondrosarcomas: A center-based study of 69 cases. Cancer 91:1201–1212, 2001.

36. Ozaki T, Flege S, Liljenqvist U, et al: Osteosarcoma of the spine: experience of the Cooperative Osteosarcoma Study Group. Cancer 94:1069–1077, 2002.

37. Spiegel DA, Richardson WJ, Scully SP, et al: Long-term survival following total sacrectomy with reconstruction for the treatment of primary osteosarcoma of the sacrum. A case report. J Bone Joint Surg Am 81:848–855, 1999.

38. Sharafuddin MJ, Haddad FS, Hitchon PW, et al: Treatment options in primary Ewing's sarcoma of the spine: Report of seven cases and review of the literature. Neurosurgery 30:610–618, 1992.

39. Pilepich MV, Vietti TJ, Nesbit ME, et al: Ewing's sarcoma of the vertebral column. Int J Radiat Oncol Biol Physiol 7:27–31, 1981.

40. Grubb MR, Currier BL, Pritchard DJ, et al: Primary Ewing's sarcoma of the spine. Spine 19:309–313, 1994.

41. Baker ND, Dorfman DM: Ewing's sarcoma of the sacrum. Skel Radiol 25:302–304, 1996.

42. Evans RG, Nesbit ME, Gehan EA, et al: Multimodal therapy for the management of localized Ewing's sarcoma of pelvic and sacral bones: A report from the second intergroup study. J Clin Oncol 9:1173–1180, 1991.

43. Yang RS, Eckardt JJ, Eilber FR, et al: Surgical indications for Ewing's sarcoma of the pelvis. Cancer 76:1388–1397, 1995.

44. Ozdemir MH, Gurkan I, Yildiz Y, et al: Surgical treatment of malignant tumours of the sacrum. Eur J Surg Oncol 25:44–49, 1999.

45. Salehi SA, McCafferty RR, Karahalios D, et al: Neural function preservation and early mobilization after resection of metastatic sacral tumors and lumbosacropelvic junction reconstruction: Report of three cases. J Neurosurg 97(1 Suppl):88–93, 2002.

46. Crowe PJ, Temple WJ, Lopez MJ, et al: Pelvic exenteration for advanced pelvic malignancy. Semin Surg Oncol 17:152–160, 1999.

47. Moffat FL Jr, Falk RE: Radical surgery for extensive rectal cancer: Is it worthwhile? Recent Results Cancer Res 146:71–83, 1998.

48. Gunterberg B, Norlen L, Stener B, et al: Neurological evaluation after resection of the sacrum. Invest Urol 13:183–188, 1975.

49. Biagini R, Ruggieri P, Mercuri M, et al: Neurologic deficit after resection of the sacrum. Chir Organi Mov 82:357–372, 1997.

50. Nakai S, Yoshizawa H, Kobayashi S, et al: Anorectal and bladder function after sacrifice of the sacral nerves. Spine 25:2234–2239, 2000.

51. Todd LT Jr, Yaszemski MJ, Currier BL, et al: Bowel and bladder function after major sacral resection. Clin Orthop 397:36–39, 2002.

52. Gunterberg B, Romanus B, Stener B: Pelvic strength after major amputation of the sacrum. An experimental study. Acta Orthop Scand 47:635–642, 1976.

53. Bridwell KH: Management of tumors at the lumbosacral junction. In Margulies JY, Floman Y, Farcy JPC, Neuwirth MG (eds): Lumbosacral and Spinopelvic Fixation. Philadelphia: Lippincott-Raven, 1996, pp 109–122.

54. Bowers R: Giant cell tumor of the sacrum. A case report. Ann Surg 1:1164–1172, 1948.

55. McDonald J, Lane JM: Surgical approaches to the sacroiliac joint. In Sundaresan N, Schmidek HH, Schiller AL, Rosenthal DI (eds): Tumors of the Spine: Diagnosis and Clinical Management. Philadelphia: WB Saunders, 1996, pp 426–431.

56. Weaver JM, Flynn MB: Hemicorporectomy. J Surg Oncol 73:117–124, 2000.

57. McCarty CS, Waugh JM, Mayo CW, et al: The surgical treatment of presacral tumors: A combined problem. Proc Staff Meet Mayo Clin 27:73–84, 1952.

58. Miles WK, Chang DW, Kroll SS, et al: Reconstruction of large sacral defects following total sacrectomy. Plast Reconstr Surg 105:2387–2394, 2000.

59. Hung SJ, Chen HC, Wei FC: Free flaps for reconstruction of the lower back and sacral area. Microsurgery 20:72–76, 2000.

60. Shikata J, Yamamuro T, Kotoura Y, et al: Total sacrectomy and reconstruction for primary tumors. Report of two cases. J Bone Joint Surg Am 70:122–125, 1988.

61. Santi MD, Mitsunaga MM, Lockett JL: Total sacrectomy for a giant sacral schwannoma: A case report. Clin Orthop 294:285–289, 1993.

62. Wuisman P, Lieshout O, Sugihara S, et al: Total sacrectomy and reconstruction: Oncologic and functional outcome. Clin Orthop 381:192–203, 2000.

63. Doita M, Harada T, Iguchi T, et al: Total sacrectomy and reconstruction for sacral tumors. Spine 28:E296–E301, 2003.

64. Ohata N, Ozaki T, Kunisada T, et al: Extended total sacrectomy and reconstruction for sacral tumor. Spine 29:E123–E126, 2004.

65. Karakousis CP, Emrich LJ, Driscoll DL: Variants of hemipelvectomy and their complications. Am J Surg 158:404–408, 1989.

66. Fourney DR, Abi-Said D, Lang FF, et al: Use of pedicle screw fixation in the management of malignant spinal disease: Experience in 100 consecutive procedures. J Neurosurg 94(1 Suppl):25–37, 2001.

67. Carson WL, Duffield RC, Arendt M, et al: Internal forces and moments in transpedicular spine instrumentation: The effect of pedicle screw angle and transfixation-the 4R-4bar linkage concept. Spine 15:893–901, 1990.

68. McCord DH, Cunningham BW, Shono Y, et al: Biomechanical analysis of lumbosacral fixation. Spine 17(8 Suppl):235–243, 1992.

69. Carlson GD, Abitbol JJ, Anderson DR, et al: Screw fixation in the human sacrum. An in vitro study of the biomechanics of fixation. Spine 17(6 Suppl):196–203, 1992.

70. Smith DA, Kumar R, Cahill DW: Sacral lesions. In Benzel EC (ed): Spine Surgery: Techniques, Complication Avoidance, and Management. New York: Churchill Livingstone, 1999, pp 741–758.

71. Krag MH, Beynnon BD, Pope MH, et al: Depth of insertion of transpedicular vertebral screws into human vertebrae: Effect upon screw-vertebra interface strength. J Spinal Disord 1:287–294, 1988.

72. Baldwin NG, Benzel EC: Sacral fixation using iliac instrumentation and a variable angle screw device. J Neurosurg 81:313–316, 1994.

73. Wuisman P, Lieshout O, van Dijk M, et al: Reconstruction after total en bloc sacrectomy for osteosarcoma using a custom-made prosthesis: A technical note. Spine 26:431–439, 2001.

74. Allen BL Jr, Ferguson RL: The Galveston technique for L rod instrumentation of the scoliotic spine. Spine 7:276–284, 1982.

Surgery of the Peripheral Nervous System

159 Thoracoscopic Sympathectomy for Hyperhidrosis

SAAD KHAIRI, PATRICK JOHNSON, and
WILLIAM C. WELCH

OVERVIEW

Sympathectomy procedures involve interrupting thoracic or lumbar sympathetic pathways to provide relief from autonomically mediated syndromes. Currently the most common disorder treated is essential hyperhidrosis,[1,2] but sympathectomies have been used extensively in the past to treat various pain syndromes that include complex regional pain syndrome (CRPS), reflex sympathetic dystrophy (RSD), causalgia, vascular insufficiency pain syndromes, and Raynaud's disease.[3-6] In the past several years pain syndromes have been treated less frequently with ablative sympathectomy procedures because of the limited success with sympathectomy and potential improvement in outcomes with neurostimulation techniques.[7,8] This chapter will focus on thoracoscopic sympathectomy as a treatment for palmar hyperhidrosis.

HISTORICAL BACKGROUND

The earliest known investigations of sympathetic nervous system surgery were described by François Parfour du Petit in 1727 reporting on the results of sympathectomy in dogs, and Biffi reported similar findings in a doctoral thesis in 1846. Budge and Walker demonstrated the clinical effects of stimulation of the cervical sympathetic chain in humans in 1852. However, it was Claude Bernard, a French physiologist who published a series of articles in the 1850s describing his observations after sectioning and stimulating the cervical sympathetic chain in rabbits, who provided a clearer understanding of clinical correlates. A well-recognized clinical correlate of Bernard's experimental observations, described by Frederick T. Horner in 1869, is now known as Horner's syndrome. However, the first clinical report of a sympathectomy causing the typical ocular changes was reported by Mitchell and colleagues in 1864, predating Horner's description by 5 years. These authors also coined the term causalgia, a condition that was treated primarily with sympathectomy for many years. Early surgical sympathectomy procedures were promoted by Jaboulay and Johnson, who stripped the periarterial sympathetics to treatment of exophthalmos, glaucoma, and tic douloureux, as well as vascular insufficiency. One of Jaboulay's students, Leriche, promoted the use of sympathectomy for ischemic vascular disease. Sympathectomy was used frequently in the 1940s for nerve injuries sustained by soldiers in World War II. Subsequently, various sympathectomy procedures we will review were refined to treat hyperhidrosis and both ischemic and neuropathic pain syndromes.

CLINICAL SYNDROMES

Hyperhidrosis

Palmar and axillary hyperhidrosis are defined as excessive sweating in the upper extremities, particularly the hands and armpits, most often noted during periods of stress. The etiology is unknown, and the incidence is approximately 1% in Western populations but may be slightly higher in Asian populations. The sympathetic nervous system innervates the eccrine sweat glands via cholinergic fibers arising from the intermediolateral column of the thoracic and upper lumbar spinal cord segments. Sympathetic stimulation causes vasoconstriction to produce cooling of the skin and, when combined with sweating, exacerbates the symptoms. Anesthetic block of the stellate ganglion results in a dramatic drying and warming effect in the ipsilateral hand and armpit due to decreasing sweating and increased blood flow through cutaneous vessels that is similar to resection of the sympathetic chain and ganglia in the upper thoracic region, which results in lasting relief from hyperhidrosis.

Neuropathic and Ischemic Pain

Chronic pain syndromes[9,10] such as causalgia and RSD (now referred to as CRPS) are thought to arise from peripheral nerve trauma that is usually ill defined. Several other related syndromes (phantom pain, shoulder-hand syndrome, post-traumatic neuralgia) are also included. Characteristic symptoms are burning pain and trophic skin changes in the extremity. Ischemic pain syndromes, including Raynaud's syndrome and other vasculitic disorders, typically have episodes of severe, painful skin blanching, primarily of the hands and fingertips.[11] Cold temperature or emotional response may exacerbate these episodes, and extreme cases may result in ischemia and gangrenous ulceration of the digits. The initial treatment is avoidance of cold and administration of alpha-adrenergic blocking agents that are useful for less severe cases. Sympathectomy procedures have been used extensively in the past and can provide significant initial relief from severe pain and digital ulcers. Recent studies show that early treatment (<3 months' duration of symptoms) with thoracoscopic sympathectomy improves outcomes.[12,13] However, the long-term outcomes of sympathectomy for relieving the episodic vasospasms associated with chronic pain syndromes and Raynaud's syndrome are less optimal.

ANATOMY AND PHYSIOLOGY

The autonomic nervous system includes both the sympathetic and the parasympathetic nervous systems. The sympathetic system mediates the "fight-or-flight" responses such as pupillary dilation, tachycardia, bronchial dilation, increased muscle blood flow, and the release of adrenergic agents from the adrenal glands. It is a two-neuron disynaptic system in which responses are mediated through autonomic ganglia and the ultimate regulation occurs in the hypothalamus. Outflow from the hypothalamus to spinal levels involves several pathways that are not clearly defined. Anatomically, the sympathetic nervous system has outflow in the thoracic and upper lumbar regions of the spinal cord. Preganglionic fibers from the intermediolateral cell column exit the spinal cord through the ventral nerve roots into spinal nerves and enter the paravertebral chain ganglia coursing through the myelinated white rami communicantes.[3,4] Once in the ganglia, the presynaptic neuron can (1) synapse with a postganglionic neuron and exit as a gray ramus to the viscera, (2) synapse with a postganglionic neuron and exit as a gray ramus in a segmental nerve, (3) travel up or down the sympathetic chain, (4) stimulate the adrenal gland, or (5) exit the sympathetic chain in the splanchnic nerves and enter peripherally located ganglia such as the mesenteric ganglia. Postganglionic fibers travel in peripheral nerves or along arteries to reach their target organs. Afferent autonomic fibers travel from receptors through the dorsal spinal roots to enter the spinal cord, where they can trigger reflexes through spinal cord interneurons and efferent autonomic fibers.

The autonomic ganglia are variable in size, number, and location. There are generally three cervical ganglia (superior, middle, and inferior). The lowest cervical ganglia can fuse with the highest thoracic ganglia to form the stellate or cervicothoracic ganglion.[3,4] Pupillary dilation occurs as a result of sympathetic output from the spinal cord ciliospinal center of Budge. The preganglionic fibers exit the spinal cord at the T1 and T2 levels and travel through the thoracic, stellate, and middle cervical ganglia to synapse in the superior cervical ganglia. Postganglionic fibers then enter the sympathetic plexus surrounding the carotid artery and travel along the third, fifth, and sixth cranial nerves to enter the orbit and pass through the ciliary ganglion to the pupillary dilators via the long anterior ciliary nerves. A lesion anywhere along this course is manifested by pupillary miosis, anhidrosis (loss of sympathetic innervation to the sweat glands of the face), ptosis (loss of innervation of the superior tarsal musculature), and, occasionally, enophthalmos. The thoracic ganglia correlate with the corresponding thoracic level, as do the upper lumbar ganglia.

Sexual function and urinary function are also influenced by the autonomic nervous system.[14] Sympathetic efferent innervation to the bladder arises from the lower thoracic and upper lumbar levels. The efferent nerves travel through a series of ganglia in the sacral region, and the postganglionic fibers travel to the vesicular plexus via the hypogastric nerves. There is also sympathetic stimulation involved in both erection and ejaculation in male patients.

It is generally believed that the presynaptic sympathetic neurons release acetylcholine and peptides that act on muscarinic, nicotinic, or peptidergic receptors of the postsynaptic neurons, which, in turn, release norepinephrine to achieve stimulatory responses in the innervated organs.

The effects of a sympathetic denervation for the treatment of hyperhidrosis presumably occur through the interruption of cutaneous sweating and vasoconstriction mediated by the sympathetic nervous system. The mechanisms of sympathectomy for treating pain and ischemic syndromes are mediated through less well understood pathways from the denervated sympathetic ganglion into the central nervous system; reducing sympathetic input by a sympathectomy will achieve at least temporary improvement in the pain symptoms.

PREOPERATIVE EVALUATION

Patients with autonomically mediated syndromes require thorough diagnostic evaluation and aggressive medical treatment before consideration for surgical treatment. A thorough history and physical examination are necessary to evaluate the possibility of underlying metabolic, infectious, or neoplastic disorders, and radiologic evaluation with plain radiographs and either computed tomography (CT) or magnetic resonance imaging (MRI) of the thorax and brachial plexus may be needed. However, most preoperative diagnostic studies are limited, and imaging studies have not demonstrated any clear diagnostic information. Psychologic evaluation should be considered, particularly in patients with chronic pain disorders.

Diagnostic sympathetic blocks with short-acting anesthetics provide temporary relief but may cause a transient Horner's syndrome. Sympathetic blocks may be useful indicators that a sympathectomy will be therapeutically successful. Occasionally, repeated blocks may provide temporary relief of pain syndromes that allow rehabilitation to proceed and preclude the need for a sympathectomy.

Medical treatment of autonomically mediated syndromes is theoretically useful and may have potential in limited cases. Medications that produce systemic sympathetic blockade include phenoxybenzamine, which blocks the alpha-adrenergic receptors.[15,16] Although there are frequently complications, including hypotension, miosis, and loss of ejaculatory function, this remains an effective test treatment for causalgia-type symptoms.

ENDOSCOPIC SYMPATHECTOMY TECHNIQUES

Thoracoscopic Approach for Cervical and Thoracic Sympathectomy

Endoscopic thoracic sympathectomy for the upper extremity was originally reported in 1951 by Kux,[17] who described treatment of hyperhidrosis with excellent results. The most frequent indication for thoracic sympathectomy is hyperhidrosis.[18-22] Thoracoscopic sympathectomy has become commonplace in most communities for the treatment of hyperhidrosis. Less frequently, RSD, CRPS, causalgia, Raynaud's syndrome, postamputation syndrome (phantom pain), and refractory cardiac tachyarrhythmias[23-25] are now treated with sympathectomy. Endoscopic techniques provide both a panoramic and magnified view for precise identification of the sympathetic chain and adjacent structures, allowing definition of the anatomy for resection of the sympathetic chain. This procedure has become the preferred method of thoracic sympathectomy, and extensive clinical experience has resulted in improvements in patient satisfaction as well as reduced hospital stays and costs. Since thoracoscopic procedures have a definite learning curve, it is necessary to understand the intrathoracic anatomy and gain endoscopic experience with a thoracoscopic surgeon initially.

Palmar hyperhidrosis is currently the main indication for a thoracic sympathectomy using minimally invasive techniques. Patients with severe axillary sweating (with or without palmar hyperhidrosis) and some patients with facial hyperhidrosis have also been treated successfully with a sympathectomy procedure. The precise sympathectomy procedure for each of these clinical syndromes (i.e., which ganglia levels should be resected) remains somewhat speculative. Most authors agree that only a T2 and T3 sympathectomy will effectively treat palmar hyperhidrosis (Fig. 159-1). However, some authors recommend either a T2 or T3 sympathectomy and cite a lowered incidence of compensatory sweating, but this has not been clearly substantiated and some data exist to the contrary.[26] Treatment of axillary sweating is generally accepted as best done with a sympathectomy at T3–T5 for good results. Facial sweating is treated with a T2 sympathectomy just below the stellate ganglion.[27] Many patients are undergoing bilateral sympathectomy for palmar hyperhidrosis on an outpatient basis with good results.[28] Others advocate sequential treatment to assess compensatory hyperhidrosis.[29]

Patients with pain syndromes and vasculitis or Raynaud's syndrome may also respond to an endoscopic T2, T3, and/or T4 sympathectomy, but results are less optimal.[30,31] Recent experience with spinal stimulation appears to have largely replaced sympathectomy procedures for several reasons,[8] including these: Pain symptoms have a high incidence of recurrence; it is a nonablative procedure; stimulation is usually a technically less demanding procedure than a sympathectomy; it is a reversible procedure; and it can be modulated after the procedure is completed.

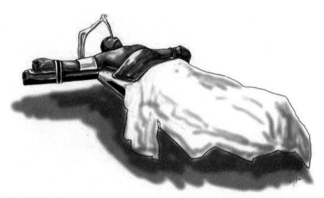

FIGURE 159-2 Supine position for bilateral thoracoscopic sympathectomy. (© J. Patrick Johnson, M.D.)

Patients with cardiac tachyarrhythmias have also been treated with sympathectomy procedures. Studies have demonstrated effectiveness in treating stress-related malignant tachyarrhythmias that may be related to disproportionate left and right sympathetic innervation. Patients treated inadequately with medical therapy can be considered for a left thoracoscopic sympathectomy; however, improved medical therapy has nearly eliminated the use of this procedure with these patients.[3–6]

OPERATIVE TECHNIQUE

Anesthesia and Positioning

The patient requires general anesthesia and placement of a double-lumen endotracheal tube to allow collapse of the lung on the operated side. The supine position (Fig. 159-2) is used, and the head of the table can be elevated and rotated.

Instruments

The equipment and instruments needed for performing a thoracoscopic sympathectomy procedure are commonly used for laparoscopic surgery. A standard endoscopic video monitor system with either a 5- or 10-mm-diameter rigid laparoscope (having either a 0- or 30-degree-angled lens) is used. The essential endoscopic instruments are: (1) 5-mm-diameter blunt-tipped (mini-Metzenbaum-type) scissors with a monopolar electrocautery, or similar dissection-cautery instrument such as a Harmonic Scalpel (Ethicon); (2) a 5-mm-diameter curved grasper (a hemostat); (3) a 5-mm-diameter suction irrigator.

Ports and Port Placement

A soft, flexible thoracic endoscopic port is inserted through a 2-cm chest wall incision similar to that used for placement of a chest tube. There is some concern that a hard port increases the incidence of intercostal neuralgia. A single port (Fig. 159-3A), or occasionally two ports (see Fig. 159-3B), can be used, and both the endoscope and other working instruments can be placed in the port.[28,32–34] The port is placed in the third or fourth intercostal space in the midaxillary line while the anesthesiologist deflates the ipsilateral lung.

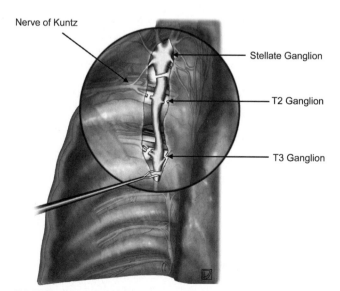

Nerve of Kuntz

Stellate Ganglion

T2 Ganglion

T3 Ganglion

FIGURE 159-1 Dissected upper thoracic sympathetic chain with T2 and T3 ganglia prepared for excision.

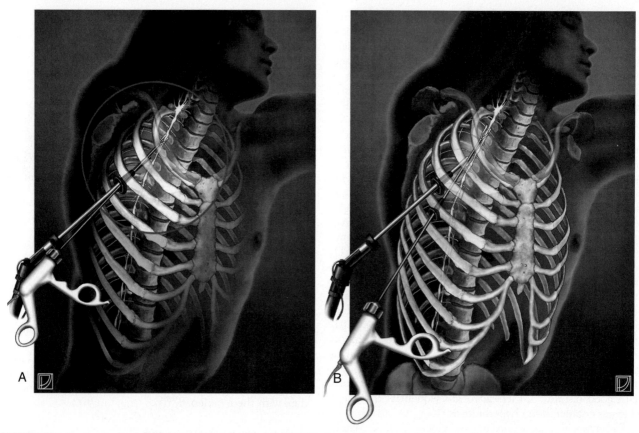

FIGURE 159-3   Access for right thoracoscopic sympathectomy. *A,* Single portal access. *B,* Double portal access. (© J. Patrick Johnson, M.D.)

THE OPERATIVE PROCEDURE

The endoscope is placed in the chest through the portal, and the lung is retracted. The lung can be further retracted with blunt instruments and rotation of the operating table, allowing the lung to fall forward and away from the vertebral column. The sympathetic chain is visualized overlying the rib heads in the upper thoracic region. The intercostal vessels course over the middle portion of each vertebral body, usually beneath the sympathetic chain. The sympathetic chain appears as a slightly pinkish white, glistening, raised, longitudinal structure. The rostral aspect of the sympathetic chain extends beneath a fat pad that envelopes the subclavian artery and obscures the first rib and stellate ganglion (Fig. 159-4).

The sympathectomy procedure begins with an incision in the pleura overlying the sympathetic chain at the T3 level using the curved scissors. The pleural incision is extended in a rostral direction over the sympathetic chain to T2, and the sympathetic ganglia and chain at T2 and T3 are then cauterized. The nerve of Kuntz (see Fig. 159-1), which can often be identified as a large branch arising from the T2 ganglion, courses laterally to the brachial plexus, probably providing much of the sympathetic innervation to the upper extremity. Thus denervation of the T2 ganglion is important.[35] Prevention of Horner's syndrome is best accomplished by avoiding injury or traction to the stellate ganglion that can occur during the dissection and denervation of the T2 ganglion. Once the sympathectomy has been completed, a portion of the sympathetic ganglion can be sent for pathologic evaluation. The surgical site is irrigated and hemostasis confirmed. A red rubber catheter is inserted through the port and aspirated while the lung is reinflated by the anesthesiologist and the port is removed; the incision is then closed with absorbable sutures and Steri-Strips. Submission of a histologic specimen of the ganglia remains an option to confirm the appropriate site of sympathectomy.

Alternate techniques have been described that do not utilize a double-lumen endotracheal tube. These techniques instead involve carbon dioxide insufflation in the chest. The usual volume necessary to adequately retract the lung is between 600 and 1000 mL.[36] Additionally, this technique requires air-sealed laparoscopic ports which theoretically tamponades bleeding in the surgical resection bed.

POSTOPERATIVE CARE

A postoperative chest radiograph is obtained in the operating room to confirm lung inflation. A small pneumothorax will resolve, but a large persistent pneumothorax suggests a parenchymal lung leak that would require chest tube placement until the leak resolves. Oral analgesics are adequate, for pain control, and hospital stay is usually only 1 or 2 days.

COMPLICATIONS

Surgical complications[37–39] from thoracoscopic sympathectomy are few, and most do not require intervention.

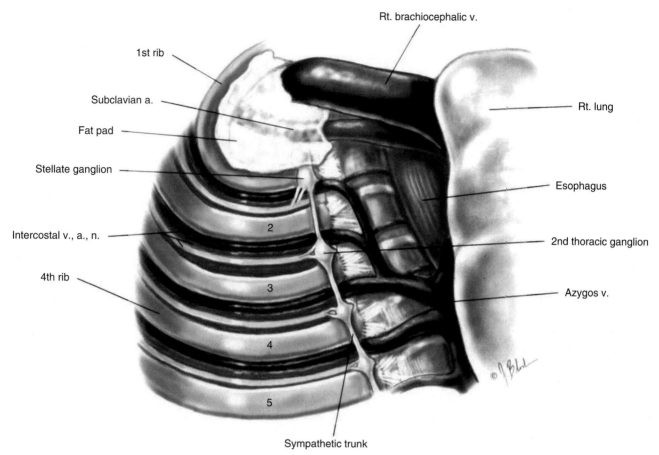

Rt. brachiocephalic v.

1st rib

Subclavian a.

Fat pad

Stellate ganglion

Intercostal v., a., n.

4th rib

Rt. lung

Esophagus

2nd thoracic ganglion

Azygos v.

2

3

4

5

Sympathetic trunk

FIGURE 159-4 Anatomy of right thoracic sympathetic chain.

Complications may include: (1) pneumothorax, (2) Horner's syndrome, (3) subcutaneous emphysema, (4) pleural effusions, (5) segmental atelectasis, and (6) intercostal neuralgia. Postoperative pneumothorax usually results from inadequate reinflation of the collapsed lung; however, a small apical pneumothorax can be observed and will spontaneously resolve. Horner's syndrome results from injury to the stellate ganglion and is infrequent and usually transient. Injury to the intercostal nerves during port placement or pressure applied during the procedure may result in intercostal neuralgia. The incidence is minimized by using soft, flexible thoracic endoscopic ports rather than rigid laparoscopic ports.

Compensatory hyperhidrosis is increased sweating, usually in the truncal areas, occurring after a sympathectomy procedure.[40] The incidence is probably higher than previously recognized and has been reported to range from 10% to 90%. The severity is also highly variable, ranging from mild to severe, and cannot be determined preoperatively. Some authors advocate a more limited sympathectomy of only T2 that may reduce the incidence of compensatory sweating while others claim that a sympathectomy of T3 only reduces the incidence.[26] However, none of these theories has been clearly substantiated. More recently, clipping of the sympathetic chain has been performed in hopes of creating a reversible lesion.[41,42] Reconstruction of the sympathetic chain has been reported, but no long-term data about reversibility are available.[36,40]

RESULTS

Success rates for thoracoscopic sympathectomies are very good overall, with patient satisfaction rates usually higher than 90%. Compensatory sweating, though common (5% to 30%), was usually not debilitating and was tolerated by most patients.

CONCLUSIONS

The indications for sympathectomy have become clearer throughout 50 years of clinical research. Surgical techniques have recently become more refined with modern endoscopy and have led to precise and minimally invasive procedures. Endoscopy allows less tissue disruption with the aid of a magnified and illuminated exposure. The technical challenges and complications of these procedures are now well understood and well defined. The surgeon can now custom-tailor the necessary procedure for optimal outcomes according to a patient's individual condition.

REFERENCES

1. Adar R, Kurchin A, Zweig A, Mozes M: Palmar hyperhidrosis and its surgical treatment. Ann Surg 186:34–41, 1977.
2. Munro PAG: Sympathectomy: An Anatomical and Physiological Study with Clinical Applications. London: Oxford University Press, 1959.

3. Hardy RW, Bay JW: Surgery of the sympathetic nervous system. In Schmidek HH, Sweet WH (eds): Operative Neurosurgical Techniques, 2nd edition. Orlando, FL: Grune and Stratton, 1988, p 1271.

4. Kleinert HE, Norberg H, McDonough JJ: Surgical sympathectomy—upper and lower extremity. In Omer GE Jr, Spinner M (eds): Management of Peripheral Nerve Problems. Philadelphia: WB Saunders, 1980, p 284.

5. Malone PS, Cameron AEP, Rennie JA: The surgical treatment of upper limb hyperhidrosis. Br J Dermatol 115:81–84, 1986.

6. Rutherford RB: Role of sympathectomy in the management of vascular disease. In Moore WS (ed): Vascular Surgery: A Comprehensive Review. Philadelphia: WB Saunders, 1993, p 300.

7. Barolat G, Schwartzman R, Woo R: Epidural spinal cord stimulation in the management of reflex sympathetic dystrophy. Stereotact Funct Neurosurg 53:29–39, 1989.

8. Oakley JC, Prager JP: Spinal cord stimulation: Mechanisms of action. Spine 27:2574–2578, 2002.

9. Bandyk DF, Johnson BL, Kirkpatrick AF, et al: Surgical sympathectomy for reflex sympathetic dystrophy syndromes. J Vasc Surg 35:269–277, 2002.

10. Bergan JJ, Conn J Jr.: Sympathectomy for pain relief. Med Clin North Am 52: 147, 1968.

11. Matsumoto Y, Ueyama T, Endo M, et al: Endoscopic thoracic sympathectomy for Raynaud's phenomenon. J Vasc Surg 36:57–61, 2002.

12. Singh B, Moodley J, Shaik AS, Robbs JV: Sympathectomy for complex regional pain syndrome. J Vasc Surg 37:508–511, 2003.

13. Schwartzman RJ, Liu JE, Smullens SN, Hyslop T, Tahmoush AJ: Long-term outcome following sympathectomy for complex regional pain syndrome type 1 (RSD). J Neurol Sci 150:149–152, 1997.

14. Burchiel KJ, Burns AS: Summary statement: Pain, spasticity, and bladder and sexual function after spinal cord injury [Comment]. Spine 26(Suppl 24):S161, 2001.

15. Ghostine SY, Comair YG, Turner DM, et al: Phenoxybenzamine in the treatment of causalgia: Report of 40 cases. J Neurosurg 60:1263–1268, 1984.

16. Weiner N: Drugs that inhibit adrenergic nerves and block adrenergic receptors. In Gilman AG, Goodman LS, Gilman A (eds): Goodman and Gilman's Pharmacological Basis of Therapeutics, 6th edition. New York: MacMillan, 1980, p 176.

17. Kux E: The endoscopic approach to the vegetative nervous system and its therapeutic possibilities. Dis Chest 20:139–147, 1951.

18. Adams DCR, Wood SJ, Tulloh BR, et al: Endoscopic transthoracic sympathectomy: Experience in the south west end of England. Eur J Vasc Surg 6:558–562, 1992.

19. Banerjee AK, Edmondson R, Rennie JA: Endoscopic transthoracic electrocautery of the sympathetic chain for palmar and axillary hyperhidrosis. Br J Surg 77:1435, 1990.

20. Byrne J, Walsh TN, Hederman WP: Endoscopic transthoracic electrocautery of the sympathetic chain for palmar and axillary hyperhidrosis. Br J Surg 77: 1046–1049, 1990.

21. Chen HJ, Liang CL, Lu K: Associated change in plantar temperature and sweating after transthoracic endoscopic T2–3 sympathectomy for palmar hyperhidrosis. J Neurosurg 95(Suppl 1):58–63, 2001.

22. Claes G, Gothberg G, Drott C: Endoscopic transthoracic electrocautery of the sympathetic chain for palmar and axillary hyperhidrosis. Br J Surg 78:760, 1991.

23. Crampton R: Preeminence of the left stellate ganglion in the long QT syndrome. Circulation 59:769–778, 1979.

24. Ouriel K, Moss AJ: Long QT syndrome: An indication for cervicothoracic sympathectomy. Cardiovasc Surg 3:475–478, 1995.

25. Schwartz PJ, Periti M, Malliani A: The long QT syndrome. Am Heart J 89:378–390, 1975.

26. Leseche G, Castier Y, Thabut G, et al: Endoscopic transthoracic sympathectomy for upper limb hyperhidrosis: Limited sympathectomy does not reduce postoperative compensatory sweating. J Vasc Surg 37:124–128, 2003.

27. Lin TS, Fang HY: Transthoracic endoscopic sympathectomy for craniofacial hyperhidrosis: Analysis of 46 cases. J Laparoendosc Adv Surg Tech A 10:243–247, 2000.

28. Lin TS, Kuo SJ, Chou MC: Uniportal endoscopic thoracic sympathectomy for treatment of palmar and axillary hyperhidrosis: Analysis of 2000 cases. Neurosurgery 51(Suppl 5):84–87, 2002.

29. Al Dohayan A: Transaxillary thoracoscopic sympathectomy experience in a hot climate: Management of the dominant hand. Surg Laparosc Endosc Percutan Tech 9:317–321, 1999.

30. Ahn SS, Machleder HI, Concepcion B, Moore WS: Thoracoscopic cervicodorsal sympathectomy: Preliminary results. J Vasc Surg 20:511–517, 1994.

31. Whitworth LA, Feler CA: Application of spinal ablative techniques for the treatment of benign chronic painful conditions: History, methods, and outcomes [Review]. Spine 27:2607–2613, 2002.

32. Johnson JP, Patel NP: Uniportal and biportal endoscopic thoracic sympathectomy. Neurosurgery 51(Suppl 5):79–83, 2002.

33. Johnson JP, Obasi C, Hahn MS, Glatleider P: Endoscopic thoracic sympathectomy. J Neurosurg 91(Suppl 1):90–97, 1999.

34. Vanaclocha V, Saiz-Sapena N, Panta F: Uniportal endoscopic superior thoracic sympathectomy. Neurosurgery 46:924–928, 2000.

35. Wang YC, Sun MH, Lin CW, Chen YJ: Anatomical location of T2–3 sympathetic trunk and Kuntz nerve determined by transthoracic endoscopy. J Neurosurg 96(Suppl 1):68–72, 2002.

36. Reisfeld R, Nguyen R, Pnini A: Endoscopic thoracic sympathectomy for hyperhidrosis: Experience with both cauterization and clamping methods. Surg Laparosc Endosc Percutan Tech 12:255–267, 2002.

37. Lin TS, Wang NP, Huang LC: Pitfalls and complication associated with transthoracic endoscopic sympathectomy for primary hyperhidrosis (analysis of 2200 cases). Int J Surg Investig 2:377–385, 2001.

38. Plas EG, Fugger R, Herbst F, Fritsch A: Complications of endoscopic thoracic sympathectomy. Surgery 118:493–495, 1995.

39. Singh B, Moodley J, Ramdial PK, Ramsaroop L, Satyapal KS: Pitfalls in thoracoscopic sympathectomy: Mechanisms for failure. Surg Laparosc Endosc Percutan Tech 11:364–367, 2001.

40. Telaranta T: Secondary sympathetic chain reconstruction after endoscopic thoracic sympathectomy. Eur J Surg 580(Suppl):17–18, 1998.

41. Beatty RA: The use of clip-suture in thoracic sympathectomy. J Neurosurg 81:482, 1994.

42. Lin TS, Huang LC, Wang NP, Lai CY: Video-assisted thoracoscopic T2 sympathetic block by clipping for palmar hyperhidrosis: Analysis of 52 cases. J Laparoendosc Adv Surg Tech A 11:59–62, 2001.

160 Superior Sulcus Tumors

MARK H. BILSKY

DEFINITION

Non–small cell lung cancer (NSCLC) arising in the superior sulcus is a relatively uncommon tumor, composing less than 5% of all primary lung cancers. First described by Hare in 1838, the clinical description of superior sulcus tumors is attributed to H. K. Pancoast from a paper published in 1932.[1] In deference to this description, these tumors are commonly referred to as "Pancoast tumors." Initially, palliative radiation was offered, but advances in thoracic surgical techniques proved these tumors to be resectable. For a number of years, preoperative radiation followed by resection was offered, with survival rates approaching 30% at 5 years.[1-4] These data excluded the majority of tumors with spinal and extensive brachial plexus involvement because these tumors could not be resected to achieve negative histologic margins. More recently, induction chemoradiation has shown up to a 65% complete or near total histologic tumor response.[5] Improvements in neoadjuvant therapy, spine surgical techniques, and segmental fixation may justify resection of superior sulcus lung tumors even with involvement of the spine and brachial plexus. In this chapter we describe the anatomy of superior sulcus tumors, evolution of multiple-modality treatment, evaluation for surgical resection, and posterior approaches with emphasis on spine resection, cervicothoracic reconstruction, and brachial plexus management.

ANATOMY

Pancoast's classic description of a superior sulcus tumor is a NSCLC arising in the apex of the chest and presenting with a clinical triad of shoulder and arm pain, atrophy of hand muscles, and Horner's syndrome. Application of computed tomography (CT) and magnetic resonance imaging (MRI) has led to earlier diagnosis of apical tumors before development of brachial plexus and stellate ganglion involvement. On this basis, Detterbeck proposed refining the definition of Pancoast tumors to emphasize their clinical and anatomic spectrum.[6] In general, Pancoast tumors arise at the apex of the lung and involve the chest wall, including but not limited to structures superior to the second rib. The chest wall involvement may be limited to the parietal pleura but does not include tumors extending only to the visceral pleura. Tumor extension through the parietal pleura may abut or infiltrate the ribs, vertebral body, nerve roots, brachial plexus, stellate ganglion, and/or subclavian vessels.

Detterbeck divided the apical lung region into three compartments based on their relationship to the first rib. Tumors may involve any or all compartments. The anterior compartment includes the sternocleidomastoid muscles and the jugular and subclavian veins. The middle compartment includes the anterior and middle scalene muscles, subclavian artery, phrenic nerve, and brachial plexus (trunks). The posterior compartment contains the vertebral body, neural foramen, nerve roots, and sympathetic chain. The posterior compartment tumors are of greatest interest to spine surgeons and will be the emphasis of the remainder of this chapter.

Pancoast tumors are staged according to the American Joint Committee on Cancer (AJCC) staging manual. As applied to superior sulcus tumors, T3 tumors involve the parietal pleura, chest wall, and/or brachial plexus. T4 tumors include the vertebral body, subclavian artery, or esophagus. The node status is delineated as N0 (no nodes), N1 (ipsilateral peribronchial or hilar), or N2 (ipsilateral mediastinal or carinal). Metastases are identified as M0 (no metastases) or M1 (metastases). The most common tumors that present for resection include Stage IIa (T1N0M0), IIIa (T3N2M0), and IIIb (T4N0M0).

PRESENTATION

Typical symptoms of lung cancer, such as cough and hemoptysis, are often absent in Pancoast tumors because of their peripheral location. In modern series, the majority of patients with apical tumors present with shoulder pain with or without radiation to the scapula, shoulder, or arm. This shoulder pain is often misinterpreted as a rotator cuff injury, and patients have often been treated with local corticosteroid injections. This pain results from chest wall involvement and radiculopathy (T2–T4) intensifying at night. The pain eventually becomes constant and on a visual analogue scale is often rated as 10/10. It is important to document the pain intensity at presentation, because the efficacy of induction therapy can often be judged by the degree of pain reduction even in the absence of radiographic changes.

Despite the proximity of many tumors to the neural foramen, it is decidedly rare for patients to present with myelopathy from spinal cord compression. In a series of 42 patients reviewed at Memorial Sloan-Kettering Cancer Center (MSKCC), only one patient (2%) presented with myelopathy at diagnosis.[7] The most common neurologic symptoms at presentation include nerve root and brachial plexus involvement. The extent of brachial plexus involvement can often be judged clinically. It is important to distinguish T1–nerve root involvement from that of C8 or lower trunk of the brachial plexus. Pain extending along the ulnar aspect of the forearm to the wrist with normal hand intrinsic muscle function suggests isolated involvement of the T1 nerve root. Conversely, pain radiating into the hand, especially the fourth and fifth digits, is indicative of involvement of the C8 nerve root or lower trunk of the brachial plexus. This pain is often associated with significant hand intrinsic weakness. CT and MRI both image the brachial plexus well but often do not show enough anatomic detail to assess T1 from C8 or lower trunk involvement. In our experience, the clinical examination is helpful and reliably correlates with intraoperative findings.

Sympathetic nerve infiltration of the stellate ganglion leads to a Horner's syndrome defined by a constellation of symptoms including ptosis, miosis, and unilateral anhydrosis. Involvement of the superior ganglion results in a warm upper extremity. Patients will often be unaware of these findings, but a physician commonly discovers them either incidentally or subsequent to the discovery of an apical mass. Horner's syndrome does not typically improve with treatment, since this is a destructive lesion of the sympathetic plexus. Although reflex sympathetic dystrophy has been described with tumor destruction of the sympathetic nerves, it is decidedly rare.

IMAGING AND WORKUP

Plain radiographs and CT scans of the chest and upper abdomen are the standard imaging modalities for most chest lesions. CT scans identify the extent of the chest lesion and nodes. Additionally, CT scan bone windows may show lytic destruction of the vertebral bodies not visualized on standard chest windowing. Consequently, axial cuts should be obtained of the lower cervical and upper thoracic spine as well as brachial plexus.

In addition to CT scans, assessment of Pancoast tumors may benefit from MRI and positron emission tomography (PET) imaging. In recent years, MRI has routinely been used to assess the spine, brachial plexus, and vascular anatomy of apical tumors.[8] MRI may show infiltration of the bone marrow in the vertebral body signified as hypointensity on T1-weighted images and hyperintensity on STIR images. This is presumed to represent disease for planning purposes even in the absence of lytic destruction on CT scans. An MRI classification of Detterbeck's posterior compartment has been applied to tumors with spinal involvement to determine the approach and type of operation required for complete tumor resection.[7] Class A tumors have periosteal involvement but do not encroach on the neural foramen. Class B tumors abut the neural foramen but do not extend to the epidural space. Class C tumors extend through the neural foramen and may cause extensive epidural compression. Class D tumors have bone infiltration (vertebral body and/or posterior elements) and may extend to cause epidural compression (Fig. 160-1). This classification is useful in determining the type of approach required to achieve a complete resection (R0/R1).

MRI and CT both show the brachial plexus relatively well, although we rely more on clinical assessment as previously described. MR neurography may improve the assessment of these nerves, although we have not used it as routine assessment. MR angiograms have also recently been used to assess the vascular anatomy of the subclavian artery.

The tumor stage is well delineated with a combination of CT and MRI. However, F18 PET scanning is increasingly being used to assess node status and metastases. The sensitivity and specificity are not currently known. Previously PET scans gave little anatomic detail, but the recently developed PET-CT fusion images give an excellent 3-dimensional rendering of hot spots. Despite improvement with PET imaging, mediastinoscopy should be used to obtain histologic confirmation of suspicious nodes (>1 cm or hot on PET). The presence of N2 nodes significantly worsens the prognosis and is considered a relative contraindication to surgery.

TREATMENT

Before the 1950s, superior sulcus tumors were considered incurable and patients were typically offered palliative radiation. Subsequent application of multiple-modality therapy has shown that these tumors are not universally fatal. The first long-term survivor was reported by Chardack and Maccallum in 1956.[9] The patient underwent en bloc resection of the tumor and chest wall followed by 6500 cGy external-beam radiation therapy. The patient died more than 5 years after the operation of unrelated causes. Postmortem examination revealed no residual tumor.

In 1956, Shaw performed a lobectomy and chest wall resection in a patient 3 weeks after completing radiation (3500 cGy). The specimen revealed scar tissue with microscopic residual tumor. Shaw and Paulson subsequently described 18 patients who underwent preoperative radiation therapy followed by surgical resection.[10] Although the median follow-up was only 1 year, this regimen became the standard for modern treatment of superior sulcus tumors. Induction radiation followed by resection results in 5-year survivals of 25% to 30%.[1-4] Following radiation doses of 30 to 45 Gy, complete pathologic responses are seen in 5% to 20% of patients,[11,12] and complete resections have been reported in various series from 15% to 81%.

A recent review of 225 patients treated at MSKCC between 1974 and 1985 showed variable application of induction therapy, with 55% receiving radiation therapy (median dose 4248 cGy) and 20% receiving chemotherapy.[13] No induction therapy was given in 35% of patients in the belief that a wide resection could be achieved followed by high-dose external-beam radiation. Among 55 patients with T4 tumors, 34 patients were defined as having T4 disease because of spinal involvement (62%). In univariate analysis, tumor stage, node status (N2), and completeness of resection were significant prognostic factors in terms of survival and local tumor control. Patients with Stage IIa tumors (T3N0) survived significantly longer than patients

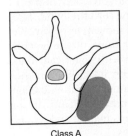
Class A

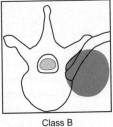
Class B

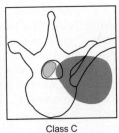
Class C

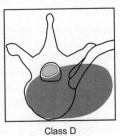
Class D

FIGURE 160-1 Artist's illustration of tumor classes. *Class A,* Extends to periosteum of the vertebral body. *Class B,* Extends to the neural foramen but does not have epidural extension. *Class C,* Encroaches through the neural foramen to compress the epidural space. *Class D,* Vertebral body or posterior element involvement with or without epidural tumor.

with Stage IIIa (T3N2) or Stage IIIb tumors (T4N0), with 5-year actuarial survivals of 46%, 0%, and 13%, respectively. The spine was most often the limiting factor in achieving a complete resection and was the most common site of locoregional relapse for all stages.

Review of the subpopulation of superior sulcus tumors with spinal involvement underscores the importance of complete tumor resection.[7] Extent of resection was evaluated as complete, defined as R0 (en bloc resection with negative margins) or R1 (gross-total resection with microscopic tumor-positive margins). Incomplete resection was defined as R2 (gross resection with positive margins). In a review of 42 patients at MSKCC undergoing resections for all radiographic classes of tumor,[6,7,13,14] complete tumor resection (R0/R1) was achieved in 27 (64%) patients and incomplete (R2) in 15 (36%) patients. For patients undergoing complete tumor resection, the 2- and 5-year survival rates were 63% and 40%, respectively. There were no 2-year survivors in patients with positive margins or gross residual disease (R2).

In an attempt to improve patient outcomes, chemoradiation followed by resection has been used in a number of recent studies.[5,15,16] In the Southwest Oncology Group Trial 9416 (Intergroup trial 0160), etoposide, cisplatin, and 45-Gy radiation were given concomitantly as induction therapy, followed by resection and two cycles of postoperative chemotherapy. Of the 111 patients enrolled, 83 were candidates for operation, but 28 patients were excluded because of complications from induction therapy, poor performance status, or the presence of unresectable disease. In 55 pathologic specimens (65%) reviewed, histologic examination showed either a complete response or minimal residual microscopic disease. Interestingly, postinduction radiographic imaging did not correlate with histologic findings. A complete histologic response or microscopic disease was found in 73% (28/38) of patients showing a partial radiographic response and 55% (22/40) showing stable disease. Complete tumor resection (R0 or R1) was achieved in 55 (92%) patients with T3 tumors and 21 (91%) of T4 tumors. The 2-year survival was 55% for all eligible patients and 70% for patients with a complete resection. Survival was not influenced by tumor status, and survival for T4 tumors was significantly better than historical controls. This finding may translate to T4 tumors that have spinal involvement. The most common site of

relapse was not locoregional as had previously been seen using preoperative radiation alone. Relapse was most commonly distant metastases, predominantly the brain (41%).

Chemoradiation will probably become standard induction therapy for superior sulcus tumors. Newer conformal radiation delivery systems, such as intensity modulated radiation therapy (IMRT), are now being used in an attempt to deliver higher doses of radiation to the tumor than are possible with conventional external-beam radiation. IMRT using dynamic field shaping may provide improved tumor control and spare toxicity to the spinal cord and brachial plexus.[15,17,18]

SURGERY

Surgical Technique: Class A and B

For tumors presenting with Class A or B radiographic appearance, the classic posterolateral thoracotomy as described by Shaw and Paulson[10,19] is used (Fig. 160-2A,B). Patients are positioned in the lateral decubitus position on a beanbag. During inflation of the beanbag, care must be taken to avoid compression of the abdomen, which may result in increased bleeding from the epidural venous plexus. The incision extends midway between the scapula and spine, extending over the tip of the scapula (Fig. 160-3A). The levator scapulae and rhomboids are sectioned to elevate the scapula off the chest wall, which is secured with an internal mammary retractor (see Fig. 160-3B). The majority of patients require extensive chest wall resections. The chest wall is cut distal to the tumor, most often involving the first through fourth ribs. The chest contents are explored for pulmonary metastases and mediastinal nodes (N2) that may preclude resection. At this point, the paraspinal muscles are dissected from the posterior elements of the spine to expose the transverse processes, pars interarticularis, and unilateral laminae. Using an osteotome or drill (e.g., 3-mm matchstick burr), the base of the transverse process is sectioned distal to the pedicle at the level of the neural foramen and fractured through the costovertebral junction using forward traction (see Fig. 160-3C). Tenotomy scissors are used to dissect the intercostal muscles and identify the nerve roots at the level of the neural foramen. Rhizotomy of the infiltrated nerve roots is accomplished by double ligation with

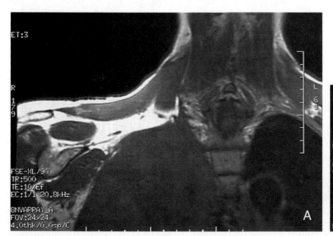
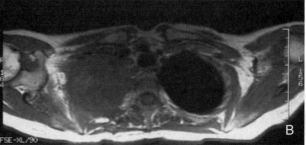

FIGURE 160-2 *A* and *B*, Coronal and axial images showing a large Class B Pancoast tumor with extension to the neural foramen, but without bone or epidural tumor extension.

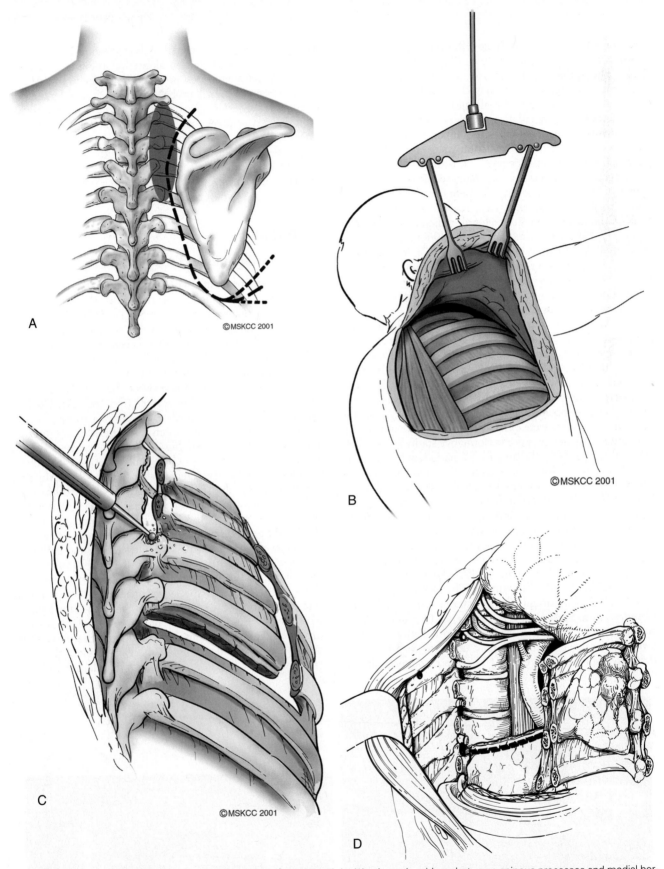

FIGURE 160-3 Artist's illustration of a posterolateral thoracotomy. *A,* Incision is made midway between spinous processes and medial border of the scapula and extending over the inferior border. *B,* The rhomboids and levator scapulae are sectioned to elevate the scapula from the chest wall using a mammary self-retaining retractor. *C,* The paraspinal muscles are dissected to expose the junction of the laminae and transverse processes. A small curved osteotome or drill is used to resect the transverse processes distal to the pedicle and pars interarticularis to expose the neural foramen. For a Class C resection the laminae, facet joints, and pedicles are resected to expose the lateral dura. *D,* En bloc resection of chest wall including transverse processes and costovertebral joint and lobectomy are completed. Multilevel rhizotomy is performed to achieve a proximal margin on the tumor. The T1 nerve root is often sacrificed with minimal residual deficit, but C8 and T1 nerve root damage will often result in diffuse intrinsic hand weakness.

(Continued)

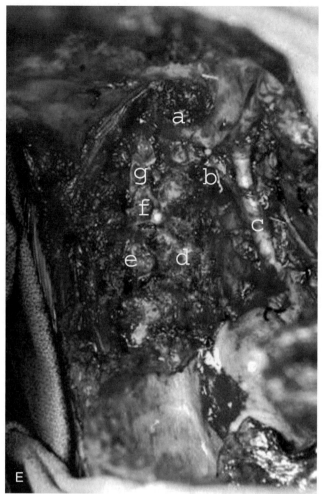

FIGURE 160-3 Cont'd *E,* Intraoperative photograph post-Pancoast tumor resection showing (a) C8 nerve root, (b) cut distal end of T1 nerve root, (c) subclavian artery, (d) vertebral body, (e/g) cut end of transverse process, (f) T2 nerve root sacrificed at the neural foramen. (*A* to *C,* © 2001 Memorial Sloan-Kettering Cancer Center, New York, NY and from Bilsky MH, Vitaz TW, Boland PJ, et al: Surgical treatment of superior sulcus tumors with spinal and brachial plexus involvement. J Neurosurg: Spine 97:305, 2002. *D,* © 2004, Memorial Sloan-Kettering Cancer Center, New York, NY.)

small vascular clips and sectioning. Proximal nerve roots should be sent for margins and re-resected more proximally if positive. The vertebral body periosteum is dissected using Bovie cautery starting from a normal plane, and segmental feeding vessels are ligated with vascular clips or 2-0 silk ligatures. Spinal instrumentation is not required with a Class A dissection as the pars interarticularis and facet joints remain intact. Following spinal resection, attention is then returned to completion of lobectomy or pneumonectomy as indicated (see Fig. 160-3D, E).

Surgical Technique: Class C

Class C tumors extend through the neural foramen to compress the epidural space without bone infiltration. Patient positioning and exposure of the spine are the same as a Class A resection. Using a 3-mm matchstick burr, the laminae and facet joints are cut proximal to the facet joint, transverse process, and pars interarticularis, and the pedicles are drilled

to the base of the vertebral body. This exposes the proximal neural foramen and lateral dura. Tumor is dissected from the dura using tenotomy scissors, and rhizotomy is performed as previously described. We have not taken dura as a margin because of a perceived increased risk of intradural seeding. Unilateral single-level facet resection is generally tolerated without instrumentation, but multilevel resection can result in a scoliosis. Although instrumentation has been described in lateral position,[20] our preference is a second posterior approach to place the instrumentation to ensure coronal and sagittal plane alignment.

Surgical Techniques: Class D

The extent of resection and spinal fixation for Class D tumors depends on the degree of vertebral body, posterior element, and epidural involvement. For patients with isolated epidural and vertebral body tumor, the procedure for a Class C tumor is performed followed by intralesional resection of the involved vertebral body level(s). Polymethyl methacrylate (PMMA) and Steinman pins or autologous rib or iliac crest bone graft are used for anterior vertebral body reconstruction. This is augmented by an anterior plate or screw-rod construct. The majority of plates designed for thoracic and lumbar application are too prominent to be used in the high thoracic spine. Single screw-rod systems (e.g., Frontier; Depuy Spine, Inc., Raynham, MA), used predominantly for anterior pediatric scoliosis correction, are the best alternative.

Additional posterior element resection and instrumentation are required for tumors that infiltrate the vertebral body and posterior elements and/or for extensive epidural tumor. We previously described a single-stage posterolateral approach, which gives excellent spine exposure for tumor resection but restricts the thoracic surgeon in performing a lobectomy because of limited visibility and access to the pulmonary hilum. Gokaslan and the M.D. Anderson group have described a very elegant single-staged resection in the lateral decubitus position, in which anterior chest and posterior elements are simultaneously exposed.[20] For some surgeons, the limitation of this approach is the technical aspect of placing posterior cervicothoracic instrumentation into a patient positioned in the lateral decubitus position. Additionally, maintaining sagittal and coronal plane balance can be problematic.

Currently our preferred operation is a two-stage posterior-anterior approach. The posterior approach is performed first. Patients are positioned prone on lateral chest supports with the head in the Mayfield fixation device. Great care is taken to maintain coronal and sagittal plane alignment. A midline incision is made from C5 to T7. A posterolateral laminectomy is performed in which the laminae, bilateral pedicles, facet joints, pars interarticularis, and transverse processes are resected using a high-speed drill. This posterolateral spine resection extends over the involved segments. Epidural tumor is resected using tenotomy scissors beginning from a normal dural plane. Multilevel rhizotomy at the thecal sac is accomplished with small vascular clips. The T1 nerve root is typically spared until histologic proof of tumor involvement is confirmed by frozen section. Scar tissue can be stripped from the nerve root starting from a normal dural plane. Following the placement of posterior instrumentation, the ribs are disarticulated from the vertebral bodies and cut distally to the tumor.

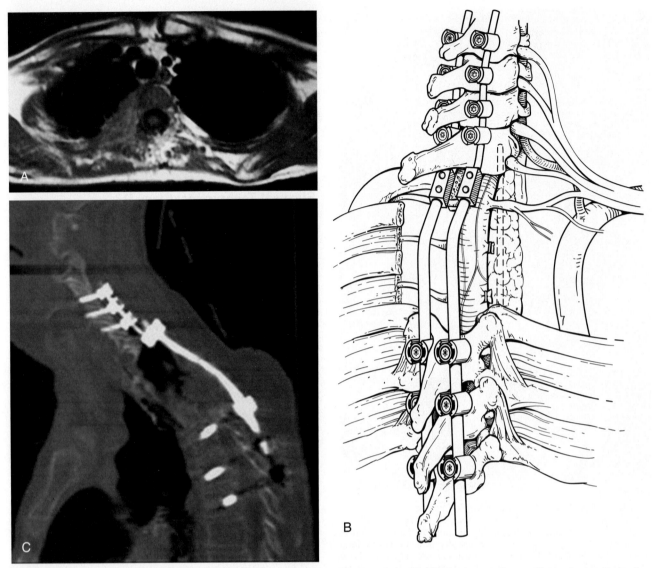

FIGURE 160-4   MRI of Class D tumor. Patient presented with right-sided back pain and T1 distribution numbness. She underwent induction chemoradiation with significant resolution of arm symptoms. Axial (*A*) MRI shows hypointense signal in the T2–T3 vertebral bodies, suggestive of marrow infiltration. The paraspinal tumor at T2–T3 shows abutment of the epidural space and involvement of the right lamina. *B*, Artist's illustration of hybrid lateral mass screw rod system connected to pedicle screw system using a wedding band connector. *C*, Postoperative CT scan showing the system described in artist's illustration. (*A*, From Bilsky MH, Vitaz TW, Boland PJ, et al: Surgical treatment of superior sulcus tumors with spinal and brachial plexus involvement. J Neurosurg: Spine 97:304, 2002. *B*, © 2004, Memorial Sloan-Kettering Cancer Center, New York, NY.)

Posterior instrumentation strategies for the cervicothoracic junction have recently evolved as both cervical and thoracic instrumentation have improved. Previous instrumentation strategies, including Wisconsin wires and sublaminar hooks, had significant limitations. The development of polyaxial pedicle screw systems (PPSSs) and lateral mass screw-rod systems (LMSRSs) have dramatically improved our ability to safely and effectively instrument the cervicothoracic junction. Because of the extensive bone removal, the general rule for posterior instrumentation is placement of at least four points of fixation above and below the level of tumor resection.

When the posterior elements or vertebral body of T1 are involved, a hybrid system using PPSS pedicle screws at T5–T6 is connected to an LMSRS using lateral mass screws at C5–C6 and a pedicle screw at C7. Hybrid systems can be created using a tapered rod or wedding band connectors (Fig. 160-4A–C).

Where there is tumor involvement below T1, a PPSS with a quarter-inch rod can be placed in most patients. This construct consists of pedicle screws placed at C7 and T1 as well as the upper thoracic spine (e.g., T5–T6). The C7 pedicle can typically accommodate a 4.5 or 4.75 × 25 mm screw available in most PPSSs. T1 is often a large pedicle that can accommodate a 5.5 or 6.5 × 30 mm screw. To place the C7 pedicle screw, a small window laminotomy is created adjacent to the C6–C7 foramen to probe the pedicle and ensure safety of the functionally important C7 and C8 roots. Ending the construct at C7 preserves motion segments in the neck. If the C7 pedicle cannot accommodate a 4.5-mm screw, the hybrid system can be used for salvage (Fig. 160-5A–C).

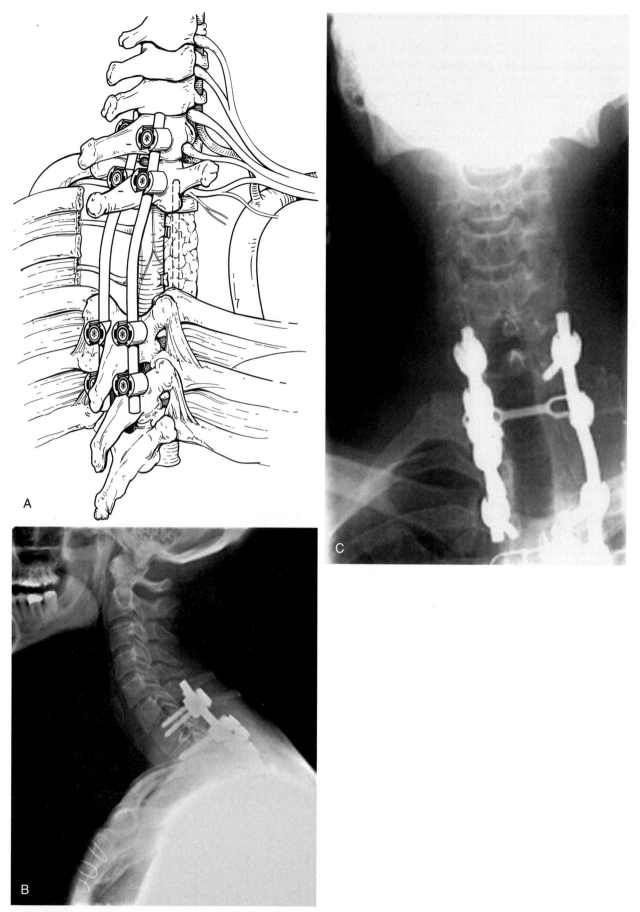

FIGURE 160-5   *A,* Artist's illustration of a short segment pedicle screw fixation with the superior screw at C7, which can be used as an alternative to hybrid systems for tumors involving T2 and below. This construct achieves two points of fixation at C7 and T1 without extending the fixation into the midcervical spine and losing motion segments. *B* and *C,* Plain radiographs showing a Pancoast tumor resection with unilateral left T1 facet and pedicle resection. The superior 4.75-mm pedicle screw was placed at C7. (*A,* © 2004, Memorial Sloan-Kettering Cancer Center, New York, NY.)

The posterior incision is closed before opening the posterolateral thoracotomy. The intrathoracic dissection, including lobectomy, is completed; the chest wall, tumor, and lobe are then resected en bloc. The vertebral body is completely resected using a high-speed drill. The posterior longitudinal ligament should be removed to ensure a clean anterior dural margin. The anterior reconstruction is done as previously noted in this section.

En bloc vertebral body resection has been entertained to obtain a wide resection on Pancoast tumors. Achieving wide margins is technically challenging in these cases because of the presence of multiple vertebral body levels, extensive epidural tumor, and a large chest wall component. The marked response of most tumors to neoadjuvant chemoradiation may ensure a complete R1 resection with curettage alone, lessening the need to place the patient at increased risk from an en bloc resection.

Brachial Plexus

The T1 nerve root is frequently involved, since it traverses the apex of the chest cavity to join the lower trunk of the brachial plexus. The T1 nerve root is resected if it is encased in tumor. This root is larger than the other thoracic nerve roots and is ligated with a suture ligature (e.g., 2-0 silk) rather than vascular clips. Resection of T1 may result in diffuse intrinsic hand weakness, but the hand typically remains functional. Return of normal hand function may occur in 3 to 6 weeks with therapy. Sacrifice of the C8 nerve root and/or lower trunk of the brachial plexus results in significant hand intrinsic muscle weakness. Every attempt is made to spare these nerves. Biopsy samples of perineural tissue may consist of scar from neoadjuvant therapy rather than viable tumor. While the hand is often significantly impaired preoperatively, extensive consent discussions should specifically address postoperative hand weakness.

The sympathetic nervous system is commonly infiltrated by tumor. The stellate ganglion traverses the T1 rib head. Tumor involvement or rib resection of T1 will result in a Horner's syndrome and is an expected outcome from this procedure.

COMPLICATIONS

The primary complications from Pancoast resection are pulmonary, particularly pneumonia and empyema. These complications result from a poor cough as sequelae of the chest wall resection and pain. The aggressive uses of systemic analgesics, epidural pain catheters, and aggressive pulmonary hygiene have decreased the risk of infectious complications. Bedside bronchoscopy to evacuate retained secretions is common. Other pulmonary complications are parenchymal air leaks and bronchopleural fistulae.

Neurologic complications have been discussed, including intrinsic hand weakness from C8 and/or lower trunk of the brachial plexus. Cerebrospinal fluid (CSF) leaks may occur if nerve roots are not identified intraoperatively and ligated. CSF leaks can result in simple CSF pleural effusions, intracranial hypotension, or tension pneumocephalus. Any of these entities may require a reoperation for nerve root ligation either via a thoracotomy or more commonly with a laminectomy. In patients who are not chest tube dependent from a pneumothorax, discontinuing chest tube suction may decrease CSF extravasation enough to resolve intracranial tension pneumocephalus.

Vascular complications can be devastating, most commonly occurring in planned resection and reconstruction of the subclavian artery. Graft reconstruction requires a minimum of 6 months of anticoagulation to prevent clot formation. Subclavian vein thrombosis can result from radiation and surgery. Thrombosis or sectioning of the vein results in upper extremity edema.

CONCLUSIONS

The evolution of treatment for superior sulcus tumors has improved survival and cure rates. These improvements have come through a combination of advances in neoadjuvant therapy and operative techniques. Currently, most patients are offered induction chemotherapy with carboplatin and etoposide and concomitant radiation. The significant histologic responses often do not correlate with radiographic responses, and many patients are subsequently resected for radiographic residual tumor. Whereas T4 tumors with spinal and brachial plexus involvement were traditionally considered unresectable for local tumor control and cure, the use of neoadjuvant therapy and aggressive surgery may change these prospects. We have described operations for posterior compartment tumors based on the MRI assessment of spine and brachial plexus involvement. Using these techniques, complete resections (R0/R1) can be achieved for these technically challenging tumors.

REFERENCES

1. Pancoast HK: Superior sulcus tumor. JAMA 99:1391–1396, 1932.
2. Ginsberg RJ, Martini N, Zaman M, et al: Influence of surgical resection and brachytherapy in the management of superior sulcus tumor. Ann Thorac Surg 57:1440–1445, 1994.
3. Maggi G, Casadio C, Pischedda F, et al: Combined radiosurgical treatment of Pancoast tumor. Ann Thorac Surg 57:198–202, 1994.
4. Martinez-Monge R, Herreros J, Aristu JJ, et al: Combined treatment in superior sulcus tumors: Influence of surgical resection and brachytherapy in the management of superior sulcus tumor. Am J Clin Oncol 17: 317–322, 1994.
5. Rusch VW, Giroux DJ, Kraut MJ, et al: Induction chemoradiation and surgical resection for non-small cell lung carcinomas of the superior sulcus: Initial results of Southwest Oncology Group Trial 9416 (Intergroup Trial 0160). J Thorac Cardiovasc Surg 121:472–483, 2001.
6. Detterbeck FC: Changes in the treatment of Pancoast tumors. Ann Thorac Surg 75:1990–1997, 2003.
7. Bilsky MH, Vitaz TW, Boland PJ, et al: Surgical treatment of superior sulcus tumors with spinal and brachial plexus involvement. J Neurosurg 97:301–309, 2002.
8. Freundlich IM, Chasen MH, Varma DG: Magnetic resonance imaging of pulmonary apical tumors. J Thorac Imaging 11:210–222, 1996.
9. Chardack WM, MacCallum JD: Pancoast tumor (five year survival without recurrence or metastases following radical resection and postoperative irradiation. J Thorac Surg 31:535–542, 1956.
10. Shaw RR, Paulson DL, Kee JL Jr: Treatment of the superior sulcus tumor by irradiation followed by resection. Ann Surg 7:29–40, 1961.
11. Ricci C, Rendina EA, Venuta F, et al: Superior pulmonary sulcus tumors: Radical resection and palliative treatment. Int Surg 74: 175–179, 1989.
12. Satori F, Rea F, Calabro F, et al: Carcinoma of the superior pulmonary sulcus: Results of irradiation and radical resection. J Thorac Cardiovasc Surg 104:679–683, 1992.
13. Rusch VW, Parekh KR, Leon L, et al: Factors determining outcome after surgical resection of T3 and T4 lung cancers of the superior sulcus. J Thorac Cardiovasc Surg 119:1147–1153, 2000.

14. Kent MS, Bilsky MH, Rusch VW: Resection of superior sulcus tumors (posterior approach). Thorac Surg Clin 14:217–228, 2004.

15. Barnes JB, Johnson SB, Dahiya RS, et al: Concomitant weekly cisplatin and thoracic radiotherapy for Pancoast tumors of the lung: Pilot experience of the San Antonio Cancer Institute. Am J Clin Oncol 25:90–92, 2002.

16. Wright CD, Menard MT, Wain JC, et al: Induction chemoradiation compared with induction radiation for lung cancer involving the superior sulcus. Ann Thorac Surg 73:1541–1544, 2002.

17. Dartevelle P, Macchiarini P: Surgical management of superior sulcus tumors. Oncologist 4:398–407, 1999.

18. Kraut MJ, Vallieres E, Thomas CR Jr: Pancoast (superior sulcus) neoplasms. Curr Probl Cancer 27:81–104, 2003.

19. Vallieres E, Karmy-Jones R, Mulligan MS, et al: Pancoast tumors. Curr Probl Surg 38:293–376, 2001.

20. Gokaslan Z, York J, Walsh G: Transthoracic vertebrectomy for metastatic spinal tumors. J Neurosurg 89:599–609, 1998.

161 Surgical Management of Brachial Plexus Injuries in Adults

JULIA K. TERZIS and MARIOS D. VEKRIS

Post-traumatic brachial plexus paralysis affects mostly young people, resulting in devastating socioeconomic and psychologic hardships for these unfortunate patients. In recent years the number of severe brachial plexus injuries has increased because of the increased survival rate after severe motor vehicle accidents due to the application of advanced resuscitation techniques. Fortunately, modern reconstruction modalities have improved dramatically in a linear relationship with the evolution of microsurgery. Avulsion injuries of the brachial plexus represent the most devastating palsies of the affected upper extremity, and the prognosis is poor. Even in these severe palsies, however, current plexus management can improve the usefulness of the affected extremity.

Precise and careful evaluation of the plexus lesion is of paramount importance, since it permits more accurate prognosis and allows more realistic planning for reconstruction. The evolution in spinal cord and plexus imaging has greatly aided in the establishment of diagnosis and surgical planning.

The difficulty in plexus reconstruction vis-à-vis peripheral nerve repair is dual: (1) the lack of adequate nerve grafts to bridge extensive and massive plexus defects and (2) in the case of avulsions, the lack of adequate proximal intraplexus donors (roots) that are in continuity with the spinal cord. These conditions make the anatomic restoration of the brachial plexus practically impossible, with the exception of partial plexus injuries. The challenge for the reconstructive microsurgeon is to identify and sacrifice less important functions so as to direct motor fibers and use them to neurotize more important targets for restoration of basic functions to the flail and anesthetic arm.

Although attempts at brachial plexus reconstruction were introduced early in the 20th century, a nonoperative approach was recommended because of disappointing results and surgery was justified only for brachial plexus exploration to determine prognosis.[1–7] For the flail and anesthetic arm, the alternatives were to amputate through the arm, fuse the shoulder, and fit the patient with a prosthesis[8] or use specialized splints (flail arm splint).[9]

This pessimistic attitude of "wait and see" changed gradually as reports accumulated of improved outcomes in brachial plexus reconstruction even in severe palsies involving root avulsions. These results were made feasible with the introduction of microsurgical techniques[10–12] and the principle of tension-free repair[13,14] in peripheral nerve surgery, the better understanding of the nature of brachial plexus injuries, and the experience gained over the years.[15]

The whole spectrum of reconstruction aims to regain important functions of the upper extremity (i.e., shoulder stability, elbow flexion, elbow extension, protective sensation in the hand and, if feasible, hand reanimation). Since no patient wants the amputation of the paralyzed limb, preferring to use it even partially, the surgeon's effort focuses on maximizing the muscle and sensory recovery by whatever means seem appropriate. The modern armamentarium in plexus surgery comprises various neurotizations both intraplexal or extraplexal, the use of nerve grafts (conventional and/or vascularized), transfer of free vascularized and neurotized muscles (powered via banked nerves or via neurotizations in a one-stage procedure), tendon transfers, bone fusions, and osteotomies. It is obvious that all these treatments require more than one procedure. The patient should be notified about the multistaged reconstruction and become familiar with the possibility of a partial return of function and use of the paralyzed extremity as an accessory extremity during daily activities.

ESTABLISHMENT OF DIAGNOSIS

Preoperative Examination

A precise preoperative assessment is of paramount importance, since it makes diagnosis and prognosis more accurate and permits the implementation of a realistic plan of reconstruction. Such an assessment should incorporate an explicit history of the injury and a comprehensive physical examination of the patient in addition to various paraclinical examinations, including neuroradiologic and electrophysiologic studies.

The history is critical because the patients usually arrive for plexus reconstruction several weeks or months after the injury. A detailed explicit history can reveal the mechanism of the injury and the velocity of the impact; high-velocity injuries indicate root avulsion. Concomitant fractures and/or dislocations around the shoulder and/or vascular injury of the subclavian or axillary vessels indicate extensive trauma to the plexus with a possible double level of injury and additional scar tissue that will complicate exploration of the plexus. The presence of a vein graft used elsewhere to bridge an arterial defect should make the surgeon more cautious, because the plexus will have to be explored through dense scar tissue with the vein graft hidden somewhere in this scar.

Loss of consciousness and admission to the intensive care unit indicate possible central nervous system damage and can complicate the paralysis pattern. Furthermore, the results of reconstruction in these patients are less satisfactory because of possible coexistent brain injury reflected to the paralyzed extremity and insufficient cooperation of the patient in the rehabilitation program.

Clinical examination commences with observation of muscle wasting, scars, contractures, neurotrophic vasomotor changes, and the presence of Horner's sign, which indicates lower root avulsion. The strength of all muscles of the upper extremity is examined, from the shoulder to the hand, and recorded according to the British Medical Council Scale of M0 to M5 using + and – between each grade (e.g., M3+). The range of motion of all joints is assessed to reveal joint contractures. The sensory status of the extremity is examined as well, in terms of light touch sensation, static and moving two-point discrimination test, and vibration modalities with tuning forks. Ninhydrin sweat test reveals damage of the sympathetic chain and is an indicator of lower root avulsion. The presence or absence of pain and its characteristics (location, frequency, duration, quality, and intensity), the degree of need for medication, and the changes of these characteristics since the accident, combined with the sensory status of the extremity, help rule out avulsion.

Laboratory examinations should include inspiration and expiration chest radiographs and/or chest fluoroscopy to rule out phrenic nerve injury, an indicator of upper root avulsion. Other plain radiographs are useful if there is evidence from the history for fractures or dislocations or ectopic ossification; the latter is not rare in coma patients with prolonged stays in the intensive care unit. Fractures and/or dislocations around the shoulder and elbow indicate possible double-level injury of specific peripheral nerves. For example, clavicle fracture indicates injury to the infraclavicular plexus, humeral head fracture and/or dislocation may involve injury to the axillary nerve, scapula neck fracture may injure the suprascapular nerve, and humeral shaft fracture may damage the radial nerve. Arteriography of the upper extremity is necessary in case of previous vessel injury and/or reconstruction with vein graft, as well as when free-muscle transfers are to be performed.

The combination of cervical myelogram, introduced by Murphey and colleagues[16] in 1947 and computed tomography (CT) myelography is considered the best method to examine the ventral and dorsal rootlets and rule out avulsions, with a low rate (3.5%) of false negative results.[17] Conventional magnetic resonance imaging (MRI) is best at showing the plexus beyond the foramina, but the recently introduced technique of MR myelography surpasses conventional myelography and is similar in accuracy to CT after myelography.[18] The presence of pseudomeningoceles indicates root avulsion.

Lately, ultrasonography[19] and 3-dimensional rotational myelography[20] have been used for demonstration of brachial plexus injury, with encouraging prospects in the diagnosis of brachial plexus lesions.

Electrodiagnostic evaluation includes electromyography,[21] nerve conduction velocities, sensory action potentials,[22] and percutaneous lamina stimulation test.[23] In the latter examination, tiny volleys of electrical stimulation are applied on each exiting root, and the patient perceives the dermatome subserved by this root. A positive response is strong evidence against avulsion. The presence of sensory nerve action potential (NAP) and normal sensory conduction velocity in the peripheral nerves innervating a flail and anesthetic extremity invariably implies root avulsion.

These preoperative data are necessary to arrive at a prognosis and establish a reasonable reconstructive plan. The final diagnosis, though, is made intraoperatively.

Brachial Plexus Exploration and Intraoperative Diagnosis

Exploration of the entire supraclavicular and infraclavicular brachial plexus is necessary to identify the roots and the injured plexus elements. In postganglionic lesions and if there is any residual function, intraoperative electrical nerve stimulation with 0.5 to 2.0 mA intensity is helpful, especially in cases of neuroma in continuity. To rule out root avulsions intraoperatively, various methods are in use.

Cross sections of the roots are sent to the pathology lab for immediate histology to identify axons, ganglion cells, and excessive scar tissue. In case of the presence of ganglion cells, the root is considered avulsed and therefore cannot be used as a donor for neurotization. Additional histochemistry of the roots with carbonic anhydrase[24] and cholinesterase[25] can be processed immediately in specialized centers to generate additional information about the sensorimotor distribution of a nerve biopsy site.

Somatosensory evoked potentials (SSEPs) record the response of the opposite brain hemisphere in electrical stimuli at the root level, utilizing superficial recording electrodes, and is reported to be a reliable method to rule out avulsion.[26] These traditional intraoperative neurophysiologic assessment methods, such as NAP and SSEP monitoring, have been used to evaluate proximal nerve stump integrity, but these methods do not allow evaluation of the integrity of motor fibers back to the anterior horn cell.

Recently, motor evoked potentials (MEPs) have been used to diagnose avulsion of the anterior rootlets (motor fibers).[27] This method records action potential at the root level after transcranial electrical stimulation of the brain. If there is a response, there is connectivity and thus no avulsion of the examined root from the spinal cord. Burkholder and co-workers[28] reported that neurogenic MEPs coupled with NAPs and SSEPs can evaluate successfully the functional status of motor fibers back to the anterior horn cell for accurate localization of the lesion sites.

The authors use a scale of intraoperative assessment of the severity of the lesion, which is called total severity score and was introduced by Terzis and colleagues.[29] Each root is graded as follows: 0 = avulsion; 1 = avulsion/rupture; 2 = rupture; 3 = rupture/traction; 4 = traction; 5 = normal. The total severity score of the normal brachial plexus is 25. The lower the severity score, the worse the injury and the prognosis, and the lesser the available intraplexus donors for neurotization.

TIMING OF RECONSTRUCTION

The optimal time for reconstruction in the treatment of closed traction injuries has been the subject of controversy in the past. The attitude of "wait and see" has no place today in the management of these injuries, since there is minimal or no benefit from late nerve reconstruction, especially if performed after 2 years of denervation.

Magalon and co-workers[30] and Brunelli and Brunelli[31] suggested an emergency repair of lesions associated with vascular trauma, while Alnot[32] advocated exploration of the plexus during vascular repair and reconstruction as a secondary stage. Sedel[33] asserts that the results obtained from repairs done up to 9 months after the injury were better than those achieved with more delayed reconstruction. We believe that aggressive early reconstruction within 6 weeks to 3 months after injury offers the most rewarding results.[29]

BRACHIAL PLEXUS RECONSTRUCTION

In postganglionic supraclavicular and infraclavicular injuries, most of the distal plexus elements can usually be reconstructed with restoration of the anatomic pathways (Fig. 161-1). Neurolysis is useful in the presence of scar tissue and in neuroma in continuity where there is response during the intraoperative electrical stimulation. Nerve grafting is the most common method of reconstruction in postganglionic injuries, utilizing conventional nerve grafts to bridge the defects. The most popular sensory nerves used as grafts are the following in order of preference: sural, saphenous, medial brachial, medial antebrachial cutaneous, and superficial radial nerves.

Vascularized nerve grafts have been added to the armamentarium of brachial plexus surgeons.[34,35] These grafts maintain their blood supply and survive transfer even if placed in a scarred bed. Thus, the intraneural environment is optimally preserved and axonal carry-through is not compromised even when a nerve trunk is transferred (e.g., ulnar nerve)[36] (Fig. 161-2).

In cases of root avulsions, the reconstructive surgeons have promoted and used various extraplexus motor donors in their effort to neurotize selected muscles to achieve essential function in the shoulder, elbow, and hand. Yeoman and Seddon[37] introduced neurotization of the musculocutaneous nerve with intercostal nerve transfer in cases of avulsion. In addition, the use of branches of the ipsilateral cervical plexus,[38] contralateral lateral pectoral nerve,[39] accessory nerve,[40] hypoglossal nerve,[41,42] phrenic nerve and contralateral C7,[43,44] and selective contralateral C7[45] are currently in use.

In C5 and C6 root avulsions of upper brachial plexus injury with the lower plexus intact, various intraplexus neurotizations have been proposed, including selective ulnar nerve to musculocutaneous,[46] medial pectoral nerve to musculocutaneous or axillary,[47] ipsilateral C7 (J.K. Terzis, personal communication, 8 December 1992),[48] nerve to the long head of the triceps to axillary,[49] and one-fascicle median nerve transfer to biceps.[50]

The evolution of end-to-side neurorrhaphy, with many publications in the experimental field, and the promising results of these studies have made possible the use of this technique in brachial plexus surgery. Mennen and colleagues[51] used end-to-side neurorrhaphy of the musculocutaneous nerve to adjacent donor nerves via an epineurial window on the donor nerve and reported encouraging results. More clinical studies with larger numbers of patients should be published to establish the usefulness of this technique.

In cases of avulsed roots, the reconstruction plan is limited to extraplexus neurotizations, because an avulsed root cannot be used as a proximal donor. In an effort to reconstruct the majority of the lost function, attempts to reunite the distal plexus elements to the spinal cord have been reported. Carlsted[52] reported experimental reinnervation through avulsed roots implanted in the spinal cord. Clinically, in root avulsions and replantations he observed muscle function, but the functional outcome was compromised by severe co-contraction. Bertelli and Ghizoni[53] demonstrated muscle reinnervation through nerve grafts implanted directly into the spinal cord. It seems that the combination of intra- and extradural neurotizations improves the proximal muscle function results. However, the extent of this improvement is limited and, according to the authors, does not justify the use of spinal implants.

There is some controversy about the level of distal coaptation of the nerve grafts during neurotization procedures. Bentolila and co-workers[54] reported better outcomes when the grafts were coapted distally to the lateral or posterior cord in relation to more distal coaptations near the distal target (e.g., musculocutaneous). On the contrary, Alnot[32] and Terzis and colleagues[29] stated that nerve grafting is more rewarding when the nerve grafts are coapted distally to the peripheral nerve than to proximal plexus elements (i.e., cords). We concur with this notion, because this method of reconstruction will result in the majority of the nerve fibers being driven to the desired target and not lost in random reinnervation.

Strategy of Reconstruction

Postganglionic Lesions

The roots are not avulsed in postganglionic lesions, and the injury extends to various lengths and can involve trunks, divisions, and/or cords. The reconstruction with neurolysis and nerve grafts can be global and anatomic. In extended injuries, direct neurotization procedures can be used if a lack of nerve grafts precludes anatomic restoration. Care should be taken to connect the anterior part of the proximal plexus elements with the lateral and medial cord and the posterior to the posterior cord to avoid cocontraction.

If the plexus injury is complicated with vascular injury of the subclavian and/or axillary artery (see Fig. 161-1), the trauma is usually extensive and a tremendous amount of scar tissue develops, especially in cases in which a vein graft was used to restore continuity of the arterial pathways immediately after injury. Therefore, it seems it would have been better to perform the brachial plexus reconstruction at the time of vascular reconstruction. The only argument against this, which is critical for the final outcome, is that in these extensive injuries usually the element of avulsion of the neural tissue is present. Hence, it is sometimes impossible to ascertain the accurate estimation of the limits of the nerve injury because the longitudinal extent of the lesion is usually much greater than the gap seen during exploration. Diagnosing the exact degree of the damage to the plexus, and thus the success of nerve repairs, have a better chance if exploration and reconstruction are done at a later stage.

To achieve reinnervation of the various distal targets in these extended injuries, long nerve grafts need to drive through a scarred bed. In these cases the use of vascularized nerve grafts is preferred, since these grafts have a better

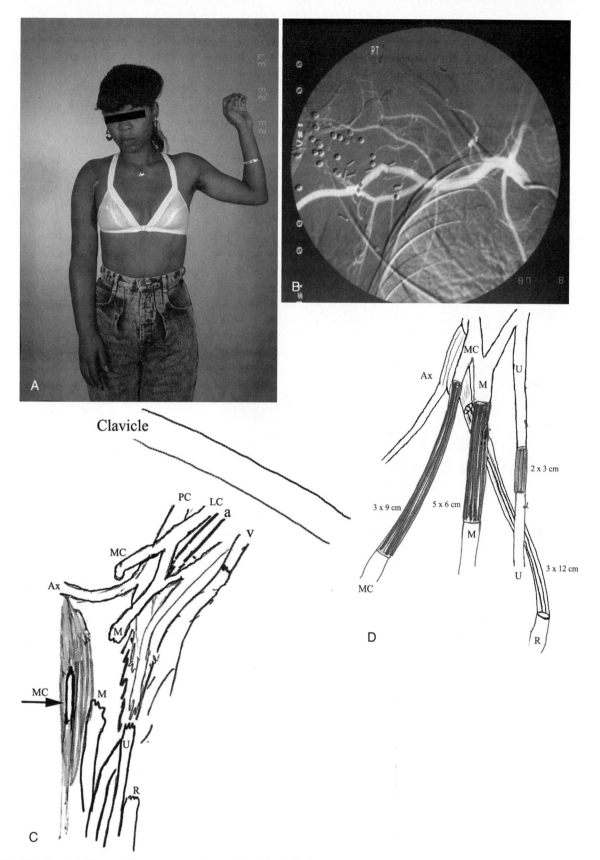

Clavicle

FIGURE 161-1 *A,* A 24-year-old woman sustained a right infraclavicular brachial plexus injury secondary to shotgun wound. The brachial plexus injury was accompanied by axillary artery injury and right humerus fracture. Preoperative view showing patient with complete motor and sensory paralysis at the right shoulder, elbow, and hand. At another facility she initially underwent open reduction and internal fixation of the right humerus fracture and vein grafting of the right axillary artery. *B,* Preoperative angiography; note interposition vein graft and multiple shotgun shell fragments. *C,* At 8 weeks the infraclavicular brachial plexus was explored. Exploration revealed a significant amount of scar surrounding torn elements of the plexus and axillary artery with interposition vein graft (V). *D,* The following microsurgical reconstruction was performed: Interposition nerve grafting of the median (M) nerve (6 cm × 5), ulnar (U) nerve (2 cm × 3), musculocutaneous (MC) nerve (9 cm × 3), and radial (R) nerve (12 cm × 3); microneurolysis of the posterior cord (PC) and axillary nerve.

(Continued)

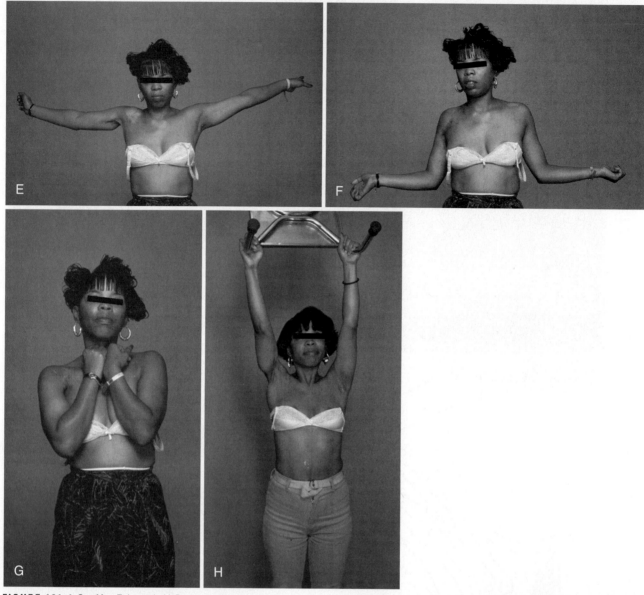

FIGURE 161-1 Cont'd   *E* through *H,* Postoperative views of the patient 4 years after surgery showing shoulder abduction and external rotation, and elbow flexion and extension. (*B* and *C,* From Terzis JK, Vekris M, Soucacos P: Brachial plexus root avulsions. World J Surg 25: 1049–1061, 2001.)

chance to survive in this hostile scarred environment and carry through the newly formed regenerating axons (see Fig. 161-2).

If there is avulsion of the peripheral nerves from the muscle, direct implantation of the nerve grafts in several places of the muscle belly is a method of reinnervation. Furthermore, free functioning muscle transfer can be used to replace the muscle that sustained avulsion of its nerve at the neuromuscular junction.

Preganglionic Lesions

The lower roots are avulsed more frequently, and in this case the others are involved to a variable degree, following the rule that the farther a root is from the avulsion the less the insult. The prognosis is better if the avulsion affects the middle plexus, because in this case the hand is spared (Fig. 161-3).

If C5 and/or C6 are avulsed, usually selective regions of the posterior division of C7 are guided to the posterior cord and parts from the anterior division of C7 are guided to the lateral cord. In adults, to date, neurotization of C8 and T1 is not justified, since the long distances do not offer any possibility for recovery of the small muscles of the hand.

If only C5 and C6 are available, the suprascapular nerve is neurotized from the terminal branch of the ipsilateral accessory nerve, while conventional nerve grafts or the ipsilateral ulnar nerve is utilized as a vascularized nerve graft to connect C5 and C6 with the musculocutaneous, axillary, median, and/or radial nerves (see Fig. 161-2). The ulnar nerve, based on the superior ulnar collateral vessels, can connect two or three targets at the same time with the proximal donor root(s), using the "loop" technique introduced by Terzis[36] in 1981 (see Fig. 161-2). Through perineurial windows the fascicles are divided, to be coapted to the root(s) and the distal

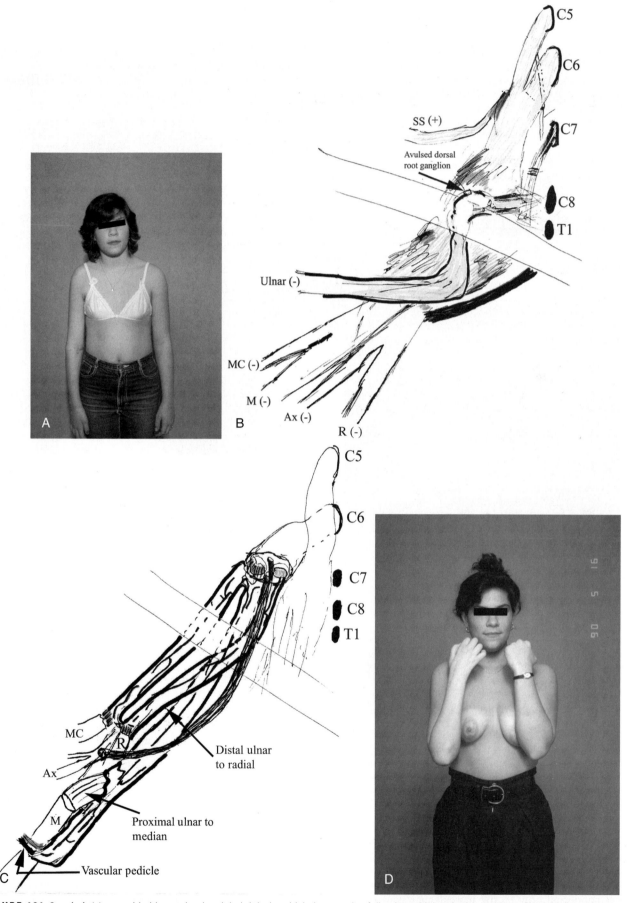

FIGURE 161-2 *A,* A 14-year-old girl sustained a global right brachial plexus palsy following a high-velocity accident. She initially underwent exploratory surgery elsewhere by vascular surgeons because of a concomitant subclavian artery injury. Preoperatively, the patient presented with a totally paretic right upper extremity. *B,* Seven months after the injury, the patient underwent exploration with intraoperative findings of C5, C6 roots rupture, C7, C8, T1 roots avulsion, and then (*C*) reconstruction.

(Continued)

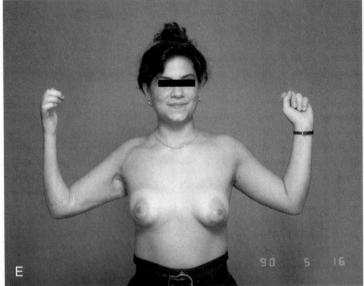

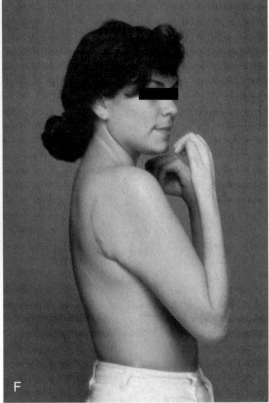

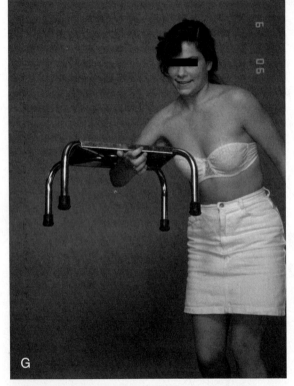

FIGURE 161-2 Cont'd   The ulnar nerve was used as a pedicled vascularized nerve graft to reconstruct the musculocutaneous (MC), median (M), and radial (R) nerves. Sural nerves were used as nonvascularized nerve grafts to repair the axillary nerve. SS, Suprascapular nerve. *D* through *G*, Postoperative presentation of the patient at 5 (*D* and *E*) and 10 years (*F* and *G*), following surgery. Note return of elbow flexion (*D* and *F*), shoulder external rotation and abduction (*E*), and the ability to use the reconstructed limb as assist arm (*G*).

targets, maintaining the nerve's epineurial blood supply (see Fig. 161-2C). If only C5 is available and the brachial plexus is prefixed, a similar strategy of reconstruction is followed.

If the brachial plexus is postfixed and C5 root is tiny, then it is connected only to the musculocutaneous nerve with conventional nerve grafts and the ulnar nerve is reserved, to be used for connection with the anterior division of the contralateral C7 and the ipsilateral median nerve at a

second stage. The posterior cord elements, including the axillary nerve, nerve to the triceps, and radial nerve, are neurotized by extraplexus motors including ipsilateral intercostals, partial phrenic, and/or cervical plexus motors.

In case of global avulsion, the lack of intraplexus donors leads the surgeon to seek alternate donor axonal pools in extraplexus ipsilateral or contralateral intraplexus donors. It is of paramount importance to assure the good status of the ipsilateral nerves, since in these devastating injuries, these may be involved to a variable degree. The most frequently used neurotizations are the following:

1. Accessory to suprascapular directly
2. Intercostals are used to neurotize either anterior or posterior targets, but not both, to avoid cocontraction. Direct coaptation to the recipient nerve is preferable. For the musculocutaneous nerve, one needs at least three intercostals.
3. The phrenic, the cervical plexus motor branches, the partial hypoglossal, and the anterior and posterior division of the contralateral C7 are used to neurotize

as many targets as possible. Sometimes, to match the axonal number of the target's nerve to the lesser number of axons offered by the donors, two or more donor nerves may be driven to the same important target (e.g., musculocutaneous nerve).

Protective sensation is given to the median nerve from sensory branches of the intercostals and/or from the sensory supraclavicular nerves. Furthermore, nerve grafts, connected proximally with various motor donors, are banked subcutaneously in the arm at elbow level for future neurotization of free-muscle transfers.

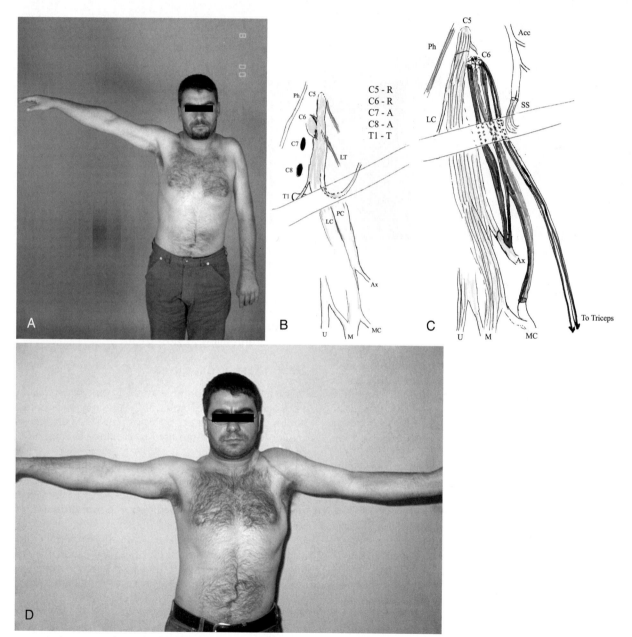

FIGURE 161-3 *A,* A 22-year-old man sustained a left brachial plexus palsy in a motorcycle accident. Preoperatively, the patient presented with a complete palsy of the left upper extremity. *B,* Intraoperative findings upon exploration were as follows: C5, C6 roots rupture (R); C7, C8 roots avulsion (A); T1 root traction (T). *C,* Microsurgical reconstruction included the following procedures: (1) Direct neurotization of the suprascapular (SS) nerve by the distal accessory (Acc); (2) C6 to musculocutaneous (MC) and triceps nerves, with interposition nerve grafts; (3) C6 to axillary (Ax) by distal end-to-side repair; (4) microneurolysis of the entire supraclavicular and infraclavicular brachial plexus. LC, lateral cord; M, median nerve; Ph, phrenic nerve. *D* through *G,* Two years postoperatively, the patient presents with excellent functional return. Note restored shoulder abduction (*D*), external rotation (*E*) and anterior flexion (*G*). In addition, patient demonstrates strong elbow flexion (*F*).

(Continued)

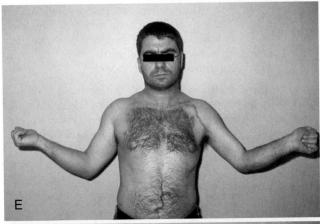

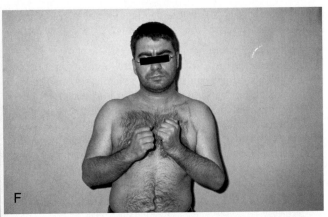

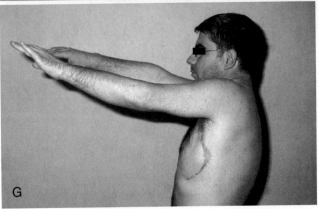

FIGURE 161-3 Cont'd

Pain Management

The extremity is totally flail and anesthetic, usually with intolerable constant pain that leads the patient to seek relief even with amputation, a method not now acceptable. Control of the pain can be achieved either by conservative methods (i.e., pharmaceutical agents and/or electrical stimulation) or, if it persists, with surgical intervention consisting of coagulation at the levels of the dorsal horn, which is the site of the avulsed dorsal root entry zones (DREZ) in the spinal cord (introduced by Nashold[55]). This procedure should precede the nerve reconstruction. Chen and colleagues[56] performed, for intractable pain, DREZ lesions made by thermocoagulation in 34 cases. The pain relief rate was good in about 75%. Combined neural reconstruction was performed in 15 cases. They concluded that combined pain control and reconstruction offer an early rehabilitation for brachial plexus avulsion injury.

After the brachial plexus microreconstruction, the pain dramatically decreases and the majority of the patients have no pain or very mild and tolerable pain.[29,32,57] The pain decrease correlates directly with sensation improvement postoperatively.

The restoration of protective sensation allows the patient to recognize the position of the extremity in space and avoid injuries, while any return of afferent input, even protective, blocks dramatically the nociceptive afferent pathways. Relief of pain permits the patient to focus on the rehabilitation of the extremity and improve its dexterity and overall function, which returns many months later.

Secondary Procedures

Procedures such as muscle transfers and wrist fusion are necessary to improve function, especially in late cases in which the muscle targets have atrophied. Pedicled muscle or tendon transfers[58–61] are used to enhance the functionality of the paretic arm.

The local muscle or tendon transfers that are utilized to restore or enhance the function of the shoulder (i.e., trapezius transfer), the elbow (i.e., Steindler flexorplasty), and the hand are motor units spared from the initial injury or reinnervated spontaneously or obtained after plexus reconstruction. In the second case, care should be taken so the transferred muscle-tendon unit has preoperatively a muscle strength of at least M4. This way, it will be strong enough to function postoperatively, since it is well known that after the transfer one grade of the initial muscle strength is lost (i.e., an M4 will be M3).

Advances in microsurgery brought the era of free functional muscle transfer for brachial plexus paralysis management.[62–64] The transferred free muscles are neurotized either by previously banked nerve grafts or directly from local motor donors (i.e., intercostal nerves; Fig. 161-4). The most commonly restored functions are elbow flexion and extension, finger flexion and extension, and, in some cases, shoulder

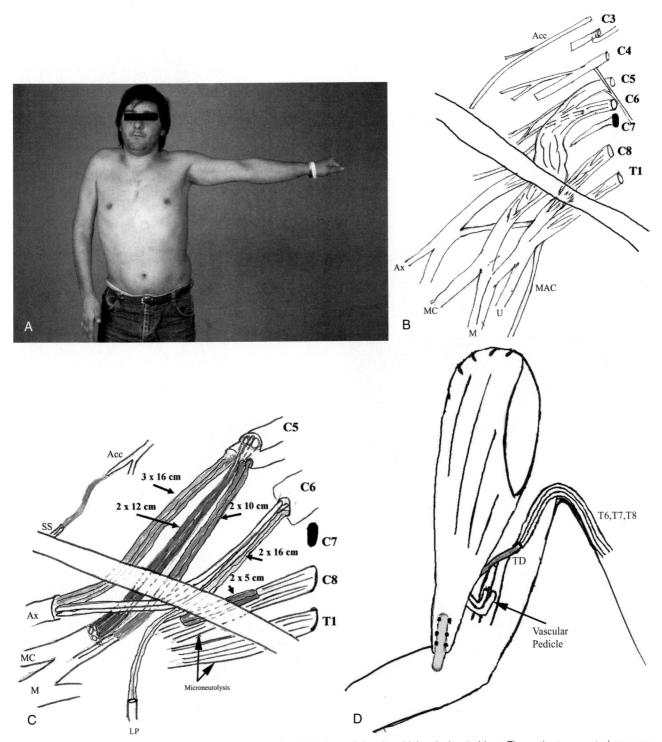

FIGURE 161-4 *A*, A 23-year-old man sustained a right brachial plexus injury in a high-velocity accident. The patient presented preoperatively with total paralysis at the shoulder and elbow. *B*, Exploration took place at 5 months following his injury. Intraoperative findings were as follows: C5, C6 roots rupture, C7 root avulsion, C8, T1 roots traction. *C*, Reconstruction included microneurolysis of C8 and T1 roots (with partial grafting of C8 root). Interposition nerve grafts connected distal accessory (Acc) to suprascapular (SS) nerve, C5 to musculocutaneous (MC), median (M), and axillary (Ax) nerves, and C6 to axillary and lateral pectoral (LP) nerves. MAC, medial antebrachial cutaneous nerve. *D*, Two years later, the patient underwent a microvascular transfer of the contralateral latissimus as a free myocutaneous flap for enhancement of elbow flexion. The thoracodorsal nerve (TD) was neurotized by T6, T7, and T8 ipsilateral intercostal nerves.

(Continued)

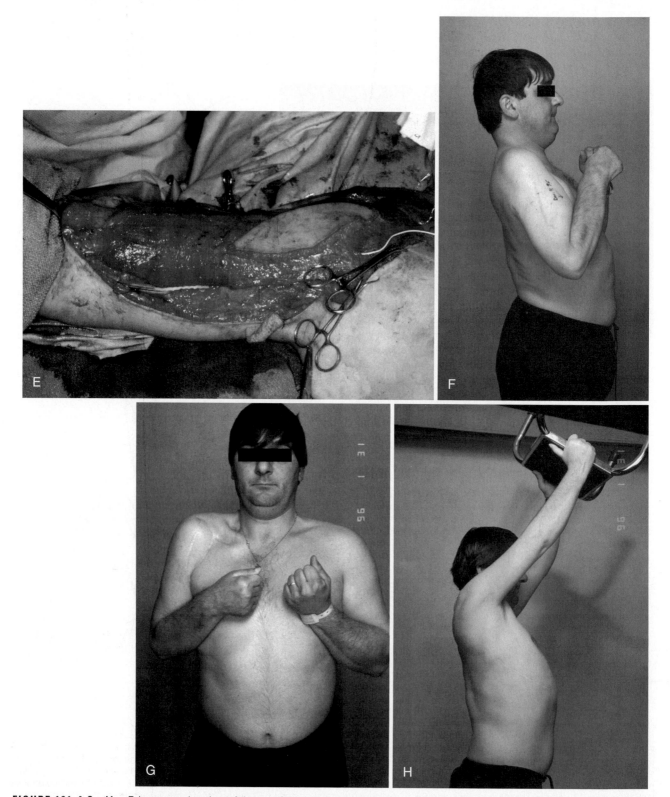

FIGURE 161-4 Cont'd   *E*, Intraoperative view of the transferred free muscle. *F* and *G*, Lateral and anterior views of the patient 6 years post-operatively. Strong elbow flexion has been achieved. *H*, Patient is easily lifting a stool over his head. Patient has returned to full-time employment as a truck driver.

abduction and intrinsic substitution. Latissimus dorsi and rectus femoris are good transfer candidates for elbow flexion restoration. For hand reanimation, gracillis and rectus femoris can be used.[29] Some surgeons prefer to restore two functions with one muscle transfer (e.g., elbow flexion and finger flexion or elbow extension and finger extension).[64,65]

In addition to the various muscle and tendon transfers, bone osteotomies (i.e., rotational osteotomy of the humerus and radius), as well as wrist fusion, are procedures that can enhance the overall function of the paretic arm, providing a better position of the extremity in space. Wrist fusion in particular provides not only stability of the wrist and increase of the hand strength, but permits tendon transfers of the wrist flexors and extensors, if strong enough, to be used for hand reanimation and thus achieve further improvement of hand function.

RESULTS

Important variables determining the prognosis of the lesion are the age of the patient, the denervation time (i.e., the time interval between the injury and the surgery), and the severity score, which is a scale introduced by Terzis to grade the degree of root injury at exploration.[29] The consensus today is that the best results are obtained in younger patients with short denervation time (<6 months) and higher severity score.[29,66–68]

Doi and co-workers[69] confirm that the patients who underwent suprascapular nerve repair demonstrated statistically significantly better ranges of motion for flexion and abduction of the shoulder, compared with the other two groups who had undergone arthrodesis of the humeroscapular joint or had undergone no procedures for shoulder function. We concur with this statement, since the results from our series[29] demonstrate that primary reconstruction gives function superior to secondary procedures alone.

Most authors report better results in upper root palsies. The reason for this is twofold. First, the hand is spared, and second, the muscle targets of reconstruction are closer to the plexus. The latter also explains the better outcome of proximal muscles (e.g., supraspinatus, biceps).

Many authors[29,57,67,70–72] prefer to use intraplexus motor donors for neurotizations, when they are available, since they give better results. The reason for this is that the intraplexus donors have a greater number of axons than do the extraplexus ones, and, therefore, there are greater chances for successful neurotization.

It seems that some of the extraplexus donors give consistently superior results when they are used with specific targets (e.g., shoulder and elbow). Merrell and colleagues,[73] in a meta-analysis of the English literature regarding neurotizations for restoration of the shoulder and elbow function, suggest that interposition nerve grafts should be avoided when possible when performing nerve transfers. Better results for restoration of elbow flexion have been obtained with direct intercostal to musculocutaneous transfers than with spinal accessory nerve transfers, which would require a nerve graft, and spinal accessory to suprascapular transfers appear to have the best outcomes for return of shoulder abduction.

The use of intercostal nerves to directly neurotize the musculocutaneous nerve continues to be a standard approach in the reconstruction of severe plexus lesions, especially avulsions. The muscle strength results are good to excellent (more than M3) in 60% to 70% of the patients.[13,29,57,72,74–76] Ogino and Naito[77] consider intercostal transfer a useful procedure to provide elbow flexion and protective sensation to the hand.

The accessory nerve is another reliable donor. Direct neurotization of the suprascapular nerve yielded results comparable to repair with intraplexus donors. Neurotization of the suprascapular nerve gave 75% good or excellent (M3+ to M4+) results.[29] Millesi[13] reported that neurotization of the suprascapular and axillary with the accessory gave stability of the shoulder in 61% of the patients. Various authors[32,54,76,78,79] reported good to excellent result (≥M3+) in 55% to 86% of the patients, with respect to recovery of biceps function after transfer of the spinal accessory nerve to the musculocutaneous nerve. Samii and colleagues[79] reported that a statistical comparison of the different preoperative time intervals (0–6 months compared with 7–12 months) showed a significantly better outcome in patients treated with early surgery ($P < 0.05$). An analysis of the impact of the length of the interposed nerve grafts revealed a statistically significant better outcome in patients with grafts 12 cm or shorter compared with that in patients with grafts longer than 12 cm ($P < 0.005$).

Other extraplexus donors give less rewarding results; the explanation for this, in the case of cervical plexus motors, is probably related to the fact that a small number of fibers destined initially for short distances are now being forced into a long journey. In the case of the contralateral C7, the length of the cross-chest nerve grafts imposes necessary delay before target connectivity. Gu and co-workers[66,80] showed good results in 75% of the musculocutaneous neurotization with the phrenic, as well as recovery of biceps up to M3 in 60% and recovery of the triceps up to M4 in 50% with contralateral C7 neurotizations. The results were good in 50% of the suprascapular and axillary neurotization with motor branches of the cervical plexus. Cervical plexus motors and contralateral C7 gave overall inferior outcome as related to hand reanimation.[15,29]

Restoration of hand function remains the most difficult task for the reconstructive microsurgeon. It must nevertheless always be pursued, even though the results of hand reanimation, as with neurotizations, are not as successful as the elbow flexion restoration. The good results range from 15% to 40% in various series addressing finger extension and flexion, regardless of the donor nerve that is used for neurotization of the radial and median nerves.[29,57,66,81] If we can find means to preserve the muscle targets, especially the distal ones, we believe that we can expect better functional restoration in the hand.

From the foregoing experience, it seems that certain muscle groups (shoulder abductors and external rotators, supinators, and extensors) present an inferior response to reconstruction. Narakas and Hentz[57] mentioned that this paradox could be explained partially on the basis of the embryologic origin of the various muscles. Thus, there seems to be an inherent preference for restoration of the flexors, which are vital for the survival of the organism.

In global avulsions, in late cases, or in the reconstruction of distal targets such as the hand, free-muscle transfers and other secondary procedures (e.g., wrist fusion) can improve the final outcome.[29,65,82]

An important point is that not only are the overall results dependent on the method of reconstruction of a specific function (e.g., hand motion), but each function is influenced by the function of the more proximal joints or the function of antagonistic muscles. Doi and colleagues[69] affirm that shoulder function is important for achieving prehensile function among patients with complete paralysis of the brachial plexus when they undergo double free-muscle transfer.

In conclusion, post-traumatic brachial plexus injuries present a challenge to the reconstructive microsurgeon. Usually these are devastating lesions produced by high-velocity injuries. Early and aggressive microsurgical reconstruction should be the method of choice in the management of these injuries. The current sophisticated techniques of nerve reconstruction (neurotizations utilizing every available ipsilateral and contralateral intraplexus and extraplexus donors, with conventional and/or vascularized nerve grafts), in combination with secondary free functional muscle transfers, offer satisfactory outcome even in multiple avulsion injuries. Amputation is no longer an option today even in the face of global avulsion.

REFERENCES

1. Stevens JH: Brachial plexus paralysis. In Godman EA (ed): The Shoulder. Brooklyn, NY: G Mill, 1934.
2. Barnes R: Traction injuries of the plexus in adults. J Bone Joint Surg 31B:10–16, 1949.
3. Larsen EH: Injuries of the brachial plexus in adults. J Bone Joint Surg 37B:733–734, 1955.
4. Tracy JF, Brannon EW: Management of brachial plexus injuries (traction type). J Bone Joint Surg 40A:1031–1042, 1958.
5. Bonney G: Prognosis in traction lesions of the brachial plexus. J Bone Joint Surg 41B:4–35, 1959.
6. Leffert RD, Seddon H: Infraclavicular brachial plexus injuries. J Bone Joint Surg 49B:9–22, 1965.
7. Nelson KG, Jolly PC, Thomas PA: Brachial plexus injuries associated with missile wounds of the chest. A report of 9 cases from Vietnam. J Trauma 8:268–275, 1968.
8. Fletcher I: Traction lesions of the brachial plexus. Hand 1:129–136, 1969.
9. Wynn Parry CB: Rehabilitation of patients following traction injuries of the brachial plexus. Hand Clin 11:517–533, 1995.
10. Kurze T: Microtechniques in neurological surgery. Clin Neurosurg 11:128–137, 1964.
11. Millesi H: Brachial plexus injuries. Management and results. Clin Plast Surg 11:115–120, 1984.
12. Narakas A: The surgical management of brachial plexus injuries. In Daniel RK, Terzis JK (eds): Reconstructive Microsurgery, Vol. 1. Boston: Little-Brown, 1977, pp 443–460.
13. Millesi H: Nerve grafting. Clin Plast Surg 11:105–113, 1984.
14. Terzis JK, Faibisoff B, Williams B: The nerve gap: Suture under tension vs. graft. Plast Reconstr Surg 56:166–170, 1975.
15. Terzis JK, Vekris MD, Soucacos PN: Brachial plexus root avulsions. World J Surg 25:1049–1061, 2001.
16. Murphey F, Hartung W, Kirklin JW: Myelographic demonstration of avulsing injury of the brachial plexus. Am J Roentgenol 58:102–105, 1947.
17. Marshall RW, De Silva RDD: Computerized axial tomography in traction injuries of the brachial plexus. J Bone Joint Surg 68B:734–738, 1986.
18. Nakamura T, Yabe Y, Horiuchi Y, et al: Magnetic resonance myelography in brachial plexus injury. J Bone Joint Surg 79B:764–769, 1997.
19. Mallouhi A, Meirer R, Bodner G: Ultrasonographic features of brachial plexus traumatic rupture. Case illustration. J Neurosurg 99:432, 2003.
20. Kufeld M, Claus B, Campi A, et al: Three-dimensional rotational myelography. Am J Neuroradiol 24:1290–1293, 2003.
21. Hodes RR, Larrabee MC, German W: The human electromyogram in response to nerve stimulation and the conduction velocity of motor axons. Arch Neurol Psychiatr 60:340–365, 1948.
22. Dawson GD, Scott JW: The recording of nerve action potentials through skin in man. J Neurol Neurosurg Psychiatr 12:259–267, 1949.
23. Liberson WT, Terzis JK: Contribution of clinical neurophysiology and rehabilitation medicine to the management of brachial plexus palsy. In Terzis JK (ed): Microreconstruction of Nerve Injuries. Philadelphia: WB Saunders, 1987, pp 555–567.
24. Carson KA, Terzis JK: Carbonic anhydrase histochemistry: A potential diagnostic method for peripheral nerve repair. Clin Plast Surg 12:227–232, 1985.
25. Kanaya F, Ogden L, Breidenbach WC, et al: Sensory and motor fiber differentiation with Karnovsky staining. J Hand Surg [Am] 16A:851–858, 1991.
26. Oberle J, Antoniadis G, Rath SA, et al: Radiological investigations and intra-operative evoked potentials for the diagnosis of nerve root avulsion: Evaluation of both modalities by intradural root inspection. Acta Neurochir (Wien) 140:527–531, 1998.
27. Turkof E, Millesi H, Turkof R, et al: Intraoperative electroneurodiagnostics (transcranial electrical motor evoked potentials) to evaluate the functional status of anterior spinal roots and spinal nerves during brachial plexus surgery. Plast Reconstr Surg 99:1632–1641, 1997.
28. Burkholder LM, Houlden DA, Midha R, et al: Neurogenic motor evoked potentials: Role in brachial plexus surgery. Case report. J Neurosurg 98:607–610, 2003.
29. Terzis JK, Vekris MD, Soucacos PN: Outcomes of brachial plexus reconstruction in 204 patients with devastating paralysis. Plast Reconstr Surg 104:1221–1240, 1999.
30. Magalon G, Bordeaux J, Legre R: Emergency versus delayed repair of severe brachial plexus injuries. Clin Orthop 237:32–35, 1988.
31. Brunelli GA, Brunelli GR: Preoperative assessment of the adult plexus patient. Microsurgery 16:17–21, 1995.
32. Alnot J: Traumatic brachial plexus lesions in the adult. Indications and results. Hand Clin 11: 623–631, 1995.
33. Sedel L: Repair of severe traction lesions of the brachial plexus. Clin Orthop 237:62–66, 1988.
34. Taylor GI, Ham FJ: The free vascularized nerve graft: A further experimental and clinical application of microvascular techniques. Plast Reconstr Surg 57:413–426, 1976.
35. Daniel RK, Terzis JK, Schwarz G: Neurovascular free flaps. A preliminary report. Plast Reconstr Surg 56:13–20, 1975.
36. Terzis JK, Breidenbach W: The anatomy of free vascularized nerve grafts. In Terzis JK (ed): Microreconstruction of Nerve Injuries. Philadelphia: WB Saunders, 1987, 101–116.
37. Yeoman PM, Seddon HJ: Brachial plexus injuries. Treatment of the flail arm. J Bone Joint Surg 43B:493–500, 1961.
38. Brunelli G: Neurotization of avulsed roots of the brachial plexus by means of anterior nerves of the brachial plexus. Int J Microsurg 2:55–58, 1980.
39. Gilbert A: Neurotization by contralateral pectoral nerve. Presented at the 10th Symposium on the Brachial Plexus, Lausanne, Switzerland, 1992.
40. Allieu Y, Privat JM Bonnel F: Paralysis in root avulsion of the brachial plexus: Neurotization by the spinal accessory nerve. Clin Plast Surg 11:133–136, 1984.
41. Narakas A: Thoughts on neurotization or nerve transfers in irreparable nerve lesions. Clin Plast Surg 11:153–159, 1984.
42. Chuang D: Neurotization procedures for brachial plexus injuries. Hand Clin 11:633–645, 1995.
43. Gu YD, Wu MM, Zhen YL, et al: Phrenic nerve transfer for brachial plexus motor neurotization. Microsurgery 10:287–289, 1989.
44. Gu YD, Zhang GM, Chen DS, et al: Cervical nerve root transfer from contralateral normal side for treatment of brachial plexus root avulsion. Chin Med J (Engl) 104:208–211, 1991.
45. Terzis JK: Contralateral C7: A powerful source of motor neurons for devastating brachial plexus paralysis. Presented at the 7th annual meeting of European Association of Plastic Surgeons, Innsbruck, Austria, 1996.
46. Loy S, Bhatia A, Asfazadourian H, Oberlin C: Ulnar nerve fascicle transfer onto the biceps muscle nerve in C5-C6 or C5-C6-C7 avulsions of the brachial plexus. Eighteen cases. Ann Chir Main Memb Super 16:275–284, 1997.
47. Samardzic M, Grujicic D, Rasulic L, et al: Transfer of the medial pectoral nerve: Myth or reality? Neurosurgery 50:1277–1282, 2002.
48. Gu YD, Cai PQ, Xu F, et al: Clinical application of ipsilateral C7 nerve root transfer for treatment of C5 and C6 avulsion of brachial plexus. Microsurgery 23:105-108, 2003.
49. Leechavengvongs S, Witoonchart K, Uerpairojkit C, et al: Nerve transfer to deltoid muscle using the nerve to the long head of the triceps, Part II: A report of 7 cases. J Hand Surg [Am] 28:633–638, 2003.

50. Sungpet A, Suphachatwong C, Kawinwonggowit V: One-fascicle median nerve transfer to biceps muscle in C5 and C6 root avulsions of brachial plexus injury. Microsurgery 23:10–13, 2003.
51. Mennen U, van der Westhuizen MJ, Eggers IM: Re-innervation of M. biceps by end-to-side nerve suture. Hand Surg 8:25–31, 2003.
52. Carlstedt TP: Spinal nerve root injuries in brachial plexus lesions: Basic science and clinical application of new surgical strategies. A review. Microsurgery 16:13–16, 1995.
53. Bertelli JA, Ghizoni MF: Brachial plexus avulsion injury repairs with nerve transfers and nerve grafts directly implanted into the spinal cord yield partial recovery of shoulder and elbow movements. Neurosurgery 52:1385–1389, 2003.
54. Bentolila V, Nizard R, Bizot P, et al: Complete traumatic brachial plexus palsy. Treatment and outcome after repair. J Bone Joint Surg 81A:20–28, 1999.
55. Friedman AH, Nashold BS, Jr, Bronec PR: Dorsal root entry zone lesions for the treatment of brachial plexus avulsion injuries: A follow-up study. Neurosurgery 22:369–373, 1988.
56. Chen HJ, Lu K, Yeh MC: Combined dorsal root entry zone lesions and neural reconstruction for early rehabilitation of brachial plexus avulsion injury. Acta Neurochir Suppl 87:95–97, 2003.
57. Narakas A, Hentz V: Neurotization in brachial plexus injuries: Indications and results. Clin Orthop 237:43–56, 1988.
58. Zancolli EA, Zancolli ER: Palliative surgical procedures in sequelae of obstetrical palsy. Hand Clin 4:643–669, 1988.
59. Marshall RW, Williams DH, Birch R, et al: Operations to restore elbow flexion after brachial plexus injuries. J Bone Joint Surg 70B:577–582, 1988.
60. Aziz W, Singer RM, Wolff TW: Transfer of the trapezius for flail shoulder after brachial plexus injury. J Bone Joint Surg 72B:701–704, 1990.
61. Brunelli GA, Vigasio A, Brunelli GR: Modified Steindler procedure for elbow flexion restoration. J Hand Surg [Am] 20A:743–746, 1995.
62. Manktelow RT, McKee NH: Free muscle transplantation to provide active finger flexion. J Hand Surg [Am] 3:416–426, 1978.
63. Terzis JK, Sweet RC, Dykes RW, et al: Recovery of function in free muscle transplants using microneurovascular anastomoses. J Hand Surg [Am] 3:37–59, 1978.
64. Doi K: New reconstructive procedure for brachial plexus injury. Clin Plast Surg 24:75–85, 1997.
65. Berger A, Becker M: Brachial plexus surgery: Our concept of the last twelve years. Microsurgery 15:760–767, 1994.
66. Gu Y, Wu M, Zheng Y, et al: Microsurgical treatment for root avulsion of the brachial plexus. Chin Med J (Engl) 100:519–522, 1987.
67. Hentz V, Narakas A: The results of microneurosurgical reconstruction in complete brachial plexus palsy. Assessing outcome and predicting results. Orthop Clin North Am 19:107–114, 1988.
68. Nagano A: Treatment of brachial plexus injury. J Orthop Sci 3:71–80, 1998.
69. Doi K, Hattori Y, Ikeda K, et al: Significance of shoulder function in the reconstruction of prehension with double free-muscle transfer after complete paralysis of the brachial plexus. Plast Reconstr Surg 112:1596–1603, 2003.
70. Allieu Y, Cenac P: Neurotization via the spinal accessory nerve in complete paralysis due to multiple avulsion injuries of the brachial plexus. Clin Orthop 237:67–74, 1988.
71. Allieu Y, Chammas M, Picot MC: Paralysis of the brachial plexus caused by supraclavicular injuries in the adult. Long-term comparative results of nerve grafts and transfers. Rev Chir Orthop Reparatrice Appar Mot 83:51–59, 1997.
72. Kawai H, Kawabata H, Masada K, et al: Nerve repairs for traumatic brachial plexus palsy with root avulsion. Clin Orthop 237:75–86, 1988.
73. Merrell GA, Barrie KA, Katz DL, et al: Results of nerve transfer techniques for restoration of shoulder and elbow function in the context of a meta-analysis of the English literature. J Hand Surg [Am] 26:303–314, 2001.
74. Nagano A, Tsuyama N, Ochiai N, et al: Direct nerve crossing with the intercostal nerve to treat avulsion injuries of the brachial plexus. J Hand Surg [Am] 14:980–985, 1989.
75. Malessy MJ, Thomeer RT: Evaluation of intercostal to musculocutaneous nerve transfer in reconstructive brachial plexus surgery. J Neurosurg 88:266–271, 1998.
76. Waikakul S, Wongtragul S, Vanadurongwan V: Restoration of elbow flexion in brachial plexus avulsion injury: Comparing spinal accessory nerve transfer with intercostal nerve transfer. J Hand Surg [Am] 24A:571–577, 1999.
77. Ogino T, Naito T: Intercostal nerve crossing to restore elbow flexion and sensibility of the hand for a root avulsion type of brachial plexus injury. Microsurgery 16:571–577, 1995.
78. Songcharoen P, Mahaisavariya B, Chotigavanich C: Spinal accessory neurotization for restoration of elbow flexion in avulsion injuries of the brachial plexus. J Hand Surg [Am] 21A:387–390, 1996.
79. Samii A, Carvalho GA, Samii M: Brachial plexus injury: Factors affecting functional outcome in spinal accessory nerve transfer for the restoration of elbow flexion. J Neurosurg 98:307–312, 2003.
80. Gu YD, Chen DS, Zhang GM, et al: Long-term functional results of contralateral C7 transfer. J Reconstr Microsurg 14:57–59, 1998.
81. Sedel L: The results of surgical repair of brachial plexus injuries. J Bone Joint Surg 64B: 54–66, 1982.
82. Chuang DC, Carver N, Wei FC: Results of functioning free muscle transplantation for elbow flexion. J Hand Surg [Am] 21A:1071–1077, 1996.

162 Surgical Management of Spinal Nerve Root Injuries

THOMAS P. CARLSTEDT

Spinal nerve root injury is considered a type of central nervous system (CNS) lesion and, hence, not amenable to operative repair.[1] However, the ventral root, containing the first extramedullary part of the spinal motor neuron, can be expected to regenerate like a peripheral nerve, whereas nerve fibers in the dorsal root regenerate toward the spinal cord but do not enter it[2] (Fig. 162-1). Ventral roots would therefore regenerate functionally with respect to both somatic and autonomic systems,[3] but regeneration in the dorsal root would be of no functional value. Occasional reports on root repair are available.[4,5] This chapter describes surgical means to repair ruptured or avulsed spinal nerve roots, particularly after traction injury to the nerve plexus.

RELEVANT ANATOMIC AND PATHOPHYSIOLOGIC DETAILS

The spinal nerve roots are the intraspinal parts of the peripheral nervous system (PNS) that link the spinal cord with the peripheral nerves. There are well-known structural differences between the nerve root and the peripheral nerve.[6] For the PNS, there is a unique functional segregation of sensory and motor nerve fibers into the dorsal and ventral roots.[7] The roots traverse the subarachnoid space

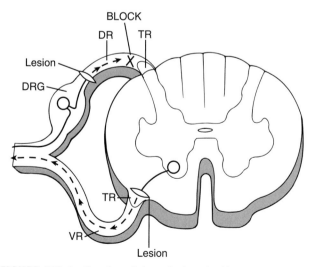

FIGURE 162-1 Drawing of the spinal cord with ventral (VR) and dorsal root (DR) and dorsal root ganglion (DRG). At the root–spinal cord junction, spinal cord tissue extends into the root. TR, transitional region. Regeneration in the DR is blocked at the TR. Motor neurons regenerate peripherally to the intramedullary lesion through the spinal cord and farther peripherally in the VR.

surrounded by a root sheath and bathed in cerebrospinal fluid (CSF). The root sheath consists of an outer layer that resembles the arachnoid and an inner layer that resembles the perineurium.[8] The outer layer consists of loosely arranged cells with intervening spaces, and it is reflected back onto the arachnoid in the subarachnoid angle at the distal end of the root. At the root–spinal cord junction, this layer is continuous with the pia mater.[9] The inner layer consists of flattened cells closely associated with an overlying basal lamina. This layer is continuous with the perineurium distally and terminates close to the root–spinal cord junction proximally, being open-ended toward the spinal cord. Most of the peripheral nerve perineurium separates from the spinal nerve and continues along the inner aspect of the dura mater.[10] The epineurium of the spinal nerve becomes continuous with the dura, which is adherent to the dorsal root ganglion in the intervertebral foramen. In the event of a distal traction force on the spinal nerve, as in a classic brachial plexus injury, the spinal nerve together with the ganglion is displaced laterally. Traction on the nerve sheath tears the dura-arachnoid, and CSF leaks out through the foramen. This is seen as a pseudomeningocele on the myelogram.

The diffusion barrier in the perineurium of a peripheral nerve is not present in the root sheath.[11] Thus there is direct continuity between the endoneurial space of the root and the CSF. The chemical environment of nerve fibers in the root is, therefore, directly influenced by the composition of the CSF. The blood supply to the nerve roots is less developed than in the peripheral nerve,[12] so that nerve fibers in the roots seem to depend on diffusion from the CSF for some of their nutrition as well as oxygen supply.[13,14]

The thin root sheath makes the root less resistant than the peripheral nerve to tearing forces. Studies on stress-strain phenomena showed that the maximum load before rupture of the medial and ulnar nerves was approximately 10 times higher than that for a root, but that the maximum tensile stress calculated on the cross-sectional area was less than half for the root compared with the nerve. The ventral root is more fragile than the dorsal root.[15] Thus, the root sheath does not provide much mechanical or physiologic integrity for the nerve elements in the root. It affords little protection from traction and is not suitable for use in suturing stumps of a severed root together.

The nerve root occupies less than 50% of the intervertebral foramen. The residual space between the wall of the intervertebral canal and the nerve structure is filled with loose areolar connective tissue. Throughout the spine, the nerve root is only weakly fixated to the wall of the foramen, where there is some exchange of connective tissue fibers from the nerve root and the capsule of the intervertebral joint.[16] At the lower cervical spine, however, the spinal nerves of C5, C6, and C7 are attached to the overlying transverse processes of C4, C5, and C6 by the transverse radicular ligaments.[16,17] Nowhere else are the nerve roots so firmly anchored to the spine, which certainly offers protection to the brachial plexus against traction strain.

The spinal nerve roots are supplied by a collateral vascular system that derives from two sets of arteries: the proximal radicular arteries, arising from the medullary artery and situated on the spinal cord surface; and the distal radicular arteries, which are branches of the spinal or segmental arteries and are located extraspinally. The capillaries in the root are of the continuous type, which maintain a blood-nerve or blood-root barrier.[18] In contrast to the peripheral nerve, there are no lymphatic vessels in the root.

The patency of the collateral vascular system in the roots can vary. Thus, the medullary artery is not always able alone to maintain adequate circulation in a pertinent root or spinal cord segment if the extraspinal artery has been compromised.[19,20] Impaired blood supply through the extraspinal artery at, for example, the intervertebral foramen might lead to an infarct and deterioration of function in the spinal cord. Sometimes this appears as a Brown-Séquard syndrome after root avulsion where the spinal artery together with the root has been torn, or in cases of severe vascular damage (i.e., proximal rupture of the subclavian or the vertebral vessels in conjunction with brachial plexus lesions).

The endoneurial content of the roots resembles that of the peripheral nerves but with less collagen. The myelinated and unmyelinated nerve fibers of the dorsal root are the central processes of the primary sensory neurons in the dorsal root ganglion, whereas in the ventral root they represent the final common pathway of spinal cord motor neurons for motor command. However, in humans the ventral roots comprise approximately 30% unmyelinated fibers, which are not postganglionic autonomic fibers but have been found to be "recurrent sensory fibers."[21] There also is evidence for the existence of myelinated afferent fibers in the ventral root.

The attachment of spinal roots to the cord is characterized by a specialized transitional region[22,23] (see Fig. 162-1) containing elements of both the PNS and the CNS. Thus, spinal nerve roots contain a proximal, short, cone-shaped CNS part, and distal to that, the longer PNS part. At the PNS-CNS interface, the axon–Schwann cell units suspended in a collagen-containing extracellular space cross to an environment where the extracellular space is exceedingly small, collagen is lacking, and the axons are embedded in a complex network of oligodendrocyte and astrocyte processes. The vessels of the PNS part of the root do not cross this interface into the CNS part of the root.

In animal experiments, root injury, particularly avulsion of the root from the spinal cord, is especially hazardous for neurons in the spinal cord. Proximity of the lesion and disconnection from the periphery with interrupted supply of neurotrophic factors seem to be incompatible with cell survival.[24,25] The response to injury is quite different in the PNS and the CNS parts of the root. Tissue components such as neurotrophic factors and extracellular matrix molecules

of the PNS support nerve fiber regrowth, but these elements are not present in the CNS.[26] There is a drastic difference in regeneration at the very PNS-CNS interface in the root where the growing nerve fibers are impeded (see Fig. 162-1).[27] In a long series of animal experiments, it has been demonstrated that regrowing nerve fibers do not enter the spinal cord, but neurons in the spinal cord extend new axons peripherally if offered a PNS conduit.[27] Thus after ventral root avulsion from the spinal cord, functional restitution is possible if the detached roots are replanted back to the spinal cord. Recovery of function depends on regrowth of new nerve fibers through the white matter in the spinal cord and the scar from avulsion and implantation, as well as among the leptomeningeal cells along the surface of the spinal cord. The leptomeningeal cells on the spinal cord or the root support nerve fiber growth because of their expression of nerve growth factor receptors.[28] The new neuronal growth in the spinal cord depends on the up-regulation of key trophic factors, their receptors, and matrix molecules among the CNS glial cells and in the scar tissue.[29] Technically, therefore, it is not necessary to implant the nerves back into the motor neuron pool in the gray matter of the spinal cord to induce regeneration. An implantation just deep to the pia mater and the surface layer of the spinal cord does not interfere with long fiber tracts but is sufficient to promote regeneration from motor neurons.[27,30]

ROOT INJURY

Spinal nerve roots are compromised by such closed lesions as tumors or fractures of the spine, or in open injuries from missiles or stabbing. The most common spinal nerve root injury follows closed traction to the brachial or lumbosacral plexus. In a comprehensive review, Huittinen[31] reported that in approximately half of patients with persisting neurologic symptoms after pelvic fractures with sacroiliac joint dislocation, there were ruptures of the lumbosacral roots. No avulsion of the roots from the spinal cord was observed. Nerve roots to the brachial plexus are more susceptible to injury than the lumbosacral roots because of the loose attachment of the shoulder girdle compared with the rigid bony pelvis. The first description of a root avulsion was by Flaubert,[32] but it was first confirmed at operation after laminectomy by Frazier and Skillern.[33] Their report remains up to date by advocating early surgery (10 days after injury) as well as by its clear description of the severe pain experienced by patients with root avulsion lesions. At that time, root injury in brachial plexus lesions was quite rare, whereas it is now reported to occur in most cases of severe brachial plexus trauma (75% of severe supraclavicular lesions[34]).

The lower spinal nerve roots, C8 and T1, are more susceptible to tear probably because of the unique ligamentous fixations between the transverse processes and the C5, C6, and C7 spinal nerves.[17] The ventral root is more susceptible to injury than the dorsal root because it is thinner and has a lower tensile strength.[15] Although the exact mechanical events leading to brachial plexus root avulsion injuries have not been completely defined, two mechanisms for producing different types of root injuries have been described. In the peripheral mechanism, there is lateral traction of the spinal nerve that, if forceful enough, displaces the roots and the ganglion out of the intervertebral foramen. In the central

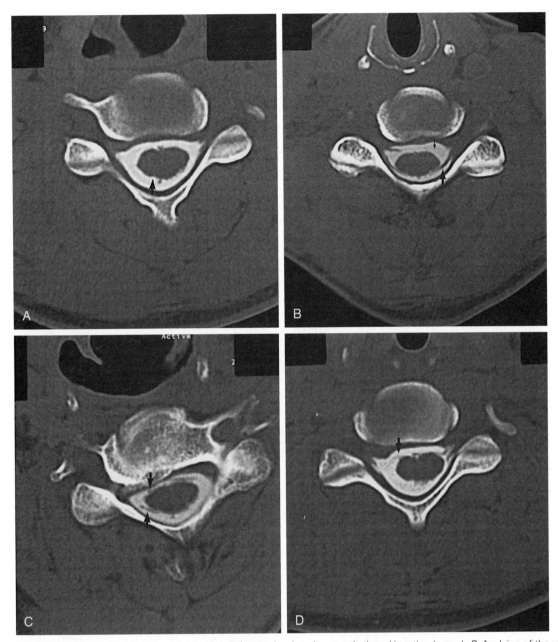

FIGURE 162-2 CT myelograms. *A,* Total avulsion with a defect at the dorsal root–spinal cord junction (*arrow*). *B,* Avulsion of the ventral root (*small arrow*) and an intact dorsal root (*large arrow*). *C,* The remaining dorsal root and the stump of the ventral root (*arrows*). *D,* The avulsed dorsal root with the stump of the ventral root (*arrow*).

mechanism, there is no displacement of the spinal nerve and ganglion from the intervertebral foramen, but a shift of the spinal cord, probably in a longitudinal direction, causes avulsion of the roots. In this situation, the detached roots remain in the subdural space.[16] Because the root–spinal cord junction is the weakest point of the root,[35] an avulsion rather than a rupture is most likely. However, as we found at intraspinal explorations of the injured brachial plexus, and as described by others,[36,37] there is great variation with regard to the type of root injury. Combinations occur of total and partial ruptures and avulsions, leaving either the

dorsal or ventral root intact. The most frequent pattern is complete avulsion of both dorsal and ventral roots, mostly of the lower roots to the plexus. The combination of intact dorsal and avulsed ventral root was more common than spared ventral and torn dorsal root. Most of the partial root avulsions occurred for the upper (C5, C6) part of the plexus.[38,39] (For descriptions of different types of root lesions, see Birch and colleagues.[40])

More rare than the brachial plexus injuries are lesions of the lumbosacral plexus because of its protected position within the bony pelvis. In severe pelvic fractures, usually with dissociation of the sacroiliac joint together with fractures of the pubic bones, there are traction lesions to the lumbosacral plexus[31] or its spinal nerve roots—the cauda equina.[41,42]

Diagnosis

Root avulsion is suspected with a history of high-energy injury, such as a motor bike accident at high speed in which the forequarter is violently dislocated from the trunk. Absence of Tinel's sign in the posterior triangle of the neck also indicates a serious proximal lesion. An electrophysiologic investigation showing sensory conduction despite no perception of sensation is a sign of a dorsal root lesion ganglion and the peripheral nerve intact and functioning but without central connection and the possibility of sensation.[43] Tests of axon reflexes such as the histamine flare response and cold vasodilatation tests would be intact in root lesions because the sensory ganglion and the distal neurites are functioning,[44] quite unlike the situation in peripheral nerve lesions. With imaging techniques it is possible to appreciate signs of root injury. Plain radiographs demonstrating fractures of cervical transverse processes and upper ribs are consistent with root avulsion injuries.

Myelography with computed tomography (CT) is still superior to magnetic resonance imaging (MRI) for resolving intraspinal plexus injuries[36] (Fig. 162-2). In none of these assessments, however, is it possible to obtain an accurate and consistent diagnosis of the root lesion. A precise diagnosis is possible only by such invasive methods as endoscopy or open inspection of the intraspinal parts of the plexus after hemilaminectomy.

Inspection of the spinal canal and its content by introducing a small-caliber endoscope through the intervertebral foramen can give information about root stumps or complete avulsions (Fig. 162-3). This procedure has been possible only in cases in which the plexus has been explored shortly after the injury, when the ganglion has been displaced out of its location in the intervertebral canal.

A diagnosis of level of injury is difficult in a lumbosacral plexus injury. A Tinel's test cannot be performed. A sign of a proximal, possibly intraspinal or cauda equina lesion is loss of function in the superior gluteal nerve, which emerges from the L5 spinal nerve or the lumbosacral trunk as well as from the S1 spinal nerve proximal to the plexus. Paralysis of the gluteal muscles with impaired pelvic stability (e.g., a positive Trendelenburg's test) could indicate an intraspinal or cauda equina lesion. CT together with contrast myelogram demonstrates traumatic meningoceles (Fig. 162-4). In series of transverse scans individual roots can be followed and the site of rupture defined. Electrophysiology with H-reflex and F-response studies can be useful.

Surgical Exposure and Repair of the Intraspinal Part of the Plexus

An ideal approach permits the simultaneous exploration of both the intraspinal and extraspinal parts of the plexus. In the conventional approach to the plexus, the patient is positioned in a supine, "beach-chair" position, and the intraspinal part can be reached only after excision of parts of the vertebral bodies.[45] This approach risks profuse bleeding, making any detailed microsurgical work on the spinal cord impossible; in addition, stabilization of the operated segment of the cervical spine is necessary. Two other approaches to explore the intraspinal and extraspinal parts of the plexus have been used in humans: the dorsal subscapular approach and the extreme lateral approach.

Kline and associates[46] have described the dorsal subscapular approach to the proximal extraspinal part of the brachial plexus. This approach, slightly modified, has been used for intraspinal exploration.[38] With the head in a

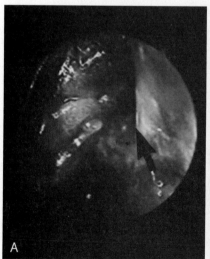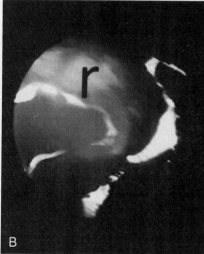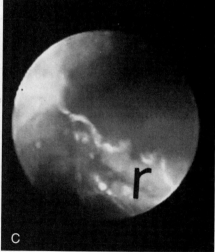

FIGURE 162-3   Endoscopy of an intradural lesion. *A*, At the entrance of the intervertebral canal. *B*, The root stump (r). *C*, The root stump (r) at the junction with the spinal cord.

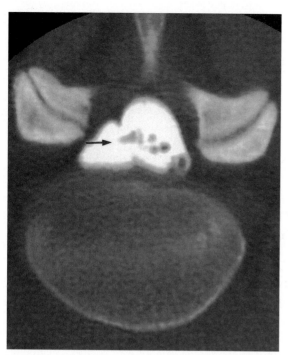

FIGURE 162-4 A CT myelogram at L5–S1 level showing a few remaining roots and anterior cysts in continuity with the subarachnoid space. Note proximal root stump at the transition between the subarachnoid space and cyst (*arrow*) available for reconstruction by means of nerve grafting. (From Lang E, Borges J, Carlstedt T: Surgical treatments of lumbosacral plexus injuries. J Neurosurg Spine 1:64–71, 2004.)

Mayfield clamp and the neck maximally flexed, a midline incision from the occiput to the midthoracic level (T6) is made. The trapezius and rhomboid muscles are detached from their insertions on the spinous processes. The scapula is retracted laterally to facilitate reaching the plexus, which is deep in the wound lying in a fat pad between the medial and anterior scalene and sternocleidomastoid muscles. To prepare for a hemilaminectomy, the cervical paravertebral muscles are detached from the pertinent hemilaminae of C4–T1 and pushed laterally.

More recently, Crockard and colleagues[47,48] described the extreme lateral approach. This approach is preferred because it gives easy access to both the intraspinal and extraspinal parts of the plexus (Fig. 162-5). The patient is placed in a straight and lateral position. The head rests in a Mayfield headrest with the neck slightly flexed laterally to the opposite side. The head-up position of the operating table is used to prevent venous congestion, particularly of the epidural veins. During the procedure, the operating table's tilting facility can be used when going from medial to lateral exposures of the plexus. A skin incision is made from the region of the sternoclavicular joint continuing in the posterior triangle of the neck in a lateral and cranial direction toward the C4–C5 spinous processes in the back of the neck (see Fig. 162-5A). This provides access to both the supraclavicular part of the plexus and to the lower cervical spine. The skin, platysma, and subcutaneous tissue

are raised as two flaps. The accessory nerve is identified and protected as it emerges from the dorsal aspect of the cranial part of the sternocleidomastoid muscle (see Fig. 162-5B). The posterior tubercles of the transverse processes of C4–C7 can be palpated, and they are followed in dissecting through a connective tissue plane between the levator scapulae and the posterior and medial scalene muscles (see Fig. 162-5C). The longissimus muscle deep to this plane must be split longitudinally to expose the posterior tubercles of the transverse processes and the hemilaminae (see Fig. 162-5C, D). The paravertebral muscles are freed from the hemilaminae and pushed dorsomedially (see Fig. 162-5D). After a standard hemilaminectomy using the drill or rongeurs, with hemostasis of epidural veins, the dura mater is incised longitudinally. Sometimes a rent in the dura has been produced by the trauma. The denticulate ligaments, which are mostly preserved, are cut and held with stay sutures. It is then possible to maneuver and slightly twist the cord to reach as ventral a position as feasible (Fig. 162-6).

The intraspinal plexus lesion may appear as a complete avulsion of the roots from their attachments to the spinal cord or as ruptures with the remaining root stumps attached to the spinal cord (Fig. 162-7). The avulsed or ruptured roots may be found in the subdural space or completely displaced from the spinal canal and lodged between the scalene muscles or even further distally (see Fig. 162-7). Only in patients operated on shortly after the injury is it possible to retrieve the avulsed roots back into the spinal canal by pulling them through the intervertebral canal using a catheter or tube. This must be done with great care to avoid injury to the vertebral vessels. This maneuver is not possible if the surgery is delayed more than 2 weeks, because the displaced roots will be scarred and the intervertebral foramen sealed by scar tissue. If the roots cannot be relocated into the subdural space, nerve grafts, usually taken from the ipsilateral arm (superficial radial nerve and medial cutaneous nerve of forearm), are used to connect the roots to the site of the lesion inside the subdural space. If the foramen is blocked, the grafts are passed from the outside through the incision in the dura.

The injured ventral roots are repaired. In cases of ventral root rupture with a remaining central stump, the distal root stump, if available, or a nerve graft, is joined to the central stump. The position of the apposed ends is maintained by tissue glue (Tisseal). Stitching the two ends together is difficult because of the fine root sheath (see earlier). In cases of avulsion, the ventral root is implanted into the ventrolateral aspect of the spinal cord. By gently tilting the cord using the stay sutures in the denticulate ligaments, the surgeon approaches the ventrolateral part of the spinal cord. This is easier with a pure lateral approach than with the patient in a prone position. The root or the nerve graft to be implanted is split into individual fascicles. Small slits in the pia mater are made without penetrating into the white matter of the spinal cord (see Fig. 162-6). The tips of the fascicles are pushed into the pial slits (see Fig. 162-6). Because the pia is somewhat elastic, it closes around the introduced tips of the implanted nerves or nerve grafts. To stabilize further and maintain the position of the implanted nerves, Tisseal glue is applied around the site of implantation (see Fig. 162-6). During intraspinal manipulations,

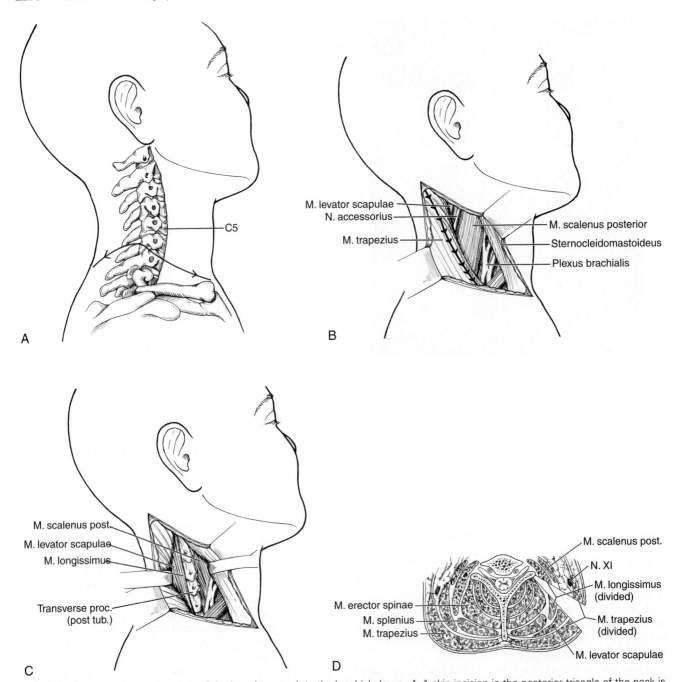

FIGURE 162-5 Schematic drawings of the lateral approach to the brachial plexus. *A*, A skin incision in the posterior triangle of the neck is extended toward the spinous process of the C5 vertebra. *B*, The trapezius muscle is divided according to the line with the *arrows* so that the accessory nerve is protected. *C* and *D*, Through a plane in between the levator scapulae and the scalenus muscles, the longissimus is reached and split longitudinally. The posterior tubercles of the transverse processes can now be seen.

monitoring of sensory as well as motor tract function is recorded so as to detect any impairment of spinal cord function. The dura can be closed using a vein graft as a patch. If the nerve grafts have not been passed through the intervertebral foramina but into the subdural space through the incision in the dura, closure can be done on either side of the grafts, with CSF leakage prevented by sealing with Tisseal glue. If the dura is not closed, a lumbar drain is necessary.

In cases of lumbosacral plexus injury with cauda equina ruptures, a hemilaminectomy of the pertinent lumbar and sacral vertebrae is performed as indicated by the CT myelogram. A direct repair of ruptured ventral roots by means of sural nerve grafts can be performed (Fig. 162-8A). If the distal stumps are not possible to retrieve (Fig. 162-8B), nerve grafts connect the proximal ventral root stumps to the superior gluteal nerve only or, if possible, also to the

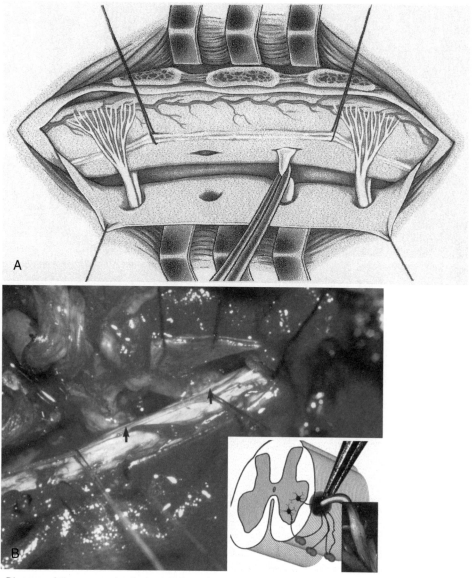

FIGURE 162-6 *A,* Diagram of the exposed spinal cord after a lateral approach and a hemilaminectomy. The dura mater is opened, and by stay sutures in the denticulate, the spinal cord has been rotated slightly for access to its ventral part. Through slits in the pia mater and spinal cord surface, nerve grafts are implanted superficially into the spinal cord. *B,* An intraoperative picture of spinal cord implantation of nerve grafts (*arrows*). Note the stay sutures in the denticulate ligament to tilt the cord. The *inset* shows that the implanted root or nerve graft should be positioned superficially. There will be regeneration through the spinal cord as well as in the pia mater along the surface of the cord. (*A,* from Carlstedt T, Anand P, Hallin R, et al: Spinal nerve root repair and reimplantation of avulsed ventral roots into the spinal cord after brachial plexus injury. J Neurosurg Spine 93:237–247, 2000. *B,* Courtesy of M. Risling, MD.)

sciatic nerve (see Fig. 162-8C, *D*) for extrapelvic repair of key leg functions.

OUTCOME AND COMMENTS

Spinal nerve root injury is amenable to surgery with a functional outcome.[38,39,49,50] In most patients in whom ventral roots had been avulsed and reconnected to the spinal cord, there were signs of functional restitution as well as beneficial effects on pain. In approximately 30% of cases with complete brachial plexus avulsion, useful muscle power returned.[50] Regeneration of function was in most cases limited to the

proximal part of the arm and the shoulder, with no return of hand function. Among the unfavorable conditions that interfered with functional recovery were a delay of surgery of more than 1 month after injury, and presence of associated vascular or severe brain or spinal cord injuries.[50] Recovery of function in the entire upper extremity including the hand is possible, as was noted in a remarkable case of complete C5–T1 avulsion injury with reconnection of all parts of the avulsed plexus to the spinal cord in a preadolescent boy.[51] The recovered function is in many cases compromised by muscle synkinesis with antagonistic as well as breathing muscles ("breathing arm" phenomenon),

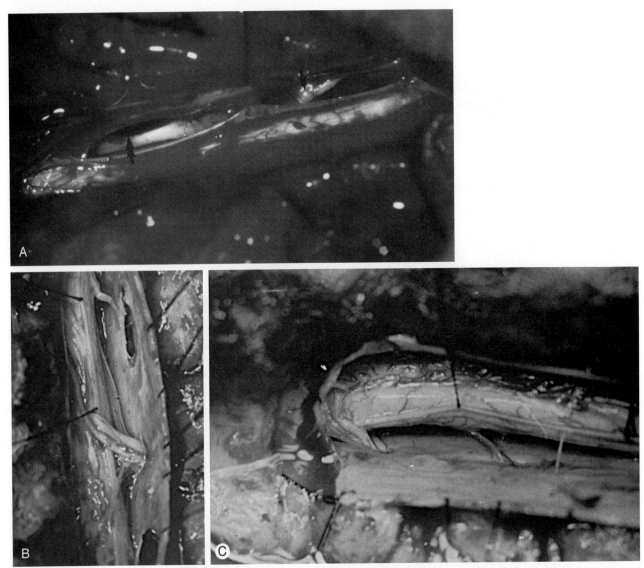

FIGURE 162-7   Intraoperative pictures of various root lesions. *A,* C6 (*arrow*) and C7 avulsed. C6 is located in the vicinity of the cord, but C7 has been torn out from the subdural space through the intervertebral foramen (*double arrows*). *B,* Intact C6 and dorsal root stump at C5. (Courtesy of Mr. George Bonney.) *C,* Intact C6; C7 dorsal root avulsed; and partial avulsion of ventral root at C7. (Courtesy of Mr. George Bonney.)

probably due to nondirectional regrowth of the new nerve fibers. The lack of proprioception also reduces the usefulness of the recovered function.

Indications for root repair or spinal cord implantation include cases in which at least four roots have been avulsed or those involving partial lesions with spared function in the lower roots but avulsion of two or three of the C5–C7 roots. Contraindications are associated CNS lesions from head or spine injury with, for example, a Brown-Séquard syndrome. If a preoperative CT myelogram or MRI show displacement of the cord from hematoma, or if there has been a severe vascular insult to the subclavian or vertebral vessels, root reimplantation should not be performed.

A surgical strategy for repair of root injuries outside the region of the brachial plexus has also been applied. Thus in lesions of the cauda equina, after fracture-dislocation of the

lumbar spine, as well as in lumbosacral plexus injuries, repair of ruptured roots with functional restitution has been performed. The surgical strategy after such injuries is to restore the key functions in the leg for standing and walking. Regeneration of function in the gluteal muscles in cases of sacral plexus injury that have undisturbed femoral nerve function will restore the ability to stand and walk without much restoration in the sciatic nerve. With the short distance from the ruptured cauda equina to the hip muscles this is a realistic objective, and in several cases of severe sacral plexus injury restoration of standing and locomotion has been possible.[52]

Spinal nerve root repair or reimplantation of avulsed roots in the spinal cord has the potential to produce functional restitution if the surgery is performed early after the lesion occurs.

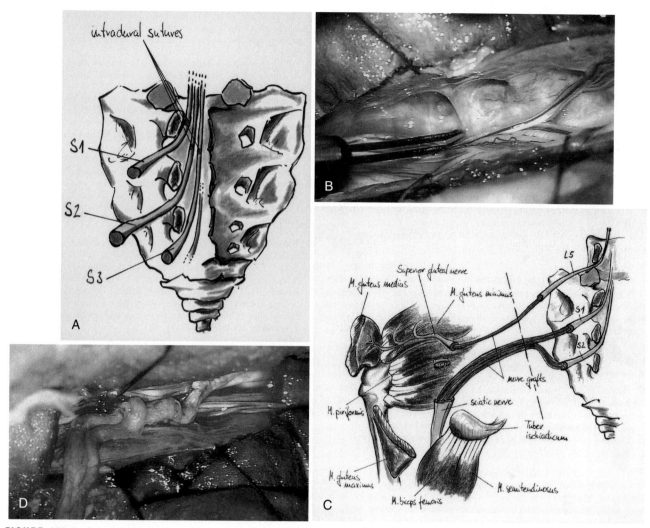

FIGURE 162-8 Intraspinal lumbosacral plexus or cauda equina injury and repair. *A,* Diagram of cauda equina repair with nerve grafts. *B,* Intraoperative picture of avulsed nerve roots with empty foramina for L5 and S1. *C,* Intraspinal and extrapelvic reconstruction of sacral plexus by means of nerve grafts to the gluteal and sciatic nerves. *D,* Intraoperative picture of sacral spinal canal after sural nerve grafting to proximal stump of S1 ventral root. (From Lang E, Borges J, Carlstedt T: Surgical treatments of lumbosacral plexus injuries. J Neurosurg Spine 1:64–71, 2004.)

REFERENCES

1. Seddon HF: Surgical Disorders of the Peripheral Nerves. Baltimore: Williams & Wilkins, 1972.
2. Cajal SR: Degeneration and Regeneration of the Nervous System. London: Oxford University Press, 1928.
3. Kilvington B: An investigation on the regeneration of nerves, with regard to surgical treatment of certain paralysis. BMJ 1:988–990, 1907.
4. Carlsson CA, Sundin T: Reconstruction of efferent pathways to the urinary bladder in a paraplegic child. Rev Surg 24:73–76, 1967.
5. Bonney G, Jamison A: Reimplantation of C7 and C8: Communication au symposium sur le plexus brachial. Int Microsurg 1:103–106, 1979.
6. Key A, Retzius G: Studien in der Anatomie des Nerven Systems und des Bindgewebes. Stockholm: Sammon & Wallin, 1876.
7. Magendie F: Experiences sur les functions des racines des nerfs rachidiens. J Physiol Exp Pathol 2:276–279, 1822.
8. Haller FR, Low FN: The fine structure of peripheral nerve root sheath in the subarachnoid space in the rat and other laboratory animals. Am J Anat 131:1–20, 1971.
9. Nabeshima S, Reese TS, Landis DMD, Brightman MW: Junction in the meninges and marginal glia. J Comp Neurol 164:127–170, 1975.
10. Pease DC, Schultz RL: Electron microscopy of rat cranial meninges. Am J Anat 102:301–321, 1958.
11. Rydevik B, Brown MD, Lundborg G: Pathoanatomy and pathophysiology of nerve root compression. Spine 9:7–15, 1984.
12. Yoshizawa H, Kobayashi S, Hachiya Y: Blood supply of nerve roots and dorsal root ganglia. Orthop Clin North Am 22:195–211, 1991.
13. Rydevik B, Holm B, Brown MD, Lundborg G: Diffusion from the cerebrospinal fluid as a nutritional pathway for spinal nerve roots. Acta Physiol Scand 138:247–248, 1990.
14. Ukai T: Effect of stagnant cerebrospinal fluid on spinal cord. Bull Fujita Gakuen Med Soc 10:155–176, 1996.
15. Sunderland S, Bradley KC: Stress-strain phenomenon in human spinal nerve roots. Brain 84:120–124, 1961.
16. Sunderland S: Mechanisms of cervical nerve root avulsion in injuries of the neck and shoulder. J Neurosurg 41:705–714, 1974.
17. Narakas A, Herzberg G: Les transfers neuro-nerveux intraplexuels dans les avulsions radiculaire traumatiques du plexus brachial. Ann Chir Main 4:211–218, 1985.
18. Kobayashi S, Yoshizawa H, Hachiya Y, et al: Vasogenic edema induced by compression injury to the spinal nerve root: Distribution of

intravenously injected protein tracers and gadolinium-enhanced resonance imaging. Spine 18:1410–1424, 1993.

19. Dommisse GF: The Arteries and Veins of the Human Spinal Cord from Birth. Edinburgh: Churchill Livingstone, 1975.

20. Park WW, Gamell K, Rothman RH: Arterial vascularization of the cauda equina. J Bone Joint Surg Am 63:53–61, 1981.

21. Coggeshal RE: Afferent fibres in ventral roots. Neurosurgery 4:443–448, 1993.

22. Obersteiner H, Redlich E: Über Wesen und Pathogenese der tabischen Hinterstrangsdegeneration. Arb Neurologischen Inst Wiener Univ 1:158–172, 1894.

23. Berthold C-H, Carlsted T, Corneliusson O: The central-peripheral transition zone. In Dyck PJ, Thomas PK (eds): Peripheral Neuropathy, 3rd edition. Philadelphia: WB Saunders, 1993, pp 73–91.

24. Linda H, Risling M, Shupliakov O, Cullheim S: Changes in the Synaptic Input to Lumbar Motorneurons after Intramedullary Axotomy in the Adult Cat. Thesis. Stockholm: Karolinska Institutet, 1993.

25. Koliatsos VE, Price CA, Padro DL: Ventral root avulsion: An experimental model of death of motorneurons. J Comp Neurol 342:35–44, 1994.

26. Korsching S: The neurotrophic factor concept: A re-examination. J Neurosci 13:2739–2748, 1993.

27. Carlstedt T: Nerve fiber regeneration across the peripheral-central transitional zone. J Anat 190:51–56, 1997.

28. Risling M, Carlstedt T, Linda H, Cullheim S: The pia mater: A conduit for regenerating axons after ventral root replantation. Restor Neurol Neurosci 3:157–160, 1991.

29. Frisen J, Risling M, Korhonen L, et al: Nerve growth factors induces process formation in meningeal cells: Implantation for scar formation in the injured CNS. J Neurosci 18:5714–5722, 1998.

30. Cullheim S, Carlstedt T, Risling M: Axon regeneration of spinal mononeurons following a lesion at the cord-ventral root interface: From basic animal research to a new surgical approach in human cases of ventral root avulsion lesions. Spinal Cord 37:811–819, 1999.

31. Huittinen VM: Lumbosacral nerve injury in fracture of the pelvis: A postmortem radiographic and patho-anatomical study. Acta Chir Scand Suppl 429:3–43, 1972.

32. Flaubert G: Memoire sur plusieurs cas de luxation dans lesquelles les effort pour la reduction ont ete suivis d'accident grave. Rep Gen Anat Physiol Pathol 3:55–79, 1827.

33. Frazier CH, Skillern PG: Supraclavicular subcutaneous lesions of the brachial plexus not associated with skeletal injuries. JAMA 57:1957–1963, 1911.

34. Narakas AO, Henz VR: Neurotization in brachial plexus injuries: Indications and results. Clin Orthop 237:43–56, 1988.

35. Livesey FJ, Fraher JP: Experimental traction injury of the cervical spinal nerve roots: A scanning EM study of rupture pattern in fresh tissue. Neuropathol Appl Neurobiol 18:376–386, 1992.

36. Carvalho GA, Nikkhah G, Matthies C, et al: Diagnosis of root avulsions in traumatic brachial plexus injuries: Value of computerized tomography myelography and magnetic resonance imaging. J Neurosurg 86:69–76, 1997.

37. Privat JM, Mailhe D, Bonnel F: Hemilaminectomie cervicale exploratice et neurotisation precoce du plexus brachial. Neurochirurgie 28:107–113, 1982.

38. Carlstedt T, Noren G: Repair of ruptured spinal nerve roots in a brachial plexus lesion. J Neurosurg 82:661–663, 1995.

39. Carlstedt T, Grane P, Hallin RG, Noren G: Return of function after spinal cord implantation of avulsed spinal nerve roots. Lancet 346:1323–1335, 1995.

40. Birch R, Bonney G, Wynn Parry CB: Surgical Disorders of the Peripheral Nerves. Edinburgh: Churchill Livingstone, 1998.

41. Barnett HG, Conolly ES: Lumbosacral nerve root avulsion: Report of a case and review of the literature. J Trauma 15:532–535, 1975.

42. Harris WB, Rathbun JB, Wortzman G, et al: Avulsion of lumbar roots complicating fracture of the pelvis. J Bone Joint Surg 55A:1436–1442, 1973.

43. Bonney G, Gilliat RW: Sensory nerve conduction after traction lesions of the brachial plexus. Proc R Soc Med 51:365–367, 1958.

44. Bonney G: The value of axon responses in determining the site of lesion in traction injuries of the brachial plexus. Brain 77:588–609, 1954.

45. Fournier H-D, Mercier P, Menei P: Lateral interscalenic multilevel oblique corpectomies to repair ventral root avulsions after brachial plexus injury in humans: Anatomical study and first clinical experience. J Neurosurg Spine 95:202–207, 2001.

46. Kline DG, Kott J, Barnes G: Exploration of selected brachial plexus lesions by the posterior subscapular approach. J Neurosurg 49:872–880, 1978.

47. Crockard HA, Kratimenos GP: The far lateral approach for ventrally placed foramen magnum and upper cervical spine tumors. Br J Neurosurg 7:129–140, 1993.

48. Crockard HA, Rogers M: Open reduction of traumatic atlanto-axial rotatory dislocation with use of the extreme lateral approach. J Bone Joint Surg Am 78:431–436, 1996.

49. Bertelli JA, Ghizoni MF: Brachial plexus avulsion injury repairs with nerve transfers and nerve grafts directly implanted into the spinal cord yield partial recovery of shoulder and elbow movements. Neurosurgery 52:1385–1390, 2003.

50. Carlstedt T, Anand P, Hallin R, et al: Spinal nerve root repair and reimplantation of avulsed ventral roots into the spinal cord after brachial plexus injury. J Neurosurg Spine 93:237–247, 2000.

51. Carlstedt T, Anand P, Htut M, Misra P, Svensson M: Restoration of hand function and so called "breathing arm" after intraspinal repair of C5–T1 brachial plexus avulsion injury. Case report. Neurosurg Focus 16:1–5, 2004.

52. Lang E, Borges J, Carlstedt T: Surgical treatments of lumbosacral plexus injuries. J Neurosurg Spine 1:64–71, 2004.

163 Surgical Management of Peripheral Nerve Tumors

AURANGZEB NAGY, DAVID G. KLINE,
ALAN R. HUDSON, and DANIEL H. KIM

INTRODUCTION

The incidence of tumors originating in a nerve or an extrinsic tumor compressing nerve is far less than that of entrapments or nerve injuries.[1] These lesions, which can be vexatious to manage, are by no means rare, however.[2,3] Every neurosurgeon should understand the pathogenesis of these lesions, and those undertaking their management need experience with the surgical anatomy of the area involved by the tumor as well as the internal structure of the involved nerve itself.[4,5] Surgical removal of a nerve tumor can be difficult, as can its pathologic diagnosis. As a result, these are not cases for the occasional surgeon. Significant neurologic loss and increased or new pain can occur. Thus inadequate surgery or an aggressive operation without regard to maintenance of function or even misinterpreted histology can result in serious disability. When in doubt, the physician should refer at least the more difficult nerve tumors to a center with surgeons and pathologists specializing in such cases.

DIAGNOSIS

Patients with peripheral nerve tumors can present with primary symptomatology of pain, weakness, paresthesias, mass, or with no symptoms at all, the tumor having been found incidentally.[6] Recognizing that the cause of a particular patient's symptom complex is due to a peripheral nerve tumor is sometimes very difficult, and patients will sometimes see several physicians before the correct diagnosis is made.[7] A nerve tumor has frequently not been considered in their differential diagnosis. Aids to diagnosis and preoperative evaluation of peripheral nerve tumors are discussed.

When evaluating a patient with neurogenic symptoms, effort should be made to tap sharply along the entire course of a nerve suspected to be involved. If, as a result of the tapping, the patient reports paresthesias in a sensory distribution appropriate to the particular nerve tapped, it may indicate the presence of a mass at the site of percussion.[8] When a mass is able to be palpated, the finding that it can be displaced at right angles to the course of the peripheral nerve but not in a longitudinal manner is a classic finding associated with peripheral nerve tumors.[9] While the surgeon is palpating the mass, the patient may likewise complain of appropriate sensory phenomena. If a peripheral nerve tumor is suspected in a patient, evidence of other nerve tumors and evidence of von Recklinghausen's disease (VRD) should be sought (Fig. 163-1). If such findings are noted, the tumor is likely to be of neural sheath origin. Absence of such findings, however, does not exclude neural sheath tumor because the

majority of such tumors involving a major nerve are solitary and not associated with the neurophakomatoses.[10]

Magnetic resonance imaging is very important in delineating the true extent of a tumor and often aids in inference of a tumor's pathologic classification[11,12] (Table 163-1; Fig. 163-2). With any suspected nerve tumor situated close to the spine, the medial extent of the tumor should be carefully defined by computed tomography or occasionally with myelography (Fig. 163-3). Conventional angiography may be indicated if the tumor is intimately involved with large vessels.[5,13] Positron emission tomography has been shown to be useful in identifying malignant change within benign peripheral nerve sheath tumors.[14] Unfortunately, no scan or other imaging study can definitively differentiate schwannoma from neurofibroma or be used to diagnose a malignant peripheral nerve sheath tumor (MPNST) with 100% certainty. A precise diagnosis requires histologic study of tumor tissue and, preferably, as much of the lesion as possible.[15]

The cellular pathology of nerve tumors has immense range and complexity, but the commonly encountered neoplasms, such as schwannomas, neurofibromas, plexiform neurofibromas, and MPNSTs, have characteristic gross and microscopic features.[16,17] Study of a few of the texts delineating these differences is of great help to the surgeon attempting to manage these lesions.[18,19] Knowledge of the

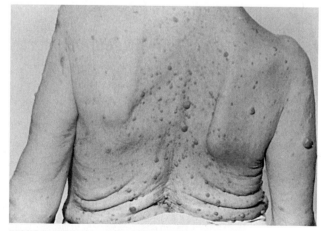

FIGURE 163-1 von Recklinghausen's disease. The patient was referred for management of a brachial plexus tumor. In fact, the initial symptoms and signs were related to cervical syringomyelia. Thus the central manifestations of this disease must always be kept in mind when planning therapy for more peripheral tumors.

TABLE 163-1 ▪ Magnetic Resonance Imaging Appearance of Various Nerve Tumors

Tumor Type	T1 Weighting	T2 Weighting	Enhancement Pattern
Schwannoma/neurofibroma*	Dark	Bright	Central
Malignant nerve sheath tumor	Dark	Bright	Invasive margins
Neuroblastoma	Dark	Bright	Homogeneous
Hemangioma	Dark	Bright	Homgeneous, sustained
Desmoid	Dark/isodense	Mildly bright	Inconsistent, irregular
Hypertrophic neuropathy	Dark/isodense	Flash of brightness	Enhances
Breast/lung metastasis	Dark	Bright	May reveal lymph nodes

*Schwannoma can sometimes be differentiated from neurofibroma by the presence of a capsule sometimes seen around schwannomas on T2-weighted images.

gross appearance of different tumor types often helps the surgeon to determine how best to approach the dissection and resection of the tumor he or she is facing.

Table 163-2 lists the peripheral nerve tumors commonly encountered but is by no means an exhaustive list of the various diagnostic possibilities. These are tumors for which surgery has been performed at Louisiana State University Medical School over a 25-year period.

If the diagnosis of a peripheral nerve tumor is based on clinical grounds, the surgeon must appreciate that he or she cannot ascertain at that stage whether the diagnosis is a schwannoma, neurofibroma, or even an MPNST. Depending on the surgeon's experience with nerve tumors, it may be best to refer such a patient to an appropriate center where a more definitive diagnosis can be made, and, if necessary, definitive surgery can be performed.

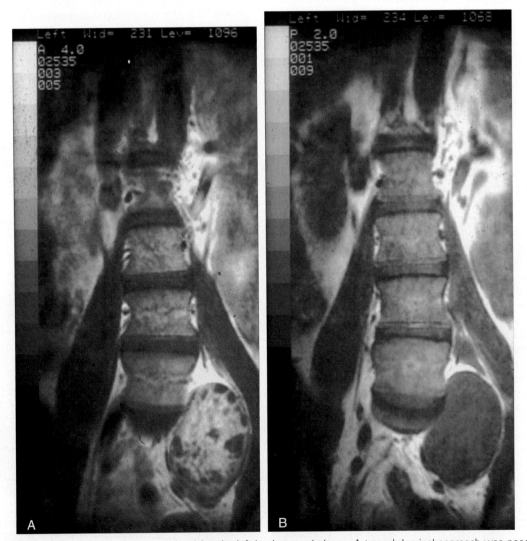

FIGURE 163-2 MRI of pelvic schwannoma involving the left lumbrosacral plexus. A transabdominal approach was needed to resect this lesion. T1 phase is to the left (*A*) and T2 phase to the right (*B*).

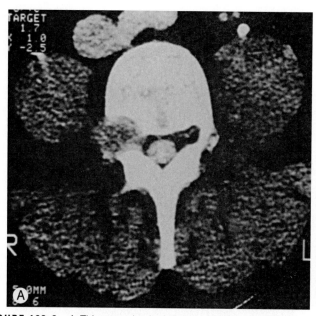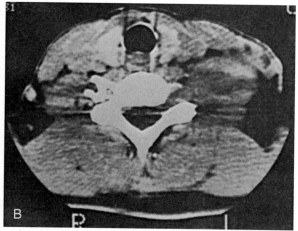

FIGURE 163-3 *A,* This scan clearly delineates the position of a schwannoma within the intervertebral foramen (on the patient's right side). This patient presented with pain and neurologic disability. The myelogram was normal. *B,* The figure shows a larger tumor involving not only the intraforaminal spinal nerve but also a good deal of the extraforaminal plexus (on the patient's left side).

SURGICAL MANAGEMENT

Benign Neural Sheath Tumors

Schwannomas

Neural sheath tumors are the most common subset of tumors affecting a nerve and include the most common specific tumor of a nerve—the schwannoma.[6] The usual presentation of a schwannoma is as a painless but palpable mass. Rarely, an unoperated schwannoma presents with

neurologic deficit or causes abnormal electromyographic results.[20] Conversely, if biopsy or a previous attempt at removal has been performed, presenting symptoms are more likely to be pain, paresthesias, deficit, or all these.[21] Tapping over the lesion, if superficial, almost always causes paresthesias in the distribution of the nerve. If the tumor is symptomatic, our practice has been to remove such lesions, providing that the general risks of an anesthetic are not considerable. For asymptomatic tumors, we defer resection until development of the symptoms or signs that are often harbingers of malignant transformation and then advocate resection. These are listed in Table 163-3. Close follow-up of these patients has always, in our experience, led to the removal of a tumor before malignant spread was detectable.

Most investigators agree that the schwannoma's cell of origin has a basement membrane and is most likely a Schwann cell.[15,22] The compact Antoni type A tissue differs from the less compact and more myxomatous matrix of a neurofibroma. Sometimes, Antoni type B tissue with a somewhat loose stroma is present in the schwannoma, but the matrix does not stain positively with a mucopolysaccharide stain as it does for a neurofibroma.[16]

TABLE 163-2 ▪ Commonly Encountered Peripheral Nerve Tumors

Benign neural sheath tumors
  Schwannomas
  Solitary neurofibromas
  von Recklinghausen's disease–associated neurofibromas
  Plexiform neurofibromas
Benign nonneural sheath tumors or masses involving nerve
  Desmoids and myositis ossificans
  Myoblastomas and lymphangiomas
  Hemangiomas, venous aneurysms, fistulas, and
    hemangiopericytomas
  Ganglion and epidermoid cysts
  Lipomas and lipohamartomas
  Hypertrophic neuropathy or onion bulb disease
Malignant neural sheath tumors
  Neurogenic sarcomas
  Fibrosarcomas
Malignant nonneural sheath tumors
  Carcinomas
    Lung (Pancoast)
    Breast
    Other
  Sarcomas of joint origin

TABLE 163-3 ▪ Signs and Symptoms Associated with Malignant Transformation of Peripheral Nerve Sheath Tumors

Pain
Rapid increase in size
Development/worsening of neurologic deficit
Change in consistency from soft to hard tumor

PROCEDURE

After induction of anesthesia, the patient is positioned so that the involved limb's response to stimulation can be observed. Surgical exposure (Table 163-4) includes the nerve and related structures both proximal and distal to the lesion itself (Fig. 163-4). Exceptions may be schwannomas involving the pelvic plexus or the proximal spinal nerve level of the brachial plexus, where exposure either proximal or distal to the lesion may be difficult. The tumor is usually found nestled within a nerve, with the nerve's fascicles "bundled" around the mass (Fig. 163-5).[13,20,23]

As a schwannoma grows larger, it may bulge out from the nerve eccentrically, leaving fascicles less symmetrically arrayed around the mass itself. Schwannomas have a capsule, and by dissecting longitudinally along the mass and splitting apart the fascicles, the surgeon can dissect them from the capsule. These fascicles can then be gently dissected away from the tumor capsule, much like pulling down a bucket or basket handle. Often, the capsule is quite thin but can be used when opened longitudinally to help peel back the fascicles in groups. This is done by grasping the edge of the split capsule with a forceps with teeth, such as Cushing's or Gerald's, and rolling the capsule with embedded lateral fascicles out and away from both sides of the enclosed solid tumor. Further dissection at the proximal and distal poles of the tumor usually reveals a relatively small fascicle entering and leaving the tumor (Table 163-5).

Nerve action potential recording across such a lesion by stimulating and recording from the entering and exiting fascicle produces a flat trace, and no nerve action potential is conducted. Stimulation alone of the proximal and, less frequently, the distal tumor fascicle sometimes causes muscle contraction in the distribution of the nerve, but the contraction results from retrograde stimulation of more healthy peripheral fascicles. Division of the entering

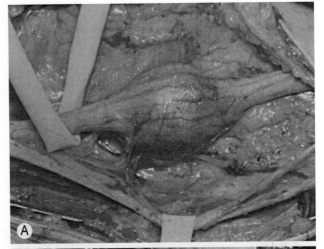

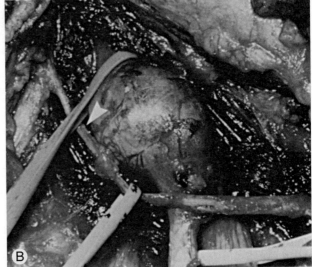

FIGURE 163-4 Typical operative appearance of a benign neural sheath tumor. *A,* Note the fascicles displaced to the periphery of the lesion. (*A,* From Kline D, Hudson A: Nerve Injuries: Operative Results for Major Nerve Injuries, Entrapments, and Tumors. Philadelphia: WB Saunders, 1995, p 527.) *B,* A brachial plexus neural sheath tumor arising from C6 to the upper trunk region. The macroscopic dissection of the region clearly defined the adjacent structures, and these are identified and maneuvered with the aid of Silastic slings or a Penrose drain. (*Arrowhead,* phrenic nerve.)

TABLE 163-4 ■ Operative Steps for Removal of Solitary Benign Neural Sheath Tumors

1. Expose nerve well proximal and distal to the mass itself, whenever possible.
2. Dissect away and preserve other nerves or plexus elements and major vessels.
3. Dissect down to capsule in a longitudinal direction, splitting away fascicles surrounding the mass.
4. Work fascicles over mass of tumor, mobilizing them to the inferior aspect of the mass. Capsule can be opened if needed to work off fascicles.
5. Dissect fascicles at both poles of the tumor. Fascicles exterior to or entering leaves of the capsule need to be dissected away from the mass of the tumor and preserved. Any fascicles entering and exiting the mass of the lesion should be tested by stimulation and recording across the fascicle(s). If nonfunctional, these fascicles can be sectioned at one end or the other, and then, by working under the tumor mass, they can be dissected away from surrounding fascicles. Finally, the fascicle at the opposite pole is sectioned.
6. In some large tumors or previously operated lesions, opening any capsule, enucleating the contents, and then gently dissecting the capsule away from preserved fascicles may be necessary.

and exiting fascicle usually permits removal of the tumor and sometimes its capsule as a single, solitary mass (Fig. 163-6). Alternatively, the capsule of the schwannoma can be opened longitudinally, and its relatively soft, usually homogeneous, and sometimes cystic contents can be evacuated. Then, the capsule can be gently dissected away from the fascicles to which it is usually mildly adherent.

Most schwannomas can be totally removed as a single mass, but some large tumors involving the pelvic or brachial plexus are best removed piecemeal. Not all schwannomas can be totally removed. The procedure with several very large pelvic tumors in our series had to be subtotal, particularly when the sacral plexus was involved. Some brachial plexus tumors involving both spinal nerves and more proximal plexus elements have been removed through a

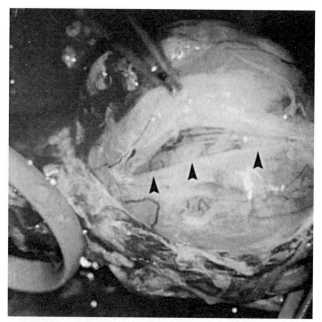

FIGURE 163-5 Schwannoma. A fascicular group is being mobilized (*arrowheads*). A few individual fascicles will be dissected subsequently and moved around the periphery of the underlying schwannoma.

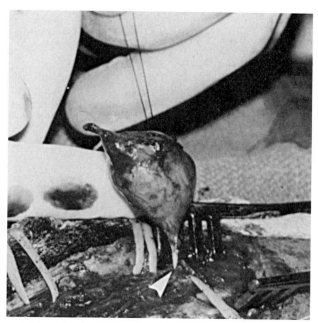

FIGURE 163-6 Schwannoma of the peroneal nerve. The schwannoma is being removed. A single fascicle has been transected proximally, and a single fascicle continuous with the distal pole of the tumor is about to be divided (*arrowhead*). These fascicular inputs and outputs for schwannomas and most neurofibromas do not transmit a nerve action potential and can be sacrificed to permit complete removal of the tumor.

posterior subscapular approach after resection of the first rib (Fig. 163-7).[24]

Solitary Neurofibromas Not Associated with von Recklinghausen's Disease

Solitary neurofibromas are more likely to be associated with either local or radicular pain than schwannomas.[25] A neurologic deficit at the time of presentation is slightly more likely than with schwannomas but is greatly increased in patients who have undergone previous biopsy or attempted but incomplete removal.[6]

TABLE 163-5 ▪ Operative Steps for Decompression of Plexiform Tumors

1. Expose, if possible, the involved nerve or plexus element and related structures proximal, distal, and circumferential to the lesion.
2. Plexiform tumors that are symptomatic and involve only sensory nerves or branches (e.g., saphenous, sural, superficial sensory radial, and antebrachial cutaneous) can be resected en masse along with the nerve of origin.
3. An attempt can be made to decompress the bulk of the tumor when it involves major nerves or a plexus element by dissecting it between fascicles and important branches. This process may require opening the capsule, if present, and debulking the interior of multiple interlacing and interconnecting but interweaving masses.
4. Unfortunately, a capsule may not be present, and much of the nerve or element often interweaves within the tumor mass. Even an attempt at partial removal may lead to reduction or complete loss of function, but such a procedure may be necessary in cases in which size of the mass threatens the function of adjacent, compressed nerves or those in which significant pain is a problem or massive size may predispose to malignant change.

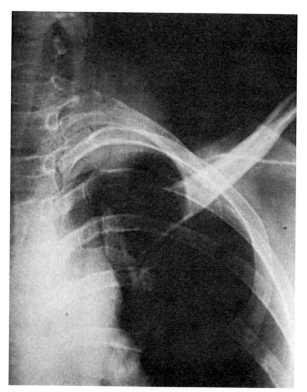

FIGURE 163-7 A large schwannoma is seen at the apex of the lung on a chest radiograph. This lesion, which involved the T1 spinal nerve and the lower trunk of the plexus, was removed by a posterior subscapular approach and resection of the posterior and lateral portions of the first rib.

The cells of a neurofibroma are generally thought to be schwannian in origin, although these cells may be more primitive than those giving rise to a schwannoma.[15] Histologically, the tumor background is less compact and more myxomatous, has more axons, and stains more positively with a mucopolysaccharide stain, such as Alcian blue, than does the schwannoma.[16] No histologic difference exists between a neurofibroma associated with VRD and one that is not.

PROCEDURE

The surgical approach is much the same as that for a schwannoma. In most cases, the nerve fascicles are basketed around the main mass and must be dissected and levered away from the main tumor mass (Fig. 163-8). These tumors often have a capsule, even though it is more adherent to the central mass of the tumor than in a schwannoma. Some of these peripheral fascicles, especially at the poles of the tumor, may be ensheathed or encapsulated by this capsule-like layer. The key steps for removal of a neurofibroma include dissecting the fascicles at both poles or ends of the tumor. If solitary, the fascicle entering and leaving a neurofibroma is larger than that in a comparably sized schwannoma.

In other lesions, several fascicles approach and leave the tumor. Despite these findings, the nerve action potential recording obtained across the tumor by stimulating the entering fascicles and recording from the leaving fascicles is usually flat, and these fascicles can be sectioned just as in a schwannoma.[25,26] Nerve action potential recording after the mass is removed confirms maintenance of most function, just as in a schwannoma (Fig. 163-9). Great care must be taken to determine the fascicular anatomy at each pole, however. Sometimes it is more efficacious to section an entering or leaving fascicle or fascicles at one or the other pole and then gently elevate the mass of the tumor and dissect beneath it to clear the mass away from remaining fascicles and, at times, any capsule left on the underside. Nonetheless, occasionally, the neurofibroma requires partial graft repair after resection because of damage to

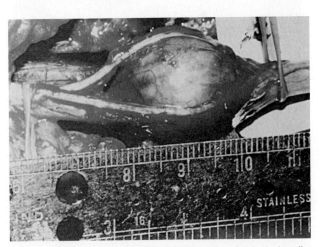

FIGURE 163-8 It was possible to isolate surface fascicular bundles and dissect them from around the mass of this neural sheath tumor. The mass proved to be a neurofibroma and was resected. Entering and exiting fascicles at each pole were tested and were found not to transmit a nerve action potential.

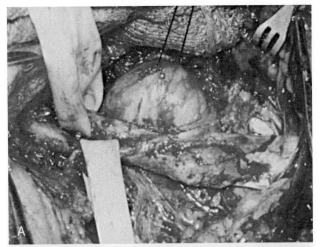

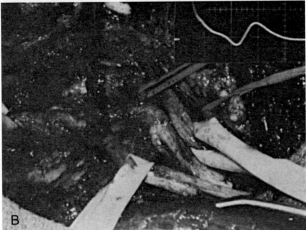

FIGURE 163-9 *A,* A large benign neural sheath tumor involving the middle trunk of plexus. The upper Penrose drain is around C6, and the lower one is around C5 and the area of takeoff of the subclavian branch. *B,* Exposure of a neurofibroma involving the plexus (*arrow*) involving C8 and T1 to medial cord. A recording of nerve action potential at the top was made by stimulation of T1, and a recording from the medial cord. A similar response was recorded after excision of the tumor. (From Lusk M, Kline D, Garcia C: Tumors of the brachial plexus. Neurosurgery 21:439–453, 1987.)

functional fascicles. Very large tumors may require piecemeal removal and decompression by a Cavitron ultrasonic aspirator.

Neurofibromas Associated with von Recklinghausen's Disease

Even though it sometimes requires a more difficult dissection, in most cases the solitary and somewhat globular neurofibroma associated with VRD can also be excised without serious deficit (Fig. 163-10), even when the tumor involves a major nerve. The approach is the same as that for a neurofibroma unassociated with VRD. Peripherally located fascicles are dissected away. Then, the proximal and distal poles of the tumor are dissected at a fascicular level and nonconducting fascicles are sectioned. If functioning fascicles are found entering the tumor, they must be dissected through the tumor or replaced by grafts once the mass is removed. The latter method is less likely to be efficacious if separate but smaller neurofibromas involve fascicles proximal

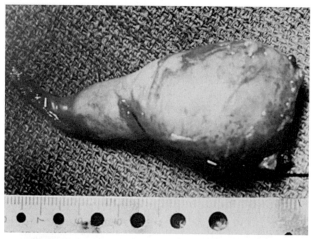

FIGURE 163-10 Neurofibroma. This operative specimen is an example of what can sometimes be achieved. Only a minor neurologic deficit followed resection of this mass from the parent trunk.

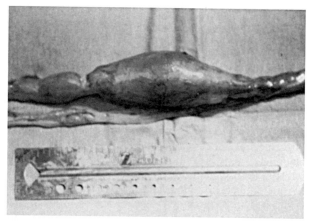

FIGURE 163-11 Surgical specimen typical of a plexiform neurofibroma. This lesion involved a sensory nerve as well as a less involved branch and was totally resected.

or distal to the main tumor mass and do so in a plexiform fashion.

Plexiform Neurofibromas

Plexiform neurofibromas are histologically identical to solitary neurofibromas but involve a length of nerve in an interweaving fashion.[27] Tumor masses are both intrafascicular and extrafascicular. Operation on these plexiform lesions is difficult but possible when the indications are good (see Table 163-3). Complete removal, however, is not usually possible without loss of function. When such a tumor gets quite large or when severe pain is a dominant symptom, decompression with partial removal of some of the tumorous bulk may be helpful to the patient. The lesion cannot, however, be completely resected without total or near-total loss of function when involving a nerve containing motor fibers. At times, even an attempt at subtotal removal of a plexiform tumor may lead to serious loss of function. Section of a nerve both proximal and distal to such a lesion and repair of the gap, which is lengthy, does not usually restore function. By contrast, such tumors involving less important sensory nerves or branches, such as antebrachial cutaneous, superficial sensory radial, sural, and saphenous nerves, can be removed in toto, along with the nerve of origin (Fig. 163-11).

Plexiform neurofibromas are more likely to be associated with VRD, especially its regionalized form but surprisingly can also be encountered as solitary non-VRD–associated lesions. Sometimes, a sizable plexiform tumor is accompanied by hundreds of smaller neurofibromas involving the nerve of origin of the larger lesion. These associated tumors involve the nerve well proximal and distal to the large lesion and occasionally are present in other nerves in the same limb. This phenomenon is called regionalized VRD, or neurofibromatosis type 5 and is thought to occur due to genetic mosaicism.[28,29] Under these circumstances, only a palliative operative procedure can be performed. If the plexiform tumor is quite large, and especially if it is firm, removal may be performed to ensure that a malignant peripheral nerve sheath tumor (MPNST) has not occurred or will not occur.

Secondary operations for neural sheath tumors for which repair is necessary require frozen-section biopsy of nerves or elements of origin to ensure that residual tumor is not incorporated into the repair (Fig. 163-12). If malignancy is found and radiation is necessary, then we generally wait 3 months before attempting a repair. Nerve grafting in this situation is generally less likely to give good results than repairs performed in the setting of trauma. The rate of malignant transformation of VRD-related neurofibromas into MPNSTs has been observed to be between 2% and 5%.[30]

Benign Nonneural Sheath Tumors or Masses Involving Nerve

These types of tumors occur less frequently than lesions of neural sheath origin. Nonetheless, these lesions can be

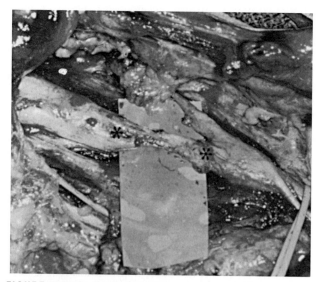

FIGURE 163-12 The brachial plexus, upper trunk. Resection of an unidentified mass resulted in almost complete destruction of the upper trunk of the plexus. Advice based on the result of quick sections and expert neuropathologic input are required to distinguish between scarring of the proximal and distal stumps (*stars*) and the tumor before reconstructive grafting.

responsible for pain and, in some instances, loss of nerve function. A few examples of such lesions follow.

Desmoids and Myositis Ossificans

Desmoids and myositis ossificans are thought to arise from muscle, and although they are more common on the abdominal wall than elsewhere, they can be present in the neck, shoulder, or upper or lower extremity. When located at extra-abdominal sites, they tend to involve surrounding soft tissue and can compress, incorporate, or be adherent to major nerves as well as vessels. They are benign in the sense that they do not metastasize to other parts of the body, but they are difficult to cure. Recurrence after a presumed gross total resection is common.[3]

Operation requires a relatively wide exposure of the lesion and early identification of any nerve or nerves involved. Tumor usually needs to be sharply dissected away from the nerve, and involved epineurium usually requires resection. The tumor can invade the nerve fascicles, requiring fascicular resection and graft repair.[31] Both the firmness of these lesions and their adherence to nerves and vessels make removal without deficit difficult unless great care is taken during the dissection. Despite careful and patient dissection, deficit can still occur.[32]

Myositis ossificans is a poorly defined disorder that may be related to previous trauma or surgery. It usually produces a very firm to hard mass of tissue with calcification and, like a desmoid, can envelop contiguous soft tissues, including vessels and bone. If it is symptomatic because of neural involvement, vascular involvement, or both, removal of such masses can be technically demanding. Again, no substitute exists for performing wide exposure, dissecting neural elements, displacing them away from the pathologic mass, and preserving as many major vessels as possible. Complete removal is only seldom possible and is usually not indicated.

Myoblastomas and Lymphangiomas

These two unusual lesions are grouped together because, when they involve a nerve, they behave similarly and have a somewhat similar appearance at the operating table. Myoblastomas, also called granular cell tumors, are formed of plump and somewhat angular cells with acidophilic granules, whereas lymphangiomas have cells of a lymphoid nature. These tumors tend to spread as a sheet of tumorous tissue and are less likely to form a globular mass than a desmoid tumor or a hemangioma.[3,33] Both tumors can also become adherent to nerves and, in some cases, envelop or invade them.[34] If care is not taken in skeletonizing the involved nerve or nerves, severe deficits can occur. As a result, it is best to plan a wide as well as a lengthy exposure and to determine normal anatomy distal and proximal to the lesion, if possible.[35]

Lipomas and Lipofibromas

Lipomas do not usually involve major nerves because they are mostly subcutaneous. Exceptions occur when a large lipoma envelops or compresses a nerve or when one originates at a deeper level in the limb and compresses or entraps a nerve and produces symptoms.[3,36] The latter behavior can occur at forearm or popliteal levels, with resultant posterior interosseous or peroneal palsy. Larger lipomas in the

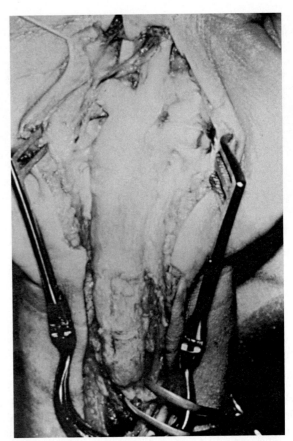

FIGURE 163-13   The median nerve. The patient had carpal tunnel syndrome. The operation revealed diffuse fatty infiltration of the median nerve. The symptoms were helped by the division of the transverse carpal ligament (lipofibromatous hamartoma).

supraclavicular fossa can involve the brachial plexus. Large lipomas in the buttocks, leg, or arm can less frequently involve median, sciatic, or ulnar nerves. Their adherence to epineurium can sometimes make their safe removal challenging.[37]

Lipofibromas (also called lipohamartomas, intraneural lipoma, fibrofatty infiltration lipomatous, or lipofibromatous hamartoma) are intrinsic to a nerve and usually involve the median nerve at the wrist or palmar levels (Fig. 163-13).[15,38] When pain and paresthesias occur, decompression, including section of both the transverse carpal ligament in the palm and its extension covering the nerve and the lipomatous mass at the wrist level, is necessary. When serious loss of median function occurs, more extensive surgery is required. An internal neurolysis with reduction of the bulk of the tumor from around individual fascicles can be performed or, for a more focal lipohamartoma, resection of the tumor and nerve repair can be performed.[39]

Hemangiomas and Hemangiopericytomas

Hemangiomas and hemangiopericytomas, as well as aneurysms and arteriovenous fistulas, can originate close to nerves and compress or envelop them.[40] Operation for these lesions, especially if a nerve is involved, is never easy. Preoperative angiography is of some help in planning surgery, but the key surgical steps include isolating vessels on the periphery of the lesion and ligating or clipping them if they are not the major supply to an extremity and, once again, dissecting nerves away from the lesion while protecting them as much as possible. Occasionally, a hemangioma, hemangioblastoma, venous aneurysm, or fistula directly involves a nerve or appears to originate in it. Then, if symptoms warrant, a careful interfascicular dissection is necessary for removal. Each fascicle or group of fascicles needs to be stripped of the abnormal vascular tissue.

The hemangiopericytoma, which usually arises in the mediastinum and secondarily involves the brachial plexus, can behave malignantly and metastasize to other sites, rarely including the brain. It cannot usually be removed entirely, and the surgeon must be content with a subtotal but, one hopes, decompressive procedure for the plexus.

Ganglions, Epidermoid Cysts, and Tumors of Bone

Most ganglions arise from joints and at sites that do not usually involve nerves, such as the dorsum or the side of the wrist.[41] Less frequently, this cystic tumor arises from a joint and causes compression of a nerve. At the area of the wrist joint, a ganglion can arise that compresses the thenar sensory branch of the median or whole median nerve itself or ulnar nerve in Guyon's canal. Other sites in which these ganglions are clearly of joint origin include the forearm, where they arise from radioulnar joints and compress the posterior interosseous nerve; the knee, involving the peroneal nerve; the ankle, involving the posterior tibial nerve; and the hip, involving the sciatic nerve. Ganglions at the elbow level can involve radial, and, less frequently, median or ulnar nerves, whereas those in the shoulder can involve the brachial plexus, particularly its suprascapular branch in the region of the scapular notch.[42]

Ganglions can be found within the substance of the nerve, such as those found in the peroneal nerve over the surgical neck of the fibula (Fig. 163-14).[43] It is believed that these ganglions form because of a one-way valve that develops in the articular branch of the nerve and allows synovial fluid to dissect along the path of least resistance within the nerve.[44] The original connection to the cyst is sometimes not evident.

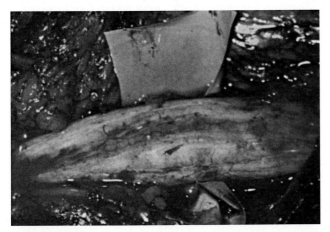

FIGURE 163-14 The typical appearance of a ganglion cyst involving the peroneal nerve. Interfascicular dissection is necessary to remove this type of tumor. Although function was maintained in this patient, this is not always the case when the lesion is large and extends up and down the nerve.

Ganglions may extend great distances along the course of a nerve and can gradually produce paralysis.[42] Less extensive lesions are resectable without serious loss of function, but exceptions exist.

For ganglions extrinsic to a nerve but compressing it, the surgeon must dissect around such lesions after dissecting away and protecting the involved nerve. The origin of the cystic lesion should be ligated or otherwise secured close to the joint to reduce recurrence. For ganglions within a nerve, interfascicular dissection seems to work best because fascicles are cleared of the cyst and then its capsule and its contents are excised. In a patient with the usual intraneural ganglion involving the peroneal nerve, a connection with the knee joint should always be sought, isolated, and ligated, if present.[45] In some large lesions, it may be necessary to evacuate the synovium-like contents of the cyst and then dissect the capsule away from the decompressed and split fascicles, but this is not always necessary. Recurrence is a possibility, and some larger lesions require several operations before they are obliterated.

Epidermoid cysts can also compress a nerve, although unlike ganglions, they usually do not extend within the nerve itself. These extraneural lesions may involve the sciatic nerve close to the sciatic notch or may be behind the knee, involving the posterior tibial nerve.[3] The surgeon can usually dissect these and deliver them as a solitary mass after performing neurolysis on and gently retracting involved nerves. Occasionally, a large lesion at the hip or pelvic level requires evacuation initially and then dissection of the capsule away from adjacent tissues, including nerves.

Other benign lesions, such as those arising from bone, may involve a nerve secondarily. Although benign, such tumors may incorporate or severely deform the nerve, making tumor removal without deficit difficult (Fig. 163-15).

Localized Hypertrophic Neuropathy

Localized hypertrophic mononeuropathy, also called onion bulb disease or intraneural perineuroma, is of unknown etiology and pathogenesis. Fascicles and individual nerve fibers become encased by connective tissue in a circular fashion, as if the endoneurium has proliferated. This phenomenon results in a hypertrophic nerve with, on microscopy, an "onion bulb" appearance to its nerve fibers. These strange, tumor-like lesions tend to affect children or young adults more frequently than adults. Patients are exclusively white in our experience, and the tumors have some preference for the peroneal nerve in the leg or the median nerve in the arm.[46–48] Nonetheless, in our clinics, the disease has also been found in the brachial plexus as well as the ulnar, radial, and sciatic nerves.[49,50] The lesion results in a progressive loss of function and tends to involve a fairly lengthy segment of the nerve.[51] It does not spread to other nerves or metastasize elsewhere in the body. Some of its histologic features seem to suggest either a contusive stretch injury or a chronically compressive etiology, but a history of significant trauma is usually missing and surgical exploration reveals no obvious entrapment or irritative environment.

Pain or progressive loss of function leads to exploration. Function is usually partially spared distal to the lesion; as a result, some nerve action potential conduction across the lesion is present. Because of these observations, surgeons

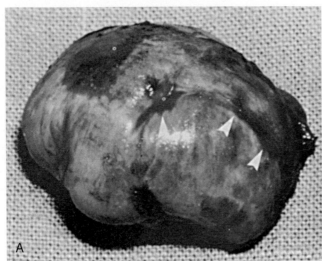

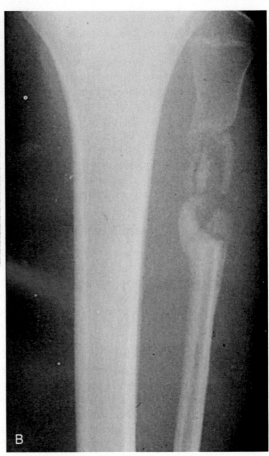

FIGURE 163-15 *A,* Osteoma of the neck of the radius. The patient had a posterior interosseous nerve (PIN) syndrome, and at surgery, the nerve was found to occupy a groove on the surface of this benign bone tumor (*arrowheads*). Removal required extensive mobilization of the PIN well proximal and distal to the tumor site as well as over the top of the tumor. *B,* A benign tumor of the proximal fibula. The patient had a normal preoperative neurologic examination. Postoperative footdrop was found to be the result of a total division of the peroneal nerve, which occurred during surgery of the bone.

have tended to perform either external or external and internal neurolysis on these lesions. Unfortunately, function usually continues to deteriorate. Manipulation of the lesion, particularly by internal neurolysis, may produce additional and even complete loss despite the fact that neurolysis is less invasive than resection. An alternative is to proceed with resection of the lesion, despite the attendant loss, and to replace the lost segment by grafts. This procedure has been performed in 20 cases encountered at the Louisiana State University Medical School in more recent years. As a result, some degree of recovery has occurred in some of these patients.[49]

Malignant Neural Sheath Tumors

Neurogenic fibrosarcomas and malignant schwannomas arising from or involving a nerve can be suspected if a mass increases rapidly in size, especially if it is associated with a progressive loss of function.[52,53] These lesions tend to be firmer on palpation than benign neural sheath tumors and are relatively adherent to surrounding structures. They are often painful but not always (Table 163-6). The incidence of MPNSTs is increased in patients with VRD, but these lesions can occur as solitary lesions in patients without VRD.[54]

Even though malignancy may be suggested by the preoperative symptoms and findings, the clinician cannot be certain of the diagnosis without a thorough biopsy, which usually requires an operation. Positron emission tomography has been shown to be a sensitive test for the detection of MPNSTs and can be used to select for biopsy the most metabolically active areas within a large tumor.[14]

If previous biopsy or operation has been performed and a diagnosis of neurogenic sarcoma or malignant schwannoma is in hand, the surgeon must make certain that metastasis has

TABLE 163-6 ■ Clinical Presentation of Patients Harboring Malignant Peripheral Nerve Tumors as Reported to University of Toronto Pathology Registry (N = 37)

Clinical Presentation	No. of Patients	Percentage (%)
Painless mass	24	55
Painful mass	12	28
Nerve dysfunction	12	28
History of lump excision	12	28
Associated with neurofibromatosis	12	28

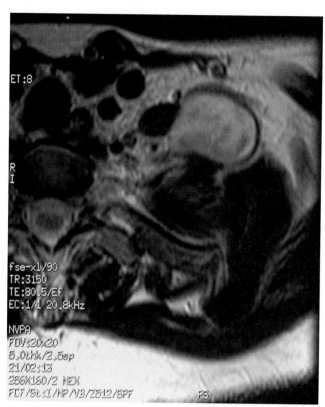

FIGURE 163-16 MRI of malignant schwannoma of brachial plexus.

the level of the plexus spinal nerves.[57] Proximal lower limb lesions may require hip disarticulation with section of the proximal sciatic and femoral nerves. It is preferable to rule out metastatic disease to lung, liver, spleen, and bone before amputation is done.

If we do not know the diagnosis based on previous biopsy or operation, our practice has been to remove such lesions just as with any other lesion of neural sheath origin, but to do so widely, especially when frozen section suggests a malignancy. The surgeon (in conjunction with the patient, the family, and an oncologic surgeon) can subsequently make a decision for proximal amputation versus irradiation with or without chemotherapy.

The essential step in managing these lesions is to obtain as thorough a neuropathologic examination of as much tissue as possible. As a result, further treatment depends heavily on the nature of the malignancy as determined by permanent sections. Fairly often, the tissue blocks and slides must also be evaluated by extramural experts to obtain additional opinions.

The recurrence rate of these malignancies is high, even after wide local excision and irradiation, but some patients have survived beyond 5 years with proper management.[3,53] Although patients have died despite forequarter amputation or hip disarticulation performed when evidence of metastasis was negative, the largest percentage of survivors beyond 5 years is in this category in the Louisiana State University Medical School series.[3,58] In recent years, however, we have performed limb-sparing procedures, including wide local resection, placement of x-ray rods, and sometimes external radiographic treatment, in conjunction with a surgical oncologist in carefully screened and selected patients.[58,59] Survival rates to date seem excellent, but this subset of patients needs additional and longer follow-up before this approach can be used more extensively (Fig. 163-17).

not already occurred. These tumors commonly metastasize to the lungs, liver, brain, soft tissue, bone, regional lymph tissue, skin, and retroperitoneum.[15] In addition to obtaining magnetic resonance images of the involved area (Fig. 163-16), a thorough workup requires a chest radiograph, CT with contrast medium of the head and chest as well as radionucleotide liver, spleen, and bone scans.[55]

If metastasis has occurred, palliative surgery may be offered to those patients with severe neurogenic pain caused by the tumor. More extensive surgery is unwarranted in this situation. These patients and patients without metastasis who refuse surgical treatment should discuss the option of chemotherapy with an oncologist because these types of tumors are moderately sensitive to that treatment modality. Radiation therapy should also be discussed, although little effect has been shown on long-term survival.

In the absence of metastasis, survival depends on complete tumor removal.[56] Options are wide local resection or amputation. A wide local resection should include removal of adjacent as well as adherent soft tissues. Resection should include a several-centimeter margin of entering and exiting nerve shown to be free of malignant changes on frozen and subsequent permanent sections. At that time, some surgical oncologists favor placement of tissue rods for irradiation locally for mid- or high-grade tumors, whereas others favor external irradiation.

Limb amputation, if done, should be done well above the level of the lesion. Proximal upper limb lesions can also be managed by forequarter amputation of shoulder and arm at

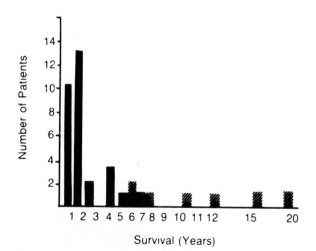

FIGURE 163-17 Survival rates of patients in the University of Toronto Malignant Peripheral Nerve Tumor Pathology Registry. Patients surviving longer intervals (*crosshatched columns*) may display specific histologic characteristics on biopsy, but this issue is not yet settled.

Metastatic Carcinoma

This diverse group of tumors usually involves nerves by direct extension from the primary site, but occasionally a malignancy metastasizes to a nerve or tissues adjacent to it. The presentation and extent of involvement related to the individual behavior of each type of cancer is so varied that management must be individualized. The largest group of metastatic lesions involving a nerve in our series was related to breast carcinoma.[3,58] Most of these lesions involved the brachial plexus. Those at an infraclavicular axillary level appeared to arise by direct extension, although lymph node origin was a possibility, as it was for breast cancer involving the supraclavicular plexus. Because most of these patients had previously undergone mastectomy followed by irradiation, differentiation between metastatic breast cancer and irradiation plexitis is difficult. This is the subject of many papers.[60,61]

If a mass is palpable or visible on a scan in a patient with a history of breast cancer, decompression of involved neural elements may be in order. Unlike malignant neural sheath tumors, nerves involved by this disease receive external neurolysis and are carefully and thoroughly cleaned of tumor. As much of the adjacent mass as possible is also removed. Usually, this type of cancer does not invade the nerve beyond the epineurial level, but exceptions exist. Then, if pain is a problem, resection of the involved elements may be palliative.

Another type of cancer involving a nerve, particularly the plexus, is pulmonary metastatic disease (Fig. 163-18). Pulmonary cancer can involve the brachial plexus by direct extension, and most often produces Pancoast's syndrome. Sometimes if pain is a severe problem, a palliative approach can consist of posterior subscapular resection of the first rib and subtotal resection of the apical tumor to decompress the lower elements of the plexus.[12] Also palliative is this procedure combined with cervical laminectomy for associated epidural metastatic disease. Occasionally, high contralateral open cervical cordotomy also helps control the pain associated with Pancoast's syndrome. Although palliative, the main focus for operation is adequate decompression of the compressed or entrapped nerve or plexus element.[33,62]

True metastatic disease involving a nerve is less common than breast cancer or pulmonary cancer involvement by direct extension but has occurred with lymphoma, bladder cancer, and melanoma. With melanomas involving the plexus, removing the tumor from any epineurial attachments has sufficed. The surgical procedure is then followed by local irradiation. A similar approach has also sufficed for lymphoma, at least for palliative purposes. One lymphoma, however, metastasized to an intraneural locus within the radial nerve, necessitating resection and repair by grafts. Local irradiation at the graft site and the subsequent course of the disease did not augur any significant recovery of radial function.

SUMMARY

Peripheral nerve tumors present a challenging problem for the neurosurgeon. Severe chronic pain or paralysis can be produced by inadvertent fascicular damage. Complex cases should be referred to surgeons who are experienced in the treatment of these difficult tumors. History, examination, and magnetic resonance imaging are sufficient for preoperative evaluation of most cases. Imaging is not able to definitively differentiate between different tumor types so positive identification of the tumor generally must await tissue diagnosis. Needle and especially open biopsy should be minimized in tumors suspected to involve a nerve because of the risk of permanent injury or neuropathic pain. Surgical management differs depending on the type of tumor encountered, so accurate diagnosis of frozen pathology can sometimes be important. The final decision of how much to resect, which fascicles to sacrifice, and whether to repair rests on the clinical judgment of the surgeon based on his or her knowledge and experience with these types of tumors. Because much of what will be done for a patient can change once the tumor has been exposed, surgeons attempting peripheral nerve tumor surgery should have a firm understanding of nerve action potential recording, nerve grafting procedures, and the gross pathologic characteristics of these tumors as well as a mastery of the most useful surgical approaches.

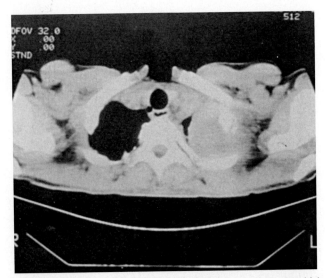

FIGURE 163-18 A computed tomography scan of the brachial plexus demonstrates invasion by an apical thoracic malignancy arising from the lung. This left-sided mass resulted in a severe pain syndrome with associated loss of hard intrinsic muscle function and anesthesia of the left hand.

REFERENCES

1. Seddon H, Livingstone C: Nerve Tumours in Surgical Disorders of the Peripheral Nerves. Edinburgh: ES Livingstone, 1972, pp 153–170.
2. Brooks D: Clinical presentation and treatment of peripheral nerve tumors. In Bunge R, Dyck P, Lambert E, Thomas P (eds): Peripheral Neuropathy, vol 2. Philadelphia: WB Saunders, 1984, pp 2236–2251.
3. Kline DG, Hudson AR: Nerve Injuries: Operative Results of Major Nerve Injuries, Entrapments, and Tumors. Philadelphia: WB Saunders, 1995.
4. Hudson AR: Peripheral nerve surgery. In Bunge R, Dyck P, Lambert E, Thomas P (eds): Peripheral Neuropathy, Vol 2. Philadelphia: WB Saunders, 1984, pp 420–438.

5. Rizzoli H, Horowitz N: Peripheral nerve tumors. In Horowitz N, Rizzoli H (eds): Postoperative Complications of Extracranial Neurological Surgery. Baltimore: Williams & Wilkins, 1977.

6. Ganju A, Roosen N, Kline DG, Tiel RL: Outcomes in a consecutive series of 111 surgically treated plexal tumors: A review of the experience at the Louisiana State University Health Sciences Center. J Neurosurg 95:51–60, 2001.

7. Ghaly RF: A posterior tibial nerve neurilemmoma unrecognized for 10 years: Case report. Neurosurgery 48:668–672, 2001.

8. Pearce JMS: Tinel's sign of formication. J Neurol Neurosurg Psychiatry 61:61, 1996.

9. Campbell R: Tumors of peripheral and sympathetic nerves. In Youmans JR (ed): Neurologic Surgery, 3rd ed. Philadelphia: WB Saunders, 1990.

10. Seppala MT, Sainio MA, Haltia MJJ, et al: Multiple schwannomas: Schwannomatosis or neurofibromatosis type 2. J Neurosurg 89:36–41, 1998.

11. Kichari JR, Hussain SM, Den Hollander JC, Krestin GP: MR imaging of the brachial plexus: Current imaging sequences, normal findings, and findings in a spectrum of focal lesions with MR-pathologic correlation. Curr Probl Diagn Radiol 32:88–101, 2003.

12. Ogose A, Hotta T, Morita T, et al: Tumors of peripheral nerves: Correlation of symptoms, clinical signs, imaging features, and histologic diagnosis. Skeletal Radiol 28:183–188, 1999.

13. Craviato H: Neoplasms of peripheral nerve. In Wilkins R, Rengachary E (eds): Neurosurgery. Baltimore: Williams & Wilkins, 1988.

14. Ferner RE, Lucas JD, O'Doherty MJ, et al: Evaluation of 18-fluorodeoxyglucose positron emission tomography in the detection of malignant peripheral nerve sheath tumours arising from within plexiform neurofibromas in neurofibromatosis 1. Clin Nucl Med 26:525–528, 2001.

15. Ferner RE, Gutmann DH: International consensus statement on malignant peripheral nerve sheath tumours in neurofibromatosis I. Cancer Res 62:1573–1577, 2002.

16. Harkin JC, Reed RJ: Tumours of the Peripheral Nervous System. Fascicle 3, Atlas of Tumour Pathology. Armed Forces Institute of Pathology, 1969.

17. Urich H, Tien RD: Tumors of the cranial, spinal and peripheral nerve sheaths. In Bigner DD, McLendon RE, Bruner JM (eds): Russel's and Rubenstein's Pathology of Tumors of the Nervous System, vol 2, 6th ed. London: Arnold, 1998.

18. Weller R, Cervos-Navarro J: Tumours of the peripheral nervous system. In Asbury A, Johnson P (eds): Pathology of Peripheral Nerves. London: Butterworths, 1977, pp 144–207.

19. Asbury A, Johnson P: Tumours of the peripheral nerve. In Asbury A, Johnson P (eds): Pathology of Peripheral Nerves. Philadelphia: WB Saunders, 1978, pp 206–249.

20. Thomas JE, Piepgras DG, Scheithauer B: Neurogenic tumors of the sciatic nerve: A clinical and clinicopathologic study of 35 cases. Mayo Clin Proc 58:640–647, 1983.

21. Kehoe NJ, Reid RP, Semple JC: Solitary benign peripheral-nerve tumours. Review of 32 years experience. J Bone Joint Surg Br 77:497–500, 1995.

22. Ferner RE, O'Doherty MJ: Neurofibroma and schwannoma. Curr Opin Neurol 15:679–684, 2002.

23. Kang HJ, Shin SJ, Kang ES: Schwannomas of the upper extremity. J Hand Surg [Br] 25:604–607, 2000.

24. Dubuisson A, Kline D, Weinshel S: Posterior subscapular approach to the brachial plexus: Report of 100 cases. J Neurosurg 79:319–330, 1993.

25. Woodhall B: Peripheral nerve tumors. Surg Clin North Am 34:1167–1172, 1954.

26. Kline DG, Happel LT: Penfield Lecture. A quarter century's experience with intraoperative nerve action potential recording. Can J Neurol Sci 20:3–10, 1993.

27. Donner T, Voorhies R, Kline D: Benign neural sheath tumors of major peripheral nerves. J Neurosurg 81:362–373, 1994.

28. Byrne JJ: Nerve tumors. In Gelberman R (ed): Operative Nerve Repair and Reconstruction. Philadelphia: JB Lippincott, 1991.

29. Ruggeri M, Polizzi A: Segmental neurofibromatosis [letter]. J Neurosurg 93:530–531, 2000.

30. Ducatman B, Scheithauer B, Piepgras D, et al: Malignant peripheral nerve sheath tumors: A clinicopathologic study of 120 cases. Cancer (Phila) 57:2006–2021, 1986.

31. Ferraresi S, Garozzo D, Bianchini E: Aggressive fibromatosis (desmoid tumor) of the radial nerve: Favorable resolution. Case report. J Neurosurg 95:332–333, 2001.

32. Gaposchkin CG, Bilsky MH, Ginsberg R, Brennan MF: Function-sparing surgery for desmoid tumors and other low-grade fibrosarcomas involving the brachial plexus. Neurosurgery 42:1297–1303, 1998.

33. Kim DH, Cho Y, Tiel R, Kline DG: Operative management of brachial plexus injuries and tumors. Neurosurg Q 13:1–19, 2003.

34. Yasutomi T, Koike H, Nakatsuchi Y: Granular cell tumour of the ulnar nerve. J Hand Surg [Br] 24:122–124, 1999.

35. Sun JC, Maguire J, Zwimpfer TJ: Traumatically induced lymphangioma of the ulnar nerve. Case report. J Neurosurg 93:1069–1071, 2000.

36. Goldstein LJ, Helfend LK, Kordestani RK: Postoperative edema after vascular access causing nerve compression secondary to the presence of a perineuronal lipoma: Case report. Neurosurgery 50:412–414, 2002.

37. Woodruff J: The pathology and treatment of peripheral nerve tumors and tumor-like conditions. Cancer J Clin 43:290–308, 1993.

38. Mackinnon SE, Dellon AL: Tumors of the peripheral nerve. In Mackinnon SE, Dellon AL (eds): Surgery of the Peripheral Nerve. New York: Thieme, 1988.

39. Lowenstein J, Chandnani V, Tomaino MM: Fibrolipoma of the median nerve: A case report and review of the literature. Am J Orthop 29:797–798, 2000.

40. Curtis RM, Clark GL: Tumors of the blood and lymphatic vessels. In Gelberman R (ed): Operative Nerve Repair and Reconstruction. Philadelphia: JB Lippincott, 1991.

41. Tindall SC: Ganglion cysts of peripheral nerves. In Wilkins RH, Rengachary SS (eds): Neurosurgery. New York: McGraw-Hill, 1985, p 1900.

42. Harbaugh K, Tiel R, Kline D: Ganglion cyst involvement of peripheral nerve. J Neurosurg 87:403–408, 1997.

43. Scherman BM, Bilbao JM, Hudson AR: Intraneural ganglion: A case report with electron-microscopic observations. Neurosurgery 8:487–490, 1981.

44. Spinner RJ, Atkinson JLD, Tiel RL: Peroneal intraneural ganglia: The importance of the articular branch. A unifying theory. J Neurosurg 99:330–343, 2003.

45. Spinner RJ, Atkinson JLD, Scheithauer BW, et al: Peroneal intraneural ganglia: The importance of the articular branch. Clinical series. J Neurosurg 99:319–329, 2003.

46. Bilbao JM, Briggs SJ, Hudson AR, et al: Perineurioma (localized hypertrophic neuropathy). Arch Pathol Lab Med 108:557–560, 1984.

47. Heilburn ME, Tsuruda JS, Townsend JJ, et al: Intraneural perineurioma of the common peroneal nerve. Case report and review of the literature. J Neurosurg 94:811–815, 2001.

48. Kline DG, Gruen JP, Cummings TJ: Letter on Heilburn ME, Tsuruda JS, Townsend JJ, et al.: Intraneural perineurioma of the common peroneal nerve. Case report and review of the literature. J Neurosurg 97:238–240, 2002.

49. Gruen P, Mitchell W, Kline D: Resection and graft repair for localized hypertrophic neuropathy. Neurosurgery 43:78–83, 1998.

50. Hudson AR, Tranmer B: Brachial plexus injuries. In Wilkins RH, Rengachary SS (eds): Neurosurgery. New York: McGraw-Hill, 1985, pp 1817–1832.

51. Simmons Z, Mahadeen ZI, Kothari MJ, et al: Localized hypertrophic neuropathy: Magnetic resonance imaging findings and long-term follow-up. Muscle Nerve 22:28–36, 1999.

52. Vieta JO, Pack GT: Malignant neurilemmomas of peripheral nerve. Am J Surg 82:416–431, 1951.

53. Gentili F, Rewcastle B: Malignant peripheral nerve tumours. Paper presented at the Eighth International Congress of Neurological Surgery, 1985, Toronto, Canada.

54. D'Agostino AN, Soule EH, Miller RH: Primary malignant neoplasm of nerves (malignant neurilemmomas) in patients without manifestations of multiple neurofibromatosis (von Recklinghausen's disease). Cancer 16:1003–1014, 1963.

55. Patel SR, Benjamin RS: Soft tissue and bone sarcomas and bone metastasis. In Braunwald E, Fauci AS, et al (eds): Harrison's Principles of Internal Medicine, 15th ed. New York: McGraw-Hill, 2001, pp 625–628.

56. Casanova M, Ferrari A, et al: Malignant peripheral nerve sheath tumors in children: A single-institution twenty-year experience. J Pediatr Hematol Oncol 21:509–513, 1999.

57. Wittig JC, Bickels J, Kollender Y, et al: Palliative forequarter amputation for metastatic carcinoma to the shoulder girdle region: Indications, preoperative evaluation, surgical technique, and results. J Surg Oncol 77:105–114, 2001.

58. Lusk M, Kline D, Garcia C: Tumors of the brachial plexus. Neurosurgery 21:439–453, 1987.

59. Bickels J, Wittig JC, Kollender Y, et al: Sciatic nerve resection: Is that truly an indication for amputation? Clin Orthop 399:201–204, 2002.

60. Kori SH, Foley FM, Posner JB: Brachial plexus lesions in patients with cancer: 100 cases. Neurology 31:45–50, 1981.

61. Lederman RJ, Wilbourn AJ: Brachial plexopathy: Recurrent cancer or radiation? Neurology 34:1331–1335, 1984.

62. Hudson AR, Berry H, Mayfield F: Chronic injuries of peripheral nerves by entrapment. In Youmans JR (ed): Neurological Surgery, 2nd ed. Philadelphia: WB Saunders, 1982, pp 2430–2474.

164 Thoracic Outlet Syndrome

JOHN E. McGILLICUDDY

The thoracic outlet syndrome is the most controversial and least understood of all nerve compression syndromes. Although it has been studied and described by four surgical specialties—neurosurgery, thoracic surgery, vascular surgery, and orthopedics—for over 70 years, there is still no agreement as to what symptoms and signs constitute the syndrome, its etiology and pathophysiology, and its appropriate treatment. The unifying theme of these disparate syndromes is their alleged origin from structural abnormalities in the region bounded by the cervical spine, the scalene muscles, the first rib, and in some cases, the clavicle. This broad area between the base of the neck and the axilla is termed by many as the thoracic outlet. It includes the "true" thoracic outlet surrounded by the first rib, as well as the costoclavicular space and subcoracoid space.

Historically, these syndromes were at first described in terms of their presumed site of local static or dynamic neurovascular compression: the scalenus anticus syndrome, cervical rib syndrome, costoclavicular syndrome, and hyperabduction syndrome. Each had its own specific treatment, and none were particularly successful. In 1956, Peet brought all these syndromes together under one common diagnosis—the thoracic outlet syndrome—to indicate that all the syndromes had in common neurovascular compression at the level of the thoracic outlet.[1] Although some of the symptom complexes described may be caused by compression between the clavicle and the first rib (the costoclavicular space) or in the subcoracoid space beneath the tendon of the pectoralis minor, the vast majority are believed to be due to vascular or neural compression in the area bounded medially by the transverse processes of the cervical spine, laterally by the anterior and middle scalene muscles, and inferiorly by the superior surface of the first rib—the scalene triangle or the true thoracic outlet.

A brief examination of the syndromes reveals that they may be initially grouped into vascular (arterial and venous) and neurogenic types.[2] The arterial syndrome is rare, comprising about 2% of all thoracic outlet syndromes, and is due to compression of the subclavian artery in the scalene triangle. This compression is usually due to a bony abnormality such as a large cervical rib or an abnormally developed first rib. Compression here can lead to post-stenotic dilatation of the artery and aneurysm formation, to distal arterial embolization, and to occlusion of the artery. Retrograde thrombosis of the subclavian artery can lead to vertebral or carotid artery occlusion and stroke. Prompt surgical attention is necessary when symptoms occur. Angiography—contrast or magnetic resonance imaging (MRI)—is the diagnostic procedure of choice and surgery is often required.

Venous thoracic outlet syndrome, also called effort thrombosis or Paget-Schroetter syndrome, is markedly different symptomatically from the other types and is usually included in discussions of thoracic outlet syndrome by virtue of its location. The syndrome often follows heavy exercise. Here, occlusion of the subclavian or axillary vein is associated with upper extremity edema, venous engorgement, distal cyanosis, and severe deep-seated limb pain.[3] Anticoagulation and occasionally thrombectomy and first rib resection is indicated. These vascular syndromes are well covered in the thoracic and vascular surgical literature and will not be further considered here. Vascular and neurogenic syndromes rarely occur in the same patient.

The neurogenic type of outlet syndrome itself has diverse presentations, is much more common than vascular types, and is the source of considerable confusion and controversy.[4–7] There is great variability as to what symptoms and signs should be included in the diagnosis and in how the diagnosis should be treated.

ANATOMY

The thoracic outlet is most often considered to be the area circumscribed by the first rib on each side. Within this area the most important structure in the genesis of the thoracic outlet syndrome is the interscalene triangle. The triangle is made up of the anterior and middle scalene muscles as the sides of the triangle and the superior surface of the first rib between the insertions of the scalenes as the base. The anterior scalene originates from the anterior tubercles of the transverse processes of C3 through C6, while the middle scalene takes its origin from the posterior tubercles of the transverse processes of C2 through C6. Both scalene muscles insert on the superior surface of the first rib—the anterior scalene at the scalene tubercle and the middle scalene about 2 cm posterolaterally.

The anterior and posterior tubercles of the transverse processes are, respectively, the anterior and posterior limits of the lateral extensions of the cervical foramina. Thus, the cervical spinal nerves that comprise the brachial plexus must exit their foramina between the scalenes and cross the interscalene triangle in a caudal and lateral direction. The T1 spinal nerve takes a different course, leaving its foramen below the first rib and passing anteriorly and superiorly around the neck of this rib to join with the C8 spinal nerve and form the lower trunk of the plexus near the costovertebral junction (Fig. 164-1). The origins of the lower trunk, therefore, embrace the neck of the first rib. The course of the T1 spinal nerve thus leads the lower trunk of the plexus to be tethered inferiorly and therefore causes the lower trunk to be vulnerable to pressure from inferiorly since it cannot ascend in response to this pressure and will be compressed or deformed by it. This is an important fact in the etiology of the neurogenic thoracic outlet syndrome.

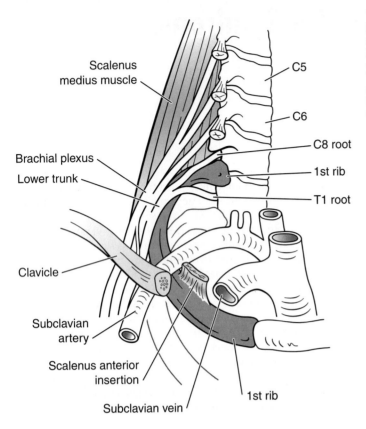

FIGURE 164-1 An oblique view of the right thoracic outlet shows the relationships between the C8 and T1 spinal nerves, lower trunk, subclavian artery, and first rib. The T1 spinal nerve courses medial to the first rib as it ascends to join the C8 nerve. The lower trunk and the subclavian artery rest on the first rib laterally. The distance between the anterior and medial scalene has been increased for clarity. The artery and the lower trunk are actually in contact in the narrow interscalene space.

The subclavian artery ascends from the thorax to exit between the scalenes just anterior to the lower trunk of the brachial plexus. While the entire brachial plexus has traversed the interscalene triangle to reach the axilla, only the lower trunk and the subclavian artery come into direct contact with the lateral first rib between the insertions of the scalenes. It is in this location in the lateral and inferior interscalene triangle that the vast majority of neural and vascular compressions occur. Anomalies of scalene muscle insertion, fused scalene muscles, cervical ribs, anomalous first ribs, and fibrous bands arising from ribs and cervical vertebrae have all been implicated. The lower trunk and the subclavian artery are affected. Although upper plexus (C5, C6, C7) thoracic outlet syndromes have been described, it is most unlikely that the upper or middle trunk could be compressed by structural anomalies in the scalene triangle.[8]

In many descriptions of the thoracic outlet syndrome, two other areas—the costoclavicular space between the clavicle and the first rib, and the subcoracoid space, bounded anteriorly by the tendinous insertion of the pectoralis minor—are considered to be part of the thoracic outlet. While the subclavian-axillary artery, and perhaps the brachial plexus, can be transiently stretched or compressed by retraction of the shoulders or hyperabduction of the arms in these areas, there is scant evidence linking these areas to any chronic plexus compression.

Chronic compression, however, can occur in the costoclavicular space if the clavicle is fractured.[9] This is the traumatic thoracic outlet syndrome. The majority of clavicular fractures occur in the middle third of the clavicle. The lateral fragment is left deep to and inferior to the proximal. If this malalignment persists, the space between the clavicle and the first rib will be narrowed. The medial cord of the plexus is usually the structure compressed. A malaligned, healing clavicular fracture with a large callous can cause compression here and has been frequently described.[10] Easily recognized on x-ray by the deformity and the exuberant callus, it can be relieved by resection of the clavicle, removal of the callus, or removal of the first rib. Rarely, an acute fracture of the clavicle can produce a similar plexus compression.[11]

PATHOPHYSIOLOGY

A wide variety of postural and dynamic factors have been implicated in the development of stretch and compression of the brachial plexus.[12] Their importance is disputed. The shoulder girdle gradually descends from childhood to adulthood, perhaps due to our upright posture. This descent may cause some traction on the lower plexus elements as they pass over the first rib. Descent is more common in women who also tend to have weaker shoulder suspensory muscles. These factors may account for the nearly fourfold greater prevalence of outlet syndrome in females. Cervicothoracic scoliosis has also been implicated. Transient but prolonged postural changes associated with certain occupations have been cited as causative factors. Prolonged hyperabduction of the arms and a forward flexed position of the head and neck can result in muscle imbalances with tight contracted muscles, especially the scalenes, and weakened, slack muscles leading to abnormal postures that may, in turn, lead to neck and shoulder pain and possible nerve compression or stretch in the thoracic outlet.[13]

The importance of these abnormalities of posture is debatable, but there is little doubt that certain anatomic anomalies can elevate and kink the lower trunk of the brachial plexus

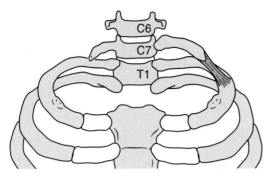

FIGURE 164-2 The bony anomalies associated with stretching or kinking of the lower trunk of the plexus are seen. The typical elongated downward-pointing and "beaked" transverse process is on the left. A short cervical rib with the associated fibrous band attached to the first rib is on the right.

within the scalene triangle. These anomalies include cervical ribs, anomalous first ribs, and fibrous bands originating from the tips of short cervical ribs and from the tips of the abnormally elongated and beaked C7 transverse processes (Fig. 164-2). Very often these bands appear as a thickening and fibrosis of the medial edge of the scalenus medius. The distortion of the lower trunk caused by these anomalies is in turn responsible for the neurologic deficits characteristic of thoracic outlet syndrome.[14] A wide variety of additional fibrotic bands have been described as being associated with thoracic outlet syndromes. These bands between structures in the thoracic outlet are believed to compress or distort the plexus.[15] They have not been as clearly associated with objective neurologic findings, and their importance is uncertain.

SIGNS AND SYMPTOMS

The signs and symptoms attributed to the neurogenic thoracic outlet syndrome in the vast majority of cases are many and varied. Virtually all patients complain of pain in the arm and often the shoulder. The pain is deep, aching, and diffuse, not conforming to dermatomal distributions. It is frequently made worse by exercise or by working with the arms above shoulder level. Paresthesias are also a common complaint and usually involve the medial forearm and the ulnar side of the hand, implicating involvement of the lower trunk of the plexus or the medial cord. While these paresthesias can progress to numbness, objective and well-defined sensory loss is found in only a small number of patients.

Sensory symptoms predominate and motor complaints are less prominent. The most common symptoms are subjective weakness of grip and clumsiness of the hand. Objective evidence of weakness, atrophy, or denervation is rare, but a subset of patients do demonstrate clear atrophy of the thenar eminence, especially the abductor pollicis brevis and the hypothenar eminence.[14,16] Since muscles innervated by both the median and ulnar nerves are affected here, a proximal, plexus level, lesion must be responsible.

Vasomotor findings are frequently prominent with blanching, hyperemia, coldness, and cyanosis of the hands.

These changes are not necessarily related to activity or the ambient temperature. These changes are likely due to involvement of the postganglionic sympathetic fibers distributed to the upper extremity via the T1 root.

The symptomatology often appears to be precipitated by trauma. Whiplash injury in auto collisions accounts for the most thoracic outlet syndromes with an identifiable cause.[17,18] Cumulative trauma or repetitive strain injury from head and neck positioning during work is becoming more frequently indicted.[13] Whether these injuries contribute directly to the thoracic outlet syndrome is controversial; in one series, two thirds of over 5000 patients referred for thoracic outlet syndrome had a history of neck or shoulder trauma prior to the onset of symptoms.[19] Acute trauma is thought to act via direct injury to the plexus or via injury to the scalene muscle, which leads to persistent spasm and eventually to permanent changes in the fine structure of the muscle.[20] While some investigators have identified significant changes within the muscle, others have been unable to do so. In cumulative trauma injuries, abnormal head and neck positioning is thought to cause nerve compression. Many of these injuries and cumulative trauma incidents appear to have been trivial, and the role of litigation and secondary gain cannot be discounted.

THE TWO NEUROGENIC THORACIC OUTLET SYNDROMES

Review of literature and experience leads to the conclusion that there are two distinct types of thoracic outlet syndrome with very little overlap between them. Although the same area and similar structures are presumed to be involved in the production of these syndromes, the clinical symptoms and signs are distinctly different. The first syndrome, termed the "true" or "classic" thoracic outlet syndrome, is rare, occurring in about one per million population and almost exclusively affecting young to middle-aged females; the female:male ratio is 9:1. This syndrome was first separated from the rest of the thoracic outlet syndrome by Gilliatt in 1970.[14] These patients present with moderate medial arm and forearm pain rarely severe enough to seek medical attention and often present for years before definitive diagnosis of thoracic outlet syndrome. Shoulder and arm pain is uncommon. Sensory loss is modest and patchy in the medial arm and forearm; it may extend into the ulnar two fingers. There are no vasomotor signs or symptoms. The most impressive complaint is progressive hand weakness and atrophy of the intrinsic hand muscles. Medial forearm muscles are also often atrophied. Characteristically the thenar muscles, especially the abductor pollicis brevis, are the most wasted, producing the so-called Gilliatt-Sumner hand with "guttering" of the lateral thenar area (Fig. 164-3). This syndrome is, in virtually every case, associated with and caused by radiologically demonstrable bony anomalies at the thoracic outlet-cervical ribs, abnormal first ribs, or elongated, downward-sloping, and "beaked" C7 transverse processes (Fig. 164-4). A firm fibrous band runs from the tip of these structures to its insertion on the first rib, just anterior to the insertion of the scalenus medius. The lower trunk of the brachial plexus is stretched over this band, producing the neurologic symptoms indicative of lower trunk plexopathy[21] (Fig. 164-5).

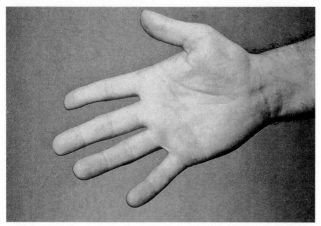

FIGURE 164-3 Atrophy or hollowing out (guttering) of the lateral thenar eminence can be seen along the lateral margin of the base of the thumb. This is the result of atrophy of the abductor pollicis brevis with relative preservation of other thenar muscles. This appearance is characteristic of the "true" thoracic outlet syndrome and is one piece of evidence of the greater involvement of median motor fibers than ulnar motor fibers in this syndrome.

Cervical ribs are rare, occurring in less than 1% of the population, and abnormal C7 transverse processes may be rarer still. Both can be demonstrated by oblique cervical spine studies or an apical lordotic chest film, but both may be quite small and can be easily overlooked. Cervical ribs are three times more common in females, which likely accounts for their higher incidence of "true" thoracic outlet syndrome. Nearly two thirds of cervical ribs are bilateral,

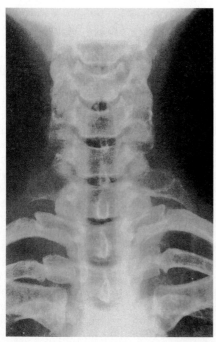

FIGURE 164-4 A patient with right thoracic outlet syndrome who has hand intrinsic muscle atrophy. A beaked, elongated, downward-pointing transverse process is seen on this side. A larger abnormality, a small cervical rib, is on the left. Both may be very difficult to see unless an apical lordotic chest film is used. It is not uncommon for the symptomatic side in bilateral cervical ribs to be the smaller one.

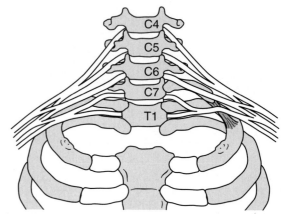

FIGURE 164-5 The mechanism of production of the neurologic deficits in thoracic outlet syndrome. The lower trunk is elevated by a fibrous band running from the tip of the cervical rib. In the majority of instances of the "true" outlet syndrome, the lower trunk is elevated by a fibrous band and not a cervical rib.

but the smaller rib is more often the symptomatic one. The size of the bony anomaly is unimportant. It is nearly always the attached fibrous band that compresses the plexus. Cervical ribs may also be thought to be the first rib; the tip-off to prevent this error is that the transverse process at C7 points downward (caudally) when associated with a cervical rib, whereas all thoracic transverse processes point upward (cranially). The "true" thoracic outlet syndrome is thus defined clinically by a combination of intrinsic hand muscle atrophy and typical bony anomalies visualized on imaging studies.

The second type of thoracic outlet syndrome is far more prevalent. The overwhelming majority of the literature on thoracic outlet syndrome concerns this syndrome. Patients with this syndrome present primarily with combinations of arm, shoulder, and neck pain that is often quite disabling. This pain is typically made worse by exertion and/or by elevation of the arms. It is deep, dull, and diffuse and does not follow a dermatomal pattern. Paresthesias are frequent and are usually in the medial forearm and the ulnar side of the hand, suggesting involvement of the lower trunk of the plexus. Patients complain of weakness and clumsiness of the hand, but objective weakness and atrophy are rare. Autonomic instability in the affected arm is common, with coolness, blanching, hyperemia, and cyanosis resembling Raynaud's disease; this could be due to disturbance of the T1 sympathetic fibers. The radiologic abnormalities universally seen in the "true" thoracic outlet syndrome are rarely seen in this type, occurring in only 5% to 8% of patients in several large series.

This syndrome, with a wide variety of symptoms (including headaches and chest pain), which usually has no radiologic abnormalities nor any demonstrable neurologic deficits, has been called the "disputed" or "common" type of thoracic outlet syndrome. Many of its basic tenets are in dispute, even among surgeons who treat it frequently. The paucity of objective findings makes the diagnosis very physician dependent, but even among experts in this syndrome, there are considerable differences as to which set of symptoms and which diagnostic tests reliably diagnose thoracic outlet syndrome. One experienced surgeon believes that electrodiagnostic studies are unnecessary and basically useless. The results are usually nondiagnostic and normal. The diagnosis thus can be made on the basis of a "typical" history and a neurologic examination.[22] Another equally experienced surgeon does not accept a diagnosis of thoracic outlet syndrome unless ulnar or median nerve conduction studies show slowing of conduction across the thoracic outlet.[23] Each surgeon treating this syndrome appears to have a unique personal set of diagnostic criteria.

Although this syndrome is extremely subjective, without a unifying history and with no predictable incidence of neurologic abnormalities, there may indeed be an element of plexus compression; a Tinel's sign on percussion in the supraclavicular area is a frequent finding in patients with the "disputed" syndrome. In the midst of confusing data on the thoracic outlet syndromes, it is important to remember that the thoracic outlet syndrome is a diagnosis of exclusion. The diagnoses of cervical radiculopathy, ulnar entrapment at the elbow, and carpal tunnel syndrome—all of which have characteristic physical findings and abnormal ancillary study results—must be considered and ruled out before making the diagnosis of thoracic outlet syndrome. One study of patients referred to a thoracic surgery clinic with a diagnosis of thoracic outlet syndrome found that 64% had a different diagnosis.[24]

ANCILLARY STUDIES

Imaging studies, electrodiagnostics, and so-called provocative tests have been widely used to make or confirm the diagnosis of thoracic outlet syndromes. The lack of objective neurologic findings increases the importance of these tests. The first tests used to attempt to diagnose thoracic outlet syndrome were the provocative tests used to produce obliteration of the radial pulse. If the radial pulse disappeared, this was considered to mean that there was vascular and therefore also neural compression at the thoracic outlet. The Adson's maneuver was the first provocative test. Described in 1926, it consisted of turning the head toward the affected side, elevating the chin, and taking a deep breath. Later researchers turned the head toward the contralateral side (modified Adson's) and also abolished the pulse. Other provocative tests include the hyperabduction maneuver in which radial pulse obliteration is sought when the arm is elevated 180 degrees from the side, and the costoclavicular maneuver in which the shoulders are drawn back in an exaggerated military position while the arm is pulled down. The most frequently used maneuver today was described by Roos as the elevated arm stress test (EAST), in which the arm is elevated 90 degrees at the shoulder and externally rotated—the "hold-up" position. Initially a radial pulse–centered maneuver, the result is now considered positive if opening and closing the hands repeatedly in this position reproduces the patient's symptoms in less than 3 minutes.[15]

These provocative tests are not specific. At least 50% of normal people have a positive Adson's test result and a similar percentage of false-positive results is seen with the other maneuvers.[25] Even the EAST maneuver reproduces pain of paresthesia in 57% to 74% of asymptomatic controls in two separate trials.[26,27] Provocative tests are testing the wrong system (the vascular system) and are prone to a high percentage of false positive results. They are of no proven value in diagnosing neurogenic thoracic outlet syndrome.

Electrodiagnostic studies have an unusual position in the diagnosis of thoracic outlet syndrome. On the one hand, the "true" thoracic outlet syndrome has a very characteristic set of findings, while the "disputed" type is not associated with any abnormalities on standard testing. The findings of the "classic" thoracic outlet syndrome are those of a chronic axonal neuropathy of the lower trunk of the plexus.[14,16] Nerve conduction studies show (1) a low-amplitude median motor response measured at the abductor pollicis brevis, (2) a low-amplitude ulnar sensory response, (3) a normal to slightly low ulnar motor response, and (4) a normal median sensory response. There are usually denervation changes in the intrinsic hand muscles, especially the abductor pollicis brevis.[28] In many cases the ulnar intrinsics also show denervation. The median sensory responses are normal since the involved axons to the median sensory distribution in the hand are derived from the C6 and C7 spinal nerves and travel in the upper and middle trunks at plexus level and therefore are not involved in the lower trunk compression. Recent studies have shown that the sensory potential in the medial antebrachial cutaneous nerve is also reduced. The nerve conduction velocities in the median and ulnar nerve are normal.[29] Somatosensory evoked potentials (SSEPs) may show reduction on ulnar nerve stimulation but are normal on median stimulation. Neither SSEP nor evaluation of F-responses are of much value in this situation since the findings on nerve conduction and electromyography (EMG) studies are so characteristic.

In contrast, the situation in the "disputed" thoracic outlet syndrome shows no reproducible abnormalities in nerve conduction or EMG studies. The search for an objective electrophysiologic finding in this syndrome has not been successful. SSEPs have been heavily utilized; some observers have found ulnar nerve SSEPs to be delayed, but an equal number have not found this a reliable test.[30–32] Attempts to find differences in latency when the arm is in the normal position and in the abducted externally rotated position (EAST) have not shown significant differences.[33] Slowed ulnar nerve conduction velocity across the thoracic outlet was described as characteristic of this syndrome in 1972 and continues to be used by some surgeons.[34] This finding has not been reproduced by others, and the reality of these findings has been questioned. In the "disputed" thoracic outlet syndrome, electrophysiologic studies have been more useful in identifying or ruling out other peripheral neuropathies, such as carpal tunnel or ulnar neuropathy and cervical radiculopathies, than in confirming a diagnosis of outlet syndrome.

Imaging studies have not been helpful in most cases. One of the bony abnormalities enumerated earlier is present in all cases of "true" syndrome, while only about 9% to 10% of the disputed cases show any abnormalities. It is important, in this context, to remember that many cervical ribs are asymptomatic. Up to 50% are bilateral, and bilateral thoracic outlet syndrome of any type is very unusual. Computed tomography has not been of much use in evaluation for thoracic outlet syndrome. It can occasionally help in better defining an abnormal C7 or cervical rib, but is not more specific than plain x-rays.[35] Computed tomography may be helpful in confirming a diagnosis of thoracic outlet syndrome when other criteria support it, but it is inconclusive at excluding this diagnosis. Magnetic resonance imaging (MRI) scans of the brachial plexus are purported by some to be able to identify compressive bands through their distortion of the lower plexus, but these findings have not been widely replicated.[36] MRI is not commonly useful in the diagnosis of thoracic outlet syndrome. MRI of the cervical spine, however, has been useful to search for signs of cervical radiculopathy in instances of diagnostic uncertainty. The use of MR neurography may be able to demonstrate plexus distortion clearly. Adequate data to evaluate this new technology are not yet available.

The lack of positive findings on the ancillary studies in the "disputed" thoracic outlet syndrome have led many researchers to describe this syndrome as an early form of the "true" or "classic" syndrome. It is thought that the symptomatology in this former syndrome, while subjectively severe, is not associated with enough nerve compression to effect changes in electrodiagnostic studies or in the neurological examination. Given enough time, these patients will then evolve into the "true" syndrome. In fact, this does not appear to be the case. There have been very few, if any, patients with the "true" syndrome who have had prior complaints of severe, disabling pain characteristic of the "disputed" syndrome. In addition, a substantial portion of the "true" syndrome patients are young females in their late teens or twenties; the "true" syndrome is not one of elderly patients with a long history of unilateral upper extremity pain and paresthesias.

TREATMENT

If there are two types of thoracic outlet syndrome, a separate management strategy would seem to be indicated for each. An accurate diagnosis of the type of thoracic outlet syndrome is essential before proceeding with treatment. In those patients without a clear structural abnormality or a definite abnormal neurologic findings, a conservative approach initially should be adopted.[1,12,37] Physical therapy may be very useful in this situation. Strengthening of the shoulder girdle muscles is the primary focus of treatment.[38] This is combined with improvement of posture, relaxation of the scalenes, and strengthening of the trapezius. The program should be continued for a minimum of 1 month and ideally for 3 months. Improvement in the short term has been reported to occur in 60% to 90% of patients. Continued attention to posture and a continued exercise program may often bring permanent relief. In this group of patients—usually those with "disputed" thoracic outlet syndrome—evaluation of psychological factors prior to surgery is also wise.

Patients not relieved by conservative therapy will be considered for surgery. Choosing the patients who will profit from surgery and choosing the surgical approach varies widely from surgeon to surgeon. Historically, the focus of the surgical approach has shifted from the first rib in the early 20th century to the anterior scalene muscles as advocated by Adson and Coffey in 1927, and back to the first rib again. The return to the first rib as the "common denominator" of the thoracic outlet syndrome was emphasized by Clagett in 1962, and first rib resection has been the principal treatment for most cases of thoracic outlet syndrome since that time.[39]

Those patients with clear anatomic abnormalities and neurologic deficits—the "true" thoracic outlet syndrome—will not be helped by physical therapy. Theirs is a pure mechanical problem, with chronic compression of the lower trunk by structures whose position cannot be changed by physical therapy. The first, best, and only option in these cases is resection of the offending cervical rib or fibrous band. Unfortunately, these patients often come to surgical attention late in their course with major weakness and atrophy, and further delay only worsens their deficit.

SURGICAL TREATMENT

There are three surgical approaches to the thoracic outlet currently in use: they are the supraclavicular, the transaxillary, and the posterior.

Supraclavicular Approach

The supraclavicular approach is the oldest of the three approaches. It was described by Adson and Coffey in 1926 and popularized by Falconer and Li in 1962.[40] It was eventually eclipsed by the transaxillary approach in the 1970s, but it has become more frequently used in the past 10 years. The return to this approach has been brought about by the evidence of a gradual but definite deterioration in the results of the transaxillary approach on long-term follow-up and by the recognition of the serious complications occurring with that approach.[4] This approach is best for displaying the proximal plexus at the scalene triangle, for identification and excision of cervical ribs, identification and resection of congenital bands, and for division and resection of the scalene muscles.

The approach begins with the patient supine and with the neck, ipsilateral anterior hemithorax, shoulder, and upper arm prepared and draped in continuity. The forearm and hand are sheathed in an impervious sleeve and rested on the abdomen so that motor responses to stimulation may be observed. A linear supraclavicular incision is opened about 2 cm cranial to the clavicle and extending from the lateral border of the sternocleidomastoid to the junction of the middle and lateral thirds of the clavicle[21] (Fig. 164-6). The wound edges are retracted after the platysma is divided, and a subplatysmal dissection mobilizes the edges. The omohyoid muscle is identified and transected in its tendinous midportion. A combination of blunt and sharp dissection then mobilizes the scalene fat pad from medial to lateral. The internal jugular vein must be sought and protected in developing the medial edge of this dissection. As the fat pad is mobilized, the transverse cervical artery is identified, ligated, and divided. With the fat pad retracted, the scalenus anterior is readily seen with the phrenic nerve running from lateral to medial on its surface. Immediately posterior to the anterior scalene is the brachial plexus; its upper and middle trunks are easily seen (Fig. 164-7). Working caudally along the lateral border of the anterior scalene brings the first rib, the subclavian artery, and the lower trunk of the plexus into view. If the phrenic nerve is freed from the fascia atop the scalene, retracted medially, and protected, the scalene can be divided at the clavicle.

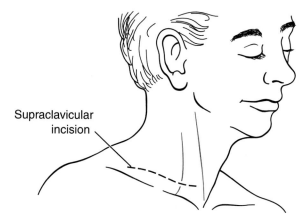

FIGURE 164-6 A linear incision is used for a supraclavicular exposure of the plexus and the surgery on congenital bands, cervical ribs, the scalenes, and the first rib. This exposure is essentially the one used for exploration of the brachial plexus for tumors and trauma as well. The clavicular head of the sternocleidomastoid can be transected for increased exposure.

This will better expose the artery and lower trunk if needed. Transection of the anterior scalene is usually not necessary if this procedure is used in the "true" thoracic outlet syndrome. In this situation, the subclavian artery can be retracted caudally and slightly anteriorly and the lower trunk moved carefully in the same direction. The typical fibrous band of the "true" syndrome can be seen and felt posterolateral to the plexus. It often appears to be a fibrous strip at the anterior edge of the scalenus medius (Fig. 164-8). Transection of this band may suffice to decompress the lower trunk, but a section of the band and medial scalene can be removed to ensure full freeing up of the plexus.

There is generally no need to resect the elongated C7 transverse process or a short cervical rib. It is nearly always the fibrotic band alone that is compressing the lower trunk. If the cervical rib is long and is in contact with the plexus, however, it may be removed piecemeal with Leksell or Kerrison rongeurs while protecting the plexus elements.

If it is felt necessary to remove the first rib, the scalenus anterior should be transected close to the rib while protecting the subclavian artery and vein. The subclavian vein will be found anterior to the anterior scalene between the first rib and the clavicle. It must be carefully freed from the first rib; the subclavius muscle may need to be identified and transected at its medial end to fully mobilize the vein. The rib can be transected anteriorly near the anterior scalene while retracting and protecting the subclavian vein. The scalenus medius is then also divided close to the rib while protecting the plexus. The rib can then be transected more posteriorly near the insertion of the scalenus medius while retracting the plexus and artery anteriorly. This segment of rib is then removed carefully, freeing it from the surrounding soft tissue and the pleura. The rib is then removed piecemeal with rongeurs, working anteriorly to the costochondral junction and posteriorly to the costovertebral junction. The posterior removal can be difficult by this approach, and great care must be taken to protect the lower plexus and especially the T1 root as it courses superiorly on the inner edge of the first rib to join the C8 root. A small stump of first rib approximately 1 to 1.5 cm in length may be left if it does not impinge on the T1 spinal nerve. Extraperiosteal removal of the first rib is absolutely critical. Persistence of the periosteum may lead to reformation of the rib or to intense scarring in this area and bring about recurrence of the thoracic outlet syndrome.

FIGURE 164-7 Retraction of the scalene fat pad (not shown) reveals the anterior scalene and the phrenic nerve. Tracing the phrenic nerve proximally establishes the position of the C5 spinal nerve where the phrenic joins it. Once C5 and the upper trunk are identified, the remainder of the plexus can be clearly identified and it can be followed distally to visualize the lower trunk.

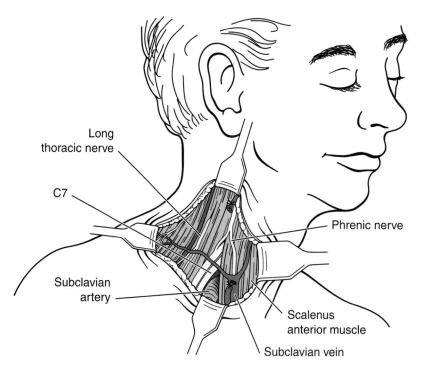

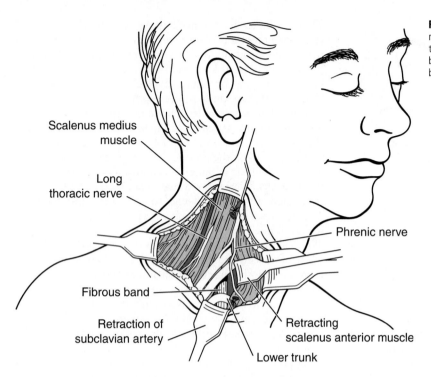

FIGURE 164-8 When the subclavian artery is retracted, the fibrous band elevating the lower trunk can be seen and felt. The fibrous band can be transected either above (as shown here) or below the subclavian artery.

Scalenus medius muscle

Long thoracic nerve

Phrenic nerve

Fibrous band

Retraction of subclavian artery

Retracting scalenus anterior muscle

Lower trunk

Recent data suggest that supraclavicular excision of the scalene muscles has as good a long-term outcome as first rib removal. Reports in the thoracic and vascular surgical literature, where virtually all reports of treatment of the "disputed" thoracic outlet syndrome appear, have also advocated a supraclavicular approach in order to perform both a first rib resection and a wide removal of the anterior, and in some cases, the middle scalene muscle.[4,41,42] This scalenectomy approach is felt to reduce the likelihood of recurrence of symptoms. Some reports indicate that a combined middle and anterior scalenectomy has results that are as good as supraclavicular first rib resection.[43,44] This approach is familiar to neurosurgeons—it is the standard approach for supraclavicular plexus exploration—and is the preferred approach for the "true" thoracic outlet syndrome.

Transaxillary Approach

The transaxillary approach was developed by Roos in 1966 and rapidly became widely used. Its introduction is credited with a marked increase in the rate of surgery for the thoracic outlet syndrome.[45] The transaxillary approach has the advantage of allowing the removal of the entire first rib through one exposure under direct vision. Another attraction not to be discounted is its nearly invisible and well-concealed incisional scar. This approach is preferred by vascular and thoracic surgeons, who perform the vast majority of thoracic outlet surgeries in the United States. The prevailing view in these specialties is that the first rib is the culprit—the "common denominator"—in the thoracic outlet syndrome and must be removed to effect relief.

Surgery is performed with the patient in the lateral decubitus position and rolled back 30 to 45 degrees toward the surgeon. The arm, shoulder, and axilla are prepared and the axilla draped out. The entire arm is covered in layers of sterile stockinette. As described by Roos, the third rib lies subcutaneously in the axilla just as the axillary skin separates from the chest wall. A transverse incision 8 to 10 cm in length is made here at the inferior margin of the axillary hairline. The incision is carried directly down to the rib. Dissection then proceeds up along the surface of the rib cage bluntly toward the apex of the axilla. This exposes the first and second ribs (Fig. 164-9). The intercostobrachial nerve crosses the field here and should be preserved. Damage to the nerve can cause pain in the axilla and medial upper arm postoperatively.

Once the first rib is identified, an assistant lifts the arm, which is abducted 90 degrees at the shoulder, vertically. This opens the apex of the axilla and the thoracic outlet at the level of the first rib. Further access depends critically on the abduction and distraction created by the assistant, who must be both strong and tireless. In order to prevent damage to the plexus, which is on mild stretch during positioning, the vertical vector must be released for a few minutes every 15 to 20 minutes. Roos emphasizes the great importance of adequate but gentle distraction of the arm. An experienced assistant is important here. Roos believes that most plexus injuries incurred during this procedure are due to prolonged or excessive stretch of the plexus.[45] When the arm is fully abducted and raised, the brachial plexus and subclavian artery and vein are raised up off the first rib and compressed against the humerus. The scalene muscles are transected at their insertion on the first rib and retract out of the way (Fig. 164-10). As in all middle scalenectomies, the long thoracic nerve, which travels through the muscle and emerges on its superficial surface several centimeters cranial to the first rib, must be identified and preserved. An extraperiosteal excision of the first rib is then carried out. The rib is sectioned at the costochondral junction and then freed by blunt dissection back to the transverse process

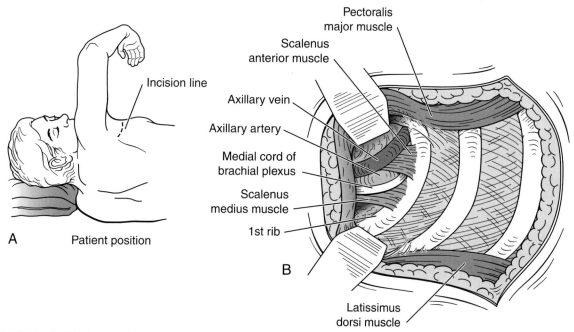

FIGURE 164-9 Positioning is critical for the transaxillary approach. *A,* The arm must be gently but fully abducted 180 degrees and maintained in the axial plane. Incision is at the base of the axillary hairline and is carried straight down to the third rib. *B,* Blunt dissection along the chest wall exposes the first rib. Careful blunt dissection along the first rib establishes the position of the scalenes. The lower trunk–medial cord and the subclavian artery veer upward from the superior edge of the first rib.

and removed. The maneuvers to free up the first rib are complex and critical; careful, blunt dissection circumferentially around the rib releases the intercostal muscle, the apical pleura, and any remaining scalene musculature while preserving the periosteum on the rib. The operative description of Roos should be read and thoroughly understood before attempting this procedure.[45]

This is a technically challenging procedure. The exposure is deep and narrow. The subclavian vein may be torn during exposure anteriorly. The plexus is not well seen until late in the dissection. The T1 root is at risk as the posterior portion of the rib is freed up and transected. Severe plexus injuries

have occurred as a result of this approach.[46] Although a low incidence of complications is claimed for this operation, nearly 300 cases of plexus injury were reported by 1982.[47] One fourth of these were permanent; the lower trunk is the usual injured element, with devastating consequences for hand function and often with severe causalgic pain.[48] The transaxillary approach is nonetheless useful for the rare vascular thoracic outlet syndrome and in cases of failure of the supraclavicular approach for thoracic outlet syndrome. It must be performed with meticulous attention to the neural and vascular elements exposed and retracted at the apex of this deep exposure.

FIGURE 164-10 The scalenes have been transected and have retracted. The subclavian artery and the lower trunk–medial cord of the plexus are well visualized, especially when the abducted arm is distracted vertically. The lines across the first rib indicate the initial transection boundaries. Removal of rib anteriorly and posteriorly from these points is done piecemeal.

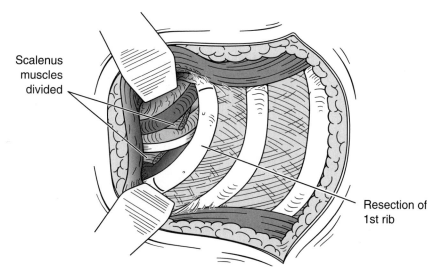

Posterior Approach

The posterior subscapular approach proposed by Clagett in 1962 and refined by Kline is not frequently employed but is very useful, especially in cases of recurrent thoracic outlet syndrome when the problem is due to a persistent posterior stump of rib impinging on the lower plexus.[49] This approach gives excellent exposure of the posterior first rib, any cervical rib, and the proximal lower trunk of the plexus. It is a technically demanding procedure; the trapezius must be transected, leading to the possibility of scapular instability and significant postoperative pain.

The patient is positioned prone with the arm on the operative side abducted and placed on a padded Mayo stand beside the table.[50] A skin incision extending from approximately the C6 level to below the inferior angle of the scapula is opened halfway between the spinous processes and the medial border of the scapula (Fig. 164-11). The trapezius muscle is divided along the same line and is extended up into the lower cervical area. The rhomboids and often the levator scapulae are also divided. The Mayo stand is then lowered, allowing the scapula to retract laterally and exposing the upper three ribs and their costotransverse junctions. The first rib is deep and the second rib may be mistaken for it. Careful palpation is essential.

The posterior scalene muscle is transected, exposing the posterior first rib. Cautious, blunt dissection around the first rib superiorly and inferiorly frees it from the deeper endothoracic fascia and the intercostal muscles. The C8 nerve root and its junction with the T1 nerve must be felt and seen and carried laterally to the formation of the lower trunk. With these elements thus identified and protected, the rib can be transected at the costovertebral junction. There is no need to remove the most proximal rib head at its attachment to the transverse process, pedicle, and vertebral body.

The rib is then removed piecemeal, but extraperiosteally from medial to lateral while protecting the plexus. The medial scalene will be transected. The most proximal parts of the lower plexus from the cervical foramina to the distal trunks are thus exposed. The view of the C8 and T1 roots is better in this exposure than in any other. Full visualization of the lower trunk is possible in a relatively shallow operative field. Access to the proximal first rib is also the most direct with this approach. If the lower spinal nerves or the lower trunk are impinged on by the first rib, the posterior approach provides the safest, most direct means of separating these structures and further resecting the first rib. Thorough repair of the rhomboids and trapezius at closure is essential to prevent scapular instability and pain. Use of a postoperative sling for 3 weeks is recommended.

This is an excellent procedure for exploration of the proximal lower plexus but comes at a high cost in terms of potential postoperative shoulder instability and pain. It is ideal for treatment of cervicothoracic paraspinal tumors. In the setting of a thoracic outlet syndrome, it is most useful in, and best reserved for, re-exploration of failed thoracic outlet surgery, especially after the transaxillary approach. The posterior approach for re-exploration avoids the scarring around the thoracic outlet caused by the first procedure and allows surgery in a clear field beginning in normal, unaltered anatomy.

RESULTS

The results of surgery for the "true" thoracic outlet syndrome patients who have been reported are rather discouraging. The arm pain—usually not a major issue—generally decreases, but the weakness and atrophy in the hand persist.[14,21] The weakness and atrophy are arrested, halting the progressive deterioration. The failure to reverse these

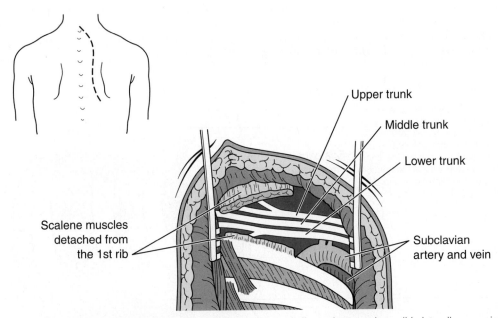

FIGURE 164-11   The posterior parascapular approach splits the trapezius and allows the scapula to slide laterally, exposing the upper ribs. The first rib may be hidden above and behind the second. It must be searched for and identified. Resection of the posterior scalene will expose the proximal lower trunk. This is the best view of the proximal lower plexus.

latter findings is no doubt due to the long delay before patients are correctly diagnosed and presented for surgery, leading to severe atrophy and permanent change in muscles and nerves.

The results of surgery for the "disputed" thoracic outlet syndrome have varied widely. Good initial results are reported in a wide range from 43% to 92%.[51] This great variability is likely due to the lack of objective diagnostic criteria and outcome criteria. Each paper reporting results has its own system for defining the diagnosis and the outcome. There is no agreement on a set of standards to investigate this syndrome. Patient selection and outcome are frequently evaluated by the operating surgeon, and objective criteria and rigorous analysis are lacking. Even though an excellent result in up to 90% of patients is reported initially, the percentage of good results decreases with longer follow-up. Good result reports can drop from 90% at 1 month postsurgery to 70% at 2-year follow-up.[44] A recurrence rate of about 20% has been reported in many series of transaxillary procedures done for the "disputed" thoracic outlet syndrome.

Except for the well-delineated "true" thoracic outlet syndrome, the thoracic outlet syndrome is a vaguely defined grouping based on quite variable criteria. The diagnosis is based almost entirely on subjective complaints. There are few, if any, objective findings to evaluate outcome. When considered in combination with the risk for serious complications and the high recurrence rate, these factors should prompt a careful approach to treatment of this problem. Surgery for the symptoms of thoracic outlet syndrome in the absence of objective physical findings or structural abnormalities should be approached cautiously.

Nonetheless, there appear to be a number of patients with an upper limb pain syndrome consistent with the "disputed" thoracic outlet syndrome. Some have a cervical rib and no electrophysiologic or clinical evidence of nerve compression. Some have minor neurophysiologic changes but no clear abnormalities around the thoracic outlet. Advocates of the "disputed" syndrome believe that these patients can be, and are, helped by surgery; doubtless some are helped. Determining which patients will be helped and which sign, symptom, or combination of both will predict success is the critical problem and a question which has yet to be definitively answered.

REFERENCES

1. Peet RM, Henricksen JD, Anderson TP, et al: Thoracic-outlet syndrome: Evaluation of a therapeutic exercise program. Mayo Clin Proc Staff Meet 31:231–287, 1956.
2. Pang D, Wessel H: Thoracic outlet syndrome. Neurosurgery 22:105–121, 1988.
3. Glass BA: The relationship of axillary vein thrombosis to the thoracic outlet syndrome. Ann Thorac Surg 19:613–621, 1975.
4. Reilly LM, Stoney RJ: Supraclavicular approach for thoracic outlet decompression. J Vasc Surg 8:329–334, 1988.
5. Roos DB: Congenital anomalies associated with thoracic outlet syndrome: Anatomy, symptoms, diagnosis, treatment. Ann J Surg 132:771–778, 1976.
6. Urschel HC Jr, Razzuk MA: Upper plexus thoracic outlet syndrome: Optimal therapy. Ann Thorac Surg 63:935–939, 1997.
7. Wilbourn AJ, Porter JM: Neurogenic thoracic outlet syndrome: Surgical vs. conservative therapy. J Vasc Surg 15:881–891, 1992.
8. Roos DB: The place for scalenectomy and first rib resection in thoracic outlet syndrome. Surgery 92:1077–1085, 1982.
9. Connolly JF, Deane R: Non-union of the clavicle and thoracic outlet syndrome. J Trauma 29:1127–1133, 1989.
10. DellaSanta D, Narakas A, Bonnard C: Late lesions of the brachial plexus after fracture of the clavicle. Ann Hand Surg 10:531–540, 1991.
11. Barbier O, Malghem J, Delaere O, et al: Injury to the brachial plexus by a fragment of bone after fracture of the clavicle. J Bone Joint Surg Br 79:534–536, 1997.
12. Novak CB: Thoracic outlet syndrome. Clin Plastic Surg 30:175–188, 2003.
13. Mackinnon SE, Novak CB: Evaluation of the patient with thoracic outlet syndrome. Semin Thorac Cardiovasc Surg 8:190–200, 1996.
14. Gilliatt RW, Lequesne PM, Logue V, Sumner AJ: Wasting of the hand associated with a cervical rib or band. J Neurol Neurosurg Psychiatry 33:615–626, 1970.
15. Roos DB: New concepts of thoracic outlet syndrome that explain etiology, symptoms, diagnosis and treatment. Vasc Surg 13:313–321, 1979.
16. Wilbourn AJ: Thoracic outlet syndromes. Neurol Clin 17:477–497, 1999.
17. Kai Y, Oyama M, Kurose S, et al: Neurogenic thoracic outlet syndrome in whiplash injury. J Spinal Disord 14:487–493, 2001.
18. Sanders RJ, Jackson CGR, Banchero N, Pearce WH: Scalene muscle abnormalities in traumatic thoracic outlet syndrome. Am J Surg 159:231–236, 1990.
19. Roos DB: Thoracic outlet syndromes: Update 1987. Am J Surg 154:568–573, 1987.
20. Machleder HI, Moll F, Verity A: The anterior scalene muscle in thoracic outlet compression syndrome: Histochemical and morphometric studies. Arch Surg 121:1141–1144, 1986.
21. Hardy RW Jr, Wilbourn A, Hanson M: Surgical treatment of compressive cervical band. Neurosurgery 7:10–13, 1980.
22. Roos DB: Thoracic outlet syndrome is underdiagnosed. Muscle Nerve 22:126–129, 1999.
23. Urschel HC Jr, Razzuk MA: Neurovascular compression at the thoracic outlet. Changing management over 50 years. Ann Surg 228:609–617, 1998.
24. Sobey AVF, Grewal RP, Hutchinson KJ, Urschel JD: Investigation of nonspecific neurogenic thoracic outlet syndrome. J Cardiovasc Surg 34:343–345, 1993.
25. Gergoudis R, Barnes RW: Thoracic outlet compression: Prevalence in normal persons. Angiology 31:538–541, 1980.
26. Costigan DA, Wilbourn AJ: The elevated arm stress test: Specificity in the diagnosis of thoracic outlet syndrome. Neurology 35 (Suppl 1): 74, 1985.
27. Plewa MC, Delinger M: The false-positive rate of thoracic outlet syndrome shoulder maneuvers in healthy subjects. Acad Emerg Med 5:337–342, 1998.
28. LeForestier N, Moulonguet A, Maisonobe T, et al: True neurogenic thoracic outlet syndrome: Electrophysiological diagnosis in six cases. Muscle Nerve 21:1129–1134, 1998.
29. Kothari MJ, Macintosh K, Heistant M, Logigian EL: Medial antebrachial cutaneous sensory studies in the evaluation of neurogenic thoracic outlet syndrome. Muscle Nerve 21:647–649, 1998.
30. Jerrett SA, Cuzzone LJ, Pasternak BM: Thoracic outlet syndrome. Electrophysiologic reappraisal. Arch Neurol 41:960–963, 1984.
31. Machleder HI, Moll F, Nuwer M, Jordan SL: Somatosensory evoked potentials in the assessment of thoracic outlet compression syndrome. J Vasc Surg 6:177–184, 1987.
32. Veilleux M, Stevens JC, Campbell JK: Somatosensory evoked potentials: Lack of value for diagnosis of thoracic outlet syndrome. Muscle Nerve 11:571–575, 1998.
33. Komanetsky RM, Novak CB, Mackinnon SE, et al: Somatosensory evoked potentials fail to diagnose thoracic outlet syndrome. J Hand Surg Am 21:662–666, 1996.
34. Urschel HC, Razzuk MA: Management of the thoracic outlet syndrome. N Engl J Med 286:1140–1143, 1972.
35. Bilbey JH, Muller NL, Connell DG, et al: Thoracic outlet syndrome: Evaluation with CT. Radiology 171:381–384, 1989.
36. Panegyres PK, Moore N, Gibson R, et al: Thoracic outlet syndromes and magnetic resonance imaging. Brain 116:823–841, 1993.
37. Lindgren KA: Conservative treatment of thoracic outlet syndrome: A 2 year follow-up. Arch Phys Med Rehabil 78:373–378, 1997.
38. Kenny RA, Traynor GB, Withington D, Keegan DJ: Thoracic outlet syndrome: A useful exercise treatment option. Am J Surg 165:282–284, 1993.

39. Clagett OT: Presidential address: Research and prosearch. J Thorac Cardiovasc Surg 44:153–166, 1962.

40. Falconer MA, Li FWP: Resection of the first rib in costoclavicular compression of the brachial plexus. Lancet 13:59–63, 1962.

41. Maxey TS, Reece TB, Ellman PI, et al: Safety and efficacy of the supraclavicular approach to thoracic outlet decompression. Ann Thorac Surg 76:396–400, 2003.

42. Maxwell-Armstrong CA, Noorpuri BSW, Abdul-Haque S, Bake DM, et al: Long-term results of surgical decompression of the thoracic outlet compression syndrome. J R Coll Surg Edinb 46:35–38, 2001.

43. Cheng SWK, Reilly LM, Nelken NA, et al: Neurogenic thoracic outlet decompression: Rationale for sparing the first rib. Cardiovasc Surg 3:617–623, 1995.

44. Sanders RJ, Pearce WH: The treatment of thoracic outlet syndrome. A comparison of different operations. J Vasc Surg 10:626–634, 1989.

45. Roos DB: Essentials and safeguards of surgery for thoracic outlet syndrome. Angiology 32:187–193, 1981.

46. Horowitz SH: Brachial plexus injuries with causalgia resulting from transaxillary rib resection. Arch Surg 120:1189–1191, 1985.

47. Dale WA: Thoracic outlet compression syndrome: Critique in 1982. Arch Surg 117:1437–1445, 1982.

48. Melliere D, Becquemin JP, Etienne G, LeCheviller B: Severe injuries resulting from operations for thoracic outlet syndrome: Can they be avoided? J Cardiovasc Surg 32:599–603, 1991.

49. Kline DG, Kott J, Barnes G, et al: Exploration of selected brachial plexus lesions by the posterior subscapular approach. J Neurosurg 49:872–880, 1978.

50. Dubuisson A, Kline DG, Weinshel SS: Posterior subscapular approach to the brachial plexus. Report of 102 patients. J Neurosurg 79:319–330, 1993.

51. Lindgren KA, Oksala I: Long term outcome of surgery for thoracic outlet syndrome. Am J Surg 169:358–360, 1995.

165 Surgical Management of Median Nerve Compression at the Wrist by Open Technique

ALEXANDRA K. SCHMIDEK and JONATHAN M. WINOGRAD

INTRODUCTION

Carpal tunnel syndrome is the most common compressive neuropathy of the upper extremity. The prevalence of electrophysiologically confirmed, symptomatic carpal tunnel syndrome is approximately 3% among women and 2% among men, with a peak prevalence in women older than 55 years of age.[1] Because carpal tunnel syndrome can be effectively treated by division of the transverse carpal ligament, carpal tunnel release is the most common hand operation performed, with 300,000 to 500,000 operations each year at a total cost of more than $2 billion.[2]

Sir James Paget[3] first described carpal tunnel syndrome in 1854. However, the first surgical release of the transverse carpal ligament for median nerve compression was not described until 1924, when Drs. Herbert Galloway and Andrew Mackinnon performed the procedure in a patient with post-traumatic neuropathy.[4] The patient continued to have pain, and hospital records report that in the following year "Dr. Galloway reoperated and found that the palmar cutaneous nerve was excised." Injury to the palmar cutaneous branch of the median nerve remains a significant and relatively common complication of carpal tunnel surgery in the modern era.

PATHOPHYSIOLOGY

Carpal tunnel syndrome is caused by elevated pressure in the carpal tunnel, with subsequent median nerve ischemia resulting in impaired nerve conduction, paresthesia, and pain.[5] The earliest manifestation of a low-grade peripheral nerve compression is reduced epineurial blood flow, which occurs at 20 to 30 mm Hg of compression. At 30 mm Hg of compression, axonal transport is impaired, and at 30 to 40 mm Hg of median nerve compression, neurophysiologic changes and symptoms of paresthesias have been induced in human volunteers.[6] Experimental compression of 50 mm Hg for 2 hours induces axonal transport block, and pressures greater than 60 mm Hg cause complete intraneural ischemia, exhibited as complete sensory block followed by complete motor block. Although short periods of nerve compression are well tolerated, recovery after chronic nerve compression may be slow or nonexistent, suggesting that the initial vascular insult is compounded by other mechanical processes, such as fibrosis of the nerve, that diminish the potential for recovery.[7] Nerve compression lesions therefore exist along a spectrum that can be divided into early, intermediate, and late categories. In early stages of compression, no morphologic changes are observable in the median nerve, and symptoms may respond to nonoperative forms of therapy such as splinting or steroid injection. Intermediate stages result from persistent interference of intraneural microcirculation, with resultant segmental demyelination. The attendant paresthesias and numbness can be alleviated by mechanical decompression of the nerve, as in carpal tunnel release. In advanced stages of nerve compression, long-standing ischemia results in endoneural fibrosis, and nerve dysfunction may be irreversible.

PRESENTATION

Idiopathic carpal tunnel syndrome is a chronic, progressive neuropathy of the median nerve at the carpal tunnel. Up to one-third of cases of idiopathic carpal tunnel syndrome are associated with a variety of medical conditions. Some of these conditions lead directly to compression by causing a decrease in the size or an increase in the contents of the carpal tunnel, whereas others are multifactorial. These conditions include pregnancy, renal failure, inflammatory arthritis, Colles' fracture, amyloidosis, hypothyroidism, diabetes mellitus, acromegaly, and the use of corticosteroids and estrogens.[8] Screening for metabolic abnormalities and common coexistent medical conditions should therefore be a routine part of the diagnostic evaluation. In the absence of anatomic or metabolic anomalies, compression of the median nerve in carpal tunnel syndrome is generally attributed to hypertrophy of the synovium of the flexor tendons within the carpal canal. Recently, Talmor and colleagues[9] found upregulation of cyclooxygenase-2 in the tenosynovium of patients with carpal tunnel syndrome, suggesting that cyclooxygenase-2 may play a role in the pathologic tissue remodeling of tenosynovitis, thereby offering a therapeutic target for inhibition.

Carpal tunnel syndrome has been reported to be more prevalent among patients who use excessive force or who sustain repeated trauma to their hands.[10] Occupations associated with a high incidence of carpal tunnel syndrome include food-processing, manufacturing, logging, and construction work, although there has not been conclusive evidence that repetitive stress is a major etiologic factor in the development of the syndrome.[11]

Finally, acute carpal tunnel syndrome may occur in the setting of severe trauma, most commonly with fractures of the distal radius. This progressive condition is a subset of acute compartment syndromes and must be surgically decompressed within 6 to 8 hours to prevent irreversible nerve damage.

Idiopathic carpal tunnel syndrome occurs more commonly in women 40 to 60 years of age and is often bilateral. The clinical evaluation of the patient with suspected carpal tunnel syndrome should begin with a careful history. The classic clinical presentation consists of the insidious onset of pain and paresthesias in the median nerve distribution, which includes the palmar aspect of the thumb, index, and long fingers and the radial half of the ring finger. These symptoms are often worse at night, and patients may note that their fingers seem to "go to sleep" when their wrists are in the positions used for driving, sleeping, or typing. On detailed questioning, patients may be able to relate that symptoms do not affect the small finger, although some patients may complain of involvement of the entire hand, with radiation as proximal as the shoulder. A diagram of the hand may be useful to enable patients to localize their symptoms. Some patients will also report clumsiness of the hand, including a tendency to drop small objects. This can be due to decreased median nerve sensibility, decreased oil secretion of the palmar skin from denervation of sympathetic nerves to the skin adnexa, or thenar weakness in advanced cases. In work-related carpal tunnel syndrome, symptoms are elicited by certain activities and are relieved by cessation of these motions.

In addition to a careful history, several provocative maneuvers may assist in the diagnosis of carpal tunnel syndrome. However, no one clinical test has been universally accepted as diagnostic. In Phalen's maneuver, the wrist is flexed for 60 seconds and the patient reports whether this elicits pain or paresthesia in the median nerve distribution. In Phalen's original description[12] of 654 patients with carpal tunnel syndrome, he reported a sensitivity of 74% for the wrist flexion test. Tinel's sign is present if light percussion over the volar wrist causes radiating paresthesia in the digits innervated by the median nerve. The sensitivity of Tinel's sign ranges from 23% to 67%, although its specificity is higher (67% to 93%).[13-15] In the pressure provocation test, the examiner's thumb is pressed over the carpal tunnel for 30 seconds,[16] and in the tourniquet test, a blood pressure cuff is inflated around the arm above systolic blood pressure for 60 seconds. Both of these tests are positive if they elicit paresthesias in the median nerve distribution. Flexion of the wrist with pressure over the median nerve for 20 seconds had sensitivity of 82% and specificity of 99%.[17] As there is no gold standard clinical test with both high sensitivity and specificity, a combination of provocative tests may be most useful when attempting to diagnose carpal tunnel syndrome.[13] Additionally, Semmes-Weinstein monofilament and vibration testing have been found to be more sensitive than two-point discrimination when assessing early median nerve dysfunction.[18] Thenar atrophy and abnormal two-point discrimination suggest late-stage median nerve compression.

Electrodiagnostic testing is the only objective means of localizing and quantifying nerve dysfunction and thus remains the diagnostic gold standard. Such testing may be used in conjunction with the patient history and clinical examination to diagnose carpal tunnel syndrome, or it can be used to document the progress or resolution of a neuropathy. However, electrodiagnostic testing is highly operator dependent and should therefore be done by the same operator and equipment each time. In general, distal motor latencies of more than 4.5 milliseconds and distal sensory latencies of more than 3.5 milliseconds are considered abnormal. Nerve conduction latencies and velocities can be compared with established population norms, with the contralateral nerve, or with previous tests in the same patient. Asymmetry of conduction between both hands of more than 1 millisecond for motor conduction and 0.5 millisecond for sensory conduction is considered abnormal.

THE DOUBLE-CRUSH SYNDROME

The "double-crush" hypothesis was introduced by Upton and McComas[19] in 1973 to describe the concept that compression of a nerve at one site decreases its ability to withstand additional compression distally (Fig. 165-1).

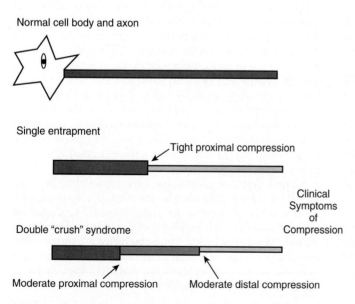

FIGURE 165-1 Schematic of axonal involvement in double-crush syndrome. (Redrawn from Simpson RL, Fern SA: Multiple compression neuropathies and the double-crush syndrome. Orthop Clin North Am 27:381–388, 1996.)

Normal cell body and axon

Single entrapment

Tight proximal compression

Clinical
Symptoms
of
Compression

Double "crush" syndrome

Moderate proximal compression   Moderate distal compression

It has become an accepted theory that a decrease in axonal flow at one site that may be insufficient to cause clinical symptoms will render the nerve more susceptible to symptomatic compression at a second site along the course of the same nerve. Mackinnon[20] has extended this concept, noting that multiple compressions along a nerve have a cumulative effect on conduction. This concept is particularly applicable to forearm compression syndromes and certain job-related overuse syndromes in which repetitive maneuvers of the arm can produce multiple levels of compression.[21] Clinical correlation of the double-crush phenomenon is also demonstrated by the high incidence of concurrent carpal tunnel syndrome in patients with cervical radiculopathy; in one study by Yu and colleagues,[22] 11% of patients with carpal tunnel syndrome showed signs of cervical radiculopathy. Certain metabolic abnormalities such as diabetes, myxedema, uremia, and pyridoxine deficiency can be thought of as the proximal "crush" that renders the nerve more susceptible to a compressive insult.[23] Accordingly, approximately 17% of patients with carpal tunnel syndrome have a history of diabetes mellitus.[24] Dellon[25] is an advocate of early peripheral nerve decompression in patients with diabetes if there is clinical evidence of specific-site compression, reporting 100% improvement after nerve decompression in cases of peripheral diabetic neuropathy and localized nerve entrapment.

With this in mind, the diagnosis of carpal tunnel syndrome should consider the possibility of coexistent cervical root compression, thoracic outlet syndrome, or a similar more proximal lesion of the same nerve. Operative release of the carpal tunnel may relieve the patient's symptoms without the need to release all sites. Alternatively, coexistent cervical root compression is one of the reasons for persistent residual symptoms after carpal tunnel release. Of note, the intraoperative findings of a narrowing of the median nerve may be quite minimal because the overall symptomatology is being created by the summation of the effects of several different sites of nerve compression.

ANATOMY OF THE CARPAL TUNNEL

The carpal tunnel is an inelastic structure located at the base of the palm, just distal to the distal wrist crease (Fig. 165-2). The tunnel itself is approximately 5 cm long, with its narrowest portion abutting the hook of the hamate (Fig. 165-3). Although the carpal tunnel is open ended proximally and distally, it behaves like a closed compartment physiologically.[26] It is bounded on three sides by the carpal bones, which form a concave arch, and on the palmar side by the unyielding transverse carpal ligament. Nine flexor tendons and the median nerve traverse the carpal tunnel. The flexor retinaculum has three components: the deep forearm fascia, the transverse carpal ligament, and, most distally, the palmar aponeurosis between the thenar and hypothenar muscles. At the distal edge of the retinaculum, the nerve normally divides into six branches: the recurrent motor branch, two common digital nerves, and three proper digital nerves. Iatrogenic nerve injury during carpal tunnel surgery usually involves one of the branches of the median nerve, most commonly the palmar cutaneous branch, which originates from the radiopalmar aspect of the median nerve approximately 8 cm proximal to the wrist crease. This branch courses directly beneath the thenar crease and can be inadvertently transected during exposure of the transverse carpal ligament, leading to a painful neuroma of the surgical scar.[27] Anatomic variations of median nerve anatomy have been

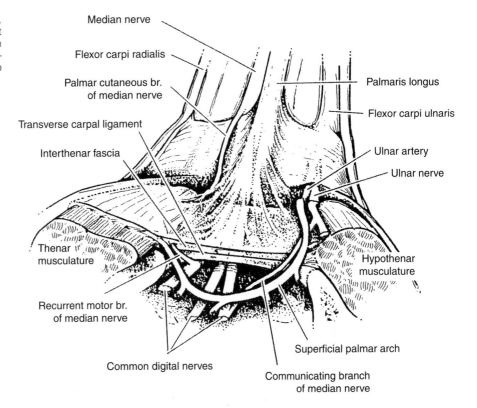

FIGURE 165-2 The carpal tunnel, located at the base of the palm, is just distal to the distal wrist crease. (Redrawn from Mirza MA, King ET: Newer techniques of carpal tunnel release. Orthop Clin North Am 27:357–371, 1996.)

Median nerve
Flexor carpi radialis
Palmar cutaneous br. of median nerve
Transverse carpal ligament
Interthenar fascia
Thenar musculature
Recurrent motor br. of median nerve
Common digital nerves
Palmaris longus
Flexor carpi ulnaris
Ulnar artery
Ulnar nerve
Hypothenar musculature
Superficial palmar arch
Communicating branch of median nerve

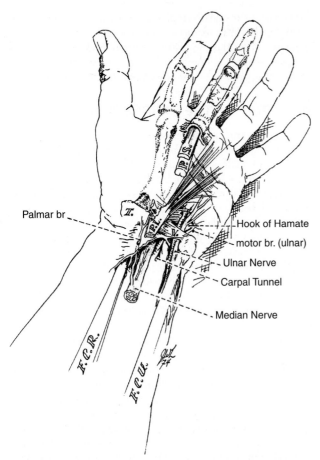

Palmar br.
Hook of Hamate
motor br. (ulnar)
Ulnar Nerve
Carpal Tunnel
Median Nerve

FIGURE 165-3 The carpal tunnel is approximately 5 cm long; its narrowest portion abuts the hook of the hamate. (Redrawn from Burton RI, Littler JW: Nontraumatic soft tissue afflictions of the hand. Curr Probl Surg 12:1–56, 1975.)

described by Lanz.[28] The recurrent motor branch of the median nerve has three major variants: extraligamentous (46%), subligamentous (31%), and transligamentous (23%) (Fig. 165-4).[29] A communicating branch between the ulnar and median nerves is present in as many as 90% of cases and may lie close to the distal edge of the transverse carpal ligament.[30] The superficial palmar arch is located from 2 to 26 mm from the distal edge of the transverse carpal ligament and is often hidden within a fat pad, making it vulnerable to iatrogenic injury.[31] A useful estimation of the location of the superficial palmar arch may be obtained with Kaplan's cardinal line, a transverse line drawn from the base of the thumb web space across the palm. Finally, the proximal entrance to Guyon's canal lies just ulnar to the carpal tunnel at the level of the distal wrist flexion crease. The introduction of devices into this area during endoscopic techniques may lead to inadvertent release of Guyon's canal (and unrecognized failure to release the transverse carpal ligament) or injury to the ulnar neurovascular bundle.[32]

CONSERVATIVE TREATMENT

When carpal tunnel syndrome is associated with an underlying medical condition, such as inflammatory arthritis, hypothyroidism, and diabetes mellitus, treatment of the associated condition is appropriate and may alleviate carpal tunnel symptoms. Nonoperative management also includes splinting and corticosteroid injection. More than 80% of patients with carpal tunnel syndrome report that splinting the wrist in a neutral position while sleeping alleviates symptoms, often within days.[33] Splinting has been demonstrated to reduce sensory latency and may alter the underlying course of carpal tunnel syndrome.[34]

Although there is no evidence that oral nonsteroidal antiinflammatory medications, diuretics, or pyridoxine (vitamin B_6) are efficacious in alleviating the symptoms of carpal tunnel syndrome, local corticosteroid injection has been found to be superior to injection of placebo, and more than 75% of patients experience an improvement in their symptoms.[35,36] Local steroid injection is associated

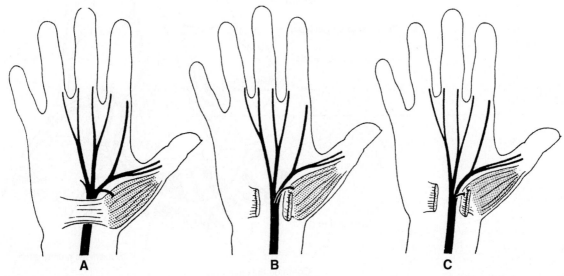

A   B   C

FIGURE 165-4 The recurrent motor branch of the median nerve has three major variants: extraligamentous (46%), subligamentous (31%), and transligamentous (23%). (Redrawn from Lanz U: Anatomic variations of the median nerve in the carpal tunnel. J Hand Surg [Am] 2:44–53, 1977.)

with improvement in median nerve conduction, but symptoms generally recur within 1 year.[37] A 25-gauge needle is used to inject a solution of 1 mL (8 mg) of dexamethasone acetate (Decadron) and 2 mL of 1% lidocaine into the carpal tunnel 1 cm proximal to the distal wrist flexion crease between the palmaris longus and flexor carpi radialis tendons. If the patient complains of sudden paresthesias, the needle should be redirected before injecting the steroid solution. Dexamethasone (Decadron) has been shown experimentally to be better tolerated than other steroids such as triamcinolone acetonide (Kenalog) if inadvertently injected into the nerve in an intrafascicular location.[38] Within a few minute, numbness from the lidocaine in the median distribution confirms proper placement. Steroid injection may be followed by splinting in the neutral position. It should be noted that steroid injection is not an entirely benign procedure: Injection of steroid agents into the nerve itself can result in severe and lasting damage to the involved nerve.[39] Nonetheless, steroid injection can offer significant symptomatic relief from carpal tunnel syndrome. A strong correlation has been demonstrated between patients with a good response to steroid injection and those with good results after surgical management, with relief from steroid injection as the best predictor for success of surgery.[40,41]

SURGICAL MANAGEMENT

There are several surgical approaches to carpal tunnel release. The open method remains the standard approach for patients who have failed conservative management. In the traditional open procedure, the surgeon makes a 4- to 6-cm long incision extending distally from the distal wrist crease and releases the transverse carpal ligament under direct visualization. The open method of carpal tunnel release affords the advantage of direct visualization of the structures within the carpal tunnel and confirmation of complete release of the transverse carpal ligament. It is a reliable, reproducible procedure that can be performed quickly and safely under regional or local anesthesia. Inherent in this technique is the ability to identify and address anomalous anatomy or pathology. The most frequent patient complaint after the open technique is a painful scar or persistent symptoms. Kushner and colleagues[42] reviewed 14 studies on open carpal tunnel release, including 3035 cases. A nerve injury rate of 0.8% was reported, with the palmar cutaneous branch being most commonly involved. The overall complication rate of the open technique is approximately 1% to 2%. Two alternate approaches have been reported: limited incision techniques and the endoscopic carpal tunnel release.

Endoscopic technology is increasingly being applied to a variety of surgical conditions within the majority of surgical subspecialties. Although endoscopy is typically performed in a joint, viscus, or hollow body cavity, the carpal tunnel is none of these and is remarkable for both its anatomic intricacy and limited size.[43] Several endoscopic methods have been described in carpal tunnel surgery, each of which relies heavily on topographic landmarks to define the location of surgical anatomy and to compensate for reduced operative exposure. The first of these endoscopic carpal tunnel procedures were reported by Chow[44] and Okutsu and colleagues[45] in 1989 and by Agee and colleagues[46] in 1994.

These techniques avoid making incisions on the palmar aspect of the hand in an attempt to decrease postoperative morbidity.[47] Currently, there are two commonly used endoscopic techniques: the Chow[48-50] two-portal technique and the Agee single-portal incision technique.[51,52] Both of these techniques involve the placement of a specially designed blunt instrument beneath the transverse carpal ligament, with division of that structure by endoscopic visualization. These techniques have been reported to be equivalent to traditional techniques in alleviating the symptoms of carpal tunnel syndrome.[53] The benefits and drawbacks of endoscopic release remain controversial. Even proponents of endoscopic techniques do not claim better long-term results; rather, they cite less postoperative pain, a more rapid recovery, and earlier return to activities of daily living and work.[54] Thus the main advantage of endoscopic carpal tunnel release is that patients have decreased incision pain for the first 3 weeks postoperatively.[55] However, endoscopic techniques have a steep learning curve, higher complications such as neurovascular and tendon injuries, and extra expense in equipment and operating time. As visualization is limited, it may be difficult to distinguish between synovium and nerve tissue, putting critical structures at risk. Injury to the recurrent motor branch, particularly with an aberrant branch pattern, continues to be a drawback. Also, there seems to be a statistically higher incidence of recurrence of carpal tunnel syndrome after endoscopic release compared with the traditional open release.[56] According to recent studies, the overall complication rate is probably between 1% and 2% in experienced hands for both endoscopic and open carpal tunnel release.[57] However, it should be noted that the nature of these complications is different. Although a complete laceration of the median or ulnar nerve is a devastating and exceedingly rare complication of open carpal tunnel release, it is a reported complication of endoscopic carpal tunnel release even when done by experienced surgeons.[58]

In an attempt to combine the benefits of open and endoscopic techniques, Lee and Strickland[59] developed a limited open technique using a small palmar incision and a set of specially designed instruments known as the Indiana Tome system (Fig. 165-5). In this technique, a 1.5-cm palmar incision is made over the transverse carpal ligament, and a set of three specially designed strippers (Biomet, Warsaw, IN) is used to sequentially develop the spaces superficial and deep to the transverse carpal ligament. The blade of a front-cutting scalpel, the Indiana Tome, is then advanced through the length of the ligament. In a study comparing two-portal endoscopic release and limited open release using Indiana Tome system in patients with bilateral carpal tunnel system, the patients in the limited open group had significantly less scar tenderness and postoperative pain and expressed a subjective preference for limited open versus endoscopic release.[60] Despite this relative advantage, the increased risk inherent in this alternative limited exposure technique remains a challenge.

Surgical Technique

Approximately 15 mL of local anesthetic (a 1:1 mixture of 0.5% bupivacaine and 1% lidocaine) is infiltrated subcutaneously over the median nerve at the wrist and palm in the

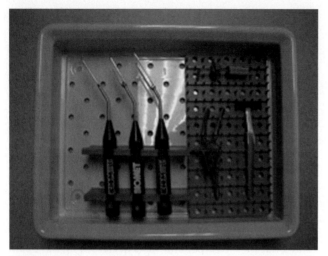

FIGURE 165-5 The Indiana Tome carpal tunnel release system. (Courtesy of Biomet, Warsaw, IN.)

area of the incision and also directly into the carpal tunnel. A nonsterile pneumatic tourniquet is placed on the forearm, and the limb is prepped and draped to the elbow in the standard fashion.

The proposed incision is marked 4 mm ulnar to and parallel with the intrathenar crease (Fig. 165-6). As opposed to incisions within the thenar crease, this more ulnar incision is well away from the course of the palmar cutaneous branch of the median nerve. Its ulnar location also attempts to avoid the anomalous recurrent motor branch of the median nerve and ensures that wound healing is not occurring directly over the median nerve.[61] The beginning of the incision is just proximal to Kaplan's cardinal line (a transverse line drawn from the ulnar border of the maximally abducted and extended thumb) and ends proximally at the distal wrist crease.

After adequate anesthesia has been achieved, the arm is exsanguinated with an Esmark bandage, and the tourniquet is inflated to 250 mm Hg. The skin incision is made with

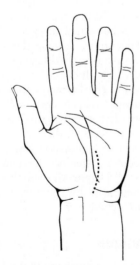

FIGURE 165-6 The proposed incision is marked 4 mm ulnar to and parallel with the intrathenar crease. (Redrawn from Mackinnon SE: Carpal tunnel syndrome. Surg Neurol 47:105–114, 1997.)

a no. 15 blade under loupe magnification. The incision is extended through the subcutaneous tissue and the silvery fibers of superficial palmar fascia using a combination of sharp and transverse blunt dissection until the transverse carpal ligament is visualized. Care is taken to avoid any crossing sensory branches from the palmar cutaneous nerve, and the fat is handled gently to provide a cushion between the scar and the median nerve. Muscle fibers of the abductor pollicis brevis may be seen crossing the midline. A bipolar electrocautery is used to achieve meticulous hemostasis. The transverse carpal ligament is scored with a no. 15 blade until it has been divided. The division is then extended distally until the distal edge has been divided, just proximal to the superficial palmar arch, often denoted by the presence of a fat pad. The release is then extended proximally to the edge of the antebrachial fascia. Blunt retractors are used to expose the fascia, which is cleared of soft tissue superficially and the median nerve deeply and divided under direct vision with a Stevens tenotomy scissors. A finger should pass easily into the forearm proximally and the palmar subcutaneous tissues distally without restriction at the completion of the release. A tenosynovectomy is then performed if necessary, and the carpal tunnel is carefully inspected for space-occupying lesions or bony prominences. The wound is then irrigated with normal saline and careful hemostasis is achieved. The skin is closed with a single layer of interrupted 4-0 nylon horizontal mattress sutures. This is followed by a bulky dressing and a volar plaster splint to keep the wrist in a neutral position. The tourniquet is deflated after the dressing has been applied, and the hand is strictly elevated to minimize postoperative edema and hematoma formation. The wrist is splinted for 1 week to prevent bowstringing of the flexor tendons during the early postoperative period. Early finger and thumb motion is encouraged to prevent stiffness and adhesions and to promote tendon gliding. Sutures are removed after 2 weeks. Gradual progression to full strength and motion should occur by 1 month postoperatively.

Bilateral Carpal Tunnel Release

In patients with bilateral carpal tunnel entrapment, a bilateral surgical release is efficient and cost-effective, compressing the usual 2- to 3-week recuperation into one period. Excluding patients who are dependent on walkers or canes for support, operating both sides simultaneously was found to be well tolerated in one study that used a closed technique for carpal tunnel release.[62] Nonetheless, having both hands immobilized postoperatively would represent a significant hardship for most patients, and bilateral procedures should probably be offered only after significant preoperative discussion and patient education.

Technical Controversies

The issue of neurolysis in primary and secondary carpal tunnel surgery is somewhat controversial.[63] In response to concerns that chronic compression of the median nerve results in internal fibrosis and a tight epineurial envelope, internal neurolysis and epineurotomy have been advocated as a standard part of open carpal tunnel release. Controlled clinical studies have shown no difference in the results of patients treated

TABLE 165-1 ■ Complications Associated with Carpal Tunnel Release

Complication	Clayburgh et al.[1]	Kulick et al.[2]	Fissette and Onkelinx[3]	Lichtman et al.[4]	MacDonald et al.[5]	Gainer and Nugent[6]	Ariyan and Watson[7]	Das and Brown[8]*	Hybbinette and Mannerfelt[9]	Semple and Cargill[10]	Doyle and Carroll[11]	Cseuz et al.[12]	Phalen[13]	Downie[14]
No. of cases	60	130	95	100	186	430	429	113	506	150	100	489	212	35
Nerve injury														
Palmar cutaneous	1	1	—	2	11	—	—	3	2	—	—	—	—	—
Motor branch	—	—	—	—	—	—	—	—	1	—	—	—	—	—
Digital nerve	—	—	—	—	—	—	—	—	—	3	—	—	—	—
Infection (unspecified)														
Superficial	2	—	—	—	—	26	1	—	—	—	1	—	1	—
Incomplete division of Transverse carpal Ligament	—	—	—	—	12	—	—	—	—	—	—	—	—	—
Persistence of symptoms, i.e.,	31	15	—	—	—	—	—	6	4	—	—	—	1	1
residual symptoms; hypesthesia; persistent nocturnal discomfort; pain other than incisional	—	—	—	—	—	—	—	—	13	38	2	28	—	—
Recurrence of symptoms	—	—	—	—	—	—	4	—	—	—	—	—	—	—
Painful or hypertrophic scar	7	—	5	—	2	18	—	1	6	—	—	—	1	—
Reflex sympathetic dystrophy	3	—	1	5	4	—	1	—	3	31	—	113	1	—
Hematoma	—	—	—	—	—	—	1	—	—	—	—	—	1	—
Bowstringing of flexor tendons	—	—	—	—	2	—	—	—	—	—	—	—	—	—
Adherence of flexor tendons	—	—	—	—	1	—	—	—	—	—	—	—	—	—
Weakness of wrist	—	—	24	—	—	—	—	—	—	—	—	—	—	—
Damage to superficial palmar arch	—	—	—	—	2	—	—	—	—	—	—	—	—	—

*Does not include seven cases with complications from surgery performed elsewhere, then referred to author.

From Kuschner SK, Brien WW, Johnson D, Gellman H: Complications associated with carpal tunnel release. Orthop Rev 20: p. 346, 1991.

1. Clayburgh RM, Beckenbaugh RD, Dobyns JH: Carpal tunnel release in patients with diffuse peripheral neuropathy. J Hand Surg 12(A):380–383, 1987.
2. Kulick MII, Gordillo G, Javid T, et al: Long-term analysis of patients having surgical treatment for carpal tunnel syndrome. J Hand Surg [AM] 11:59–66, 1986.
3. Fissette J, Onkelinx A: Treatment of carpal tunnel syndrome: Comparative study with and without epineurolysis. Hand 11:206–210, 1979.
4. Lichtman DM, Florio RL, Mack GR: Carpal tunnel release under local anesthesia: Evaluation of outpatient procedure. J Hang Surg 6:544–546, 1979.
5. MacDonald RI, Lichtman DM, Hanlon JJ, Wilson JN: Complications for surgical release of carpal tunnel syndrome. J Hand Surg 3:70–76, 1978.
6. Gainer JV Jr, Nugent GR: Carpal tunnel syndrome: Report of 430 operations. South Med J 70:325–328, 1977.
7. Ariyan S, Watson HK: The palmar approach for the visualization and release of the carpal tunnel: An analysis of 429 cases. Plast Reconstr Surg 60:539–547, 1977.
8. Das SK, Brown HG: In search of complications in carpal tunnel decompression. Hand 8:243–249, 1976.
9. Hybbinette CH, Mannerfelt L: The carpal tunnel syndrome: A retrospective study of 400 operated patients. Acta Othop Scand 46:610–620, 1975.
10. Semple JC, Cargill AO: Carpal-tunnel syndrome: Results of surgical decompression. Lancet 1:918–919, 1969.
11. Doyle JR, Carroll RE: The carpal tunnel syndrome: A review of 100 patients treated surgically. Calif Med 108:263–267, 1968.
12. Cseuz KA, Thomas JE, Lambert EH, et al: Long-term results of operation for carpal tunnel syndrome. Mayo Clin Proc 41:232–241, 1966.
13. Phalen GS: The carpal-tunnel syndrome. Seventeen years' experience in diagnosis and treatment of six hundred fifty-four hands. J Bone Joint Surg Am 48:211–228,1966.
14. Downie AW: "Misery in the hand"—the carpal tunnel syndrome. NC Med J 26:487–493, 1965.

with either simple decompression or decompression combined with internal neurolysis.[64-66] Epineurotomy, making a longitudinal incision into the volar surface of the nerve to release any thickened epineurium, has also not been shown to improve results compared with simple decompression and may cause neuritis or neuralgia.[67]

Thickening or enlargement of the synovium within the carpal tunnel is clearly a contributing factor to many cases of median nerve compression. However, tenosynovectomy should not necessarily be considered a benign addition to the procedure. The resultant hematoma, swelling, and inflammation may prolong the postoperative course and contribute to tendon adhesions. Therefore, the need for synovectomy should be assessed on a case-by-case basis and may best be reserved for cases in which the synovium impinges on surrounding structures, as in rheumatoid arthritis.

RESULTS

Carpal tunnel release successfully relieves symptoms in most patients. More than 70% of patients report being completely satisfied or very satisfied with the results of carpal tunnel surgery, and 70% to 90% of patients report being free of nocturnal pain postoperatively.[68] However, a small group of patients continue to have problems after carpal tunnel release. Complications after carpal tunnel surgery generally fall into one of three groups: persistent symptoms, recurrent symptoms, and new symptoms (Table 165-1). The persistence of preoperative complaints is the most common complication after carpal tunnel release, with an incidence of 7% to 20%.[63] This is most frequently due to incomplete release of the transverse carpal ligament, usually in its most distal portion. This is a complication of inadequate exposure, as may be the case in endoscopic or limited incision techniques. Secondary surgery to complete the decompression is generally curative. Preoperative symptoms may also persist because of more proximal compression of the median nerve or misdiagnosis.

Patients may do well initially after surgery, only to have their preoperative symptoms recur, usually several months after surgery. This may be due to scar formation around the median nerve or scarring with subsequent reformation of the transverse carpal ligament. Meticulous hemostasis and appropriate postoperative range-of-motion exercises can theoretically reduce morbidity associated with excessive postoperative scarring.

Finally, patients may experience new symptoms after carpal tunnel surgery. Neurologic complications usually involve one of the branches of the median nerve, or less commonly, the median nerve itself. As previously noted, iatrogenic injury to the palmar cutaneous branch of the median nerve is most frequently the problem, although other branches that may be injured include the recurrent motor branch and common digital nerves. Direct injury to the median nerve may also occur. The most superficial or anteriorly located fascicles of the median nerve are most vulnerable to injury and usually supply sensation to the third web space; injury may result in burning and numbness in the long and ring fingers. Complete median nerve transection has also been reported after carpal tunnel surgery.[69] Other neurologic complications include injury to the ulnar nerve, neuroma formation, and complex regional pain syndrome.[70,71] Vascular complications of carpal tunnel surgery include

injury to the superficial palmar arch or ulnar artery. Such injuries may be subclinical or may lead to hematoma accumulation in the palm. If unrecognized, this may ultimately progress to the devastating complication of massive necrosis of the palmar skin. Finally, wrist and tendon problems have been reported after carpal tunnel release. Carpal arch alterations are a reported complication of sectioning the transverse carpal ligament.[72] Attempts to reconstruct the carpal ligament have been associated with reformation of the carpal tunnel and recurrent symptoms. Tendon problems include anterior dislocation or bowstringing of the flexor tendons, flexor tendon adhesions, and a higher incidence of trigger finger after carpal tunnel surgery, perhaps due to the transmission of greater forces to the first annular pulley.[73]

CONCLUSION

Compression of the median nerve in the carpal tunnel is common clinical entity that can be effectively treated with surgical release of the carpal tunnel. In the words of George Phalen, "few operations indeed are as successful and rewarding both to the patient and to the surgeon as the operation for carpal-tunnel syndrome."[74] However, the inherent simplicity of carpal tunnel release should not overshadow the potential pitfalls of surgical management. Although the role of minimally invasive techniques in carpal tunnel surgery remains somewhat controversial, it is generally acknowledged that complications of carpal tunnel release can be reduced by familiarity with surgical anatomy, division of the transverse carpal ligament under direct vision, and the use of an appropriate skin incision.

REFERENCES

1. Atroshi I, Gummesson C, Johnsson R, et al: Prevalence of carpal tunnel syndrome in a general population. JAMA 282:153–158, 1999.
2. Palmer DH, Hanrahan LP: Social and economic costs of carpal tunnel surgery. Instr Course Lect 44:167–172, 1995.
3. Paget J: Lectures on Surgical Pathology, 2nd ed. Philadelphia: Lindsay and Blakiston, 1854, p 42–48.
4. Amadio PC: The Mayo Clinic and carpal tunnel syndrome. Mayo Clin Proc 67:42, 1992.
5. Gelberman R, Rydevik BL, Pess GM, et al: Carpal tunnel syndrome: A scientific basis for clinical care. Orthop Clin North Am 19:115–124, 1988.
6. Gelberman RH, Szabo RM, Williamson RV, et al: Tissue perfusion threshold for peripheral nerve viability. Clin Orthop 178:285–291, 1983.
7. Szabo RM: Entrapment and compression neuropathies. In Green DP, Hotchkiss RN, Pederson WC (eds): Green's Operative Hand Surgery, 4th ed. Philadelphia: Churchill Livingstone, 1999, pp 1404–1447.
8. Stevens JC, Beard CM, O'Fallon WM, Kurland LT: Conditions associated with carpal tunnel syndrome. Mayo Clin Proc 67:541–548, 1992.
9. Talmor M, Patel PP, Spann MD, et al: COX-2 upregulation in idiopathic carpal tunnel syndrome. Plast Reconstr Surg 112:1807–1814, 2003.
10. Silverstein BA, Fine LJ, Armstrong TJ: Occupational factors and carpal tunnel syndrome. Am J Ind Med 11: 343–358, 1987.
11. Katz JN, Simmons BP: Carpal tunnel syndrome. N Engl J Med 346: 1807–1812, 2002.
12. Phalen GS: The carpal tunnel syndrome: Seventeen years experience in diagnosis and treatment of six hundred and fifty four hands. J Bone Joint Surg Am 48:211–228, 1966.
13. Katz JN, Larson MG, Sabra A, et al: The carpal tunnel syndrome: Diagnostic utility of the history and physical examination findings. Ann Intern Med 112:321–327, 1990.
14. D'Arcy CA, McGee S: The rational clinical examination: Does this patient have carpal tunnel syndrome? JAMA 3110–3117, 2000.

15. Wiesman IM, Novak CB, Mackinnon SE, Winograd JM: Sensitivity and specificity of clinical testing for carpal tunnel syndrome. Can J Plast Surg 11:70–72, 2003.
16. Durkan JA: A new diagnostic test for carpal tunnel syndrome. J Bone Joint Surg Am 73:535–538, 1991.
17. Tetro A, Evanoff BA, Hollstien SB, Gelberman RH: A new provocative test for carpal tunnel syndrome: Assessment of wrist flexion and nerve compression. J Bone Joint Surg Br 80:493–498, 1998.
18. Gelberman H, Szabo RM, Williamson RV, Dimick MP: Sensibility testing in peripheral nerve compression syndromes: An experimental study in humans. J Bone Joint Surg Am 65:632–638, 1983.
19. Upton ARM, McComas AJ: The double crush in nerve entrapment syndromes. Lancet ii:359–362, 1973.
20. Macinnon SE: Double and multiple "crush" syndromes. Hand Clin 8:369–390, 1992.
21. Simpson RL, Fern SA: Multiple compression neuropathies and the double-crush syndrome. Orthop Clin 27:381–388, 1996.
22. Yu J, Bendler E, Montari A: Neurological disorders associated with carpal tunnel syndrome. Electromyogr Clin Neurophysiol 19:27–32, 1979.
23. Dellon AL, Mackinnon SE, Seiler WA: Susceptibility of the diabetic nerve to chronic compression. Ann Plast Surg 20:117–119, 1988.
24. Phalen GS: Reflection on 21 years experience with carpal tunnel syndrome. JAMA 212:1365–1367, 1970.
25. Dellon AL: Treatment of symptomatic diabetic neuropathy by surgical decompression of multiple peripheral nerves. Plast Reconstr Surg 89:689–697, 1992.
26. Cobb TK, Dalley BK, Posteraro RH, Lewis RC: The carpal tunnel as a compartment. An anatomic perspective. Orthop Rev 21:451–453, 1992.
27. Watchmaker GP, Weber D, Mackinnon SE: Avoidance of transection of the palmar cutaneous branch of the median nerve in carpal tunnel release. J Hand Surg [Am] 21:644–650, 1996.
28. Lanz U: Anatomical variations of the median nerve in the carpal tunnel. J Hand Surg [Am] 2:44–53, 1977.
29. Tountas CP, Bihrle DM, MacDonald CJ, Bergman RA: Variations of the median nerve in the carpal canal. J Hand Surg [Am] 12:708–712, 1987.
30. Meals RA, Shaner M: Variations in digital sensory patterns: A study of the ulnar nerve-median nerve palmar communicating branch. J Hand Surg [Am] 8:411–414, 1983.
31. Cobb TK, Knudson GA, Cooney WP: The use of topographical landmarks to improve the outcome of Agee endoscopic carpal tunnel release. Arthroscopy 11:165–172, 1995.
32. Luallin SR, Toby EB: Incidental Guyon's canal release during attempted endoscopic carpal tunnel release: An anatomical study and report of two cases. Arthroscopy 9:382–386, 1993.
33. Burke DT, Burke MM, Steward GW, Cambre A: Splinting for carpal tunnel syndrome: In search of the optimal angle. Arch Phys Med Rehabil 75:1241–1244, 1994.
34. Walker WC, Metzler M, Cifu DX, Swartz Z: Neutral wrist splinting in carpal tunnel syndrome: A comparison of night-only versus full-time wear instructions. Arch Phys Med Rehabil 81:424–429, 2000.
35. Chang MH, Chiang HT, Lee SS, et al: Oral drug of choice in carpal tunnel syndrome. Neurology 51:390–393, 1998.
36. Dammers JWHH, Cerring MM, Vermeulen M: Injection with methylprednisolone proximal to the carpal tunnel: Randomized double blind trial. BMJ 319:884–886, 1999.
37. Ayhan-Ardic FF, Erdem HR: Long-term clinical and electrophysiological results of local steroid injection in patients with carpal tunnel syndrome. Funct Neurol 15:157–165, 2000.
38. Mackinnon SE, Hudson AR, Gentili F, et al: Peripheral nerve injection injury with steroid agents. Plast Reconstr Surg 69:482–489, 1982.
39. Gentili F, Hudson AR, Kline D, et al: Peripheral nerve injection injury. Neurosurgery 4:244–253, 1979.
40. Green DP: Diagnostic and therapeutic value of carpal tunnel injection. J Hand Surg [Am] 9:850–854, 1984.
41. Edgell SE, McCabe SJ, Breidennack WC, et al: Predicting the outcome of carpal tunnel release. J Hand Surg [Am] 28:255–261, 2003.
42. Kuschner SK, Brien WW, Johnson D, Gellman H: Complications associated with carpal tunnel release. Orthop Rev 20:346–352, 1991.
43. Mirza MA, King ET: Newer techniques of carpal tunnel release. Orthop Clin 27:355–371, 1996.
44. Chow JC: Endoscopic release of the carpal ligament: A new technique for carpal tunnel syndrome. Arthroscopy 5:679–683, 1989.
45. Okutsu I, Ninomiya S, Takatori Y, et al: Endoscopic management of carpal tunnel syndrome. Arthroscopy 5:11–18, 1989.

46. Agee JM, McCarroll HR, North ER: Endoscopic carpal tunnel release using the single proximal incision technique. Hand Clin 10:647–659, 1994.
47. Agee JM, McCarroll HR, Tortosa R, et al: Endoscopic release of the carpal tunnel: A randomized prospective multicenter study. J Hand Surg [Am] 17:987–995, 1992.
48. Chow JC: Endoscopic release of the carpal ligament: A new technique for carpal tunnel syndrome. Arthroscopy 5:19–24, 1989.
49. Chow JC: Endoscopic release of the carpal ligament for carpal tunnel syndrome: 22-month clinical result. Arthroscopy 6:288–296, 1990.
50. Chow JC: Endoscopic carpal tunnel release. Two-portal technique. Hand Clin 10:637–646, 1994.
51. Agee JM, McCarroll HR, Tortosa R, et al: Endoscopic release of the carpal tunnel: A randomized prospective multicenter study. J Hand Surg [Am] 17:987–995, 1992.
52. Agee JM, Peimer CA, Pyrek JD, Walsh WE: Endoscopic carpal tunnel release: A prospective study of complications and surgical experience. J Hand Surg [Am] 20:165–171, 1995.
53. Palmer DH, Paulson JC, Lane-Larson CL, et al: Endoscopic carpal tunnel release: A comparison of two techniques with open release. Arthroscopy 9:498-508, 1993.
54. Einhorn N, Leddy JP: Pitfalls of endoscopic carpal tunnel release. Orthop Clin North Am 27:373–380, 1996.
55. Agee JM, McCarroll HRK, Tortosa RD, et al: Endoscopic release of the carpal tunnel: A randomized prospective multicenter study. J Hand Surg [Am] 17:987–995, 1992.
56. Concannon MJ, Brownfield ML, Puckett CL: The incidence of recurrence after endoscopic carpal tunnel release. Plast Reconstr Surg 105:1662–1665, 2000.
57. Einhorn N, Leddy JP: Pitfalls of endoscopic carpal tunnel release. Orthop Clin North Am 27:373–380, 1996.
58. Feinstein PA: Endoscopic carpal tunnel release in a community-based series. J Hand Surg [Am] 18:451–454, 1993.
59. Lee WP, Strickland JW: Safe carpal tunnel release via a limited palmar incision. Plast Reconstr Surg 101:418–424, 1998.
60. Wong KC, Hung LK, Ho PC, Wong JMW: Carpal tunnel release: A prospective, randomized study of endoscopic versus limited-open methods. J Bone Joint Surg Br 85:863–868, 2003.
61. Mackinnon SE: Carpal tunnel syndrome. Surg Neurol 47:105–114, 1997.
62. Pagnanelli DM, Barrer SJ: Bilateral carpal tunnel release at one operation: Report of 228 patients. Neurosurgery 31:1030–1034, 1992.
63. Tung THH, Mackinnon SE: Secondary carpal tunnel surgery. Plast Reconstr Surg 107:1830–1843, 2001.
64. Holmgreen-Larsson H, Leszniewsji W, Linden U, et al: Internal neurolysis or ligament division only in carpal tunnel syndrome: Results of a randomized study. Acta Neurochir 74:118–121, 1985.
65. Lowry WE Jr, Follender AB: Interfascicular neurolysis in the severe carpal tunnel syndrome: A prospective, randomized, double-blind, controlled study. Clin Orthop 227:251–254, 1988.
66. Mackinnon SE, McCabe S, Murray JF, et al: Internal neurolysis fails to improve the results of primary carpal tunnel syndrome. J Hand Surg [Am] 16:211–218, 1991.
67. Foulkes GD, Atkinson RE, Beuchel C, et al: Outcome following epineurotomy in carpal tunnel syndrome: A prospective randomized clinical trial. J Hand Surg [Am] 19:539–547, 1994.
68. Katz JN, Keller RB, Simmons BP, et al: Maine Carpal Tunnel Study: outcomes of operative and nonoperative therapy for carpal tunnel syndrome in a community-based cohort. J Hand Surg [Am] 23:697–710, 1998.
69. Cartotto RC, McCabe S, Mackinnon SE: Two devastating complications of carpal tunnel surgery. Ann Plast Surg 28:472–474, 1992.
70. May JW: Division of the sensory ramus communicans between the ulnar and median nerves, a complication following carpal tunnel release: A case report. J Bone Joint Surg Am 63:836–838, 1981.
71. Nath RK, Mackinnon SE, Stelnicki E: Reflex sympathetic dystrophy: The controversy continues. Clin Plast Surg 23:435–436, 1996.
72. Gartsman GM, Kovach JC, Crouch CC, et al: Carpal arch alteration after carpal tunnel release. J Hand Surg [Am] 11:372–374, 1986.
73. Tung THH, Mackinnon SE: Secondary carpal tunnel surgery. Plast Reconstr Surg 107:1830–1843, 2001.
74. Phalen GS. Reflections on 21 years' experience with carpal tunnel syndrome. JAMA 212:1365–1367, 1970.

166 Entrapment Neuropathies of the Lower Extremities

S. SCOTT LOLLIS and DIMITRIOS C. NIKAS

Entrapment neuropathies (ENs) are a group of peripheral nerve disorders caused by compression. This occurs where the nerves are normally confined to a narrow anatomic passageway, a fibro-osseous tunnel, or a superficial course that provides little protection and renders the nerves susceptible to constricting pressures. The source of the pressure may be external (such as the peroneal palsy due to pressure from a cast or brace) or internal (compression or angulation by adjacent tissues within the body, from a compromised space, or directional changes causing angulation or stretching of the nerve). Symptoms depend on the location and internal anatomy of the affected nerve and generally consist of paresthesias, pain, and motor deficits in the area supplied. The compression and thus the symptoms can be acute, continuous, or intermittent.

ENs in the lower extremity (LE) can be as disabling as ENs in the upper extremity. They occur in several different but predictable locations. They produce a spectrum of sensory and motor deficits in the foot and lower extremity and can present a challenge in differential diagnosis. A careful clinical examination in conjunction with electromyography (EMG) and nerve conduction studies can usually identify the site of entrapment. Prognosis depends on the degree of nerve injury, which is related to both the cause and duration of the entrapment.

Although many LE ENs have been described, these neuropathies are relatively uncommon, with the exception of meralgia paresthetica and common peroneal nerve palsy.

The general features of the most common LE ENs and various treatment modalities are summarized here.

TARSAL TUNNEL SYNDROME: ENTRAPMENT OF THE POSTERIOR TIBIAL NERVE

Anatomy

The components of the tibial nerve are derived from the ventral divisions of the primary rami of spinal nerves L4–S3. The tibial nerve and the common peroneal nerve run as a single trunk (the sciatic nerve) in the pelvis and thigh, since they are surrounded by a common connective tissue sheath. They separate above the knee joint in the popliteal fossa. Then the tibial nerve runs deep to the gastrocnemius muscle, then beneath the tendinous arch of the soleus muscle, and distally between the flexor hallucis longus and flexor digitorum longus muscles. It then turns around the back of the medial malleolus and enters the tarsal tunnel beneath the flexor retinaculum of the medial aspect of the ankle. Below the malleolus it divides into its terminal branches,

the medial and lateral plantar nerves that form the interdigital nerves supplying the toes, and the calcaneal branches that supply the skin of the medial and plantar surfaces of the heel.

The tarsal tunnel contains the tibial nerve, the tibial artery and vein, and tendons from the tibialis posterior, flexor digitorum longus, and flexor hallucis longus muscles. The floor is formed by the flexor retinaculum (lancinate ligament) that covers the contents of the canal as they pass the ankle at a point between the medial malleolus and the medial tubercle of the calcaneus. Unlike the carpal tunnel, with which it is often compared, the tarsal tunnel contains numerous fibrous septa running between the roof and floor that serve to subdivide it.

An entrapment neuropathy of the posterior tibial nerve can occur behind and immediately below the medial malleolus.

Mechanism

Most cases of tarsal tunnel syndrome are idiopathic with no clear precipitating event. Involvement of the posterior tibial nerve usually occurs after a fracture or dislocation involving the malleoli or calcaneus. Delayed post-traumatic effects can result from tendon injury that can cause tenosynovitis and can act as a space-occupying lesion within the tarsal tunnel. Increased vascular compromise during standing and walking account for the crises experienced by patients with tarsal tunnel syndrome.

Clinical Presentation

Pain in the plantar aspect of the foot is the main complaint in the majority of patients. It is of burning quality and occasionally radiates up the calf. It is elicited or exacerbated by standing or walking. The motor disturbance is manifested by weakness and postural change in the foot. It assumes a pes cavus configuration, with clawing of the toes. The muscular weakness is revealed by a loss of flexion at the metatarsophalangeal joints and extension at the interphalangeal joints. Since the long flexors of the foot and toes are preserved, patients have no difficulty standing or walking, and muscular dysfunction can be difficult to detect.

Usually Tinel's sign (in which percussion causes paresthesias that radiate distally) is elicited at the site of greatest entrapment.

Evaluation

The history may uncover a traumatic event or vascular deficiency. In patients with diabetes or arterial insufficiency, care should be taken not to attribute the syndrome exclusively to an entrapment neuropathy. Pressure over the nerve in the retro- and inferomalleolar region usually causes local and radiating pain. Occasionally forcing the heel into valgus (away from the midline) will aggravate the symptoms, while forcing the heel into varus may cause sufficient slack in the lancinate ligament and decrease symptoms.

EMG in the initial stages exhibits a prolonged or dispersed sensory potential, and in advanced stages prolonged motor distal latencies in the medial plantar nerves, lateral plantar nerves, or both. Magnetic resonance imaging (MRI) has become a valuable tool in identifying mass lesions within the tarsal tunnel.

Treatment

Treatment depends on the identification of external forces acting on the ankle, such as repetitive local trauma versus disorders intrinsic to the tarsal tunnel. In case of venous engorgement or tenosynovitis, extrinsic correction of these disorders may solve the problem. If abnormal foot mechanics or standing posture is the problem, an external ankle support is indicated with special attention to decrease valgus position of the heel. When surgical decompression is necessary, unroofing the tarsal tunnel should be accompanied by exploration of the entrapment points for the medial and lateral plantar nerves, which should be followed into the abductor hallucis muscle, and transaction of any tight fascial bands. Surgery is performed with the patient in the supine position, with an incision made along the course of the posterior tibial nerve starting approximately 2 to 3 cm above the medial malleolus. The flexor retinaculum is identified and divided, with attention to include deep fibrous septa that surround the nerve. If the incision is close to the medial malleolus (not posterior enough) injury to the terminal branches of the saphenous nerve might occur. Care should also be taken to preserve the calcaneal nerve, particularly when it arises from the medial plantar nerve and courses posteriorly to reach the heel. There it crosses superficially to the lateral plantar nerve. If scarring is encountered, a complete external neurolysis should be performed. Surgery should not be taken lightly, and the decision to proceed should be made after thoughtful conservative management has failed. Patients with identifiable mass lesions intrinsic to the tarsal tunnel have the best prognosis. Patients who have undergone previous exploration, those with a diagnosis of associated plantar fasciitis, or those with an associated autoimmune inflammatory disorder do less well.

COMMON PERONEAL NERVE ENTRAPMENT

Anatomy of the Common Peroneal Nerve and Its Divisions

The common peroneal nerve originates from the L4–S2 nerve roots and the posterior division of the lumbosacral plexus. It comprises the posterior component of the sciatic nerve, which then exits the infrapiriform region of the greater sciatic foramen and courses inferiorly in the posterior compartment of the thigh. High in the popliteal fossa, the common peroneal nerve separates from the tibial nerve

and immediately gives off two minor branches, the articular branch and the lateral sural cutaneous nerve. The latter provides sensory innervation to the proximal lateral calf. The common peroneal nerve continues along the lateral border of the popliteal fossa, just medial to the tendinous insertion of the biceps femoris muscle. It descends obliquely across the plantaris muscle and wraps laterally around the fibular head; in so doing, it assumes a relatively superficial position and is thus vulnerable to compression injury and laceration.

The common peroneal nerve then pierces the tendinous origin of the peroneus longus muscle and enters a confined space bound medially by the periosteum of the fibular neck and laterally by the peroneus longus muscle—the so-called peroneal tunnel. Within the confines of the peroneal tunnel, the nerve is particularly susceptible to entrapment. Plantar flexion or inversion of the ankle causes a relative narrowing of the tunnel as well as a stretching of the nerve over its tendinous arch and can be an important clue to the cause of a patient's dysesthetic symptoms.

Division of the common peroneal nerve into the deep and superficial peroneal nerves usually occurs at the level of the fibular head (67%) but can also occur more proximally, in the popliteal fossa (22%), or distally, at the level of the fibular neck (11%).[1] The superficial peroneal nerve then descends inferiorly, usually in the lateral compartment, between the peroneus longus muscle laterally and the anterior intermuscular septum medially; approximately 14% of patients will demonstrate an anomalous course down the anterior compartment. The superficial peroneal nerve innervates the foot-everting muscles of the lateral compartment, the peroneus longus and peroneus brevis, and provides sensory innervation to the distal lateral calf. A variable amount of the leg's more proximal lateral aspect receives its sensory innervation from the lateral sural cutaneous nerve, mentioned previously. In the distal one-third of the leg, the superficial peroneal nerve pierces the fascia before giving off an intermediate dorsal cutaneous nerve and a medial dorsal cutaneous nerve, which together innervate the dorsum of the foot, save its most lateral aspect and the first web space.

The deep peroneal nerve continues deep to the fibrous lateral edge of the peroneus longus muscle and enters the anterior compartment. It courses inferiorly with the tibial artery and vein along the anterior surface of the interosseus membrane. It provides motor innervation to the muscles of the anterior compartment, the tibialis anterior, the extensor digitorum longus, the extensor hallucis longus, and the peroneus longus. It is thus responsible for dorsiflexion and eversion of the foot, as well as extension of the toes. The deep peroneal nerve then passes deep to the superior extensor retinaculum and inferior extensor retinaculum (also called the cruciform ligament) before projecting onto the dorsum of the foot. The space beneath the Y-shaped cruciform ligament is commonly referred to as the anterior tarsal tunnel and is another common site of entrapment.

In the foot, the deep peroneal nerve runs with the dorsalis pedis artery, bounded medially by the prominent extensor hallucis longus tendon, and laterally by the extensor hallucis brevis muscle. A lateral branch provides motor innervation only to the extensor digitorum brevis muscle, and a medial branch provides sensory innervation to the web space between the first and second toes.

Common Peroneal Neuropathy and Peroneal Tunnel Syndrome

A focal neuropathy affecting the dermatomes and myotomes of both the superficial and deep peroneal nerves is most likely to originate either from the area of the fibular head or the peroneal tunnel. In the former case, the nerve's superficial location makes it particularly susceptible to blunt or sharp trauma. Intoxicated patients from the community and obtunded patients in the hospital can develop a common peroneal neuropathy after spending a prolonged time with their lateral leg resting against a hard surface, such as a hospital bedrail. Above-knee and below-knee casts can also cause compression. Compression in the peroneal tunnel is more commonly the result of traction on the nerve, which is tethered by the fibrous tissue of the proximal peroneus longus. This can occur with distracting trauma to the leg or ankle as well as prolonged periods spent squatting or in the lithotomy position. Spontaneous entrapment can occur in patients with congenitally narrow peroneal tunnels and is usually exacerbated by extended periods of inversion or plantar flexion (Table 166-1).

Peroneal tunnel syndrome classically presents with pain over the fibular neck, spreading distally to involve the dermatomes of the superficial and deep peroneal nerves. In the advanced stages, there is marked weakness of dorsiflexion and eversion, manifested by the need to lift the affected leg higher when walking to avoid dragging the toes (drop foot). Exam reveals muscle tenderness over the area of compression, often with a positive Tinel's sign; this distinguishes the syndrome from lumbar radiculopathy and more proximal sciatic nerve compression. Weakness is often accompanied by atrophy of anterior and lateral compartments. In severe cases, there can be secondary trophic changes in surrounding bone. The condition known as restless legs syndrome is thought to be a variant presentation of peroneal tunnel syndrome.

TABLE 166-1 ▪ Causes of Focal Common Peroneal Neuropathy

External compression (casts, obtundation)
Laceration
Fracture of fibular head
Osteophytes
Exostosis
Superior tibiofibular dislocation (paratrooper's injury)
Traction injury (trauma, lithotomy position, prolonged squatting)
Laceration
Iatrogenic (vascular/orthopedic surgery)
Masses
   Ganglionic cyst: intraneural < extraneural
   Schwannoma
   Neurofibroma
   Neurogenic sarcoma
   Focal hypertrophic neuropathy
   Osteochondroma
Aneurysm
Repetitive inversion/pronation (running, pedaling)

Evaluation

Electromyography and nerve conduction studies (both sensory and motor) are helpful in corroborating clinical exam findings and precisely determining the anatomic location of the lesion. Equally important, they can rule out a more proximal lesion, such as piriformis muscle syndrome or lumbar radiculopathy, before surgical exploration. MRI is helpful in ruling out a mass lesion.

Treatment

Once a mass lesion or nerve transection has been excluded, a trial of conservative therapy is appropriate. This involves removing any obvious compressive causes, minimizing plantar flexion (an ankle orthosis worn at night is often helpful, as is a lateral sole wedge for the shoe), minimizing repetitive movements (i.e., cycling), and physical therapy. Nonsteroidal anti-inflammatory drugs are often helpful for relief of symptoms. If this is not effective, sensory symptoms are often relieved with corticosteroid injection at the site of compression.

If conservative therapy is ineffective, then operative neurolysis is indicated. Except for sharp lacerations and mass lesions, which benefit from early operative intervention, there is a dearth of data regarding timing of surgery. Most authors recommend a trial of 3 to 4 months of conservative therapy before surgical intervention on a suspected common peroneal nerve entrapment. When a prominent fibular head is believed to be contributory, it is partially rongeured off and bone wax applied to minimize nerve angulation.[2]

Results

In a recent article, Kim and colleagues describe their 32-year operative experience with 318 patients with knee-level common peroneal nerve lesions of all types. In it, they advocate intraoperative nerve action potential recordings (NAPs) as an essential guide to operative therapy; the presence of NAPs indicates residual function and is therefore an indication for external neurolysis and decompression only. The absence of NAP transmission is an indication of complete nerve injury and is an indication for nerve graft repair. Using this technique, Kim and co-workers document at least moderate improvement in motor function in 88% of patients undergoing neurolysis, 84% of patients undergoing end-to-end suture repair, and 42% undergoing graft repair. Outcome data specific to entrapment syndromes are not available, but of the 21 patients undergoing surgery for compression, 16 required neurolysis only and 5 required graft placement.[2]

There is a clear relationship between graft length and restoration of motor activity. Among patients with complete loss of common peroneal nerve function, 75% of patients receiving grafts 6 cm and shorter regain a moderate degree of function, in contrast to 38% of patients with grafts between 6 and 12 cm in length.[2]

Superficial Peroneal Nerve Entrapment

Clinical Presentation

Isolated superficial peroneal neuropraxia usually results from a lesion in the distal one-third of the leg, where the sensory component of the superficial peroneal nerve pierces the crural fascia. Causes can include direct trauma, fibrosis and/or scarring from previous surgery or trauma, lipoma, muscular hernia, or stretch injury after forced inversion–plantar flexion at the ankle.

Patients typically report burning paresthesias or anesthesia along the distal lateral leg and along the dorsum of the foot. These sensory disturbances spare the most lateral aspect of the foot and the web space between the first and second toes. Retrograde pain distribution is also possible. In the rare case of a more proximal injury to the superficial peroneal nerve, there might be weakness of ankle eversion.

Dysesthesia or worsened pain can be elicited with passive plantar flexion and inversion or resisted dorsiflexion and eversion. Symptoms can be exacerbated further if direct pressure is simultaneously applied over the suspected site of nerve compression. In thin patients, a palpable nodule can sometimes be appreciated at the site of compression.

When patients complain of pain or dysesthesia associated with exercise, consideration should be given to the possibility of a chronic lateral compartment syndrome, which can cause the syndrome of superficial peroneal nerve entrapment.

Evaluation

Sensory NAPs will demonstrate slowed conduction across the compressive lesion, as well as decreased amplitude along the entire course of the nerve, if compression has been prolonged and severe. However, normal sensory NAPs at rest do not exclude the possibility of a chronic compartment syndrome causing intermittent superficial peroneal nerve entrapment.[3] Diagnosis of this condition requires assessment of lateral compartment pressure after exercise.

EMG and motor nerve conduction studies are helpful in excluding deep peroneal nerve involvement as well as more proximal neuropathies, plexopathies, and radiculopathies. As mentioned previously, steroid injection at the site of compression is both diagnostic and palliative. Finally, imaging can be undertaken when a mass lesion is suspected.

Treatment

Again, a lateral sole wedge and shoe flare can be helpful in maintaining eversion and thus minimizing nerve traction. If this and other conservative measures fail, operative intervention is indicated. First, a local fascial release is attempted. If this fails, resection of the involved portion of the nerve will ameliorate the dysesthesias but leave behind an area of anesthesia on the lateral leg.

Results

Styf and colleagues performed superficial peroneal decompression and lateral fasciotomy for 21 patients with superficial peroneal nerve entrapment; of 19 patients followed for 37 months, 9 were satisfied with the result, 6 were improved but unsatisfied because of persistent athletic limitations, 3 exhibited no change, and 1 was worse.[3] A subsequent observational study by the same author followed 17 patients with clinical exam findings consistent with superficial peroneal nerve entrapment but negative electrophysiologic studies. Among these patients, 14 underwent decompression of the superficial peroneal tunnel and 3 underwent local fasciectomy. In this study, 80% of the patients demonstrated resolution or improvement of symptoms. These studies confirm that neurolysis and fasciectomy, when indicated, constitute

an appropriate treatment for superficial peroneal nerve entrapment, and that negative electrophysiologic studies should not rule out the diagnosis when clinical exam is highly suggestive.

Anterior Tarsal Tunnel Syndrome

Clinical Presentation

Anterior tarsal syndrome usually results from compression of the deep peroneal nerve as it passes deep to the inferior extensor retinaculum, a Y-shaped connective tissue band that extends from the sinus tarsi of the calcaneus to the medial malleolus superiorly and the navicular and first cuneiform bones inferiorly. Causes of nerve entrapment in the area are outlined in Table 166-2. Typically, patients complain of paresthesias involving the first web space that are often worse at night. If compression is relatively proximal, the lateral branch of the nerve can be involved as well, producing weakness of the extensor digitorum brevis and extensor hallucis brevis muscles as well as a diffuse aching sensation across the lateral midfoot.

On exam, patients will often demonstrate a Tinel's sign over the cruciform ligament. Paresthesias can also be elicited by passive plantar flexion of the ankle or dorsiflexion of the toes. Localization can be complicated by retrograde pain. The extensor digitorum brevis muscle can be assessed by having the patient dorsiflex the ankle and then attempt to further dorsiflex the toes.

Evaluation

Nerve conduction studies will reveal a prolonged latency across the lesion. EMG reveals denervation of the extensor digitorum brevis. If the lesion is more distal, involving only the medial (sensory) branch, an isolated increase in sensory NAP latency can also be seen.

Treatment

Conservative treatment of anterior tarsal syndrome involves minimization of plantar flexion. A splint can be used at night to maintain the ankle in a neutral position and thus minimize nocturnal symptoms. Patients should also be counseled to avoid tight or high-heeled shoes.

Surgical treatment involves division of the retinaculum and/or excision of any suspected mass lesions, fibrous bands, or osteophytes. If this fails and resection of the nerve is necessary, it should be performed proximal to the extensor

---

TABLE 166-2 ▪ Causes of Anterior Tarsal Tunnel Syndrome

Impingement
  Osteophytes
  Synovial pseudocysts
  Tendon sheath or retinaculum ganglions
  Neuromas
  Anomalous/hypertrophic muscle
  Fracture
  Aneurysm of dorsalis pedis artery
Repetitive compression (e.g., shoe straps)
Repetitive stretching (e.g., high-heeled shoes)
Trauma involving violent plantar flexion and/or inversion of the ankle

retinaculum; this minimizes the risk of a neuroma interfering with tendon function.

MERALGIA PARESTHETICA

Anatomy of the Lateral Femoral Cutaneous Nerve

The lateral cutaneous nerve of the thigh is a purely sensory nerve that originates from the posterior divisions of the L2–L4 nerve roots and then emerges from the lateral border of the psoas muscle at the level of L4–L5. It courses laterally across the iliacus muscle to the anterior-superior iliac spine and then passes through or beneath the inguinal ligament, 1 to 2 cm medial to the anterior superior iliac spine. This is the common point of entrapment. Here, the nerve is tethered to both iliac fascia and the inguinal ligament proximally and the fascia lata of the thigh distally; it is thus susceptible to traction with truncal movements or adduction of the leg. The lateral femoral cutaneous nerve emerges medial to the sartorius muscle origin, still beneath the deep fascia. Approximately 5 cm inferior to the inguinal ligament, it moves superficially to become subcutaneous; approximately 10 cm inferior to the inguinal ligament, it divides into an anterior branch, which provides sensory innervation to the anterolateral thigh as far as the knee, and a posterior branch, which provides sensory innervation to the lateral buttock over the greater trochanter. The posterior thigh is supplied by the posterior cutaneous nerve of the thigh, derived from the sacral plexus and roots S1–S3.

Lateral Femoral Cutaneous Nerve Entrapment or Meralgia Paresthetica

Clinical Presentation

Meralgia paresthetica has a 3:1 male-to-female predominance. Obesity and chronic cough are frequently contributory comorbidities. In obese people and pregnant women, the abdominal pannus tends to cause downward traction on the inguinal ligament, causing chronic stretching of the nerve. In people with chronic cough or constipation, repeated Valsalva maneuvers draw the inguinal ligament down against the nerve. Other contributory factors include habitually long periods of standing (policemen, mail carriers, etc.) and the wearing of abdominal binders, large belts, and corsets.

Patients will typically describe a paresthesia of the anterolateral thigh, which can range from "pins and needles" to a painful burning sensation. The area involved is usually in the dermatome of the anterior branch only and is much smaller than the actual area innervated by this nerve. Symptoms are relieved by recumbency and hip flexion. Meralgia paresthetica is commonly progressive, and the discomfort may progress to a more severe, constant pain that is not relieved by any position. Point tenderness is often present just medial to the anterior superior iliac spine. There are no associated motor or reflex deficits. Occasionally there is associated hair loss in this region of the thigh.

Evaluation

In classic cases, the diagnosis is a clinical one. However, if there are any other signs or symptoms not consistent with the diagnosis, such as back pain, weakness, reflex asymmetry, or sensory changes in other dermatomes, additional workup with computed tomography (CT) or MRI is warranted. Infiltration of 1 to 5 mL of 1% lidocaine just medial to the anterior superior iliac spine can confirm the diagnosis.

Treatment

Conservative treatment involves weight loss and removal of restrictive belts or corsets. If this fails, or if symptoms are sufficiently severe that the patient is unwilling to wait for relief, surgical treatment can be undertaken. Two options exist: neurolysis and sectioning of the nerve. Decompression can be undertaken with either an infrainguinal or a suprainguinal approach. In both cases, the nerve is dissected free of surrounding fascial bands, and its course through the inguinal ligament is bluntly freed of impinging connective tissue.

Sectioning of the nerve itself is a more definitive procedure but has two drawbacks: possible neuroma formation at the inguinal ligament and persistent anesthesia in the dermatome of the sectioned nerve. Previously, sectioning was used only after a trial of neurolysis had failed.

Results

In a clinical trial comparing the two techniques in patients for whom conservative therapy had failed, van Eerten and colleagues demonstrate significantly improved relief of symptoms following nerve sectioning. Of 11 patients undergoing this procedure, 9 showed complete relief and 2 partial relief. By contrast, neurolysis seemed to offer no significant benefit over conservative therapy, with 4 of 9 patients complaining of worsened symptoms after surgery.[4] Neuroma formation and long-term dissatisfaction with thigh anesthesia were not assessed. On the basis of this trial, it seems that sectioning of the nerve is a more appropriate surgical option for patients with intractable meralgia paresthetica; however, there continues to be considerable variability in practice.

FEMORAL AND SAPHENOUS NERVES

Anatomy

The femoral nerve is the largest branch of the lumbar plexus. It arises from the nerve roots L2–L4 and the posterior division of the lumbar plexus. The femoral nerve emerges from the posterolateral edge of the psoas muscle at the junction of the upper two-thirds and lower one-third of that muscle and then courses deep to the fascia of the iliacus muscle around the pelvic inlet. It then passes beneath the inguinal ligament to reside lateral to the femoral vessels in the femoral triangle. It is surrounded by a fascial sheath within the iliopectineal fascia, deep to the fascia lata. In the upper thigh, the femoral nerve gives off numerous small branches to supply the musculature of the anterior compartment of the thigh. The femoral nerve provides motor innervation to the iliopsoas, the quadriceps femoris, the pectineus, and the sartorius muscles. A sensory branch, the anterior femoral cutaneous nerve, sends multiple projections through the fascia to supply sensory innervation to the anteromedial aspect of the thigh.

The continuation of the femoral nerve in the lower leg is known as the saphenous nerve and is purely sensory. The saphenous nerve joins the superficial femoral artery and vein in the upper thigh and with them, enters the adductor canal (also called Hunter's canal). It does not traverse the entire canal but exits medially from the roof of the canal along with the descending genicular artery. It pierces the subsartorial fascia approximately 10 cm above the knee joint. It then courses inferiorly behind the sartorius muscle before emerging from the deep fascia between the sartorius and gracilis tendons. An infrapatellar branch supplies sensory innervation to the medial leg below the knee, while a descending branch courses inferiorly and supplies sensory innervation to the distal anteromedial leg and foot, including the medial malleolus.

Femoral Nerve Entrapment

Clinical Presentation

The femoral nerve can become entrapped anywhere along its course. Table 166-3 divides possible causes into those occurring more proximally, in the retroperitoneum and pelvis, and those occurring distal to the inguinal ligament.

Presentation usually involves sensory loss or dysesthesia in the anterior thigh and medial calf. Weakness of knee extension is more common than weakness of the hip flexion. Since both the afferent and efferent limbs of the patellar reflex are mediated by the femoral nerve, the knee jerk may be reduced or absent.

Evaluation

Motor nerve conduction studies demonstrate decreased amplitudes along the course of the nerve. While the intrapelvic portions of the nerve are difficult to assess because of their location, a lesion at the level of the inguinal ligament can sometimes be confirmed when a prolonged motor latency is noted in this area. EMG will confirm denervation of the quadriceps muscles and sparing of other muscles not innervated by the femoral nerve. Sensory NAPs will demonstrate decreased amplitudes in the saphenous nerve. As usual, the real value of nerve conduction studies lies in their ability to rule out other, more proximal nerve lesions. If a mass lesion is suspected in the lower extremity, MRI is a useful adjunct; if a retroperitoneal or pelvic cause is suspected, CT scan with contrast is a more appropriate first step.

Treatment

Treatment is usually conservative, unless a mass lesion can be confirmed. A knee-ankle-foot orthosis is helpful if gait

---

TABLE 166-3 ▪ Causes of Femoral Nerve Neuropraxia/Entrapment

Psoas region

Retroperitoneal mass or hematoma
Penetrating trauma
Retropsoas abscess
Iatrogenic

Inguinal region

Iatrogenic (arteriography/central line placement)
Lithotomy position
Pregnancy (secondary to fetal pressure)
Kidney transplant
Mass lesion

---

instability and knee buckling are a significant problem. A cane or walker is often necessary to minimize the risk of falling.

Saphenous Nerve Entrapment

Clinical Presentation

Entrapment of the saphenous nerve usually occurs at the point of penetrance of the fascia of the adductor canal. It can occur spontaneously or after trauma. Spontaneous entrapment is most common in women, obese patients, and patients with some degree of genu varum. Causative trauma is usually significant enough to also cause injury to the knee joint. Other possible causes of an isolated saphenous neuropathy are primarily iatrogenic; these should be considered in patients with a history of saphenous vein harvest or medial arthrotomy.

Patients with saphenous neuropathy usually complain of radiating pain along the entire medial calf. Pain is often exacerbated by attempts to climb stairs. There is usually tenderness and a positive Tinel's sign over the site of entrapment. Extension of the knee will increase patient discomfort, and thus walking is often problematic and patients are often misdiagnosed as having vascular claudication. Because the saphenous nerve is purely sensory, there is no associated weakness or muscle atrophy.

Evaluation

Since an L3 or L4 root lesion can present similarly, MRI of the lumbosacral spine should be performed to rule out herniated disc or other spinal mass lesion. If a patient is unable to undergo MRI, EMG can be helpful in demonstrating intact neuromuscular function in the L3 and L4 myotomes. When compression is present, sensory NAPs will show prolonged latency across the region of the adductor canal.

Injection of corticosteroid in the vicinity of the nerve's exit from the adductor canal can be both diagnostic and therapeutic. Because of the proximity to the femoral vessels, this should only be undertaken by experienced hands.

Treatment

Intractable cases of saphenous neuralgia can be treated with division of the subsartorial fascia. If this fails, division of the nerve will relieve painful dysesthesias but obviously results in permanent anesthesia along the medial leg. For both surgeries, the nerve is approached at the point of its emergence from the subsartorial fascia. Dissection occurs in the plane between the sartorius and vastus medialis muscles. The subsartorial fascia, once identified, can be opened generously, with care to avoid the underlying femoral vessels. Nerve sectioning, when performed, should be done as proximally as possible.

Results

Large-scale studies of the efficacy of surgery for saphenous neuralgia are not available. Luerssen and co-workers describe six patients treated surgically. Of these, three demonstrated improvement following external neurolysis, and three required neurectomy for recurrent symptoms.[5] Thus it appears reasonable to undertake decompression as a first step and reserve nerve sectioning for those in whom the initial surgery fails.

OBTURATOR NERVE

Anatomy of the Obturator Nerve

The obturator nerve originates from the L2–L4 nerve roots and the anterior division of the lumbar plexus. It courses caudally along the posteromedial aspect of the psoas, emerging at the level of L5. It then passes around the pelvic outlet and exits the pelvis through the obturator foramen with the obturator artery. It immediately bifurcates into two mixed nerves, the anterior branch and the posterior branch; these are separated by the adductor brevis muscle. The anterior branch projects anterior to the obturator externus and adductor brevis muscles and deep to the adductor longus muscle. It supplies motor innervation to the adductor longus muscle, the adductor brevis muscle, and the gracilis muscle, and sensory innervation to a small patch of skin on the medial thigh. The posterior branch passes through the obturator externus muscle. It supplies motor innervation to the obturator externus muscle and portions of the pectineus and adductor magnus muscles. Its sensory innervation is limited to a few small twigs innervating the hip joint.

Obturator Nerve Entrapment

Clinical Presentation

Isolated obturator neuropathy is rare and usually the result of penetrating trauma or iatrogenic injury; compressive neuropathy can result from pelvic mass lesions, particularly in the iliac fossa or anterior inferior pelvic wall. When the compression is proximal, there is frequently compromise of the femoral nerve as well; the resultant weakness of both knee extension and hip adduction is far more debilitating than an isolated obturator nerve lesion.

Entrapment of the obturator nerve by normal anatomic structures is rare and usually results from either an obturator hernia or impingement by fascia as the nerve traverses the obturator foramen. Patients will typically report exercise-induced medial thigh pain or paresthesias. On exam, weakness of thigh adduction can sometimes be demonstrated. If weakness is marked, patients will have difficulty stabilizing the hip joint and thus adopt a wide-based gait. Absence of the adductor reflex can sometimes be demonstrated.

Evaluation

Electromyography and nerve conduction studies are helpful confirmatory tests. CT scan should be used to rule out a pelvic mass lesion.

Treatment

Treatment involves blunt decompression of the nerve as it traverses the fibroses tunnel within the obturator foramen. Dissection is carried down between the adductor longus and pectineus muscles. The fascia is split along the course of the nerve's anterior branch. The obturator foramen is then identified and its fascia bluntly dissected free of the nerve.

REFERENCES

1. Bogdanović D, Ilić A, Marenić S: Peroneal tunnel syndrome. Acta Orthoped Ingos 3:357, 1972.
2. Kim DH, Murovic JA, Tiel RL, et al: Management and outcomes in 318 operative common peroneal nerve lesions at the Louisiana State University Health Sciences Center. Neurosurgery 54:1421–1429, 2004.
3. Styf J: Entrapment of the superficial peroneal nerve: Diagnosis and results of decompression. J Bone Joint Surg 71B:131–135, 1989.
4. Van Eerten PV, Polder TW, Broere CAJ, et al: Operative treatment of meralgia paresthetica: Transection versus neurolysis. Neurosurgery 37:63–65, 1995.
5. Luerssen TG, Campbell RL, Defalque RJ, et al: Spontaneous saphenous neuralgia. Neurosurgery 13: 238–241, 1983.

167 Surgical Management of Sciatic Nerve Lesions

SUSAN R. DURHAM and JASON H. HUANG

Proper management of lesions of the sciatic nerve can prevent profound and disabling pain, as well as motor and sensory deficits of the lower extremity. Management of these lesions can be challenging because most surgeons have only a limited experience of the natural history and management of lesions of the sciatic nerve. The largest nerve in the human body, the sciatic nerve, innervates the flexors of the knee, dorsiflexors and plantar flexors of the foot, evertors and invertors of the foot, and all intrinsic foot musculature. It is responsible for sensation of the posterior thigh, lateral lower leg, and entire foot. The correct diagnosis and management of sciatic nerve lesions is vital to maximize recovery and avoid severe functional deficits and disability.

SURGICAL ANATOMY

The sciatic nerve is formed from the anterior and posterior divisions of L4, L5, S1, and S2 spinal roots and the anterior division of the S3 spinal root. The anterior divisions combine to form the tibial division of the sciatic nerve, and the posterior divisions combine to form the peroneal division of the sciatic nerve. The tibial and peroneal divisions of the sciatic nerve combine within the pelvis on the anterior surface of the piriformis muscle to form the sciatic nerve (Fig. 167-1). The newly formed sciatic nerve courses distally over the anterior surface of the piriformis muscle and exits the pelvis below the piriformis muscle through the greater sciatic notch. Prior to exiting the pelvis through the greater sciatic notch, the superior gluteal nerve, along with the superior gluteal artery and vein, pass above the pyriformis muscle to supply the gluteus medius and minimus muscles and the tensor fascia lata. The inferior gluteal nerve, which supplies the gluteus maximus muscle, is closely applied to the sciatic nerve as it exits the greater sciatic notch. The region of the greater sciatic notch and the association of the sciatic nerve to the piriformis muscle can be complex because the piriformis muscle can lie either superficial or deep to the nerve or even between the two divisions of the nerve. Great care must be taken not to damage the superior or inferior gluteal vessels close to the sciatic notch as they can retract into the pelvis leading to a pelvic hematoma which can be difficult to evacuate and control.

After passing through the greater sciatic notch, the sciatic nerve courses distally dorsal to the obturator internus, gemelli, and quadratus femoris muscles directly beneath the gluteus maximus muscle. It enters the thigh lateral to the biceps femoris and courses distally between the biceps femoris and the semitendinosus muscle. Upon entering the thigh, the tibial division branches supply the long head of the biceps

femoris, semitendinosus, semimembranosus, and adductor magnus muscles. The short head of the biceps femoris is innervated by a proximal thigh branch of the peroneal division. As the sciatic nerve proceeds distally into the lower thigh, it bifurcates into the tibial and common peroneal nerves, which continue distally to innervate the lower leg.

SCIATIC NERVE LESIONS

Tumors

Schwannomas and neurofibromas are the most common tumors affecting the sciatic nerve. Less common tumors

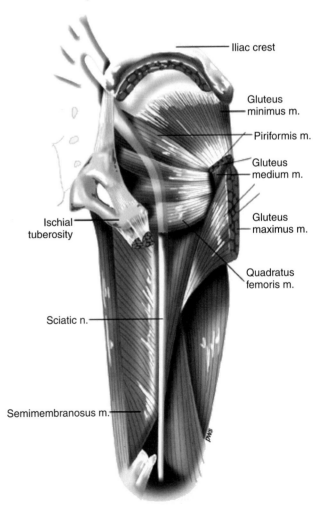

FIGURE 167-1 Dorsal view of the course of the sciatic nerve in the pelvis, buttock, and proximal thigh.

include malignant peripheral nerve sheath tumor (MPNST), ganglion cyst, lipoma, desmoid tumor, or metastatic tumor.

Schwannomas are indolent tumors that arise eccentrically from the nerve sheath. They are generally painless but may present with paresthesias or pain secondary to nerve compression by the tumor mass. Microscopic pathology classically reveals a distinctive pattern of Schwann cells organized into two contrasting components: Antoni A areas consist of a compact collection of spindle-shaped cells arranged in sheets and palisades with the pathognomic Verocay bodies; Antoni B areas, by contrast, possess a loose myxoid matrix with collagen fibrils and only rare spindle cells and lymphocytes.[1]

Neurofibromas arise from the perineurial cells of the nerve sheath and therefore are not encapsulated tumors.[2,3] They are often solitary, but are sometimes multiple, especially in those cases associated with neurofibromatosis (NF) type I. Neurofibromas are usually oval or fusiform in shape and pale white or gray in color. Plexiform neurofibromas are pathognomic for NF type I, and are composed of a thick, convoluted, bulbous mass similar to a bag of worms. Histologically, neurofibromas are composed of intercalated bundles of fusiform, elongated cells with darkly staining nuclei surrounded by an insubstantial matrix containing collagen fibrils, mucoid deposits, lymphocytes, and xanthoma cells. Infrequently, neurofibromas may have cystic, hemorrhagic, or fatty changes.

Malignant peripheral nerve sheath tumors may arise de novo from degeneration of an existing solitary neurofibroma affecting the sciatic nerve or, less commonly, from a schwannoma. The most common type of MPNST affecting the sciatic nerve is a neurofibrosarcoma. Other MPNSTs include malignant neurilemmoma, malignant schwannoma, and neurogenic sarcoma. MPNSTs present with a painful, enlarging mass and patients often have progressive neurologic deficits. Histologically, most MPNSTs are composed of spindle cells, showing markedly increased cellularity, nuclear pleomorphism, mitotic figures, hemorrhage, and necrosis.[1]

Trauma

Trauma to the sciatic nerve at buttock level may be a result of needle injury caused by injection, hip fracture-dislocation, hip arthroplasty surgery, contusion secondary to blunt trauma, or gunshot wounds (GSWs).[4–10] In the largest series of surgically treated sciatic nerve injuries, Kim and colleagues reported in their series of 175 patients with buttock-level sciatic nerve trauma that 37% of injuries were caused by injection, 15% by fracture-dislocation, and 10% by GSWs.[10] Sciatic nerve injuries at the thigh level are commonly caused by GSWs, femoral fracture, laceration from stab injury, contusion from blunt trauma, or iatrogenic injuries.[7–11] In Kim and colleagues' series of 178 patients with thigh-level sciatic nerve injury, 35% were caused by GSWs and 19% were caused by femoral fracture.[10]

Entrapment

Piriformis syndrome is a controversial clinical entity characterized by symptoms referable to the sciatic nerve distribution. The diagnosis is often difficult to establish with certainty, and patients may have associated lumbosacral spine disease. Classically, piriformis syndrome is believed to be caused by an inflamed or irritable piriformis muscle, or the variable anatomic relationship of the sciatic nerve to the muscle. Patients with piriformis syndrome often report symptoms similar to those with L5 or S1 radiculopathy due to herniated lumbar disc and/or lower lumbar facet arthropathy with foraminal narrowing. They complain mainly of a "sciatica" type of pain with sensory impairment in the distribution of the sciatic nerve. Weakness and atrophy are often difficult to detect on physical examination. Tenderness over the belly of the piriformis muscle can be elicited by external lateral palpation or medial internal palpation via rectal examination. Provocative testing using inward hip rotation often reproduces the pain.

DIAGNOSTIC TESTING

Clinical evaluation of sciatic lesions includes a thorough neurologic and electrophysiologic examination of the sciatic nerve, including motor and sensory function of the distal tibial and peroneal territories.

Neurologic Examination

Motor function of the sciatic nerve can be divided into the tibial and peroneal components. The tibial division function is tested by examining motor function of the long head of the biceps femoris, semitendinosus, and semimembranosus muscles (knee flexion), gastrocnemius and soleus muscles (plantar flexion), posterior tibialis muscle (foot inversion), flexor digitorum longus muscle (toe flexion), and flexor hallicus longus muscle (great toe flexion). The proximal or common peroneal division is tested by examining motor function of the short head of the biceps femoris muscle (knee flexion). Distal peroneal nerve function can be tested by evaluating the superficial peroneal nerve–innervated muscles, which include the peroneus longus and brevus muscles (foot eversion), as well as the deep peroneal branch–innervated muscles, which include the anterior tibialis muscle (dorsiflexion of the foot), extensor hallicus longus muscle (great toe extension), and extensor digitorum brevis muscle (toe extension). Motor function of the short head of the biceps femoris muscle is important in differentiating proximal versus distal involvement of the peroneal nerve.

Sensory function of the sciatic nerve can be tested in the posterior thigh, lateral leg, and foot and the plantar surface of the foot. Diminished or absent deep tendon reflexes at the ankle can also be seen in sciatic nerve lesions.

Electrophysiologic Evaluation

Electrophysiologic evaluation of sciatic nerve lesions typically includes sensory action potentials, compound muscle action potentials, nerve conduction velocities, and electromyography. Electrophysiologic evaluation is often useful in differentiating pelvic plexus from sciatic nerve lesions because the surgical management of the former can be quite involved. Clinical or electrophysiologic evidence of gluteal or femoral distribution loss favors pelvic-level involvement of the pelvic plexus. Electrophysiologic studies of sciatic nerve lesions can demonstrate significant axonal loss, based on low-amplitude sensory actions potentials and compound muscle action potentials as well as findings of denervation on electromyography. The presence of a recordable compound muscle action potential from the extensor digitorum brevis has been reported to be the best electrophysiologic predictor of recovery from sciatic nerve injury.[12] Electrophysiologic studies, although helpful in the localization and characterization of sciatic lesions, should not be used primarily for surgical decision making.

Magnetic Resonance Neurography

Conventional techniques for magnetic resonance imaging of the lumbosacral spinal cord are well established and provide excellent visualization of the spinal axis, including the central canal and foramina. However, these techniques do not adequately examine lesions of the lumbosacral plexus or the sciatic nerve. Recently, novel magnetic resonance protocols have been reported to increase the visibility of peripheral nerves outside of the spinal axis.[13-17] Magnetic resonance neurography (MRN) has the potential ability to study peripheral nerves along their length and identify areas of compression, entrapment, neoplastic processes, nerve rupture, or avulsion. In addition to identifying structural abnormalities of the nerve itself, MRN has also been reported to demonstrate signal change within the nerve adjacent to the region of injury. Early methods of MRN showed promise; however, visibility of the nerve was difficult relative to the surrounding fat and muscle. It has now been demonstrated in a variety of peripheral nerve lesions that MRN can demonstrate excellent clinical images of the peripheral nerves in a variety of pathologic conditions utilizing high-resolution coils and appropriate image processing. High-resolution peripheral nerve imaging requires careful consideration of coil selection, pulse sequence, method of fat suppression, section thickness, and field of view. Unfortunately, there has not been widespread acceptance of this technique, presumably due to the great variability of published protocols and difficulty in interpretation of the data.

SURGICAL TREATMENT

Indications and Timing of Surgery

As with most peripheral nerve injuries, there is disagreement on the optimal period of time one should allow for spontaneous recovery before contemplating surgical exploration. Sharp transactions of the sciatic nerve should be repaired as acutely as possible to achieve optimal results. For stretch or contusional-type injuries, most researchers recommend surgical exploration for complete or very serious deficits that fail to improve spontaneously over several months.[10,18,19] The majority of patients with partial deficits or improvement in function will have recovery of useful function if treated conservatively.

Conservative management is appropriate for small, nonpainful, indolent tumors of the sciatic nerve that do not cause neurologic dysfunction. For patients with genetic tumor predisposition syndromes such as neurofibromatosis or schwannomatosis, these often asymptomatic tumors need to be monitored with serial MRI studies, usually at a yearly interval.[20,21] Surgery is indicated for any tumors that cause neurologic dysfunction or severe pain or for any rapidly growing tumors with a suspicion of malignancy.

Given the controversial etiology of piriformis syndrome, conservative management, including a trial of nonsteroidal anti-inflammatory medication and resting, should precede any surgical treatment. In a selective group of patients who failed conservative therapy, surgical intervention may be considered. Symptoms of buttock pain, gluteal weakness, and atrophy have been shown to improve with surgical decompression and piriformis sectioning in some series.

Surgical Exposure

Pelvic-level exposure of the sciatic nerve from its origin in the lumbosacral plexus is quite difficult and requires combined expertise from general surgery colleagues through a retroperitoneal or transperitoneal approach. For the purposes of this chapter, the sciatic nerve exposure will be divided into buttock-level and thigh-level approaches. It is important to preoperatively differentiate pelvic-level, buttock-level, and thigh-level sciatic nerve lesions for adequate surgical planning.

Buttock-Level Exposure

The patient is placed prone with elevation of the ipsilateral hip and the knee slightly bent. If sural nerve grafting is anticipated, the lower leg (ipsilateral and contralateral) should be included in the surgical field. The buttock incision is started inferior to the posterior iliac crest, directed laterally over the mass of the buttock, and turned medially along the buttock crease (Fig. 167-2A). At the midpoint of the proximal thigh, the incision can be continued inferiorly if needed. The gluteus maximus is incised 2 to 3 cm medial to its greater trochanter insertion, leaving a tagged cuff for reattachment (Fig. 167-2B). The gluteus maximus and some gluteus medius muscle is then reflected and retracted medially along with the inferior gluteal nerve and vasculature to expose the sciatic nerve (Fig. 167-2C). The sciatic nerve is then followed superiorly toward the sciatic notch, being careful to preserve the hamstring and posterior femoral cutaneous branches and gluteal nerves and vessels. The region of the sciatic notch can be anatomically complex, and great care must be taken to prevent inadvertent injury to the surrounding nerve branches and vasculature. The piriformis muscle may be sectioned to facilitate exposure of the sciatic notch region. After adequate exposure of the sciatic nerve at the buttock level, the nerve may be split into its two divisions and each division can be electrophysiologically evaluated before proceeding with neurolysis or nerve grafting/repair.

Thigh-Level Exposure

The patient is placed prone with the knee and lower leg supported. A posterior curvilinear incision is started at the midportion of the buttock crease, extending inferiorly and laterally toward the lateral popliteal fossa (Fig. 167-3A). This can be extended superiorly or inferiorly as needed. The sciatic nerve is located beneath the gluteus maximus muscle and between the semitendinosus and biceps femoris muscle (Fig. 167-3B). The biceps femoris muscle, which angles across the upper thigh, is identified and retracted laterally to expose the proximal thigh-level sciatic nerve as it courses underneath

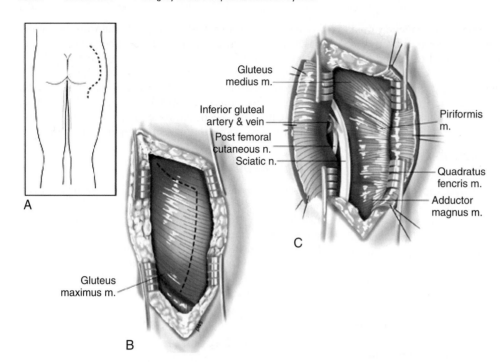

FIGURE 167-2 *A,* Incision for buttock-level exposure of the sciatic nerve. *B,* Exposure and incision of the gluteus maximus muscle. *C,* Exposure of the sciatic nerve after reflection of the gluteus maximus muscle medially to expose the sciatic nerve exiting the pelvis beneath the piriformis muscle.

(Fig. 167-3C). Care is taken to preserve the branches to the short head of the biceps femoris muscle from the peroneal division of the sciatic nerve just distal to the buttock crease. Once the lesion of the sciatic nerve has been exposed between the biceps femoris and the semitendinosus and semimembranosus muscles, sharp dissection of the nerve is performed to gain circumferential exposure of the nerve above and below the lesion. It is often necessary to split the nerve into the tibial and peroneal divisions above and below the lesion in order to allow independent electrophysiologic assessment and repair if necessary.

Intraoperative Evaluation

Basic to the approach of a sciatic nerve lesion is to split the nerve into the tibial and peroneal divisions both proximal and distal to the lesion and perform independent electrophysiologic evaluation of each division. After exposure of the sciatic nerve lesion, each division is then stimulated proximal and recorded distal to the lesion and monitored for a nerve action potential (NAP). A recordable NAP across the lesion denotes either significant sparing of function or adequate regeneration, and neurolysis alone is adequate. Absence of an NAP several months postinjury signifies a minimal chance

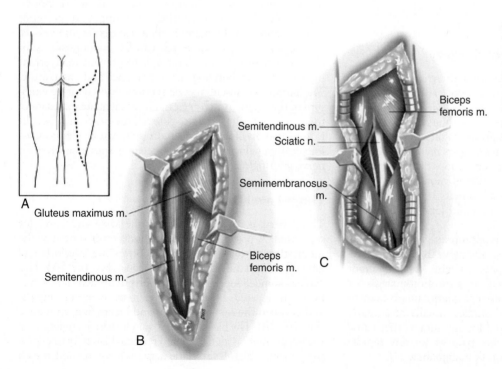

FIGURE 167-3 *A,* Incision for thigh-level exposure of the sciatic nerve. *B,* Exposure of the gluteus maximus, semitendinosus, and biceps femoris muscles in the thigh. *C,* Exposure of the sciatic nerve after retraction of the biceps femoris, semitendinosus, and semimembranosus muscles in the thigh.

of recovery without resection of the lesion and repair. Often a split repair can be established where a section of the nerve that transmits an NAP can be identified through internal neurolysis and spared, while the remainder of the nerve that does not transmit an NAP is resected and repaired.[10]

Nerve resection and repair can be accomplished by primary end-to-end epineurial repair if the nerve can be mobilized sufficiently and brought together without tension. In most causes, nerve grafts are needed between the prepared proximal and distal stumps. Numerous materials have been used as grafting materials, most commonly the sural nerve harvested from the lower leg. Other materials such as collagen-based nerve guide tubes and vein grafts have been used with varying levels of success. The success of the grafting procedure drops considerably with increasing graft length.

OUTCOME AND RESULTS

The two largest series of surgically treated sciatic nerve lesions are from Louisiana State University Medical Center.[10,19] Originally published in 1998 and updated in 2004, these reports constitute the largest published experience of surgical management of sciatic nerve lesions, with 353 patients over a 31-year period. These patients were categorized into buttock- or thigh-level lesions as well as mechanism of injury. Injection injury for buttock-level and missile injury for thigh-level lesions were the most common. Tibial division injuries had better outcomes than peroneal division for each injury mechanism and type of surgical repair. This proclivity of the peroneal division to injury is postulated to be due to its lateral and more susceptible position to compression forces, relative fixed position at the surgical head of the fibula, smaller blood supply, and less surrounding connective tissue.

Recently, the authors of these extensive series proposed an algorithm for surgical management of sciatic nerve injuries for both open and closed injuries.[10] Open, sharp injuries should be primarily repaired within 72 hours. In blunt, open injuries, the nerve ends should be identified and tacked to surrounding fascial tissue and undergo secondary repair at 2 to 3 weeks. Closed injuries should undergo clinical assessment, including neurologic examination, serial EMG, radiographic evaluation, and physical therapy. If regeneration is noted either clinically or electrophysiologically, conservative management is recommended. In cases with no evidence of regeneration or recovery, surgical exploration is recommended in 2 to 3 months for focal lesions and 4 to 6 months for lengthy lesions to allow time for adequate regeneration to be noted. Intraoperative exploration with NAP recordings is recommended to differentiate regenerative versus nonregenerative lesions and to guide intraoperative decision making. Lesions in continuity with a recordable NAP had the best clinical outcomes after neurolysis alone, followed by primary suture repair.

Graft repair resulted in the lowest number of good outcomes, but the researchers felt it was still worthwhile.[10]

REFERENCES

1. Skovronsky DM, Oberholtzer JC: Pathologic classification of peripheral nerve tumors. Neurosurg Clin N Am 15(2):157–166, 2004.
2. Haraida S, Nerlich AG, Bise K, et al: Comparison of various basement membrane components in benign and malignant peripheral nerve tumors. Virchows Arch A Pathol Anat Histopathol 421(4):331–338, 1992.
3. Nerlich AG, Haraida S, Wiest I: Basement membrane components as differential markers for mesenchymal tumors of various origins. Anticancer Res 14(2B):683–692, 1994.
4. Haidukewych GJ, Scaduto J, Herscovici D, et al: Iatrogenic nerve injury in acetabular fracture surgery: A comparison of monitored and unmonitored procedures. J Orthop Trauma 16(5):297–301, 2002.
5. Cornwall R, Radomisli T: Nerve injury in traumatic dislocation of the hip. Clin Orthop 377:84–91, 2000.
6. Hillyard RF, Fox J: Sciatic nerve injuries associated with traumatic posterior hip dislocations. Am J Emer Med 21(7):545–548, 2003.
7. Samardzic MM, Rasulic LG, Vuckovic CD: Missile injuries of the sciatic nerve. Injury Int J Care Injured 30:15–20, 1999.
8. Taha A, Taha J: Results of suture of the sciatic nerve after missile injury. J Trauma 45:340–344, 1998.
9. Plewnia C, Wallace C, Zochodne D: Traumatic sciatic neuropathy. A novel cause, local experience and review of the literature. J Trauma 47:986–991, 1999.
10. Kim DH, Murovic JA, Tiel R, Kline DG: Management and outcomes in 353 surgically treated sciatic nerve lesions. J Neurosurg 101(1):8–17, 2004.
11. Takami H, Takahashi S, Ando M: Sciatic nerve injury associated with fracture of the femoral shaft. Arch Orthop Trauma Surg 119:103–104, 1999.
12. Yuen EC, Yuen TS, Olney RK: The electrophysiologic features of sciatic neuropathy in 100 patients. Muscle Nerve 18:414–420, 1995.
13. Cudlip SA, Howe FA, Griffiths JR, et al: Magnetic resonance neurography of peripheral nerve following experimental crush injury, and correlation with functional deficit. J Neurosurg 96:755–759, 2002.
14. Hans FJ, Reinges MH, Krings T: Lumbar nerve root avulsion following trauma: Balanced fast field-echo MRI. Neuroradiology 46:144–147, 2004.
15. Cudlip SA, Howe FA, Clifton A, et al: Magnetic resonance neurography studies of the median nerve before and after carpal tunnel release. J Neurosurg 96:1046–1051, 2002.
16. Gupta R, Villablanca PJ, Jones NF: Evaluation of an acute nerve compression injury with magnetic resonance neurography. J Hand Surg 26:1093–1099, 2001.
17. Moore KR, Tsuruda JS, Dailey AT: The value of MR neurography for evaluating extraspinal neuropathic leg pain: A pictorial essay. Am J Neuroradiol 22:787–794, 2001.
18. Omer GE: The prognosis for untreated traumatic injuries. In Omer GE, Spinner M, Van Beek AL (eds): Management of Peripheral Nerve Problems. Philadelphia: WB Saunders, 1998, pp 365–370.
19. Kline DG, Kim D, Midha R, et al: Management and results of sciatic nerve injuries: A 24-year experience. J Neurosurg 89:12–23, 1998.
20. Brooks DG: The neurofibromatoses: Hereditary predisposition to multiple peripheral nerve tumors. Neurosurg Clin N Am 15(2):145–155, 2004.
21. Huang JH, Simon SL, Nagpal S, et al: Management of patients with schwannomatosis: Report of six cases and review of the literature. Surg Neurol 62(4):353–361, 2004.

Safety Measures in Surgery

168 Ensuring Patient Safety in Surgery—"First Do No Harm"

GEORGE T. BLIKE

Primum non nocere—first do no harm. This often-quoted phrase epitomizes the importance the medical community places on avoiding iatrogenic complications.[1] In the process of providing care, patients, physicians, and the entire clinical team join to use all available medical weapons to combat disease to avert the natural history of pathologic processes. Iatrogenic injury or, simply, "treatment related harm" occurs when this implicit rule to "first do no harm" is violated. Both society and the medical community have historically been intolerant of medical mistakes, associating them with negligence. The fact is that complex medical care is prone to failure. Medical mistakes are much like "friendly fire" incidents in which soldiers in the high-tempo, complex fog of war mistakenly kill comrades rather than the enemy. Invariably, medical error and iatrogenic injury are associated with multiple latent conditions (constraints, hazards, system vulnerabilities, etc.) that predisposed front-line clinicians to err. This chapter will review the science of human error in medicine and surgery. The specific case of wrong-sided brain surgery will be used as an illustration for implementation of emerging new strategies for enhancing patient safety.

THE NATURE OF IATROGENIC INJURY IN MEDICINE AND SURGERY

The earliest practitioners of medicine recognized and described iatrogenic injury. Iatrogenic (Greek, *iatros* = doctor, *genic* = arising from or developing from) literally translates to "disease or illness caused by doctors." Famous examples exist of likely iatrogenic deaths, such as that of George Washington, who died while being treated for pneumonia with blood letting. The Royal Medical and Surgical Society, in 1864, documented 123 deaths that "could be positively assigned to the inhalation of chloroform."[2] Throughout history, physicians have reviewed unexpected outcomes related to the medical care they provided to learn and improve that care. The "father" of modern neurosurgery, Harvey Cushing, and his contemporary Sir William Osler modeled the practice of learning from error by publishing their errors openly so as to warn others on how to avert future occurrences.[3-5] However, the magnitude of iatrogenic morbidity and mortality was not quantified across the spectrum of health care until the Harvard Practice Study, published in 1991.[6] This seminal study estimated that iatrogenic failures occur in approximately 4% of all hospitalizations and is the eighth leading cause of death in America—responsible for up to 100,000 deaths per year in the United States alone.[7]

A subsequent review of over 14,700 hospitalizations in Colorado and Utah identified 402 surgical adverse events, producing an annual incidence rate of 1.9%.[8] The nature of surgical adverse events were categorized by type of injury and by preventability (Table 168-1).

These two studies were designed to characterize iatrogenic complications in health care. While not statistically powered to allow surgical subspecialty analysis, it is likely that the types of failures and subsequent injuries this study identified can be generalized to the neurosurgical patient population. More recent literature supports the findings of these landmark studies.[9-11]

The Institute of Medicine used the Harvard Practice Study as the basis for its report, which endorsed the need to discuss and study errors openly with the goal of improving patient safety.[7] One might argue that morbidity and mortality reviews already achieve this aim. The "M&M" conference has a long history of reviewing negative outcomes in medicine. The goal of this traditional conference is to learn how to prevent future patients from suffering similar harm, and thus incrementally improve care. However, frank discussion of error is limited in M&M conferences. Also, the actual review practices fail to support deep learning regarding systemic vulnerabilities[12]; indeed, since M&M conferences do not explicitly require medical errors to be reviewed,

TABLE 168-1 ▪ Surgical Adverse Events Categorized by Type of Injury and Preventability

Type of Event	Percentage of Adverse Events	Percentage Preventable
Technique-related complication	24	68
Wound infection	11	23
Postoperative bleeding	11	85
Postpartum/neonatal related	8	67
Other infection	7	38
Drug-related injury	7	46
Wound problem (noninfectious)	4	53
Deep venous thrombosis	4	18
Nonsurgical procedure injury	3	59
Diagnostic error/delay	3	100
Pulmonary embolus	2	14
Acute myocardial infarction	2	0
Inappropriate therapy	2	100
Anesthesia injury	2	45
Congestive heart failure	1	33
Stroke	1	0
Pneumonia	1	65
Fall	.5	50
Other	5.5	32

errors are rarely addressed. One prospective investigation of four U.S. academic hospitals found that a resident vigilantly attending weekly internal medicine M&M conferences for an entire year would discuss errors only once. The surgical version of the M&M conference was better with error discussion. However, while surgeons discussed adverse events associated with error 77% of the time, individual provider error was the focus of the discussion and cited as causative of the negative outcome in 8 of 10 conference discussions.[12] Surgical conference discussion rarely identified structural defects, resource constraints, team communication, or other system problems. Further limiting its utility, the M&M conference is reactive by nature and highly subject to hindsight bias. This is the basis for most clinical outcome reviews, focusing solely on medical providers and their decision making.[13] In their report on "Nine Steps to Move Forward from Error" in medicine, human factors experts Cook and Woods challenged the medical community to resist the temptation to simplify the complexities practitioners face when reviewing accidents post hoc. Premature closure by blaming the closest clinician hides the deeper patterns and multiple contributors associated with failure and ultimately leads to naïve "solutions" that are weak or even counterproductive.[14] The Institute of Medicine has also cautioned against blaming an individual and recommending training as the sole outcome of case review.[7] While the culture within medicine is to learn from failure, the M&M conference does not typically achieve this aim.

A HUMAN FACTORS APPROACH TO IMPROVING PATIENT SAFETY

Murphy's Law—that whatever can go wrong will—is the common-sense explanation for medical mishaps. The science of safety (and how to create it), however, is not common sense. The field of human factors engineering grew out of a focus on human interaction with physical devices, especially in military or industrial settings. This initial focus on how to improve human performance addressed the problem of workers that are at high risk for injury while using a tool or machine in high hazard industries. In the past several decades, the scope of this science has broadened. Human factors engineering is now credited with advancing safety and reliability in aviation, nuclear power, and other high hazard work settings. Membership in the Human Factors and Ergonomics Society in North America alone has grown to over 15,000 members. Human factors engineering and related disciplines are deeply interested in modeling and understanding mechanisms of complex system failure. Furthermore, these applied sciences have developed strategies for designing error prevention and building error tolerance into systems to increase reliability and safety, and these strategies are now being applied to the health care industry.[15–20] The specialty of anesthesiology has employed this science to reduce the anesthesia-related mortality rate from approximately 1 in 10,000 in the 1970s to over 1 in 250,000 three decades later.[21] Critical incident analysis was used by a bioengineer (Jeffrey Cooper, Ph.D.) to identify preventable anesthesia mishaps in 1978.[22] Dr. Cooper's seminal work was supplemented by the "closed claim" liability studies, which delineated the most common and severe modes of failure and factors that contributed to those failures. The specialty of anesthesiology and its leaders

endorsed the precepts that safety stems more from improved system design than from increasing vigilance of individual practitioners. As a direct result, anesthesiology was the first specialty to adopt minimal standards for care and monitoring, preanesthesia equipment checklists similar to those used in commercial aviation, standardized medication labels, interlocking hardware to prevent gas mix-ups, international anesthesia machine standards, and the development of high-fidelity human simulation to support crisis team training in the management of rare events. Lucien Leape, M.D., a former surgeon, one of the lead authors of the Harvard Practice Study, and a national advocate for patient safety, has stated, "Anesthesia is the only system in healthcare that begins to approach the vaunted 'six sigma' (a defect rate of 1 in a million) level of clinical safety perfection that other industries strive for. This outstanding achievement is attributable not to any single practice or development of new anesthetic agents or even any type of improvement (such as technological advances) but to application of a broad array of changes in process, equipment, organization, supervision, training, and teamwork. However, no single one of these changes has ever been proven to have a clear-cut impact on mortality. Rather, anesthesia safety was achieved by applying a whole host of changes that made sense, were based on an understanding of human factors principles, and had been demonstrated to be effective in other settings."[23] The Anesthesia Patient Safety Foundation, which has become the clearinghouse for patient safety successes in anesthesiology, was used as a model by the American Medical Association to form the National Patient Safety Foundation in 1996.[24] Over the subsequent decade, the science of safety has begun to permeate health care.

The human factors psychologist James Reason, Ph.D., has characterized accidents as evolving over time and as virtually never being the consequence of a single cause.[25,26] Rather, he describes accidents as the net result of local triggers that initiate and then propagate an incident though a hole in one layer of defense after another until irreversible injury occurs (Fig. 168-1). This model has been referred to as the "Swiss cheese" model of accident causation. Surgical care consists of thousands of tasks and subtasks. Errors in the execution of these tasks need to be prevented, detected and managed, or tolerated. The layers of Swiss cheese represent the system of defenses against such error. *Latent conditions* is the term used to describe "accidents waiting to happen" that are the holes in each layer that will allow an error to propagate until it ultimately causes injury or death. The goal in human factors system engineering is to know all the layers of Swiss cheese and create the best defenses possible (i.e., make the holes as small as possible). This very approach has been the centerpiece of incremental improvements in anesthesia safety.

One structured approach designed to identify all of the holes in the major layers of cheese in medical systems has been described by Vincent.[27,28] He classifies the major categories of factors that contribute to error as follows:

1. Patient factors: condition, communication, availability and accuracy of test results and other contextual factors that make a patient challenging
2. Task factors: using an organized approach in reliable task execution, availability and use of protocols, and other aspects of task performance

FIGURE 168-1 Reason's model of accident causation. Accidents (adverse outcomes) require a combination of latent failures, psychological precursors, event triggers, and failures in several layers of the system's "defense in depth." Copyright Dr. Reason.

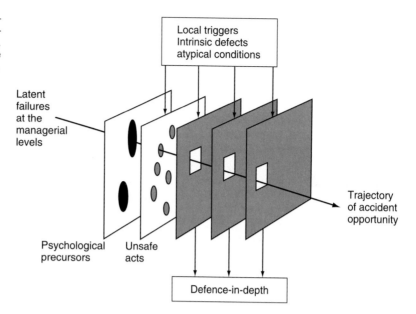

3. Practitioner factors: deficits and failures by any individual member of the care team that undermines management of the problem space in terms of knowledge, attention, strategy, motivation, physical or mental health, and other factors that undermine individual performance
4. Team factors: verbal/written communication, supervision/seeking help, team structure and leadership, and other failures in communication and coordination among members of the care team such that management of the problem space is degraded
5. Working conditions: staffing levels, skills mix and workload, availability and maintenance of equipment, administrative and managerial support, and other aspects of the work domain that undermine individual or team performance
6. Organization and management factors: financial resources, goals, policy standards, safety culture and priorities, and other factors that constrain local microsystem performance
7. Societal and political factors*: economic and regulatory issues, health policy and politics, and other societal factors that set thresholds for patient safety

If this schema is used to structure a review of a morbidity or mortality, that review will be extended beyond myopic attention to the singular practitioner. Furthermore, the array of identified factors that undermine safety can then be countered systematically by tightening each layer of defense, one hole at a time. I have adapted active error management as described by Reason and others into a set of steps for making incremental systemic improvements to increase safety and reliability. In this adaptation, a cycle of active error management consists of (a) surveillance to identify potential threats; (b) investigation of all contributory factors; (c) prioritization of failure modes; (d) development of countermeasures to eliminate or mitigate individual

*Author modified the "institutional" category to "societal and political" to capture factors external to the hospital that resource or constrain practice.

threats; and (e) broad implementation of validated countermeasures (Fig. 168-2).

The goal is to move from a reactive approach based on review of actual injuries toward a proactive approach that anticipates threats based on a deep understanding of human capabilities and system design that aids human performance rather than undermines it.

A comprehensive review of the science of human factors and patient safety is beyond the scope of this chapter; neurosurgical patient safety has been reviewed, including ethical issues and the impact of legal liability.[29] Safety in aviation and nuclear power has taken over four decades to achieve the cultural shift that supports a robust system of countermeasures and defenses against human error. However, it is practical to use an example to illustrate some of the human factors principles introduced. Consider this case example as a window into the future of managing the most common preventable adverse events associated with surgery (Table 168-1).

EXAMPLE OF MEDICAL ERROR: "WRONG-SIDED BRAIN SURGERY"

Wrong site surgery is an example of an adverse event that seems as though it should "never happen." However, given over 40 million surgical procedures annually, we should not be surprised when it occurs. The news media has diligently reported wrong site surgical errors, especially when they involve neurosurgery. Headlines such as "Brain Surgery Was Done on the Wrong Side, Reports Say" (*New York Daily News*, 2001) and "Doctor Who Operated on the Wrong Side of Brain Under Scrutiny" (*New York Times*, 2000), are inevitable when wrong site brain surgery occurs.[30–32] As predicted, these are not isolated stories. A recent report from the state of Minnesota found 13 instances of wrong site surgery in a single year during which time approximately 340,000 surgeries

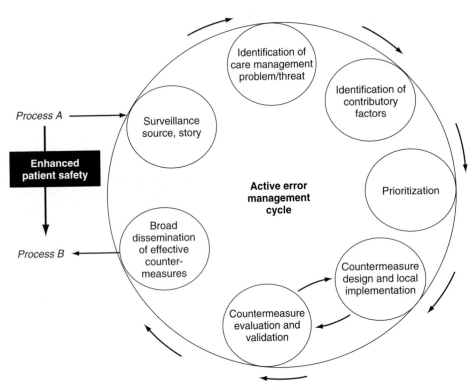

FIGURE 168-2 Sequence of steps for identifying vulnerabilities and then implementing corrective measures. Copyright Blike 2002.

were performed.[33] No hospital appeared to be immune to what appears on the surface to be such a blatant mistake. Indeed, an incomplete registry collecting data on wrong site surgery since 2001 now includes over 150 cases. Of 126 instances that have been reviewed, 41% relate to orthopedic surgery, 20% relate to general surgery, 14% to neurosurgery, 11% to urologic surgery, and the remaining to the other surgical specialties.[34]

The sensational "front page news" media fails to identify the deeper second story behind these failures and how to prevent future failures through creation of safer systems.[35] In this example, we provide an analysis of contributory factors associated with wrong site surgery to reveal the myriad of holes in the defensive layers of "cheese." These holes will need to be eliminated to truly impact the frequency of this already rare event and create more reliable care for our patients.

CONTRIBUTORY FACTOR ANALYSIS

Patient Factors Associated with Wrong Site Surgery

Patient Condition (Medical Factors That If Not Known Increase the Risk for Complications)

Neurosurgical patients are at higher risk for wrong patient surgery than average. Patients and their surgical conditions contribute to error. When patients are asked what surgery they are having done on the morning of surgery, only 70% can correctly state and point to the location of the planned surgical intervention.[36] Patients are a further source of misinformation of surgical intent when the pathology and symptoms are contralateral to the site of surgery, a common condition in neurosurgical cases. Patients scheduled for brain surgery and carotid surgery often confuse the side of the surgery with the side of the symptoms. Patients with

educational or language barriers or cognitive deficits are more vulnerable since they are unable to accurately communicate their surgical condition or the planned surgery.

Certain operations in the neurosurgical population pose higher risk for wrong site surgery. While left-right symmetry and sidedness represents one high-risk class of surgeries, spinal procedures in which there are multiple levels is another.[37]

Patients with anatomy and pathology that disorient the surgical team to side or level are especially at risk. Anterior cervical discectomies can be approached by surgeons from either side. This lack of a consistent cue for the rest of the surgical team as to the approach for the same surgery makes it unlikely anyone would trap an error in positioning or draping. It is known that patient position and opaque draping can remove external cues as to left and right orientation of the patient and thus predispose surgeons to wrong-sided surgery. When a patient is lateral, fully draped, and the table rotated 180 degrees prior to the attending surgeon entering the operating theater, it is difficult to verify right from left. Furthermore, the language for positioning creates ambiguity since the terminology of left lateral decubitus, right side up, and left side down are used interchangeably by the surgical team to specify the position. A patient with bilateral disease, predominant right-sided symptoms, and left-sided pathology having a left-sided craniotomy in the right lateral decubitus position with the table turned 180 degrees and fully draped obviously creates more confusion than a gallbladder surgery in the supine position.

Communication (Factors That Undermine the Patient's Ability to Be a Source of Information Regarding Conditions That Increase the Risk for Complications and Need to Be Managed)

Obviously, patients with language barriers or cognitive deficits represent a group that may be unable to communicate their understanding of the surgical plan. This can increase the chance of patient identification errors that lead to wrong site surgery. In a busy practice, patients requiring the same surgery might be scheduled in the same operating room (OR). It is not uncommon to perform five carotid endarterectomies in a single day.[38] When one patient is delayed and the order switched to keep the OR moving, this vulnerability is expressed. Patients with common names are especially at risk. A 500-bed hospital will have approximately 1,000,000 patients in the medical record system. About 10% of patients will have the same first and last names. Five percent will have a first, middle, and last name in common with one other individual. Only by cross-checking the name with one other patient identifier (either birth date or a medical record number) can wrong patient errors be trapped.[39]

Another patient communication problem that increases risk for wrong site surgery consists of patients marking themselves. Marking the skin on the side of the proposed surgery with a pen is now common practice by the surgical team and part of the Universal Protocol. However, some patients have placed an X on the site not to be operated on. The surgical team has then confused this patient mark with their own in which an X specifies the side to be operated on. Patients are often not given information of what to expect and will seek outside information. For example, a neurosurgeon on a popular daytime talk show discussing medical mistakes stated incorrectly that patients should mark themselves with an X on the side that should not be operated on.[40] This error in information reached millions of viewers, and was in direct violation of recommendations for marking provided by the Joint Commission on Accreditation of Healthcare Organizations (and endorsed by the American College of Surgeons, American Society of Anesthesiology, and Association of Operating Room Nurses). Patients who watched this show and took the advice of the physician are now at higher risk than average for a wrong-sided surgical error.

Availability and Accuracy of Test Results (Factors That Undermine Awareness of Conditions That Increase the Risk for Complications and Need to Be Managed)

Radiologic imaging studies can be independent markers of surgical pathology and anatomy. However, films and/or reports are not always available. Films may be lost or misplaced. Also, they may be unavailable because they were performed at another facility. New digital technology has created electronic imaging systems that virtually eliminate lost studies. However, space constraints have led many hospitals to remove old view boxes to make room for digital radiologic monitors. When patients bring films from an outside hospital, this decision to eliminate view boxes prevents effective use of the studies. Even when available, x-rays and diagnostic studies are not labeled with 100% reliability. Imaging studies have been mislabeled and/or oriented backward, leading to wrong-sided surgery.[41]

Task Factors Associated with Wrong Site Surgery

Tasks are the steps that need to be executed to accomplish a work goal. It is especially important to structure tasks and task execution procedures when work domains are complex, the task must be executed under time pressure, and the

consequence of errors in task execution are severe. Typical tools for structuring task execution are protocols, checklists, and algorithms.

Task Design and Clarity of Structure (Consider This to Be an Issue When Work Is Being Performed in a Manner That Is Inefficient and Not Well Thought Out)

In large hospitals, ORs do not execute a consistent set of checks and balances to verify that the right patient, the surgical intent, and critical equipment and implants are present. If surgical team members think that they can announce the patient name and procedure aloud and that this will reliably prevent wrong site surgery, they are mistaken. Structuring tasks for reliability such that current failure rates will be moved from approximately 1 in 30,000 to 1 in 1 million will take the kind of task structure and consistency seen on the flight decks of commercial planes. For decades, pilots have used well-organized preflight checklists to perform the tasks to start up an engine and verify that all mission critical equipment is present and functional.

An example of a mature use of checklists exists in anesthesiology. An anesthesia machine (and other critical equipment) must be present and functional prior to the induction of anesthesia and initiation of paralysis so that a patient can have an airway as well as breathing and circulatory support provided within seconds to avoid hypoxia and subsequent cardiovascular complications. Until 1990, equipment failures were a significant problem leading to patient injury in anesthesia, even though anesthesia machines and equipment had been standardized and were being used on thousands of patients in a given facility.[42] At this time, a preanesthesia checklist was established to structure the verification of mission critical components required to provide the anesthetic state and to verify that these components functioned nominally.[43] This checklist includes over 40 items and has included redundancy for checking critical components. It has been introduced as a standard operating procedure for the discipline of anesthesia and is now mandated by the U.S. Food and Drug Association[44] (Fig. 168-3).

Availability and Use of Protocols (If Standard Protocols Exist, Are They Well Accepted and Are They Being Used Consistently?)

The universal protocol for preventing wrong patient, wrong site errors is based on checklist principles; but it is not yet a validated comprehensive checklist that will trap errors in the way aviation checklists do. This is largely due to the lack of consistent execution of the checklists in a challenge-response format that is identical in procedure and practice throughout a single hospital's ORs. This protocol is a first step, but the barriers to effective implementation are extensive at present and hinder improved safety.[45,46]

Another hazard is the lack of clarity for marking surgical sites. Marking the surgical site has been endorsed to improve safety and is a major component of the Universal Protocol. However, as described previously, the mark can be a source of error when placed inappropriately by the patient or any other member of the surgical team. Some specifics regarding the details of what, when, and how to mark are lacking. Do you mark the incision site or the target of the surgery? What constitutes a unique and definitive mark? What shape and color should be used? What type of pen should be used? Does the ink pose any risk for infection or

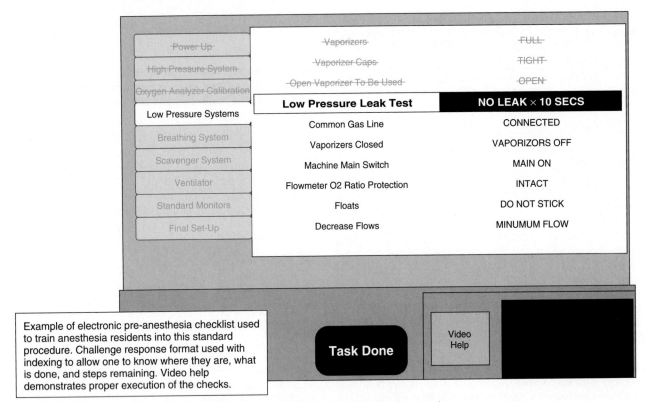

~~Power Up~~	~~Vaporizers~~ — ~~FULL~~
~~High Pressure System~~	~~Vaporizer Caps~~ — ~~TIGHT~~
~~Oxygen Analyzer Calibration~~	~~Open Vaporizer To Be Used~~ — ~~OPEN~~
Low Pressure Systems	**Low Pressure Leak Test** — NO LEAK × 10 SECS
~~Breathing System~~	Common Gas Line — CONNECTED
~~Scavenger System~~	Vaporizers Closed — VAPORIZORS OFF
~~Ventilator~~	Machine Main Switch — MAIN ON
~~Standard Monitors~~	Flowmeter O2 Ratio Protection — INTACT
~~Final Set-Up~~	Floats — DO NOT STICK
	Decrease Flows — MINUMUM FLOW

Example of electronic pre-anesthesia checklist used to train anesthesia residents into this standard procedure. Challenge response format used with indexing to allow one to know where they are, what is done, and steps remaining. Video help demonstrates proper execution of the checks.

Task Done   Video Help

FIGURE 168-3 Example of computer implementation.

is it washed off during the course of preparation? Who should place the mark? What are the procedures that get marked and which should not? Are there any patients for whom the mark is dangerous? How do you mark for a left liver lobe resection or other procedures like brain surgery in which there is a single organ but still sidedness that is critical? I worked with over 10 surgical specialties to develop specific answers to these questions. Multiple marks and pens were tested. Not all symbols and pens were equally effective. Many inks did not withstand preparation and remain visible in the operative field. We now use specific permanent pens (Carter fine and Sharpie very fine) and a green circle to mark only "sided" procedures. We specified that the target is marked rather than the incision, the mark must be done by the surgeon, and the mark must be placed in a manner in which it is visible during the preincision check after the position, preparation, and drape have been completed. For example, a procedure requiring cystoscopy to inject the right ureteral orifice to treat reflux is now marked on the right thigh so that the green circle mark is a cue to all members of the surgical team and can be seen even when the patient is prepared and draped. Again, we used the mark to specify the target, not the incision or body entry point. In addition, we have had every procedure in our booking system labeled as "mark required" or "mark not required," because this was not always clear. Even with this level of specificity, we have found marking to be erroneous and inconsistent during our initial implementation. Marking the skin for spine surgery to indicate the level may increase the risk of wrong site errors.[47] A superior method for "marking" to verify the correct spinal level to be operated upon is to perform an intraoperative radiologic study with a

radiopaque marker. We expect that many revisions to this type of safety measure will be needed before the marking procedure is robust and truly adds safety value. Cross-checking procedures in aviation were developed and matured over decades to achieve the reliability and consistency now observed.[48]

Practitioner Factors Associated with Wrong Site Surgery

Knowledge, Skills, and Rules (Individual Deviation from Standard of Care Due to Lack of Knowledge, Poor Skills, or a Failure to Use Rules Associated with Best Practice)

Knowledge deficits are often due to overreliance on memory for information used rarely. Measures that increase availability of referent knowledge when needed would be helpful. Unfortunately, references at the point of care on the day of surgery are not standard or reliable. Three descriptions of the surgery often exist. The operative consent lists the planned surgery in lay language patients should be able to understand. The surgical preoperative note may provide a technical description of the planned surgery but often is incomplete, failing to include such information as the specific reason for surgery, sidedness, target, approach, position, need for implants, and/or special equipment. The booking system will often use a third nomenclature to describe the planned surgery that is administrative and linked to billing codes. The use of three different references for the same surgical procedure creates ambiguity. A "right L3–4 facetectomy in the prone position" may be listed on the consent form as a "right third lumbar vertebrae joint surgery" on the consent and a CPT code "LUMBAR FACETECTOMY 025-36047."[49]

Subtle knowledge deficits are more likely to reach a patient and cause harm when individuals are charged to do work that is at the limits of their competency. The culture of medicine does not encourage knowledge calibration, the term used to describe how well individuals know what they know and know what they do not know.[50] At our institution, when preoperative nurses were assigned the role of marking patients to identify sidedness, they routinely marked the wrong site or marked in a manner such that the mark was not visible after the position, prep, and drape. These nurses accepted this assigned role because our medical culture encourages guessing and assertiveness. On further review we have found that only the surgeon has knowledge required to specify the surgical plan in detail and to mark patients correctly. Other members of the surgical team often have subtle knowledge deficits regarding surgical anatomy, terminology, and technical requirements such that they are prone to err in marking or positioning patients. Similarly, nurses and anesthesiologists in the presurgical areas are not able to verify or reconcile multiple differing sources of information as to the surgical plan. Instead they often propagate errors and/or enter new misinformation into scheduling systems and patient records.

Attention (Factors That Undermine Attention)

Task execution is degraded when attention is pulled away from the work being performed. Distraction and noise are significant problems in the operating theater that can dramatically affect performance and vigilance. Because the wall and floor surfaces are designed to be cleaned easily, noise levels in the OR are similar to those on a busy highway.[51,52] The preincision interval is a very active time, when the patient is being given anesthesia, being positioned, and being prepared. These parallel activities represent competing priorities that conflict with a coordinated effort by the entire surgical team to verify surgical intent.

Strategy (Given Many Alternatives, Was the Strategy Optimized to Minimize Risks Through Preventive Measures and Through Recovery Measures That Use Contingency Planning and Anticipatory Behaviors?)

Strategic planning is not a major contributory factor for wrong site surgery in my opinion. However, we have found that our initial attempts to use the exact same preincision checklist for all types of surgical populations was a strategic error and overly simplistic.

Motivation/Attitude (Motivational Failures and Poor Attitudes Can Undermine Individual Performance— the Psychology of Motivation Is Complex)

Because wrong site surgery is a rare event, motivating the operative team to invest significant energy into preventive measures can be challenging. Even though the career risk for performing a wrong site surgery is significant, the rarity of this complication predisposes surgeons to deny this complication as a significant problem. Part of the problem is that surgeons do not have an adequate understanding of human vulnerabilities and the potential for error. Many surgeons see wrong site surgery as purely a failure in vigilance by an individual surgeon. The motivation to lead a team

effort and accept cross-checking is therefore low. Human error training in surgery is just now beginning to address the decreased performance associated with fatigue, personal stress, production pressure, and so forth. Motivational barriers are not limited to the surgeon. Many nurses and anesthesiologists see wrong site surgery as an isolated surgeon failure and believe they should have no responsibility for verifying patient and/or procedure. Individual training about human error is needed across all members of the operative team to increase motivation to change behavior and use new methods (such as a team-executed checklist) to prevent wrong site surgery.

Physical/Mental Health (Provider Performance Deviations from Standard "Competencies" Can Be Due to Physical or Mental Illness)

Industries that have come to accept the human component as having requirements for optimal man-machine system performance have thus promoted regular "fit for duty" examinations.[53] In the aviation industry, job screening includes a "color-blindness" test for air traffic controllers since many of the monitors encode critical information in color.[54] Some specific provider health conditions can predispose to wrong site surgery. Surgeons and other members of the perioperative team with dyslexia and related neuropsychiatric deficits have particular difficulty with sidedness and left-right orientation.

Team Factors Associated with Wrong Site Surgery

A complex work domain will overwhelm the cognitive abilities of any one individual and not permit expertise of the entire field of practice. A common strategy for managing the excess demands that complex systems (like that of human physiology and pathophysiology) place on any individual is to subspecialize. Breaking a big problem into smaller parts that are then more manageable by a group of individuals is rational. However, by "fixing" the problem of individual cognitive work overload, a new class of problems manifest— those due to team communication and coordination failure. Many human factors experts consider team failures to be the most common contributory factor associated with error in complex sociotechnical work systems.[55] Crisis resource management training and team training in aviation is considered to have played a major role in improving aviation safety.[56] These methods are just now being applied in medicine.[57]

Verbal/Written Communication (Any Communication Mode That When It Fails Leads to a Degradation in Team Performance)

Verbal communications fail due to noise (just do not hear) or content comprehension (mismatch between what was intended and what was understood). Noise should be minimized to support verbal communication in the OR. Comprehension problems have many mechanisms. Human to human communication requires "grounding," which is the process whereby both parties frame the communication episode based on how the one conveying a message discovers the frame of reference of the one receiving the message. This activity represents a significant part of effective communication. Agreeing on a common language and structuring communication goes a long way toward increasing accuracy and speed of communication of mission-critical information.[16,17,58] While isolated examples of structured communication across members of the operative team exist, it is usually confined to individuals knowledgeable in safety science and the use of structured communication in the military and in aviation.

Supervision/Seeking Help (Any Member of the Team Who Fails to Mobilize Help When Getting into a Work Overload Situation, or a Team Member in a Supervisory Role Failing to Provide Adequate Oversight, Especially in Settings in Which There Are Learners and/or Transient Rotating Team Members)

True team performance is only realized when a group of individuals share a common goal, divide work tasks between individuals to create role delineation and role clarity within the team, and know each other's roles well enough to provide cross-checks of mission-critical activities.[59] On medical teams, data gathering and treatment implementation tend to be nursing roles, and diagnostic decision making and treatment selection tend to be physician roles.[60] A myriad of supporting clinicians and nonclinicians are vital in medical teams. The nurse, nurse practitioner, medical student, physicians, and others must be able to detect problem states or deviations from the "expected course" and activate control measures. When a practitioner fails to work within his or her competencies or is on the learning curve for his or her role on the team, failure to get or provide supervision comes into play. For wrong site surgery errors, this issue manifests when one surgeon does the preoperative consultation and operative planning and the other starts the surgery with incomplete knowledge. For example, a resident or fellow may fail to call an attending physician to seek clarification of the operative plan.

Team Structure and Leadership (Teams That Do Not Have Structure, Role Delineation, and Clarity, and Methods for Flattening Hierarchy While Resolving Conflict Will Have Suboptimal Team Performance)

Teams will inevitably have to face ambiguous situations that need immediate action. Authority gradients prevent junior members of the team from questioning the decision making and action planning of the leader (a nurse might be hesitant to tell a senior surgeon that he or she is violating a safety procedure, and/or the surgeon might disregard the nurse).[59] Methods for flattening hierarchy will lead to more robust team situational awareness and support cross-checking behavior. In contrast, it is essential to have efficient ways of resolving conflict, especially under emergency conditions. Some surgeons view the Universal Protocol as a ridiculous requirement forced upon them by regulatory bodies responding to liability pressure. This can create a void in leadership regarding team behaviors that would otherwise help to trap errors that predispose to wrong site surgery.

Working Conditions Associated with Wrong Site Surgery

Individuals and teams cannot perform optimally when they have inadequate resources to manage the work at hand. Typically, workers have little control over the conditions in which they are required to work. Managers make decisions that ultimately aid or constrain practitioners in terms of ratios of patients per provider, the physical space available, and the tools and/or technology available to front-line workers.

Staffing Levels, Skills Mix, and Workload (Managers Facing Financial Pressures, a Nursing Shortage, and Increasing Patient Acuity Can Choose to Institute Hiring Freezes and Reduce Staffing Ratios to Decrease the Costs Associated with Care)

While institutions and providers that have high surgical case volumes have been noted to have the best surgical outcomes, medical mishaps occur even in these institutions. Providing exceptional care to a few patients is easier that providing reliable care to everyone.[61] Indeed, excessive production pressure and patient volumes are associated with safety violations due to cutting corners when productivity goals are unrealistic. Over two thirds of wrong site surgeries occurred in ambulatory surgery settings in which patient acuity is the lowest but productivity pressures are high.[62] Financial constraints have forced more ORs to be staffed by temporary traveling position nurses, have resulted in nursing orientations that have been reduced, and have increased production pressure on surgeons to increase their utilization of OR time. Unfortunately, such aggressive measures to utilize all the capacity of the OR resources conflicts with the need for some reserve capacity to manage the inherent uncertainty and variability associated with medical disease and surgical care. As a result, emergency situations can easily overwhelm care systems that lack reserve resources. Providers calling in sick during flu season and/or a flurry of surgical emergencies can create dangerous conditions for elective surgery due to the need to redirect those resources that might otherwise be available.

Availability and Maintenance of Equipment (Technology and Tools Vary in their Safety Features and Usability: Equipment Must Be Maintained or It Can Become a Liability)

For preventing wrong site surgery, we have found that the specific marking pen we are utilizing needs to be stocked and available throughout the hospital to allow surgeons to perform the safety practice we have required. Surgeons unable to find a green marker will use alternative pens, resulting in a variation in practice that degrades the value of the safety measure. Other aspects of our wrong site surgery safeguards have proved difficult to maintain. A computerized scheduling system had triggers to cue the operative team as to the marking protocol and special equipment needs. When a new procedure was added to the scheduling system, the programmers overlooked the "needs to be marked" trigger, and for a period of time these patients were not marked. The operative team had been using technology designed to support their work, but that technology was not maintained. The best team of practitioners can perform even better when provided state-of-the-art working conditions. For example, patient identification technology that utilizes bar coding and radiofrequency identification tags will virtually eliminate wrong patient errors.[63] Although this technology is currently available, few organizations have been able to afford this technology to prevent wrong site errors due to patient misidentification.

Administrative and Managerial Support (In Complex Work Settings, Domain Experts That Perform the Work Need to Be Supported by Personnel Who Are Charged with Managing Resources, Scheduling, Transcription, Billing, etc.)

Clinical information systems (e.g., an OR scheduling system) are not reliable or robust at confirming operative intent early in the process or planning for surgery.[45] Busy surgical clinics often do not have efficient and reliable mechanisms for providing a scheduling secretary with the information they need or for verifying that booking information is accurate. Secretaries may be using a form that is illegible or may simply be working from a verbal description of the planned surgery. Because these support personnel may not understand the terminology, errors are common. In addition, busy surgeons may forget that other information, such as the operative position required, the need for surgical implants, or the requirement for special equipment, is not obvious, and thus fail to be explicit. In addition, this work and the expertise required is often undervalued. The result can be to hire inexperienced secretaries and accept high support staff turnover.

Organizational Factors Associated with Wrong Site Surgery

Organizations must make safety a priority. If production pressure and economic goals are in conflict with safety, organizations must have structure and methods for ensuring safety as the priority.[64] Independent offices of patient safety and patient safety officers with the authority to stop operations when necessary are examples of organizational structures designed to maintain safety in the face of economic pressure.

Financial Resources (Safety Is Not Free; the Costs Associated with Establishing Safe Practices and Acquiring Safety Technology May Be Prohibitive)

Many organizations have implemented the Universal Protocol, but have done so in an incomplete manner doing the minimum to pass a regulatory review. Given the rarity of wrong site surgery, the cost of preventing each instance would appear significant (although good safety habits or practice can or should be generalizable). The financial impact of correcting computer system flaws, improving secretarial support, and slowing down throughput to perform safety checks is unknown. Costs are a significant barrier to implementing safeguards robustly.

Goals and Policy Standards (Practice of Front-line Workers Is Shaped by Clear Goals and Consistent Policies That Are Clinically Relevant)

Policies and procedures regarding prevention of wrong site surgery are difficult to develop. Legal liability tends to constrain medical policy makers to be purposely vague. Explicit procedures that are standardized would be helpful. Unfortunately, newly developed procedures may be recommended as policy prior to proper testing and validation for effectiveness. For example, the Universal Protocol has not been fully validated and yet this protocol has been mandated.

Safety Culture and Priorities (A Safety Culture of an Organization May Be Pathologic, Reactive, Proactive, or Generative.)

Most hospitals today are reactive in their culture of safety.[26] The result is that those institutions that have had the most public wrong site surgeries have done the most to establish safety countermeasures to prevent future wrong site surgery. Proactive action to invest in creating safeguards is beyond the capability or commitment of most health care organizations as of 2005.

Sociopolitical Factors Associated with Wrong Site Surgery

Economic, Regulatory Issues, Health Policy, and Politics

We practice medicine within large national health care systems. Currently, third-party payers wish for safety to be a priority. However, organizations that invest in safety technologies to avert error do not typically get a return on that investment. In fact, hospital investment to prevent iatrogenic injury directly benefits third-party payers, not the hospital. Similarly, our legal system does not serve as a strong incentive for safety because jury verdicts do not accurately identify and punish negligent care. Rather, patients with negative outcomes that were not preventable still win jury verdicts, while patients that truly suffered a preventable adverse event commonly fail to seek legally allowed compensation.[65]

Summary of Contributory Factor Analysis

This example of wrong site surgery was used to illustrate the multiple contributory factors that allow error to propagate and evolve into an injury causing accident. Even with an error as blatant as wrong brain surgery, one can identify multiple vulnerabilities in the multiple layers of our complex medical care systems (Fig. 168-4). While hind-site bias tempts one to blame the individuals involved as the sole causative factor, it is clear that the individuals are part of a complex system with mul-tiple latent conditions (hazards and "accidents waiting to happen"). High reliability organizations are notable for their dedication to systematically identify all hazards and then counter each one. These organizations understand that failure is multidimensional and so is maximizing safety.

SUMMARY

Reducing iatrogenic injury has become a priority in health care. The scientific disciplines that have advanced safety in other high hazard industries such as aviation and nuclear power are just beginning to be used to help advance safety in health care. The causes of iatrogenic injury are complex, as are robust solutions. Success in other industries has been achieved through the use of a global strategy based on small incremental changes to identify threats and then systematically counter each one. Aviation started using this approach over 40 years ago. This strategy appears viable in

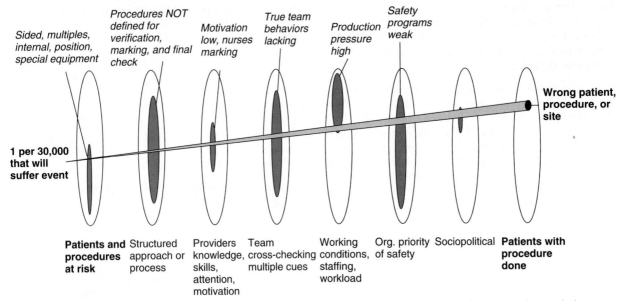

FIGURE 168-4   This graphic summarizes the major vulnerabilities identified as contributory toward wrong site surgical error.

health care but requires a long-term commitment. In addition, the battle to improve reliability and safety will be ongoing. Eliminating one set of vulnerabilities always reveals new ones that did not previously exist. Thus, the goal is to trade in the old problems for new ones that are more bearable. The future is hopeful as new safety sciences support medicine's quest to "first do no harm."

REFERENCES

1. Smith CM: Origin and uses of *primum non nocere*—above all, do no harm! J Clin Pharmacol 45:371–377, 2005.
2. Cushing H: The establishment of cerebral hernia as a decompressive measure for inaccessible brain tumors; with the description of intramuscular methods of making the bone defect in temporal and occipital regions. Surg Gynecol Obstet 1:297–314, 1905.
3. Pinkus RL: Mistakes as a social construct: An historical approach. Kennedy Inst Ethics J 11:117–133, 2001.
4. Bliss M: William Osler: A Life in Medicine. Toronto: University of Toronto Press, 1999.
5. Report of the Committee Appointed by the Royal Medical and Surgical Society to Inquire into the Uses and Physiological, Therapeutical and Toxical Effects of Chloroform. London: JR Adlarto, 1864.
6. Brennan TA, Leape LL, Laird NM, et al: Incidence of adverse events and negligence in hospitalized patients—Results of the Harvard Medical Practice Study I. N Engl J Med 324(6):370–376, 1991.
7. Kohn LT, Corrigan JM, Donaldson MS (eds): (2000). To Err is Human: Building a Safer Health System. Washington, DC: National Academy Press.
8. Gawande AA, Thomas EJ, Zinner MJ: The incidence and nature of surgical adverse events in Colorado and Utah in 1992. Surgery 126(1):66–75; 1999.
9. Leape LL, Rennan Ta, Laird N, et al: The nature of adverse events in hospitalized patients. Results of the Harvard Medical Practice Study II. N Engl J Med 324:377–384, 1991.
10. Vincent C, Neale G, Woloshynowych M: Adverse events in British hospitals: Preliminary retrospective record review. BMJ 322:517–519, 2001.
11. Wilson RM, Harrison BT, Gibberd RW, Hamilton JD: An analysis of the causes of adverse events from the Quality of Australian Health Care Study. Med J Aust 170:411–415, 1999.
12. Pierluissi E, Fischer MA, Campbell AR, Landefeld CS: Discussion of medical errors in morbidity and mortality conferences. JAMA 290(21):2838–2842, 2003.
13. Woods DD, Cook RI: Perspectives on human error: Hindsight bias and local rationality. In Durso FT, Nickerson RS (eds). Handbook of Applied Cognition. New York: John Wiley & Sons, 1999.
14. Woods DD, Cook RI: Nine steps to move forward from error. Cognition Technol Work 4:137–144, 2002.
15. Gawande A: Complications: A Surgeon's Notes on an Imperfect Science. New York: Picador, 2002.
16. Wickens CD, Gordon SE, Liu Y: An Introduction to Human Factors Engineering. Reading, MA: Addison-Wesley, 1998.
17. Sanders MS, McCormick EJ: Human Factors in Engineering and Design, 7th ed. New York: McGraw-Hill, 1993.
18. Bogner MS: Human Error in Medicine. Mahwah, NJ: Lawrence Erlbaum, 1994.
19. deLeval MR, Carthey J, Wright DJ, et al: All United Kingdom Pediatric Cardiac Centers. Human factors, and cardiac surgery: A multicenter study. J Thorac Cardiovasc Surg 119:661–672.
20. Douchin Y, Gopher D, Olin M, et al: A look into the nature and causes of human errors in the intensive care unit. Crit Care Med 23:298, 1995.
21. Keats AS: Anesthesia mortality in perspective. Anesth Analg 71:113–119, 1990.
22. Cooper JB, Newbower RS, Long CD, McPeek B: Preventable anesthetic mishaps: A study of human factors. Anesthesiology 49:399–406, 1978.
23. Leape L, Berwick DM, Bates DW: What practices will most improve safety? JAMA 288:501–507, 2002.
24. National Patient Safety Foundation: The NPSF is an independent, nonprofit research and education organization. http://www.npsf.org/html/research/rfp.html
25. Reason J: Human Error. New York: Cambridge University Press, 1990.
26. Reason J: Managing the risks of organizational accidents. Ashgate, 1997.
27. Vincent C, Taylor-Adams S, Chapman EJ, et al: How to investigate and analyze clinical incidents: Clinical risk unit and association of litigation and risk management protocol. BMJ 320:777–781, 2000.
28. Vincent N, et al: Patient safety: Understanding and responding to adverse events. N Engl J Med 348(11):1051–1056, 2003.
29. Bernstein M, Hebert PC, Etchells E: Patient safety in neurosurgery: Detection of errors, prevention of errors, and disclosure of errors. Neurosurg Q 13(2):125–137, 2003.
30. Brain surgery was done on the wrong side, reports say. New York Daily News 2001.
31. Brain surgeon cited in bungled '95 case faces a new inquiry. New York Times, February 18, 2000.
32. Altman LK: State issues scathing report on error at Sloan-Kettering. New York Times, November 16, 1995.
33. Report details Minnesota hospital errors. Wall Street Journal, January 20, 2005.
34. Joint Commission of Accreditation of Healthcare Organizations: Sentinel event statistics. 2003. Available at http://www.jcaho.org/accredited+organizations/hospitals/sentinel+events/sentinel+events+statistics.htm

35. Cook RI, Woods DD, Miller C: A tale of two stories: Contrasting views of patient safety. Chicago, IL: National Patient Safety Foundation, 1998. Available at *http://www.npsf.org/exec/front.html*
36. Schlosser E: Dartmouth-Hitchcock Medical Center Wrong Site Surgery Observational Study. Unpublished report, 2004.
37. Joint Commission of Accreditation of Healthcare Organizations: Lessons learned: Wrong site surgery, sentinel event, No. 6, 2001. Available at *http://www.jcaho.org/edu_pub/sealert/sea6.html*
38. Harbaugh R: Developing a neurosurgical carotid endarterectomy practice. Am Assoc Neurol Surg Bull 4(2), 1995.
39. Campion P: Dartmouth-Hitchcock Medical Center report on patient misidentification risk. Unpublished report, 2004.
40. Gupta S: Patient checklist. Outrageous medical mistakes—Oprah Winfrey Show, October 2003. Available at *http://www2.oprah.com/health/yourbody/health_yourbody_gupta.jhtml*
41. Warnke JP, Kose A, Schienwind F, Zierski J: Erroneous laterality marking in CT of head. A case report. Zentralbl Neurochir 50:190–192, 1989.
42. Cooper JB, Newbower RS, Kitz RJ: An analysis of major errors and equipment failures in anesthesia management: Considerations for prevention and detection. Anesthesiology 60:34–42, 1984.
43. U.S. Food and Drug Administration: Anesthesia apparatus checkout recommendations. Federal Registry 59:35373–35374, 1994.
44. Blike G, Biddle C: Preanesthesia detection of equipment faults by anesthesia providers at an academic hospital: Comparison of standard practice and a new electronic checklist. AANA J 68:497–505, 2000.
45. Rogers ML, Cook RI, Bower R, et al: Barriers to implementing wrong site surgery guidelines: A cognitive work analysis. IEEE Trans Systems Man Cybernetics 34(6):757–763, 2004.
46. Agency for Healthcare Research and Quality: Prevention of misidentifications: Strategies to avoid wrong-site surgery. Chapter 43.2, 2003. Available at *http://www.ahrq.gov/clinic/ptsafety/chap43b.htm*
47. Adverse Health Events in Minnesota Hospitals: First Annual Public Report 2004. Includes Hospital Events Reported July 2003–October 2004. Available at *http://www.health.state.mn.us/patientsafety/aereport0105.pdf*
48. Degani A, Wiener EL: Cockpit checklists—concepts, design, and use. Hum Factors 35:345–359, 1993.
49. Current procedural terminology CPT ICD9-CM. AMA Press, 2005. Available at *https://catalog.ama-assn.org/Catalog/cpt/cpt_home.jsp*
50. Cook R, Woods DD: Chapter x Bogner MS. Human error in medicine. Mahwah, NJ: Lawrence Erlbaum, 1994.
51. Shapiro RA, Berland T: Noise in the operating room. N Engl J Med 287(24):1236–1238, 1972.
52. Firth-Cozens J: Why communication fails in the operating room. Quality Safety Health Care 13:327, 2004.
53. Federal Aviation Administration, Aerospace Medical Certification Division: Pilot medical certification questions and answers, AAM-300. Available at *http://www.cami.jccbi.gov/AAM-300/amcdfaq.html*
54. Can corrective lenses effectively improve a color vision deficiency when normal color vision is required? J Occup Environ Med 40(6):518–519, 1998.
55. Helmreich RL, Foushee HC: Why crew resource management? The history and status of human factors training programs in aviation. In Wiener E, Kanki, Helmreich R (eds): Cockpit Resource Management. New York: Academic Press, 1993.
56. Helmreich RL, Wilhelm JA: Outcomes of crew resource management training. Int J Aviat Psychol 1:287–300, 1991.
57. Howard SK, Gaba DM, Fish KJ, et al: Anesthesia crisis resource management training: Teaching anesthesiologists to handle critical incidents. Aviat Space Environ Med 63(9):763–770, 1992.
58. Monan B: Readback hearback. Aviation Safety Reporting System Directline, No. 1, March 1991. Available at *http://asrs.arc.nasa.gov/directline_issues/dl1_read.htm*
59. Salas E, Dickinson DL, Converse SA, et al: Toward an understanding of team performance and training. In Swezey RW, Salas E (eds): Teams: Their training and performance. Norwood, NJ: Ablex, 1992.
60. Surgenor SD, Blike GT, Corwin HL: Teamwork and collaboration in critical care: Lessons from the cockpit [Editorial]. Crit Care Med 31:992–993, 2003.
61. Berwick DM: Errors today and errors tomorrow. N Engl J Med 348(25):2570–2572, 2003.
62. Joint Commission on Accreditation of Healthcare Organizations: Sentinel event alert: Follow-up review of wrong site surgery. No. 24, 2001.
63. VeriChip expands hospital infrastructure: Hackensack University Medical Center becomes the second major medical center to adopt the VeriChip system. Delray Beach, FL. Business Wire, March 14, 2005.
64. Cook R, Rasmussen J: "Going solid": A model of system dynamics and consequences for patient safety. Qual Safety Health Care 2005 (in press).
65. Studdert DM, Mello MM, Brennan TA: Medical malpractice. N Engl J Med 350:283–292, 2004.

INDEX

Note: Page numbers followed by f indicate figures; those followed by t indicate tables; those followed by b indicate boxed material.

A

AADI (anterior atlanto-dens interval), in rheumatoid arthritis, 1779–1780
ABC(s), of resuscitation
for cervical spine injury, 1738
for traumatic brain injury, 46–47
ABC plate, 1830–1831
ABCD (amphotericin B colloidal dispersion), for fungal infections, 1667
Abdominal fat graft, for endoscopic transsphenoidal surgery, 341, 342f
Abdominal pseudocysts, due to shunt infection, 499
Abducens nerve, surgical anatomy of, 167f
Abductor pollicis brevis, neurophysiologic mapping of, 603f
Abelcet (amphotericin B lipid complex), for fungal infections, 1667
ABLC (amphotericin B lipid complex), for fungal infections, 1667
Abscess
brain, 1591–1597
clinical course of, 1596
clinical presentation of, 1593–1594
defined, 1591
diagnosis of, 1594–1595
epidemiology of, 1591
fungal, 1637, 1660, 1661f
historical background of, 1591
nonoperative management of, 1595–1596, 1595t
pathogenesis and bacteriology of, 1591–1593, 1592t
postoperative, 63, 1601f, 1603
prognosis for, 1596–1597
rupture of, 1596
stereotactic biopsy of, 634–635, 634f
surgical management of, 1596
tubercular, 1618
brain stem, 1592
cranial epidural, 1597–1598
intrasellar or suprasellar, 470, 1592
lung, pyogenic brain abscess due to, 1592t, 1595t
postoperative subdural, 1603
spinal epidural, 1687–1700
antibiotic therapy for, 1695
clinical presentation of, 1691–1692
epidemiology of, 1687
immobilization for, 1695–1696
laboratory findings in, 1692
microbiology of, 1690–1691, 1690t
pathogenesis and pathophysiology of, 1687–1689
radiographic studies of, 1692–1693, 1693f–1695f
risk factors for, 1689, 1689t

Abscess (Continued)
surgery for, 1696–1700, 1699f–1700f
outcome of, 1700
Absence seizures, corpus callosotomy for, 1417, 1418t
ACA. See Anterior cerebral artery (ACA).
Academy of Royal Medical Colleges, 3
Accessory nerve, for brachial plexus reconstruction, 2261
Accidents, evolution over time of, 2328
Accuray Treatment Planning System, 1958
Acellular cadaver dermal matrix (ACDM), for CSF leak, 141
ACHO. See Anterior choroidal (ACHO) artery.
Acipimox–growth hormone–releasing hormone (GHRH) stimulation test, 311
ACoA. See Anterior communicating artery(ies) (ACoA).
Acoustic neuroma. See Vestibular schwannoma(s).
Acoustic neuropathy, due to gamma knife surgery, 533
Acoustic tubercle, 881f, 882
Acquired immunodeficiency syndrome (AIDS). See also Human immunodeficiency virus (HIV).
primary CNS lymphoma with
diagnosis of, 655, 656–657, 657f
epidemiology of, 652, 653–654
prognosis for, 662
stereotactic biopsy of, 1608f, 1611–1613, 1619t
treatment of, 657f, 658, 662
Acromegaly
assessment of cure of, 375
clinical manifestations of, 374–375
follow-up of, 378
medical management of, 315–318, 316t, 376–377
pathogenesis of, 374
perioperative evaluation of, 308
postoperative evaluation of, 312t, 313
preoperative evaluation of, 302t, 303
radiation therapy for, 377–378
stereotactic radiosurgery for, 294
surgical management of, 375
Acrylic cranioplasty, 24–25, 27f, 28b
ACTH. See Adrenocorticotropic hormone (ACTH).
Actinomycosis, 1656–1659
characteristics of, 1639t, 1656
clinical presentation of, 1639t, 1657–1658, 1657f, 1658f
diagnosis of, 1639t, 1658
epidemiology of, 1636t

Actinomycosis (Continued)
granulomas due to, 1661, 1662f
neuropathology of, 1640t, 1657
pathogenesis of, 1639t
prognosis for, 1639t
risk factors for, 1656
spinal, 1658, 1658f
treatment for, 1639t, 1658–1659
Acute cerebrovascular events, due to fungal infection, 1662–1665, 1666f
Adamantinoma, 425
Adenocarcinoma
of ethmoid sinus, 190
ethmoidosphenoidal, 187f
Adenoma(s)
gonadotroph, 303
intrasellar, sella turcica repair after transsphenoidal surgery for, 397, 398f
pituitary. See Pituitary adenoma(s).
thyroid-stimulating hormone (thyrotropin-secreting)
medical management of, 318–319
preoperative evaluation of, 302t
Administrative support, and patient safety, 2335
ADPKD (autosomal dominant polycystic kidney disease), cerebral aneurysm in, 1089, 1096
Adrenal insufficiency
perioperative evaluation of, 307
postoperative evaluation of, 309–310
preoperative evaluation of, 300–301, 301t
Adrenalectomy, for Cushing's disease, 421–422
Adrenocorticotropic hormone (ACTH)
"big," 409
diurnal rhythms of, 411f–412f
Adrenocorticotropic hormone (ACTH) insufficiency
perioperative evaluation of, 307
postoperative evaluation of, 309–310
preoperative evaluation of, 300–301, 301t
Adrenocorticotropic hormone (ACTH)-producing tumors
Cushing's disease due to, 409–410, 409t, 410f, 412–414, 414f–417f
gamma knife surgery for, 293–294, 551t, 552, 552t
medical management of, 314–315, 314t
perioperative evaluation of, 307–308
postoperative evaluation of, 312–313, 312t
preoperative evaluation of, 302–303, 302t, 303b
Adrenocorticotropic hormone (ACTH) stimulation test, 300–301, 309
Adson's maneuver, 2293
Advance Trauma Life Support, 46
for penetrating brain injury, 90